Effects of Disease on Clinical Laboratory Tests

Richard B. Friedman, MD, FACP
Professor and Vice Chairman
Department of Medicine
University of Wisconsin
Madison, Wisconsin

Donald S. Young, MB, PhD
Director, Division of Laboratory Medicine
Department of Pathology and Laboratory Medicine
University of Pennsylvania
Philadelphia, Pennsylvania

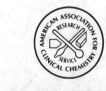

AACC PRESS

2029 K Street, NW
Seventh Floor
Washington, DC 20006

W9-CHC-284

ISBN 0-915274-52-3

Book assembly and typography
by Lexi-Comp Inc, Hudson, Ohio

INTRODUCTION

This compilation is a markedly expanded version of the *Effects of Disease on Clinical Laboratory Tests* previously published in 1980 as a supplemental issue of *Clinical Chemistry*, the journal of the American Association for Clinical Chemistry (Volume 26, Number 4, March 1980). Many new tests and diseases have occurred since that publication and the most important ones have been added to this edition.

This compilation of the effect of diseases on clinical laboratory tests is an attempt to bring together, in one resource, information that is scattered in many textbooks and specialty journals. This listing is neither exhaustive nor selective. While I have attempted to review the major texts and journals for information in this area, it is clear that, with any task as large as this, some important interactions must have been omitted. The major criterion for inclusion in this listing is citation in a major text or journal. No attempts have been made to verify the information or to select only the most significant interactions. Where possible, information concerning the frequency and degree of the abnormality has been included. In those cases where there is reported information as to when in the disease course the test result changes, I have included this information. The author is a specialist in internal medicine, and the file clearly reflects his clinical interest. Disorders from many other clinical specialties are included, but the majority of entries clearly fall within the concerns of internal medicine.

Some may criticize the non-selective nature of the file, and the fact that an abnormal increase and decrease for the same test is often listed in association with a single disease. This, in reality, reflects what has been observed clinically. When a test result can be either increased or decreased at the same time in the course of the disease, or at different times during the course of the disease, this information is included. Where authors differ on the direction of the abnormality, both entries have been included to highlight this discrepancy. So that the user can make his/her own decision about which abnormality is appropriate in their clinical situation, part of the original text is included along with the appropriate reference.

This file is meant as a companion to *Effects of Drugs on Clinical Laboratory Tests*, authored by Dr. Donald S. Young, to be published by the American Association for Clinical Chemistry. Given these two volumes, one should be able to generate a comprehensive listing of the possible causes of any laboratory test abnormality encountered in clinical practice.

In attempting to determine the cause of a test abnormality, one should always be aware that normality is a statistical concept and therefore a certain percentage of "abnormal" results is to be expected in patients with no discernible pathology. One should also remember that many patients have more than one disease, and therefore a reported test-disease relationship may really be ascribable to a co-existent disease, or to the interaction of multiple diseases.

If an abnormal test-disease relationship is not reported in the file, then either published reports show that this test is usually normal in that disease or no report of abnormality could be found. Only in those cases where authors have made a specific effort to study the results of a particular test in a disease and have found it to be normal is a normal result listed.

Structure of the File

The file is divided into five parts:

Laboratory Test Index (Alphabetical*)
Disease Keyword Index (Alphabetical)
Laboratory Test Listings (Alphabetical*)
Disease Listings by ICD-9-CM Classification
References

Laboratory Test Index

This in an alphabetized listing of all tests contained in the file. Where a test has two or more acceptable names, additional names are included with a reference to the preferred name (e.g., SGOT [see aspartate aminotransferase]). The user will find the test in the alphabetic listing by test file under the *preferred* name (e.g., aspartate aminotransferase).

---

*Test names beginning with a **numeral** are listed first

Some test names represent groupings of individual tests (e.g., amino acids). In these cases, entries will be included under the more general heading (e.g., amino acids) if the reference article only referred to the general grouping, and under the more specific test name if the article described the effect of a specific test (e.g., alanine). To assist the user in finding specific tests contained in a general group, but listed separately, entries in this category are listed after the term *see also* following the general heading (e.g., amino acids [*see also* alanine, asparagine, arginine, leucine, etc).

Disease Keyword Index

This file includes an alphabetized keyword listing of all diseases in the file. Included as a keyword is any major term in all the commonly used names for that particular disease. After each entry one will find the ICD-9-CM (The International Classification of Disease—9th revision—Clinical Modification) code for the disease. Since the *Disease Listings by ICD-9-CM Classification* file is arranged by ICD-9-CM code, this number should be used to find entries in that file. If the user cannot find a disease in the file, he/she is encouraged to consult an ICD-9-CM manual for a more exhaustive indexing of disease names. Because the *Disease Listings by ICD-9-CM Classification* is compatible with ICD-9-CM coding, one can go directly from that index to the file. Where no ICD-9-CM code exists for a disease (i.e., Acquired Immunodeficiency Syndrome [AIDS]—279.31), a code has been created to place that disease in the relevant section of the listing.

Laboratory Test Listings

The file contains information on over 450 of the most commonly administered clinical laboratory tests listed in alphabetical order. I have attempted to prepare a comprehensive listing of diseases associated with abnormalities in results of the most commonly administered tests; however, the listing of diseases associated with the less commonly administered tests may not be as exhaustive. No attempt has been made to differentiate by technique used to conduct a laboratory test. Therefore, the listing for acid phosphatase includes the techniques of Bodansky, King-Armstrong, etc. The user is encouraged to check which technique is used in his/her own laboratory and then compare this with the technique cited in the reference article before assuming that a true association exists.

I have included information on some tests that are no longer commonly reported by clinical laboratories (i.e., Thymol Turbidity, Cephalin Flocculation, etc). These tests are included because some laboratories may still include them in their test offering and for historical perspective.

For a particular test, the associated diseases are arranged by ICD-9-CM code. This should facilitate cross checking between diseases of common etiology or similar organ system as well as provide access to the *Disease Listings by ICD-9-CM Classification.* file.

Entries for a particular test are arranged first by specimen type and then direction of the abnormality. For each individual entry, a discussion of the course, extent, and frequency of the abnormality is included, when available, as well as a reference to the appropriate literature.

Disease Listings by ICD-9-CM Classification

How best to organize a disease file requires considerable thought. If one organized it by common disease name, then the choice of preferred name becomes crucial and associations by etiology or organ system are lost. I, therefore, decided to organize this listing by ICD-9-CM code number. This method makes the file compatible with the most commonly used classification system. The advantages of such compatibility are considerable; it not only permits use of existing comprehensive ICD-9-CM indexes, but also makes the file compatible with many existing disease and laboratory data bases.

The ICD-9-CM coding system is not perfect. It condenses several diseases into a single classification when they should be separate. It separates into different categories some diseases which should be combined. Because it requires approval of many groups, it is never totally current and therefore does not reflect the latest thinking in disease etiology. In addition, some of the most recently identified diseases are not included. Where necessary, new classification numbers have been created for diseases that are not in the existing coding system. Some categories in which two or more diseases have been lumped under a single classification number have been subdivided. Such "new" diseases and subdivided categories can usually be identified by the presence of a two-decimal place number.

No one will be totally satisfied with the ICD-9-CM coding system but, given its widespread use and the opportunity to make this listing compatible with a wealth of existing files, I elected this procedure. It may represent the best possible compromise.

For a particular disease, all tests are listing in alphabetical order. If more than one entry exists for a test it is re-sorted, first by specimen type then by direction. Each entry consists of the test name, the specimen type, the direction of the abnormality and if available, an explanation about that abnormality. This explanation will contain any data found about the occurrence, extent, and frequency of the abnormality. After each entry, a number is included. This number can be used to look up the source of this information in the reference file.

References

References are listed in alphabetical order. Each entry consists of the name of the author, the title of the article, and the journal or text citation.

Units

The Système International d'Unités (SI) as adopted by the 30th World Assembly of the World Health Organization in April 1977 is utilized wherever possible. These units may be somewhat confusing to some users and required conversion from the more traditional units and used in many of the reference texts. For those users not familiar with SI units, it is suggested that they review the text, *SI Units in Medicine*, by Lippert and Lehmann (Urban and Schwarzenberg, Baltimore-Munich, 1978).

Interpretation of Data

This file is intended to provide assistance in the interpretation of laboratory data, in particular to assist in explaining unexpected results or changes in data. It should not be assumed that, because an entry exists in the file, it necessarily explains an abnormal test result in a given patient. Nor should it be assumed that, because no entry exists, a disease is not the cause of an abnormal laboratory result.

I have tried to include most of the relevant information in the file, although it is unlikely that I have been able to obtain all pertinent literature or facts. I would be pleased to receive any additional information that users of the file possess. Although the author has attempted to ensure that information has been entered correctly into the file, errors may occur, and I would be most grateful if these could be pointed out to me. All correspondence should be sent to: Dr. Richard B. Friedman, Room H4/416, Clinical Sciences Center, University of Wisconsin, 600 Highland Ave., Madison, WI 53792.

Acknowledgement

The original idea for this file came as a result of an earlier collaboration with Dr. Donald S. Young on the first edition of *Effects of Drugs on Clinical Laboratory Tests, Clin. Chem.* 18: 1041-1303 (1972). Dr. Young's work served an inspiration for the present effort, and his encouragement, counsel and collaboration were instrumental in bringing this endeavor to fruition. Dr. Young is probably the only living soul who could have read this file not once but twice. If it were not for his collaboration, this project would have been impossible. Mr. Lenne P. Miller and Mr. Scott Hunt of the American Association for Clinical Chemistry advised and encouraged us in this effort, and there were periods when only this determination and constant encouragement kept the project moving forward. Mr. David K. Ream and Mr. Thomas A. Haught of Lexi-Comp Inc, Hudson, Ohio, were instrumental in bringing this project to fruition. Their contributions extended well beyond that of a typesetting service.

Mrs. Carol Schwartz assisted me by entering much of the material into the computer. Mr. Steve Entine performed the truly Herculean task of maintaining the computerized data base. Without his long hours and total dedication, the project could never have been completed. It is not altogether clear to me which of us contributed more to this project.

Each section of this file was sent to a medical specialist at the University of Wisconsin Medical School for review. While many were called, only a few truly rose to the task. Among these were: Dr. Wolfram Nolten—Endocrinology; Dr. Donald Harkness—Hematology; Dr. Ford Ballantyne—Cardiology; Dr. John Hamilton—Gastroenterology; Dr. Richard Day—General Internal Medicine; Dr. Lawrence Fleming—General Internal Medicine; Dr. Dennis Maki—Infectious Disease; Dr. Carolyn Bell—Rheumatology; and Dr. Aaron Friedman—Pediatrics. While these individuals contributed to the accuracy of the file, the final responsibility for any material in the file must rest solely with the author.

During my original work on this file, I served on the faculty of the Wisconsin Clinical Cancer Center. The late Dr. Harold Rusch, the first Director of the Center, and Dr. Paul Carbone, his successor, both advised and encouraged me in the original effort. Because the facilities used in the earlier effort were partly funded by a comprehensive Cancer Center Core Grant, the support of the National Cancer Institute Grant, CA-14520-04, is gratefully acknowledged.

While working on the current edition, I received support from Dr. Donald Harkness, Chairman of the Department of Medicine at the University of Wisconsin. Mrs. Trena Teela assisted me in preparing the introduction and facilitating the review by our expert panel.

Finally, I would like to acknowledge the assistance of my wife, Margaret Friedman, and of Mr. Entine's wife, Lynn Entine, who shouldered additional burdens while Mr. Entine and I spent countless nights and weekends revising and re-revising the data base files.

— Richard B. Friedman
May, 1989

1 LABORATORY TEST INDEX

^{131}I Uptake
1,25-Dihydroxy-Vitamin D$_3$
1-Methylhistidine
   see Methylhistidine
2,3-Diphosphoglycerate
2,5-Dihydroxyphenylacetic Acid
   see Homogentisic Acid
3,4-Dihydroxyphenylalanine
   see Dopa (3,4-
     Dihydroxyphenylalanine)
3,4-Dihydroxyphenylethylamine
   see Dopamine
3-Methylhistidine
   see Methylhistidine
5-Hydroxyindoleacetic Acid (5-HIAA)
5-Hydroxytryptamine (Serotonin)
5'-Nucleotidase
11-Hydroxycorticosteroids
   see also
     Deoxycorticosterone
17-Hydroxycorticosteroids
17-Hydroxyprogesterone
17-Ketogenic Steroids
17-Ketosteroids
17-KGS
   see 17-Ketogenic Steroids
17-KS
   see 17-Ketosteroids
17-OHCS
   see 17-Hydroxycorticosteroids
25-Hydroxy-Vitamin D
   see 25-Hydroxy Vitamin D$_3$
25-Hydroxy Vitamin D$_3$

A

ACE
   see Angiotensin-Converting Enzyme
     (ACE)
Acetoacetate
   see also
     Ketones
Acetone
   see also
     Ketones
Acetylcholinesterase
Acid Alpha-D-Glucoside Glucohydrolase
   see Alpha-Glucosidase
Acid Phosphatase
ACP
   see Acid Phosphatase
ACTH
   see Corticotropin
Activated Partial Thromboplastin Time
   see Partial Thromboplastin Time
Acute Phase Proteins
   see Alpha$_1$-Antitrypsin
Acute Phase Reactant
   see C-Reactive Protein

Acylcholine Acyl Hydrolase
   see Pseudocholinesterase
Adenosine Deaminase
Adenosine Monophosphate
   see Cyclic Adenosine Monophosphate
Adenylate Kinase
Adrenaline
   see Epinephrine
Adrenocorticotropic Hormone
   see Corticotropin
AFP
   see Alpha-Fetoprotein
Agglutination Tests
   see also
     Hemagglutination Inhibition
     Rheumatoid Factor
     VDRL
     Weil-Felix Reaction
AHF-Like Antigen
ALA
   see Aminolevulinic Acid
Alanine
   see also
     Amino Acids
Alanine Aminopeptidase
Alanine Aminotransferase
Albumin
Aldolase
Aldosterone
Alkaline Phosphatase
Alkaline Phosphatase Isoenzymes
Alkaloids
Alloisoleucine
Alpha$_1$-Antichymotrypsin
Alpha$_1$-Antitrypsin
Alpha$_1$-Globulin
Alpha$_1$-Glycoprotein
Alpha$_1$-Lipoprotein
Alpha$_2$-Antiplasmin
Alpha$_2$-Globulin
Alpha$_2$-Macroglobulin
Alpha-Aminobutyrate
   see Alpha-Amino-N-Butyric Acid
Alpha-Amino-N-Butyric-Acid
   see also
     Amino Acids
Alpha-Amino-Nitrogen
Alpha-Fetoprotein
Alpha-Glucosidase
Alpha-Hydroxybutyrate Dehydrogenase
   see Lactate Dehydrogenase
     Isoenzymes
Alpha-Ketoglutarate
Alpha$_1$-Lipoprotein
   see also
     Lipoproteins
ALT
   see Alanine Aminotransferase
Aluminum
Aminoacid Arylpeptidase

Amino Acids
   see also
     Alanine
     Alpha-Amino-N-Butyric Acid
     Arginine
     Asparagine
     Aspartic Acid
     Beta-Amino-Isobutyric-Acid
     Citrulline
     Cystathionine
     Cysteine
     Cystine
     Glutamic Acid
     Glutamine
     Glycine
     Histidine
     Homocitrulline
     Homocystine
     Hydroxyproline
     Isoleucine
     Leucine
     Lysine
     Methionine
     Methylhistidine
     Ornithine
     Phenylalanine
     Proline
     Sarcosine
     Serine
     Taurine
     Threonine
     Tryptophan
     Tyrosine
     Valine
Aminoisobutyric Acid
   see Beta-Amino-Isobutyric-Acid
Aminolevulinic Acid
Aminolevulinic Acid Dehydrase
Ammonia
AMP
   see Cyclic Adenosine Monophosphate
Amylase
Androgens
   see also
     Androstenedione
     Androsterone
     Testosterone
Androstenedione
   see also
     Androgens
Androsterone
   see also
     Androgens
Angiotensin
Angiotensin-Converting Enzyme (ACE)
Angiotensin II
Anisocytes
Antibodies to Centromeres
   see also
     Antibody Titer

Lipoprotein, Very Low Density
    see Cholesterol, Very Low Density
        Lipoprotein
Lithocholic Acid
Long Acting Thyroid Stimulating Hormone
    (LATS)
Long Acting Thyroid Stimulator
    see Long Acting Thyroid Stimulating
        Hormone (LATS)
Low Density Lipoprotein Cholesterol
    see Cholesterol, Low Density
        Lipoprotein
Lupus Erythematosus Cells
    see LE Cells
Luteinizing Hormone (LH)
    see also
        Gonadotropin, Pituitary
Lymphocyte B-Cell
Lymphocytes
Lymphocyte T-Cell
Lysine
    see also
        Amino Acids
Lysolecithin
Lysozyme

M

Macroglobulins, Alpha$_2$
    see Alpha$_2$-Macroglobulin
Macroglobulins, Beta$_2$
    see Beta$_2$-Macroglobulin
Magnesium
Malate Dehydrogenase
Manganese
MB
    see Creatine Kinase
MCH
MCHC
MCV
Melanin
Metamyelocytes
Metanephrine
    see Metanephrines, Total
Metanephrines, Total
    see also
        Catecholamines
Methemalbumin
Methionine
    see also
        Amino Acids
Methylene Blue (Sabin-Feldman) Dye Test
Methylhistidine
    see also
        Amino Acids
Methylmalonate
Mg
    see Magnesium
Monoamine Oxidase
Monocytes
Mucopolysaccharides
Mucoprotein
Muramidase
    see Lysozyme
Myelocytes
Myoglobin

N

Na
    see Sodium
NBT Test
NEFA
    see Fatty Acids, Free (FFA)
Neutralizing Antibodies
    see also
        Antibody Titer
Neutral Sterols
Neutrophils

N-Formiminoglutamic Acid
    see FIGLU (N-Formiminoglutamic
        Acid)
Nickel
Nicotinamide
Nitrogen
Nonceruloplasmin Copper
    see Copper, Nonceruloplasmin
Non-esterified Fatty Acids
    see Fatty Acids, Free (FFA)
Noradrenaline
    see Norepinephrine
Norepinephrine
    see also
        Catecholamines
Normetanephrine
    see Metanephrines, Total

O

Occult Blood
Ornithine
    see also
        Amino Acids
Ornithine Carbamoyl Transferase (OCT)
Orosomucoid
    see Alpha$_1$-Glycoprotein
Orthophosphoric Monoester
    Phosphohydrolase
    see Acid Phosphatase
Osmolality
Osmotic Fragility
Osteocalcin
O$_2$ Saturation
    see Oxygen Saturation
Oval Fat Bodies
Oxalate
Oxygen Saturation
Oxytocin

P

paCO$_2$
    see pCO$_2$
paO$_2$
    see pO$_2$
Parathyroid Hormone
Partial Thromboplastin Time
Pb
    see Lead
PCE
    see Pseudocholinesterase
pCO$_2$
Pepsin
Pepsinogen
pH
Phenylalanine
    see also
        Amino Acids
Phosphatase, Acid
    see Acid Phosphatase
Phosphatase, Alkaline
    see Alkaline Phosphatase
Phosphate
Phosphoethanolamine
Phosphoglucomutase
Phospholipids, Total
    see also
        Lecithin
        Lipids
Phosphorus
    see Phosphate
Phytanic Acid
Plasma Cells
Plasma Thromboplastin Antecedent
    see Factor XI
Plasma Thromboplastin Component
    see Factor IX
Plasminogen
Platelet Adhesiveness
Platelet Aggregation

Platelet Count
Platelet Survival
pO$_2$
Poikilocytes
Porphobilinogen
Porphyrins
    see also
        Coproporphyrin
        Protoporphyrin
        Uroporphyrin
Porter-Silber Chromogens
    see 17-Hydroxycorticosteroids
Potassium
Prealbumin
Precipitins
    see also
        Antibody Titer
Pregnanediol
Pregnanetriol
Proaccelerin
    see Factor V
Progesterone
Proinsulin
Prolactin
Proline
    see also
        Amino Acids
Proline Hydroxylase
Properidin
Prostaglandin E2
Prostaglandins
Protein
Protein Bound Iodine (PBI)
Protein Casts
Prothrombin
    see Factor II
Prothrombin Consumption
Prothrombin Time
Protoporphyrin
    see also
        Porphyrins
Pseudocholinesterase
PTA
    see Factor XI
PTC
    see Factor IX
Pyridoxine
Pyrophosphate
Pyruvate
Pyruvate Kinase

R

Recalcification Time
Reduced Glutathione
Renin Activity
Reptilase Time
Reticulocytes
Retinol
    see Vitamin A
Reverse Triiodothyronine
    see Tri-iodothyronine, Reverse
Rheumatoid Factor
    see also
        Agglutination Tests
Riboflavin
Ribonuclear Protein Antibodies
    see Antibodies to RNP
Ribose

S

Sarcosine
    see also
        Amino Acids
SCL-70 Antibodies
    see Antibodies to SCL-70
Scleroderma Antibody
    see Antibodies to SCL-70
Sedimentation Test
    see Erythrocyte Sedimentation Rate

Selenium
Serine
　　see also
　　　　Amino Acids
Serologic Test for Syphilis
　　see VDRL
Serotonin
　　see 5-Hydroxytryptamine (Serotonin)
SGOT
　　see Aspartate Aminotransferase
SGPT
　　see Alanine Aminotransferase
Sialic Acid
Sickle Cells
Single Stranded DNA Antibodies
　　see Antibodies to ss-DNA
Sjögren Syndrome A Antibodies
　　see Antibodies to Sjögren Syndrome
　　　　A
Sjögren Syndrome B Antibodies
　　see Antibodies to Sjögren Syndrome
　　　　B
Smith Antigen Antibodies
　　see Antibodies to SmAg
Sodium
Somatomedin
Somatomedin-C
Somatostatin
Somatotropin
　　see Growth Hormone
Sorbitol Dehydrogenase
Specific Gravity
ssDNA Antibodies
　　see Antibodies to ss-DNA
Stuart Factor
　　see Factor X
Sulfate

T

T_3 Uptake
Taurine
　　see also
　　　　Amino Acids
Testosterone
　　see also
　　　　Androgens
Tetrahydroaldosterone
Thiamine
Threonine
　　see also
　　　　Amino Acids
Thrombin Time
Thromboglobulin, Beta
Thromboplastin Generation
Thromboxane B_2
Thymol Turbidity
Thyro-Binding Index
Thyroglobulin Antibodies
　　see Antithyroglobulin Antibodies
Thyroid Stimulating Hormone (TSH)
Thyrotropin
　　see Thyroid Stimulating Hormone
　　　　(TSH)
Thyroxine Binding Globulin
Thyroxine Binding Prealbumin
Thyroxine, Free
Thyroxine Index, Free (FTI)
Thyroxine (T_4)
TIBC
　　see Iron-Binding Capacity, Total
　　　　(TIBC)
T Lymphocyte
　　see Lymphocyte T-Cell
Tocopherol
　　see Vitamin E (Tocopherol)
Total Hemolytic Complement
　　see Complement, Total
Total Iron-Binding Capacity
　　see Iron-Binding Capacity, Total
　　　　(TIBC)
Transcortin

Transferrin Saturation
　　see Iron Saturation
Trehalase
Triglycerides
　　see also
　　　　Lipids
Tri-iodothyronine, Free
Tri-iodothyronine, Reverse
Tri-iodothyronine (T_3)
Triiodothyronine Uptake
　　see T_3 Uptake
Triolein ^{131}I Test
Trypsin
Trypsin Inhibitor
Tryptophan
　　see also
　　　　Amino Acids
Tryptophan, Free
TSH
　　see Thyroid Stimulating Hormone
　　　　(TSH)
T_3
　　see Tri-iodothyronine (T_3)
T_4
　　see Thyroxine (T_4)
Tyrosine
　　see also
　　　　Amino Acids
Tyrosine Crystals

U

Unconjugated Bilirubin
　　see Bilirubin, Indirect
Urea Nitrogen
Uric Acid
Uric Acid Clearance
Urobilin
Urobilinogen
Urocanic Acid
Uropepsinogen
Uroporphyrin
　　see also
　　　　Porphyrins

V

Valine
　　see also
　　　　Amino Acids
Vanillylamine
Vanillylmandelic Acid
　　see also
　　　　Catecholamines
Vasopressin
　　see Antidiuretic Hormone
VDRL
　　see also
　　　　Agglutination Tests
Very Low Density Lipoprotein Cholesterol
　　see Cholesterol, Very Low Density
　　　　Lipoprotein
Viscosity
Vitamin A
Vitamin B_{12}
Vitamin B_{12} Binding Capacity
Vitamin B_1
　　see Thiamine
Vitamin C
　　see Ascorbic Acid
Vitamin D_3
　　see 1,25-Dihydroxy-Vitamin D_3
　　see 25-Hydroxy Vitamin D_3
Vitamin E (Tocopherol)
Vitamin K
VLDL Cholesterol
　　see Cholesterol, Very Low Density
　　　　Lipoprotein
Volume

W

Wasserman Reaction
　　see VDRL
Weil-Felix Reaction
　　see also
　　　　Agglutination Tests

X

Xanthine
Xanthurenic Acid
Xylose Tolerance Test

Z

Zimmerman Reaction
　　see 17-Ketosteroids
Zinc

2 DISEASE KEYWORD INDEX

A

Abetalipoproteinemia
Abetalipoproteinemia 272.52

Abortion
Threatened Abortion 640.00

Abscess
Abscess of Lung 513.00
Intracranial Abscess 324.00
Intraspinal Abscess 324.10
Liver Abscess (Pyogenic) 572.00

Acid
Folic Acid Deficiency Anemia 281.20

Acidosis
Diabetic Acidosis 250.10
Distal Renal Tubular Acidosis 588.82
Metabolic Acidosis 276.20
Proximal Renal Tubular Acidosis 588.81

Acne
Acne 706.10

Acquired
Acquired Hemolytic Anemia (Autoimmune) 283.00
Acquired Hydrocephalus 331.40
Acquired Immunodeficiency Syndrome (AIDS) 279.31
Pyloric Stenosis, Acquired 537.00

Acquired [Immunodeficiency (Common Variable)]
Immunodeficiency (Common Variable) 279.06

Acromegaly
Acromegaly 253.00

Actinomycosis
Actinomycosis 39.90

Active
Chronic Active Hepatitis 571.49

Activity (Muscular)
Exercise 994.50

Acute
Acute Alcoholic Intoxication 303.00
Acute and Subacute Necrosis of Liver 570.00
Acute Appendicitis 540.90
Acute Arthritis (Pyogenic) 711.00
Acute Cholecystitis 575.00
Acute Intermittent Porphyria 277.14
Acute Myocardial Infarction 410.90
Acute Myocarditis 422.00
Acute Pancreatitis 577.00
Acute Pericarditis 420.00
Acute Poliomyelitis 45.90
Acute Poststreptococcal Glomerulonephritis 580.00
Acute Pyelonephritis 590.10
Acute Renal Failure 584.00
Acute Tonsillitis 463.00
Lymphocytic Leukemia (Acute) 204.00
Myelocytic Leukemia (Acute) 205.00

Acute (Gastritis)
Gastritis 535.00

Addison's (Disease)
Adrenal Cortical Hypofunction 255.40

Adenomatous
Adenomatous Polyp 211.41

Adrenal
Adrenal Cortical Hyperfunction (Glucocorticoid Excess) 255.00
Adrenal Cortical Hyperfunction (Mineralocorticoid Excess) 255.10
Adrenal Cortical Hypofunction 255.40
Benign Neoplasm of Adrenal Cortex 227.00
Malignant Neoplasm of Adrenal Gland 194.00

Afibrinogenemia
Congenital Afibrinogenemia 286.34

African (Sleeping Sickness)
Trypanosomiasis 86.90

Agammaglobulinemia
Agammaglobulinemia (Congenital Sex-linked) 279.04

Agnogenic (Myeloid Metaplasia)
Myelofibrosis 289.80

Agranulocytosis
Agranulocytosis 288.00

AIDS
Acquired Immunodeficiency Syndrome (AIDS) 279.31

Alcoholic
Acute Alcoholic Intoxication 303.00
Laennec's or Alcoholic Cirrhosis 571.20

Alcoholism
Alcoholism 303.90

Aldosteronism [Adrenal Cortical Hyperfunction (Mineralocorticoid Excess)]
Adrenal Cortical Hyperfunction (Mineralocorticoid Excess) 255.10

Alkalosis
Metabolic Alkalosis 276.30

Alkaptonuria
Alkaptonuria 270.21

Allergic
Allergic Alveolitis 495.90
Allergic Purpura 287.00

Alpha
Alpha$_1$-Antitrypsin Deficiency 496.01
Heavy Chain Disease (Alpha) 273.22

Alveolar
Pulmonary Alveolar Proteinosis 516.00

Alveolitis
Allergic Alveolitis 495.90

Alzheimer's
Alzheimer's Disease 331.00

Amaurotic (Idiocy)
Tay-Sach's Disease 330.11

Amebiasis
Amebiasis 6.00

Amyloidosis
Amyloidosis 277.30

Amyotonia
Amyotonia Congenita 358.80

Amyotrophic
Amyotrophic Lateral Sclerosis   335.20

Analbuminemia
Analbuminemia   273.80

Ancinariasis [Ancylostomiasis (Hookworm Infestation)]
Ancylostomiasis (Hookworm Infestation)   126.90

Ancylostomiasis
Ancylostomiasis (Hookworm Infestation)   126.90

Anderson's
Anderson's Disease   272.71

Anemia
Aplastic Anemia   284.90
Congenital Aplastic Anemia   284.01
Folic Acid Deficiency Anemia   281.20
Hereditary Nonspherocytic Hemolytic Anemia   282.31
Iron Deficiency Anemia   280.90
Pernicious Anemia   281.00
Sideroblastic Anemia   285.00
Vitamin B_6 Deficiency Anemia   281.30

Anemias
Acquired Hemolytic Anemia (Autoimmune)   283.00
Anemias Due To Disorders of Glutathione
    Metabolism   282.20
Sickle Cell Anemia   282.60

Aneurysm
Dissecting Aortic Aneurysm   441.00
Ruptured Aortic Aneurysm   441.50

Angina
Angina Pectoris   413.90

Ankylosing
Rheumatoid (Ankylosing) Spondylitis   720.00

Anterior
Anterior Pituitary Hypofunction   253.40

Anthracosis
Anthracosis   500.00

Anus
Benign Neoplasm of Rectum and Anus   211.40

Anxiety
Anxiety Neurosis   300.00

Aortic
Dissecting Aortic Aneurysm   441.00
Pulseless Disease (Aortic Arch Syndrome)   446.70
Ruptured Aortic Aneurysm   441.50

Aplastic
Aplastic Anemia   284.90
Congenital Aplastic Anemia   284.01

Appendicitis
Acute Appendicitis   540.90

Arch
Pulseless Disease (Aortic Arch Syndrome)   446.70

Arrhenoblastoma
Arrhenoblastoma   220.95

Arterial
Arterial Embolism and Thrombosis   444.90

Arteriosclerosis
Arteriosclerosis   440.00

Arteritis
Cranial Arteritis and Related Conditions   446.50

Artery
Mesenteric Artery Embolism   557.01

Arthritis
Acute Arthritis (Pyogenic)   711.00
Juvenile Rheumatoid Arthritis   714.30
Rheumatoid Arthritis   714.00

Arthropod-Borne
Arthropod-Borne Hemorrhagic Fever   65.00

Asbestosis
Asbestosis   501.00

Ascariasis
Ascariasis   127.00

Aseptic
Aseptic Meningitis   47.00

Aspergillosis
Aspergillosis   117.30

Asthma
Asthma (Intrinsic)   493.10

Ataxia
Friedreich's Ataxia   334.00

Ataxia-Telangiectasia
Ataxia-Telangiectasia   334.80

Atelectasis (Pulmonary Collapse)
Pulmonary Collapse   518.00

Atopic
Atopic Eczema   691.80

Atrial (Myxoma)
Benign Neoplasm of Cardiovascular Tissue   212.70

Atrophica
Myotonia Atrophica   359.21

Atrophic (Gastritis)
Gastritis   535.00

Atrophy
Cerebral and Cortical Atrophy   331.90
Familial Progressive Spinal Muscular Atrophy   335.11

Autoimmune
Acquired Hemolytic Anemia (Autoimmune)   283.00

Autoimmune (Hepatitis)
Chronic Active Hepatitis   571.49

Autoimmune (Thyroiditis)
Hashimoto's Thyroiditis   245.20

Autonomic (Neuroblastoma)
Neuroblastoma   192.50

B

Bacillary
Bacillary Dysentery   4.90

Bacterial
Bacterial Endocarditis   421.00
Bacterial Pneumonia   482.90
Meningitis (Bacterial)   320.90

Bartonellosis
Bartonellosis   88.00

Becker (Dystrophy)
Progressive Muscular Dystrophy   359.11

Benign
Benign Neoplasm of Adrenal Cortex   227.00
Benign Neoplasm of Brain and CNS   225.90
Benign Neoplasm of Breast   217.00
Benign Neoplasm of Cardiovascular Tissue   212.70
Benign Neoplasm of Ovary   220.00
Benign Neoplasm of Pancreas   211.60
Benign Neoplasm of Rectum and Anus   211.40
Benign Neoplasm of Stomach   211.10
Benign Neoplasm of Testis   222.00
Benign Prostatic Hypertrophy   600.00
Essential Benign Hypertension   401.10

Benign (Arrhenoblastoma)
Arrhenoblastoma   220.95

Benign (Granulosa Cell Tumor of Ovary)
Granulosa Cell Tumor of Ovary   220.92

Benign (Lutein Cell Tumor of Ovary)
Lutein Cell Tumor of Ovary   220.93

Benign (Theca Cell Tumor of Ovary)
Theca Cell Tumor of Ovary   220.94

Beriberi (Thiamine (B_1) Deficiency)
Thiamine (B_1) Deficiency   265.00

Berylliosis
Berylliosis   503.01

Bile
Malignant Neoplasm of Intrahepatic Bile Ducts   155.10

Biliary
Biliary Cirrhosis   571.60
Extrahepatic Biliary Obstruction   576.20

Bladder
Malignant Neoplasm of Bladder   188.90

Blastomycosis
Blastomycosis   116.00

Bone
Fracture of Bone   829.00
Malignant Neoplasm of Bone   170.90
Secondary Malignant Neoplasm of Bone   198.50

Bone (Marble)
Osteopetrosis 756.52
Bone (Osteitis Deformans)
Osteitis Deformans 731.00
Bone (Osteopetrosis)
Osteopetrosis 756.52
Brain
Benign Neoplasm of Brain and CNS 225.90
Brain Infarction 434.90
Malignant Neoplasm of Brain 191.90
Secondary Malignant Neoplasm of Brain 198.30
Brain (Cerebral Thrombosis)
Cerebral Thrombosis 434.00
Breast
Benign Neoplasm of Breast 217.00
Malignant Neoplasm of Breast 174.90
Brill's
Brill's Disease 81.10
Brill-zinsser (Brill's Disease)
Brill's Disease 81.10
Bronchiectasis
Bronchiectasis 494.00
Bronchitis
Chronic Bronchitis 491.00
Bronchus
Malignant Neoplasm of Bronchus and Lung 162.90
Bronzed (Diabetes)
Hemochromatosis 275.00
Brucellosis
Brucellosis 23.00
Bruton's [Agammaglobulinemia (Congenital Sex-linked)]
Agammaglobulinemia (Congenital Sex-linked) 279.04
Bubo (Climatic)
Lymphogranuloma Venereum 99.10
Burn
Burns 948.00

C

Calculus
Kidney Calculus 592.00
Ureter Calculus 592.10
Candidiasis (Moniliasis)
Moniliasis 112.90
Carbon
Toxic Effects of Carbon Monoxide 986.00
Carcinoid
Carcinoid Syndrome 259.20
Carcinoma
Medullary Carcinoma of Thyroid 193.01
Carcinoma (Disseminated)
Secondary Malignant Neoplasm (Disseminated) 199.00
Carcinomatosis [Secondary Malignant Neoplasm (Disseminated)]
Secondary Malignant Neoplasm (Disseminated) 199.00
Cardiomyopathies
Cardiomyopathies 425.40
Cardiovascular
Benign Neoplasm of Cardiovascular Tissue 212.70
Carrion's (Disease)
Bartonellosis 88.00
Celiac
Celiac Sprue Disease 579.00
Cell
Granulosa Cell Tumor of Ovary 220.92
Lutein Cell Tumor of Ovary 220.93
Non-Hodgkins Lymphoma 202.80
Sickle Cell Anemia 282.60
Theca Cell Tumor of Ovary 220.94
Cell (Chronic Active Hepatitis)
Chronic Active Hepatitis 571.49
Cell (Giant, Thyroiditis)
Subacute Thyroiditis 245.10
Cell (Large, Lymphoma)
Non-Hodgkins Lymphoma 202.80

Cell (Plasma, Hepatitis)
Chronic Active Hepatitis 571.49
Ceramide (Glucosyl Lipidosis)
Gaucher's Disease 272.72
Cerebral
Cerebral and Cortical Atrophy 331.90
Cerebral Embolism 434.10
Cerebral Hemorrhage 431.00
Cerebral Thrombosis 434.00
Transient Cerebral Ischemia 435.90
Cerebral (Metachromatic Leukodystrophy)
Metachromatic Leukodystrophy 330.00
Cervix
Malignant Neoplasm of Cervix 180.90
Chain
Heavy Chain Disease (Alpha) 273.22
Heavy Chain Disease (Gamma) 273.23
Chickenpox
Chickenpox 52.00
Cholangitis
Cholangitis 576.10
Cholecystitis
Acute Cholecystitis 575.00
Cholera
Cholera 1.00
Chondrodystrophy
Chondrodystrophy 756.40
Chorea
Huntington's Chorea 333.40
Choriocarcinoma
Malignant Neoplasm of Trophoblast (Choriocarcinoma) 181.00
Choriomeningitis
Lymphocytic Choriomeningitis 49.00
Christmas
Christmas Disease 286.10
Chromosome
Syndromes Due to Sex Chromosome Abnormalities 758.80
Chronic
Chronic Active Hepatitis 571.49
Chronic Bronchitis 491.00
Chronic Ischemic Heart Disease 414.00
Chronic Obstructive Lung Disease 496.00
Chronic Pancreatitis 577.10
Chronic Pyelonephritis 590.00
Chronic Renal Failure 585.00
Chronic Sinusitis 473.90
Lymphocytic Leukemia (Chronic) 204.10
Myelocytic Leukemia (Chronic) 205.10
Cirrhosis
Biliary Cirrhosis 571.60
Cirrhosis of Liver 571.90
Laennec's or Alcoholic Cirrhosis 571.20
Citrullinemia
Citrullinemia 270.61
Climatic (Bubo)
Lymphogranuloma Venereum 99.10
CNS
Benign Neoplasm of Brain and CNS 225.90
CNS (Syphilis)
Syphilis 97.90
Coagulopathy
Disseminated Intravascular Coagulopathy 286.60
Coccidioidomycosis
Coccidioidomycosis 114.90
Colitis
Gastroenteritis and Colitis 9.00
Ulcerative Colitis 556.00
Colon
Diverticulitis of Colon 562.11
Colon (Carcinoma)
Malignant Neoplasm of Large Intestine 153.90
Colorado (Tick-Borne Fever)
Tick-Borne Fever 66.10
Combined
Severe Combined Immunodeficiency 279.20

Common
Immunodeficiency (Common Variable) 279.06

Congenita
Amyotonia Congenita 358.80
Myotonia Congenita 359.22

Congenital
Agammaglobulinemia (Congenital Sex-linked) 279.04
Congenital Afibrinogenemia 286.34
Congenital Aplastic Anemia 284.01
Congenital Dysfibrinogenemia 286.31
Congenital Erythropoietic Porphyria (Günther's Disease) 277.11
Congenital Rubella 771.00
Hereditary (Congenital) Spherocytosis 282.00

Congestion
Pulmonary Congestion and Hypostasis 514.00

Congestive
Congestive Heart Failure 428.00

Connective
Mixed Connective Tissue Disease 711.10

Constrictive
Constrictive Pericarditis 423.10

Convulsions
Convulsions 780.30

Coproporphyria
Erythropoietic Coproporphyria 277.13
Hereditary Coproporphyria 277.17

Cor
Cor Pulmonale 415.00

Corpus
Malignant Neoplasm of Corpus Uteri 182.00

Cortex
Benign Neoplasm of Adrenal Cortex 227.00

Cortex (Adrenal)
Adrenal Cortical Hyperfunction (Glucocorticoid Excess) 255.00

Cortical
Adrenal Cortical Hyperfunction (Glucocorticoid Excess) 255.00
Adrenal Cortical Hyperfunction (Mineralocorticoid Excess) 255.10
Adrenal Cortical Hypofunction 255.40
Cerebral and Cortical Atrophy 331.90
Infantile Cortical Hyperostosis 756.55

Cough
Whooping Cough 33.00

Cranial
Cranial Arteritis and Related Conditions 446.50

Crescentic [Glomerulonephritis (Rapidly Progressive)]
Glomerulonephritis (Rapidly Progressive) 580.40

Crigler-Najjar
Crigler-Najjar Syndrome 277.44

Crohn's (Disease)
Regional Enteritis or Ileitis 555.90

Crush
Crush Injury (Trauma) 929.00

Cryoglobulinemia
Cryoglobulinemia (Essential Mixed) 273.21

Cryptococcosis
Cryptococcosis 117.50

Current
Effects of Electric Current 994.80

Cushing's (Syndrome)
Adrenal Cortical Hyperfunction (Glucocorticoid Excess) 255.00

Cutanea
Porphyria Cutanea Tarda 277.16

Cyst
Ovarian Cyst 620.20
Pancreatic Cyst and Pseudocyst 577.20

Cystathioninuria
Cystathioninuria 270.41

Cystic
Cystic Fibrosis 277.00
Medullary Cystic Disease 753.12
Polycystic Kidney Disease 753.10

Cystinosis
Cystinosis 270.03

Cystinuria
Cystinuria 270.01

Cytomegalic
Cytomegalic Inclusion Disease 78.50

D

Deficiency
Alpha$_1$-Antitrypsin Deficiency 496.01
Deficiency State (Unspecified) 269.90
Dysgammaglobulinemia (Selective Immunoglobulin Deficiency) 279.07
Factor II Deficiency 286.38
Factor V Deficiency 286.35
Factor VII Deficiency 286.37
Factor X Deficiency 286.36
Factor XI Deficiency 286.20
Factor XII Deficiency 286.32
Factor XIII Deficiency 286.33
Folic Acid Deficiency Anemia 281.20
IgA Deficiency (Selective) 279.01
Immunodeficiency (Common Variable) 279.06
Iron Deficiency Anemia 280.90
Thiamine (B$_1$) Deficiency 265.00
Vitamin B$_6$ Deficiency Anemia 281.30
Vitamin C Deficiency 267.00
Vitamin D Deficiency Rickets 268.00
Vitamin K Deficiency 269.00

Deficiency (Factor VIII)
Congenital Dysfibrinogenemia 286.31

Deficiency (Factor IX)
Christmas Disease 286.10

Deficiency (Glucose-6-Phosphatase)
Von Gierke's Disease 271.01

Deficiency (Iodine, Goiter)
Simple Goiter 240.00

Deficiency (Pyruvate-Kinase)
Hereditary Nonspherocytic Hemolytic Anemia 282.31

Deficiency (Simple Goiter)
Simple Goiter 240.00

Deficiency (Vasopressin)
Diabetes Insipidus 253.50

Deformans
Osteitis Deformans 731.00

Degeneration
Hepatolenticular Degeneration 275.10

Dehydration
Dehydration 276.50

Delirium
Delirium Tremens 291.00

Dependence
Drug Dependence (Opium and Derivatives) 304.90

Depressive
Depressive Neurosis 300.40
Manic Depressive Disorder 296.80

De Quervain's (Thyroiditis)
Subacute Thyroiditis 245.10

Dermatitis
Dermatitis Herpetiformis 694.00

Dermatomyositis
Dermatomyositis/Polymyositis 710.40

Dermatomyositis/Polymyositis
Dermatomyositis/Polymyositis 710.40

Dermoid
Teratoma (Dermoid) 220.01

Dermoid (Benign Neoplasm of Ovary)
Benign Neoplasm of Ovary 220.00

Diabetes
Diabetes Insipidus 253.50
Diabetes Mellitus 250.00

Diabetes (Bronzed)
Hemochromatosis 275.00

Diabetic
Diabetic Acidosis 250.10

Diaphragm
Hernia Diaphragmatic 553.30

Diarrhea
Diarrhea 558.90

Diet
Diet 1013.00
Diet (High Sodium) 1013.01
Diet (Low Sodium) 1013.02

Differenciated Progressive Histiocytosis
Histiocytosis X 202.52

Diffuse (Histiocytic Lymphoma)
Non-Hodgkins Lymphoma 202.80

Diffuse (Hyperthyroidism)
Hyperthyroidism 242.90

Diffuse (Nontoxic Goiter)
Simple Goiter 240.00

Diffuse (Reticulum Cell Sarcoma)
Non-Hodgkins Lymphoma 202.80

Diffuse (Simple Goiter)
Simple Goiter 240.00

Diffuse (Toxic Goiter)
Hyperthyroidism 242.90

DiGeorge's
DiGeorge's Syndrome 279.11

Digestive
Secondary Malignant Neoplasm of Digestive System 197.50

DiGuglielmo's (Syndrome)
Erythroleukemia 207.00

Diphtheria
Diphtheria 32.00

Diphyllobothriasis
Diphyllobothriasis (Intestinal) 123.40

Disease
Alzheimer's Disease 331.00
Anderson's Disease 272.71
Brill's Disease 81.10
Celiac Sprue Disease 579.00
Christmas Disease 286.10
Chronic Ischemic Heart Disease 414.00
Chronic Obstructive Lung Disease 496.00
Congenital Erythropoietic Porphyria (Günther's Disease) 277.11
Cytomegalic Inclusion Disease 78.50
Diverticular Disease of Intestine 562.00
Forbes Disease 271.03
Gaucher's Disease 272.72
Gilbert's Disease 277.42
Hartnup Disease 270.02
Heavy Chain Disease (Alpha) 273.22
Heavy Chain Disease (Gamma) 273.23
Hemoglobin C Disease 282.71
Hemoglobin E Disease 282.72
Hemoglobin H Disease 282.73
Hemolytic Disease of Newborn (Erythroblastosis Fetalis) 773.00
Hodgkin's Disease 201.90
Lyme Disease 104.10
Maple Syrup Urine Disease 270.31
McArdle's Disease 271.02
Medullary Cystic Disease 753.12
Mixed Connective Tissue Disease 711.10
Niemann-Pick Disease 272.73
Parkinsons's Disease 332.00
Polycystic Kidney Disease 753.10
Pulseless Disease (Aortic Arch Syndrome) 446.70
Refsum's Disease 356.30
Reiter's Disease 99.30
Tangier Disease 272.51
Tay-Sach's Disease 330.11
Von Gierke's Disease 271.01
Von Willebrand's Disease 286.40
Whipple's Disease 40.20

Disease (Addison's)
Adrenal Cortical Hypofunction 255.40

Disease (Bartonellosis)
Bartonellosis 88.00

Disease (Carrion's)
Bartonellosis 88.00

Disease (Crohn's)
Regional Enteritis or Ileitis 555.90

Disease (Durand-Nicolas-Favre)
Lymphogranuloma Venereum 99.10

Disease (Gastritis)
Gastritis 535.00

Disease (Grave's)
Hyperthyroidism 242.90

Disease (Hansen's)
Leprosy 30.00

Disease (Hookworm)
Ancylostomiasis (Hookworm Infestation) 126.90

Disease (Hyaline Membrane)
Respiratory Distress Syndrome 770.80

Disease (Letterer-Siwe)
Histiocytosis X 202.52

Disease (Marble Bone)
Osteopetrosis 756.52

Disease (Ménétrier's)
Gastritis 535.00

Disease (Oppenheim's)
Amyotonia Congenita 358.80

Disease (Osteitis Deformans)
Osteitis Deformans 731.00

Disease (Osteopetrosis)
Osteopetrosis 756.52

Disease (Paget's)
Osteitis Deformans 731.00

Disease (Steinert's)
Myotonia Atrophica 359.21

Disease (Striatopallidal System)
Huntington's Chorea 333.40

Disease (Thomsen's)
Myotonia Congenita 359.22

Disease (Weil's)
Leptospirosis 100.00

Disease (Wilson's)
Hepatolenticular Degeneration 275.10

Dissecting
Dissecting Aortic Aneurysm 441.00

Disseminated
Disseminated Intravascular Coagulopathy 286.60
Disseminated Tuberculosis 18.00
Secondary Malignant Neoplasm (Disseminated) 199.00

Distal
Distal Renal Tubular Acidosis 588.82

Distal (Muscular Dystrophy)
Progressive Muscular Dystrophy 359.11

Distress
Respiratory Distress Syndrome 770.80

Diverticular
Diverticular Disease of Intestine 562.00

Diverticulitis
Diverticulitis of Colon 562.11

Diverticulosis (Diverticular Disease of Intestine)
Diverticular Disease of Intestine 562.00

Down's
Down's Syndrome 758.00

Drug
Drug Dependence (Opium and Derivatives) 304.90

Dubin-Johnson
Dubin-Johnson Syndrome 277.41

Duchenne (Progressive Muscular Dystrophy)
Progressive Muscular Dystrophy 359.11

Dumping
Postgastrectomy (Dumping) Syndrome 564.20

Duodenum
Fistula of Stomach and Duodenum 537.40

Durand-Nicolas-Favre (Disease)
Lymphogranuloma Venereum 99.10

Dwarfism
Renal Dwarfism 588.00

Dysentery
Bacillary Dysentery 4.90

Dysfibrinogenemia
Congenital Dysfibrinogenemia 286.31

Dysfunction (Ovarian)
Ovarian Hyperfunction 256.00
Ovarian Hypofunction 256.30
Polycystic Ovaries 256.40

Dysgammaglobulinemia
Dysgammaglobulinemia (Selective Immunoglobulin Deficiency)   279.07

Dysplasia
Polyostotic Fibrous Dysplasia   756.54

Dystrophy
Progressive Muscular Dystrophy   359.11

Dystrophy (Myotonic)
Myotonia Atrophica   359.21

E

Eastern
Eastern Equine Encephalitis   62.20

Echinococcosis (Hydatidosis)
Hydatidosis   122.90

Eclampsia
Eclampsia   642.60

Ectopic
Ectopic Pregnancy   633.90

Eczema
Atopic Eczema   691.80

Edema
Pulmonary Edema   518.40

Effects
Effects of Electric Current   994.80
Effects of X-Ray Irradiation   990.00
Toxic Effects of Carbon Monoxide   986.00
Toxic Effects of Lead and Its Compounds (including Fumes)   984.00
Toxic Effects of Non-medicinal Metals   985.00
Toxic Effects of Venom   989.50

Electric
Effects of Electric Current   994.80

Elliptocytosis
Hereditary Elliptocytosis   282.10

Embolism
Arterial Embolism and Thrombosis   444.90
Cerebral Embolism   434.10
Fat Embolism   958.10
Mesenteric Artery Embolism   557.01
Pulmonary Embolism and Infarction   415.10

Emphysema
Pulmonary Emphysema   492.80

Empyema
Empyema   510.00

Encephalitis
Eastern Equine Encephalitis   62.20
Western Equine Encephalitis   62.10

Encephalomyelitis
Encephalomyelitis   323.92

Encephalopathy
Hepatic Encephalopathy   572.20

Endemic
Endemic Typhus   81.00

Endocarditis
Bacterial Endocarditis   421.00
Loeffler's Endocarditis   421.91

Enteritis
Regional Enteritis or Ileitis   555.90

Enteropathy
Protein-Losing Enteropathy   579.01

Eosinophilic (Gastritis)
Gastritis   535.00

Epidemic
Epidemic Typhus   80.00

Epidemic (Hemorrhagic Fever)
Arthropod-Borne Hemorrhagic Fever   65.00

Epilepsy
Epilepsy   345.90

Equine
Eastern Equine Encephalitis   62.20
Western Equine Encephalitis   62.10

Erythema
Erythema Multiforme   695.10

Erythematosus
Systemic Lupus Erythematosus   710.00

Erythremia (Erythroleukemia)
Erythroleukemia   207.00

Erythremic myelosis (Erythroleukemia)
Erythroleukemia   207.00

Erythroblastosis
Hemolytic Disease of Newborn (Erythroblastosis Fetalis)   773.00

Erythroleukemia
Erythroleukemia   207.00

Erythropoietic
Congenital Erythropoietic Porphyria (Günther's Disease)   277.11
Erythropoietic Coproporphyria   277.13
Erythropoietic Protoporphyria   277.12

Esophagus
Malignant Neoplasm of Esophagus   150.90

Essential
Cryoglobulinemia (Essential Mixed)   273.21
Essential Benign Hypertension   401.10

Excess
Adrenal Cortical Hyperfunction (Glucocorticoid Excess)   255.00
Adrenal Cortical Hyperfunction (Mineralocorticoid Excess)   255.10

Exercise
Exercise   994.50

Externa
Otitis Externa   380.10

Extrahepatic
Extrahepatic Biliary Obstruction   576.20

F

Facio-scapulohumeral (Progressive Muscular Dystrophy)
Progressive Muscular Dystrophy   359.11

Factor
Factor II Deficiency   286.38
Factor V Deficiency   286.35
Factor VII Deficiency   286.37
Factor X Deficiency   286.36
Factor XI Deficiency   286.20
Factor XII Deficiency   286.32
Factor XIII Deficiency   286.33

Factor (VIII)
Congenital Dysfibrinogenemia   286.31

Factor (IX)
Christmas Disease   286.10

Failure
Acute Renal Failure   584.00
Chronic Renal Failure   585.00
Congestive Heart Failure   428.00
Hepatic Failure   572.40

Familial
Familial Periodic Paralysis   275.34
Familial Progressive Spinal Muscular Atrophy   335.11

Familial (Amaurotic Idiocy)
Tay-Sach's Disease   330.11

Familial (Hypercholesterolemia)
Type IIA Hyperlipoproteinemia   272.00
Type IIB Hyperlipoproteinemia   272.21

Familial (Hyperphosphatasia)
Hyperphosphatasia   275.31

Familial (Hypophosphatemic Rickets)
Vitamin D Resistant Rickets   275.35

Familial (Osteoectasia)
Hyperphosphatasia   275.31

Familial (Vitamin D Resistant Rickets)
Vitamin D Resistant Rickets   275.35

Fat
Fat Embolism   958.10

Felty's
Felty's Syndrome   714.10

Fetalis
Hemolytic Disease of Newborn (Erythroblastosis Fetalis) 773.00

Fever
Arthropod-Borne Hemorrhagic Fever 65.00
Hay Fever 477.90
Phlebotomus Fever 66.00
Relapsing Fever 87.00
Rheumatic Fever 390.00
Rocky Mountain Spotted Fever 82.00
Scarlet Fever 34.10
Tick-Borne Fever 66.10
Typhoid Fever 2.00
Yellow Fever 60.00

Fever (Heat stroke)
Heat stroke 992.00

Fever (Oroya)
Bartonellosis 88.00

Fever (Parrot)
Psittacosis 73.90

Fever (Verruga)
Bartonellosis 88.00

Fibrinogen
Congenital Afibrinogenemia 286.34
Congenital Dysfibrinogenemia 286.31

Fibrosis
Cystic Fibrosis 277.00

Fibrous
Polyostotic Fibrous Dysplasia 756.54

Fistula
Fistula of Stomach and Duodenum 537.40

Flea-borne (Endemic Typhus)
Endemic Typhus 81.00

Focal
Glomerulonephritis (Focal) 580.01

Folic
Folic Acid Deficiency Anemia 281.20

Forbes
Forbes Disease 271.03

Fracture
Fracture of Bone 829.00

Fragilitis (Ossium)
Osteogenesis Imperfecta 756.51

Franklin's (Disease)
Heavy Chain Disease (Alpha) 273.22

Friedreich's
Friedreich's Ataxia 334.00

Fructose
Hereditary Fructose Intolerance 271.20

Fumes
Toxic Effects of Lead and Its Compounds (including Fumes) 984.00

Fungoides
Mycosis Fungoides 202.10

G

Galactosemia
Galactosemia 271.10

Gallbladder
Malignant Neoplasm of Gallbladder 156.00

Gamma
Heavy Chain Disease (Gamma) 273.23

Gangrene
Gangrene 785.40

Gastritis
Gastritis 535.00

Gastroenteritis
Gastroenteritis and Colitis 9.00

Gaucher's
Gaucher's Disease 272.72

German (Measles)
Rubella 56.00

Giant-Cell (Arteritis)
Cranial Arteritis and Related Conditions 446.50

Giant-Cell (Thyroiditis)
Subacute Thyroiditis 245.10

Giardia
Giardiasis 7.10

Giardiasis
Giardiasis 7.10

Gierke's
Von Gierke's Disease 271.01

Gilbert's
Gilbert's Disease 277.42

Gland
Malignant Neoplasm of Adrenal Gland 194.00
Malignant Neoplasm of Thyroid Gland 193.00

Glands
Diseases of the Salivary Glands 527.90

Glanzmann's
Thrombasthenia (Glanzmann's) 287.10

Glomerulonephritis
Acute Poststreptococcal Glomerulonephritis 580.00
Glomerulonephritis (Focal) 580.01
Glomerulonephritis (Membranoproliferative) 580.05
Glomerulonephritis (Membranous) 580.04
Glomerulonephritis (Minimal Change) 580.02
Glomerulonephritis (Rapidly Progressive) 580.40

Glucocorticoid
Adrenal Cortical Hyperfunction (Glucocorticoid Excess) 255.00

Glucose-6-Phosphatase (Deficiency)
Von Gierke's Disease 271.01

Glucosyl (Ceramide Lipidosis)
Gaucher's Disease 272.72

Glutathione
Anemias Due To Disorders of Glutathione Metabolism 282.20

Glycogen (Storage Disease)
Anderson's Disease 272.71
Forbes Disease 271.03
McArdle's Disease 271.02
Von Gierke's Disease 271.01

Goiter
Simple Goiter 240.00

Goiter (Toxic)
Hyperthyroidism 242.90

Goodpasture's
Goodpasture's Syndrome 446.20

Gout
Gout 274.00

Granulomatous (Thyroiditis)
Subacute Thyroiditis 245.10

Granulosa
Granulosa Cell Tumor of Ovary 220.92

Grave's (Disease)
Hyperthyroidism 242.90

Gravis
Myasthenia Gravis 358.00

Guillain-Barré
Guillain-Barré Syndrome 357.00

Günther's
Congenital Erythropoietic Porphyria (Günther's Disease) 277.11

H

Hageman (Trait)
Factor XII Deficiency 286.32

Hairy cell (Leukemic Reticuloendotheliosis)
Leukemic Reticuloendotheliosis 202.40

Hansen's (Disease)
Leprosy 30.00

Hartnup
Hartnup Disease 270.02

Hashimoto's
Hashimoto's Thyroiditis 245.20

Hay
Hay Fever 477.90

Heart
Chronic Ischemic Heart Disease   414.00
Congestive Heart Failure   428.00

Heat
Heat stroke   992.00

Heavy
Heavy Chain Disease (Alpha)   273.22
Heavy Chain Disease (Gamma)   273.23

Hemochromatosis
Hemochromatosis   275.00

Hemoglobin
Hemoglobin C Disease   282.71
Hemoglobin E Disease   282.72
Hemoglobin H Disease   282.73

Hemolytic
Acquired Hemolytic Anemia (Autoimmune)   283.00
Hemolytic Disease of Newborn (Erythroblastosis Fetalis)   773.00
Hereditary Nonspherocytic Hemolytic Anemia   282.31

Hemolytic (Congenital Jaundice)
Hereditary (Congenital) Spherocytosis   282.00

Hemolytic (Hereditary Elliptocytosis)
Hereditary Elliptocytosis   282.10

Hemophilia
Hemophilia   286.01

Hemophilia (B)
Christmas Disease   286.10

Hemophilia (Congenital Dysfibrinogenemia)
Congenital Dysfibrinogenemia   286.31

Hemophilia (Vascular)
Von Willebrand's Disease   286.40

Hemorrhage
Cerebral Hemorrhage   431.00

Hemorrhagic
Arthropod-Borne Hemorrhagic Fever   65.00

Hemosiderosis
Idiopathic Pulmonary Hemosiderosis   516.10

Hepatic
Hepatic Encephalopathy   572.20
Hepatic Failure   572.40

Hepatitis
Chronic Active Hepatitis   571.49
Toxic Hepatitis   573.30
Viral Hepatitis   70.00

Hepatocellular
Jaundice Due to Hepatocellular Damage (Newborn)   774.40

Hepatolenticular
Hepatolenticular Degeneration   275.10

Hereditary
Hereditary (Congenital) Spherocytosis   282.00
Hereditary Coproporphyria   277.17
Hereditary Elliptocytosis   282.10
Hereditary Fructose Intolerance   271.20
Hereditary Nonspherocytic Hemolytic Anemia   282.31

Hereditary (Friedreich's Ataxia)
Friedreich's Ataxia   334.00

Hernia
Hernia Diaphragmatic   553.30

Herpes
Herpes Simplex   54.00
Herpes Zoster   53.00

Herpetiformis
Dermatitis Herpetiformis   694.00

High
Diet (High Sodium)   1013.01

Histidinemia
Histidinemia   270.51

Histiocytic (Diffuse, Lymphoma)
Non-Hodgkins Lymphoma   202.80

Histiocytic Lymphoma
Non-Hodgkins Lymphoma   202.80

Histiocytic (Medullary Reticulosis)
Non-Hodgkins Lymphoma   202.80

Histiocytic (Mixed Lymphocytic Lymphoma)
Non-Hodgkins Lymphoma   202.80

Histiocytic (Reticulum Cell Sarcoma)
Non-Hodgkins Lymphoma   202.80

Histiocytosis X
Histiocytosis X   202.52

Histoplasmosis
Histoplasmosis   115.00

Hodgkin's
Hodgkin's Disease   201.90

Homocystinuria
Homocystinuria   270.42

Hookworm
Ancylostomiasis (Hookworm Infestation)   126.90

Huntington's
Huntington's Chorea   333.40

Hyaline (Membrane Disease)
Respiratory Distress Syndrome   770.80

Hydatidiform
Hydatidiform Mole   630.00

Hydatidosis
Hydatidosis   122.90

Hydrocephalus
Acquired Hydrocephalus   331.40

Hydronephrosis
Hydronephrosis   591.00

Hydroxyprolinemia
Hydroxyprolinemia   270.82

Hyperbetalipoproteinemia (Type IIA Hyperlipoproteinemia)
Type IIA Hyperlipoproteinemia   272.00

Hyperfunction
Adrenal Cortical Hyperfunction (Glucocorticoid Excess)   255.00
Adrenal Cortical Hyperfunction (Mineralocorticoid Excess)   255.10
Ovarian Hyperfunction   256.00

Hyperglyceridemia (Mixed)
Type V Hyperlipoproteinemia   272.32

Hyperhidrosis
Hyperhidrosis   780.80

Hyperlipoproteinemia
Type I Hyperlipoproteinemia   272.31
Type IIA Hyperlipoproteinemia   272.00
Type IIB Hyperlipoproteinemia   272.21
Type III Hyperlipoproteinemia   272.22
Type IV Hyperlipoproteinemia   272.10
Type V Hyperlipoproteinemia   272.32

Hypernephroma (Malignant Neoplasm of Kidney)
Malignant Neoplasm of Kidney   189.00

Hyperostosis
Infantile Cortical Hyperostosis   756.55

Hyperparathyroidism
Hyperparathyroidism   252.00

Hyperphosphatasia
Hyperphosphatasia   275.31

Hyperprebetalipoproteinemia (Type IV Hyperlipoproteinemia)
Type IV Hyperlipoproteinemia   272.10

Hyperprolinemia
Hyperprolinemia   270.81

Hypersensitivity Angiitis
Goodpasture's Syndrome   446.20

Hypersplenism
Hypersplenism   289.40

Hypertension
Essential Benign Hypertension   401.10
Malignant Hypertension   401.00
Renovascular Hypertension   405.91

Hypertension (Eclampsia)
Eclampsia   642.60

Hypertension (Pre-Eclampsia)
Pre-Eclampsia   642.40

Hyperthyroidism
Hyperthyroidism   242.90

Hypertrophic (Gastritis)
Gastritis   535.00

Hypertrophy
Benign Prostatic Hypertrophy   600.00

Hyperventilation
Hyperventilation Syndrome   306.10

Hypervitaminosis
Hypervitaminosis D   278.40

Hypocomplementemic [Glomerulonephritis (Membranoproliferative)]
Glomerulonephritis (Membranoproliferative)   580.05

Hypofunction
Adrenal Cortical Hypofunction   255.40
Anterior Pituitary Hypofunction   253.40
Ovarian Hypofunction   256.30
Testicular Hypofunction   257.20

Hypogammaglobulinemia [Immunodeficiency (Common Variable)]
Immunodeficiency (Common Variable)   279.06

Hypoglycemia,
Hypoglycemia, Unspecified   251.20

Hypokalemia
Hypokalemia   276.80

Hypomagnesia
Hypomagnesemia   275.21

Hypoparathyroidism
Hypoparathyroidism   252.10

Hypophosphatasemia (Hypophosphatasia)
Hypophosphatasia   275.32

Hypophosphatasia
Hypophosphatasia   275.32

Hypophosphatemic (Familial Rickets)
Vitamin D Resistant Rickets   275.35

Hypostasis
Pulmonary Congestion and Hypostasis   514.00

Hypothermia
Hypothermia   991.60

Hypothyroidism
Hypothyroidism   244.90

I

Idiocy (Amaurotic)
Tay-Sach's Disease   330.11

Idiopathic
Idiopathic Pulmonary Hemosiderosis   516.10
Idiopathic Thrombocytopenic Purpura   287.30

Idiopathic (Polyneuritis)
Guillain-Barré Syndrome   357.00

IgA
IgA Deficiency (Selective)   279.01

Ileitis
Regional Enteritis or Ileitis   555.90

Immunodeficiency
Acquired Immunodeficiency Syndrome (AIDS)   279.31
Immunodeficiency (Common Variable)   279.06
Severe Combined Immunodeficiency   279.20

Immunoglobulin
Dysgammaglobulinemia (Selective Immunoglobulin Deficiency)   279.07

Immunoglobulin [Agammaglobulinemia (Congenital Sex-linked)]
Agammaglobulinemia (Congenital Sex-linked)   279.04

Immunoglobulin [Immunodeficiency (Common Variable)]
Immunodeficiency (Common Variable)   279.06

Imperfecta
Osteogenesis Imperfecta   756.51

Inclusion
Cytomegalic Inclusion Disease   78.50

Infantile
Infantile Cortical Hyperostosis   756.55

Infarction
Acute Myocardial Infarction   410.90
Brain Infarction   434.90
Prostatic Infarction   602.80
Pulmonary Embolism and Infarction   415.10
Renal Infarction   593.81

Infarction (Cerebral Thrombosis)
Cerebral Thrombosis   434.00

Infection
Urinary Tract Infection   599.00

Infectious
Infectious Mononucleosis   75.00

Infertility
Infertility in Males   606.90

Inflammation
Inflammation of Optic Nerve and Retina   363.20

Influenza
Influenza   487.10

Injury
Crush Injury (Trauma)   929.00

Insipidus
Diabetes Insipidus   253.50

Intermittent
Acute Intermittent Porphyria   277.14

Intestinal
Diphyllobothriasis (Intestinal)   123.40
Intestinal Obstruction   560.90

Intestine
Diverticular Disease of Intestine   562.00
Malignant Neoplasm of Large Intestine   153.90
Malignant Neoplasm of Small Intestine   152.90

Intolerance
Hereditary Fructose Intolerance   271.20

Intoxication
Acute Alcoholic Intoxication   303.00

Intracranial
Intracranial Abscess   324.00

Intrahepatic
Malignant Neoplasm of Intrahepatic Bile Ducts   155.10

Intraspinal
Intraspinal Abscess   324.10

Intra-Uterine
Pregnancy Complicated by Intrauterine Death   656.40

Intravascular
Disseminated Intravascular Coagulopathy   286.60

Intrinsic
Asthma (Intrinsic)   493.10

Iodine (Deficiency Goiter)
Simple Goiter   240.00

Iron
Iron Deficiency Anemia   280.90

Irradiation
Effects of X-Ray Irradiation   990.00

Ischemia
Transient Cerebral Ischemia   435.90

Ischemic
Chronic Ischemic Heart Disease   414.00

J

Jaundice
Jaundice Due to Hepatocellular Damage (Newborn)   774.40

Jaundice (Congenital Hemolytic)
Hereditary (Congenital) Spherocytosis   282.00

Juvenile
Juvenile Rheumatoid Arthritis   714.30

K

Kala-azar (Leishmaniasis)
Leishmaniasis   85.00

Keratoconjunctivitis (Sjögren's Syndrome)
Sjögren's Syndrome   710.20

Kidney
Kidney Calculus   592.00
Malignant Neoplasm of Kidney   189.00
Medullary Sponge Kidney   753.13
Polycystic Kidney Disease   753.10

Kidney (Nephrotic Syndrome)
Nephrotic Syndrome   581.90

Klinefelter's
Klinefelter's Syndrome (XXY)   758.70

Kwashiorkor (Protein Malnutrition)
Protein Malnutrition   260.00

Kyphoscoliosis
Kyphoscoliosis   737.30

L

Lactosuria
Lactosuria 271.30

Laennec's
Laennec's or Alcoholic Cirrhosis 571.20

Lambliasis
Giardiasis 7.10

Large
Malignant Neoplasm of Large Intestine 153.90

Large Cell Lymphoma
Non-Hodgkins Lymphoma 202.80

Larva
Larva Migrans (Visceralis) 128.00

Lateral
Amyotrophic Lateral Sclerosis 335.20

Lead
Toxic Effects of Lead and Its Compounds (including Fumes) 984.00

Leishmaniasis
Leishmaniasis 85.00

Leprosy
Leprosy 30.00

Leptospirosis
Leptospirosis 100.00

Lesch-Nyhan
Lesch-Nyhan Syndrome 277.22

Letterer-Siwe
Histiocytosis X 202.52

Leucinosis (Maple Syrup Urine Disease)
Maple Syrup Urine Disease 270.31

Leukemia
Lymphocytic Leukemia (Acute) 204.00
Lymphocytic Leukemia (Chronic) 204.10
Monocytic Leukemia 206.00
Myelocytic Leukemia (Acute) 205.00
Myelocytic Leukemia (Chronic) 205.10

Leukemia (Hairy Cell)
Leukemic Reticuloendotheliosis 202.40

Leukemic
Leukemic Reticuloendotheliosis 202.40

Leukodystrophy
Metachromatic Leukodystrophy 330.00

Leydig (Cell Tumor)
Arrhenoblastoma 220.95

Limb-Girdle (Dystrophy)
Progressive Muscular Dystrophy 359.11

Lipid (Nephrosis)
Glomerulonephritis (Minimal Change) 580.02

Lipidosis (Gaucher's Disease)
Gaucher's Disease 272.72

Lipidosis (Glucosyl Ceramide)
Gaucher's Disease 272.72

Lipidosis (Sphingomyelin)
Niemann-Pick Disease 272.73

Lipoid [Glomerulonephritis (Minimal Change)]
Glomerulonephritis (Minimal Change) 580.02

Liver
Acute and Subacute Necrosis of Liver 570.00
Cirrhosis of Liver 571.90
Liver Abscess (Pyogenic) 572.00
Malignant Neoplasm of Liver 155.00
Secondary Malignant Neoplasm of Liver 197.70

Loeffler's
Loeffler's Endocarditis 421.91

Louse-borne (Epidemic Typhus)
Epidemic Typhus 80.00

Lung
Abscess of Lung 513.00
Chronic Obstructive Lung Disease 496.00
Malignant Neoplasm of Bronchus and Lung 162.90

Lupoid (Hepatitis)
Chronic Active Hepatitis 571.49

Lupus
Systemic Lupus Erythematosus 710.00

Lutein
Lutein Cell Tumor of Ovary 220.93

Lyme
Lyme Disease 104.10

Lymphocytic
Lymphocytic Choriomeningitis 49.00
Lymphocytic Leukemia (Acute) 204.00
Lymphocytic Leukemia (Chronic) 204.10

Lymphocytic (Mixed Histiocytic, Lymphoma)
Non-Hodgkins Lymphoma 202.80

Lymphocytic (Reticulum Cell Sarcoma)
Non-Hodgkins Lymphoma 202.80

Lymphocytic (Thyroiditis)
Hashimoto's Thyroiditis 245.20

Lymphogranuloma
Lymphogranuloma Venereum 99.10

Lymphoma
Non-Hodgkins Lymphoma 202.80

Lymphoma (Diffuse Histocytic)
Non-Hodgkins Lymphoma 202.80

Lymphoma (Histiocytic)
Non-Hodgkins Lymphoma 202.80

Lymphoma (Large Cell)
Non-Hodgkins Lymphoma 202.80

Lymphoma (Mixed)
Non-Hodgkins Lymphoma 202.80

Lymphoma (Reticulum Cell Sarcoma)
Non-Hodgkins Lymphoma 202.80

Lymphomatosa (Struma)
Hashimoto's Thyroiditis 245.20

Lymphosarcoma
Non-Hodgkins Lymphoma 202.80

M

Macroglobulinemia
Waldenström's Macroglobulinemia 273.30

Major
Thalassemia Major 282.41

Malabsorption,
Malabsorption, Cause Unspecified 579.90

Malaria
Malaria 84.00

Malignant
Malignant Hypertension 401.00
Malignant Melanoma of Skin 172.90
Malignant Neoplasm of Adrenal Gland 194.00
Malignant Neoplasm of Bladder 188.90
Malignant Neoplasm of Bone 170.90
Malignant Neoplasm of Brain 191.90
Malignant Neoplasm of Breast 174.90
Malignant Neoplasm of Bronchus and Lung 162.90
Malignant Neoplasm of Cervix 180.90
Malignant Neoplasm of Corpus Uteri 182.00
Malignant Neoplasm of Esophagus 150.90
Malignant Neoplasm of Gallbladder 156.00
Malignant Neoplasm of Intrahepatic Bile Ducts 155.10
Malignant Neoplasm of Kidney 189.00
Malignant Neoplasm of Large Intestine 153.90
Malignant Neoplasm of Liver 155.00
Malignant Neoplasm of Other Parts of Nervous System 192.90
Malignant Neoplasm of Ovary 183.00
Malignant Neoplasm of Pancreas 157.90
Malignant Neoplasm of Pituitary 194.30
Malignant Neoplasm of Prostate 185.00
Malignant Neoplasm of Rectum 154.10
Malignant Neoplasm of Small Intestine 152.90
Malignant Neoplasm of Stomach 151.90
Malignant Neoplasm of Testis 186.90
Malignant Neoplasm of Thyroid Gland 193.00
Malignant Neoplasm of Trophoblast (Choriocarcinoma) 181.00
Secondary Malignant Neoplasm (Disseminated) 199.00
Secondary Malignant Neoplasm of Bone 198.50
Secondary Malignant Neoplasm of Brain 198.30
Secondary Malignant Neoplasm of Digestive System 197.50
Secondary Malignant Neoplasm of Liver 197.70

Secondary Malignant Neoplasm of Respiratory
System 197.00

Malignant [Glomerulonephritis (Rapidly Progressive)]
Glomerulonephritis (Rapidly Progressive) 580.40

Malignant (Medullary Carcinoma of Thyroid)
Medullary Carcinoma of Thyroid 193.01

Malignant (Neuroblastoma)
Neuroblastoma 192.50

Malnutrition
Protein Malnutrition 260.00

Manic
Manic Depressive Disorder 296.80

Maple
Maple Syrup Urine Disease 270.31

Marasmus (Protein Malnutrition)
Protein Malnutrition 260.00

Marble (Bone)
Osteopetrosis 756.52

Marie-Strumpell (Spondylitis)
Rheumatoid (Ankylosing) Spondylitis 720.00

McArdle's
McArdle's Disease 271.02

Measles
Measles 55.00

Measles (Rubella)
Rubella 56.00

Media
Otitis Media 381.00

Medullary
Medullary Carcinoma of Thyroid 193.01
Medullary Cystic Disease 753.12
Medullary Sponge Kidney 753.13

Medullary (Histiocytic Reticulosis)
Non-Hodgkins Lymphoma 202.80

Medullary (Reticulum Cell Sarcoma)
Non-Hodgkins Lymphoma 202.80

Melanoma
Malignant Melanoma of Skin 172.90

Mellitus
Diabetes Mellitus 250.00

Membrane (Hyaline, Disease)
Respiratory Distress Syndrome 770.80

Membranoproliferative
Glomerulonephritis (Membranoproliferative) 580.05

Membranous
Glomerulonephritis (Membranous) 580.04

Ménétrier's (Disease)
Gastritis 535.00

Meningitis
Aseptic Meningitis 47.00
Meningitis (Bacterial) 320.90
Meningococcal Meningitis 36.00
Tuberculosis Meningitis 13.00

Meningococcal
Meningococcal Meningitis 36.00

Menopausal
Menopausal and Postmenopausal Symptoms 627.90

Mental
Mental Retardation 319.00

Mesangiocapillary [Glomerulonephritis (Membranoproliferative)]
Glomerulonephritis (Membranoproliferative) 580.05

Mesenteric
Mesenteric Artery Embolism 557.01

Metabolic
Metabolic Acidosis 276.20
Metabolic Alkalosis 276.30

Metabolism
Anemias Due To Disorders of Glutathione
Metabolism 282.20

Metachromatic
Metachromatic Leukodystrophy 330.00

Metals
Toxic Effects of Non-medicinal Metals 985.00

Metaplasia (Myelofibrosis)
Myelofibrosis 289.80

Metastases (Disseminated)
Secondary Malignant Neoplasm (Disseminated) 199.00

Migraine
Migraine 346.00

Migrans
Larva Migrans (Visceralis) 128.00

Milk-Alkali
Milk-Alkali Syndrome 275.41

Mineralocorticoid
Adrenal Cortical Hyperfunction (Mineralocorticoid
Excess) 255.10

Minimal
Glomerulonephritis (Minimal Change) 580.02

Minor
Thalassemia Minor 282.42

Mite-Borne
Mite-Borne Typhus 81.20

Mixed
Cryoglobulinemia (Essential Mixed) 273.21
Mixed Connective Tissue Disease 711.10

Mixed (Histiocytic-Lymphocytic Lymphoma)
Non-Hodgkins Lymphoma 202.80

Mixed (Hyperglyceridemia)
Type V Hyperlipoproteinemia 272.32

Mixed Lymphoma
Non-Hodgkins Lymphoma 202.80

Molar (Pregnancy)
Hydatidiform Mole 630.00

Mongolism (Down's Syndrome)
Down's Syndrome 758.00

Moniliasis
Moniliasis 112.90

Monocytic
Monocytic Leukemia 206.00

Mononucleosis
Infectious Mononucleosis 75.00

Monoxide
Toxic Effects of Carbon Monoxide 986.00

Moschcowitz's (Syndrome)
Thrombotic Thrombocytopenic Purpura 446.60

Mucoviscidosis (Cystic Fibrosis)
Cystic Fibrosis 277.00

Multiforme
Erythema Multiforme 695.10

Multinodular (Simple Goiter)
Simple Goiter 240.00

Multinodular (Toxic Goiter)
Hyperthyroidism 242.90

Multiple
Multiple Myeloma 203.00
Multiple Sclerosis 340.00

Mumps
Mumps 72.00

Murine (Endemic Typhus)
Endemic Typhus 81.00

Muscular
Familial Progressive Spinal Muscular Atrophy 335.11
Progressive Muscular Dystrophy 359.11

Muscular (Activity)
Exercise 994.50

Myasthenia
Myasthenia Gravis 358.00

Mycoplasma
Mycoplasma Pneumoniae 483.01

Mycosis
Mycosis Fungoides 202.10

Myelitis
Myelitis 323.91

Myelocytic
Myelocytic Leukemia (Acute) 205.00
Myelocytic Leukemia (Chronic) 205.10

Myelofibrosis
Myelofibrosis 289.80

Myeloid (Metaplasia)
Myelofibrosis 289.80

Myeloma
Multiple Myeloma   203.00

Myeloproliferative (Myelofibrosis)
Myelofibrosis   289.80

Myelosclerosis (Myelofibrosis)
Myelofibrosis   289.80

Myelosis (Erythroleukemia)
Erythroleukemia   207.00

Myocardial
Acute Myocardial Infarction   410.90

Myocarditis
Acute Myocarditis   422.00

Myoglobinuria
Myoglobinuria   791.30

Myotonia
Myotonia Atrophica   359.21
Myotonia Congenita   359.22

Myotonic (Dystrophy)
Myotonia Atrophica   359.21

Myotonic (Myotonia Atrophica)
Myotonia Atrophica   359.21

Myxoma (Atrial)
Benign Neoplasm of Cardiovascular Tissue   212.70

N

Necrosis
Acute and Subacute Necrosis of Liver   570.00

Neoplasm
Benign Neoplasm of Adrenal Cortex   227.00
Benign Neoplasm of Brain and CNS   225.90
Benign Neoplasm of Breast   217.00
Benign Neoplasm of Cardiovascular Tissue   212.70
Benign Neoplasm of Ovary   220.00
Benign Neoplasm of Pancreas   211.60
Benign Neoplasm of Rectum and Anus   211.40
Benign Neoplasm of Stomach   211.10
Benign Neoplasm of Testis   222.00
Malignant Neoplasm of Adrenal Gland   194.00
Malignant Neoplasm of Bladder   188.90
Malignant Neoplasm of Bone   170.90
Malignant Neoplasm of Brain   191.90
Malignant Neoplasm of Breast   174.90
Malignant Neoplasm of Bronchus and Lung   162.90
Malignant Neoplasm of Cervix   180.90
Malignant Neoplasm of Corpus Uteri   182.00
Malignant Neoplasm of Esophagus   150.90
Malignant Neoplasm of Gallbladder   156.00
Malignant Neoplasm of Intrahepatic Bile Ducts   155.10
Malignant Neoplasm of Kidney   189.00
Malignant Neoplasm of Large Intestine   153.90
Malignant Neoplasm of Liver   155.00
Malignant Neoplasm of Other Parts of Nervous
   System   192.90
Malignant Neoplasm of Ovary   183.00
Malignant Neoplasm of Pancreas   157.90
Malignant Neoplasm of Pituitary   194.30
Malignant Neoplasm of Prostate   185.00
Malignant Neoplasm of Rectum   154.10
Malignant Neoplasm of Small Intestine   152.90
Malignant Neoplasm of Stomach   151.90
Malignant Neoplasm of Testis   186.90
Malignant Neoplasm of Thyroid Gland   193.00
Malignant Neoplasm of Trophoblast
   (Choriocarcinoma)   181.00
Secondary Malignant Neoplasm (Disseminated)   199.00
Secondary Malignant Neoplasm of Bone   198.50
Secondary Malignant Neoplasm of Brain   198.30
Secondary Malignant Neoplasm of Digestive System   197.50
Secondary Malignant Neoplasm of Liver   197.70
Secondary Malignant Neoplasm of Respiratory
   System   197.00

Neoplasm (Medullary Carcinoma of Thyroid)
Medullary Carcinoma of Thyroid   193.01

Neoplasm (Neuroblastoma)
Neuroblastoma   192.50

Nephrolithiasis (Kidney Calculus)
Kidney Calculus   592.00

Nephrosis [Glomerulonephritis (Minimal Change)]
Glomerulonephritis (Minimal Change)   580.02

Nephrotic
Nephrotic Syndrome   581.90

Nerve
Inflammation of Optic Nerve and Retina   363.20

Nervous (Neuroblastoma)
Neuroblastoma   192.50

Neuroblastoma
Neuroblastoma   192.50

Neurosis
Anxiety Neurosis   300.00
Depressive Neurosis   300.40

Newborn
Hemolytic Disease of Newborn (Erythroblastosis
   Fetalis)   773.00
Jaundice Due to Hepatocellular Damage (Newborn)   774.40

Nezeloff's
Nezeloff's Syndrome   279.13

Niemann-Pick
Niemann-Pick Disease   272.73

Nocturnal
Paroxysmal Nocturnal Hemoglobinuria   283.21

Non-Hodgkins
Non-Hodgkins Lymphoma   202.80

Non-medicinal
Toxic Effects of Non-medicinal Metals   985.00

Nonspherocytic
Hereditary Nonspherocytic Hemolytic Anemia   282.31

Nontoxic (Goiter)
Simple Goiter   240.00

Nontropical (Sprue)
Celiac Sprue Disease   579.00

O

Obesity
Obesity   278.00

Obstruction
Extrahepatic Biliary Obstruction   576.20
Intestinal Obstruction   560.90

Obstructive
Chronic Obstructive Lung Disease   496.00

Ocular (Muscular Dystrophy)
Progressive Muscular Dystrophy   359.11

Opium
Drug Dependence (Opium and Derivatives)   304.90

Oppenheim's (Disease)
Amyotonia Congenita   358.80

Optic
Inflammation of Optic Nerve and Retina   363.20

Ornithosis (Psittacosis)
Psittacosis   73.90

Oroya (Fever)
Bartonellosis   88.00

Ossium (Fragilitis)
Osteogenesis Imperfecta   756.51

Osteitis
Osteitis Deformans   731.00

Osteoarthritis
Osteoarthritis   715.90

Osteoectasia (Familial)
Hyperphosphatasia   275.31

Osteogenesis
Osteogenesis Imperfecta   756.51

Osteomalacia
Osteomalacia   268.20

Osteomyelitis
Osteomyelitis   730.00

Osteopetrosis
Osteopetrosis   756.52

Osteoporosis
Osteoporosis   733.00

Otitis
Otitis Externa   380.10

Otitis Media   381.00

Ovarian
Ovarian Cyst   620.20
Ovarian Hyperfunction   256.00
Ovarian Hypofunction   256.30

Ovaries
Polycystic Ovaries   256.40

Ovary
Benign Neoplasm of Ovary   220.00
Granulosa Cell Tumor of Ovary   220.92
Lutein Cell Tumor of Ovary   220.93
Malignant Neoplasm of Ovary   183.00
Theca Cell Tumor of Ovary   220.94

Ovary (Arrhenoblastoma)
Arrhenoblastoma   220.95

Ovary (Polycystic Ovaries)
Polycystic Ovaries   256.40

P

Paget's (Disease)
Osteitis Deformans   731.00

Pancreas
Benign Neoplasm of Pancreas   211.60
Malignant Neoplasm of Pancreas   157.90

Pancreatic
Pancreatic Cyst and Pseudocyst   577.20

Pancreatitis
Acute Pancreatitis   577.00
Chronic Pancreatitis   577.10

Paralysis
Familial Periodic Paralysis   275.34

Paralysis Agitans
Parkinsons's Disease   332.00

Paranoid
Paranoid States and Other Psychoses   297.90

Parkinsons's
Parkinsons's Disease   332.00

Parotitis (Mumps)
Mumps   72.00

Paroxysmal
Paroxysmal Nocturnal Hemoglobinuria   283.21

Parrot (Fever)
Psittacosis   73.90

Pasturella Pestis Infection
Typhoid Fever   2.00

Pectoris
Angina Pectoris   413.90

Pemphigus
Pemphigus   694.40

Peptic
Peptic Ulcer, Site Unspecified   533.90

Pericarditis
Acute Pericarditis   420.00
Constrictive Pericarditis   423.10

Periodic
Familial Periodic Paralysis   275.34

Peritonitis
Peritonitis   567.90

Pernicious
Pernicious Anemia   281.00

Pertussis (Whooping Cough)
Whooping Cough   33.00

Pharyngeal Pouch Syndrome
DiGeorge's Syndrome   279.11

Phenylketonuria
Phenylketonuria   270.10

Pheochromocytoma
Pheochromocytoma   227.91

Phlebitis
Phlebitis and Thrombophlebitis   451.90

Phlebotomus
Phlebotomus Fever   66.00

Pituitary
Anterior Pituitary Hypofunction   253.40

Malignant Neoplasm of Pituitary   194.30

Plague
Plague   20.00

Plasma (Cell Hepatitis)
Chronic Active Hepatitis   571.49

Plasma (Chronic Active Hepatitis)
Chronic Active Hepatitis   571.49

Plummer-Vinson
Plummer-Vinson Syndrome   280.81

Pneumomediastinum
Pneumomediastinum   518.10

Pneumonia
Bacterial Pneumonia   482.90
Resolving Pneumonia   486.01
Viral Pneumonia   480.90

Pneumoniae
Mycoplasma Pneumoniae   483.01

Poliomyelitis
Acute Poliomyelitis   45.90

Polyarteritis-Nodosa
Polyarteritis-Nodosa   446.00

Polycystic
Polycystic Kidney Disease   753.10
Polycystic Ovaries   256.40

Polycythemia
Polycythemia, Secondary   289.00
Polycythemia Vera   238.40

Polymyalgia (Rheumatica)
Cranial Arteritis and Related Conditions   446.50

Polymyositis
Dermatomyositis/Polymyositis   710.40

Polyneuritis
Polyneuritis   357.90

Polyneuritis (Idiopathic)
Guillain-Barré Syndrome   357.00

Polyostotic
Polyostotic Fibrous Dysplasia   756.54

Polyp
Adenomatous Polyp   211.41

Polyradiculitis (Polyneuritis)
Polyneuritis   357.90

Porphyria
Acute Intermittent Porphyria   277.14
Congenital Erythropoietic Porphyria (Günther's Disease)   277.11
Erythropoietic Coproporphyria   277.13
Erythropoietic Protoporphyria   277.12
Hereditary Coproporphyria   277.17
Porphyria Cutanea Tarda   277.16
Porphyria Variegata   277.15

Postcardiotomy
Postcardiotomy Syndrome   429.40

Postcholecystectomy
Postcholecystectomy Syndrome   576.00

Postgastrectomy
Postgastrectomy (Dumping) Syndrome   564.20

Postmenopausal
Menopausal and Postmenopausal Symptoms   627.90

Postnecrotic (Cirrhosis of Liver)
Cirrhosis of Liver   571.90

Poststreptococcal
Acute Poststreptococcal Glomerulonephritis   580.00

Pre-Eclampsia
Pre-Eclampsia   642.40

Pregnancy
Ectopic Pregnancy   633.90
Pregnancy   650.00
Pregnancy Complicated by Intrauterine Death   656.40

Pregnancy (Eclampsia)
Eclampsia   642.60

Pregnancy (Pre-Eclampsia)
Pre-Eclampsia   642.40

Primary [Immunodeficiency (Common Variable)]
Immunodeficiency (Common Variable)   279.06

Progressive
Familial Progressive Spinal Muscular Atrophy   335.11
Glomerulonephritis (Rapidly Progressive)   580.40

Progressive Muscular Dystrophy 359.11
Progressive Systemic Sclerosis 710.10

Progressive (Metachromatic Leukodystrophy)
Metachromatic Leukodystrophy 330.00

Prostate
Malignant Neoplasm of Prostate 185.00

Prostatic
Benign Prostatic Hypertrophy 600.00
Prostatic Infarction 602.80

Prostatitis
Prostatitis 601.00

Protein
Protein Malnutrition 260.00

Protein-Losing
Protein-Losing Enteropathy 579.01

Proteinosis
Pulmonary Alveolar Proteinosis 516.00

Prothrombin (Deficiency)
Factor V Deficiency 286.35

Protoporphyria
Erythropoietic Protoporphyria 277.12

Proximal
Proximal Renal Tubular Acidosis 588.81

Pseudocyst
Pancreatic Cyst and Pseudocyst 577.20

Pseudohypoparathyroidism
Pseudohypoparathyroidism 275.42

Psittacosis
Psittacosis 73.90

Psoriasis
Psoriasis 696.10

Psychoses
Paranoid States and Other Psychoses 297.90

Pulmonale
Cor Pulmonale 415.00

Pulmonary
Idiopathic Pulmonary Hemosiderosis 516.10
Pulmonary Alveolar Proteinosis 516.00
Pulmonary Collapse 518.00
Pulmonary Congestion and Hypostasis 514.00
Pulmonary Edema 518.40
Pulmonary Embolism and Infarction 415.10
Pulmonary Emphysema 492.80
Pulmonary Tuberculosis 11.00

Pulmonary (Chronic Obstructive Lung Disease)
Chronic Obstructive Lung Disease 496.00

Pulseless
Pulseless Disease (Aortic Arch Syndrome) 446.70

Purpura
Allergic Purpura 287.00
Idiopathic Thrombocytopenic Purpura 287.30
Thrombotic Thrombocytopenic Purpura 446.60

Pyelonephritis
Acute Pyelonephritis 590.10
Chronic Pyelonephritis 590.00

Pyloric
Pyloric Stenosis, Acquired 537.00

Pyogenic
Acute Arthritis (Pyogenic) 711.00
Liver Abscess (Pyogenic) 572.00

Pyogenic (Osteomyelitis)
Osteomyelitis 730.00

Pyridoxine-Responsive (Anemia)
Vitamin B$_6$ Deficiency Anemia 281.30

Pyruvate-Kinase (Deficiency)
Hereditary Nonspherocytic Hemolytic Anemia 282.31

R

Rabies
Rabies 71.00

Rapidly
Glomerulonephritis (Rapidly Progressive) 580.40

Rectum
Benign Neoplasm of Rectum and Anus 211.40
Malignant Neoplasm of Rectum 154.10

Refsum's
Refsum's Disease 356.30

Regional
Regional Enteritis or Ileitis 555.90

Reiter's
Reiter's Disease 99.30

Relapsing
Relapsing Fever 87.00

Related
Cranial Arteritis and Related Conditions 446.50

Renal
Acute Renal Failure 584.00
Chronic Renal Failure 585.00
Distal Renal Tubular Acidosis 588.82
Proximal Renal Tubular Acidosis 588.81
Renal Dwarfism 588.00
Renal Infarction 593.81

Renovascular
Renovascular Hypertension 405.91

Resistant
Vitamin D Resistant Rickets 275.35

Resolving
Resolving Pneumonia 486.01

Respiratory
Respiratory Distress Syndrome 770.80
Secondary Malignant Neoplasm of Respiratory System 197.00

Retardation
Mental Retardation 319.00

Reticuloendotheliosis
Leukemic Reticuloendotheliosis 202.40

Reticuloendotheliosis (Histiocytosis X)
Histiocytosis X 202.52

Reticulolymphocytic Leukemia (Chronic)
Leukemic Reticuloendotheliosis 202.40

Reticulosis (Histiocytic Medullary)
Non-Hodgkins Lymphoma 202.80

Reticulum Cell Sarcoma
Non-Hodgkins Lymphoma 202.80

Retina
Inflammation of Optic Nerve and Retina 363.20

Reye's
Reye's Syndrome 331.81

Rheumatic
Rheumatic Fever 390.00

Rheumatica (Polymyalgia)
Cranial Arteritis and Related Conditions 446.50

Rheumatoid
Juvenile Rheumatoid Arthritis 714.30
Rheumatoid (Ankylosing) Spondylitis 720.00
Rheumatoid Arthritis 714.00

Rickets
Vitamin D Deficiency Rickets 268.00
Vitamin D Resistant Rickets 275.35

Rickets (Renal Dwarfism)
Renal Dwarfism 588.00

Rickettsialpox
Rickettsialpox 83.20

Rocky
Rocky Mountain Spotted Fever 82.00

Rotor's
Rotor's Syndrome 277.43

Rubella
Congenital Rubella 771.00
Rubella 56.00

Ruptured
Ruptured Aortic Aneurysm 441.50

S

Salivary
Diseases of the Salivary Glands 527.90

Sandfly (Fever)
Phlebotomus Fever 66.00

Sarcoidosis
Sarcoidosis 135.00

Scapuloperoneal (Progressive Muscular Dystrophy)
Progressive Muscular Dystrophy 359.11

Scarlet
Scarlet Fever 34.10

Schistosomiasis
Schistosomiasis 120.00

SCID
Severe Combined Immunodeficiency 279.20

Scleroderma (Progressive Systemic Sclerosis)
Progressive Systemic Sclerosis 710.10

Sclerosing [Glomerulonephritis (Focal)]
Glomerulonephritis (Focal) 580.01

Sclerosis
Amyotrophic Lateral Sclerosis 335.20
Multiple Sclerosis 340.00
Progressive Systemic Sclerosis 710.10

Scrub (Typhus)
Mite-Borne Typhus 81.20

Scurvy (Vitamin C Deficiency)
Vitamin C Deficiency 267.00

Secondary
Polycythemia, Secondary 289.00
Secondary Malignant Neoplasm (Disseminated) 199.00
Secondary Malignant Neoplasm of Bone 198.50
Secondary Malignant Neoplasm of Brain 198.30
Secondary Malignant Neoplasm of Digestive System 197.50
Secondary Malignant Neoplasm of Liver 197.70
Secondary Malignant Neoplasm of Respiratory System 197.00

Segmental [Glomerulonephritis (Focal)]
Glomerulonephritis (Focal) 580.01

Selective
Dysgammaglobulinemia (Selective Immunoglobulin Deficiency) 279.07
IgA Deficiency (Selective) 279.01

Septicemia
Septicemia 38.00

Sertoli-Leydig (Cell Tumor)
Arrhenoblastoma 220.95

Severe
Severe Combined Immunodeficiency 279.20

Shigellosis (Bacillary Dysentery)
Bacillary Dysentery 4.90

Shingles (Herpes Zoster)
Herpes Zoster 53.00

Shock
Shock 785.50

Sicca (Keratoconjunctivitis)
Sjögren's Syndrome 710.20

Sickle
Sickle Cell Anemia 282.60

Sickness (Sleeping, African)
Trypanosomiasis 86.90

Sideroblastic
Sideroblastic Anemia 285.00

Silicosis
Silicosis 502.00

Simple
Simple Goiter 240.00

Simplex
Herpes Simplex 54.00

Sinusitis
Chronic Sinusitis 473.90

Site
Peptic Ulcer, Site Unspecified 533.90

Sjögren's
Sjögren's Syndrome 710.20

Skin
Malignant Melanoma of Skin 172.90

Sleeping (Sickness, African)
Trypanosomiasis 86.90

Small
Malignant Neoplasm of Small Intestine 152.90

Smallpox
Smallpox 50.00

Sodium
Diet (High Sodium) 1013.01
Diet (Low Sodium) 1013.02

Spasm
Spasm of Sphincter of Oddi 576.50

Spherocytosis
Hereditary (Congenital) Spherocytosis 282.00

Sphincter
Spasm of Sphincter of Oddi 576.50

Sphingomyelin (Lipidosis)
Niemann-Pick Disease 272.73

Spinal
Familial Progressive Spinal Muscular Atrophy 335.11

Spondylitis
Rheumatoid (Ankylosing) Spondylitis 720.00

Sponge
Medullary Sponge Kidney 753.13

Sporotrichosis
Sporotrichosis 117.10

Spotted
Rocky Mountain Spotted Fever 82.00

Sprue
Celiac Sprue Disease 579.00

Steatorrhea (Celiac Sprue Disease)
Celiac Sprue Disease 579.00

Steinert's (Disease)
Myotonia Atrophica 359.21

Stein-Leventhal
Stein-Leventhal Syndrome 256.41

Stenosis,
Pyloric Stenosis, Acquired 537.00

Stomach
Benign Neoplasm of Stomach 211.10
Fistula of Stomach and Duodenum 537.40
Malignant Neoplasm of Stomach 151.90

Stone (Kidney Calculus)
Kidney Calculus 592.00

Stone (Ureter Calculus)
Ureter Calculus 592.10

Storage (Glycogen)
Anderson's Disease 272.71
Forbes Disease 271.03
McArdle's Disease 271.02
Von Gierke's Disease 271.01

Stress
Stress 308.00

Striatopallidal (System Disorders)
Huntington's Chorea 333.40

Stroke
Heat stroke 992.00

Strongyloidiasis
Strongyloidiasis 127.20

Struma (Lymphomatosa)
Hashimoto's Thyroiditis 245.20

Stuart (Factor Deficiency)
Factor X Deficiency 286.36

Subacute
Acute and Subacute Necrosis of Liver 570.00
Subacute Thyroiditis 245.10

Subacute [Glomerulonephritis (Rapidly Progressive)]
Glomerulonephritis (Rapidly Progressive) 580.40

Subacute (Hepatitis)
Chronic Active Hepatitis 571.49

Syndrome
Acquired Immunodeficiency Syndrome (AIDS) 279.31
Carcinoid Syndrome 259.20
Crigler-Najjar Syndrome 277.44
DiGeorge's Syndrome 279.11
Down's Syndrome 758.00
Dubin-Johnson Syndrome 277.41
Felty's Syndrome 714.10
Goodpasture's Syndrome 446.20
Guillain-Barré Syndrome 357.00
Hyperventilation Syndrome 306.10
Klinefelter's Syndrome (XXY) 758.70
Lesch-Nyhan Syndrome 277.22
Milk-Alkali Syndrome 275.41
Nephrotic Syndrome 581.90
Nezeloff's Syndrome 279.13
Plummer-Vinson Syndrome 280.81

Postcardiotomy Syndrome 429.40
Postcholecystectomy Syndrome 576.00
Postgastrectomy (Dumping) Syndrome 564.20
Pulseless Disease (Aortic Arch Syndrome) 446.70
Respiratory Distress Syndrome 770.80
Reye's Syndrome 331.81
Rotor's Syndrome 277.43
Sjögren's Syndrome 710.20
Stein-Leventhal Syndrome 256.41
Wiskott-Aldrich Syndrome 279.12
Zollinger-Ellison Syndrome 251.50

Syndrome (Cushing's)
Adrenal Cortical Hyperfunction (Glucocorticoid Excess) 255.00

Syndrome (Digugleilmo's)
Erythroleukemia 207.00

Syndrome (Familial Progressive Spinal Muscular Atrophy)
Familial Progressive Spinal Muscular Atrophy 335.11

Syndrome (Moschcowitz's)
Thrombotic Thrombocytopenic Purpura 446.60

Syndromes
Syndromes Due to Sex Chromosome Abnormalities 758.80

Syndrome (Werdnig-Hoffman)
Familial Progressive Spinal Muscular Atrophy 335.11

Syphilis
Syphilis 97.90

Syringobulbia
Syringomyelia and Syringobulbia 336.00

Syrup
Maple Syrup Urine Disease 270.31

Systemic
Progressive Systemic Sclerosis 710.10
Systemic Lupus Erythematosus 710.00

T

Takayasu's [Pulseless Disease (Aortic Arch Syndrome)]
Pulseless Disease (Aortic Arch Syndrome) 446.70

Tangier
Tangier Disease 272.51

Tarda
Porphyria Cutanea Tarda 277.16

Tay-Sach's
Tay-Sach's Disease 330.11

Telangiectasia
Ataxia-Telangiectasia 334.80

Temporal (Arteritis)
Cranial Arteritis and Related Conditions 446.50

Teratoma
Teratoma (Dermoid) 220.01

Teratoma (Benign Neoplasm of Ovary)
Benign Neoplasm of Ovary 220.00

Testicular
Testicular Hypofunction 257.20

Testis
Benign Neoplasm of Testis 222.00
Malignant Neoplasm of Testis 186.90

Tetanus
Tetanus 37.00

Thalassemia
Thalassemia Major 282.41
Thalassemia Minor 282.42

Theca
Theca Cell Tumor of Ovary 220.94

Thiamine
Thiamine (B_1) Deficiency 265.00

Thomsen's (Disease)
Myotonia Congenita 359.22

Thrombasthenia
Thrombasthenia (Glanzmann's) 287.10

Thrombocytopenic
Idiopathic Thrombocytopenic Purpura 287.30
Thrombotic Thrombocytopenic Purpura 446.60

Thrombophlebitis
Phlebitis and Thrombophlebitis 451.90

Thrombosis
Arterial Embolism and Thrombosis 444.90
Cerebral Thrombosis 434.00

Thrombotic
Thrombotic Thrombocytopenic Purpura 446.60

Thyroid
Malignant Neoplasm of Thyroid Gland 193.00
Medullary Carcinoma of Thyroid 193.01

Thyroiditis
Hashimoto's Thyroiditis 245.20
Subacute Thyroiditis 245.10

Thyrotoxicosis (Hyperthyroidism)
Hyperthyroidism 242.90

Tick
Tick-Borne Fever 66.10

Tissue
Benign Neoplasm of Cardiovascular Tissue 212.70
Mixed Connective Tissue Disease 711.10

Tonsillitis
Acute Tonsillitis 463.00

Toxic
Toxic Effects of Carbon Monoxide 986.00
Toxic Effects of Lead and Its Compounds (including Fumes) 984.00
Toxic Effects of Non-medicinal Metals 985.00
Toxic Effects of Venom 989.50
Toxic Hepatitis 573.30

Toxic (Diffuse Goiter)
Hyperthyroidism 242.90

Toxic (Multinodular Goiter)
Hyperthyroidism 242.90

Toxoplasmosis
Toxoplasmosis 130.00

Tract
Urinary Tract Infection 599.00

Transient
Transient Cerebral Ischemia 435.90

Trauma
Crush Injury (Trauma) 929.00

Tremens
Delirium Tremens 291.00

Trichinosis
Trichinosis 124.00

Trichuriasis
Trichuriasis 127.30

Trisomy
Trisomy 13 758.10

Trisomy (Down's Syndrome)
Down's Syndrome 758.00

Trophoblast
Malignant Neoplasm of Trophoblast (Choriocarcinoma) 181.00

Trypanosomiasis
Trypanosomiasis 86.90

Tuberculosis
Disseminated Tuberculosis 18.00
Pulmonary Tuberculosis 11.00
Tuberculosis Meningitis 13.00

Tubular
Distal Renal Tubular Acidosis 588.82
Proximal Renal Tubular Acidosis 588.81

Tularemia
Tularemia 21.00

Tumor
Granulosa Cell Tumor of Ovary 220.92
Lutein Cell Tumor of Ovary 220.93
Theca Cell Tumor of Ovary 220.94

Tumor (Arrhenoblastoma)
Arrhenoblastoma 220.95

Tumor (Sertoli-Leydig Cell)
Arrhenoblastoma 220.95

Turner's (Syndrome)
Syndromes Due to Sex Chromosome Abnormalities 758.80

Type I
Type I Hyperlipoproteinemia 272.31

Type I (Distal Renal Tubular Acidosis)
Distal Renal Tubular Acidosis 588.82

Type I [Glomerulonephritis (Rapidly Progressive)]
Glomerulonephritis (Rapidly Progressive)   580.40
Type I (Glycogen-Storage)
Von Gierke's Disease   271.01
Type IIA
Type IIA Hyperlipoproteinemia   272.00
Type IIB
Type IIB Hyperlipoproteinemia   272.21
Type III
Type III Hyperlipoproteinemia   272.22
Type III (Glycogen Storage Disease)
Forbes Disease   271.03
Type II (Proximal Renal Tubular Acidosis)
Proximal Renal Tubular Acidosis   588.81
Type IV
Type IV Hyperlipoproteinemia   272.10
Type IV (Glycogen Storage Disease)
Anderson's Disease   272.71
Type I (Von Gierke's Disease)
Von Gierke's Disease   271.01
Type V
Type V Hyperlipoproteinemia   272.32
Type V (Glycogen Storage)
McArdle's Disease   271.02
Typhoid
Typhoid Fever   2.00
Typhus
Endemic Typhus   81.00
Epidemic Typhus   80.00
Mite-Borne Typhus   81.20

U

Ulcer
Peptic Ulcer, Site Unspecified   533.90
Ulcerative
Ulcerative Colitis   556.00
Ureter
Ureter Calculus   592.10
Urethritis
Urethritis   597.80
Urinary
Urinary Tract Infection   599.00
Urine
Maple Syrup Urine Disease   270.31
Uroporphyria (Erythropoietic)
Congenital Erythropoietic Porphyria (Günther's Disease)   277.11
Urticaria
Urticaria   708.90
Uteri
Malignant Neoplasm of Corpus Uteri   182.00

V

Variable
Immunodeficiency (Common Variable)   279.06
Varicella (Chickenpox)
Chickenpox   52.00
Variegata
Porphyria Variegata   277.15
Vascular (Hemophilia)
Von Willebrand's Disease   286.40
Vasopressin (Diabetes Insipidus)
Diabetes Insipidus   253.50
Venereum
Lymphogranuloma Venereum   99.10
Venom
Toxic Effects of Venom   989.50
Vera
Polycythemia Vera   238.40
Verruga (Fever)
Bartonellosis   88.00

Viral
Viral Hepatitis   70.00
Viral Pneumonia   480.90
Visceralis
Larva Migrans (Visceralis)   128.00
Vitamin
Vitamin B_6 Deficiency Anemia   281.30
Vitamin C Deficiency   267.00
Vitamin D Deficiency Rickets   268.00
Vitamin D Resistant Rickets   275.35
Vitamin K Deficiency   269.00
Vomiting
Vomiting   787.00

W

Waldenström's
Waldenström's Macroglobulinemia   273.30
Warm antibody [Acquired Hemolytic Anemias (Autoimmune)]
Acquired Hemolytic Anemia (Autoimmune)   283.00
Weil's (Leptospirosis)
Leptospirosis   100.00
Werdnig-Hoffman (Disease)
Familial Progressive Spinal Muscular Atrophy   335.11
Western
Western Equine Encephalitis   62.10
Whipple's
Whipple's Disease   40.20
Whipworm (Infection)
Trichuriasis   127.30
Whooping
Whooping Cough   33.00
Willebrand's
Von Willebrand's Disease   286.40
Wilson's Disease
Hepatolenticular Degeneration   275.10
Wiskott-Aldrich
Wiskott-Aldrich Syndrome   279.12

X

Xanthinuria
Xanthinuria   277.21
XXY
Klinefelter's Syndrome (XXY)   758.70

Y

Yaws
Yaws   102.90
Yellow
Yellow Fever   60.00
Yersinia Pestis Infection
Typhoid Fever   2.00

Z

Zollinger-Ellison
Zollinger-Ellison Syndrome   251.50
Zoster
Herpes Zoster   53.00

3 LABORATORY TEST LISTINGS

^{131}I Uptake

Serum Decrease

244.90 Hypothyroidism Usually low but may be normal or in a rare patient slightly elevated at 2 or 4 h. *0999*

245.10 Subacute Thyroiditis The association of a very low uptake with a normal or high serum T_4 concentration is characteristic of the early phase of disease. Subnormal values for thyroid ^{131}I uptake are usually found. *2540* Extremely low. *0962 2104*

245.20 Hashimoto's Thyroiditis Markedly depressed. *0992* Subnormal values are usually found early in the disease. *2540* In the far advanced stage of thyroid destruction, all tests show the results of hypothyroidism: radioiodide uptake is low normal to low. *2035* May be normal, elevated, or low. *0962*

253.40 Anterior Pituitary Hypofunction *0995*

428.00 Congestive Heart Failure *2104*

580.00 Acute Poststreptococcal Glomerulonephritis In renal disease. *2104*

584.00 Acute Renal Failure In renal disease. *2104*

585.00 Chronic Renal Failure In renal disease. *2104*

Serum Increase

155.00 Malignant Neoplasm of Liver In hepatic disease. *2104*

240.00 Simple Goiter In some patients, elevated to the 70-95% range. *0151 0962*

242.90 Hyperthyroidism Thyroid uptake is increased. It is relatively more affected at 1, 2, or 6 h than at 24 h. It may be normal in presence of recent iodine ingestion. *2467* Uptake is > 30% in 6 h, > 40% in 12 h, and > 55% in 24 h, with rapid release. *0619* Mean uptake = 63.6% in patients over 60 y of age. *0512* May be present. *0962*

245.20 Hashimoto's Thyroiditis An early abnormality is a relative impairment of the process of organification of iodide trapped by the thyroid cell. Radioiodide uptake studies from 20 min to 6 h after administration may be relatively high, compared to the 24 h uptake. *2035* May be normal or elevated in euthyroid patients. *1106* May be slightly elevated in chronic patients. *0999* May be normal, elevated, or low. *0962*

428.00 Congestive Heart Failure *2104*

570.00 Acute and Subacute Necrosis of Liver In hepatic disease. *2104*

571.90 Cirrhosis of Liver In hepatic disease. *2104*

581.90 Nephrotic Syndrome Urinary loss of TBG results in lowering of most blood thyroid hormones and increased T_3 uptake. *0962 2104*

1013.00 Diet Low-iodine diets. *2104*

Serum Normal

240.00 Simple Goiter Usually normal. *2540*

245.20 Hashimoto's Thyroiditis *0962*

253.40 Anterior Pituitary Hypofunction The thyroidal uptake is often inexplicably normal even when the patient is clinically hypothyroid. *0151*

1,25-Dihydroxy-Vitamin D_3

Serum Decrease

202.80 Non-Hodgkins Lymphoma In five patients with adult T-Cell Lymphoma. All had levels at or below the normal range. These data show that calcitriol levels are not uniformly elevated in this order and may not be the usual cause of hypercalcemia. *0574*

252.10 Hypoparathyroidism *0062*

275.35 Vitamin D Resistant Rickets *0062*

275.42 Pseudohypoparathyroidism *0062*

585.00 Chronic Renal Failure *0062*

Serum Increase

11.00 Pulmonary Tuberculosis *0062*

18.00 Disseminated Tuberculosis *0062*

135.00 Sarcoidosis *0062*

202.80 Non-Hodgkins Lymphoma Three patients had elevated levels (56,72,77 pg/mL) compared to normal (< 50). *0280*

252.00 Hyperparathyroidism *0062*

502.00 Silicosis *0062*

Serum Normal

202.80 Non-Hodgkins Lymphoma In five patients with adult T-Cell Lymphoma. All had levels at or below the normal range. These data show that calcitriol levels are not uniformly elevated in this order and may not be the usual cause of hypercalcemia. *0574*

2,3-Diphosphoglycerate

Urine Increase

250.00 Diabetes Mellitus *0503*

Red Blood Cells Decrease

276.20 Metabolic Acidosis Concentration will be low. *0158*

770.80 Respiratory Distress Syndrome *0236*

Red Blood Cells Increase

162.90 Malignant Neoplasm of Bronchus and Lung Synthesis is increased in response to hypoxia. *0159*

242.90 Hyperthyroidism Results in reduced oxygen affinity. *1596*

250.00 Diabetes Mellitus Increased to 15.0 μmol/g (normal = 13.7). Concentrations vary in response to plasma inorganic phosphate levels. *0567*

277.00 Cystic Fibrosis A study of 35 patients demonstrated that increasing severity of pulmonary involvement was associated with a mild but definite increase in erythrocyte 2,3-DPG and a decrease in hemoglobin affinity for oxygen. *1988*

280.90 Iron Deficiency Anemia Synthesis is increased in response to hypoxia. *0159*

281.00 Pernicious Anemia Synthesis is increased in response to hypoxia. *0159*

283.00 Acquired Hemolytic Anemia (Autoimmune) Synthesis is increased in response to hypoxia. *0159*

2,3-Diphosphoglycerate *(continued)*

Red Blood Cells   Increase *(continued)*

284.90 Aplastic Anemia   Synthesis is increased in response to hypoxia. *0159*

493.10 Asthma (Intrinsic)   In acute untreated attacks. *1228*

496.00 Chronic Obstructive Lung Disease   Synthesis is increased. *0159*

585.00 Chronic Renal Failure   Intracellular concentration is appropriately increased in response to anemia. *2538 0389*

785.50 Shock   Disturbed RBC 2,3-DPG metabolism results in reduced oxygen affinity and delivery to tissues. *0151*

5-Hydroxyindoleacetic Acid (5-HIAA)

Urine   Decrease

202.80 Non-Hodgkins Lymphoma   Absent from urine. *0619*

270.02 Hartnup Disease   Low; may represent a slight diversion of tryptophan from serotonin formation. *2246*

270.10 Phenylketonuria   *2468*

Urine   Increase

162.90 Malignant Neoplasm of Bronchus and Lung   Oat-cell carcinoma of the bronchus and bronchial adenoma of carcinoid type may cause excess secretion. *0619*   Rarely a carcinoid syndrome is associated with bronchogenic carcinoma with the laboratory manifestation of abnormal urinary levels of 5-HIAA. *0962*

259.20 Carcinoid Syndrome   Diagnostic of a carcinoid tumor. *1108*   Normally there are 2-9 mg/24h while levels up to 1 g/24h may occur in the carcinoid syndrome. *0962*   75% of 75 patients with this disorder had elevated levels *0719*   Excretions > 130 mmol/24h is diagnostic provided walnuts and bananas have been excluded from the diet for 24 h. *2612*   Usually associated with 5-HIAA urinary concentrations 25 mg/24h. *2404*   Increased, usually when tumor is far advanced, but may not be increased despite massive metastases. Useful in confirming diagnosis in only 5-7% *2468*

346.00 Migraine   Levels are increased during acute attacks. *0996*

579.00 Celiac Sprue Disease   Abnormal tryptophan metabolism may result in elevated urinary excretion in patients with malabsorption. *2199*   Slightly increased level (12-16 mg/24h). *0995*

1013.00 Diet   With ingestion of plums or pineapples; high serotonin content. *0984*

Urine   Normal

259.20 Carcinoid Syndrome   Hyperserotoninemia with normal urinary 5-HIAA in ileal carcinoid tumors. *2404*

CSF   Decrease

331.00 Alzheimer's Disease   Lower than in an aged matched control group. *1765*

CSF   Increase

53.00 Herpes Zoster   Has been reported. *1167*

CSF   Normal

335.20 Amyotrophic Lateral Sclerosis   *1495*

5-Hydroxytryptamine (Serotonin)

Blood   Decrease

270.02 Hartnup Disease   Low; may represent a slight diversion of tryptophan from serotonin formation. *2246*

270.51 Histidinemia   In the 3 cases in which serotonin concentration has been determined, values were found to be 50% of the normal concentration. *2246*

Blood   Increase

162.90 Malignant Neoplasm of Bronchus and Lung   Oat-cell carcinoma of the bronchus and bronchial adenoma of carcinoid type may cause excessive secretion. *0619*   Rarely a carcinoid syndrome is associated with bronchogenic carcinoma with the laboratory manifestation of abnormal urinary levels of 5-HIAA. *0962*

193.01 Medullary Carcinoma of Thyroid   In medullary cancer. *0962*

259.20 Carcinoid Syndrome   Systemic symptoms appear only after metastasis to the liver; the serotonin released from the metastasis passes directly to the systemic circulation, avoiding hepatic metabolism. *0962*   Carcinoid tumors differ widely in their ability to produce or store 5-HT. Excessive production remains their most characteristic chemical abnormality. *2199*   Usually associated with an excess of circulating 5-HT. *2612*   Serotonin and related products are the biochemical markers of this disorder. *2404*

Urine   Increase

259.20 Carcinoid Syndrome   Systemic symptoms appear only after metastasis to the liver; the serotonin released from the metastasis passes directly to the systemic circulation, avoiding hepatic metabolism. *0962*   Carcinoid tumors differ widely in their ability to produce or store 5-HT. Excessive production remains their most characteristic chemical abnormality. *2199*   Usually associated with an excess of circulating 5-HT. *2612*

5'-Nucleotidase

Serum   Increase

6.00 Amebiasis   With liver involvement. *1058*

18.00 Disseminated Tuberculosis   2 cases were reported in which the tests were 25 and 118 U/L (Normal = 2-11 U/L). *1312*   Serum 5'-nucleotidase was significantly elevated in 2 of 3 patients with liver granulomata. *1312*

23.00 Brucellosis   Significantly elevated in 2 of 3 patients with liver granulomata. *1312*

38.00 Septicemia   4 patients with extrahepatic infection showed elevated levels, ranging from 21-75 U/L (Normal = 3-17). *1681*

70.00 Viral Hepatitis   Elevations ranging from 8-103 U/L (normal = 2-11) were observed in 24 patients. *1312   0151*

115.00 Histoplasmosis   Significantly elevated in 2 of 3 patients with liver granulomata. *1312*

120.00 Schistosomiasis   Elevated above normal upon admission and rose to 2 X normal during treatment. *2026*   Significantly elevated in 2 of 3 patients with live granulomata. *1312*

135.00 Sarcoidosis   Levels ranging from 14.5-91.3 U/L were observed in 5 cases. *1312*   Significantly elevated in 2 of 3 patients with liver granulomata. *1312*

155.00 Malignant Neoplasm of Liver   88.4% of 51 hepatoma patients had values > 10% above the normal upper limit. *1115 0503*

157.90 Malignant Neoplasm of Pancreas   Due to biliary tract obstruction, values range from 28.0-40.0 U/L (normal = 4.0). *2576*   Values are elevated when there is an element of obstruction of the common bile duct or metastases to the liver. *0151   1312*

197.70 Secondary Malignant Neoplasm of Liver   Five patients with carcinoma of head of pancreas metastatic to liver showed elevations ranging from 20-118 U/L (normal = 2-11). *1312*

201.90 Hodgkin's Disease   Six patients showed elevations varying from 18.8-126.2 U/L (normal = 2-11). *1312*

202.80 Non-Hodgkins Lymphoma   Ten patients with lymphosarcoma, showed 5'-nucleotidase activities ranging from 16-59 U/L (normal = 2-11). *1312*

272.72 Gaucher's Disease   May be abnormal with liver involvement. *0995*

275.00 Hemochromatosis   With liver involvement. *0962*

275.10 Hepatolenticular Degeneration   With liver involvement. *0995*

570.00 Acute and Subacute Necrosis of Liver   Increased (although low levels have been reported with very severe liver damage), especially if intrahepatic cholestasis present. *0619*

571.20 Laennec's or Alcoholic Cirrhosis   Elevations ranging from 32.7-265 U/L (normal = 2-11) were observed in 36 patients. In 20 cases of Laennec's cirrhosis with acute fatty infiltration the range was 18.8-56.9. *1312*

571.60 Biliary Cirrhosis   In 18 patients levels ranged from 32.7-265 U/L, mean = 127.8 ± 79.5. *1312   0151*

571.90 Cirrhosis of Liver   Increased in 50% of patients. *2467*

573.30 Toxic Hepatitis   Six cases of toxic drug hepatitis showed activities ranging from 91.3-155.7 U/L (normal = 2-11 U/L). *1312*

575.00 Acute Cholecystitis   Slight hepatic inflammation and partial biliary obstruction. *0186*

576.10 Cholangitis   Elevated levels indicate extrahepatic obstruction. *0151*

576.20 Extrahepatic Biliary Obstruction   Increased in extra-hepatic biliary obstruction. *0619*

577.00 Acute Pancreatitis   Six patients showed elevations ranging from 16.1-67.1 U/L (normal = 2-11). *1312*

710.00 Systemic Lupus Erythematosus   In 2 cases elevated to 13 and 26 U/L. *1312*

714.00 Rheumatoid Arthritis   May be found in up to 33% of patients with a greater increase in enzyme activity in the synovial fluid. *0619*

Serum   Normal

275.00 Hemochromatosis   Over 50% of patients have no laboratory evidence of liver dysfunction. *0995*

650.00 Pregnancy   Normal in pregnancy and the postpartum period (in contrast to serum leucine aminopeptidase and alkaline phosphatase); therefore may aid in differential diagnosis of hepatobiliary disease occurring during pregnancy. *2467*

Synovial Fluid   Increase

714.00 Rheumatoid Arthritis   In 58% with reduction to normal following corticosteroid therapy. *0619*   Slightly increased in cases showing more advanced x-ray changes. *2320*

Lymphocytes   Decrease

204.10 Lymphocytic Leukemia (Chronic)   Reduced or absent in the lymphocytes of most patients. *1429   2538*

11-Hydroxycorticosteroids

Plasma   Decrease

255.40 Adrenal Cortical Hypofunction   *0619*

Plasma   Increase

244.90 Hypothyroidism   Due to slow disposal of circulating cortisol. *0619*

255.00 Adrenal Cortical Hyperfunction (Glucocorticoid Excess)   Cortisol-binding globulin becomes saturated at the upper limit of normal for plasma cortisol, resulting in a disproportionately high unbound cortisol concentration. *0999*   Increased free plasma concentration and failure to reduce secretion with dexamethasone. *2612*

303.00 Acute Alcoholic Intoxication   Alcohol excess in nonalcoholics. No rise in chronic alcoholics. *0619*

650.00 Pregnancy   Rises progressively throughout pregnancy. *2084*

991.60 Hypothermia   Increase in accidental hypothermia. *0619*

Urine   Increase

194.00 Malignant Neoplasm of Adrenal Gland   Usually very high. *2612*

227.00 Benign Neoplasm of Adrenal Cortex   In Cushingoid patients. *2612*

255.00 Adrenal Cortical Hyperfunction (Glucocorticoid Excess)   Raised and relatively constant urinary excretions usually occur, but values may fluctuate from normal to elevated over a period of days. *0978*   Increased in all forms of the syndrome. *2612   0999*

Urine   Normal

242.90 Hyperthyroidism   *2540*

791.30 Myoglobinuria   Endocrine studies are normal. *2467*

17-Hydroxycorticosteroids

Urine   Decrease

40.20 Whipple's Disease   Reduced 24-h excretion of 17-hydroxycorticosteroids and 17-ketosteroids has been found in debilitated patients. *2199*

242.90 Hyperthyroidism   *0503*

244.90 Hypothyroidism   As a result of decreased rate of turnover of cortisol. *2540*   Low in untreated disease. Does not necessarily indicate pituitary origin. *2612*

250.00 Diabetes Mellitus   *0503*

253.40 Anterior Pituitary Hypofunction   *0999*

255.40 Adrenal Cortical Hypofunction   Low for males in the diagnosis of Addison's Disease. *0999*

257.20 Testicular Hypofunction   Decreased with castration in men. *2467*

260.00 Protein Malnutrition   *2467*

274.00 Gout   *0503*

579.00 Celiac Sprue Disease   In patients with sufficient malabsorption to cause pituitary or adrenal insufficiency. *2540*

581.90 Nephrotic Syndrome   *0503*

585.00 Chronic Renal Failure   *0503*

Urine   Increase

38.00 Septicemia   Increased due to severe stress. *2467*

162.90 Malignant Neoplasm of Bronchus and Lung   Ectopic ACTH production. *0536*

186.90 Malignant Neoplasm of Testis   *2467*

194.00 Malignant Neoplasm of Adrenal Gland   *0503*

220.01 Teratoma (Dermoid)   *0503*

220.95 Arrhenoblastoma   *0503*

242.90 Hyperthyroidism   Normal or slightly increased. *2540*

253.00 Acromegaly   *0503*

255.00 Adrenal Cortical Hyperfunction (Glucocorticoid Excess)   Increased excretion of 17-OHCS and 17-KS is characteristic. *0842*   Elevated values at a time when the patient is not under acute exogenous stress strongly favor the diagnosis. Confirmed by demonstrating nonsuppressibility of urinary 17-OHCS to low-dose dexamethasone. *1108*

255.10 Adrenal Cortical Hyperfunction (Mineralocorticoid Excess)   May cause high excretion with feminization and no Cushing's syndrome involved. *0999*   Urine 17-hydroxycorticosteroids and 17-KS excretion levels are always within normal range in patients with aldosteronomas but may occasionally be elevated in more rare instances of primary aldosteronism due to adrenal carcinoma. *0995*

256.41 Stein-Leventhal Syndrome   *0503*

259.20 Carcinoid Syndrome   May be 10 X normal. *0151*

277.14 Acute Intermittent Porphyria   In acute attacks. *2246*

277.17 Hereditary Coproporphyria   In acute attacks. *2246*

278.00 Obesity   Increased 24 hour hydroxycorticoid excretion. *0062*

308.00 Stress   *2467*

401.00 Malignant Hypertension   Slightly increased. *2467*

410.90 Acute Myocardial Infarction   *1108*

577.00 Acute Pancreatitis   May be marked; increased due to severe stress. *2467*

584.00 Acute Renal Failure   Both free and glucuronide fraction of 17 OHCS are elevated in acute but not chronic failure. *0219*

642.60 Eclampsia   Increased due to severe stress. *2467*

650.00 Pregnancy   Primarily during 3rd trimester. *0071*

785.50 Shock   *0164*

929.00 Crush Injury (Trauma)   Due to severe stress. *0995*

948.00 Burns   Increased due to severe stress. *2467*

994.50 Exercise   The normal output after daily routine activity is twice the resting output. *0619*   Effect most marked in well trained individuals. *0089*   Response to stress of exercise. *0342*

Urine   Normal

194.00 Malignant Neoplasm of Adrenal Gland   Can be normal to moderately elevated in masculinizing or feminizing tumors. *0995*

253.40 Anterior Pituitary Hypofunction   *2467*

255.10 Adrenal Cortical Hyperfunction (Mineralocorticoid Excess)   Urine 17-hydroxycorticosteroids and 17-KS excretion levels are always within normal range in patients with aldosteronomas but may occasionally be elevated in more rare instances of primary aldosteronism due to adrenal carcinoma. *0995*

255.40 Adrenal Cortical Hypofunction   *2467*

758.70 Klinefelter's Syndrome (XXY)   Usually normal. *1090*

791.30 Myoglobinuria   *2467*

17-Hydroxyprogesterone

Plasma   Increase

255.10   **Adrenal Cortical Hyperfunction (Mineralocorticoid Excess)**   Congenital Adrenal Hyperplasia. *2596*

17-Ketogenic Steroids

Urine   Decrease

40.20   **Whipple's Disease**   Reduced 24 h excretion of 17-hydroxycorticosteroids and 17-ketosteroids has been found in debilitated patients. *2199*

242.90   **Hyperthyroidism**   May be moderately reduced. *2540*

244.90   **Hypothyroidism**   As a result of decreased rate of turnover of cortisol. *2540*   Low in untreated disease. Does not necessarily indicate pituitary origin. *2612*

250.00   **Diabetes Mellitus**   *0503*

253.40   **Anterior Pituitary Hypofunction**   Low or low normal levels are suggestive but not diagnostic. *2612*

255.40   **Adrenal Cortical Hypofunction**   Markedly decreased. *2468*

257.20   **Testicular Hypofunction**   Decreased with castration in men. *2467*

260.00   **Protein Malnutrition**   *2467*

274.00   **Gout**   *0503*

581.90   **Nephrotic Syndrome**   *2467*

585.00   **Chronic Renal Failure**   *0503*

Urine   Increase

38.00   **Septicemia**   Increased due to severe stress. *2467*

162.90   **Malignant Neoplasm of Bronchus and Lung**   Ectopic ACTH production. *0536*

186.90   **Malignant Neoplasm of Testis**   *2467*

194.00   **Malignant Neoplasm of Adrenal Gland**   Very high values in Cushing's suggests ectopic ACTH production or adrenocortical carcinoma. *2612*

220.01   **Teratoma (Dermoid)**   *0503*

220.93   **Lutein Cell Tumor of Ovary**   Increased in lutein cell tumor of the ovary if androgenic *2467* .

220.95   **Arrhenoblastoma**   *0503*

222.00   **Benign Neoplasm of Testis**   The 17-ketosteroids occasionally are elevated when a Leydig cell tumor is present. *0433*

227.00   **Benign Neoplasm of Adrenal Cortex**   May be normal or raised. *2612*

242.90   **Hyperthyroidism**   Normal or slightly increased. *2540*

253.00   **Acromegaly**   *0433*

255.00   **Adrenal Cortical Hyperfunction (Glucocorticoid Excess)**   Over 4 X normal in 50% of adrenal carcinomas, 15% of extrapituitary tumors that secrete ACTH, 3% of adrenal hyperplasias without tumors with Cushing's Syndrome. *2467*   Diagnosis is confirmed by demonstrating nonsuppressibility of 17-KS to low-dose dexamethasone. *1108*   Very high values suggest ectopic ACTH production or adrenocortical carcinoma. *2612*   *0151*

259.20   **Carcinoid Syndrome**   *0151*

277.14   **Acute Intermittent Porphyria**   In acute attacks. *2246*

277.17   **Hereditary Coproporphyria**   In acute attacks. *2246*

308.00   **Stress**   *2467*

401.00   **Malignant Hypertension**   Slightly increased. *2467*

410.90   **Acute Myocardial Infarction**   *1108*

577.00   **Acute Pancreatitis**   May be marked; increased due to severe stress. *2467*

584.00   **Acute Renal Failure**   Both free and glucuronide fraction of 17 OHCS are elevated in acute but not chronic failure. *0219*

642.60   **Eclampsia**   Increased due to severe stress. *2467*

650.00   **Pregnancy**   *2467*

785.50   **Shock**   *2246*

929.00   **Crush Injury (Trauma)**   Due to severe stress. *0995*

948.00   **Burns**   Increased due to severe stress. *2467*

994.50   **Exercise**   The normal output after daily routine activity is twice the resting output. *0619*   Effect most marked in well trained individuals. *0089*   Response to stress of exercise. *0342*

Urine   Normal

194.00   **Malignant Neoplasm of Adrenal Gland**   Can be normal to moderately elevated in masculinizing or feminizing tumors. *0995*

253.40   **Anterior Pituitary Hypofunction**   *2467*

255.00   **Adrenal Cortical Hyperfunction (Glucocorticoid Excess)**   May be normal in pituitary-dependent Cushing's syndrome. *2612*

758.70   **Klinefelter's Syndrome (XXY)**   Usually normal. *1090*

791.30   **Myoglobinuria**   *2467*

17-Ketosteroids

Serum   Increase

220.92   **Granulosa Cell Tumor of Ovary**   Ketosteroids are increased in virilizing ovarian tumors (e.g., adrenal rest tumor, granulosa cell tumor, hilar cell tumor, Brenner tumor, and most frequently, arrhenoblastoma) increased in 50% of patients and normal in 50% of the patients. *2467*

220.93   **Lutein Cell Tumor of Ovary**   Ketosteroids are increased in virilizing ovarian tumors (e.g., adrenal rest tumor, granulosa cell tumor, hilar cell tumor, Brenner tumor, and most frequently, arrhenoblastoma) increased in 50% of the patients and normal in 50% of the patients. *2467*

220.94   **Theca Cell Tumor of Ovary**   Ketosteroids are increased in virilizing ovarian tumors (e.g., adrenal rest tumor, granulosa cell tumor, hilar cell tumor, Brenner tumor, and most frequently, arrhenoblastoma) increased in 50% of the patients and normal in 50% of the patients. *2467*

Urine   Decrease

40.20   **Whipple's Disease**   Reduced 24-h excretion of 17-hydroxycorticosteroids and 17-ketosteroids has been found in debilitated patients. *2199*

174.90   **Malignant Neoplasm of Breast**   Total 17-ketosteroids and the sum of the fractions were significantly decreased in comparison with controls. *0390*

244.90   **Hypothyroidism**   Low in untreated disease. Does not necessarily indicate pituitary origin. *2612*

253.00   **Acromegaly**   Varies from low, normal to high. *0503*

253.40   **Anterior Pituitary Hypofunction**   Low or low normal levels are suggestive but not diagnostic. *2612*   *0151*

255.40   **Adrenal Cortical Hypofunction**   Markedly decreased. *2467*   *0999*

257.20   **Testicular Hypofunction**   Decreased in primary and secondary hypogonadism. *2467*

274.00   **Gout**   Moderate decrease. *0503*

359.11   **Progressive Muscular Dystrophy**   *0995*

359.21   **Myotonia Atrophica**   Primary testicular failure in males. *0878*   *2467*

579.00   **Celiac Sprue Disease**   In patients with sufficient malabsorption to cause pituitary or adrenal insufficiency. *2540*

581.90   **Nephrotic Syndrome**   Marked decrease. *0503*

627.90   **Menopausal and Postmenopausal Symptoms**   *2468*

758.70   **Klinefelter's Syndrome (XXY)**   May be normal or decreased. *0962*

Urine   Increase

194.00   **Malignant Neoplasm of Adrenal Gland**   Usually very high. *2612*   *2467*   *0619*

220.00   **Benign Neoplasm of Ovary**   May be slightly increased in arrhenoblastoma. May be moderately increased in Leydig cell tumors in masculinizing ovarian tumors. *2467*

220.92   **Granulosa Cell Tumor of Ovary**   Urine 17-KS may be slightly increased in arrhenoblastoma. May be markedly increased in adrenal tumors of ovary. May be moderately increased in Leydig cell tumors in masculinizing ovarian tumors. *2467*

220.93   **Lutein Cell Tumor of Ovary**   Urine 17-KS may be slightly increased in arrhenoblastoma. May be markedly increased in adrenal tumors of ovary. May be moderately increased in Leydig cell tumors in masculinizing ovarian tumors. *2467*

220.94   **Theca Cell Tumor of Ovary**   Urinary 17-KS may be slightly increased in arrhenoblastoma. May be markedly increased in adrenal tumors of ovary. May be moderately increased in Leydig cell tumors in masculinizing ovarian tumors. *2467*

220.95   **Arrhenoblastoma**   May be slightly increased in arrhenoblastoma. May be moderately increased in Leydig cell tumors in masculinizing ovarian tumors. *2467*

222.00 **Benign Neoplasm of Testis** *0619*

227.00 **Benign Neoplasm of Adrenal Cortex** In Cushing patients with adrenocortical adenoma. *2612*

253.00 **Acromegaly** Varies from low, normal to high. *0503* *0151*

255.00 **Adrenal Cortical Hyperfunction (Glucocorticoid Excess)** Characteristic. *0842* May be very high in Cushing's syndrome with adrenocortical carcinoma. *2612*

255.10 **Adrenal Cortical Hyperfunction (Mineralocorticoid Excess)** Urine 17-hydroxycorticosteroids and 17-KS excretion levels are always within normal range in patients with aldosteronomas but may occasionally be elevated in more rare instances of primary aldosteronism due to adrenal carcinoma. *0995* *0999*

256.41 **Stein-Leventhal Syndrome** *2540*

275.34 **Familial Periodic Paralysis** In the most severe attacks. *0903 2246*

308.00 **Stress** *0503*

650.00 **Pregnancy** Last trimester. *0503*

Urine   Normal

253.00 **Acromegaly** Varies from low, normal to high. *0503*

255.00 **Adrenal Cortical Hyperfunction (Glucocorticoid Excess)** Usually normal in hyperplasia and adenoma of adrenal cortex. *2612*

25-Hydroxy Vitamin D$_3$

Serum   Decrease

268.20 **Osteomalacia** Vitamin D deficiency. *0995*

277.00 **Cystic Fibrosis** Patients supplemented with multivitamins still presented a 36% decrease in 25-OH vitamin D concentration. *0959*

303.90 **Alcoholism** Lower mean value (15.0 ± 7.6 ng/mL) was found in 13 chronic alcoholics with no evidence of cirrhosis on biopsy. Normal = 23.6 ± 9.8 ng/mL. *2424*

571.90 **Cirrhosis of Liver** In patients with stable cirrhosis, values were slightly depressed, mean = 18.9 ± 8.9 ng/mL. Lower normal limit = 21 ng/mL. *2077*

579.00 **Celiac Sprue Disease** *2238*

579.90 **Malabsorption, Cause Unspecified** 66% of patients with malabsorption had low (< 21 ng/mL) serum concentrations. Only 1 of 31 patients had a value > 21 ng/mL and 20 had assays < 12 ng/mL. *2077*

581.90 **Nephrotic Syndrome** Range in 26 patients was 1-18.6 ng/mL, mean = 8.6 ± 1. Normal value = 21.8 ± 2.3 ng/mL. Values were inversely correlated with degree of proteinuria and directly related to serum albumin. *0882*

592.00 **Kidney Calculus** Significantly lower in 29 untreated patients with recurrent calcium containing kidney stones (15.8 ± 9.8 ng/mL) than in controls (23.6 ± 9.8 ng/mL). Deficiency is possible due to low milk diet followed by recurrent stone patients. *2424*

Acetoacetate

Serum   Increase

253.00 **Acromegaly** Elevated levels. *2356*

Acetylcholinesterase

Red Blood Cells   Decrease

281.20 **Folic Acid Deficiency Anemia** Megaloblastic Anemia during relapse. *1443*

281.30 **Vitamin B$_6$ Deficiency Anemia** Megaloblastic Anemia during relapse. *1443*

283.21 **Paroxysmal Nocturnal Hemoglobinuria** *1443*

Acid Phosphatase

Serum   Decrease

758.00 **Down's Syndrome** May be low. *2468*

Serum   Increase

70.00 **Viral Hepatitis** Closely parallels serum bilirubin. *2104*

162.90 **Malignant Neoplasm of Bronchus and Lung** In a series of 25 cases of lung cancer 36% had elevated levels. Acid phosphatase is of no value as a marker for lung cancer. *1637*

170.90 **Malignant Neoplasm of Bone** The multinucleated giant cells of giant cell tumors are rich in acid phosphatase yet only rarely is this enzyme elevated in the patient's serum. *0536*

174.90 **Malignant Neoplasm of Breast** Female patients with metastatic breast cancer, selected at random and including both treated and untreated cases, had a mean serum activity which was significantly (P < 0.001) above that seen in females with benign disease. *1921* *0812 1157*

185.00 **Malignant Neoplasm of Prostate** May be raised, especially if the tumor has extended outside the gland. Anaplastic tumors secrete minimal enzyme. *0619* Useful in detecting metastases but is of no value in detecting the presence of resectable carcinoma. 50-75% of patients with carcinoma extended beyond the capsule have elevated levels. Patients with carcinoma still confined within the capsule usually have normal serum levels. *0812 0503* Normal levels do not exclude possibility of carcinoma. 26% of proved cases *0944 1175 0433*

197.70 **Secondary Malignant Neoplasm of Liver** Closely parallels serum bilirubin. *2104*

198.50 **Secondary Malignant Neoplasm of Bone** Especially from breast carcinoma; concentrations > 9 U/L indicate active invasion. *0619* Often slightly increased, especially in prostatic metastases (osteolytic metastases), and especially in primary tumor of bronchus, breast, kidney, and thyroid. *2467* Occurred in 61% of cases. Normal levels were found in 39% of cases when bone metastases were present. *1954*

202.80 **Non-Hodgkins Lymphoma** In a few patients, a striking increase has been noted. *2523* A patient with histiocytic medullary reticulosis was found to have up to 60 X the normal upper limit, which then paralleled the activity of disease during temporary responses to therapy. *2523*

203.00 **Multiple Myeloma** May be elevated even in the absence of prostatic carcinoma. *0433* 2 patients showed elevated levels of both total and prostatic fraction of the serum acid phos. *0775 0812 0948 1375*

205.10 **Myelocytic Leukemia (Chronic)** 9 of 16 patients with myeloid metaplasia or chronic granulocytic leukemia were found to have slight but significant elevations. *0129*

250.00 **Diabetes Mellitus** In 90 diabetics, an increased activity 137%, P < 0.001) was found. The increase was moderate (55%) in uncomplicated diabetics with slightly elevated glycemia (148 ± 24 mg/dL), and about twice normal levels in diabetics with either vasculopathies or marked hyperglycemia (343 ± 108 mg/dL). *0154* Increased activity correlated with blood sugar concentration. *0155*

252.00 **Hyperparathyroidism** Found in 28 cases with definite skeletal changes. Activity was increased in every instance from 1.4-16 X the normal maximum. *0948* *0812*

272.72 **Gaucher's Disease** Commonly elevated or high normal serum concentrations, irrespective of the patient's clinical status. The excess is caused by spillage from tissue accumulations, primarily from the spleen. *0474* In 12 proved cases, there was a range of 12-25 U/L , with a mean of 16.8 U/L, (normal range = 7-9 U/L). *2382* A 5-50 fold elevation in serum activity in 8 patients with the adult, non-neuropathic form of Gaucher's Disease was found. *0363* *1571*

272.73 **Niemann-Pick Disease** Ranging from 35-45 U/L over a 4 month period in a patient with this disease. *1000* Increased levels have been documented in only a few cases. *0473* *0474*

275.31 **Hyperphosphatasia** Increased in this uncommon inherited disorder showing painful swelling of the periosteal soft tissue and spontaneous fractures. *2467* The lesions show pronounced increases in the amount of alkaline and acid phosphatase, aminopeptidase and lactic dehydrogenase, acid mucopolysaccharides and reticulin. *2259*

277.30 **Amyloidosis** Increased in 66% of 14 patients tested. The tartrate inhibition (< 20%) was within normal limits. *1334*

282.60 **Sickle Cell Anemia** Marked rise may occur during a severe hemolytic episode. *2104*

287.30 **Idiopathic Thrombocytopenic Purpura** 13 of 15 patients had elevations. In 15 of 16 patients, serum gave higher values than plasma. *1743* Only 2 out of 9 cases showed plasma levels to be of diagnostic value. Results of previous studies could not be reproduced successfully. *0444* Plasma beta-glycerol acid phosphatase may be elevated in any form of thrombocytopenia due to accelerated plasma destruction. *2552*

Acid Phosphatase *(continued)*

Serum Increase *(continued)*

289.80 Myelofibrosis 9 of 16 patients with myeloid metaplasia or chronic granulocytic leukemia were found to have slight but significant elevations of serum acid phos. *0129* A patient with histiocytic medullary reticulosis was found to have up to 60 X the normal upper limit, which then paralleled the activity of disease during temporary responses to therapy. *2523*

334.00 Friedreich's Ataxia One pair of siblings displayed a slight elevation. *1956*

410.90 Acute Myocardial Infarction Ten cases of acute transmural infarction were accompanied by a rise of 50-400% in serum concentration several h after onset of symptoms and lasted 3-5 days. *2078* Significant increases evident within 2-3 h and persist 3-5 days in some cases. *2104 0812*

415.10 Pulmonary Embolism and Infarction *0812*

444.90 Arterial Embolism and Thrombosis Acid hyperphenylphosphatasia which lasted from 3-6 days and reached a maximum of 4.1, 5.8, and 7 U/L, respectively, was noted after each of the 3 episodes of thromboembolism. *2079* Peak activity is reached 2-3 days after onset of symptoms. *2104 0812*

451.90 Phlebitis and Thrombophlebitis 8 of 9 female patients with thrombophlebitis of the lower extremities had elevations. Activities of 11-16.1 U/L during the acute phase of disease, a fall to borderline values of 9 U/L during convalescence, and a return to normal values of 1.6-6.5 U/L after recovery. *2080 0812*

487.10 Influenza In some cases, even in the absence of discernible complications. *2368*

557.01 Mesenteric Artery Embolism Peak activity is reached 2-3 days after onset of symptoms. *2104*

570.00 Acute and Subacute Necrosis of Liver Up to 16 U/L. *2467 0812* With jaundice. *0169 1033*

571.20 Laennec's or Alcoholic Cirrhosis Up to 16 U/L in Laennec's cirrhosis. *0812* Closely parallels serum bilirubin. *2104*

576.20 Extrahepatic Biliary Obstruction Closely parallels serum bilirubin. *2104*

584.00 Acute Renal Failure Not related to degree of azotemia. *2467*

585.00 Chronic Renal Failure Marked increase in activity in urine, erythrocytes, and serum in the terminal stage of renal failure. *1290*

600.00 Benign Prostatic Hypertrophy May have slight elevations after vigorous prostatic massage. *0503* Ordinary digital rectal palpation of the prostate produced significantly raised activities in 3 of 24 patients. *0492* Elevated in 7% of 141 cases. *1647*

602.80 Prostatic Infarction Sometimes to high levels. *2467 1085*

731.00 Osteitis Deformans Seen occasionally in advanced disease. *2104* Elevated in very advanced cases and rare in early to moderate cases. *0948 0945*

756.51 Osteogenesis Imperfecta Much higher than normal in all 8 patients (37-77 U/L). *0822 0812*

756.52 Osteopetrosis Sometimes increased. *2467*

Serum Normal

185.00 Malignant Neoplasm of Prostate Percentage of patients with normal levels varied from 14-96% depending upon the stage of disease. *1052* Normal levels do not exclude possibility of this cancer. *1175* Some patients with known metastatic carcinoma have low values, possibly due to a recent episode of hyper- or hypothermia, as the enzyme is subject to common serum inhibitors. *0433 1426*

272.73 Niemann-Pick Disease Eleven measurements on 6 different patients all fell within the normal range for their respective age groups. Observations of increased concentration have not been able to be confirmed. *0473 0474 1000*

731.00 Osteitis Deformans Normal in a high percentage of patients. *2104*

756.51 Osteogenesis Imperfecta The levels in patients did not differ significantly from those in controls of the same age. *1135*

Urine Increase

585.00 Chronic Renal Failure Activity in urine, erythrocytes, and serum was increased in patients with renal failure. Marked increases occur in all 3 specimens in the terminal stage. *1290*

CSF Increase

331.90 Cerebral and Cortical Atrophy Increased in lumbar CSF in relation to the degree of cerebral atrophy and duration of dementia. *2592*

Synovial Fluid Increase

714.00 Rheumatoid Arthritis Of 155 patients with different joint disorders, patients with rheumatoid arthritis showed significantly higher levels than those with bacterial arthritis, osteoarthritis and noninflammatory joint effusions. About 70% of the patients with RA had higher concentrations than those found among the patients with nonrheumatoid diseases. *0147*

Ascitic Fluid Increase

577.00 Acute Pancreatitis Ranged from 0.3-11.2 mmol p-nitrophenol/h/mL. *0827*

Bone Marrow Increase

185.00 Malignant Neoplasm of Prostate Significant in detecting unsuspected metastases before they become radiologically apparent. Bone marrow levels elevate at an earlier stage in the disease than serum levels. *1513* Of the 25 patients with histologically confirmed malignancy, 18 had an elevation in bone marrow while only 11 had serum elevations. *1261 0404 2422*

198.50 Secondary Malignant Neoplasm of Bone Early bone metastases were detected by an increased activity in the bone marrow before any serum elevation or discernible radiographic changes occurred. Bone marrow activity was consistently much higher than in the serum in patients with histologically confirmed bone metastases. *0404 1261*

Leukocyte Decrease

202.80 Non-Hodgkins Lymphoma *1388*
204.10 Lymphocytic Leukemia (Chronic) *1388*

Leukocyte Increase

75.00 Infectious Mononucleosis *1388*
202.40 Leukemic Reticuloendotheliosis *1388*
273.30 Waldenström's Macroglobulinemia *1388*

Leukocyte Normal

203.00 Multiple Myeloma *1388*

Red Blood Cells Increase

585.00 Chronic Renal Failure A 2-fold increase was found in uremic patients compared to normal controls. After hemodialysis both the serum phosphate and acid phosphatase activity were reduced. *1567* Activity in urine, erythrocytes, and serum was increased. Marked increase occurred in all 3 specimens in the terminal stage. *1290*

Adenosine Deaminase

Serum Decrease

279.06 Immunodeficiency (Common Variable) Decreased in Severe Combined Immunodeficiency Disease. *0655 1737 2235*

Serum Increase

2.00 Typhoid Fever Found to be significantly elevated in children. *1873*

70.00 Viral Hepatitis Found to be significantly elevated in children. *1873*

155.00 Malignant Neoplasm of Liver Increased in obstructive jaundice seen with neoplastic disease. *0655 1737 2235*

185.00 Malignant Neoplasm of Prostate Increased. *0655 1737 2235*

188.90 Malignant Neoplasm of Bladder Increased. *0655 1737 2235*

274.00 Gout Increased. *0655 1737 2235*

275.00 Hemochromatosis Increased. *0655 1737 2235*

282.41 Thalassemia Major Significantly elevated and related to the transfusion schedule of the patient. *1873*

283.00 Acquired Hemolytic Anemia (Autoimmune) Increased in hemolytic anemia. *0655 1737 2235*

390.00 Rheumatic Fever Increased. *0655 1737 2235*

571.90 Cirrhosis of Liver Increased. *0655 1737 2235*

Serum   Normal

279.20   **Severe Combined Immunodeficiency**   Normal levels. *0793*

Lymphocytes   Decrease

189.00   **Malignant Neoplasm of Kidney**   Decreased concentration in lymphocyte adenosine deaminase is found in renal cell carcinoma. Progression of disease is associated with a fall in lymphocyte values in all patients. RBC concentrations are low only in blood types B and O. *2292*

Lymphocytes   Increase

188.90   **Malignant Neoplasm of Bladder**   Lymphocyte concentrations were elevated in all patients with transitional cell bladder carcinoma and correlated with stage, activity, clinical course and tumor resection but not with grade. Erythrocyte levels were also elevated in all cases but showed no correlation to disease parameters. *2293*

Red Blood Cells   Increase

188.90   **Malignant Neoplasm of Bladder**   Lymphocyte concentrations were elevated in all patients with transitional cell bladder carcinoma and correlated with stage, activity, clinical course and tumor resection but not with grade. Erythrocyte levels were also elevated in all cases but showed no correlation to disease parameters. *2293*

Adenylate Kinase

Serum   Increase

994.50   **Exercise**   Observed after protracted exercise. *0589*

Agglutination Tests

Serum   Positive

2.00   **Typhoid Fever**   The diagnostic value of the Widal reaction has been diminished by the widespread use of TAB vaccination. In an unimmunized patient, it does not become positive until after 7-10 days of illness. *0433*

21.00   **Tularemia**   Positive between the 1st and 3rd weeks, and a rising titer is usually demonstrable between acute and convalescent sera. *0962*   Agglutination reaction becomes positive in 2nd week of infection. Significant titer is 1:40; usually it becomes > 1:320 by 3rd week. Peaks at 4-7 weeks 1:100), then gradually decreases during next year. *2468*

23.00   **Brucellosis**   Of 200 cases of symptomatic brucella infection, 198 had titers of 160 or > in the standard tube agglutination test. *0307*   Agglutinins appear 1-2 weeks after onset of infection. *0962*   Becomes positive during 2nd to 3rd week of illness; 90% of patients have titers of > 1:320, and may remain positive long after infection has been cured. *2468*

33.00   **Whooping Cough**   These antibodies are produced in low titer and appear only after the second week of disease. *0962*

100.00   **Leptospirosis**   Antibodies appear during 2nd week of illness. *0962*   Tests reach peaks in 4-7 weeks and may last for many years. An individual titer of 1:300 is suggestive of this disease. *2468*

112.90   **Moniliasis**   Serum agglutinin and precipitin titers against Candida are of little value, as many normal individuals harbor the organism without tissue invasion. A low titer probably makes esophageal candidiasis unlikely. *2199*

115.00   **Histoplasmosis**   Antibodies are demonstrable, but cross reactions with Blastomyces and Coccidioides are seen in these tests. *0962*

117.50   **Cryptococcosis**   With CNS involvement about 66% of patients have antigen in their serum, CSF or both. *1058*

CSF   Positive

117.50   **Cryptococcosis**   With CNS involvement about 66% of patients have antigen in their serum, CSF or both. *1058*

AHF-Like Antigen

Plasma   Increase

286.01   **Hemophilia**   Plasma contains normal or even elevated amounts of antigenic material detected by heterologous antiserum. *2617*

994.50   **Exercise**   Increased in proportion to extent. *0166*

Alanine

Serum   Decrease

250.00   **Diabetes Mellitus**   Decreased. *0094 0269 2149*

270.51   **Histidinemia**   *0995*

333.40   **Huntington's Chorea**   19 patients showed a significantly lower concentration of proline, alanine, valine, leucine, isoleucine, and tyrosine compared to 38 normal controls. *0534*

585.00   **Chronic Renal Failure**   Decreased. *0094 0269 2149*

Serum   Increase

38.00   **Septicemia**   Concentrations determined in 10 burned patients with gram-negative sepsis and 9 burned patients without sepsis revealed an increase in the gluconeogenic precursors alanine, glycine, methionine and phenylalanine in those patients with sepsis. *2543*

255.00   **Adrenal Cortical Hyperfunction (Glucocorticoid Excess)**   Increased. *0094 0269 2149*

270.61   **Citrullinemia**   Mild elevations have been found. *2246*

274.00   **Gout**   Increased. *0094 0269 2149*

Urine   Increase

270.02   **Hartnup Disease**   5-20 X normal values. *2246   0995*

270.10   **Cystinosis**   Nonspecific pattern of aminoaciduria. Fanconi's syndrome. *0995*

270.51   **Histidinemia**   Moderate increase. *0831 2246*

275.10   **Hepatolenticular Degeneration**   *0503*

585.00   **Chronic Renal Failure**   Increases up to 4 X normal value. *0192*

714.00   **Rheumatoid Arthritis**   *2104*

984.00   **Toxic Effects of Lead and Its Compounds (including Fumes)**   With lead intoxication. *0889*

Alanine Aminopeptidase

Serum   Increase

70.00   **Viral Hepatitis**   *1443*

275.31   **Hyperphosphatasia**   Increased in the uncommon inherited disorder showing painful swelling of the periosteal soft tissue and spontaneous fractures. *2467*   Pronounced increase. *2259*

570.00   **Acute and Subacute Necrosis of Liver**   *1443*

572.40   **Hepatic Failure**   *1443*

573.30   **Toxic Hepatitis**   *1443*

650.00   **Pregnancy**   *1443*

Alanine Aminotransferase

Serum   Decrease

994.50   **Exercise**   Effect of physical training. *0804   1930*

Serum   Increase

6.00   **Amebiasis**   With liver involvement. *1058*

18.00   **Disseminated Tuberculosis**   In 5 cases of hepatic granuloma, ALT was 70 U/L with a range of 50-115 U/L. *1452*

23.00   **Brucellosis**   In 5 cases of hepatic granuloma, ALT was elevated to a mean value of 70 U/L (normal = 50 U/L) and a range of 50-115 U/L. *1452*

37.00   **Tetanus**   Mainly in the more severe cases. *0433*

38.00   **Septicemia**   Elevations observed in 6 cases of extrahepatic sepsis. *1681*

39.90   **Actinomycosis**   Liver involvement. *1058*

Alanine Aminotransferase (continued)

Serum Increase (continued)

60.00 Yellow Fever Activity was above normal in all sera tested, the degree of increase approximately proportional to the severity of disease. *1179*

70.00 Viral Hepatitis Appears to reflect acute hepatic disease somewhat more specifically than is true of AST. Striking elevations of 220-1,800 U/L. *0503* May be elevated 2-4 weeks before the onset of jaundice and may reach peak levels after 1-2 weeks. Reflects organelle injury rather than necrosis or alteration of the permeability of the plasma membranes. Elevations as high as 2,000-3,000 U/L may be seen. *0433* Increases provide early indication of impending relapse, before clinically apparent. *2368* Marked elevation in nearly all patients. *2260   2576 0962 0781*

73.90 Psittacosis With severe liver involvement. *0433*

75.00 Infectious Mononucleosis Reflected the presence and extent of hepatic damage, and the severity of subjective symptoms in 36 patients. *1912* Show abnormal results in most cases. *1319* Elevations occur in 80-100% during acute illness and return to normal in 3-5 weeks. *2538   0619 2467 0962*

78.50 Cytomegalic Inclusion Disease Slight increase which becomes more marked with clinical hepatitis in some cases. *2468*

84.00 Malaria Moderate increase. *2468*

99.10 Lymphogranuloma Venereum May indicate severe liver impairment. *0433*

100.00 Leptospirosis Increased in 50% of the patients but average levels are not as high as in hepatitis. *2468*

115.00 Histoplasmosis In 5 cases of hepatic granuloma, ALT was elevated to a mean value of 70 U/L (normal = 50 U/L) and a range of 50-115 U/L. *1452*

120.00 Schistosomiasis May be mild elevations, but jaundice is uncommon. *0962* In 5 cases of hepatic granuloma, ALT was elevated to a mean value of 70 U/L (normal = 50 U/L) and a range of 50-115 U/L. *1452*

122.90 Hydatidosis With liver involvement. *1058*

124.00 Trichinosis May show a moderate rise. *0433   0962*

135.00 Sarcoidosis In 5 cases of hepatic granuloma, ALT was elevated to a mean value of 70 U/L (normal = 50 U/L) and a range of 50-115 U/L. *1452*

155.00 Malignant Neoplasm of Liver In all cases of intrahepatic malignant disease, values were above normal, and all but 1 showed higher AST than ALT. ALT values ranged from 31-43 U/L. *2576* Elevated in only 34% of 32 patients with primary hepatoma (normal = 2.4-17 U/L). *0029*

155.10 Malignant Neoplasm of Intrahepatic Bile Ducts Found in all cases of malignant disease of biliary tract; ranging from 65.5-87 U/L. *2576*

157.90 Malignant Neoplasm of Pancreas Elevated due to extrahepatic biliary tract obstruction. *2576* In 40% of 10 patients at initial hospitalization for this disorder. *0781*

197.00 Secondary Malignant Neoplasm of Respiratory System In 24% of 33 patients at initial hospitalization for this disorder. *0781*

197.70 Secondary Malignant Neoplasm of Liver Generally parallels AST but the increase is less marked. *2467* Modestly elevated (145 U/L). All cases of intrahepatic disease showed elevations. Values ranged from 12.5-116 U/L. *2576* 83% of 12 patients showed increase. Mean elevation 72 U/L (normal = 24). *1452* Raised in 33% of cases of liver metastases. *2093* Occasional elevation. *2260   0503 0962*

201.90 Hodgkin's Disease May be a systemic sign of active disease or may indicate involvement of liver or bone. *0433* In 30% of 10 patients at initial hospitalization for this disorder. *0781*

202.80 Non-Hodgkins Lymphoma May be a systemic sign of active disease or may indicate involvement of liver or bone. *0433* In 30% of 10 patients at initial hospitalization for this disorder. *0781*

205.00 Myelocytic Leukemia (Acute) Infiltration of the liver. *0619* Moderate elevation observed in lymphomas and leukemia but less frequently than in other hepatic disease. *0503*

205.10 Myelocytic Leukemia (Chronic) Less elevation than in acute leukemia. *2468*

242.90 Hyperthyroidism Slight rise (mean = 12.1 U/L, normal = 8.1). The differences between hyper- and euthyroid groups were statistically significant but individually, minor changes would be of little positive diagnostic significance. *1320*

250.10 Diabetic Acidosis In some instances, mostly in severe cases, especially with severe circulatory failure and liver enlargement. *0155*

271.03 Forbes Disease There may be some mild abnormalities of liver function. Elevations of AST and ALT are common, especially in Type III. *0433*

271.10 Galactosemia Deranged liver function. *2246*

271.20 Hereditary Fructose Intolerance Marked rise was noted within 1.5 h after a single large dose of fructose. *2246*

272.52 Abetalipoproteinemia Two subjects. *2246*

272.71 Anderson's Disease Liver involvement. *2246*

272.72 Gaucher's Disease May be abnormal with liver involvement. *0995*

272.73 Niemann-Pick Disease Seen in type B disease. *2246*

275.10 Hepatolenticular Degeneration Minimal elevation in 14% (5 of 37 patients). Mean = 30 U/L. *2278*

277.16 Porphyria Cutanea Tarda Liver function is highly variable. May be mildly elevated. *2552*

277.41 Dubin-Johnson Syndrome May be normal or moderately increased. *0602*

282.00 Hereditary (Congenital) Spherocytosis *0962*

283.00 Acquired Hemolytic Anemia (Autoimmune) *0962*

291.00 Delirium Tremens *0962*

303.90 Alcoholism Above the normal limit (18 U/L) in 30% of 67 alcoholics, during or immediately after a heavy bout of drinking. *1781* 50% of 182 male chronic alcoholics had raised values. Highest values were found after 5-20 y of confirmed alcoholism. Patients with > 20 y duration displayed a tendency to normalization of enzyme activity. *2196*

304.90 Drug Dependence (Opium and Derivatives) This and other liver function tests are increased in 75% of patients. *2468*

331.81 Reye's Syndrome Reflects hepatic damage. *0151* High serum transaminases. *0962*

335.11 Familial Progressive Spinal Muscular Atrophy Elevations of serum enzymes are frequently encountered but never reach the magnitude seen in Duchenne muscular dystrophy. *0433*

359.11 Progressive Muscular Dystrophy Particularly during the early and middle stages of the disease. In the late stage of the disease when the muscle mass has been severely reduced, serum enzyme levels may be only minimally elevated. *0433   0962*

359.21 Myotonia Atrophica Usually normal or minimally elevated. *0433*

410.90 Acute Myocardial Infarction Normal or only minimally elevated. *0503* Generally parallels AST but the increase is less marked. *2467* Observed only when resulting cardiac tissue necrosis is great enough to cause a rise in AST equivalent to 150 spectrophotometric U. *2577* In 49% of 18 patients hospitalized for this disorder. *0781   0962*

415.10 Pulmonary Embolism and Infarction Slight increase. *0962*

420.00 Acute Pericarditis *0962*

428.00 Congestive Heart Failure Heart failure or shock with attendant hepatic necrosis may lead to elevated values. *0503* Depending on the severity and chronicity of cardiac failure. *0433* Increased in about 12% of patients. *2467* 33% of 9 patients showed increases (range = 6.3-76.3 U/L). *1452*

434.90 Brain Infarction *0962*

496.01 Alpha$_1$-Antitrypsin Deficiency Related to liver disease. *1636*

555.90 Regional Enteritis or Ileitis Liver abnormalities are common. *0995*

556.00 Ulcerative Colitis With liver involvement. *0433*

570.00 Acute and Subacute Necrosis of Liver A marked increase occurs which is relatively higher than the rise in AST. The level is raised in nonicteric attacks. In liver disease results of ALT and sorbitol dehydrogenase run parallel with AST results. *0619* Sometimes reaches levels of 2,000 U/L. It falls slowly reaching normal levels in about 2-3 months, unless complications occur. *2467 0812* Levels are higher in acute hepatitis than in obstructive jaundice. *0503* Peak values between 200-1,500 U/L are typical. *0992   2576*

571.20 Laennec's or Alcoholic Cirrhosis Ranged from 20-258 U/L (35 = maximum normal limit). *2576* Usually much lower than the AST. *0999*

571.49 Chronic Active Hepatitis   Usually increased (up to 10 X normal range). *2467*   Continuing or phasic release of transaminase enzymes from damaged liver cells, depending upon the degree of hepatocellular necrosis: serum levels range from 300-1000 U/L during exacerbations. *1922*   Mild elevation. *0962*   In 90% of 15 patients at initial hospitalization for this disorder. *0781 2035*

571.60 Biliary Cirrhosis   Modestly elevated (300 U/L) in most of these patients. Values are as high or higher than those of AST. *0503*   Usually only mildly elevated. *0962*

571.90 Cirrhosis of Liver   Values are modestly elevated (300 U/L). Much lower than the respective values for AST. In cirrhosis of the liver, even with jaundice, the moderate AST level and the lower ALT level are in contrast with the high levels of both transaminases observed in acute viral hepatitis. *0503*   Slight elevation occurred in 33% of patients with cirrhosis. Values ranged from 11-77 U/L. *1452*   In 52% of 48 patients at initial hospitalization for this disorder. *0781   0962 2576*

572.00 Liver Abscess (Pyogenic)   Increases during preicteric phase to peaks 500 U/L) by the time jaundice appears; then rapid fall in several days; become normal 2-5 weeks after onset of jaundice. *2467*

572.40 Hepatic Failure   May be increased or normal. *0503*

573.30 Toxic Hepatitis   Rises precipitously. *0433*   Levels depend upon severity. In severe toxic hepatitis, serum enzymes may be 10-20 X higher than in acute hepatitis and show a different pattern, i.e., increase in LD > AST > ALT > (acute icteric period). *2467*   Elevations in toxic hepatitis due to carbon tetrachloride occur within 24 h and may reach peaks of up to 27,000 U/L. Other toxins (chlorpromazine salicylates, azaserine and pyrazinamide) will cause smaller elevations. *2577*

575.00 Acute Cholecystitis   4 of 8 patients showed elevated levels. Mean value = 44, range = 8-154 U/L. *1452*   Occasionally increased. *0995*   May be mildly elevated even in the absence of intrahepatic infection or common bile duct obstruction. *2199*

576.10 Cholangitis   With parenchymal cell necrosis and malfunction. *2467*   77% of 13 patients showed mild elevation with a mean of 46 and range of 11-96 U/L. *1452*

576.20 Extrahepatic Biliary Obstruction   10-100 U/L; returns to normal within 1 week after obstruction is relieved. *2467*   Increased activity in all cases of biliary tract obstruction. Common duct obstruction due to stones, pancreatitis, tumor, duct carcinoma, and leukemia nodes showed values of 64-400 U/L. Calculous biliary obstruction was associated with ALT activity of 42-45 U/L. *2576*   In obstruction due to benign or malignant disease. *2260   0962*

577.00 Acute Pancreatitis   4 of 10 patients showed elevations. Values ranged from 10-50 U/L,mean = 26.5 U/L (upper limit of normal = 24 U/L). *1452   0962*

577.10 Chronic Pancreatitis   *2199*

585.00 Chronic Renal Failure   In 38% of 142 patients at initial hospitalization for this disorder. *0781*

593.81 Renal Infarction   Increased if area of infarction is large; peak by 2nd day; return to normal by 5th day with arterial infarction of kidney. *2468*

642.40 Pre-Eclampsia   In about 20% of patients with mild cases. *0387*   Degree of abnormality closely parallels the severity. *0472 2311 1635*

642.60 Eclampsia   Degree of abnormality closely parallels the severity. *1635*   All 14 patients had normal activities on the day of convulsion. On the 2nd day, the test became progressively abnormal and peaked on the 5-7th day postpartum. *0500*   Presumably due to ischemic damage to liver cells. *0322*

710.00 Systemic Lupus Erythematosus   May be found in patients with myositis. *0433*

710.40 Dermatomyositis/Polymyositis   In general, serum enzymes correlate well with the disease activity and are useful therapeutic and prognostic indicators. *0244   0962*   Elevated at some time in nearly every patient. *0244   0962*

714.30 Juvenile Rheumatoid Arthritis   Mild elevation is common in untreated and aspirin-treated children but increases are sporadic. *1870*

785.40 Gangrene   *0962*

785.50 Shock   Heart failure or shock with attendant hepatic necrosis may lead to elevated values. *0503*

929.00 Crush Injury (Trauma)   *0962*

948.00 Burns   Rises soon after burn. *2104*

985.00 Toxic Effects of Non-medicinal Metals   Hepatotoxicity may occur with arsenicals. *1446*

989.50 Toxic Effects of Venom   Found in 6 of 14 patients admitted for bee stings. *1822*

990.00 Effects of X-Ray Irradiation   May be increased in cases of radiation injury, indicating major cell and tissue damage. *0151*

991.60 Hypothermia   14 of 24 patients with accidental hypothermia showed elevated values. *1472*

992.00 Heat stroke   Increases (mean = 10 X normal) to a peak on the 3rd day and returns to normal by the 2nd week. Very high levels are associated with lethal outcome. *2468*

Serum   Normal

238.40 Polycythemia Vera   Normal in uncomplicated cases. *1379 2538*

271.01 Von Gierke's Disease   Liver may be massively enlarged but liver function tests are normal. *2246*

272.31 Type I Hyperlipoproteinemia   *2246*

277.30 Amyloidosis   Usually normal. *0125*

277.41 Dubin-Johnson Syndrome   Routine liver function tests are normal. *0962*

277.42 Gilbert's Disease   *0995*

277.43 Rotor's Syndrome   Routine liver function tests are normal. *0962*

277.44 Crigler-Najjar Syndrome   Liver function tests were uniformly normal. *2246   0469*

333.40 Huntington's Chorea   No abnormalities in 8 patients. *0534*

390.00 Rheumatic Fever   Usually normal unless the patient has cardiac failure with liver damage. *2467*

410.90 Acute Myocardial Infarction   Usually not increased unless there is liver damage due to congestive heart failure, drug therapy, etc. *2467*

441.00 Dissecting Aortic Aneurysm   Unless complications occur. *2467*

571.20 Laennec's or Alcoholic Cirrhosis   Normal in most cases of portal cirrhosis. *2260*

572.00 Liver Abscess (Pyogenic)   Transaminase levels are often normal in the absence of biliary tract infections in acute liver abscess. *0151*

642.40 Pre-Eclampsia   Usually are not elevated. When transaminases are found to be elevated, either pronounced hepatic or marked myocardial alterations have occurred. *0433*

650.00 Pregnancy   Incidence of abnormal activities is < 5%. *0387 2359*

714.00 Rheumatoid Arthritis   Generally normal. *0962*

994.50 Exercise   No significant change after 12 min on cycle-ergometer. *0804*

Urine   Increase

580.00 Acute Poststreptococcal Glomerulonephritis   Increased. *1807 1199 2534*

580.01 Glomerulonephritis (Focal)   Increased. *1807 1199 2534*

580.02 Glomerulonephritis (Minimal Change)   Increased. *1807 1199 2534*

580.04 Glomerulonephritis (Membranous)   Increased. *1807 1199 2534*

580.05 Glomerulonephritis (Membranoproliferative)   Increased. *1807 1199 2534*

580.40 Glomerulonephritis (Rapidly Progressive)   Increased. *1807 1199 2534*

590.00 Chronic Pyelonephritis   Increased. *1807 1199 2534*

591.00 Hydronephrosis   Increased. *1807 1199 2534*

Albumin

Serum   Decrease

9.00 Gastroenteritis and Colitis   Hypoalbuminemia and persistent diarrhea in cytomegalovirus enteritis. *2401*

11.00 Pulmonary Tuberculosis   Tends to be reduced to a degree proportional to the severity of the lesions. *1821 2104*   In 36% of 26 patients at initial hospitalization for this disorder. *0781*

30.00 Leprosy   Markedly decreased in lepromatous leprosy and lepra reaction. *2045*

38.00 Septicemia   Decreased in 6 cases of extrahepatic sepsis. *1681*   In 54% of 11 patients at initial hospitalization for this disorder. *0781*

Albumin *(continued)*

Serum   Decrease *(continued)*

40.20 Whipple's Disease   Excessive loss into GI tract and decreased production. *0995*   A low serum albumin will reflect possible malabsorption of protein or protein-losing enteropathy. *0962*   In patients with severe diarrhea and malabsorption. *2199 0999*

52.00 Chickenpox   May be decreased with increased beta and gamma globulins. *2468*

53.00 Herpes Zoster   In 32% of 18 patients at initial hospitalization for this disorder. *0781*

70.00 Viral Hepatitis   Levels may be normal in the early stages of the disease process and may gradually decrease only after parenchymal damage has occurred. In severe and prolonged cases, levels bear a close relation to the clinical state and are helpful prognostically and in following results of treatment. *2339*   In 32% of 24 patients at initial hospitalization for this disorder. *0781 0724*

82.00 Rocky Mountain Spotted Fever   Common. *0433*

84.00 Malaria   *2468*

85.00 Leishmaniasis   Decreased with reversed A/G ratio. *2468*

86.90 Trypanosomiasis   *1058*

99.10 Lymphogranuloma Venereum   A common finding during active infection. Often reversal of the A/G ratio. *0962   2199*

100.00 Leptospirosis   May occur with jaundice after the 1st week of fever. *2368*

115.00 Histoplasmosis   Concentrations of < 3.0 g/dL occur in 60% of patients with disseminated disease. *0999*

120.00 Schistosomiasis   A significant decrease associated with a compensatory increase in globulin throughout the course of the disease. The drop may be due to decreased anabolism or increased catabolism. *2026*

124.00 Trichinosis   Decrease occurs in severe cases between 2-4 weeks and may last for years. *2468*   In severe cases there may be hypoalbuminemia. *0962   0433*

126.90 Ancylostomiasis (Hookworm Infestation)   *2199*

127.20 Strongyloidiasis   Has been observed. *2199*

135.00 Sarcoidosis   Associated with increased globulin in 'sarcoid step' characteristic patterns. *2468*

150.90 Malignant Neoplasm of Esophagus   In 35% of 40 patients at initial hospitalization for this disorder. *0781*

151.90 Malignant Neoplasm of Stomach   Found occasionally, due to leakage into stomach. *0992*   In 38% of 47 patients at initial hospitalization for this disorder. *0781*

153.90 Malignant Neoplasm of Large Intestine   Significantly reduced (median = 35.7 g/L compared to controls (44.0 g/L). *1025*   In 28% of 149 patients at initial hospitalization for this disorder. *0781*

155.00 Malignant Neoplasm of Liver   Mean values were found to be highest in the healthy subjects followed by acute viral hepatitis, primary hepatocellular carcinoma and cirrhosis, in that order. Both the mean albumin and mean total globulin of each group of subjects were significantly different from the respective means of the other 3 groups. *0724*   Reversed A/G ratio in 54% of 51 hepatoma patients. *1115*   In 42% of 14 patients at initial hospitalization for this disorder. *0781*

157.90 Malignant Neoplasm of Pancreas   In 44% of 46 patients at initial hospitalization for this disorder. *0781*

162.90 Malignant Neoplasm of Bronchus and Lung   Significantly reduced (median = 35.7 g/L) in patients with carcinoma compared to controls (44.0 g/L). *1025*

174.90 Malignant Neoplasm of Breast   Significantly reduced (median = 35.7 g/L) in patients with carcinoma compared to controls (44.0 g/L). *1025*

182.00 Malignant Neoplasm of Corpus Uteri   Significantly reduced (median = 35.7 g/L ± 2.6 g/L) compared to controls (44.0 g/L ± 3.4 g/L). *1025*

185.00 Malignant Neoplasm of Prostate   In 31% of 86 patients at initial hospitalization for this disorder. *0781*

188.90 Malignant Neoplasm of Bladder   In 27% of 45 patients at initial hospitalization for this disorder. *0781*

189.00 Malignant Neoplasm of Kidney   *0151*

197.00 Secondary Malignant Neoplasm of Respiratory System   In 30% of 601 patients at initial hospitalization for this disorder. *0781*

199.00 Secondary Malignant Neoplasm (Disseminated)   Serum concentration of albumin and transferrin were significantly reduced while haptoglobin was increased in disseminated carcinoma compared with localized. *1025*

201.90 Hodgkin's Disease   With active disease. *2538 0073*   In 22% of 72 patients at initial hospitalization for this disorder. *0781 2552*

202.80 Non-Hodgkins Lymphoma   In patients with advanced disease, reduction in serum protein concentration with hypoalbuminemia and hypogammaglobulinemia is frequent. *2462*   In 40% of 74 patients at initial hospitalization for this disorder. *0781 2538*

203.00 Multiple Myeloma   In 57% of 33 patients at initial hospitalization for this disorder. *0781   2467*

204.00 Lymphocytic Leukemia (Acute)   Normal at diagnosis and declines as disease advances. *0689 2552*   In 30% of 44 patients at initial hospitalization for this disorder. *0781*

204.10 Lymphocytic Leukemia (Chronic)   In 47% of 27 patients at initial hospitalization for this disorder. *0781   2467*

205.00 Myelocytic Leukemia (Acute)   Normal at diagnosis, but falls as disease progresses. *0689 2552*   In 34% of 36 patients at initial hospitalization for this disorder. *0781*

205.10 Myelocytic Leukemia (Chronic)   Electrophoresis shows decrease. *2468*   In 46% of 21 patients at initial hospitalization for this disorder. *0781*

206.00 Monocytic Leukemia   In 33% of 23 patients at initial hospitalization for this disorder. *0781*

211.10 Benign Neoplasm of Stomach   Secondary to protein-losing enteropathy in adenocarcinoma. *2104*

242.90 Hyperthyroidism   Possibly due to rapid turnover in severe thyrotoxicosis. *0619   2467*

250.00 Diabetes Mellitus   Tends to be low with increased $alpha_2$-globulins, particularly with vascular complications. *2104*   In 29% of 105 patients at initial hospitalization for this disorder. *0781*

250.10 Diabetic Acidosis   *0619*

251.50 Zollinger-Ellison Syndrome   Serum concentration in 20 patients with proved or presumed ZE syndrome (4.1 ± 0.8 g/dL) were significantly lower than observed in 40 normal controls (5.1 ± 0.3). 40 duodenal ulcer patients (5.1 ± 0.4 g/dL). Total gastrectomy induced a rise in serum albumin in 8 patients studied. *1345*   A low serum albumin will reflect possible malabsorption of protein or protein-losing enteropathy. *0962*

259.20 Carcinoid Syndrome   Commonly observed in patients with carcinoid tumor. *1508*

260.00 Protein Malnutrition   Usually 1.5-2.5 g/dL but may be < I g/dL. Correlates with the degree of fatty liver and of edema; becomes normal after 3 weeks of normal diet; standard test for diagnosis of kwashiorkor and to monitor response to treatment. *2468*   Albumin, prealbumin and transferrin concentrations were found to be lower in cases of protein-energy malnutrition associated with infection than the corresponding values for a group of healthy preschool children. *2065*

267.00 Vitamin C Deficiency   Decreased in scurvy. *0619*

269.90 Deficiency State (Unspecified)   Serum concentration falls before other indicators change. *0619*

271.30 Lactosuria   A low serum albumin will reflect possible malabsorption of protein or protein-losing enteropathy. *0962*

272.00 Type IIA Hyperlipoproteinemia   Reduced, while the serum gamma globulin fraction is increased. *0619 2467*

272.21 Type IIB Hyperlipoproteinemia   Reduced, while the serum gamma globulin fraction is increased. *0619 2467*

273.22 Heavy Chain Disease (Alpha)   Usually reduced with reversed A/G ratio. *2538*

273.23 Heavy Chain Disease (Gamma)   Usually reduced with reversed A/G ratio. *2538*

273.30 Waldenström's Macroglobulinemia   *2467*

273.80 Analbuminemia   Marked decrease due to impaired synthesis. *2104*   Cannot be detected by routine lab methods. *0433*

275.10 Hepatolenticular Degeneration   Reduced in 27% or 10 of 37 patients. *2278*

277.00 Cystic Fibrosis   With advanced lung disease the development of hypoalbuminemia suggests expansion of plasma volume secondary to Cor Pulmonale. *0433*   May be found before cardiac involvement is clinically apparent. *2467*   In 56% of 12 patients at initial hospitalization for this disorder. *0781   2284*

277.30 Amyloidosis Found to be < 3.0 g/dL in 76% of patients. *1334* Frequently found with liver involvement. *0962* Has been observed. No correlation with severity or duration of disease. *0120 2246*

281.00 Pernicious Anemia *0619*

287.00 Allergic Purpura Hypoalbuminemia occurs in patients with gastrointestinal involvement. *1184 2538*

308.00 Stress *2467*

340.00 Multiple Sclerosis 12.5% of 64 patients had concentrations < 45% of total protein. 10.9% had concentrations > 65% of total proteins. *1295*

390.00 Rheumatic Fever Impaired hepatic synthesis. Decreased serum albumin with strikingly increased alpha₂ and gamma globulins. *2104*

401.10 Essential Benign Hypertension *2467*

410.90 Acute Myocardial Infarction In 22% of 111 patients hospitalized for this disorder. *0781 2531*

421.00 Bacterial Endocarditis Mildly depressed, mean = 3.0 ± 0.1 g/dL. Lowest values found in pneumococcal infection 2.4 ± 0.4 g/dL. *1798*

423.10 Constrictive Pericarditis Decreased with normal total protein. *2467 0999*

428.00 Congestive Heart Failure Common with cardiac fibrosis of liver. *2467* Increase in plasma volume without increase in total protein. *0619*

446.00 Polyarteritis-Nodosa Hypoalbuminemia occurs only in those patients with the nephrotic syndrome. *0962*

446.50 Cranial Arteritis and Related Conditions In 30% of 16 patients hospitalized for this disorder. *0781*

482.90 Bacterial Pneumonia In 50% of 17 patients at initial hospitalization for this disorder. *0781 2467*

496.01 Alpha₁-Antitrypsin Deficiency Related to liver disease. *1636*

513.00 Abscess of Lung *0186*

533.90 Peptic Ulcer, Site Unspecified *2467*

535.00 Gastritis May be low in patients with giant hypertrophic gastritis who exude protein into the lumen. *0433* Secondary to protein-losing enteropathy in atrophic gastroenteritis. *2104*

555.90 Regional Enteritis or Ileitis In 32 patients, 13 fell into a distinct group of low tryptophan sera levels. Patients in this group ate less, had lower albumin levels and greater intestinal protein loss than normal tryptophan patients. *0150* Occurs frequently and is probably due largely to the leakage of protein from the diseased gut. *2466* A reasonably accurate indication of the patient's overall condition. *2199 1160 2035*

556.00 Ulcerative Colitis Deficiency may result in anemia. *0532* Occurs frequently and is probably due largely to the leakage of protein from the diseased gut. *2466* Portends a worse prognosis, probably because the degree of abnormality parallels clinical severity. *2199 1160 2035*

557.01 Mesenteric Artery Embolism *0433*

560.90 Intestinal Obstruction 6% mortality in cases with > 3 g/dL; 33% mortality with < 3 g/dL. *0619* In 35% of 42 patients at initial hospitalization for this disorder. *0781*

567.90 Peritonitis Increase in plasma volume without increase in total protein. *0619*

570.00 Acute and Subacute Necrosis of Liver *2467 0619*

571.20 Laennec's or Alcoholic Cirrhosis In 95 patients, there was a significant decrease in mean albumin concentration, increase in mean gamma globulins, while mean alpha and beta globulins were normal. Characteristic electrophoresis pattern revealed a lack of demarcation between beta and gamma peaks (beta-gamma bridging). *2296*

571.49 Chronic Active Hepatitis Active phases with hepatocellular necrosis are marked by signs of hepatic dysfunction. *2035* In 36% of 19 patients at initial hospitalization for this disorder. *0781 0962*

571.60 Biliary Cirrhosis Normal or slightly decreased early; later more markedly decreased. *2467 2238*

571.90 Cirrhosis of Liver Mean values were found to be highest in the healthy subjects followed by acute viral hepatitis, primary hepatocellular carcinoma and cirrhosis, in that order. Both the mean albumin and mean total globulin of each group, were significantly different from the respective means of the other 3 groups. *0724* Parallels functional status of parenchymal cells and may be useful for following progress of liver disease; but it may be normal in the presence of considerable liver damage. *2467* In 51% of 69 patients at initial hospitalization for this disorder. *0781*

572.00 Liver Abscess (Pyogenic) Levels below 3.0 g/dL are common. *0433* Decreased synthesis and increased catabolism of albumin cause hypoproteinemia in the majority of patients with acute liver abscess. *0151*

572.20 Hepatic Encephalopathy Marked decrease. *1733*

572.40 Hepatic Failure *1733 0503*

575.00 Acute Cholecystitis *2467*

577.00 Acute Pancreatitis In 66% of 21 patients at initial hospitalization for this disorder. *0781 1119*

577.10 Chronic Pancreatitis In 27% of 11 patients at initial hospitalization for this disorder. *0781* Mild depression may occur. *2199*

579.00 Celiac Sprue Disease Reflects possible malabsorption of protein or protein-losing enteropathy. *0962* May be diminished owing to excessive leakage of serum protein into the gut lumen. *2199*

579.01 Protein-Losing Enteropathy Excessive enteric loss usually leads to the development of edema. *2104*

579.90 Malabsorption, Cause Unspecified Marked hypoproteinemia. *0433* Decreased in malabsorption syndrome. *0151 0962*

580.00 Acute Poststreptococcal Glomerulonephritis May be low as a result of urinary loss and excessive catabolism of protein. *0995*

580.02 Glomerulonephritis (Minimal Change) Occurs as a result of heavy protein loss, especially low molecular weight plasma proteins such as albumin and transferrin in the urine. *0151*

581.90 Nephrotic Syndrome Invariably reduced to < 3 g/dL, usually between 1-3 g/dL, with occasional values of < 0.5 g/dL in hypovolemia. *0151* Massive loss in urine results in low serum concentration despite increased synthesis. *2104 0962*

585.00 Chronic Renal Failure Concentrations are normal or low in chronic uremia. *1038* In 43% of 141 patients at initial hospitalization for this disorder. *0781* Tend to be diminished as a result of urinary protein loss

642.40 Pre-Eclampsia Significantly reduced below the levels for normal pregnancy. *0433*

642.60 Eclampsia Significantly reduced below the levels for normal pregnancy. *0433*

650.00 Pregnancy Decreased 22% and total globulins were unchanged. *2287 2286* Usually falls abruptly in early pregnancy and then more slowly during late. *1755* Levels decreased progressively after the first trimester *0517 0387*

694.40 Pemphigus In untreated patients in the advanced stage of disease. Often drops to 25% of normal. *0743*

710.00 Systemic Lupus Erythematosus Found in 50-66% of patients. *0677* Low serum concentration (2.5 g/dL) were found in 8% of 39 patients. *2081* Indicates the severity of excessive protein loss; tends to rise in the improving patient. *0782*

710.20 Sjögren's Syndrome Common. *0433*

714.00 Rheumatoid Arthritis Frequent finding attributed to generalized hypermetabolism. Corticosteroid administration accentuates hypoalbuminemia. *2104 0962*

714.30 Juvenile Rheumatoid Arthritis In acute systemic form. *0136*

730.00 Osteomyelitis *2467*

773.00 Hemolytic Disease of Newborn (Erythroblastosis Fetalis) *0433*

948.00 Burns Superficial burns reduce capillary membrane semipermeability and cause a disproportionate loss of albumin. *2104*

Serum Increase

85.00 Leishmaniasis In tropical splenomegaly, increased plasma volume occurs mainly due to raised intravascular pools of albumin IgG and IgM. The variance in plasma volume was attributable to increases in these 3 pools, IgM and IgG accounting for 42% of the total and albumin for 28%. *0466*

135.00 Sarcoidosis Some cases when active. *0619*

244.90 Hypothyroidism Increase in total pool may occur. *2540* In 37% of 13 patients at initial hospitalization for this disorder. *0781*

276.50 Dehydration By approximately 11.6% after heat exposure for 2-11 h. *2114*

340.00 Multiple Sclerosis 12.5% of 64 patients had concentrations < 45% of total protein. 10.9% had concentrations > 65% of total proteins. *1295*

571.20 Laennec's or Alcoholic Cirrhosis *0619*

Albumin (continued)

Serum Increase (continued)

992.00 Heat stroke   By approximately 11.6% after heat exposure for 2-11 h. *2114*

994.50 Exercise   Significant increase after 12 min on cycle-ergometer. *0804*   Approximately 10% increase immediately, then a delayed fall. *1837*

Serum Normal

70.00 Viral Hepatitis   Normal in acute hepatitis; a decrease suggests chronic liver disease. *0962*

204.10 Lymphocytic Leukemia (Chronic)   Usually within normal limits. *0241 2552*

205.10 Myelocytic Leukemia (Chronic)   Usually normal. *2552*

279.04 Agammaglobulinemia (Congenital Sex-linked)   *2467*

279.06 Immunodeficiency (Common Variable)   *2467*

280.90 Iron Deficiency Anemia   *2467*

282.20 Anemias Due To Disorders of Glutathione Metabolism   *2467*

335.20 Amyotrophic Lateral Sclerosis   *0665*

496.01 Alpha$_1$-Antitrypsin Deficiency   *2467*

560.90 Intestinal Obstruction   *0619*

570.00 Acute and Subacute Necrosis of Liver   *2467*

571.90 Cirrhosis of Liver   Usually parallels functional status of parenchymal cells, but it may be normal in the presence of considerable liver cell damage. *2467*

710.00 Systemic Lupus Erythematosus   In patients with low grade activity and those in remission the serum concentration remain within the normal range. *0354*   In 39 patients serum concentrations were stable throughout the course of SLE. *2081*

Urine Increase

2.00 Typhoid Fever   Common during the febrile period. *0151 0433*

21.00 Tularemia   Mild albuminuria may occur at the height of illness. *0151*

32.00 Diphtheria   Common, particularly in severe forms of the disease. *0433*

36.00 Meningococcal Meningitis   May occur. *2468*

37.00 Tetanus   Some patients show proteinuria. *0433*

38.00 Septicemia   Transient slight increase. *2468*

50.00 Smallpox   With the elimination of toxic material. *0433*

60.00 Yellow Fever   Sudden development of intense albuminuria about day 3-4 is characteristic, often reaching levels of 3-5 g/L or higher. *0151*   Most marked on the 3rd-4th day of illness and declined thereafter. *1179*

70.00 Viral Hepatitis   A few RBC or mild proteinuria. *0433*

71.00 Rabies   May be present. *2468*

72.00 Mumps   Proteinuria should suggest a diagnosis of mumps nephritis. *0433*

73.90 Psittacosis   Frequently seen. *0433*

80.00 Epidemic Typhus   During the febrile period. *0433*

81.10 Brill's Disease   Transient albuminuria may occur. *0433*

82.00 Rocky Mountain Spotted Fever   Varying degrees. *0433*

84.00 Malaria   In uncomplicated infection, mild. *0433*

87.00 Relapsing Fever   Noted occasionally. *0433*

124.00 Trichinosis   In severe cases. *2468*   Possibly due to capillary leakage. *0992*

153.90 Malignant Neoplasm of Large Intestine   24 h excretion and renal clearance were significantly increased in localized tumor patients compared to normals and disseminated cancer cases. Increased high molecular weight protein excretion implies glomerular injury in these patients. *1025*

162.90 Malignant Neoplasm of Bronchus and Lung   24 h excretion and renal clearance were significantly increased in localized tumor patients compared to normals and disseminated cancer cases. Increased high molecular weight protein excretion implies glomerular injury in these patients. *1025*

174.90 Malignant Neoplasm of Breast   24 h excretion and renal clearance were significantly increased in localized tumor patients compared to normals and disseminated cancer cases. Increased high molecular weight protein excretion implies glomerular injury in these patients. *1025*

182.00 Malignant Neoplasm of Corpus Uteri   24 h excretion and renal clearance were significantly increased in localized tumor patients compared to normals and disseminated cancer cases. Increased high molecular weight protein excretion implies glomerular injury in these patients. *1025*

188.90 Malignant Neoplasm of Bladder   May be completely negative or may show microscopic evidence of hematuria, pyuria, albumin, and threads of mucus. *0433*

189.00 Malignant Neoplasm of Kidney   Albuminuria often accompanies hematuria but may occur alone in metastatic renal tumors, especially those of lymphatic or leukemic origin. *0433*

203.00 Multiple Myeloma   Occurs in 90% of patients. *0433*   Frequent proteinuria due to albumin and globulins. *2468*   Greater than 1.0 g/day. *0518*

238.40 Polycythemia Vera   Occasionally. *2552*

244.90 Hypothyroidism   Urinalysis commonly demonstrates mild proteinuria without significant formed elements, and there is preservation of normal concentrating ability. *0433*

250.00 Diabetes Mellitus   An early sign of diabetic nephropathy. *2104*

250.10 Diabetic Acidosis   *0962*

271.10 Galactosemia   Manifestation of a renal toxicity syndrome. *1067*

271.20 Hereditary Fructose Intolerance   Characteristic symptom in small children. *0177*   Develops rapidly after ingestion. *2246*

273.21 Cryoglobulinemia (Essential Mixed)   Common. *0433*

277.30 Amyloidosis   Frequently seen. Massive proteinuria (over 10 g/24h) and other manifestations of the nephrotic syndrome may also be present. *0433*

282.60 Sickle Cell Anemia   May develop. *0433*

283.21 Paroxysmal Nocturnal Hemoglobinuria   Has been demonstrated immediately before and after an episode of hemoglobinuria, but usually there is none between attacks. *0477 2552*

287.00 Allergic Purpura   Mild proteinuria associated with normal Addis count signifies renal involvement. *0433*

288.00 Agranulocytosis   Urine may contain traces of albumin but is otherwise normal. *2552*

390.00 Rheumatic Fever   Slight febrile albuminuria. Indicates mild focal nephritis. Concomitant glomerulonephritis appears in up to 2.5% of cases. *2467* . A high percentage of patients show some proteinuria. *0151*

401.00 Malignant Hypertension   May occur from leaking glomerular capillaries. significant proteinuria 500 mg/24h or > 1+ by qualitative estimation) occurs very rarely in benign essential hypertension; their presence suggests the malignant phase or primary renal parenchymal disease. *0433*

421.00 Bacterial Endocarditis   Almost invariably present, even when no renal lesions are found with bacterial endocarditis. *2468*

428.00 Congestive Heart Failure   The urinalysis frequently demonstrates reversible proteinuria. *0433*   Slight albuminuria (< 1 g/day) is common. *2467*

444.90 Arterial Embolism and Thrombosis   Constant finding among 31 patients. *1108*

446.00 Polyarteritis-Nodosa   Abnormal urinalysis is far more frequent (70-80%) than azotemia (25-30%). *0433*

482.90 Bacterial Pneumonia   Common. *2368*

487.10 Influenza   Mild albuminuria will be found in most febrile conditions. *0433*   Febrile albuminuria may occur. *2368*

513.00 Abscess of Lung   Frequent. *2467*

580.00 Acute Poststreptococcal Glomerulonephritis   Common although it rarely exceeds 3 g/24h. *0433*   Usually occurs, with size of proteins indicating degree of glomerular damage. Albumin is nearly always present. *2545 0995*

580.01 Glomerulonephritis (Focal)   Noted to have slight but persistent proteinuria. *0433*

580.02 Glomerulonephritis (Minimal Change)   Characterized by heavy proteinuria, consisting almost entirely of low molecular weight plasma proteins, especially albumin and transferrin. Values are > 5 g/24h. *0151*

580.04 Glomerulonephritis (Membranous)   In excess of 3 g/24h is characteristic. *0433*   Usually occurs, with size of proteins indicating degree of glomerular damage. *2545*

580.40 Glomerulonephritis (Rapidly Progressive)   Usually occurs; with size of proteins indicating degree of glomerular damage. *2545*

581.90 Nephrotic Syndrome   The principal protein found in the urine. Despite the fact that its concentration may be greatly reduced in the plasma. *0999*   Massive loss in urine. *2104*

585.00 Chronic Renal Failure   Proteinuria and granular casts suggest chronic parenchymal renal disease. *0433*

590.00 Chronic Pyelonephritis   Qualitative proteinuria may be absent but if present is mild. *0433*

590.10 Acute Pyelonephritis   Often present but minimal in degree. *0433*

592.10 Ureter Calculus   The urinalysis often shows no significant alteration from normal but may progress through the stages of mild pyuria to moderate pyuria with albuminuria and onto frank infection or passage of renal casts. *0433*

600.00 Benign Prostatic Hypertrophy   The urinalysis may be completely normal or may reveal albuminuria, pyuria, and hematuria as a result of obstruction with infection or stone formation. *0433*

642.40 Pre-Eclampsia   Characteristic but may appear late in the course of the disease. Fluctuates from day to day. *0387*

642.60 Eclampsia   Characteristic finding. Reflects severity of disease. *0387*

710.00 Systemic Lupus Erythematosus   The most common abnormality ranging from mild to intermittent to nephrotic levels (> 3.56 g/24h). *0433   0962*

710.10 Progressive Systemic Sclerosis   Appears during renal failure. *0433   0962*

714.00 Rheumatoid Arthritis   No abnormalities are found in the urinalysis except for proteinuria. *0433*

753.10 Polycystic Kidney Disease   Progressive albuminuria. *0151*

985.00 Toxic Effects of Non-medicinal Metals   Common in mercury intoxication. *0151*

994.80 Effects of Electric Current   Albuminuria and hemoglobinuria occurs in presence of severe burns. *2468*   Characteristic. *0995*

Urine   Normal

591.00 Hydronephrosis   In uninfected hydronephrosis the urine is negative. If infection supervenes, WBC and albumin are noted. *0433*

CSF   Decrease

340.00 Multiple Sclerosis   18.7% of patients had concentrations < 45% of total proteins; 7.8% had values > 65% of total proteins. *1295*

345.90 Epilepsy   Slightly decreased in CSF of patients with grand mal epilepsy. *1625*

CSF   Increase

320.90 Meningitis (Bacterial)   CSF IgG and albumin are increased due to defect in the blood-CSF barrier. *0809*   Often 100-200 mg/dL. *0433*

340.00 Multiple Sclerosis   18.7% of patients had concentrations < 45% of total proteins; 7.8% had > 65% of total proteins. *1295*

357.00 Guillain-Barré Syndrome   Usually elevated between 65 and 1000 mg/dL but may not peak until four to six weeks after onset of neurologic signs. Elevation may persist for several months. Elevation is primarily albumin. *1307*   IgG and Albumin increased probably result from blood/CSF barrier damage *1099*

357.90 Polyneuritis   CSF shows a gradual increase in protein, almost all of which is albumin in postinfectious polyneuritis, without a concomitant rise in cells. *0999*

CSF   Normal

331.00 Alzheimer's Disease   No significant difference in levels compared with controls. *0372*

Pleural Effusion   Increase

577.00 Acute Pancreatitis   *0186*

Ascitic Fluid   Increase

577.00 Acute Pancreatitis   Elevated level (> 2.9 g/dL) is characteristic. *2199*

577.10 Chronic Pancreatitis   Elevation (> 2.9 g/dL) is characteristic. *2199*

Duodenal Contents   Increase

277.00 Cystic Fibrosis   In excess of that found in the duodenal fluid of controls. *0392*

Aldolase

Serum   Decrease

303.90 Alcoholism   *0126*

401.10 Essential Benign Hypertension   *0126*

Serum   Increase

37.00 Tetanus   Very high serum levels are found in severe cases. *0619   1643*

70.00 Viral Hepatitis   Increased in 90% of patients up to 10 X normal. It parallels transaminase with a sharp rise before serum bilirubin rises and a return to normal 2-3 weeks after jaundice begins (acute icteric period). *2467   0962*

75.00 Infectious Mononucleosis   *0962*

124.00 Trichinosis   Moderate rise probably related to myositis. *0992   0962*

150.90 Malignant Neoplasm of Esophagus   Significantly elevated in tumors of the gastrointestinal tract. Mean = 4.9 ± 0.8 U/L compared to normal, 1.6 ± 0.21. *1201*

151.90 Malignant Neoplasm of Stomach   Significantly elevated in tumors of the gastrointestinal tract. Mean = 4.9 ± 0.8 U/L compared to normal, 1.6 ± 0.21. *1201*

152.90 Malignant Neoplasm of Small Intestine   Significantly elevated in tumors of the gastrointestinal tract. Mean = 4.9 ± 0.8 U/L compared to normal, 1.6 ± 0.21. *1201*

153.90 Malignant Neoplasm of Large Intestine   Significantly elevated in tumors of the gastrointestinal tract. Mean = 4.9 ± 0.8 U/L compared to normal, 1.6 ± 0.21. *1201*

154.10 Malignant Neoplasm of Rectum   Significantly elevated in tumors of the gastrointestinal tract. Mean = 4.9 ± 0.8 U/L compared to normal, 1.6 ± 0.21. *1201*

155.00 Malignant Neoplasm of Liver   *0962*

162.90 Malignant Neoplasm of Bronchus and Lung   Slightly elevated in bronchogenic carcinomas. Mean = 2.8 ± 0.6 U/L compared to normal, 1.6 ± 0.21. *1201*

172.90 Malignant Melanoma of Skin   Markedly elevated in melanoblastomas. Mean = 9.0 ± 2.9 compared to 1.6 ± 0.21 U/L. *1201*

174.90 Malignant Neoplasm of Breast   Significantly elevated; mean = 4.8 ± 0.7 U/L compared to normal, 1.6 ± 0.21. *1201*

180.90 Malignant Neoplasm of Cervix   Mildly elevated in uterine cervix and corpus carcinomas. Mean = 2.9 ± 1.1 U/L compared to normal, 1.6 ± 0.21 U/L. *1201*

183.00 Malignant Neoplasm of Ovary   Mildly elevated. Mean = 3.8 ± 1.0 U/L compared to normal, 1.6 ± 0.21. *1201*

185.00 Malignant Neoplasm of Prostate   Cell destruction. *2467 0962*

186.90 Malignant Neoplasm of Testis   Mildly elevated in tumors of the testicle and kidney. Mean = 4.1 ± 0.5 U/L compared to normal, 1.6 ± 0.21. *1201*

189.00 Malignant Neoplasm of Kidney   Mildly elevated in tumors of the testicle and kidney. Mean = 4.1 ± 0.5 U/L compared to normal, 1.6 ± 0.21. *1201*

191.90 Malignant Neoplasm of Brain   The serum of cancer patients contains a greater proportion of aldolase A (muscle-type) than serum from normal persons. Gliomas and normal brain tissue contain aldolase C (nerve and brain variant), but in meningiomas or tissue metastatic to brain, only aldolase A (liver and fetal form) is detected. *2093*

197.70 Secondary Malignant Neoplasm of Liver   Elevated in 75% of cases of liver metastases. *2093*

198.30 Secondary Malignant Neoplasm of Brain   The serum of cancer patients contains a greater proportion of aldolase A (muscle-type) than serum from normal persons. Gliomas and normal brain tissue contain aldolase C (nerve and brain variant), but in meningiomas or tissue metastatic to brain, only aldolase A (liver and fetal form) is detected. *2093*

199.00 Secondary Malignant Neoplasm (Disseminated)   Variable rises in serum levels may be found in carcinomatosis. Serum aldolase and phosphohexose isomerase are roughly parallel. *0619*

201.90 Hodgkin's Disease   Markedly elevated in malignant lymphomas. Mean = 5.0 ± 0.4 U/L compared to normal, 1.6 - 0.21. *1201*

Aldolase *(continued)*

Serum Increase *(continued)*

202.80 Non-Hodgkins Lymphoma Markedly elevated in malignant lymphomas. Mean = 5.0 ± 0.4 U/L compared to normal, 1.6 ± 0.21. *1201*

205.00 Myelocytic Leukemia (Acute) Slight elevation in 50% of patients. *2468*

205.10 Myelocytic Leukemia (Chronic) Less elevation than in acute leukemia. *2468*

225.90 Benign Neoplasm of Brain and CNS The serum of cancer patients contains a greater proportion of aldolase A (muscle-type) than serum from normal persons. Gliomas and normal brain tissue contain aldolase C (nerve and brain variant), but in meningiomas or tissue metastatic to brain, only aldolase A (liver and fetal form) is detected. *2093*

244.90 Hypothyroidism May be elevated. *0433*

271.02 McArdle's Disease Increases dramatically within h after strenuous exercise. *0970 2246*

271.20 Hereditary Fructose Intolerance Marked rise was noted within 1.5 h after a single large dose of fructose. *2246*

275.34 Familial Periodic Paralysis Occasional patients with paramyotonia congenita. *0760*

281.00 Pernicious Anemia Increased less consistently and to a lesser degree than LD. *0652 2552*

281.20 Folic Acid Deficiency Anemia 12 of 16 patients had levels elevated from 2-20 X the normal mean. *1023* Increased less consistently and to a lesser degree than LD. *2552 0652*

282.00 Hereditary (Congenital) Spherocytosis *0962*

282.60 Sickle Cell Anemia Slightly elevated in a group of 15 patients. The range was 1.0-7.3 U/L with a mean of 2.7 U/L (normal = 1.8 U/L). *1023*

283.00 Acquired Hemolytic Anemia (Autoimmune) *0962*

291.00 Delirium Tremens *0962*

297.90 Paranoid States and Other Psychoses The increased activity of CK or aldolase or both, was generally present at the onset of a psychotic episode in acute patients and lasted about 5-10 days. Increased activities ranged from 5-50 fold above control limits. *1569*

334.00 Friedreich's Ataxia Elevated in 11 cases but markedly so in only 5 of 23 cases. *1956*

335.11 Familial Progressive Spinal Muscular Atrophy Elevations of serum enzymes are frequently encountered but never reach the magnitude seen in Duchenne muscular dystrophy. *0433*

335.20 Amyotrophic Lateral Sclerosis Rises in the early stages, falling to normal later. This pattern occurs in any primary neurogenic muscular dystrophy. *0619* Normal or slightly increased. *0962*

359.11 Progressive Muscular Dystrophy Serum enzymes reach extremely high levels, particularly during the early and middle stages of the disease. In the late stage of the disease when the muscle mass has been severely reduced, serum enzyme levels may be only minimally elevated. *0433* Increases in the early stages to 10-15 X normal in 90% of cases. Levels are normal in the later and terminal stages. *0619* Strikingly elevated. *0962*

359.21 Myotonia Atrophica Usually normal or minimally elevated. *0433* Due to cell destruction. Increased in about 20% of the patients. *2467*

410.90 Acute Myocardial Infarction With cell destruction. *2467* Rises after 3 h to a peak by 24 h (2-15 X normal), falling to normal by 4-7 days. There is a semiquantitative relation between the amount of necrosis and the peak level in the serum. *0619 0962*

415.10 Pulmonary Embolism and Infarction Moderate increase found, with no sharp peak as in myocardial infarction. *0619 0962*

434.90 Brain Infarction *0962*

482.90 Bacterial Pneumonia *0962*

570.00 Acute and Subacute Necrosis of Liver Cell destruction. Normal or may be slightly increased. *2467 0619*

571.90 Cirrhosis of Liver Normal or slightly increased. *0962*

573.30 Toxic Hepatitis Due to carbon tetrachloride and other poisons. *0619*

576.20 Extrahepatic Biliary Obstruction Normal or slightly increased. *0962*

577.00 Acute Pancreatitis Other nonspecific serum enzymes may also be increased. *2467 0962*

710.00 Systemic Lupus Erythematosus May be found in patients with myositis. *0433*

710.40 Dermatomyositis/Polymyositis Elevated at some time in nearly every patient. *0244* Released as a result of destructive myopathy. Almost invariably elevated in the acute or subacute stages. *1791 2035 0962*

785.40 Gangrene *0962*

791.30 Myoglobinuria Found in paroxysmal myoglobinuria due to muscle destruction. *0619*

929.00 Crush Injury (Trauma) *0995*

948.00 Burns Cell destruction. *2467*

984.00 Toxic Effects of Lead and Its Compounds (including Fumes) *0962*

986.00 Toxic Effects of Carbon Monoxide Often elevated. *0262*

994.50 Exercise An effect of physical training. *1930*

994.80 Effects of Electric Current *0995*

Serum Normal

358.00 Myasthenia Gravis *2057*

359.21 Myotonia Atrophica Usually normal or minimally elevated. *0433*

446.50 Cranial Arteritis and Related Conditions *0186*

570.00 Acute and Subacute Necrosis of Liver Normal or may be slightly increased. *2467*

571.90 Cirrhosis of Liver Normal or slightly increased. *0962*

994.50 Exercise Strenuous physical activity has no effect. *1930*

CSF Increase

272.73 Niemann-Pick Disease *0619*

330.00 Metachromatic Leukodystrophy Increased initially, then diminishes. *0078*

Red Blood Cells Increase

282.60 Sickle Cell Anemia Mean red cell concentrations were slightly elevated in 15 patients. Mean = 2.2 U/L (normal = 1.2 U/L) and range = 0.9-3.9 U/L. *1023*

Aldosterone

Plasma Decrease

250.00 Diabetes Mellitus Commonly found, a result of reduced renin secretion or a specific defect in synthesis are common. *1854*

253.40 Anterior Pituitary Hypofunction *2467*

255.40 Adrenal Cortical Hypofunction Adrenal cortex destruction results in deficiency of glucocorticoids, androgens, and mineralocorticoids. *2612*

303.00 Acute Alcoholic Intoxication Decreased during ethanol intoxication, but increased greatly during hangover. *1412*

642.40 Pre-Eclampsia The secretory rate is somewhat depressed, but often falls within the lower range of normal for pregnancy. In severe cases, concentration was found to be within the range for nonpregnant women (10% of that of normal pregnancy). *2495* Significantly suppressed during the last trimester despite levels of renin substrate and progesterone that were not significantly different from those observed in normotensive pregnancy. *2507 0387*

Plasma Increase

194.00 Malignant Neoplasm of Adrenal Gland In tumors of the zona glomerulosa. *0536*

255.10 Adrenal Cortical Hyperfunction (Mineralocorticoid Excess) If the secretion rate is elevated, it may be assumed that the patient has either primary or secondary aldosteronism. *0151 0433*

308.00 Stress Emotional crises or extreme anxiety elicit increased secretion in normal subjects. *2104*

401.00 Malignant Hypertension Most patients. *0995*

401.10 Essential Benign Hypertension Decreased metabolic clearance rate. *1708*

428.00 Congestive Heart Failure In far-advanced failure, or in moderate failure under vigorous therapy with diuretics, increases in production and excretion, ranging from detectable to very striking, have been noted. *1108* Enhanced ADH and aldosterone activity. *2104*

496.00 Chronic Obstructive Lung Disease Plasma renin and aldosterone tended to have higher than normal baseline values, especially in hypercapnic patients. *0698*

567.90 **Peritonitis** Increased adrenal production. *0995*

571.20 **Laennec's or Alcoholic Cirrhosis** Increased secretion. *2104*

571.90 **Cirrhosis of Liver** Increased levels. *1887* Increased secretion *2104*

580.00 **Acute Poststreptococcal Glomerulonephritis** The decreased GFR and increased aldosterone secretion lead to retention of sodium and water with resultant hypervolemia. *1108*

581.90 **Nephrotic Syndrome** Secretion is augmented in response to decreased plasma values. *0995* Excess contributes to the development of edema. *2104*

585.00 **Chronic Renal Failure** Observed in some patients. *0995*

642.40 **Pre-Eclampsia** At term, hypertensive, toxemic pregnant women had elevated aldosterone and plasma renin activity, which remained elevated > 1 week after delivery. *0066*

642.60 **Eclampsia** At term, hypertensive, toxemic pregnant women had elevated aldosterone and plasma renin activity, which remained elevated > 1 week after delivery. *0066*

650.00 **Pregnancy** Among the normotensive subjects plasma renin activity, aldosterone and progesterone concentrations were elevated as early as the 6th week of gestation. While consistent, progressive, further increases were noted in renin substrate, aldosterone and progesterone during pregnancy. *2507* In hypertensive patients. *2494* *0387*

992.00 **Heat stroke** Increases by 76% after 1 week of thermal stress. *0100*

1013.02 **Diet (Low Sodium)** Increased secretion with a reduced salt diet. *2104*

Plasma Normal

242.90 **Hyperthyroidism** *1448*

244.90 **Hypothyroidism** *1448*

642.40 **Pre-Eclampsia** In hypertensive groups, plasma renin activity and aldosterone concentration were significantly suppressed during the last trimester despite levels of renin substrate and progesterone that were not significantly different from those observed in normotensive pregnancy. *2507* During normal pregnancy, plasma levels of renin, angiotensin II, and aldosterone are increased. Paradoxically with pregnancy-induced hypertension they commonly decrease towards the normal. *1859*

Urine Decrease

250.00 **Diabetes Mellitus** Commonly found, a result of reduced renin secretion or a specific defect in synthesis are common. *1854*

253.40 **Anterior Pituitary Hypofunction** *2467*

255.40 **Adrenal Cortical Hypofunction** Decreased as a result of the progressive destruction of the adrenal cortex. *0619*

401.10 **Essential Benign Hypertension** Decreased metabolic clearance rate of aldosterone. *1708*

580.00 **Acute Poststreptococcal Glomerulonephritis** Occurs in the presence of edema in children. *2468*

642.40 **Pre-Eclampsia** The secretory rate is somewhat depressed, but often falls within the lower range of normal for pregnancy. In severe cases, concentration was found to be within the range for nonpregnant women (10% of that of normal pregnancy). *2495* Significantly suppressed during the last trimester despite levels of renin substrate and progesterone that were not significantly different from those observed in normotensive pregnancy. *2507* *0387*

642.60 **Eclampsia** Less than concentrations usually found in normal pregnancy. *0619*

1013.01 **Diet (High Sodium)** Reduced excretion with increased concentration of salt in diet. *1274*

Urine Increase

194.00 **Malignant Neoplasm of Adrenal Gland** In tumors of the zona glomerulosa. *0536*

255.40 **Adrenal Cortical Hyperfunction (Mineralocorticoid Excess)** Increased on normal salt diet (not detectable on all days); cannot be reduced by high sodium intake and DOCA administration. Increased in primary and secondary hyperaldosteronism due to adrenal adenoma and adrenal carcinoma. *2468*

275.34 **Familial Periodic Paralysis** Striking change noted prior to attack. *2246*

428.00 **Congestive Heart Failure** May be increased in edematous states of cardiac failure. *0619* In far-advanced failure, or in moderate failure under vigorous therapy with diuretics, increases in production and excretion, ranging from detectable to very striking, have been noted. *1108*

567.90 **Peritonitis** Increased adrenal production. *0995*

571.20 **Laennec's or Alcoholic Cirrhosis** May be increased in edematous states of hepatic cirrhosis. *0619* High renal output is due to increased secretion and decreased catabolism. Renal clearance rate may be reduced. *2104*

571.90 **Cirrhosis of Liver** May be increased in edematous states of hepatic cirrhosis. *0619*

580.00 **Acute Poststreptococcal Glomerulonephritis** The decreased GFR and increased aldosterone secretion lead to retention of sodium and water with resultant hypervolemia. *1108*

581.90 **Nephrotic Syndrome** *2104*

585.00 **Chronic Renal Failure** Observed in some patients. *0995*

642.40 **Pre-Eclampsia** At term, hypertensive, toxemic pregnant women had elevated aldosterone and plasma renin activity, which remained elevated > 1 week after delivery. *0066*

650.00 **Pregnancy** In the 3rd trimester of normal pregnancy. *0619*

Urine Normal

359.11 **Progressive Muscular Dystrophy** The differences between the patient group and the control group for sodium and potassium in serum and urine and for urinary aldosterone were not significant. The pathologically elevated sodium:potassium ratio in skeletal muscle is not due to increased aldosterone or other causes of renal wastage of potassium. *0816*

642.40 **Pre-Eclampsia** In hypertensive groups, plasma renin activity and aldosterone concentration were significantly suppressed during the 1st trimester despite levels of renin substrate and progesterone that were not significantly different from those observed in normotensive pregnancy. *2507* During normal pregnancy, plasma levels of renin, angiotensin II, and aldosterone are increased. Paradoxically with pregnancy-induced hypertension, they commonly decrease towards the normal. *1859*

Alkaline Phosphatase

Serum Decrease

40.20 **Whipple's Disease** An indication of vitamin D and calcium malabsorption. *0962*

244.90 **Hypothyroidism** Characteristically low in infantile and juvenile cases. *2540* *2468*

251.50 **Zollinger-Ellison Syndrome** An indication of vitamin D and calcium malabsorption. *0962*

252.10 **Hypoparathyroidism** Normal or slightly low. *2540*

260.00 **Protein Malnutrition** Marked reductions are recognized characteristics. *0151* Decreased unless dehydration is present with marasmus. *2468*

267.00 **Vitamin C Deficiency** *0619*

269.90 **Deficiency State (Unspecified)** Decreased in malnutrition. *2467* *0503*

271.30 **Lactosuria** An indication of vitamin D and calcium malabsorption. *0962*

275.32 **Hypophosphatasia** Marked reduction in activity is one of the cardinal features of hypophosphatasia. Reduced to 25% of the lower limit of normal, the mean levels varying widely with individual cases between almost no activity to 40% activity. There is no correlation between the degree of serum depression and the severity of the clinical manifestations. *0769* *0503*

275.41 **Milk-Alkali Syndrome** *2467*

278.40 **Hypervitaminosis D** *0503*

281.00 **Pernicious Anemia** 33% of patients. *2467* Decreased activity. *2410*

281.20 **Folic Acid Deficiency Anemia** *2538* *2410*

756.40 **Chondrodystrophy** Following arrest of growth in childhood, falls rapidly to adult levels. *0619*

Serum Increase

2.00 **Typhoid Fever** Increased due to complications. *2468*

6.00 **Amebiasis** Becomes elevated earliest with liver abscess. *0433*

Alkaline Phosphatase (continued)

Serum   Increase (continued)

11.00 Pulmonary Tuberculosis   Isolated elevation suggests liver involvement in the absence of other causes. *0433*   Elevated in 50% of cases, ranging from 25-270 U/L, with only 10% of cases having values > 100. *0503*   In 25% of 26 patients at initial hospitalization for this disorder. *0781*

18.00 Disseminated Tuberculosis   Constant chemical finding due to diffuse involvement of the liver with granulomas. *0962*   Marked elevation in all 5 cases of granuloma of liver. Maximum upper limit of normal = 85 U/L. Average elevated value = 425 U/L. Range = 191-700 U/L. *1452   0999*

23.00 Brucellosis   Marked elevation in all 5 cases of granuloma of liver. Maximum upper limit of normal = 85 U/L. Average elevated value = 425 U/L. Range = 191-700 U/L. *1452*

38.00 Septicemia   Elevated in 5 of 6 cases of extrahepatic sepsis, with levels as high as 460 U/L recorded. *1681*   In 27% of 11 patients at initial hospitalization for this disorder. *0781*

39.90 Actinomycosis   May be elevated in cases with osteomyelitis. *0433*

40.20 Whipple's Disease   An indication of vitamin K malabsorption. *0962*

53.00 Herpes Zoster   In 31% of 18 patients at initial hospitalization for this disorder. *0781*

70.00 Viral Hepatitis   Approximately 90% of patients have elevated values. *0503*   40% of cases have values > 210 U/L. *2104*   In 72% of 25 patients at initial hospitalization for this disorder. *0781   2576 1312*

73.90 Psittacosis   With severe liver involvement. *0433*

75.00 Infectious Mononucleosis   Increased in many cases, with maximum values during the 3rd week of the disease. 60-70% of cases are elevated ranging from 25-215 U/L. Only 20% of cases had values > 107 U/L. *0619*   30 (65%) had dissociation with serum bilirubin concentration. Occasionally high levels, even with normal bilirubin concentration. *2156*   May occur; hepatic involvement is usually mild. *2538   1687 0962*

78.50 Cytomegalic Inclusion Disease   Increased in infants. *0619*

84.00 Malaria   Moderate increase. *2468*

100.00 Leptospirosis   Increased in 50% of the patients. *2468*   Jaundice may appear at the end of the 1st week of fever. Liver tests show hepatic decompensation of the intrahepatic type. *2368*

115.00 Histoplasmosis   Present in 50% of patients with disseminated disease. *0999*   Marked elevation in all 5 cases of granuloma of liver. Maximum upper limit of normal = 85 U/L. Average elevated value = 425 U/L. Range = 191-700 U/L. *1452*

116.00 Blastomycosis   May be increased with bone lesions. *2468*

120.00 Schistosomiasis   Found in 50% of adult patients but is not useful in children. *2468*   Consistently elevated and remains high for 1 month after treatment. *2026*   Marked elevation in all 5 cases of granuloma of liver. Maximum upper limit of normal = 85 U/L. Average elevated value = 425 U/L. Range = 191-700 U/L. *1452   0151 0962*

122.90 Hydatidosis   May increase with obstruction of biliary system. *0812*   With bone involvement. *1058*

135.00 Sarcoidosis   Elevated in 40% of cases involving the liver, usually ranging from 25-97 U/L, with < 15% presenting values > 107 U/L. *0503*   Marked elevation in all 5 cases of granuloma of liver. Maximum upper limit of normal = 85 U/L. Average elevated value = 425 U/L. Range = 191-700 U/L. *1452   1312 0999*

150.90 Malignant Neoplasm of Esophagus   In 29% of 40 patients at initial hospitalization for this disorder. *0781*

151.90 Malignant Neoplasm of Stomach   In 38% of 45 patients at initial hospitalization for this disorder. *0781*

153.90 Malignant Neoplasm of Large Intestine   In 24% of 150 patients at initial hospitalization for this disorder. *0781   0992*

155.00 Malignant Neoplasm of Liver   Due to obstruction, elevated in 88% of patients with primary cancer. *0029*   Elevated in 95-100% of primary cancers, usually ranging from 80-215 U/L, with only 80% having values 107 U/L. *0503*   Usually moderately elevated; 40-50% of patients have concentration between 20-75 U/L and 15-30% are above 81 U/L. *0364*   Elevated in 80.5% of 62 patients with hepatoma. *1115*   In about 80% of cases. *0962*   In 90% of 12 patients at initial hospitalization for this disorder. *0781   0151*

155.10 Malignant Neoplasm of Intrahepatic Bile Ducts   In all cases; elevated from 94-263 U/L (normal = 25 U/L) due to common duct obstruction. *2576*

157.90 Malignant Neoplasm of Pancreas   Due to biliary tract obstruction values range from 150-215 U/L (normal = 21 U/L). *2576*   Elevated without marked abnormalities in all liver function tests. *0267*   Elevated in 85 of 100 patients with histologically proven disease. *0932*   In 82% of 46 patients at initial hospitalization for this disorder. *0781   0151*

162.90 Malignant Neoplasm of Bronchus and Lung   Elevated shortly before death or with tumor extension. Little diagnostic use but helpful in detecting metastases to bone. *0819*   In 9 patients, initial values ranged from 43-263 U/L (normal < 105 U/L). *2267*

170.90 Malignant Neoplasm of Bone   Marked increase up to 40 X normal in osteogenic forms, parallels clinical course. *2467*   In predominantly osteolytic forms remains normal or only moderately increased. *0619*   All groups of bone tumors showed a significant increase when compared to the norm. Maximum values were found in the group of osteosarcomas and minimum in that of fibrosarcomas. *0301*   In 39% of 26 patients at initial hospitalization for this disorder. *0781   0503*

174.90 Malignant Neoplasm of Breast   Mean level in patients without bone metastases was above the normal range. The mean levels with metastases to bone was even higher, with 56% of all cases above the normal range. *2566*

183.00 Malignant Neoplasm of Ovary   In 5 cases, the initial value was 45-190 U/L (normal < 107 U/L). *0326*

185.00 Malignant Neoplasm of Prostate   Levels were elevated above the normal range in cases without bone metastases. With bone metastases, levels were much higher and 90% of patients showed marked elevations. *2566*   In 54% of 83 patients at initial hospitalization for this disorder. *0781   0870 1863*

197.00 Secondary Malignant Neoplasm of Respiratory System   In 49% of 588 patients at initial hospitalization for this disorder. *0781*

197.70 Secondary Malignant Neoplasm of Liver   Degree of elevation may at times be striking with little or no rise in bilirubin. Occurs in 80% of cases, usually ranging from 25-375 U/L with 20% of cases showing values > 107 U/L. *0503*   Useful index of partial obstruction of the biliary tree when serum bilirubin is usually normal and urine bilirubin is increased. Increased in 80% of patients with metastatic carcinoma. *2467*   Consistent elevation with metastases. *1312*

198.50 Secondary Malignant Neoplasm of Bone   Rises in proportion to the formation of new bone cells. *0812*   Usually increased in osteoblastic metastases (especially from primary tumor in prostate). *2467*   Especially secondary to prostate *1954* and breast carcinoma. *2566*   23% of patients with bone metastasis showed normal concentrations. *2062   0503*

201.90 Hodgkin's Disease   Progressive increase in patients over 20 y of age with elevated concentrations found with advancing clinical stage. Patients < 20 had frequent (50%) occurrence of elevations but this did not correlate with stage of disease. More sensitive than GGT in following the clinical course. *0160*   May be a systemic sign of active disease or may indicate involvement of liver or bone. *2538 1204*   Lymphoma associated with hyperbilirubinemia is accompanied by elevations from 43-331 U/L. In some cases, reflects osteoblastic lesions as well as metastases. *2576   0433 0781*

202.80 Non-Hodgkins Lymphoma   In 10 patients with lymphosarcoma involving the liver, value was 69 ± 28 U/L. *1312*   May be increased as a result of liver and less frequently bone disease. *0025*   May be a systemic sign of active disease or may indicate involvement of liver or bone. *0433*   Lymphoma associated with hyperbilirubinemia is accompanied by elevations from 43-331 U/L. In some cases, reflects osteoblastic lesions as well as metastases. *2576*

203.00 Multiple Myeloma   In the absence of fracture with callus formation, the level is usually normal, although elevated levels have been reported. *0433*   Normal or slightly elevated, even in patients with extensive bone lesions. *2538*   In 27% of 31 patients at initial hospitalization for this disorder. *0781*

204.00 Lymphocytic Leukemia (Acute)   Infiltration of the liver may result in obstruction of biliary system. *2468*   Elevations > 95 U/L. *1322*   In 56% of 42 patients at initial hospitalization for this disorder. *0781*

204.10 Lymphocytic Leukemia (Chronic)   Infiltration of the liver may result in obstruction of the biliary system. *2468*   Elevations > 95 U/L. *1322*   In 42% of 27 patients at initial hospitalization for this disorder. *0781*

205.00 Myelocytic Leukemia (Acute) Infiltration of the liver may result in obstruction of the biliary system. *2468* Elevations > 95 U/L. *1322*

205.10 Myelocytic Leukemia (Chronic) Infiltration of the liver may result in obstruction of the biliary system. *2468* 21 of 54 patients had levels > 95 U/L. *1322* In 54% of 21 patients at initial hospitalization for this disorder. *0781*

206.00 Monocytic Leukemia In 34% of 21 patients at initial hospitalization for this disorder. *0781*

242.90 Hyperthyroidism Mean level was 42.5 U/L or 55% higher in the hyperthyroid than in the euthyroid group. *1320 0999*

244.90 Hypothyroidism Excess enzyme originates from the bone. *2468* In 24% of 12 patients at initial hospitalization for this disorder. *0781*

245.10 Subacute Thyroiditis Elevated in 3 of 10 patients; no apparent relation to degree of T_4 elevation and of unknown origin. *0489*

245.20 Hashimoto's Thyroiditis Elevated in 3 patients, suggesting hepatic origin of the enzymes. *0489*

250.00 Diabetes Mellitus Occurred in 11-17% of the patients. Ketoacidosis and death occurred more often among patients with elevated serum enzymes than those with normal levels. *0873* In 24% of 105 patients at initial hospitalization for this disorder. *0781* Elevated by 40% in 44% of 166 untreated patients. Activity did not correlate with blood sugar concentration. *0155*

252.00 Hyperparathyroidism Found to be elevated in only 30%, and each of these showed normal results for other liver function tests. Correlated well with serum calcium, but only significant in female patients. *1492* Following the removal of the parathyroid tumor, the increased serum concentration persists and may even rise temporarily, falling gradually over a period of months as bone repair is completed. *0619*

253.00 Acromegaly May indicate secretory activity of tumor. *2467* Increased bone turnover found in this condition may result in elevation. *0962*

255.00 Adrenal Cortical Hyperfunction (Glucocorticoid Excess) Presumably due to excess ACTH. *0619*

268.00 Vitamin D Deficiency Rickets The earliest and most reliable biochemical abnormality; until bone healing is complete. *2467* Increased in active rickets, the degree of elevation corresponding to the severity of the disease. The average phosphatase in 9 cases of uncomplicated rickets was 0.75, with a range of 0.3-1.4. *2213* Consistently elevated. *2246 0503 0441 0442*

268.20 Osteomalacia In adults this test represents the single most sensitive indicator of active disease. The earliest biochemical alteration. *2467* Persistently raised concentration despite evident relief of symptoms. *0441* Typically. *2199 0503 0999*

270.03 Cystinosis With the appearance of rickets. *2246*

272.72 Gaucher's Disease With bone resorption. *0619 0812*

272.73 Niemann-Pick Disease Seen in type B disease. *2246*

275.00 Hemochromatosis With liver involvement. *0962*

275.10 Hepatolenticular Degeneration With liver involvement. *0995*

275.31 Hyperphosphatasia Pronounced increase. *2259*

275.35 Vitamin D Resistant Rickets In older infants or children. *0503* Many children and patients continued to show persistently raised concentration, despite evident relief of symptoms in those with rickets or osteomalacia and increased growth rate in the school children. *0441* As skeletal changes develop. *2246*

277.00 Cystic Fibrosis Noted in 40% of 36 children. Serum activity as a whole is fairly insensitive to occurrence and degree of disease because of high upper limits for normal children. *0578* In 65% of 12 patients at initial hospitalization for this disorder. *0781*

277.30 Amyloidosis Frequently elevated, usually ranging from 25-535 U/L. No jaundice. In patients with space-occupying lesions such as amyloidosis the degree of elevation at times may be striking with little or no rise in the serum bilirubin values. *2467 0138 0140* Increased in almost 50% of patients with primary disease, mean value = 108 U/L. *1334* Frequently found with liver involvement. *0962* With hepatic involvement. *0125 0503*

277.41 Dubin-Johnson Syndrome May be normal or moderately increased. *0602*

282.60 Sickle Cell Anemia Serum concentration and the isoenzyme pattern appear to be in concordance with severity of sickle cell crisis. Bone isoenzyme is the principal enzyme fraction that increases during symptomatic crises. Serum concentration may be an additional indicator of degree, frequency, and persistence of tissue i injuries. Increased during crisis, representing vaso-occlusive bone injury as well as liver damage with sickle cell disease. *2467 0288*

289.80 Myelofibrosis *0151 2538*

303.90 Alcoholism Elevation occurred in 10.4% of cases. *1781* Mild elevation occurred in 80% of 5 cases with range 75-140 U/L. Maximum upper limit for normal 84 U/L. *1452* In 28% of 14 patients hospitalized for this disorder. *0781*

334.00 Friedreich's Ataxia One pair of siblings displayed a slight elevation. *1956*

410.90 Acute Myocardial Infarction Some patients; usually during phase of organization. *2467* Increased in conjunction with normal levels of bilirubin indicate congestive heart failure or myocardial infarction-28%, carcinoma-25%, hepatobiliary-16%, and other miscellaneous diseases. *0191*

415.10 Pulmonary Embolism and Infarction Elevation is temporary and found at maximum value within 1-3 weeks after embolism. *0562* In 30% of 19 patients at initial hospitalization for this disorder. *0781*

428.00 Congestive Heart Failure Usually elevated with cardiac cirrhosis. *0433* Mild to moderate increase (30-135 U/L) in 45% of cases. *2467* Increase in conjunction with normal levels of bilirubin indicate congestive heart failure or myocardial infarction in 28% of cases. *0191*

446.50 Cranial Arteritis and Related Conditions Abnormal liver test results, have been found, but biopsies have shown only minor nonspecific changes. *0557 2035*

451.90 Phlebitis and Thrombophlebitis In 28% of 51 patients at initial hospitalization for this disorder. *0781*

480.90 Viral Pneumonia In 70% of 10 patients at initial hospitalization for this disorder. *0781*

496.01 Alpha₁-Antitrypsin Deficiency Related to liver disease. *1636*

537.40 Fistula of Stomach and Duodenum Leading to secondary osteomalacia. *0619*

555.90 Regional Enteritis or Ileitis Indicates hepatic involvement. *0433* Frequently abnormal in patients who otherwise show no indication of liver disease. *2199*

556.00 Ulcerative Colitis Often increased slightly. *2467 0433*

557.01 Mesenteric Artery Embolism A selective elevation of the intestinal isoenzyme has been described in acute intestinal ischemia. *0433*

560.90 Intestinal Obstruction In 31% of 42 patients at initial hospitalization for this disorder. *0781*

570.00 Acute and Subacute Necrosis of Liver Higher in obstructive jaundice than in acute hepatitis. The basis for elevation in patients with hepatobiliary disease is obscure. Increased formation by hepatic parenchymal or ductal cells, perhaps supplemented by impaired excretion, is the apparent mechanism. *0503* Most commonly between 65-160 U/L. *0619* Incidence of elevation is 80-100%; usual range 25-80 U/L. *0503 2576 0999*

571.20 Laennec's or Alcoholic Cirrhosis Incidence of elevation: 40%; usual range of values: 25-85 U/L; 5% incidence of values > 107 U/L. Jaundice may be absent or present. Usually normal or only mildly elevated. *0503* Associated with jaundice. *2576 1312*

571.49 Chronic Active Hepatitis Only slight increases. *2035* Occasionally. *0962* In 60% of 19 patients at initial hospitalization for this disorder. *0781* Moderately elevated (X 2) or normal. *0992* Approximately 90% of patients with toxic hepatocellular jaundice have elevated values. Almost always < 88 U/L and in most < 50. Approximately 5% of patients with hepatocellular jaundice may have levels of 88-135 U/L. In jaundiced patients with higher levels, posthepatic jaundice should be suspected. *0503*

571.60 Biliary Cirrhosis Striking elevations. Incidence of elevation is 100%. Usual range of values 270-375 U/L. *1312 0151 0999 2035*

571.90 Cirrhosis of Liver Nonspecifically elevated in cirrhosis but often reaches levels exceeding 160 U/L. *0433* Average elevation in 6 cases = 3.5 X normal upper limit. *1452* In 47% of 67 patients at initial hospitalization for this disorder. *0781* 50% incidence of elevation usually in the range of 25-188 U/L in postnecrotic cirrhosis. *0503 2576*

Alkaline Phosphatase (continued)

Serum   Increase (continued)

572.00 Liver Abscess (Pyogenic)   In patients with space-occupying lesions such as liver abscess, the degree of elevation may be striking (270-535 U/L) with little or no rise in the serum bilirubin values. This pattern of hepatic dysfunction is useful in the recognition of these space-occupying lesions particularly in the recognition of metastasis to the liver in patients with carcinomatosis. *0812 0503*   25-80 U/L in over 80% of cases; 80-375 U/L in 100% of cases during obstructive phase. *2467*   Elevated in 75% of cases. *2199   0433*

572.40 Hepatic Failure   May be normal or increased. *0503*

573.30 Toxic Hepatitis   Elevated to > 3 X normal. *0433*   Found in 6 patients with toxic drug hepatitis with values of 134 ± 19.8 U/L. *1312*   Drugs particularly likely to produce this type of jaundice are chlorpromazine or organic arsenicals. Alk phos values are at least as high as in posthepatic jaundice. *0503*   Striking increase. *2104*

575.00 Acute Cholecystitis   Increased in some cases, even if serum bilirubin is normal. *2467*   Average elevation = 3 X maximum normal limit in 75% of 8 cases studied. *1452*   May be mildly elevated even in the absence of intrahepatic infection or common bile duct obstruction. *2199*   In 30% of 16 patients at initial hospitalization for this disorder. *0781*

576.10 Cholangitis   Elevation (mean = 255 U/L) observed in 100% of 13 cases. *1452*   Values indicate extrahepatic obstruction. *0151 0433*

576.20 Extrahepatic Biliary Obstruction   Markedly increased, related to the completeness of obstruction. Up to 376 U/L in complete biliary obstruction. *2467*   Associated with increase of 53-240 U/L. Common duct obstruction due to stones had values of 53-110 U/L. *2576*   95% - 100% incidence of elevation usually ranging from 60-140 U/L. Incidence of values > 105 U/L = 40%. *0503*   May become elevated in attack in the absence of hyperbilirubinemia. *0433*

577.00 Acute Pancreatitis   Parallels serum bilirubin. *2467*   Anicteric cases had normal levels. Cases with some degree of common bile duct obstruction were all elevated. *1312*   In 45% of 21 patients at initial hospitalization for this disorder. *0781*

577.10 Chronic Pancreatitis   Jaundice may occur not only during acute attacks but also during the silent stage. Usually due to extrahepatic cholestasis an elevated alkaline phosphatase and normal AST at the early stages tend to support this. *0433*   In each of 6 male alcoholic patients with calcific disease, a marked elevation was associated with minimal elevation in serum bilirubin or BSP excretion. *2217*   In 40% of 12 patients at initial hospitalization for this disorder. *0781*

577.20 Pancreatic Cyst and Pseudocyst   Increased in 10% of patients. *2467*

579.00 Celiac Sprue Disease   Leading to secondary osteomalacia. *0619*   Suggestive of secondary hyperparathyroidism. *0433*

579.90 Malabsorption, Cause Unspecified   An indication of vitamin D and calcium malabsorption. *0962   0151*

581.90 Nephrotic Syndrome   In 40% of 25 patients at initial hospitalization for this disorder. *0781*

585.00 Chronic Renal Failure   In 29% of 139 patients at initial hospitalization for this disorder. *0781*

588.00 Renal Dwarfism   Usually elevated. *0151*

588.81 Proximal Renal Tubular Acidosis   Increased in Albright-type renal tubular acidosis, as in Fanconi Syndrome, but no aminoaciduria. *0619   0503 0433 2246*

590.10 Acute Pyelonephritis   Significant elevation can be found in some patients. This occurs in cases with clinical or histological evidence of severe disease, occasionally associated with papillary necrosis and gram-negative septicemia. Widespread renal inflammatory destruction results in release of enzyme from the tubular cells into the blood stream. *0753*   In 29% of 13 patients at initial hospitalization for this disorder. *0781*

642.40 Pre-Eclampsia   May be elevated above the normal increase found in pregnancy. This is due to a rise in the heat-stable (placental) isoenzyme. *2034*   Exaggerated increases may occur and could indicate placental as well as hepatic damage. *0387*

650.00 Pregnancy   Increase is due entirely to the heat stable form of the enzyme produced exclusively in the placenta. *1557*   Marked increase to term *0517   0503 0387 2020*

714.00 Rheumatoid Arthritis   Characteristically abnormal when the arthritis is active. *0433*

720.00 Rheumatoid (Ankylosing) Spondylitis   Elevation in 47.5% of 40 patients and in most cases was derived from bone. *1250*

730.00 Osteomyelitis   In 36% of 24 patients at initial hospitalization for this disorder. *0781*

731.00 Osteitis Deformans   Gradually rises with the extension of the disease, rising rapidly if osteogenic sarcoma develops. ACTH or cortisone causes a transitory fall, often followed by a sharp rebound increase. *0619*   Marked increase directly related to severity and extent of disease. *2467*   20 cases were reported in which all patients showed elevated serum concentration. *1312 1986 0999*

733.00 Osteoporosis   In hypermetabolic osteopenia. *0999*

756.51 Osteogenesis Imperfecta   Increase observed in 2 cases. *1312   2467*

756.54 Polyostotic Fibrous Dysplasia   In some cases. *0619 2467 0503 1156*

785.40 Gangrene   In 45% of 32 patients hospitalized for this disorder. *0781*

829.00 Fracture of Bone   Rises in proportion to the formation of new bone cells. *0812 0503*

985.00 Toxic Effects of Non-medicinal Metals   Hepatotoxicity may occur with arsenicals. *1446*

Serum   Normal

170.90 Malignant Neoplasm of Bone   Usually normal in Ewing's sarcoma and other osteolytic tumors. *2467*

174.90 Malignant Neoplasm of Breast   No significant elevation was found in patients without bone metastases. *1312*

203.00 Multiple Myeloma   Usually normal. *0433   0992*

252.10 Hypoparathyroidism   Normal or slightly low. *2540*

275.00 Hemochromatosis   Over 50% of patients have no laboratory evidence of liver dysfunction. *0995*

275.35 Vitamin D Resistant Rickets   Normal in most patients without radiologic signs of rickets. *2246*

277.41 Dubin-Johnson Syndrome   Routine liver function tests are normal. *0962*

277.42 Gilbert's Disease   *0995*

277.43 Rotor's Syndrome   Routine liver function tests are normal. *0962*

277.44 Crigler-Najjar Syndrome   *0469*

642.40 Pre-Eclampsia   Usually not elevated. When elevated, either pronounced hepatic or marked myocardial alterations have occurred. *0433   2034*

714.00 Rheumatoid Arthritis   Generally normal. *0962*

730.00 Osteomyelitis   Normal in all 39 cases. *2464*

733.00 Osteoporosis   *0433 2467*

756.52 Osteopetrosis   *2467*

994.50 Exercise   Insignificant change after physical activity. *0804*

Urine   Increase

188.90 Malignant Neoplasm of Bladder   Elevated in 43% of 35 patients. *0817*   Elevated in 10 of 26 (38.5%) of active transitional cell carcinomas. *1843   0818*

189.00 Malignant Neoplasm of Kidney   Occurs mainly when a tumor has extended beyond the renal parenchyma or into bladder muscle. *0818*   Elevated in 55% of patients. *0817*

580.00 Acute Poststreptococcal Glomerulonephritis   *0619*

585.00 Chronic Renal Failure   69% of cases showed elevation. *0817*

590.00 Chronic Pyelonephritis   Almost invariably elevated in a group of 10 patients. *0817*

Synovial Fluid   Decrease

274.00 Gout   *0619*

Leukocyte   Decrease

151.90 Malignant Neoplasm of Stomach   Low activity is present irrespective of tumor category, activity of disease, or type of therapy. In 11 patients, median activity was 5 U/L (normal = 55). *1423*

153.90 Malignant Neoplasm of Large Intestine   Low activity is present irrespective of tumor category, activity of disease, or type of therapy. In 11 patients median value was 18 U/L (normal = 55). *1423*

157.90 Malignant Neoplasm of Pancreas Low activity is present irrespective of tumor category, activity of disease, or type of therapy. In 11 patients, median activity was 5 U/L (normal = 55). *1423*

162.90 Malignant Neoplasm of Bronchus and Lung Low activity is present irrespective of tumor category, activity of disease, or type of therapy. In 12 patients median activity was 8 U/L (normal = 55). *1423*

172.90 Malignant Melanoma of Skin Low activity is present irrespective of tumor category, activity of disease, or type of therapy. In 11 patients, median activity was 5 U/L (normal = 55). *1423*

174.90 Malignant Neoplasm of Breast Low activity is present irrespective of tumor category, activity of disease, or type of therapy. In 21 patients, median value = 25 U/L (normal = 55). *1423*

185.00 Malignant Neoplasm of Prostate Low activity is present irrespective of tumor category, activity of disease, or type of therapy. In 11 patients, median activity was 5 U/L (normal = 55). *1423*

197.00 Secondary Malignant Neoplasm of Respiratory System Patients with metastases of the lung, bone and skin all showed decreased activity, with median values of 6.4 20.5, and 10.0 U/L respectively (normal = 55 U). *1423*

198.50 Secondary Malignant Neoplasm of Bone Patients with metastases of the lung, bone and skin all showed decreased activity, with median values of 6.4, 20.5, and 10.0 U/L respectively (Normal = 55 U). *1423*

199.00 Secondary Malignant Neoplasm (Disseminated) Patients with metastases of the lung, bone, and skin all showed decreased activity, with median values of 6.4, 20.5, and 10.0 U/L respectively (Normal = 55 U). *1423*

201.90 Hodgkin's Disease Activity is low irrespective of tumor category, activity of disease, or type of therapy. In 17 cases of malignant lymphoma, median LAP was 17 U/L (Normal = 55). *1423*

202.80 Non-Hodgkins Lymphoma Activity is low irrespective of tumor category, activity of disease, or type of therapy. In 17 cases of malignant lymphoma, median LAP was 17 U/L (Normal = 55). *1423*

205.00 Myelocytic Leukemia (Acute) The range of activity per 10^{10} leukocytes was 0.0-6.2 U/L, the mean being 1.6 U/L. The tendency toward low levels for both alkaline and acid phosphatase activity suggests that the blast form is poor in phosphatase; the activity being attributable chiefly to the more mature cells in acute leukemia. *0144* leukemia. *1949 1563 2552*

205.10 Myelocytic Leukemia (Chronic) In 60 patients, mean = 33 U/L, ranging from 0-294 U/L. In untreated cases, the mean score was 6.6 U/L, ranging from 0-28 U/L. Mean in 19 treated cases was 45.15 U/L with a range of 3-294 U/L. Leukopenic cases showed the average score as 104 U/L, ranging from 52-208 U/L. *1563* 25% of 38 patients who achieved remission had normal activity. *1991* A striking decrease can be demonstrated; about 20% of normal mature granulocytes give a positive reaction. *2538* Abnormally low and may actually be absent *0525 2552*

268.00 Vitamin D Deficiency Rickets *0151*

275.32 Hypophosphatasia In untreated hereditary hypophosphatasia. *2467*

281.30 Vitamin B₆ Deficiency Anemia Score is reduced in about 50% of the patients. *1327*

282.60 Sickle Cell Anemia Decreased activity. *2468* Low levels found. *2454*

283.21 Paroxysmal Nocturnal Hemoglobinuria Usually decreased. *2538* Often very low or absent. *1385*

285.00 Sideroblastic Anemia Score is reduced in about 50% of the patients. *1327 2538*

289.80 Myelofibrosis Significantly elevated in most cases but in 10% of the cases in myelofibrosis the levels were in the CML range (markedly decreased or absent). *0433* In myelofibrosis, variable with normal, high, and low figures being found. Level tends to fall as the disease progresses. *2538*

359.11 Progressive Muscular Dystrophy Untreated disease. *2467*

581.90 Nephrotic Syndrome Untreated disease. *2467*

Leukocyte Increase

38.00 Septicemia Usually increased in untreated disease. *2467 0619*

70.00 Viral Hepatitis *2467*

197.70 Secondary Malignant Neoplasm of Liver Parallel alkaline phosphatase but is not affected by bone disease. *2467* Liver metastases appear to be the only metastatic site which tends to increase activity. Patients with liver metastases had a median value of 65 U/L (normal = 55). Other primary and secondary malignancies usually present significantly low levels. *1423*

201.90 Hodgkin's Disease In 4 cases, mean value was 135, ranging from 92-182. Activities were elevated in patients in spite of good remission with no clinical and radiological sign of disease. *1563* 22 of 23 patients with active disease had significant LAP elevations, mean score of 164 ± 51. Of 19 patients with inactive disease, 15 had normal scores, 63 ± 17, and the 4 with elevated scores soon redeveloped symptoms of activity. *0167* Elevated during active phases. Normal during remission. *2538 0151*

202.80 Non-Hodgkins Lymphoma Usually increased in untreated diseases. Increased in lymphoma (including Hodgkin's disease and reticulum cell sarcoma). *2467*

203.00 Multiple Myeloma Over a 13 y period, 60 of 62 patients had consistently elevated levels. One patient had a normal level, and one had an initially normal level which later increased. Elevations could not be correlated with age, hemoglobin, WBC, or BUN. *0292*

204.00 Lymphocytic Leukemia (Acute) The mean activity score was 159.4 ranging from 83-308 (12 cases). *1563* Tend to be high, in contrast to acute myelogenous leukemia. *1011*

204.10 Lymphocytic Leukemia (Chronic) Mean score of 139.4 with a range of 73-180. *1563* The range of actual enzyme levels per 10^{10} leukocytes was 2.5-68.2 with a mean of 20.8. Only 3 determinations were higher than 26.5. Normal = 25.8, ranging from 13.4-58.0. *0144*

205.00 Myelocytic Leukemia (Acute) Slightly elevated in > 50% of cases. *2552*

205.10 Myelocytic Leukemia (Chronic) Occasionally can be elevated if some complicating condition (ulcerative colitis, a second neoplasm, or an acute infection) is present. *0433*

206.00 Monocytic Leukemia Mean value in 13 cases of acute monomyelocytic leukemia was 103.4 with a range of 12-208. *1563*

207.00 Erythroleukemia In 2 cases of erythroleukemia, the scores from polymorphonuclears were 24 and 78. Normal mean = 61.9. *1563 2538*

238.40 Polycythemia Vera Three polycythemic patients showed elevations the mean = 82, compared with the mean of the normal group (25.8) and that of the group with chronic myelocytic leukemia (4.0). *0144* 70-90% of patients have above the upper limits of normal, while a small number of patients have normal values. No clinical or hematologic differences are apparent in patients with normal activity as compared with those with increased activity. *0069* Strikingly increased. *1610 2468 1563 2538*

284.90 Aplastic Anemia Usually increased in untreated disease. *2467*

288.00 Agranulocytosis Usually increased in untreated disease. *2467*

289.80 Myelofibrosis Usually high but in 10% of cases, scores were in the CML range (markedly decreased or absent). *0433* Findings tend to be inconsistent. Generally elevated in the majority of patients. *2317* In agnogenic myeloid metaplasia, 41 of 78 patients had scores > 1.00. A significant negative correlation was found between LAP and absolute percentage of immature cells. *2167* Variable; tends to fall as the disease progresses. *2538 1563*

555.90 Regional Enteritis or Ileitis Markedly increased. *1297*

556.00 Ulcerative Colitis Markedly increased. *1297*

570.00 Acute and Subacute Necrosis of Liver Markedly increased; may remain increased for years after jaundice has disappeared. *2467*

571.90 Cirrhosis of Liver Slightly increased in 30% of patients. *2467*

576.20 Extrahepatic Biliary Obstruction Parallels alkaline phosphatase. *2467*

650.00 Pregnancy Increases are directly proportion to period of gestation and returned to normal after 4th week postpartum. *0081* Elevation of score has been found in high risk pregnancies due to diabetes mellitus, toxemia, renal diseases and 3rd trimester hemorrhage, but not in pregnancies complicated by cardiac disease. *1610* Activities obtained from 20 pregnant women were markedly elevated in all cases. Mean value was 187 with a range of 98-242. *1563 1424*

758.00 Down's Syndrome *2467*

758.70 Klinefelter's Syndrome (XXY) *2467*

Alkaline Phosphatase (continued)

Leukocyte   Normal

202.80   Non-Hodgkins Lymphoma   In 10 cases, mean activity was found to be in the normal range or slightly below, irrespective of treatment. *1563   2467*

282.20   Anemias Due To Disorders of Glutathione Metabolism *2467*

289.00   Polycythemia, Secondary   *2467*

Alkaline Phosphatase Isoenzymes

Serum   Decrease

340.00   Multiple Sclerosis   Preliminary studies indicate a depression of serum alk phos of intestinal origin (serum type PP2) especially in blood group O. Comparisons were made with normal sera after matching blood groups, a factor not previously taken into account. *1759*

Serum   Increase

2.00   Typhoid Fever   Increased incidence of the Regan (placental) isoenzyme. *0740*

70.00   Viral Hepatitis   Isoenzyme I was elevated in 12 of 12 patients. Isoenzyme IV was elevated in only 5 cases. *1221*

75.00   Infectious Mononucleosis   An electrophoretically distinct isoenzyme (phosphatase N) was found in the serum of all 22 patients. Values ranged from 13-100% of the total activity, with 6 cases having > 80% phos-N activity. *1687*

135.00   Sarcoidosis   Elevated hepatic isoenzyme is characteristically present. *0999*

151.90   Malignant Neoplasm of Stomach   Concentration of Regan isoenzyme was 12.5-34.2 U/L. *0549*

153.90   Malignant Neoplasm of Large Intestine   Increased incidence of the Regan (placental) isoenzyme. *0740*   13.25% had increased concentration of the Regan isoenzyme, ranging from 7.17-24.3 U/L. *0549*

155.00   Malignant Neoplasm of Liver   Of 15 cases all had increased values of isoenzyme-I and 6 had increased isoenzyme-IV as well. *1221*

155.10   Malignant Neoplasm of Intrahepatic Bile Ducts   Regan isoenzyme concentration was 27.6 U/L. *0549*

157.90   Malignant Neoplasm of Pancreas   Highest concentrations were found in sera of patients with cancer of the pancreas. Ranges were 11.8-81.4 U/L. *0549*

174.90   Malignant Neoplasm of Breast   Cancer of the ovary, endometrium, cervix and breast as a group exhibited the highest frequency of Regan isoenzyme (placental). *0326*

180.90   Malignant Neoplasm of Cervix   Cancer of the ovary, endometrium, cervix and breast as a group exhibited the highest frequency of Regan isoenzyme (placental). *0326*

183.00   Malignant Neoplasm of Ovary   In 5 cases, the initial value was 44.7-191 (normal 106.5 U/L). The Regan isoenzyme was found in all cases and ranged from 99-264 U/L placental isoenzyme units. *2267*   Cancer of the ovary, endometrium, cervix and breast as a group exhibited the highest frequency of Regan isoenzyme (placental) in malignancies. *0326*

186.90   Malignant Neoplasm of Testis   Gonadal neoplasms (ovary and testis) showed the greatest frequency of Regan isoenzymes (placental) in cancers. *0740*

189.00   Malignant Neoplasm of Kidney   Increased incidence of the Regan (placental) isoenzyme. *0740*

197.70   Secondary Malignant Neoplasm of Liver   23 of 24 patients with metastatic carcinoma of liver had markedly elevated liver $alpha_1$ and $alpha_2$ alkaline phosphatase isoenzyme levels. Mean values were 19 ± 18 U/L and 45 ± 28 U/L respectively. *1926*

198.50   Secondary Malignant Neoplasm of Bone   5 of 7 patients with metastatic lesions of bone had elevated isoenzyme-II. Isoenzymes I and IV were elevated in 2 of the 7 cases. *1221*

204.00   Lymphocytic Leukemia (Acute)   In all 6 patients, an electrophoretically distinct isoenzyme (phosphatase N) was present in the serum. The range of phosphatase N was 26-100% of the total alkaline phosphatase activity. *1687*

204.10   Lymphocytic Leukemia (Chronic)   A distinct isoenzyme (phosphatase N) was found in the serum of 5 patients. Values ranged from 35-39% of the total activity. *1687*

277.00   Cystic Fibrosis   Liver fraction. *2246*

282.60   Sickle Cell Anemia   Serum concentration and the isoenzyme pattern appear to be in concordance with severity of sickle cell crisis. Bone isoenzyme is the principal enzyme fraction that increases during symptomatic crises. *2467*

428.00   Congestive Heart Failure   All 5 patients showed elevations of isoenzyme I. *1221*

557.01   Mesenteric Artery Embolism   A selective elevation of the intestinal isoenzyme has been described in acute intestinal ischemia. *0433*

571.20   Laennec's or Alcoholic Cirrhosis   Alkaline phosphatase-I was the major elevated isoenzyme in 12 of 14 cases. Isoenzyme-IV was raised in 5 of the 14 patients. *1221*

575.00   Acute Cholecystitis   All 11 patients with biliary tree disease, including 5 with cholecystitis and 6 with pericholangitis, showed elevated isoenzyme I. 7 of the 11 had raised isoenzyme-IV. *1221*

576.10   Cholangitis   All 11 patients with biliary tree disease, including 5 with cholecystitis and 6 with pericholangitis, showed elevated isoenzyme I. 7 of the 11 had raised isoenzyme-IV. *1221*

576.20   Extrahepatic Biliary Obstruction   10 jaundiced patients with extrahepatic biliary obstruction had elevated isoenzyme-I and 8 of the 10 had raised isoenzyme-IV. *1221*   15 of 17 patients with obstructive jaundice showed a couplet of liver isoenzymes in the $alpha_1$ and $alpha_2$ areas. Mean levels were 4.7 and 20.5 respectively. *1926*   Two main isoenzymes are present: $alpha_2$-globulin, derived directly from the liver cells, which contributed the major fraction, and the 2nd, present in smaller proportions and represents the regurgitation of bile alkaline phosphatase as a result of obstruction to the normal flow of bile. *1855*

642.40   Pre-Eclampsia   May be elevated above the normal increase found in pregnancy, due to a rise in the heat-stable (placental) isoenzyme. *2034*

650.00   Pregnancy   Elevation is due to circulating placental isoenzyme. *0213*   Heat-stable isoenzyme progressively increases as pregnancy approaches term. If > 50% of total serum concentration is heat stable, placenta size is compatible with mature fetus in maternal serum. *2467   2020*

731.00   Osteitis Deformans   All 7 patients had elevations of isoenzyme II. *1221*

Pleural Effusion   Increase

183.00   Malignant Neoplasm of Ovary   59% (13 of 22) patients had detectable regan isoenzyme in malignant effusions. *2268*

Ascitic Fluid   Increase

183.00   Malignant Neoplasm of Ovary   59% (13 of 22) patients had detectable regan isoenzyme. *2268*

Alkaloids

Serum   Increase

156.00   Malignant Neoplasm of Gallbladder   Increased. *0655 1737*

Alloisoleucine

Serum   Increase

270.31   Maple Syrup Urine Disease   Alloisoleucine, an amino acid not normally present in plasma, is elevated. *0433*

Alpha$_1$-Antichymotrypsin

Serum   Increase

199.00   Secondary Malignant Neoplasm (Disseminated)   Increased with any kind of invasive tumor. *1262   1248*

205.00   Myelocytic Leukemia (Acute)   Increased 24-48 hours after chemotherapy in patients with or without DIC. *1262   0807*

260.00   Protein Malnutrition   Elevated in children with clinical protein malnutrition. *2067*

277.00   Cystic Fibrosis   Increase compared to matched controls. *2504*

297.90   Paranoid States and Other Psychoses   Schizophrenic patients do exhibit a marked and rapid increase during acute phase reaction. *0234 0235*

410.90   Acute Myocardial Infarction   Following myocardial infarction, a large rapid increase was noted to a maximum at day 5. *1168*

491.00   Chronic Bronchitis   A study of patients with emphysema, bronchitis or asthma revealed there was no deficiency similar to that of alpha$_1$-antitrypsin. In fact, the levels were increased in all the disease states studied. *0461*

493.10   Asthma (Intrinsic)   A study of patients with emphysema, bronchitis or asthma revealed there was no deficiency similar to that of alpha$_1$-antitrypsin. In fact, the levels were increased in all the disease states studied. *0461*

510.00   Empyema   A study of patients with emphysema, bronchitis or asthma revealed there was no deficiency similar to that of alpha$_1$-antitrypsin. In fact, the levels were increased in all the disease states studied. *0461*

555.90   Regional Enteritis or Ileitis   Serum concentrations were associated with increasing severity. *2505*

556.00   Ulcerative Colitis   Serum concentrations were associated with increasing severity. *2505*

650.00   Pregnancy   Many acute phase reactants are elevated during pregnancy, but pregnancy has been associated with only a slight elevation of this enzyme. *1248*

710.00   Systemic Lupus Erythematosus   Collagen vascular diseases. *1248   1168*

710.10   Progressive Systemic Sclerosis   Collagen vascular diseases. *1248   1168*

710.20   Sjögren's Syndrome   Collagen vascular diseases. *1248 1168*

714.00   Rheumatoid Arthritis   Significant rise. *1306 0268*

948.00   Burns   Acutely burned children exhibited a rapid rise to a maximum on day 10 postburn, which remained elevated after 60 days. *1168*

Serum   Normal

297.90   Paranoid States and Other Psychoses   Serum and plasma levels in acutely psychotic patients and schizophrenic patients are comparable to normals. *0234 0235*

CSF   Increase

297.90   Paranoid States and Other Psychoses   Detected in the CSF of patients suffering from various psychotic and neurological disorders. *0234*

320.90   Meningitis (Bacterial)   Increased in patients with meningitis or mild hemorrhage, but equal to normal in patients with encephalitis, epilepsy, degenerative disorders or diseases of the CNS. *0079*

431.00   Cerebral Hemorrhage   Increased in patients with meningitis or mild hemorrhage, but equal to normal in patients with encephalitis, epilepsy, degenerative disorders or diseases of the CNS. *0079*

CSF   Normal

323.92   Encephalomyelitis   Increased in patients with meningitis or mild hemorrhage, but equal to normal in patients with encephalitis, epilepsy, degenerative disorders or diseases of the CNS. *0079*

345.90   Epilepsy   Increased in patients with meningitis or mild hemorrhage, but equal to normal in patients with encephalitis, epilepsy, degenerative disorders or diseases of the CNS. *0079*

Synovial Fluid   Increase

714.00   Rheumatoid Arthritis   Significant rise. *1306 0268*

Duodenal Contents   Increase

579.90   Malabsorption, Cause Unspecified   Concentration in duodenal juice from children with malabsorption disease is elevated relative to children with pancreatic insufficiency. *1248*

Alpha$_1$-Antitrypsin

Serum   Decrease

197.50   Secondary Malignant Neoplasm of Digestive System   Increased levels of alpha$_1$ antitrypsin and alpha$_1$ acid glycoprotein are associated with metastases to the large bowel. *2480*

245.10   Subacute Thyroiditis   These conditions reduce activity. *2633*

245.20   Hashimoto's Thyroiditis   Reduced activity. *2633*

260.00   Protein Malnutrition   Decreased. *1866 0042 1946 1947 2129*   These conditions reduce activity *2633*

492.80   Pulmonary Emphysema   alpha$_1$ antitrypsin deficiency trait may account for up to 10% of emphysema cases. *1609*

496.00   Chronic Obstructive Lung Disease   Homozygotes for alpha$_1$ antitrypsin deficiency traits usually develop chronic obstructive lung disease by age 40. Heterozygotes have levels intermediate between normals and homozygotes, and frequently develop this disease. *1609*

496.01   Alpha$_1$-Antitrypsin Deficiency   *2467*

577.00   Acute Pancreatitis   Decreased. *1866 0042 1946 1947 2129*

579.90   Malabsorption, Cause Unspecified   These conditions reduce activity. *2633*

581.90   Nephrotic Syndrome   These conditions reduce activity. *2633*

770.80   Respiratory Distress Syndrome   Decreased. *1866 0042 1946 1947 2129*

948.00   Burns   Decreased during acute phase of thermal burn. *1866 0042 1946 1947 2129*

Serum   Increase

70.00   Viral Hepatitis   Increased. *1866 0042 1946 1947 2129*

155.00   Malignant Neoplasm of Liver   Significant elevation compared with controls (n = 58). *0700*

157.90   Malignant Neoplasm of Pancreas   Significantly higher than controls. Pancreatic Ca. patients average 487 mg/dL, Controls average 434 mg/dL. *2370*   Only 3 of 16 patients had elevated levels. *1856*

180.90   Malignant Neoplasm of Cervix   Increased. *1866 0042 1946 1947 2129*

197.50   Secondary Malignant Neoplasm of Digestive System   Increased levels of alpha$_1$ antitrypsin and alpha$_1$ acid glycoprotein are associated with metastases to the large bowel. *2480*

199.00   Secondary Malignant Neoplasm (Disseminated)   Increased. *1866 0042 1946 1947 2129*

202.80   Non-Hodgkins Lymphoma   Increased. *1866 0042 1946 1947 2129*

245.20   Hashimoto's Thyroiditis   There was an increase in serum C3, IgM, alpha$_1$-acid glycoprotein and alpha$_1$-antitrypsin levels found in 40 patients. *1715*   Increased *1866   0042 1946 1947 2129*

272.21   Type IIB Hyperlipoproteinemia   *2246*

277.30   Amyloidosis   In patients with rheumatoid arthritis complicated by amyloidosis. *1526*

410.90   Acute Myocardial Infarction   Showed a significant increase when compared to controls and remained elevated for 3 months after ischemic episode. *1438*   Significantly elevated in patients with AMI (n = 48) compared with controls (n = 19). *0845*

434.00   Cerebral Thrombosis   Increased. *1866 0042 1946 1947 2129*

434.90   Brain Infarction   High molecular weight fibrinogen complexes, native fibrinogen, alpha$_1$ antitrypsin and alpha$_2$ macroglobulin were significantly increased in cerebral infarction patients. *0747*

556.00   Ulcerative Colitis   Increased compared to control subjects. There was a correlation between the level and disease activity. *0205*

571.49   Chronic Active Hepatitis   Increased. *1866 0042 1946 1947 2129*

571.90   Cirrhosis of Liver   Increased. *1866 0042 1946 1947 2129*

573.30   Toxic Hepatitis   Increased. *1866 0042 1946 1947 2129*

581.90   Nephrotic Syndrome   Increased. *1866 0042 1946 1947 2129*

650.00   Pregnancy   Increased in advanced stages. *1866 0042 1946 1947 2129*   Increased in 96% in late normal pregnancy *2286 2287*

710.00   Systemic Lupus Erythematosus   Increased. *1866 0042 1946 1947 2129   2467*

714.00   Rheumatoid Arthritis   In patients with RA complicated by Amyloidosis. *1526*

948.00   Burns   Increased. *1866 0042 1946 1947 2129*

994.50   Exercise   Significant increase within 15 min partial return by 1 day. *0985*

Alpha$_1$-Antitrypsin *(continued)*

Serum   Normal

273.30 **Waldenström's Macroglobulinemia** *2467*

273.80 **Analbuminemia** *2467*

279.01 **IgA Deficiency (Selective)** No deficiency was found in children with this disorder. *1747*

279.04 **Agammaglobulinemia (Congenital Sex-linked)** *2467*

280.90 **Iron Deficiency Anemia** *2467*

282.20 **Anemias Due To Disorders of Glutathione Metabolism** *2467*

570.00 **Acute and Subacute Necrosis of Liver** *2467*

571.49 **Chronic Active Hepatitis** No differences with controls noted. *0700*

580.00 **Acute Poststreptococcal Glomerulonephritis** *2467*

994.50 **Exercise** No significant change was noted. *1837*

Synovial Fluid   Increase

714.00 **Rheumatoid Arthritis** Elevated in 36 patients with involvement of the knee joint. *1953*

Ascitic Fluid   Decrease

577.00 **Acute Pancreatitis** Ranged from 15-170 mg/dL in ascites (normal serum value = 200-400 mg/dL). *0827*

Alpha$_1$-Globulin

Serum   Decrease

30.00 **Leprosy** Decreased in dimorphic leprosy. *2045*

70.00 **Viral Hepatitis** Indicates acute hepatocellular damage. *2467*

274.00 **Gout** alpha$_1$ and alpha$_2$-globulins reduced in many gouty patients. *0050*

496.01 **Alpha$_1$-Antitrypsin Deficiency** Low alpha$_1$ globulin fraction in a patient with cirrhosis of the liver suggests the diagnosis. *0962*

570.00 **Acute and Subacute Necrosis of Liver** Tend to be low in hepatocellular disease falling in parallel with serum albumin. *2339*

581.90 **Nephrotic Syndrome** Normal or decreased. *2085*

Serum   Increase

162.90 **Malignant Neoplasm of Bronchus and Lung** Increased in squamous, large and small cell carcinoma and adenocarcinoma of lung. A 2-fold decrease in trypsin inhibitory capacity was also found in association. *0989*

199.00 **Secondary Malignant Neoplasm (Disseminated)** *2467*

201.90 **Hodgkin's Disease** In the presence of fever. *2552* Increased alpha$_1$ and alpha$_2$-globulins suggest disease activity. *2468*

204.00 **Lymphocytic Leukemia (Acute)** Often reflects the presence of fever or infection. *0689 2552*

205.00 **Myelocytic Leukemia (Acute)** Often reflects the presence of fever or infection. *0689 2552*

205.10 **Myelocytic Leukemia (Chronic)** Increased alpha and gamma globulins. *2468*

308.00 **Stress** *2467*

340.00 **Multiple Sclerosis** 7.8% of 64 patients had concentration 8% of total proteins. *1295*

390.00 **Rheumatic Fever** Moderate increase in the early stages. *0619*

446.00 **Polyarteritis-Nodosa** Moderate increase. *0619*

533.90 **Peptic Ulcer, Site Unspecified** May be increased. *2467*

556.00 **Ulcerative Colitis** Serum orosomucoid was well correlated with clinical activity, intestinal protein loss, serum albumin, fractional catabolic rates of albumin, and IgG synthesis rate. *1161*

579.01 **Protein-Losing Enteropathy** In protein-losing enteropathy. *2467*

580.00 **Acute Poststreptococcal Glomerulonephritis** Moderate increase. *0619*

585.00 **Chronic Renal Failure** Moderate increases. *0619*

590.00 **Chronic Pyelonephritis** Moderate increases. *0619*

590.10 **Acute Pyelonephritis** Moderate increases. *0619*

642.40 **Pre-Eclampsia** Significantly elevated. *0433*

642.60 **Eclampsia** Significantly elevated. *0433*

650.00 **Pregnancy** Markedly increased during last 2 trimesters of pregnancy. *2468* Rises about 0.1 g/dL. *2533*

694.40 **Pemphigus** *0151*

710.00 **Systemic Lupus Erythematosus** Moderate increase. *0619*

714.00 **Rheumatoid Arthritis** Moderate increase. *0619*

990.00 **Effects of X-Ray Irradiation** *0619*

Serum   Normal

204.10 **Lymphocytic Leukemia (Chronic)** Usually within normal limits. *0241*

273.80 **Analbuminemia** *2467*

279.04 **Agammaglobulinemia (Congenital Sex-linked)** *2538*

279.06 **Immunodeficiency (Common Variable)** *2467*

571.20 **Laennec's or Alcoholic Cirrhosis** *2467*

714.00 **Rheumatoid Arthritis** Generally not significantly changed. *0962*

Urine   Increase

581.90 **Nephrotic Syndrome** Significant quantities are found. *0995*

CSF   Increase

340.00 **Multiple Sclerosis** Concentrations > 79% of total proteins found in 10.9% of cases. *1295*

Alpha$_1$-Glycoprotein

Serum   Increase

70.00 **Viral Hepatitis** It was found to have a sensitivity of 65% and a specificity of 80% with severe liver disease. *0709*

155.00 **Malignant Neoplasm of Liver** It was found to have a sensitivity of 65% and a specificity of 80% with severe liver disease. *0709*

197.00 **Secondary Malignant Neoplasm of Respiratory System** Elevated with metastases and larger tumor mass. *1239 1672 1866 1947 2096 2170*

197.50 **Secondary Malignant Neoplasm of Digestive System** Elevated with metastases and larger tumor mass. *1239 1672 1866 1947 2096 2170*

197.70 **Secondary Malignant Neoplasm of Liver** It was found to have a sensitivity of 65% and a specificity of 80% with severe liver disease. *0709*

199.00 **Secondary Malignant Neoplasm (Disseminated)** Elevated with metastases and larger tumor mass. *1239 1672 1866 1947 2096 2170*

204.00 **Lymphocytic Leukemia (Acute)** Elevated levels in states associated with cell proliferation. *1239 1672 1947 2096 2170 1866*

204.10 **Lymphocytic Leukemia (Chronic)** Elevated levels in states associated with cell proliferation. *1239 1672 1947 2096 2170 1866*

205.00 **Myelocytic Leukemia (Acute)** Elevated levels in states associated with cell proliferation. *1239 1672 1947 2096 2170 1866*

410.90 **Acute Myocardial Infarction** One of the most reliable indicators of acute inflammation. *1239 1672 1866 1947 2096 2170*

555.90 **Regional Enteritis or Ileitis** One of the most reliable indicators of acute inflammation. *1239 1672 1866 1947 2096 2170*

570.00 **Acute and Subacute Necrosis of Liver** It was found to have a sensitivity of 65% and a specificity of 80% with severe liver disease. *0709*

571.90 **Cirrhosis of Liver** It was found to have a sensitivity of 65% and a specificity of 80% with severe liver disease. *0709*

573.30 **Toxic Hepatitis** It was found to have a sensitivity of 65% and a specificity of 80% with severe liver disease. *0709*

696.10 **Psoriasis** Elevated levels in states associated with cell proliferation. *1239 1672 1866 1947 2096 2170*

710.00 **Systemic Lupus Erythematosus** One of the most reliable indicators of acute inflammation. *1239 1672 1866 1947 2096 2170*

714.00 Rheumatoid Arthritis One of the most reliable indicators of acute inflammation. *1239 1672 1866 1947 2096 2170*

929.00 Crush Injury (Trauma) One of the most reliable indicators of acute inflammation. *1239 1672 1866 1947 2096 2170*

948.00 Burns One of the most reliable indicators of acute inflammation. *1239 1672 1866 1947 2096 2170*

992.00 Heat stroke One of the most reliable indicators of acute inflammation. *1239 1672 1866 1947 2096 2170*

994.50 Exercise One of the most reliable indicators of acute inflammation. *1239 1672 1866 1947 2096 2170*

Pleural Effusion Increase

162.90 Malignant Neoplasm of Bronchus and Lung Highest levels found in malignant exudates. *1239 1672 1866 1947 2096 2170*

197.00 Secondary Malignant Neoplasm of Respiratory System Highest levels found in malignant exudates. *1239 1672 1866 1947 2096 2170*

Alpha$_1$-Lipoprotein

Serum Decrease

272.22 Type III Hyperlipoproteinemia There is generally a decrease in alpha and beta lipoproteins. *0774*

272.31 Type I Hyperlipoproteinemia There is generally a decrease in alpha and beta lipoproteins. *0774*

272.32 Type V Hyperlipoproteinemia Hyperprebeta-lipoproteinemia accompanied by low alpha and beta lipoproteins. *2177*

Alpha$_2$-Antiplasmin

Serum Decrease

286.60 Disseminated Intravascular Coagulopathy Measured values in 9 patients with DIC. Subnormal values in 6, normal in 2 and increased in 1. *2337* Significantly decreased levels in 25 patients with acute, subacute and chronic compensated and uncompensated DIC. *2032*

571.90 Cirrhosis of Liver Significant decrease in hepatic cirrhosis and in several other liver diseases. Mean value of 73 ± 15% compared to 100 ± 8% for controls. *2337* Values of 4.24 and 2.56 mg/dL for compensated and decompensated liver cirrhosis compared to 6.2 mg/dL for controls. *0070 2032*

581.90 Nephrotic Syndrome A slight decrease in patients with nephrotic syndrome, but a normal level in patients with chronic latent glomerulonephritis. *2312*

Serum Increase

250.00 Diabetes Mellitus High fast-antiplasmin levels and low or missing slow-antiplasmin levels. *0051*

Serum Normal

580.05 Glomerulonephritis (Membranoproliferative) A slight decrease in patients with nephrotic syndrome, but a normal level in patients with chronic latent glomerulonephritis. *2312*

650.00 Pregnancy No significant change in pregnant woman or those taking contraceptive pills compared with age and sex related controls. *2337*

Alpha$_2$-Globulin

Serum Decrease

70.00 Viral Hepatitis Indicates acute hepatocellular damage. *2467*

274.00 Gout alpha$_1$ and alpha$_2$-globulins reduced in many gouty patients. *0050*

570.00 Acute and Subacute Necrosis of Liver Alpha and beta globulins decrease when hepatocellular failure impairs their synthesis. *0151*

Serum Increase

70.00 Viral Hepatitis Slight to moderate increase (related to the increase in alpha-lipoprotein). *0619*

99.10 Lymphogranuloma Venereum Elevated with a reversal of the A/G ratio. In such cases, the increase occurs in the alpha$_2$ and gamma globulin regions. *0433*

99.30 Reiter's Disease Evidence of nonspecific inflammation. *0433*

100.00 Leptospirosis May occur with jaundice after the 1st week of fever. *2368*

124.00 Trichinosis *0433*

135.00 Sarcoidosis Stepwise increase of alpha$_2$, beta, and gamma globulin 'sarcoid steps' helps differentiate from other lung disease *2467* Marked increase is frequent. *0619*

153.90 Malignant Neoplasm of Large Intestine Increased plasma concentrations in primary cancer. Haptoglobin values were especially useful to indicate tumor activity. *0450*

154.10 Malignant Neoplasm of Rectum alpha$_2$-globulins, especially haptoglobins, were generally increased in primary colorectal cancer, and the liver. Haptoglobin values were useful to indicate tumor activity. *0450*

155.00 Malignant Neoplasm of Liver alpha$_2$-globulins, especially haptoglobins, were generally increased in primary colorectal cancer, and the liver. Haptoglobin values were useful to indicate tumor activity. *0450*

189.00 Malignant Neoplasm of Kidney *0151*

199.00 Secondary Malignant Neoplasm (Disseminated) *2467*

201.90 Hodgkin's Disease Frequently increased in later stages of disease. *2450* With active disease. *2538 0073* Often quite high. *2552*

202.80 Non-Hodgkins Lymphoma Moderate increase. *0619*

203.00 Multiple Myeloma Marked increase. *0619* Homogeneous component seen in some patients. *0992*

204.00 Lymphocytic Leukemia (Acute) Often reflects the presence of fever or infection. *0689 2552*

205.00 Myelocytic Leukemia (Acute) Often reflects the presence of fever or infection. *0689 2552*

205.10 Myelocytic Leukemia (Chronic) Increased alpha and gamma globulins. *2468*

250.00 Diabetes Mellitus *2467*

252.00 Hyperparathyroidism Slightly increased but return to normal after parathyroidectomy. *2467*

255.00 Adrenal Cortical Hyperfunction (Glucocorticoid Excess) May be moderately increased. *2467*

273.22 Heavy Chain Disease (Alpha) Markedly elevated broad peak. *2035*

273.80 Analbuminemia *2467*

277.30 Amyloidosis Hyperglobulinemia occurs in 15% of cases of cardiac amyloidosis; alpha$_2$ and gamma fractions moderately increased. *0151*

308.00 Stress *2467*

320.90 Meningitis (Bacterial) *2467*

340.00 Multiple Sclerosis Concentrations > 14% of total protein occurred in 14% of patients. *1295*

390.00 Rheumatic Fever Serum proteins are altered, with decreased serum albumin and increased alpha$_2$ and gamma globulins. Streptococcus A infections do not increase alpha$_2$ globulin. *2467* Increases occur in the acute phase (parallel with the serum C-reactive protein), and fall during quiescence or following steroid therapy. *0619*

414.00 Chronic Ischemic Heart Disease Rapid increase occurs before the rise in the gamma fraction. *0619*

446.00 Polyarteritis-Nodosa Marked increase. *0619*

446.50 Cranial Arteritis and Related Conditions Parallels the rapid ESR. *2035*

482.90 Bacterial Pneumonia *2467*

533.90 Peptic Ulcer, Site Unspecified May be increased. *2467*

556.00 Ulcerative Colitis May be increased. *2467*

570.00 Acute and Subacute Necrosis of Liver If the necrosis is not too extensive there may be a slight increase. *0619*

571.20 Laennec's or Alcoholic Cirrhosis Moderate increase. *0619*

571.60 Biliary Cirrhosis Moderate increases. *0619*

576.20 Extrahepatic Biliary Obstruction In cholestasis, the increase in alpha$_2$ and beta globulin components correlates with the height of serum lipid values and is a useful point in distinguishing between biliary obstructive lesions and other nonobstructive types of jaundice. *2339*

Alpha$_2$-Globulin *(continued)*

Serum Increase *(continued)*

579.01 Protein-Losing Enteropathy In protein-losing enteropathy. *2467*

580.00 Acute Poststreptococcal Glomerulonephritis There is a moderate increase appearing in the early stages. *0619*

581.90 Nephrotic Syndrome There is an increase with poor separation from the beta globulin band. *0619* Hypoproteinemia is primarily due to a decrease in the albumin fraction and an increase in the alpha$_2$-globulin fraction. *0962* *0433*

585.00 Chronic Renal Failure There is a moderate increase. *0619* Biochemical abnormalities are those seen in the nephrotic syndrome. *0962*

590.00 Chronic Pyelonephritis Moderate increase. *0619*

590.10 Acute Pyelonephritis Moderate increase. *0619*

642.40 Pre-Eclampsia Significantly elevated. *0433*

642.60 Eclampsia Significantly elevated. *0433*

650.00 Pregnancy Increased in last 2 trimesters of pregnancy. *2468* Rises about 0.1 g/dL. *2286*

694.40 Pemphigus *0151*

710.00 Systemic Lupus Erythematosus A less specific but frequent abnormality. *0433* Marked increase. *0619* May be elevated in lupus nephritis. *0962*

710.40 Dermatomyositis/Polymyositis Commonly elevated. *0151*

714.00 Rheumatoid Arthritis Alpha$_2$ or beta globulin fractions are often elevated in the acute active phase, whereas during the chronic active phase, gamma globulin fractions are elevated. *0433* Elevation occurs in some 50% of all patients and in the majority with progressive chronic disease. *0999* Elevated and does not fall with steroid therapy. *0619*

730.00 Osteomyelitis *2467*

990.00 Effects of X-Ray Irradiation *0619*

Serum Normal

204.10 Lymphocytic Leukemia (Chronic) Usually within normal limits. *0241* *2552*

279.04 Agammaglobulinemia (Congenital Sex-linked) *2538*

279.06 Immunodeficiency (Common Variable) *2467*

571.20 Laennec's or Alcoholic Cirrhosis *2467*

Urine Increase

580.04 Glomerulonephritis (Membranous) *0995*

CSF Increase

340.00 Multiple Sclerosis Values of > 8% of total proteins found in 26.5% of patients. *1295*

Alpha$_2$-Macroglobulin

Serum Decrease

203.00 Multiple Myeloma Mild. *1141*

260.00 Protein Malnutrition Found to be lower in cases of protein-energy malnutrition associated with preschool children. *2065*

496.00 Chronic Obstructive Lung Disease *2629*

642.40 Pre-Eclampsia Mild. *1074*

714.30 Juvenile Rheumatoid Arthritis In acute systemic form. *0136*

Serum Increase

70.00 Viral Hepatitis *2640*

155.00 Malignant Neoplasm of Liver Moderate elevation. *1082*

199.00 Secondary Malignant Neoplasm (Disseminated) *1438*

250.00 Diabetes Mellitus All age groups. *1142* Extent of elevation is usually found to directly correlate with duration of disease and presence of vascular complications. *2630* *1203* *0107*

277.30 Amyloidosis Has been observed. No correlation with severity or duration of disease. *0120* *2246*

434.90 Brain Infarction High molecular weight fibrinogen complexes, native fibrinogen, alpha$_1$ antitrypsin, and alpha$_2$ macroglobulin were significantly increased in cerebral infarction patients. *0747*

440.00 Arteriosclerosis *1438*

496.01 Alpha$_1$-Antitrypsin Deficiency Patients with all types of this disorder were found to have significantly elevated levels. *0284*

571.20 Laennec's or Alcoholic Cirrhosis Significantly increased. *1654*

571.49 Chronic Active Hepatitis Moderate elevation. *1082* *2640* Significant increase *1654*

571.90 Cirrhosis of Liver Significantly increased in patients with cryptogenic cirrhosis, alcoholic cirrhosis and chronic active hepatitis. *1654* High concentrations were found in decompensated hepatic cirrhosis, 2.8 ± 0.8 g/L compared to normal, 2.3 ± 0.6 g/L. *2064* Moderate elevation *1082*

573.30 Toxic Hepatitis *2640*

577.00 Acute Pancreatitis *2640*

577.10 Chronic Pancreatitis *2640*

580.00 Acute Poststreptococcal Glomerulonephritis *2632*

580.01 Glomerulonephritis (Focal) *2632*

580.02 Glomerulonephritis (Minimal Change) *2632*

580.04 Glomerulonephritis (Membranous) *2632*

580.05 Glomerulonephritis (Membranoproliferative) *2632*

580.40 Glomerulonephritis (Rapidly Progressive) *2632*

581.90 Nephrotic Syndrome Marked elevations. *1692* *0046* Elevations as high as 1.0 g/dL have been noted. *1355* Primarily due to decreased plasma values and selective retention of the high molecular weight protein. Increased synthesis may also be a factor. *2635*

642.40 Pre-Eclampsia Low concentration of albumin and other small proteins may stimulate almost indiscriminate synthesis of many proteins. Larger molecules cannot leak through the glomeruli and accumulate in the blood. *2287* *2286* *0387*

650.00 Pregnancy *2614* *2412*

994.50 Exercise Significant increase within 15 min partial return by 1 day. *0985* Approximately 5% rise immediately after. *1837*

CSF Increase

320.90 Meningitis (Bacterial) *2069*

CSF Normal

97.90 Syphilis Neurosyphilis. *2069*

191.90 Malignant Neoplasm of Brain Neurotumors. *2069*

340.00 Multiple Sclerosis *2069*

Ascitic Fluid Decrease

577.00 Acute Pancreatitis Ascites had concentrations from 44-400 mg/dL. Normal serum level is 200-400 mg/dL. *0827*

Alpha-Amino-Nitrogen

Plasma Decrease

260.00 Protein Malnutrition Abnormally low. *0151*

Urine Increase

275.10 Hepatolenticular Degeneration Increased in 79% of patients. *2278*

984.00 Toxic Effects of Lead and Its Compounds (including Fumes) With lead intoxication. *0889*

Alpha-Fetoprotein

Serum Increase

70.00 Viral Hepatitis Levels > 30 ng/mL were found in 87% of patients with acute hepatitis and in 58% with chronic active hepatitis. *0036* Among 51 patients with fulminant hepatitis and coma, AFP was detected in 17 (85%) of 20 who survived and in only 12 (38.7%) of 31 fatal cases, (p = 0.002). Positivity was related to the severity of the disease and its appearance was followed by recovery. High values in severe forms are a favorable prognostic sign. *1231* In some cases. *1255*

78.50 Cytomegalic Inclusion Disease Among 54 patients with verified infection, 8 (15%) had raised levels in sera taken after the onset of infection. *0802* In the newborn, the level was abnormal but disappeared by the end of the 1st month. *1598*

130.00 Toxoplasmosis In newborn but disappeared by the end of the 1st month. *1598*

151.90 Malignant Neoplasm of Stomach Elevated in 18% of cases. *1348*

153.90 Malignant Neoplasm of Large Intestine Elevated in 5% of cases. *1348*

155.00 Malignant Neoplasm of Liver Detectable in 14 of 19 (76%) patients. *0029* Incidence of positivity varies with geographical area from 50-90%; in this country 50% is a more accurate estimate. Serum concentration > 500 ng/mL indicates hepatoma 97% of the time. Postoperative serial determinations show an exponential fall to normal when the tumor has been completely excised. Recurrence of elevated levels indicates tumor recurrence. *2583* Above 30 ng/mL in 69%. Levels declined as age increased. Appeared to be related to the tumor cell type: the relatively immature *0036 0383 2116*

157.90 Malignant Neoplasm of Pancreas Over 50 ng/mL in 10-15% of cases. *2116*

174.90 Malignant Neoplasm of Breast Elevated *1348*

180.90 Malignant Neoplasm of Cervix CEA, AFP and hCG were measured in 253 patients with gynecologic malignancies and in 317 patients with benign gynecologic diseases. Concentrations of each of these antigens were elevated in a significantly greater number of patients with invasive cancer. *0580*

183.00 Malignant Neoplasm of Ovary Present in embryonal carcinoma (in 27% of cases) or malignant teratoma (60% of cases) of ovary and testis. *2467* 15 out of 20 cases of teratoblastoma of testis and ovary showed raised levels. *0007* Over 50 ng/mL in 33% of cases of gonadal teratoblastoma. *2116 0580*

186.90 Malignant Neoplasm of Testis Present in embryonal carcinoma (in 27% of cases) or malignant teratoma (in 60% of cases). Concentrations > 40 g/L are found in 75% of patients with teratocarcinoma *2467* Elevated in 60% of stage A and B cases and all patients with stage 3 disease *0756* In patients with nonseminomatous testicular germ cell malignant growths during and after therapeutic interventions, an elevated marker assay indicated the presence of active disease. A normal marker assay does not exclude active disease. *1621* 15 out of 20 cases of teratoblastoma of testis and ovary showed raised levels. *0007* Over 50 ng/mL in 33% of cases of gonadal teratoblastoma. *2116 2337*

188.90 Malignant Neoplasm of Bladder Of 112 cases, 59 (52.8%) showed positive results, and no false positive results occurred. *0045*

197.70 Secondary Malignant Neoplasm of Liver Present in some patients with liver metastases from carcinoma of the stomach or pancreas. *2467*

334.80 Ataxia-Telangiectasia Present in inordinately high concentration in a majority of patients. *0151* Has been reported. *2459*

570.00 Acute and Subacute Necrosis of Liver 10-20% of nonmalignant liver diseases of all types have elevated serum levels, which tend to be fluctuating or transient. Steady or rising levels indicate malignancy. *2583* Increased in hepatitis, especially in infants (when levels exceed 40 ng/mL). *0619* Up to 40% of patients with massive hepatic necrosis. *2199 0036*

571.20 Laennec's or Alcoholic Cirrhosis Concentration above 30 ng/mL were found in 14% of patients. *0036*

571.49 Chronic Active Hepatitis Concentration above 30 ng/mL, were found in 58% of patients. *0036* Elevated in 42% of cases *2111 0351*

571.90 Cirrhosis of Liver 10-20% of nonmalignant liver diseases of all types have elevated serum concentration, which tend to be fluctuating or transient. Steady or rising levels indicate malignancy. *2583* Elevated above 10 ng/mL in 34% of cases *2111*

572.00 Liver Abscess (Pyogenic) 10-20% of nonmalignant liver diseases of all types have elevated serum AFP levels, which tend to be fluctuating or transient. Steady or rising levels indicate malignancy. *2583*

572.20 Hepatic Encephalopathy In fulminant hepatic failure, 15 of the 64 patients (23%) had raised levels but in only 2 did they exceed 50 ng/mL. Of the 23 survivors, 11 (48%) had elevated levels. This rise was found early after the development of a grade IV coma and constitutes an encouraging prognostic sign at a time when the liver function tests and EEG are not helpful. *1655*

572.40 Hepatic Failure In fulminant hepatic failure, 15 of the 64 patients (23%) had raised levels but in only 2 did they exceed 50 ng/mL. Of the 23 survivors, 11 (48%) had elevated levels. This rise was found early after the development of a grade IV coma and constitutes an encouraging prognostic sign at a time when the liver function tests and EEG are unhelpful. *1655 0503*

581.90 Nephrotic Syndrome Markedly raised maternal serum and amniotic fluid AFP levels were found in 2 cases of congenital nephrotic syndrome of the fetus. *2117*

650.00 Pregnancy In a screening study 1.2 % had raised levels. Of these 25/249 had babies with neural tube defects, an additional 13/249 had other congenital defects. *1599* Substantial increase in concentration in the maternal circulation during pregnancy*1195* Ranged from 10-80 ng/mL in 18 of 23 normal pregnancy *1575 2116*

774.40 Jaundice Due to Hepatocellular Damage (Newborn) Elevations occur in many cases of neonatal hepatitis and may be helpful in differentiating this condition from biliary atresia. *2609*

Serum Normal

181.00 Malignant Neoplasm of Trophoblast (Choriocarcinoma) In pure choriocarcinomas, human chorionic gonadotropins are always elevated and AFP is absent. *2583*

183.00 Malignant Neoplasm of Ovary No elevations are seen in conjunction with pure dysgerminomas of the ovary. *2583*

186.90 Malignant Neoplasm of Testis No elevations are found in conjunction with pure seminomas of the testis. In teratoblastoma, both AFP and hCG are usually absent, but may be increased in tumors with small areas of extra-embryonic tumor tissue. *2583*

189.00 Malignant Neoplasm of Kidney Not elevated. *1348*

220.01 Teratoma (Dermoid) *2468*

277.00 Cystic Fibrosis In 30 patients, the highest value obtained was 10.2 ng/mL and in a control 10.8 ng/mL. These are within published normal limits. Previously reported large increases in CF patients and in heterozygote carriers have not been confirmed. *0285* In CF patients 97.5% and in normal children 95% of the values were within the normal range for healthy adults (1-9 ng/mL). *1288*

573.30 Toxic Hepatitis Curiously absent. *2199*

630.00 Hydatidiform Mole Undetectable in 100% of patients with intact mole, but > 10 ng/mL in 18 of 23 normal pregnancies. *1613*

640.00 Threatened Abortion In patients with premature labor, the majority of concentrations were significantly below the normal range, and the peak levels were achieved approximately 1 month earlier than normal. In patients whose pregnancies were terminated by abortion, the levels exhibited a significant rise within a few h after induction because of resorption of fetal elements into the maternal circulation. *1008*

Pleural Effusion Increase

155.00 Malignant Neoplasm of Liver Positive results were most frequently found in samples derived from patients with liver tumors. The highest levels (6 and 30 ng/mL), were determined in samples of two hepatoma patients. *0622*

197.70 Secondary Malignant Neoplasm of Liver Positive results were most frequently found in samples derived from patients with secondary or primary liver tumors. The highest levels (6 and 30 ng/mL) were determined in samples of 2 hepatoma patients. *0622*

Alpha-Glucosidase

Serum Decrease

271.02 McArdle's Disease Absence of activity in skeletal muscle or liver biopsy tissue or in the blood leukocytes. *1108 1097*

Serum Increase

174.90 Malignant Neoplasm of Breast The elevations were observed when the disease was in an early clinical stage. *0808*

277.00 Cystic Fibrosis Acutely ill patients with cystic fibrosis demonstrated significant increases compared with cystic fibrosis outpatients. *1842*

577.00 Acute Pancreatitis Patients with pancreatitis associated with trauma or complicated by severe necrosis, hemorrhage, or abscess also displayed greater increases. *1842*

Alpha-Ketoglutarate

Serum Increase

205.10 Myelocytic Leukemia (Chronic) Increased in the vast majority of patients with myeloproliferative disorders, reflective of the WBC pool size. *0337*

Alpha-Ketoglutarate (continued)

Serum   Increase (continued)

340.00   **Multiple Sclerosis**   High concentrations noted in these patients imply a defect in carbohydrate metabolism. 2104

Aluminum

Serum   Increase

585.00   **Chronic Renal Failure**   Accumulates in all patients with renal failure. 2430

Aminoacid Arylpeptidase

Serum   Increase

994.50   **Exercise**   With exertion. 0985

Amino Acids

Plasma   Decrease

66.00   **Phlebotomus Fever**   Basal hypoaminoacidemia. After intravenous glucose administration the total amino acid concentration rapidly decreased as much as or more than the original decline. 2479

255.00   **Adrenal Cortical Hyperfunction (Glucocorticoid Excess)**   Cortisol accelerates the catabolism of protein and stimulates the hepatic uptake and deamination of amino acids. 0151

259.20   **Carcinoid Syndrome**   Decreased tryptophan, valine, isoleucine, lysine and ornithine were found. All others were normal except methionine, which was elevated. The low plasma levels were not due to hyperexcretion, as urinary levels were normal. 0718

270.02   **Hartnup Disease**   Reduced about 30% due to increased excretion and reduced absorption. 2246

333.40   **Huntington's Chorea**   19 patients showed a significantly lower concentration of proline, alanine, valine, leucine, isoleucine, and tyrosine compared to 38 normal controls. 0534

577.00   **Acute Pancreatitis**   In patients with acute hemorrhagic necrotizing pancreatitis. 1994

580.01   **Glomerulonephritis (Focal)**   Mean concentration of essential amino acids and tyrosine were significantly lower, resulting in a low essential/total ratio. 1545

580.04   **Glomerulonephritis (Membranous)**   Mean concentration of essential amino acids and tyrosine were significantly lower, resulting in a low essential/total ratio. 1545

581.90   **Nephrotic Syndrome**   0619

714.00   **Rheumatoid Arthritis**   Frequent hypoaminoacidemia. Arginine, glutamine, tyrosine, and histidine are low. 2104

753.10   **Polycystic Kidney Disease**   Mean concentration of essential amino acids and tyrosine were significantly lower, resulting in a low essential/total ratio. 1545

Plasma   Increase

60.00   **Yellow Fever**   Increased in severe cases. 0619

242.90   **Hyperthyroidism**   Slight increase. 0619

250.00   **Diabetes Mellitus**   Found with ketosis, probably associated with gluconeogenesis. 0619

270.10   **Phenylketonuria**   Phenylalanine is increased. 0619

270.31   **Maple Syrup Urine Disease**   The branched-chain amino acids valine, leucine, and isoleucine, are increased to 10-30 X above normal levels. 0433   Large excess of branched-chain amino acids and keto acids in blood and urine in the untreated patient. 2246

270.82   **Hydroxyprolinemia**   Other amino acids (excluding hydroxyproline) are normal. 2246

271.10   **Galactosemia**   Frequent in patients receiving a milk diet. 2104

271.20   **Hereditary Fructose Intolerance**   Excess amino acids in serum and urine. 0151

331.81   **Reye's Syndrome**   Markedly elevated reflecting hepatic injury. 0435

428.00   **Congestive Heart Failure**   Slight increase. 0619

570.00   **Acute and Subacute Necrosis of Liver**   In acute yellow atrophy, the plasma concentration is roughly proportional to the degree of liver damage. Methionine and tyrosine show the highest increase. 0619

571.20   **Laennec's or Alcoholic Cirrhosis**   Increased amino acids (gly, glu, ser, thr, tyr, and ala) in portal cirrhosis. 2049

579.00   **Celiac Sprue Disease**   Found in celiac disease and idiopathic steatorrhea if liver damage is also present. 0619

579.90   **Malabsorption, Cause Unspecified**   0619

584.00   **Acute Renal Failure**   Increased total concentration due to rise in nonessential amino acids. Proline, hydroxyproline, glycine, citrulline, ornithine, were increased. Valine and tryptophan were decreased. 0533

585.00   **Chronic Renal Failure**   Increased total concentration due to rise in nonessential amino acids. Proline, hydroxyproline, glycine, citrulline, ornithine were increased. Valine, and tryptophan were decreased. 0533

642.60   **Eclampsia**   0619

785.50   **Shock**   In severe shock. 0619

948.00   **Burns**   In severe burns the peptides derived from the burnt tissues appear in the plasma. 0619

Plasma   Normal

260.00   **Protein Malnutrition**   In starvation, the amino acid level in the blood does not usually fall below the normal fasting level. Protein level is maintained at the expense of body protein. 0619   Severe protein deficiency alters the qualitative pattern, not the total amount. 2104

277.30   **Amyloidosis**   2246

Urine   Increase

70.00   **Viral Hepatitis**   Amount of urinary loss reflects degree of hepatic involvement. 2104

203.00   **Multiple Myeloma**   Aminoaciduria may be nonselective and associated with renal glycosuria and mild renal acidosis. 0962

250.00   **Diabetes Mellitus**   In severe diabetic ketosis. 0619

252.00   **Hyperparathyroidism**   Quite common. 2540

268.00   **Vitamin D Deficiency Rickets**   Decreased net reabsorption, probably due to increased circulating parathyroid hormone. 2246

268.20   **Osteomalacia**   Aminoaciduria secondary to PTH excess is seen. 0999

270.01   **Cystinuria**   Cystine, lysine, arginine, and ornithine are increased in urine. 0619

270.02   **Hartnup Disease**   Aminoaciduria is the single most important diagnostic finding; it is constantly present, even between episodes of symptoms. An increased urinary excretion of the monoamino-monocarboxylic amino acids with neutral or aromatic side chains, i.e., alanine, serine, threonine, valine, leucine, isoleucine, phenylalanine, tyrosine, histidine, asparagine, glutamine, and tryptophan is characteristic. 0433   Usually at least a 10-fold increase. 2246   0995

270.03   **Cystinosis**   Aminoaciduria with increased cystine. 0619   May be masked by severely reduced GFR, so that total urinary amino acids are in the normal range. 2246

270.10   **Phenylketonuria**   Phenylalanine and ketoderivatives are increased. 0619

270.31   **Maple Syrup Urine Disease**   Valine, leucine, and isoleucine are present in the urine. 0619   Large excess of branched-chain amino acids and keto acids in blood and urine in the untreated patient. 2246

270.41   **Cystathioninuria**   Elevated cystathionine. 0631 2246

270.42   **Homocystinuria**   Increased homocystine. 0631

270.51   **Histidinemia**   Slight increase in several amino acids other than histidine. 0831 2246

270.61   **Citrullinemia**   Generalized hyperaminoaciduria may be found in severely affected infants. 2246

270.81   **Hyperprolinemia**   Hyperaminoaciduria of proline, glycine and hydroxyproline is specific. 2246

271.10   **Galactosemia**   General aminoaciduria - identified by chromatography. 2468   Manifestation of a renal toxicity syndrome. 1066

271.20   **Hereditary Fructose Intolerance**   During acute intoxication, signs of a proximal tubular syndrome and of liver failure are common. 0433   Characteristic symptom in small children. 0177   Develops rapidly after ingestion. 2246

275.10 Hepatolenticular Degeneration   77% of patients tested before penicillamine therapy had hyperaminoaciduria. Urinary excretion of amino acids decreased after therapy. *2278*

275.35 Vitamin D Resistant Rickets   Generalized aminoaciduria is present. *0433*

277.14 Acute Intermittent Porphyria   *1565*

281.00 Pernicious Anemia   Amino aciduria with an excess excretion of taurine, especially if there is associated subacute combined degeneration of the spinal cord. Amino aciduria does not occur in other megaloblastic anemias. *2468*   May be slight excess of urinary amino acids, especially taurine. *0755 2364*

281.20 Folic Acid Deficiency Anemia   Aminoaciduria reportedly occurs, but observers differ on its frequency and significance. *2538*   May be slight excess of urinary amino acids, especially taurine. *0755 2364*

282.41 Thalassemia Major   Found to be markedly increased in children. *0395*

345.90 Epilepsy   Transient rise due to disturbed renal function during grand mal seizure. *2104*

359.11 Progressive Muscular Dystrophy   *0995*

570.00 Acute and Subacute Necrosis of Liver   In massive liver necrosis the amount present in urine is proportional to the degree of liver damage. *2104*

571.60 Biliary Cirrhosis   Aminoaciduria, especially cystine and threonine, may be found. *2467*

571.90 Cirrhosis of Liver   Increased in advanced cirrhosis in proportion to the degree of liver damage. *0619*   Mean amino acid clearance (glycine, glumine, serine, threonine, alanine, and tyrosine) were raised in Indian childhood cirrhosis patients. *2049*

572.40 Hepatic Failure   *0503*

577.00 Acute Pancreatitis   In some patients with familial pancreatitis the urine may contain an excess amount of amino acids, especially cystine and lysine. *0433*

580.01 Glomerulonephritis (Focal)   May be found. *0951*

585.00 Chronic Renal Failure   As GFR decreases, amino acid clearance and excretion increases. Increased levels of alanine (4 X normal), threonine, cystine, valine, and leucine (2-3 X normal), and proline are found in urine. *0192*

588.81 Proximal Renal Tubular Acidosis   Found in children. *0433*

650.00 Pregnancy   During normal pregnancy increased amounts of histidine and threonine are excreted, returning to normal during lactation. *0619*   Much larger quantities. *0400 2619*

948.00 Burns   Amino acids and peptides from burnt tissues are excreted in urine. *0619*

984.00 Toxic Effects of Lead and Its Compounds (including Fumes)   Results from changes in the epithelium of the proximal convoluted tubules in lead poisoning. *0151*   Transient finding. *0294*

Urine   Normal

270.03 Cystinosis   Aminoaciduria with increased cystine. *0619*   May be masked by severely reduced GFR, so that total urinary amino acids are in the normal range. *2246*

275.35 Vitamin D Resistant Rickets   Normal, in contrast to Vitamin D deficient rickets. *2246*

335.20 Amyotrophic Lateral Sclerosis   *0665*

CSF   Increase

570.00 Acute and Subacute Necrosis of Liver   In massive liver necrosis the amount present in CSF is proportional to the degree of liver damage. *0619*

571.90 Cirrhosis of Liver   Increased in advanced cirrhosis in proportion to the degree of liver damage. *0619*

Feces   Increase

270.02 Hartnup Disease   Closely mirrors the pattern in urine. *2246*

Saliva   Normal

270.02 Hartnup Disease   *2246*

Sweat   Normal

270.02 Hartnup Disease   *2246*

Aminolevulinic Acid

Serum   Increase

277.14 Acute Intermittent Porphyria   Severe attacks. *2246*

984.00 Toxic Effects of Lead and Its Compounds (including Fumes)   In 50 cases, brain levels increased 4-fold, urine 8-fold and plasma only 2-fold compared to controls. *0487*   Concentration > 20 mg/dL indicates poisoning. *0294*

Urine   Increase

70.00 Viral Hepatitis   May occur. *0503*

155.00 Malignant Neoplasm of Liver   May occur. *0503*

197.70 Secondary Malignant Neoplasm of Liver   May occur. *0503*

277.14 Acute Intermittent Porphyria   In the hereditary hepatic porphyrias. *0145*   A reduction in the activity of the enzyme uroporphyrinogen I synthetase appears to explain the accumulation in body fluids and increased amounts in the urine. Excessive accumulation is further aggravated by an increased ALA synthetase activity. *2271*   May contain as much as 180 mg/24h. *1529*   In 21 symptomatic patients, an average of 43 mg ALA/24h was excreted. Tends to decrease somewhat during remission. *2254   0962 2552*

277.15 Porphyria Variegata   May appear during acute attacks. *2552*   Normal or moderate increase in asymptomatic patients. Sharp rise with acute attacks. *0613   0995*

277.16 Porphyria Cutanea Tarda   During acute stage. *0995*   Rarely occurs. *0613 2246*

277.17 Hereditary Coproporphyria   Mild increase during latent and acute stage. *0995*   Only during acute attacks. *2552   2246*

984.00 Toxic Effects of Lead and Its Compounds (including Fumes)   Delta-aminolevulinic acid is increased. *2468*   In 50 cases, brain levels increased 4-fold, urine 8-fold and plasma only 2-fold compared to controls. *0487*   In lead poisoning. *0889*

Urine   Normal

277.11 Congenital Erythropoietic Porphyria (Günther's Disease)   With chromatographic methods, within normal limits. *0867   0995 2426*

277.12 Erythropoietic Protoporphyria   *0995 1478*

277.13 Erythropoietic Coproporphyria   *0995 1478*

277.16 Porphyria Cutanea Tarda   *1344*

Aminolevulinic Acid Dehydrase

Red Blood Cells   Decrease

984.00 Toxic Effects of Lead and Its Compounds (including Fumes)   RBC concentration correlates negatively with serum lead concentration. *0294*

Ammonia

Blood   Decrease

270.02 Hartnup Disease   *0433*

401.00 Malignant Hypertension   Decreased arterial ammonia in azotemic patients, (mean = 34 mmol/L). *1853*

401.10 Essential Benign Hypertension   Decreased arterial ammonia in azotemic patients, mean = 34 mmol/L ± 1.4. *1853*

584.00 Acute Renal Failure   Decreased arterial ammonia in azotemic patients mean = 34 mmol/L ± 1.4. *1853*

585.00 Chronic Renal Failure   Decreased arterial ammonia in azotemic patients, (mean = 34 mmol/L ± 1.4). *1853*

753.10 Polycystic Kidney Disease   Decreased arterial ammonia in azotemic patients, (mean = 34 mmol/L) due to reduced synthesis by diseased kidney. *1853*

Blood   Increase

270.51 Histidinemia   Postprandial elevation. *0995*

270.61 Citrullinemia   Characteristic elevation. May rise to 400-1,000 mg/dL postprandial. *2246*

331.00 Alzheimer's Disease   Post prandial blood ammonia levels were significantly higher in 22 patients with Alzheimer's than in 37 control subjects. *0742*

Ammonia (continued)

Blood Increase (continued)

331.81 Reye's Syndrome Elevated in most patients. *1473* Reflects hepatic damage. *0151* Hyperammonemia results from excess waste nitrogen that overwhelms the ability of reduced ornithine transcarbamylase to detoxify the ammonia load. *2222* Increased ammonia may reflect accumulation of octopamine. *0339 0962*

415.00 Cor Pulmonale Due to hepatic congestion. *2411*

428.00 Congestive Heart Failure In patients with azotemia, arterial levels were elevated to 88 mmol/L. *1853*

492.80 Pulmonary Emphysema Found in high percentage of patients without evidence of congestive failure or liver disease. *2104*

496.00 Chronic Obstructive Lung Disease Venous levels were significantly influenced by pH and pCO_2. *0538*

570.00 Acute and Subacute Necrosis of Liver In acute hepatic necrosis and cirrhosis; may increase after portacaval anastomosis. *2467*

571.20 Laennec's or Alcoholic Cirrhosis Increased in terminal portal cirrhosis. *0619*

571.90 Cirrhosis of Liver Increased in liver coma and cirrhosis and with portacaval shunting of blood. *2467*

572.20 Hepatic Encephalopathy Elevated in most patients. *1473* Elevated in about 60% of patients. Poor correlation between the level of blood ammonia and the depth of the hepatic coma. *0962 0339*

572.40 Hepatic Failure Characteristic of liver failure. *2104 0503*

585.00 Chronic Renal Failure Despite reduced excretion, renal failure does not usually lead to arterial excess, unless hepatic failure occurs. *2104*

773.00 Hemolytic Disease of Newborn (Erythroblastosis Fetalis) There is some evidence associating hyperammonemia with the pathogenesis of kernicterus. *2104*

994.50 Exercise Tissue catabolism. *0811*

Urine Decrease

255.40 Adrenal Cortical Hypofunction *0619*

580.00 Acute Poststreptococcal Glomerulonephritis Decreased in nephritis with damage to the distal renal tubules. *0619*

584.00 Acute Renal Failure With severe renal damage. May be < 1% of the urea nitrogen. *2104*

585.00 Chronic Renal Failure With severe renal damage may be < 1% of the urea nitrogen. *2104*

588.81 Proximal Renal Tubular Acidosis *2246 2552*

Urine Increase

250.00 Diabetes Mellitus Reflects severity of acidosis and parallels the degree of ketonuria. *0619*

255.10 Adrenal Cortical Hyperfunction (Mineralocorticoid Excess) In primary hyperaldosteronism, possibly due to hormone action on the renal tubule cells or to the associated potassium depletion. *0619* Exaggerated ammonia production results in a tendency to a persistently alkaline urine. *1108*

260.00 Protein Malnutrition *0619*

270.03 Cystinosis Increased ammonium ion. *2246*

558.90 Diarrhea In prolonged diarrhea. *0619*

787.00 Vomiting Increase in urine ammonia in prolonged vomiting with associated achlorhydria and ketosis. *0619*

CSF Increase

572.20 Hepatic Encephalopathy Elevated in most patients. *1473*

Amylase

Serum Decrease

157.90 Malignant Neoplasm of Pancreas Slightly increased in early stages (< 10% of cases). With later destruction of pancreas, normal or decreased. *2467*

242.90 Hyperthyroidism Severe thyrotoxicosis. *0619* When accompanied by severe liver damage. *2467*

250.00 Diabetes Mellitus Both abnormally high and low values have been observed. *2104*

260.00 Protein Malnutrition Marked reductions are recognized characteristics. *0151* Circulating concentration appears consistent with the amount of structural damage to the pancreas, characteristic of kwashiorkor. *2104*

303.90 Alcoholism 20% of 182 male chronic alcoholics had decreased activity of serum pancreatic isoamylase, whereas only 6% had low total serum amylase activity. *2196*

428.00 Congestive Heart Failure Possibly decreased in some cases. *0619*

570.00 Acute and Subacute Necrosis of Liver Decrease possible due to liver damage. *0619*

572.00 Liver Abscess (Pyogenic) Severe liver damage. *2467*

573.30 Toxic Hepatitis Severe liver damage. *2467*

575.00 Acute Cholecystitis Decreased in some cases. *0619*

577.00 Acute Pancreatitis Extensive marked destruction of pancreas. Decreased levels are clinically significant only in occasional cases of fulminant pancreatitis. *2467*

642.60 Eclampsia Severe liver damage. *2467*

948.00 Burns Decreased in severe burns. *0619*

Serum Increase

70.00 Viral Hepatitis Mild pancreatitis may occur and is a contributing factor in mortality. Morphological evidence of pancreatitis found in 44% of 19 hepatitis patients at autopsy. *2031* Moderate elevation found in some patients. *2104*

72.00 Mumps Increased during the period of swelling and for about 10 days thereafter in 90% of patients. *0433* 96.2% of 224 patients showed elevations during the course of the disease. In 83.77% of patients the elevations occurred in the first week and fell progressively. *0336 1319*

75.00 Infectious Mononucleosis May be associated with hyperamylasemia. *1386*

150.90 Malignant Neoplasm of Esophagus *0062*

157.90 Malignant Neoplasm of Pancreas May be slightly increased in early stages (< 10% of cases). With later destruction of pancreas, normal or decreased. *2467* Early obstruction of pancreatic duct. *0151* Elevated serum and urinary S-amylase has been reported. *2151* Hyperamylasemia found in only 9% of 100 histologically proven cases. *0932* May be mildly elevated in a few patients as a result of pancreatitis secondary to an obstructing tumor. *2199* In 35% of 14 patients at initial hospitalization for this disorder. *0781*

162.90 Malignant Neoplasm of Bronchus and Lung May occur. *0178* Markedly increased in serum, urine and tumor tissue. *2598*

183.00 Malignant Neoplasm of Ovary Hyperamylasemia may occur in ovarian papillary cystadenocarcinoma. *1373*

185.00 Malignant Neoplasm of Prostate Reported in 95% of patients with benign hypertrophy and 70% of carcinomas. Similar results have not been reported elsewhere. *0973*

250.00 Diabetes Mellitus High incidence of pancreatic abnormality in patients with no clinical evidence of pancreatic acinar disease. *2406* Increased activity correlated with blood sugar concentration. *0155*

250.10 Diabetic Acidosis Raised in ketoacidosis. *2485* Occurs frequently; 21 of 35 patients (60%) had elevated concentrations. Occurs most often when blood sugar > 500 mg/dL. *0869* 21 of 35 patients were hyperamylasemic, with 6 showing values > 1,000 Somogyi U. No relation was found between degree of elevation and morbidity and mortality or acidosis or azotemia. Relation was found with degrees of hyperglycemia. *1286* Elevated levels *2646*

272.31 Type I Hyperlipoproteinemia During bouts of abdominal pain. *2246*

272.32 Type V Hyperlipoproteinemia During bouts of abdominal pain. *2246*

303.00 Acute Alcoholic Intoxication Increased in serum and urine in 8.5% of 129 patients after acute intoxication, due to changes in salivary isoenzyme, not as a result of pancreatic damage. *0178* Common as a result of vomiting and increased peptic stimulation of the pancreas. *2104*

303.90 Alcoholism Rises after gross ethanol intake (in the chronic alcoholic). *0619 2104*

304.90 Drug Dependence (Opium and Derivatives) Large doses of morphine or codeine will provoke a sharp rise. *2104* Increased levels were found in 19% of 91 addicts admitted after overdose. The rise was due to elevated salivary-type isoenzyme. *0178*

323.92 Encephalomyelitis If amylase levels are elevated, mumps or Coxsackie virus may be indicated. *0433*

441.00 Dissecting Aortic Aneurysm Hyperamylasemia has been reported, although mechanism is unclear. *0653 1546*

527.90 Diseases of the Salivary Glands Salivary gland disease: mumps, suppurative inflammation, duct obstruction due to calculus. *2467*

533.90 Peptic Ulcer, Site Unspecified Mild-moderate elevation with active ulcer and no associated pancreatitis. Rise is directly related to the size and duration of perforation, and amount of fluid accumulated in peritoneal cavity. Free perforations not in contact with pancreas may lead to hyperamylasemia also. *2031* Extremely high values found in any condition in which the GI tract is perforated or loses viability. *2104*

540.90 Acute Appendicitis 57 of 149 cases had increased concentration. Highest value was 1,480 U/L in a patient with an obstructed gangrenous appendix. *0320*

557.01 Mesenteric Artery Embolism May occur with mesenteric infarction. *0320*

560.90 Intestinal Obstruction Moderate hyperamylasemia without evidence of associated pancreatitis. Values > 1,850 U/L may indicate strangulated or necrotic bowel. *2031* Often marked elevation. *2104*

567.90 Peritonitis Hyperamylasemia up to 405 U/L without appreciable pancreatic disease. *1871*

571.90 Cirrhosis of Liver High incidence of pancreatic abnormality in patients with no clinical evidence of pancreatic acinar disease. *2406*

575.00 Acute Cholecystitis May exceed 1,000 U/L. May or may not indicate concomitant acute pancreatitis, because elevations in this range may be seen in acute cholecystitis without any changes in the pancreas. *2199 2038*

576.00 Postcholecystectomy Syndrome If tests are performed repeatedly, immediately after attacks, some abnormalities will appear if there is an organic cause of the syndrome. *0995*

576.20 Extrahepatic Biliary Obstruction Occurs in calculus common duct obstruction without pancreatitis due to an increase in pancreatic isoenzyme. *2486* Marked elevations should point to the diagnosis of acute pancreatitis of primary nature or secondary to calculus biliary tract disease. *0433* Values > 1,000 U/L usually indicate choledocholithiasis. *0017*

576.50 Spasm of Sphincter of Oddi Obstruction of the pancreatic duct by drug-induced spasm of sphincter (e.g., opiates, codeine, methyl choline, chlorothiazide). *2467*

577.00 Acute Pancreatitis Increase begins in 3-6 h, rises to over 250 U/L within 8 h in 75% of patients, reaches maximum in 20-30 h, and may persist for 48-72 h. May be up to 40 X normal, but the height of the increase does not correlate with the severity of the disease. More than 10% of patients may have normal values even in terminal stage. *2467* Amylase isoenzyme, P3, is elevated in acute pancreatitis but not in other conditions. *0789* Rises within 24-48 h of acute onset, normalizing within 3-5 days. *2031 0827*

577.10 Chronic Pancreatitis Hyperamylasemia in acute exacerbation sometimes accompanied by a transient elevation in salivary type isoamylase (S-amylase). *2456* May be found, especially if the blood is drawn early in the attack. With each succeeding episode, however, pancreatic exocrine function decreases and the likelihood of finding an elevated amylase diminishes. *0999* Usually normal during quiescent phase. Rises as chronic damage progresses, but tends to become less pronounced. May actually be normal during relapse. *2031 2199*

577.20 Pancreatic Cyst and Pseudocyst Laboratory findings preceding acute pancreatitis are present (mild and unrecognized in 33% of cases). Persistent increase after an acute episode may indicate formation of a pseudocyst. *2467* Persistent increase 4-6 weeks following onset of pancreatitis suggests pseudocyst. 77% of 78 patients had hyperamylasemia at diagnosis. *2031 0581*

579.90 Malabsorption, Cause Unspecified Increased in chronic malabsorption with intestinal villous atrophy. *0619*

584.00 Acute Renal Failure May be increased without evidence of pancreatitis in early stage. *2468* Mild elevation may occur with renal insufficiency but rarely more than twice the normal upper limit. *2031*

585.00 Chronic Renal Failure Patients with severe failure may have significant hyperamylasemia in the absence of clinical symptoms or signs of acute pancreatitis. *2336* Mild elevation may occur with renal insufficiency but rarely more than twice the normal upper limit. *2031*

600.00 Benign Prostatic Hypertrophy Reported in 95% of patients with benign disease and 70% of carcinomas. Similar results have not been reported elsewhere. *0973*

601.00 Prostatitis Moderate increase in total concentration. *2486*

633.90 Ectopic Pregnancy Associated with ruptured ectopic pregnancy. *1247* Values of 2,000 U/L have been reported. *0744* Elevated levels *2646*

650.00 Pregnancy Salivary amylase, present in small quantities in nonpregnant women as well as in men, show a substantial increase in concentration in the maternal circulation during pregnancy. *1195* May be associated with hyperamylasemia. *1386 1209*

785.50 Shock May be associated with hyperamylasemia. *1386*

929.00 Crush Injury (Trauma) Crush injury to abdomen resulting in contusion, rupture or hemorrhage provokes hyperamylasemia. *2104*

948.00 Burns May be associated with hyperamylasemia. *1386*

990.00 Effects of X-Ray Irradiation Sharp rise following salivary gland irradiation. Peak values range from 9-18 X preirradiation values. Steady decline to normal within 2-3 days. *0384*

991.60 Hypothermia About 10% of cases of severe accidental hypothermia develop acute pancreatitis. *0619*

Serum   Normal

157.90 Malignant Neoplasm of Pancreas May be slightly increased in early stages (< 10% of cases). With later destruction of pancreas, normal or decreased. *2467*

577.00 Acute Pancreatitis Occasionally seen; probably following a transient rise and fall, extensive necrosis or acute exacerbation of chronic pancreatitis in which the pancreas cannot produce amylase. *2031*

577.10 Chronic Pancreatitis Usually normal during quiescent phase. Rises as chronic damage progresses but tends to become less pronounced. May actually be normal during relapse. *2031* As disease progresses and more of the gland is destroyed, acute pancreatitis may occur without elevation. *2199*

650.00 Pregnancy *0323*

994.50 Exercise No effect even with strenuous exercise. *1838*

Urine   Increase

72.00 Mumps Increased during first week. *2468*

157.90 Malignant Neoplasm of Pancreas 1 h excretion is increased in up to 30% of patients. *0992* Elevated serum and urinary S-amylase has been reported. *2151* May be mildly elevated in a few patients as a result of pancreatitis secondary to an obstructing tumor. *2199*

162.90 Malignant Neoplasm of Bronchus and Lung Markedly increased in serum, urine and tumor tissue. *2598*

250.00 Diabetes Mellitus High incidence of pancreatic abnormality in patients with no clinical evidence of pancreatic acinar disease. *2406*

303.00 Acute Alcoholic Intoxication Increased in serum and urine in 8.5% of 129 patients after acute intoxication, due to changes in salivary isoenzyme, not as a result of pancreatic damage. *0178*

571.90 Cirrhosis of Liver High incidence of pancreatic abnormality in patients with no clinical evidence of pancreatic acinar disease. *2406*

576.20 Extrahepatic Biliary Obstruction Increased excretion in obstruction due to stone in common bile duct. *0619*

577.00 Acute Pancreatitis Often elevated and persists up to the 3rd day after the onset of the disease. *0433* Tends to reflect serum changes by a time lag of 6-10 h, but sometimes increased urine levels are higher and of longer duration than serum levels. *2467* Elevation has been used to diagnose acute pancreatitis in the absence of renal failure. Levels higher than 6,000 U/24h or 300 U/h are usually seen in patients with acute attacks. *0151* Increased renal clearance. *0178*

577.20 Pancreatic Cyst and Pseudocyst Persistent increase 4-6 weeks after onset of pancreatitis suggests pseudocyst. Hyperamylasuria is usual but not invariable. *2031*

585.00 Chronic Renal Failure In patients with severe renal insufficiency, the amylase to creatinine ratios were significantly raised. Clearance ratios of pancreatic and salivary isoamylase to creatinine changed in parallel to that of total amylase. The results suggest that in severe renal failure the loss of nephrons results in decreased fractional reabsorption of amylase in the tubules. *1779*

Amylase *(continued)*

Pleural Effusion   Increase

11.00   Pulmonary Tuberculosis   Pleural fluid levels may be high. *1584*

157.90   Malignant Neoplasm of Pancreas   Carcinoma of the pancreas and other organs. *1405*

162.90   Malignant Neoplasm of Bronchus and Lung   High pleural fluid concentrations may occur. *0662*   Elevated in primary or metastatic lung cancer, pancreatitis, or esophageal perforation. *2031*

183.00   Malignant Neoplasm of Ovary   Rare occurrence of ovarian carcinoma producing amylase-rich ascites and pleural effusions. Salivary type amylase has been identified in tumor tissue. *0457*

415.10   Pulmonary Embolism and Infarction   *2017*   May occur *1584*

428.00   Congestive Heart Failure   May occur. *1584*

577.00   Acute Pancreatitis   Pleural effusions occur in about 10% of patients, with amylase commonly elevated. *1403*   Elevated in primary or metastatic lung cancer, pancreatitis, or esophageal perforation. *2031*   May contain very high concentration, even with normal serum level. If the concentrations are lower than the serum, pancreatitis is virtually excluded as the cause. *2199*   Pleural effusion has been reported in about 6% of patients with acute pancreatitis. These effusions contain pleural fluid amylase. May occur in other conditions including metastatic carcinoma. *0503*   With pancreatic pseudocyst *1405 2017*

577.10   Chronic Pancreatitis   Pleural effusions occur in about 10% of pancreatitis patients, with amylase commonly elevated. *1403*   Elevated in primary or metastatic lung cancer, pancreatitis, or esophageal perforation. *2031*   Pleural fluid pH of < 7.20 or 0.15 below arterial pH frequently occurs in parapneumonic effusion *1403*   With Pancreatic pseudocyst *2017 1405*

577.20   Pancreatic Cyst and Pseudocyst   *2017*

710.00   Systemic Lupus Erythematosus   Elevation in pleural fluid may occur. *1584*

Pleural Effusion   Normal

162.90   Malignant Neoplasm of Bronchus and Lung   Usually less than or equal to serum level. *2017*

197.00   Secondary Malignant Neoplasm of Respiratory System   Usually less than or equal to serum level. *2017*

415.10   Pulmonary Embolism and Infarction   Usually less than or equal to serum level. *2017*

428.00   Congestive Heart Failure   Usually less than or equal to serum level. *2017*

482.90   Bacterial Pneumonia   Usually less than or equal to serum level. *2017*

571.90   Cirrhosis of Liver   Usually less than or equal to serum level. *2017*

714.00   Rheumatoid Arthritis   Usually less than or equal to serum level. *2017*

Ascitic Fluid   Increase

183.00   Malignant Neoplasm of Ovary   Rare occurrence of ovarian carcinoma producing amylase-rich ascites and pleural effusions was reported; salivary type amylase was identified in tumor tissue. *0457*

199.00   Secondary Malignant Neoplasm (Disseminated)   With carcinomatous peritonitis 91% of the increased amylase activity was of salivary type and the remainder of pancreatic type. *1364*   Parallels the degree of metastatic involvement of the peritoneum. *2104*

560.90   Intestinal Obstruction   *0186*

567.90   Peritonitis   *0186*

577.00   Acute Pancreatitis   Concentration in ascitic fluid is usually 1,000 U/L. *0080*   Varied from 1,060-48,000 U/L in ascites. *0827*   Ascites may develop, 0.5-2 liters in volume, containing increased amylase with a level higher than that of serum. *2467 2199*

577.10   Chronic Pancreatitis   Greatly increased in pancreatic ascites. *2199*

577.20   Pancreatic Cyst and Pseudocyst   Greatly increased in pancreatic ascites. *2199*

Gastric Material   Decrease

260.00   Protein Malnutrition   Activity is lowered almost to zero in kwashiorkor. *0151*

Peritoneal Fluid   Increase

533.90   Peptic Ulcer, Site Unspecified   With perforation. *2467*

Saliva   Decrease

577.10   Chronic Pancreatitis   Salivary output, amylase, and HCO_3 concentration decreased in 88% of patients. *1210*

Saliva   Increase

277.00   Cystic Fibrosis   In healthy adults and children the value for pancreatic:salivary amylase is > 1. In 80% of gene carriers, the P:S is < 1 with a mean of 0.68 ± 0.13. In addition to the higher total amylase activity, in homozygotes P:S is < 0.1, and even 0.001. The phenomenon is explained by a compensatory enhancement of salivary activity. *2316*   Submaxillary saliva is turbid, with increased calcium, total protein, and amylase. These changes are not generally found in parotid saliva. *2467*

577.00   Acute Pancreatitis   Increased alpha-amylase in parotid saliva. *0922   0080*

Androgens

Plasma   Decrease

253.00   Acromegaly   Testosterone has been reported to be low in the presence of normal gonadotropin levels. *0433*

253.40   Anterior Pituitary Hypofunction   Decreased testosterone in hypopituitarism and hypogonadism. *0619*

255.40   Adrenal Cortical Hypofunction   Adrenal cortex destruction results in deficiency of glucocorticoids, androgens, and mineralocorticoids. *2612*

257.20   Testicular Hypofunction   Decreased testosterone in primary and secondary hypogonadism. *2467*

275.00   Hemochromatosis   Decreased testosterone found in 12 of 12 patients. *0199*

282.60   Sickle Cell Anemia   Deficient as a result of primary rather than secondary hypogonadism in 29 of 32 adult male patients. *0005*

303.90   Alcoholism   *1805*

758.70   Klinefelter's Syndrome (XXY)   Testosterone reported to be low in most studies, although there is considerable overlap between normal males and Klinefelter males. Generally higher in mosaics than in pure Klinefelter patients. *1090*   Quite variable but often tends to be midway between the normal male and female. *0962*

Plasma   Increase

174.90   Malignant Neoplasm of Breast   Plasma testosterone concentrations were measured in sequential samples from 6 women and were compared to concentrations in 6 control women matched for age, y since menopause, and parity. Concentrations in each cancer patient were significantly higher than in each matched control. *1543*

194.00   Malignant Neoplasm of Adrenal Gland   Excessive androgen secretion in adrenocortical carcinoma. *2612*

220.00   Benign Neoplasm of Ovary   *0433*

255.00   Adrenal Cortical Hyperfunction (Glucocorticoid Excess)   Secretion may be increased and may be a factor in hirsutism, but virilization is rare. *2612*

256.40   Polycystic Ovaries   Women with polycystic ovary had significantly higher plasma androgen levels than women with 'simple' amenorrhea both before treatment and during induction of ovulation. *1356*

256.41   Stein-Leventhal Syndrome   Plasma levels of androstenedione and dehydroepiandrosterone are elevated. *0995*

600.00   Benign Prostatic Hypertrophy   Increased testosterone; especially in older patients. *0972*

650.00   Pregnancy   Mean testosterone concentration in pregnant women with female fetuses was 597 ± 167 pg/mL, and in women with male fetuses, mean value was 828 ± 298 pg/mL, significantly higher (p = < 0.01). Increases began in week 7, reaching a maximum by 9-11. *1284*

706.10   Acne   Elevated in 38% of 26 females with acne between ages 27 and 42 y. *2074*   In a group of 34 women with this condition 80% had an androgen excess *2082*

758.80 Syndromes Due to Sex Chromosome Abnormalities
High plasma testosterone in XYY males. *0619*

Plasma   Normal

255.40 Adrenal Cortical Hypofunction   *2612*

Urine   Decrease

151.90 Malignant Neoplasm of Stomach   Both androsterone and etiocholanolone were significantly lower in 18 male patients than in controls and patients with rectal cancer. *2333*

154.10 Malignant Neoplasm of Rectum   Significantly decreased, 1.86 ± 0.20 mg/g creatinine in 16 male patients. *2333*

174.90 Malignant Neoplasm of Breast   Significantly decreased in comparison with controls. *0390*

Androstenedione

Serum   Decrease

282.60 Sickle Cell Anemia   Basal serum testosterone, dihydrotestosterone, and androstenedione were lower in 32 adult male patients. Secondary sex characteristics were abnormal in 29 of 32 patients. *0005*

Serum   Increase

256.41 Stein-Leventhal Syndrome   Plasma levels of androstenedione and dehydroepiandosterone are elevated. *0995*

706.10 Acne   Elevated in 38% of 26 females with acne between ages 27 and 42 y. *2074*

Androsterone

Urine   Decrease

151.90 Malignant Neoplasm of Stomach   Both androsterone and etiocholanolone were significantly lower in 18 male patients than in controls and patients with rectal cancer. *2333*

154.10 Malignant Neoplasm of Rectum   Significantly decreased, 1.86 ± 0.20 mg/g creatinine in 16 male patients. *2333*

174.90 Malignant Neoplasm of Breast   Significantly decreased in comparison with controls. *0390*

Angiotensin

Plasma   Decrease

253.40 Anterior Pituitary Hypofunction   Both plasma renin substrate and angiotensin are low and unresponsive to adequate stimulation *0103*

Angiotensin-Converting Enzyme (ACE)

Serum   Decrease

162.90 Malignant Neoplasm of Bronchus and Lung   In 141 patients with newly diagnosed primary lung cancer it was found to be lower than in the control group. This suggests that low levels may be associated with a poor prognosis in this condition. *1967 1501*

199.00 Secondary Malignant Neoplasm (Disseminated)   Most cancer patients present with normal to low levels. *1501*

201.90 Hodgkin's Disease   No relationship was found between enzyme activity and stage, activity, histo- pathology, etc. Levels were lower than healthy controls but not significantly *0258 1969*

202.80 Non-Hodgkins Lymphoma   Patients with low values had a poorer prognosis. *1969*

203.00 Multiple Myeloma   Depression of activity. Significant decrease *1969*

204.10 Lymphocytic Leukemia (Chronic)   Significant decrease. Depression of Activity *1969*

205.00 Myelocytic Leukemia (Acute)   Mean value for group 19.9 U/L compared with 24.4 U/L for control group. *1969*

244.90 Hypothyroidism   Levels 13.9 U/mL in hypothyroid patients versus 17.0 U/mL in controls. In 12 hypothyroid patients levels rose from 11.6 to 15.8 U/mL after thyroid replacement therapy. Patients with thyroxine index less than 5.0 had significantly lower levels than normal controls *0278   2202*

555.90 Regional Enteritis or Ileitis   Significantly depressed compared with normal controls and those with inactive disease. *0483*

584.00 Acute Renal Failure   Level increased with normalization of renal function. *1970*

650.00 Pregnancy   It is thought to be caused by enzyme consumption in the kinin system which is activated by pregnancy. *0608*

Serum   Increase

30.00 Leprosy   *1398 2014*

114.90 Coccidioidomycosis   Decreased. *1398*

115.00 Histoplasmosis   Elevated in 25% of 86 patients. *2015* Rises acutely in all patients with Histo and then falls gradually towards baseline (n = 44). *0506*

135.00 Sarcoidosis   Most frequently elevated in patients with pulmonary parenchymal involvement. *1968*   Elevated in 33% of patients with Sarcoidosis. *0941*   Elevated in 60-80% of cases. *0560*   Increased levels in 67.2% of 100 patients. *2041*   Elevated in 75% of patients. *2118   1400*

242.90 Hyperthyroidism   Significantly elevated in 21 patients with hyperthyroidism (mean 65 U/mL) compared with healthy control subjects (mean 30 U/mL). *2600*   Consistently elevated in untreated patients compared with controls. *1673 2165 0278*   Significantly higher than hypothyroid or normal subjects. Higher than all other groups but fell from 30.8 to 17.4 U/mL with therapy in 35 patients studied *0901 2202*

250.00 Diabetes Mellitus   Elevated levels were detected in 24% of 265 patients with this disease. *1399*   Elevated in 32% of 81 patients. *2068*

272.72 Gaucher's Disease   Elevated. *1398*

502.00 Silicosis   Elevated and associated with a progression of the disease. *1464 1705*

533.90 Peptic Ulcer, Site Unspecified   Significant increase regardless of whether ulceration was gastric or duodenal. *0483*

571.20 Laennec's or Alcoholic Cirrhosis   In patients with alcoholic liver disease mean 30.8 U/mL compared with 22.8 in controls. 30% of patients had elevated levels. *0255*

585.00 Chronic Renal Failure   It is thought that an enlarged pulmonary vascular bed and accelerated cellular breakdown were the cause. *0608*   Significantly higher than that of an age - matched control group *1611*   Elevated regardless of severity of disease *2164*

710.00 Systemic Lupus Erythematosus   *1398 2014*

710.20 Sjögren's Syndrome   A study of 21 cases of this syndrome revealed that only 2 cases had elevated levels and these were only modest increases. *1464 1398 2014*

710.40 Dermatomyositis/Polymyositis   *1398 2014*

714.00 Rheumatoid Arthritis   *1398 2014*

Serum   Normal

11.00 Pulmonary Tuberculosis   No difference in levels found between control group of 108 and TB group of 100. *0907*

73.90 Psittacosis   Not elevated in active hypersensitivity pneumonitis. *1539*

199.00 Secondary Malignant Neoplasm (Disseminated)   Most cancer patients present with normal to low levels. *1501*

244.90 Hypothyroidism   Patients had levels within the normal range. *0309   1673*

401.10 Essential Benign Hypertension   No difference was detected between men and woman and between normotensives and hypertensives. *0608*   Normal levels for 14 patients with this disorder *2041 0608 2417*

555.90 Regional Enteritis or Ileitis   No significant difference was noted between active Crohn's, inactive Crohn's, and normal controls. However, patients who had active disease and were receiving steroid therapy had significantly lower levels. *1710*   Wide variation. *0483*

556.00 Ulcerative Colitis   Similar levels as controls. *0483*

650.00 Pregnancy   Levels didn't change throughout pregnancy. *0609*

696.10 Psoriasis   Not significantly different in Psoriatic arthritis (n = 12) from normal controls. *1443*   . Normal in cutaneous Psoriasis. *2346*   Levels remained normal *2346*

710.20 Sjögren's Syndrome   Raised activity isn't usually associated with this syndrome. *1464*

714.00 Rheumatoid Arthritis   Not significantly different (n = 48) from normal controls (n = 26). *1443*

Angiotensin-Converting Enzyme (ACE)
(continued)

Serum   Normal *(continued)*

715.90   Osteoarthritis   Not significantly different (n = 11) from normal controls (n = 26). *1443*

720.00   Rheumatoid (Ankylosing) Spondylitis   Not significantly different (n = 24) from normal controls (n = 26). *1443*

Urine   Increase

592.00   Kidney Calculus   Activity was found to be significantly elevated. *0256*

599.00   Urinary Tract Infection   Activity was found to be significantly elevated. *0256*

CSF   Decrease

297.90   Paranoid States and Other Psychoses   Both treated and drug free patients had low activity when compared with controls *0148*

331.00   Alzheimer's Disease   Decreased 41% of cases compared to age and sex matched controls. *2620*

332.00   Parkinsons's Disease   Decreased in 27% of cases compared to matched control group. *2620*   Level decrease 27% compared with an age and sex matched control group *2620*

Angiotensin II

Plasma   Decrease

255.00   Adrenal Cortical Hyperfunction (Glucocorticoid Excess)   In 4 patients with Cushing's Syndrome values were extremely low in renal venous blood. *1331*

255.10   Adrenal Cortical Hyperfunction (Mineralocorticoid Excess)   In 8 patients with primary aldosteronism values were extremely low in renal venous blood. *1331*

Anisocytes

Blood   Increase

202.40   Leukemic Reticuloendotheliosis   Usually normochromic, normocytic anemia; mild anisocytosis and poikilocytosis were common. *2390*

238.40   Polycythemia Vera   Mild anisocytosis and poikilocytosis may be seen in the peripheral blood. *2538*

244.90   Hypothyroidism   A minor degree of anisocytosis and also acanthocytosis (32 of 172) was demonstrated. *1078*

272.72   Gaucher's Disease   If splenectomy has been carried out, severe anisocytosis and poikilocytosis occur, with many target cells, some nucleated red cells, and Howell-Jolly bodies usually present. *2538*

280.90   Iron Deficiency Anemia   Usually there is moderate to marked anisocytosis and poikilocytosis. *0999*   Characteristic of well-developed iron deficiency. *0962   0151*

281.30   Vitamin B$_6$ Deficiency Anemia   Blood smear shows anisocytosis with many bizarre forms, target cells, hypochromia with pyridoxine-responsive anemia. *2467*   Prominent findings on blood smear. *2552*

282.00   Hereditary (Congenital) Spherocytosis   Anisocytosis is marked. *2468*

282.41   Thalassemia Major   The red cells show marked aniso-poikilocytosis, with hypochromia, target-cell formation, and a variable degree of basophilic stippling. *2538   2246*

282.42   Thalassemia Minor   Defective globin synthesis. *0962*   Aniso- and poikilocytosis may be very striking and far out of proportion to the degree of anemia. *2552*

282.60   Sickle Cell Anemia   Blood film reveals marked poikilocytosis and anisocytosis, target cells, some macrocytes, and occasional sickled erythrocytes. Nucleated red cells are frequently seen, particularly in children. *0999*

282.73   Hemoglobin H Disease   Anisopoikilocytosis of RBC. *2246*

285.00   Sideroblastic Anemia   Blood smear shows anisocytosis with many bizarre forms, target cells, hypochromia with pyridoxine-responsive anemia. *2467*   Prominent findings on blood smear. In hereditary x-linked sideroblastic anemia. *2552*

289.80   Myelofibrosis   In myelofibrosis is usually pronounced. *2538*

516.10   Idiopathic Pulmonary Hemosiderosis   Peripheral blood displays the classic changes of severe iron depletion: anisocytosis, poikilocytosis, microcytosis, and hypochromia. *2538*

Antibodies to Centromeres

Serum   Increase

710.10   Progressive Systemic Sclerosis   Found in 10% of cases (77% with CREST syndrome). *2204*

Serum   Normal

714.00   Rheumatoid Arthritis   Found in 0% of cases. *2204*

Antibodies to dsDNA

Serum   Increase

710.00   Systemic Lupus Erythematosus   Found in 49% of cases. *2204*

710.40   Dermatomyositis/Polymyositis   Found in 25% of cases of dermatomyositis. *2204*

711.10   Mixed Connective Tissue Disease   Found in 25% of cases. *2204*

714.00   Rheumatoid Arthritis   Found in 2% of cases. *2204 0186*

714.30   Juvenile Rheumatoid Arthritis   Found in 5% of cases. *2204*

Serum   Normal

710.10   Progressive Systemic Sclerosis   Found in 0% of cases. *2204*

710.20   Sjögren's Syndrome   Found in 0% of cases. *2204*

714.10   Felty's Syndrome   Found in 0% of cases. *2204*

Antibodies to Histones

Serum   Increase

710.00   Systemic Lupus Erythematosus   Found in 46% of cases. *2204*   Found in 50% of patients. *1503*   Found in 100% of patients with drug induced SLE. *0062*

714.00   Rheumatoid Arthritis   Found in 10% of cases. *2204*   Found in 15-20% of cases *0062*

Antibodies to RNP

Serum   Increase

710.00   Systemic Lupus Erythematosus   Found in 34% of cases. *2204*

710.10   Progressive Systemic Sclerosis   Found in 5% of cases. *2204*

710.20   Sjögren's Syndrome   Found in 5% of cases. *2204*

711.10   Mixed Connective Tissue Disease   Found in 100% of cases. *2204*

714.00   Rheumatoid Arthritis   Found in 1% of cases. *2204*

714.30   Juvenile Rheumatoid Arthritis   Found in 3% of cases. *2204*

Serum   Normal

710.40   Dermatomyositis/Polymyositis   Found in 0% of cases. *2204*

Antibodies to SCL-70

Serum   Increase

710.10   Progressive Systemic Sclerosis   Found in 23% of cases (10% with CREST syndrome). *2204*

Serum   Normal

714.00   Rheumatoid Arthritis   Found in 0% of cases. *2204*

Antibodies to Sjögren Syndrome A

Serum   Increase

710.00   Systemic Lupus Erythematosus   Found in 35% of cases.
2204   Found in 100% of neonatal SLE cases. *0062*

710.10   Progressive Systemic Sclerosis   Found in 33% of cases.
2204

710.20   Sjögren's Syndrome   Found in 70% of cases. *2204*

714.00   Rheumatoid Arthritis   Found in 4% of cases. *2204*

Serum   Normal

714.30   Juvenile Rheumatoid Arthritis   Found in 0% of cases.
2204

Antibodies to Sjögren Syndrome B

Serum   Increase

710.00   Systemic Lupus Erythematosus   Found in 5% of cases.
2204   15% of cases. *1670*

710.10   Progressive Systemic Sclerosis   Found in 6% of cases.
2204

710.20   Sjögren's Syndrome   Found in 60% of cases. *2204*

714.00   Rheumatoid Arthritis   Found in 1% of cases. *2204*

Serum   Normal

714.30   Juvenile Rheumatoid Arthritis   Found in 0% of cases.
2204

Antibodies to SmAg

Serum   Increase

710.00   Systemic Lupus Erythematosus   Found in 23% of cases.
2204   Present in 30% of cases. Highly diagnostic. *1670*

711.10   Mixed Connective Tissue Disease   Found in 8% of
cases. *2204*

714.00   Rheumatoid Arthritis   Found in 5% of cases. *2204*

Serum   Normal

710.10   Progressive Systemic Sclerosis   Found in 0% of cases.
2204

710.20   Sjögren's Syndrome   Found in 0% of cases. *2204*

710.40   Dermatomyositis/Polymyositis   Found in 0% of cases of
dermatomyositis. *2204*

Antibodies to ss-DNA

Serum   Increase

710.00   Systemic Lupus Erythematosus   Found in 42% of cases.
2204

710.10   Progressive Systemic Sclerosis   Found in 14% of cases.
2204

714.00   Rheumatoid Arthritis   Found in 4% of cases. *2204*

714.10   Felty's Syndrome   Found in 100% of cases. *2204*

714.30   Juvenile Rheumatoid Arthritis   Found in 3% of cases.
2204

Serum   Normal

710.20   Sjögren's Syndrome   Found in 0% of cases. *2204*

Antibody Titer

Serum   Decrease

279.04   Agammaglobulinemia (Congenital Sex-linked)   Very
low levels of antibody to certain animal viruses can be demonstrated. *2035*

279.06   Immunodeficiency (Common Variable)   Antibody
responses to most antigens are low or absent. *2552*

Serum   Increase

7.10   Giardiasis   Anti-Giardia IgM and IgG by ELISA was found.
Specificity and Sensitivity was 96%. *0862*

11.00   Pulmonary Tuberculosis   Used to differentiate pulmonary
sarcoidosis from tuberculosis. Antituberculous antibodies were
found in TB in 83%; in sarcoidosis in 22%. *1309*

23.00   Brucellosis   Antibodies elicited early in natural infection
are predominantly IgM, with lesser quantities of IgG. As the disease progresses, IgM declines, and IgG increases, reaching its
height at the period of maximum resistance to reinfection. *2035*

75.00   Infectious Mononucleosis   The presence of EB virus
antibody is essential for diagnosis in heterophil-negative cases.
Antibody to early antigen and EB virus-specific IgM antibody
occurs in 75-85% of acute cases. *1028   2538*

80.00   Epidemic Typhus   Antibodies are demonstrable in significant titers by the 3rd week. *0433*   Acute phase antibodies are of
the IgM type. *0151*

81.10   Brill's Disease   Acute-phase antibodies are of the IgG
class. *0151*

100.00   Leptospirosis   The contrast between negative acute-
phase and positive convalescent phase sera is diagnostic. *2368*

115.00   Histoplasmosis   Elevated convalescent phase titer may
be the result of skin testing or of active disease. *2508*

117.50   Cryptococcosis   Several serologic tests for anticryptococcal antibody are in use. Although sometimes of value, false positive
reactions limit the utility of these tests. *1058*

135.00   Sarcoidosis   Used to differentiate pulmonary sarcoidosis
from tuberculosis. Antituberculous antibodies were found in TB in
83%; in sarcoidosis 22%. *1309*

244.90   Hypothyroidism   Antiparietal cell antibodies present in up
to 40% of cases. *0186*

245.20   Hashimoto's Thyroiditis   Characteristically present in
high titer during the active phase of chronic thyroiditis. *0999*   Virtually all patients with this disease have circulating autoantibodies.
2540   Antimicrosomal antibodies present in 78% of patients. *0992*
Almost all patients have thyroid autoantibodies in their serum, and
extremely high titers of any of the autoantibodies are inconsistent
with most other diagnoses. *2035*

250.00   Diabetes Mellitus   Antibodies to Islet cells. Present in
60% of juvenile onset diabetics of less than 1 years duration. Such
antibodies tend to disappear rapidly after the disease is recognized clinically. *1670*

252.00   Hyperparathyroidism   Parathyroid antibodies. *1670*

255.40   Adrenal Cortical Hypofunction   Antibodies to adrenocortical cell in primary Addison's Disease. *1670*

279.31   Acquired Immunodeficiency Syndrome (AIDS)   Using
the enzyme-linked immunosorbent assay (ELISA) for HTLV-III
antibodies, 82% of 88 patients with AIDS were positive, 16% borderline and 2% negative. Only 1% of 297 volunteer controls were
positive, 6% borderline and 93% negative for a specificity of 98.6%
and sensitivity of 97.3%. *2511*

281.00   Pernicious Anemia   Antibodies against parietal cells are
found in 75% of all patients. Antibodies against intrinsic factor are
seen in 50% of these patients. *0962*

286.01   Hemophilia   Titers of antibodies to cytomegalovirus were
generally higher in hemophiliac patients than in a control group of
healthy volunteers. *1378*

335.20   Amyotrophic Lateral Sclerosis   IgA and IgM antibodies
to myelin of rabbit spinal cord. Found in 70% of patients. When IgG
antimyelin antibody is present in titers greater than 1:8 it is suggestive, but not diagnostic. *1670*

340.00   Multiple Sclerosis   IgA and IgM antibodies to myelin of
rabbit spinal cord. Found in 70% of patients. When IgG antimyelin
antibody is present in titers greater than 1:8 it is suggestive, but
not diagnostic. *1670*   Serum IgE and measles antibodies were
increased more frequently in hypocomplementemic patients than
in normal populations *2375*

358.00   Myasthenia Gravis   50% of patients with this disease,
usually those with thymoma, have antibodies to striated muscle. At
times there is an increasing titer in severe disease. Generally a titer
greater than 1:60 is diagnostic. *1670*

390.00   Rheumatic Fever   Antifibrinolysin titer is increased in this
disease and in recent hemolytic streptococcus infections. 1 of the
3 titers (ASO, antihyaluronidase, antifibrinolysin elevated in 95% of
cases. If all are normal, a diagnosis is less likely. Antihyaluronidase
titer of 1,000-1,500 follows recent streptococcus A disease and up
to 4,000 with rheumatic fever. Average titer is higher in early rheumatic activity than in subsiding or inactive rheumatic fever.
Increased as often as ASO and antifibrinolysin titers. *2467*

429.40   Postcardiotomy Syndrome   Excellent correlation
between the titer of circulating antiheart antibodies and the development of this syndrome in postoperative patients. *1108   0664*

Antibody Titer *(continued)*

Serum   Increase *(continued)*

446.20   Goodpasture's Syndrome   Glomerular and alveolar basement membrane antibodies. *1670*   Circulating antibodies to glycopeptide antigen are found in over 90% of cases. *0062*

483.01   Mycoplasma Pneumoniae   IgM antibodies present in 13 of 14 patients tested. *2639*

535.00   Gastritis   Parietal cell antibody detected by CF tests using gastric mucosal homogenate or by direct immunofluorescence on sections of gastric mucosa is present in approximately 60% of patients with idiopathic atrophic gastritis. *0583*

555.90   Regional Enteritis or Ileitis   Antibodies to Reticulin. *1670*

571.49   Chronic Active Hepatitis   Increased incidence of high titers of serum autoantibodies. *2145*

571.60   Biliary Cirrhosis   Increased incidence of high titers of serum autoantibodies. *2145*

571.90   Cirrhosis of Liver   Increased incidence of high titers of serum autoantibodies. *2145*   Patients with cirrhosis appear to have antibodies to a larger number of enteric bacteria though not higher titers to individual strains. *1829*   Increased incidence of antithyroid antibodies. *2238*

579.00   Celiac Sprue Disease   Antibodies to Reticulin found in 78% of cases. *1670*

694.00   Dermatitis Herpetiformis   Reticulin antibodies. *1670*

694.40   Pemphigus   Numerous studies have confirmed the presence of autoantibodies specific for an intercellular substance of skin and mucosa in serum from patients with active pemphigus. *0642*

710.10   Progressive Systemic Sclerosis   The anticentromere antibody is thought to be closely associated with the CREST variant of Scleroderma. It may be a useful prognostic indicator. *1846*

710.20   Sjögren's Syndrome   Antibodies to Reticulin. 75% of patients exhibit antibodies to salivary duct epithelium. *1670*

710.40   Dermatomyositis/Polymyositis   Occasionally patients with dermatomyositis display antibodies to striated muscle. *1670*

714.00   Rheumatoid Arthritis   Antibodies to Reticulin. *1670*

CSF   Increase

130.00   Toxoplasmosis   Congenital infection is indicated when CSF antibody concentration is higher for toxoplasmosis than for rubeola. *1360*

Antidiuretic Hormone

Serum   Decrease

253.50   Diabetes Insipidus   Posterior pituitary insufficiency is signaled by the deficiency of ADH. *1108*

428.00   Congestive Heart Failure   *0619*

581.90   Nephrotic Syndrome   *0619*

Serum   Increase

11.00   Pulmonary Tuberculosis   Inappropriate secretion of ADH with consequent water retention can occur. *0962*

13.00   Tuberculosis Meningitis   Inappropriate secretion of ADH with consequent water retention. *0962*

162.90   Malignant Neoplasm of Bronchus and Lung   Inappropriate secretion of ADH is associated with hyponatremia, decreased serum osmolality, and inappropriately high sodium concentration in the urine. The entire syndrome resolves following resection of the tumor. *0962*

191.90   Malignant Neoplasm of Brain   Associated with excessive ADH production resulting in sodium loss. *2104*

198.30   Secondary Malignant Neoplasm of Brain   Associated with excessive ADH production resulting in sodium loss. *2104*

225.90   Benign Neoplasm of Brain and CNS   Associated with excessive ADH production resulting in sodium loss. *2104*

277.14   Acute Intermittent Porphyria   Syndrome of inappropriate ADH secretion has been documented in a number of cases. *2552*

320.90   Meningitis (Bacterial)   Associated with excessive ADH production resulting in sodium loss. *2104*

323.92   Encephalomyelitis   Associated with excessive ADH production resulting in sodium loss. *2104*

428.00   Congestive Heart Failure   Enhanced ADH and aldosterone activity. *2104*

431.00   Cerebral Hemorrhage   Associated with excessive ADH production resulting in sodium loss. *2104*

434.00   Cerebral Thrombosis   Associated with excessive ADH production resulting in sodium loss. *2104*

434.10   Cerebral Embolism   Associated with excessive ADH production resulting in sodium loss. *2104*

480.90   Viral Pneumonia   Inappropriate increase. *2540*

482.90   Bacterial Pneumonia   Inappropriate increase. *2540*

493.10   Asthma (Intrinsic)   In status asthmaticus. *1228*

570.00   Acute and Subacute Necrosis of Liver   *0992*

642.40   Pre-Eclampsia   Positive correlation between severity of toxemia and circulating ADH. *2104*

642.60   Eclampsia   Positive correlation between severity of toxemia and circulating ADH. *2104*

Urine   Increase

308.00   Stress   50% increase with mental stress. *2092*

Urine   Normal

991.60   Hypothermia   With cold exposure. *2092*

Antimitochondrial Antibodies

Serum   Increase

245.20   Hashimoto's Thyroiditis   Presence correlates with degree of lymphocytic infiltration of the gland. *0186*

571.49   Chronic Active Hepatitis   Present in 30% of patients. *2145*   Found in 10-20% of patients. *0992*   Found in 66% of patients compared to 2% of controls. *1840*

571.60   Biliary Cirrhosis   Present in > 90% of patients compared with 2-3% of obstructive bile duct patients. *2145*   Found in almost 100% of cases, while incidence is only 10% in extrahepatic biliary obstruction. *1829*   79-94% of all cases give positive results. *0619 0962 1840*

571.90   Cirrhosis of Liver   Found in 5-30% of patients with postnecrotic cirrhosis depending upon the technique used. *1829 2145*

573.30   Toxic Hepatitis   Especially in drug-induced hepatitis due to halothane or chlorpromazine. *1829*

710.00   Systemic Lupus Erythematosus   8% of patients were positive. *0619*   Found in 18% of patients and 2% of controls. *1840*

710.20   Sjögren's Syndrome   May occur. *2134*   Found in 18% of patients and 2% of controls. *1840*

Serum   Normal

70.00   Viral Hepatitis   *1840*

571.20   Laennec's or Alcoholic Cirrhosis   *1840*

576.20   Extrahepatic Biliary Obstruction   *1840*

Antinuclear Antibodies

Serum   Increase

30.00   Leprosy   Found in 30%. *2035*

70.00   Viral Hepatitis   Found in 23% of patients and 2% of controls. *1840*

75.00   Infectious Mononucleosis   65% of patients were positive. *1799*   May be present without positive LE cell test. *0619*

84.00   Malaria   An unusually high incidence was observed during chronic infection. *0916   2035*

204.00   Lymphocytic Leukemia (Acute)   Positive in 25% of patients. *1799*

204.10   Lymphocytic Leukemia (Chronic)   Positive in 20% of patients. *1799*

205.00   Myelocytic Leukemia (Acute)   Positive in 25% of patients. *1799*

245.20   Hashimoto's Thyroiditis   Present in 1-8% of cases. *0995*

273.30   Waldenström's Macroglobulinemia   Positive in 16%. *1799*

283.00   Acquired Hemolytic Anemia (Autoimmune)   Found in a significant number of patients without other features of SLE or other rheumatic disease. *2035*

358.00 Myasthenia Gravis Approximately 20% contain antinuclear factor which can occur in IgA, IgG, or IgM. *1544* There is an increased incidence of this compared to the population as a whole. *2035*

446.00 Polyarteritis-Nodosa Infrequently seen and, when present, are in low titer. *0962* Usually absent, and when present should suggest that the arteritis is part of another disorder. *2035*

571.20 Laennec's or Alcoholic Cirrhosis Low incidence of the autoimmune serological markers antinuclear antibody (13%) and smooth muscle antibody (13%). *0880* 7% of patients were positive (2% of controls). *1840 2035*

571.49 Chronic Active Hepatitis Raised more often than LE cell phenomenon positive. *0619* Common (20-60% of cases). *0992* Recognized by immunofluorescence, with an incidence of positive tests of 60%. *2201* 57% of patients were positive compared to 2% of controls. *1840* Increased incidence of high titers of serum autoantibodies. *2145 2035*

571.60 Biliary Cirrhosis Moderate incidence (24%), but the reaction is relatively weak. *2035* Found in 40% of patients and 2% of controls. *1840* Increased incidence of high titers of serum autoantibodies. *2145 1799*

571.90 Cirrhosis of Liver With postnecrotic cirrhosis. *0151* Increased incidence of high titers of serum autoantibodies. *2145*

576.20 Extrahepatic Biliary Obstruction Positive in 11% of patients (2% in controls). *1840*

585.00 Chronic Renal Failure Increased in 11 of 86 patients who had never been dialyzed and 52 of 243 chronic dialysis patients. Significantly lower Hcts and WBC counts were noted with the presence of these antibodies. *1702*

710.00 Systemic Lupus Erythematosus Present in 97.7% of patients (44 of 45) tested using immunofluorescent technique. *0321* Titers were higher in patients with nephritis than in a control group of SLE patients without nephritis but were no higher than in scleroderma. *1771* Nearly all patients with active SLE are positive. Titers vary according to the intensity of disease activity. *0999* Present in high titer but only low titers were found in other rheumatoid diseases. *1707* Appearance of antibody to DNA frequently (40% of the time) heralds an approaching clinical flare within several months. *0782* 95-100% positivity. *1799* Found in 100% of cases *2204 0713*

710.10 Progressive Systemic Sclerosis Present in 60% of 47 serum samples in titers of 1:16 or greater. *1995* Detected in low titer in 50-60% of cases and usually related to the nucleolar and ill-defined glycoprotein antigens. *0999* Found in the sera of 40-90% of patients. In most cases the titers are relatively low, as compared to those found in SLE. *2035* 75-80% positivity. *1799* Found in 58% of cases *2204 1771*

710.20 Sjögren's Syndrome Demonstrable in close to 70% of patients. *0226* Present in about 60% (fluorescent technique). *0999* 40-75% positivity. *1799 2035*

710.40 Dermatomyositis/Polymyositis 40% of patients were ANA positive and LE cell negative. *0321* Positive in 35% of patients tested, although only 2% of patients with pure disease had detectable levels. *1791* Reported to be positive in 25%, positive only in a few cases of uncomplicated disease; positive titer in 2%, contrary to other reports. Higher titers were found in patients with other complications. *0244* Found in 82% of cases of polymyositis *2204 2035 1799*

711.10 Mixed Connective Tissue Disease Usually high titers (> 1:1000), speckled pattern. *0062*

714.00 Rheumatoid Arthritis 30 of 42 (73.2%) severely affected patients were antinuclear factor positive and 19 of them were LE cell negative. *0321* Present in serum of 10-50% of patients (depending on the technique used) but is also usually in low titer compared to that in SLE. *0999* Highly sensitive tests will detect them in 60% of patients. Titers are generally lower than in SLE; predominantly IgM. *0962* 25-60% positivity. *1799* Found in 56% of cases *2204*

714.10 Felty's Syndrome Found in 75% of cases. *2204* Positive in 100% of cases. *1799*

714.30 Juvenile Rheumatoid Arthritis Frequently found in sera from patients with pauciarticular disease and children with mild disease activity. *1993*

714.30 Juvenile Rheumatoid Arthritis Found in 57% of cases. *2204* Found in 13% of cases.

Serum Normal

99.30 Reiter's Disease *0999*

117.10 Sporotrichosis Normal in all patients with Sporotrichosis arthritis. *0478*

390.00 Rheumatic Fever *1799*

446.50 Cranial Arteritis and Related Conditions Characteristically absent. *2035*

710.00 Systemic Lupus Erythematosus Of 165 patients with SLE a subgroup of 8 patients with active SLE yet with persistently negative tests for antinuclear factor and LE cells was identified. *0849* 10 patients with clinical signs of disease had persistently negative ANA tests. Raynaud's phenomenon, excessive hair fall and oral ulcers were frequent in this subgroup. *0728*

714.30 Juvenile Rheumatoid Arthritis In acute systemic form. *0136*

Synovial Fluid Increase

710.00 Systemic Lupus Erythematosus *0962*

714.00 Rheumatoid Arthritis Occasionally positive. *0962*

Pleural Effusion Increase

710.00 Systemic Lupus Erythematosus Indicates SLE. *0962*

Antismooth Muscle Antibodies

Serum Increase

60.00 Yellow Fever Occasionally positive in low titer. *1829*

70.00 Viral Hepatitis IgM smooth muscle antibody may appear as opposed to the IgG antibody found in chronic hepatitis. *1829* Transiently positive. *0703* 11% of patients were positive (6% of controls). *1840 2251 2035*

75.00 Infectious Mononucleosis IgM smooth muscle antibody may appear as opposed to the IgG antibody found in chronic hepatitis. *1829* Transiently positive. *1062 2035*

358.00 Myasthenia Gravis There is an increased incidence of this compared to the population as a whole. *2035*

493.10 Asthma (Intrinsic) In 20% of cases. *0211*

571.20 Laennec's or Alcoholic Cirrhosis Low incidence of the autoimmune serological markers - ANA (13%) and SMA (13%). *0880 2035 2528 1840*

571.49 Chronic Active Hepatitis In a high percentage of cases. More frequent in HBsAg negative cases. *0992* Reaction is highly positive (an incidence of 60-70%). True incidence could be even higher if tests were done only in phases of activity. *2035* Found in about 50-66% of patients. *0962* Positive in 85% of cases. *1840 2251*

571.60 Biliary Cirrhosis Occurs in up to 50% of patients. *1829* Reported incidence of 10-50%, depending on the titer selected for positivity. *0584* 40% positive. *1840 2251 2035*

571.90 Cirrhosis of Liver Positive in a majority of patients with postnecrotic cirrhosis, independent of the presence of HBsAg or LE cells. *1829*

576.20 Extrahepatic Biliary Obstruction 11% of patients were positive and 6% of controls. *1840 2251*

710.00 Systemic Lupus Erythematosus Positive in 12% of patients and 6% of controls. *1840 2251*

710.20 Sjögren's Syndrome May occur. *2134*

714.00 Rheumatoid Arthritis Occasionally positive in low titer. *1829* Positive in 10% of patients. *2528 2035*

Serum Normal

710.00 Systemic Lupus Erythematosus Uniformly absent. *2528 2035*

Antistreptolysin O

Serum Increase

1.00 Cholera Above normal titers may occur. *1752*

11.00 Pulmonary Tuberculosis Above normal titers may occur. *1752*

18.00 Disseminated Tuberculosis Above normal titers may occur. *1752*

38.00 Septicemia Appear in the serum 10-21 days after onset of acute streptococcal infection. *0962*

70.00 Viral Hepatitis Above normal titers may occur. *1752*

287.00 Allergic Purpura A hemolytic streptococci can be implicated both by culture and by antistreptolysin O titers. This is an inconstant finding. *0962*

Antistreptolysin O *(continued)*

Serum   Increase *(continued)*

390.00 **Rheumatic Fever**   Increased titer is found in 80% of patients within the first 2 months. Height of titer is not related to severity; rate of fall is not related to course of disease. *2467* Antibodies appear in 7 days, peak 2-4 weeks later and may remain elevated for months. Rising titer suggests infections. *2508*   Titer of 250 Todd U in adults and 333 in children is considered diagnostic of preceding streptococcal infection. *1108*   Increased titers develop after 2nd week and peak in 4-6 weeks. *0962*

482.90 **Bacterial Pneumonia**   In group A streptococcal infections. *0962*

580.00 **Acute Poststreptococcal Glomerulonephritis**   Usually raised indicating recent streptococcal infection but may fall rapidly with the use of antimicrobials. *0151*   Titer usually exhibits a rise some time during the course of the disease and may be the only evidence of antecedent beta-hemolytic streptococcal infection. *0999*

580.01 **Glomerulonephritis (Focal)**   Above normal titers may occur. *1752*

580.02 **Glomerulonephritis (Minimal Change)**   Above normal titers may occur. *1752*

580.04 **Glomerulonephritis (Membranous)**   Above normal titers may occur. *1752*

580.05 **Glomerulonephritis (Membranoproliferative)**   In about 40% of patients. *0331*

580.40 **Glomerulonephritis (Rapidly Progressive)**   May be found in 30% of patients without other evidence of streptococcal etiology. *2544*

714.00 **Rheumatoid Arthritis**   Above normal titers may occur. *1752*

714.30 **Juvenile Rheumatoid Arthritis**   Increased in 50% of cases. *0793*

Antithrombin III

Plasma   Decrease

155.00 **Malignant Neoplasm of Liver**   Decreased in parenchymatous liver disease. *2353 1482*

199.00 **Secondary Malignant Neoplasm (Disseminated)**   Seen with carcinoma. *2353 1482*

205.10 **Myelocytic Leukemia (Chronic)**   Below normal in some patients. *2318*

238.40 **Polycythemia Vera**   Below normal in some patients. *2318*

250.00 **Diabetes Mellitus**   Reports of increased and decreased levels. *2353 1482*

286.60 **Disseminated Intravascular Coagulopathy**   Early and significant decreases occur and therefore this may serve as a useful diagnostic test. *0203 2353*

410.90 **Acute Myocardial Infarction**   Found to be significantly diminished when measured by the Von Kaulla Method; otherwise found to show a significant increase 3 months after an acute ischemic episode. *1438*   Significant decrease. *1724*

451.90 **Phlebitis and Thrombophlebitis**   Significant decrease. *2025*

570.00 **Acute and Subacute Necrosis of Liver**   Decreased in parenchymatous liver disease. *2353 1482*

571.49 **Chronic Active Hepatitis**   Decreased in parenchymatous liver disease. *2353 1482*

571.90 **Cirrhosis of Liver**   Decreased. *2353 1482*

577.00 **Acute Pancreatitis**   In both survivors (n = 10) and fatal cases (n = 4) a high frequency of reduced values were found during the first week after admission. Values were significantly more reduced in the fatal cases. *0004*

581.90 **Nephrotic Syndrome**   In infants this has been suggested to explain hypercoagulability. *1437 2353   1482*   Greatly reduced concentration and activity. *2420*

642.40 **Pre-Eclampsia**   Noted in one patient with severe pre-eclampsia toxemia. *0312*

650.00 **Pregnancy**   Last trimester and early postpartum. *2353 1482*

714.00 **Rheumatoid Arthritis**   No significant correlation between low levels and thromboembolic disease. *0238*

Plasma   Increase

250.00 **Diabetes Mellitus**   Reports of increased and decreased levels. *2353 1482*

410.90 **Acute Myocardial Infarction**   Found to be significantly diminished when measured by the Von Kaulla Method; otherwise found to show a significant increase 3 months after an acute ischemic episode. *1438*

573.30 **Toxic Hepatitis**   Elevated in the acute hepatitis following renal transplantation. *1482 2353*

Plasma   Normal

250.00 **Diabetes Mellitus**   Normal levels seen with diabetic nephropathy. *0365*

Antithrombin Titer

Blood   Decrease

415.10 **Pulmonary Embolism and Infarction**   About 2% of venous thromboembolism is due to antithrombin III deficiency. *1108*

451.90 **Phlebitis and Thrombophlebitis**   About 2% of venous thromboembolism is due to antithrombin III deficiency. *1108*

Antithyroglobulin Antibodies

Serum   Increase

155.00 **Malignant Neoplasm of Liver**   Rare. *1736*

193.00 **Malignant Neoplasm of Thyroid Gland**   In 20% of cases. *0058*

242.90 **Hyperthyroidism**   High incidence reflects focal toxicity in the gland and correlates with the development of postoperative hypothyroidism. *2612*   Patients with Graves' disease often have some or all of the thyroid autoantibodies of Hashimoto's disease. *2035*

244.90 **Hypothyroidism**   May be detected in high titer if due to thyroiditis. *2612*   Found in 50% of cases of myxedema. *0058*

245.10 **Subacute Thyroiditis**   Circulating thyroid antibodies are present in low titer in a minority of cases and disappear when disease subsides. *2540*

245.20 **Hashimoto's Thyroiditis**   May be detected in high titer. *2612*   Characteristically present in high titer during the active phase of chronic thyroiditis. *0999*   Almost all patients have thyroid autoantibodies in their serum, and extremely high titers of any of the autoantibodies are inconsistent with most other diagnoses. *2035*   In over 80% of cases. *0058*   In most patients present in high titers (> 1:25,000 in tanned red cell test). Young patients may have low titers of autoantibodies. *2540*

273.30 **Waldenström's Macroglobulinemia**   Rare. *2373*

281.00 **Pernicious Anemia**   In 25% of cases. *0058*

358.00 **Myasthenia Gravis**   Serum contains at least one form of antithyroid antibody. *2035*

535.00 **Gastritis**   With atrophic gastritis. *2199*

571.90 **Cirrhosis of Liver**   Increased incidence of antithyroid antibodies. *1115   2238*

710.20 **Sjögren's Syndrome**   Rare. *0061*

Serum   Normal

585.00 **Chronic Renal Failure**   *1617*

Apolipoprotein AI

Serum   Decrease

38.00 **Septicemia**   Sepsis causes the concentration to decrease. *0049*

256.30 **Ovarian Hypofunction**   Estrogen effect. *0995*

272.22 **Type III Hyperlipoproteinemia**   There is generally a decrease in alpha and beta lipoproteins. *0774*   An excess of lipoproteins with beta mobility but abnormally low density. *0772*   Decreased concentration of both low and high density lipoproteins. *1631*   Slight to moderately decreased. *2246*

272.31 **Type I Hyperlipoproteinemia**   There is generally a decrease in alpha and beta lipoproteins in hyperlipoproteinemia. *0774*   Decreased concentration of both low and high density lipoproteins. *1631   0772*

272.32 Type V Hyperlipoproteinemia Reduced pools of alpha and beta lipoproteins. *2177* In severe affected patients. *2246*

272.51 Tangier Disease Almost none. *0151* Congenital absence or gross reduction. *0619 2467* Electrophoretically absent, irrespective of the medium used. *2246*

414.00 Chronic Ischemic Heart Disease In each major study group mean high density lipoproteins were lower in persons with coronary heart disease than in those without the disease. The average difference was small--typically 3-4 mg/dL -- but statistically significant. *0357*

440.00 Arteriosclerosis Patients with angiographically documented coronary artery disease were found to have elevated levels of Apolipoprotein B and decreased levels of A-I or A-II compared with individuals without the disease. *2221 1935 2241* An excellent predictor of this condition. *2330*

571.49 Chronic Active Hepatitis The levels of prebeta and alpha lipoprotein were decreased. *0710*

571.60 Biliary Cirrhosis Low in patients with cholestatic liver disease. *0750* In 4 female patients compared with 6 age and sex matched controls. *0127*

571.90 Cirrhosis of Liver Prebeta and alpha lipoprotein were decreased. *0710*

581.90 Nephrotic Syndrome Untreated uncomplicated nephrotic syndrome is characterized by increased low (beta) and very low (prebeta) density lipoproteins and a diminution of high density (alpha) lipoprotein. Changes correlated strictly with albumin concentrat were more pronounced with albumin concentration < 20 g/L. *0833* In severe, fully developed cases, increase in low density lipoproteins with normal or decreased alpha lipoproteins has been described. *0962*

Serum   Increase

256.00 Ovarian Hyperfunction Estrogen effect. *0995*

272.00 Type IIA Hyperlipoproteinemia *2246*

272.52 Abetalipoproteinemia Highly variable. *2246*

303.90 Alcoholism Higher in drinkers than in control subjects. *1864*

496.01 Alpha₁-Antitrypsin Deficiency In patients with liver disease all apolipoproteins were elevated. *0563*

Serum   Normal

272.52 Abetalipoproteinemia *0878*

714.00 Rheumatoid Arthritis In 54 female patients found to be in normal range. *1435*

Apolipoprotein AII

Plasma   Decrease

440.00 Arteriosclerosis Patients with angiographically documented coronary artery disease were found to have elevated levels of Apolipoprotein B and decreased levels of A-I or A-II compared with individuals without the disease. *2221 1935 2241*

571.60 Biliary Cirrhosis Low in patients with cholestatic liver disease. *0750* In 4 female patients compared with 6 age and sex matched controls. *0127*

Plasma   Increase

303.90 Alcoholism Higher in drinkers (+45%) than in control subjects. *1864*

496.01 Alpha₁-Antitrypsin Deficiency In patients with liver disease all apolipoproteins were elevated. *0563*

Apolipoprotein B

Serum   Decrease

38.00 Septicemia Sepsis causes the concentration to decrease. *0049*

272.52 Abetalipoproteinemia *0062*

Serum   Increase

414.00 Chronic Ischemic Heart Disease Patients with Coronary Artery Disease had increased levels. *1505*

440.00 Arteriosclerosis Patients with angiographically documented coronary artery disease were found to have elevated levels of Apolipoprotein B and decreased levels of A-I or A-II compared with individuals without the disease. *2221 1935 2241*

496.01 Alpha₁-Antitrypsin Deficiency In patients with liver disease all apolipoproteins were elevated. *0563*

Apolipoprotein E

Plasma   Decrease

571.60 Biliary Cirrhosis Low in patients with cholestatic liver disease. *0750*

Arginine

Plasma   Decrease

585.00 Chronic Renal Failure Children with mild renal insufficiency showed a significant decrease in tyrosine and arginine. *0192*

714.00 Rheumatoid Arthritis Frequently low. *2104*

Urine   Increase

270.01 Cystinuria Characteristic. *2246*

270.03 Cystinosis Nonspecific pattern of aminoaciduria. Fanconi's syndrome. *0995*

Arsenic

Urine   Increase

985.00 Toxic Effects of Non-medicinal Metals Patients with chronic arsenic poisoning excrete 0.1 mg/day of arsenic. Normal values average 0.015 mg/day. *0151*

Arylsulfatase

Serum   Decrease

330.00 Metachromatic Leukodystrophy Most types of leukodystrophy are associated with a basic deficiency in arylsulfatase A. *2246* Heterozygote carriers for metachromatic leukodystrophy have leukocyte arylsulfatase A concentrations of 40-60% of normal range. Patients with disease showed levels only 20% of normal value. *1190*

Serum   Increase

205.00 Myelocytic Leukemia (Acute) 30-50% increase in serum activity. *0610*

205.10 Myelocytic Leukemia (Chronic) 30-50% increase in serum activity. *0610*

494.00 Bronchiectasis 30-50% increase in activity. *0610*

580.00 Acute Poststreptococcal Glomerulonephritis 30-50% increase in activity. *0610*

650.00 Pregnancy *0919 2182* 30-50% increase in serum activity *0610*

Urine   Increase

11.00 Pulmonary Tuberculosis Considerable increase. *0610*

18.00 Disseminated Tuberculosis Considerable increase in urinary activity in pulmonary and renal tuberculosis. *1890* *0610*

153.90 Malignant Neoplasm of Large Intestine Urinary arylsulfatase B was observed in high concentrations in patients with colon carcinoma. Increased activity correlated with the extent of disease. Elevations were observed in only 28% of patients with Dukes' A disease. 55% of those with Dukes' B, and in more than 75% of patients with Dukes' C and D lesions. *2093*

188.90 Malignant Neoplasm of Bladder Up to 40-fold increase in urinary activity. *0610* Arylsulfatase A (100%) and B (82.8%) were elevated in 29 cases of active disease. *1843*

192.50 Neuroblastoma Urine arylsulfatase and homovanillic acid are inversely related in neuroblastomas. In melanotic tumors, HVA is elevated and arylsulfatase normal or slightly elevated. Amelanotic tumors have low-normal HVA and high arylsulfatase. *1630*

Arylsulfatase *(continued)*

Ascitic Fluid   Increase

577.00 **Acute Pancreatitis**   Varied from 89-5170 pmol/min/mL. *0827*

Liver   Decrease

330.00 **Metachromatic Leukodystrophy**   Just at the limit of detection in 8 patients with metachromatic leukodystrophy. *2246*

Ascorbic Acid

Serum   Decrease

242.90 **Hyperthyroidism**   Secondary to increased metabolic processes. *2540*

267.00 **Vitamin C Deficiency**   Plasma level of ascorbic acid is decreased--usually 0 in frank scurvy. Normal is 0.5-1.5 mg/dL but lower level does not prove diagnosis. *2468*   Not reliable for diagnostic purposes because tissue levels vary widely. Ascorbic acid assay of the buffy coat for the WBC and platelet count of this vitamin is more helpful, the normal level being 20-30 mg/dL. In latent or overt deficiency, this level falls to 0-2 mg/dL. *0433*

579.90 **Malabsorption, Cause Unspecified**   In steatorrhea. *0211*

650.00 **Pregnancy**   May be decreased, reaching lowest level in the postpartum period. *0211*

Serum   Normal

579.00 **Celiac Sprue Disease**   *2238*

Asparagine

Urine   Increase

270.02 **Hartnup Disease**   5-20 X normal values. *2246*   *0995*

270.03 **Cystinosis**   Nonspecific pattern of aminoaciduria. Fanconi's syndrome. *0995*

Aspartate Aminotransferase

Serum   Decrease

84.00 **Malaria**   Activity was increased in 11 patients untreated for more than 4 days. *2066*   May be elevated. *0962*

650.00 **Pregnancy**   Abnormal pyridoxal metabolism. Usual values 0-3 U/L. *0503*

Serum   Increase

2.00 **Typhoid Fever**   Frequently seen due to complications. *2468*

6.00 **Amebiasis**   With liver involvement. *1058*

11.00 **Pulmonary Tuberculosis**   In 35% of 26 patients at initial hospitalization for this disorder. *0781*

18.00 **Disseminated Tuberculosis**   In 5 cases of granuloma of liver, 100% were mildly elevated, showing a mean elevation of 36 U/L over the normal maximum limit of 24 U/L. *1452*

23.00 **Brucellosis**   In 5 cases of granuloma of liver, 100% were mildly elevated, showing a mean elevation of 36 U/L over the normal maximum limit of 24 U/L. *1452*

37.00 **Tetanus**   Mainly in the more severe cases. *0433*   Elevation occurred in 2 of 5 cases. *1677*

38.00 **Septicemia**   Elevations observed in 6 cases of extrahepatic sepsis. *1681*   In 27% of 11 patients at initial hospitalization for this disorder. *0781*

45.90 **Acute Poliomyelitis**   A mild rise was reported in all 8 cases. *1677*

53.00 **Herpes Zoster**   In 36% of 18 patients at initial hospitalization for this disorder. *0781*

60.00 **Yellow Fever**   Activity was above normal in all sera tested, the degree of increase approximately proportional to the severity of disease. *1179*

70.00 **Viral Hepatitis**   Striking elevations (145-200 U/L) are seen in patients with acute hepatic necrosis. *0503*   May be elevated 2-4 weeks before the onset of jaundice and may reach peak levels after 1-2 weeks. Reflects organelle injury rather than necrosis or alteration of the permeability of the plasma membrane. *0433*   In 92% of 25 patients at initial hospitalization for this disorder. *0781 0999 0962*

73.90 **Psittacosis**   With severe liver involvement. *0433*

75.00 **Infectious Mononucleosis**   In 80% of patients moderate (50-300 U/L) increases are observed. Usual values 25-400 U/L. *0503*   Elevations occur in 80-100% during acute illness and return to normal in 3-5 weeks. *2538*   In 90% of 11 patients at initial hospitalization for this disorder. *0781   0812 1912 0962*

78.50 **Cytomegalic Inclusion Disease**   Slight increase which becomes more marked with clinical hepatitis in some cases. *2468*

82.00 **Rocky Mountain Spotted Fever**   Common. *0433*

84.00 **Malaria**   Moderate increase. *2468*

99.10 **Lymphogranuloma Venereum**   May indicate severe liver impairment. *0433*

100.00 **Leptospirosis**   Increased in 50% of the patients but average levels are not as high as in hepatitis. *2468*   Values are rarely increased more than 2-3 X normal regardless of the degree of hyperbilirubinemia. *0151*   Elevated in patients without clinically evident liver disease. *0962*

104.10 **Lyme Disease**   May be elevated in Lyme Disease if mild hepatic involvement persists. *2639*

115.00 **Histoplasmosis**   Present in 70% of patients with disseminated disease. *0999*   In 5 cases of granuloma of liver, 100% were mildly elevated, showing a mean elevation of 36 U/L over the normal maximum limit of 24 U/L. *1452*

120.00 **Schistosomiasis**   Markedly increased without concomitant elevation of ALT. Remains elevated from admission, through nitridazole treatment, and at follow-up 1 month later. *2026*   May be mild elevations, but jaundice is uncommon. *0962*   In 5 cases of granuloma of liver, 100% were mildly elevated, showing a mean elevation of 36 U/L over the normal maximum limit of 24 U/L. *1452*

122.90 **Hydatidosis**   With liver involvement. *1058*

124.00 **Trichinosis**   Moderate to marked. *0503*   During the acute stage. *0962*

135.00 **Sarcoidosis**   In 36% of 24 patients at initial hospitalization for this disorder. *0781*   In 5 cases of granuloma of liver, 100% were mildly elevated, showing a mean elevation of 36 U/L over the normal maximum limit of 24 U/L. *1452*

150.90 **Malignant Neoplasm of Esophagus**   In 41% of 40 patients at initial hospitalization for this disorder. *0781*

151.90 **Malignant Neoplasm of Stomach**   In 28% of 47 patients at initial hospitalization for this disorder. *0781*

155.00 **Malignant Neoplasm of Liver**   Levels may be 10-100 X normal and remain elevated for long periods. *0812*   Elevated from 2-5 X the normal level in 66-70% of patients with primary carcinoma. *0029*   Elevated in 80%. *0364*   Over 10% above normal upper limit in 83.3% of 66 hepatoma patients. *1115*   In 98% of 12 patients at initial hospitalization for this disorder. *0781*

155.10 **Malignant Neoplasm of Intrahepatic Bile Ducts**   May be slightly elevated, but rarely higher than 200 U/L. *0151*

157.90 **Malignant Neoplasm of Pancreas**   Slight elevation occurred in 2 of 4 cases. Range of values was 12.5-45, while the maximum upper limit of normal is 24 U/L. *1452*   63% of patients showed elevated values. *0932*   In 74% of 46 patients at initial hospitalization for this disorder. *0781*

162.90 **Malignant Neoplasm of Bronchus and Lung**   Becomes elevated only shortly before death. In most cases, elevated values indicate the presence of metastases. *0819*

170.90 **Malignant Neoplasm of Bone**   In 32% of 25 patients at initial hospitalization for this disorder. *0781*

174.90 **Malignant Neoplasm of Breast**   In 25% of 296 patients at initial hospitalization for this disorder. *0781*

185.00 **Malignant Neoplasm of Prostate**   In 25% of 86 patients at initial hospitalization for this disorder. *0781*

191.90 **Malignant Neoplasm of Brain**   In occasional cases. *2467*   In 33% of 24 patients at initial hospitalization for this disorder. *0781*

193.01 **Medullary Carcinoma of Thyroid**   In 31% of 22 patients at initial hospitalization for this disorder. *0781*

197.00 **Secondary Malignant Neoplasm of Respiratory System**   In 48% of 592 patients at initial hospitalization for this disorder. *0781*

197.70 **Secondary Malignant Neoplasm of Liver** Approximately 50% of patients with metastatic carcinoma have elevated values, usually in the same range as patients with cirrhosis and posthepatic jaundice. Usual values < 145 U/L. *0503* All 12 cases of liver metastases showed a moderate elevation (mean = 106). Normal upper limit 24 U/L. *1452* *0962*

201.90 **Hodgkin's Disease** Minimal elevation was observed in 5 of 11 patients. *0160* May be a systemic sign of active disease or may indicate involvement of liver or bone. *0433*

202.80 **Non-Hodgkins Lymphoma** May be a systemic sign of active disease or may indicate involvement of liver or bone. *0433* In 24% of 72 patients at initial hospitalization for this disorder. *0781*

203.00 **Multiple Myeloma** In 45% of 33 patients at initial hospitalization for this disorder. *0781*

204.00 **Lymphocytic Leukemia (Acute)** Infiltration of the liver. *0619* Moderately elevated levels are observed in lymphomas and leukemia but less frequently than in other hepatic disease. *0503* In 71% of 43 patients at initial hospitalization for this disorder. *0781*

204.10 **Lymphocytic Leukemia (Chronic)** Moderately elevated levels are observed in lymphomas and leukemia but less frequently than in other hepatic disease. *0503* In 27% of 27 patients at initial hospitalization for this disorder. *0781*

205.00 **Myelocytic Leukemia (Acute)** Moderately elevated levels are observed in lymphomas and leukemia but less frequently than in other hepatic disease. *0503* In 37% of 36 patients at initial hospitalization for this disorder. *0781*

205.10 **Myelocytic Leukemia (Chronic)** Infiltration of the liver. *0619* Moderately elevated levels are observed in lymphomas and leukemia but less frequently than in other hepatic disease. *0503* Less elevation than in acute leukemia. *2468* In 54% of 21 patients at initial hospitalization for this disorder. *0781*

206.00 **Monocytic Leukemia** In 63% of 23 patients at initial hospitalization for this disorder. *0781*

212.70 **Benign Neoplasm of Cardiovascular Tissue** May reflect many small emboli to striated muscle. *2467*

225.90 **Benign Neoplasm of Brain and CNS** In 31% of 22 patients at initial hospitalization for this disorder. *0781*

242.90 **Hyperthyroidism** A slight rise in mean activity over the normal with hepatic dysfunction (mean 13.5, normal = 11.1). *1320*

244.90 **Hypothyroidism** The muscle involvement of this disease appears to be responsible for the elevation. *0503* May be elevated. *0433* In 58% of 13 patients at initial hospitalization for this disorder. *0781*

245.10 **Subacute Thyroiditis** *0151*

250.00 **Diabetes Mellitus** Of 200 untreated diabetics, 12% had unexplainable elevations. *0873*

250.10 **Diabetic Acidosis** Mild-moderate abnormalities may occur in 20-65% of patients but bears no relation to degree of abdominal pain or prognosis. *1316* In some instances, mostly in severe cases, especially with severe circulatory failure and liver enlargement. *0155*

271.02 **McArdle's Disease** Slight to moderate increase. *0503*

271.03 **Forbes Disease** There may be some mild abnormalities of liver function. Elevations of AST and ALT are common, especially in Type III. *0433*

271.10 **Galactosemia** Deranged liver function. *2246*

271.20 **Hereditary Fructose Intolerance** Marked rise was noted within 1.5 h after a single large dose of fructose. *2246*

272.71 **Anderson's Disease** Liver involvement. *2246*

272.73 **Niemann-Pick Disease** Seen in type B disease. *2246*

274.00 **Gout** Increased levels have been reported in acute stages. *0619*

275.00 **Hemochromatosis** With liver involvement. *0962*

275.10 **Hepatolenticular Degeneration** Minimally elevated in 36% (14 of 39 patients). Mean = 30 U/L. *2278*

275.34 **Familial Periodic Paralysis** Occasional patients with paramyotonia congenita. *0760*

276.20 **Metabolic Acidosis** In type II-B, with lactic acidosis. *2468*

277.00 **Cystic Fibrosis** In 56% of 12 patients at initial hospitalization for this disorder. *0781* With liver involvement. *1235*

277.16 **Porphyria Cutanea Tarda** Liver function is highly variable. May be mildly elevated. *2552*

277.30 **Amyloidosis** Elevated in > 33% of patients with primary disease. *1334*

277.41 **Dubin-Johnson Syndrome** May be normal or moderately increased. *0602*

282.00 **Hereditary (Congenital) Spherocytosis** *0962*

282.41 **Thalassemia Major** Usually elevated. *2552*

283.00 **Acquired Hemolytic Anemia (Autoimmune)** *0962*

291.00 **Delirium Tremens** Irrespective of associated hepatic disease and may arise in muscle. *0503* *0962*

297.90 **Paranoid States and Other Psychoses** In 39% of 33 patients hospitalized for this disorder. *0781*

303.90 **Alcoholism** 60% of 5 cases showed mild elevation, with a mean = 16 X the normal upper limit. *1452* 73% of 182 male chronic alcoholics had raised activities. Highest values were found after 5-20 y of confirmed alcoholism. Patients with 20 y duration displayed a tendency to normalization of activities. *2196* In 66% of 13 patients hospitalized for this disorder. *0781*

304.90 **Drug Dependence (Opium and Derivatives)** This and other liver function tests are usually increased in 75% of patients. *2468*

320.90 **Meningitis (Bacterial)** In 70% of 14 patients hospitalized for this disorder. *0781*

330.00 **Metachromatic Leukodystrophy** Invariable in initial phases of disease. Diminishes to normal range by 4th year. *0077*

331.81 **Reye's Syndrome** 2-300 times normal values. *0416* Reflects hepatic damage *0151* High serum transaminases *0962*

335.11 **Familial Progressive Spinal Muscular Atrophy** Elevations of serum enzymes are frequently encountered but never reach the magnitude seen in Duchenne muscular dystrophy. *0433*

359.11 **Progressive Muscular Dystrophy** Released from breaking down muscle. Levels tend to be increased in affected young children. *0503 0433* May have elevated levels. Usual values 145 U/L. *0503* A marked increase in CK, LD, and AST was noted. 21 of 23 cases showed moderate-high levels of AST ranging from 24-105 U/L. *1677* *0962*

359.21 **Myotonia Atrophica** Slight to moderate increase. *0503* Usually normal or minimally elevated. *0433* Increased in about 15% of the patients. *2467*

359.22 **Myotonia Congenita** Slight to moderate increase. *0503*

390.00 **Rheumatic Fever** The incidence and mechanism of occurrence is not clear. Usual values < 50 U/L. *0503* May occur as a result of chronic passive congestion in congestive heart failure or as a result of hepatotoxicity following salicylate therapy. *0962* Serum level related to severity in the early stages. *0619*

401.10 **Essential Benign Hypertension** In 29% of 101 patients hospitalized for this disorder. *0781*

415.10 **Pulmonary Embolism and Infarction** Rises later and slower than after cardiac infarction. Possibly related to associated congestive failure. *0619* Characterized by increased LD and usually by normal AST values. Incidence of elevation has varied from 0-30% and the elevations are slight to moderate. The rise is delayed for 3-5 days after onset of pain. *2467* In a small proportion of patients with this disease slightly elevated values occur by 3 or 4 days after the bout of chest pain. *0503* Slight increase. *0962* *2474 1748*

420.00 **Acute Pericarditis** 50% incidence of slightly elevated values reported. Usual values < 48.2 U/L. *0503* Modest elevations occur. This is especially likely to happen when pericardial effusion produces venous hypertension and hepatic congestion. *1108* *0962*

422.00 **Acute Myocarditis** Marked elevation signals a poor prognosis. *1108*

425.40 **Cardiomyopathies** Increased, often to extremely high levels; these may rise even further after recovery from shock in cobalt beer cardiomyopathy. *2467*

428.00 **Congestive Heart Failure** Usually < 100 U/L. *0503* Depending on the severity and chronicity of cardiac failure. *0433* Mild elevation occurred in 33% of 9 cases, levels ranged from 11-39, with the maximum upper limit of normal at 24 U/L. *1452*

434.00 **Cerebral Thrombosis** Increased the following week in 50% of cases. *2467* Values may be up to 50 U/L. *0503*

434.10 **Cerebral Embolism** Increased the following week in 50% of cases. *0619* Values may be up to 50 U/L. *0503*

434.90 **Brain Infarction** Increased the following week in 50% of cases. *0619* Values may be up to 50 U/L. *0503* *0962*

441.00 **Dissecting Aortic Aneurysm** Not helpful since modest elevations may occur in both dissection and infarction. *1108*

444.90 **Arterial Embolism and Thrombosis** In 38% of 37 patients hospitalized for this disorder. *0781*

451.90 **Phlebitis and Thrombophlebitis** In 25% of 51 patients at initial hospitalization for this disorder. *0781*

480.90 **Viral Pneumonia** In 80% of 10 patients at initial hospitalization for this disorder. *0781*

Aspartate Aminotransferase (continued)

Serum Increase (continued)

482.90 Bacterial Pneumonia In 54% of 18 patients at initial hospitalization for this disorder. 0781

486.01 Resolving Pneumonia In 40% of 65 patients at initial hospitalization for this disorder. 0781

487.10 Influenza Usually elevated. 0962

493.10 Asthma (Intrinsic) Possibly due to anoxic tissue damage in status asthmaticus. 0619 Increased in 90% of acute untreated asthma patients. 1228

496.01 Alpha₁-Antitrypsin Deficiency Related to liver disease. 1636

535.00 Gastritis In 33% of 37 patients at initial hospitalization for this disorder. 0781

555.90 Regional Enteritis or Ileitis Due to associated liver disease. 0218 Liver abnormalities are common 0995

556.00 Ulcerative Colitis With liver involvement. 0433

557.01 Mesenteric Artery Embolism After intestinal infarction. 0619 2467 0433

560.90 Intestinal Obstruction In 33% of 42 patients at initial hospitalization for this disorder. 0781

570.00 Acute and Subacute Necrosis of Liver In liver diseases, may be 10-100 X normal and remain elevated for long periods of time. 0619 0812 Higher in acute hepatitis than in obstructive jaundice. 0503 Mean elevation in 17 cases of hepatitis was 36.5 X the normal upper limit (24 U/L). All patients showed elevation, mean = 766 U/L. 1452

571.20 Laennec's or Alcoholic Cirrhosis Consistently elevated and higher than ALT activity. 2576 50-145 U/L. 0999

571.49 Chronic Active Hepatitis Usually increased (up to 10 X normal range). 2467 Continuing or phasic release of transaminase enzymes from damaged liver cells, depending upon the degree of hepatocellular necrosis: serum concentrations range from 145-500 U/L during exacerbations. 1922 Mild elevation. 0962 In 97% of 18 patients at initial hospitalization for this disorder. 0781 2035

571.60 Biliary Cirrhosis Modest elevations (usually < 145 U/L). 0503 Hepatocellular necrosis is slight as judged by low serum transaminase levels, and hepatocellular function is well preserved. 2035 Usually only mildly elevated. 0962

571.90 Cirrhosis of Liver 60-70% incidence of elevated levels. Up to 145 U/L in 65-75% of cases. 2467 Mild elevation occurred in 86% of 6 cases. Mean elevation was 2 X normal upper limit. 1452 In 89% of 69 patients at initial hospitalization for this disorder. 0781 0503 0962 2576

572.00 Liver Abscess (Pyogenic) May exhibit a mild to moderate elevation. 0433 Both rise during preicteric phase to peaks 240 U/L) by the time jaundice appears; then rapid fall in several days; become normal 2-5 weeks after onset of jaundice. 2467

572.40 Hepatic Failure May be normal or increased. 0503

573.30 Toxic Hepatitis Elevations of ALT reflects acute hepatic disease somewhat more specifically than is true of AST. 0503 Usual values seen: 240-1,900 U/L. Values > 145 U/L are usual and > 240 are frequent. 0503 Concentration depend upon severity. In severe cases, (especially carbon tetrachloride poisoning), serum enzymes may be 10-20 X higher than in acute hepatitis and show a different pattern (i.e., increase in LD > AST > ALT). 2467 Elevations in toxic hepatitis due to carbon tetrachloride exposure occur within 24 h and may reach peaks of up to 13,000 U/L. Other toxins (chlorpromazine, salicylates, azaserine, and pyrazinamide) will 2577

575.00 Acute Cholecystitis May be increased in 75% of patients. 2467 In 8 cases, 4 showed moderate elevation. The mean value for the group was 38 U/L, while the normal upper limit was 24 U/L. 1452 Occasionally increased. 0995 May be mildly elevated even in the absence of intrahepatic infection or common bile duct obstruction. 2199 In 57% of 15 patients at initial hospitalization for this disorder. 0781

576.10 Cholangitis With parenchymal cell necrosis and malfunction. 2467 Mean elevation of 48 U/L, twice the normal upper limit, was found in 13 cases. 77% of the patients had elevated levels. 1452 Usually remaining < 100 U/L, but values of 240 are found, followed by a sharp drop within 48 h. 0151 In 70% of 10 patients at initial hospitalization for this disorder. 0781

576.20 Extrahepatic Biliary Obstruction Up to 145 U/L; returns to normal within 1 week after obstruction is relieved. 2467 Increased activity in all cases of biliary tract obstruction. Common duct obstruction due to stones, pancreatitis, tumor, duct carcinoma, and leukemia nodes showed values of 31-193 U/L. 2576 0962

577.00 Acute Pancreatitis No apparent correlation with damage to pancreas, serum lipase, amylase, or calcium, but there is direct correlation with the serum bilirubin level suggesting increase due to biliary obstruction. 0619 Both normal and elevated levels have been reported. Usual values = 20-700 U/L. 2467 0503 Mild elevation (mean = 36.2 U/L) in 80% of 10 cases (normal maximum = 24 U/L). 1452 In 87% of 21 patients at initial hospitalization for this disorder. 0781 0962

577.10 Chronic Pancreatitis In 48% of 12 patients at initial hospitalization for this disorder. 0781 2199

584.00 Acute Renal Failure In 63% of 11 patients at initial hospitalization for this disorder. 0781

590.10 Acute Pyelonephritis In 28% of 14 patients at initial hospitalization for this disorder. 0781

593.81 Renal Infarction In unilateral renal arterial infarction. Reaches a peak within several days then gradually falls. 2104 Increased if area of infarction is large; peaks by 2nd day; returns to normal by 5th day with arterial infarction of kidney. 2468

601.00 Prostatitis In 26% of 15 patients at initial hospitalization for this disorder. 0781

642.40 Pre-Eclampsia In about 20% of patients with mild cases. 0387 Degree of abnormality closely parallels the severity. 0472 2311 1635

642.60 Eclampsia Degree of abnormality closely parallels the severity. 1635 0472 Presumably due to ischemic damage to liver cells. 0322

710.00 Systemic Lupus Erythematosus May be found in patients with myositis. 0433

710.10 Progressive Systemic Sclerosis Moderate to marked increase with associated myositis. 0503

710.40 Dermatomyositis/Polymyositis May be increased in the absence of clinical evidence of muscle wasting. Steroid therapy causes the level to fall towards normal. 0619 Moderate to marked increase. Usual values < 145 U/L. 0503 Elevated at some time in nearly every patient. 0244 Released as a result of destructive myopathy. Almost invariably elevated in the acute or subacute stages. 1791 2035 0962

714.00 Rheumatoid Arthritis Characteristically abnormal when the arthritis is active. 0433

714.30 Juvenile Rheumatoid Arthritis Transiently but only moderately elevated in many children receiving high dosages of aspirin; decreases to normal as the dosage of salicylates is lowered. 0433 Mild elevation is common in untreated and aspirin-treated children but increases are sporadic. 1870

715.90 Osteoarthritis In 23% of 120 patients at initial hospitalization for this disorder. 0781

730.00 Osteomyelitis In 36% of 25 patients at initial hospitalization for this disorder. 0781

785.40 Gangrene May produce slight elevations. Usual values 50 U/L. 0503 In 27% of 32 patients hospitalized for this disorder. 0781 Found with extensive necrosis 0186 0962

785.50 Shock Usual values 20-900 U/L. 0503

791.30 Myoglobinuria 0619 2467

929.00 Crush Injury (Trauma) Slightly to moderate increase. 0503 0619 0962

948.00 Burns Rises soon after burn. 2104

985.00 Toxic Effects of Non-medicinal Metals Hepatotoxicity may occur with arsenicals. 1446

986.00 Toxic Effects of Carbon Monoxide From skeletal muscle, heart muscle, and brain. 0619

989.50 Toxic Effects of Venom Elevated in 9 of 17 patients admitted for wasp/bee stings. 1822 0619

990.00 Effects of X-Ray Irradiation May be increased in cases of radiation injury, indicating major cell and tissue damage. 0151 2467 0619

991.60 Hypothermia 21 of 25 patients with accidental hypothermia had raised values. 1472 Due to hypoxia, acid-base imbalance hypotension. 1471

992.00 Heat stroke Following severe heat stroke. *0619* Increased (mean = 20 X normal) peaks on 3rd day and returns to normal in 2 weeks. Very high levels are often associated with lethal outcome. *2468* In a case of malignant hyperpyrexia, the initial elevation (after 3 h) of 110 U/L was due to muscle damage. Later elevations (12-24 h) was 1,600 and 3,440 U/L reflected damage of the liver. *0541*

994.50 Exercise Three well-trained men ran 100 km at a slow speed. After the race the clinical state was good and EKG were normal, but all three subjects had a significant rise in LD, AST, and CK. *2076* Marked increase after strenuous exercise, less in trained individuals. *1930*

994.80 Effects of Electric Current Indicates severe tissue damage. *2468* Trauma following direct current countershock to convert arrhythmia to normal rhythm (from intercostal muscle damage. *0619*

Serum Normal

238.40 Polycythemia Vera Normal in uncomplicated cases. *1379 2538*

271.01 Von Gierke's Disease Liver may be massively enlarged but liver function tests are normal. *2246*

272.31 Type I Hyperlipoproteinemia *2246*

275.00 Hemochromatosis Over 50% of patients have no laboratory evidence of liver dysfunction. *0995*

277.30 Amyloidosis Usually normal. *0125*

277.41 Dubin-Johnson Syndrome Routine liver function tests are normal. *0962*

277.42 Gilbert's Disease *0995*

277.43 Rotor's Syndrome Routine liver function tests are normal. *0962*

277.44 Crigler-Najjar Syndrome Liver function tests were uniformly normal. *2246   0469*

333.40 Huntington's Chorea No abnormalities in 8 patients. *0534*

358.00 Myasthenia Gravis *2057*

359.21 Myotonia Atrophica Usually normal in myotonic dystrophy. *2246*

413.90 Angina Pectoris *2467*

441.00 Dissecting Aortic Aneurysm Unless complications occur. *2467*

446.50 Cranial Arteritis and Related Conditions *0186*

482.90 Bacterial Pneumonia *2467*

572.00 Liver Abscess (Pyogenic) Transaminase levels are often normal in the absence of biliary tract infections in acute liver abscess. *0151*

642.40 Pre-Eclampsia Usually are not elevated. When elevated, either pronounced hepatic or marked myocardial alterations have occurred. *0433*

650.00 Pregnancy Incidence of abnormal findings is < 5%. *0387 2359*

714.00 Rheumatoid Arthritis Generally normal. *0962*

992.00 Heat stroke Normal in children. *0548*

994.50 Exercise Insignificant effect after 12 min on cycle ergometer. *0804* Normal after 2 h march. *2092*

CSF Increase

45.90 Acute Poliomyelitis Always increased but does not correlate with serum level or with severity of paralysis; reaches peak in 1 week and returns to normal by 4 weeks. *2468*

198.30 Secondary Malignant Neoplasm of Brain Elevated activities were associated with metastatic carcinoma of CNS. Patients with primary tumors generally showed normal levels. *0507* In all but 2 patients with metastatic tumors of the CNS, the activity was significantly raised. The mean for the group was 20.4 U/L. *0507*

330.00 Metachromatic Leukodystrophy Increased initially, then diminishes. *0078*

431.00 Cerebral Hemorrhage *2467*

434.90 Brain Infarction Increased for some days after infarction or cerebrovascular accident without a corresponding rise in CSF ALT. *0619*

Bacteria

Ascitic Fluid Increase

560.90 Intestinal Obstruction *0186*

Basophilic Stippling

Blood Increase

238.40 Polycythemia Vera May be found. *2552*

281.30 Vitamin B$_6$ Deficiency Anemia Prominent findings on blood smear. *2552*

282.41 Thalassemia Major The red cells show marked anisopoikilocytosiss, with hypochromia, target-cell formation, and a variable degree of basophilic stippling. *2538*

282.42 Thalassemia Minor Mild anemia, usually with microcytosis, hypochromia, stippling, and target cells usually occurs in heterozygous beta thalassemia. *0151*

285.00 Sideroblastic Anemia Prominent findings on blood smear. *2552*

984.00 Toxic Effects of Lead and Its Compounds (including Fumes) Coarse basophilic stippling occurs to an extreme degree, with involvement of up to 1-2% of cells. *2538* Occurs in 60% of childhood cases. *0294*

Basophils

Blood Decrease

242.90 Hyperthyroidism *0532*

289.80 Myelofibrosis *0532*

650.00 Pregnancy *2467 0532*

708.90 Urticaria *0532*

Blood Increase

11.00 Pulmonary Tuberculosis *2538*

50.00 Smallpox *2467*

52.00 Chickenpox *2467*

126.90 Ancylostomiasis (Hookworm Infestation) *2538*

201.90 Hodgkin's Disease *2467*

205.00 Myelocytic Leukemia (Acute) Occasionally. *0992*

205.10 Myelocytic Leukemia (Chronic) Particularly in the stage preceding acute blastic crisis. *0433* Slight to moderate persistent basophilia may occur. Often regarded as a poor prognostic sign. *2538* High absolute number in almost all patients. *2552 0992*

238.40 Polycythemia Vera Usually a mild basophilia. *0433* Increase in the absolute count (above 65/µL) is observed in about 66% of cases. *0840* Slight to moderate persistent basophilia may occur. *2538*

244.90 Hypothyroidism *2467*

250.00 Diabetes Mellitus *2538*

282.00 Hereditary (Congenital) Spherocytosis During the chronic stage of anemia. *0810 2552*

283.00 Acquired Hemolytic Anemia (Autoimmune) Punctate basophilia and normoblastemia are common in severe cases. *2035 2538*

289.80 Myelofibrosis Eosinophilia and basophilia occur in 10-30% of myelofibrosis patients. *2317   0532 2538*

473.90 Chronic Sinusitis *2467*

487.10 Influenza *2538*

556.00 Ulcerative Colitis *2538*

581.90 Nephrotic Syndrome Some cases. *2467*

650.00 Pregnancy *0532*

708.90 Urticaria *0532*

Blood Normal

289.00 Polycythemia, Secondary *2538*

Bone Marrow Increase

205.10 Myelocytic Leukemia (Chronic) May be considerably increased; usually in proportion to their number in the circulating blood. *2538*

Basophils *(continued)*

Bone Marrow Increase *(continued)*

238.40 Polycythemia Vera An unusually high number may be found. *2552*

273.30 Waldenström's Macroglobulinemia Characteristic presence of large numbers of basophils and tissue mast cells interspersed among the other cells. *2552*

Bence-Jones Protein

Serum Present

203.00 Multiple Myeloma Demonstrable in the serum or urine, or both, of over 90% of cases of overt, symptomatic myeloma, it is only the rare case in which there is not an abnormal serum or urinary protein. *2035* Electrophoresis of sera reveals a double spike. *2436*

205.00 Myelocytic Leukemia (Acute) *0619*

205.10 Myelocytic Leukemia (Chronic) *0619*

277.30 Amyloidosis May occur. *0999* Found in 21 of 22 patients with primary disease. *1745*

Urine Absent

273.22 Heavy Chain Disease (Alpha) *2468*

273.23 Heavy Chain Disease (Gamma) *2468*

Urine Present

170.90 Malignant Neoplasm of Bone Uncommon in osteogenic sarcoma. *0619*

202.80 Non-Hodgkins Lymphoma 30-40% of patients. *2478*

203.00 Multiple Myeloma Kappa or lambda light chains with no heavy chains attached found in 26 of 35 patients. 11 excreted large amounts (> 1 g/day). *0518* Demonstrable in the serum or urine, or both, of over 90% of cases of overt, symptomatic myeloma, it is only the rare case in which there is not an abnormal serum or urinary protein. *2035* The amount excreted varies from a few mg to 25-40 g/24h. Found in the urine of 70-80% of patients. *1333* Highly indicative. *2218 2538*

204.00 Lymphocytic Leukemia (Acute) *0619*

204.10 Lymphocytic Leukemia (Chronic) *0619*

238.40 Polycythemia Vera Appears in the urine uncommonly. *0619*

268.20 Osteomalacia *0619*

273.30 Waldenström's Macroglobulinemia Present in approximately 10% of cases, but renal functional impairment is much less common than in myeloma. *2035* Reported to occur in 25% of patients. *2538*

277.30 Amyloidosis Found in 57% of secondary and only 8% of primary cases. *1334* Detected in 6 of 15 cases; excretion was < 1 g/24h in all patients. *0125*

Beta₁A-Globulin

Serum Increase

994.50 Exercise Increases by approximately 14% immediately following. *1837*

Beta₂-Macroglobulin

Serum Decrease

581.90 Nephrotic Syndrome An increase in urine and a decrease in serum levels is seen. *1236 2220*

584.00 Acute Renal Failure An increase in urine and a decrease in serum levels is seen in disorders of renal tubular function. *1236*

585.00 Chronic Renal Failure An increase in urine and a decrease in serum levels is seen in disorders of renal tubular function. *1236*

588.82 Distal Renal Tubular Acidosis An increase in urine and a decrease in serum levels is seen. *1236*

Serum Increase

70.00 Viral Hepatitis An increased serum concentration is characteristic. *1236*

135.00 Sarcoidosis Elevated in 63% of patients. *1773*

201.90 Hodgkin's Disease May be increased. *1236 0388*

202.10 Mycosis Fungoides Compared with healthy controls. *1354* Elevated compared to normal controls *1353*

203.00 Multiple Myeloma Showed the best correlation with survival. May be increased. *1236*

204.00 Lymphocytic Leukemia (Acute) May be increased in leukemia of B-lymphocyte lineage. *1236*

204.10 Lymphocytic Leukemia (Chronic) May be increased in leukemia of B-lymphocyte lineage. *1236* With leukemia of B-lymphocyte lineage *2232*

273.30 Waldenström's Macroglobulinemia Marked increase. *2467*

279.31 Acquired Immunodeficiency Syndrome (AIDS) Elevated > 2.5 mg/L in 29 or 37 patients. *0646* Found frequently. *1318*

286.01 Hemophilia Significantly higher. *1318*

571.49 Chronic Active Hepatitis An increased serum concentration is characteristic. *1236*

571.90 Cirrhosis of Liver *2467*

573.30 Toxic Hepatitis An increased serum concentration is characteristic. *1236*

710.20 Sjögren's Syndrome Often elevated and correlates well with the degree of lymphocytic infiltration seen on biopsy. *2134*

714.00 Rheumatoid Arthritis *2467*

Urine Increase

199.00 Secondary Malignant Neoplasm (Disseminated) 24 h excretion and renal clearance were significantly increased in disseminated carcinoma compared with localized. *1025*

581.90 Nephrotic Syndrome An increase in urine and a decrease in serum levels is seen. *1236*

584.00 Acute Renal Failure An increase in urine and a decrease in serum levels is seen in disorders of renal tubular function. *1236*

585.00 Chronic Renal Failure An increase in urine and a decrease in serum levels is seen in disorders of renal tubular function. *1236*

588.82 Distal Renal Tubular Acidosis An increase in urine and a decrease in serum levels is seen. *1236*

CSF Increase

201.90 Hodgkin's Disease May be increased in lymphomas involving the central nervous system. *1236* With Involvement of the CNS *0388*

202.80 Non-Hodgkins Lymphoma With involvement of the CNS. *0388* May be increased in lymphomas involving the central nervous system *1236*

Synovial Fluid Increase

714.00 Rheumatoid Arthritis Increased concentration. *2302 2326*

Saliva Increase

710.20 Sjögren's Syndrome *0793*

Beta-Amino-Isobutyric-Acid

Plasma Increase

260.00 Protein Malnutrition In Kwashiorkor, there is an increase in beta-aminoisobutyric acid. During recovery ethanolamine is elevated. *0619*

990.00 Effects of X-Ray Irradiation Due to tissue destruction. *1556*

Urine Increase

260.00 Protein Malnutrition Increased beta-aminoisobutyric acid and ethanolamine in urine of patients with kwashiorkor. *0619*

984.00 Toxic Effects of Lead and Its Compounds (including Fumes) A result of the nephrotoxic effect of lead. *0618*

Beta-Galactosidase

Serum   Decrease

191.90   Malignant Neoplasm of Brain   Mean serum concentration in patients with tumors (both benign and malignant) were depressed to 0.065 ± 0.009 mmol/min/L, compared with 0.243 ± 0.038 in controls. *1099*

225.90   Benign Neoplasm of Brain and CNS   Mean serum concentration in patients with tumors (both benign and malignant) were depressed to 0.065 ± 0.009 mmol/min/L, compared to 0.243 ± 0.038 in normals. *1099*

331.90   Cerebral and Cortical Atrophy   In cerebral atrophy due to presenile dementia and/or cerebrovascular disease. *2592*

340.00   Multiple Sclerosis   In 10 patients, mean activity was 0.163 ± 0.025 U/L at pH = 4.5, normal = 0.243 ± 0.038. *1099*

357.00   Guillain-Barré Syndrome   In 10 patients, mean activity was 0.163 ± 0.025 mmol/min at pH = 4.5, normal = 0.243 ± 0.038. *1099*

710.00   Systemic Lupus Erythematosus   Mean serum concentration was 0.139 ± 0.019 mmol/min/L, compared with 0.243 ± 0.038 in controls. *1099*

714.00   Rheumatoid Arthritis   Mean serum concentration was 0.139 ± 0.019 mmol/min/L, compared with 0.243 ± 0.038 in controls. *1099*

Beta-Globulin

Serum   Decrease

199.00   Secondary Malignant Neoplasm (Disseminated)   *2467*

201.90   Hodgkin's Disease   *2467*

202.80   Non-Hodgkins Lymphoma   *2467*

204.00   Lymphocytic Leukemia (Acute)   Common. *0689 2552*

204.10   Lymphocytic Leukemia (Chronic)   *2467*

206.00   Monocytic Leukemia   *2467*

260.00   Protein Malnutrition   Tends to be both relatively and absolutely decreased. *0151*

556.00   Ulcerative Colitis   *2467*

570.00   Acute and Subacute Necrosis of Liver   Alpha and beta globulins decrease when hepatocellular failure impairs their synthesis. *0151*

Serum   Increase

52.00   Chickenpox   May be increased. *2468*

70.00   Viral Hepatitis   Increased in cholangiolitis. May reach very high levels in chronic progressive disease. *2339*   Associated with intrahepatic biliary obstruction. *0619*

135.00   Sarcoidosis   Stepwise increase of alpha$_2$, beta, and gamma globulin. 'sarcoid steps' help differentiate from other lung disease. *2467*

201.90   Hodgkin's Disease   Active disease. *0073*

203.00   Multiple Myeloma   Markedly increased. *0619*

205.00   Myelocytic Leukemia (Acute)   Common. *0689 2552*

250.00   Diabetes Mellitus   *2467*

272.00   Type IIA Hyperlipoproteinemia   Marked increase due to primary xanthomatosis. *0619*

272.21   Type IIB Hyperlipoproteinemia   Marked increase due to primary xanthomatosis. *0619*

272.22   Type III Hyperlipoproteinemia   Marked increase due to essential hyperlipemia. *0619*

272.31   Type I Hyperlipoproteinemia   Marked increase due to essential hyperlipemia. *0619*

273.22   Heavy Chain Disease (Alpha)   Markedly elevated broad peak. *2035*

273.80   Analbuminemia   *2467*

340.00   Multiple Sclerosis   Concentration > 15% of total protein was observed in 9.3% of patients. *1295*

446.00   Polyarteritis-Nodosa   Moderate increase in some cases. *0619*

571.60   Biliary Cirrhosis   Marked increase. *0619*

576.20   Extrahepatic Biliary Obstruction   In cholestasis, the increase in alpha$_2$ and beta globulin components correlates with the height of serum lipid values and is a useful point in distinguishing between biliary obstructive lesions and other nonobstructive types of jaundice. *2339*

581.90   Nephrotic Syndrome   There is a marked increase with incomplete separation from the alpha$_2$ fraction. *0619*

650.00   Pregnancy   Slightly increased in second trimester of pregnancy. *2468*   Rises progressively by about 0.3 g/dL. *0791*

714.00   Rheumatoid Arthritis   Alpha$_2$ or beta globulin fractions are often elevated in the acute phase, whereas during the chronic active phase, gamma globulin fractions are elevated. *0433*

Serum   Normal

204.10   Lymphocytic Leukemia (Chronic)   Usually within normal limits. *0241   2552*

279.04   Agammaglobulinemia (Congenital Sex-linked)   *2538*

279.06   Immunodeficiency (Common Variable)   *2467*

571.20   Laennec's or Alcoholic Cirrhosis   *2467*

585.00   Chronic Renal Failure   *2467*

714.00   Rheumatoid Arthritis   Generally not significantly changed. *0962*

Urine   Increase

581.90   Nephrotic Syndrome   Significant quantities are found. *0995*

Beta-Glucosidase

Serum   Decrease

272.72   Gaucher's Disease   At pH 4.0, individuals demonstrate a marked reduction. However, little or no reduction is found at the optimum pH, 5.5. *1808*

Beta-Glucuronidase

Serum   Decrease

570.00   Acute and Subacute Necrosis of Liver   Decreased. *0741 0866*

572.20   Hepatic Encephalopathy   Decreased. *0741 0866*

572.40   Hepatic Failure   Decreased. *0741 0866*

Serum   Increase

153.90   Malignant Neoplasm of Large Intestine   Increased. *0741 0866*

155.00   Malignant Neoplasm of Liver   Increased. *0741 0866*

157.90   Malignant Neoplasm of Pancreas   Increased. *0741 0866*

174.90   Malignant Neoplasm of Breast   Increased. *0741 0866*

180.90   Malignant Neoplasm of Cervix   Increased. *0741 0866*

197.70   Secondary Malignant Neoplasm of Liver   Increased. *0741 0866*

250.00   Diabetes Mellitus   Increased activity correlated with blood sugar concentration. *0155*

272.72   Gaucher's Disease   *1723 2538*

571.60   Biliary Cirrhosis   Increased. *0741 0866*

571.90   Cirrhosis of Liver   Increased. *0741 0866*

573.30   Toxic Hepatitis   Increased with extensive cell necrosis. *0741 0866*

650.00   Pregnancy   Increased. *0741 0866*

Urine   Increase

189.00   Malignant Neoplasm of Kidney   All 17 patients with renal adenocarcinoma had slightly elevated activity with values ranging from 32-55 U/L (mean 42.8 ± 6.1 U). Uncomplicated renal cysts revealed normal urinary enzyme activities (mean = 17.9 ±12.8). *1525*

401.10   Essential Benign Hypertension   Moderately elevated (33.7 ± 23.4 U/L). Approximately half of the values were above normal. *0885*

580.00   Acute Poststreptococcal Glomerulonephritis   31 of 38 patients with active disease had elevated activities, with a mean value of 70.0 ± 50.4. Of the 38 patients with inactive glomerulonephritis, 17 had elevated activities. *1525*

581.90   Nephrotic Syndrome   8 of 13 patients had activities > 30 U/L, mean for the entire group was 44.3 ± 25.3. *1525*

584.00   Acute Renal Failure   All 8 patients revealed high values of urinary activity above the normal limit of 30 with a mean value of 148.1 ± 158.3 U/L. *0885*

Beta-Glucuronidase (continued)

Urine Increase (continued)

590.00 Chronic Pyelonephritis All 15 patients showed elevated activity (mean 61.9 ± 39.1), whereas 11 of 13 patients with inactive disease showed normal values (mean 24.0 ± 7.8 U). *0885*

590.10 Acute Pyelonephritis All 15 patients with active disease showed elevated activity (mean 61.9 ± 39.1 U/L), whereas 11 of 13 patients with inactive disease showed normal values (mean 24.0 ± 7.8 U/L). *0885 1525*

599.00 Urinary Tract Infection Of the 13 patients with positive bladder and negative ureteral cultures, 6 showed elevated activity. The mean value was 29.5 ± 15.7. Of 25 ureteral specimens (right or left) with negative cultures, 7 showed elevated activity (mean 25.5 ± 10.8 enzyme U). *0885*

650.00 Pregnancy Moderately elevated (33.7 ± 23.4 U/L); approximately 50% of the values were above normal. 50% of the patients in the gestation period from 20-32 weeks showed elevated urinary enzyme activity. *0885* Mean activity in 17 patients was 35.2 U/L. Eight had values > the normal upper limit. *1525*

Ascitic Fluid Increase

577.00 Acute Pancreatitis Ranged from 850-16,500 µg phenolphthalein/h/dL. *0827*

Gastric Material Increase

151.90 Malignant Neoplasm of Stomach Greater than 1 U/mg protein in 90% of subjects with cancer or gastric atrophy. *0992* Elevated in gastric cancer. Overlap between noncancer and cancer patients limits usefulness and specificity. *2199 1266*

Beta-Glusosaminidase

Serum Increase

250.00 Diabetes Mellitus Increased activity correlated with blood sugar concentration. *0155*

Bicarbonate

Serum Decrease

9.00 Gastroenteritis and Colitis May be noted. *0433*

37.00 Tetanus The lowest values are found in the more severe cases. *0433*

242.90 Hyperthyroidism Respiratory alkalosis may occur. *0962*

250.00 Diabetes Mellitus *2467*

250.10 Diabetic Acidosis May be < 2 mmol/L in profound cases and 15 mmol/L in severe cases. *2540* Metabolic acidosis may occur. *0962*

252.00 Hyperparathyroidism Decreased bicarbonate in 24% of cases. *1492*

255.40 Adrenal Cortical Hypofunction Dehydration and hypotension lead to prerenal impairment of renal function. *0433* Normal or decreased. *2467 0999*

265.00 Thiamine (B_1) Deficiency Respiratory alkalosis may occur. *0962*

270.03 Cystinosis Metabolic, hyperchloremic acidosis. *0433* Reflects renal bicarbonate loss. *2246*

275.10 Hepatolenticular Degeneration Decreased serum CO_2 in 12 of 27 patients (44%). *2278*

276.20 Metabolic Acidosis Total plasma CO_2 content is decreased; < 15 mmol/L almost certainly rules out respiratory alkalosis. *2468* Serum bicarbonate falls as hydrogen ions accumulate. *0962*

276.50 Dehydration Normal or decreased. *2467*

291.00 Delirium Tremens Respiratory alkalosis may occur. *1430*

303.00 Acute Alcoholic Intoxication Plasma bicarbonate ranged from 2-10 mmol/L in acidosis following alcoholic binge. *1594*

331.81 Reye's Syndrome Due to impaired oxidative metabolism. *0435*

428.00 Congestive Heart Failure Acidosis occurs when renal insufficiency is associated or there is CO_2 retention due to pulmonary insufficiency. *2467*

486.01 Resolving Pneumonia Respiratory alkalosis may occur. *0962*

493.10 Asthma (Intrinsic) In a moderate to severe attack the partial pressure of CO_2 is reduced, while normal values are obtained for bicarbonate and pH. A the condition worsens the pCO_2 and bicarbonate will rise and pH fall. *0433* May be decreased in early stages and may be increased in later stages. *2467*

496.01 Alpha$_1$-Antitrypsin Deficiency Associated COPD. *1636*

514.00 Pulmonary Congestion and Hypostasis Respiratory alkalosis may occur. *0962*

518.00 Pulmonary Collapse Respiratory alkalosis may occur. *0962*

537.40 Fistula of Stomach and Duodenum Metabolic acidosis may occur. *0962*

558.90 Diarrhea *2467*

572.20 Hepatic Encephalopathy Respiratory alkalosis may occur. *0962*

579.00 Celiac Sprue Disease If diarrhea is severe, marked electrolyte depletion. *2199*

579.90 Malabsorption, Cause Unspecified Normal or decreased. *2467*

580.00 Acute Poststreptococcal Glomerulonephritis Metabolic acidosis. *0062*

584.00 Acute Renal Failure In 74% of 12 patients at initial hospitalization for this disorder. *0781* Metabolic acidosis. *0787* Falls 1-2 mmol/L each day during oliguric phase. *0277 0962*

585.00 Chronic Renal Failure Metabolic acidosis may occur. *0962* In 59% of 146 patients at initial hospitalization for this disorder. *0781*

588.81 Proximal Renal Tubular Acidosis Low levels in the presence of alkaline urine; very low levels with acid urine. *0186* Low Bicarbonate level *2246*

588.82 Distal Renal Tubular Acidosis Alkaline urine regardless of bicarbonate level. *0186*

597.80 Urethritis Reveals the degree of renal impairment. *0433*

642.40 Pre-Eclampsia Changes in electrolytes are usually insignificant. In severe cases, the bicarbonate may be lowered. *0387*

642.60 Eclampsia Usually reduced. Not uncommon to see values < 13.5 mmol/L. *0621*

650.00 Pregnancy Decreased markedly throughout pregnancy. *0517* An effect of progesterone; slight decrease *1460*

770.80 Respiratory Distress Syndrome Metabolic acidosis. *0570*

785.50 Shock Respiratory alkalosis may occur. *0962*

985.00 Toxic Effects of Non-medicinal Metals May be depressed in chronic mercury poisoning. *0618*

991.60 Hypothermia Especially in cases preceded by exhaustion and prolonged shivering. *0151* Due to hypoxia, acid-base imbalance hypotension. *1471*

994.50 Exercise Reduced by 3 mmol/L after vigorous 30 min exercise. *0706* Decreased to 11 mmol/L with intermittent exercise. *1254*

Serum Increase

11.00 Pulmonary Tuberculosis In 64% of 23 patients at initial hospitalization for this disorder. *0781*

37.00 Tetanus Metabolic alkalosis may occur with potassium loss. *0962*

45.90 Acute Poliomyelitis Respiratory acidosis may occur. *0962*

135.00 Sarcoidosis In 55% of 20 patients at initial hospitalization for this disorder. *0781*

191.90 Malignant Neoplasm of Brain In 74% of 21 patients at initial hospitalization for this disorder. *0781*

197.00 Secondary Malignant Neoplasm of Respiratory System In 41% of 280 patients at initial hospitalization for this disorder. *0781*

201.90 Hodgkin's Disease In 60% of 45 patients at initial hospitalization for this disorder. *0781*

217.00 Benign Neoplasm of Breast In 42% of 14 patients at initial hospitalization for this disorder. *0781*

225.90 Benign Neoplasm of Brain and CNS In 74% of 16 patients at initial hospitalization for this disorder. *0781*

244.90 Hypothyroidism Significant CO_2 retention can occur. *0433* In 60% of 13 patients at initial hospitalization for this disorder. *0781*

252.10 Hypoparathyroidism *1337*

255.00 Adrenal Cortical Hyperfunction (Glucocorticoid Excess) Metabolic alkalosis may occur with potassium loss. *0962*

255.10 Adrenal Cortical Hyperfunction (Mineralocorticoid Excess) Most patients exhibit a CO_2 content in the range of 32-38 mmol/L. *1108* Metabolic alkalosis may occur with potassium loss. *0962* *2467*

276.30 Metabolic Alkalosis Total plasma CO_2 is increased (bicarbonate > 30 mmol/L). *2468*

357.00 Guillain-Barré Syndrome Respiratory acidosis may occur. *0962*

358.00 Myasthenia Gravis Associated respiratory insufficiency. *0995*

401.00 Malignant Hypertension Metabolic alkalosis may occur with potassium loss. *0962*

401.10 Essential Benign Hypertension In 59% of 98 patients hospitalized for this disorder. *0781*

414.00 Chronic Ischemic Heart Disease In 62% of 434 patients hospitalized for this disorder. *0781*

428.00 Congestive Heart Failure Alkalosis occurs in uncomplicated failure; hyperventilation, alveolar-capillary block due to associated pulmonary fibrosis; hypochloremic alkalosis due to K^+ depletion. *2467*

435.90 Transient Cerebral Ischemia In 70% of 31 patients hospitalized for this disorder. *0781*

440.00 Arteriosclerosis In 56% of 67 patients hospitalized for this disorder. *0781*

480.90 Viral Pneumonia Increased standard bicarbonate in blood. *0619*

491.00 Chronic Bronchitis In 59% of 18 patients at initial hospitalization for this disorder. *0781*

493.10 Asthma (Intrinsic) May be decreased in early stages and increased in later stages. *2467* In 40% of 95 patients at initial hospitalization for this disorder. *0781* *0999*

496.00 Chronic Obstructive Lung Disease Suggests chronic hypoventilation. *0962* In 82% of 69 patients at initial hospitalization for this disorder. *0781*

500.00 Anthracosis CO_2 retention may occur. *0433*

501.00 Asbestosis CO_2 retention may occur. *0433*

502.00 Silicosis CO_2 retention may occur. *0433*

503.01 Berylliosis CO_2 retention may occur. *0433*

533.90 Peptic Ulcer, Site Unspecified Pyloric obstruction with vomiting and loss of gastric secretion results in hypochloremia, hyponatremia, hypokalemia, elevated serum pH and carbon dioxide content, and azotemia. *0962*

537.00 Pyloric Stenosis, Acquired Metabolic alkalosis secondary to vomiting. *0587*

560.90 Intestinal Obstruction Metabolic alkalosis secondary to vomiting. *2467* In 46% of 47 patients at initial hospitalization for this disorder. *0781*

572.40 Hepatic Failure Persistent alkalosis in patients with hepatic failure. *1775*

785.40 Gangrene In 37% of 28 patients hospitalized for this disorder. *0781*

787.00 Vomiting Metabolic alkalosis. *0619*

Serum Normal

253.50 Diabetes Insipidus *2467*

255.40 Adrenal Cortical Hypofunction Normal or decreased. *2467*

275.35 Vitamin D Resistant Rickets *2246*

276.50 Dehydration Normal or decreased. *2467*

428.00 Congestive Heart Failure *2467*

780.80 Hyperhidrosis *2467*

Urine Increase

588.82 Distal Renal Tubular Acidosis Alkaline urine regardless of bicarbonate level in blood. *0186*

650.00 Pregnancy Alkalosis is prevented by renal excretion of bicarbonate to offset the loss of CO_2 from the blood. *1460*

Pleural Effusion Increase

714.00 Rheumatoid Arthritis 60-70 mm Hg. *0797*

Duodenal Contents Decrease

157.90 Malignant Neoplasm of Pancreas Acinar destruction (as in pancreatitis) shows normal volume (20-30 mL/10 min collection period) but bicarbonate and enzyme levels may be decreased. In carcinoma, the test result depends on the relative extent and combination of acinar destruction and of duct obstruction. *2467*

533.90 Peptic Ulcer, Site Unspecified Bicarbonate level has been shown to be 1/2 of controls. *0949*

577.20 Pancreatic Cyst and Pseudocyst Duodenal contents after secretin-pancreozymin stimulation usually show decreased bicarbonate content (< 70 mmol/L) but normal volume and normal content of amylase, lipase, and trypsin. *2467*

Duodenal Contents Normal

157.90 Malignant Neoplasm of Pancreas Secretin-pancreozymin stimulation evidences duct obstruction when duodenal intubation shows decreased volume of duodenal contents (< 10 mL/10 min collection period) with usually normal bicarbonate and enzyme levels in duodenal contents. *2467*

Feces Increase

1.00 Cholera Fecal carbonate concentration is higher than in plasma. *0151*

579.00 Celiac Sprue Disease In occasional patients, significant metabolic acidosis can develop in association with bicarbonate loss in the stool. *2199*

Saliva Decrease

577.10 Chronic Pancreatitis Salivary output, amylase, and (HCO_3) concentration decreased in 88% of patients. *1210* *0080*

Bile Acids

Serum Decrease

555.90 Regional Enteritis or Ileitis In patients with Crohn's Disease whether resected or not the postprandial level of bile acids is low. *1039*

Serum Increase

70.00 Viral Hepatitis In one study with viral hepatitis type B, bile acids and transaminase were of equal sensitivity. *2199*

277.00 Cystic Fibrosis Serum bile acid determination seems to be of no value in evaluating the extent of liver disease in cystic fibrosis. Chenodeoxycholic acids are more frequent and more elevated than cholic acid. *2274*

496.01 Alpha₁-Antitrypsin Deficiency In 34 patients with this disease all patients with morphological cirrhosis. *1685*

571.20 Laennec's or Alcoholic Cirrhosis Total bile acids were elevated in all patients with alcoholic liver cirrhosis. This test was found to discriminate most efficiently between acute alcohol intoxication and liver cirrhosis. *1166* In 30 pts. with alcoholic liver cirrh. portal hypertension and bleeding esophageal varices. *1165* *0920*

571.49 Chronic Active Hepatitis Postprandial levels were significantly higher. *0920*

714.00 Rheumatoid Arthritis In a series of 20 patients with RA and without prior causes of hepatic damage. Elevated in 80% of patients. *2625*

Serum Normal

277.42 Gilbert's Disease An elevated bilirubin coexisting with a normal bile acid level suggests Gilbert's Disease. *2199* Fasting and post prandial levels were normal with reduced and normal caloric loads. *0283*

571.90 Cirrhosis of Liver Serum bile acids did not discriminate between anicteric patients with fatty liver (n = 10) and liver cirrhosis (n = 9) and normal controls (n = 27). *0638*

Urine Increase

496.01 Alpha₁-Antitrypsin Deficiency Excretion was increased. *0563*

571.90 Cirrhosis of Liver Mean values for Bile Acids in urine: Control 1.9 μg/mL, Obstructive Jaundice μg/mL and Cirrhosis 15.14 μg/mL (compensated) and 11.84 μg/mL (compensated). *2323*

Bile Acids *(continued)*

Urine   Increase *(continued)*

576.20 Extrahepatic Biliary Obstruction   Mean values for Bile Acids in urine: Control 1.9 µg/mL, Obstructive Jaundice µg/mL, Cirrhosis 15.14 µg/mL (compensated) and 11.84 (uncompensated). *2323*

Feces   Increase

496.01 Alpha₁-Antitrypsin Deficiency   Excretion was increased. *0563*

Bilirubin

Serum   Decrease

280.90 Iron Deficiency Anemia   A test of minor or incidental importance. *0433   0151*

Serum   Increase

18.00 Disseminated Tuberculosis   Bilirubin usually only minimally elevated. *0999   2538 0486*

52.00 Chickenpox   *2538 1857*

54.00 Herpes Simplex   *2538 1857*

55.00 Measles   *2538 1857*

60.00 Yellow Fever   Slightly increased. *2468*   Has been reported. *1179*

70.00 Viral Hepatitis   Jaundice becomes apparent when concentration exceeds 2 mg/dL. Usually rises for 10-14 days to an average peak of about 10 mg/dL. But much higher levels are encountered especially when hemolysis is present. The rate of decline from the peak level is more gradual and often requires 2-6 weeks. The level has no prognostic significance. *0433*   On occasion there is severe hemolytic anemia resulting in a marked rise in the serum bilirubin, this frequently occurs in patients with glucose-6-phosphate dehydrogenase deficiency. *0962*   In 78% of 24 patients at initial hospitalization for this disorder. *0781   2156 2576*

75.00 Infectious Mononucleosis   Over 1 mg/dL in 37% of patients. *0433*   May occur; hepatic involvement is usually mild. *2538   0962*

78.50 Cytomegalic Inclusion Disease   Hemolytic anemia. *2538 0767*

84.00 Malaria   Evidence of hemolysis. *2468*

85.00 Leishmaniasis   Hemolytic anemia. *2538 2568*

87.00 Relapsing Fever   Occurs late in the course of the disease. *0962*

88.00 Bartonellosis   *2538 1918*

99.10 Lymphogranuloma Venereum   May indicate severe liver impairment. *0433*

100.00 Leptospirosis   Increased in 50% of the patients. *2468*   May reach 65 mg/dL but is < 20 mg/dL in 66% of patients. *0151*   Elevated values found in patients without clinically evident liver disease. *0962*   Jaundice may appear at the end of the 1st week of fever. Liver tests show hepatic decompensation of the intrahepatic type. *2368   0992*

115.00 Histoplasmosis   Greater than 1.0 mg/dL in 25% of patients with disseminated disease. *0999*

117.30 Aspergillosis   Hemolytic anemia. *2538 1950*

120.00 Schistosomiasis   May be mild elevations, but jaundice is uncommon. *0962*

122.90 Hydatidosis   With liver involvement. *1058*

130.00 Toxoplasmosis   *2538 0486*

155.00 Malignant Neoplasm of Liver   In patients with primary tumors, values ranged from 3.5-5.2 mg/dL (normal < 1.0). *2576*   Commonly found (60-70%), but concentration > 85 mmol/L were found in only 10-25% of patients. *0364*   Over 10% above upper limit of normal in 43.2% in 67 cases of hepatoma. *1115*   In 38% of 13 patients at initial hospitalization for this disorder. *0781*

155.10 Malignant Neoplasm of Intrahepatic Bile Ducts   Markedly elevated levels, ranging from 16.0-23.2 mg/dL. *2576*   Values exceed 10 mg/dL in most cases, with a mean value of about 18 mg/dL. *0151*

157.90 Malignant Neoplasm of Pancreas   Markedly elevated with values ranging from 4.0-17.9 mg/dL. *2576*   May become significantly elevated with direct fraction greater than the indirect fraction. *0433*   Increased (12-25 mg/dL), mostly direct. Increase is persistent and nonfluctuating. *2467*   Elevated without marked abnormalities in liver all function tests. *0267*   In 39% of 46 patients at initial hospitalization for this disorder. *0781*

197.70 Secondary Malignant Neoplasm of Liver   Elevated serum bilirubin values of 2.6-12.2 mg/dL were reported in patients with carcinoma metastatic to liver. *2576*

201.90 Hodgkin's Disease   May be a systemic sign of active disease or may indicate involvement of liver or bone. *0433*

202.52 Histiocytosis X   May occur in the presence of extensive liver involvement. *0433*

202.80 Non-Hodgkins Lymphoma   May be a systemic sign of active disease or may indicate involvement of liver or bone. *0433*

204.10 Lymphocytic Leukemia (Chronic)   20% of patients develop severe hemolysis. *0992*

207.00 Erythroleukemia   Evidence of a mild or moderate increase in hemolysis is commonly observed, but the erythrokinetic findings are those of ineffective erythropoiesis. *2538*

238.40 Polycythemia Vera   Slightly elevated. *0181*   Rarely. *0995*

242.90 Hyperthyroidism   Due to hemolysis. *0151*

259.20 Carcinoid Syndrome   Rare until extensive hepatic metastases occur. *2540*

271.20 Hereditary Fructose Intolerance   Noted with the chronic syndrome found in young children and after fructose administration in adults. *2246*

272.52 Abetalipoproteinemia   Reflects increased RBC turnover. *1583*

275.00 Hemochromatosis   With liver involvement. *0962*

275.10 Hepatolenticular Degeneration   Elevated in 13 of 38 (34%) patients; mean = 1.45 mg/dL. Direct bilirubin was increased in 9 of 36 (25%) patients. *2278*

277.30 Amyloidosis   10% of patients had increased direct bilirubin and 5% had high indirect bilirubin. *1334*

277.41 Dubin-Johnson Syndrome   Characterized by chronic nonhemolytic, predominantly conjugated hyperbilirubinemia. *0180*   The total serum bilirubin ranges between 2-10 mg/24h. *0962*   Slight to marked in degree with marked fluctuations in intensity. *0602 2246*

277.42 Gilbert's Disease   Mild increase in unconjugated serum bilirubin reduced by phenobarbital and increased within 24 h of a reduced calorie diet. *0619*   Degree of elevation does not correlate with symptoms. *0180*   Highest after fasting and rarely exceeds 3 mg/dL. *0962*   Usually in range of 1.2-3 mg/dL, rarely > 5 mg/dL. *0995*

277.43 Rotor's Syndrome   The total serum bilirubin ranges between 2-10 mg/24h. *0962*   Slight to moderate direct bilirubinemia. *2246*

277.44 Crigler-Najjar Syndrome   Patients with apparent autosomal recessive pattern of inheritance with severe hyperbilirubinemia (20-31 mg/dL). *0999*   Almost invariably in the range of 15-48 mg/dL with virtually all giving an indirect van den Bergh reaction. Fluctuations are frequent, with higher values in winter and incidental illness. *2071   2246*

281.00 Pernicious Anemia   Mild due to increase in indirect fraction. *0995*

281.20 Folic Acid Deficiency Anemia   Slightly to moderately increased. *2538   0151*

282.00 Hereditary (Congenital) Spherocytosis   Primarily indirect. *2538*

282.10 Hereditary Elliptocytosis   In patients with more severe forms of this disease there may be a compensated hemolytic anemia with raised serum bilirubin. *0433*   Primarily indirect. *0995*   Hemolysis and hyperbilirubinemia have been observed in the newborn period. *0087*

282.20 Anemias Due To Disorders of Glutathione Metabolism   Varying degrees may be evident. *2538*

282.41 Thalassemia Major   Usually increased. *0999*

282.60 Sickle Cell Anemia   Intrahepatic cholestasis with extremely high circulating levels also appears to be characteristic. *2538*

282.71 Hemoglobin C Disease   Increase is minimal. *2468*

283.00 Acquired Hemolytic Anemia (Autoimmune) Although clinical jaundice is present in < 50% of patients, elevated serum bilirubin, particularly of the unconjugated fraction, is common. *2538* Increase depends on liver function and amount of hemolysis. With normal liver function, it is increased 1 mg/dL in 1-6 h to maximum in 3-12 h following hemolysis of 100 mL of blood, with hemolytic anemias. *2468*

283.21 Paroxysmal Nocturnal Hemoglobinuria *0433*

289.00 Polycythemia, Secondary Increased slightly. *0151*

303.90 Alcoholism 12% of 182 male chronic alcoholics had increased concentrations. Highest values were found after 5-20 y of confirmed alcoholism. *2196*

331.81 Reye's Syndrome Usually remains below 3 mg/dL. *0416* Normal or mildly elevated *0962*

428.00 Congestive Heart Failure Depending on the severity and chronicity of cardiac failure. *0433* Frequently increased (indirect more than direct); usually 1-5 mg/dL. It usually represents combined right- and left-sided failure with hepatic engorgement and pulmonary infarcts. May suddenly rise rapidly if superimposed myocardial infarction occurs. *2467*

446.60 Thrombotic Thrombocytopenic Purpura Elevated in 90% of patients. *2538*

482.90 Bacterial Pneumonia Occasionally present. *0962*

483.01 Mycoplasma Pneumoniae *2538 0729*

487.10 Influenza Hemolytic anemia. *2538 1857*

496.01 Alpha₁-Antitrypsin Deficiency Related to liver disease. *1636*

555.90 Regional Enteritis or Ileitis Due to associated liver disease. *0218*

570.00 Acute and Subacute Necrosis of Liver May be > 30 mg/dL. *2467* Rarely exceeds 15-20 mg/dL. *0999 0619*

571.20 Laennec's or Alcoholic Cirrhosis Elevated ranging from 2.4-9.5 mg/dL. *2576 0999*

571.49 Chronic Active Hepatitis Usually moderately increased (3-10 mg/dL) but rarely exceeds 20 mg/dL. *0992* Active phases with hepatocellular necrosis are marked by signs of hepatic dysfunction. *2035* In 51% of 19 patients at initial hospitalization for this disorder. *0781*

571.60 Biliary Cirrhosis Usually conjugated bilirubinemia and total concentration range from 3-20 mg/dL or higher. In the final stages, concentrations may exceed 50 mg/dL. *0992* Usually conjugated, representing posthepatic cell obstruction. At times, a large proportion may be unconjugated reflecting impaired hepatic function. *2238 0999*

571.90 Cirrhosis of Liver Usually elevated except in well-compensated liver disease. A direct bilirubin > 0.3 mg/dL means liver disease unless severe hemolysis or the rare congenital syndromes of bilirubin metabolism are present. *0433* Most is indirect unless cirrhosis is of the cholangiolitic type. Higher and more stable in postnecrotic cirrhosis; lower and more fluctuating levels occur in Laennec's cirrhosis. Terminal icterus may be constant and severe. *2467* In 54% of 68 patients at initial hospitalization for this disorder. *0781* Values range from 7.8-8 mg/dL in postnecrotic cirrhosis. *2576*

572.00 Liver Abscess (Pyogenic) Moderate increase in about 33% of patients. Usually indicates pyogenic rather than amebic and suggests poorer prognosis because of more tissue destruction. *2467* Elevated in 50% of cases. *2199 0433*

572.20 Hepatic Encephalopathy *0151*

572.40 Hepatic Failure May be increased or normal. *0503*

573.30 Toxic Hepatitis *0433*

575.00 Acute Cholecystitis Mild hyperbilirubinemia occasionally occurs. *0999* Usually mild (< 4.0 mg/dL). *2199*

576.10 Cholangitis Values are usually in the range of 2-4 mg/dL and are uncommonly higher than 10 mg/dL. *0151*

576.20 Extrahepatic Biliary Obstruction During or soon after an attack of biliary colic. Increased in about 33% of patients. *2467*

577.00 Acute Pancreatitis Seen in about 20% of patients. *0999* May be moderately elevated as a consequence of edema of the head of the pancreas with resultant obstruction of the common bile duct. *0962* In 32% of 21 patients at initial hospitalization for this disorder. *0781*

577.10 Chronic Pancreatitis *2199*

577.20 Pancreatic Cyst and Pseudocyst Serum direct bilirubin is increased (> 2 mg/dL) in 10% of patients. *2467* Occasionally elevated. *0433*

642.60 Eclampsia Elevated in only 3 of 134 patients, and those cases were only minimally elevated. *0429* Uncommon. In 134 women, including 45 with eclampsia, only 3 had levels > 1.2 mg/dL, with 2.3 mg/dL as the highest value. *1859 0387*

770.80 Respiratory Distress Syndrome *0702*

773.00 Hemolytic Disease of Newborn (Erythroblastosis Fetalis) After birth, the rate of rise is a reflection of both the severity of the hemolytic process and the degree of hepatic maturity. *2538* In the severely affected group, cord blood concentration may be 10 mg/dL (of which 33-66% is direct-acting bilirubin). Peak levels may climb despite treatment, into the 30 mg/dL range (of which 66% is direct- acting bilirubin). *0433* After birth, the rate of rise is a reflection of both severity of the hemolytic process and the degree of hepatic maturity. *2538 2061*

774.40 Jaundice Due to Hepatocellular Damage (Newborn) *2061*

984.00 Toxic Effects of Lead and Its Compounds (including Fumes) Hemolytic anemia may occur. *0484*

985.00 Toxic Effects of Non-medicinal Metals Hepatotoxicity may occur with arsenicals. *1446*

990.00 Effects of X-Ray Irradiation Transient hyperbilirubinemia may be observed in cases of radiation injury. *0151*

992.00 Heat stroke Clinically apparent jaundice appears 24-36 h after admission. *0995*

Serum Normal

6.00 Amebiasis With liver involvement, jaundice is uncommon and bilirubin is usually normal. *1058*

197.70 Secondary Malignant Neoplasm of Liver Common finding. *0186*

275.00 Hemochromatosis Over 50% of patients have no laboratory evidence of liver dysfunction. *0995*

281.30 Vitamin B₆ Deficiency Anemia Rarely elevated despite the mild hemolytic anemia. *0433*

285.00 Sideroblastic Anemia Rarely elevated despite the mild hemolytic anemia. *0433 1327*

410.90 Acute Myocardial Infarction *2467*

413.90 Angina Pectoris *2467*

482.90 Bacterial Pneumonia *2467*

575.00 Acute Cholecystitis Some cases. *2467*

576.20 Extrahepatic Biliary Obstruction Remains normal in the presence of serum alkaline phosphatase that is markedly increased with the obstruction of one hepatic bile duct. *2467*

577.00 Acute Pancreatitis May be increased when pancreatitis of biliary tract origin but is usually normal in alcoholic pancreatitis. *2467*

585.00 Chronic Renal Failure Within normal limits in all 26 cases. *1421*

642.60 Eclampsia Seldom elevated, even in severe eclampsia. *0387*

Urine Increase

70.00 Viral Hepatitis Appears a few days before the onset of jaundice. *0433* Seen in anicteric hepatitis. *0151 0999*

87.00 Relapsing Fever Noted occasionally. *0433*

197.70 Secondary Malignant Neoplasm of Liver Increased serum alkaline phosphatase is the most useful index of partial obstruction of the biliary tree when serum bilirubin is usually normal and urine bilirubin is increased. *2467*

277.41 Dubin-Johnson Syndrome May be seen. *0180* Patient presents with intermittent jaundice and bilirubinuria. *0962 0999*

277.43 Rotor's Syndrome Patient presents with intermittent jaundice and bilirubinuria. *0962 2467*

428.00 Congestive Heart Failure With jaundice. *2467*

516.10 Idiopathic Pulmonary Hemosiderosis Excretion may be increased by the increased porphyrin catabolism. *2538*

570.00 Acute and Subacute Necrosis of Liver May precede the onset of jaundice by several days *0999*

571.60 Biliary Cirrhosis *2467*

571.90 Cirrhosis of Liver *2467*

573.30 Toxic Hepatitis *2467*

575.00 Acute Cholecystitis Occasionally found. *0999*

Bilirubin (continued)

Urine Increase (continued)

576.20 Extrahepatic Biliary Obstruction Values of 1-5 mg/dL are common in an episode of cholecystitis. Levels higher than 5 mg/dL are usually the result of common bile duct obstruction, particularly if there is a predominance of the direct-reacting fraction of bilirubin. *0433* During or soon after an attack of biliary colic. Increased in about 33% of patients. *2467*

577.00 Acute Pancreatitis Seen in about 20% of patients. *0999*

Urine Normal

277.42 Gilbert's Disease *2246*

277.43 Rotor's Syndrome *2246*

277.44 Crigler-Najjar Syndrome None detectable. *2246*

774.40 Jaundice Due to Hepatocellular Damage (Newborn) *2467*

Feces Decrease

70.00 Viral Hepatitis *2467*

277.42 Gilbert's Disease *2467*

277.43 Rotor's Syndrome *0503*

277.44 Crigler-Najjar Syndrome *2467 0503*

573.30 Toxic Hepatitis *2467*

576.20 Extrahepatic Biliary Obstruction Marked decrease. Clay colored stools. *2467*

774.40 Jaundice Due to Hepatocellular Damage (Newborn) Normal or decreased. *2467*

Feces Increase

558.90 Diarrhea In severe diarrhea a little bilirubin may be present. *0619*

570.00 Acute and Subacute Necrosis of Liver *2467*

Bilirubin, Direct

Serum Decrease

277.44 Crigler-Najjar Syndrome *2246*

Serum Increase

70.00 Viral Hepatitis Serum bilirubin is 50-75% direct in the early stage; later, indirect bilirubin is proportionately more in acute icteric period. *2467* Direct and indirect bilirubin are equally elevated in the icteric phase. *0151* In 93% of 19 patients at initial hospitalization for this disorder. *0781 0999*

78.50 Cytomegalic Inclusion Disease Usually > 5% of total concentration and may be 50%. *2368*

100.00 Leptospirosis Hyperbilirubinemia, which is predominantly conjugated (direct) may reach 65 mg/dL but is < 20 mg/dL in 66% of patients. *0151*

157.90 Malignant Neoplasm of Pancreas In 91% of 14 patients at initial hospitalization for this disorder. *0781*

275.10 Hepatolenticular Degeneration Increased in 9 of 36 (25%) patients. *2278*

277.30 Amyloidosis 10% of patients had increased direct bilirubin and 5% had high indirect bilirubin. *1334*

277.41 Dubin-Johnson Syndrome Characterized by chronic nonhemolytic, predominantly conjugated hyperbilirubinemia associated with jaundice. *0180* Familial, conjugated hyperbilirubinemia due to a defect in the excretion of bilirubin from the liver. *0962 0999 2246*

277.43 Rotor's Syndrome Familial, conjugated hyperbilirubinemia due to a defect in the excretion of bilirubin from the liver. *0962*

283.00 Acquired Hemolytic Anemia (Autoimmune) Elevated if the total serum bilirubin exceeds 4 mg/dL; attributed to an associated hepatic injury permitting conjugated bilirubin to regurgitate into the general circulation. *2361 2538*

570.00 Acute and Subacute Necrosis of Liver Normal or slight increase (< 15% of total). *2467*

571.20 Laennec's or Alcoholic Cirrhosis Occasionally acute alcoholic disease presents with a predominant elevation in the serum conjugated bilirubin suggesting extrahepatic obstruction of the biliary system. *0999 0151*

571.49 Chronic Active Hepatitis *0992*

571.60 Biliary Cirrhosis Usually conjugated bilirubinemia and total concentrations range from 3-20 mg/dL or higher. In the final stages, concentrations may exceed 50 mg/dL. *0992* Increases in the serum bilirubin, mostly of the direct fraction. *0962* Usually conjugated, representing posthepatic cell obstruction. *2238*

571.90 Cirrhosis of Liver In 87% of 29 patients at initial hospitalization for this disorder. *0781 2467*

573.30 Toxic Hepatitis Increased early. *2467*

576.20 Extrahepatic Biliary Obstruction *0999*

577.00 Acute Pancreatitis In 80% of 10 patients at initial hospitalization for this disorder. *0781*

577.20 Pancreatic Cyst and Pseudocyst Increased (> 2 mg/dL) in 10% of patients. *2467*

773.00 Hemolytic Disease of Newborn (Erythroblastosis Fetalis) Severely affected group. *0433*

774.40 Jaundice Due to Hepatocellular Damage (Newborn) Normal or slight increase. *2467*

Serum Normal

277.42 Gilbert's Disease 20% of total bilirubin. *0995*

Bilirubin, Indirect

Serum Increase

70.00 Viral Hepatitis Serum bilirubin is 50-75% direct in the early stage; later, indirect bilirubin is proportionately more. *2467* In 75% of 18 patients at initial hospitalization for this disorder. *0781*

78.50 Cytomegalic Inclusion Disease In hemolytic anemia. *1058*

84.00 Malaria Evidence of hemolysis. *2468*

85.00 Leishmaniasis Hemolytic anemia. *2538 2568*

88.00 Bartonellosis *2538 1918*

117.30 Aspergillosis Hemolytic anemia. *2538 1950*

157.90 Malignant Neoplasm of Pancreas In 56% of 14 patients at initial hospitalization for this disorder. *0781*

204.10 Lymphocytic Leukemia (Chronic) 20% of patients develop severe hemolysis. *0992*

277.30 Amyloidosis 10% of patients had increased direct bilirubin and 5% had high indirect bilirubin. *1334*

277.41 Dubin-Johnson Syndrome *0995*

277.42 Gilbert's Disease Mild asymptomatic increase of indirect serum bilirubin, usually discovered on routine lab exam. May rise to 18 mg/dL but usually is < 4 mg/dL. *2467* Unexplained, mild, chronic elevation. *2246 0962*

277.43 Rotor's Syndrome *2467*

277.44 Crigler-Najjar Syndrome Increased; it appears on 1st or 2nd day of life, rises to 12-45 mg/dL, and persists for life. *2467* Familial unconjugated hyperbilirubinemia due to low or absent hepatic glucuronyl-transferase activity. *0962*

281.00 Pernicious Anemia Mild unconjugated hyperbilirubinemia. *0151* Slight indirect hyperbilirubinemia as a result of increased production of bile pigment. Normal values are common and values > 2 mg/dL are unusual. *2552*

281.20 Folic Acid Deficiency Anemia Slight indirect hyperbilirubinemia as a result of increased production of bile pigment. Normal values are common and values 2 mg/dL are unusual. *2552*

282.00 Hereditary (Congenital) Spherocytosis Mean = 1.6 ± 1.1 mg/dL. *1470 2538*

282.10 Hereditary Elliptocytosis *2538*

282.20 Anemias Due To Disorders of Glutathione Metabolism Indirect laboratory evidence that hemolysis is present. *0433*

282.31 Hereditary Nonspherocytic Hemolytic Anemia In some cases. *2538*

282.41 Thalassemia Major Unconjugated bilirubinemia (1-3 mg/dL) and slightly increased icterus index. *2552*

282.60 Sickle Cell Anemia Elevation is always seen but late in the course true liver function abnormalities also develop. *0433* Laboratory signs of hemolysis with increased indirect-reacting serum bilirubin. *2538*

282.71 Hemoglobin C Disease Manifested by a hemolytic state. *0962*

283.00 Acquired Hemolytic Anemia (Autoimmune) There is increased indirect serum bilirubin (< 6 mg/dL because of compensatory excretory capacity of liver). *2468* Although clinical jaundice is present in < 50% of patients, elevated serum bilirubin, particularly of the unconjugated fraction, are common. *2538*

283.21 Paroxysmal Nocturnal Hemoglobinuria Reflects hemolysis. *2552*

428.00 Congestive Heart Failure Unconjugated hyperbilirubinemia reflects reduced hepatic blood flow. *0151*

446.60 Thrombotic Thrombocytopenic Purpura In 90% of patients. *2538*

483.01 Mycoplasma Pneumoniae Occasional patients have been reported with hemolytic anemia. *0433   0729*

516.10 Idiopathic Pulmonary Hemosiderosis Occasional findings of hemolytic type of anemia. *2467*

570.00 Acute and Subacute Necrosis of Liver *2467*

571.20 Laennec's or Alcoholic Cirrhosis *2199*

571.49 Chronic Active Hepatitis *0992*

571.60 Biliary Cirrhosis Total concentration is usually 5-10 mg/dL but may vary between normal and 25 mg/dL. Usually conjugated and therefore represents posthepatic cell obstruction, but at times a large proportion of unconjugated bilirubin may be present in the serum as a reflection of impaired hepatic function. *2238*

571.90 Cirrhosis of Liver In 71% of 27 patients at initial hospitalization for this disorder. *0781   2467*

573.30 Toxic Hepatitis Increased predominantly. *2467*

576.20 Extrahepatic Biliary Obstruction Normal or slight increase. *2467*

577.00 Acute Pancreatitis In 40% of 10 patients at initial hospitalization for this disorder. *0781*

773.00 Hemolytic Disease of Newborn (Erythroblastosis Fetalis) In mild cases on the 2nd-5th day of life, depending upon the rapidity of increase in the degree of jaundice. *0433* Concentration > 4 mg/dL in cord blood suggest severe disease. Levels of > 50 mg/dL may be seen by the 3rd day of life in untreated, severely affected infants. *2538   2061*

774.40 Jaundice Due to Hepatocellular Damage (Newborn) *2467*

Serum   Normal

773.00 Hemolytic Disease of Newborn (Erythroblastosis Fetalis) Intermediate moderately affected group: rarely a baby in this group will develop jaundice. *0433*

Bleeding Time

Blood   Decrease

201.90 Hodgkin's Disease Has been reported. *2538 1087* Thrombocytopenia. *2246*

Blood   Increase

65.00 Arthropod-Borne Hemorrhagic Fever Prolonged in hemorrhagic fever caused by dengue viruses. *0151*

271.01 Von Gierke's Disease Prolonged bleeding is a major clinical problem, probably due to impaired platelet function. *2246*

273.30 Waldenström's Macroglobulinemia Evidence of impaired platelet function. *2538*

277.00 Cystic Fibrosis Secondary to vitamin K deficiency. *0551*

281.00 Pernicious Anemia May be prolonged. *2552*

281.20 Folic Acid Deficiency Anemia May be prolonged. *2552*

284.90 Aplastic Anemia Reflects low platelet count. *2538* Usually moderately prolonged. *2552*

286.01 Hemophilia In severe cases. *0995*

286.10 Christmas Disease In severe cases. *2468*

286.20 Factor XI Deficiency Variable. *2246* In severe cases. *0995*

286.31 Congenital Dysfibrinogenemia Usually prolonged, but in some cases no clot forms at all. *2538*

286.34 Congenital Afibrinogenemia Often increased (33% of patients). *2468* Prolonged bleeding times, unrelated to thrombocytopenia, are found in some patients. *2590* Variable. *2246   2538*

286.35 Factor V Deficiency Slightly prolonged in approximately 33% of cases. *2538*

286.37 Factor VII Deficiency May be abnormally long. *2246*

286.40 Von Willebrand's Disease Usually prolonged 2 h after dose of 10 grains of aspirin; bleeding time is variable without this aspirin tolerance test. *2467* Prolonged. *0227* Commonly occurs in homozygotes and heterozygotes. *1389* May be detected by Dukes' method or the standard Ivy procedure. *2538   2246*

287.10 Thrombasthenia (Glanzmann's) Deficient platelet factor III. *0433* Bleeding time is usually prolonged and aggregation of platelets by collagen or thrombin is abnormal. *0999* Often marked. *2246   2552*

287.30 Idiopathic Thrombocytopenic Purpura *2552 2246*

446.60 Thrombotic Thrombocytopenic Purpura Varies depending upon the platelet count. *2035   2552 2246*

992.00 Heat stroke *0995*

Blood   Normal

238.40 Polycythemia Vera *2468*

267.00 Vitamin C Deficiency *2467*

286.01 Hemophilia Bleeding time and prothrombin time are not significantly prolonged. *2538   2246*

286.10 Christmas Disease *2538 2246*

286.20 Factor XI Deficiency Usually normal. *2538*

286.32 Factor XII Deficiency Prothrombin and bleeding times are normal. *2538   2246*

286.33 Factor XIII Deficiency *2538 2246*

286.35 Factor V Deficiency Slightly prolonged in 33% of cases. *2538   2246*

286.36 Factor X Deficiency *0995 2246*

286.37 Factor VII Deficiency *0995 2246*

286.38 Factor II Deficiency *2246*

287.00 Allergic Purpura Tourniquet test may be positive, but other tests of hemostasis are usually normal. *2552*

288.00 Agranulocytosis Normal in most typical cases. *2552*

BSP Retention

Serum   Increase

70.00 Viral Hepatitis Useful in screening for anicteric disease and during convalescence. *0433* The earliest abnormality, followed by bilirubinuria, before serum bilirubin increases. *2467*

75.00 Infectious Mononucleosis May occur; hepatic involvement is usually mild. *2538*

115.00 Histoplasmosis Elevated in 70% of patients with disseminated disease. *0999*

120.00 Schistosomiasis 5% retention upon admission. *2026* Common. *0962*

155.00 Malignant Neoplasm of Liver Increased retention in 90% of cases. *0364*

197.70 Secondary Malignant Neoplasm of Liver Increased serum alkaline phosphatase and increased BSP retention is 65% reliable to establish this diagnosis. *2467*

201.90 Hodgkin's Disease May be a systemic sign of active disease or may indicate involvement of liver or bone. *0433*

202.80 Non-Hodgkins Lymphoma May be a systemic sign of active disease or may indicate involvement of liver or bone. *0433*

242.90 Hyperthyroidism Mild retention. *2540*

259.20 Carcinoid Syndrome May be seen in later course of disease. *2540*

271.10 Galactosemia Deranged liver function. *2246*

275.00 Hemochromatosis With liver involvement. *0962*

275.10 Hepatolenticular Degeneration Excretion was delayed in 76% of cases. Mean retention in 29 patients tested was 15%, and 9 patients had values > 20%. *2278*

277.14 Acute Intermittent Porphyria Normal liver function tests except for BSP. Over 10% BSP retained in 79% of symptomatic patients and in 55% of those in remission. *2254*

277.16 Porphyria Cutanea Tarda Usually abnormal. *2458*

277.30 Amyloidosis Retention is increased in 75% of patients with liver involvement. *2468* Found to be elevated in over 50% of patients 5% in 1 h), contrary to the suggestion that hepatomegaly with normal or only slightly abnormal liver function is characteristic. *1334* With hepatic involvement. *0125   0962*

BSP Retention *(continued)*

Serum   Increase *(continued)*

277.41 Dubin-Johnson Syndrome   Higher at 90 min than at 45 min after IV administration. *0180*   Normal or slightly impaired excretion. *2246*   Normal decrease in serum concentration 45 min after injection, followed by a rise at 2 h, due to difficulty in its excretion from the liver with leakage back into the bloodstream. *0962*

277.42 Gilbert's Disease   Mild 45 min retention has been observed in 20% of patients. *0180*   In a significant number of patients. *0179*

277.43 Rotor's Syndrome   Marked retention. *2246*   Defects in the excretion of BSP and of gallbladder dye may reveal a normal decrease in its serum concentration 45 min after injection, followed by a rise at 2 h, due to difficulty in its excretion from the live with leakage back into the bloodstream. *0962*

423.10 Constrictive Pericarditis   *2467*

425.40 Cardiomyopathies   Disordered liver function in advanced cases of obliterative cardiomyopathy. *1108*

428.00 Congestive Heart Failure   The most frequently abnormal test. It may indicate circulatory stasis as well as cellular damage. *2467*   Hepatic dysfunction, often with structural damage to the liver, may result in moderate BSP retention. *1108*

570.00 Acute and Subacute Necrosis of Liver   Commonly observed. *0992*

571.20 Laennec's or Alcoholic Cirrhosis   *0151*

571.49 Chronic Active Hepatitis   Noted even during inactive phase of disease. *0992*   Active phases with hepatocellular necrosis are marked by signs of hepatic dysfunction. *2035*

571.90 Cirrhosis of Liver   Sensitive index of liver function and is most useful in the absence of jaundice to follow the course of disease when the other liver function tests are normal. *2467*   Decreased removal of dye in advanced cirrhosis of liver. *0619*

572.40 Hepatic Failure   *0503*

573.30 Toxic Hepatitis   *0503*

575.00 Acute Cholecystitis   Increased BSP retention (some cases) even if serum bilirubin is normal. *2467*

576.20 Extrahepatic Biliary Obstruction   Normal or may later become only slightly increased. *2467*

642.40 Pre-Eclampsia   A larger proportion of hypertensive women have increased retention than normal pregnant women, (> 5% in 45 min), but many are in the range of normal. *0387*

650.00 Pregnancy   Abnormal retention occurs during last month of pregnancy. *2468*   The rate of BSP clearance is slower in normal pregnancy, but after 60 min only 4 of 20 had more than a trace left. *2214   0387*

714.00 Rheumatoid Arthritis   In a series of 20 patients with RA and without prior causes of hepatic damage. Elevated in 60% of patients. *2625*   At times increased *0433*

985.00 Toxic Effects of Non-medicinal Metals   Hepatotoxicity may occur with arsenicals. *1446*

992.00 Heat stroke   In almost 50% of patients with induced fever. *0222*   Without liver disease. *2467*

994.50 Exercise   Related to extent of activity. *0763*

Serum   Normal

271.01 Von Gierke's Disease   Liver may be massively enlarged but liver function tests are normal. *2246*

275.00 Hemochromatosis   Over 50% of patients have no laboratory evidence of liver dysfunction. *0995*

277.44 Crigler-Najjar Syndrome   Liver function tests were uniformly normal. *2246*

570.00 Acute and Subacute Necrosis of Liver   In patients with ascites, BSP dye may be lost into abdomen. Results may falsely appear normal. *2467*

572.00 Liver Abscess (Pyogenic)   BSP dye may be lost into abdomen. Results may falsely appear normal. *2467*

Butanol Extractable Iodine (BEI)

Serum   Decrease

240.00 Simple Goiter   Normal or slightly low. *0962*

244.90 Hypothyroidism   *2468*

245.20 Hashimoto's Thyroiditis   Depressed in chronic thyroiditis patients. *0999*

581.90 Nephrotic Syndrome   Urinary loss of TBG results in lowering of most blood thyroid hormones and increased T_3 uptake. *0962*

Serum   Increase

242.90 Hyperthyroidism   May be present. *0962*

Serum   Normal

240.00 Simple Goiter   Normal or slightly low. *0962*

245.20 Hashimoto's Thyroiditis   *0962*

Cadmium

Serum   Decrease

585.00 Chronic Renal Failure   Probably due to proteinuria and a loss of cadmethionein in urine. *0019*

Serum   Increase

303.90 Alcoholism   *0126*

401.10 Essential Benign Hypertension   There was a high correlation between systolic and diastolic BP and cadmium levels. *0126*   No association between subclinical cadmium exposure and hypertension but confirmed relationship with cigarette smoking. *0152*

440.00 Arteriosclerosis   The highest blood cadmium level was observed in smokers with coronary heart disc plus hypertension. *0019*

Serum   Normal

606.90 Infertility in Males   No significant difference from fertile male controls. *2247*

Calcitonin

Serum   Decrease

252.00 Hyperparathyroidism   *0619 0520*

Serum   Increase

162.90 Malignant Neoplasm of Bronchus and Lung   Elevated in 75% of patients with oat cell carcinoma. *1553*   8 of 11 patients with oat cell carcinoma (including 4 with skeletal metastases) had concentrations > 0.1 ng/mL, ranging up to 5 ng/mL. *0445*   Elevated in 54 (68%) of 79 patients with small cell carcinoma. 20 patients (25%) had levels usually associated with medullary carcinoma of the thyroid. *0980*   Increase found in both thyroid and bronchogenic carcinomas. Medullary thyroid cancer is characterized by the presence of at least 7 different fractions, ranging from fraction I (> 30,000 molecular weight) to V (2,500 molecular weight). Bronchogenic cancers had a predominance of high molecular weight fractions (I and IIa). *0146*   High levels can also be produced ectopically by small cell cancer of the lung. *0962   1589*

193.01 Medullary Carcinoma of Thyroid   Increased baseline levels or increased level after calcium infusion indicates medullary carcinoma. May be found even in absence of palpable mass in the thyroid. *2468*   Observed in 2 patients with medullary cancer of the thyroid. *1587*   Increased in both thyroid and bronchogenic carcinomas. Medullary thyroid cancer is characterized by the presence of at least 7 different fractions, ranging from fraction I to V. Bronchogenic cancers had a predominance of high molecular weight fractions (I and IIa). *0146   0962*

198.50 Secondary Malignant Neoplasm of Bone   8 patients with skeletal metastases had increased concentrations, ranging from 0.15 ng/mL - 9.0 ng/mL. *0445*

199.00 Secondary Malignant Neoplasm (Disseminated)   Elevated. *0918*

227.91 Pheochromocytoma   *1589*

251.50 Zollinger-Ellison Syndrome   In some cases. *1041*

259.20 Carcinoid Syndrome   Secreted in bronchial and intestinal carcinoid tumors. *1589*

275.42 Pseudohypoparathyroidism   *0619*

281.00 Pernicious Anemia   In some cases. *1041*

571.20 Laennec's or Alcoholic Cirrhosis   Immunoreactive calcitonin was increased in relation to raised alkaline phosphatase activity. *1040*

585.00 Chronic Renal Failure Basal plasma concentrations were increased to a mean of 185.88 ± 16.36 pg/mL. *1368*

Serum Normal

174.90 Malignant Neoplasm of Breast In 107 patients with breast cancer; CEA, ferritin and calcitonin levels were measured. CEA and ferritin but not calcitonin levels were statistically higher in those patients with metastases. *0200*

Urine Increase

193.01 Medullary Carcinoma of Thyroid Urinary calcitonin is high in medullary cancer patients. *0962*

Calcium

Serum Decrease

30.00 Leprosy Significantly decreased in all types of leprosy except tuberculoid. *2187*

40.20 Whipple's Disease An indication of vitamin D and calcium malabsorption. *0962* In patients with severe diarrhea and malabsorption. *2199 0995*

204.00 Lymphocytic Leukemia (Acute) Hypocalcemia with values of 6.6-8.3 mg/dL was observed within 24-48 h after initiation of chemotherapy. *2622*

250.00 Diabetes Mellitus Osmotic diuresis secondary to hyperglycemia. *2540*

251.50 Zollinger-Ellison Syndrome An indication of vitamin D and calcium malabsorption. *0962*

252.10 Hypoparathyroidism Rapidly reduced to a stable low level following removal of gland. *2104* Decreased PTH causes increased serum phosphate and reduced serum calcium. *0503*

253.40 Anterior Pituitary Hypofunction *0503*

256.30 Ovarian Hypofunction Estrogen effect. *0995*

260.00 Protein Malnutrition Decreased in hypoproteinemia. *0503*

268.00 Vitamin D Deficiency Rickets Decreased absorption in the gut leads to overproduction of parathyroid hormone and the resulting phosphaturia and hypophosphatemia. *1287* Concentrations < 8 mg/dL are common. *2246 0999*

268.20 Osteomalacia Advanced and sustained vitamin D deficiency. Renal tubular acidosis, hypophosphatasia, and dietary deficiency or a failure of absorption of calcium and vitamin D as well as other causes of increased loss of calcium must be considered in patients with osteomalacia. *2467 0503* Advanced disease. *2199 0999*

270.03 Cystinosis Hypocalcemic, hypophosphatemic rickets resistant to the usual doses of vitamin D. *0433*

271.30 Lactosuria An indication of vitamin D and calcium malabsorption. *0962*

273.22 Heavy Chain Disease (Alpha) Patients usually present with chronic diarrhea, hypocalcemia, and excessive fecal losses of water and electrolytes. *2538*

273.23 Heavy Chain Disease (Gamma) Patients usually present with chronic diarrhea, hypocalcemia, and excessive fecal losses of water and electrolytes. *2538*

273.80 Analbuminemia Lower limits of normal. *0433*

275.10 Hepatolenticular Degeneration Related to decreased albumin. *2280*

275.21 Hypomagnesemia Plasma ionized calcium is reduced. *0619*

275.42 Pseudohypoparathyroidism End-organ failure. A rare cause of hypocalcemia. Must be considered in osteomalacia. *0503 0999*

276.30 Metabolic Alkalosis Decrease in ionized calcium. *0791*

277.00 Cystic Fibrosis Hypoalbuminemia. *2467*

279.11 DiGeorge's Syndrome *2344*

303.00 Acute Alcoholic Intoxication Hypocalcemia is common in alcoholic subjects. *1394*

303.90 Alcoholism Hypocalcemia is common in alcoholic subjects. *1394*

306.10 Hyperventilation Syndrome Respiratory alkalosis reduces ionized Ca concentration. *2103 0995*

345.90 Epilepsy Up to 33% of epileptic children on long-term anticonvulsant therapy. *0619*

496.01 Alpha$_1$-Antitrypsin Deficiency Related to decreased Albumin. *1636*

555.90 Regional Enteritis or Ileitis *0995*

556.00 Ulcerative Colitis Usually deficient. *0995*

571.20 Laennec's or Alcoholic Cirrhosis Low concentrations correlated well with high AST activity in 78 cirrhotic patients. *1574*

571.90 Cirrhosis of Liver Low concentrations correlated well with high AST activity in 78 cirrhotic patients. *1574* In 38% of 68 patients at initial hospitalization for this disorder. *0781*

577.00 Acute Pancreatitis Decreased in severe cases 1-9 days after onset. Usually occurs after amylase and lipase levels have become normal. Values < 7.0 mg/dL indicates poor prognosis. *0151* Often found with a low serum albumin; when correction of serum calcium is made for hypoalbuminemia, most patients are found to be normocalcemic. *0039* Mean = 7.3 ± 1.5 mg/dL in the 12 patients (range = 4.6-9.9). The 5 patients who did not recover had the lowest concentrations. *0827* Total and ionized calcium were low or in the low normal range in 11 clearly documented case. *2509 1119 0962 2199*

577.10 Chronic Pancreatitis Malnutrition is the result of the malabsorption of fat, proteins, and fat-soluble vitamins which results in low concentrations. *0433*

579.00 Celiac Sprue Disease An indication of vitamin D and calcium malabsorption. *0962* Often decreased in patients with diarrhea and steatorrhea. *2199* In 50% of untreated patients, concentration may be less than 9 mg/dL. *2238*

579.01 Protein-Losing Enteropathy *0503 2467*

579.90 Malabsorption, Cause Unspecified Decreased in hypoproteinemia. *0503* Particularly in small bowel disease. *0151* An indication of vitamin D and calcium malabsorption. *0962*

580.01 Glomerulonephritis (Focal) Decreases as metabolic acidosis develops. *0962*

580.40 Glomerulonephritis (Rapidly Progressive) Decreases renal failure develops. *0962*

581.90 Nephrotic Syndrome Reduced proportionately to the fall in albumin concentration in the early stages with true hypocalcemia evident later in the disease. *1523* In 12 patients with nephrotic syndrome and 14 nephrotic patients during clinical remission, mean ionized calcium = 1.08 ± 0.10 and 1.21 ± 0.10 mmol/L ultrafiltrate respectively, significantly lower than the normal mean (1.28 ± 0.06 mmol/L). *1408* In 76% of 25 patients at initial hospitalization for this disorder. *0781*

584.00 Acute Renal Failure May occur in early stage. *2468* Hypocalcemia in acute (anuria) and chronic renal failure. *0503* In 72% of 11 patients at initial hospitalization for this disorder. *0781* In the range of 6.3-8.3 mg/dL. *1522*

585.00 Chronic Renal Failure Falls late in renal failure, often reaching 6 mg/dL and occasionally 4 mg/dL. *0151* Usually reduced primarily as a result of diminished synthesis of active metabolites of vitamin D, particularly in the setting of high levels of intracellular phosphate. *1108* Hypocalcemia in acute (anuria) and chronic renal failure. *0503* In 47% of 142 patients at initial hospitalization for this disorder. *0781*

588.00 Renal Dwarfism May lead to hypocalcemia or low normal serum calcium levels. In time there will be significant parathyroid hyperplasia, and the serum calcium may become inappropriately elevated. *0999* May be quite low but is more commonly in the low-normal range. *0151*

588.81 Proximal Renal Tubular Acidosis Renal tubular acidosis or Fanconi Syndrome. Must be considered in patients with osteomalacia. Normal to decreased values. *0503 2246*

588.82 Distal Renal Tubular Acidosis *0614*

592.00 Kidney Calculus May represent presenting manifestations. *0503*

597.80 Urethritis Reveals the degree of renal impairment. *0433*

650.00 Pregnancy Levels decreased progressively after the first trimester. *0517* Insufficient calcium, phosphorus and vitamin D ingestion *2467*

694.40 Pemphigus *0151*

733.00 Osteoporosis Hypocalcemia may be present in severe cases. *0999*

753.12 Medullary Cystic Disease Frequent, but not invariable. *0277*

756.52 Osteopetrosis Moderate hypocalcemia occasionally in children. *0995*

958.10 Fat Embolism Decreased calcium correlated with leukocytosis and low hemoglobin. *1683*

992.00 Heat stroke Initially and consistently high phosphate levels resulted in the fall of serum calcium to 5 mg/dL after 24 h in a case of malignant hyperpyrexia. *0541*

Calcium (continued)

Serum Increase

135.00 Sarcoidosis Much less frequent than hypercalciuria. Found in 6-13% of cases. *0433* Occurs in approximately 33% of patients at some stage of disease. *1083 0962 2199*

150.90 Malignant Neoplasm of Esophagus Neoplasm without evidence of direct bone involvement. Parathyroid hormone-secreting tumors. *0503*

155.00 Malignant Neoplasm of Liver A serious complication in many cases of hepatoma. *1246 1507* Sometimes present. Occasionally antedate the discovery of the tumor. *0962*

157.90 Malignant Neoplasm of Pancreas Without evidence of direct bone involvement. Parathyroid hormone-secreting tumors. *0503 1509*

162.90 Malignant Neoplasm of Bronchus and Lung In squamous cell neoplasm without evidence of direct bone involvement. Parathyroid hormone- secreting tumors. *0503* Frequent hypercalcemia in advanced cases. *0393*

170.90 Malignant Neoplasm of Bone Lytic tumors involving bone can lead to nephrocalcinosis and renal failure. The most frequent cause of hypercalcemia. *0619 2467 0503*

174.90 Malignant Neoplasm of Breast Neoplasm without evidence of direct bone involvement. Parathyroid hormone-secreting tumors. Metastatic or lytic tumors involving bone. *0503* Frequent hypercalcemia in advanced cases. *0393*

188.90 Malignant Neoplasm of Bladder Neoplasm without evidence of direct bone involvement. Parathyroid hormone-secreting tumors. *0503*

189.00 Malignant Neoplasm of Kidney 5-15% of patients with hypernephroma develop hypercalcemia usually secondary to metastases. *0836*

197.00 Secondary Malignant Neoplasm of Respiratory System In 7 cases of bronchogenic metastases, hypercalcemia was recorded (range 10.6-16.4 mg/dL). *1904*

198.50 Secondary Malignant Neoplasm of Bone May be normal or increased in osteolytic metastases (especially from primary tumor of bronchus, breast, kidney, thyroid). *2467* Elevations in patients with carcinoma of prostate metastatic to bone were negligible at first but mild hypercalcemia developed at some time in 9% of patients. *2566 1904*

201.90 Hodgkin's Disease Observed in 6 cases (range 10.6 - 16.4 mg/dL). *1904* In patients with bone and liver disease. *2538 1204* Metastatic or lytic tumor involving bone. *0503* Indicates bone involvement. *0433*

202.80 Non-Hodgkins Lymphoma Has been observed in the absence of hyperparathyroidism or of skeletal metastases. *2180* Metastatic or lytic tumor involving bone. *0503 2538*

203.00 Multiple Myeloma Found in about 21% of patients. *2566* If the renal excretory capacity for calcium is exceeded. *2035* Frequent hypercalcemia in advanced cases. *0393* Elevated above 11.0 mg/dL in about 30% of patients at the time of diagnosis, and rises above this level in an additional 30% during the course of the disease. *0176 1904 0962*

204.00 Lymphocytic Leukemia (Acute) May be increased in some cases. *0503* Elevated levels (> 11.0 mg/dL) may occur with leukemic infiltration of bone. *1322* Has been observed but is uncommon. *2552*

204.10 Lymphocytic Leukemia (Chronic) Elevations > 11 mg/dL may occur with leukemic infiltration of bone. *1322 0503*

205.00 Myelocytic Leukemia (Acute) Elevation (> 11 mg/dL) may occur with leukemic infiltration of bone. *1322* Has been observed, but is uncommon. *2552 0503*

205.10 Myelocytic Leukemia (Chronic) Elevation > 11 mg/dL may occur with leukemic infiltration of bone. *1322* Has been described occasionally. *0109 1392*

227.91 Pheochromocytoma May be caused by ectopic parathyroid hormone production in a few patients but usually results from associated parathyroid hyperplasia in the familial cases. *0433* Hypercalcemia can occur independently or in association with coexistent hyperparathyroidism. *0962* Can occur, disappearing after removal of the tumor. *0962*

238.40 Polycythemia Vera Slight rise, cause unknown. *0619*

242.90 Hyperthyroidism An incidental finding and an uncommon complication. *0999* Ionized and total calcium levels were elevated in 21 of 45 (47%) and in 12 of 45 (27%) thyrotoxic patients, respectively. Mean ionized and total calcium levels were higher in these 45 patients than in normal persons. *0319* Usually normal but may occur in as many as 20% of patients. *2540* Found in rare occasions with severe thyrotoxicosis due to increased turnover of bone. *2612 0962*

244.90 Hypothyroidism Sometimes increased. *2468*

252.00 Hyperparathyroidism Of 50 primary cases, 47 had increased concentration (> 10.3 mg/dL). *1957* In 149 samples, 0.7% of serum ionized calcium and 7.5% of total calcium determinations were within the normal range. All patients exhibited abnormally elevated values upon repeated testing. *0626* Hyperparathyroidism associated with pathologic lesions, shows hypercalcemia 10.5 mg/dL. Probably the single most important diagnostic aid. *0503 2595 1083 0812 1492 0781 0589*

253.00 Acromegaly In 20 patients with active disease, gut absorption was greater than normal and positively correlated with both the elevated serum and urine concentration. *2161* Often noted, because of increase GI absorption. *0962*

253.40 Anterior Pituitary Hypofunction *0433*

255.00 Adrenal Cortical Hyperfunction (Glucocorticoid Excess) Some cases with osteoporosis. *0619*

255.40 Adrenal Cortical Hypofunction In most instances the clinical picture is not altered by the hypercalcemia. It is not clear in all cases that the hypercalcemia reflects an increase in ionized calcium since hemoconcentration may contribute to the elevation if nausea, vomiting, and dehydration are prominent. Hypercalcemia may appear, however, with acute withdrawal of exogenous corticosteroids. It usually vanishes promptly with small doses of steroids. *0999 0503*

256.00 Ovarian Hyperfunction Estrogen effect. *0995*

272.00 Type IIA Hyperlipoproteinemia The greatest increment being in the protein-bound calcium form. *0503*

272.21 Type IIB Hyperlipoproteinemia The greatest increment being in the protein-bound calcium form. *0503*

275.32 Hypophosphatasia Intermittent hypercalcemia may be observed in these patients, who also demonstrate an increase in phosphoethanolamine in their blood and urine. *0503* Total serum concentration was elevated in 10 patients and normal or undetermined in 6. Individual readings tended to vary widely and hypercalcemic patients had normal readings occasionally. *0769*

275.41 Milk-Alkali Syndrome An unusual complication of intensive peptic ulcer therapy is the evolution of hypercalcemia from excessive intake of milk and absorbable alkali. *0999*

276.20 Metabolic Acidosis Increase in ionized calcium. *0791*

278.40 Hypervitaminosis D Especially with added calcium in the diet; hypercalcemia corrected by steroids. *0619* 4 cases with hypercalcemia (range 10.6-16.4 mg/dL). *1904 2199*

303.00 Acute Alcoholic Intoxication Increased following alcoholic binge of several days duration. *1594*

303.90 Alcoholism Increased following alcoholic binge of several days duration. *1594*

345.90 Epilepsy High in cases of idiopathic grand mal epilepsy. CSF calcium remained normal. This increase in serum calcium may be due to hyperparathyroidism because of low magnesium concentration. *0093*

503.01 Berylliosis *2467*

533.90 Peptic Ulcer, Site Unspecified Due to excessive alkali intake if the antacid contains calcium, or if milk is taken in excess. *0619*

577.00 Acute Pancreatitis Occasionally, in patients whose pancreatitis is related to hyperparathyroidism, it may be elevated even during the acute attack. *0433*

588.00 Renal Dwarfism May be normal or elevated. When both phosphate and calcium are high, metastatic calcifications in subcutaneous tissues and conjunctiva may develop. *0999*

588.81 Proximal Renal Tubular Acidosis Hypercalcemia in 5 of 17 patients with transient primary renal tubular acidosis. *1753*

714.00 Rheumatoid Arthritis After correction for hypoalbuminemia, 113/229 female and 65/135 male patients had hypercalcemia. *1251*

731.00 Osteitis Deformans Usually normal but immobilization of affected individuals produces a high risk of hypercalcemia. *0999 0503*

733.00 Osteoporosis *2467*

985.00 Toxic Effects of Non-medicinal Metals Highly significant hypercalciuria and decreased serum inorganic phosphate was found in a group of workers with cadmium intoxication. *2098*

994.50 Exercise Observed after 12 min on cycle-ergometer. *0804*

Serum Normal

170.90 Malignant Neoplasm of Bone Usually normal in Ewing's sarcoma and other osteolytic tumors. *2467*

193.01 Medullary Carcinoma of Thyroid Usually normal, in spite of very high titers of plasma calcitonin seen in medullary cancer of the thyroid. *0962*

242.90 Hyperthyroidism Significant hypercalcemia did not occur in patients over 60 years of age. *0512*

244.90 Hypothyroidism Usually. *2540*

268.00 Vitamin D Deficiency Rickets Usually normal or slightly decreased. *2467 0433*

268.20 Osteomalacia In early stages, stimulation of skeletal mobilization of calcium compensates for the high renal loss or the low intestinal absorption. Serum concentration is therefore normal or low normal. *2199*

275.35 Vitamin D Resistant Rickets Usually normal. *2246*

277.00 Cystic Fibrosis Normal unless complications occur (e.g., chronic pulmonary disease with accumulation of CO_2, massive salt loss due to sweating). *2467*

277.30 Amyloidosis Rarely elevated in primary disease. *1334*

333.40 Huntington's Chorea *1252*

410.90 Acute Myocardial Infarction Plasma concentration measured in 18 patients several days after admission showed a fall in 13 cases. Correction of values to a fixed albumin level removed the apparent tendency to hypocalcemia. *2531*

588.00 Renal Dwarfism May be normal or elevated. When both phosphate and calcium are high, metastatic calcifications in subcutaneous tissues and conjunctiva may develop. *0999*

642.60 Eclampsia *0621*

708.90 Urticaria In acute and chronic urticaria, mean serum values did not differ significantly from control groups. Only 7 cases had abnormal values. Abnormal calcium metabolism is not associated with urticaria and calcium treatment is not indicated. *1169*

714.00 Rheumatoid Arthritis Generally normal. *0962*

730.00 Osteomyelitis Normal in all 39 cases. *2464*

733.00 Osteoporosis Process is usually so gradual that homeostatic forces control the serum calcium. *1083 0433*

756.52 Osteopetrosis *2467*

948.00 Burns On average, free or ionized calcium were in the normal range. However they were weakly correlated with the severity of burn injury. *0723*

Urine Decrease

157.90 Malignant Neoplasm of Pancreas No evidence of direct bone involvement. Parathyroid hormone-secreting tumors. *0503*

198.50 Secondary Malignant Neoplasm of Bone Low in osteoblastic metastases (especially from primary tumor in prostate). *2467*

244.90 Hypothyroidism In general. *2540*

252.00 Hyperparathyroidism Although they may have hypercalciuria, compared with normal controls, they have very low rates for their serum calcium. *2540*

252.10 Hypoparathyroidism Rises acutely, then falls to low levels as plasma calcium falls. *2540*

268.00 Vitamin D Deficiency Rickets Low in the untreated state. *2246*

268.20 Osteomalacia *0503 2467*

275.35 Vitamin D Resistant Rickets In children, urinary excretion is 10-20 mg/24h whereas in adults urinary excretion ranges between 50-120 mg/24h. *0151* Usually low in untreated cases. *2246*

275.42 Pseudohypoparathyroidism *0503*

276.30 Metabolic Alkalosis *0503*

579.00 Celiac Sprue Disease *2467*

580.00 Acute Poststreptococcal Glomerulonephritis Decreased excretion in acute nephritis, partly due to decreased intestinal absorption. *0619*

581.90 Nephrotic Syndrome Low urinary excretion is common. *1523*

585.00 Chronic Renal Failure Falls early, to < 100 mg/24h, before there is any drop in serum levels, reflecting the fall of GFR. *0151*

733.00 Osteoporosis May be increased, normal, or decreased but is not influenced by intake; calcium restriction does not produce the normal fall. *2467*

Urine Increase

120.00 Schistosomiasis Increased despite normal serum levels. *0955*

135.00 Sarcoidosis 30-60% of the patients. *0503* Solitary hypercalciuria without hyperparathyroidism indicates sarcoidosis. *0503 0433* Occurs in approximately 33% of patients at some stage. Urinary levels are high, stool content low, and serum phosphate normal or low. *1083 0999 1361 2199*

170.90 Malignant Neoplasm of Bone Lytic tumors. *0503 0619*

174.90 Malignant Neoplasm of Breast *0503*

188.90 Malignant Neoplasm of Bladder No evidence of bone involvement. Parathyroid hormone-secreting tumors. *0503*

198.50 Secondary Malignant Neoplasm of Bone Patients with osteostatic metastatic neoplasms (especially with active or extensive lesions) may display hypercalcemia and hypercalciuria which can be further complicated by nephrocalcinosis and renal failure. *0503* Often increased; marked increase may reflect increased rate of tumor growth. *2467 0151*

201.90 Hodgkin's Disease *0503*

202.80 Non-Hodgkins Lymphoma Neoplasm. Metastatic tumors involving the bone. *0503*

203.00 Multiple Myeloma Skeletal destruction results in hypercalciuria in virtually all cases. *2035*

204.00 Lymphocytic Leukemia (Acute) May be increased in some cases. *0503*

204.10 Lymphocytic Leukemia (Chronic) *0503*

205.00 Myelocytic Leukemia (Acute) *0503*

205.10 Myelocytic Leukemia (Chronic) *0503*

242.90 Hyperthyroidism Urinary excretion was increased and correlated positively to degree of hyperthyroidism. *1638 0999 1083*

250.00 Diabetes Mellitus Osmotic diuresis secondary to hyperglycemia. *2540*

252.00 Hyperparathyroidism 24 h excretion is high because of significant hypercalcemia, even though the renal clearance of calcium is relatively reduced. *0151* 39 of 54 patients had elevations above the normal upper limit (250-300 mg/24h). *2161* Found in about 50% of primary cases. *1957* Most patients are hypercalcemic and hypercalciuric. *1492 0433*

252.10 Hypoparathyroidism Rises acutely, then falls to low levels as plasma calcium falls. *2540*

253.00 Acromegaly In 20 patients with active disease, gut absorption was greater than normal and positively correlated with both the elevated serum and urine concentrations. *2161 0151*

255.00 Adrenal Cortical Hyperfunction (Glucocorticoid Excess) *0503*

268.00 Vitamin D Deficiency Rickets In young persons. *0151 0503*

268.20 Osteomalacia Other factors than vitamin D in adults. *0503*

270.02 Hartnup Disease *2467*

270.03 Cystinosis Secondary from acidosis. *0995*

275.10 Hepatolenticular Degeneration Slightly increased clearance in 19% of patients. *2278*

275.32 Hypophosphatasia *2246*

275.41 Milk-Alkali Syndrome *0503*

276.20 Metabolic Acidosis *0503*

278.40 Hypervitaminosis D *2199*

335.20 Amyotrophic Lateral Sclerosis Disuse atrophy with a major portion of the body immobilized. *0503*

503.01 Berylliosis Hypercalciuria may occur. *0433 2467*

555.90 Regional Enteritis or Ileitis High levels may be found. *0282 2035*

556.00 Ulcerative Colitis High levels may be found. *0282 2035*

588.81 Proximal Renal Tubular Acidosis The hypercalciuria results in nephrocalcinosis or nephrolithiasis which, in the absence of generalized aminoaciduria, aids in the differentiation of this disease from the more common De Toni-Debre-Fanconi Syndrome. *0433 0503 2246*

Calcium *(continued)*

Urine Increase *(continued)*

588.82 Distal Renal Tubular Acidosis An almost constant feature and frequently results in the formation of renal calculi. *0151 0614*

592.00 Kidney Calculus 35% of patients have increased urinary concentration (> 250 mg/24h in females and > 300 mg/24h in males). *2468* Increased in the majority of patients with calcareous calculi, but will be normal in patients whose primary problem is infection. *0151*

731.00 Osteitis Deformans Excretion is frequently increased and may lead to stone formation. *0151* Common. *0999 0503*

733.00 Osteoporosis May be increased, normal, or decreased but is not influenced by intake; calcium restriction does not produce the normal fall. *2467 0503 0999*

753.10 Polycystic Kidney Disease Found in nonuremic medullary cystic disease. *0151*

753.12 Medullary Cystic Disease Found in nonuremic medullary cystic disease. *0151*

753.13 Medullary Sponge Kidney Hypercalciuria in 19 of 36 patients tested. *0644*

CSF Normal

345.90 Epilepsy *0093*

Feces Decrease

135.00 Sarcoidosis At some stage of disease. *1083*

278.40 Hypervitaminosis D Decreased in stool. More calcium is absorbed from the diet than normal. *0619*

Feces Increase

242.90 Hyperthyroidism Excess of thyroid hormone induces a marked increase in fecal and urinary excretion. *1083*

268.00 Vitamin D Deficiency Rickets Urine and serum concentration is low with high stool content. *2246*

275.35 Vitamin D Resistant Rickets Diminished intestinal absorption. *2246*

579.00 Celiac Sprue Disease In steatorrhea. *0619*

579.90 Malabsorption, Cause Unspecified In diarrheas of all sorts, but especially steatorrheas, large fecal calcium losses occur. One patient with steatorrhea (nontropical sprue) was observed to excrete all ingested calcium plus the amount calculated to have been derived from 8 liters of intestinal juices which are normally excreted into the tract, a deficit amounting to 500 mg of calcium daily. *1083*

581.90 Nephrotic Syndrome May be high indicating intestinal absorption. *1523*

Red Blood Cells Increase

282.00 Hereditary (Congenital) Spherocytosis RBC content of Ca^{++} is increased. *0711* In 18 cases of congenital hemolytic anemias, increased erythrocytic Ca^{++} level was observed in 10 cases. *0184* A marked increase in calcium uptake was observed in the ATP depleted red cells of the unsplenectomized patients *2643*

283.00 Acquired Hemolytic Anemia (Autoimmune) In 19 cases of acquired autoimmune hemolysis, increased erythrocytic Ca^{++} level was observed in 6 cases. *0184*

359.21 Myotonia Atrophica Erythrocytes from these patients accumulate calcium at a significantly higher rate than normals do. This increased rate of net accumulation appears related to an enhanced permeability of the membrane, rather than to an impairment in its active outward transport. *1827*

Saliva Increase

277.00 Cystic Fibrosis Submaxillary saliva is turbid, with increased calcium, total protein, and amylase. These changes are not generally found in parotid saliva. *2467*

Sweat Increase

585.00 Chronic Renal Failure Concentrations of Ca, Mg and phosphate in sweat were significantly elevated due to an increase in the secretion of these electrolytes in the secretory portion of the sweat gland, while that in the reabsorptive duct is normal. *1861*

Capillary Fragility

Blood Increase

284.90 Aplastic Anemia Reflects low platelet count. *2538*

286.01 Hemophilia Occasional patients may have positive tourniquet tests. *2552*

287.00 Allergic Purpura Tourniquet tests are, at times, positive. *2538 2552*

287.10 Thrombasthenia (Glanzmann's) *2246*

287.30 Idiopathic Thrombocytopenic Purpura Positive tourniquet test. *2552 2538*

446.60 Thrombotic Thrombocytopenic Purpura Positive tourniquet test. *2552*

Carcinoembryonic Antigen

Serum Increase

11.00 Pulmonary Tuberculosis 37% of patients had values > 2.5 ng/mL. *2199*

70.00 Viral Hepatitis 30% of patients had values > 2.5 ng/mL. *2199*

150.90 Malignant Neoplasm of Esophagus In 66% of patients with localized upper GI tract malignancy, mean = 4.9 ng/mL. *1817 2467 2035 0795*

151.90 Malignant Neoplasm of Stomach In 66% of patients with localized upper GI tract malignancy, mean = 4.9 ng/mL. *1817 2035 0795*

152.90 Malignant Neoplasm of Small Intestine In 66% of patients with localized upper GI tract malignancy, mean = 4.9 ng/mL. *1817 2035 0795*

153.90 Malignant Neoplasm of Large Intestine Increased in about 80% of the patients. *2467* 55% of patients had elevated concentrations (mean = 6.3 ng/mL). 91% of patients had positive plasma assays. *0830* In 73% of cases. *2199* In 66% of patients with localized upper GI tract malignancy, mean = 4.9 ng/mL. *1817 2035 0795*

154.10 Malignant Neoplasm of Rectum In 73% of cases. *2199* In 66% of patients with localized upper GI tract malignancy, mean = 4.9 ng/mL. *1817 2035 0795*

155.00 Malignant Neoplasm of Liver In 67% of cases. *2199 0795 2035*

157.90 Malignant Neoplasm of Pancreas Elevated levels were noted in 33% of the patients with tumors localized to the pancreas. When the carcinoma had extended beyond the pancreas or distant metastases were present, 78% of patients had elevated levels. *1767* In 92% of cases. *2199 2035 0795*

162.90 Malignant Neoplasm of Bronchus and Lung Very high titers have been found in 76% of patients. *0431* 88 of 115 (or 77%) of patients had an initial concentration > 2.5 ng/mL. Of 28 patients with concentration 15 ng/mL at the time of initial examination, 27 were found to have locally extensive or disseminated disease. *2432* Found in > 50 % of the patients *0925* Concentrations > 40 μg/L were found in 40.6% of patients with oat cell carcinoma. *1553* In 72% of cases. *2199 0795 2035*

174.90 Malignant Neoplasm of Breast 12 of 17 patients had initially elevated values. Levels in later stages of the disease were usually higher than those in earlier stages. Referring to the international TNM classification, values were particularly elevated in both the T$_3$ and T$_4$ stages, with axillary node involvement and with the presence of bone metastases. *2374* In 52% of cases. *2199 0200 0795 2035*

180.90 Malignant Neoplasm of Cervix Of the 156 patients with carcinoma in situ, 14 (9%) were positive. Progressive increase in the percentage of positive patients as stage increases, from 26% in stage I to 88% in stage IV. 52 of 61 (85%) with recurrent squamous cell carcinoma showed a positive value. *0564* 59% positivity reported. In advanced disease 84% had elevated values. *0740* Elevations found in cervical adenocarcinoma (19%) and squamous cell carcinoma of the uterine cervix (10%). *2386* Elevated (> 2.5 ng/mL) in 48% of 300 patients, and varied directly with stage of disease and histologic differentiation of the tumor. Rising of concentration indicated recurrence in 29 patients. *2413* In 42% of cases. *2199 0580*

182.00 Malignant Neoplasm of Corpus Uteri   Positive in 25 of 47 patients with adenocarcinoma of the endometrium. A tendency toward higher values in the advanced stages evidenced by 24% incidence in stage I in contrast to a 57% incidence in stage III. *0564* 67% positivity; incidence rose to 84% in advanced cases. *0740* In 27% of the cases. *2199*

183.00 Malignant Neoplasm of Ovary   Of the 132 patients with adenocarcinoma, 73 had positive values. The largest number of patients were in the stage III category where 45 of 77 patients (58%) were positive. *0564* 77% positivity. *0740* Most commonly found in ovarian cancer. Elevated levels occurred in 6 of 30 cases, all at advanced stages III or IV. *2386* In 35% of cases. *2199 0580*

185.00 Malignant Neoplasm of Prostate   30% of patients with advanced urologic tumors have elevated plasma levels. There is a good correlation between the stage of carcinoma and the degree of elevation. In general, with advanced active disease positive results exceed the normal level of 2.5 ng., whereas levels in inactive disease have been negative or at least below normal. *0433* In 40% of cases. *2199* 35% of patients. *2503* *0795 2035*

186.90 Malignant Neoplasm of Testis   In 57% of cases. *2199*

188.90 Malignant Neoplasm of Bladder   Increased in 53% of the patients (without urinary infection). No false positive results. *1304* In 33% of cases. *2199* *0795 2035*

189.00 Malignant Neoplasm of Kidney   In 35% of cases. *2199*

192.50 Neuroblastoma   In 100% of cases. *2199*

193.01 Medullary Carcinoma of Thyroid   Over 5 ng/mL in 20% of patients. All patients with medullary carcinoma had considerably elevated levels (> 25 ng/mL). *0624*

197.50 Secondary Malignant Neoplasm of Digestive System   All but 1 of the patients with metastatic disease of the GI tract had elevated concentrations of CEA. Mean value for upper GI tract disease was 21.8 ± 22.7 ng/mL, and 285.2 ± 441 ng/mL for lower GI tract disease. *1817*

197.70 Secondary Malignant Neoplasm of Liver   Markedly increased (> 25 ng/mL) values are highly suggestive of metastatic cancer, particularly hepatic metastasis. *0859*

199.00 Secondary Malignant Neoplasm (Disseminated)   High preoperative values had been shown to be associated with an increased risk of metastases or recurrence in patients who apparently had a successful resection of a carcinoma of the large bowel. Measurements after surgery provide an earlier warning of metastases and recurrence often with a lead time of many months. *0450*

201.90 Hodgkin's Disease   In 22% of cases. *2199*

202.80 Non-Hodgkins Lymphoma   In 22% of cases. *2199*

204.00 Lymphocytic Leukemia (Acute)   Above 2.5 ng/mL in 38% of patients with acute and chronic leukemia. *0211*

204.10 Lymphocytic Leukemia (Chronic)   Above 2.5 ng/mL in 38% of patients with acute and chronic leukemia. *0211*

205.00 Myelocytic Leukemia (Acute)   Above 2.5 ng/mL in 38% of patients with acute and chronic leukemia. *0211*

205.10 Myelocytic Leukemia (Chronic)   Above 2.5 ng/mL in 38% of patients with acute and chronic leukemia. *0211*

211.40 Benign Neoplasm of Rectum and Anus   14 (15%) of 93 adult patients with sporadic colorectal adenomata had concentration > 2.5 ng/mL. No associations were found with age, polyp volume, or villous histology. *0587* 19% of patients had values > 2.5 ng/mL. *2199*

217.00 Benign Neoplasm of Breast   15% of patients had values > 2.5 ng/mL. *2199*

244.90 Hypothyroidism   32% of patients had values > 2.5 ng/mL. *0979*

250.00 Diabetes Mellitus   38% of patients had values > 2.5 ng/mL. *2199*

358.00 Myasthenia Gravis   18% of patients had values > 2.5 ng/mL. *2199*

401.10 Essential Benign Hypertension   28% of patients had values > 2.5 ng/mL. *2199*

414.00 Chronic Ischemic Heart Disease   39% of patients had values > 2.5 ng/mL. *2199*

482.90 Bacterial Pneumonia   47% of patients had values > 2.5 ng/mL. *2199*

491.00 Chronic Bronchitis   33% of patients had values > 2.5 ng/mL. *2199*

492.80 Pulmonary Emphysema   57% of patients had values > 2.5 ng/mL. *2199*

516.10 Idiopathic Pulmonary Hemosiderosis   *0795 2035*

533.90 Peptic Ulcer, Site Unspecified   14% of patients had positive assay (values > 12.5 ng/mL). *0253* 45% of patients had values > 2.5 ng/mL. *0979 2199*

537.40 Fistula of Stomach and Duodenum   Found in 15% (2.5 ng/mL). *0587*

555.90 Regional Enteritis or Ileitis   14% of 58 patients had positive assay. There was no correlation between CEA concentration and extent or activity of disease, but those with elevated levels all had the disease for > 7 y, mean = 18.1 y duration. *0253* 40% of patients had values > 2.5 ng/mL. *2199 0979*

556.00 Ulcerative Colitis   Elevated in as many as 27% of patients. *2005* 11% of 61 patients had positive assays. There was no correlation between CEA and length of history, degree of activity, or extent of colonic involvement. *0253* Serial measurements done of 57 patients yield significant correlations between peak CEA concentration and disease severity and extent of colonic involvement. *0815* 31% of patients had values > 2.5 ng/mL. *0979 0795 2035 2199*

562.00 Diverticular Disease of Intestine   41% of patients had values > 2.5 ng/mL. *0979 2199*

562.11 Diverticulitis of Colon   27% of patients had values > 2.5 ng/mL. *0979 0795 2035*

570.00 Acute and Subacute Necrosis of Liver   Found in 50% of 16 patients with acute liver damage. Levels increased with increasing clinical severity. In acute damage, peak CEA occurs later than the time of maximum liver necrosis, suggesting that the rise is associated with regeneration. Higher levels occur in those patients with greater disturbance of liver function suggesting altered metabolism or excretion of CEA. *0311*

571.20 Laennec's or Alcoholic Cirrhosis   Positive assays were obtained in 40 of 88 patients with severe alcoholic liver disease but in none of 14 patients with nonalcoholic liver disease. Values usually were lower than in colonic or pancreatic cancer. *1623* About 50% of patients with severe alcoholic liver disease have elevated (> 2.5 ng/mL) values, usually < 5 and rarely 10 ng/mL. *1624* 70% of patients had values > 2.5 ng/mL. *0979 2199*

571.49 Chronic Active Hepatitis   4 of 7 patients showed elevated values (> 12.5 ng/mL). *0253*

571.90 Cirrhosis of Liver   *0795 2035*

575.00 Acute Cholecystitis   23% of patients had values > 2.5 ng/mL. *2199*

576.20 Extrahepatic Biliary Obstruction   Circulating levels are elevated in benign extrahepatic biliary tract obstruction and inflammation. *2290* 43% of patients had values > 2.5 ng/mL. *0979 2199*

577.00 Acute Pancreatitis   May be found. *0537* 53% of patients had values > 2.5 ng/mL. *0979 0795 2035 2199*

579.00 Celiac Sprue Disease   In adult celiac disease, 2 of 9 patients had concentrations > 12.5 ng/mL (normal < 12.5 ng/mL). *0253*

584.00 Acute Renal Failure   Increased in about 50% of the patients. *2467*

714.00 Rheumatoid Arthritis   In seropositive cases. *0619*

715.90 Osteoarthritis   30% of patients had values > 2.5 ng/mL. *2199*

Serum   Normal

201.90 Hodgkin's Disease   Levels are low in this malignancy, remaining within the normal range or just above it. *2374*

571.90 Cirrhosis of Liver   Positive assays were obtained in 40 of 88 patients with severe alcoholic liver disease but in none of 14 patients with nonalcoholic liver disease. Values usually were lower than in colonic or pancreatic cancer. *1623*

630.00 Hydatidiform Mole   Only 1 of 17 patients had a value > 2.5 ng/mL in serum. In all cases, the hydatid fluid had values > 2.5 and the range was 3-40 ng/mL. *0564*

Pleural Effusion   Increase

11.00 Pulmonary Tuberculosis   Benign inflammatory effusions (tuberculosis, empyema, pneumonia) had mean CEA activity of 6.2 ± 3.4 ng/mL, higher than effusions caused by congestive heart failure (2.9 ± 1.5) and other noninflammatory effusions. *1945*

150.90 Malignant Neoplasm of Esophagus   The highest levels (> 1,000 ng/mL) were found in samples from patients with gastrointestinal carcinomas. *0622* 24 (34%) of 70 malignant effusions had levels 12 ng/mL. *1945*

Carcinoembryonic Antigen (continued)

Pleural Effusion   Increase (continued)

151.90 **Malignant Neoplasm of Stomach**   The highest levels (> 1,000 ng/mL) were found in samples from patients with gastrointestinal carcinomas. *0622*   24 (34%) of 70 malignant effusions had levels 12 ng/mL. *1945*

152.90 **Malignant Neoplasm of Small Intestine**   The highest levels (> 1,000 ng/mL) were found in samples from patients with gastrointestinal carcinomas. *0622*   24 (34%) of 70 malignant effusions had levels > 12 ng/mL. *1945*

153.90 **Malignant Neoplasm of Large Intestine**   The highest levels (> 1,000 ng/mL) were found in patients with gastrointestinal carcinomas. *0622*   24 (34%) of 70 malignant effusions had levels > 12 ng/mL. *1945*

154.10 **Malignant Neoplasm of Rectum**   The highest levels (> 1,000 ng/mL) were found in samples from patients with gastrointestinal carcinomas. *0622*   24 (34%) of 70 malignant effusions had levels > 12 ng/mL. *1945*

162.90 **Malignant Neoplasm of Bronchus and Lung**   24 (34%) of 70 malignant effusions had levels > 12 ng/mL. *1945*

174.90 **Malignant Neoplasm of Breast**   24 (34%) of 70 malignant effusions had levels > 12 ng/mL. *1945*

480.90 **Viral Pneumonia**   Benign inflammatory effusions (tuberculosis, empyema, pneumonia) had mean activity of 6.2 ± 3.4 ng/mL, higher than effusions caused by congestive heart failure (2.9 ± 1.5 ng/mL) and other noninflammatory effusions. *1945*

482.90 **Bacterial Pneumonia**   Benign inflammatory effusions (tuberculosis, empyema, pneumonia) had mean activity of 6.2 ± 3.4 ng/mL, higher than effusions caused by congestive heart failure (2.9 ± 1.5) and other noninflammatory effusions. *1945*

510.00 **Empyema**   Benign inflammatory effusions (tuberculosis, empyema, pneumonia) had mean activity of 6.2 ± 3.4 ng/mL, higher than effusions caused by congestive heart failure (2.9 ± 1.5) and other noninflammatory effusions. *1945*

Ascitic Fluid   Increase

150.90 **Malignant Neoplasm of Esophagus**   CEA > 10 ng/mL ascites indicating cancerous effusion. *1420*

151.90 **Malignant Neoplasm of Stomach**   CEA > 10 ng/mL ascites indicating cancerous effusion. *1420*

152.90 **Malignant Neoplasm of Small Intestine**   CEA > 10 ng/mL ascites indicating cancerous effusion. *1420*

153.90 **Malignant Neoplasm of Large Intestine**   Ascitic fluid assays detected 11 of 13 cases; (CEA > 10 ng/mL ascites indicating cancerous effusion). *1420*

154.10 **Malignant Neoplasm of Rectum**   CEA > 10 ng/mL ascites indicating cancerous effusion. *1420*

155.00 **Malignant Neoplasm of Liver**   In malignant effusions. *2199*

155.10 **Malignant Neoplasm of Intrahepatic Bile Ducts**   In malignant effusions. *2199*

157.90 **Malignant Neoplasm of Pancreas**   In malignant effusions. *2199*

174.90 **Malignant Neoplasm of Breast**   4 of 6 breast cancer patients were detected by CEA estimations in ascitic fluid. Values > 10 ng/mL were considered cancerous effusions. *1420*

183.00 **Malignant Neoplasm of Ovary**   In malignant effusions. *2199*

188.90 **Malignant Neoplasm of Bladder**   In malignant effusions. *2199*

189.00 **Malignant Neoplasm of Kidney**   In malignant effusions. *2199*

197.00 **Secondary Malignant Neoplasm of Respiratory System**   In malignant effusions. *2199*

197.70 **Secondary Malignant Neoplasm of Liver**   In malignant effusions. *2199*

Peritoneal Fluid   Increase

150.90 **Malignant Neoplasm of Esophagus**   The highest levels (> 1,000 ng/mL) were found in samples from patients with gastrointestinal carcinomas. *0622*

151.90 **Malignant Neoplasm of Stomach**   The highest levels (> 1,000 ng/mL) were found in samples from patients with gastrointestinal carcinomas. *0622*

152.90 **Malignant Neoplasm of Small Intestine**   The highest levels (> 1,000 ng/mL) were found in samples from patients with gastrointestinal carcinomas. *0622*

153.90 **Malignant Neoplasm of Large Intestine**   The highest levels (> 1,000 ng/mL) were found in patients with gastrointestinal carcinomas. *0622*

154.10 **Malignant Neoplasm of Rectum**   The highest levels (> 1,000 ng/mL were found in patients with gastrointestinal carcinomas. *0622*

Carotene

Serum   Decrease

40.20 **Whipple's Disease**   A useful indication of fat malabsorption low levels are found in as many 80% of patients with steatorrhea. *0962*   Common. *2199*   *0999*

157.90 **Malignant Neoplasm of Pancreas**   Secondary to malabsorption. *2199*

251.50 **Zollinger-Ellison Syndrome**   A useful indication of fat malabsorption, low levels are found in as many as 80% of patients with steatorrhea. *0962*

259.20 **Carcinoid Syndrome**   Secondary to malabsorption or steatorrhea. *2540*

260.00 **Protein Malnutrition**   Extremely low in children with kwashiorkor. *0151*

271.30 **Lactosuria**   A useful indication of fat malabsorption, low levels are found in as many as 80% of patients with steatorrhea. *0962*

272.51 **Tangier Disease**   Tends to be low, probably due to the absence of high and low density lipoproteins, not malabsorption. *2246*   Occasionally low. *0878*

272.52 **Abetalipoproteinemia**   Very low. *0878*

555.90 **Regional Enteritis or Ileitis**   With malabsorption. *2199*

570.00 **Acute and Subacute Necrosis of Liver**   *2467*

577.10 **Chronic Pancreatitis**   With malabsorption. *2238*

579.00 **Celiac Sprue Disease**   At the time of the initial diagnosis, most patients have steatorrhea, low serum carotene levels, abnormal d-xylose absorption, and an abnormal small bowel x-ray pattern. *0999*   A useful indication of fat malabsorption low levels are found in as many as 80% of patients with steatorrhea. *0962*   Usually depressed in patients with sufficient intestinal involvement to produce steatorrhea. *2199*   *0433*

579.90 **Malabsorption, Cause Unspecified**   Decreased in malabsorption syndrome. *0151*   A useful indication of fat malabsorption low levels are found in as many as 80% of patients with steatorrhea. *0962*

992.00 **Heat stroke**   *2467*

Serum   Increase

244.90 **Hypothyroidism**   *2468*

245.10 **Subacute Thyroiditis**   *0151*

250.00 **Diabetes Mellitus**   *2467*

272.00 **Type IIA Hyperlipoproteinemia**   Increased concentration carried in beta lipoproteins are easily visible. *0992*

272.21 **Type IIB Hyperlipoproteinemia**   Increased concentration carried in beta lipoproteins are easily visible. *0992*

272.31 **Type I Hyperlipoproteinemia**   *2467*

650.00 **Pregnancy**   Increased. *0299 1030 1032*

Casts

Urine   Increase

32.00 **Diphtheria**   Frequently present. *2468*

82.00 **Rocky Mountain Spotted Fever**   Varying degrees. *0433*

100.00 **Leptospirosis**   Urine is abnormal in 75% of patients. *2468*   During the leptospiremic phase. *0962*

238.40 **Polycythemia Vera**   Occasionally. *2552*

250.10 **Diabetic Acidosis**   *2468*

390.00 **Rheumatic Fever**   Often mild abnormality of Addis count (protein, casts, RBC WBC) indicates mild focal nephritis. Concomitant glomerulonephritis appears in up to 2.5% of cases. *2467*

446.60 **Thrombotic Thrombocytopenic Purpura**   With kidney involvement. *0962*

580.40 **Glomerulonephritis (Rapidly Progressive)**   *2545*

581.90 Nephrotic Syndrome Sediment may be abnormal early in the disease before clinical signs of the syndrome become manifest, characterized by hyaline, granular, and waxy casts and plain casts with inclusions of RBC, WBC, tubular cells, and refractile fat bodies. *0962*

585.00 Chronic Renal Failure With renal parenchymal disease. *0838*

590.00 Chronic Pyelonephritis As in acute pyelonephritis, the leukocyte cast in the absence of other cellular casts is a most helpful finding and strongly supports the diagnosis. The urine sediment may be normal but repeated examination will usually reveal pyuria and cylindruria *0433* With Renal Parenchymal Disease *0838*

590.10 Acute Pyelonephritis Generally interpreted as indicative of renal parenchymal inflammation and which in the absence of other types of cellular casts provides strong support for a diagnosis of pyelonephritis. *0433* Essentially diagnostic. *0962* With renal parenchymal disease *0838*

599.00 Urinary Tract Infection In uncomplicated acute symptomatic infections, urine sediment usually contains numbers of pus cells and WBC casts. *0962*

985.00 Toxic Effects of Non-medicinal Metals Nephrotoxicity may occur with therapeutic doses of arsenicals. *1514 0651 0889*

994.50 Exercise Hyaline and granular; both increased with increased exercise. *1205*

Urine Normal

753.12 Medullary Cystic Disease Normal urinary sediment. *0277*

Catalase

Red Blood Cells Decrease

280.90 Iron Deficiency Anemia Has been demonstrated to be decreased in RBCs. *0104*

Catecholamines

Plasma Decrease

242.90 Hyperthyroidism Decreased plasma levels correlate inversely with total T_4. *2139*

250.00 Diabetes Mellitus Common. *1854* Long-term diabetics with neuropathy showed significant reductions. Diabetics without neuropathy had normal concentrations. *0399*

Plasma Increase

37.00 Tetanus Found in patients with severe disease. It is believed that this increase is caused by autonomic nervous system overactivity. *0433*

38.00 Septicemia Severe stress resulting from sepsis, hypovolemia or hypercapnia causes hypersecretion. *2236*

192.50 Neuroblastoma Catecholamine secretion is as high or higher than in pheochromocytoma. *2612*

227.91 Pheochromocytoma In pediatric cases, venous catheterization showed a great increase in catecholamine efflux from the left adrenal vein, while dopamine-beta-hydroxylase (DBH) was only slightly elevated. Circulating catecholamines fluctuated greatly during removal of tumors, but DBH decreased gradually. *1021* Twice upper limit of normal. *0999* Usually very high, there is significant overlap with values that may be obtained with excitement, emotional disturbance, essential hypertension and depression. *0151*

244.90 Hypothyroidism *2139*

250.10 Diabetic Acidosis *2540*

296.80 Manic Depressive Disorder Patients with a 6 month or longer history of anxiety and depression had total plasma catecholamine concentration significantly above normal. *1300*

300.40 Depressive Neurosis Patients with a 6 month or longer history of anxiety and depression had total plasma catecholamine concentration significantly above normal. *1300*

308.00 Stress Normal metabolic response. *2315*

401.10 Essential Benign Hypertension Raised plasma catecholamines in some patients with primary hypertension. *0522*

410.90 Acute Myocardial Infarction The adrenal medulla can release circulating catecholamines as the result either of the generalized sympathetic stress reaction or of arterial hypoxia. Patients with higher plasma levels of catecholamines and free fatty acids may have a higher incidence of severe arrhythmias, shock, and death than patients with lower levels. *1108*

414.00 Chronic Ischemic Heart Disease Epinephrine and norepinephrine increase in proportion to the severity of circulatory failure. Catecholamine excretion, especially norepinephrine, is significantly raised in grades 3 and 4 of hemodynamic disturbance. *2572*

415.00 Cor Pulmonale Epinephrine and norepinephrine increase in proportion to the severity of circulatory failure. Catecholamine excretion, especially norepinephrine, is significantly raised in grades 3 and 4 of hemodynamic disturbance. *2572*

556.00 Ulcerative Colitis Circulating levels. *0995*

567.90 Peritonitis Increased adrenal production. *0995*

585.00 Chronic Renal Failure Moderate increase. *0649*

Plasma Normal

242.90 Hyperthyroidism *2540*

244.90 Hypothyroidism *2540*

Urine Decrease

250.00 Diabetes Mellitus Common. *1854* Long-term diabetics with neuropathy showed significant reductions. Diabetics without neuropathy had normal concentrations. *0399*

300.40 Depressive Neurosis Documented decrease in urinary excretion of catecholamine and indolamine metabolites reported in depressed patients. Not used as a clinical tool at this time. *0433*

714.00 Rheumatoid Arthritis The more severe the stage and class of the arthritis, the lower the epinephrine, and the closer to normal norepinephrine values. Norepinephrine seems to reflect a compensation in catecholamine metabolism rather than adrenal cortex system influence. *1114*

Urine Increase

37.00 Tetanus Usually found in patients with severe disease. It is believed that this increase is caused by autonomic nervous system overactivity. *0433*

38.00 Septicemia Increased due to severe stress. *2467* Severe stress resulting from sepsis, hypovolemia or hypocapnia causes hypersecretion. *2236*

227.91 Pheochromocytoma Of the 3 different types of catecholamines present in the urine - the metanephrine test is positive in more than 97% of patients with the disease and is rarely falsely positive in hypertensive subjects who do not have the disease. *1223* Most excrete > 300 μg/24h. *1108* *0999 0962*

244.90 Hypothyroidism *2139*

259.20 Carcinoid Syndrome Catecholamines and their metabolites have been elevated in the urine of some patients. This abnormality is unusual and to date has not been correlated with specific symptoms or origins of the tumors. *2199 1568*

296.80 Manic Depressive Disorder Patients with a 6 month or longer history of anxiety and depression had total plasma catecholamine concentration significantly above normal. *1300*

300.40 Depressive Neurosis Patients with a 6 month or longer history of anxiety and depression had total plasma catecholamine concentration significantly above normal. *1300*

308.00 Stress With physical or emotional stress. *2092*

358.00 Myasthenia Gravis Some cases. *2467*

359.11 Progressive Muscular Dystrophy *2467*

390.00 Rheumatic Fever Epirephrine and norepinephrine increase in proportion to the severity of circulatory failure. Catecholamine excretion, especially norepinephrine, is significantly raised in grades 3 and 4 of hemodynamic disturbance. *2572*

401.00 Malignant Hypertension Slightly increased. *2467*

401.10 Essential Benign Hypertension Up to 100 μg/24h may be excreted. *0619*

410.90 Acute Myocardial Infarction Total urinary catecholamines were significantly elevated in the first 48 h. *0529*

414.00 Chronic Ischemic Heart Disease Epinephrine and norepinephrine increase in proportion to the severity of circulatory failure. Catecholamine excretion, especially norepinephrine, is significantly raised in grades 3 and 4 of hemodynamic disturbance. *2572*

Catecholamines *(continued)*

Urine   Increase *(continued)*

415.00   Cor Pulmonale   Epinephrine and norepinephrine increase in proportion to the severity of circulatory failure. Catecholamine excretion, especially norepinephrine, is significantly raised in grades 3 and 4 of hemodynamic disturbance. *2572*

556.00   Ulcerative Colitis   Circulating levels. *0995*

567.90   Peritonitis   Increased adrenal production. *0995*

577.00   Acute Pancreatitis   May be marked; increased due to severe stress. *2467*

642.60   Eclampsia   Increased due to severe stress. *2467*

785.50   Shock   *0164*

929.00   Crush Injury (Trauma)   Due to severe stress. *0995*

948.00   Burns   Increased due to severe stress. *2467*   With physical or emotional stress. *2092*

994.50   Exercise   May be increased by vigorous exercise prior to urine collection (up to 7 fold). *0212*   The normal output after daily routine activity is twice the resting output. *0619*

Urine   Normal

242.90   Hyperthyroidism   *2540*

994.50   Exercise   After mild or moderate exercise. *2092*

Cells

Blood   Increase

282.71   Hemoglobin C Disease   One of the most striking features of homozygous disease is the marked increase in the number of target cells in the peripheral blood. *2538*

Urine   Increase

580.00   Acute Poststreptococcal Glomerulonephritis   36% renal epithelial cells were found in tubular nephrosis (necrosis) and in glomerulonephritis. *1411*   Granular and epithelial cell casts are found. *2468*

585.00   Chronic Renal Failure   Renal epithelial cells were increased to 49% of total cells in benign endemic nephropathy. *1411*

994.50   Exercise   Epithelial cells increase with heavy exercise. *1205*

CSF   Increase

13.00   Tuberculosis Meningitis   25-500/μL; chiefly lymphocytes. *0962*

18.00   Disseminated Tuberculosis   Spinal fluid shows predominantly mononuclear pleocytosis (up to several hundred cells/μL). *0999*

32.00   Diphtheria   With neuritis, a pleocytosis can occur. *1058*

36.00   Meningococcal Meningitis   Cell count is elevated to thousands/μL, mostly neutrophils. *0151*

45.90   Acute Poliomyelitis   Is usually 25-500/μL. At first most are polymorphonuclear leukocytes; after several days most are lymphocytes. *2468*   Chiefly lymphocytes. *0962*

47.00   Aseptic Meningitis   A pleocytosis of up to 3,000/μL may occur. In the first day or two of illness, polymorphonuclears may predominate, but the cell differential then shifts to one predominantly of lymphocytes. *0999*

52.00   Chickenpox   Encephalitis. *2467*

53.00   Herpes Zoster   40% of patients show increased cells (< 300 mononuclear cells/μL). *2468*   *0962*

54.00   Herpes Simplex   Up to 500/μL, with lymphocytes or mononuclear cells predominating. *0151*

55.00   Measles   *2467*

56.00   Rubella   *2467*

71.00   Rabies   Usually < 1,000/μL but counts between 1,500-4,000/μL have been observed. *1319*

72.00   Mumps   In meningitis and meningoencephalitis fewer than 500/μL with only occasional cell counts exceeding 2,000/μL. In most cases the cells are almost exclusively mononuclear from the onset: polymorphonuclear leukocytes predominate for the first few days in only a small percentage of patients. Pleocytosis may continue for as long as 5 weeks. *0433*

78.50   Cytomegalic Inclusion Disease   Pleocytosis in congenital disease. *1319*

80.00   Epidemic Typhus   With severe encephalitis manifestations. *0433*

87.00   Relapsing Fever   Mononuclear cells sometimes increased. *2468*

97.90   Syphilis   Increased in meningovascular syphilis. *0999*   First sign of asymptomatic syphilis arising from latency is pleocytosis of > 4 cells/μL, followed by increase in protein. With progress to parenchymatous neurosyphilis, 150 cells/μL and marked increase in protein (globulin) is found. *0151*   *0962*

100.00   Leptospirosis   Increased up to 500/μL in about 66% of patients. Indicates meningeal involvement. *2468*   Pleocytosis of 25-500 cells/μL in > 75% of cases. *0962*

112.90   Moniliasis   Pleocytosis in all patients with Candida meningitis, predominantly lymphocytic. *0138*

114.90   Coccidioidomycosis   CSF cell and chemistry are indistinguishable from tuberculous meningitis. *2368*

130.00   Toxoplasmosis   In congenital, both RBC and WBC with a predominance of mononuclear elements. In acquired predominantly mononuclear cells, 30-2000/μL. *1319*

135.00   Sarcoidosis   In granulomatous basilar meningitis affecting cranial nerves. *0992*

191.90   Malignant Neoplasm of Brain   Mononuclear cells are increased. *0999*

198.30   Secondary Malignant Neoplasm of Brain   Increased cells which are not usually recognized as blast cells because of poor preservation (meningeal infiltration of leukemic cells). *2467*

204.00   Lymphocytic Leukemia (Acute)   Pleocytosis with meningeal infiltration. *2538*

205.00   Myelocytic Leukemia (Acute)   Pleocytosis with meningeal infiltration. *2538*

225.90   Benign Neoplasm of Brain and CNS   Elevated from 5-100/μL in 33% of cases. May exceed 1,000, particularly if the tumor involves the ventricular wall and has undergone necrosis. *0151*   *0962*

320.90   Meningitis (Bacterial)   Increased polymorphonuclear cells are found in CSF. Mononuclear cells appear later in the disease. *0999*   CSF cells are always elevated, ranging from 100-100,000/μL initially polymorphonuclear leukocytes predominate; these are replaced by lymphocytes as the inflammatory process progresses. *0151*

323.91   Myelitis   Spinal fluid may be normal or may show increased protein and cells (20-1,000/μL - lymphocytes and mononuclear cells). *2467*   Increased WBCs, mononuclear, and polymorphonuclear cells are found. *0999*

323.92   Encephalomyelitis   Usually increased (< 100/μL), mostly polymorphonuclear leukocytes. After the third day cell count is > 90% lymphocytes. *2468*

324.00   Intracranial Abscess   Usually < 500/μL with polymorphonuclears predominating in chronic encapsulating infections. *0999*   May vary from 0 to many thousands, depending on the degree of meningitic involvement, and may be particularly high if the abscess has ruptured into the ventricles. In most chronic abscesses, the cell count is usually > 100, and the cells are usually mononuclear in the type. *0433*

340.00   Multiple Sclerosis   About 50% of patients have mononuclear cells in the CSF during an acute episode in the range of 10-50 cells. *0999*

357.90   Polyneuritis   Characteristically, fewer than 10 cells/μL usually lymphocytes, are present in the CSF, and the presence of > 40/μL raises other diagnostic considerations, such as herpes simplex myelitis and poliomyelitis. *0433*

CSF   Normal

356.30   Refsum's Disease   High CSF protein concentration in the absence of pleocytosis has been found in all cases. *2246*

357.00   Guillain-Barré Syndrome   Characteristic findings are elevated protein concentration but no increase in number of cells in CSF. *0151*

Synovial Fluid   Present

99.30   Reiter's Disease   Reiter's Cells (macrophages with partially digested neutrophils). *0186*

Pericardial Fluid   Decrease

420.00   Acute Pericarditis   Few lymphocytes or RBCs. *0758*

Bone Marrow   Decrease

260.00   Protein Malnutrition   Normally cellular or slightly hypocellular, and the erythroid/myeloid ratio was decreased. *2538*

283.21   Paroxysmal Nocturnal Hemoglobinuria   The cellularity of the marrow may be decreased and may even appear aplastic. *2538*

284.01   Congenital Aplastic Anemia   Marrow is described as fatty and hypocellular or normocellular. *0695*

284.90   Aplastic Anemia   Marked hypocellularity of the marrow fragments with a predominance of reticulum cells, mast cells, lymphocytoid cells, and plasma cells. Cells of the myeloid series are often grossly reduced in numbers. *0151   0415*

Bone Marrow   Increase

202.80   Non-Hodgkins Lymphoma   Erythrocytic and granulocytic hyperplasia may develop in the bone marrow. *2538*

204.00   Lymphocytic Leukemia (Acute)   Almost always hypercellular and heavily infiltrated or replaced by abnormal lymphoid elements. *2538*

205.00   Myelocytic Leukemia (Acute)   Marked occurrence of either sea-blue histiocytes or Gaucher like cells, or of both, was observed in bone marrow smears and the hematopoietic tissues of 23 patients with chronic disease and in acute, but with lower frequency and degree. *2319*   Blast cells are present even when none are found in the peripheral blood. *2468*

205.10   Myelocytic Leukemia (Chronic)   Occurrence of either sea-blue histiocytes or Gaucher like cells, or of both, was observed in bone marrow smears of 23 patients and in the hematopoietic tissues of 44 of the examined cases; particularly marked in chronic disease and in acute forms, though less in frequency or degree. *2319*   Bone marrow aspirated from almost any site usually yields a grossly hypercellular specimen in which the fat is practically absent. *2538*

207.00   Erythroleukemia   Marrow is nearly always hypercellular and characteristically shows a selective hyperplasia of the erythroid cells, with a myeloid/erythroid ratio of 1.0 or even lower. *2538*

238.40   Polycythemia Vera   Hyperplasia of erythroid, myeloid and megakaryocytic elements within those areas of the skeleton that normally contain active marrow. Marrow differential count may be normal or may reveal a reduction in the myeloid/erythroid ratio, reflecting a predominant normoblastic hyperplasia. *2538*

267.00   Vitamin C Deficiency   Normoblastic hyperplasia in the bone marrow. *2538*

272.73   Niemann-Pick Disease   Bone marrow contains typical foam cells, containing small droplets throughout the cytoplasm. *2538*

273.30   Waldenström's Macroglobulinemia   Bone marrow sections are always hypercellular and show extensive infiltration with atypical lymphocytes and also plasma cells, with macroglobulinemia. *2468*   Bone marrow punctures may result in dry tap due to great cellularity of the marrow combined with increased viscosity of the tissue fluid. *1225*

280.90   Iron Deficiency Anemia   Characterized by erythroid hyperplasia of mild-moderate degree. *2552*

281.20   Folic Acid Deficiency Anemia   Bone marrow shows megaloblastic dysplasia that varies from mild to marked in megaloblastic anemia of infancy. *2467*   Aspirated bone marrow is cellular and often hyperplastic. *2538*

281.30   Vitamin B$_6$ Deficiency Anemia   Bone marrow is characterized by intense erythroid hyperplasia, often associated with a shift to younger forms, particularly polychromatophilic normoblasts, some of which show megaloblastic nuclear changes. *2538*

282.31   Hereditary Nonspherocytic Hemolytic Anemia   Erythroid hyperplasia. *2538*

282.41   Thalassemia Major   Bone marrow is cellular and shows erythroid hyperplasia. *2468*

282.42   Thalassemia Minor   Bone marrow is cellular and shows erythroid hyperplasia and contains stainable iron with thalassemias. *2468*

285.00   Sideroblastic Anemia   Bone marrow is characterized by intense erythroid hyperplasia, often associated with a shift to younger forms, particularly polychromatophilic normoblasts, some of which show megaloblastic nuclear changes. *2538*

287.30   Idiopathic Thrombocytopenic Purpura   Normal or increased numbers of megakaryocytes, many of which are smooth in contour, are found in the bone marrow. *2538*

446.60   Thrombotic Thrombocytopenic Purpura   Increased number of megakaryocytes but with marginal platelets. *2468*

571.20   Laennec's or Alcoholic Cirrhosis   Normal or increased. *1268*

571.90   Cirrhosis of Liver   Normal or increased. *1268*

585.00   Chronic Renal Failure   Tends to be moderately hypercellular. *2552 0329*

733.00   Osteoporosis   The iliac bone marrow specimens showed infiltrates consisting of elongated mast cells, eosinophils, plasma cells, and varying numbers of lymphocytes. *2334*

Bone Marrow   Normal

115.00   Histoplasmosis   Marrow smears reveal no cellular abnormalities. *2368*

Peritoneal Fluid   Increase

11.00   Pulmonary Tuberculosis   Cell count in the peritoneal fluid varies from 2,000-10,000/μL and shows a marked predominance of lymphocytes. *0962*

Sputum   Increase

55.00   Measles   Wright's stain of sputum shows measles multinucleated giant cells, especially during prodrome and early rash. *2468*

482.90   Bacterial Pneumonia   Gram's stain of sputum reveals many polymorphonuclear leukocytes, and many gram-positive cocci in pairs and singly in pneumonoccal pneumonia. *2468*

491.00   Chronic Bronchitis   *0433*

494.00   Bronchiectasis   Polymorphonuclear and lymphocytic, as well as bronchial epithelial cells with varying degrees of metaplasia. *0433*

Cellular Casts

Urine   Increase

446.00   Polyarteritis-Nodosa   Found in patients with glomerular disease. *0999   0962*

710.00   Systemic Lupus Erythematosus   *0433*

Cephalin Flocculation

Serum   Increase

70.00   Viral Hepatitis   Occurs frequently; concurrent with increase in direct bilirubin. *2467*

75.00   Infectious Mononucleosis   Maximal by 2nd week and normal by 5th week. *0619*   Reflected the presence and extent of hepatic damage, and paralleled the severity of subjective symptoms in 36 patients. *1912*   In most cases. *1319   2368*

78.50   Cytomegalic Inclusion Disease   Slight increase which becomes more marked with clinical hepatitis in some cases. *2468*

120.00   Schistosomiasis   Positive in acute disease. *2468*

273.23   Heavy Chain Disease (Gamma)   *2468*

273.30   Waldenström's Macroglobulinemia   In some cases. *1225   0020 2035*

277.41   Dubin-Johnson Syndrome   May be positive. *2467*

304.90   Drug Dependence (Opium and Derivatives)   Cephalin flocculation or thymol turbidity tests are increased in 75% of patients. *2468*

421.00   Bacterial Endocarditis   Positive due to altered serum proteins and increase in gamma globulin. *2467*

428.00   Congestive Heart Failure   Hepatic dysfunction, often with structural damage to the liver, may result in positive flocculation test. *1108*   Positive in about 20% of cases. *2467*

571.20   Laennec's or Alcoholic Cirrhosis   *0992*

571.90   Cirrhosis of Liver   *2467*

572.00   Liver Abscess (Pyogenic)   *2467*

572.40   Hepatic Failure   *0503*

573.30   Toxic Hepatitis   Normal or slight increase. *2467*

576.20   Extrahepatic Biliary Obstruction   Normal or may later become only slightly increased. *2467*

642.40   Pre-Eclampsia   34 of 72 women with mild disease had abnormal reactions. *0777   0387*

642.60   Eclampsia   11 of 16 cases were reported to be abnormal. *2447*   Higher incidence of abnormal reactions in hypertensive than in normotensive pregnancies. *0387*

Cephalin Flocculation *(continued)*

Serum   Increase *(continued)*

650.00   Pregnancy   Reported prevalence of abnormal reactions in normal pregnancy range from 0-35%, the average in 986 cases is 12%. *0387*

710.00   Systemic Lupus Erythematosus   Positive; reflects nonspecific serum protein abnormalities. *0962*

714.00   Rheumatoid Arthritis   Characteristically abnormal when the arthritis is active. *0433*

985.00   Toxic Effects of Non-medicinal Metals   Hepatotoxicity may occur with arsenicals. *1446*

Serum   Normal

157.90   Malignant Neoplasm of Pancreas   Usually normal. *2467*

Ceruloplasmin

Serum   Decrease

256.30   Ovarian Hypofunction   Estrogen effect. *0995*

260.00   Protein Malnutrition   Moderate transient deficiencies in patients with nephrosis. *2467*

275.10   Hepatolenticular Degeneration   Most patients are deficient; concentration is usually 15 mg/dL, but patients are seen with concentration within the normal range (25-45 mg/dL). This is particularly likely to be the case when liver damage predominates. *0433* Low ceruloplasmin and elevated copper are characteristic. This is the result of an impaired ability to incorporate copper into protein, particularly ceruloplasmin, which causes unbound copper to be deposited in tissues and fluids throughout the body. *0999*

340.00   Multiple Sclerosis   Slight elevation of serum copper with significant reduction of serum ceruloplasmin. *1830*

579.00   Celiac Sprue Disease   Moderate transient deficiencies in patients with nephrosis. *2467*

581.90   Nephrotic Syndrome   Found regularly with hypoproteinemia. *0350*   Moderate transient deficiencies *2467*

Serum   Increase

151.90   Malignant Neoplasm of Stomach   High only in gastric and pulmonary cancer. In 58 cases there was a correlation between copper and ceruloplasmin levels in the same subject; significant only in gastric forms. *2058*

162.90   Malignant Neoplasm of Bronchus and Lung   High in gastric and pulmonary cancer. *2058*

170.90   Malignant Neoplasm of Bone   A highly significant increase over normal levels in sera from patients with osteosarcoma. *2155*

201.90   Hodgkin's Disease   *0151*

256.00   Ovarian Hyperfunction   Estrogen effect. *0995*

297.90   Paranoid States and Other Psychoses   Elevated serum copper and ceruloplasmin blood levels were reported. It is postulated that this may be an important pathognomonic feature. *0027 0065*

345.90   Epilepsy   Slightly elevated (62.30 ± 6.62 mg/dL) in patients with grand mal epilepsy. *1625*

440.00   Arteriosclerosis   High concentrations of Zn, Cu and ceruloplasmin were found in 13 patients when compared with controls. The Zn:Cu ratio is much higher in arteriosclerotic patients than in healthy subjects. *0324*

571.20   Laennec's or Alcoholic Cirrhosis   *1654*

571.49   Chronic Active Hepatitis $Alpha_2$ glycoproteins, ceruloplasmin, and transferrin were elevated. *1654*

571.60   Biliary Cirrhosis   Elevated in 46 of 46 cases. *0526*

571.90   Cirrhosis of Liver   Elevated in various forms of acute and chronic liver disease. *0931*

580.00   Acute Poststreptococcal Glomerulonephritis   *1064*

580.01   Glomerulonephritis (Focal)   *1064*

580.02   Glomerulonephritis (Minimal Change)   *1064*

580.04   Glomerulonephritis (Membranous)   *1064*

580.05   Glomerulonephritis (Membranoproliferative)   *1064*

580.40   Glomerulonephritis (Rapidly Progressive)   *1064*

590.00   Chronic Pyelonephritis   Found in 84 patients with exacerbated disease. Raised levels indicate the amount of activity of the pathologic process and distinguishes it from glomerulonephritis. *2362*

650.00   Pregnancy   Approximately twice normal at term. Mechanism not known. *2636*   Normal pregnancy *0304*   Increased in last trimester of pregnancy *2468*

710.10   Progressive Systemic Sclerosis   Mean level of ceruloplasmin, but not copper were raised in these patients, although both were raised in the 2 patients with the most aggressive disease. *1155*   Believed to occur as a nonspecific response (acute phase reactant). *2035*

714.00   Rheumatoid Arthritis   May cause green color of plasma. *2467*   Significantly raised in rheumatoid disease in both sexes. *2100*

720.00   Rheumatoid (Ankylosing) Spondylitis   Raised significantly, with the greatest increases in the worst cases. *1155*

994.50   Exercise   Generally occurs within 15 min and persists for 24 h. *0985*

Serum   Normal

275.10   Hepatolenticular Degeneration   Normal in 5% of patients with overt disease. *2467*

335.20   Amyotrophic Lateral Sclerosis   *0665*

CSF   Decrease

345.90   Epilepsy   Slightly decreased in grand mal epilepsy. *1625*

Synovial Fluid   Increase

714.00   Rheumatoid Arthritis   Characteristic of rheumatoid effusions. *2101*

Chenodeoxycholic Acid

Serum   Increase

70.00   Viral Hepatitis   Increased serum bile acids in anicteric viral hepatitis from either A or B virus. Elevated postprandial levels may persist even after transaminase and BSP retention have returned to normal. *1154*

277.00   Cystic Fibrosis   Fifteen patients had elevated levels not correlated to liver morphology.

496.01   Alpha$_1$-Antitrypsin Deficiency   In 34 patients with this disease all patients with morphological cirrhosis. *1685*

571.49   Chronic Active Hepatitis   Degree of elevation is related to the severity of illness as judged by other biochemical and clinical parameters. Bile acids return to normal in patients who respond to therapy. *1154*   3-Beta-Hydroxy-5-Cholenoic Acid was elevated in hepatobiliary disease. Normal 0.184 mmol/L, Chronic Active Hepatitis 2.364. *2325*

571.60   Biliary Cirrhosis   In 15 patients with primary biliary cirrhosis 13 had increased fasting levels. *2036*   Severe Cholestasis *1154*

571.90   Cirrhosis of Liver   3-Beta-Hydroxy-5-cholenoic acid was elevated in hepatobiliary disease. Normal -- 0.184 mmol/L; Cirrhosis: compensated 0.433 and uncompensated 1.636. *2325*   Raised fasting levels were found in 29 of 49 patients. *2363*

576.20   Extrahepatic Biliary Obstruction   3-Beta-Hydroxy-5-cholenoic acid was elevated in hepatobiliary disease. Normal = 0.184 mmol/L, Obstructive Jaundice 6.783. *2325*   Serum bile acids elevate promptly during the acute episode and indicate biliary tract disease *1154*

Serum   Normal

277.42   Gilbert's Disease   Normal levels in hyperbilirubinemic patients. *2642 0751*

555.90   Regional Enteritis or Ileitis   Fasting values were in the normal range but post prandial increase was lower than in healthy controls. *1039*

Chloride

Serum   Decrease

4.90   Bacillary Dysentery   Fluid and electrolyte loss may be quite significant, particularly in pediatric and geriatric populations. *1058*

9.00   Gastroenteritis and Colitis   Either elevated or diminished may be noted. *0433*

13.00   Tuberculosis Meningitis   Fall may be due to vomiting. *0619*

135.00 Sarcoidosis Suggests the presence of sarcoidosis or malignancy in conjunction with other tests. *0433*

250.00 Diabetes Mellitus Osmotic diuresis secondary to hyperglycemia. *2540*

250.10 Diabetic Acidosis *0962*

255.00 Adrenal Cortical Hyperfunction (Glucocorticoid Excess) *0995*

255.10 Adrenal Cortical Hyperfunction (Mineralocorticoid Excess) May be seen. *0962* Depressed reciprocally with the bicarbonate elevation. *1108*

255.40 Adrenal Cortical Hypofunction *2467*

256.00 Ovarian Hyperfunction Progesterone effect. *0995*

276.30 Metabolic Alkalosis Is relatively lower than sodium. *2468*

277.14 Acute Intermittent Porphyria Hyponatremia, hypochloremia, hypokalemia, hypomagnesemia, and alkalosis associated with azotemia of variable degree are often present on admission but may also develop acutely during the course of the attack. The electrolyte disorders are attributable in many patients to electrolyte depletion with inappropriate and injudicious overhydration. *0433 2538*

320.90 Meningitis (Bacterial) The chloride content is reduced but not as dramatically as in tubercular meningitis. *0433* Slight decrease. *0503* In 33% of 18 patients hospitalized for this disorder. *0781*

428.00 Congestive Heart Failure Tends to fall but may be normal before treatment. *2467*

496.00 Chronic Obstructive Lung Disease Suggests chronic hypoventilation. *0962* In 44% of 71 patients at initial hospitalization for this disorder. *0781*

496.01 Alpha₁-Antitrypsin Deficiency Seen with associated hyperventilation. *1636*

533.90 Peptic Ulcer, Site Unspecified May fall below 100 mmol/L in an ulcer complicated by obstruction. With persistent marked obstruction, may reach as low as 60 mmol/L. *0433* Pyloric obstruction with vomiting and loss of gastric secretion results in hypochloremia, hyponatremia, hypokalemia, elevated serum pH and carbon dioxide content, and azotemia. *0962*

537.00 Pyloric Stenosis, Acquired Metabolic alkalosis secondary to vomiting. *0587*

537.40 Fistula of Stomach and Duodenum In gastric fistula, hypokalemic, hypochloremic alkalosis may result. *2199*

556.00 Ulcerative Colitis *0433*

558.90 Diarrhea *2467*

560.90 Intestinal Obstruction Metabolic alkalosis secondary to vomiting. *2467*

579.00 Celiac Sprue Disease If diarrhea is severe, marked electrolyte depletion. *2199*

580.00 Acute Poststreptococcal Glomerulonephritis Seen in azotemic or oliguric patients. *0062*

585.00 Chronic Renal Failure Decreased or normal. *2467*

642.60 Eclampsia With marked edema. *0621*

694.40 Pemphigus *0151*

780.80 Hyperhidrosis *2467*

785.40 Gangrene In 39% of 28 patients hospitalized for this disorder. *0781*

Serum Increase

1.00 Cholera Due to marked loss of fluid and electrolytes. *2468*

9.00 Gastroenteritis and Colitis Reflects the loss of greater volumes of fluid than salt. Either elevated or diminished may be noted. *0433*

151.90 Malignant Neoplasm of Stomach In 34% of 29 patients at initial hospitalization for this disorder. *0781*

203.00 Multiple Myeloma Typical hyperchloremic acidosis with respiratory compensation in 9 of 35 patients. *0518*

252.00 Hyperparathyroidism The chloride values were higher (mean = 107 mmol/L) and phosphate, lower (mean = 2.6 mg/dL mL) in the 25 hyperparathyroid patients, whereas the chloride concentrations were lower (mean = 98 mmol/L) and phosphate, higher (mean = 4.5 mg/dL) in the 27 patients with hypercalcemia from other causes. The chloride to phosphate ratio ranged from 31.8-80 in hyperparathyroidism, with 96% more than 33, and from 17.1-32.3 in those with hypercalcemia from other causes, with 92% < 30. *1766* Increases and phosphate decreases resulting in a Cl/PO₃ ratio > 33. *1957* Hyperchloremic acidosis occurs as a result of renal effects *2541 0781*

253.50 Diabetes Insipidus *2467*

255.10 Adrenal Cortical Hyperfunction (Mineralocorticoid Excess) The electrolyte pumps respond to mineralocorticoids by conserving sodium and chloride and by wasting bodily potassium. *2540*

255.40 Adrenal Cortical Hypofunction *2468*

256.30 Ovarian Hypofunction Estrogen effect. *0995*

268.00 Vitamin D Deficiency Rickets Mild acidosis and hyperchloremia may be observed. *2246*

270.03 Cystinosis Metabolic, hyperchloremic acidosis. *0433*

271.10 Galactosemia Hyperchloremic acidosis. May be secondary to GI disturbance, poor food intake, or renal tubular dysfunction. *2246 1797*

275.10 Hepatolenticular Degeneration Frequent hyperchloremia; occurred in 13 of 31 patients (42%). *2278*

276.50 Dehydration *2467*

277.00 Cystic Fibrosis *0619*

405.91 Renovascular Hypertension Acidosis which is out of proportion to the degree of azotemia. *0962*

560.90 Intestinal Obstruction With dehydration. *2199*

580.05 Glomerulonephritis (Membranoproliferative) 16 patients with membranoproliferative glomerulonephritis had a mean value significantly higher than that in normal subjects or patients with nephrotic syndrome. *0598*

584.00 Acute Renal Failure *2467*

588.81 Proximal Renal Tubular Acidosis *2246*

588.82 Distal Renal Tubular Acidosis Normal anion gap. *0186*

590.00 Chronic Pyelonephritis Hyperchloremia frequently accompanies chronic pyelonephritis. *0962*

597.80 Urethritis Reveals the degree of renal impairment. *0433*

992.00 Heat stroke Normal to high in severe cases. *0151*

994.50 Exercise Vigorous exercise for 30 min results in 2 mmol/L rise. *0706*

Serum Normal

252.00 Hyperparathyroidism Appears to be more reliable than inorganic phosphate for differentiating hyperparathyroidism from other causes of hypercalcemia. *2542*

260.00 Protein Malnutrition *2467*

277.00 Cystic Fibrosis Serum electrolytes are normal unless complications occur (e.g., chronic pulmonary disease with accumulation of CO₂, massive salt loss due to sweating). *2467*

428.00 Congestive Heart Failure Tends to fall but may be normal before treatment. *2467*

579.90 Malabsorption, Cause Unspecified *2467*

585.00 Chronic Renal Failure Decreased or normal. *2467*

650.00 Pregnancy Throughout pregnancy. *0517*

Urine Decrease

252.10 Hypoparathyroidism May occur. *2540*

253.50 Diabetes Insipidus Urine chloride concentration is very low, but because of the large urine volume, the daily output is normal. *0619*

255.40 Adrenal Cortical Hypofunction Inability of the renal tubules to reabsorb sodium chloride and water and relative inability to excrete potassium. *0619*

275.34 Familial Periodic Paralysis Precedes attack. *2246*

482.90 Bacterial Pneumonia Excretion of chlorides is decreased. *2368*

558.90 Diarrhea Excessive loss, due to severe diarrhea. *0619*

787.00 Vomiting Excessive chloride loss, due to vomiting. *0619*

Urine Increase

250.00 Diabetes Mellitus Osmotic diuresis secondary to hyperglycemia. *2540*

253.40 Anterior Pituitary Hypofunction Diminished tubular sodium reabsorption because of adrenal cortical steroid deficiency. The urine volume is increased, with loss of the normal diurnal variation, and an increased sodium and chloride concentration. *0619*

Urine Normal

252.10 Hypoparathyroidism Usually. *2540*

Chloride (continued)

CSF   Decrease

13.00   Tuberculosis Meningitis   May be due mainly to the associated fall in the plasma level following vomiting, but may be associated with alteration in the plasma/CSF barrier. *0619*   525-675 mg/dL. *0962*

45.90   Acute Poliomyelitis   670-750 mg/dL. *0962*

97.90   Syphilis   Usually slightly decreased. *0962*

225.90   Benign Neoplasm of Brain and CNS   *0962*

320.90   Meningitis (Bacterial)   Characteristically reduced. *2368*

324.00   Intracranial Abscess   600-750 mg/dL. *0962*

CSF   Increase

323.92   Encephalomyelitis   Usually normal or increased. *0433*

CSF   Normal

45.90   Acute Poliomyelitis   *2368*

62.10   Western Equine Encephalitis   *1058*

62.20   Eastern Equine Encephalitis   *1058*

Feces   Increase

1.00   Cholera   Fecal concentrations are above normal, but are consistently lower than the plasma values. *0151*

273.22   Heavy Chain Disease (Alpha)   Patients usually present with chronic diarrhea, hypocalcemia, and excessive fecal losses of water and electrolytes. *2538*

273.23   Heavy Chain Disease (Gamma)   Patients usually present with chronic diarrhea, hypocalcemia, and excessive fecal losses of water and electrolytes. *2538*

558.90   Diarrhea   During moderate diarrhea the output may increase to 60 mmol/day. In very severe diarrhea the fecal composition approaches that of ileal fluid, and up to 500 mmol of chloride can be lost in 24 h. *0619*

Saliva   Decrease

428.00   Congestive Heart Failure   *2467*

Saliva   Increase

277.00   Cystic Fibrosis   Submaxillary saliva has slightly increased chloride and sodium but not potassium; however, considerable overlap with normal individuals prevents diagnostic usage. *2467*

Sweat   Increase

277.00   Cystic Fibrosis   A value > 60 mmol/L is consistent with the diagnosis. *0433*   Striking increase in sweat sodium and chloride 60 mmol/L) and to a lesser extent potassium is present in virtually all homozygous patients. It is present throughout life from time of birth and is not related to severity of disease or organ involvement. *2467   0151*

493.10   Asthma (Intrinsic)   High concentrations found in sweat of chronic asthmatics and their relatives. *2275*

Cholecystokinin (CCK)

CSF   Decrease

297.90   Paranoid States and Other Psychoses   Significant decrease in cholecystokinin in untreated schizophrenics (1.4 pmol/L) compared with controls (4.0). *1440*

332.00   Parkinsons's Disease   Significant decreased cholecystokinin (1.9 pmol/L) versus control (4.0). *1440*

Cholesterol

Serum   Decrease

11.00   Pulmonary Tuberculosis   In 34% of 26 patients at initial hospitalization for this disorder. *0781*

30.00   Leprosy   Slightly decreased. *2468*

38.00   Septicemia   May fall, during convalescence the level rises, sometimes above the normal range. *0619*   May fall. *0049*   In 54% of 11 patients at initial hospitalization for this disorder. *0781*

40.20   Whipple's Disease   Common. *2199   0999*

53.00   Herpes Zoster   In 21% of 18 patients at initial hospitalization for this disorder. *0781*

60.00   Yellow Fever   Infections associated with liver damage. *0619*

70.00   Viral Hepatitis   Magnitude of depression is directly related to degree of hepatic damage. A progressive fall is a grave prognostic sign. *2104*   In 25% of 19 patients at initial hospitalization for this disorder. *0781*   Normal or mildly depressed in hepatitis; but markedly depressed in severe hepatitis. *0503*

75.00   Infectious Mononucleosis   In 60% of 10 patients at initial hospitalization for this disorder. *0781*

100.00   Leptospirosis   May occur with jaundice. *2368*

153.90   Malignant Neoplasm of Large Intestine   The mean levels were lower (202.2 mg/dL) than controls (219.5). Patients with Duke B stage cancer accounted for most of the difference. *1686*

155.00   Malignant Neoplasm of Liver   The close relationship between serum levels of cholesterol and bile acids has been confirmed in 46 patients with primary hepatoma, serum levels of cholesterol and bile acids are roughly correlated with serum AFP. Because the relationship between serum cholesterol and bile acids did not exist in common hepatocellular diseases, the results suggest a peculiar sterol metabolism occurring in human hepatoma. *1050*   20-30% incidence. *0364*

157.90   Malignant Neoplasm of Pancreas   In 27% of 43 patients at initial hospitalization for this disorder. *0781*

185.00   Malignant Neoplasm of Prostate   Pretreatment levels (196 ± 1.3 mg/dL) (normal = 1093) were significantly lower than those reported for age-matched controls. *2102*

197.70   Secondary Malignant Neoplasm of Liver   *0503*

199.00   Secondary Malignant Neoplasm (Disseminated)   Among 150 men who died of cancer, cholesterol level fell 22.7 mg/dL more than in survivors over the equivalent period. *2148*

201.90   Hodgkin's Disease   In 27% of 72 patients at initial hospitalization for this disorder. *0781*

202.80   Non-Hodgkins Lymphoma   In 24% of 74 patients at initial hospitalization for this disorder. *0781*

203.00   Multiple Myeloma   150 mg/dL in 25% of patients while only 5% have a level > 300 mg/dL. *0433*   In 27% of 31 patients at initial hospitalization for this disorder. *0781*

204.00   Lymphocytic Leukemia (Acute)   In 37% of 42 patients at initial hospitalization for this disorder. *0781*

204.10   Lymphocytic Leukemia (Chronic)   In 43% of 27 patients at initial hospitalization for this disorder. *0781*

205.00   Myelocytic Leukemia (Acute)   In 51% of 36 patients at initial hospitalization for this disorder. *0781*

206.00   Monocytic Leukemia   In 51% of 23 patients at initial hospitalization for this disorder. *0781*

242.90   Hyperthyroidism   Direct stimulation of synthesis and metabolism. *2540*   Falls, but not in simple relation to the associated rise in the BMR. Diet has a variable effect on the blood level. *0812*

252.00   Hyperparathyroidism   Hypercalcemia due to hyperparathyroidism is linked with low cholesterol levels and high parathyroid hormone and calcitonin production. An average increase of 41 µg/dL occurred after corrective surgery. *0520*   About 8-10% lower in both females and males compared with corresponding control cases. *0401*

256.00   Ovarian Hyperfunction   Estrogen effect. *0995*

259.20   Carcinoid Syndrome   Secondary to malabsorption or steatorrhea. *2540*

260.00   Protein Malnutrition   With protein malnutrition. *2468*   In kwashiorkor. *0151*

272.51   Tangier Disease   Ranges from 30-125 mg/dL. *2246*   Unique combination of low cholesterol and high triglycerides is indicative. Ranges from 40-125 mg/dL.

272.52   Abetalipoproteinemia   Diagnosis is established by finding very low cholesterol concentration (about 50 mg/dL). The lowest serum cholesterol level in any disease. *0619*   Markedly reduced. Averages < 50 mg/dL. *0172 2246   0999*

275.10   Hepatolenticular Degeneration   Related to liver disease. *2280*

280.90   Iron Deficiency Anemia   *0812*

281.00   Pernicious Anemia   Decreases in relapse; during remission, or following treatment the serum cholesterol increases as the reticulocyte count rises. *0812*   In relapse, increased fatty acid and triglyceride concentrations but decreased concentrations of total cholesterol, unesterified cholesterol and all examined phospholipid fractions. *2471*

281.20 Folic Acid Deficiency Anemia   Hypocholesterolemia occurred consistently in 10 patients with anemia. Values ranged from 80-180 mg/dL. *2519   0140*

282.00 Hereditary (Congenital) Spherocytosis   Observed in 8 patients. Values ranged from 110-170 mg/dL. *1942*   Low serum values correlated well with hemoglobin concentration. *2109*

282.20 Anemias Due To Disorders of Glutathione Metabolism   *0812*

282.60 Sickle Cell Anemia   Hypocholesterolemia was found in 8 cases. Values ranged from 2.6-4.3 mmol/L. *2519*   Plasma lipids are significantly reduced. *0028*

286.01 Hemophilia   May be below normal in this condition. *0619*

304.90 Drug Dependence (Opium and Derivatives)   Significantly decreased in heroin addiction. *1053*

319.00 Mental Retardation   Serum values from over 1,400 patients were significantly lower than corresponding results from normal subjects. Male patients had significantly lower results than the female patients. There appeared to be no significant correlation between serum cholesterol values and IQ, systolic or diastolic blood pressures, drugs used in treatment, presence or absence of epilepsy. *0617*

428.00 Congestive Heart Failure   With severe hepatic congestion. *0619   2467*

434.90 Brain Infarction   In all patients a significant reduction in total lipids, cholesterol, triglyceride and all lipoproteins was demonstrated after the acute cerebrovascular accident presumably due to the stress situation. *1192*

480.90 Viral Pneumonia   In 40% of 10 patients at initial hospitalization for this disorder. *0781*

482.90 Bacterial Pneumonia   Infections associated with liver damage; possibly severe pneumonia. *0619*   In 45% of 17 patients at initial hospitalization for this disorder. *0781*

496.00 Chronic Obstructive Lung Disease   Decreased in decompensated patients. Amount of decrease correlates with degree of hypoxemia. *2044*

496.01 Alpha₁-Antitrypsin Deficiency   Related to liver disease. *1636*

556.00 Ulcerative Colitis   *0995*

557.01 Mesenteric Artery Embolism   *0433*

560.90 Intestinal Obstruction   In 39% of 42 patients at initial hospitalization for this disorder. *0781*

570.00 Acute and Subacute Necrosis of Liver   Due to severe liver damage. *0619   0503*

571.49 Chronic Active Hepatitis   Significantly reduced. *0710*

571.90 Cirrhosis of Liver   Significantly reduced. Prebeta and alpha lipoprotein were decreased also. *0710*   In 24% of 61 patients at initial hospitalization for this disorder. *0781*

572.40 Hepatic Failure   *0503*

573.30 Toxic Hepatitis   Liver damage due to cinchophen, chloroform, carbon tetrachloride, or phosphate. *0619*   Normal or mildly depressed in hepatitis; but markedly depressed in severe hepatitis. *0503*

577.00 Acute Pancreatitis   In 42% of 21 patients at initial hospitalization for this disorder. *0781*

579.00 Celiac Sprue Disease   Malnutrition due to malabsorption. *0619*   Usually depressed in patients with sufficient intestinal involvement to produce steatorrhea. *2199*

579.90 Malabsorption, Cause Unspecified   Decreased in malabsorption syndrome. *0151*

581.90 Nephrotic Syndrome   Normal or low cholesterol suggests poor nutrition and suggests a poor prognosis. *0186*

714.00 Rheumatoid Arthritis   Reduced; appears to be related to the severity and activity of the disease; not affected by therapy. *0962*

730.00 Osteomyelitis   In 32% of 24 patients at initial hospitalization for this disorder. *0781*

Serum   Increase

126.90 Ancylostomiasis (Hookworm Infestation)   *2199*

155.10 Malignant Neoplasm of Intrahepatic Bile Ducts   Averages about 400 mg/dL. *0151*

157.90 Malignant Neoplasm of Pancreas   May remain normal until late in the disease. *0433*   Increased (usually > 300 mg/dL) with esters not decreased. *2467*

185.00 Malignant Neoplasm of Prostate   Nonesterified cholesterol hyperexcretion occurred in 44.8% of stage A and B and in 52.6% of stage C and D. Total cholesterol was elevated in 52.2% and 63.2% respectively. *1196*

203.00 Multiple Myeloma   150 mg/dL in 25% of patients while only 5% have a level > 300 mg/dL. *0433*

205.10 Myelocytic Leukemia (Chronic)   In 65% of 21 patients at initial hospitalization for this disorder. *0781*

244.90 Hypothyroidism   A moderate elevation that may reflect depression in overall metabolism is almost always demonstrable. *0503*   In true myxedema, level is usually > 200 mg/dL, but may be normal if there is also associated malnutrition. *0619*   Values ranged from 143-556 in 10 patients. *0905*   In pituitary hypothyroidism, may be normal or low. *2540*   In 58% of 12 patients at initial hospitalization for this disorder. *0781*

245.10 Subacute Thyroiditis   If hypothyroid. *0151*

250.00 Diabetes Mellitus   Moderate increase. *0503*   Mean levels in children (205 ± 78 mg/dL) were significantly higher than for controls (155 ± 27 mg/dL), as were mean triglyceride levels. 8 with diabetes had hypercholesterolemia, 5 had hypertriglyceridemia, and 9 had combined hypercholesterolemia and hypertriglyceridemia. *0377*

253.40 Anterior Pituitary Hypofunction   In some cases due to secondary hypothyroidism. *0433*

255.00 Adrenal Cortical Hyperfunction (Glucocorticoid Excess)   Slight elevations. *0503*

256.30 Ovarian Hypofunction   Estrogen effect. *0995*

271.01 Von Gierke's Disease   Striking elevation. *1086 2246*   Significant elevations generally occur in the glycogen storage diseases. *2104*

271.02 McArdle's Disease   Significant elevations generally occur in the glycogen storage diseases. *2104*

271.03 Forbes Disease   Concentrations vary from 200 to > 1,400 mg/dL. Extreme variability of cholesterol and triglyceride concentration is a diagnostic feature and in distinct contrast to the steady elevations in Type II. *0772*   Increased in all 49 cases. *1631*   Significant elevations generally occur in the glycogen storage diseases. *2104*

272.00 Type IIA Hyperlipoproteinemia   The plasma is clear even with extremely elevated cholesterol. *0962*   Manifested by high cholesterol concentration in low density lipoproteins. Generally 2 X normal mean for heterozygotes and 6 X normal in homozygotes. *2246   1108*

272.10 Type IV Hyperlipoproteinemia   An increase in cholesterol of about 1 mg/dL for each 5 mg/dL increase in triglyceride concentration. *0773*   The percentage of esterified cholesterol in plasma and the esterification rate were always reduced when the triglyceride concentration exceeded 600 mg/dL and the rate of esterification rose significantly with appropriate triglyceride-lowering therapy in patients with hypertriglyceridemia. *0897   0151 0962*

272.21 Type IIB Hyperlipoproteinemia   The plasma is clear even with extremely elevated cholesterol. *0962*   Manifested by high cholesterol concentration in low density lipoproteins. Generally 2 X normal mean for heterozygotes and 6 X normal in homozygotes. *2246   1108*

272.22 Type III Hyperlipoproteinemia   Usually > 300 mg/dL. *2246*

272.31 Type I Hyperlipoproteinemia   Moderate elevation. *0433*

272.32 Type V Hyperlipoproteinemia   In 11 patients with Type V hyperlipoproteinemia, concentration ranged from 212-1,512 mg/dL. *2177*   Usually abnormally high, although initial normal values are frequently found. *2246*

272.71 Anderson's Disease   Significant elevations generally occur in the glycogen storage diseases. *2104*

273.80 Analbuminemia   Often elevated. *0433*

274.00 Gout   Many patients. *0991*   Frequently elevated in individual patients; no correlation has been shown between urate and cholesterol. *2246*

277.00 Cystic Fibrosis   In 91% of 12 patients at initial hospitalization for this disorder. *0781*

277.30 Amyloidosis   High concentrations found in 33% of primary cases and < 20% of secondary cases. *1334*

278.00 Obesity   Hyperlipidemia. *0996 2641*

308.00 Stress   With mental stress. *2092*   Concentrations rise during heavy stress periods. *2113*

334.00 Friedreich's Ataxia   In Friedreich's patients, the relative proportion of cholesterol and triglycerides was increased while the relative protein content was greatly reduced. *1091*

Cholesterol (continued)

Serum Increase (continued)

401.00 Malignant Hypertension Mean concentration was 199.7 ± 7.5 mg/dL in 24 male patients compared to 170.9 ± 6.3 in controls. *0381*

401.10 Essential Benign Hypertension Frequently elevated. *0995*

405.91 Renovascular Hypertension Predisposes to development of arteriosclerosis. *0992*

410.90 Acute Myocardial Infarction Very significantly elevated. Mean value was 212.2 ± 15.0 mg/dL in females and 209.1 ± 4.4 in males. Normal was 168.3 ± 4.2 and 170.9 ± 6.3 in females and males, respectively. *0381* Tends to slowly decrease for a few weeks after infarction. *1108*

414.00 Chronic Ischemic Heart Disease Studies of patients with coronary atherosclerotic heart disease and of their families have indicated a significantly higher incidence (16-44%) of elevated plasma cholesterol and/or triglyceride levels, usually classified as type II or type IV. *1108*

440.00 Arteriosclerosis Correlates highly with the risk of myocardial infarction. *0992* Elevated fasting plasma concentration was frequently found in 219 male and 63 female patients. *0108* Severity of disease correlated (not significantly) with plasma cholesterol concentration. *0508* Nonfasting levels are related to the development of coronary heart disease in both men and women aged 19 years and older *0358*

446.00 Polyarteritis-Nodosa Leading to nephrosis. *2467*

496.01 Alpha₁-Antitrypsin Deficiency Average 604 mg/dL. *0563*

570.00 Acute and Subacute Necrosis of Liver In patients with obstructive jaundice or intrahepatic cholestasis concentration is usually elevated to 250-500 mg/dL; greater elevations occur occasionally. *0619 0503* Greater elevations are more characteristic of hepatocanalicular jaundice (intrahepatic cholestasis) than of posthepatic jaundice. *0503*

571.20 Laennec's or Alcoholic Cirrhosis In fatty infiltration of the liver the serum concentration was significantly increased, as compared with the normal values and with the figures obtained in the cases of chronic inflammatory liver disease. *0710*

571.60 Biliary Cirrhosis Moderate to marked elevations up to 1,800 mg/dL. *0503* Marked increase in total cholesterol and phospholipids takes place, with normal triglycerides; serum is not lipemic. The increase is associated with xanthomas and xantholasmas. *2467* Hypercholesterolemia of an extreme degree (2,000 mg/dL) may be present. *0999 2035*

573.30 Toxic Hepatitis *2467*

576.20 Extrahepatic Biliary Obstruction Continues to rise for some time after obstruction has been established, reaching extreme heights. Persists for a long period, falling when the obstruction is relieved. *1494* In 15 patients, (aged 16-78), compared to controls, there was an increase in total cholesterol due to an increase in the unesterified fraction. *1606*

577.10 Chronic Pancreatitis Some cases. *0619*

580.00 Acute Poststreptococcal Glomerulonephritis Sometimes elevated even when serum albumin is not greatly decreased. *0995*

580.02 Glomerulonephritis (Minimal Change) Usually occurs. *0151*

580.04 Glomerulonephritis (Membranous) Occurs, but is less frequent than in minimal change glomerulonephritis. *0151*

581.90 Nephrotic Syndrome Typically elevated. *0962* In 50% of 14 patients at initial hospitalization for this disorder. *0781*

585.00 Chronic Renal Failure May be elevated. *1038* Most studies show only a modest increase. *1108 1243*

600.00 Benign Prostatic Hypertrophy In patients with residual urine, nonesterified cholesterol was elevated in 42.1% and total levels in 61.4%. Patients with no residual urine had normal cholesterol. *1196*

650.00 Pregnancy Third trimester of pregnancy with sustained elevations until several weeks after delivery. *0503* Increases after 8th week to maximum by 30th week in pregnancy. *2468 0913*

710.00 Systemic Lupus Erythematosus Leading to nephrosis. *2467*

758.70 Klinefelter's Syndrome (XXY) Hyperlipidemia found in 8 of 24 patients; in 6, only cholesterol was elevated. *1454*

985.00 Toxic Effects of Non-medicinal Metals Hepatotoxic effects of arsenicals may be marked. *1446*

994.50 Exercise Occasionally. *0342*

Serum Normal

227.91 Pheochromocytoma No characteristic changes. *1108*

272.10 Type IV Hyperlipoproteinemia Usually found to be normal or only moderately elevated. *1108 0151*

758.00 Down's Syndrome Plasma lipid levels were measured in 20 mongoloid and 16 nonmongoloid mentally retarded subjects. Significant elevations of plasma triglyceride levels were found in patients with Down's syndrome compared with mentally retarded controls. However, no significant difference was found in plasma cholesterol, phospholipid and free fatty acid levels between the mongoloids and control subjects. *1698*

994.50 Exercise Normal, with relative reduction of unsaturated acid. *1109 0342*

Urine Increase

180.90 Malignant Neoplasm of Cervix Nonesterified cholesterol hyperexcretion (values > 1.5 mg/24h) occurred in 65 of 68 women with active carcinoma including 13 with carcinoma in situ. *0012*

182.00 Malignant Neoplasm of Corpus Uteri Hyperexcretion in 42 of 45 women with active carcinoma, sequential studies demonstrated an almost perfect correlation between excretion and the clinical status of the patient following surgical and/or radiation therapy. *0012*

183.00 Malignant Neoplasm of Ovary Hyperexcretion in 18 of 19 cystadenocarcinomas of the serous and/or mucinous types; 1 of 1 endometrial carcinoma; 4 of 4 malignant granulosa cell tumors; two of two mixed malignant germ cell tumors; and one of one malignant mixed Müllerian tumor. A normal excretion was characteristic of 19 of 21 surviving patients treated by surgery and adjunctive therapy. The 94% correlation between the presence of proven active ovarian carcinomas and urinary hyperexcretion is significant. *0013*

185.00 Malignant Neoplasm of Prostate In 42 patients, 62% were found to have levels 2.6 mg/24h. *0403*

277.14 Acute Intermittent Porphyria *0151*

277.15 Porphyria Variegata *0151*

277.17 Hereditary Coproporphyria *0151*

CSF Decrease

331.90 Cerebral and Cortical Atrophy Significantly low CSF values for cholesterol and total lipids were found in a group of patients with brain atrophy in comparison with a control group. It is possible that these changes are a function of reduced brain mass or of defect in brain lipid metabolism in brain atrophy patients. *1035*

CSF Increase

340.00 Multiple Sclerosis Raised in several neurologic diseases including multiple sclerosis. *0912*

Pleural Effusion Increase

11.00 Pulmonary Tuberculosis Rarely. *0418*

Pericardial Fluid Increase

18.00 Disseminated Tuberculosis High levels (2.6-5.2 mmol/L; 100 to 200 mg/dL). *0274*

199.00 Secondary Malignant Neoplasm (Disseminated) High levels (2.6-5.2 mmol/L; 100 to 200 mg/dL). *0274*

244.90 Hypothyroidism High levels (2.6-5.2 mmol/L; 100 to 200 mg/dL). *0274*

714.00 Rheumatoid Arthritis High levels (2.6-5.2 mmol/L; 100 to 200 mg/dL). *0274*

Feces Increase

153.90 Malignant Neoplasm of Large Intestine Fecal excretion of cholesterol, coprostanol, coprostanone, total bile acids, deoxycholic acid, lithocholic acid was higher in colonic cancer and adenomatous polyps compared to normal controls as well as in patients with other digestive diseases. *1896*

211.40 Benign Neoplasm of Rectum and Anus The fecal excretion of cholesterol, coprostanol, coprostanone, total bile acids, deoxycholic acid, lithocholic acid was higher in patients with colon cancer and patients with adenomatous polyps compared to normal American and Japanese controls as well as in patients with other digestive diseases. *1896* Although the total fecal neutral sterol concentrations were not different between the groups, the patients with familial polyposis excreted a high amount of cholesterol and low levels of coprostanol and coprostanone compared with other groups. Increased cholesterol and decreased lithocholic acid is excreted in patients with familial polyposis. *1895*

556.00 Ulcerative Colitis The fecal excretion of cholesterol, coprostanol, and cholestane-38 beta, 5 alpha, 6 beta-triol was higher in these patients than in other control and patient groups. *1897*

Liver Increase

272.73 Niemann-Pick Disease Usually elevated, may be more prominent than sphingomyelin in type D. *2246*

Peritoneal Fluid Increase

183.00 Malignant Neoplasm of Ovary Markedly increased in active cases. *1547*

Red Blood Cells Increase

70.00 Viral Hepatitis 25-50% increase in the membrane concentration, resulting in the characteristic target cell. *2552*

282.60 Sickle Cell Anemia Plasma lipids are significantly reduced and RBC cholesterol is higher in sickle cell patients than in normal subjects. *0028*

570.00 Acute and Subacute Necrosis of Liver An increase was detected in most patients with hepatocellular disease or cholestatic jaundice but the alteration in RBC lipid content did not correlate with RBC survival. *1848* 25-50% increase in the membrane concentration, resulting in the characteristic target cell. *2552*

571.20 Laennec's or Alcoholic Cirrhosis 25-50% increase in the membrane concentration, resulting in the characteristic target cell. *2552*

576.20 Extrahepatic Biliary Obstruction 25-50% increase in the membrane concentration, resulting in the characteristic target cell. *2552* An increase in RBC cholesterol and phospholipid was detected in most patients with hepatocellular disease or cholestatic jaundice but the alteration in RBC lipid content did not correlate with RBC survival. *1848*

Red Blood Cells Normal

272.51 Tangier Disease *2246*

Cholesterol Esters

Serum Decrease

70.00 Viral Hepatitis Striking decrease as liver involvement progresses. *2104*

244.90 Hypothyroidism No significant difference in rate of esterification between hypo-, hyper- and euthyroid subjects. The fractional rates were highly significant, decreased in hypo- and increased in hyperthyroid patients. *1336*

428.00 Congestive Heart Failure *2467*

496.01 Alpha₁-Antitrypsin Deficiency Greatly depressed as was cholesterol absorption. *0563*

571.90 Cirrhosis of Liver Decreased esters reflect more severe parenchymal cell damage. *2467*

Serum Increase

242.90 Hyperthyroidism *1336*

401.00 Malignant Hypertension Mean concentration was 118.0 ± 8.4 mg/dL in 24 male patients (normal = 101.7 ± 6.3). *0381*

410.90 Acute Myocardial Infarction Mean concentration was 134.0 ± 13.6 mg/dL compared to 92.6 ± 6.7 in women, and 129.2 ± 3.7 compared to 101.7 ± 5.6 in men. *0381*

CSF Increase

340.00 Multiple Sclerosis Significantly higher. *0912*

Cholesterol, Free

Serum Decrease

281.00 Pernicious Anemia In relapse, increased free fatty acid and triglyceride concentrations but decreased concentrations of total cholesterol, unesterified cholesterol and all examined phospholipid fractions. *2471*

Serum Increase

272.31 Type I Hyperlipoproteinemia The proportion of free cholesterol is elevated to about 50% instead of 30%. *0774* The unesterified cholesterol proportion may be as high as 50%. *2246*

576.20 Extrahepatic Biliary Obstruction In simple biliary obstruction the increase is greater in the free fraction. *0619*

Cholesterol, High Density Lipoprotein

Serum Decrease

38.00 Septicemia Sepsis causes the concentration to decrease. *0049*

250.00 Diabetes Mellitus Decreased. *0131 1519 2556*

272.10 Type IV Hyperlipoproteinemia Decreased. {0131,1519,2556}

272.31 Type I Hyperlipoproteinemia *2614*

272.32 Type V Hyperlipoproteinemia *2614*

440.00 Arteriosclerosis Non fasting HDL is inversely related to the development of coronary heart disease in both men and women aged 49 years and older. *0358*

571.90 Cirrhosis of Liver Decreased. *0131 1519 2556*

581.90 Nephrotic Syndrome Decreased. *0131 1519 2556*

714.00 Rheumatoid Arthritis In 54 female patients 36% reduction was noted. *1435*

Serum Increase

303.90 Alcoholism Higher in drinkers. *1864* Increased. *0131 1519 2556*

571.49 Chronic Active Hepatitis Increased. *0131 1519 2556*

571.60 Biliary Cirrhosis In 7 female patients compared to 6 normal age matched controls. *0127 0131 1519 2556*

572.40 Hepatic Failure Increased. *0131 1519 2556*

Serum Normal

272.00 Type IIA Hyperlipoproteinemia *2614*

272.21 Type IIB Hyperlipoproteinemia *2614*

272.22 Type III Hyperlipoproteinemia *2614*

308.00 Stress No change in pilot flying high performance aircraft. *0430*

359.11 Progressive Muscular Dystrophy Within normal limits in 15 patients with this disorder. *2328*

710.00 Systemic Lupus Erythematosus Total lipid concentration was found to be low but HDL fraction was normal. *1435*

720.00 Rheumatoid (Ankylosing) Spondylitis Total lipid concentration was found to be low but HDL fraction was normal. *1435*

Cholesterol, Low Density Lipoprotein

Serum Decrease

272.52 Abetalipoproteinemia Absent. *0062*

714.00 Rheumatoid Arthritis In 54 female patients 26% reduction was noted. *1435*

Serum Increase

155.00 Malignant Neoplasm of Liver Moderate increase secondary to lack of feedback inhibition of hepatic cholesterol synthesis by dietary cholesterol. *0062*

244.90 Hypothyroidism Marked elevation secondary to decreased catabolism. *0062 2614*

255.00 Adrenal Cortical Hyperfunction (Glucocorticoid Excess) Moderate elevation secondary to increased conversion of VLDL to LDL. *0062*

272.00 Type IIA Hyperlipoproteinemia *2614*

Cholesterol, Low Density Lipoprotein
(continued)

Serum Increase *(continued)*

272.21 Type IIB Hyperlipoproteinemia Serum cholesterol level is elevated, equal to, or greater than the triglyceride level; both LDL and VLDL are increased. *0151 2614*

272.22 Type III Hyperlipoproteinemia *2614*

277.14 Acute Intermittent Porphyria Moderate elevation. *0062*

581.90 Nephrotic Syndrome Marked elevation secondary to direct secretion by liver and decrease catabolism. *0062*

Serum Normal

272.10 Type IV Hyperlipoproteinemia *2614*

272.31 Type I Hyperlipoproteinemia *2614*

272.32 Type V Hyperlipoproteinemia *2614*

Cholesterol, Very Low Density Lipoprotein

Serum Decrease

272.52 Abetalipoproteinemia Absent. *0062*

Serum Increase

70.00 Viral Hepatitis Marked elevation. *0062*

201.90 Hodgkin's Disease Moderate increase due to presence of IgG or IgM that forms complexes with chylomicron remnants and/or VLDL thereby decreasing catabolism. *0062*

202.80 Non-Hodgkins Lymphoma Moderate increase due to presence of IgG or IgM that forms complexes with chylomicron remnants and/or VLDL thereby decreasing catabolism. *0062*

203.00 Multiple Myeloma Moderate increase due to presence of IgG or IgM that forms complexes with chylomicron remnants and/or VLDL thereby decreasing catabolism. *0062*

244.90 Hypothyroidism *2614*

250.00 Diabetes Mellitus Marled elevation due to increased secretion and decreased catabolism secondary to reduced lipoprotein lipase activity. *0062 2614*

253.00 Acromegaly Minimal elevation due to increased secretion. *0062*

255.00 Adrenal Cortical Hyperfunction (Glucocorticoid Excess) Minimal elevation due to increased secretion. *0062*

271.01 Von Gierke's Disease Marked elevation due to increased secretion and decreased catabolism due to reduced lipoprotein lipase activity. *0062*

272.10 Type IV Hyperlipoproteinemia *2614*

272.21 Type IIB Hyperlipoproteinemia Serum cholesterol level is elevated, equal to,or greater than triglyceride level Both LDL and VLDL are increased. *0151 2614*

272.22 Type III Hyperlipoproteinemia *2614*

272.32 Type V Hyperlipoproteinemia *2614*

273.30 Waldenström's Macroglobulinemia Moderate increase due to presence of IgG or IgM that forms complexes with chylomicron remnants and/or VLDL thereby decreasing catabolism. *0062*

308.00 Stress Moderate increase secondary to increased secretion and decreased catabolism. *0062*

571.49 Chronic Active Hepatitis Marked elevation. *0062*

573.30 Toxic Hepatitis Marked elevation. *0062*

581.90 Nephrotic Syndrome Marked elevation with uremia. *0062*

585.00 Chronic Renal Failure Marked elevation with uremia. *0062*

948.00 Burns Moderate increase secondary to increased secretion and decreased catabolism. *0062*

Serum Normal

272.00 Type IIA Hyperlipoproteinemia *2614*

272.31 Type I Hyperlipoproteinemia *2614*

Cholic Acid

Serum Decrease

277.42 Gilbert's Disease Significantly reduced in hyperbilirubinemic patients. *2642*

359.11 Progressive Muscular Dystrophy In 15 patients with this disorder the serum values were usually low (0.16 μmol/L) compared with controls (1.47 μmol/L). *2328*

Serum Increase

70.00 Viral Hepatitis Increased serum bile acids in anicteric viral hepatitis from either A or B virus. Elevated postprandial levels may persist even after transaminase and BSP retention have returned to normal. *1154*

277.00 Cystic Fibrosis Of cystic fibrosis patients with steatorrhea, 38% had fasting levels greater than 3 standard deviation above mean fasting control levels. *0505* Eight patients had elevated levels not correlated with liver pathology.

496.01 Alpha₁-Antitrypsin Deficiency In 34 patients with this disease all patients with morphological cirrhosis. *1685*

571.49 Chronic Active Hepatitis Degree of elevation is related to the severity of illness as judged by other biochemical and clinical parameters. Bile acids return to normal in patients who respond to therapy. *1154* Mean fasting and 3h total cholic acid conjugates were significantly higher *1183* Elevated in 80% of Patients *1039*

571.60 Biliary Cirrhosis In 15 patients with primary biliary cirrhosis 13 had increased fasting levels. *2036* Severe Cholestasis *1154*

571.90 Cirrhosis of Liver Raised fasting levels were found in 19 of 49 patients (39%). *2363* Elevated in 97% of patients. *1039*

576.20 Extrahepatic Biliary Obstruction Serum bile acids elevate promptly during the acute episode indicate biliary tract disease. *1154*

Serum Normal

277.42 Gilbert's Disease Fasting levels were normal in all 24 patients studied. *2642*

555.90 Regional Enteritis or Ileitis Fasting values were in the normal range but post prandial increase was lower than in healthy controls. *1039*

Chromium

Serum Decrease

650.00 Pregnancy Compared to non pregnant. *0966*

Chylomicrons

Serum Decrease

272.52 Abetalipoproteinemia Complete absence of chylomicrons. *0151* Totally absent. *2246* None present. *0878*

Serum Increase

201.90 Hodgkin's Disease Moderate increase due to presence of IgG or IgM that forms complexes with chylomicron remnants and/or VLDL thereby decreasing catabolism. *0062*

202.80 Non-Hodgkins Lymphoma Moderate increase due to presence of IgG or IgM that forms complexes with chylomicron remnants and/or VLDL thereby decreasing catabolism. *0062*

203.00 Multiple Myeloma Moderate increase due to presence of IgG or IgM that forms complexes with chylomicron remnants and/or VLDL thereby decreasing catabolism. *0062*

244.90 Hypothyroidism Increased. *1380 1936 1948*

250.00 Diabetes Mellitus Increased. *1380 1936 1948* Minimal elevation secondary to decreased catabolism due to reduced lipoprotein lipase activity. *0062*

253.40 Anterior Pituitary Hypofunction Increased. *1380 1936 1948*

255.10 Adrenal Cortical Hyperfunction (Mineralocorticoid Excess) Increased. *1380 1936 1948*

271.01 Von Gierke's Disease Minimal elevation secondary to decreased catabolism due to reduced lipoprotein lipase activity. *0062*

272.31 Type I Hyperlipoproteinemia Chylomicronemia develops as soon as fat is ingested, and the disorder has been diagnosed during the 1st week of life. *0151* Characterized by the presence of chylomicrons in high concentration in plasma 14 h or more after the last meal of normal diet. *0774* Heavy chylomicronemia and subnormal concentrations of all other lipoproteins. A qualitative abnormality which is not a specific marker for a single genetic disease. Occurs in familial lipoprotein lipase deficiency. *2246*

272.32 Type V Hyperlipoproteinemia In severely affected patients. *2246* Chylomicronemia and hyperprebeta-lipoproteinemia. *2177*

272.51 Tangier Disease Frequently. *2246*

273.30 Waldenström's Macroglobulinemia Moderate increase due to presence of IgG or IgM that forms complexes with chylomicron remnants and/or VLDL thereby decreasing catabolism. *0062*

280.90 Iron Deficiency Anemia Increased. *1380 1936 1948*

303.90 Alcoholism Increased. *1380 1936 1948*

577.00 Acute Pancreatitis Increased. *1380 1936 1948*

581.90 Nephrotic Syndrome Increased. *1380 1936 1948*

710.10 Progressive Systemic Sclerosis Moderate increase secondary to presence of IgG or IgM that binds heparin and thereby decreases the activity of lipoprotein lipase. *0062*

Synovial Fluid   Decrease

714.00 Rheumatoid Arthritis Cylous effusions have been reported. *1689 2012*

Synovial Fluid   Increase

710.00 Systemic Lupus Erythematosus Chylous effusions have been reported. *1689 2012*

Peritoneal Fluid   Increase

571.90 Cirrhosis of Liver Present. *1486*

Chymotrypsin

Serum   Decrease

277.00 Cystic Fibrosis *1901*

Feces   Decrease

277.00 Cystic Fibrosis Fecal concentrations may be related to the severity of pancreatic insufficiency. *0113*

577.10 Chronic Pancreatitis Found to be a more reliable measure of pancreatic function than trypsin activity. False-positives have been noted in 10% of controls, and normal values may occur in patients. *0052*

579.90 Malabsorption, Cause Unspecified Found to be a more reliable measure of pancreatic function than trypsin activity. False-positives have been noted in 10% of controls, and normal values may occur in patients. *0052*

Citrate

Serum   Decrease

252.10 Hypoparathyroidism *2540*

Serum   Increase

252.00 Hyperparathyroidism Elevated in the high normal range. *2540*

Urine   Increase

252.00 Hyperparathyroidism High or in high normal range. *2540* Often elevated. *0992*

984.00 Toxic Effects of Lead and Its Compounds (including Fumes) Citraturia results from changes in the proximal convoluted tubules. *0151*

Citrulline

Serum   Increase

270.61 Citrullinemia Marked accumulation. Increased to 1-4.5 μmol/L, at least 40 X normal. Concentration does not correlate with severity of symptoms. *2246*

Urine   Increase

270.02 Hartnup Disease 5-20 X normal values. *2246*

270.61 Citrullinemia Ranges from several hundred mg/24h in infants to several g/24h in adults. *2246   2468*

CSF   Increase

270.61 Citrullinemia Greatly increased. Ranges between 0.1-0.3 μmol/L (normal < 0.003). CSF concentrations are lower than in blood. *2246*

Clot Retraction

Blood   Normal

286.40 Von Willebrand's Disease *2538*

Blood   Poor

201.90 Hodgkin's Disease With thrombocytopenia. *2246*

238.40 Polycythemia Vera A common defect has been the excessive number of untrapped RBCs after clot retraction (the escape phenomenon of excessive red cell fallout). An increased rate of retraction has also been observed. *2538 1883 1989* Bleeding time and coagulation time are normal but clot retraction may be poor *2468*

273.30 Waldenström's Macroglobulinemia Evidence of impaired platelet function. *2538*

281.00 Pernicious Anemia May be poor. *2552*

281.20 Folic Acid Deficiency Anemia May be poor. *2552*

284.90 Aplastic Anemia Reflects low platelet count. *2538   2552*

286.31 Congenital Dysfibrinogenemia *2538*

287.10 Thrombasthenia (Glanzmann's) Due to platelet function abnormalities. *2246*

287.30 Idiopathic Thrombocytopenic Purpura Absent or deficient due to thrombocytopenia. *2552   0433*

446.60 Thrombotic Thrombocytopenic Purpura Varies depending upon the platelet count. *2035* Absent or deficient due to thrombocytopenia. *2552*

Clot Solubility

Blood   Poor

286.33 Factor XIII Deficiency *0433*

Clotting Time

Blood   Decrease

642.60 Eclampsia Markedly reduced. *1012*

Blood   Increase

85.00 Leishmaniasis Normal early in the disease but later becomes prolonged. *0151*

286.01 Hemophilia May be 24 h or longer and show spontaneous irregular variations. *2552   0995 2246*

286.10 Christmas Disease In severe deficiencies. *2538   0995 2246*

286.20 Factor XI Deficiency *2246*

286.31 Congenital Dysfibrinogenemia The clotting time of whole blood or the recalcification time of platelet-poor plasma has usually been normal or prolonged. *2538*

286.32 Factor XII Deficiency In severe deficiencies. *0995   2246*

286.34 Congenital Afibrinogenemia Corrected by the addition of normal plasma or normal fibrinogen to the patient's plasma. *2538* Infinite. *2246*

286.35 Factor V Deficiency *2538 2246*

286.36 Factor X Deficiency *0995 2246*

286.38 Factor II Deficiency *2246*

286.40 Von Willebrand's Disease Variable. *2246*

989.50 Toxic Effects of Venom Increased clotting time indicates severe envenomation from snake bite. *0151*

992.00 Heat stroke *0995*

Blood   Normal

286.31 Congenital Dysfibrinogenemia The clotting time of whole blood or the recalcification time of platelet-poor plasma has usually been normal or prolonged. *2538*

286.33 Factor XIII Deficiency *2246*

Clotting Time (continued)

Blood   Normal (continued)

286.37   Factor VII Deficiency   Clotting time of recalcified plasma is normal, distinguishing this from Stuart factor deficiency. *2246 2538*

287.10   Thrombasthenia (Glanzmann's)   *2246*

287.30   Idiopathic Thrombocytopenic Purpura   *2246*

446.60   Thrombotic Thrombocytopenic Purpura   *0054 2246*

Coagulation Time

Blood   Increase

50.00   Smallpox   Commonly found in hemorrhagic smallpox. *0433*

286.01   Hemophilia   In severe cases. *2552*

286.10   Christmas Disease   In severe cases. *2468*

286.20   Factor XI Deficiency   *2468*

286.32   Factor XII Deficiency   *2468*

286.35   Factor V Deficiency   Increase in coagulation time is not corrected by administration of vitamin K. *2468*

710.00   Systemic Lupus Erythematosus   Circulating anticoagulants are not rare but do not usually cause bleeding. *0962*

Blood   Normal

238.40   Polycythemia Vera   *2468*

287.30   Idiopathic Thrombocytopenic Purpura   *2552*

288.00   Agranulocytosis   Normal in most typical cases. *2552*

Cold Agglutinins

Serum   Increase

70.00   Viral Hepatitis   Elevated titers may persist for weeks or months. *2035*

72.00   Mumps   Increased titer. *0186*

75.00   Infectious Mononucleosis   Occur frequently; they are present mostly in the IgM fraction and have anti-I specificity. *0502* Elevated titers may persists for weeks or months. *2035 0330 2538*

78.50   Cytomegalic Inclusion Disease   *2468*

84.00   Malaria   An unusually high incidence was observed during chronic infection. *0916   2035 1826*

86.90   Trypanosomiasis   *2035 1826*

202.80   Non-Hodgkins Lymphoma   *2035*

203.00   Multiple Myeloma   Cold agglutinin or cryoglobulins with lymphocytes. *2468*

204.00   Lymphocytic Leukemia (Acute)   Tends to rise. *1752*

204.10   Lymphocytic Leukemia (Chronic)   Tends to rise. *1752*

238.40   Polycythemia Vera   *2035*

273.21   Cryoglobulinemia (Essential Mixed)   *2035*

273.30   Waldenström's Macroglobulinemia   *2035*

283.00   Acquired Hemolytic Anemia (Autoimmune)   In hemolytic anemias. *2468*

415.10   Pulmonary Embolism and Infarction   Implicated as cause of intravascular thrombosis, but their role is neither clear nor constant. *1108*

423.10   Constrictive Pericarditis   *2035*

446.00   Polyarteritis-Nodosa   Have been reported. *0962*

483.01   Mycoplasma Pneumoniae   Fourfold or greater rise in titer during the illness is considered diagnostic. *0433*   Significant titers in 50% of patients during the 2nd to 4th weeks, disappearing by the 6th to 8th weeks. *2508*   50% of patients, mostly severely ill, will develop reaction at the end of the 1st or the beginning of the 2nd week. *0151*   Elevated titers may persist for weeks or months. *2035 0715*   In over 50% of patients and is related to the *2368*

494.00   Bronchiectasis   Elevated titers may persist for weeks or months. *2035*

571.20   Laennec's or Alcoholic Cirrhosis   Elevated titers may persist for weeks or months. *2035 2001*

650.00   Pregnancy   Occasionally. *2468*

710.00   Systemic Lupus Erythematosus   Have been detected. *0962   2035*

710.10   Progressive Systemic Sclerosis   Increased titer. *0186*

Serum   Normal

73.90   Psittacosis   *2468*

Complement C1q

Serum   Decrease

260.00   Protein Malnutrition   *1732*

273.21   Cryoglobulinemia (Essential Mixed)   Low levels of early components (C1q, C1s, and C4). *2329*

580.00   Acute Poststreptococcal Glomerulonephritis   Particularly during diuretic phase. *0062*

710.00   Systemic Lupus Erythematosus   *2090*

Serum   Increase

714.00   Rheumatoid Arthritis   *2090*

Serum   Normal

38.00   Septicemia   Normal concentrations of C1, C3, and C4. *2522*

Complement C1r

Serum   Decrease

710.00   Systemic Lupus Erythematosus   *2090*

714.00   Rheumatoid Arthritis   {793} {2522}

Complement C1s

Serum   Decrease

260.00   Protein Malnutrition   *1732*

710.00   Systemic Lupus Erythematosus   *2090*

948.00   Burns   {793} {2522}

Complement C2

Serum   Decrease

260.00   Protein Malnutrition   {793} {2522}

579.01   Protein-Losing Enteropathy   *1732*

579.90   Malabsorption, Cause Unspecified   {793} {2522}

710.00   Systemic Lupus Erythematosus   *2090*

Serum   Increase

714.00   Rheumatoid Arthritis   *2090*

Serum   Normal

38.00   Septicemia   Normal concentrations of C1, C2, and C4. *2522*

Complement C3

Serum   Decrease

38.00   Septicemia   In severe gram-negative infection associated with shock, depression of C3, C5, C6, and C9 may occur, with normal concentrations of C1, C2, and C4. Abnormalities develop early, before shock. C3 concentration correlates with mortality. *2522 0452 1275 0375*

84.00   Malaria   Only in patients with defective hemoglobin synthesis. *2240*

260.00   Protein Malnutrition   All complement components except C4 and C5 were significantly lower in children with protein-calorie malnutrition: C3 and C9 were the most severely depressed. C5 was the only complement that was significantly higher in malnourished children than in normal children. *1732*   C3 was the only fraction which is significantly diminished in marasmic infants. *0956*

281.00   Pernicious Anemia   Significantly reduced in patients with vitamin B_{12} deficiency. Levels correlate with the degree of anemia but not with serum vitamin B_{12} levels at diagnosis. *1079*

281.20 Folic Acid Deficiency Anemia Significantly reduced in patients with vitamin B$_{12}$ deficiency. Levels correlate with the degree of anemia but not with serum vitamin B$_{12}$ levels at diagnosis. *1079*

283.00 Acquired Hemolytic Anemia (Autoimmune) Caused by hypercatabolism. *0375 0793 1275 0509 0452*

283.21 Paroxysmal Nocturnal Hemoglobinuria Caused by hypercatabolism. *0375 0793 1275 0509 0452*

340.00 Multiple Sclerosis Hypocomplementemia (fall in factor C3 related to a fall in total hemolytic activity) was found in 29.5% of the patients not on corticotherapy at the first assay, and in 36% of the patients when repeated assays were carried out. Hypocomplementemia is significantly more frequent in MS than in the normal population (0%) and in neurological patients (9.6%). *2375* Mean level was slightly lower than normal. *0068*

421.00 Bacterial Endocarditis Decreased total C3 and C4, with conversion products of both, in subacute endocarditis. *2522* Decreased total hemolytic complement or C3 in 8 of 17 or 47% of patients tested. 7 of the 8 had evidence of renal disease. *1798*

482.90 Bacterial Pneumonia Mean concentrations in acute infection was slightly decreased. *0449*

571.20 Laennec's or Alcoholic Cirrhosis Low levels of C3, C4 and factor B were common with cirrhosis and confined to those cases with severe reduction in serum albumin and/or prothrombin index. *0376*

571.90 Cirrhosis of Liver Low levels of C3, C4, and factor B were common with cirrhosis and confined to those cases with severe reduction in serum albumin and/or prothrombin time. *0376*

579.00 Celiac Sprue Disease Found in 28% of patients. *1614*

580.00 Acute Poststreptococcal Glomerulonephritis Persistently low with C3 conversion products and normal C4. *2522*

580.05 Glomerulonephritis (Membranoproliferative) Permanent depression of C3 is found in 60-80% of patients. *2468* Profound prolonged depression ascribed to anticomplementary factors. *0995* In 70% of cases. *0331*

710.00 Systemic Lupus Erythematosus Concentration 63 ± 8 mg/dL in patients with subendothelial deposits, compared to 142 ± 27 mg/dL in controls. *0168* Reduced levels arise from increased catabolism and reduced synthesis which always occurs at some stage of active SLE. *1550 2198* 21 children had 52 episodes of C3 depression (mean duration 25 weeks); only 11 had active nephritis when concentrations were depressed. *2186* Especially low in patients with active nephritis. C5 is usually normal. *2090* Caused by hypercatabolism *0375 1275 0509*

710.20 Sjögren's Syndrome Caused by hypercatabolism. *0375 0793 1275 0509 0452*

714.00 Rheumatoid Arthritis Caused by hypercatabolism. *0375 0793 1275 0509 0452*

770.80 Respiratory Distress Syndrome Neonatal- Caused by hypercatabolism. *0375 0793 1275 0509 0452*

948.00 Burns Caused by hypercatabolism. *0375 0793 1275 0509 0452*

Serum Increase

30.00 Leprosy High levels of both C2 and C3 have been recorded. *2035 2387*

150.90 Malignant Neoplasm of Esophagus Increased in patients with local disease. Very closely linked to the stage of the disease. Patients in remission had normal levels, but further increases were noted in distant metastases. Levels dropped significantly in the terminal phase of the disease. *2427*

151.90 Malignant Neoplasm of Stomach Increased in patients with local disease. Very closely linked to the stage of the disease. Patients in remission had normal levels, but further increases were noted in distant metastases. Levels dropped significantly in the terminal phase of disease. *2427*

152.90 Malignant Neoplasm of Small Intestine Increased in patients with local disease. Very closely linked to the stage of the disease. Patients in remission had normal levels, but further increases were noted in distant metastases. Levels dropped significantly in the terminal phase of the disease. *2427*

153.90 Malignant Neoplasm of Large Intestine Increased in patients with local disease. Found to be very closely linked to the stage of the disease. Patients in remission had normal levels, but further increases were noted in distant metastases. Dropped significantly in the terminal phase of disease. *2427*

154.10 Malignant Neoplasm of Rectum Increased in patients with local disease. Found to be very closely linked to the stage of the disease. Patients in remission had normal levels, but further increases were noted in distant metastases. Dropped significantly in the terminal phase of disease. *2427*

157.90 Malignant Neoplasm of Pancreas Increased in patients with local disease. Very closely linked to the stage of the disease, patients in remission had normal levels, but further increases were noted in distant metastases. Dropped significantly in the terminal phase of disease. *2427*

162.90 Malignant Neoplasm of Bronchus and Lung Increased in patients with local disease. Very closely linked to the stage of the disease. Patients in remission had normal levels, but further increases were noted in distant metastases. Levels dropped significantly in the terminal phase of disease. *2427*

174.90 Malignant Neoplasm of Breast Increased in patients with local disease. Very closely linked to the stage of the disease. Patients in remission had normal levels, but further increases were noted in distant metastases. Dropped significantly in the terminal phase of the disease. *2427*

180.90 Malignant Neoplasm of Cervix Increased in patients with local disease. Closely linked to the stage of the disease. Patients in remission had normal levels, but further increases were noted in distant metastases. Dropped significantly in the terminal phase of disease. *2427*

183.00 Malignant Neoplasm of Ovary Increased in patients with local disease. Closely linked to the stage of the disease. Patients in remission had normal levels, but further increases were noted in distant metastases. Levels dropped significantly in the terminal phase of disease. *2427*

185.00 Malignant Neoplasm of Prostate 26% had raised levels ranging from 208-440 mg/dL. *0008* Levels were found to be very closely linked to the stage of the disease. Patients in remission had normal levels, but further increases were noted in distant metastases. Levels dropped significantly in the terminal phase of disease. *2427*

188.90 Malignant Neoplasm of Bladder Increased in patients with local disease. Closely linked to the stage of the disease. Patients in remission had normal levels, but further increases were noted in distant metastases. Dropped significantly in the terminal phase of disease. *2427*

245.10 Subacute Thyroiditis Increased serum C3, IgM, alpha$_1$-acid glycoprotein and alpha$_1$-antitrypsin levels in 40 patients. *1715*

245.20 Hashimoto's Thyroiditis There was an increase in serum C3, IgM, alpha$_1$-acid glycoprotein and alpha$_1$-antitrypsin levels found in 40 patients. *1715*

277.00 Cystic Fibrosis Found in 13 patients. *1834*

277.30 Amyloidosis Found mostly in the recovery phase. *0793 0452 1275 0509 0375*

283.21 Paroxysmal Nocturnal Hemoglobinuria May, on occasion, be detected in the direct Coombs' test. *2538*

390.00 Rheumatic Fever Elevated during the acute stages of disease, coinciding with other indices of acute inflammation. *2035*

570.00 Acute and Subacute Necrosis of Liver *2467*

580.00 Acute Poststreptococcal Glomerulonephritis Particularly during diuretic phase. *0062*

710.00 Systemic Lupus Erythematosus Early in active disease the acute inflammatory response may cause increased C3 and C4 production. *1550*

714.00 Rheumatoid Arthritis The mean plasma C3e level in these samples (3.0 ± 1.3 mg/dL) was significantly increased as compared to patients with degenerative joint disease (0.9 ± 0.4 mg/dL) and healthy blood donors (0.8 ± 0.5 mg/dL). C3d levels were increased by more than 2 SD in 79% of RA samples. In most RA patients, the C3d levels were higher in synovial fluid than in plasma. *1712*

714.30 Juvenile Rheumatoid Arthritis Serum C2, C4, and C9 were elevated, but only C9 correlated well with ESR. *2090*

Serum Normal

273.21 Cryoglobulinemia (Essential Mixed) In 26 patients affected by essential cryoglobulinemia, a peculiar pattern was observed which was characterized by: low levels of early components (C1q, C1s and C4), normal levels of C3 and high concentrations of late components (C5,C9) and CH50 values significantly lower than normal. *2329* May be normal in mixed cryoglobulinemia. *2522*

273.30 Waldenström's Macroglobulinemia *2467*

273.80 Analbuminemia *2467*

Complement C3 *(continued)*

Serum   Normal *(continued)*

277.00   Cystic Fibrosis   *1397*

279.04   Agammaglobulinemia (Congenital Sex-linked)   *2467*

280.90   Iron Deficiency Anemia   *2467*

282.20   Anemias Due To Disorders of Glutathione Metabolism   *2467*

287.30   Idiopathic Thrombocytopenic Purpura   In one series. *1259*

446.20   Goodpasture's Syndrome   Almost always normal. *0062*

496.01   Alpha₁-Antitrypsin Deficiency   *2467*

580.01   Glomerulonephritis (Focal)   *0419*

580.02   Glomerulonephritis (Minimal Change)   *1383*

580.04   Glomerulonephritis (Membranous)   Nearly always. *0419*

580.40   Glomerulonephritis (Rapidly Progressive)   *1383*

708.90   Urticaria   Patients with hereditary angioedema have decreased levels of C1 esterase inhibitor and C4 in the presence of normal amounts of C3 and C1q. Normal values for these complement components are found in persons with allergic angioedema. *0272*

Synovial Fluid   Decrease

710.00   Systemic Lupus Erythematosus   Complement levels are very low. *0433*

714.00   Rheumatoid Arthritis   Marked reduction of C1, C2, C3 and C4 in seropositive patients. Only C4 was significantly decreased in seronegative patients. *2090*

714.30   Juvenile Rheumatoid Arthritis   Synovial fluid levels C1q, C3, C4 and C9 were consistently depressed in all seropositive patients, and in 5 of 14 seronegative patients. *2090*

Synovial Fluid   Increase

714.00   Rheumatoid Arthritis   The mean plasma C3e level in these samples (3.0 ± 1.3 mg/dL) was significantly increased as compared to patients with degenerative joint disease (0.9 ± 0.4 mg/dL). C3d levels were increased by more than 2 SD in 79% of RA samples. In most patients, the C3d levels were higher in synovial fluid than in plasma. *1712*

Pleural Effusion   Decrease

710.00   Systemic Lupus Erythematosus   *0062*

714.00   Rheumatoid Arthritis   In about 5% of cases. *0062*

Pericardial Fluid   Decrease

710.00   Systemic Lupus Erythematosus   Low or absent *0764 0877*

714.00   Rheumatoid Arthritis   Low or absent *0764 0877*

Red Blood Cells   Increase

283.00   Acquired Hemolytic Anemia (Autoimmune)   Only fractions of the complement system of proteins, principally C3 and C4 components, are detected on the red cells by antiglobulin sera having anti-C specificity. *0485   2538*

Complement C4

Serum   Decrease

205.10   Myelocytic Leukemia (Chronic)   Occasionally occurs. *1120*

273.21   Cryoglobulinemia (Essential Mixed)   In 26 patients affected by essential cryoglobulinemia, a peculiar pattern was observed which was characterized by: low levels of early components (C1q, C1s and C4), normal levels of C3 and high concentrations of late components (C5, C9) and CH50 values significantly lower than normal. *2329*   C1q, C2, and C4 are especially decreased whereas C3 may be normal in mixed cryoglobulinemia. *2522*

421.00   Bacterial Endocarditis   Decreased total C3 and C4, with conversion products of both, in subacute endocarditis. *2522*

493.10   Asthma (Intrinsic)   Decreased serum concentrations of C4 and factor B were found in 3 of 15 skin-test positive asthmatic children. Confirming the involvement of complement in the pathogenesis of immediate type reaction. *1088*

571.20   Laennec's or Alcoholic Cirrhosis   Low levels of C3, C4 and factor B were common with cirrhosis and confined to those cases with severe reduction in serum albumin and/or prothrombin index. *0376*

571.90   Cirrhosis of Liver   Decreased C3 and C4 occasionally occur. *1120*   Low levels of C3, C4, and factor B were common with cirrhosis and confined to those cases with severe reduction in serum albumin and/or prothrombin time. *0376*

580.00   Acute Poststreptococcal Glomerulonephritis   Usually less than that of C3. *0277*

708.90   Urticaria   Patients with hereditary angioedema have decreased levels of C1 esterase inhibitor and C4 in the presence of normal amounts of C3 and C1q. Normal values for these complement components are found in persons with allergic angioedema. *0272*   Low C4 or C1 esterase confirms clinical diagnosis of hereditary angioedema. *0766*

710.00   Systemic Lupus Erythematosus   Serum C4 levels was 8 ± 2 mg/dL in patients with subendothelial deposits, compared to 27 ± 6 mg/dL in patients with deposits. *0168*   Reduced levels arise from increased catabolism synthesis which always occurs at some stage of active disease. *2198 1550*   C4 occasionally remained depressed longer than C3, perhaps reflecting continuing subclinical disease activity. *2186*   Especially low in patients with active nephritis. C5 is usually normal. *2090*

Serum   Increase

150.90   Malignant Neoplasm of Esophagus   Increased in patients with local disease. Very closely linked to the stage of the disease. Patients in remission had normal levels, but further increases were noted in distant metastases. Levels dropped significantly in the terminal phase of disease. *2427*

151.90   Malignant Neoplasm of Stomach   Increased in patients with local disease. Very closely linked to the stage of the disease. Patients in remission had normal levels, but further increases were noted in distant metastases. Levels dropped significantly in the terminal phase of disease. *2427*

152.90   Malignant Neoplasm of Small Intestine   Increased in patients with local disease. Very closely linked to the stage of the disease. Patients in remission had normal levels, but further increases were noted in distant metastases. Levels dropped significantly in the terminal phase of disease. *2427*

153.90   Malignant Neoplasm of Large Intestine   Increased in patients with local disease. Very closely linked to the stage of the disease. Patients in remission had normal levels, but further increases were noted in distant metastases. Levels dropped significantly in the terminal phase of disease. *2427*

154.10   Malignant Neoplasm of Rectum   Increased in patients with local disease. Very closely linked to the stage of the disease. Patients in remission had normal levels, but further increases were noted in distant metastases. Levels dropped significantly in the terminal phase of disease. *2427*

157.90   Malignant Neoplasm of Pancreas   Increased in patients with local disease. Very closely linked to the stage of the disease. Patients in remission had normal levels, but further increases were noted in distant metastases. Levels dropped significantly in the terminal phase of disease. *2427*

162.90   Malignant Neoplasm of Bronchus and Lung   Increased in patients with local disease. Very closely linked to the stage of the disease. Patients in remission had normal levels, but further increases were noted in distant metastases. Levels dropped significantly in the terminal phase of disease. *2427*

174.90   Malignant Neoplasm of Breast   Increased in patients with local disease. Very closely linked to the stage of the disease. Patients in remission had normal levels, but further increases were noted in distant metastases. Levels dropped significantly in the terminal phase of the disease. *2427*

180.90   Malignant Neoplasm of Cervix   Increased in patients with local disease. Very closely linked to the stage of the disease. Patients in remission had normal levels, but further increases were noted in distant metastases. Levels dropped significantly in the terminal phase of disease. *2427*

183.00   Malignant Neoplasm of Ovary   Increased in patients with local disease. Very closely linked to the stage of the disease. Patients in remission had normal levels, but further increases were noted in distant metastases. Levels dropped significantly in the terminal phase of the disease. *2427*

185.00 Malignant Neoplasm of Prostate Increased in patients with local disease. Very closely linked to the stage of the disease. Patients in remission had normal levels, but further increases were noted in distant metastases. Levels dropped significantly in the terminal phase of disease. *2427*

188.90 Malignant Neoplasm of Bladder Increased in patients with local disease. Very closely linked to the stage of the disease. Patients in remission had normal levels, but further increases were noted in distant metastases. Levels dropped significantly in the terminal phase of the disease. *2427*

710.00 Systemic Lupus Erythematosus Early in active disease the acute inflammatory response may cause increased C3 and C4 production. *1550*

714.30 Juvenile Rheumatoid Arthritis Serum C2, C3, C4, and C9 were elevated, but only C9 correlated well with ESR. *2090*

720.00 Rheumatoid (Ankylosing) Spondylitis Mean levels of C4 and IgA were significantly elevated in patients with sporadic disease. *1273* Raised concentration of C4 and complement inactivation products. *2152*

Serum Normal

38.00 Septicemia In severe gram-negative infection associated with shock, depression of C3, C5, C6, and C9 may occur, with normal concentrations of C1, C2, and C4. Abnormalities develop early, before shock. C3 concentration correlates with mortality. *2522*

260.00 Protein Malnutrition All complement components except C4 and C5 were significantly lower in children with protein-calorie malnutrition: C3 and C9 were the most severely depressed. C5 was the only complement that was significantly higher in malnourished children than in normal children. *1732*

446.20 Goodpasture's Syndrome Almost always normal. *0062*

493.10 Asthma (Intrinsic) Usually normal. *1228*

580.00 Acute Poststreptococcal Glomerulonephritis C3 was persistently low with C3 conversion products and normal C4. *2522*

580.02 Glomerulonephritis (Minimal Change) *1383*

580.04 Glomerulonephritis (Membranous) Nearly always. *0419*

580.05 Glomerulonephritis (Membranoproliferative) *0277*

580.40 Glomerulonephritis (Rapidly Progressive) *1383*

CSF Decrease

710.00 Systemic Lupus Erythematosus Low CSF levels of C4 occur in patients with CNS involvement, due to in vivo immune reaction. *2090*

Synovial Fluid Decrease

710.00 Systemic Lupus Erythematosus Complement levels are very low. *0433*

714.00 Rheumatoid Arthritis Marked reduction of C1, C2, C3, and C4 in seropositive patients. Only C4 was significantly decreased in seronegative patients. *2090*

714.30 Juvenile Rheumatoid Arthritis Synovial fluid levels of C1q, C3, C4, and C9 were consistently depressed in all seropositive patients and in 5 of 14 seronegative patients. *2090*

Pleural Effusion Decrease

710.00 Systemic Lupus Erythematosus *0062*

714.00 Rheumatoid Arthritis In about 5% of cases. *0062*

Pericardial Fluid Decrease

710.00 Systemic Lupus Erythematosus Low or absent *0764 0877*

714.00 Rheumatoid Arthritis Low or absent *0764 0877*

Red Blood Cells Increase

283.00 Acquired Hemolytic Anemia (Autoimmune) Only fractions of the complement system of proteins, principally C3 and C4 components, are detected on the red cells by antiglobulin sera having anti-C specificity. *0485 2538*

Complement Fixation

Serum Increase

6.00 Amebiasis Usually positive during active (especially hepatic) disease. Significant positive titer is > 1:16. *2468*

11.00 Pulmonary Tuberculosis Used to differentiate pulmonary sarcoidosis from tuberculosis. Antituberculous antibodies were found in TB is 83%; in sarcoidosis 22%. *1309*

23.00 Brucellosis In late active disease, usually 1:16 or higher. *1058*

33.00 Whooping Cough These antibodies are produced in low titer and appear only after the second week of disease. *0962*

45.90 Acute Poliomyelitis *1058*

49.00 Lymphocytic Choriomeningitis Develops within 2-4 weeks. *2368 1058*

50.00 Smallpox Highly significant in an unvaccinated patient or when vaccination was performed years previously. *0433* A rising antibody titer is seen in paired sera. *0962*

53.00 Herpes Zoster A significant (4-fold or greater) anamnestic response usually occurs. *1058* 11 of 12 children showed a rise in CF antibody during convalescence. *0302*

54.00 Herpes Simplex Increased titer of complement-fixation and neutralizing antibodies is shown in convalescent-phase compared with acute-phase sera in primary infections. *2468*

55.00 Measles Antibodies tend to decrease with time but may be used for diagnosing recent infection. *0433* Becomes positive 1 week after onset. *2468* CF antibody appeared at the same time as the rash and rose to a maximum titer of 1:512 between the 5th and 16th days after the axanthem. *2368*

56.00 Rubella Antibodies appear within 1 week after rash; therefore acute-phase serum must be collected promptly or the rise in titer may not be detected. They may last for 8 months to years. *2468*

60.00 Yellow Fever Can be confirmed by CF antibody rises in paired sera. *1179*

66.10 Tick-Borne Fever Increased in sera taken during acute and convalescent phases. *2468*

72.00 Mumps Antibodies against the S and V antigens are the most widely used serologic test. The S antibodies usually rise within the first week of illness, the V antibodies appearing 1-2 weeks later. A presumptive diagnosis can therefore be made when elevated S antibodies are found in the absence of V antibodies. *0433* Positive during 2nd week and remains elevated > 6 weeks; paired sera showing a 4-fold increase in titer confirm recent infection. *2368 1319*

73.90 Psittacosis Positive but not conclusive tests are presumptive in diagnosis because of false positives with other infections and cross reactions with lymphogranuloma venereum. *2468* A low titer is highly suspicious during the acute phase of the illness, and the diagnosis is confirmed by a 4-fold increase in titer. *0962 2368*

78.50 Cytomegalic Inclusion Disease Requires use of multiple serologic types and is too time consuming and not very practical. *1319*

80.00 Epidemic Typhus Antibodies first appear in the serum between the 7-12 days. *0151* A demonstration of a 4-fold increase is considered significant. *1319* Antibodies develop which are both group- and species- specific. *0962 0433*

81.00 Endemic Typhus Antibodies develop which are both group- and species- specific. Appear during the 2nd week of illness and reach a peak during the 4th week. *0962*

81.10 Brill's Disease The diagnosis can be made by demonstrating a rising titer of antibodies which fix complement in the presence of epidemic typhus antigen or agglutinate suspensions of washed Rickettsia prowazekii. The antibody occurs earlier (4-6th day) and peaks between the 8-10th day. *0433 2368*

81.20 Mite-Borne Typhus Available antigens detect complement fixing antibody in only about 50% of the cases. *0962* Irregular results. *2368*

82.00 Rocky Mountain Spotted Fever Antibodies develop which are both group- and species- specific. Appear during the 2nd week of illness and reach a peak during the 4th week. *0962* A 4-fold or greater rise is considered confirmatory. *0151* Significant rise in titer occurs by the 3rd week. *1319*

83.20 Rickettsialpox A 4-fold or greater rise in antibody titer in paired sera. Because of cross reactions, the Rocky Mountain spotted fever test will also be positive. *1319*

84.00 Malaria In natural infections, the complement-fixation and indirect hemagglutination tests detect malarial antibodies equally efficiently for the first 2 months after onset, but titers obtained by complement-fixation rapidly decline with time, while the indirect hemagglutination titers remain elevated. *2547*

85.00 Leishmaniasis Positive but is also positive in tuberculosis. *2468*

Complement Fixation (continued)

Serum   Increase (continued)

86.90 Trypanosomiasis *1058*

87.00 Relapsing Fever   Antibodies develop but antigens are not sufficiently well standardized to be useful. *0962*

97.90 Syphilis   Kolmer test. *1058*

99.10 Lymphogranuloma Venereum   Early in the course of the disease, in symptomatic and asymptomatic patients, titers of 1:40-1:160 will occur. Later stages may produce titers as high as 1:640 in most patients. *0433*   This test is nonspecific and may be positive following infections with other chlamydiae. *0962*   A rising titer strongly indicates acute disease. May remain positive after antimicrobial therapy and an apparent clinical remission. *2199*   Much more sensitive than the Frei test, but cross reacts with other chlamydiae infections, such as psittacosis. *2060 2368   2468*

100.00 Leptospirosis   Antibodies appear during second week of illness. *0962*

114.90 Coccidioidomycosis   Highly specific and has prognostic significance. Positive in about 60% of cases with chronic coccidioidal cavities, but often negative in patients with asymptomatic coccidioidomas. *0151*   Positive 4-6 weeks following onset of symptoms with maximum response at 2-3 months. Titers > 1:2 may indicate active disease and 80% with disseminated infection have titers > 1:16. *2508*   Titer correlates with increasing severity of the disease. A rising titer may indicate spread of the disease to extrapulmonary sites. *0433 2207 0962 2368*

115.00 Histoplasmosis   Of 79 consecutive patients with positive test 28 (35%) were false-positive results. 12 patients (15%) had titers of > 1:32, without cultural or histological evidence of active infection. Using histoplasmin as antigen detected antibodies in the sera of 72.8% of the 70 proven cases, while yeast antigen detected antibodies in 94%. *2343*   Initially positive in 74% of 228 cases (titers > 1:64). *0892*   In primary pulmonary infection, antibodies to yeast antigen appear 10-21 days following fungus exposure. Histoplasmin antibodies are of greater importance in chronic infection, in which antibodies to yeast antigen may be decreased or absent. Titer of > 1:8 is presumed to indicate active infection, most patients have titers > 1:16. *2508*   CF antibodies are produced in a high percentage of patients in the acute phase, and fade out as the infection becomes asymptomatic or inactive. *2368   0962*

116.00 Blastomycosis   Titers of 1:8 or greater may be present in 33-50% of the patients. Positive titers of 1:32 or higher are highly suggestive of active disease. *0433*   High titer is correlated with poor prognosis. *2468*   Reactions are transient and inconsistent with poor sensitivity and high incidence of cross-reactivity. *2508*

117.50 Cryptococcosis   With CNS involvement about 66% of patients have antigen in their serum, CSF or both. *1058*

120.00 Schistosomiasis   The best serologic procedure to diagnose chronic disease (100% specific and 95% sensitive). *2468*

122.90 Hydatidosis *1058*

124.00 Trichinosis   Becomes positive about 2 weeks after occurrence of eosinophilia and may remain positive for 6 months. *2468*   Using bentonite particles, become positive later in the disease and are most helpful when they exhibit a significant change in titer. *0962*

128.00 Larva Migrans (Visceralis)   Positive in 75% of patients. *0992*

130.00 Toxoplasmosis   Antibody is present within 1-2 months of infection and is usually negative within 2 y. *2035*   Becomes positive later than the other serologic tests, and its titer declines earlier. *0962*   In 26 patients with congenital infection and in 22 of their mothers, tests results were positive on all specimens from the patients younger than 2 y of age and on 69% of specimens collected from older patients. *1244*   CF antibodies appear later than Sabin-Feldman or hemagglutinating antibodies and diminish more rapidly. *2368   1319*

135.00 Sarcoidosis   Used to differentiate pulmonary sarcoidosis from tuberculosis. Antituberculous antibodies were found in TB in 83%; in sarcoidosis 22%. *1309*

245.20 Hashimoto's Thyroiditis   Virtually all patients with this disease have circulating autoantibodies. *2540*   Antimicrosomal antibodies present in 78% of patients. *0992*   Positive for cytoplasmic microsomal antigen in > 80% of cases. High titers of 1:256 usually occur in chronic thyroiditis. *0999*

357.00 Guillain-Barré Syndrome   30 patients (33%) had markedly elevated levels of complement-fixing antibody to cytomegalovirus and in 21, a 4-fold or more alteration in titer was demonstrated. *0595*

422.00 Acute Myocarditis   Positive in helminthic myocarditis. *1108*

483.01 Mycoplasma Pneumoniae   A 4-fold or greater rise in titer of paired sera obtained during acute and convalescent phases is diagnostic of recent mycoplasma infection. *2508*   Proved to be inappropriate for the early etiological diagnosis of infections, since the high titers were distributed undifferentially among the various patient groups and many sera (38%) showed anticomplementary activity. *0352*   Demonstration of CF antibodies of IgM type in week 2 provides early specific diagnosis. *0661*

487.10 Influenza   A very high titer is suggestive of recent infection. Recent immunization with inactivated influenza virus vaccine has little effect upon titer obtained when S antigen is used. A 4-fold or greater rise between paired sera is accepted as evidence of infection. *0433*   May become positive during the 2nd week of illness. *0962   0999*

571.49 Chronic Active Hepatitis   Incidence of positivity to anticytoplasmic antibodies (titer > 8) was reported to be 27-30% in contrast to an incidence of 3-4% in controls and 7-12% in other types of liver disease. *1466   2035*

694.40 Pemphigus   50-75% of bullous pemphigoid patients have serum antibodies capable of fixing complement to the basement membrane. *2035*

Serum   Positive

480.90 Viral Pneumonia   Complement-Fixing antibodies appear 8-9 days after onset. *1905*

CSF   Increase

86.90 Trypanosomiasis *1058*

114.90 Coccidioidomycosis   Generally the titer is lower than in the serum. *2207*   Pleural, joint, and CSF fluids contain complement-fixing antibody but in lower titer than in serum. *0151*   In 75% of patients with coccidioidal meningitis. *2368   2035*

117.50 Cryptococcosis   With CNS involvement about 66% of patients have antigen in their serum, CSF or both. *1058*

Synovial Fluid   Increase

114.90 Coccidioidomycosis   Pleural, joint, and CSF fluids contain complement-fixing antibody but in lower titer than in serum. *0151*

Pleural Effusion   Increase

114.90 Coccidioidomycosis   Generally the titer is lower than in the serum. *2207*   Pleural, joint, and CSF fluids contain complement-fixing antibody but in lower titer than in serum. *0151   2035*

Peritoneal Fluid   Increase

114.90 Coccidioidomycosis   Generally the titer is lower than in the serum. *2207   2035*

Complement, Total

Serum   Decrease

38.00 Septicemia   In severe gram-negative infection associated with shock, depression of C3, C5, C6, and C9 may occur, with normal concentrations of C1, C2, and C4. Abnormalities develop early, before shock. C3 concentration correlates with mortality. *2522*   In 51 patients, 24% had decreased values. *2223*

205.10 Myelocytic Leukemia (Chronic)   Occasionally occurs. *1120*

260.00 Protein Malnutrition   Individual components of the complement system were significantly lower in kwashiorkor than in normal controls. *0956*   All complement components except C4 and C5 were significantly lower in children with protein-calorie malnutrition: C3 and C9 were the most severely depressed. C5 was the only complement that was significantly higher in malnourished children than in normal children. *1732*   Mean activity in children with kwashiorkor was significantly less on hospital days 1 and 4 than in control subjects. On day 8 it rose to normal, and by day 50 it was significantly higher than the controls. 11 (40%) evidence anticomplementary activity in their serum on either day 1 or day 4. *2298*

273.21 Cryoglobulinemia (Essential Mixed)   In 26 patients affected by essential cryoglobulinemia, peculiar pattern was observed which was characterized by: low levels of early components (C1q, C1s and C4), normal levels of C3 and high concentrations of late components (C5,C9) and CH50 values significantly lower than normal. *2329*

273.30 Waldenström's Macroglobulinemia   In some cases. *0020*

274.00 Gout   Depleted in serum by urate crystals. *1664*

283.00 Acquired Hemolytic Anemia (Autoimmune)   Low serum titers have been reported in patients with warm antibody hemolytic disease. *1804 2035*

340.00 Multiple Sclerosis   Hypocomplementemia was found in 29.5% of the patients not on corticotherapy at the first assay, and in 36% of the patients when repeated assays were carried out. Hypocomplementemia is significantly more frequent than in the normal population (0%) and in neurological patients (9.6%). *2375*

358.00 Myasthenia Gravis   40 of 68 patients had activity below normal at some time in the course of disease. On the basis of clinical correlations, 15 patients with subnormal levels were judged to be in exacerbation. *1680 2035*

390.00 Rheumatic Fever   In general, normal or elevated. A small number of patients have reduced levels during the acute phase without any clear relation to severity or particular clinical manifestation. *0962*

421.00 Bacterial Endocarditis   Decreased total hemolytic complement in 8 of 17 or 47% of patients tested. 7 of the 8 had evidence of renal disease. *1798*   Decreased total C3 and C4, with conversion products of both, in subacute endocarditis. *2522*

446.00 Polyarteritis-Nodosa   Depression of titers may be found in early, acute phases. *0642*   Subsides with remission. *2090*

571.20 Laennec's or Alcoholic Cirrhosis   Low levels of C3, C4 and factor B were common with cirrhosis and confined to those cases with severe reduction in serum albumin and/or prothrombin index. *0376*

571.49 Chronic Active Hepatitis   Normal or mildly decreased. *0992*

571.90 Cirrhosis of Liver   Decreased C3 and C4 occasionally occurs. *1120*   Depressed in patients with chronic liver disease; does not correlate with immune phenomena, but appears to be related to impaired hepatic protein synthesis. *0151*

580.00 Acute Poststreptococcal Glomerulonephritis   Marked reduction coincident with development of nephritis. *0151*

580.05 Glomerulonephritis (Membranoproliferative)   Characteristic of membranoproliferative glomerulonephritis. *2545*

694.40 Pemphigus   Cryoproteins observed in patients with pemphigus have been shown to contain IgG, complement components, and other serum proteins. *1612*

708.90 Urticaria   Patients with hereditary angioedema have decreased levels of C1 esterase inhibitor and C4 in the presence of normal amounts of C3 and C1q. Normal values for these complement components are found in persons with allergic angioedema. *0272*   10 of 72 patients were found to have decreased total complement hemolytic activity. *1524 0743*

710.00 Systemic Lupus Erythematosus   Reduced in about 75% of patients with active disease. Reduction may be correlated with the activity of the illness and varies inversely with ANA titers. *2089*   Reduced levels arise from increased catabolism and reduced synthesis which always occurs at some stage of active SLE. *2198 1550*   Low C1 (C1q and C1s), C2, C3, and C4 occur in active SLE. Especially low in patients with active nephritis. C5 is usually normal. *2090*   Found in 80 (57%) patients. *0713*   In 35 patients, 77% had decreased values. In discoid lupus, 57% had elevated levels. *2223 0999*

710.10 Progressive Systemic Sclerosis   Occasionally. *2090*   In 27 patients, 44% had decreased values. *2223*

710.20 Sjögren's Syndrome   Occasionally decreased, especially with cryoglobulinemia. *2090*

710.40 Dermatomyositis/Polymyositis   In 15 patients, 20% had decreased values. *2223*

711.10 Mixed Connective Tissue Disease   In 30% of cases. *0062*

714.00 Rheumatoid Arthritis   In rare instances and with a highly acute onset, may be low. *0962*   In 64 patients, 19% had decreased values. *2223*

714.10 Felty's Syndrome   Hypocomplementemia usually occurs. *1605*

714.30 Juvenile Rheumatoid Arthritis   In 22 patients, 32% had decreased values. *2223*

Serum   Increase

30.00 Leprosy   Sarcoidosis, leprosy, and Wegener's granulomatosis have elevated levels. *1699*

38.00 Septicemia   In 51 patients, 27% had increased values. *2223*

99.30 Reiter's Disease   Elevated during active inflammation and subsides with remission. *2090*   In 14 patients, 64% had increased values. *2223*

135.00 Sarcoidosis   *0151 1699*

150.90 Malignant Neoplasm of Esophagus   Found to be very closely linked to the stage of the disease. Patients in remission had normal levels, but further increases were noted in distant metastases. Levels dropped significantly in the terminal phase of the disease. *2427*

151.90 Malignant Neoplasm of Stomach   CH50, C1q, C3, and C4 were significantly higher in cancer patients than in matched controls. The increase was dependent upon the stage of disease and the therapy. *2427*

153.90 Malignant Neoplasm of Large Intestine   Found to be very closely linked to stage of disease. Patients in remission had normal levels, but further increases were noted in distant metastases. Levels dropped significantly in the terminal phase of disease. *2427*

157.90 Malignant Neoplasm of Pancreas   Very closely linked to the stage of the disease. Patients in remission had normal levels, but further increases were noted in distant metastases. Dropped significantly in the terminal phase of disease. *2427*

162.90 Malignant Neoplasm of Bronchus and Lung   Closely linked to the stage of the disease. Patients in remission had normal levels, but further increases were noted in distant metastases. Levels dropped significantly in the terminal phase of disease. *2427*

170.90 Malignant Neoplasm of Bone   Levels from sera of 21 bone tumors showed normal or slightly elevated titers. *0369*

174.90 Malignant Neoplasm of Breast   Very closely linked to the stage of the disease. Patients in remission had normal levels, but further increases were noted in distant metastases. Levels dropped significantly in the terminal phase of disease. *2427*

180.90 Malignant Neoplasm of Cervix   Closely linked to the stage of the disease, patients in remission had normal levels, but further increases were noted in distant metastases. Levels dropped significantly in the terminal phase of the disease. *2427*

183.00 Malignant Neoplasm of Ovary   Closely linked to the stage of the disease. Patients in remission had normal levels, but further increases were noted in distant metastases. Dropped significantly in the terminal phase of disease. *2427*

185.00 Malignant Neoplasm of Prostate   Closely linked to the stage of the disease. Patients in remission had normal levels, but further increases were noted in distant metastases. Dropped significantly in the terminal phase of the disease. *2427*

188.90 Malignant Neoplasm of Bladder   Closely linked to the stage of the disease. Patients in remission had normal levels, but further increases were noted in distant metastases. Dropped significantly in the terminal phase of disease. *2427*

201.90 Hodgkin's Disease   58 of 72 patients had elevated total complement levels which were associated with C-reactive protein, ESR and beta globulin levels. *1998*   A highly significant increase of the mean total serum hemolytic complement activity was found in stages III-A and IV-A and all stages with systemic symptoms in Hodgkin's disease. *2450*

273.21 Cryoglobulinemia (Essential Mixed)   In 26 patients affected by essential cryoglobulinemia, a peculiar pattern was observed which was characterized by: low levels of early components (C1q, C1s and C4), normal levels of C3 and high concentrations of late components (C5,C9) and CH50 values significantly lower than normal. *2329*

274.00 Gout   Elevated during active inflammation and subsides with remission. *2090*

390.00 Rheumatic Fever   In general, normal or elevated. A small number of patients have reduced levels during the acute phase without any clear relation to severity or particular clinical manifestation. *0962*   During the acute stage. *2035*   Elevated during activity inflammation and subsides with remission. *2090*

446.00 Polyarteritis-Nodosa   In some patients. *0030*   Possibly the result of low utilization or a rapid rate of production. *0962*   Elevated during active inflammation and subsides with remission. *2090 0999*

446.50 Cranial Arteritis and Related Conditions   In 6 patients, 50% had increased values. *2223*

556.00 Ulcerative Colitis   Mean titer in 16 increased in 16 patients. *0752*

642.40 Pre-Eclampsia   Significantly higher than in late normal pregnancy. *2286 0409*

Complement, Total *(continued)*

Serum Increase *(continued)*

650.00 Pregnancy Beta-1 A-C component of complement was increased in 39% of late normal pregnancies. *2287 2286*

710.00 Systemic Lupus Erythematosus Normal or elevated. *0151* Early in active SLE the acute inflammatory response may cause increased C3 and C4 production. *1550* In discoid lupus, 57% had elevated levels. *2223*

710.10 Progressive Systemic Sclerosis In 27 patients, 19% had increased values. *2223*

710.40 Dermatomyositis/Polymyositis Elevated during active inflammation and subsides with remission. *2090* In 15 patients, 13% had increased values. *2223*

714.00 Rheumatoid Arthritis In 64 patients, 16% had increased values. *2223* Activity tends to be elevated in patients with mild disease, lower levels were found in seropositive than seronegative patients. *2090*

714.30 Juvenile Rheumatoid Arthritis Serum C2, C3, C4, and C9 were elevated, but only C9 correlated well with ESR. RF positive patients tend to have lower CH50 than do RF negative patients, but both groups show increased titers during active disease. *2090* In 22 patients, 13% had increased values. *2223* Normal or increased *0136*

Serum Normal

117.10 Sporotrichosis Normal in all patients with Sporotrichosis arthritis. *0478*

279.04 Agammaglobulinemia (Congenital Sex-linked) Other serum constituents involved in resistance to infection are normal. *2246* Normal *2539 2035*

287.00 Allergic Purpura Usually normal. *0962*

390.00 Rheumatic Fever In general, normal or elevated. A small number of patients have reduced levels during the acute phase without any clear relation to severity or particular clinical manifestation. *0962* During the acute stage. *2035* Elevated during activity inflammation and subsides with remission. *2090*

446.20 Goodpasture's Syndrome Almost always normal. *0062*

446.50 Cranial Arteritis and Related Conditions *2035*

493.10 Asthma (Intrinsic) In the absence of any immunoglobulin deficiency, the levels of the other immunoglobulins as well as complement are within normal limits. *2035*

571.49 Chronic Active Hepatitis No characteristic alterations have been reported for levels of complement or complement components. *1844 2035*

580.04 Glomerulonephritis (Membranous) Nearly always. *0419*

580.40 Glomerulonephritis (Rapidly Progressive) *0962 1383*

642.60 Eclampsia *1764*

650.00 Pregnancy *1764*

710.10 Progressive Systemic Sclerosis Normal in all but a few patients. *2372 2035*

714.00 Rheumatoid Arthritis *0186*

714.30 Juvenile Rheumatoid Arthritis Normal or increased. *0136*

CSF Decrease

340.00 Multiple Sclerosis Significantly lower. *1330*

710.00 Systemic Lupus Erythematosus Abnormally low C4 levels. *1700*

CSF Increase

357.00 Guillain-Barré Syndrome Oligoclonal IgG bands, specific elevation of IgM and complement activation products have been reported during the acute phase of the disease. *1307*

Synovial Fluid Decrease

390.00 Rheumatic Fever The early and late components of the complement system are decreased. *2300*

710.00 Systemic Lupus Erythematosus May be markedly reduced below the complement level of serum. *1700* Marked decrease in synovial fluids. *1796* Low levels may occur in some patients. *2090* Compared to total protein, levels are low in 60-70% of joint effusions *0314*

711.00 Acute Arthritis (Pyogenic) Compared to total protein, levels are low in 60-70% of joint effusions. *0314*

714.00 Rheumatoid Arthritis Low compared to that in other types of inflammatory joint effusions, especially in relation to the total protein concentration. *0999* Whole complement activity is reduced. *1014* Intra-articular depletion of whole complement activity in the presence of normal or elevated serum levels is in proportion to the titer of rheumatoid factor in serum or synovial fluid. *2090* Marked reduction of C1, C2, C3, and C4 in seropositive patients. Only C4 was significantly decreased in seronegative patients. *2090* Low values associated with more severe disease and poorer prognosis. *0313* Compared to total protein, levels are low in 60-70% of joint effusions *0314*

714.30 Juvenile Rheumatoid Arthritis Synovial fluid levels of C1q, C3, C4, and C9 were consistently depressed in all seropositive patients and in 5 of 14 negative patients. *2090*

Synovial Fluid Increase

99.30 Reiter's Disease Usually higher than in most other types of effusions in contrast to the very low levels in rheumatoid arthritis. *0433* Elevated levels appear to be directly related to the severity and duration of joint inflammation. *2090*

274.00 Gout Frequently occurs. *2090*

720.00 Rheumatoid (Ankylosing) Spondylitis Frequently occurs. *2090*

Synovial Fluid Normal

282.60 Sickle Cell Anemia Total hemolytic complement ranged from 22-80 U/L, usually at the upper limit of normal. *0676*

Pleural Effusion Decrease

710.00 Systemic Lupus Erythematosus 5 of 7 cases showed reduced levels of CH50, C1, C1 inhibitor and C2 in pleural fluid. *0854* Low complement (< 10 U/mL) in 11 of 12 patients with SLE or rheumatoid pleuritis. *1403*

714.00 Rheumatoid Arthritis Seropositive patients had decreased CH50, C1, C2, and C1 inhibitor in pleural and pericardial fluids. *0854* Low complement (< 10 U/mL) in 11 of 12 patients with SLE or rheumatoid pleuritis. *1403*

Pericardial Fluid Decrease

710.00 Systemic Lupus Erythematosus Low or absent *0764 0877*

714.00 Rheumatoid Arthritis Low or absent *0764 0877*

Congo Red Test

Blood Positive

277.30 Amyloidosis Of 20 patients with amyloidosis, only 9 had > 60% disappearance of congo red from blood in 1 h. False-negative tests may be expected in > 50% of cases. *0341* Positive in 33% of patients with primary and in 66% of patients with secondary amyloidosis. *2468* Positive in up to 50% of patients with cardiac amyloidosis. *0151*

Coombs' Test

Blood Negative

203.00 Multiple Myeloma Usually. *2538*

207.00 Erythroleukemia *2538*

272.52 Abetalipoproteinemia *0130*

273.30 Waldenström's Macroglobulinemia Almost always negative. *2538*

282.00 Hereditary (Congenital) Spherocytosis Usually negative. *2552*

282.10 Hereditary Elliptocytosis In uncomplicated cases. *2552*

283.21 Paroxysmal Nocturnal Hemoglobinuria Usually negative. *2538*

446.00 Polyarteritis-Nodosa *0642*

446.60 Thrombotic Thrombocytopenic Purpura *2552*

773.00 Hemolytic Disease of Newborn (Erythroblastosis Fetalis) Infant RBCs show a negative direct Coombs' test (by standard methods) with ABO erythroblastosis. *2468* Negative or only weakly positive in cases of hemolytic disease due to ABO incompatibility. *2538* Usually negative when due to anti-A antibodies. It becomes negative within a few days of effective exchange transfusion. *2468*

Blood   Positive

23.00   Brucellosis   The modified Coombs' test overcomes the blocking antibody and prozone phenomenon. *2035*

84.00   Malaria   Patients occasionally have a Coombs'-positive hemolytic anemia. *0151*

201.90   Hodgkin's Disease   Usually negative, but on occasion it is positive. *0641 2538*

202.80   Non-Hodgkins Lymphoma   Autoimmune hemolytic anemia, with a positive Coombs' test, occurs in a few patients. *1186* May occur. *2552   2538*

204.10   Lymphocytic Leukemia (Chronic)   20% of patients develop severe hemolysis. *0992*

205.10   Myelocytic Leukemia (Chronic)   Positive in 33% of patients. *2468*

283.00   Acquired Hemolytic Anemia (Autoimmune)   May or may not be positive, depending on the total amount of autoantibody present and its binding affinity for the red cell mass. *2538*

287.30   Idiopathic Thrombocytopenic Purpura   In chronic ITP when autoimmune hemolytic anemia and ITP occur together (Evans' syndrome). *0682*

289.80   Myelofibrosis   Positive in 6 of 29 myelofibrosis patients. Positivity tends to develop in later stages of disease. *2317*

421.00   Bacterial Endocarditis   Rarely there is hemolytic anemia with a positive Coombs' test. *2467*

446.60   Thrombotic Thrombocytopenic Purpura   Rarely. *1706*

483.01   Mycoplasma Pneumoniae   May occur. *0151*   Direct test may be positive in convalescence. *2368*

556.00   Ulcerative Colitis   Has been described. *2199*

571.49   Chronic Active Hepatitis   Sometimes present. *2467 0992*

710.00   Systemic Lupus Erythematosus   A positive test is frequently associated with active hemolysis but may be seen in individuals without markedly shortened RBC survival. *0999*   Positive in 18-65% of patients in different studies, but only 10% of these manifest significant hemolysis. *0309*   About 5% of patients may develop hemolytic anemia. Direct Coombs' test is almost always positive in these cases. *0962   0713*

710.20   Sjögren's Syndrome   May occur. *2134*

773.00   Hemolytic Disease of Newborn (Erythroblastosis Fetalis)   Strongly positive in infants sensitized by Rh(D) red cells and by red cells with most of the rarely involved blood group antigens. Negative or only weakly positive in cases of hemolytic disease due to ABO incompatibility. *2538*   Direct test is strongly positive on cord blood RBC when due to Rh, Kel, Kidd, Duffy antibodies. *2468*

Copper

Serum   Decrease

256.30   Ovarian Hypofunction   Estrogen effect. *0995*

260.00   Protein Malnutrition   Serum, erythrocyte and urinary copper levels showed decline in marasmic malnutrition and kwashiorkor. Marked fall of serum and erythrocyte copper level in children suffering from kwashiorkor. *1140*

275.10   Hepatolenticular Degeneration   The serum concentration is directly related to that of the ceruloplasmin, for the protein binds the majority of the metal. Estimation of the serum copper seldom gives additional diagnostic information unless there is a discrepancy indicating a higher level of serum copper than can be accounted for by that present in ceruloplasmin. The normal serum concentration is between 90-140 µg/dL; in untreated disease it is commonly between 40-60 µg/dL but the range of variation is enormous. *0433   2467*

280.90   Iron Deficiency Anemia   Decreases in some iron-deficiency anemias of childhood (that require copper as well as iron therapy). *2467*   Ceruloplasmin lost in urine *2467*

414.00   Chronic Ischemic Heart Disease   Epidemiologic and metabolic data are consistent with the hypothesis that a metabolic imbalance in regard to zinc and copper is a major factor in the etiology of coronary heart disease. A metabolic imbalance is either a relative or an absolute deficiency of copper characterized by a high ratio of zinc to copper. The imbalance results in hypercholesterolemia and an increased mortality due to coronary heart disease. *1280*

579.00   Celiac Sprue Disease   Plasma zinc and copper depression was found in 10 adult patients. These findings further indicate that trace metal deficiency is another common nutritional complication. *2225*   Decreased in sprue and celiac disease in infants as a result of the inability to synthesize the apoprotein. *0619*

581.90   Nephrotic Syndrome   Found regularly with hypoproteinemia. *0350*

606.90   Infertility in Males   Infertile men (n = 8) had higher mean concentrations than those of proven fertility (n = 38) The difference was statistically significant. (P < 0.01) but was of small magnitude (about 1.5 µmol). *2247*

Serum   Increase

2.00   Typhoid Fever   Before the onset of overt clinical illness. *1795*

11.00   Pulmonary Tuberculosis   Characteristically elevated in whole blood, plasma, and erythrocytes. *0239*

38.00   Septicemia   Increased in acute and chronic infections. *2467*

70.00   Viral Hepatitis   Significant P < 0.001. *2429*

151.90   Malignant Neoplasm of Stomach   A correlation between copper and ceruloplasmin was reported in 58 cases of gastric neoplasm. *2058*   In 35 cases of primary malignant tumors of the digestive organs, plasma copper was increased (1.24 ± 0.34 ppm). *1125*

153.90   Malignant Neoplasm of Large Intestine   Increased in 35 cases of primary malignant tumors of the digestive organs, (mean = 1.24 ± 0.34 ppm). *1125*

162.90   Malignant Neoplasm of Bronchus and Lung   Extremely high in 82% of the 34 patients. *1296*   Increased in stomach, lung and large intestine neoplasm. Serum ceruloplasmin was high in gastric and lung cancer but not in the large intestine. *2058*

170.90   Malignant Neoplasm of Bone   12 cases of osteosarcoma at various stages were analyzed. Elevations occurred in primary and metastatic cases. Patients with advanced cases had the highest levels. *0735*   Significantly elevated in 18 patients with primary untreated osteogenic sarcoma (173 ± 30 µg/dL). *0276*

174.90   Malignant Neoplasm of Breast   All 23 patients demonstrated elevations (299 ± 34 mg/dL) compared to normal (108 ± 10 mg/dL). *0519   2094*

180.90   Malignant Neoplasm of Cervix   Elevations are related to the stage of the disease and decrease in response to treatment. *1719   2094*

183.00   Malignant Neoplasm of Ovary   Does not result from a shift of zinc into or release of copper out of malignant tumor tissue. *1406*

197.70   Secondary Malignant Neoplasm of Liver   High in advanced carcinoma with liver metastases. *1125*

198.50   Secondary Malignant Neoplasm of Bone   12 cases of osteosarcoma at various stages were analyzed for Cu and Zn serum levels. Elevated Cu occurred in primary and metastatic cases, while elevated Zn occurred only in primary osteosarcoma and depressed serum Zn in metastases. Patients with advanced cases had the highest serum Cu:Zn ratios. *0735*

201.90   Hodgkin's Disease   Correlates significantly to stage of disease and amount of tumor tissue. Varies with activity of the disease--increases with progression and decreases with improvement. *2354*   Has been reported. *2538 1087*   In all 50 patients with lymphoma, invariably found to be raised. After radiotherapy, the level was significantly lowered. *1888*

202.80   Non-Hodgkins Lymphoma   Invariably raised in all 50 patients with lymphoma. Significantly lowered after radiotherapy. *1888*

204.00   Lymphocytic Leukemia (Acute)   Significant increase observed in 16 children with acute leukemias. Drop in concentration occurs in cases who respond to quadruple chemotherapy while those who failed to respond showed persistently high serum levels. *0645*

204.10   Lymphocytic Leukemia (Chronic)   In acute and chronic leukemias. *2468*

205.00   Myelocytic Leukemia (Acute)   Significant increase observed in 16 cases of acute leukemia. Drop occurs in cases who respond to quadruple chemotherapy while those who failed to respond showed persistently high levels. *0645*

242.90   Hyperthyroidism   *2467 0619*

244.90   Hypothyroidism   *2467*

252.00   Hyperparathyroidism   Slightly > normal mean. *1490*

256.00   Ovarian Hyperfunction   Estrogen effect. *0995*

Copper *(continued)*

Serum   Increase *(continued)*

275.00 Hemochromatosis *0999*

280.90 Iron Deficiency Anemia *0433 0619*

281.00 Pernicious Anemia *2467 0619*

281.20 Folic Acid Deficiency Anemia   A secondary finding. *0151* Due to intramedullary hemolysis found in megaloblastic anemias. *2467*

282.41 Thalassemia Major   In 42 patients (age 3 mo. to 22 y.) with homozygous beta-thalassemia and thalassemia intermedia, serum zinc was significantly decreased while Cu and Fe were increased. *0072*   May be increased. *2552*

282.42 Thalassemia Minor   In 42 patients (age 3 mo-22 y) with homozygous beta-thalassemia and thalassemia intermedia, serum zinc was significantly decreased while Cu and Fe were increased. *0072*   May be increased on occasion. *0349*

282.60 Sickle Cell Anemia   Significantly increased in patients with SS compared to controls P < 0.001 Increased. *2052 1729*

284.90 Aplastic Anemia *2467*

297.90 Paranoid States and Other Psychoses   Elevated serum copper and ceruloplasmin blood levels were reported. It is postulated that this may be an important pathognomonic feature. *0027 0065*

303.90 Alcoholism *0998*

333.40 Huntington's Chorea   Some studies show elevated levels while others did not. *0878*

340.00 Multiple Sclerosis   Slight elevation of serum copper with significant reduction of serum ceruloplasmin. *1830*

390.00 Rheumatic Fever   In acute disease. *2467*   Has been used as an index of disease activity. *0619*   Statistically significant *2188*

410.90 Acute Myocardial Infarction   After infarction, a significant increase in serum copper and a decrease in zinc were observed. *2428*   Mean concentration = 123 μg/dL in 27 patients. *2502*

428.00 Congestive Heart Failure   Statistically significant. *2188*

434.90 Brain Infarction   Abnormally high concentrations in plasma and CSF. The plasma Cu:Zn ratio was also significantly elevated. *0240*

440.00 Arteriosclerosis   High concentrations found in 13 patients when compared with controls. The Zn:Cu ratio is much higher in arteriosclerotic patients than in healthy subjects. *0324*   Statistically significant *2188*

482.90 Bacterial Pneumonia   Statistically significant. *2188*

491.00 Chronic Bronchitis   Statistically significant. *2188*

493.10 Asthma (Intrinsic)   Statistically significant. *2188*

571.90 Cirrhosis of Liver   Elevated in various forms of acute and chronic liver disease. *0931 0619*

580.00 Acute Poststreptococcal Glomerulonephritis *1064*

580.01 Glomerulonephritis (Focal) *1064*

580.02 Glomerulonephritis (Minimal Change) *1064*

580.04 Glomerulonephritis (Membranous) *1064*

580.05 Glomerulonephritis (Membranoproliferative) *1064*

580.40 Glomerulonephritis (Rapidly Progressive) *1064*

606.90 Infertility in Males   The mean concentrations were higher than in men of proven fertility (P < 0.01) but the increases were of small magnitude. *2247*

650.00 Pregnancy   During normal pregnancy the concentration in maternal serum may almost double due to increased synthesis of ceruloplasmin. Value were lower in abnormal pregnancies than in normal ones. *0304*   Higher in early and late pregnancy. *0969* Approximately twice normal at term. Mechanism not known. *2636 0576*

710.00 Systemic Lupus Erythematosus   Increased. *2052 1729* Increase in collagen diseases *2467 0619*

710.10 Progressive Systemic Sclerosis   Increased. *2052 2188 1729*

710.20 Sjögren's Syndrome   Increased. *2052 2188 1729*

710.40 Dermatomyositis/Polymyositis   Increased. *2052 2188 1729*

714.00 Rheumatoid Arthritis   Both serum Cu and ceruloplasmin were measured 189 RA patients and were found to be significantly elevated. An inverse relation was found between serum iron and copper and a strong direct correlation between serum antioxidant activity and ceruloplasmin. *2100*   Elevated in excess of the binding capacity of ceruloplasmin, resulting in raised free copper levels. *1433*

720.00 Rheumatoid (Ankylosing) Spondylitis   Raised significantly, with the greatest increases in the worst cases. *1155*

Serum   Normal

333.40 Huntington's Chorea   Some studies show elevated levels while others did not. *0878*

Urine   Decrease

260.00 Protein Malnutrition   Serum, erythrocyte, and urinary copper levels showed decline in marasmic malnutrition and kwashiorkor. *1140*

Urine   Increase

252.00 Hyperparathyroidism   Mean 24 h urinary excretion was greater than normal in 17 patients with untreated disease. *1490*

275.10 Hepatolenticular Degeneration   In untreated disease the amount is usually > 200 μg/24h but occasionally much lower, particularly in young presymptomatic siblings. *0433*   A good indirect indicator of the copper concentration in the liver. *1506*   The ceruloplasmin fraction is defective. Copper is excreted in the urine, bound to amino acids which act as chelating agents. *0619*

571.60 Biliary Cirrhosis   Elevated in 42 of 46 patients. A correlation was found (R = 0.68) between urinary and hepatic copper. *0526   1944*

714.00 Rheumatoid Arthritis   Patients show an abnormal copper excretion pattern compared with nonrheumatoid subjects. *1558*

CSF   Increase

332.00 Parkin?on's Disease   Although there was considerable overlap between the 24 Parkinsonian and 34 control subjects, the former had significantly higher levels (P < 0.001). *1763*

434.90 Brain Infarction   Patients with cerebral infarctions had abnormally high concentrations in plasma and CSF. The plasma Cu:Zn ratio was also significantly elevated. *0240*

Synovial Fluid   Increase

714.00 Rheumatoid Arthritis   Characteristic of rheumatoid effusions. *2101*

Liver   Increase

135.00 Sarcoidosis   Increased in hepatocytes in 5 patients. *2004*

275.10 Hepatolenticular Degeneration   Liver biopsy shows high copper concentration 250 μg/g of dry liver). *2467*   Hepatic copper concentration is the most exact criterion in the diagnosis. In the course of the penicillamine therapy the copper content in the liver decreases, but normal values are achieved only after 5 or more y of treatment. The urinary copper excretion is a good indicator of the copper concentration in the liver. *1506*

571.60 Biliary Cirrhosis   Elevated in 43 of 45 patients, > 400 μg/g dry weight were found almost exclusively in patients with advanced histological disease. *0526*   8 of 13 patients had liver copper content as high as seen in patients with hepatolenticular degeneration (250 μg/g dry wt). *1944*

Red Blood Cells   Decrease

260.00 Protein Malnutrition   Serum, erythrocyte, and urinary copper levels showed decline in marasmic malnutrition and kwashiorkor. Marked fall of serum and erythrocyte copper level in children suffering from kwashiorkor. *1140*

Red Blood Cells   Increase

11.00 Pulmonary Tuberculosis   Characteristically elevated levels. *0239*

984.00 Toxic Effects of Lead and Its Compounds (including Fumes)   RBC concentration may increase with poisoning. *0618*

Copper, Nonceruloplasmin

Serum   Increase

275.10   Hepatolenticular Degeneration   Heterozygotes and treated homozygotes had nonceruloplasmin copper concentration ± 5.9 and 9.8 ± µg/dL, respectively) which did not differ significantly from normal (10.1 ± 1.6 µg/dL). Untreated patients had very significantly raised free copper concentration (22.9 ± 4.5 µg/dL). *1296*   There is a complete absence of ceruloplasmin in this condition, and copper is deposited in the liver, brain, and renal tubules. The copper-carrying protein present is abnormal. *0619*

Coproporphyrin

Urine   Increase

45.90   Acute Poliomyelitis   Possibly derived from nervous system. *0619*

70.00   Viral Hepatitis   *0619*

75.00   Infectious Mononucleosis   *0151*

277.11   Congenital Erythropoietic Porphyria (Günther's Disease)   Large amounts but less than the uroporphyrin. *2072*

277.14   Acute Intermittent Porphyria   Excessive amounts. *0995*

277.15   Porphyria Variegata   Characteristic finding in urine and feces. *1940*   Sharp rise in acute attacks. *0613*   During acute attacks. *2246   2538*

277.16   Porphyria Cutanea Tarda   Average in 66 patients was 560 µg/24h (normal < 200 µg/24h). *0611   2552*

277.17   Hereditary Coproporphyria   May occur during symptomatic periods but is usually normal during remission. *2552   2538   2246*

277.41   Dubin-Johnson Syndrome   Increases in the urinary excretion of coproporphyrin I have been found not only in patients with this syndrome but also in close relatives. *0962*   Mean excretion is 3-4 X that of normal subjects. *2561*   Total excretion is normal or slightly increased, but 84-90% in type I isomer, strikingly different from normal. *2246*

277.43   Rotor's Syndrome   Increases in the urinary excretion of coproporphyrin I have been found not only in patients with this syndrome but also in close relatives. *0962*   Marked increase in some patients. *2465*

280.90   Iron Deficiency Anemia   *0619*

282.00   Hereditary (Congenital) Spherocytosis   Increased hemopoiesis. *0619   0151*

283.00   Acquired Hemolytic Anemia (Autoimmune)   *0151*

289.00   Polycythemia, Secondary   Increased hemopoiesis. *0619*

303.90   Alcoholism   *0619 0151*

390.00   Rheumatic Fever   *0619*

570.00   Acute and Subacute Necrosis of Liver   In liver disease, coproporphyrinuria may not indicate increased formation of the pigment, but rather its diversion from bile to urine. *0151*

571.90   Cirrhosis of Liver   In liver disease, coproporphyrinuria may not indicate increased formation of the pigment, but rather its diversion from bile to urine. *0151*

984.00   Toxic Effects of Lead and Its Compounds (including Fumes)   A reliable sign of intoxication and is often demonstrable before basophilic stippling. *2468*   Increase in urine coproporphyrin III is associated with an increase in urine uroporphyrin and red cell protoporphyrin. *0619   0151 0889*

985.00   Toxic Effects of Non-medicinal Metals   Increased markedly in chronic arsenic poisoning. *0151*

Urine   Normal

277.12   Erythropoietic Protoporphyria   *1478*

277.13   Erythropoietic Coproporphyria   *0619*

277.41   Dubin-Johnson Syndrome   Total excretion is normal or slightly increased, but 84-90% in type I isomer, strikingly different from normal. *2246*

Bone Marrow   Increase

277.11   Congenital Erythropoietic Porphyria (Günther's Disease)   *2072*

Feces   Increase

277.11   Congenital Erythropoietic Porphyria (Günther's Disease)   Large amounts. *2073   2538 2246*

277.12   Erythropoietic Protoporphyria   At times. *2538*   In some carriers, elevated even with normal RBC porphyrins. Fluctuates markedly from one time period to another in the same patient. *0579   2246*

277.14   Acute Intermittent Porphyria   Slight to moderate increase. *2498*   Small increases may be found. *2246*

277.15   Porphyria Variegata   The most characteristic and consistent abnormality. *2254*   Ranges from 70 - > 1,000 µg/g dry weight (normal < 100 µg/g). *2552*   Large amounts. *0524*   Even when clinical manifestations are minimal. *0928*

277.16   Porphyria Cutanea Tarda   Large amounts. *0995*   Highly variable, but never as high as in variegata porphyria. *2314   2246*

277.17   Hereditary Coproporphyria   Between 100-3,000 µg/g dry weight (normal < 40). *2552*   Unremitting excretion of large amounts. *2538*   Striking abnormality, large excess of coproporphyrin III. *2246*

Feces   Normal

277.12   Erythropoietic Protoporphyria   *2538*

277.13   Erythropoietic Coproporphyria   *2538*

Liver   Increase

277.14   Acute Intermittent Porphyria   Has been isolated from hepatic tissue in some cases. *2072 2246*

Red Blood Cells   Increase

277.11   Congenital Erythropoietic Porphyria (Günther's Disease)   Elevated, but lower than uroporphyrins. *2246*   Variable. *2246 2072*

277.12   Erythropoietic Protoporphyria   *0619*

277.13   Erythropoietic Coproporphyria   Large amounts. *0619*

285.00   Sideroblastic Anemia   Conflicting reports from marked elevation to normal. *1326*

984.00   Toxic Effects of Lead and Its Compounds (including Fumes)   Free erythrocyte coproporphyrin ranges from 1-20 µg/dL (Normal = 0-2 µg/dL) in lead poisoning. *0151*

Red Blood Cells   Normal

277.14   Acute Intermittent Porphyria   *0995*

277.15   Porphyria Variegata   *0995 2246*

277.16   Porphyria Cutanea Tarda   *0995*

277.17   Hereditary Coproporphyria   No increase demonstrable. *2246 0868   0995*

277.41   Dubin-Johnson Syndrome   Total concentration is normal but the isomer percentages are reversed. Normally, coproporphyrin III constitutes 75%, while in homozygous patients it is over 80% of the total. *0180*

Corticosterone

Plasma   Decrease

255.40   Adrenal Cortical Hypofunction   Adrenal cortex destruction results in deficiency of glucocorticoids, androgens, and mineralocorticoids. *2612*

Plasma   Increase

194.00   Malignant Neoplasm of Adrenal Gland   In tumors of the zona glomerulosa or zona fasciculata. *0536*

Corticotropin

Plasma   Decrease

194.00   Malignant Neoplasm of Adrenal Gland   Very low or undetectable in Cushing's patients with adrenocortical tumors. *2612*

227.00   Benign Neoplasm of Adrenal Cortex   Very low or undetectable in Cushing's patients with adrenocortical tumor. *2612*

253.40   Anterior Pituitary Hypofunction   May be deficient and lead to secondary adrenocortical hypofunction. *2612   0995*

255.00   Adrenal Cortical Hyperfunction (Glucocorticoid Excess)   Very low or undetectable in Cushing's patients with primary adrenocortical tumor. *2612*

275.00   Hemochromatosis   9 of 15 patients had pituitary dysfunction. *2265*   A frequent complication. *2246*

Corticotropin *(continued)*

Plasma   Increase

157.90 Malignant Neoplasm of Pancreas   Uncommon. *1562*

193.01 Medullary Carcinoma of Thyroid   May occur. *0995*

255.00 Adrenal Cortical Hyperfunction (Glucocorticoid Excess)   Loss of the diurnal rhythm, with 6 P.M. levels abnormally raised in spite of increased cortisol concentration. Secondary disease (pituitary) *0619*

255.40 Adrenal Cortical Hypofunction   Results from the lack of cortisol-suppression feedback mechanism. *2612*

308.00 Stress   Excess secretion. *2113*

CSF   Increase

194.30 Malignant Neoplasm of Pituitary   21 of 22 patients with suprasellar extension of a pituitary tumor had elevations of one or more CSF adenohypophyseal hormones. *1189*

Cortisol

Plasma   Decrease

253.40 Anterior Pituitary Hypofunction   Low or low normal levels are suggestive but not diagnostic. *2612*

255.40 Adrenal Cortical Hypofunction   Markedly decreased (< 5 $\mu g/dL$) and fails to rise to more than twice this level 1 h after injection of ACTH. This is a reliable easy screening test to establish primary adrenocortical insufficiency. *2467*   Adrenal cortex destruction results in deficiency of glucocorticoids, androgens, and mineralocorticoids. *2612   0433*

359.21 Myotonia Atrophica   Abnormal diurnal variation with decreased 8 A.M. values in 4 of 7 patients. *1029*

493.10 Asthma (Intrinsic)   In 36 asthmatic children 8:00 A.M. plasma concentrations were compared with changes in their total eosinophil count (TEC) from 8:00 A.M. to 9:30 A.M. All children with low cortisol levels had decreases in TEC of $< 2\%$, whereas 78% of children with normal cortisol had decreases $> 15\%$. All children with decreases 15% had normal cortisol levels. *0232*

770.80 Respiratory Distress Syndrome   18 newborn infants of $<$ 37 weeks gestation who developed moderate to severe disease had a significantly lower mean cord plasma cortisol concentration at birth than that observed in 67 unaffected infants of similar gestational age; mean values were 3.36 ± 0.42 and 5.58 ± 0.43 $\mu g/dL$, respectively. *2307*

994.50 Exercise   Slight. *0763*

Plasma   Increase

194.00 Malignant Neoplasm of Adrenal Gland   Both 9 h and 23 h basal plasma concentrations are very high. *2612*   In tumors of the zona fasciculata. *0536*

227.00 Benign Neoplasm of Adrenal Cortex   Basal plasma concentrations may be normal or raised at 9 h and raised at 23 h. *2612*

250.10 Diabetic Acidosis   *2425*

255.00 Adrenal Cortical Hyperfunction (Glucocorticoid Excess)   Untreated patients almost always have concentrations in excess of 15 $\mu g/dL$ at all times. *0151*   All forms demonstrate some degree of autonomous secretion of excessive amounts of cortisol. *0999*   Increased due to adrenal hyperplasia and adrenal neoplasia. *1450*   Elevated night values or the lack of significant day-night variation is a consistent feature. *0978   2612*

255.10 Adrenal Cortical Hyperfunction (Mineralocorticoid Excess)   Untreated patients almost always have concentration in excess of 15 $\mu g/dL$ at all times. *0151*   All forms demonstrate some degree of autonomous secretion of excessive amounts of cortisol. *0999*   Increased due to adrenal hyperplasia and adrenal carcinoma. *1450*   Elevated night values or the lack of significant day-night variation is a consistent feature. *0978*

259.20 Carcinoid Syndrome   *0151*

278.00 Obesity   *0062*

303.00 Acute Alcoholic Intoxication   Increased following alcoholic binge of several days duration. *1594*

303.90 Alcoholism   Increased following alcoholic binge of several days duration. *1594*

308.00 Stress   Marked; in response to emotional stress. *2092*

410.90 Acute Myocardial Infarction   *1108*

584.00 Acute Renal Failure   Normal or slightly elevated. *0667*

585.00 Chronic Renal Failure   Normal or slightly elevated. *0667*

650.00 Pregnancy   Most plasma proteins decrease with the exception of alpha$_1$ globulins which account for elevation of protein-bound iodine and blood cortisol. *0433*

Plasma   Normal

244.90 Hypothyroidism   *2540*

493.10 Asthma (Intrinsic)   In 36 asthmatic children 8:00 A.M. plasma concentrations were compared with changes in their total eosinophil count (TEC) from 8:00 A.M. to 9:30 A.M. All children with low cortisol levels had decreases in TEC of $< 2\%$, whereas 78% of children with normal cortisol had decreases 15%. All children with decreases $> 15\%$ had normal cortisol levels. *0232*

994.50 Exercise   Usually normal in most people. *1363*

C-Reactive Protein

Serum   Increase

11.00 Pulmonary Tuberculosis   Increased inconsistently. *2467*

21.00 Tularemia   Elevated in proportion to the activity of the disease. *0433   1058*

38.00 Septicemia   Increased inconsistently. *2467*

174.90 Malignant Neoplasm of Breast   14 of 16 patients with overt metastases had elevated C-reactive proteins (> 10 mg/L). *0446*

201.90 Hodgkin's Disease   Increased during active stages; may be normal during remission. *2468*

212.70 Benign Neoplasm of Cardiovascular Tissue   May be increased in myxoma of left atrium. *2467*

320.90 Meningitis (Bacterial)   Markedly elevated. *1337*

390.00 Rheumatic Fever   Test is frequently positive and is not influenced by anemia, but is frequently positive with congestive heart failure of any cause. *1108*   Almost always positive in the early stages of untreated disease and the most sensitive indicator of activity. Remains positive in the presence of active carditis. *0962*

410.90 Acute Myocardial Infarction   Appear within 24-48 h, begin to fall by the 3rd day and become negative after 1-2 weeks. *2467*   Significant increase *1724*

446.50 Cranial Arteritis and Related Conditions   *0186*

482.90 Bacterial Pneumonia   Nonspecific indicator of acute infection. *0186*

590.10 Acute Pyelonephritis   Marked increase indicates an acute infection. *0186*

593.81 Renal Infarction   With large infarction. *0186*

710.00 Systemic Lupus Erythematosus   C-reactive proteins and other acute phase reactants are elevated and remain elevated to some degree during periods of apparent remission. *0999   0962*

714.00 Rheumatoid Arthritis   Increased inconsistently. *2467*   Nearly always abnormal and generally reflects the degree of disease activity. *2035*

714.30 Juvenile Rheumatoid Arthritis   In acute systemic form. *0136*

720.00 Rheumatoid (Ankylosing) Spondylitis   90% of cases. *0186*

730.00 Osteomyelitis   Indicates active disease. *0186*

785.40 Gangrene   Precedes the rise in ESR; with recovery disappearance precedes the return to normal of the ESR. Also disappears when inflammatory process is suppressed by steroids or salicylates. *2467*

Creatine

Serum   Increase

45.90 Acute Poliomyelitis   *0619*

204.00 Lymphocytic Leukemia (Acute)   Increased formation. *0619*

242.90 Hyperthyroidism   Excess T_4 or TSH stimulates creatinuria. *2104*

250.00 Diabetes Mellitus   Increased formation and decreased renal absorption. *0619*

253.00 Acromegaly   Accelerated rate of synthesis may result in high serum and urine concentrations. *2104*

255.00 Adrenal Cortical Hyperfunction (Glucocorticoid Excess)   Increased formation. *0619*

359.11 **Progressive Muscular Dystrophy** Decreased transport into muscle and leakage out of muscle occur in muscular dystrophies. *2246*

359.21 **Myotonia Atrophica** Decreased transport into muscle and leakage out of muscle occur in muscular dystrophies. *2246*

584.00 **Acute Renal Failure** High concentrations in blood and CSF have been associated with azotemia. *2104*

585.00 **Chronic Renal Failure** High concentrations in blood and CSF have been associated with azotemia. *2104*

710.00 **Systemic Lupus Erythematosus** Correlates well with severity of morphologic lesions. *1047*

714.00 **Rheumatoid Arthritis** *2467 0619*

791.30 **Myoglobinuria** Muscle destruction after crush injury. *0619*

Urine Decrease

244.90 **Hypothyroidism** *2467*

Urine Increase

38.00 **Septicemia** Increased breakdown of muscle. *2467*

45.90 **Acute Poliomyelitis** Increased formation; myopathy. *2467*

124.00 **Trichinosis** Constant finding. *0433*

197.70 **Secondary Malignant Neoplasm of Liver** Increased formation. *0619*

204.00 **Lymphocytic Leukemia (Acute)** Pronounced increase in children and adult males with acute leukemias. *2104* Extremely variable. *2453*

204.10 **Lymphocytic Leukemia (Chronic)** Increased breakdown. *2468*

205.00 **Myelocytic Leukemia (Acute)** Pronounced increase in children and adult males with acute leukemias. *2104* Extremely variable. *2453*

205.10 **Myelocytic Leukemia (Chronic)** Increased breakdown. *2467 2468*

242.90 **Hyperthyroidism** Increased excretion when the muscle mass is reduced, or is unable to take up creatine due to muscle catabolism. *0619*

250.00 **Diabetes Mellitus** Creatinuria occurs with gonadal dysfunction in males and females. *2104*

253.00 **Acromegaly** Accelerated rate of synthesis may result in high serum and urine concentrations. *2104*

255.00 **Adrenal Cortical Hyperfunction (Glucocorticoid Excess)** Increased formation. *2468*

256.30 **Ovarian Hypofunction** Creatinuria occurs with gonadal dysfunction in males and females. *2104*

257.20 **Testicular Hypofunction** Increased formation. *2467*

358.00 **Myasthenia Gravis** Increased formation; myopathy. *2467*

358.80 **Amyotonia Congenita** Increased formation; myopathy. *2467 0619*

359.11 **Progressive Muscular Dystrophy** Urine creatine is increased; urine creatinine is decreased. These changes are less marked in limb-girdle and fascioscapulohumeral types than in the Duchenne type. May occur irregularly. *2467* Decreased transport into muscle and leakage out of muscle occur in muscular dystrophies. *2246* Excessive concentrations appearing in urine are newly synthesized and do not originate from muscle cells. *2104*

359.21 **Myotonia Atrophica** Decreased transport into muscle and leakage out of muscle occur in muscular dystrophies. *2246*

359.22 **Myotonia Congenita** May be increased in some patients (Thomsen's disease). *2467*

650.00 **Pregnancy** It has been suggested that renal tubular reabsorption is depressed. *0619*

710.00 **Systemic Lupus Erythematosus** Increased breakdown. *2467*

710.40 **Dermatomyositis/Polymyositis** Urine shows a moderate increase in creatine and a decrease in creatinine. *2467*

791.30 **Myoglobinuria** *2467*

829.00 **Fracture of Bone** Increased breakdown. *2467*

929.00 **Crush Injury (Trauma)** Increased formation myopathy. *2467*

948.00 **Burns** Increased breakdown. *2467*

990.00 **Effects of X-Ray Irradiation** Due to tissue destruction. *1556*

CSF Increase

584.00 **Acute Renal Failure** High concentrations in blood and CSF have been associated with azotemia. *2104*

585.00 **Chronic Renal Failure** High concentrations in blood and CSF have been associated with azotemia. *2104*

Creatine Kinase

Serum Decrease

242.90 **Hyperthyroidism** Below normal but increased after treatment. *0573*

282.00 **Hereditary (Congenital) Spherocytosis** *2538*

650.00 **Pregnancy** Decreased during 8th-20th week (maximum at 12th week). *2468*

Serum Increase

2.00 **Typhoid Fever** Occurs in some patients. *2468*

37.00 **Tetanus** Levels were found to be elevated in 75 cases and related to the clinical severity of disease. Values higher than 2.97 mU/mL were found to be highly suggestive of disease. *2407 1643*

45.90 **Acute Poliomyelitis** Mild elevation was reported in 50% of 8 cases. *1677*

100.00 **Leptospirosis** Increased in 33% of patients during the 1st week. Differentiates the condition from hepatitis. *2468*

122.90 **Hydatidosis** With bone involvement. *1058*

124.00 **Trichinosis** Moderate to marked increase. *0503* Is observed as the consequence of muscular necrosis. *0433* During the acute stage. *0962*

153.90 **Malignant Neoplasm of Large Intestine** Highest activity of CK-BB in brain and smooth muscle. *1347*

162.90 **Malignant Neoplasm of Bronchus and Lung** Highest activity of CK-BB in brain and smooth muscle. *1347*

185.00 **Malignant Neoplasm of Prostate** *1347*

191.90 **Malignant Neoplasm of Brain** Highest activity of CK-BB in brain and smooth muscle. *1347* In necrotic glioma *0619*

244.90 **Hypothyroidism** Abnormally high serum levels found. *0619* Muscle involvement appears to be responsible for the elevation. *0503* Significantly higher than in normal controls in patients with primary hypothyroidism. *0573* Found in 66% of 15 patients. Values returned to normal after restoration of thyroid function. *0905* Slight increase. *0962* Often raised, but of no diagnostic value. *2612 0642*

245.10 **Subacute Thyroiditis** If hypothyroid. *0151*

250.10 **Diabetic Acidosis** Mild-moderate abnormalities may occur in 20-65% of patients but bears no relation to degree of abdominal pain or prognosis. *1316*

271.02 **McArdle's Disease** During myoglobinuric attacks. *0619* Increases dramatically within h after strenuous exercise. *0970 2246 0503*

276.80 **Hypokalemia** Patients with severe hypokalemia such as that occurring in hyperaldosteronism with muscle weakness may have elevated CK directly related to their hypokalemia. In other patients with hypokalemia, 10% may have increased CK but this is related to other disease processes. *0467*

286.01 **Hemophilia** Increases when bleeding occurs into the muscles. Serum activity returns to normal after 10 days following treatment with cryoprecipitate. The test is useful in distinguishing between hemorrhage into the psoas muscle (raised levels) and into the hip joint only (no increase). *0619*

286.10 **Christmas Disease** Increases when bleeding occurs into the muscles. Serum activity returns to normal after 10 days following treatment with cryoprecipitate. The test is useful in distinguishing between hemorrhage into the psoas muscle (raised levels) and into the hip joint only (no increase). *0619*

291.00 **Delirium Tremens** High elevations irrespective of associated hepatic disease and may arise in muscle. *0812 0503 1942 0962*

296.80 **Manic Depressive Disorder** Return towards normal following successful lithium therapy. *0619*

297.90 **Paranoid States and Other Psychoses** Increased in 24 of 37 acutely psychotic patients, some of whom had had repeated admissions. Activity was 20 X the upper limits of normal in some specimens. There were no increases in nonpsychotic psychiatric patients, but patients with toxic psychoses and with some acute brain diseases, such as brain trauma, had increased activity. *1569 0503*

Creatine Kinase *(continued)*

Serum Increase *(continued)*

303.00 Acute Alcoholic Intoxication *1942*

303.90 Alcoholism In 21 alcoholic patients, mean values were found to be elevated to 35.1 U/L (normal value = 7.0). *1803   0503*

304.90 Drug Dependence (Opium and Derivatives) Following intravenous adulterated heroin associated with myopathy and myoglobinuria. *0619* Concentrations up to 14,000 U/L were recorded in heroin addicts. *1929*

320.90 Meningitis (Bacterial) *0962*

323.92 Encephalomyelitis Enzyme studies may help suggest certain causes, (e.g., CK is elevated with myopathy, particularly in Coxsackie A infections and leptospirosis). *0433   0962*

331.81 Reye's Syndrome Especially muscle (CPK-MM) fraction. In severely affected children. *0435* Markedly abnormal *1887*

335.11 Familial Progressive Spinal Muscular Atrophy Elevations of CK and other serum enzymes are frequently encountered but never reach the magnitude seen in Duchenne muscular dystrophy. *0433*

345.90 Epilepsy Especially after status epilepticus. *0619* Increases in necrosis or acute atrophy of striated muscle in status epilepticus. *2467* In 50% of 10 patients hospitalized for this disorder. *0781*

359.11 Progressive Muscular Dystrophy Range of values up to 50 X normal upper limit with higher results in the younger patients. Abnormal results are accentuated if vasoconstriction is applied for 10 min before venesection. (Muscular atrophy of neurogenic origin shows no such increase in serum levels). *0619* Especially Duchenne type. The most sensitive reflection of certain types of muscular dystrophy. *0812 0503* Extremely high concentrations, particularly during the early and middle stages of the disease. In the late stage of the disease when the muscle mass has been severely reduced, may be only *0433 1677 1071 2418*

359.21 Myotonia Atrophica Slight to moderate increase. *0503* Increased in about 50% of the patients. *2467   0433*

359.22 Myotonia Congenita Slight to moderate increase. *0503*

410.90 Acute Myocardial Infarction Rises in 3 h reaching peak by 36 h (10-25 X normal), returning to normal by 4 days. Prolonged elevation indicates bad prognosis. *0619* Peak levels may be 50-100 X normal. *0812* The incidence of elevation is approximately equal to AST and LD, but is more specific. *0503* Increased in > 90% of patients when blood is drawn at appropriate time. *2467* Allows early diagnosis because increases appear within the appearance of CK-MB in the serum, the isoenzyme found only in the myocardium, is specific for myocardial damage. *0999   1264 2205*

415.10 Pulmonary Embolism and Infarction For reasons that are still unclear some cases may have high levels. *0812*

422.00 Acute Myocarditis Elevated cardiac enzymes may be the earliest evidence of myocarditis. *1108*

425.40 Cardiomyopathies Increased, often to extremely high levels; may rise even further after recovery from shock in cobalt beer cardiomyopathy. *2467*

434.00 Cerebral Thrombosis Increases in 50% of patients with extensive brain infarction. Maximum levels in 3 days; increase may not appear before 2 days; levels usually < in acute myocardial infarction and remain increased for longer time; return to normal within 14 days; high mortality associated with levels > 300 U/L. *2467* 15 of 21 patients with acute stroke had raised levels at some time during the 1st week after ictus. Values ranged from 28.3-710 U/L. *0603   0639 2560*

434.10 Cerebral Embolism Peak values occur at 48 h, falling in 3-4 days. Bad prognosis is indicated by an early rise, and by its magnitude. No increase is associated with brain stem infarction and angiomata. *0619*

434.90 Brain Infarction Peak values occur at 48 h, falling in 3-4 days. Bad prognosis is indicated by an early rise, and by its magnitude. No increase is associated with brain stem infarction or angiomata. *0619   0962*

444.90 Arterial Embolism and Thrombosis *2079 0992*

487.10 Influenza Higher in the acute stage than during the convalescence out of bed, while the controls showed higher activities when ambulant than during bed rest. *0784*

493.10 Asthma (Intrinsic) Increases correlated with severity of symptoms (subjective) and objective measurement of airway obstruction. *0318* High in 38% of acute untreated asthma patients. *1228*

518.40 Pulmonary Edema For reasons that are still unclear some cases may have high levels. *0812 0503*

577.00 Acute Pancreatitis Was found to indicate a more severe or prolonged course than in cases with normal levels, but to have little diagnostic value. *1942*

650.00 Pregnancy Increased during the last few weeks and remains elevated through parturition, becoming normal approximately 5 days postpartum. *0962*

710.00 Systemic Lupus Erythematosus May be found in patients with myositis. *0433*

710.10 Progressive Systemic Sclerosis Moderate to marked increase with associated myositis. *0503*

710.40 Dermatomyositis/Polymyositis Elevated at some time in nearly every patient. Most consistent of the serum enzymes and correlated best with clinical course and parameters of activity. *0244* Released as a result of destructive myopathy. *1791* Almost invariably elevated in the acute stages, whereas in the clinically inactive cases or in those in remission they are often normal. *2035   2219 0962*

780.30 Convulsions Raised levels have been reported following convulsive seizures. *0962*

785.40 Gangrene Found with extensive necrosis. Predominantly CPK-MM. *0186*

791.30 Myoglobinuria Increases in necrosis or acute atrophy of striated muscle. *2467*

929.00 Crush Injury (Trauma) Raised for approximately 15 days, especially if associated arterial obstruction. *0619* Increases in necrosis or acute atrophy of striated muscle. *2467* Most reliable measure of skeletal muscle damage. *0503   0812 0962*

948.00 Burns In 8 thermal burn patients there was a significant increase (P < 0.01). *0933*

986.00 Toxic Effects of Carbon Monoxide 11 of 13 cases of carbon monoxide poisoning showed elevation, often accompanied by aldolase and transaminase elevation as well. *0262*

989.50 Toxic Effects of Venom 14 of 17 patients admitted for wasp/bee stings showed elevated activities, indicating presence of damage to muscle fibers. *1822*

991.60 Hypothermia High concentrations have been found during a study of 25 patients with accidental hypothermia. Profound cellular damage, especially in cardiac and skeletal muscle, was recorded. *1472* In response to cold exposure. *2092*

992.00 Heat stroke Biochemical estimations in a fatal case of malignant hyperpyrexia showed very high serum CK, phosphate, and potassium. *0541   0542*

994.50 Exercise Extent of elevation depends upon severity of exercise and conditioning of patient. *1711* Maximum effect observed the following day. *0985   2076 2160 1930*

994.80 Effects of Electric Current Rose to abnormal levels in 5 of 8 patients, while the AST values showed no rise in patients undergoing D.C. countershock. *1103* Electrical cardiac defibrillation or countershock in 50% of patients; returns to normal in 48-72 h. *2467* Electrocautery used within the preceding days to the test may also produce elevated levels. *0812*

Serum Normal

70.00 Viral Hepatitis *0962*

275.10 Hepatolenticular Degeneration Normal. *2280*

281.00 Pernicious Anemia *2467*

282.00 Hereditary (Congenital) Spherocytosis *0962*

283.00 Acquired Hemolytic Anemia (Autoimmune) *0962*

333.40 Huntington's Chorea No abnormalities in 8 patients. *0534*

335.20 Amyotrophic Lateral Sclerosis *0962*

358.00 Myasthenia Gravis *2057*

413.90 Angina Pectoris *2467*

415.10 Pulmonary Embolism and Infarction The absence of elevated CK and the presence of increased LD in conjunction with other diagnostic techniques can be used to distinguish pulmonary from myocardial infarction. *2467   0437 0962*

420.00 Acute Pericarditis *2467*

441.00 Dissecting Aortic Aneurysm Unless complications occur. *2467*

446.50 Cranial Arteritis and Related Conditions *0186*

570.00 Acute and Subacute Necrosis of Liver *2467*

571.90 Cirrhosis of Liver *0962*

576.20 Extrahepatic Biliary Obstruction *0962*

593.81 Renal Infarction *0186*

Pleural Effusion   Increase

991.60   **Hypothermia**   Due to hypoxia, acid-base imbalance hypotension. *1471*

Creatinine

Serum   Decrease

275.10   **Hepatolenticular Degeneration**   Definitely elevated in 4 of 30 (13%) but decreased in 3 others. *2278*

642.40   **Pre-Eclampsia**   Low BUN (9 ± 2 mg/dL) and low creatinine (0.75 ± 0.2 mg/dL) in late pregnancy are indicative of toxemia. *0151*

642.60   **Eclampsia**   Low BUN (9 ± 2 mg/dL) and low creatinine (0.75 ± 0.2 mg/dL) in late pregnancy are indicative of toxemia. *0151*

650.00   **Pregnancy**   Slightly lower in the pregnant state than the nonpregnant state. *0433*   Decreases approximately 25%, especially during first 2 trimesters. Creatinine of 1.2 mg/dL is definitely abnormal in pregnancy although normal in nonpregnant women. *2468*   Level in pregnancy 0.46 mg ± 0.13 mg/dL compared to 0.67 mg ± 0.14 mg/dL for controls. *2179*   Decreased markedly throughout pregnancy *0517*

Serum   Increase

38.00   **Septicemia**   In 49% of 12 patients at initial hospitalization for this disorder. *0781*

53.00   **Herpes Zoster**   In 15% of 17 patients at initial hospitalization for this disorder. *0781*

73.90   **Psittacosis**   With severe renal involvement. *0433*

80.00   **Epidemic Typhus**   With varying degrees of renal involvement. *0433*

84.00   **Malaria**   In all patients, independent of the duration of the acute infection, levels were significantly raised. *2066*

100.00   **Leptospirosis**   Marked oliguria or anuria develops after the 1st week of disease and is attended by severe azotemia and electrolyte imbalance characteristic of lower nephron nephrosis. *2368*

135.00   **Sarcoidosis**   In 38% of 13 patients at initial hospitalization for this disorder. *0781*

153.90   **Malignant Neoplasm of Large Intestine**   In 34% of 63 patients at initial hospitalization for this disorder. *0781*

182.00   **Malignant Neoplasm of Corpus Uteri**   In 35% of 35 patients at initial hospitalization for this disorder. *0781*

185.00   **Malignant Neoplasm of Prostate**   In 59% of 59 patients at initial hospitalization for this disorder. *0781*

186.90   **Malignant Neoplasm of Testis**   In 53% of 13 patients at initial hospitalization for this disorder. *0781*

188.90   **Malignant Neoplasm of Bladder**   In 70% of 37 patients at initial hospitalization for this disorder. *0781*

201.90   **Hodgkin's Disease**   In 36% of 37 patients at initial hospitalization for this disorder. *0781*

202.80   **Non-Hodgkins Lymphoma**   In 42% of 47 patients at initial hospitalization for this disorder. *0781*

203.00   **Multiple Myeloma**   Not uncommon. *0433*   Ranged from 53.0-981 µmol/L in 35 patients. *0518*   In 68% of 28 patients at initial hospitalization for this disorder. *0781*

204.00   **Lymphocytic Leukemia (Acute)**   In 49% of 16 patients at initial hospitalization for this disorder. *0781*

204.10   **Lymphocytic Leukemia (Chronic)**   In 49% of 24 patients at initial hospitalization for this disorder. *0781*

205.00   **Myelocytic Leukemia (Acute)**   In 55% of 27 patients at initial hospitalization for this disorder. *0781*

205.10   **Myelocytic Leukemia (Chronic)**   In 83% of 13 patients at initial hospitalization for this disorder. *0781*

206.00   **Monocytic Leukemia**   In 49% of 22 patients at initial hospitalization for this disorder. *0781*

242.90   **Hyperthyroidism**   *0503*

250.00   **Diabetes Mellitus**   High levels may be the result of interference by the high levels of glucose and acetone present. *1003*   In 49% of 102 patients at initial hospitalization for this disorder. *0781*

252.00   **Hyperparathyroidism**   Mean concentration was 4.8 ± 1.8 mg/dL. *1475*   In 45% of 11 patients at initial hospitalization for this disorder. *0781*

253.00   **Acromegaly**   Increased rate of formation. *2467*

255.40   **Adrenal Cortical Hypofunction**   Dehydration and hypotension lead to prerenal impairment of renal function. *0433*

270.03   **Cystinosis**   Elevated with advanced renal disease as early as 2 y of age in some patients. *2246*

274.00   **Gout**   Rises with renal failure, but these changes may be subtle and slow. *0433*

275.10   **Hepatolenticular Degeneration**   Definitely elevated in 4 of 30 (13%) but decreased in 3 others. *2278*

276.50   **Dehydration**   Leading to reduced renal blood flow (prerenal azotemia). *2467*

277.30   **Amyloidosis**   Increased in > 50% of patients at time of diagnosis due to renal insufficiency. *1334*

279.12   **Wiskott-Aldrich Syndrome**   Increased incidence of renal failure. *0793*

283.00   **Acquired Hemolytic Anemia (Autoimmune)**   In 72% of 11 patients hospitalized for this disorder. *0781*

287.00   **Allergic Purpura**   Increase is mild and transitory. *0433*   Elevated in the presence of renal failure. *2538*

320.90   **Meningitis (Bacterial)**   Dehydration. *0995*

331.81   **Reye's Syndrome**   Markedly elevated reflecting renal injury. *0435*

335.20   **Amyotrophic Lateral Sclerosis**   Severe muscle disease. *0503*

359.21   **Myotonia Atrophica**   In severe muscle disease. *0503*

401.10   **Essential Benign Hypertension**   In 49% of 106 patients hospitalized for this disorder. *0781*

410.90   **Acute Myocardial Infarction**   9 of 22 patients showed elevations within 6 days of infarction. Initial and peak means were 0.101 ± 0.022 and 0.117 ± 0.025 µmol/L, respectively. *2530*   In 59% of 98 patients at initial hospitalization for this disorder. *0781*

413.90   **Angina Pectoris**   In 60% of 50 patients hospitalized for this disorder. *0781*

414.00   **Chronic Ischemic Heart Disease**   In 58% of 312 patients hospitalized for this disorder. *0781*

421.00   **Bacterial Endocarditis**   Elevated in patients with diffuse glomerulonephritis and chronic infective endocarditis. *0433*   Increase parallels BUN elevation; higher concentration found in fatal cases than in survivors. *1798*

428.00   **Congestive Heart Failure**   Diminished renal excretion. *0619*   Causes reduced blood flow leading to prerenal azotemia. *0619 2467*

440.00   **Arteriosclerosis**   In 64% of 36 patients hospitalized for this disorder. *0781*   May occur with kidney involvement. *0503*

444.90   **Arterial Embolism and Thrombosis**   In 50% of 21 patients hospitalized for this disorder. *0781*

446.00   **Polyarteritis-Nodosa**   With renal involvement. *0995*

446.20   **Goodpasture's Syndrome**   Progressive renal failure. *0062*

446.60   **Thrombotic Thrombocytopenic Purpura**   Renal function may be impaired. *0962*

558.90   **Diarrhea**   Leading to reduced renal blood flow (prerenal azotemia). *2467*

560.90   **Intestinal Obstruction**   With dehydration. *2199*

572.40   **Hepatic Failure**   High values (> 1.6 mg/dL) in 22 of 50 cases of hepatic failure due to decompensated cirrhosis or attacks of acute viral hepatitis. *0379*

577.00   **Acute Pancreatitis**   In 42% of 14 patients at initial hospitalization for this disorder. *0781*

580.00   **Acute Poststreptococcal Glomerulonephritis**   Mild renal failure with plasma values of 1.5-4.0 mg/dL is very common in the initial stages. *0151   0999*

580.05   **Glomerulonephritis (Membranoproliferative)**   BUN and creatinine rise as GFR decreases. *0962*

580.40   **Glomerulonephritis (Rapidly Progressive)**   Over 2.5 mg/dL at time of biopsy in all cases. *1633*   BUN and creatinine rise as GFR decreases. *0962*

581.90   **Nephrotic Syndrome**   In 48% of 24 patients at initial hospitalization for this disorder. *0781*

584.00   **Acute Renal Failure**   Characteristic. *1607*   In 99% of 12 patients at initial hospitalization for this disorder. *0781 0787*

585.00   **Chronic Renal Failure**   In late failure. *0151*   Appears to rise more slowly in the presence of renal disease than the BUN. It is less useful than the BUN to assess effectiveness of hemodialysis in the treatment of renal failure, since it does not decrease as rapidly as BUN. *0503*   In 97% of 144 patients at initial hospitalization for this disorder. *0781 0787*

590.00   **Chronic Pyelonephritis**   *2468*

Creatinine *(continued)*

Serum   Increase *(continued)*

590.10 Acute Pyelonephritis   In 48% of 16 patients at initial hospitalization for this disorder. *0781   2468*

591.00 Hydronephrosis   In 70% of 10 patients at initial hospitalization for this disorder. *0781*

597.80 Urethritis   Reveals the degree of renal impairment. *0433*

600.00 Benign Prostatic Hypertrophy   In 53% of 58 patients at initial hospitalization for this disorder. *0781*

642.40 Pre-Eclampsia   If the hypertension has reached relatively severe levels, may be elevated, indicating renal damage. *0433*

642.60 Eclampsia   If the hypertension has reached relatively severe levels, may be elevated, indicating renal damage. *0433*

710.00 Systemic Lupus Erythematosus   Serum creatinine and BUN were increased, indicating uremia. *1269*   Most reliable variable for estimation of renal involvement. *0782*

710.10 Progressive Systemic Sclerosis   Renal function may be impaired. *0962*

753.10 Polycystic Kidney Disease   Common. *0186*

780.80 Hyperhidrosis   Leading to reduced renal blood flow (prerenal azotemia). *2467*

785.50 Shock   Causes reduced renal blood flow leading to prerenal azotemia. *2467*

787.00 Vomiting   Leading to reduced renal blood flow (prerenal azotemia). *2467*

985.00 Toxic Effects of Non-medicinal Metals   Nephrotoxicity is common with therapeutic doses of arsenicals. *0811*

992.00 Heat stroke   Renal failure is a common complication. *0995*

1013.00 Diet   Ingestion of creatinine (roast meat). *2467*   The observation has been made that with substantial protein ingestion healthy young men have a urinary creatinine excretion in the range of 2.5-2.7 g/24h specimen but normal blood levels (0.6-1.2 mg/dL of serum). *2467 0503*

Serum   Normal

273.30 Waldenström's Macroglobulinemia   *0062*

994.50 Exercise   The observation has been made that after intensive exercise over extended periods the urinary creatinine excretion in healthy young men is in the range of 2.5-2.7 g/24h but normal blood levels (0.6-1.2 mg/dL of serum). *0503*   Observed effect with 12 min cycle-ergometer. *0804*

Urine   Decrease

242.90 Hyperthyroidism   With associated rise in urine creatine. *0619*

260.00 Protein Malnutrition   Decreased 24 hour urinary creatinine. *0186*

335.20 Amyotrophic Lateral Sclerosis   Roughly in proportion to loss of muscle mass. *0665*

359.11 Progressive Muscular Dystrophy   Urine creatine is increased; urine creatinine is decreased. These changes are less marked in limb-girdle and fascioscapulohumeral types than in the Duchenne type. *2467*   Reduced excretion in any myopathic or neurogenic condition which decreases muscle mass. *2246   0995*

359.21 Myotonia Atrophica   Reduced excretion in any myopathic or neurogenic condition which decreases muscle mass. *2246*

710.40 Dermatomyositis/Polymyositis   Active disease. As the urine creatine increases, so the urine creatinine falls. *0619*

Urine   Increase

244.90 Hypothyroidism   Occasionally increased. *0619*   Usually normal. *2540*

253.00 Acromegaly   *0619*

405.91 Renovascular Hypertension   Confirmatory evidence of greater water reabsorption as a cause of the decreased volume from the suspected kidney. *1108   0590*

994.50 Exercise   The observation has been made that after intensive exercise over extended periods the urinary creatinine excretion in healthy young men is in the range of 2.5-2.7 g/24h but normal blood levels (0.6-1.2 mg/dL of serum). *0503*

Urine   Normal

244.90 Hypothyroidism   Usually normal. *2540*

Creatinine Clearance

Urine   Decrease

120.00 Schistosomiasis   Significantly decreased in 35 children with hepatic bilharziasis. *0955*

203.00 Multiple Myeloma   Clearance ranged from 0.03-2.02 mL/s (2-121 mL/min) in 35 cases. 19 had rates > 0.83 mL/s. Mean clearance was significantly lower in the patients with Bence-Jones proteinuria. *0518*

252.00 Hyperparathyroidism   Strong negative correlation between creatinine clearance and serum calcium. *1492*

275.10 Hepatolenticular Degeneration   Reduced in 7 of 24 patients (29%). *2278*

276.50 Dehydration   Following overnight dehydration. *2114*

405.91 Renovascular Hypertension   Renal functional impairment. *0962*

428.00 Congestive Heart Failure   Diminished renal excretion with severe failure. *0619*

580.04 Glomerulonephritis (Membranous)   Progression of the disease is characterized by declining creatinine clearance. *0433*

584.00 Acute Renal Failure   *0619*

585.00 Chronic Renal Failure   Less than 20 mL/min. *1374*

590.00 Chronic Pyelonephritis   Decreased 24 h clearance. *2468*

590.10 Acute Pyelonephritis   Decreased 24 h clearance. *2468*

710.00 Systemic Lupus Erythematosus   Mean decrease in clearance of 18% was accompanied by a 14% inulin clearance fall, and correlated with the prostaglandin E levels. *1269*

753.10 Polycystic Kidney Disease   Diminished clearance with acidosis. *0433*

753.12 Medullary Cystic Disease   Diminished with acidosis. *0433*

994.50 Exercise   Decrease with heavy exercise. *1205*

Urine   Increase

650.00 Pregnancy   *2179*

948.00 Burns   Mean clearance in 20 burned patients, measured between the 4-35 postburn day, was 172.1 ± 48.4 mL/min/1.73 m^2. 13 patients had values > 2 S.D. above the normal. *1422*

994.50 Exercise   40% decrease with severe exercise. Mild, walking at 5.6 km/h produced 20% increase. *2092*   Slight but consistent increase. *2104*

1013.00 Diet   On high protein diet. *2104*

Cryofibrinogen

Serum   Increase

151.90 Malignant Neoplasm of Stomach   *2035 1551*

152.90 Malignant Neoplasm of Small Intestine   *2035 1551*

153.90 Malignant Neoplasm of Large Intestine   *2035 1551*

155.00 Malignant Neoplasm of Liver   *2035 1551*

155.10 Malignant Neoplasm of Intrahepatic Bile Ducts   *2035 1551*

157.90 Malignant Neoplasm of Pancreas   *2035 1551*

162.90 Malignant Neoplasm of Bronchus and Lung   *2035 1551*

183.00 Malignant Neoplasm of Ovary   *2035 1551*

185.00 Malignant Neoplasm of Prostate   *2035 1551*

188.90 Malignant Neoplasm of Bladder   *2035 1551*

189.00 Malignant Neoplasm of Kidney   *2035 1551*

199.00 Secondary Malignant Neoplasm (Disseminated)   *2035 1551*

201.90 Hodgkin's Disease   *2035 1551*

203.00 Multiple Myeloma   *2035 1551*

204.10 Lymphocytic Leukemia (Chronic)   *2035 1551*

244.90 Hypothyroidism   *2035 0856 1551 2046*

250.00 Diabetes Mellitus   *2035 0856 1551 2046*

273.30 Waldenström's Macroglobulinemia   *0186*

287.30 Idiopathic Thrombocytopenic Purpura   *2035 0856 1551 2046*

289.80 Myelofibrosis   *2035 1551*

320.90 Meningitis (Bacterial)   *2035 1138*

390.00 Rheumatic Fever   *2035 0856 1551*

410.90 Acute Myocardial Infarction   *2035 0856 1551 2046*

415.10 Pulmonary Embolism and Infarction Implicated as a cause of intravascular thrombosis, but their role is neither clear nor constant. *1108*

482.90 Bacterial Pneumonia *2035 1138*

533.90 Peptic Ulcer, Site Unspecified *2035 0856 1551 2046*

571.90 Cirrhosis of Liver *2035 0856 1551 2046*

642.40 Pre-Eclampsia Suggest that slow, chronic, intravascular clotting is taking place. *2538 2035 1549*

650.00 Pregnancy *0856*

710.00 Systemic Lupus Erythematosus *2035 1138 1551*

710.10 Progressive Systemic Sclerosis Small amounts. *1112 2035 0856 1551*

Cryoglobulins

Serum Increase

30.00 Leprosy Found in 95%. *2035*

104.10 Lyme Disease May be detected in Lyme Disease. *2639*

201.90 Hodgkin's Disease May be associated with cryoglobulinemia. *2468*

202.80 Non-Hodgkins Lymphoma May be associated with cryoglobulinemia. *2468*

203.00 Multiple Myeloma Associated cryoglobulinemia. *2468*

204.10 Lymphocytic Leukemia (Chronic) May be associated with cryoglobulinemia. *2468*

238.40 Polycythemia Vera Variable elevation of cryoglobulins. *2104*

273.30 Waldenström's Macroglobulinemia Demonstrated in the sera of 37% of the tested patients. *2538* Marked elevation of cryoglobulins. *2104*

283.00 Acquired Hemolytic Anemia (Autoimmune) Variable elevation of cryoglobulins. *2104*

414.00 Chronic Ischemic Heart Disease Variable elevation of cryoglobulins. *2104*

415.10 Pulmonary Embolism and Infarction Implicated as a cause of intravascular thrombosis, but their role is neither clear nor constant. *1108*

421.00 Bacterial Endocarditis Variable elevation of cryoglobulins. *2104*

446.00 Polyarteritis-Nodosa Cryoglobulinemia is rarely reported, but this may reflect late collection or improper handling of specimens. *2035* Variable elevation of cryoglobulins. *2104*

571.60 Biliary Cirrhosis Found in high concentration in 90% of patients (undetectable in controls). Composed of IgM (60%), IgG-IgM (25%), and IgA-IgM (5%). *2477*

694.40 Pemphigus When observed in patients with pemphigus have been shown to contain IgG, complement components, and other serum proteins. Appeared in the clinically active stage and disappeared subsequent to clinical improvement. *1612*

710.00 Systemic Lupus Erythematosus Increased cryoglobulins were found in patients with severe lesions and in no instance did it occur simultaneously with rheumatoid factor which was found in milder lesions. *1047* Found in 7-90% of patients in various studies; associated with disease activity especially nephritis. *0402* Variable elevations of cryoglobulins. *2104*

710.20 Sjögren's Syndrome Variable elevation of cryoglobulins. *2104*

714.00 Rheumatoid Arthritis Demonstrated occasionally but do not appear to have diagnostic significance. *0962* Variable elevation of cryoglobulins. *2104*

720.00 Rheumatoid (Ankylosing) Spondylitis Variable elevation of cryoglobulins. *2104*

785.40 Gangrene Marked elevation of cryoglobulins. *2104*

Cryomacroglobulins

Serum Increase

70.00 Viral Hepatitis *0863*

75.00 Infectious Mononucleosis *0863*

97.90 Syphilis *0863*

238.40 Polycythemia Vera *0863*

415.10 Pulmonary Embolism and Infarction Implicated as a cause of intravascular thrombosis, but their role is neither clear nor constant. *1108*

440.00 Arteriosclerosis *0863*

580.00 Acute Poststreptococcal Glomerulonephritis *0863*

710.20 Sjögren's Syndrome *0863*

Cyclic Adenosine Monophosphate

Plasma Decrease

304.90 Drug Dependence (Opium and Derivatives) Significantly decreased in heroin addiction. *1053*

Plasma Increase

584.00 Acute Renal Failure Elevated in uremia. *0968*

585.00 Chronic Renal Failure Elevated in uremia. *0968*

Urine Decrease

135.00 Sarcoidosis *0575*

170.90 Malignant Neoplasm of Bone *0575*

244.90 Hypothyroidism Lack of primary messenger necessary to activate adenyl cyclase system resulting in decreased levels. No hormonal effect noted. *2356*

300.40 Depressive Neurosis Lack of primary messenger necessary to activate adenyl cyclase system resulting in decreased levels. No hormonal effect noted. *2356*

Urine Increase

252.00 Hyperparathyroidism Parathyroid hormone action on the kidney leads to increased cAMP excretion. Mean urinary concentration was almost twice that of normals. *1492*

994.50 Exercise Modest increase in normal people. *0464*

994.80 Effects of Electric Current Mean change from 4.2 μmol/24h to 14.2 μmol/24h. *2520*

Urine Normal

252.00 Hyperparathyroidism In 21 patients, mean urinary excretion of cAMP/24h was 5.0 ± 1.9 μmol uncorrected. When correlated to albumin-corrected serum calcium, this overlap between hyperparathyroidism and normality disappears completely. Excretion is influenced to a considerable degree by the biological activity of circulating parathyroid hormone. *1475 1492*

275.35 Vitamin D Resistant Rickets Reported to be normal in untreated heterozygotes and homozygotes, with normal response to PTH infusion. *0853 2246*

CSF Increase

345.90 Epilepsy CSF concentration was measured in 62 neurological patients, 46 of whom were epileptics and 16 with CNS damage. In epileptic patients the CSF concentration was significantly elevated for 3 days after an attack when compared with those free from attacks for at least 2 weeks. *1660*

Lymphocytes Decrease

691.80 Atopic Eczema Individuals in the severe eczema group were shown to have a significant diminution in their unstimulated lymphocyte cAMP concentrations and absolute responses. *1770*

Cystathionine

Serum Increase

270.41 Cystathioninuria *0151*

Urine Increase

270.01 Cystinuria Has been reported. *0785 2246*

270.03 Cystinosis Nonspecific pattern of aminoaciduria. Fanconi's syndrome. *0995*

270.41 Cystathioninuria *0151 2246*

Cysteine

Urine Decrease

714.00 Rheumatoid Arthritis *2104*

Cysteine (continued)

Urine   Increase

270.03 **Cystinosis**   Nonspecific pattern of aminoaciduria. Fanconi's syndrome. *0995*

Cystine

Serum   Decrease

260.00 **Protein Malnutrition**   *0151*

Serum   Increase

585.00 **Chronic Renal Failure**   Children with renal failure showed a decrease in most amino acids but an increase in cystine and glycine. 14 of 31 children (45%) had cystine concentrations above the normal upper limit. *0192*

Urine   Increase

270.01 **Cystinuria**   Increased (20-30 X normal) with cystinuria. *2468*   Characteristic. *2246*

270.03 **Cystinosis**   Generally increased in the same proportion as other amino acids. *2246*   Nonspecific pattern of aminoaciduria. Fanconi's syndrome. *0995*

Dehydroepiandrosterone (DHEA)

Serum   Decrease

272.00 **Type IIA Hyperlipoproteinemia**   *0299 2356 2540*

272.10 **Type IV Hyperlipoproteinemia**   *0299 2356 2540*

272.21 **Type IIB Hyperlipoproteinemia**   *0299 2356 2540*

272.22 **Type III Hyperlipoproteinemia**   *0299 2356 2540*

272.31 **Type I Hyperlipoproteinemia**   *0299 2356 2540*

272.32 **Type V Hyperlipoproteinemia**   *0299 2356 2540*

297.90 **Paranoid States and Other Psychoses**   *0299 2356 2540*

696.10 **Psoriasis**   *0299 2356 2540*

Serum   Increase

194.00 **Malignant Neoplasm of Adrenal Gland**   Virilizing adrenal tumors. *0995*

256.41 **Stein-Leventhal Syndrome**   Plasma levels of androstenedione and dehydroepiandosterone are elevated. *0995*

Dehydroepiandrosterone Sulfate (DHEA-S)

Serum   Decrease

255.40 **Adrenal Cortical Hypofunction**   *0046 1692*

Serum   Increase

194.00 **Malignant Neoplasm of Adrenal Gland**   *0046 1692*

227.00 **Benign Neoplasm of Adrenal Cortex**   *0046 1692*

255.00 **Adrenal Cortical Hyperfunction (Glucocorticoid Excess)**   *0046 1692*

255.10 **Adrenal Cortical Hyperfunction (Mineralocorticoid Excess)**   *0046 1692*

256.41 **Stein-Leventhal Syndrome**   *0046 1692*

706.10 **Acne**   Elevated in 38% of 26 females with acne between ages 27 and 42 y. *2074*   Women with acne and hirsutism had increased levels compared to a group with acne only. *1020*

Dehydroisoandrosterone

Urine   Increase

194.00 **Malignant Neoplasm of Adrenal Gland**   *2467*

Deoxycholic Acid

Feces   Increase

153.90 **Malignant Neoplasm of Large Intestine**   The fecal excretion of cholesterol, coprostanol, coprostanone, total bile acids, deoxycholic acid, lithocholic acid was higher in colonic cancer and adenomatous polyps compared to normal controls as well as in patients with other digestive diseases. *1896*

211.40 **Benign Neoplasm of Rectum and Anus**   The fecal excretion was higher in patients with colon cancer and patients with adenomatous polyps compared to normal American and Japanese controls as well as patients with other digestive diseases. *1896*

Deoxycorticosterone

Plasma   Decrease

642.40 **Pre-Eclampsia**   Plasma concentrations averaged 10.2 ± 2.7 ng/dL, which is about half the value found in normal pregnant women. *2510   0387*

Plasma   Increase

650.00 **Pregnancy**   Plasma concentration is double the normal value in late pregnancy. *2510   0387*

Deoxycytidine

Urine   Increase

990.00 **Effects of X-Ray Irradiation**   Due to tissue destruction. *1556*

Dopa (3,4-Dihydroxyphenylalanine)

Serum   Increase

172.90 **Malignant Melanoma of Skin**   Significantly increased (P < 0.001) in plasma of all 65 patients with active disease (stage II), 2.08 µg/L compared with 32 normal control values of 1.23 µg/L. *0696*

192.50 **Neuroblastoma**   Increased production by neuroblastoma cell system. *1630*

Urine   Increase

192.50 **Neuroblastoma**   Elevated levels receded toward normal after treatment. *1511*

197.70 **Secondary Malignant Neoplasm of Liver**   Found to be elevated in the urine of patients with metastatic disease. Excretion appears to be proportional to the tumor burden. *1511*

199.00 **Secondary Malignant Neoplasm (Disseminated)**   Found to be elevated in the urine of patients with metastatic disease. Excretion appears to be proportional to the tumor burden. *1511*

Dopamine

Serum   Increase

192.50 **Neuroblastoma**   Excess secretion in some tumors. *2612*

Urine   Increase

192.50 **Neuroblastoma**   Elevated levels receded toward normal after treatment. *1511*

Dopamine Hydroxylase

Serum   Decrease

277.22 **Lesch-Nyhan Syndrome**   Decreased although norepinephrine is normal. *1300*

572.20 **Hepatic Encephalopathy**   A decrease in H3-dopamine uptake was demonstrated in the blood platelets of 22 hepatic encephalopathy patients when compared to that of patients with liver cirrhosis but without hepatic encephalopathy, and controls. There was a direct correlation between the stage of hepatic encephalopathy and the decrease in H3-dopamine uptake. *1627*

758.00 Down's Syndrome Present in abnormally low plasma concentrations although norepinephrine is not reduced. *1300*

Serum Increase

227.91 Pheochromocytoma In pediatric cases, venous catheterization showed a great increase in catecholamine efflux from the left adrenal vein, while dopamine-beta-hydroxylase (DBH) was only slightly elevated. Circulating catecholamines fluctuated greatly during removal of tumors, but DBH decreased gradually. *1021*

333.40 Huntington's Chorea *1395*

715.90 Osteoarthritis 2 X normal value. *2037*

Serum Normal

994.50 Exercise No effect observed. *2520*

994.80 Effects of Electric Current *2520*

Synovial Fluid Increase

715.90 Osteoarthritis 3 X normal value. *2037*

Endorphin, Beta

Plasma Increase

278.00 Obesity Baseline concentrations were two times higher than in nonobese adolescents and children. *0824*

CSF Decrease

346.00 Migraine Closely correlated with severity of disease. Decreased significantly in patients with common migraine (38.5 fmol/mL) compared with healthy controls (86.1 fmol/mL). *0825*

CSF Normal

331.00 Alzheimer's Disease No difference from controls. *1881*

Eosinophils

Blood Decrease

2.00 Typhoid Fever *0151*

80.00 Epidemic Typhus Absent or rare in the early stages. *2368*

84.00 Malaria During acute infections. *0433*

250.10 Diabetic Acidosis Often a polymorphonucleocytosis with a lymphopenia and eosinopenia. *0962*

255.00 Adrenal Cortical Hyperfunction (Glucocorticoid Excess) Eosinopenia is frequent (usually < 100/μL). *2468* Patients with hypercortisolism often have neutrophilia, lymphopenia, and eosinophilia. *0962* Below 100/μL in 90% of cases. *0995* *0433*

275.34 Familial Periodic Paralysis Occasionally during attacks. *2246*

308.00 Stress A drop in eosinophils with increased corticoid and epinephrine production are manifestations of stress. *2113*

694.40 Pemphigus In severely ill patients the percentage, even if previously high, drops off - often to 0%. *0743*

785.50 Shock *2467*

Blood Increase

6.00 Amebiasis *2538*

34.10 Scarlet Fever *0779*

84.00 Malaria Depressed during acute infections but may become elevated during convalescence. *0433* *2538*

114.90 Coccidioidomycosis Occasional eosinophilia during either the primary or the disseminated stages. *0433* In the initial infection. *2368*

117.30 Aspergillosis Mean percentage was 16.2, ranging from 8-29% in 20 cases of allergic bronchopulmonary aspergillosis. *1983*

120.00 Schistosomiasis Eosinophilia occurs and may be 20-60%. *2468* In 64 patients (22%) showed eosinophil counts > 1,000/μL. *2028* Tends to decrease with chronicity. *2199*

122.90 Hydatidosis Occurs in parasitic infestation especially with tissue invasion. *2467* *0433*

123.40 Diphyllobothriasis (Intestinal) May be a mild eosinophilia, between 5-10%. *2199*

124.00 Trichinosis May reach 8,000/μL and persists for several weeks. In fatal cases, it is the only sign of disease. *0433* The most constant finding and one of significance early in the course of disease. Generally appears before the end of the 2nd week. *0992* Characteristic. *2508* Marked; ranging from 15-50% of the total WBC. Highest during the active stage of the disease. *0962* *2199*

126.90 Ancylostomiasis (Hookworm Infestation) Very characteristic. *0433* Generally an eosinophilia of 7-15%, and it may exceed 50% in severe cases. *2199* Common in hookworm anemia. *1924* *2538*

127.00 Ascariasis May occur, but this finding is more characteristic of hookworm infection and strongyloidiasis. *0433* Increased during symptomatic phase, especially pulmonary phase. *2468* May be a mild eosinophilia ranging between 5-10%. *1105* *2199* *0151* *2538*

127.20 Strongyloidiasis 10% eosinophilia is usual and counts of 50% or even higher are occasionally found. *0433* Increase is almost always present, but the number usually decreased with chronicity. *2468* Typically, an eosinophilia between 8-10% and in very severe infections, up to 50%. *2199* *2538*

127.30 Trichuriasis May be > 25%. *2468* *0433*

128.00 Larva Migrans (Visceralis) Highest level of eosinophilia has been described due to Toxocara canis or catis infection in children. *2035* Severe eosinophilia, splenomegaly, and lymphadenopathy in several members of the same family were infected from a common environmental source. *0585* Characteristic feature. *2368* *2538*

130.00 Toxoplasmosis *2538*

135.00 Sarcoidosis Occurs in 15% of patients. *2468* In 44% of 25 patients at initial hospitalization for this disorder. *0781* *2538*

170.90 Malignant Neoplasm of Bone Increases in tumors involving the bone. *2467*

172.90 Malignant Melanoma of Skin *2538*

183.00 Malignant Neoplasm of Ovary *2467*

186.90 Malignant Neoplasm of Testis In 46% of 27 patients at initial hospitalization for this disorder. *0781*

191.90 Malignant Neoplasm of Brain In 41% of 23 patients at initial hospitalization for this disorder. *0781*

199.00 Secondary Malignant Neoplasm (Disseminated) *2538*

201.90 Hodgkin's Disease Occasionally seen. *0433* Eosinophilia, usually < 10%, may be seen in 10-20% of cases. *0999* Tends to occur in patients with severe and longstanding pruritus. *0151* A striking eosinophilia is the outstanding characteristic. *1484* In 29% of 77 patients at initial hospitalization for this disorder. *0781* *0532* *2538*

202.10 Mycosis Fungoides Eosinophilia. *2539*

205.00 Myelocytic Leukemia (Acute) Occasionally. *0992*

205.10 Myelocytic Leukemia (Chronic) Increased in percentage, which means a striking absolute increase. *0151* Characteristic shift toward immaturity of the granulocytes and the increase in eosinophils and basophils. *0151* Often regarded as a poor prognostic sign. *2538* Absolute increase in almost all cases. *2552* *0992*

238.40 Polycythemia Vera Sometimes eosinophilia. *0433*

240.00 Simple Goiter In 50% of 19 patients at initial hospitalization for this disorder. *0781*

242.90 Hyperthyroidism Often occurs. *2540*

253.40 Anterior Pituitary Hypofunction With reduced adrenal cortical or pituitary function eosinophilia may be seen. *0433*

255.40 Adrenal Cortical Hypofunction A total count of 50/μL is evidence against severe adrenocortical hypofunction. *2468* With reduced adrenal cortical or pituitary function. *0433* May be a relative lymphocytosis and moderate eosinophilia. *0962*

273.23 Heavy Chain Disease (Gamma) Eosinophilia sometimes marked with relative lymphocytosis. *2468* Often associated with mild to marked leukopenia and eosinophilia. *2538*

273.30 Waldenström's Macroglobulinemia *2035* *0128*

279.20 Severe Combined Immunodeficiency Commonly elevated. *2539*

281.00 Pernicious Anemia Occurs in some hematopoietic diseases. *2467*

287.00 Allergic Purpura May be a polymorphonuclear leukocytosis and an increase in eosinophils. *2538* Slight leukocytosis and occasional eosinophilia may be seen. *0962* *2552*

287.30 Idiopathic Thrombocytopenic Purpura Originally thought to be common, has not been a constant finding. *1538* Described in many patients, but has not been confirmed as a prognostic indicator. *2552* *2538*

Eosinophils *(continued)*

Blood   Increase *(continued)*

288.00 Agranulocytosis   May occur. *0992*

289.80 Myelofibrosis   Eosinophils and basophils may be increased in agnogenic myeloid metaplasia. *2468*   Eosinophilia and basophilia occur in 10-30% of myelofibrosis patients. *2317 0532*

304.90 Drug Dependence (Opium and Derivatives)   Eosinophilia occurs in 25% of drug addicts. *2468*

381.00 Otitis Media   In 48% of 70 patients hospitalized for this disorder. *0781*

421.91 Loeffler's Endocarditis   Eosinophilia up to 70%; may be absent at first but appears sooner or later. *2467*   Marked eosinophilia of the blood associated with diffuse organ infiltration by eosinophils. *1108 2538*

422.00 Acute Myocarditis   Characteristic of helminthic myocarditis. *1108*

425.40 Cardiomyopathies   Mild to moderate eosinophilia. Marked in Loeffler's eosinophilic cardiomyopathy. *1108 2227*

431.00 Cerebral Hemorrhage   In 45% of 13 patients hospitalized for this disorder. *0781*

446.00 Polyarteritis-Nodosa   Hallmark of patients with allergic granulomatosis and angiitis is eosinophilia > 400/µL, and usually > 1,500/µL. This degree of eosinophilia is rarely seen in patients with polyarteritis in whom the lungs are spared. *0642*   Eosinophilia is almost exclusively related to the variants of necrotizing angiitis with pulmonary involvement, it is uncommonly seen in classical polyarteritis. *0962   0999 0532 2538*

446.60 Thrombotic Thrombocytopenic Purpura   WBC generally normal or slightly increased, often with a relative lymphocytosis and eosinophilia. *2035*

451.90 Phlebitis and Thrombophlebitis   In 40% of 49 patients at initial hospitalization for this disorder. *0781*

477.90 Hay Fever   May occur during the season, but its presence or absence has little diagnostic value, since it is variable. *0433*   Characterized by a mild, persistent eosinophilia despite rather profound tissue involvement. *2538*

480.90 Viral Pneumonia   In 32% of 15 patients at initial hospitalization for this disorder. *0781*

482.90 Bacterial Pneumonia   *2538*

483.01 Mycoplasma Pneumoniae   May be observed. *0063*

491.00 Chronic Bronchitis   Increased if there is allergic basis or component. *2467*   In 36% of 24 patients at initial hospitalization for this disorder. *0781*

493.10 Asthma (Intrinsic)   Tended to increase after bronchial provocation test but the increase did not correlate with the occurrence of the immediate type bronchial provocation test reaction. *1088*   In more than 60% of patients tested. *0405*   In 52 patients with active bronchial asthma (not on steroid therapy), total eosinophil counts were > 350/µL. Counts showed inverse correlation (R = -0.74) with specific airway conductance. *1072*   In 55% of 122 patients at initial hospitalization for this disorder. *0781 2538*

495.90 Allergic Alveolitis   Eosinophilia is exceptional. *0433*   Eosinophilia up to 45%. *2467*

496.00 Chronic Obstructive Lung Disease   In 37% of 79 patients at initial hospitalization for this disorder. *0781*

516.10 Idiopathic Pulmonary Hemosiderosis   In up to 20% of patients. *2467*   Eosinophilia of moderate degree occurs in about 12% of the cases. *2538*

518.00 Pulmonary Collapse   *0433*

535.00 Gastritis   Peripheral eosinophilia in eosinophilic gastritis. *2199*

555.90 Regional Enteritis or Ileitis   *2538*

556.00 Ulcerative Colitis   *2538*

579.01 Protein-Losing Enteropathy   Occasional eosinophilia. *2467*

580.00 Acute Poststreptococcal Glomerulonephritis   Occasionally. *2538*

581.90 Nephrotic Syndrome   In 42% of 26 patients at initial hospitalization for this disorder. *0781*

584.00 Acute Renal Failure   In 32% of 12 patients at initial hospitalization for this disorder. *0781*

601.00 Prostatitis   In 45% of 13 patients at initial hospitalization for this disorder. *0781*

691.80 Atopic Eczema   *2538*

694.00 Dermatitis Herpetiformis   Occurs in some skin diseases. *2467*   In 36% of 11 patients at initial hospitalization for this disorder. *0781   0532 2538*

694.40 Pemphigus   Slight or absent eosinophilia in pemphigus foliaceous. *0743*   Moderately increased percentage in pemphigus vulgaris. *0743   0532 2538*

695.10 Erythema Multiforme   Occurs in some infectious diseases. *2467   0532*

696.10 Psoriasis   *2538*

708.90 Urticaria   Characterized by a mild, persistent eosinophilia despite rather profound tissue involvement. *2538*   In 34% of 28 patients at initial hospitalization for this disorder. *0781*

710.10 Progressive Systemic Sclerosis   Early in the disease, the blood count is normal save for rare eosinophilia. *1700*   Eosinophilia has been observed but is uncommon. *0962*

710.20 Sjögren's Syndrome   Occurs in about 25% of the patients. *2134*

710.40 Dermatomyositis/Polymyositis   Frequently increased. *2467*

714.00 Rheumatoid Arthritis   Eosinophilia has been reported in patients with pleural or pulmonary manifestations. *0962*

984.00 Toxic Effects of Lead and Its Compounds (including Fumes)   Increases in poisoning. *2467*

985.00 Toxic Effects of Non-medicinal Metals   Usually 10-20% in arsenic poisoning. *0977   0811*

989.50 Toxic Effects of Venom   Increases in poisoning (e.g., phosphate, black widow spider bite). *2467*

990.00 Effects of X-Ray Irradiation   After repeated irradiation. *0134*

Blood   Normal

202.52 Histiocytosis X   No associated eosinophilia. *2552*

289.00 Polycythemia, Secondary   *0995*

Pleural Effusion   Increase

480.90 Viral Pneumonia   Eosinophilia greater than 10% may be present. *0062*

482.90 Bacterial Pneumonia   Eosinophilia greater than 10% may be present. *0062*

577.00 Acute Pancreatitis   Eosinophilia greater than 10% may be present. *0062*

577.10 Chronic Pancreatitis   Eosinophilia greater than 10% may be present. *0062*

Ascitic Fluid   Increase

567.90 Peritonitis   Ascites associated with eosinophilic enteritis and peritonitis has a high eosinophil count. *2199*

Bone Marrow   Increase

205.10 Myelocytic Leukemia (Chronic)   Particularly in the stage preceding acute blastic crisis. *0433*   May be considerably increased; usually in proportion to their number in the circulating blood. *2538*

238.40 Polycythemia Vera   An unusually high number may be found. *2552*

273.23 Heavy Chain Disease (Gamma)   Bone marrow aspirations and lymph node biopsies have demonstrated a proliferation of plasmacytic and lymphocytic forms, along with eosinophils and large reticulum or reticuloendothelial cells, (the pattern of a pleomorphic reticular neoplasm). *2035*   Bone marrow may be normal, but usually there is an increased proportion of plasma cells or lymphocytes or both, often accompanied by eosinophilia. *2538*

446.60 Thrombotic Thrombocytopenic Purpura   Increased numbers of young megakaryocytes and often an increase in eosinophils. *1456   2035*

733.00 Osteoporosis   The iliac bone marrow specimens showed infiltrates consisting of elongated mast cells, eosinophils, plasma cells, and varying numbers of lymphocytes. *2334*

Liver   Increase

201.90 Hodgkin's Disease   Eosinophilic predominance occurs mainly in the fibrotic types of Hodgkin's disease. The survival time of patients with eosinophilic predominance was significantly shorter than that of the controls. *2369*

Sputum   Increase

127.00 Ascariasis   *0151*

491.00 Chronic Bronchitis More than 3% eosinophils indicates an allergic state. *0433* *1718*

492.80 Pulmonary Emphysema *1718*

493.10 Asthma (Intrinsic) Stained sputum is usually found to contain eosinophils; pointed elongated crystals derived from eosinophilic granules (Charcot-Leyden crystals) and spiral mucocellular bronchial casts (Curschmann's spirals) are also found. *0999* Often found; although suggestive of asthma in both allergic and infective types, they are not pathognomonic. *2035* *1718*

Epinephrine

Plasma Decrease

410.90 Acute Myocardial Infarction Significantly reduced the first few days. *1289*

Plasma Increase

38.00 Septicemia In patients with septicemic, traumatic or hemorrhagic shock, plasma epinephrine and norepinephrine concentrations were increased above the normal range. *0164*

250.10 Diabetic Acidosis *2425*

260.00 Protein Malnutrition Marasmic and normal weight infants excreted proportionally 3-4 X less epinephrine than norepinephrine (ratio: 0.20-0.38). Children with kwashiorkor excreted nearly similar amounts of epinephrine and norepinephrine (ratio: 0.88). In marasmus, norepinephrine may predominate and in kwashiorkor epinephrine may predominate, in the regulation of the metabolic adaptations to assure survival. *1877*

308.00 Stress A drop in eosinophils with increased corticoid and epinephrine production are manifestations of stress. *2113*

401.10 Essential Benign Hypertension *0765*

410.90 Acute Myocardial Infarction Correlates with fasting plasma free fatty acids, which are associated with increased incidence of serious arrhythmias after infarctions. *0937* Evidence for a sympathoadrenal response is found in the increased blood and urinary concentration of norepinephrine, epinephrine, or their metabolic products. *1108* *1163* *1451*

431.00 Cerebral Hemorrhage Plasma concentrations were 0.65 ± 0.11 ng/mL in subarachnoid hemorrhage patients. *0163*

577.00 Acute Pancreatitis Increased circulating epinephrine. *0619*

585.00 Chronic Renal Failure Moderate increase. *0649*

785.50 Shock In patients with septicemic, traumatic or hemorrhagic shock. Plasma epinephrine and noradrenaline concentrations were increased above the normal range. *0164*

929.00 Crush Injury (Trauma) *0995*

948.00 Burns A drop in eosinophils with increased corticoid and epinephrine production are manifestations of stress. *2113*

994.50 Exercise Significant effect after physical stress. *0768*

Urine Increase

227.91 Pheochromocytoma In almost all patients, analysis of any 24 h urine collection will reveal increased excretion. *0151* *0962*

308.00 Stress With physical or emotional stress. *2092* Urinary excretion of epinephrine and its metabolites are rough indicators of degree of stress. *2113*

390.00 Rheumatic Fever Epinephrine and norepinephrine increase in proportion to the severity of circulatory failure. Catecholamine excretion, especially norepinephrine, is significantly raised in grades 3 and 4 of hemodynamic disturbance. *2572*

410.90 Acute Myocardial Infarction Evidence for a sympathoadrenal response is found in the increased blood and urinary concentration of norepinephrine, epinephrine, or their metabolic products. *1108* In patients developing heart failure or cardiogenic shock, the urinary level of both free catecholamines rose notably in the 1st week after infarction. in uncomplicated cases, a moderate rise in the norepinephrine level in the 1st week was associated with only a transient rise in the epinephrine level. *1163* *1451*

414.00 Chronic Ischemic Heart Disease Increased in proportion to the severity of circulatory failure. Catecholamine excretion is significantly raised in grades 3 and 4 of hemodynamic disturbance. *2572*

415.00 Cor Pulmonale Increased in proportion to the severity of circulatory failure. Catecholamine excretion is significantly raised in grades 3 and 4 of hemodynamic disturbance. *2572*

948.00 Burns With physical or emotional stress. *2092* Urinary excretion of epinephrine and its metabolites are rough indicators of degree of stress. *2113*

994.50 Exercise If strenuous may be increased 10-fold. *0161*

Urine Normal

991.60 Hypothermia With cold exposure. *2092*

Erythrocyte Casts

Urine Increase

38.00 Septicemia Transient slight increase. *2468*

72.00 Mumps Suggests a diagnosis of mumps nephritis. *0433*

287.00 Allergic Purpura Indicate active glomerulitis. *0962* Common but often transient. *2552* *2538*

421.00 Bacterial Endocarditis Found in 12% of patients. *1798* Casts are seen in the occasional patient with diffuse glomerulonephritis. *0433*

446.00 Polyarteritis-Nodosa *0962*

580.00 Acute Poststreptococcal Glomerulonephritis Microscopic examination reveals numerous red blood cells and variable numbers of casts. Indicate bleeding from the glomerulus. *0151* *0999*

580.40 Glomerulonephritis (Rapidly Progressive) *2468*

584.00 Acute Renal Failure Associated with active glomerulonephritis. *0433*

592.10 Ureter Calculus The urinalysis often shows no significant alteration from normal but may progress through the stages of mild pyuria to moderate pyuria with albuminuria and onto frank infection or passage of renal casts. *0433*

710.00 Systemic Lupus Erythematosus In lupus glomerulonephritis it is not unusual to find a sediment in which all the formed elements and casts seen in various stages. *0962*

710.10 Progressive Systemic Sclerosis Appears during renal failure. *0433*

Urine Absent

599.00 Urinary Tract Infection A variable number of RBCs may be present, but there are no RBC casts. *0962*

Urine Normal

592.10 Ureter Calculus The urinalysis often shows no significant alteration from normal. *0433*

Erythrocytes

Blood Decrease

18.00 Disseminated Tuberculosis Pancytopenia is a common feature. *2538*

84.00 Malaria Anemia with an average 2.5 million/µL is usually hypochromic; may be macrocytic in severe chronic cases. *2468* Pancytopenia is a common feature. *2538* *0151*

126.90 Ancylostomiasis (Hookworm Infestation) May be reduced. *2368*

127.30 Trichuriasis In children can be accompanied by a microcytic hypochromic anemia. *0433*

130.00 Toxoplasmosis Anemia is present. *2468*

135.00 Sarcoidosis Pancytopenia is a common feature. *2538*

198.50 Secondary Malignant Neoplasm of Bone Depression of all formed elements of the blood is often seen in disseminated neoplastic disease. *0999*

201.90 Hodgkin's Disease Pancytopenia is a common feature. *2538*

202.40 Leukemic Reticuloendotheliosis Pancytopenia was found in almost 50% of all patients (102). *2390*

203.00 Multiple Myeloma Overgrowth of plasma cells may produce pancytopenia, or may evoke a leukoerythroblastic reaction. *2538*

204.10 Lymphocytic Leukemia (Chronic) Reduced production plus shortened survival. *2538*

272.72 Gaucher's Disease Pancytopenia is a common feature. *2538*

272.73 Niemann-Pick Disease Pancytopenia is a common feature. *2538*

Erythrocytes *(continued)*

Blood Decrease *(continued)*

280.90 Iron Deficiency Anemia *2467*

281.20 Folic Acid Deficiency Anemia Pancytopenia is a common feature in vitamin B_{12} and folic acid deficiency. *2538* Depressed to a greater degree than other parameters. *0962*

281.30 Vitamin B_6 Deficiency Anemia Reported to be low in about 80% of patients. *0433*

282.00 Hereditary (Congenital) Spherocytosis Anemia may be absent, moderate or severe. The RBC is reduced proportionately to the hemoglobin concentration. *0433* Reductions in RBC may not be proportional to hemoglobin. *2552*

282.41 Thalassemia Major With the more severe expression of the disease, homozygote or heterozygote, all parameters of erythrocyte numbers are depressed. *0962* Count is often between 2-3 million/μL, with great variation in size and shape of cells. *2552*

282.42 Thalassemia Minor With the more severe expression of the disease, homozygote or heterozygote, all parameters of erythrocyte numbers are depressed. *0962*

282.60 Sickle Cell Anemia Usually between 2.0-3.5 million/μL. *2538 0999*

283.21 Paroxysmal Nocturnal Hemoglobinuria Pancytopenia is a common feature. *2538*

284.90 Aplastic Anemia RBC and all cellular elements are decreased. *0151* Peripheral pancytopenia associated with hypocellular bone marrow. *0415* Invariable finding. *2538*

285.00 Sideroblastic Anemia Reported to be low in about 80% of patients. *0433*

287.00 Allergic Purpura The RBC is generally within normal limits except if severe gastrointestinal blood loss has occurred. *0433*

289.40 Hypersplenism Pancytopenia is a common feature. *2538* As much as 38% may be trapped in the enlarged spleen. *1824*

289.80 Myelofibrosis Pancytopenia is a common feature. *2538*

571.90 Cirrhosis of Liver Anemia reflects increased plasma volume and some increased destruction of RBCs. If more severe, rule out hemorrhage in gastrointestinal tract, folic acid deficiency, excessive hemolysis, etc. *2467*

579.90 Malabsorption, Cause Unspecified *0151*

585.00 Chronic Renal Failure In chronic renal insufficiency, anemia is commonly caused by a relative or absolute deficiency of red cell production. *1669*

650.00 Pregnancy Decreased < 10-15% because of increased plasma volume during pregnancy. *2468*

756.52 Osteopetrosis Anemia and pancytopenia. *2468*

773.00 Hemolytic Disease of Newborn (Erythroblastosis Fetalis) Generally parallels the fall of hemoglobin. *2061*

785.50 Shock Hemoconcentration (dehydration, burns) or hemodilution (hemorrhage, crush injuries, and skeletal trauma) takes place. *2467* Disturbed RBC 2,3-DPG metabolism results in reduced oxygen affinity and delivery to tissues. *0151*

984.00 Toxic Effects of Lead and Its Compounds (including Fumes) Hemolytic anemia. *0484*

985.00 Toxic Effects of Non-medicinal Metals Pancytopenia may occur in arsenic intoxication. *0484*

990.00 Effects of X-Ray Irradiation Predominant only after large doses. *0995*

Blood Increase

1.00 Cholera Due to severe dehydration. *0992*

155.00 Malignant Neoplasm of Liver In the absence of systemic hypoxia, erythrocytosis may develop in hepatocellular carcinoma as a compensatory response to local liver hypoxia. *2377* Erythrocytosis occurs in about 11% of hepatoma patients with increased red cell mass and bone marrow erythroid hyperplasia. *0300 1507* Occasional erythrocytosis. *0962*

189.00 Malignant Neoplasm of Kidney Erythrocytosis is common; disappears after nephrectomy if no metastases are present. *1391* Erythrocytosis has been associated with hypernephromas. *1982 1992*

191.90 Malignant Neoplasm of Brain Erythrocytosis seen in association with cerebellar hemangioblastomas appears to be due to the secretion of erythropoietin by these lesions. *1992*

203.00 Multiple Myeloma Has been found in a small number of patients. *1357*

227.91 Pheochromocytoma Erythrocytosis associated with pheochromocytoma. *2461*

238.40 Polycythemia Vera RBC is 7-12 million; may increase to > 15 million/μL. *2468* RBC > 6.5 million/μL in men and 5.6 million in women. *0532*

255.00 Adrenal Cortical Hyperfunction (Glucocorticoid Excess) Mild erythrocytosis in some patients. *2538 0151*

277.00 Cystic Fibrosis Slight, in older children. *0338*

280.90 Iron Deficiency Anemia In infants and children, hypochromia may occur earlier in the course of iron deficiency and counts > 5.5 million/μL are sometimes encountered. *2538*

282.42 Thalassemia Minor Typically, the RBC are increased in number but are microcytic hypochromic and show prominent poikilocytosis and targeting. *0433* Over 5.7 million/μL and MCV is < 75 fL are most often due to thalassemia trait. *2468* In many heterozygotes the hematocrit and hemoglobin are slightly depressed but the erythrocyte number is normal or increased. *0962*

282.71 Hemoglobin C Disease Seen in large numbers in Hemoglobin C disease. *0999*

289.00 Polycythemia, Secondary Frequently 7-10 million or more/μL when patients are first seen. *0151* Absolute erythrocytosis caused by an enhanced stimulation of RBC production. *2538*

415.00 Cor Pulmonale Secondary polycythemia. *2467* Erythrocytosis, secondary to chronic hypoxemia may be prominent, especially in bronchitic patients. *1108*

425.40 Cardiomyopathies Increased, often to extremely high levels; may rise even further after recovery from shock in cobalt beer cardiomyopathy. *2467*

440.00 Arteriosclerosis True polycythemia with a considerable increase of red cell volume may occur. *1669*

492.80 Pulmonary Emphysema Secondary polycythemia. *2467*

496.00 Chronic Obstructive Lung Disease Erythrocytosis, secondary to chronic hypoxemia may be prominent, especially in bronchitic patients. *1108*

500.00 Anthracosis May become progressively elevated. *0433* Secondary polycythemia. *2467*

501.00 Asbestosis May become progressively elevated. *0433* Secondary polycythemia. *2467*

502.00 Silicosis May become progressively elevated. *0433*

503.01 Berylliosis Secondary polycythemia. *2467* May become progressively elevated. *0433*

591.00 Hydronephrosis True polycythemia with a considerable increase of red cell volume may occur. *1669*

785.50 Shock Hemoconcentration (e.g., dehydration, burns) or hemodilution (e.g., hemorrhage, crush injuries, and skeletal trauma) takes place. *2467*

Blood Normal

4.90 Bacillary Dysentery Anemia is uncommon. *0992*

20.00 Plague Usually normal. *0996*

282.42 Thalassemia Minor In many heterozygotes the hematocrit and hemoglobin are slightly depressed but the erythrocyte number is normal or increased. *0962*

287.00 Allergic Purpura The RBC is generally within normal limits except if severe gastrointestinal blood loss has occurred. *0433*

Urine Increase

36.00 Meningococcal Meningitis May show increase. *2468*

72.00 Mumps Suggests a diagnosis of mumps nephritis. *0433*

80.00 Epidemic Typhus Microscopic hematuria can be expected. *0433*

85.00 Leishmaniasis Frequent. *2468*

87.00 Relapsing Fever There may be blood in urine during the febrile period. *0962*

100.00 Leptospirosis In 75% of patients. *2468* During the leptospiremic phase. *0962* Hemorrhagic manifestations may occur in the first few days of fever. *2368* Hematuria, pyuria, and cylindruria in most cases. *2368*

117.30 Aspergillosis With urinary tract obstruction. *1058*

188.90 Malignant Neoplasm of Bladder By far the most common symptom; may be intermittent or persistent, gross or microscopic. The urine can be completely negative or may show microscopic evidence of hematuria, pyuria, albumin, and threads of mucus. *0433*

189.00 Malignant Neoplasm of Kidney 95% of patients with this disease will have either gross or microscopic hematuria at some time. *0433* Intermittent hematuria found in 60%, occasionally causes colic. *1391* Urinalysis in malignant tumors usually reveals only painless hematuria. *0962*

227.91 Pheochromocytoma Gross or microscopic hematuria may occur early. *0433*

270.03 Cystinosis As glomerular damage progresses. *2246*

273.21 Cryoglobulinemia (Essential Mixed) Urinary sediment contains erythrocytes and finely granular casts. *0433*

275.10 Hepatolenticular Degeneration Microscopic hematuria may occur. *2278*

277.22 Lesch-Nyhan Syndrome Hematuria often occurs. *2246*

277.30 Amyloidosis Microscopic hematuria is frequently seen. *0433*

282.60 Sickle Cell Anemia Hematuria is frequent. *2467* *2538* *1001*

286.01 Hemophilia Hematuria may persist for weeks or months. *0999* Bleeding from the kidneys is often caused by trauma, but usually the cause cannot be determined. May occasionally be due to infection. Occurs in approximately 20% of the moderate and severe cases and in 5% of the mild cases. *2538*

286.10 Christmas Disease Hematuria may persist for weeks or months. *0999* Bleeding from the kidneys is often caused by trauma, but usually the cause cannot be determined. May occasionally be due to infection. Occurs in approximately 20% of the moderate and severe cases and in 5% of the mild cases. *2538*

286.37 Factor VII Deficiency Hematuria has been observed. *2246*

287.00 Allergic Purpura In varying degrees signify renal involvement. *0433* An early feature of urinalysis is macroscopic hematuria. *0962*

323.92 Encephalomyelitis Hematuria may occur with viremia but is transient. *0433*

390.00 Rheumatic Fever Often mild abnormality of Addis count (protein, casts, RBC, WBC) indicates mild focal nephritis. Concomitant glomerulonephritis appears in up to 2.5% of cases. *2467* Moderate increase. *0151*

401.00 Malignant Hypertension Malignant phase of hypertension. May occur from leaking glomerular capillaries. Hematuria occurs very rarely in benign essential hypertension; its presence suggests the malignant phase or primary renal parenchymal disease. *0433*

421.00 Bacterial Endocarditis Hematuria (usually microscopic) occurs at some stage in many cases due to glomerulitis or renal infarct or focal embolic glomerulonephritis. *2467* Microscopic hematuria found in 55% of patients. *1798* Hematuria even without renal involvement *2488* *0433*

428.00 Congestive Heart Failure There are isolated RBC and WBC, hyaline and sometimes granular casts. *2467*

446.00 Polyarteritis-Nodosa Abnormal urinalysis is far more frequent (70-80%) than azotemia (25-30%). *0433* Microscopic hematuria is found in patients with glomerular disease. *0999* Hematuria is likely to be intermittent. *0962*

446.60 Thrombotic Thrombocytopenic Purpura Gross or microscopic hematuria. *0962*

516.10 Idiopathic Pulmonary Hemosiderosis Microscopic hematuria in some cases. Gross hematuria occurs infrequently. *2538*

540.90 Acute Appendicitis Small numbers are found in the urine in about 25% of patients. *2199*

562.11 Diverticulitis of Colon Although urinalysis may be normal hematuria may signal involvement of the bladder or ureter. *0433*

570.00 Acute and Subacute Necrosis of Liver In a few patients, slight hematuria. *0992*

572.40 Hepatic Failure WBC, RBC, and hyaline casts were found in 26% of patients with hepatic failure due to decompensated cirrhosis or attacks of acute viral hepatitis. *0379*

580.00 Acute Poststreptococcal Glomerulonephritis Hematuria, gross or only microscopic. May occur during the initial febrile upper respiratory infection then reappear with nephritis in 1-2 weeks. It lasts 2-12; usual duration is 2 months. *2468* Hematuria usually occurs in conjunction with proteinuria, but may occur alone in some cases. *2545* *0151*

580.01 Glomerulonephritis (Focal) Noted to have slight persistent proteinuria accompanied by microscopic hematuria. *0433* Microscopic or massive hematuria. *0962*

580.02 Glomerulonephritis (Minimal Change) Microscopic hematuria is seen in a minority of patients. *2544*

580.04 Glomerulonephritis (Membranous) Gross hematuria is uncommon even though microscopic hematuria is observed in 40% of the patients. *0433* Hematuria usually occurs in conjunction with proteinuria, but may occur alone in some cases. *2545* Microscopic hematuria is common. *0332*

580.05 Glomerulonephritis (Membranoproliferative) *0331*

580.40 Glomerulonephritis (Rapidly Progressive) Hematuria usually occurs in conjunction with proteinuria, but may occur alone in some cases. *2545* Microscopic hematuria in 15 of 29 patients. *1633* Hematuria is usually microscopic, and it is a rather constant feature indicating activity. *0962*

581.90 Nephrotic Syndrome Microscopic hematuria is present in 33% of cases but casts are rare and there is no evidence of prior streptococcal infection. *0999*

584.00 Acute Renal Failure In the early stage. *2468*

585.00 Chronic Renal Failure With renal parenchymal disease. *0838*

590.00 Chronic Pyelonephritis With renal parenchymal disease. *0838* Microscopic hematuria may be present *0433*

590.10 Acute Pyelonephritis The finding of gross or microscopic hematuria is variable but not uncommon. *0433* With renal parenchymal disease {838}

592.00 Kidney Calculus Microscopic hematuria is found. *0151*

592.10 Ureter Calculus *0277*

593.81 Renal Infarction Common. *0186*

599.00 Urinary Tract Infection A variable number of RBCs may be present, but there are no RBC casts. *0962*

600.00 Benign Prostatic Hypertrophy The urinalysis may be completely normal or may reveal albuminuria, pyuria, and hematuria as a result of obstruction with infection or stone formation. *0433*

695.10 Erythema Multiforme *0151*

710.00 Systemic Lupus Erythematosus Levels of hematuria and proteinuria correlate well with severity of morphologic lesions. *1047* *0433* *0962*

710.10 Progressive Systemic Sclerosis Appears during renal failure. *0433* *0962*

753.10 Polycystic Kidney Disease Progressive hematuria. *0151* Intermittent hematuria is common, and gross hematuria may be seen occasionally. *0962*

984.00 Toxic Effects of Lead and Its Compounds (including Fumes) Renal damage may occur. *0889*

985.00 Toxic Effects of Non-medicinal Metals Common in mercury poisoning. *0151* Marked hematuria may occur in arsenic intoxication. *0850* *1514* *0651* *0889*

986.00 Toxic Effects of Carbon Monoxide Occurs in severe cases. *0151*

Urine Present

267.00 Vitamin C Deficiency Microscopic hematuria is present is 33% of patients with scurvy. *2468*

Urine Normal

600.00 Benign Prostatic Hypertrophy The urinalysis may be completely normal or may reveal albuminuria, pyuria, and hematuria as a result of obstruction with infection or stone formation. *0433*

CSF Increase

54.00 Herpes Simplex RBC or xanthochromia frequently found, reflecting hemorrhagic nature of the lesions. *0151*

324.00 Intracranial Abscess *2467*

431.00 Cerebral Hemorrhage RBCs reach the CSF by seeping into the ventricle after hypertensive hemorrhage. CSF may remain clear if hemorrhage was small and wholly confined to the brain substance. *0999* In 75% of the patients with intracerebral hemorrhage, the CSF was either grossly bloody or xanthochromic: in 25%, the CSF was clear. *1369* All 17 patients with hemorrhagic vascular lesions had RBC counts > 5,000/μL. *2560*

434.10 Cerebral Embolism Usually findings are the same as in cerebral thrombosis. 33% of patients develop hemorrhagic infarction, usually producing slight xanthochromia several days later; some cases may have grossly bloody CSF (10,000 RBC/μL). *2467*

994.80 Effects of Electric Current Bloody spinal fluid as a result of widespread vascular injury. *0995*

Erythrocytes *(continued)*

CSF   Normal

434.00   Cerebral Thrombosis   Never causes blood in the spinal fluid unless the infarct is especially congested, then a very faint xanthochromia may occur. *0992*

Pleural Effusion   Increase

11.00   Pulmonary Tuberculosis   < 10,0000/μL. *2017 0962*

162.90   Malignant Neoplasm of Bronchus and Lung   1000-> 100,000/μL. *2017 0962*

197.00   Secondary Malignant Neoplasm of Respiratory System   1000-> 100,000/μL. *2017 0962*

415.10   Pulmonary Embolism and Infarction   Pleural effusions in association with infarction often are bloody. *1108*   In about 10% of cases. *0503*   1000-100,000/μL *2017*

428.00   Congestive Heart Failure   May be present. *0062*

482.90   Bacterial Pneumonia   *0962*

501.00   Asbestosis   Often blood pleural effusions. *0151*

577.00   Acute Pancreatitis   1000-10,000/μL. *2017*

577.10   Chronic Pancreatitis   1000-10,000/μL. *2017*

714.00   Rheumatoid Arthritis   *0962*

Ascitic Fluid   Increase

18.00   Disseminated Tuberculosis   > 10,000 cells/μL seen in about 5% of patients. *2626*

151.90   Malignant Neoplasm of Stomach   > 10,000 cells/μL seen in 20% of cases. *2626*

152.90   Malignant Neoplasm of Small Intestine   > 10,000 cells/μL seen in 20% of cases. *2626*

153.90   Malignant Neoplasm of Large Intestine   > 10,000 cells/μL seen in 20% of cases. *2626*

155.00   Malignant Neoplasm of Liver   Strongly suggests neoplasm, especially hepatoma. *0151*   A large number of RBC, especially grossly bloody ascites, suggests a neoplasm, particularly hepatoma or ovarian cancer. *2199*   > 10,000 cells/μL seen in 20% of cases *0696*

157.90   Malignant Neoplasm of Pancreas   Grossly bloody ascites suggests neoplasm. *2199*

183.00   Malignant Neoplasm of Ovary   A large number of RBC, especially grossly bloody ascites, suggests a neoplasm, particularly hepatoma or ovarian cancer. *2199*

189.00   Malignant Neoplasm of Kidney   Grossly bloody ascites suggests neoplasm. *2199*

197.70   Secondary Malignant Neoplasm of Liver   > 10,000 cells/μL seen in 20% of cases. *2626*

425.40   Cardiomyopathies   Ascitic fluid and pericardial fluid are usually blood-stained or serous and contain leukocytes in obliterative cardiomyopathies. *1108*

428.00   Congestive Heart Failure   > 10,000 cells/μL seen in 10% of cases. *2626*

560.90   Intestinal Obstruction   Bloody ascitic fluid. *0186*

567.90   Peritonitis   May be bloody. *0186*   < 10,000 cells/μL is unusual. Normally more seen *2626*

571.90   Cirrhosis of Liver   > 10,000 cells/μL seen in 1% of cases. *2626*

577.00   Acute Pancreatitis   In hemorrhagic pancreatitis. *0186*

581.90   Nephrotic Syndrome   > 10,000 cells/μL is unusual. *2626*

Ascitic Fluid   Normal

577.00   Acute Pancreatitis   Variable amount noted. *2626*

577.10   Chronic Pancreatitis   Variable amount noted. *2626*

Pericardial Fluid   Increase

425.40   Cardiomyopathies   Ascitic fluid and pericardial fluid are usually blood-stained or serous and contain leukocytes in obliterative cardiomyopathies. *1108*

Bone Marrow   Decrease

202.80   Non-Hodgkins Lymphoma   In histiocytic medullary reticulosis, severe cytopenias may be associated with the abnormal phagocytosis of erythrocytes, platelets or leukocytes seen in the bone marrow. *2538*

284.90   Aplastic Anemia   Nucleated red cells are decreased in number, but may be the most numerous cell type. *2538   2552*

Peritoneal Fluid   Increase

567.90   Peritonitis   Bloody ascites may be seen with tuberculous peritonitis. *2199*

Saliva   Increase

71.00   Rabies   May be bloody. *2368*

Sputum   Increase

73.90   Psittacosis   Occasionally bloody. *2368*

415.10   Pulmonary Embolism and Infarction   Blood-streaked or grossly bloody sputum. *1108*

Sputum   Present

480.90   Viral Pneumonia   Sputum in acute pneumonia is rusty, blood-streaked and mucopurulent. *0999*

482.90   Bacterial Pneumonia   Sputum in acute pneumonia is rusty, blood-streaked and mucopurulent. *0999*

Erythrocyte Sedimentation Rate

Blood   Decrease

2.00   Typhoid Fever   *2468*

75.00   Infectious Mononucleosis   Low readings may reflect the intracellular nature of the offending organism or liver involvement that causes decreased synthesis of fibrinogen. *0962*

124.00   Trichinosis   Characteristically slow. *0992*

238.40   Polycythemia Vera   Characteristically decreased and may be 0. *2538*

260.00   Protein Malnutrition   With cachexia. *2231*

272.52   Abetalipoproteinemia   High percentage of acanthocytes results in low ESR. *2246*

273.21   Cryoglobulinemia (Essential Mixed)   Rare finding of a rate approaching 0 mm/h (in the absence of marked hypofibrinogenemia). *2035*

282.00   Hereditary (Congenital) Spherocytosis   Very low rate. *2231*

282.60   Sickle Cell Anemia   Decreased ESR becomes normal after blood is aerated. *2467*   Consistently decreased. *2552*

286.34   Congenital Afibrinogenemia   *2538*

286.35   Factor V Deficiency   Nearly 0; RBC remain suspended even after 24 h. *2246*

289.00   Polycythemia, Secondary   *2231*

390.00   Rheumatic Fever   May be decreased in the presence of congestive heart failure. *1108*

428.00   Congestive Heart Failure   May be decreased because of decreased serum fibrinogen. *2467*   As a result of decreased synthesis of fibrinogen by the liver which is passively congested. *0962 1108*

580.05   Glomerulonephritis (Membranoproliferative)   Normal or low. *1017*

710.10   Progressive Systemic Sclerosis   Decreased in 33% of patients. *2468*

Blood   Increase

6.00   Amebiasis   The general rule. *1058*   Increased with liver abscess. *2468*

11.00   Pulmonary Tuberculosis   Usually elevated. *0433*   Normal rates may be seen on occasion in patients with active tuberculosis. *0962*

13.00   Tuberculosis Meningitis   Over 100 mm/h indicate serious disease. *0532*

18.00   Disseminated Tuberculosis   Increased in disseminated or advanced tuberculosis but is not used as an index of activity. *2468*

21.00   Tularemia   Elevated in proportion to the activity of the disease. *0433*   During the active stages. *0151   1058*

23.00   Brucellosis   Occurs in < 25% of patients and usually in nonlocalized type. *2468*

30.00   Leprosy   ESR directly correlates with the increase in plasma fibrinogen in lepromatous leprosy. *1878*

32.00   Diphtheria   *0962*

37.00   Tetanus   Is often increased. *0433*

38.00   Septicemia   Increased in most bacterial infections; reflects the activity of the infectious process. *0962*

39.90 Actinomycosis Almost always elevated. *0433*

40.20 Whipple's Disease *0999*

54.00 Herpes Simplex 26 patients with vulval and cervical herpetic lesions showed highly significant elevations compared to normals. *1272*

70.00 Viral Hepatitis High (mean = 24.1 ± 10.7 mm/h) in cases of uncomplicated HBsAg-negative hepatitis and normal (mean < 10 mm/h) in HBsAG positive cases. *1575* Nonspecific. *1900*

72.00 Mumps May occur with mumps arthritis and orchitis. *0433*

73.90 Psittacosis Usually is increased but may be normal. *2468*

78.50 Cytomegalic Inclusion Disease Slightly increased. *2468*

84.00 Malaria *2468*

85.00 Leishmaniasis Increased due to increased serum globulin. *2468*

87.00 Relapsing Fever Common. *0433*

97.90 Syphilis Raised in 66.6% of seronegative primary cases, 80% of seropositive cases, 100% secondary cases, 80% early latent cases, and 73.9% of late latent cases. Also raised in 16/17 cases of neurosyphilis and 11/11 cases of cardiovascular syphilis. *0759*

99.10 Lymphogranuloma Venereum Is often increased. *0433* *0962 2199*

99.30 Reiter's Disease The increased ESR parallels clinical course. *2468* Common. *0999*

100.00 Leptospirosis Increased in > 50% of the patients but is usually < 50 mm/h. *0151*

104.10 Lyme Disease Often mildly elevated in Lyme Disease. *2639*

114.90 Coccidioidomycosis In active infection. *2368*

116.00 Blastomycosis Most common hematologic abnormality. *0433*

117.10 Sporotrichosis Elevated in all 4 patients studied. *1459* Elevated in all patients with Sporotrichosis arthritis (average 55 mm/h). *0478*

120.00 Schistosomiasis Increased in acute disease. *2468*

124.00 Trichinosis Normal or moderately increased in some patients. *0433*

135.00 Sarcoidosis May reflect raised immunoglobulin levels, or associated erythema nodosum or secondary infection. *0151* *0433*

151.90 Malignant Neoplasm of Stomach Normal in peptic ulcer, but accelerated in carcinoma of the stomach. *0962*

153.90 Malignant Neoplasm of Large Intestine Increased in significant tissue necrosis. Extreme elevation frequently occurs. Indicates inflammation. *2467 0962*

155.00 Malignant Neoplasm of Liver Sometimes increased. *2467*

174.90 Malignant Neoplasm of Breast Extreme elevation frequently occurs. *2467* In 385 patients, the frequency distribution curve was found to be distorted when compared to controls. *1939 0962*

189.00 Malignant Neoplasm of Kidney Unusually high rates of up to 150 mm/h are characteristic. *0151* Common. *0836* Values over 100 mm/h found in 16 of 34 patients. *0894*

198.50 Secondary Malignant Neoplasm of Bone *0962*

199.00 Secondary Malignant Neoplasm (Disseminated) ESR > 100 mm in the 1st h indicates serious disease, as in tuberculosis and carcinomatosis. *0532*

201.90 Hodgkin's Disease Commonly elevated in patients with active disease. *0151* Increases with stage of disease. *2450* Increased in significant tissue necrosis, especially neoplasms - most frequently malignant lymphoma, cancer of the colon and breast. *2468*

202.52 Histiocytosis X Correlates with the prognosis and extent of disease. *2348*

202.80 Non-Hodgkins Lymphoma Increased in significant tissue necrosis, especially neoplasms - most frequently malignant lymphoma, cancer of the colon and breast. *2467*

203.00 Multiple Myeloma Typically increased but a normal or modestly elevated rate does not exclude the diagnosis. Approximately 25% of patients have a ESR > 50 mm/h (Westergren). *0433* Over 100 mm/h in almost 50% of patients. *1980* A result of hyperglobulinemia. *2538 0962*

212.70 Benign Neoplasm of Cardiovascular Tissue Reflection of abnormal serum proteins. *2467* Occurs with myxoma, possibly reflecting tumor emboli or tumor breakdown products. *1108*

242.90 Hyperthyroidism Raised in 12% of patients over 60. *0512*

244.90 Hypothyroidism *2467*

245.10 Subacute Thyroiditis Consistently increased, normal rate mitigates against the diagnosis. *0433* Invariably elevated in the 1st month, reaching very high levels that appear out of proportion to the degree of inflammation and remain so long after symptoms disappear. *1106* Frequently greatly elevated. *0962*

245.20 Hashimoto's Thyroiditis In 50% of chronic thyroiditis patients. *0999* May be mildly elevated. *0962*

252.00 Hyperparathyroidism Raised in 48%, without apparent explanation. *1492* *0999*

270.03 Cystinosis Usually. *2246*

273.21 Cryoglobulinemia (Essential Mixed) May be increased at 37 C. *2468*

273.23 Heavy Chain Disease (Gamma) *0186*

273.30 Waldenström's Macroglobulinemia Markedly increased. *2552* The presence of cryomacroglobulins may give the appearance of a normal ESR. *0433 2035*

273.80 Analbuminemia Usually elevated owing to the increased globulin level. *0433*

274.00 Gout Frequently elevated with acute gout. *0433* Increased in gouty arthritis. *0962* *0999*

275.10 Hepatolenticular Degeneration May be increased, particularly if liver damage is present. *0433*

277.30 Amyloidosis Over 55 mm/h (Westergren) in 50% of patients. *1334*

282.60 Sickle Cell Anemia Elevated in 6 of 18 patients. *0676*

287.00 Allergic Purpura During the acute illness. *0433* Usually elevated. *2538*

288.00 Agranulocytosis Greatly accelerated. *2552*

320.90 Meningitis (Bacterial) *0433*

324.00 Intracranial Abscess Usually elevated, as in other chronic infections, and when present with symptoms and signs of an intracranial mass lesion one should consider the possibility of brain abscess. *0433*

357.00 Guillain-Barré Syndrome Moderately elevated. *0878*

381.00 Otitis Media *0433*

390.00 Rheumatic Fever Sensitive test of rheumatic activity; returns to normal with adequate treatment with ACTH or salicylates. It may remain increased after WBC becomes normal. Becomes normal with onset of congestive heart failure even in the presence of rheumatic activity. *2467* Almost always elevated early in the course of untreated cases. May be decreased in the presence of congestive heart failure but not usually to the normal range. *1108* Typically seen in the myocarditis of rheumatic fever. *0962*

410.90 Acute Myocardial Infarction Increased, usually by 2-3 days; peaks in 4-5 days; persists for 2-6 months. Sometimes more sensitive than WBC as it may occur before fever and persists after temperature and WBC have returned to normal. Degree of increase does not correlate with severity or prognosis. *2467* Rises slowly and may persist for weeks even though no complications are present. *0999* May be a crude indication of the extent of myocardial damage. A normal ESR during the 2nd week suggests absence of or small myocardial infarction. *0962* *1108 1828*

415.10 Pulmonary Embolism and Infarction Elevated in most patients. *0999*

421.00 Bacterial Endocarditis Usually elevated with a mean of 57.3 ± 3.6 mm/h. Mean ESR in survivors, 77.5, was significantly higher than in fatalities, 40.7 mm/h. *1798* Elevated in 90% of cases but is of no differential aid in the work-up of fever of unknown origin. *1108* Increased in 90% of cases. A normal ESR is useful in excluding this diagnosis. *0962* *2488*

425.40 Cardiomyopathies Often elevated in Loeffler's disease. *1108*

429.40 Postcardiotomy Syndrome *2467*

431.00 Cerebral Hemorrhage *2467 0992*

441.00 Dissecting Aortic Aneurysm *2467*

441.50 Ruptured Aortic Aneurysm *0186*

444.90 Arterial Embolism and Thrombosis *2079 0992*

446.00 Polyarteritis-Nodosa Almost a prerequisite for diagnosis. *0433* Generally reflects the intensity of the disease activity. *0999* Almost always elevated in active untreated polyarteritis. *2035* Generally elevated (often exceeding 80 mm/h Westergren). *0962*

Erythrocyte Sedimentation Rate *(continued)*

Blood   Increase *(continued)*

446.50 Cranial Arteritis and Related Conditions   A striking elevation of ESR is characteristic. *0969*   Elevated to > 80 mm/h (Westergren) in polymyalgia rheumatica. *0151*   The only laboratory abnormality of significance is a very rapid ESR, often reaching 100 mm/h (Westergren method). *2035   0962*

446.70 Pulseless Disease (Aortic Arch Syndrome)   May be present. *2086*   Consistently elevated to high levels. *2035*

482.90 Bacterial Pneumonia   Nonspecific indicator of acute infection. *0186*

483.01 Mycoplasma Pneumoniae   Usually elevated. *0151 2368*

487.10 Influenza   *2368*

491.00 Chronic Bronchitis   Present during the course of infection. *0433*

494.00 Bronchiectasis   Nonspecific elevation seen with acute infections. *2220*

495.90 Allergic Alveolitis   *2467*

500.00 Anthracosis   Increased ESR generally indicates secondary infection. *0433*

501.00 Asbestosis   Increased ESR generally indicates secondary infection. *0433*

502.00 Silicosis   Increased ESR generally indicates secondary infection. *0433*

503.01 Berylliosis   Increased ESR generally indicates secondary infection. *0433*

513.00 Abscess of Lung   Markedly elevated. *0433*

533.90 Peptic Ulcer, Site Unspecified   Elevation of the WBC, increased ESR and related phenomena are, to be expected in the event of perforation, massive hemorrhage, and toxic or infectious complications. *0962*

540.90 Acute Appendicitis   With abscess formation or peritonitis, the rate increases rapidly. *0962*

555.90 Regional Enteritis or Ileitis   Elevation takes place during acute exacerbations. *0433*   Tend to suggest that the inflammatory process is active. *2199   2035*

556.00 Ulcerative Colitis   Often normal or only slightly increased. *2467   2035*

562.00 Diverticular Disease of Intestine   May be mildly elevated. *0433*

562.11 Diverticulitis of Colon   *2467*

570.00 Acute and Subacute Necrosis of Liver   *2467*

571.20 Laennec's or Alcoholic Cirrhosis   Extreme elevation is found. *2467   0992*

571.90 Cirrhosis of Liver   Extreme elevation is found. *2467*

575.00 Acute Cholecystitis   Increased ESR, WBC (up to 20,000/μL) and other evidences of acute inflammatory process. *2467*

577.00 Acute Pancreatitis   *2199*

580.00 Acute Poststreptococcal Glomerulonephritis   Usually moderately raised. *0151*

580.01 Glomerulonephritis (Focal)   High ESR may be found in patients with abnormal plasma protein levels. *0962*

581.90 Nephrotic Syndrome   Due to increased fibrinogen. *0186*

585.00 Chronic Renal Failure   Characteristic increase as a result of increased plasma fibrinogen. *0151*

633.90 Ectopic Pregnancy   Rises in the first 24 h *0962*

650.00 Pregnancy   Increased from the 3rd month to about 3 weeks postpartum. Due to increased fibrinogen during pregnancy. *2468   0433*

694.40 Pemphigus   Increased globulin, especially fibrinogen, probably accounts for the increased ESR. *0151*

710.00 Systemic Lupus Erythematosus   Frequently and markedly elevated, even in the presence of apparently mild disease activity due to the presence of abnormal globulins. *0962   0433   0999*

710.10 Progressive Systemic Sclerosis   Increased in 33% of patients. *2468   0433*

710.20 Sjögren's Syndrome   In approximately 66% of patients. *2134   0999*

710.40 Dermatomyositis/Polymyositis   Moderately to markedly increased; may be normal. *2467   0433 0151*

711.00 Acute Arthritis (Pyogenic)   *2467*

714.00 Rheumatoid Arthritis   In 100 patients, correlated with disease activity and stage of disease. *1634*   Nearly always abnormal and generally reflects the degree of disease activity. *2035*   At times, although joint inflammation has subsided, ESR will remain accelerated because of the continued elevation of serum globulins. *0962   0999*

714.30 Juvenile Rheumatoid Arthritis   Are usually elevated moderately when inflammatory disease is severe, but is often normal in the presence of disease activity and is not a constant laboratory parameter. *0433*   Moderately increased; mean = 68 mm/h, and range = 38-104 in 6 children with chronic polyarthritis. *0463*

715.90 Osteoarthritis   Occurs only during rare episodes of acute inflammation of the joints. *0962*

720.00 Rheumatoid (Ankylosing) Spondylitis   Elevated in most but not in all patients with active disease. May be normal in patients who are symptomatic. *0433*   Occurs in about 80% of patients but other acute phase reactants tend to be absent. *0666 0999*

730.00 Osteomyelitis   May be elevated or normal. *2464*

756.55 Infantile Cortical Hyperostosis   Increased (Caffey's disease). *2467*

773.00 Hemolytic Disease of Newborn (Erythroblastosis Fetalis)   Of 70 infants showing accelerated rate, 49 had signs of hemolytic disease. The test was found to be very sensitive, detecting ABO incompatibilities even in absence of marked bilirubinemia. *2150*

984.00 Toxic Effects of Lead and Its Compounds (including Fumes)   With arsenic and lead intoxication. *2467*

985.00 Toxic Effects of Non-medicinal Metals   With arsenic and lead intoxication. *2467*

Blood   Normal

2.00 Typhoid Fever   *0186*

73.90 Psittacosis   Frequently normal. *2368*

117.50 Cryptococcosis   Even in extensive infection, the blood WBC, hct, and ESR remain normal. *1058*

273.21 Cryoglobulinemia (Essential Mixed)   Normal at room temperature. *2468*

273.30 Waldenström's Macroglobulinemia   The presence of cryomacroglobulins may give the appearance of a normal ESR. *2467*

287.00 Allergic Purpura   Unlike with other necrotizing angiitis, the ESR is often normal. *0962*

358.00 Myasthenia Gravis   Complete blood count and ESR are normal. *2467*

359.21 Myotonia Atrophica   Usually normal. *2467*

413.90 Angina Pectoris   May be helpful in distinguishing this entity from acute myocardial infarction. *0962*

533.90 Peptic Ulcer, Site Unspecified   Normal in peptic ulcer, but accelerated in carcinoma of the stomach. *0962*

540.90 Acute Appendicitis   In unruptured acute appendicitis, the ESR is normal during the first 24 h, even when the appendix is suppurative or gangrenous. *0962*

710.10 Progressive Systemic Sclerosis   Normal in 33%, decreased in 33%, and increased in 33% of patients. *2468*

714.00 Rheumatoid Arthritis   Elevated when the classic case is active, normal when the disease is quiet because of its natural course or as a result of therapy. *0433*   The majority of patients who are in complete remission will have a normal ESR. *0962*

714.30 Juvenile Rheumatoid Arthritis   Are usually elevated moderately when inflammatory disease is severe, but is often normal in the presence of disease activity and is not a constant laboratory parameter. *0433*

715.90 Osteoarthritis   Usually normal. *0962*

Erythrocyte Survival

Red Blood Cells   Decrease

86.90 Trypanosomiasis   Hematological studies indicate the presence of a hemolytic process. *2569   2035*

117.30 Aspergillosis   Hemolytic anemia. *1950 2538*

201.90 Hodgkin's Disease   Mild or moderate hemolytic anemia, with a negative Coombs' test, is common in disseminated lymphoma. *0433*

202.80 Non-Hodgkins Lymphoma Characteristically short in patients with bulky lymph nodes or with enlargement of the liver and spleen. *1186 2538*

204.10 Lymphocytic Leukemia (Chronic) Characteristically short even when there is no evidence of autoimmunity. *2489 2538*

205.10 Myelocytic Leukemia (Chronic) Some shortening of survival occurs in the presence of gross splenomegaly and hepatomegaly. *2538*

207.00 Erythroleukemia Evidence of a mild or moderate increase in hemolysis is commonly observed, but the erythrokinetic findings are those of ineffective erythropoiesis. *2538*

212.70 Benign Neoplasm of Cardiovascular Tissue Hemolytic anemia and mechanical in origin (due to local turbulence of blood) may occur and may be severe. The anemia is recognized in about 50% of the patients. *2467* Occurs with myxoma, possibly reflecting tumor emboli or tumor breakdown products. *1108*

238.40 Polycythemia Vera As the disease progresses, there are increasing degrees of extramedullary ineffective hematopoiesis with progressive shortening of the red cell life-span secondary to increasing splenic sequestration. *2538 1835*

242.90 Hyperthyroidism In patients with thyrotoxicosis, a moderate shortening. *2538 1537*

272.52 Abetalipoproteinemia Usually shortened, but may be normal. *2501 2091 2246 1583*

273.30 Waldenström's Macroglobulinemia Found in 6 of 8 patients. *0413 2538*

275.10 Hepatolenticular Degeneration Reduced and found to correlate with splenic enlargement. *2279*

277.11 Congenital Erythropoietic Porphyria (Günther's Disease) With moderate to severe anemia. *2552* Hemolysis occurs in most patients. *2073 2246*

277.42 Gilbert's Disease Mild, but fully compensated hemolysis in a significant number of patients. *0754*

279.04 Agammaglobulinemia (Congenital Sex-linked) Hemolytic anemia. *2035*

280.90 Iron Deficiency Anemia Slight to moderate shortening. *2538 1436* Somewhat shortened. High correlation with the number of morphologically abnormal cells. Only severe changes can be detected by the ^{53}Cr method. *0561 2552*

281.00 Pernicious Anemia Moderately reduced. *2552* Ranged from 27-75 days in 5 patients (normal 120 days). *1442 2181*

281.20 Folic Acid Deficiency Anemia Moderately reduced. *2552* Ranged from 27-75 days in 5 patients (normal = 120 days). *1442 2181*

282.10 Hereditary Elliptocytosis *2538*

282.20 Anemias Due To Disorders of Glutathione Metabolism *2538*

282.41 Thalassemia Major Usually shortened. *2538* Generally ranges from 7-22 days as measured by ^{51}Chromium-labeling. *2289*

282.42 Thalassemia Minor Normal or slightly shortened. *1792*

282.60 Sickle Cell Anemia Mean red cell life span was 17.32 ± 4.51 days and half-life was 10.11 ± 2.82 days. Mean life span was inversely correlated with number of sickled cells. *1541* Shortened in all the varieties of sickle cell disease. *2538*

282.71 Hemoglobin C Disease Mean life span 30-55 days. *2347*

283.00 Acquired Hemolytic Anemia (Autoimmune) Shortened survival of both the patient's own red cell population and normal donor cells. *1615 2538*

284.90 Aplastic Anemia There may be evidence of premature red cell destruction. *1384* May be somewhat shortened but evidence of blood destruction is lacking. *2552 2538*

289.40 Hypersplenism May or may not be reduced. *1824 2246*

483.01 Mycoplasma Pneumoniae Occasional patients have been reported with hemolytic anemia. *0433*

487.10 Influenza Hemolytic anemia. *2538 1857*

570.00 Acute and Subacute Necrosis of Liver Decreased survival; mild to moderate hemolysis. *1849*

571.20 Laennec's or Alcoholic Cirrhosis Moderately shortened in 48 of 68 alcoholic liver disease patients. *1268 2137 2552* Especially in patients with predominant indirect bilirubinemia. *0722*

571.90 Cirrhosis of Liver Mild to moderate hemolysis. *1849* Moderately shortened in 48 of 68 alcoholic liver disease patients. *1268 2137 2552* Especially in patients with predominant indirect bilirubinemia. *0722*

572.00 Liver Abscess (Pyogenic) Decreased RBC survival; mild to moderate hemolysis. *1849*

580.05 Glomerulonephritis (Membranoproliferative) *0331*

584.00 Acute Renal Failure *0277*

585.00 Chronic Renal Failure Shortened to about half normal when the blood urea exceeds 200 mg/dL. *0151* Shortened RBC life span and inhibitor of heme synthesis cause anemia in renal insufficiency. *0736* Slightly to moderately reduced. *2552*

984.00 Toxic Effects of Lead and Its Compounds (including Fumes) Red cell life span and osmotic fragility are decreased. *0151* Hemolysis. *0618*

Red Blood Cells   Increase

255.00 Adrenal Cortical Hyperfunction (Glucocorticoid Excess) *0999*

Red Blood Cells   Normal

238.40 Polycythemia Vera Red cell life span is normal as is arterial oxygen saturation. *0999*

277.14 Acute Intermittent Porphyria Suggests that the decreased RBC mass results from reduced effective erythropoiesis. *0230*

284.01 Congenital Aplastic Anemia Shortened survival has been described in some cases but earlier reports indicate no evidence of a hemolytic process. *2552*

284.90 Aplastic Anemia Red cell survival is normal or only slightly reduced. *0999*

Erythropoietin

Serum   Decrease

201.90 Hodgkin's Disease The most frequent finding is a normochromic anemia, most often a result of decreased erythropoiesis *0999*

238.40 Polycythemia Vera Usually lower than normal or undetectable. *0999* In 21 proved cases, concentrations were all < 5 mU/mL (the limit of sensitivity) whereas 35 control subjects had a mean of 7.8 mU/mL. *0673*

585.00 Chronic Renal Failure Reduced in chronic failure causing relative hypoplasia of the marrow. *0151* Decreased secretion of erythropoietin of renal origin. *1669*

Serum   Increase

155.00 Malignant Neoplasm of Liver Increased plasma concentrations are found in patients with erythrocytosis associated with several types of tumor, especially lung, kidney and liver. *0263 1416 1507*

162.90 Malignant Neoplasm of Bronchus and Lung Increased plasma concentrations are found in patients with erythrocytosis associated with several types of tumor, especially lung, kidney and liver. *0263 1416 1507*

189.00 Malignant Neoplasm of Kidney Increased in 49 of 92 patients with renal cell carcinoma or renal cysts. Highest values were found in patients developing metastases after removal of renal carcinoma. *1609* Elevated in 63% of patients but did not correlate with tumor grade, type, stage, prognosis. *2291* Increased plasma concentrations are found in patients with erythrocytosis associated with several types of tumor, especially lung, kidney, and liver. *0263 1416 1507*

191.90 Malignant Neoplasm of Brain Erythrocytosis seen in association with cerebellar hemangioblastomas appears to be due to the secretion of erythropoietin by these lesions. *1992*

204.00 Lymphocytic Leukemia (Acute) Found to be increased and negatively correlated with hemoglobin concentration. *1785*

205.00 Myelocytic Leukemia (Acute) Increased and negatively correlated with hemoglobin concentration. *1785*

227.91 Pheochromocytoma Large amounts. *1992*

284.90 Aplastic Anemia Titers in plasma and the 24 h urinary excretion rates usually exceed those found in most other types of anemia at the same hemoglobin concentration. *2538* Activity of erythropoietin is high, in fact, higher than observed in patients with anemia of comparable severity due to other causes. *0999 0151*

289.00 Polycythemia, Secondary Secondary polycythemia caused by excessive release of erythropoietin. *2538*

584.00 Acute Renal Failure *0277*

Erythropoietin *(continued)*

Serum   Increase *(continued)*

585.00   Chronic Renal Failure   May be elevated to varying degrees in patients with anemia associated with end-stage renal disease. The increase in erythropoietin titer was apparently not sufficient to meet the increase in demand for new RBCs created by their shortened life span and the inhibitors of heme synthesis. *0736*

650.00   Pregnancy   Striking increase. *1113*

753.10   Polycystic Kidney Disease   Increased values were found in 49 plasma samples and 14 cyst fluids of 92 patients with renal cell carcinoma or renal cyst. Highest values were found in patients developing metastases after removal of renal carcinoma. *1609*

Urine   Decrease

238.40   Polycythemia Vera   Poor sensitivity of the assay techniques prevents a reliable method to differentiate secondary polycythemia from polycythemia vera. *0433   0999*

Urine   Increase

204.00   Lymphocytic Leukemia (Acute)   Urine levels are usually increased in lymphoblastic but not myeloblastic leukemia. *1785*

284.90   Aplastic Anemia   Activity is high, in fact higher than observed in patients with anemia of comparable severity due to other causes. *0999*   Titers in plasma and the 24-h urinary excretion rates usually exceed those found in most other types of anemia at the same hemoglobin concentration. *2538   0151*

Estradiol

Plasma   Decrease

758.80   Syndromes Due to Sex Chromosome Abnormalities   In Turner's Syndrome. *0002 0605 0046*

Plasma   Increase

183.00   Malignant Neoplasm of Ovary   In estrogen producing tumors estradiol is the most active estrogen. *0002   1720 0046*

220.00   Benign Neoplasm of Ovary   In estrogen producing tumors estradiol is the most active estrogen. *0002   1720 0046*

571.90   Cirrhosis of Liver   Estradiol is the most active estrogen. *0002 0605 0046*

Estriol

Urine   Decrease

650.00   Pregnancy   The predominant urinary estrogen during pregnancy is E3. Declining values indicate fetal jeopardy. *0002 0605 0046*

Estrogens

Serum   Decrease

256.30   Ovarian Hypofunction   Decreased in primary and secondary hypofunction of ovary. *2467*

642.40   Pre-Eclampsia   Average serum and urinary estrogens were reduced in pre-eclampsia compared to normal pregnancy, but there was considerable overlap in values. *2332*

642.60   Eclampsia   *2212*

758.80   Syndromes Due to Sex Chromosome Abnormalities   In Turner's syndrome. *0503*

770.80   Respiratory Distress Syndrome   The average concentrations of estradiol in umbilical cord plasma from newborns with the syndrome with or without hyaline membrane disease were lower by 25% than in controls. *2306*

Serum   Increase

181.00   Malignant Neoplasm of Trophoblast (Choriocarcinoma)   May be much increased with primary chorionepithelioma of ovary. *2467*

182.00   Malignant Neoplasm of Corpus Uteri   Mean value was 76.65 ng/dL in 28 patients with endometrial carcinoma. Highest elevations were found in obese patients. *0034*

220.92   Granulosa Cell Tumor of Ovary   Estrogens are increased in granulosa cell tumor of ovary. *2468*

220.93   Lutein Cell Tumor of Ovary   Estrogens are increased in luteoma of ovary. *2467   2468*

220.94   Theca Cell Tumor of Ovary   Estrogens are increased in theca-cell tumor of ovary. *2467   2468*

244.90   Hypothyroidism   Increased estradiol. *1731*

257.20   Testicular Hypofunction   The average daily production of estrogen is increased and the circulating levels of estrogen are relatively constant. *0151*

410.90   Acute Myocardial Infarction   34 of 35 male survivors of myocardial infarction, aged 24-48, had higher plasma concentration of estradiol than age matched controls. 29 of 35 had elevated concentration of estrone. *0669*

571.90   Cirrhosis of Liver   Inability to conjugate estrogens. *2238*

630.00   Hydatidiform Mole   Plasma unconjugated estradiol was greater than normal in 6 of 13 patients with intact mole, ranging from 1.82-8.10 ng/mL at 15-19 weeks gestation. *1613*

650.00   Pregnancy   *0484*

758.70   Klinefelter's Syndrome (XXY)   Total and free plasma concentrations of estradiol are normal or increased. Does not correlate with clinical findings such as gynecomastia or hypoandrogenicity. *1090*

780.30   Convulsions   The incidence of epileptic seizures was higher in women during the high estrogen period of the menstrual cycle. Number of seizures correlated positively to estrogen/progesterone ratio and negatively to progesterone levels. *0096*

Serum   Normal

242.90   Hyperthyroidism   Estradiol is normal. *1731*

286.31   Congenital Dysfibrinogenemia   *2538*

Urine   Decrease

256.30   Ovarian Hypofunction   *2467 0619*

627.90   Menopausal and Postmenopausal Symptoms   The urinary excretion of total estrogens will be below 10 μg/24h. Values above 20 μg/24h are suggestive of a pathologic process such as a granulosa cell tumor. *0433*

642.40   Pre-Eclampsia   Average serum and urinary estrogens were reduced in pre-eclampsia compared to normal pregnancy, but there was considerable overlap in values. *2332*   In a series of 794 patients, hypoglycemia had a significant association with low estriol excretion, fetal growth retardation, and perinatal mortality. *1427*   In 99 pre-eclamptic patients, the incidence of subnormal concentrations was 76%. *2543*   Low values were found in 36% (23 of 64) patients. *2270*

656.40   Pregnancy Complicated by Intrauterine Death   *0619*

758.80   Syndromes Due to Sex Chromosome Abnormalities   Doesn't increase with administration of hCG. *0186*

Urine   Increase

186.90   Malignant Neoplasm of Testis   *2467*

194.00   Malignant Neoplasm of Adrenal Gland   Principally due to increments in estriol and also to increments in estradiol and estrone. *0995*

220.00   Benign Neoplasm of Ovary   *2467*

220.92   Granulosa Cell Tumor of Ovary   Normal urinary excretion of total estrogens will be below 10 μg/24h. Values > 20 μg/24h are suggestive of a granulosa cell tumor. *0433*

220.93   Lutein Cell Tumor of Ovary   *2467*

220.94   Theca Cell Tumor of Ovary   *0619*

222.00   Benign Neoplasm of Testis   *0619*

570.00   Acute and Subacute Necrosis of Liver   *2467*

650.00   Pregnancy   Increase from 6 months to term 100 μg/24h). *2468   0484*

Estrone

Serum   Increase

650.00   Pregnancy   Ten fold increase during pregnancy. *1177 1432 2385*

Etiocholanolone

Urine   Decrease
151.90   **Malignant Neoplasm of Stomach**   Both androsterone and etiocholanolone were significantly lower in 18 male patients than in controls and patients with rectal cancer. *2333*

Euglobulin Clot Lysis Time

Blood   Increase
496.01   **Alpha₁-Antitrypsin Deficiency**   Increased. *0295 2353*
785.50   **Shock**   Increased in circulatory collapse. *0295 2353*

Factor II

Plasma   Decrease
38.00   **Septicemia**   May be associated with defibrination resulting in platelet and coagulation factor consumption in severe gram-positive septicemia. *2538*

54.00   **Herpes Simplex**   May be associated with defibrination resulting in platelet and coagulation factor consumption. *2538*

65.00   **Arthropod-Borne Hemorrhagic Fever**   May be associated with defibrination resulting in platelet and coagulation factor consumption (Korean and Thai fever). *2538*

82.00   **Rocky Mountain Spotted Fever**   May be associated with defibrination resulting in platelet and coagulation factor consumption. *2538*

84.00   **Malaria**   May be associated with defibrination resulting in platelet and coagulation factor consumption (in overwhelming parasitemia). *2538*

197.00   **Secondary Malignant Neoplasm of Respiratory System**   May be associated with defibrination resulting in platelet and coagulation factor consumption. *2538*

197.50   **Secondary Malignant Neoplasm of Digestive System**   May be associated with defibrination resulting in platelet and coagulation factor consumption. *2538*

199.00   **Secondary Malignant Neoplasm (Disseminated)**   May be associated with defibrination resulting in platelet and coagulation factor consumption. *2538*

205.10   **Myelocytic Leukemia (Chronic)**   Low levels found. *2318*

256.30   **Ovarian Hypofunction**   Estrogen effect. *0995*

273.30   **Waldenström's Macroglobulinemia**   A number of patients have reduced activity of one or more coagulation factors. *2538*

487.10   **Influenza**   May be associated with defibrination resulting in platelet and coagulation factor consumption. *2538*

572.40   **Hepatic Failure**   Low levels of clotting factors found in fulminant hepatic failure are due to decrease in liver synthesis aggravated by increased consumption. *0821*

579.90   **Malabsorption, Cause Unspecified**   Malabsorption of fat-soluble vitamin K results in hypoprothrombinemia. *0151*

630.00   **Hydatidiform Mole**   May be associated with defibrination resulting in platelet and coagulation factor consumption. *2538*

Plasma   Increase
256.00   **Ovarian Hyperfunction**   Estrogen effect. *0995*
650.00   **Pregnancy**   Increased in late pregnancy. *2468*
994.50   **Exercise**   Observed effect in exercise. *1839*

Plasma   Normal
286.31   **Congenital Dysfibrinogenemia**   *2538*

Factor IV

Plasma   Decrease
38.00   **Septicemia**   May be associated with defibrination resulting in platelet and coagulation factor consumption in severe gram-positive septicemia. *2538*

54.00   **Herpes Simplex**   May be associated with defibrination resulting in platelet and coagulation factor consumption. *2538*

65.00   **Arthropod-Borne Hemorrhagic Fever**   May be associated with defibrination resulting in platelet and coagulation factor consumption (Korean and Thai fever). *2538*

82.00   **Rocky Mountain Spotted Fever**   May be associated with defibrination resulting in platelet and coagulation factor consumption. *2538*

84.00   **Malaria**   May be associated with defibrination resulting in platelet and coagulation factor consumption (in overwhelming parasitemia). *2538*

197.00   **Secondary Malignant Neoplasm of Respiratory System**   May be associated with defibrination resulting in platelet and coagulation factor consumption. *2538*

197.50   **Secondary Malignant Neoplasm of Digestive System**   May be associated with defibrination resulting in platelet and coagulation factor consumption. *2538*

199.00   **Secondary Malignant Neoplasm (Disseminated)**   May be associated with defibrination resulting in platelet and coagulation factor consumption. *2538*

487.10   **Influenza**   May be associated with defibrination resulting in platelet and coagulation factor consumption. *2538*

630.00   **Hydatidiform Mole**   May be associated with defibrination resulting in platelet and coagulation factor consumption. *2538*

Plasma   Increase
410.90   **Acute Myocardial Infarction**   A mean of 95 ng/mL was found in 21 patients, compared to normal 16 ± 4 in controls. Patients with chest pain but without evidence of infarction had a mean of 29 ng/mL. Elevation persisted for 1 week and returned to normal. *0974*

413.90   **Angina Pectoris**   Patients with chest pain but without evidence of infarction had a mean of 29 ng/mL. Elevation persisted for 1 week and returned to normal. *0974*

415.10   **Pulmonary Embolism and Infarction**   Markedly elevated in patients with embolic or cardiorespiratory failure. *0974*

Factor V

Plasma   Decrease
205.00   **Myelocytic Leukemia (Acute)**   Intravascular clotting has been documented in occasional patients. *0890*

205.10   **Myelocytic Leukemia (Chronic)**   Low levels found. *2318* Intravascular clotting has been documented for rare patients. *0890*

206.00   **Monocytic Leukemia**   With disseminated intravascular clotting. *1552*

238.40   **Polycythemia Vera**   Low levels found. *2318*

273.30   **Waldenström's Macroglobulinemia**   A number of patients have reduced activity of one or more coagulation factors. *2538*

286.35   **Factor V Deficiency**   *2538*

286.60   **Disseminated Intravascular Coagulopathy**   *2538*

446.60   **Thrombotic Thrombocytopenic Purpura**   Slight decrease in 2 cases. *1376*

571.90   **Cirrhosis of Liver**   Impaired hepatic synthesis. *0424*

572.40   **Hepatic Failure**   Low levels of clotting factors found in fulminant hepatic failure are due to decrease in liver synthesis aggravated by increased consumption. *0821*

585.00   **Chronic Renal Failure**   Occasionally observed. *0151*

Plasma   Increase
581.90   **Nephrotic Syndrome**   May occur. *2322*
948.00   **Burns**   Factor V and VIII may be 4-8 X normal for up to 3 months. *2468*

Plasma   Normal
286.31   **Congenital Dysfibrinogenemia**   *2538*
994.50   **Exercise**   Observed effect in exercise. *1839*

Factor VII

Plasma   Decrease
269.00   **Vitamin K Deficiency**   Synthesized in the liver by a process that requires vitamin K. *0992*

273.30   **Waldenström's Macroglobulinemia**   A number of patients have reduced activity of 1 or more coagulation factors. *2538*

Factor VII (continued)

Plasma Decrease (continued)

286.37 Factor VII Deficiency Some patients appear to synthesize a nonfunctional variant, and other patients are truly deficient. *2246 2538*

572.20 Hepatic Encephalopathy All 7 patients with values < 8% of normal failed to regain consciousness from hepatic coma due to fulminant hepatic failure. *0821*

572.40 Hepatic Failure All 7 patients with values 8% of normal failed to regain consciousness from hepatic coma due to fulminant hepatic failure. *0821*

585.00 Chronic Renal Failure Occasionally observed. *0151*

Plasma Increase

581.90 Nephrotic Syndrome May occur. *2322*

650.00 Pregnancy Increased in late pregnancy. *2468*

Plasma Normal

286.31 Congenital Dysfibrinogenemia *2538*

Factor VIII

Plasma Decrease

205.00 Myelocytic Leukemia (Acute) Intravascular clotting has been documented in occasional patients. *0890*

205.10 Myelocytic Leukemia (Chronic) Intravascular clotting has been documented for rare patients. *0890*

206.00 Monocytic Leukemia With disseminated intravascular clotting. *1552*

244.90 Hypothyroidism May occur. *2175*

260.00 Protein Malnutrition During 10 days of total fasting in healthy normal weight males, a reduction of plasma activity with a concomitant decrease in factor VIII antigen was found, without other laboratory evidence for a disseminated intravascular coagulation. *0632*

273.30 Waldenström's Macroglobulinemia A number of patients have reduced activity of one or more coagulation factors. *2538*

286.01 Hemophilia Varies from 0% of normal in severe to 25% in mild cases. *2552* The basic defect appears to be a failure to synthesize functional AHF. *2246* May be due to decreased or absent synthesis of factor VIII or to the synthesis of a functionally inactive factor VII molecule. *1572 0962*

286.40 Von Willebrand's Disease Characteristically reduced, usually from 20-40%. A wide range may be seen and a normal concentration is not incompatible with the diagnosis. *0433* Commonly occurs in both homozygotes and heterozygotes. *1389* Activity is usually higher than in classic hemophilia, but values of 1-5% of normal may sometimes be found. May show wide fluctuation in the same person on repeated testing. *2538* A true decrease in amount of AHF protein accompanied by a proportional or even more severe decrease in AHF-like antigens. *2617 2246 0227 0962*

286.60 Disseminated Intravascular Coagulopathy *2538*

642.40 Pre-Eclampsia In the ratio between factor VIII-related antigen and factor VIII activity a highly significant increase was observed during the 3rd trimester. The highest ratios were associated with either a perinatal death or with the delivery of a severely growth retarded infant. *2355*

Plasma Increase

242.90 Hyperthyroidism May reflect increased adrenergic activity. *2540* Increased activity in hyperthyroid states. *0636*

250.00 Diabetes Mellitus Increased activity has been reported. *0635*

282.60 Sickle Cell Anemia May be increased. *1931 2552*

308.00 Stress Postoperative stress. *0544*

440.00 Arteriosclerosis In atherosclerosis. *0453*

571.20 Laennec's or Alcoholic Cirrhosis Increased activity in alcoholic liver disease. *0911*

571.90 Cirrhosis of Liver Increased activity in alcoholic liver disease. *0911*

580.00 Acute Poststreptococcal Glomerulonephritis Patients who made a complete recovery upon 4 year follow-up had normal initial values, while those who developed persistent renal damage had high factor VIII values. Other coagulation factors are of no prognostic significance. *0642*

581.90 Nephrotic Syndrome May occur. *2322*

585.00 Chronic Renal Failure Dramatic increase in both factor VIII/von Willebrand antigen and activity (315 ± 30% vs. 104 ± 9% in control, and 402 ± 48% activity in patients vs. 111 ± 5% controls). *2484* Increased activity has been reported. *0633*

650.00 Pregnancy Increased activity has been reported. *1194*

948.00 Burns Factor V and VIII may be 4-8 X normal for up to 3 months. *2468*

990.00 Effects of X-Ray Irradiation Increased activity after total body irradiation. *2189*

992.00 Heat stroke Increased activity as a result of fever. *0634*

994.50 Exercise Striking increase in titer after exercise. *2011* In proportion to extent of exercise and antigen. *0166 0544 1839*

Plasma Normal

286.31 Congenital Dysfibrinogenemia *2538*

Factor IX

Plasma Decrease

244.90 Hypothyroidism May occur. *2175*

269.00 Vitamin K Deficiency Synthesized in the liver by a process that requires vitamin K. *0992*

272.72 Gaucher's Disease Clotting factor abnormalities may be present. Factor IX deficiency seems to be particularly common, and it does not appear to be related to liver disease. *2538*

286.10 Christmas Disease Present in carriers in approximately half the concentration of that found in patients. *2538* Titers < 5% of normal are usual, and may be undetectable in severe cases. In mildly affected patients, values may be > 30%. *0121*

287.10 Thrombasthenia (Glanzmann's) Deficient platelet factor III. *0433*

572.40 Hepatic Failure *0503*

Plasma Increase

650.00 Pregnancy Concentration rises during pregnancy. *0035*

Plasma Normal

282.60 Sickle Cell Anemia *1931 2552*

286.31 Congenital Dysfibrinogenemia *2538*

Factor X

Plasma Decrease

269.00 Vitamin K Deficiency Synthesized in the liver by a process that requires vitamin K. *0992*

273.30 Waldenström's Macroglobulinemia A number of patients have reduced activity of one or more coagulation factors. *2538*

286.36 Factor X Deficiency True deficiency in some patients and deficiency of functional factor X in others. *2246 2538*

572.40 Hepatic Failure *0503*

642.40 Pre-Eclampsia Factor XII was significantly higher in 12 patients than in the normal group, while factors XI and X were slightly lower. *0432*

Plasma Increase

581.90 Nephrotic Syndrome May occur. *2322*

650.00 Pregnancy Normally increase as pregnancy advances. A secondary increase in XI and X may occur in the puerperium. Cord levels of all 3 factors are decreased. *0432*

Plasma Normal

286.31 Congenital Dysfibrinogenemia *2538*

Factor XI

Plasma   Decrease

286.20 **Factor XI Deficiency**   Definitive diagnosis is by a factor XI assay using blood from a patient with established factor XI deficiency. *2538*   Plasma thromboplastin antecedent (factor XI) deficiency. *2246*

581.90 **Nephrotic Syndrome**   In part due to excessive urinary loss. *2352*

642.40 **Pre-Eclampsia**   Factor XII was significantly higher in 12 patients than in the normal group, while factors XI and X were slightly lower. *0432*

650.00 **Pregnancy**   Decreased in late pregnancy. *2468*

Plasma   Increase

650.00 **Pregnancy**   Factor X, XI, and XII normally increase as pregnancy advances. A secondary increase in XI and X may occur in the puerperium. Cord levels of all 3 factors are decreased. *0432*

Plasma   Normal

282.60 **Sickle Cell Anemia**   *1931 2552*

Factor XII

Plasma   Decrease

82.00 **Rocky Mountain Spotted Fever**   May be associated with defibrination resulting in platelet and coagulation factor consumption. *2538*   Hypofibrinogenemia in 2 of 5 cases with marked reduction of factor XII. *2589*

286.32 **Factor XII Deficiency**   Definitive diagnosis is made by testing against plasma from an established case. *2538* Nondetectable. *1885*

581.90 **Nephrotic Syndrome**   In part due to excessive urinary loss. *2352*

Plasma   Increase

642.40 **Pre-Eclampsia**   Factor XII was significantly higher in 12 patients than in the normal group, while factors XI and X were slightly lower. *0432*

650.00 **Pregnancy**   Factor X, XI, and XII normally increase as pregnancy advances. A secondary increase in XI and X may occur in the puerperium. Cord levels of all 3 factors are decreased. *0432*

Plasma   Normal

282.60 **Sickle Cell Anemia**   *1931 2552*

Factor XIII

Plasma   Decrease

286.60 **Disseminated Intravascular Coagulopathy**   Substantial depression of factor XIII concentrations developed with concomitant significant increases in the proportion and concentration of plasma high molecular weight fibrinogen complexes (HMWFC). In inverse correlation between factor XIII and percentage of HMWFC was demonstrated in the early stages of the illness. *1491*

410.90 **Acute Myocardial Infarction**   Substantial depression developed with concomitant significant increases in the proportion and concentration of plasma high molecular weight fibrinogen complexes (HMWFC). An inverse correlation between factor XIII and percentage of HMWFC was demonstrated in the early stages of the illness. *1491*

434.90 **Brain Infarction**   Substantial depression developed together with concomitant significant increases in the proportion and concentration of plasma high molecular weight fibrinogen complexes (HMWFC). An inverse correlation between factor XIII and percentage of HMWFC was demonstrated in the early stages of the illness. *1491*

Plasma   Normal

286.31 **Congenital Dysfibrinogenemia**   *2538*

Factor B

Plasma   Decrease

260.00 **Protein Malnutrition**   *1979 2356*

282.60 **Sickle Cell Anemia**   *1979 2356*

579.01 **Protein-Losing Enteropathy**   *1979 2356*

580.04 **Glomerulonephritis (Membranous)**   *1979 2356*

710.00 **Systemic Lupus Erythematosus**   *1979 2356*

948.00 **Burns**   *1979 2356*

Synovial Fluid   Decrease

714.00 **Rheumatoid Arthritis**   *1443*

Fat

Serum   Increase

308.00 **Stress**   A rise in blood fats is characteristic. *2113*

Serum   Present

829.00 **Fracture of Bone**   Fat globules in 42-67% of cases. *2468*

Urine   Increase

303.00 **Acute Alcoholic Intoxication**   Significant lipuria occurred in a group of acutely intoxicated patients with neurological symptoms. *0289*

303.90 **Alcoholism**   Significant lipuria occurred in a group of acutely intoxicated patients with neurological symptoms. *0289*

829.00 **Fracture of Bone**   In 60% of cases. *2468*

929.00 **Crush Injury (Trauma)**   *0619*

958.10 **Fat Embolism**   In 60% of cases. *2468*

Bone Marrow   Decrease

205.10 **Myelocytic Leukemia (Chronic)**   Bone marrow aspirated from almost any site usually yields a grossly hypercellular specimen in which the fat is practically absent. *2538*

Bone Marrow   Increase

284.01 **Congenital Aplastic Anemia**   Marrow is described as fatty and hypocellular or normocellular. *0695*

Feces   Increase

40.20 **Whipple's Disease**   In small intestinal disease. *2199*

70.00 **Viral Hepatitis**   May be excessive amounts of fecal fat. *2104*

157.90 **Malignant Neoplasm of Pancreas**   Steatorrhea is found in approximately 10% of the cases as judged by abnormal chemical fat excretion. *0151*   Deficient intraluminal pancreatic enzymes. *2199*

250.00 **Diabetes Mellitus**   Defects of multiple stages of digestion-absorption. *2199*

251.50 **Zollinger-Ellison Syndrome**   Hyperacidity in duodenum inactivates pancreatic enzymes. *0962*

259.20 **Carcinoid Syndrome**   Secondary to malabsorption or steatorrhea. *2540*

272.52 **Abetalipoproteinemia**   Marked impairment of GI fat absorption. *2467*   By 4th or 5th year of life, steatorrhea becomes less marked. *2246*

277.00 **Cystic Fibrosis**   Deficient intraluminal pancreatic enzymes. *2199*   In this study of 12 patients, average was 41 g/day, compared to < 7 g/day for controls. *2246*

277.30 **Amyloidosis**   In small intestinal disease. *2199*

279.06 **Immunodeficiency (Common Variable)**   In small intestinal disease. *2199*

340.00 **Multiple Sclerosis**   Malabsorption tests were studied in 52 patients. Fat and undigested meat fibers content were found to be abnormal in 41.6 and 40.9% respectively. *0938*

537.40 **Fistula of Stomach and Duodenum**   Excessively rapid passage of intestinal contents. Increased fat in feces with gastrocolic fistula. *0619*

555.90 **Regional Enteritis or Ileitis**   Deficient intraluminal bile acids. *2199*

557.01 **Mesenteric Artery Embolism**   Excessive fecal fat loss from recurrent ischemic damage to the intestinal mucosal function resulting in malabsorption. *1108*

Fat *(continued)*

Feces   Increase *(continued)*

558.90   Diarrhea   Excessively rapid passage of intestinal contents. With severe diarrhea. *0619*

564.20   Postgastrectomy (Dumping) Syndrome   Malabsorption from poor mixing and rapid transit. *0995*

571.90   Cirrhosis of Liver   May be excessive amounts of fecal fat. *2104*

576.20   Extrahepatic Biliary Obstruction   Deficient intraluminal bile acids. *2199*   May be excessive amounts of fecal fat. *2104*

577.10   Chronic Pancreatitis   The number and size of fecal fat globules correlate with the degree of steatorrhea. *0600*   Deficiency intraluminal pancreatic enzymes. *2199*

579.00   Celiac Sprue Disease   Due to allergy to gluten (wheat protein). *0619*   If the coefficient of fat absorption is < 93%, steatorrhea is present. *2199*   In small intestinal disease. *2199*

579.90   Malabsorption, Cause Unspecified   In malabsorption syndrome. *0151*   The number and size of fecal fat globules correlates with the degree of steatorrhea. *0600*

694.00   Dermatitis Herpetiformis   In small intestinal disease. *2199*

696.10   Psoriasis   Steatorrhea has been reported in association with psoriasis; degree correlated with extent of involvement. *2157 0743*

710.10   Progressive Systemic Sclerosis   Defects of multiple stages of digestion-absorption. *2199*

Sputum   Increase

829.00   Fracture of Bone   Fat globules found in sputum of some patients. *2468*

958.10   Fat Embolism   Fat globules found in sputum of some patients. *2468*

Fatty Acids, Free (FFA)

Serum   Decrease

272.52   Abetalipoproteinemia   Slightly diminished or at low normal concentrations. *1583 0095*

277.00   Cystic Fibrosis   Analyses of children with this disease have indicated a deficiency in essential fatty acids. Arachidonic acid was found only in trace amounts or was absent. *1987*   The oleate fatty acids increase while the linoleatic portion decreases. The basis for this seems to be that oleic and linoleic acid differ in changes in oxygen pressure. The oxygen complex of linoleic acid dissociates at relatively high pressures, whereas that of oleic dissociates only at low pressures. *0334*

571.49   Chronic Active Hepatitis   In 11 cases a depression of the essential fatty acid concentration (linoleic and arachidonic) was noted with concomitant elevation of oleic, palmitic, and palmitoleic acids. *0800*

585.00   Chronic Renal Failure   Elevated in acute renal failure, but normal or low in chronic failure. *1439*

994.50   Exercise   Approximately 15% decrease with bicycle pedalling. *0909*

Serum   Increase

227.91   Pheochromocytoma   Plasma insulin levels are inappropriately low and free fatty acids are correspondingly high. *0433*   May be elevated. *0962*

242.90   Hyperthyroidism   Increased lipid degradation. *2540*

250.00   Diabetes Mellitus   Marked elevation in circulating concentration due to release of fatty acids from fat stores. *2104*

253.00   Acromegaly   May be elevated because of decreased lipogenesis. *0962*

260.00   Protein Malnutrition   *0619*

271.01   Von Gierke's Disease   Due to hypoglycemia. *1086 2246*

278.00   Obesity   Increased turnover. *0996*   Significantly higher *0864*

281.00   Pernicious Anemia   In relapse, increased free fatty acid and triglyceride concentrations but decreased concentrations of total cholesterol, unesterified cholesterol and all examined phospholipid fractions. *2471*

303.00   Acute Alcoholic Intoxication   Increased following alcoholic binge of several days duration. *1594*

303.90   Alcoholism   Increased following alcoholic binge of several days duration. *1594*   Rises only after the acute ingestion of large doses of alcohol. *0962*

308.00   Stress   Normal response. *2315*   Fear, anxiety, or hostility elicit marked increases. *2104*

331.81   Reye's Syndrome   Commonly elevated. *0151*

333.40   Huntington's Chorea   High fasting concentrations. The elevation was maintained under hypoglycemic conditions, but not in hyperglycemic states. *1816*

410.90   Acute Myocardial Infarction   Maximum values occurred within 8 h after infarction. Patients with values > 1,200 μmol/L had increased prevalence of serious arrhythmias and disorder of conductance. *2185*   Tend to rise in the first 48 h. *0529*   May be partially related to pituitary-sympathoadrenal stimulation. Patients with higher plasma levels of catecholamines and free fatty acids may have a higher incidence of severe arrhythmias, shock, and death than patients with lower levels. *1108*   High values (> 1,000 μmol/L) were associated with an increased incidence of serious cardiac arrhythmias after infarction. *0937   1451*

571.49   Chronic Active Hepatitis   The pattern in 11 cases of hepatitis accompanied by jaundice showed elevated levels of oleic, palmitic, and palmitoleic acids attributed to the decreased ability of the liver to desaturate the endogenous saturated and monounsaturated acids to polyunsaturated ones. *0800*

572.20   Hepatic Encephalopathy   Significant elevation. *1733*   Short and medium chain fatty acids with lengths C5-C8 are often elevated in blood and CSF. *1473*   Plasma free fatty acids are commonly elevated. *0151*

584.00   Acute Renal Failure   Elevated in acute renal failure, but normal or low in chronic failure. *1439*

650.00   Pregnancy   Significant use in the 36th and 40th week of gestation. *2104*

829.00   Fracture of Bone   *2468*

958.10   Fat Embolism   Not of diagnostic value. *2467*

991.60   Hypothermia   Due to hypoxia, acid-base imbalance hypotension. *1471*

994.50   Exercise   Marked increase after strenuous exercise. *1109*   Following initial depression, concentrations gradually increase during exercise. *2104*

Serum   Normal

496.01   Alpha₁-Antitrypsin Deficiency   Normal. *0563*

758.00   Down's Syndrome   Plasma lipid levels were measured in 20 mongoloid and 16 nonmongoloid mentally retarded subjects. Significant elevations of plasma triglyceride levels were found in patients with Down's syndrome compared with mentally retarded controls. However, no significant difference was found in plasma cholesterol, phospholipid and free fatty acid concentrations between the mongoloids and control subjects. *1698*

CSF   Increase

572.20   Hepatic Encephalopathy   Short and medium chain fatty acids with lengths C5- C8 are often elevated in blood and CSF. *1473*

Fatty Casts

Urine   Increase

580.00   Acute Poststreptococcal Glomerulonephritis   May appear within the first few weeks. *0995*

580.02   Glomerulonephritis (Minimal Change)   Hyaline, granular, and fatty casts are found. *0151*

581.90   Nephrotic Syndrome   *0433*

Ferritin

Serum   Decrease

280.90   Iron Deficiency Anemia   Invariably reduced. *0999*   Concentration < 10 ng/mL is characteristic. The usefulness of the assay is limited by the fact that when iron deficiency and inflammatory disease coexist, concentration may be within the normal range. *2538*

579.00   Celiac Sprue Disease   The most discriminating test to distinguish between untreated celiac disease and other gastrointestinal disorders in the pediatric age group. *2229*

Serum Increase

162.90 Malignant Neoplasm of Bronchus and Lung Increased levels were found in more than 50% of patients. *0925*

174.90 Malignant Neoplasm of Breast In 107 patients with breast cancer; CEA, ferritin and calcitonin levels were measured. CEA and ferritin but not calcitonin levels were statistically higher in those patients with metastases. *0200*

180.90 Malignant Neoplasm of Cervix In 98 patients with untreated disease 51% had elevated serum levels. *1129*

201.90 Hodgkin's Disease Serum levels are raised due to increased production by splenic tumor tissue. *2047* A high circulating concentration is characteristic. *2538 1185* Significant elevation *2244*

202.80 Non-Hodgkins Lymphoma Significant elevation. *2244*

203.00 Multiple Myeloma Significant elevation. *2244*

204.00 Lymphocytic Leukemia (Acute) Significant elevation. *2244*

205.00 Myelocytic Leukemia (Acute) Significant elevation. *2244*

205.10 Myelocytic Leukemia (Chronic) Significant elevation. *2244*

275.00 Hemochromatosis Concentration was grossly raised in all 41 patients, ranging from 670-4,100 μg/L. *1850* Markedly increased due to gross increase in iron stores. *0141* Plasma concentration of > 1,000 ng/mL is indicative of increased body iron stores, although it does not differentiate between reticuloendothelial and parenchymal storage. Correlates well with iron stores in cirrhotic patients with primary disease. *2246 2538*

285.00 Sideroblastic Anemia *0186*

570.00 Acute and Subacute Necrosis of Liver Increased in acute hepatitis. Exceeded the upper limit of the normal values in most cases. *2624* Increased in acute hepatocellular damage due to acetaminophen overdosage. *0616*

706.10 Acne 19 of 24 males had increased levels. *1387*

714.30 Juvenile Rheumatoid Arthritis Markedly increased, ranging from 120-2000 μg/dL (mean = 822) compared to normals, 35-155 μg/dL. Fluctuations correlated closely with disease activity (R = 0.954, P < 0.05). *0463*

990.00 Effects of X-Ray Irradiation Occurs within 2 h of deep x-ray therapy. *0618*

Serum Normal

275.00 Hemochromatosis Normal or marginal elevation in the precirrhotic stage. *2246*

280.90 Iron Deficiency Anemia Concentration < 10 ng/mL is characteristic. The usefulness of the assay is limited by the fact that when iron deficiency and inflammatory disease coexist, concentration may be within the normal range. *2538*

282.42 Thalassemia Minor *0186*

Bone Marrow Absent

280.90 Iron Deficiency Anemia The amount is not as important diagnostically as presence or absence. The presence is strong evidence against the diagnosis of clinically significant iron deficiency. *0962*

Fibrinogen

Serum Increase

410.90 Acute Myocardial Infarction Significant increase. *1724*

Plasma Decrease

38.00 Septicemia May be associated with defibrination resulting in platelet and coagulation factor consumption in severe gram-positive septicemia. *2538*

54.00 Herpes Simplex May be associated with defibrination resulting in platelet and coagulation factor consumption. *2538*

65.00 Arthropod-Borne Hemorrhagic Fever Indicates occurrence of intravascular coagulation in dengue hemorrhagic fever patients experiencing shock. *0247* May be associated with defibrination resulting in platelet and coagulation factor consumption (Korean and Thai fever). *2538*

82.00 Rocky Mountain Spotted Fever May be associated with defibrination resulting in platelet and coagulation factor consumption. *2538* Hypofibrinogenemia in 2 of 5 cases with marked reduction of factor XII. *2589*

84.00 Malaria May be associated with defibrination resulting in platelet and coagulation factor consumption (overwhelming parasitemia). *2538*

197.00 Secondary Malignant Neoplasm of Respiratory System May be associated with defibrination resulting in platelet and coagulation factor consumption. *2538*

197.50 Secondary Malignant Neoplasm of Digestive System May be associated with defibrination resulting in platelet and coagulation factor consumption. *2538*

199.00 Secondary Malignant Neoplasm (Disseminated) May be associated with defibrination resulting in platelet and coagulation factor consumption. *2538*

205.00 Myelocytic Leukemia (Acute) Moderate depression occurs. *0619* Intravascular clotting has been documented in occasional patients. *0890*

205.10 Myelocytic Leukemia (Chronic) Moderate depression. *0619* Intravascular clotting has been documented for rare patients. *0890*

206.00 Monocytic Leukemia With disseminated intravascular clotting. *1552*

238.40 Polycythemia Vera Usually normal although a moderate decrease (115-200 mg/dL) was found in one study. *2491 2538*

267.00 Vitamin C Deficiency Moderate depression occurs in scurvy. *0619*

273.30 Waldenström's Macroglobulinemia A number of patients have reduced activity of one or more coagulation factors. *2538*

286.31 Congenital Dysfibrinogenemia Reduced level by any technique. The discordant values suggest that abnormal fibrinogen molecules are inhibitory to coagulation of the normal fibrinogen or have a markedly delayed clotting time and are present in sufficient concentration to give a falsely low level of fibrinogen. *2538* Concentration is usually normal or only slightly depressed, but is functionally defective. *2246*

286.34 Congenital Afibrinogenemia Undetectable by almost all physicochemical measurements or functional assays. *2538*

286.60 Disseminated Intravascular Coagulopathy Substantial depression of factor XIII concentrations developed together with concomitant significant increases in the proportion and concentration of plasma high molecular weight fibrinogen complexes (HMWFC). In inverse correlation between factor XIII and percentage of HMWFC was demonstrated in the of the illness. *1491* Low or falling levels. *0433 2538*

428.00 Congestive Heart Failure Decreased secondary to impaired liver function. *1108*

446.60 Thrombotic Thrombocytopenic Purpura *0556*

487.10 Influenza May be associated with defibrination resulting in platelet and coagulation factor consumption. *2538*

570.00 Acute and Subacute Necrosis of Liver Formation is depressed in liver failure, resulting in decreased plasma levels. *0619*

571.60 Biliary Cirrhosis Formation is depressed in liver failure, resulting in decreased plasma levels. *0619*

571.90 Cirrhosis of Liver Impaired hepatic synthesis. *0424*

572.20 Hepatic Encephalopathy Low levels of clotting factors found in fulminant hepatic failure are due to decrease in liver synthesis aggravated by increased consumption. *0821*

572.40 Hepatic Failure Low levels of clotting factors found in fulminant hepatic failure are due to decrease in liver synthesis aggravated by increased consumption. *0821*

630.00 Hydatidiform Mole Decreased as a result of excess utilization due to release of tissue thromboplastin. *0619* May be associated with defibrination resulting in platelet and coagulation factor consumption. *2538*

642.60 Eclampsia A serious complication. *1012*

785.50 Shock Decreased after severe shock during operation or after trauma, as a result of excessive utilization due to release of tissue thromboplastin. *0619*

948.00 Burns Falls during first 36 h, then rises steeply for up to 3 months. *2468*

989.50 Toxic Effects of Venom *0995*

992.00 Heat stroke Formation is moderately depressed in severe heat stroke. *0619*

994.50 Exercise Observed effect in exercise. *1839*

Fibrinogen (continued)

Plasma Increase

30.00 Leprosy Significant increases were noted in cases with lepra reaction, particularly those manifesting necrotizing skin, kidney, and sclerodermic lesions. *1878*

84.00 Malaria In 25 patients with acute renal failure due to falciparum malaria, marked increase in fibrinogen and fibrin degradation products were observed. The other coagulation parameters were within the normal limits. *2190*

135.00 Sarcoidosis Indicates active disease. *1964*

201.90 Hodgkin's Disease Increases with stage of disease. *2450*

204.00 Lymphocytic Leukemia (Acute) Frequently elevated when the disease is in relapse. The absolute levels vary considerably from individual to individual. *0270 2538*

205.10 Myelocytic Leukemia (Chronic) Either elevated or normal. *2318*

250.00 Diabetes Mellitus Significantly higher in both juvenile and maturity onset diabetics. *0149*

281.00 Pernicious Anemia Moderate depression of fibrinogen formation occurs. *0619*

390.00 Rheumatic Fever *0962*

410.90 Acute Myocardial Infarction Substantial depression of factor XIII developed with concomitant significant increases in the proportion and concentration of plasma high molecular weight fibrinogen complexes (HMWFC). An inverse correlation between factor XIII and percentage of HMWFC was demonstrated in the early stages of the illness. *1491*

415.10 Pulmonary Embolism and Infarction Implicated as a cause of intravascular thrombosis, but their role is neither clear nor constant. *1108 0347*

431.00 Cerebral Hemorrhage The greater the degree of initial neurological deficit the greater were plasma high molecular weight fibrinogen complex (HMWFC) values, which were associated with poor clinical outcome. Values were significantly higher in patients with intracerebral hemorrhage, subarachnoid hemorrhage and cerebral embolism. *0747*

434.00 Cerebral Thrombosis Significant increase was noted in cerebral thromboembolic stroke in young patients. *2127*

434.10 Cerebral Embolism The greater the degree of initial neurological deficit the greater were plasma high molecular weight fibrinogen complexes values, which were associated with poor clinical outcome. Values were significantly higher in patients with intracerebral hemorrhage, subarachnoid hemorrhage and cerebral embolism. *0747*

434.90 Brain Infarction High molecular weight fibrinogen complexes, native fibrinogen, alpha$_1$ antitrypsin and alpha$_2$ macroglobulin were significantly increased in cerebral infarction patients. *0747* Substantial depression of factor XIII concentrations developed together with concomitant significant increases in the proportion and concentration of plasma high molecular weight fibrinogen complexes (HMWFC). An inverse correlation between factor XIII and percentage of HMWFC was demonstrated in the early stages of the illness. *1491*

446.50 Cranial Arteritis and Related Conditions Parallels the rapid ESR. *2035*

570.00 Acute and Subacute Necrosis of Liver Patients with severe acute hepatic necrosis may have findings compatible with intravascular coagulation, thrombocytopenia and increased levels of fibrinogen/fibrin degradation products. *1048 2538*

581.90 Nephrotic Syndrome Plasma clotting factors, especially fibrinogen, have been elevated in many patients and returned to normal when remission was induced by adrenal corticosteroids. *1108 1396 2322*

585.00 Chronic Renal Failure Usually raised about 30%, resulting in characteristic rise of ESR. *0151*

642.40 Pre-Eclampsia Increased by about 70% and 145% in preeclampsia and eclampsia, respectively. *0380*

642.60 Eclampsia Increased by about 70% and 145% in preeclampsia and eclampsia, respectively. *0380*

650.00 Pregnancy Increases progressively as the pregnancy Moderately increased by 4th month; increased 33% by term. *2468* Rises from 0.38 g/dL to 0.58 g/dL. *1892*

694.40 Pemphigus *0151*

710.00 Systemic Lupus Erythematosus Frequently elevated. *0962*

714.00 Rheumatoid Arthritis Can be used to assess disease activity. *0619*

948.00 Burns Falls during the first 36 h and then rises steeply for up to 3 months. *2468*

990.00 Effects of X-Ray Irradiation Indicates tissue damage. *0618*

Plasma Normal

286.10 Christmas Disease *0186*

286.31 Congenital Dysfibrinogenemia In most cases determined by immunologic assays, fibrin tyrosine content, or gravimetric methods have been normal. *2538 0186*

286.40 Von Willebrand's Disease *0228*

335.20 Amyotrophic Lateral Sclerosis *0665*

571.20 Laennec's or Alcoholic Cirrhosis Fibrinolytic activity is significantly increased in advanced cirrhosis. Total fibrinogen concentration was normal. *1414*

571.49 Chronic Active Hepatitis Fibrinolytic activity is increased but total fibrinogen is normal. *1414*

571.90 Cirrhosis of Liver Fibrinolytic activity is significantly increased in advanced cirrhosis and chronic aggressive hepatitis. Total fibrinogen concentration was normal. *1414*

642.40 Pre-Eclampsia Levels of fibrinogen and of other clotting factors do not differ from those found in normal late pregnancy. *0806* In essential hypertension, the level remains more or less the same as in normal pregnancy. *0380 2538*

Liver Increase

642.40 Pre-Eclampsia Fibrin outlining the hepatic sinusoids was found in all 12 cases; in 2 of them there were also large nodular deposits of fibrin and to a lesser extent of IgG, IgM, and C3 in areas of necrosis. *0074*

Fibrinopeptide A

Plasma Increase

581.90 Nephrotic Syndrome Marked increase. *0996*

Fibrin Split Products (FSP)

Plasma Decrease

30.00 Leprosy In lepromatous leprosy. *1878*

286.60 Disseminated Intravascular Coagulopathy Deposition of fibrin usually stimulates local secondary fibrinolysis producing reduced circulating plasminogen level due to consumption and a decrease in systemic fibrinolytic activity. *2538*

434.00 Cerebral Thrombosis A decrease in fibrinolytic activity was noticed. *0112*

642.40 Pre-Eclampsia Plasma fibrinolytic activity may be more depressed than in normal pregnancy. *0250 2538*

Plasma Increase

38.00 Septicemia Raised levels are common with other evidence of enhanced fibrinolysis. *1253* Elevation is much more common in fatal cases than in survivors. *2193*

47.00 Aseptic Meningitis Elevation is much more common in fatal cases than in survivors. *2193*

65.00 Arthropod-Borne Hemorrhagic Fever Indicates occurrence of intravascular coagulation in Dengue hemorrhagic fever patients experiencing shock. *0247*

84.00 Malaria In 25 patients with acute renal failure due to falciparum malaria, marked increase in plasma fibrinogen and elevation of serum fibrin degradation products were observed. The other coagulation parameters were within the normal limits. *2190*

157.90 Malignant Neoplasm of Pancreas *1253*

185.00 Malignant Neoplasm of Prostate Especially with metastases. *1253* Fibrinolysins are found in 12% of patients. *2468*

205.00 Myelocytic Leukemia (Acute) Intravascular clotting has been documented in occasional patients. *0890*

205.10 Myelocytic Leukemia (Chronic) Intravascular clotting has been documented for rare patients. *0890*

206.00 Monocytic Leukemia With disseminated intravascular clotting. *1552*

286.60 Disseminated Intravascular Coagulopathy If large amounts are present, the thrombin time will be markedly prolonged; latex agglutination test for fibrin degradation products will be positive. *2538*

287.30 Idiopathic Thrombocytopenic Purpura During the acute stage in this series. *1666*

410.90 Acute Myocardial Infarction Clinical severity of infarction is related to the degree of elevation. Mortality rate was 22% among patients with values 20 μg/dL and 11% in those < 20 μg/dL. *1728*

415.10 Pulmonary Embolism and Infarction 42% of 24 patients suspected of acute thrombophlebitis and 50% of 14 patients with documented pulmonary emboli had positive fibrinogen tests. *0347*

451.90 Phlebitis and Thrombophlebitis 42% of 24 patients suspected of acute thrombophlebitis had positive fibrinogen tests. *0347*

482.90 Bacterial Pneumonia Elevation is much more common in fatal cases than in survivors in acute respiratory infection. *2193*

570.00 Acute and Subacute Necrosis of Liver Patients with severe acute hepatic necrosis may have findings compatible with intravascular coagulation, thrombocytopenia and increased levels of fibrinogen/fibrin degradation products. *1048 2538*

571.20 Laennec's or Alcoholic Cirrhosis Fibrinolytic activity is significantly increased in advanced cirrhosis. Total fibrinogen concentration was normal. *1414*

571.49 Chronic Active Hepatitis Significantly increased. *1414*

571.90 Cirrhosis of Liver Fibrinolytic activity is significantly increased in advanced cirrhosis and chronic aggressive hepatitis. Total fibrinogen concentration was normal. *1414 1048 2538*

580.00 Acute Poststreptococcal Glomerulonephritis Increased (> 10 μg/mL) in 28% of acute cases. Mean value was 8.4 ± 5.6 μg/mL (Normal = 3.2 ± 1.2 μg/mL). *1325* Raised serum or urine levels are common without other evidence of enhanced fibrinolysis. *1253*

584.00 Acute Renal Failure In 25 patients with acute failure due to falciparum malaria, marked increase in plasma fibrinogen fibrin degradation products were observed. The other coagulation parameters were within the normal limits. *2190*

585.00 Chronic Renal Failure Elevated levels (> 10 μg/mL) occurred in 73% of chronic nephritic patients. Mean value was 16.0 ± 5.9 μg/mL. *1325*

599.00 Urinary Tract Infection Elevation is much more common in fatal cases than in survivors. *2193*

630.00 Hydatidiform Mole Increased circulating amounts with associated prolonged thrombin time indicate hypercoagulability. *1430*

642.40 Pre-Eclampsia Suggest that slow, chronic, intravascular clotting is taking place. *2538* Elevated levels (> 10 μg/mL) occurred in all patients. Mean level was 35 μg/mL. *1325*

710.00 Systemic Lupus Erythematosus Elevated levels (> 10 μgl/mL) occurred in 100% of lupus nephritis patients. Mean value was 21.4 ± 7.6 μg/mL. *1325*

785.50 Shock Raised serum or urine levels are common without other evidence of enhanced fibrinolysis. *1253*

994.50 Exercise Observed effect in exercise. *1176*

Urine   Increase

188.90 Malignant Neoplasm of Bladder A high degree of accuracy (90%) was found in correlating cytology and urinary fibrinogen degradation products with the activity of the disease. *2455*

250.00 Diabetes Mellitus With diabetic nephropathy the greater the degree of proteinuria the greater the loss of fibrinogen degradation product in the urine. *0365*

580.00 Acute Poststreptococcal Glomerulonephritis Raised serum or urine levels are common without other evidence of enhanced fibrinolysis. *1253*

581.90 Nephrotic Syndrome The greater the degree of proteinuria the greater the level of fibrinogen degradation product in the urine. *0365*

785.50 Shock Raised serum or urine levels are common without other evidence of enhanced fibrinolysis. *1253*

Ascitic Fluid   Increase

155.00 Malignant Neoplasm of Liver In malignant effusions. *2199*

155.10 Malignant Neoplasm of Intrahepatic Bile Ducts In malignant effusions. *2199*

157.90 Malignant Neoplasm of Pancreas In malignant effusions. *2199*

183.00 Malignant Neoplasm of Ovary In malignant effusions. *2199*

189.00 Malignant Neoplasm of Kidney In malignant effusions. *2199*

197.70 Secondary Malignant Neoplasm of Liver In malignant effusions. *2199*

FIGLU (N-Formiminoglutamic Acid)

Urine   Increase

260.00 Protein Malnutrition Increased in some cases of marasmus. *2467*

269.90 Deficiency State (Unspecified) Some patients. *2467*

281.00 Pernicious Anemia Increased urinary formiminoglutamate after an oral histidine load. *0433*

281.20 Folic Acid Deficiency Anemia Urine FIGLU is increased; disappears after folic acid treatment in megaloblastic anemia of infancy. *2467* Less specific than the serum folate assay. It becomes abnormal later and thus gives a better measure of tissue coenzyme levels. *2538* Increased excretion is a consistent feature of folate deficiency but is not confined to that situation. *0962*

282.00 Hereditary (Congenital) Spherocytosis *2467*

570.00 Acute and Subacute Necrosis of Liver *2467*

650.00 Pregnancy Increased in pregnancy, especially with toxemia and increased age, parity, and multiple pregnancy. *2467*

Folate

Serum   Decrease

40.20 Whipple's Disease In some cases. *2199*

199.00 Secondary Malignant Neoplasm (Disseminated) Decreased with extensive skin disease. *0299 2357 0367*

244.90 Hypothyroidism May occur. *2540*

260.00 Protein Malnutrition *2468*

267.00 Vitamin C Deficiency Decreased. *0299 2357 0367*

272.52 Abetalipoproteinemia Secondary to malabsorption of fat. *2030*

277.22 Lesch-Nyhan Syndrome Decreased. *0299 2357 0367*

281.20 Folic Acid Deficiency Anemia Low; < 4 ng/mL. *0999* When intake is reduced, the serum level falls promptly and precedes evidence of tissue deficiency. *0962*

281.30 Vitamin B$_6$ Deficiency Anemia Reported to be low in about 80% of patients. *1462 2538*

282.20 Anemias Due To Disorders of Glutathione Metabolism Excessive utilization due to marked cellular proliferation. *2467*

282.42 Thalassemia Minor Reflects increased marrow utilization of folate. *0186*

283.00 Acquired Hemolytic Anemia (Autoimmune) Decreased with extensive skin disease. *0299 2357 0367*

285.00 Sideroblastic Anemia Reported to be low in about 80% of patients. *1462 2538*

289.80 Myelofibrosis Macrocytic anemia was reported in over 50% of the patients, the probable cause was folic acid deficiency secondary to chronic excessive cell proliferation (in myelofibrosis). *1059* Decrease with extensive skin disease *0299 2357 0367 2538*

345.90 Epilepsy Reduced in 33 of 68 institutionalized patients with severe epilepsy. *0514*

555.90 Regional Enteritis or Ileitis Decreased with extensive skin disease. *0299 2357 0367* Deficiency may result in anemia *0532*

556.00 Ulcerative Colitis May be the cause of anemia. *0433*

570.00 Acute and Subacute Necrosis of Liver Decreased in some cases of liver disease due to inadequate intake. *2467*

579.00 Celiac Sprue Disease Patients may show a megaloblastic anemia and leukopenia secondary to folic acid or vitamin B$_{12}$ deficiency. In these instances low serum folate and B$_{12}$ levels will be found. *0433* Folic acid deficiency occurring in idiopathic steatorrhea (up to 80 mg/h). *2467 0151*

579.90 Malabsorption, Cause Unspecified Particularly in small bowel disease. *0151* Macrocytic anemia may occur due to vitamin B$_{12}$ or folate deficiency. MCV > 100 fL. *0532*

650.00 Pregnancy *2538*

696.10 Psoriasis Decreased with extensive skin disease. *0299 2357 0367*

Folate *(continued)*

Serum   Decrease *(continued)*

758.00   Down's Syndrome   Mean serum folate was normal in this group, these individuals displayed decreasing concentrations with age. *0828*

Serum   Increase

70.00   Viral Hepatitis   Increased. *0741 0866*

281.00   Pernicious Anemia   Normal or high. *0999*

Red Blood Cells   Decrease

281.20   Folic Acid Deficiency Anemia   A better measure of tissue folate and is less dependent on recent intake than serum. *0962*

758.00   Down's Syndrome   Red cell values were very low. *0828*

Follicle Stimulating Hormone (FSH)

Serum   Decrease

253.40   Anterior Pituitary Hypofunction   Characterized by absent or reduced production and release. *1108*   Compatible with stage of sexual development, not with age. *0399*

256.41   Stein-Leventhal Syndrome   *0151*

275.00   Hemochromatosis   Frequently occurs in idiopathic hemochromatosis. *2473*

282.60   Sickle Cell Anemia   Consistent with primary testicular failure in all 14 adult male patients tested. *0005*

Serum   Increase

303.90   Alcoholism   48 male chronic alcoholics classified in 2 groups according to the presence (22) or absence (26) of clinically evident sexual disorders. The level was significantly higher in the group with sexual disorders. *2169*

627.90   Menopausal and Postmenopausal Symptoms   *0433*

758.70   Klinefelter's Syndrome (XXY)   Commonly elevated; a result of deficient testicular function. *1090*   Always increased as a result of the extensive tubular disease. *0151*

758.80   Syndromes Due to Sex Chromosome Abnormalities   In Turner's syndrome. *2467   2468*

Serum   Normal

650.00   Pregnancy   Upper end of normal range. *0690*

Urine   Decrease

183.00   Malignant Neoplasm of Ovary   *0211*

194.00   Malignant Neoplasm of Adrenal Gland   *0211*

220.00   Benign Neoplasm of Ovary   Inhibited by increased estrogen. *2467*

220.92   Granulosa Cell Tumor of Ovary   Inhibited by increased estrogen. *2467*

220.93   Lutein Cell Tumor of Ovary   Inhibited by increased estrogen. *2467*

220.94   Theca Cell Tumor of Ovary   Inhibited by increased estrogen. *2467*

Urine   Increase

186.90   Malignant Neoplasm of Testis   Increased with seminoma. *0619*

275.34   Familial Periodic Paralysis   During attack. *0362*

758.70   Klinefelter's Syndrome (XXY)   *0619*

758.80   Syndromes Due to Sex Chromosome Abnormalities   In Turner's syndrome. *0619*

CSF   Increase

194.30   Malignant Neoplasm of Pituitary   21 of 22 patients with suprasellar extension of a pituitary tumor had elevations of one or more CSF adenohypophyseal hormones. *1189*

Frei Test

Skin   Positive

99.10   Lymphogranuloma Venereum   Diagnostic skin test. A 6 mm nodule with surrounding erythema 48 h after intradermal injection is positive reaction. *2368*   May be up to 60% false-negative reactions even in established cases. *2060*

Fructose

Serum   Increase

271.20   Hereditary Fructose Intolerance   Noted with the chronic syndrome found in young children and after fructose administration in adults. *2246*

Urine   Increase

271.20   Hereditary Fructose Intolerance   Noted with the chronic syndrome found in young children and after fructose administration in adults. *2246*

984.00   Toxic Effects of Lead and Its Compounds (including Fumes)   Occurs as a result of changes in the epithelium of the proximal convoluted tubules. *0151*

Fucose

Serum   Increase

151.90   Malignant Neoplasm of Stomach   Total concentration was increased in patients with both malignant and benign tumors of breast, lung and stomach. The glycoprotein-bound fraction was markedly elevated in cases of malignancy and not in benign disease. Mucoprotein fraction was raised in both diseases. *2331* Mean value = 13.52 ± 0.65 in 35 patients. (normal = 6.84 ± 0.13 mg/dL). *1342*

153.90   Malignant Neoplasm of Large Intestine   In 17 patients, mean value was 11.79 ± 0.72 (normal = 6.84 ± 0.13 mg/dL). *1342*

155.00   Malignant Neoplasm of Liver   Markedly increased. *1342*

157.90   Malignant Neoplasm of Pancreas   Markedly increased. *1342*

162.90   Malignant Neoplasm of Bronchus and Lung   Increased in patients with both malignant and benign tumors of breast, lung and stomach. The glycoprotein-bound fraction was very markedly elevated in cases of malignancy and not in benign disease. Mucoprotein fraction was raised in both diseases. *2331*   In 15 patients, mean = 15.98 ± 1.43. Normal value = 6.84 ± 0.13 mg/dL. *1342*

174.90   Malignant Neoplasm of Breast   Increased in patients with both malignant and benign tumors of breast, lung and stomach. The glycoprotein-bound fraction was very markedly elevated in cases of malignancy and not in benign disease. Mucoprotein fraction was raised in both diseases. *2331*   Mean elevation in 15 cases was 11.12 ± 0.68 (normal = 6.84 ± 0.13 mg/dL). Elevation was less significant in early and locally restricted breast cancer. *1342*

180.90   Malignant Neoplasm of Cervix   Markedly elevated and correlated with clinical stage of disease. Values ranged from 12.2-32.2 mg/dL. *0607*

193.01   Medullary Carcinoma of Thyroid   Elevation was less significant in early and locally restricted disease. Mean value was 10.36 ± 0.41 (normal = 6.48 ± 0.13 mg/dL). *1342*

199.00   Secondary Malignant Neoplasm (Disseminated)   Markedly increased. *1342*

201.90   Hodgkin's Disease   Markedly elevated and correlated with clinical stage of disease. Values ranged from 13 mg/dL in stage 1 to 29.5 mg/dL in stage 4. *0607*

202.80   Non-Hodgkins Lymphoma   Markedly elevated and correlated with clinical stage of disease. Values ranged from 13 mg/dL in stage 1 to 29.5 mg/dL in stage 4. *0607*

211.10   Benign Neoplasm of Stomach   Total concentration was increased in patients with both malignant and benign tumors. The glycoprotein-bound fraction was very markedly elevated in cases of malignancy and not in benign disease. Mucoprotein fraction was raised in both diseases. *2331*

217.00   Benign Neoplasm of Breast   Total concentration was increased in patients with both malignant and benign tumors. The glycoprotein-bound fraction was very markedly elevated in cases of malignancy and not in benign disease. Mucoprotein fraction was raised in both diseases. *2331*

Galactose

Serum   Increase

271.10   Galactosemia   Galactosemia (equal to total reducing sugar minus glucose oxidase sugar) with galactosemia. *2468 1067 2246*

Urine   Increase

271.10   Galactosemia   Galactosuria--detected by nonspecific reducing tests; identified by chromatography with galactosemia. *2468*   May be intermittent. *1067 2246*

Gamma Globulin

Serum   Increase

421.00   Bacterial Endocarditis   *2488*

711.10   Mixed Connective Tissue Disease   Diffuse hypergammaglobulinemia. *0062*

CSF   Increase

45.90   Acute Poliomyelitis   Especially IgG. *0186*

97.90   Syphilis   In active disease. *2174*

Pericardial Fluid   Increase

714.00   Rheumatoid Arthritis   Gamma Globulin complexes found to be present in Rheumatoid Pericarditis. *0107*

Gamma Glutamyl Transferase (GGT)

Serum   Increase

6.00   Amebiasis   With liver involvement. *1058*

18.00   Disseminated Tuberculosis   In 5 patients with liver granulomas, including miliary tuberculosis and sarcoidosis, serum GGT levels were all elevated, mean = 303, range = 116-740 U/L. *1452*

39.90   Actinomycosis   Liver involvement. *1058*

70.00   Viral Hepatitis   The mean elevation (152 U/L) in 17 patients was 5.2 X the upper limit of normal. *1452*   In 77% of 14 patients at initial hospitalization for this disorder. *0781*

73.90   Psittacosis   With severe liver involvement. *0433*

75.00   Infectious Mononucleosis   Levels correlate with serum alkaline phosphatase and 5'-nucleotidase levels. *0619*

104.10   Lyme Disease   With liver involvement. *1503*

115.00   Histoplasmosis   In 5 patients with liver granulomas, including miliary tuberculosis and sarcoidosis, serum GGT levels were all elevated, mean = 303, range = 116-740 U/L. *1452*

120.00   Schistosomiasis   In 5 patients with liver granulomas, including miliary tuberculosis and sarcoidosis, serum GGT levels were all elevated, mean = 303, range = 116-740 U/L. *1452*

122.90   Hydatidosis   With liver involvement. *1058*

135.00   Sarcoidosis   In 5 patients with liver granulomas, including miliary tuberculosis and sarcoidosis, serum GGT levels were all elevated, mean = 303, range = 116-740 U/L. *1452*

155.00   Malignant Neoplasm of Liver   *0503*

157.90   Malignant Neoplasm of Pancreas   Greatest in cases of primary carcinoma of the head of the pancreas and adenocarcinoma of bile duct. In 4 patients range was 264-1,040 U/L, mean = 590. *1452*   In 100% of 10 patients at initial hospitalization for this disorder. *0781*

174.90   Malignant Neoplasm of Breast   In 49% of 41 patients at initial hospitalization for this disorder. *0781*

185.00   Malignant Neoplasm of Prostate   In 48% of 12 patients at initial hospitalization for this disorder. *0781*

189.00   Malignant Neoplasm of Kidney   *1739*

191.90   Malignant Neoplasm of Brain   Elevated preoperatively in 13 of 23 patients. Those showing elevations included 7 of 13 patients with astrocytomas, grades I-IV, 4 of 6 patients with metastatic brain tumors, and 2 of 4 patients with cerebral meningiomas. *0684*

197.00   Secondary Malignant Neoplasm of Respiratory System   In 62% of 106 patients at initial hospitalization for this disorder. *0781*

197.70   Secondary Malignant Neoplasm of Liver   Parallels alkaline phosphatase; elevation precedes positive liver scans. *2467*   Marked elevations were observed in 12 patients. Mean 396 U/L was 13.2 X the normal upper limit (range = 208-820). *1452*

198.50   Secondary Malignant Neoplasm of Bone   In 4 patients with carcinoma metastatic to bone, 25% (1) had a slightly elevated concentration (54 U/L). *1452*

201.90   Hodgkin's Disease   Elevated in 36% (4 of 11) patients. *0160*   In 73% of 12 patients at initial hospitalization for this disorder. *0781*

202.80   Non-Hodgkins Lymphoma   In 67% of 16 patients at initial hospitalization for this disorder. *0781*

245.10   Subacute Thyroiditis   Elevated in 3 patients, suggesting hepatic origin of the enzymes. *0489*

250.00   Diabetes Mellitus   A study of 228 patients has shown a significant positive association between serum GGT and triglyceride levels. Both fall with treatment, the most marked reduction occurring in patients on insulin. This association may reflect hepatic triglyceride levels in new diabetics may reflect hepatic microsomal enzyme induction of the rate-limiting enzymes of triglyceride synthesis. Serum GGT does not seem to correlate with hepatomegaly in diabetes mellitus. *1517*   In 50% of 20 patients at initial hospitalization for this disorder. *0781   0876*

272.10   Type IV Hyperlipoproteinemia   Both GGT and pseudocholinesterase were increased in hypertriglyceridemic subjects. Both strongly correlated with the logarithm of serum triglyceride and the prebeta electrophoretic fraction. Increase of GGT was rather characteristic for gross hypertriglyceridemia. *0480*

272.72   Gaucher's Disease   May be abnormal with liver involvement. *0995*

275.00   Hemochromatosis   With liver involvement. *0962*

275.10   Hepatolenticular Degeneration   With liver involvement. *0995*

303.90   Alcoholism   In 5 cases of chronic alcoholism, range 27-850 U/L. The highest activities were seen in the patients with the most extensive hepatic damage. *1452*   69% of 182 male chronic alcoholics had increased GGT activities. Highest values were found in patients with 5-20 y of alcoholism. Patients with > 20 y duration had a tendency toward normalization of enzyme activity. *2196*

340.00   Multiple Sclerosis   6 of 33 patients had concentrations elevated above normal (40 U/L). *0684*

345.90   Epilepsy   Elevated in the sera of 64 of 75 patients (85.4%) with epilepsy. Enzyme activity usually remains at a constant level, characteristic of the patients, with some peaks and depressions in activity. *0684*

410.90   Acute Myocardial Infarction   Usually remains in the normal range for 3-4 days, then increases to reach a peak about the 8-11th day after infarction. *0684*   Activity is raised in association with anoxic damage to the liver, and also in association with recovery and repair. *0619*   Increased in 50% of patients with shock or acute right heart failure, may have early peak within 48 h with rapid decline followed by later rise. *2467   0439 0675*

413.90   Angina Pectoris   *1016*

428.00   Congestive Heart Failure   Due to anoxic damage to the liver. *0619*   All 9 patients had elevated activity, secondary to hepatic damage. Mean = 180, range = 58-568 U/L. *1452*

496.01   Alpha₁-Antitrypsin Deficiency   Related to liver disease. *1636*

555.90   Regional Enteritis or Ileitis   In the presence of pericholangitis. *2199   0619*

556.00   Ulcerative Colitis   Increased with associated liver damage and correlates with other liver enzymes. *0619   0433*

570.00   Acute and Subacute Necrosis of Liver   The estimation may be useful in monitoring duration of the disease, since raised activity persists longer than do ALT or AST activities. *0619*   In acute hepatitis, elevation is less marked than that of other liver enzymes, but it is the last to return to normal. *2467   0503*

571.20   Laennec's or Alcoholic Cirrhosis   Increases with liver damage. *0619*

571.49   Chronic Active Hepatitis   In 90% of 10 patients at initial hospitalization for this disorder. *0781*

571.60   Biliary Cirrhosis   Elevation is marked. *2467*

571.90   Cirrhosis of Liver   In inactive cases, average values are lower than in chronic hepatitis. Increases > 10-20 X in cirrhotic patients suggest superimposed primary carcinoma of the liver. *2467*   In 5 patients with cirrhosis of liver, the mean GGT elevation (132) was 4.4 X the normal upper limit. *1452*   In 79% of 34 patients at initial hospitalization for this disorder. *0781*

Gamma Glutamyl Transferase (GGT)
(continued)

Serum Increase *(continued)*

572.00 Liver Abscess (Pyogenic) In 5 patients with liver granulomas, including miliary tuberculosis and sarcoidosis, serum GGT levels were all elevated, mean = 303, range = 116-740 U/L. *1452*

573.30 Toxic Hepatitis Raised enzyme activity may be the only evidence of moderate liver damage due to drugs. *0619*

575.00 Acute Cholecystitis In 8 patients, the mean (210 U/L) was 7.0 X the normal upper limit. *1452*

576.10 Cholangitis A mean elevation of 249 U/L (8.3 X normal maximum) was found in 13 patients. *1452*

576.20 Extrahepatic Biliary Obstruction Increased with obstructive jaundice. *0619* Increase is faster and greater than that of serum alkaline phosphatase and LAP. *2467*

577.00 Acute Pancreatitis Always elevated. *2467* Was elevated to a mean level of 300 U/L (10 X normal) in all 10 cases. *1452 2010*

577.10 Chronic Pancreatitis Increased when there is involvement of the biliary tract or active inflammation. *2467 2010*

581.90 Nephrotic Syndrome *1739*

714.00 Rheumatoid Arthritis In a series of 20 patients with RA and without prior causes of hepatic damage. Elevated in 55% of patients. *2625*

Serum Normal

275.00 Hemochromatosis Over 50% of patients have no laboratory evidence of liver dysfunction. *0995*

Urine Decrease

189.00 Malignant Neoplasm of Kidney The only renal disorder to demonstrate a decreased value in urine. *1005*

Saliva Increase

155.00 Malignant Neoplasm of Liver Significantly higher (10.4 units/L) versus controls (5.12 U/L). *1164*

250.10 Diabetic Acidosis Significantly higher (11.6 U/L) versus controls (5.12 U/L). *1164*

571.90 Cirrhosis of Liver Significantly higher (8.3 units/L) versus normal controls (5.12 U/L). *1164*

575.00 Acute Cholecystitis Significantly higher (18.3 U/L) versus controls (5.12 U/L). *1164*

577.00 Acute Pancreatitis Significantly higher (15.1 U/L) versus controls (5.12 U/L). *1164*

710.20 Sjögren's Syndrome Significantly higher (19.6 U/L) versus controls (5.12 U/L). *1164*

Saliva Normal

70.00 Viral Hepatitis Infectious Hepatitis. *1164*

72.00 Mumps *1164*

Gastrin

Serum Decrease

244.90 Hypothyroidism Mean fasting plasma level was 64 ± 5 pg/mL compared to normal, 89 ± 4 pg/mL. No correlation was found between gastrin and any other parameters of thyroid function. *2121*

Serum Increase

151.90 Malignant Neoplasm of Stomach Found to be normal in 26 patients with gastric cancer. Elevated levels may occur in some patients, due to the accompanying atrophy of the oxyntic glands. *1130*

227.91 Pheochromocytoma In a few patients, elevated concentrations have become normal after tumor resection. *2199*

242.90 Hyperthyroidism Mean fasting levels in untreated hyperthyroid patients was 356 ± 26 pg/mL, (normal = 89 ± 4 pg/mL). No correlation was apparent between gastrin level and any parameter of thyroid function. *2108*

251.50 Zollinger-Ellison Syndrome Significant correlation between basal levels and malignant gastrinoma but not with benign tumors. *2244* Concentrations reach 2,800-300,000 pg/mL associated with non-insulin producing pancreatic tumors *0619*

252.00 Hyperparathyroidism Elevated in patients without ulcer and fell to normal after parathyroidectomy. *2277* Mean preoperative concentration in 18 uncomplicated patients was 122 ± 39 pg/mL. *0545* Patients may be hypergastrinemic. Some of these patients also have gastric hypersecretion. In these the hypergastrinemia can be consider pathologic. *2199* Gastrin levels above normal occurred in 22% of patients with primary hyperparathyroidism *2606*

281.00 Pernicious Anemia High level may approach that in the Zollinger-Ellison Syndrome. *2467* Concentration in the serum is high, probably because of the high pH within the lumen of the stomach. *0999* May be due to G cell hyperplasia in the pyloric antral mucosa. *1382 1534*

533.90 Peptic Ulcer, Site Unspecified Tends to be elevated in gastric ulcer and correlates with decreased acid secretion. *0151* May occur after meals. *1533*

535.00 Gastritis Increased in chronic atrophic gastritis. *2281* The combination of high serum gastrin and low pepsinogen is commonly found in patients with atrophic gastritis. *2199 2033*

571.90 Cirrhosis of Liver Mean fasting concentration was elevated (41.6 ± 3.1 pmol/L) compared to normal (26.3 ± 3.4 pmol/L) in cirrhotic patients. *1341*

584.00 Acute Renal Failure In both acute and chronic failure. *0546*

585.00 Chronic Renal Failure Elevated; no apparent correlation with calcitonin levels. *1368* In both acute and chronic failure. *1302*

714.00 Rheumatoid Arthritis Patients tend to have higher than normal serum concentration. There appears to be poor correlation with acid secretion. *1973 2199*

Serum Normal

151.90 Malignant Neoplasm of Stomach Found to be normal in 26 patients with gastric cancer. Elevated levels may occur in some patients, due to the accompanying atrophy of the oxyntic glands. *1130*

533.90 Peptic Ulcer, Site Unspecified Fasting concentration is generally normal despite hypersecretion of gastric acid. May occur after meals. *1533* Fasting serum concentrations are normal in patients with ordinary duodenal ulcer disease. Although the mean increase in concentration after a meal is higher in duodenal ulcer than in normal subjects, this test is not helpful diagnostically. *2199*

Globulin

Serum Decrease

60.00 Yellow Fever Decreased percentage during the course of the disease. *1750*

201.90 Hodgkin's Disease Infrequent. Concentrations < 200 mg/dL are rarely documented. *1061* Rare occasions. *1060*

202.80 Non-Hodgkins Lymphoma In patients with advanced disease, reduction in serum protein concentration with hypoalbuminemia and hypogammaglobulinemia is frequent. *2462 2538*

203.00 Multiple Myeloma *0615*

204.00 Lymphocytic Leukemia (Acute) *2467*

204.10 Lymphocytic Leukemia (Chronic) Concentration of 0.7-0.8 g/dL are common in early and uncomplicated disease. As disease advances, may fall to 0.3-0.4 g/dL, at which time patients become vulnerable to infections. *2399 2538 0692*

255.00 Adrenal Cortical Hyperfunction (Glucocorticoid Excess) May be decreased. *2468*

260.00 Protein Malnutrition Minimal reduction. *0995*

273.23 Heavy Chain Disease (Gamma) Almost absent on electrophoresis. *2467* In 50% of patients the concentration of the anomalous protein is > 2.0 g/dL and marked hypogammaglobulinemia is present. *2538*

277.30 Amyloidosis In 25% of patients. *1334* Hypogammaglobulinemia was found in patients with Bence-Jones proteinuria but not in any other patients. *0125* A low Albumin and globulin profile *0433*

279.04 Agammaglobulinemia (Congenital Sex-linked) The total serum globulins are decreased (100-200 mg/dL). Paper electrophoresis of serum shows complete absence of gamma globulins. *0433* Serum contains < 100 mg gamma G globulin/dL. Gamma A & M globulins are present in concentrations < 1% of normal *2246*

279.06 Immunodeficiency (Common Variable) *2467*

334.80 Ataxia-Telangiectasia May be decreased, resulting in increased susceptibility to infection. *0999*

359.21 Myotonia Atrophica *2618*

494.00 Bronchiectasis Seen when chronic uncontrolled infection persists. *0433* May be increased with chronic infection or decreased if congenital agammaglobulinemia is the underlying disease. *0999*

555.90 Regional Enteritis or Ileitis May be elevated in some patients but are normal or low in others. *2199*

570.00 Acute and Subacute Necrosis of Liver Alpha and beta globulins decrease when hepatocellular failure impairs their synthesis. *0151*

579.00 Celiac Sprue Disease May be diminished owing to excessive leakage of serum protein into the gut lumen. *2199*

579.01 Protein-Losing Enteropathy In protein-losing enteropathies. *2467*

581.90 Nephrotic Syndrome *2468*

642.40 Pre-Eclampsia Significantly reduced below the levels for normal pregnancy. *0433*

642.60 Eclampsia Significantly reduced below the levels for normal pregnancy. *0433*

650.00 Pregnancy May decrease slightly in last trimester. *2468* Falls about 0.1 g/dL. *2533* *2286 2287*

Serum Increase

2.00 Typhoid Fever Moderate hypergammaglobulinemia, especially IgA. *0880* *2035*

11.00 Pulmonary Tuberculosis Advanced pulmonary and extrapulmonary tuberculosis. *2104*

13.00 Tuberculosis Meningitis Advanced pulmonary and extrapulmonary tuberculosis. *2104*

18.00 Disseminated Tuberculosis *0999*

30.00 Leprosy In 50 cases of leprosy, (10 tuberculoid, 25 lepromatous leprosy, 10 lepra reaction, 5 dimorphic leprosy, all showed a rise). *2045* Lepromatous leprosy. *2104* Often present *0962*

32.00 Diphtheria May occur *0433* .

38.00 Septicemia Increased in 6 cases of extrahepatic sepsis. *1681*

52.00 Chickenpox May be increased. *2468*

70.00 Viral Hepatitis Mean total serum values were highest in acute viral hepatitis, primary hepatocellular carcinoma and cirrhosis, in that order. *0724* Frequent transiently elevated *0962*

73.90 Psittacosis Often associated with hypergammaglobulinemia. *2104*

75.00 Infectious Mononucleosis Often associated with hypergammaglobulinemia. *2104*

80.00 Epidemic Typhus Often associated with hypergammaglobulinemia. *2104*

84.00 Malaria Often associated with hypergammaglobulinemia. *2104* Especially euglobulin fraction *2468* *1058*

85.00 Leishmaniasis Increased with reversed A/G ratio. *2468* Often associated with hypergammaglobulinemia *2104*

86.90 Trypanosomiasis *1058*

97.90 Syphilis All 3 stages. *2104*

99.10 Lymphogranuloma Venereum Are increased with reversed A/G ratio A common finding during active infection. Often reversal of the albumin:globulin ratio. *0962* Elevated with a reversal of the A/G ratio. In such cases, the increase occurs in the alpha₂ and gamma globulin regions. *0433* Often associated with hypergammaglobulinemia *2104* *2199*

99.30 Reiter's Disease Increased in long-standing disease. *2468*

100.00 Leptospirosis May occur with jaundice after the 1st week of fever. *2368*

115.00 Histoplasmosis Levels > 3.0 g/dL occur in 50% of patients with disseminated disease. *0999* Often associated with Hypergammaglobulinemia *2104*

116.00 Blastomycosis Slightly increased. *2468*

120.00 Schistosomiasis Significant increase throughout the course of the disease. The increase in gamma globulin, the main isoenzyme causing the total elevation, may be due to the parasite's presence. The increase in gamma globulin, the main isoenzyme causing the total elevation may be due to the parasite's presence *2026* May be Present *2199*

124.00 Trichinosis Increase in relative and absolute concentrations parallels titer of serologic tests and of thymol turbidity. The increase occurs between 5-8 weeks and may last 6 months or more. *2468* Often associated with hypergammaglobulinemia. *2104*

127.20 Strongyloidiasis Has been observed. *2199*

128.00 Larva Migrans (Visceralis) Often increased. *2104* Characteristic feature. *2368*

130.00 Toxoplasmosis *2468*

135.00 Sarcoidosis Has been observed in 23.5-61% of cases. *0433* Increased in 75% of patients, producing reduced A/G ratio and increased total protein in 30% of patients. *2468* Increase of Alpha 2, and gamma globulins help differentiate from other lung disease *2467*

155.00 Malignant Neoplasm of Liver Mean values were found to be lowest in controls followed by acute viral hepatitis, primary hepatocellular carcinoma, and cirrhosis, in that order. *0724* Reversed A/G ratio in 54% of 51 hepatoma patients. *1115*

162.90 Malignant Neoplasm of Bronchus and Lung Good correlation between hypergammaglobulinemia and neoplastic disease, especially bronchogenic carcinoma. *2104*

201.90 Hodgkin's Disease May be increased with macroglobulins present and evidence of autoimmune process. *2468* With active disease. *2538 0073* Electrophoretic studies of serum proteins are often normal early in the course of the disease but may show a hyperglobulinemia (commonly alpha₂) *0999*

203.00 Multiple Myeloma Very elevated serum total protein is due to increase in globulins (with decreased A/G ratio) in 50-66% of the patients. *2468* Plasma cell dyscrasias are among the most common causes of serum elevations, which may exceed 5 g/dL. *0999* Greater than 32 g/L in 27 of 35 patients and reduced 20 g/L) in 1 case. *0518* Over 80 g/L in 60% of patients. *1980* A Homogeneous protein component ranging from slow gamma to alpha₂-globulin is seen in 60% of patients *0992*

205.00 Myelocytic Leukemia (Acute) Diffuse hypergammaglobulinemia is common. *0689 2552*

205.10 Myelocytic Leukemia (Chronic) Increased alpha and gamma globulins. *2468* Often moderately elevated. *2552*

206.00 Monocytic Leukemia An increased concentration of heterogeneous or polyclonal gamma globulin in the plasma occurs frequently. *2538 2467*

212.70 Benign Neoplasm of Cardiovascular Tissue Occurs with myxoma, possibly reflecting tumor emboli or tumor breakdown products. *1108* Recognized to be increased in about 50% of patients *2467*

245.20 Hashimoto's Thyroiditis Occurs in approximately 50% of chronic patients, and may reflect the degree of thyroiditis or autoantibody production. *0999* May be present *0962*

260.00 Protein Malnutrition Relatively high as a result of concurrent infectious process. *0151* Slightly increased with marasmus. *2468*

272.00 Type IIA Hyperlipoproteinemia Serum albumin is reduced, while the serum gamma globulin fraction is increased. *0619 2467*

272.21 Type IIB Hyperlipoproteinemia Serum albumin is reduced, while the serum gamma globulin fraction is increased. *0619 2467* *0088*

273.30 Waldenström's Macroglobulinemia Electrophoresis shows an intense sharp peak in globulin fraction, usually in the gamma zone, and takes PAS stain. Total serum protein and globulin are markedly increased. Immunoelectrophoresis identifies IgM as a component of increased globulin *2468*

273.80 Analbuminemia Usually present in increased concentration *0433* *2467*

277.00 Cystic Fibrosis Rises with progressive pulmonary disease, mainly due to IgG and IgA; IgM and IgD are not appreciably increased. *2467*

277.14 Acute Intermittent Porphyria Constant finding. *0433*

277.15 Porphyria Variegata Constant finding. *0433*

277.17 Hereditary Coproporphyria Constant finding. *0433*

277.30 Amyloidosis Increased concentration with reversed A/G ratio is frequent. *2468* Hyperglobulinemia occurs in 15% of cases of cardiac amyloidosis; alpha₂ and gamma fractions moderately increased. *0151* Has been observed. No correlation with severity or duration of disease *0120 2246*

288.00 Agranulocytosis In some patients. *0992*

333.40 Huntington's Chorea In 23 of 27 patients. *0303*

Globulin *(continued)*

Serum Increase *(continued)*

340.00 Multiple Sclerosis Increased to > 20% of total protein in 14% of 64 patients. *1295*

390.00 Rheumatic Fever Serum proteins are altered, with decreased serum albumin and increased alpha$_2$ and gamma globulins. *2467 0962 2104*

421.00 Bacterial Endocarditis Seen in about 50% of patients *0999* . Mean = 3.7 ± 0.1 g/dL in 125 cases of various types of infection. *1798 2104*

425.40 Cardiomyopathies May be found and are probably the result of hepatic insufficiency due to heart failure. *1108*

428.00 Congestive Heart Failure *2467*

446.00 Polyarteritis-Nodosa Frequently found *0962 2468*

446.50 Cranial Arteritis and Related Conditions May occur in temporal arteritis. *2468*

446.70 Pulseless Disease (Aortic Arch Syndrome) Serum proteins abnormal with increased gamma globulins, mostly composed of IgM. *2467* May be present. *2086 2035*

494.00 Bronchiectasis Seen when chronic uncontrolled infection persists. *0433* May be increased with chronic infection or decreased if congenital agammaglobulinemia is the underlying disease. *0999*

495.90 Allergic Alveolitis Elevation in the range of 2-3 g/dL. *0433*

503.01 Berylliosis Occasional transient hypergammaglobulinemia. *2467*

555.90 Regional Enteritis or Ileitis May be elevated in some patients but are normal or low in others *2199 0995*

570.00 Acute and Subacute Necrosis of Liver Mildly elevated due to increased gamma globulin. *0992*

571.20 Laennec's or Alcoholic Cirrhosis In 95 patients, there was a significant increase in mean concentration, while mean alpha and beta globulins were normal. Characteristic electrophoresis pattern reveals a lack of demarcation between beta and gamma peaks (beta-gamma bridging). *2296* Usually increased; it reflects inflammation and parallels the severity of the inflammation *2467* Mean total globulin values were found to be lowest in the healthy subjects followed by acute viral hepatitis, primary hepatocellular carcinoma and cirrhosis in that order *0724*

571.49 Chronic Active Hepatitis Elevated and remain raised without normalizing late in convalescence. *2339* Levels (> 2 g/dL) common, particularly with abundant plasma cell infiltration of liver. *0992* Hyperglobulinemia is usually found Provide a good index of activity and remission; fluctuations are synchronous with those of transaminase enzymes. *1465 0999 0962*

571.60 Biliary Cirrhosis Hypergammaglobulinemia is mainly due to an elevation of IgM. *0716* Usually elevated, particularly IgM. *0962* Serum globulins (especially beta and alpha$_2$) are increased *2467 2238 2035*

571.90 Cirrhosis of Liver Hypergammaglobulinemia exceeding 3 g/dL. Suggests chronic active hepatitis or primary biliary cirrhosis. *0433* The increase in gamma fraction is polyclonal in nature and is due first to increase in IgM fraction followed by an increase in IgG fraction. *2339* Usually increased; it reflects inflammation and parallels the severity of the inflammation *2467* Mean total values were found to be lowest in the healthy subjects followed by acute viral hepatitis primary hepatocellular carcinoma and cirrhosis in that order *0724*

572.00 Liver Abscess (Pyogenic) *2467*

572.40 Hepatic Failure *0503*

576.20 Extrahepatic Biliary Obstruction Alpha and beta globulins increase in infection or obstructive jaundice. *0151*

580.00 Acute Poststreptococcal Glomerulonephritis *2104*

694.40 Pemphigus *0151*

710.00 Systemic Lupus Erythematosus A less specific but frequent abnormality. *0433* Serum globulin concentrations in excess of 4.0 g/dL are seen in over 50% of cases. *0999* Increase in about 70% of patients *0677* Marked increase occur in patient with proteinuria *1902 2087*

710.10 Progressive Systemic Sclerosis Frequently found but is nonspecific. *0433* Occurs in about 50% of patients; usually only moderate (1.4-2.0 g/dL), values of 3.5 g/dL and higher have been observed. *2035 2250*

710.20 Sjögren's Syndrome Hypergammaglobulinemia characterized by a diffuse increase in IgG, IgA, and IgM is found especially in those patients with the sicca complex not accompanied by a connective tissue disease. *0934* Electrophoresis shows increase globulins largely due to 7S gamma globulin. *2468* Present in most cases *0999 2035*

710.40 Dermatomyositis/Polymyositis Commonly elevated. *0151 0433*

711.10 Mixed Connective Tissue Disease Diffuse hypergammaglobulinemia. *0062*

714.00 Rheumatoid Arthritis Alpha$_2$ or beta globulin fractions are often elevated in the acute active phase, whereas during the chronic active phase, gamma globulin fractions are elevated. *0433* Elevation occurs in some 50% of all patients and in the majority with progressive chronic disease. *0999*

720.00 Rheumatoid (Ankylosing) Spondylitis Electrophoresis may show an elevation of the globulin fractions without any specific pattern. *0433* 25% of 40 Patients showed elevated and abnormal globulins, alkaline phosphatase and hemogloblin *1250*

990.00 Effects of X-Ray Irradiation Some cases. *0618*

Serum Normal

204.00 Lymphocytic Leukemia (Acute) Most often normal in contrast to acute myelogenous leukemia. *0689 2552*

242.90 Hyperthyroidism *2467*

446.00 Polyarteritis-Nodosa *2467*

555.90 Regional Enteritis or Ileitis May be elevated in some patients but are normal or low in others. *2199*

575.00 Acute Cholecystitis *2467*

585.00 Chronic Renal Failure *2467*

650.00 Pregnancy Albumin was decreased and total globulins were unchanged in late normal pregnancy. *2286 2287*

Urine Increase

203.00 Multiple Myeloma *2468*

270.03 Cystinosis Over 50 X the normal excretion of light chain gamma globulin. *2460*

581.90 Nephrotic Syndrome Significant quantities are found. *0995*

CSF Increase

49.00 Lymphocytic Choriomeningitis May be found in the 2nd week. *2368*

86.90 Trypanosomiasis In 22% of cases. *0846*

97.90 Syphilis Reflected in an abnormal Lange curve. *0151*

203.00 Multiple Myeloma Increased in about 66% of patients, with corresponding colloidal gold curve. *0151*

320.90 Meningitis (Bacterial) Elevated in all forms of meningeal inflammation. *2368*

340.00 Multiple Sclerosis An increase, particularly the IgG fraction, may develop. An elevation to over 15% of the total protein and an abnormal colloidal gold curve are found in more than 75% of the patients. No relationship has been drawn with degree, type or duration of disease, or any other clinical criteria. *2075* 79.3% of patients had concentrations 12% of total protein. Over 50% had concentrations > 16%, and 9.5% of cases were > 30%. *1295* 4.5-23.8% of total protein in 13 patients. *2158*

357.90 Polyneuritis Rarely elevated. *0433*

CSF Normal

357.90 Polyneuritis Rarely elevated. *0433*

Duodenal Contents Increase

277.00 Cystic Fibrosis In excess of that found in the duodenal fluid of controls. *0392*

Glomerular Filtration Rate (GFR)

Urine Decrease

84.00 Malaria In acute renal failure due to falciparum malaria. *2190*

203.00 Multiple Myeloma Renal function is decreased. There is no correlation between the degree of Bence-Jones proteinuria and renal functional impairment. *0962* Marked reduction in PAH clearance in patients with Bence-Jones proteinuria 3.22 ± 0.65 mL/s. Diminished out of proportion to the GFR. *0518*

244.90 **Hypothyroidism** *2540*

255.40 **Adrenal Cortical Hypofunction** Dehydration may result in hemoconcentration. *0962* Fluid depletion leads to reduced circulating blood volume and renal circulatory insufficiency. *2612*

270.03 **Cystinosis** Diminishes with advancing renal disease. *2246*

274.00 **Gout** Moderate but significant reduction in all age groups. *0943*

275.10 **Hepatolenticular Degeneration** Significantly reduced. *0143*

275.35 **Vitamin D Resistant Rickets** Characteristic of the 1st few months of life. May result in a normal phosphate concentration even if the tubular defect is already present. *0994*

277.30 **Amyloidosis** Decreased due to reduced filtration surface (fewer functioning glomeruli). *0619*

405.91 **Renovascular Hypertension** Renal functional impairment. *0962*

428.00 **Congestive Heart Failure** With a fall in effective cardiac output, a commensurate reduction in renal blood flow generally occurs. *1108 2104*

446.60 **Thrombotic Thrombocytopenic Purpura** Renal function may be impaired. *0962*

496.00 **Chronic Obstructive Lung Disease** Hypercapnic patients showed low effective renal plasma flow, impaired water and sodium excretion compared to normocapnic patients and normal controls. *0698*

572.40 **Hepatic Failure** GFR varied from 1-24 mL/min in 25 of 43 hepatic failure patients. Only 1 of these survived. *2536* Reduced GFR was highly significant in 6 and mild-moderate in 14 of 50 cases of hepatic failure due to decompensated cirrhosis of liver. *0379*

580.00 **Acute Poststreptococcal Glomerulonephritis** The decreased GFR and increased aldosterone secretion lead to retention of sodium and water with resultant hypervolemia. *1108*

580.05 **Glomerulonephritis (Membranoproliferative)** BUN and creatinine rise as GFR decreases. *0962* In 50% of cases. *0331*

580.40 **Glomerulonephritis (Rapidly Progressive)** BUN and creatinine rise as GFR decreases *0962*

581.90 **Nephrotic Syndrome** Increased total body sodium and water occurs as a result of reduced GFR and causes the characteristic edema. *0151*

584.00 **Acute Renal Failure** Decreased due to reduced number of functioning glomeruli. *0619* Decreased cortical renal blood flow was noted in acute failure due to falciparum malaria. *2190*

585.00 **Chronic Renal Failure** BUN and creatinine rise as GFR decreases. *0962*

588.81 **Proximal Renal Tubular Acidosis** Usually reduced. *2246*

590.00 **Chronic Pyelonephritis** Decreased due to reduced filtration surface (fewer functioning glomeruli). *0619* A decrease proportional to progress of renal disease. *2468*

590.10 **Acute Pyelonephritis** Decreased due to reduced filtration surface (fewer functioning glomeruli). *0619*

642.40 **Pre-Eclampsia** Reduced 25-30% below the rate in normal pregnancy. *2104*

642.60 **Eclampsia** Reduced 25-30% below the rate in normal pregnancy. *2104*

710.10 **Progressive Systemic Sclerosis** Renal function may be impaired. *0962* The earliest demonstrable change in renal scleroderma. *0962*

785.50 **Shock** Decreased after shock due to decreased renal blood flow. *0619*

994.50 **Exercise** Observed with heavy treadmill exercise. *1205*

Urine   Increase

191.90 **Malignant Neoplasm of Brain** Associated excess ADH may tend to accelerate GFR. *2104*

198.30 **Secondary Malignant Neoplasm of Brain** Associated excess ADH may tend to accelerate GFR. *2104*

225.90 **Benign Neoplasm of Brain and CNS** Associated excess ADH may tend to accelerate GFR. *2104*

253.00 **Acromegaly** May be abnormally high. *0962 0433*

320.90 **Meningitis (Bacterial)** Associated excess ADH may tend to accelerate GFR. *2104*

323.92 **Encephalomyelitis** Associated excess ADH may tend to accelerate GFR. *2104*

431.00 **Cerebral Hemorrhage** Associated excess ADH may tend to accelerate GFR. *2104*

434.00 **Cerebral Thrombosis** Associated excess ADH may tend to accelerate GFR. *2104*

434.10 **Cerebral Embolism** Associated excess ADH may tend to accelerate GFR. *2104*

650.00 **Pregnancy** Renal plasma flow is increased during pregnancy. *2468*

948.00 **Burns** May rise to very high values. *1422*

986.00 **Toxic Effects of Carbon Monoxide** Occurs 12-24 h after exposure. *2256*

994.50 **Exercise** Mild exercise. *1205*

Urine   Normal

238.40 **Polycythemia Vera** GFR is kept to almost normal levels by an increased renal blood flow. *2483 2552*

994.50 **Exercise** Moderate exercise. *1205*

Glucagon

Plasma   Decrease

157.90 **Malignant Neoplasm of Pancreas** Decreased. *0306 0620 0513*

277.00 **Cystic Fibrosis** Both alpha and beta cell function is disrupted resulting in low insulin and glucagon concentration in contrast to diabetes mellitus. *1633*

577.10 **Chronic Pancreatitis** Decreased. *0306 0620 0513*

Plasma   Increase

250.10 **Diabetic Acidosis** Frequently observed. *1644*

251.20 **Hypoglycemia, Unspecified** *0619*

272.10 **Type IV Hyperlipoproteinemia** *0619*

272.22 **Type III Hyperlipoproteinemia** *0619*

564.20 **Postgastrectomy (Dumping) Syndrome** Hypoglycemia following gastrectomy, gut glucagon levels in the plasma are raised. *0619*

571.20 **Laennec's or Alcoholic Cirrhosis** May occur. *2146*

571.90 **Cirrhosis of Liver** Concentration was raised 2-6 fold in patients with spontaneous portal systemic shunting or surgically induced portacaval shunting. Increased levels were due to hypersecretion rather than decreased catabolism. *2147*

577.00 **Acute Pancreatitis** Increased concentrations lead to the release of calcitonin and resultant depression of serum calcium. *0999*

584.00 **Acute Renal Failure** Elevated 2-10 X above normal and remains essentially unchanged by dialysis. *0208*

585.00 **Chronic Renal Failure** Glucagon is elevated 2-10 X above normal and remains essentially unchanged by dialysis. *0208* Fasting immunoreactive glucagon was elevated to 534 ± 2 pg/mL in chronic failure. Normal value was 113 ± 9 pg/mL. *1321   1108*

948.00 **Burns** Increased. *0306 0620 0513*

994.50 **Exercise** Moderate to severe exercise. *0619* May increase 20%, facilitates hepatic glycogenolysis. *0721*

Plasma   Normal

278.00 **Obesity** Similar levels were obtained in 10 nonobese patients. *0864*

Glucaric Acid

Urine   Increase

70.00 **Viral Hepatitis** A 3 fold increase of D-glucaric acid was found in the early stages of disease (37.13 µmol/24h ± 3.08 vs. 9.91 ± 1.18 in controls) when serum transaminases and bilirubin were very high. A lower but significantly raised level was found during recovery when the transaminases and bilirubin were greatly reduced. *0346*

Glucocerebroside Beta-Glucosidase

Serum   Increase

272.72 **Gaucher's Disease** Frequently increased, with highly variable range of values. *2246*

Glucocerebroside Beta-Glucosidase
(continued)

Liver   Increase

272.72   Gaucher's Disease   Many times the normal concentration. *2246*

Red Blood Cells   Increase

272.72   Gaucher's Disease   Frequently increased, with highly variable range of values. *2246*

Glucocorticoids

Plasma   Decrease

255.40   Adrenal Cortical Hypofunction   Baseline plasma and urinary corticosteroids will be low in Addison's disease. *0962*   Adrenal cortex destruction results in deficiency of glucocorticoids, androgens, and mineralocorticoids. *2612*

Plasma   Increase

255.00   Adrenal Cortical Hyperfunction (Glucocorticoid Excess)   In most cases of hypercortisolism, the baseline plasma and urinary corticosteroids are elevated. Loss of the normal diurnal rhythm is usually noted. *0962*   Diagnosed by demonstrating an excessive secretion of glucocorticoid hormone. *1108*

308.00   Stress   A drop in eosinophils with increased corticoid and epinephrine production are manifestations of stress. *2113*

567.90   Peritonitis   Increased adrenal production. *0995*

Urine   Decrease

253.40   Anterior Pituitary Hypofunction   *0151*

255.40   Adrenal Cortical Hypofunction   Baseline plasma and urinary corticosteroids will be low in Addison's disease. *0962*

Urine   Increase

253.00   Acromegaly   *0151*

255.00   Adrenal Cortical Hyperfunction (Glucocorticoid Excess)   In most cases of hypercortisolism, the baseline plasma and urinary corticosteroids are elevated. Loss of the normal diurnal rhythm is usually noted. *0962*

Glucose

Serum   Decrease

9.00   Gastroenteritis and Colitis   Of 868 infants with dehydration from gastroenteritis, 7.9% of cases had blood sugar levels of 0-50 mg/dL. A high mortality rate was found in patients with hypoglycemia. *0857*

32.00   Diphtheria   Occurs frequently. *2468*

60.00   Yellow Fever   Deficiency in available glycogen. *0619*

70.00   Viral Hepatitis   Can occur with various types of liver disease. Hepatic hypoglycemia is a fasting hypoglycemia and often only transiently relieved by food. *0962*   *2104*

71.00   Rabies   May be somewhat below normal. *0433*

72.00   Mumps   *0619*

151.90   Malignant Neoplasm of Stomach   *2467*

155.00   Malignant Neoplasm of Liver   5-25% incidence. *0364*   Hypoglycemia noted in about 30% of hepatoma patients in some studies. *1507*   Sometimes present. Occasionally antedates the discovery of the tumor. *0962*   Can occur with various types of liver disease. Hepatic hypoglycemia is a fasting hypoglycemia and often only transiently relieved by food. *0962*   *2104*

157.90   Malignant Neoplasm of Pancreas   In children. Decreased due to excess insulin. *0619*   *0812*

162.90   Malignant Neoplasm of Bronchus and Lung   Occasionally, bronchogenic carcinoma is associated with insulin-like activity which may be reflected by hypoglycemia. *0962*

197.70   Secondary Malignant Neoplasm of Liver   Can occur with various types of liver disease. Hepatic hypoglycemia is a fasting hypoglycemia and often only transiently relieved by food. *0962*   *2104*

205.10   Myelocytic Leukemia (Chronic)   Artifactual hypoglycemia may be due to leukocyte glucose utilization in vitro. *0730* *2552*

211.60   Benign Neoplasm of Pancreas   Decreased glucose due to excess insulin in pancreatic islet cell. *0619*   *0812*

244.90   Hypothyroidism   Fasting blood sugar is decreased. *2468*

245.10   Subacute Thyroiditis   Severe hyponatremia and hypoglycemia may occur as a manifestation of primary or secondary thyroid failure. *0151*

251.20   Hypoglycemia, Unspecified   Insulin excess probably due to excessively rapid absorption as in postgastrectomy. This may occur particularly in: underweight, poorly nourished babies; twins; premature infants. A low birth-weight baby with a proportionally large head is very prone to hypoglycemia. Infants of diabetic mothers (fetal blood glucose is controlled by the maternal blood glucose level, but at term the newborn infant's pancreas may respond to maternal hyperglycemia by secretion of insulin and hence hypoglycemia). *0619*

253.40   Anterior Pituitary Hypofunction   May result from growth hormone and cortisol deficiency. *2612*   *0433 0151*

255.40   Adrenal Cortical Hypofunction   Patients with diminished glucocorticoid secretion commonly manifest low levels of blood glucose, and symptomatic hypoglycemia may follow a period of fasting. Occasionally, patients with glucocorticoid deficiency exhibit hypoglycemic symptoms late in the postprandial period. *0999*   Fasting blood sugar may be low, and the glucose tolerance test may be flat. *0962*   May occur due to insulin hypersensitivity in the hypoadrenal state. *2612*

259.20   Carcinoid Syndrome   *2540*

260.00   Protein Malnutrition   In kwashiorkor. *0151*   Decreased due to excess insulin resulting from deficiency in available glycogen. *0619*

269.90   Deficiency State (Unspecified)   *2467*

270.31   Maple Syrup Urine Disease   Hypoglycemic episodes are probably caused by the high concentrations of leucine. *1797 2246*

271.01   Von Gierke's Disease   Decreased glucose due to excess insulin as a result of deficiency in available glycogen. *0619*   Degree of hypoglycemia is variable. *2246*   Usually low. *2104*   *0812*

271.02   McArdle's Disease   Usually low. *2104*

271.03   Forbes Disease   Usually low. *2104*

271.10   Galactosemia   In children; following ingestion of galactose blood glucose falls (as blood galactose rises) to dangerously low levels. *0619 2467*   On rare occasions. *2246*   Replacement or destruction of functioning hepatic tissue may evoke hypoglycemia. *2104*

271.20   Hereditary Fructose Intolerance   The causes of hypoglycemia are complex and include impairment of glycogenolysis. *0433*   Frequent severe attacks of hypoglycemia. *2246*

272.71   Anderson's Disease   Usually low. *2104*

275.10   Hepatolenticular Degeneration   In 5% of patients related to malnutrition. *2280*

303.90   Alcoholism   Due to depletion of glycogen stores, and an inhibitory effect of alcohol on gluconeogenesis. *0962*

331.81   Reye's Syndrome   Hypoglycemia with decreased CSF glucose is common in patients < 5 years of age, but is rare in older children. *0151*   Occasionally hypoglycemia. *0962*   Replacement or destruction of functioning hepatic tissue may evoke hypoglycemia. *2104*

428.00   Congestive Heart Failure   May occur if cardiac output is severely curtailed and liver congestion is marked. *0151*

533.90   Peptic Ulcer, Site Unspecified   A high frequency of spontaneous hypoglycemia occurs in these patients. *2104*

564.20   Postgastrectomy (Dumping) Syndrome   Rapid absorption of carbohydrate by smaller intestine leads to release of insulin which continues to act after most of the carbohydrate has been absorbed and stored. *0619*

570.00   Acute and Subacute Necrosis of Liver   Diffuse severe disease-primary or metastatic tumor. *2467*   Lowered levels result from massive hepatic necrosis or a deficiency of enzymes necessary for glycogenolysis. *0151*   *0619 2104*

571.20   Laennec's or Alcoholic Cirrhosis   Replacement or destruction of functioning hepatic tissue may evoke hypoglycemia. *2104*

571.49   Chronic Active Hepatitis   Replacement or destruction of functioning hepatic tissue may evoke hypoglycemia. *2104*

571.60   Biliary Cirrhosis   Replacement or destruction of functioning hepatic tissue may evoke hypoglycemia. *2104*

571.90   Cirrhosis of Liver   Can occur with various types of liver disease. Hepatic hypoglycemia is a fasting hypoglycemia and often only relieved by food. *0962*   *2104*

572.00 Liver Abscess (Pyogenic) Replacement or destruction of functioning hepatic tissue may evoke hypoglycemia. *2104*

572.40 Hepatic Failure The incidence is low. *0503* Replacement or destruction of functioning hepatic tissue may evoke hypoglycemia. *2104*

573.30 Toxic Hepatitis Due to organic arsenic, carbon tetrachloride, chloroform, cinchophen, phosphate, alcohol, acute paracetamol poisoning. *0619* Can occur with various types of liver disease. Hepatic hypoglycemia is a fasting hypoglycemia and often only transiently relieved by food. *0962* *2104*

576.10 Cholangitis Often accompanies mental changes. *2199*

642.40 Pre-Eclampsia In the total series of 794 patients, hypoglycemia had a significant association with low estriol excretion, fetal growth retardation, and perinatal mortality. *1427* The patients with severe pre-eclampsia had significantly lower fasting plasma glucose levels than those with mild pre-eclampsia and normal pregnancies. *2183*

650.00 Pregnancy Occasionally decreased. *2468*

711.00 Acute Arthritis (Pyogenic) Low in most cases. *0999*

773.00 Hemolytic Disease of Newborn (Erythroblastosis Fetalis) In the more severely affected infants. *2538* *2061*

985.00 Toxic Effects of Non-medicinal Metals Hepatotoxicity may occur with arsenicals. *1446*

992.00 Heat stroke Has been observed. *0067*

994.50 Exercise Occurs with strenuous exercise. *0067*

Serum Increase

9.00 Gastroenteritis and Colitis Of 868 infants with dehydration from gastroenteritis, blood sugar levels in 10.2% were > 200 mg/dL. High mortality rate was found in patients with hyperglycemia. *0857*

21.00 Tularemia *2123* *1889*

38.00 Septicemia Fasting hyperglycemia, impaired glucose tolerance and relative hyperinsulinemia are found. *1889* *2123* In 56% of 12 patients at initial hospitalization for this disorder. *0781*

66.00 Phlebotomus Fever Impaired glucose tolerance with relative hyperinsulinemia was observed in sandfly fever. *2479*

97.90 Syphilis *0619*

157.90 Malignant Neoplasm of Pancreas 59% of 100 patients had fasting hyperglycemia. *0932* Diabetes mellitus occurs in 25-50% of cases and is manifest most frequently as an abnormal glucose tolerance test rather than overt glucosuria or fasting hyperglycemia. *2199* In 46% of 46 patients at initial hospitalization for this disorder. *0781*

185.00 Malignant Neoplasm of Prostate In 36% of 86 patients at initial hospitalization for this disorder. *0781*

205.10 Myelocytic Leukemia (Chronic) In 49% of 21 patients at initial hospitalization for this disorder. *0781*

227.91 Pheochromocytoma Fasting level is elevated in about 50% the patients, usually only slightly above normal values. *1108* May be elevated. *0962* Attacks may be accompanied by hyperglycemia and glucosuria. *2612*

242.90 Hyperthyroidism Possibly due to increased circulating epinephrine in thyrotoxicosis. Increased rate of absorption from intestine. *0619* Significantly elevated in 42 untreated patients, mean concentration was 92 ± 8 mg/dL. *0056*

244.90 Hypothyroidism In 35% of 14 patients at initial hospitalization for this disorder. *0781*

250.00 Diabetes Mellitus Diagnosis can be readily made when there is an unequivocal and persistent elevation of the fasting plasma glucose. For venous plasma, the fasting glucose is normally between 60-100 mg/100 mL and values consistently > 120 should be considered diagnostic of diabetes. *0999* *0812* *0433*

250.10 Diabetic Acidosis Increased, usually > 300 mg/dL. *2467* Seldom in excess of 800 mg/dL. *1316* *0999*

253.00 Acromegaly Overt diabetes is found manifested by fasting hyperglycemia. *0962*

255.00 Adrenal Cortical Hyperfunction (Glucocorticoid Excess) Frequently complicated by an insulin resistant diabetes. *2467* Abnormally high amounts of cortisol tend to raise the blood glucose. *0151*

265.00 Thiamine (B₁) Deficiency *0619*

272.10 Type IV Hyperlipoproteinemia Hyperglycemia is only occasionally severe enough to produce symptoms of diabetes. *0151*

272.22 Type III Hyperlipoproteinemia Fasting hyperglycemia and ketosis are uncommon. *2246*

272.32 Type V Hyperlipoproteinemia *0995*

275.00 Hemochromatosis About 82% of all patients with this disorder develop diabetes mellitus. *0995*

275.10 Hepatolenticular Degeneration Fasting glucose consistently elevated. *2278*

277.00 Cystic Fibrosis Fasting hyperglycemia and glycosuria occurred in only 8% of patients. *1633* In 45% of 13 patients at initial hospitalization for this disorder. *0781*

308.00 Stress Decreased tolerance, with excessive peak and decreased formation of glycogen with low fasting levels and subsequent hypoglycemia. Caused by increased adrenalin as in stress and pheochromocytoma (normal return to fasting level). *2467* Normal response. *2315*

320.90 Meningitis (Bacterial) In 32% of 18 patients hospitalized for this disorder. *0781*

401.10 Essential Benign Hypertension Significant increase in glucose and insulin response to a 75 gram oral glucose challenge. *2017*

405.91 Renovascular Hypertension Associated with diabetes mellitus. *0992*

410.90 Acute Myocardial Infarction Glycosuria and hyperglycemia occur in up to 50% of patients. *2467* May be partially related to pituitary-sympathoadrenal stimulation. May occur in patients who are not obviously diabetic; attributed to adrenal stimulation secondary to stress and shock. *1108* Patients have higher fasting concentrations and dispose of an oral glucose load less efficiently than controls. *2104* In 70% of 119 patients hospitalized for this disorder. *0781* *1451* *0962*

415.10 Pulmonary Embolism and Infarction In 44% of 21 patients at initial hospitalization for this disorder. *0781*

428.00 Congestive Heart Failure Abnormal increases in the fasting blood sugar are common. *0962*

431.00 Cerebral Hemorrhage In 29% of 13 patients hospitalized for this disorder. *0781*

482.90 Bacterial Pneumonia In 48% of 18 patients at initial hospitalization for this disorder. *0781*

493.10 Asthma (Intrinsic) May be due to epinephrine or corticosteroids. *0433* May be found in corticosteroid-treated patients. *2035*

540.90 Acute Appendicitis In 34% of 52 patients at initial hospitalization for this disorder. *0781*

560.90 Intestinal Obstruction In 42% of 46 patients at initial hospitalization for this disorder. *0781*

564.20 Postgastrectomy (Dumping) Syndrome Rapid and prolonged alimentary hyperglycemia with subsequent delayed absorption. *0995*

577.00 Acute Pancreatitis Transient hyperglycemia is not rare. *2199* Often found and signifies involvement of pancreatic islet cells. *0433* Seen in about 25% of patients. *0999* In 45% of 21 patients at initial hospitalization for this disorder. *0781*

577.10 Chronic Pancreatitis Some cases. *2467* Increased circulating epinephrine. *0619* In 27% of 11 patients at initial hospitalization for this disorder. *0781*

577.20 Pancreatic Cyst and Pseudocyst Occasionally there is an associated elevation of the fasting blood sugar level. *0433*

580.04 Glomerulonephritis (Membranous) Chemical or overt diabetes appears more common than might be expected by chance. *0406*

584.00 Acute Renal Failure Hyperglycemia and impaired glucose tolerance are common. Elevated ratio of insulin/glucose during glucose tolerance testing is found consistently. *0787*

585.00 Chronic Renal Failure Hyperglycemia and impaired glucose tolerance are common in renal failure. Elevated ratio of insulin/glucose during glucose tolerance testing is found consistently. *0787* Increased mean plasma concentration in chronic failure. *1243*

633.90 Ectopic Pregnancy In 45% of 11 patients at initial hospitalization for this disorder. *0781*

642.60 Eclampsia Occasionally following eclamptic fit. *0621*

758.70 Klinefelter's Syndrome (XXY) Mild diabetes is found in 10%. *0962*

785.50 Shock Increased circulating epinephrine. *0619* Hyperglycemia occurs early. *2467*

929.00 Crush Injury (Trauma) *0995*

Glucose *(continued)*

Serum   Increase *(continued)*

948.00 **Burns**   A syndrome of glycosuria, dehydration, coma, and severe glycosuria without ketosis has been recognized in patients recovering from major burns. This syndrome is distinct from the transient hyperglycemia that occurs immediately after burns or acute trauma. *2104*

991.60 **Hypothermia**   High, especially when preceded by shivering and exhaustion. *0151*

994.50 **Exercise**   Rise due to adrenal activity. *0618*

Serum   Normal

250.00 **Diabetes Mellitus**   May be normal in mild diabetes. *0812* A large percentage of patients with early diabetes have perfectly normal fasting blood glucose levels. When elevated this test is very helpful, but when normal it is of little consequence. This is a poor screening test for diabetes. *0433*

270.03 **Cystinosis**   *0995*

271.02 **McArdle's Disease**   The blood sugar level, glucose tolerance, and galactose tolerance are normal, as is the response to injected glucagon and epinephrine. *1108*   Type V patients are not hypoglycemic. *2246*

275.35 **Vitamin D Resistant Rickets**   Found in excess quantities in the urine but not in the plasma. *0433*

434.10 **Cerebral Embolism**   *2467*

650.00 **Pregnancy**   *1542*

994.50 **Exercise**   Observed effect with 12 min cycle-ergometer. *0804*

Urine   Increase

38.00 **Septicemia**   *0619*

157.90 **Malignant Neoplasm of Pancreas**   Diabetes mellitus occurs in 25-50% of cases and is manifest most frequently as an abnormal glucose tolerance test rather than overt glucosuria or fasting hyperglycemia. *2199*

203.00 **Multiple Myeloma**   Aminoaciduria may be nonselective and associated with renal glycosuria and mild renal acidosis. *0962*

227.91 **Pheochromocytoma**   Usually intermittent. *1108*   Attacks may be accompanied by hyperglycemia and glucosuria. *2612* *0999*

242.90 **Hyperthyroidism**   *2468*

250.00 **Diabetes Mellitus**   Urine testing as a preliminary screening procedure for diabetes is the cheapest method available, however, it is not very productive. *0433*   Glycosuria is characteristic of the diabetic state, but its presence is neither necessary nor sufficient for the diagnosis. *1919*

250.10 **Diabetic Acidosis**   *0999 0962*

253.00 **Acromegaly**   Increase in glucose tolerance because of glycosuria. *0619*

255.00 **Adrenal Cortical Hyperfunction (Glucocorticoid Excess)**   Glycosuria appears in 50% of patients. *2468   0433*

268.20 **Osteomalacia**   Reflects variable degree of disturbance of proximal tubular function. *0995*

270.03 **Cystinosis**   May be scanty and intermittent or profuse and constant. *0995*   Up to 5 g/dL. *2246*

271.20 **Hereditary Fructose Intolerance**   During acute intoxication, signs of a proximal tubular syndrome and of liver failure are common. *0433*

275.10 **Hepatolenticular Degeneration**   Tubular reabsorption of glucose is frequently impaired. *0143*

275.34 **Familial Periodic Paralysis**   Occasional patients. *2246*

275.35 **Vitamin D Resistant Rickets**   Found in excess quantities in the urine but not in the plasma. *0433*   Mild renal glycosuria has been reported in a few cases. *2246*

277.00 **Cystic Fibrosis**   Urinalysis reveals glycosuria due to chemical diabetes. *0433*   Fasting hyperglycemia and glycosuria occurred in only 8% of patients. *1633*

410.90 **Acute Myocardial Infarction**   Glycosuria and hyperglycemia occur in up to 50% of patients. *2467*   May occur in patients who are not obviously diabetic; attributed to adrenal stimulation secondary to stress and shock. *1108*

431.00 **Cerebral Hemorrhage**   Transient glucosuria. *0992*

564.20 **Postgastrectomy (Dumping) Syndrome**   *0619*

577.00 **Acute Pancreatitis**   Routine urinalysis is usually normal but there may be glucose in the urine. *0433*   Appears in 25% of the patients. *2467*

580.00 **Acute Poststreptococcal Glomerulonephritis**   Occasional glycosuria occurs. *0151*

580.01 **Glomerulonephritis (Focal)**   May be found. *0951*

585.00 **Chronic Renal Failure**   With renal parenchymal disease. *0838*

588.81 **Proximal Renal Tubular Acidosis**   Found in children. *0433*

590.00 **Chronic Pyelonephritis**   With renal parenchymal disease. *0838*

590.10 **Acute Pyelonephritis**   With renal parenchymal disease. *0838*

650.00 **Pregnancy**   The renal threshold for glucose may decrease, and some patients may show glycosuria without elevated blood sugar levels. *0433*   Incidence about 35%. *0386*

948.00 **Burns**   A syndrome of glycosuria, dehydration, coma, and severe glycosuria without ketosis has been recognized in patients recovering from major burns. This syndrome is distinct from the transient hyperglycemia that occurs immediately after burns or acute trauma. *2104*

984.00 **Toxic Effects of Lead and Its Compounds (including Fumes)**   Nephrotoxic effect of lead. *0618*

CSF   Decrease

9.00 **Gastroenteritis and Colitis**   In children with severe dehydration. *0433*

13.00 **Tuberculosis Meningitis**   Falls to < 50% of blood glucose. *2468*   40 mg/dL. *0999*   Normal or moderately decreased. *0962   1894*

18.00 **Disseminated Tuberculosis**   *0999*

36.00 **Meningococcal Meningitis**   Usually < 35 mg/dL. *1058 2400*

72.00 **Mumps**   Usually normal, however, recent reports have emphasized that depressed CSF concentrations (< 40 mg/dL) may be present initially and persist for several days. *0433   1319*

97.90 **Syphilis**   Decreased in 50% of the patients. *0962*   10-45 mg/dL. *2368*

99.10 **Lymphogranuloma Venereum**   In the early stages of infection. *0433*   Characteristically low. *1319*

114.90 **Coccidioidomycosis**   Often an early significant change with CNS involvement. *0151*

117.50 **Cryptococcosis**   In about 50% of cases of symptomatic meningoencephalitis. *1058*

135.00 **Sarcoidosis**   Due to multiple tumors in the meninges, in rare cases, involving the central nervous system. *0619*

192.90 **Malignant Neoplasm of Other Parts of Nervous System**   Due to multiple tumors in the meninges, but these are rare causes. *0619*

198.30 **Secondary Malignant Neoplasm of Brain**   Less than 50% of blood level (meningeal infiltration of leukemic cells). *2467*

204.00 **Lymphocytic Leukemia (Acute)**   With meningeal infiltration. *2538*

205.00 **Myelocytic Leukemia (Acute)**   With meningeal infiltration. *2538*

225.90 **Benign Neoplasm of Brain and CNS**   Values are characteristically < 40 mg/dL in patients with diffuse neoplastic involvement of the meninges, but are normal in other tumors of the brain. *0151*

251.20 **Hypoglycemia, Unspecified**   *0619*

320.90 **Meningitis (Bacterial)**   CSF glucose is < 50% blood sugar. *0999*   Decreased in children with transverse myelitis and mycoplasma pneumoniae meningoencephalitis. *1281*   CSF/blood sugar ratios were of diagnostic and prognostic value, especially in suboptimally treated cases. *1894*   Usual values < 40 mg/dL, and may be close to 0. Low CSF sugar distinguishes bacterial from viral meningitides. *0151*   Usually well below 50% the blood sugar and may be entirely absent. *0962*

323.91 **Myelitis**   Decreased in children with transverse myelitis and mycoplasma pneumoniae meningoencephalitis. *1281*

331.81 **Reye's Syndrome**   Hypoglycemia with decreased CSF glucose is common in patients < 5 years of age, but is rare in older children. *0151*   Low levels of glucose and protein found in the CSF *0416*

CSF   Increase

114.90 Coccidioidomycosis   CSF cell and chemistry are indistinguishable from tuberculous meningitis. *2368*

324.00 Intracranial Abscess   Elevated in lumbar CSF in all patients with subdural empyema. Moderate-marked elevation in lumbar CSF in 14 of 17 patients. *1238*

CSF   Normal

45.90 Acute Poliomyelitis   *0962 2368*

47.00 Aseptic Meningitis   Normal but may be depressed in mumps meningitis. *0962*

49.00 Lymphocytic Choriomeningitis   Normal or low normal. *2368*

52.00 Chickenpox   *1058*

53.00 Herpes Zoster   *0962*

62.10 Western Equine Encephalitis   *1058*

62.20 Eastern Equine Encephalitis   *1058*

100.00 Leptospirosis   *0992 0962*

130.00 Toxoplasmosis   In acquired, usually normal. *1319*

324.00 Intracranial Abscess   Usually normal; however, in the meningitic phase it may be low. *0433*   Usually normal until the process extends to actively involve the meninges. *0962   0995*

434.10 Cerebral Embolism   *0992*

510.00 Empyema   In subdural empyema. *0186*

Synovial Fluid   Decrease

99.30 Reiter's Disease   Usually normal but may be decreased when leukocyte count is increased. *0186*

274.00 Gout   Typical of inflammatory reactions sometimes showing a slight reduction in glucose. *0999*

710.00 Systemic Lupus Erythematosus   Less than 25 mg/dL, lower than blood. *0666*

711.00 Acute Arthritis (Pyogenic)   *0650*

714.00 Rheumatoid Arthritis   Normal or low. *0186*   Slightly reduced glucose content *0999*

714.30 Juvenile Rheumatoid Arthritis   *0136*

720.00 Rheumatoid (Ankylosing) Spondylitis   Lower than blood. *0666*

Synovial Fluid   Normal

99.30 Reiter's Disease   Usually normal but may be decreased when leukocyte count is increased. *0186*

714.00 Rheumatoid Arthritis   Normal or low. *0186*

715.90 Osteoarthritis   Nearly equal to blood. *0666*

Pleural Effusion   Decrease

11.00 Pulmonary Tuberculosis   Levels less than 3.3 mmol/L (60 mg/dL). *1444*

162.90 Malignant Neoplasm of Bronchus and Lung   Approximately 15% of malignancies have low concentrations in pleural fluids. *1403*   Markedly reduced, 20 mg/dL or less, is very suggestive and virtually diagnostic of rheumatoid disease. A low level in the range of 40 mg/dL can be found in infectious processes and in malignant pleural effusions. *0962   0174*

197.00 Secondary Malignant Neoplasm of Respiratory System   Markedly reduced, 20 mg/dL or less, is very suggestive and virtually diagnostic of rheumatoid disease. A low level in the range of 40 mg/dL can be found in infectious processes and in malignant pleural effusions. *0962*

480.90 Viral Pneumonia   Exudate. *0062*

482.90 Bacterial Pneumonia   Levels less than 3.3 mmol/L (60 mg/dL). *0174*

510.00 Empyema   Levels less than 3.3 mmol/L (60 mg/dL). *0174* 0-60 mg/dL. *2017*

577.10 Chronic Pancreatitis   Usually decreased in an exudate. *0062*

714.00 Rheumatoid Arthritis   Concentrations are invariably < 30 mg/dL. *1403*   Markedly reduced, 20 mg/dL or less, is very suggestive and virtually diagnostic of rheumatoid disease. A low level in the range of 40 mg/dL can be found in infectious processes and in malignant pleural effusions. *0962*

Pleural Effusion   Normal

415.10 Pulmonary Embolism and Infarction   Pleural Fluid = Serum level. *2017*

428.00 Congestive Heart Failure   Pleural Fluid = Serum level. *2017*

571.90 Cirrhosis of Liver   Pleural Fluid = Serum level. *2017*

577.20 Pancreatic Cyst and Pseudocyst   Pleural Fluid = Serum level. *2017*

710.00 Systemic Lupus Erythematosus   *0962*

Ascitic Fluid   Decrease

11.00 Pulmonary Tuberculosis   Seen with tuberculous peritonitis. *0186*

567.90 Peritonitis   Seen with tuberculous peritonitis. *0186*

Pericardial Fluid   Decrease

714.00 Rheumatoid Arthritis   With rheumatoid pericarditis a low concentration (often < 1.7 mmol/L- 30 mg/dL) is seen. *0764*

Pericardial Fluid   Normal

420.00 Acute Pericarditis   Same as serum level. *0758*

Peritoneal Fluid   Decrease

18.00 Disseminated Tuberculosis   Usually < 1.7 mmol/L. *0298*

Peritoneal Fluid   Increase

428.00 Congestive Heart Failure   High concentrations. *1831*

571.90 Cirrhosis of Liver   High concentrations. *1831*

Glucose-6-Phosphatase

Serum   Increase

571.90 Cirrhosis of Liver   Moderate rise. *0619*

573.30 Toxic Hepatitis   After liver damage with carbon tetrachloride the serum level reaches its peak values by 6 h. *0619*

585.00 Chronic Renal Failure   Slight rise with renal disease. *0619*

Liver   Decrease

271.01 Von Gierke's Disease   Deficient enzyme in the liver. *2246*

Glucose-6-Phosphate Dehydrogenase

Serum   Increase

281.20 Folic Acid Deficiency Anemia   Elevated in 12 of 12 patients from 2.5-20 X the normal mean. *1023*   Increased to about the same extent as LD. *0652 2552   2538 1022*

282.60 Sickle Cell Anemia   Elevated in 15 cases. Values ranged from 10-14 with a mean of 4.8 (normal = 1.6). *1023*

Red Blood Cells   Increase

281.00 Pernicious Anemia   Increased to about the same extent as LD. *0652 2552*

281.20 Folic Acid Deficiency Anemia   Elevated in 5 of 9 patients. Upper limit of normal = 4.6. *1023*

282.60 Sickle Cell Anemia   Mean concentrations in red cells were slightly increased to a mean of 5.4 (range = 1.5-9.8). *1023*

Glucose Tolerance

Serum   Decrease

21.00 Tularemia   *2123 1889*

38.00 Septicemia   Fasting hyperglycemia, impaired glucose tolerance and relative hyperinsulinemia are found. *2123 1889*

66.00 Phlebotomus Fever   Impaired glucose tolerance with relative hyperinsulinemia was observed in sandfly fever. *2479*

70.00 Viral Hepatitis   Subnormal insulin response to oral glucose tolerance test was found in 5 of 14 patients in the icteric phase. *1548*

157.90 Malignant Neoplasm of Pancreas   Test is abnormal in 25-50% of patients and is a more frequent abnormality than frank glycosuria or fasting hyperglycemia. *0151*   Abnormal in 25-50% of patients. More frequently than frank glucosuria or fasting hyperglycemia. *2199*

Glucose Tolerance *(continued)*

Serum Decrease *(continued)*

227.91 Pheochromocytoma Impaired glucose tolerance which may be misdiagnosed as diabetes mellitus. *0151* May be decreased because of suppressed insulin release and catecholamine-induced insulin resistance. *0962*

242.90 Hyperthyroidism Early high peak due to increased intestinal absorption (normal IV curve) with normal return to fasting level. Decreased formation of glycogen with low fasting levels and subsequent hypoglycemia. *2467* Oral test resulted in significantly increased responses in 20 untreated patients. *0056*

250.00 Diabetes Mellitus Decreased tolerance; decreased utilization with slow fall to fasting level. *2467* The responses in nondiabetic and diabetic population do not describe a bimodal distribution, but constitute a single curve skewed in the direction of higher blood sugar values. *0999*

253.00 Acromegaly Impaired in most patients with acromegaly and gigantism. *2468* In 50% of these patients, the oral administration of glucose will demonstrate decreased tolerance. *0962*

255.00 Adrenal Cortical Hyperfunction (Glucocorticoid Excess) Decreased in < 50% of patients. *2467* Frequently abnormal. *0962*

271.01 Von Gierke's Disease Decreased tolerance:excessive peak decreased formation of glycogen with low fasting levels and subsequent hypoglycemia. *2467* Decreased because of inability to form glycogen from administered glucose. *0619* Characteristically diabetic. *1086*

272.10 Type IV Hyperlipoproteinemia Present in 19 of 36 patients (52%). *0855* Occurs in most patients but not with sufficient constancy to indicate a role in causing the disorder. *2246* *0995*

272.22 Type III Hyperlipoproteinemia In roughly 55% of cases. *2246*

272.31 Type I Hyperlipoproteinemia May follow pancreatitis, but is not a feature of uncomplicated disease. *2246*

272.32 Type V Hyperlipoproteinemia More than 75% of patients. *0855* Abnormal in 80%. *2246*

275.00 Hemochromatosis Decreased tolerance:excessive peak decreased utilization with slow fall to fasting level. *2467*

275.10 Hepatolenticular Degeneration Abnormal in some patients. Fasting blood sugar levels are consistently increased. *2278*

277.00 Cystic Fibrosis Up to 40% of patients are known to have varying degrees of intolerance. Probably secondary to strangulation of the islets by fibrosis. More common with advancing age. *1633* Found in 36% of 31 patients. *0976*

282.41 Thalassemia Major 50% of patients had some abnormality in their oral test, 5 falling into the diabetic category. Intolerance correlated with number of transfusions received and age. *2054*

303.90 Alcoholism Decrease in glucose tolerance because of inability of tissues to utilize glucose. *0619*

308.00 Stress Decreased tolerance, excessive peak and decreased formation of glycogen with low fasting levels and subsequent hypoglycemia. Caused by increased epirephrine (normal returns to fasting level). *2467*

335.20 Amyotrophic Lateral Sclerosis In 30% of patients with the disease and is related to decreased muscle mass. *0665*

340.00 Multiple Sclerosis Many patients have impaired carbohydrate metabolism exhibited by abnormal curves. *2104*

410.90 Acute Myocardial Infarction Some patients will have abnormal curves when checked months later. *1108*

414.00 Chronic Ischemic Heart Disease Reported in as many as 50% of patients with coronary artery disease. *0962*

533.90 Peptic Ulcer, Site Unspecified Significantly greater rise in glucose concentration and higher output of insulin was observed in patients with duodenal ulcer. *1101*

564.20 Postgastrectomy (Dumping) Syndrome Characteristically the curve consists of a rise in blood glucose to between 200-300 mg/dL, 30 min after oral administration of glucose. This is followed by a rapid fall in the next hour to hypoglycemic levels, at which point symptoms occur. *0962*

570.00 Acute and Subacute Necrosis of Liver Decreased tolerance:excessive peak-decreased formation of glycogen with low fasting levels and subsequent hypoglycemia. *2467* Decreased because of inability to form glycogen from administered glucose. *0619*

571.20 Laennec's or Alcoholic Cirrhosis A diabetic curve may occur and is a reflection of endogenous insulin resistance. *0992*

571.90 Cirrhosis of Liver A diabetic-type curve may occur and is a reflection of endogenous insulin resistance. *0992*

572.40 Hepatic Failure There is a rapid rise of the blood sugar abnormal levels and a slow return to normal. *0503*

577.10 Chronic Pancreatitis There will be a diabetic oral test in 65% of patients and frank diabetes in > 10% of patients. *2467* Of 50 patients with chronic relapsing pancreatitis, 66% had evidence of glucose intolerance. *0962*

584.00 Acute Renal Failure Hyperglycemia and impaired glucose tolerance are common in renal failure. Elevated ratio of insulin/glucose during glucose tolerance testing is found consistently. *0787* *0098*

585.00 Chronic Renal Failure More than 50% of patients in late renal failure have glucose intolerance as severe as in mild diabetes but with normal fasting blood dextrose and often without glycosuria. *0151*

642.60 Eclampsia Due to either hepatic dysfunction or relative insulin resistance. *0322*

650.00 Pregnancy In 124 pregnant women during the 4th quartile of pregnancy, 9-21% of women were abnormal, and using the H index, 43% would have been declared diabetic. There was no evidence of a progressive change in the glucose curve detectable by the H index nor association between actual or potential fetal morbidity. *0481*

714.00 Rheumatoid Arthritis Characteristically depressed with active disease; easy to produce hypoglycemia if this abnormality is treated with oral hypoglycemic agents. *0433* Moderate intolerance in most patients. More severe in patients with associated infection and inflammation. *2104*

758.70 Klinefelter's Syndrome (XXY) Decreased 25%. *0962*

Serum Increase

40.20 Whipple's Disease Flat peak. Poor absorption from the GI tract (normal IV GTT curve). *2467*

211.60 Benign Neoplasm of Pancreas Flat peak. Late hypoglycemia. *2467*

244.90 Hypothyroidism Curve may be flat. *2612*

252.10 Hypoparathyroidism Flat peak. Poor absorption from the GI tract (normal IV GTT curve). *2467*

253.40 Anterior Pituitary Hypofunction Late hypoglycemia. *2467*

255.40 Adrenal Cortical Hypofunction Flat peak. Poor absorption from the GI tract (normal IV GTT curve). *2467* Fasting blood sugar may be low, and the glucose tolerance test may be flat. *0962* Curve is flat in adrenal hypofunction. *2612*

260.00 Protein Malnutrition In kwashiorkor. *0151*

359.21 Myotonia Atrophica Biphasic response was found in 19 patients (49%) compared with 12 of the control population (24%). In 9 patients (23%), the height of the 2nd peak was 20 mg/dL. *2008*

579.00 Celiac Sprue Disease Flat curve in celiac disease and diseases of intestinal wall and in monosaccharide malabsorption. *0151*

579.90 Malabsorption, Cause Unspecified Flat curve in celiac disease and diseases of intestinal wall and in monosaccharide malabsorption. *0151*

650.00 Pregnancy Decreased formation of glycogen with low fasting levels and subsequent hypoglycemia. Normal return to fasting level. *2467* In 124 pregnant women during the 4th quartile of pregnancy, 9-21% of women were abnormal, and using the H index 43% would have been declared diabetic. There was no evidence of a progressive change in the glucose curve detectable by the H index nor association between actual or potential fetal morbidity. *0481*

Serum Normal

259.20 Carcinoid Syndrome *2540*

271.02 McArdle's Disease The blood sugar level, glucose tolerance, and galactose tolerance are normal, as is the response to injected glucagon and epinephrine. *1108*

272.00 Type IIA Hyperlipoproteinemia *0962 0992*

272.21 Type IIB Hyperlipoproteinemia *0962 0992*

Glutamate Dehydrogenase

Serum   Decrease

994.50   **Exercise**   Observed effect with 12 min cycle-ergometer. *0804*

Serum   Increase

250.10   **Diabetic Acidosis**   In some instances, mostly in severe cases, especially with severe circulatory failure and liver enlargement. *0155*

Serum   Normal

994.50   **Exercise**   Physical activity has no effect. *1930*

Glutamic Acid

Serum   Decrease

270.51   **Histidinemia**   *0995*

585.00   **Chronic Renal Failure**   Mean concentration of serine, threonine, and glutamic acid decreased with deteriorating renal function in children with renal failure. *0192*

Serum   Increase

157.90   **Malignant Neoplasm of Pancreas**   High levels of glutamic acid and normal glutamine levels were found in 9 of 10 patients. Mean value = 3.40 ± 2.22 mg/dL. *0359*

274.00   **Gout**   Remains elevated even after casein loading. Fasting values range from 68-72 μmol (45-51 in controls). *1758*

319.00   **Mental Retardation**   Increased glutamic acid with associated decrease in glutamine may occur in De Lange Syndrome and other mental retardation syndromes. *0493*

714.00   **Rheumatoid Arthritis**   Usually the only elevated serum amino acid. *2104*

Urine   Decrease

714.00   **Rheumatoid Arthritis**   *2104*

Urine   Increase

270.03   **Cystinosis**   Nonspecific pattern of aminoaciduria. Fanconi's syndrome. *0995*

CSF   Decrease

270.51   **Histidinemia**   In some reports. *0831 1065 2246*

Red Blood Cells   Increase

274.00   **Gout**   Average values range from 214-243 μmol compared to 216 in controls. *1758*

280.90   **Iron Deficiency Anemia**   Raised RBC L-glutamate levels occur in iron deficiency anemias in the presence of a large population of young cells. *2411*

496.00   **Chronic Obstructive Lung Disease**   Erythrocyte l-glutamate was significantly elevated only in hypercapnic patients. *2411*

Glutamine

Serum   Decrease

66.00   **Phlebotomus Fever**   Most free serum amino acids are depressed in sandfly fever and other mild-moderate infections. *0122*

319.00   **Mental Retardation**   Increased glutamic acid with associated decrease in glutamine may occur in De Lange Syndrome and other mental retardation syndromes. *0493*

714.00   **Rheumatoid Arthritis**   Frequently low. *2104*

Serum   Increase

270.61   **Citrullinemia**   Mild elevations have been found. *2246*

572.20   **Hepatic Encephalopathy**   An end product in ammonia metabolism. *1473*

Serum   Normal

157.90   **Malignant Neoplasm of Pancreas**   High levels of glutamic acid and normal glutamine levels were found in 9 of 10 patients. Mean value = 3.40 ± 2.22 mg/dL. *0359*

274.00   **Gout**   *2246*

Urine   Increase

270.02   **Hartnup Disease**   Urine chromatography shows greatly increased amount of glutamine. *2468*   5-20 X normal values. *2246*

714.00   **Rheumatoid Arthritis**   *2104*

CSF   Increase

270.51   **Histidinemia**   In some reports. *0831 1065 2246*

572.20   **Hepatic Encephalopathy**   An end product in ammonia metabolism. *1473*

Glutathione

Serum   Normal

642.60   **Eclampsia**   *0621*

Red Blood Cells   Increase

289.80   **Myelofibrosis**   RBC reduced glutathione occurred in 16 of 17 myelofibrosis patients. *2317*   In myelofibrosis, usually increased. *0900*

Glutathione Reductase

Serum   Increase

197.70   **Secondary Malignant Neoplasm of Liver**   Raised in 47% of cases. *2093*

Glycerol

Serum   Increase

242.90   **Hyperthyroidism**   Increased lipid degradation. *2540*

271.01   **Von Gierke's Disease**   Has been observed. *1722*

585.00   **Chronic Renal Failure**   Increased mean plasma concentration in chronic failure. *1243*

994.50   **Exercise**   Approximately 10-30% increase with bicycle pedalling. *0909*

Glycine

Serum   Decrease

274.00   **Gout**   Distinct reduction. *2604*

Serum   Increase

38.00   **Septicemia**   Concentrations determined in 10 burned patients with gram-negative sepsis and 9 burned patients without sepsis revealed an increase in the gluconeogenic precursors alanine, glycine, methionine and phenylalanine in those patients with sepsis. *2543*

251.20   **Hypoglycemia, Unspecified**   Persistently elevated and is generally higher than in secondary hyperglycinemias. *0433*

585.00   **Chronic Renal Failure**   A significant rise in mean concentration occurred in children whose GFR was < 15 mL/min/1.73 m^3. 34% had values above normal upper limit. *0192*

Serum   Normal

275.35   **Vitamin D Resistant Rickets**   Found in excess quantities in the urine but not in the plasma. *0433*

Urine   Increase

251.20   **Hypoglycemia, Unspecified**   Persistently elevated and are generally higher than in secondary hyperglycinemias. *0433*

270.01   **Cystinuria**   *0786*

270.02   **Hartnup Disease**   5-20 X normal values. *2246*

270.41   **Cystathioninuria**   *2468*

270.81   **Hyperprolinemia**   Hyperaminoaciduria of proline, glycine and hydroxyproline is specific. *2246   2468*

275.35   **Vitamin D Resistant Rickets**   Found in excess quantities in the urine but not in the plasma. *0433*

714.00   **Rheumatoid Arthritis**   *2104*

984.00   **Toxic Effects of Lead and Its Compounds (including Fumes)**   Transient increase. *0294*

Glycine *(continued)*

Urine   Normal

270.02   **Hartnup Disease**   *0631*

Glycoproteins

Serum   Decrease

70.00   **Viral Hepatitis**   In acute fulminant hepatitis, the values showed a statistically significant difference between fatal (21.9 mg/dL) and surviving cases (37.4 mg/dL). *1291*

714.00   **Rheumatoid Arthritis**   Significant lowering of beta-2 glycoprotein concentrations found. *1305*

Serum   Increase

84.00   **Malaria**   Serum alpha$_1$ glycoproteins are increased and alpha$_2$ glycoproteins are decreased. *0151*

162.90   **Malignant Neoplasm of Bronchus and Lung**   Increased levels found in > 50% of patients. *0925*

174.90   **Malignant Neoplasm of Breast**   Significant preoperative elevation of beta$_2$ glycoprotein in cancer patients compared to patients with benign breast tumors. *1810*

197.50   **Secondary Malignant Neoplasm of Digestive System**   Metastases are indicated when levels increase in patients with large intestinal cancer. *2480*

199.00   **Secondary Malignant Neoplasm (Disseminated)**   Metastases are indicated when levels increase in patients with large intestinal cancer. *2480*

245.10   **Subacute Thyroiditis**   Increased serum C3, alpha$_1$-acid glycoprotein and alpha$_1$-antitrypsin levels found in 40 patients. *1715*

571.49   **Chronic Active Hepatitis**   Alpha$_2$ glycoproteins, ceruloplasmin, and transferrin were elevated. *1654*

642.40   **Pre-Eclampsia**   Concentration of alpha$_1$ easily precipitable glycoprotein increased greatly despite large urinary losses, indicating augmented synthesis. *2287 2286*

710.00   **Systemic Lupus Erythematosus**   Have been found to be elevated but are nonspecific. *0962*

994.50   **Exercise**   Increased alpha$_1$ acid glycoprotein occurs within 15 min and persists for 1 day. *0985*

Serum   Normal

994.50   **Exercise**   No change was observed in alpha$_1$ acid glycoprotein after exercise. *1837*

Urine   Increase

642.40   **Pre-Eclampsia**   Large urinary losses of alpha$_1$ easily precipitable glycoprotein. *2287 2286   0387*

Gonadotropin, Chorionic

Serum   Decrease

185.00   **Malignant Neoplasm of Prostate**   Patients with seminomas and teratomas should have a low titer. *0536*

633.90   **Ectopic Pregnancy**   82.6% of 23 women with proven ectopic pregnancies had abnormally low first trimester hCG levels. *0273*   Decreased *0001 0265 1691 2115*

640.00   **Threatened Abortion**   Decreased. *0001 0265 0299 1691*

Serum   Increase

151.90   **Malignant Neoplasm of Stomach**   Ectopic production. *0001 0265 0299 1691*

153.90   **Malignant Neoplasm of Large Intestine**   Ectopic production. *0001 0265 0299 1691*

155.00   **Malignant Neoplasm of Liver**   Ectopic production. *0001 0265 0299 1691*

157.90   **Malignant Neoplasm of Pancreas**   Elevated immunoreactive hCG was found in 33% of patients. *0740*

162.90   **Malignant Neoplasm of Bronchus and Lung**   Ectopic production. *0001 0265 0299 1691 0536*

180.90   **Malignant Neoplasm of Cervix**   CEA, AFP and hCG were measured in 253 patients with gynecologic malignancies and in 317 patients with benign gynecologic diseases. Concentrations of each of these antigens were elevated in a significantly greater number of patients with invasive cancer. *0580*

181.00   **Malignant Neoplasm of Trophoblast (Choriocarcinoma)**   In pure choriocarcinomas, human chorionic gonadotropins are always elevated and AFP is absent. *2583*

183.00   **Malignant Neoplasm of Ovary**   The highest incidence was found in patients with carcinoma of testis (61%), adenocarcinoma of ovary (42%), and pancreas (33%). *0740*   In 22 patients, 30% had hCG positive serum. *2268*   Elevated with invasive carcinoma. *0580*

186.90   **Malignant Neoplasm of Testis**   Elevated marker assay indicates active disease in nonseminomatous testicular germ cell tumors, during and after therapeutic interventions. Normal does not exclude active disease being present. *1621*   The highest incidence of immunoreactive hCG (61%) found in cancers. *0740*   This is an effective tumor marker in the staging and management of testicular cancer and potentially of nontrophoblastic cancers *1111*   Elevated in 60% of stage A and B cases and all patients with stage C disease *0756*

251.50   **Zollinger-Ellison Syndrome**   Significant correlation between basal levels and malignant gastrinoma but not with benign tumors. *2244*

630.00   **Hydatidiform Mole**   High concentrations of chorionic gonadotropin and reduced pregnanediol indicate diagnosis. *2104*   Human chorionic somatomammotropin was > normal in 8 of 13 patients with intact mole, ranging from 10-910 ng/mL. *1613*   0.5-2,830 IU/mL and less than 200 IU/mL in 36% of the patients. *1667*

642.40   **Pre-Eclampsia**   Severe cases often are associated with high urinary and serum concentrations, and mild cases are not. *1431*

642.60   **Eclampsia**   Not demonstrable in all cases. *2211*

650.00   **Pregnancy**   Multiple pregnancies. *0001 0265 0299 1691*

Serum   Normal

642.40   **Pre-Eclampsia**   Average serum and urinary concentrations were the same in pre-eclamptic as in normal pregnant women. *2332*

Urine   Decrease

633.90   **Ectopic Pregnancy**   Low values for the stage of pregnancy. *0619*

640.00   **Threatened Abortion**   Low values for stage of pregnancy. Low values in early pregnancy are found in habitual abortion. *0619*

Urine   Increase

181.00   **Malignant Neoplasm of Trophoblast (Choriocarcinoma)**   Markedly increased with primary chorionepithelioma of ovary. *2467*

186.90   **Malignant Neoplasm of Testis**   90% of patients with testicular tumors are positive; useful in gauging efficacy of chemotherapy. *2467*   An elevation of the gonadotropins usually indicates the presence of a tumor containing chorionic tissue and indicates poor prognosis. *0433*

630.00   **Hydatidiform Mole**   A rising titer at the end of t trimester is significant. Titers can rise to 1,000 IU/L or more. *0619*

642.40   **Pre-Eclampsia**   Severe cases often are associated with high urinary and serum concentrations, and mild cases are not. *1431*

642.60   **Eclampsia**   Not demonstrable in all cases. *2211*

650.00   **Pregnancy**   *0294*

Urine   Normal

642.40   **Pre-Eclampsia**   Average concentrations in urine and sera were the same in pre-eclamptic as in normal pregnant women. *2332*

656.40   **Pregnancy Complicated by Intrauterine Death**   *2467*

Pleural Effusion   Increase

183.00   **Malignant Neoplasm of Ovary**   In 22 patients, 30% had positive serum while 68% had positive pleural and ascites effusions. *2268*

Ascitic Fluid   Increase

183.00   **Malignant Neoplasm of Ovary**   In 22 patients, 30% had positive serum while 68% had positive pleural and ascites effusions. *2268*

Gonadotropin, Pituitary

Serum   Decrease

185.00   Malignant Neoplasm of Prostate   Patients with prostatic carcinoma and benign prostatic hypertrophy showed lower levels of LH when compared with age-matched controls. *0971*

242.90   Hyperthyroidism   *2035*

253.00   Acromegaly   Serum and urinary gonadotropins may be diminished; azoospermia and amenorrhea may ensue. *0962*

253.40   Anterior Pituitary Hypofunction   Decreased in secondary hypogonadism. *2467*

256.41   Stein-Leventhal Syndrome   *0151*

275.00   Hemochromatosis   Basal gonadotropin levels and/or their response to LHRH were low in 9 of 12 patients. *0199*

282.41   Thalassemia Major   Markedly impaired gonadotropin response to LH releasing hormones in beta thalassemia. *1346*

282.60   Sickle Cell Anemia   Serum LH and FSH before and after stimulation with gonadotropin releasing hormone were consistent with primary testicular failure in all 14 adult male patients tested. *0005*

600.00   Benign Prostatic Hypertrophy   Patients with both malignant and benign prostatic disease showed lower concentrations of luteinizing hormone when compared with age-matched controls. *0971*

Serum   Increase

151.90   Malignant Neoplasm of Stomach   Can cause the syndrome of ectopic gonadotropin production. *0962*

162.90   Malignant Neoplasm of Bronchus and Lung   Gonadotropin activity is clinically manifested by gynecomastia and by elevated gonadotropin blood levels. *0962*   All cell types of bronchogenic cancer can cause the syndrome of ectopic gonadotropin production. *0962*   Anaplastic large cell carcinoma. *0799*

181.00   Malignant Neoplasm of Trophoblast (Choriocarcinoma) *0962*

189.00   Malignant Neoplasm of Kidney   Can cause the syndrome of ectopic gonadotropin production. *0962*

194.00   Malignant Neoplasm of Adrenal Gland   Feminizing adrenal tumor can cause the syndrome of ectopic gonadotropin production. *0962*

244.90   Hypothyroidism   *0962*

245.20   Hashimoto's Thyroiditis   In the far advanced stage of thyroid destruction, all tests show the results of hypothyroidism. *2035*

256.40   Polycystic Ovaries   Elevated in polycystic ovary disease. *0879*

256.41   Stein-Leventhal Syndrome   Slightly elevated levels of LH in Stein-Leventhal syndrome. *0151*

303.90   Alcoholism   48 male chronic alcoholics classified in 2 groups according to the presence (22) or absence (26) of clinically evident sexual disorders. The level was significantly higher in the group with sexual disorders. *2169*

630.00   Hydatidiform Mole   *0962*

758.70   Klinefelter's Syndrome (XXY)   *0962*

758.80   Syndromes Due to Sex Chromosome Abnormalities   In Turner's syndrome. *2468*

Urine   Decrease

220.00   Benign Neoplasm of Ovary   Inhibited by increased estrogen. *2467*

253.00   Acromegaly   Serum and urinary gonadotropins may be diminished; azoospermia and amenorrhea may ensue. *0962*

253.40   Anterior Pituitary Hypofunction   Deficiency leads to amenorrhea and genital atrophy. *2612*   *0995*

256.30   Ovarian Hypofunction   Increased or decreased depending on whether it is primary or secondary failure. *2540*

257.20   Testicular Hypofunction   Decreased in secondary hypogonadism. *2468*

275.00   Hemochromatosis   9 of 15 patients had pituitary dysfunction. *2265*   A frequent complication. *2246*

Urine   Increase

186.90   Malignant Neoplasm of Testis   Increased with seminoma. *0619*

256.30   Ovarian Hypofunction   Increased or decreased depending on whether it is primary or secondary failure. *2540*   *2467*

257.20   Testicular Hypofunction   Increased in primary hypogonadism. *2468*

275.34   Familial Periodic Paralysis   During attack. *0362*

627.90   Menopausal and Postmenopausal Symptoms   *0433*   *2468*

758.70   Klinefelter's Syndrome (XXY)   Almost invariably increased. *0151*   Commonly elevated; a result of deficient testicular function. *1090*   *0962*

758.80   Syndromes Due to Sex Chromosome Abnormalities   In Turner's syndrome. *0619*

Granular Casts

Urine   Increase

70.00   Viral Hepatitis   During the early icteric phase may reflect renal abnormalities. *0151*

250.00   Diabetes Mellitus   With diabetic nephropathy. *0186*

270.03   Cystinosis   As glomerular damage progresses. *2246*

273.21   Cryoglobulinemia (Essential Mixed)   Urinary sediment contains erythrocytes and finely granular casts. *0433*

287.00   Allergic Purpura   May be seen. *2538*

428.00   Congestive Heart Failure   There are isolated RBC and WBC, hyaline and sometimes granular casts. *2467*

446.00   Polyarteritis-Nodosa   Abnormal urinalysis is far more frequent (70-80%) than azotemia (25-30%). *0433*   Hyaline and granular casts indicate renal involvement. *0151*

482.90   Bacterial Pneumonia   Protein, WBC, hyaline and granular casts in small amounts are common. *2467*

580.00   Acute Poststreptococcal Glomerulonephritis   Usually present. *0151*

580.02   Glomerulonephritis (Minimal Change)   Hyaline, granular, and fatty casts are found. *0151*

580.04   Glomerulonephritis (Membranous)   Usually present. *0433*

585.00   Chronic Renal Failure   Proteinuria and granular casts suggest chronic parenchymal renal disease. *0433*

710.00   Systemic Lupus Erythematosus   In lupus glomerulonephritis it is not unusual to find a sediment in which all the formed elements and casts seen in various stages. *0962*   *0433*

Granulocytes

Blood   Decrease

279.13   Nezeloff's Syndrome   *2344*

Growth Hormone

Serum   Decrease

253.40   Anterior Pituitary Hypofunction   Characterized by absent or reduced production and release. *1108*   Deficiency may lead to dwarfism in children and contribute to hypoglycemia in children and adults. *2612*   *0995*

255.00   Adrenal Cortical Hyperfunction (Glucocorticoid Excess)   Basal levels are often low and respond poorly to stimuli. *0962*

275.00   Hemochromatosis   9 of 15 patients had pituitary dysfunction. *2265*   A frequent complication. *2246*

277.00   Cystic Fibrosis   *0914*

579.00   Celiac Sprue Disease   Insulin-induced growth hormone is inadequate in most cases during the active phase, but returns to normal on recovery provided the diet is gluten-free. *2415*

1013.00   Diet   Fluctuates rapidly during the day in response to nutritional factors. Generally low after food ingestion and high during a fast. *2104*

Serum   Increase

151.90   Malignant Neoplasm of Stomach   Elevated. *0918*

162.90   Malignant Neoplasm of Bronchus and Lung   Elevated. *0918*

217.00   Benign Neoplasm of Breast   Elevated. *0918*

250.00   Diabetes Mellitus   In insulin-dependent diabetics high values are usually observed. *0858*   Often abnormally high. *2104*

250.10   Diabetic Acidosis   *2540*

Growth Hormone (continued)

Serum Increase (continued)

251.20 Hypoglycemia, Unspecified *0619*

253.00 Acromegaly The definitive test for diagnosis is an increase of 10 ng/mL, which is not suppressible by glucose. *0433* Usually basal levels > 20 ng/mL. High basal growth hormone levels and failure of suppression by glucose at 1 or 2 h are the definitive criteria for the diagnosis. *0962 0151*

259.20 Carcinoid Syndrome Elevated. *0918*

260.00 Protein Malnutrition Elevated fasting plasma concentrations in all groups of malnourished children. *1955*

278.00 Obesity Secretory response to a variety of stimuli is attenuated. *0062*

303.00 Acute Alcoholic Intoxication Increased following alcoholic binge of several days duration. *1594*

303.90 Alcoholism Increased following alcoholic binge of several days duration. *1594*

308.00 Stress Normal response. *0217*

584.00 Acute Renal Failure Consistently occurring hypersecretion may be induced by severe uremia. *0787*

585.00 Chronic Renal Failure Increased mean plasma concentration in chronic failure. *1243* Consistently occurring hypersecretion may be induced by severe uremia. *0787 1108*

994.50 Exercise Effect more marked in untrained than trained athletes. *1176 0619*

Serum Normal

270.03 Cystinosis Growth failure is characteristic even though growth hormone concentrations are normal. *2246*

278.00 Obesity Similar levels were obtained in 10 nonobese patients. *0864*

650.00 Pregnancy *2593*

758.70 Klinefelter's Syndrome (XXY) Usually normal. *1090*

Urine Increase

275.00 Hemochromatosis Marked elevation. *1445*

584.00 Acute Renal Failure Marked elevation. *1445*

585.00 Chronic Renal Failure Marked elevation. *1445*

CSF Increase

194.30 Malignant Neoplasm of Pituitary 21 of 22 patients with suprasellar extension of a pituitary tumor had elevations of one or more CSF adenohypophyseal hormones. *1189*

Guanase

Serum Increase

985.00 Toxic Effects of Non-medicinal Metals Hepatotoxicity may occur with arsenicals. *1446*

Haptoglobin

Serum Decrease

78.50 Cytomegalic Inclusion Disease Hemolytic anemia. *1058*

84.00 Malaria Intravascular hemolysis due to parasites. *2467*

85.00 Leishmaniasis Intravascular hemolysis due to parasites. *2467* Hemolytic anemia. *2568*

86.90 Trypanosomiasis Intravascular hemolysis due to parasites. *2467*

87.00 Relapsing Fever Intravascular hemolysis due to parasites. *2467*

88.00 Bartonellosis Intravascular hemolysis due to parasites. *2467*

204.10 Lymphocytic Leukemia (Chronic) 20% of patients develop severe hemolysis. *0992*

207.00 Erythroleukemia Evidence of a mild or moderate increase in hemolysis is commonly observed, but the erythrokinetic findings are those of ineffective erythropoiesis. *2538*

271.01 Von Gierke's Disease Reflects chronic hemolysis. *0186*

272.52 Abetalipoproteinemia Reflects increased red cell turnover. *2171*

275.10 Hepatolenticular Degeneration Hemolytic anemia. *0995*

281.00 Pernicious Anemia Probably due at least partly to impaired formation. *0619 0433*

281.30 Vitamin B$_6$ Deficiency Anemia Decreased in hemoglobinemias (related to the duration and severity of hemolysis) due to extravascular hemolysis. *2467*

282.00 Hereditary (Congenital) Spherocytosis Decreased in hemoglobinemia (related to the duration and severity of hemolysis) due to extravascular hemolysis. Seen in hereditary spherocytosis with marked hemolysis. Becomes normal in 4-6 days after treatment with splenectomy. *2467*

282.10 Hereditary Elliptocytosis In patients with more severe forms of this disease there may be a compensated hemolytic anemia with reduced serum haptoglobin. *0433 2538*

282.20 Anemias Due To Disorders of Glutathione Metabolism *2467*

282.31 Hereditary Nonspherocytic Hemolytic Anemia Reflects chronic hemolysis. *0186*

282.41 Thalassemia Major Decreased in hemoglobinemias (related to the duration and severity of hemolysis) due to extravascular hemolysis. *2467*

282.60 Sickle Cell Anemia RBC destruction is partially intravascular, producing elevated plasma heme proteins and decreased haptoglobin concentration. *0476 2552 2538*

282.71 Hemoglobin C Disease Substantially reduced or even absent. *2538*

282.72 Hemoglobin E Disease Substantially reduced or even absent. *2538*

282.73 Hemoglobin H Disease Substantially reduced or even absent. *2538*

283.00 Acquired Hemolytic Anemia (Autoimmune) Decreased in hemoglobinemia (related to the duration and severity of hemolysis) due to extravascular hemolysis. *2467* Usually depleted; the return to normal is a valuable indicator of remission. *2538*

283.21 Paroxysmal Nocturnal Hemoglobinuria Absent during a hemolytic episode. *2468 0041*

286.60 Disseminated Intravascular Coagulopathy Decreases in 6-10 h and lasts for 2-3 days after lysis of 20-30 mL of blood. Determination is relatively reliable and very sensitive. *2468*

446.60 Thrombotic Thrombocytopenic Purpura May accompany elevated indirect bilirubin, indicating intravascular RBC destruction. *2552*

483.01 Mycoplasma Pneumoniae Usually normal but, in some cases, decreases rapidly with bacteremia. *2368 0729*

570.00 Acute and Subacute Necrosis of Liver Mild to moderate hemolysis usually occurs. *1849*

571.49 Chronic Active Hepatitis The only protein to be significantly reduced. *1654*

572.40 Hepatic Failure *0503*

650.00 Pregnancy Decreased 16% in late normal pregnancy. *2286 2287*

710.00 Systemic Lupus Erythematosus Decreased if associated with hemolytic anemia. *2467*

994.50 Exercise Mean effect of 18 mg/dL from pre-exercise. *2092*

Serum Increase

151.90 Malignant Neoplasm of Stomach *0992*

153.90 Malignant Neoplasm of Large Intestine Increased in primary cancer, and rises in metastatic cancer especially involving the liver. Values are useful to indicate tumor activity. *0450* Increased in patients (2.2 g/L) compared to normals (1.1 g/L). *1025*

162.90 Malignant Neoplasm of Bronchus and Lung Increased to 2.2 g/L, compared to normals, 1.1 g/L. *1025*

174.90 Malignant Neoplasm of Breast Increased to 2.2 g/L compared to normals (1.1 g/L). *1025*

182.00 Malignant Neoplasm of Corpus Uteri Increased (2.2 g/L) compared to normals (1.1 g/L). *1025*

189.00 Malignant Neoplasm of Kidney May be elevated without metastases. *0836*

197.50 Secondary Malignant Neoplasm of Digestive System High levels of haptoglobin may suggest involvement of the bowel wall by recurrent cancer. *2480*

197.70 Secondary Malignant Neoplasm of Liver alpha$_2$-globulins, especially haptoglobins were generally increased in primary colorectal cancer, and rose in metastatic cancer especially when it involved the liver. Haptoglobin values were useful to indicate tumor activity. *0450*

199.00 Secondary Malignant Neoplasm (Disseminated) Serum concentration of albumin and transferrin were significantly reduced while haptoglobin was increased in disseminated carcinoma compared with localized. *1025*

201.90 Hodgkin's Disease Increased in disseminated neoplasms; conditions associated with increased ESR and alpha$_2$-globulin. *2467 0151*

202.80 Non-Hodgkins Lymphoma Conditions associated with increased ESR and alpha$_2$-globulin. *2467*

267.00 Vitamin C Deficiency Conditions associated with increased ESR and alpha 2 globulin; increases in collagen diseases. *2467*

277.30 Amyloidosis Conditions associated with increased ESR and alpha$_2$-globulin. *2467*

303.90 Alcoholism Mean value = 99.85 mg/dL for the alcoholic group. Normal value was 71.66 mg/dL. *0523*

390.00 Rheumatic Fever Conditions associated with increased ESR and alpha 2 globulin; increases in collagen disease. *2467*

410.90 Acute Myocardial Infarction Significant increase. *1724*

555.90 Regional Enteritis or Ileitis Haptoglobin concentrations rise with increasing clinical activity of the disease, while the prealbumin fraction declines. *1510 2035*

556.00 Ulcerative Colitis Haptoglobin concentrations rise with increasing clinical activity of the disease, while the prealbumin fraction declines. *1510 2035*

576.20 Extrahepatic Biliary Obstruction Can be variable or increased. Increased in 33% of patients with obstructive biliary disease. *2467*

581.90 Nephrotic Syndrome Conditions associated with increased ESR and alpha$_2$-globulin. *2467*

590.00 Chronic Pyelonephritis Increased serum levels found in 84 chronic patients correlated with activity of pathologic process and distinguished it from glomerulonephritis. *2362*

710.40 Dermatomyositis/Polymyositis Conditions associated with increased ESR and alpha 2 globulin; increases in collagen diseases. *2467*

714.00 Rheumatoid Arthritis Usually parallel the activity of the ESR. *0962*

994.50 Exercise Approximately 17% increase immediately after exercise. *1837*

Serum   Normal

273.30 Waldenström's Macroglobulinemia *2467*

273.80 Analbuminemia *2467*

279.04 Agammaglobulinemia (Congenital Sex-linked) *2467*

280.90 Iron Deficiency Anemia *2467*

496.01 Alpha$_1$-Antitrypsin Deficiency *2467*

580.00 Acute Poststreptococcal Glomerulonephritis *2467*

Urine   Increase

153.90 Malignant Neoplasm of Large Intestine 24 h excretion and renal clearance were significantly increased in localized tumor patients compared to normals and disseminated cancer cases. Increased high molecular weight protein excretion implies glomerular injury in these patients. *1025*

162.90 Malignant Neoplasm of Bronchus and Lung 24 h excretion and renal clearance were significantly increased in localized tumor patients compared to normals and disseminated cancer cases. Increased high molecular weight protein excretion implies glomerular injury in these patients. *1025*

174.90 Malignant Neoplasm of Breast 24 h excretion and renal clearance were significantly increased in localized tumor patients compared to normals and disseminated cancer cases. Increased high molecular weight protein excretion implies glomerular injury in these patients. *1025*

182.00 Malignant Neoplasm of Corpus Uteri 24 h excretion and renal clearance were significantly increased in localized tumor patients compared to normals and disseminated cancer cases. Increased high molecular weight protein excretion implies glomerular injury in these patients. *1025*

Hemagglutination Inhibition

Serum   Increase

1.00 Cholera *1058*

4.90 Bacillary Dysentery Generally demonstrable. *1058*

6.00 Amebiasis Positive test is > 1:128. *2468* Usually positive in the presence of tissue invasion and approach 100% with extracolonic disease such as liver abscess. *0999* Test for E. histolytica has been found to be positive in over 90% of patients with proven amebic liver abscess. *0962*

23.00 Brucellosis When a series of known positive sera were submitted to 6 recognized laboratories highly variable reports were received, ranging from negative to titers as high as 1:640 for the same serum. In view of many variables there can hardly be a titer considered to be diagnostic. In general a titer of 1:320 or higher in the presence of significant symptoms and a reasonable exposure history may be considered presumptive evidence of the disease. *0433 2035*

32.00 Diphtheria Assays antitoxin titer of patient's serum. 4-fold increase between titer in acute and convalescent sera confirms diagnosis. *2468*

50.00 Smallpox Only titers above 1,:1000 or a great increase in titer is significant. *0433* A rising antibody titer is seen in paired sera. *0962*

55.00 Measles Circulating antibody is present by the time the rash develops. HI antibodies and neutralizing antibodies remain indefinitely. *0433*

56.00 Rubella Change in titer from acute-phase to convalescent-phase sera is the most useful technique to demonstrate a rise in antibody titer. With rubella rash, diagnosis is established if acute sample titer is > 1:10 or if convalescent-phase serum taken 7 days after rash shows a 4-fold increase in titer. *2468* Does not distinguish between IgM and IgG antibodies but absence of HI antibodies in cord blood makes diagnosis unlikely. *2508*

72.00 Mumps Develops later and persists longer by several months than complement-fixation test. *2468* A 4-fold difference in titer between the 1st and 3rd week is diagnostic. *2368*

82.00 Rocky Mountain Spotted Fever May be superior to complement-fixation procedure in typhus and Rocky Mountain spotted fever. *1813*

84.00 Malaria Antibody to malarial parasites may be detected by the indirect fluorescent antibody test and by hemagglutination tests. *0962* In natural infections, the complement-fixation and indirect hemagglutination tests detect malarial antibodies equally efficiently for the first 2 months after onset, but titers obtained by complement-fixation rapidly decline within a year, while the indirect hemagglutination titers remain elevated. *2547*

85.00 Leishmaniasis Used for diagnosis but requires fuller development for routine use. *0503*

120.00 Schistosomiasis Indirect hemagglutination. *1058*

122.90 Hydatidosis *1058*

124.00 Trichinosis Tannic acid hemagglutination proved to be very sensitive; antibodies were detected in 6 days. *1207*

127.00 Ascariasis *0503*

128.00 Larva Migrans (Visceralis) Tests with Ascaris and Toxocara antigen are helpful, but are rarely diagnostic because cross reactions with other helminths are common. *1058*

130.00 Toxoplasmosis Specific and sensitive. *0433* Hemagglutinating antibody appears later and rises more slowly than IFA antibody. *2035* Marked elevations of antibody to toxoplasmosis. *2538 2571*

410.90 Acute Myocardial Infarction Using the passive hemagglutination reaction, a 4-fold or greater rise in antibodies to saline extracts of human heart in 46% of 50 patients was found. Highest titers and highest frequency of elevated titers occurred 2-4 weeks after onset. *1018 2035*

483.01 Mycoplasma Pneumoniae Titer of at least 1:128 (preferably 1:512) points to the presence of a M. pneumoniae infection, especially if clinical, radiological, and laboratory data suggest a nonbacterial or mixed pneumonia. *0352*

487.10 Influenza May become positive during the second week of illness. *0962* A 4-fold or greater rise in antibody level between paired sera is accepted as evidence of infection. *0433* Appears to be more useful in detecting influenza A than complement-fixation tests (CF). 23% of cases verified by HI were missed by CF. *1867*

771.00 Congenital Rubella The finding of antibody after 6-8 months of age may be taken as evidence of congenital rubella. *0433* Persistently elevated titers during 1st y of life. *2508*

Hematocrit

Blood   Decrease

2.00   Typhoid Fever   Normochromic anemia usually develops and may be aggravated by blood loss in stools. *0151* Normochromic anemia is common present late in illness and during convalescence. *0962   1058*

6.00   Amebiasis   Normochromic or hypochromic anemia is found in 75% of cases. *1058*   Mild degree of anemia is common, either normochromic or hypochromic. Severity is related to duration of symptoms. *0015*

11.00   Pulmonary Tuberculosis   Anemia is common because of the effects of the infection on RBC production and survival and because of coexistent iron and nutritional deficiencies. *0433*

18.00   Disseminated Tuberculosis   *2538 0486*

30.00   Leprosy   Anemia, when present, is usually mild. *0962*

32.00   Diphtheria   Moderate anemia persisting into convalescence is common. *0433*

38.00   Septicemia   Mild to moderate anemia may occur during the course of chronic infections. *0433*

39.90   Actinomycosis   A mild to moderate normocytic, normochromic anemia frequently accompanies this disease. *0433*

40.20   Whipple's Disease   Anemia is common and is usually associated with iron deficiency. *2199*

52.00   Chickenpox   *2538 1857*

53.00   Herpes Zoster   In 37% of 18 patients at initial hospitalization for this disorder. *0781*

54.00   Herpes Simplex   *2538 1857*

55.00   Measles   *2538 1857*

66.10   Tick-Borne Fever   Anemia develops in some patients. *1058*

70.00   Viral Hepatitis   May develop late in the course of the disease. *0151*   A mild degree of transient anemia. *0962*

75.00   Infectious Mononucleosis   Anemia is rare. *1319*

78.50   Cytomegalic Inclusion Disease   Anemia usually present in congenital disease. *1319*   Hemolytic anemia. *0767   2538*

80.00   Epidemic Typhus   Normal early, falls significantly during the illness. *0433*   May develop in the 2nd or 3rd week. *2368*

82.00   Rocky Mountain Spotted Fever   Anemia may develop in the 2nd-3rd weeks. *2368*

84.00   Malaria   With disease progression a normocytic, normochromic anemia may become apparent. *0433*   Marked anemia was found only in the patients with defective hemoglobin synthesis. *2240*   Anemia is present in proportion to the severity of the infection. *0962*

85.00   Leishmaniasis   Normochromic, normocytic anemia develops slowly but becomes severe later in the disease. *0151*   Hemolytic anemia. *2568   2538*

86.90   Trypanosomiasis   Anemia is a characteristic feature. *2569*   Mild normocytic normochromic anemia associated with reduced marrow activity. *1058   2035*

87.00   Relapsing Fever   Moderate anemia may occur later in the disease. *0962*   Intravascular hemolysis due to parasites. *2467*

88.00   Bartonellosis   Intravascular hemolysis due to parasites. *2467   2538 1918*

97.90   Syphilis   Secondary anemia. *1058*

99.10   Lymphogranuloma Venereum   Anemia and leukopenia are most common when enlargement of the liver and spleen and generalized lymphadenopathy occur. *0433   2199*

99.30   Reiter's Disease   There may be a mild anemia. *0433*

100.00   Leptospirosis   With jaundice, anemia may be severe due to intravascular hemolysis. Anemia is unusual in anicteric patients. *0992*

115.00   Histoplasmosis   50% of the patients with disseminated disease may have anemia. *0999*   A marked to moderate hypochromic anemia occurs in most cases. *0962*   Usually an iron deficient normochromic normocytic anemia. *2199*   Normochromic anemia. *2368*

116.00   Blastomycosis   Present in < 50% of patients. *0433*

117.30   Aspergillosis   Hemolytic anemia. *2538 1950*

123.40   Diphyllobothriasis (Intestinal)   When present, anemia is macrocytic. *2199*

124.00   Trichinosis   Prolonged infection may result in secondary anemia. *2368*

126.90   Ancylostomiasis (Hookworm Infestation)   A microcytic, hypochromic anemia attributed directly to blood loss; when the patient has severe malnutrition, however, the anemia may be macrocytic hypochromic anemia. *0433*   Anemia occurring in hookworm disease is a classic iron deficiency anemia. *2199*   Development of hypochromic, microcytic anemia depends on the number of worms, recency of infection, and host nutrition. *2368*

127.20   Strongyloidiasis   Anemia, when it occurs, is usually iron deficiency in type. *2199*

127.30   Trichuriasis   In children can be accompanied by a microcytic hypochromic anemia. *0433*

130.00   Toxoplasmosis   Anemia is present. *2468   2538 0486*

150.90   Malignant Neoplasm of Esophagus   In 24% of 40 patients at initial hospitalization for this disorder. *0781*

151.90   Malignant Neoplasm of Stomach   The amount of bleeding and the degree of anemia will vary widely. Anemia of more than moderate degree is a late consequence of gastric malignancy. *0962*   Anemia may be of several types. The most common is iron deficiency anemia caused by chronic occult blood loss. *2199*   In 43% of 47 patients at initial hospitalization for this disorder. *0781*

152.90   Malignant Neoplasm of Small Intestine   Anemia may be of several types. The most common is iron deficiency anemia caused by chronic occult blood loss. *2199*

153.90   Malignant Neoplasm of Large Intestine   Anemia; may be the only symptom of carcinoma of the right side of colon (present in > 50% of these patients, usually hypochromic). *2467*   Iron deficiency anemia is common, because of either gross or occult bleeding. *2199*   In 35% of 154 patients at initial hospitalization for this disorder. *0781*   Incidence of anemia between 22-74.6%. *2199*

154.10   Malignant Neoplasm of Rectum   Iron deficiency anemia is common, because of either gross or occult bleeding. *2199*

155.00   Malignant Neoplasm of Liver   In 35% of 14 patients at initial hospitalization for this disorder. *0781*

157.90   Malignant Neoplasm of Pancreas   34% of patients were anemic. *0932*   In 33% of 46 patients at initial hospitalization for this disorder. *0781*

170.90   Malignant Neoplasm of Bone   In 24% of 24 patients at initial hospitalization for this disorder. *0781*

182.00   Malignant Neoplasm of Corpus Uteri   In 25% of 155 patients at initial hospitalization for this disorder. *0781*

185.00   Malignant Neoplasm of Prostate   In 43% of 87 patients at initial hospitalization for this disorder. *0781*

188.90   Malignant Neoplasm of Bladder   May show anemia secondary to iron deficiency or secondary to a diffuse metastatic disease. *0433*   In 22% of 46 patients at initial hospitalization for this disorder. *0781*

189.00   Malignant Neoplasm of Kidney   Anemia occurs in approximately 30% of patients, secondary to bone marrow depression. *0836*   30 of 34 patients with hypernephroma were anemic, due mainly to urinary blood loss. Hemoglobin values varied from 7-12%. *0894*   Anemia is a frequent presenting symptom. *1391*

197.00   Secondary Malignant Neoplasm of Respiratory System   In 28% of 603 patients at initial hospitalization for this disorder. *0781*

198.50   Secondary Malignant Neoplasm of Bone   Depression of all formed elements of the blood is often seen in disseminated neoplastic disease. *0999*

201.90   Hodgkin's Disease   Mild or moderate hemolytic anemia, with a negative Coombs' test, is common in disseminated lymphoma. *0433*   Present in 33% of all patients at diagnosis. Develops in nearly every patient who has fever, sweats, or other systemic manifestations. Becomes worse as the disease advances and improves with remission. *2538 0414*   In 38% of 76 patients at initial hospitalization for this disorder. *0781*

202.40   Leukemic Reticuloendotheliosis   Usually normochromic, normocytic anemia; mild anisocytosis and poikilocytosis were common. *2390*

202.52   Histiocytosis X   A normocytic, normochromic anemia, sometimes severe and sometimes hemolytic in nature, may be present, especially in patients with disseminated disease. Aplastic anemia has also been described. *0433*

202.80   Non-Hodgkins Lymphoma   Anemia may result from blood loss, hemolysis, or bone marrow infiltration. *2538*   Present in < 50% of cases and is rarely severe at time of diagnosis. *2552*   In 22% of 74 patients at initial hospitalization for this disorder. *0781*

203.00 Multiple Myeloma   A normocytic, normochromic anemia is present in 66% of patients at the time of diagnosis. *0433*   Virtually all patients exhibit anemia of varying severity, either at the time of diagnosis or subsequently with disease progression. *2035*   In 69% of 33 patients at initial hospitalization for this disorder. *0781*

204.00 Lymphocytic Leukemia (Acute)   Most patients will have anemia. *0433*   Often severe, usually normochromic, normocytic. *2552*   In 81% of 36 patients at initial hospitalization for this disorder. *0781*

204.10 Lymphocytic Leukemia (Chronic)   Characteristically normochromic normocytic anemia. *0433*   Anemia is not a feature of early disease; it may begin to develop when 50% or more of the bone marrow is usurped by lymphoid tissue. *2489*   Anemia, usually mild, was present at diagnosis in 50% of patients. *2552*   In 76% of 27 patients at initial hospitalization for this disorder. *0781* *2538*

205.00 Myelocytic Leukemia (Acute)   Most patients will have anemia. *0433*   Often severe, may be macrocytic. *2552*   In 90% of 35 patients at initial hospitalization for this disorder. *0781*

205.10 Myelocytic Leukemia (Chronic)   Anemia, when present, is characteristically normochromic normocytic. *0433*   Anemia is almost always a feature of active disease, and generally increases in severity as the disease advances. Usually normocytic and normochromic with little evidence of iron deficiency, accelerated RBC hemolysis, or erythrocyte abnormality. *2538*   In 75% of 20 patients at initial hospitalization for this disorder. *0781* *2552*

206.00 Monocytic Leukemia   Anemia is often quite severe, usually normochromic and normocytic. *2552*   In 90% of 24 patients at initial hospitalization for this disorder. *0781*

207.00 Erythroleukemia   Anemia is nearly always present, but its severity is variable. Usually normocytic and normochromic. *2538*

211.10 Benign Neoplasm of Stomach   With occult bleeding, iron deficiency anemia may be present, in which case the bone marrow will not contain iron. *2199*

212.70 Benign Neoplasm of Cardiovascular Tissue   Hemolytic anemia, and mechanical in origin (due to local turbulence of blood) may occur and may be severe. The anemia is recognized in about 50% of patients. *2467*   Occurs with myxoma, possibly reflecting tumor emboli or tumor breakdown products. *1108*

242.90 Hyperthyroidism   Patients occasionally develop a mild hypochromic anemia. *2540*

244.90 Hypothyroidism   Seldom < 30%. *0433*   Mild to moderate normochromic, normocytic, or slightly macrocytic anemia with normal leukocyte and platelet counts. *0433*   Of 202 patients, anemia was present on diagnosis in 39 of 172 women and 14 of 30 men. Microcytic anemia was present in only 9 patients in the entire series. *1078*   Many patients have a hypoplastic anemia which is unresponsive to therapy with iron, vitamin B_{12}, or folic acid. The degree is mild to moderate. *2538*   Anemia observed in 21-60% of patients. *2552* *0532 0781*

252.00 Hyperparathyroidism   Unexplained anemia found in 21% of 57 patients. *1492*

253.40 Anterior Pituitary Hypofunction   In some cases slight anemia is seen. *0433*   Reduced thyroid, adrenal cortical, pituitary or testicular function can produce anemia. The hematocrit is seldom < 30%. The RBC is normochromic and normocytic. *0433*

255.00 Adrenal Cortical Hyperfunction (Glucocorticoid Excess)   Normal or occasionally slightly elevated unless a malignancy is present in which case it may be depressed. *0433*   Patients with ectopic ACTH syndrome may be anemic. *0962*

255.10 Adrenal Cortical Hyperfunction (Mineralocorticoid Excess)   An increased volume, with slight decrease of the Hct value, is usual. *1108* *0962*

255.40 Adrenal Cortical Hypofunction   Reduced thyroid, adrenal cortical, pituitary or testicular function can produce anemia. Hematocrit is seldom < 30%. The RBC is normochromic and normocytic. *0433*

257.20 Testicular Hypofunction   Reduced testicular function can produce anemia. Hematocrit is seldom < 30%. The RBC is normochromic and normocytic. *0433*

260.00 Protein Malnutrition   There may be moderate anemia. *0433*   Mild or moderate normocytic normochromic anemia occurs after 24 weeks of controlled semistarvation. *2538*

265.00 Thiamine (B_1) Deficiency   Characteristic. *1108*

267.00 Vitamin C Deficiency   Associated with anemia of normocytic, macrocytic, or hypochromic variety in about 80% of cases. *2538*

270.03 Cystinosis   Often significant anemia before renal failure is substantial. *2246*

271.01 Von Gierke's Disease   *0995*

272.52 Abetalipoproteinemia   Anemia has been described. *2246*   Severe anemia with hemoglobin as low as 4-8 g/dL is common in children. Most adult patients do not have significant anemia. *2246* *1583*

272.72 Gaucher's Disease   Unexplained splenomegaly with mild-moderate anemia and thrombocytopenia. *1808*   A normocytic, normochromic anemia is frequently present, but Hb levels rarely fall below 8 g/dL. *2538*

272.73 Niemann-Pick Disease   May be normal or mild anemia may be present. *2538*

273.23 Heavy Chain Disease (Gamma)   Normochromic, normocytic anemia present in all cases. *0999*   Presumably related to hypersplenism. *2035*   All patients have mild to moderate anemia. *2538*

273.30 Waldenström's Macroglobulinemia   Anemia is the most common presenting manifestation and is frequently profound. Usually due to a combination of factors including accelerated RBC destruction, blood loss, and especially decreased erythropoiesis. *2035*   A normochromic, normocytic anemia is usually present. *2538*

275.10 Hepatolenticular Degeneration   Mild normochromic anemia with anisocytosis and poikilocytosis. *0433*   Pancytopenia occurred frequently; hematocrit, platelets, WBC were often decreased. *2278*

277.00 Cystic Fibrosis   In late stages of chronic lung disease, decreased serum electrolytes, hemoglobin, hematocrit, etc. may reflect hemodilution. *2467*

277.11 Congenital Erythropoietic Porphyria (Günther's Disease)   Anemia is normohromic and normocytic and tends to be mild in degree. *2552*   Normochromic anemia, only rarely severe. *2073*

277.12 Erythropoietic Protoporphyria   A moderate hypochromic or normochromic anemia is frequently observed. *2538*

277.13 Erythropoietic Coproporphyria   Microcytic hypochromic anemia may occur due to blood loss or increased demand. *0532*

277.14 Acute Intermittent Porphyria   Microcytic hypochromic anemia may occur due to blood loss or increased demand. *0532*

277.16 Porphyria Cutanea Tarda   Microcytic hypochromic anemia may occur due to blood low or increased demand. *0532*

277.17 Hereditary Coproporphyria   Microcytic hypochromic anemia may occur due to blood loss or increased demand. *0532*

277.22 Lesch-Nyhan Syndrome   Many patients are anemia prior to the occurrence of renal insufficiency. *2246*

277.30 Amyloidosis   Mild anemia present in < 50% of patients. *1334*

279.04 Agammaglobulinemia (Congenital Sex-linked)   Hemolytic anemia. *2035*   Hemolytic anemia frequently occurs. *2246*

279.06 Immunodeficiency (Common Variable)   High incidence of pernicious anemia. *2538*

279.07 Dysgammaglobulinemia (Selective Immunoglobulin Deficiency)   Not uncommon. *0433*

280.81 Plummer-Vinson Syndrome   Hypochromic anemia associated with dysphagia and cardiospasm in women. *2467*

280.90 Iron Deficiency Anemia   *0999 0151*

281.00 Pernicious Anemia   Classical anemia, leukopenia (primarily granulopenia) and thrombocytopenia. Occasionally, the primary reduction may be in only 1 of these 3 major formed elements of the blood. Although patients usually present primarily with anemia they may occasionally present initially with infection associated with granulocytopenia or with bleeding associated with thrombocytopenia. *0433*   In 5 cases, hematocrit varied from 12-20% (normal = 37-54%). *2253*   Anemia may be very severe or very mild. *2552*

281.20 Folic Acid Deficiency Anemia   Hematocrit levels ranged from 12-25% in 10 patients. *2519*   Anemia is normochromic (unless iron deficiency coexists) and macrocytic, with MCV ranging from 100 to 150 fL. *2538*   Anemia ranges from absent to severe. *0962*   Anemia may be very severe or very mild. *2552*

281.30 Vitamin B_6 Deficiency Anemia   The anemia is normocytic or slightly macrocytic. *2538*

282.00 Hereditary (Congenital) Spherocytosis   Anemia may be absent, moderate or severe. RBC is reduced proportionately to the hemoglobin concentration. *0433*   Hct values ranged from 21-36% in 8 patients. *2519*   In 91% of 12 patients at initial hospitalization for this disorder. *1404* *2538 0781*

282.10 Hereditary Elliptocytosis   In severe cases. *2538*

Hematocrit *(continued)*

Blood Decrease *(continued)*

282.31 Hereditary Nonspherocytic Hemolytic Anemia Anemia. *2538*

282.41 Thalassemia Major Anemia is severe, microcytic and hypochromic. *0995*

282.42 Thalassemia Minor Mild anemia, usually with microcytosis, hypochromia, stippling, and target cells usually occurs in heterozygous beta thalassemia. *0151* In periods of stress such as pregnancy or during severe infection, a moderate degree of anemia may be present. *2538*

282.60 Sickle Cell Anemia Decreased in 7 cases, ranging from 17-24%. *2519*

282.71 Hemoglobin C Disease Mild anemia, Hct usually between 30-35. *0433*

282.72 Hemoglobin E Disease Exhibits mild or no anemia. *0433* Homozygotes for hemoglobin E have a relatively mild anemia characterized by microcytosis and targeting of the red cells. *0385 2538*

282.73 Hemoglobin H Disease Life-long anemia with variable splenomegaly and bone changes. *2538* Variable degree of anemia. *2246*

283.00 Acquired Hemolytic Anemia (Autoimmune) In cases with more active hemolysis, anemia may be moderate to severe (with hematocrit's in the 10-25% range) and the reticulocyte count markedly elevated to 50% or more. *2035*

283.21 Paroxysmal Nocturnal Hemoglobinuria May be moderate or severe. *0433* Degree of anemia may vary from none to very severe. *2538*

284.01 Congenital Aplastic Anemia The anemia is normochromic or slightly macrocytic, and macrocytes and target cells may be seen in the blood. *2552*

284.90 Aplastic Anemia A severe anemia may be found at the time of presentation. The RBC are usually normocytic or slightly macrocytic. *0433* Peripheral pancytopenia associated with hypocellular bone marrow. *0415* In 100% of 20 patients hospitalized for this disorder. *0781*

285.00 Sideroblastic Anemia The anemia is normocytic or slightly macrocytic. *2538*

286.01 Hemophilia Presence or absence of anemia depends on the severity and frequency of bleeding. *2552*

287.00 Allergic Purpura Anemia is not usually present unless the hemorrhagic manifestations have been severe. *2538 0962 2552*

287.30 Idiopathic Thrombocytopenic Purpura An anemia from blood loss may be present, but the red blood cell morphology is normal. *0433*

288.00 Agranulocytosis Depending on the underlying process the patient may also manifest moderate to severe anemia. *0433*

289.40 Hypersplenism Apparent anemia is often due to expansion of plasma volume in the presence of normal RBC volume. *1824*

289.80 Myelofibrosis Usually there is a mild to moderate anemia with a mean Hct of 32%. *0433* Anemia mostly normochromic is found in a majority of cases. Hemoglobin < 12 g/dL occurred in 73% of cases. *2317* Anemia is present in 66% of all patients when they are first seen. Usually normochromic and moderate in degree but may become severe in advanced disease in myelofibrosis. *2538*

300.40 Depressive Neurosis Anemia is often present. *0433*

320.90 Meningitis (Bacterial) In 54% of 18 patients hospitalized for this disorder. *0781*

358.00 Myasthenia Gravis Occasional cases of macrocytic anemia. *2467*

390.00 Rheumatic Fever Anemia is common, gradually improves as activity subsides; microcytic types. Anemia may be related to increased plasma volume that occurs in early phase. *2467* Usually normochromic and normocytic and resolves without specific treatment. *1108* Anemia correlates closely with the degree of inflammation; persistence of anemia suggests continued rheumatic activity. *0962*

401.00 Malignant Hypertension Many patients show evidence of microangiopathic hemolytic anemia. *0995*

410.90 Acute Myocardial Infarction After an initial small increase, decreased 12% until day 9 and remained constant thereafter. *2215* Significant increases in plasma volume, reflected by changes in hct. Average change was 12%. For the patients with accompanying pulmonary edema, the change was 17%. *2554*

421.00 Bacterial Endocarditis Anemia is more common in long-standing infection and has no specificity. *0433* Rarely there is a hemolytic anemia with a positive Coombs' test. *2467* Normocytic normochromic anemia commonly presents with mean hct = 35.5 ± 0.6%. Lowest hcts found in gram-negative (29.8 ± 3.1%) and culture-negative cases (30.4 ± 1.6%). Degree of anemia is related to duration of illness, not virulence of organism. *1798* Normochromic, normocytic anemia occurs in 60-70% of cases. *1108*

425.40 Cardiomyopathies A slight degree of anemia with obliterative cardiomyopathies. *1108*

428.00 Congestive Heart Failure Slightly decreased but red cell mass may be increased. *2467*

446.00 Polyarteritis-Nodosa Almost a prerequisite for diagnosis. *0433* Mild anemia is frequently present due either to blood loss or to chronic renal insufficiency. *0642* Anemia is found chiefly in cases complicated by renal insufficiency or blood loss. *0962*

446.20 Goodpasture's Syndrome Secondary to prolonged pulmonary bleeding. *0062*

446.50 Cranial Arteritis and Related Conditions Mild anemia is common, especially in older patients, in polymyalgia rheumatica. *0151* Hypoproliferative anemia is common and may be significant, with Hcts in the 25-30% range. *1013* In 30% of 16 patients hospitalized for this disorder. *0781 2035*

446.60 Thrombotic Thrombocytopenic Purpura Anemia secondary to blood loss may be present. *2035*

480.90 Viral Pneumonia In 49% of 16 patients at initial hospitalization for this disorder. *0781*

482.90 Bacterial Pneumonia In 40% of 19 patients at initial hospitalization for this disorder. *0781* Anemia is common in pneumococcal but not in staphylococcal pneumonia. *2368*

483.01 Mycoplasma Pneumoniae Occasional patients have been reported with hemolytic anemia. *0433* Sometimes seen in convalescence. *0726 2538 0729*

486.01 Resolving Pneumonia In 47% of 79 patients at initial hospitalization for this disorder. *0781*

487.10 Influenza Hemolytic anemia. *2538 1857*

494.00 Bronchiectasis When chronic uncontrolled infection persists, normochromic normocytic anemia is common. *0433*

496.00 Chronic Obstructive Lung Disease Even minor degrees of anemia are poorly tolerated by patients. Because of the high incidence of peptic ulcer associated with this disease, an anemia may be due to occult or clinically evident gastrointestinal bleeding. *0962*

496.01 Alpha$_1$-Antitrypsin Deficiency With associated hypersplenism. *1636*

500.00 Anthracosis Secondary anemia. *2467*

501.00 Asbestosis Secondary anemia. *2467*

502.00 Silicosis Secondary anemia. *2467*

503.01 Berylliosis Secondary anemia. *2467*

513.00 Abscess of Lung Normochromic normocytic anemia in chronic stage. *2467*

533.90 Peptic Ulcer, Site Unspecified A few patients will have anemia because of chronic blood loss. *0433* An ulcer that bleeds chronically will cause a varying degree of iron deficiency anemia. *0962*

535.00 Gastritis May be low in patients with bleeding. *0433*

537.40 Fistula of Stomach and Duodenum Anemia and hypoproteinemia reflect malnutrition and chronic disease. *2199*

553.30 Hernia Diaphragmatic Microcytic anemia (due to loss of blood) may be present. *2467*

555.90 Regional Enteritis or Ileitis Anemia when present can be a result of iron loss or of reduced absorption of vitamin B$_{12}$. *0433* Anemia in approximately 70% of cases. *2035* Iron deficiency is common. *0962* Frequently moderate anemia, most often iron deficiency, but occasionally macrocytic caused by poor diet or failure to absorb vitamin B$_{12}$ normally. *2199*

556.00 Ulcerative Colitis Anemia may be due to blood loss, simple iron deficiency, deficiencies in folic acid, pyridoxine, or vitamin B$_{12}$. *0433* Anemia in approximately 70% of cases. *2035* Anemia secondary to colonic blood loss. Severity varies, depending on the rate and duration of bleeding. *2199*

562.00 Diverticular Disease of Intestine Blood loss is usually minimal but massive bleeding may occur. *2199*

564.20 Postgastrectomy (Dumping) Syndrome Iron deficiency and vitamin B$_{12}$ deficiency are common following subtotal gastrectomy. *0962*

570.00 Acute and Subacute Necrosis of Liver Mild to moderate hemolysis usually occurs. *1849*

571.20 Laennec's or Alcoholic Cirrhosis Approximately 75% of chronic liver disease patients have anemia, usually mild. *1268 2137*

571.49 Chronic Active Hepatitis Anemia, leukopenia and thrombocytopenia occur in 40-60% of patients. *2467* Slight to moderate anemia with leukopenia and thrombocytopenia are seen, particularly in patients with splenomegaly. *2035*

571.90 Cirrhosis of Liver Anemia reflects increased plasma volume and some increased destruction of RBCs. *2467* Approximately 75% of chronic liver disease patients have anemia, usually mild. *1268 2137* In 34% of 70 patients at initial hospitalization for this disorder. *0781*

572.00 Liver Abscess (Pyogenic) Mild to moderate anemia. *0433* A mild normochromic anemia is common. *2199*

577.00 Acute Pancreatitis *2199*

579.00 Celiac Sprue Disease Characteristic iron-deficiency anemia. The peripheral blood smear may show hypochromia. In some cases iron-deficiency anemia may be the predominant abnormality indicative of malabsorption. *0433*

579.01 Protein-Losing Enteropathy There may be a moderate anemia. *0433*

579.90 Malabsorption, Cause Unspecified There may be moderate anemia in idiopathic hypoproteinemia. *0433*

580.00 Acute Poststreptococcal Glomerulonephritis Dilutional anemia. *1108* Normocytic, normochromic anemia occurs as a result of hemodilution. *0433*

580.05 Glomerulonephritis (Membranoproliferative) Mild anemia which is normocytic and normochromic develops as azotemia occurs. *0962* In over 50% of the cases. *0331*

580.40 Glomerulonephritis (Rapidly Progressive) Anemia which is normocytic and normochromic develops as azotemia occurs. *0962*

584.00 Acute Renal Failure May fall to the low 20's. *0277*

585.00 Chronic Renal Failure Anemia occurs in almost all chronic patients. Uremia without anemia suggests acute renal failure. RBCs are normochromic or have slightly reduced MCHC, about 30-31. *0151* Characteristically normocytic and normochromic, and is associated with a normal or slightly decreased number of reticulocytes. *2538* Hydremia and dehydration are common. Changes will exaggerate or minimize the degree of anemia. *2552* In 89% of 146 patients at initial hospitalization for this disorder. *0781*

590.00 Chronic Pyelonephritis A normocytic, normochromic anemia may be present as in other forms of renal insufficiency. May be more severe, since chronic infection will act synergistically with renal insufficiency to depress bone marrow function. *0433*

591.00 Hydronephrosis In cases of advanced renal damage elevation of the BUN and secondary anemia may be noted secondary to uremia. *0433*

600.00 Benign Prostatic Hypertrophy Anemia may be present secondary to uremia. *0433*

650.00 Pregnancy Blood volume increases with a disproportionate increase in plasma volume so that the hematocrit will fall slightly as pregnancy progresses. *0433* Anemia is most often caused or aggravated by a concomitant iron deficiency. *2538 0165*

694.40 Pemphigus Anemia is common and may be due to inanition, serum loss and infection. *0151*

706.10 Acne 25% of patients with severe nodulocystic disease had mild anemia. *1387*

710.00 Systemic Lupus Erythematosus Significant anemia, usually normocytic, normochromic, found in 58% (81) of cases. *0713* The most common hematologic abnormality occurring in 57-78% of patients. May be caused by hypersplenism, iron deficiency, renal disease, drugs, antierythrocyte antibody and complement. *0309* Reflects disease activity in patients both with and without renal disease. *0782* Less than 30% in 53% of patients. *0714*

710.10 Progressive Systemic Sclerosis A mild hypochromic microcytic anemia may be present. *0433* Found in up to 25% of patients. *0962*

710.20 Sjögren's Syndrome Mild normochromic, normocytic anemia occurs in about 25% of patients. *0433* Anemia is seen in 33% of patients. *2134*

710.40 Dermatomyositis/Polymyositis Mild anemia may be expected. *0433*

711.10 Mixed Connective Tissue Disease Anemia. *0062*

714.00 Rheumatoid Arthritis Normocytic, normochromic, or perhaps hypochromic anemia which may be severe when the disease is very active. *0433* Mild anemia occurs in approximately 40% of cases. *0999* Anemia may occur. *0532*

714.30 Juvenile Rheumatoid Arthritis Moderate anemia is common with Hct concentrations of 30-34%. *0433*

720.00 Rheumatoid (Ankylosing) Spondylitis Anemia is occasionally present in more severe cases and is usually normocytic. *0433* Anemia occurs in < 33% of cases. *0666*

730.00 Osteomyelitis Patients with initial episodes tended to be more anemic and have a more marked leukocytosis than patients with recurrent disease. *2464*

753.10 Polycystic Kidney Disease Most of the patients show some degree of anemia. *0433* Characteristic. *0277*

753.12 Medullary Cystic Disease Most of the patients show some degree of anemia. *0433* Characteristic anemia. *0277*

756.52 Osteopetrosis Anemia and pancytopenia. *2468*

773.00 Hemolytic Disease of Newborn (Erythroblastosis Fetalis) Mild cases may develop mild anemia in the first 4-6 weeks of life from which they recover spontaneously. *0433* Intermediate moderately affected group will become severely anemic in the first 7-10 days of life (anemia neonatoium). *2199 2538 1742*

984.00 Toxic Effects of Lead and Its Compounds (including Fumes) Acute hemolytic anemia with hemoglobinemia and hemoglobinuria occasionally occur in acute lead poisoning. *0151 0484*

985.00 Toxic Effects of Non-medicinal Metals Mild to moderate anemia occurs in chronic arsenic poisoning. *0151* Pancytopenia may occur. *0484*

989.50 Toxic Effects of Venom A drop indicates severe envenomization following snake bite. *0151*

990.00 Effects of X-Ray Irradiation After large doses. *0995*

Blood Increase

1.00 Cholera Due to severe dehydration. *0151*

9.00 Gastroenteritis and Colitis Normal to elevated, depending on the amount of dehydration. *0433*

65.00 Arthropod-Borne Hemorrhagic Fever Values may reach 70% in the hypotensive phase of epidemic hemorrhagic fever. *0151*

75.00 Infectious Mononucleosis In 27% of 11 patients at initial hospitalization for this disorder. *0781*

189.00 Malignant Neoplasm of Kidney Occurs occasionally due to erythropoietin formation by the tumor. *0186*

205.10 Myelocytic Leukemia (Chronic) In a small percentage of patients there may be a mild elevation. *0433*

225.90 Benign Neoplasm of Brain and CNS In 22% of 22 patients at initial hospitalization for this disorder. *0781*

227.91 Pheochromocytoma Occasionally found and may be due to a decreased plasma volume, a true increase in RBC mass, or both. *0433* Hemoconcentration is not uncommon. *0962* Hemoconcentration can cause increased hematocrit and plasma proteins. *0962*

238.40 Polycythemia Vera Over 60% in males and 55% in females. *0433* Before treatment, Hct values range between 55-80. *0999*

250.10 Diabetic Acidosis Secondary to dehydration. *0999* May be moderately increased because of hemoconcentration. *0962*

255.00 Adrenal Cortical Hyperfunction (Glucocorticoid Excess) Normal or occasionally slightly elevated unless a malignancy is present in which case it may be depressed. *0433*

255.40 Adrenal Cortical Hypofunction Dehydration and hemoconcentration due to severe renal sodium loss. *2612 0433 0962*

276.50 Dehydration *2467*

289.00 Polycythemia, Secondary *2538*

410.90 Acute Myocardial Infarction Volume may be decreased, together with a slight increase in hct. *1108* After an initial small increase, decreased 12% until day 9 and remained constant thereafter. *2215 2554 0316*

415.00 Cor Pulmonale Secondary polycythemia. *2141*

435.90 Transient Cerebral Ischemia In 29% of 48 patients hospitalized for this disorder. *0781*

473.90 Chronic Sinusitis In 54% of 11 patients at initial hospitalization for this disorder. *0781*

492.80 Pulmonary Emphysema Rises in later stages. *0433*

493.10 Asthma (Intrinsic) In 37% of 122 patients at initial hospitalization for this disorder. *0781*

Hematocrit *(continued)*

Blood Increase *(continued)*

496.00 Chronic Obstructive Lung Disease Polycythemia, suggesting a significant degree of chronic hypoxemia. *0962* In 42% of 80 patients at initial hospitalization for this disorder. *0781*

496.01 Alpha₁-Antitrypsin Deficiency With associated polycythemia secondary to hypoxemia. *1636*

500.00 Anthracosis May become progressively elevated. *0433*

501.00 Asbestosis May become progressively elevated. *0433*

502.00 Silicosis May become progressively elevated. *0433*

503.01 Berylliosis Secondary polycythemia. *2467* May become progressively elevated. *0433*

537.40 Fistula of Stomach and Duodenum Will reflect the degree of hemoconcentration. *2199*

557.01 Mesenteric Artery Embolism Will reflect the hemoconcentration secondary to fluid loss into the bowel and peritoneal cavity following bowel infarction. *0433*

558.90 Diarrhea When salt and water are lost in isotonic proportions, a contraction of the extracellular fluid compartment occurs and hemoconcentration develops. *2199*

560.90 Intestinal Obstruction Normal early, but later increased, with dehydration. *2467*

567.90 Peritonitis Secondary; may be increased owing to hemoconcentration from extracellular fluid loss into the peritoneal cavity. *0433*

577.00 Acute Pancreatitis Occasionally because of hemoconcentration. *0433* Probably reflects intravascular volume contraction. *0962* *2467*

642.40 Pre-Eclampsia Usually thrombocytopenia and high Hct values. *0887* Hemoconcentration is an index of severity; with grave prognosis if it increases or persists. *0387*

642.60 Eclampsia Hemoconcentration is an index of severity; with grave prognosis if it increases or persists. *0387*

994.50 Exercise 6% increase immediately after exercise; normal in 30 min. *1837*

994.80 Effects of Electric Current Immediately following major injury. *0995*

Blood Normal

4.90 Bacillary Dysentery Anemia is uncommon. *0992*

81.00 Endemic Typhus *0433*

115.00 Histoplasmosis The anemia of chronic disease is conspicuously absent. Normal values found in 91% of patients. Differentiates chronic pulmonary histoplasmosis from pulmonary tuberculosis. *0892*

117.50 Cryptococcosis Even in extensive infection, the blood WBC, hct, and ESR remain normal. *1058*

202.80 Non-Hodgkins Lymphoma Anemia is often conspicuously lacking, especially early in the disease. *1984*

255.00 Adrenal Cortical Hyperfunction (Glucocorticoid Excess) Normal or occasionally slightly elevated unless a malignancy is present in which case it may be depressed. *0433*

272.31 Type I Hyperlipoproteinemia *2246*

275.00 Hemochromatosis Anemia is not usually present with primary hemochromatosis; when present, anemia suggests secondary causes such as alcoholic cirrhosis, transfusion-induced iron overload, sideroblastic anemia, or thalassemia. *0433*

277.12 Erythropoietic Protoporphyria In most reported patients, there have been no quantitative blood abnormalities. *2552*

277.44 Crigler-Najjar Syndrome No evidence of hemolytic anemia or splenomegaly. *2246* *0469*

287.00 Allergic Purpura Anemia is not usually present unless the hemorrhagic manifestations have been severe. *2538* *2552* *0962*

288.00 Agranulocytosis Typically normal; some cases have had anemia but this was most often pre-existing. *2552*

533.90 Peptic Ulcer, Site Unspecified Uncomplicated peptic ulcer is not associated with anemia. *0962*

570.00 Acute and Subacute Necrosis of Liver Anemia is not a feature. *0992*

633.90 Ectopic Pregnancy May be normal, even in view of acute rupture of an ectopic pregnancy, as the patient has not had time for fluid stabilization. *0433*

Pleural Effusion Increase

441.50 Ruptured Aortic Aneurysm Values approaching those found in blood are more indicative of frank hemorrhage, and such levels would be found in traumatic hemothorax or bleeding associated with pneumothorax or ruptured aortic aneurysm. *0962*

Hemoglobin

Blood Decrease

2.00 Typhoid Fever Normochromic anemia usually develops and may be aggravated by blood loss in the stools. *0151* Commonly present late in illness and during convalescence. *0962* *1058*

6.00 Amebiasis Normochromic or hypochromic anemia is found in 75% of cases. *1058* Mild degree of anemia is common, either normochromic or hypochromic. Severity is related to duration of symptoms. *0015*

11.00 Pulmonary Tuberculosis Anemia is common because of the effects of the infection on RBC production and survival and because of coexistent iron and nutritional deficiencies. *0433*

30.00 Leprosy Anemia, when present, is usually mild. *0962*

32.00 Diphtheria Moderate anemia persisting into convalescence is common. *0433*

38.00 Septicemia Mild to moderate anemia may occur during the course of chronic infections. *0433*

39.90 Actinomycosis A mild to moderate normocytic, normochromic anemia frequently accompanies this disease. *0433*

40.20 Whipple's Disease Anemia is common and is usually associated with iron deficiency. *2199*

53.00 Herpes Zoster In 38% of 18 patients at initial hospitalization for this disorder. *0781*

66.10 Tick-Borne Fever Anemia develops in some patients. *1058*

70.00 Viral Hepatitis Mild anemia may appear late in the course of acute disease. *0151* A mild degree of transient anemia. *0962*

75.00 Infectious Mononucleosis Anemia is rare. *1319*

78.50 Cytomegalic Inclusion Disease Anemia usually present in congenital disease. *1319* Hemolytic anemia. *0767* *2538*

80.00 Epidemic Typhus Normal early, falls significantly during the illness. *0433* May develop in the 2nd or 3rd week. *2368*

82.00 Rocky Mountain Spotted Fever Anemia may develop in the 2nd-3rd weeks. *2368*

84.00 Malaria With disease progression, a normocytic, normochromic anemia may become apparent. *0433* Marked anemia was found in patients with defective hemoglobin synthesis. *2240* Anemia is present in proportion to the severity of the infection. *0962*

85.00 Leishmaniasis Hemolytic anemia. *2568* Normocytic, normochromic anemia develops slowly but becomes severe later in the disease. *0151*

86.90 Trypanosomiasis Anemia is a characteristic feature. Hematological studies indicate the presence of a hemolytic process. *2569* Mild normocytic normochromic anemia associated with reduced marrow activity. *1058*

87.00 Relapsing Fever Moderate anemia may occur later in the disease. *0962*

97.90 Syphilis Secondary anemia. *1058*

99.10 Lymphogranuloma Venereum Anemia and leukopenia are most common when enlargement of the liver and spleen and generalized lymphadenopathy occur. *0433* *2199*

99.30 Reiter's Disease There may be a mild anemia. *0433*

100.00 Leptospirosis With jaundice, anemia may be severe due to intravascular hemolysis. Anemia is unusual in anicteric patients. *0992*

115.00 Histoplasmosis 50% of the patients may have anemia in disseminated disease. *0999* A marked to moderate hypochromic anemia occurs in most cases. *0962* Usually an iron deficient normochromic normocytic anemia. *2199* Normochromic anemia. *2368*

116.00 Blastomycosis Present in < 50% of patients. *0433*

117.30 Aspergillosis Hemolytic anemia. *2538* *1950*

123.40 Diphyllobothriasis (Intestinal) When present, anemia is macrocytic. *2199*

124.00 Trichinosis Prolonged infection may result in secondary anemia. *2368*

126.90 Ancylostomiasis (Hookworm Infestation) A microcytic, hypochromic anemia attributed directly to blood loss; when the patient has severe malnutrition, however, the anemia may be macrocytic hypochromic anemia. *0433* Anemia occurring in hookworm disease is a classic iron deficiency anemia. *2199* Development of hypochromic, microcytic anemia depends on the numbers of worms, recency of infection, and host nutrition. *2368   0151*

127.20 Strongyloidiasis Anemia, when it occurs, is usually iron deficiency in type. *2199*

127.30 Trichuriasis In children can be accompanied by a microcytic hypochromic anemia. *0433*

130.00 Toxoplasmosis Anemia is present. *2468*

150.90 Malignant Neoplasm of Esophagus In 27% of 39 patients at initial hospitalization for this disorder. *0781*

151.90 Malignant Neoplasm of Stomach The amount of bleeding and the degree of anemia will vary widely. Anemia of more than moderate degree is a late consequence of gastric malignancy. *0962* Anemia may be of several types. The most common is iron deficiency anemia caused by chronic occult blood loss. *2199* In 46% of 46 patients at initial hospitalization for this disorder. *0781*

152.90 Malignant Neoplasm of Small Intestine Anemia may be of several types. The most common is iron deficiency anemia caused by chronic occult blood loss. *2199*

153.90 Malignant Neoplasm of Large Intestine Anemia; may be the only symptom of carcinoma of the right side of colon (present in > 50% of these patients; usually hypochromic. *2467* Incidence of anemia between 22-74.6%. Iron deficiency anemia is common, because of either gross or occult bleeding. *2199* In 45% of 153 patients at initial hospitalization for this disorder. *0781*

154.10 Malignant Neoplasm of Rectum Iron deficiency anemia is common, because of either gross or occult bleeding. *2199*

155.00 Malignant Neoplasm of Liver In 49% of 14 patients at initial hospitalization for this disorder. *0781*

157.90 Malignant Neoplasm of Pancreas In 41% of 45 patients at initial hospitalization for this disorder. *0781*

170.90 Malignant Neoplasm of Bone In 36% of 24 patients at initial hospitalization for this disorder. *0781*

182.00 Malignant Neoplasm of Corpus Uteri In 30% of 154 patients at initial hospitalization for this disorder. *0781*

185.00 Malignant Neoplasm of Prostate In 43% of 87 patients at initial hospitalization for this disorder. *0781*

188.90 Malignant Neoplasm of Bladder May show anemia secondary to iron deficiency or secondary to a diffuse metastatic disease. *0433* In 26% of 45 patients at initial hospitalization for this disorder. *0781*

189.00 Malignant Neoplasm of Kidney Anemia occurs in approximately 30% of patients with renal cell carcinoma, secondary to bone marrow depression by tumor. *0836* 30 of 34 patients with hypernephroma were anemic. Due mainly to urinary blood loss. Values varied from 7-12%. *0894* A frequent presenting symptom. *1391*

197.00 Secondary Malignant Neoplasm of Respiratory System In 37% of 597 patients at initial hospitalization for this disorder. *0781*

198.50 Secondary Malignant Neoplasm of Bone Depression of all formed elements of the blood is often seen in disseminated neoplastic disease. *0999*

201.90 Hodgkin's Disease Mild to moderate hemolytic anemia, with a negative Coombs' test, is common in disseminated lymphoma. *0433* Present in 33% of all patients at diagnosis. Develops in nearly every patient who has fever, sweats, or other systemic manifestations. Becomes worse as the disease advances and improves with remission. *2538 0414* In 44% of 76 patients at initial hospitalization for this disorder. *0781*

202.40 Leukemic Reticuloendotheliosis Usually normochromic, normocytic anemia; mild anisocytosis and poikilocytosis were common. *2390*

202.52 Histiocytosis X A normocytic, normochromic anemia, sometimes severe and sometimes hemolytic in nature, may be present, especially in patients with disseminated disease. Aplastic anemia has also been described. *0433*

202.80 Non-Hodgkins Lymphoma Anemia occurs frequently and may be due to blood loss, bone marrow infiltration, or hemolysis. *2538* Present in < 50% of patients and is rarely severe at the time of diagnosis. *2552* In 51% of 73 patients at initial hospitalization for this disorder. *0781*

203.00 Multiple Myeloma A normocytic, normochromic anemia is present in 66% of patients at the time of diagnosis. *0433* High tumor mass is indicated if hemoglobin < 8.5 g/dL, low tumor mass is present in hemoglobin > 10.5 g/dL. *2467* Virtually all patients exhibit anemia of varying severity, either at the time of diagnosis or subsequently with disease progression. *2035* Reduced to < 12.0 g/dL in 62% of the patients. *1333* In 78% of 33 patients at initial hospitalization for this disorder. *0781   2468 2538*

204.00 Lymphocytic Leukemia (Acute) Most patients will have anemia. *0433* Often severe, usually normochromic, normocytic. *2552* In 82% of 37 patients at initial hospitalization for this disorder. *0781*

204.10 Lymphocytic Leukemia (Chronic) Characteristically normochromic normocytic anemia. *0433* Anemia is not a feature of early disease; it may begin to develop when 50% or more of the bone marrow is usurped by lymphoid tissue. *2489* Anemia, usually mild, was present at diagnosis in 50% of patients. *2552* In 76% of 27 patients at initial hospitalization for this disorder. *0781 2538*

205.00 Myelocytic Leukemia (Acute) Most patients will have anemia. *0433* Often severe, may be macrocytic. *2552* In 90% of 35 patients at initial hospitalization for this disorder. *0781*

205.10 Myelocytic Leukemia (Chronic) Anemia, when present, is characteristically normochromic normocytic. *0433* Anemia is almost always a feature of active disease, and generally increases in severity as the disease advances. Usually normocytic and normochromic with little evidence of iron deficiency, accelerated RBC hemolysis, or erythrocyte abnormality. *2538* In 85% of 22 patients at initial hospitalization for this disorder. *0781 2552*

206.00 Monocytic Leukemia Anemia is often quite severe, usually normochromic and normocytic. *2552* In 91% of 24 patients at initial hospitalization for this disorder. *0781*

207.00 Erythroleukemia Anemia is nearly always present, but its severity is variable. Usually normocytic and normochromic. *2538*

211.10 Benign Neoplasm of Stomach With occult bleeding, iron deficiency anemia may be present, in which case the bone marrow will not contain iron. *2199*

212.70 Benign Neoplasm of Cardiovascular Tissue Hemolytic anemia, mechanical in origin (due to local turbulence of blood) is usual and may be severe. The anemia is recognized in about 50% of patients with this tumor. *2467* Occurs with myxoma, possibly reflecting tumor emboli or tumor breakdown products. *1108*

242.90 Hyperthyroidism In 239 patients with uncomplicated disease, the concentration was < 12.0 g/dL in 37 of 207 women and < 13.0 g/dL in 9 of 32 men. A small fall is usual and it may sometimes be sufficient to cause a mild degree of anemia. *1696* Often patients develop a normochromic and normocytic anemia with 9-11 g/dL. *0151   2540*

244.90 Hypothyroidism Seldom < 9 g/dL. Of 202 patients, anemia was present on diagnosis in 39 of 172 women and 14 of 30 men. Microcytic anemia was present in only 9 patients in the entire series. *1078* Anemia may occur, hemoglobin < 13 g/dL. *0532* Many patients have a hypoplastic anemia which is unresponsive to therapy with iron, vitamin B_{12}, or folic acid. The degree is mild to moderate, with concentration rarely < 8-9 g/dL. *2538* Anemia observed in 21-60% of patients. *2552* In 42% of 14 patients at initial hospitalization for this disorder. *0781*

252.00 Hyperparathyroidism Unexplained anemia found in 21% of 57 patients. *1492*

253.40 Anterior Pituitary Hypofunction In some cases slight anemia is seen. *0433* Reduced thyroid, adrenal cortical, pituitary or testicular function can produce anemia. The hemoglobin is seldom < 9 g/dL. The RBC is normochromic and normocytic. *0433*

255.00 Adrenal Cortical Hyperfunction (Glucocorticoid Excess) Normal or occasionally slightly elevated unless a malignancy is present in which case it may be depressed. *0433* Patients with ectopic ACTH syndrome may be anemic. *0962*

255.10 Adrenal Cortical Hyperfunction (Mineralocorticoid Excess) An increased volume, with slight decrease of the Hct value, is usual. *1108   0962*

255.40 Adrenal Cortical Hypofunction Reduced thyroid, adrenal cortical, pituitary or testicular function can produce anemia. Hemoglobin is seldom < 9 g/dL. *0433*

257.20 Testicular Hypofunction Reduced testicular function can produce anemia. The hemoglobin is seldom < 9 g/dL. The RBC is normocytic and normochromic. *0433*

Hemoglobin (continued)

Blood Decrease (continued)

260.00 Protein Malnutrition Mild anemia. *0433* In infants and children, may fall to 8-10 g/dL of blood, but some children are admitted with normal levels, probably due to a shrunken plasma volume. *2538* Mild or moderate normocytic normochromic anemia occurs after 24 weeks of controlled semistarvation. Fall was 11 g/dL in males and 9.5 g/dL in females. *2538*

265.00 Thiamine (B₁) Deficiency Characteristic. *1108*

267.00 Vitamin C Deficiency Associated with anemia of normocytic, macrocytic, or hypochromic variety in about 80% of cases. *2538*

270.03 Cystinosis Often significant anemia before renal failure is substantial. *2246*

271.01 Von Gierke's Disease *0995*

272.52 Abetalipoproteinemia Severe anemia with hemoglobin as low as 4-8 g/dL is common in children. Most adult patients do not have significant anemia. *2246 1583*

272.72 Gaucher's Disease Unexplained splenomegaly with mild-moderate anemia and thrombocytopenia. *1808* A normocytic, normochromic anemia is frequently present, but concentrations rarely fall below 8 g/dL. *2538*

272.73 Niemann-Pick Disease May be normal, or mild anemia may be present. *2538*

273.23 Heavy Chain Disease (Gamma) Normochromic, normocytic anemia present in all cases of gamma heavy chain disease. *0999* Presumably related to hypersplenism. *2035* All patients have mild to moderate anemia. *2538*

273.30 Waldenström's Macroglobulinemia Anemia is the most common presenting manifestation and is frequently profound, with Hb levels in the range of 6-9 g/dL. Usually due to a combination of factors including accelerated RBC destruction, blood loss, and especially decreased erythropoiesis. *2035* A normochromic, normocytic anemia is usually present. *2538*

275.10 Hepatolenticular Degeneration Mild normochromic anemia with anisocytosis and poikilocytosis. *0433 0530*

277.00 Cystic Fibrosis In late stages of chronic lung disease, decreased serum electrolytes, hemoglobin, hematocrit, etc., may reflect hemodilution. *2467*

277.11 Congenital Erythropoietic Porphyria (Günther's Disease) Anemia is normochromic and normocytic and tends to be mild in degree. *2552* In most patients, reduction was only slight and hemolysis was compensated by increased RBC production. *2073 2246*

277.12 Erythropoietic Protoporphyria A moderate hypochromic or normochromic anemia is frequently observed. *2538*

277.13 Erythropoietic Coproporphyria Microcytic hypochromic anemia may occur due to blood loss or increased demand. *0532*

277.14 Acute Intermittent Porphyria Microcytic hypochromic anemia may occur due to blood loss or increased demand. *0532*

277.16 Porphyria Cutanea Tarda Microcytic hypochromic anemia may occur due to blood low or increased demand. *0532*

277.17 Hereditary Coproporphyria Microcytic hypochromic anemia may occur due to blood loss or increased demand. *0532*

277.22 Lesch-Nyhan Syndrome Many patients are anemic prior to the occurrence of renal insufficiency. *2246*

277.30 Amyloidosis Mild anemia present in < 50% of patients. *1334*

279.04 Agammaglobulinemia (Congenital Sex-linked) Hemolytic anemia. *2035* Hemolytic anemia frequently occurs. *2246*

279.06 Immunodeficiency (Common Variable) High incidence of pernicious anemia. *2538*

279.07 Dysgammaglobulinemia (Selective Immunoglobulin Deficiency) Not uncommon. *0433*

280.81 Plummer-Vinson Syndrome Hypochromic anemia associated with dysphagia and cardiospasm in women. *2467*

280.90 Iron Deficiency Anemia Reduced to a mean of 7.6 g/dL in 371 patients. *0198 0999 0151*

281.00 Pernicious Anemia Classical anemia, leukopenia (primarily granulocytopenia) and thrombocytopenia. Occasionally, the primary reduction may be in only 1 of these 3 major formed elements of the blood. Although patients usually present primarily with anemia they may occasionally present initially with infection associated with granulocytopenia or with bleeding associated with thrombocytopenia. *0433* Concentration ranges from very severe to near normal. Usually 7-8 g/dL at presentation. *2552*

281.20 Folic Acid Deficiency Anemia Anemia is normochromic (unless iron deficiency coexists) and macrocytic, with MCV ranging from 100 to > 150 fL. *2538* Anemia ranges from absent to severe. *0962* Concentration ranges from very severe to near normal. Usually < 7-8 g/dL at presentation. *2552*

282.00 Hereditary (Congenital) Spherocytosis The mean value of the hemoglobin concentration in a large series is usually 11.5 g/dL rarely 7 g/dL. *0433* Concentrations between 9-12 g/dL are most common. Rapid fall to 3-4 g/dL may occur during a crisis. *2552* In 91% of 12 patients at initial hospitalization for this disorder. *0781 2538*

282.10 Hereditary Elliptocytosis In severe cases, levels rarely fall below 9-10 g/dL. *2538*

282.20 Anemias Due To Disorders of Glutathione Metabolism As the hemoglobin level falls, reticulocytosis occurs and polychromasia is seen. *2538*

282.31 Hereditary Nonspherocytic Hemolytic Anemia In most subjects, the range is 5-11.5 g/dL. *2538*

282.41 Thalassemia Major Common very low in untransfused patients usually below 7 g/dL. *0433* Severe hemolytic anemia, hypochromic and microcytic in type, is found. *0999* May be in the 2-3 g/dL range or even lower. *2538*

282.42 Thalassemia Minor Tends to be 1-2 g/dL lower than in normal subjects. *0433* Mild anemia, usually with microcytosis, hypochromia, stippling, and target cells usually occurs. *0151* In periods of stress such as pregnancy or during severe infection, a moderate degree of anemia may be present in these patients. *2538* Hypochromic microcytic anemia in thalassemia minor can be distinguished from iron deficiency by a normal or even elevated serum iron concentration and by the failure of the anemia to respond to iron. *0999*

282.60 Sickle Cell Anemia Mild anemia. *0433* Steady-state is usually between 5-11 g/dL. The anemia is normochromic. *2538*

282.71 Hemoglobin C Disease Mild anemia. *0433* Hemoglobin concentration of 8-12 g/dL. *2538*

282.72 Hemoglobin E Disease Exhibits mild or no anemia. *0433* Homozygotes for hemoglobin E have a relatively mild anemia characterized by microcytosis and targeting of the red cells. *0385 2538*

282.73 Hemoglobin H Disease Concentration in these patients usually range from about 7-10 g/dL. Both higher and lower levels have been observed. *0433* Life-long anemia with variable splenomegaly and bone changes. *2538* Variable degree of anemia. Hb A constitutes the majority and Hb H varies from 5-30%. *2246*

283.00 Acquired Hemolytic Anemia (Autoimmune) In cases with more active hemolysis, anemia may be moderate to severe and the reticulocyte count markedly elevated to 50% or more. *2035*

283.21 Paroxysmal Nocturnal Hemoglobinuria May be moderate or severe. *0433* Degree of anemia may vary from none to very severe. *2538*

284.01 Congenital Aplastic Anemia The anemia is normochromic or slightly macrocytic, and macrocytes and target cells may be seen in the blood. *2552*

284.90 Aplastic Anemia A severe anemia may be found at the time of presentation. The RBC are usually normocytic or slightly macrocytic. *0433* Usually > 7 g/dL. *2552* In 100% of 20 patients hospitalized for this disorder. *0781 0151*

285.00 Sideroblastic Anemia The degree of anemia is variable, ranging from concentrations as low as 5 g/dL, in severely affected boys with sex-linked sideroblastic anemia to almost normal levels in the milder cases. Older people with idiopathic or secondary forms of this disease usually have moderate anemias with concentrations ranging from 7-10 g/dL. *0433* The anemia is normocytic or slightly macrocytic. *2538 0151*

286.01 Hemophilia Presence or absence of anemia depends on the severity and frequency of bleeding. *2552*

287.00 Allergic Purpura Anemia is not usually present unless the hemorrhagic manifestations have been severe. *2538 0962 2552*

287.30 Idiopathic Thrombocytopenic Purpura An anemia from blood loss may be present, but the RBC morphology is normal. *0433*

288.00 Agranulocytosis Depending on the underlying process the patient may also manifest moderate to severe anemia. *0433*

289.40 Hypersplenism Apparent anemia is often due to expansion of plasma volume in the presence of normal RBC volume. *1824*

289.80 Myelofibrosis Usually there is a mild to moderate anemia. *0433* Anemia mostly normochromic is found in a majority of cases. 12 g/dL occurred in 73% of cases. *2317* Anemia is present in 66% of all patients when they are first seen. Usually normochromic and moderate in degree but may become severe in advanced disease in myelofibrosis. *2538*

300.40 Depressive Neurosis Anemia is often present. *0433*

320.90 Meningitis (Bacterial) In 66% of 18 patients hospitalized for this disorder. *0781*

358.00 Myasthenia Gravis Occasional cases of macrocytic anemia. *2467*

390.00 Rheumatic Fever Anemia is common (hemoglobin usually 8-12 g/dL); gradually improves as activity subsides; microcytic type. May be related to increased plasma volume that occurs in early phase. *2467* Usually normochromic and normocytic and resolves without specific treatment. *1108* Anemia correlates closely with the degree of inflammation; persistence of anemia suggests continued rheumatic activity. *0962*

401.00 Malignant Hypertension Many patients show evidence of microangiopathic hemolytic anemia. *0995*

421.00 Bacterial Endocarditis Anemia is more common in longstanding infection and has no specificity. *0433* Rarely there is a hemolytic anemia with a positive Coombs' test. *2467* Normocytic normochromic anemia commonly present with mean hct = 35.5 ± 0.6%. Lowest hcts found in gram-negative (29.8 ±3.1%) and culture-negative cases (30.4 ± 1.6%). Degree of anemia is related to duration of illness, not virulence of organism. *1798* Normochromic, normocytic anemia occurs in 60-70% of cases. *1108*

425.40 Cardiomyopathies A slight degree of anemia in obliterative cardiomyopathies. *1108*

446.00 Polyarteritis-Nodosa Almost a prerequisite for diagnosis. *0433* Mild anemia is frequently present due either to blood loss or to chronic renal insufficiency. *0642* Anemia is found chiefly in cases complicated by renal insufficiency or blood loss. *0962*

446.20 Goodpasture's Syndrome Secondary to prolonged pulmonary bleeding. *0062*

446.50 Cranial Arteritis and Related Conditions Mild anemia is common, especially in older patients, in polymyalgia rheumatica. *0151* Hypoproliferative anemia is common and may be significant. *1013* In 49% of 16 patients hospitalized for this disorder. *0781* *2035*

446.60 Thrombotic Thrombocytopenic Purpura Anemia secondary to blood loss may be present. *2035* 5.5 g/dL in 33% of patients. *2538* *2552*

480.90 Viral Pneumonia In 55% of 16 patients at initial hospitalization for this disorder. *0781*

482.90 Bacterial Pneumonia In 38% of 18 patients at initial hospitalization for this disorder. *0781* Anemia is common in pneumococcal but not in staphylococcal pneumonia. *2368*

483.01 Mycoplasma Pneumoniae Occasional patients have been reported with hemolytic anemia. *0433* Sometimes seen in convalescence. *0726*

486.01 Resolving Pneumonia In 42% of 79 patients at initial hospitalization for this disorder. *0781*

494.00 Bronchiectasis When chronic uncontrolled infection persists, normochromic normocytic anemia is common. *0433* Leukocytosis and anemia are common. *0999*

496.00 Chronic Obstructive Lung Disease Even minor degrees of anemia are poorly tolerated by patients. Because of the high incidence of peptic ulcer associated with this disease, an anemia may be due to occult or clinically evident gastrointestinal bleeding. *0962*

496.01 Alpha₁-Antitrypsin Deficiency With associated hypersplenism. *1636*

500.00 Anthracosis Secondary anemia. *2467*

501.00 Asbestosis Secondary anemia. *2467*

502.00 Silicosis Secondary anemia. *2467*

503.01 Berylliosis Secondary anemia. *2467*

513.00 Abscess of Lung Characteristic leukocytosis and moderate or even severe anemia. *0999* Normochromic normocytic anemia in chronic stage. *2467*

533.90 Peptic Ulcer, Site Unspecified A few patients will have anemia because of chronic blood loss. *0433* An ulcer that bleeds chronically will cause a varying degree of iron deficiency anemia. *0962*

535.00 Gastritis May be low in patients with bleeding. *0433* Hypochromic microcytic anemia due to blood loss. *2467*

537.40 Fistula of Stomach and Duodenum Anemia and hypoproteinemia reflect malnutrition and chronic disease. *2199*

553.30 Hernia Diaphragmatic Microcytic anemia (due to loss of blood) may be present. *2467*

555.90 Regional Enteritis or Ileitis Anemia when present can be a result of iron loss or of reduced absorption of vitamin B_{12}. *0433* Anemia in approximately 70% of cases. *2035* Iron deficiency is common. *0962* Frequently moderate anemia, most often iron deficiency, but occasionally macrocytic caused by poor diet or failure to absorb vitamin B_{12} normally. *2199*

556.00 Ulcerative Colitis Anemia may be due to blood loss, simple iron deficiency, deficiencies in folic acid, pyridoxine, or vitamin B_{12} (frequently 6 g/dL). *2467* Anemia in approximately 70% of cases. *2035* Anemia secondary to colonic blood loss. Severity varies, depending on the rate and duration of bleeding. *2199*

562.00 Diverticular Disease of Intestine Blood loss is usually minimal but massive bleeding may occur. *2199*

564.20 Postgastrectomy (Dumping) Syndrome Iron deficiency and vitamin B_{12} deficiency are common following subtotal gastrectomy. *0962*

570.00 Acute and Subacute Necrosis of Liver Mild to moderate hemolysis usually occurs. *1849*

571.20 Laennec's or Alcoholic Cirrhosis Approximately 75% of chronic liver disease patients have anemia, usually mild. *1268 2137*

571.49 Chronic Active Hepatitis Anemia, leukopenia, and thrombocytopenia occur in 40-60% of patients. *2467* Slight to moderate anemia with leukopenia and thrombocytopenia are seen, particularly in patients with splenomegaly. *2035*

571.90 Cirrhosis of Liver Anemia reflects increased plasma volume and some increased destruction of RBCs. *2467* Approximately 75% of chronic liver disease patients have anemia, usually mild. *1268 2137* In 36% of 69 patients at initial hospitalization for this disorder. *0781*

572.00 Liver Abscess (Pyogenic) Mild to moderate anemia. *0433* A mild normochromic anemia is common. *2199*

577.00 Acute Pancreatitis *2199*

579.00 Celiac Sprue Disease Characteristic iron-deficiency anemia. The peripheral blood smear may show hypochromia. In some cases iron-deficiency anemia may be the predominant abnormality indicative of malabsorption. *0433*

579.01 Protein-Losing Enteropathy There may be a moderate anemia. *0433* *2467*

579.90 Malabsorption, Cause Unspecified Mild anemia. *0433*

580.00 Acute Poststreptococcal Glomerulonephritis Anemia is usually present, its severity varying directly with the severity of the azotemia. *0999* Slightly reduced to 11-12 g/dL as a result of dilution. *0151* *1108*

580.05 Glomerulonephritis (Membranoproliferative) Mild anemia which is normocytic and normochromic develops as azotemia occurs. *0962* In over 50% of the cases. *0331*

580.40 Glomerulonephritis (Rapidly Progressive) Anemia which is normocytic and normochromic develops as azotemia occurs. *0962*

584.00 Acute Renal Failure *0277*

585.00 Chronic Renal Failure Anemia is characteristic of chronic failure, normal hemoglobin suggests acute failure. *0151* Normocytic and normochromic, and associated with a normal or slightly decreased number of reticulocytes. *2538* Hydremia and dehydration are common. Changes will exaggerate or minimize the degree of anemia. *2552* In 89% of 146 patients at initial hospitalization for this disorder. *0781*

590.00 Chronic Pyelonephritis A normocytic, normochromic anemia may be present as in other forms of renal insufficiency. May be more severe, since chronic infection will act synergistically with renal insufficiency to depress bone marrow function. *0433*

591.00 Hydronephrosis In cases of advanced renal damage elevation of the BUN and secondary anemia may be noted secondary to uremia. *0433*

600.00 Benign Prostatic Hypertrophy Anemia may be present secondary to uremia. *0433*

650.00 Pregnancy Decreases slightly to as low as 10 g/dL, with corresponding decrease of hematocrit during pregnancy. *2468* Anemia is most often caused or aggravated by a concomitant iron deficiency. *2538 0165*

694.40 Pemphigus Anemia is common and may be due to inanition, serum loss and infection. *0151*

706.10 Acne 25% of patients with severe nodulocystic disease had mild anemia. *1387*

Hemoglobin (continued)

Blood Decrease (continued)

710.00 Systemic Lupus Erythematosus Anemia, usually normocytic, is present in the majority of cases and is frankly hemolytic with a positive Coombs' test in < 10% of the cases. *0433* Significant anemia, usually normocytic, normochromic, found in 58% (81) of cases. *0713* The most common hematologic abnormality occurring in 57-78% of patients. May be caused by hypersplenism, iron deficiency, renal disease, drugs, antierythrocyte antibody and complement. *0309*

710.10 Progressive Systemic Sclerosis A mild hypochromic microcytic anemia may be present *0433*. Found in up to 25% of patients. *0962*

710.20 Sjögren's Syndrome Mild normochromic, normocytic anemia occurs in about 25% of patients. *0433* Anemia is seen in 33% of patients. *2134*

710.40 Dermatomyositis/Polymyositis Mild anemia may be expected. *0433*

711.10 Mixed Connective Tissue Disease Anemia. *0062*

714.00 Rheumatoid Arthritis Normocytic, normochromic, or perhaps hypochromic anemia which may be severe when the disease is very active. *0433* Mild anemia occurs in approximately 40% of cases. *0999* Anemia may occur, hemoglobin < 13 g/dL. *0532*

714.30 Juvenile Rheumatoid Arthritis Moderate anemia is common with hemoglobin concentrations of 9-11 g/dL. *0433*.

720.00 Rheumatoid (Ankylosing) Spondylitis Anemia is occasionally present in more severe cases and is usually normocytic. *0433* Anemia occurs in < 33% of cases. *0666*

730.00 Osteomyelitis Patients with initial episodes tended to be more anemic and have a more marked leukocytosis than patients with recurrent disease. *2464*

753.10 Polycystic Kidney Disease Most of the patients show some degree of anemia. *0433* Characteristic anemia. *0277*

753.12 Medullary Cystic Disease Most of the patients show some degree of anemia. *0433* Characteristic anemia. *0277*

756.52 Osteopetrosis Anemia and pancytopenia. *2468*

773.00 Hemolytic Disease of Newborn (Erythroblastosis Fetalis) In mild cases, mild anemia may develop in the first 4-6 weeks of life with spontaneous recovery. Intermediate group will become severely anemic in the first 7-10 days of life (anemia neonatorum). Hemoglobin may drop below 2 g/dL and the child may die unless given a transfusion. Because hydrops fetalis is due to hepatic dysfunction, not anemia, some fetuses become hydropic with hemoglobin levels of 7-8 g/dL. Others are not hydropic with levels of 3-4 g/dL. *0433* Adult hemoglobin is increased with hemolytic disease of the newborn. *2468 2538 1742 2061*

829.00 Fracture of Bone Unexplained fall after traumatic fracture. *2468*

958.10 Fat Embolism Decreased hemoglobin correlates with leukocytosis and hypocalcemia. *1683*

984.00 Toxic Effects of Lead and Its Compounds (including Fumes) Acute hemolytic anemia with hemoglobinemia and hemoglobinuria occasionally occur in acute lead poisoning. *0151 0484*

985.00 Toxic Effects of Non-medicinal Metals Mild to moderate anemia occurs in chronic arsenic poisoning. *0151*

989.50 Toxic Effects of Venom A drop indicates severe envenomization following snake bite. *0151*

990.00 Effects of X-Ray Irradiation After large doses. *0995*

Blood Increase

1.00 Cholera Due to severe dehydration. *0992*

9.00 Gastroenteritis and Colitis Hemoglobin and Hct are normal to elevated, depending on the amount of dehydration. *0433*

75.00 Infectious Mononucleosis In 45% of 11 patients at initial hospitalization for this disorder. *0781*

189.00 Malignant Neoplasm of Kidney Occurs occasionally due to erythropoietin formation by the tumor. *0186*

205.10 Myelocytic Leukemia (Chronic) In a small percentage of patients there may be a mild elevation. *0433*

212.70 Benign Neoplasm of Cardiovascular Tissue Often elevated without arterial hypoxemia in right atrial myxoma. *1108*

225.90 Benign Neoplasm of Brain and CNS In 31% of 22 patients at initial hospitalization for this disorder. *0781*

227.91 Pheochromocytoma Hemoconcentration is not uncommon. *0962*

255.00 Adrenal Cortical Hyperfunction (Glucocorticoid Excess) Normal or occasionally slightly elevated unless a malignancy is present in which case it may be depressed. *0433*

276.50 Dehydration *2467*

281.30 Vitamin B₆ Deficiency Anemia The degree of anemia is variable, ranging from concentrations as low as 5 g/dL, severely affected boys with sex-linked sideroblastic anemia to almost normal levels in the milder cases. Older people with idiopathic or secondary forms of this disease usually have moderate anemias with concentration ranging from 7-10 g/dL. *0433* Normocytic or slightly macrocytic. *2538 0151*

289.00 Polycythemia, Secondary May be increased less, in proportion, than the erythrocyte level because of a low MCV and MCH. *0151*

415.00 Cor Pulmonale Secondary polycythemia. *2141*

435.90 Transient Cerebral Ischemia In 25% of 48 patients hospitalized for this disorder. *0781*

473.90 Chronic Sinusitis In 63% of 11 patients at initial hospitalization for this disorder. *0781*

492.80 Pulmonary Emphysema Rises in later stages. *0433*

493.10 Asthma (Intrinsic) In 37% of 121 patients at initial hospitalization for this disorder. *0781*

496.00 Chronic Obstructive Lung Disease In 25 patients with severe disease, blood hemoglobin exhibited a significant increase indicating an improved oxygen transport. In most patients a leftward shifting of the oxygen dissociation curve occurred. Hemoglobin was significantly increased in all patients, regardless of degree of hypoxia. *1092* Polycythemia, suggesting a significant degree of chronic hypoxemia. *0962* In 39% of 80 patients at initial hospitalization for this disorder. *0781*

496.01 Alpha₁-Antitrypsin Deficiency With associated polycythemia secondary to hypoxemia. *1636*

500.00 Anthracosis May become progressively elevated. *0433*

501.00 Asbestosis May become progressively elevated. *0433*

502.00 Silicosis May become progressively elevated. *0433*

503.01 Berylliosis Secondary polycythemia. *2467* May become progressively elevated. *0433*

558.90 Diarrhea When salt and water are lost in isotonic proportions, a contraction of the extracellular fluid compartment occurs and hemoconcentration develops. *2199*

560.90 Intestinal Obstruction Normal early, but later increased, with dehydration. *2467*

567.90 Peritonitis May be increased owing to hemoconcentration from extracellular fluid loss into the peritoneal cavity. *0433*

577.00 Acute Pancreatitis Usually normal but may be high occasionally due to hemoconcentration. *0433*

992.00 Heat stroke In children. *0548*

994.50 Exercise Mild exercise causes transient decrease in blood volume. *1031*

Blood Normal

4.90 Bacillary Dysentery Anemia is uncommon. *0992*

115.00 Histoplasmosis The anemia of chronic disease is conspicuously absent. Normal values found in 91% of patients. differentiate chronic pulmonary histoplasmosis from pulmonary tuberculosis. *0892*

202.80 Non-Hodgkins Lymphoma Anemia is often conspicuously lacking, especially early in the disease. Hemoglobin above 12 g/dL found in 90% of 1269 cases. *1984*

255.00 Adrenal Cortical Hyperfunction (Glucocorticoid Excess) Normal or occasionally slightly elevated unless a malignancy is present in which case it may be depressed. *0433*

272.31 Type I Hyperlipoproteinemia *2246*

275.00 Hemochromatosis Anemia is not usually present with primary hemochromatosis; when present, anemia suggests secondary causes such as alcoholic cirrhosis, transfusion-induced iron overload, sideroblastic anemia, or thalassemia. *0433*

277.12 Erythropoietic Protoporphyria In most reported patients, there have been no quantitative blood abnormalities. *2552*

277.44 Crigler-Najjar Syndrome No evidence of hemolytic anemia or splenomegaly. *2246 0469*

282.00 Hereditary (Congenital) Spherocytosis In approximately 10-20% of patients, particularly young men. *2246*

287.00 Allergic Purpura Anemia is not usually present unless the hemorrhagic manifestations have been severe. *2538 0962 2552*

288.00 Agranulocytosis Typically normal; some cases have had anemia but this was most often pre-existing. *2552*

533.90 Peptic Ulcer, Site Unspecified Uncomplicated peptic ulcer is not associated with anemia. *0962*

570.00 Acute and Subacute Necrosis of Liver Anemia is not a feature. *0992*

994.50 Exercise No effect with normal activity. *1134*

Urine Increase

88.00 Bartonellosis Intravascular hemolysis parasites (Oroya fever); due to Bartonella bacilliformis. *2467*

994.80 Effects of Electric Current In many cases, probably secondary to severe burns. *0995*

Pleural Effusion Increase

441.50 Ruptured Aortic Aneurysm Values approaching those found in blood are more indicative of frank hemorrhage, and such levels would be found in traumatic hemothorax or bleeding associated with pneumothorax or ruptured aortic aneurysm. *0962*

Hemoglobin A$_{1C}$

Blood Decrease

282.10 Hereditary Elliptocytosis Significantly lower (P < 0.0005) in patients with hemolytic anemia (n = 20) compared to patients with nonhemolytic anemia and normal controls. *1769*

282.20 Anemias Due To Disorders of Glutathione Metabolism Significantly lower (P < 0.0005) in patients with hemolytic anemia (n = 20) compared to patients with nonhemolytic anemia and normal controls. *1769*

282.41 Thalassemia Major *2539*

282.60 Sickle Cell Anemia Due to increased RBC turnover.

283.00 Acquired Hemolytic Anemia (Autoimmune) Significantly lower (P < 0.0005) in patients with hemolytic anemia (n = 20) compared to patients with nonhemolytic anemia and normal controls. *1769*

Blood Increase

250.00 Diabetes Mellitus All patients classified as diabetic were found to have values greater than 9.9%. *1171* 2-3 fold increase in the red cells of diabetic patients. By providing an integrated measurement of blood glucose, Hb A$_{1C}$ is useful in assessing the degree of diabetic control. *0315*

272.10 Type IV Hyperlipoproteinemia Triglyceride concentrations greater than 1750 mg/dL would falsely raise the HbA1 levels. *1498*

272.31 Type I Hyperlipoproteinemia Triglyceride concentrations greater than 1750 mg/dL would falsely raise the HbA1 levels. *1498*

272.32 Type V Hyperlipoproteinemia Triglyceride concentrations greater than 1750 mg/dL would falsely raise the HbA1 levels. *1498*

280.90 Iron Deficiency Anemia *2539*

282.60 Sickle Cell Anemia Significantly elevated in children with this disease (13.1% n = 36) compared with normal children (6.25% n = 27). *1197*

303.90 Alcoholism *2539*

581.90 Nephrotic Syndrome *2539*

650.00 Pregnancy *0794*

984.00 Toxic Effects of Lead and Its Compounds (including Fumes) *2539*

Hemoglobin Casts

Urine Increase

283.21 Paroxysmal Nocturnal Hemoglobinuria May be present. *2538*

580.00 Acute Poststreptococcal Glomerulonephritis Indicate bleeding from the glomerulus. *0151*

Hemoglobin, Fetal

Blood Decrease

773.00 Hemolytic Disease of Newborn (Erythroblastosis Fetalis) *2468*

Blood Increase

203.00 Multiple Myeloma *2467*

205.00 Myelocytic Leukemia (Acute) Increased in some leukemias (especially juvenile myeloid leukemia); with HbF of 30-60%, absence of Philadelphia chromosome, rapid fatal course, more pronounced thrombocytopenia, and lower total WBC count. *2468*

281.00 Pernicious Anemia In 50% of untreated patients; increases after treatment and then gradually decreases during next 6 months; some patients still have slight elevation thereafter. *2467*

281.20 Folic Acid Deficiency Anemia Minimal elevation occurs in about 15% of patients with megaloblastic anemia. *2467*

282.41 Thalassemia Major The proportion is usually between 20-60%, but values as high as 90% may occur. *0151* Increased, ranging from 10-90% is characteristic and there may be a total deficiency of hemoglobin A synthesis. *2538*

282.42 Thalassemia Minor Elevated in about 50% of patients, usually to 1-3% and rarely to more than 5%. *2538*

282.60 Sickle Cell Anemia Increased in various hemoglobinopathies; HBF over 30% protects the cell from sickling; therefore, infants with homozygous S have few problems before age of 3 months. *2467* Electrophoresis of the hemoglobin confirms the diagnosis by showing the typical pattern of homozygous sickle inheritance: Hb S with variable amounts of Hb F and no Hb A. *0999*

282.71 Hemoglobin C Disease Slightly increased. *2468*

282.72 Hemoglobin E Disease Sometimes slightly increased. *2468*

283.21 Paroxysmal Nocturnal Hemoglobinuria Elevated levels have been reported. *1883 2538*

284.90 Aplastic Anemia Returns to normal only after complete remission, and therefore is reliable indicator of complete recovery. Better prognosis in patients with higher initial level 400 mg/dL. *2467* In adults, substantial increases are rare, but in children the concentration has been reported to be as high as 1.5 g/dL. *2122 2538*

630.00 Hydatidiform Mole *2467*

758.00 Down's Syndrome Patients with an extra G chromosome. *2467*

758.10 Trisomy 13 Patients with an extra D chromosome. *2467*

Blood Normal

758.10 Trisomy 13 Translocation - normal mosaicism in D$_1$ trisomy. *2548*

CSF Increase

431.00 Cerebral Hemorrhage Increased percentage in CSF indicates neonatal subarachnoid hemorrhage. *0373*

Hemoglobin, Free

Serum Increase

18.00 Disseminated Tuberculosis *2538 0486*

52.00 Chickenpox *2538 1857*

54.00 Herpes Simplex *2538 1857*

55.00 Measles *2538 1857*

78.50 Cytomegalic Inclusion Disease Hemolytic anemia. *0767 2538*

84.00 Malaria Intravascular hemolysis due to parasites. *2467*

85.00 Leishmaniasis Hemolytic anemia. *2568 2538*

86.90 Trypanosomiasis Intravascular hemolysis due to parasites. *2467*

87.00 Relapsing Fever Intravascular hemolysis due to parasites. *2467*

88.00 Bartonellosis Intravascular hemolysis due to parasites. *2467 2538 1918*

117.30 Aspergillosis Hemolytic anemia. *2538 1950*

130.00 Toxoplasmosis *2538 0486*

204.10 Lymphocytic Leukemia (Chronic) On occasion, severe hemolytic anemia is present at diagnosis. *0092 2258 2552*

Hemoglobin, Free *(continued)*

Serum Increase *(continued)*

275.10 Hepatolenticular Degeneration Hemolytic episodes frequently occur several years prior to onset of other symptoms; due to increased oxidative stress on RBC from excess copper. *0530*

277.42 Gilbert's Disease Mild, but fully compensated hemolysis in a significant number of patients. *0754*

279.04 Agammaglobulinemia (Congenital Sex-linked) Hemolytic anemia frequently occurs. *2246*

282.10 Hereditary Elliptocytosis In 10-15% of patients the rate of hemolysis is substantially increased with red cell half-life times as short as 5 days. *2538* Hemolysis and hyperbilirubinemia have been observed in the newborn period. *0087*

282.20 Anemias Due To Disorders of Glutathione Metabolism Indirect laboratory evidence that hemolysis is present. *0433*

282.31 Hereditary Nonspherocytic Hemolytic Anemia During acute hemolysis. *0433*

282.41 Thalassemia Major Moderate increase. *2467*

282.60 Sickle Cell Anemia Seen between as well as during crises, and no consistent increase in this value occurs in crises. *0433*

282.71 Hemoglobin C Disease Slight to moderate increase. *2467* Manifested by a hemolytic state. *0962*

283.00 Acquired Hemolytic Anemia (Autoimmune) Moderate increase when hemolysis is very rapid. *2468* Common. *2035*

283.21 Paroxysmal Nocturnal Hemoglobinuria At times of active hemolysis. *0433* Increases during sleep. *2468*

286.60 Disseminated Intravascular Coagulopathy Increases transiently with return to normal in 8 h. *2468*

446.60 Thrombotic Thrombocytopenic Purpura May accompany elevated indirect bilirubin, indicating intravascular RBC destruction. *2552*

483.01 Mycoplasma Pneumoniae Hemolysis has been reported in severe cases. *1483 2368 2538 0729*

487.10 Influenza Hemolytic anemia. *2538 1857*

570.00 Acute and Subacute Necrosis of Liver Mild to moderate hemolysis usually occurs. *1849*

571.90 Cirrhosis of Liver Mild to moderate hemolysis usually occurs. *1849*

572.00 Liver Abscess (Pyogenic) Mild to moderate hemolysis usually occurs. *1849*

585.00 Chronic Renal Failure Mild hemolysis may occur. *1669*

948.00 Burns Intravascular hemolysis due to thermal burns; injuring RBCs. *2467*

984.00 Toxic Effects of Lead and Its Compounds (including Fumes) With acute hemolytic crisis. *0151*

994.50 Exercise Light activity causes increase X 3-5, heavy increase X 10-13. *1930*

Serum Normal

282.00 Hereditary (Congenital) Spherocytosis Very little or none. Hemoglobin released during hemolysis is catabolized at the site of destruction. *2246*

Urine Increase

84.00 Malaria In severe falciparum infection may be demonstrable. *0433* Intravascular hemolysis due to parasites. *2467*

282.20 Anemias Due To Disorders of Glutathione Metabolism Indirect laboratory evidence that hemolysis is present. *0433* Intravascular hemolysis due to antibodies. *2467*

282.31 Hereditary Nonspherocytic Hemolytic Anemia During acute hemolysis. *0433* Hemosiderinuria and hemoglobinuria, particularly when oxidative stresses have been induced by drugs or other environmental factors. *2538*

283.00 Acquired Hemolytic Anemia (Autoimmune) In those patients with hyperacute hemolysis. *2538* Rarely encountered, although it is seen in occasional cases with intense hemolysis. *2035*

283.21 Paroxysmal Nocturnal Hemoglobinuria Worse at night and remits during the day; probably observed initially in < 25% of all patients. Parallels changes in pH, circadian variation in cortisol excretion, complement levels, activation of the alternative pathway of complement, and other variable components of plasma. *1632 2538*

286.60 Disseminated Intravascular Coagulopathy Occurs 1-2 h after severe hemolysis and lasts 24 h. It is a transient finding and is relatively insensitive. False positive is due to myoglobinuria or to lysis of RBCs in urine with intravascular hemolysis. *2468*

584.00 Acute Renal Failure May appear in the urine of a patient with intravascular hemolysis or myoglobin in trauma. *0433*

948.00 Burns Intravascular hemolysis due to thermal burns; injuring RBCs. *2467*

984.00 Toxic Effects of Lead and Its Compounds (including Fumes) With acute hemolytic crisis. *0850*

994.50 Exercise Intravascular hemolysis due to march hemoglobinuria and strenuous exercise. *2467*

Hemopexin

Serum Decrease

642.40 Pre-Eclampsia Found to be significantly lower than in normal pregnancy. *2286*

Serum Normal

642.40 Pre-Eclampsia No change was found compared to normal late pregnancy. *0409*

650.00 Pregnancy Unchanged in late normal pregnancies. *2286 2287*

Hepatitis B Surface Antigen

Serum Increase

70.00 Viral Hepatitis Can be present during incubation period and acute phase; occasionally may persist. *2467* About 80% of patients with clinical signs of viral hepatitis type B have been found to have the antigen in their blood when multiple timed sample were taken. *0962*

155.00 Malignant Neoplasm of Liver Reported incidence varies from 5-80%. *0364* Prevalence of antigen in sera varies with geographic location; 40% incidence was found in an African study and 80% in a study in Taiwan. *1507*

304.90 Drug Dependence (Opium and Derivatives) Found in 10% of drug patients. *2468*

446.00 Polyarteritis-Nodosa In cases associated with hepatitis B infection the hepatitis B surface antigen is persistently detectable, usually at high titers, throughout the illness. *2035* Found in approximately 25% of patients, independent of apparent liver involvement. *0962*

570.00 Acute and Subacute Necrosis of Liver 31 of 59 patients with acute uncomplicated hepatitis had detectable hepatitis B antigen. *0376*

571.49 Chronic Active Hepatitis 25-30% of patients. Occurring more frequently in men than women. *0151*

Heterophil Antibody

Serum Decrease

204.00 Lymphocytic Leukemia (Acute) Positive presumptive test but negative differential test if Forsman antigen is used. *1752*

205.00 Myelocytic Leukemia (Acute) Positive presumptive test but negative differential test if Forsman antigen is used. *1752*

238.40 Polycythemia Vera Positive presumptive test but negative differential test if Forsman antigen is used. *1752*

Serum Increase

75.00 Infectious Mononucleosis Elevated titers which agglutinate sheep RBCs; 40% have positive tests during 1st week of illness and 80% by the 3rd week. *2508* Elevated titers may persist longer than a year in 75% of patients. Over 95% of typical cases is heterophil antibody positive if followed long enough. *0679* Develop in the 1st week of illness in most patients and ultimately appear in 80-90% of patients and persist for 3-6 months. *0962 2538 0151*

201.90 Hodgkin's Disease Very rare. *0503*

204.00 Lymphocytic Leukemia (Acute) Positive presumptive test but negative differential test if Forsman antigen is used. *1752*

205.00 Myelocytic Leukemia (Acute) Positive presumptive test but negative differential test if Forsman antigen is used. *1752*

238.40 **Polycythemia Vera** Positive presumptive test but negative differential test if Forsman antigen is used. *1752*

570.00 **Acute and Subacute Necrosis of Liver** May be positive but guinea pig kidney cell absorption removes the antibody. *0992*

714.00 **Rheumatoid Arthritis** One case. *0503*

Hexokinase

Serum Increase

150.90 **Malignant Neoplasm of Esophagus** Increased in gastrointestinal tumors. Mean 15.3 ± 3.5 compared to normal, 0.93 ± 0.28 U/L. *1201*

151.90 **Malignant Neoplasm of Stomach** Increased in gastrointestinal tumors. Mean = 15.3 ± 3.5 compared to normal, 0.93 ± 0.28 U/L. *1201*

152.90 **Malignant Neoplasm of Small Intestine** Increased in gastrointestinal tumors. Mean = 15.3 ± 3.5 compared to normal, 0.93 ± 0.28 U/L. *1201*

153.90 **Malignant Neoplasm of Large Intestine** Increased in gastrointestinal tumors. Mean = 15.3 ± 3.5 compared to normal, 0.93 ± 0.28 U/L. *1201*

154.10 **Malignant Neoplasm of Rectum** Increased in gastrointestinal tumors. Mean = 15.3 ± 3.5 compared to normal, 0.93 ± 0.28 U/L. *1201*

162.90 **Malignant Neoplasm of Bronchus and Lung** Significantly increased. Mean = 20.4 ± 5.4 compared to normal, 0.93 ± 0.28 U/L. *1201*

172.90 **Malignant Melanoma of Skin** Significantly increased in melanoblastomas. Mean 17.4 ± 3.5 compared to normal 0.93 ± 0.28 U/L. *1201*

174.90 **Malignant Neoplasm of Breast** Markedly increased. Mean = 22.8 ± 3.7 U/L compared to 0.93 ± 0.28 U/L in normals. *1201*

180.90 **Malignant Neoplasm of Cervix** Markedly increased. Mean = 32.0 ± 4.7 U/L. *1201*

183.00 **Malignant Neoplasm of Ovary** Markedly increased. Mean = 22.8 ± 4.0 U/L compared to normal, 0.93 ± 0.28 U/L. *1201*

186.90 **Malignant Neoplasm of Testis** Markedly increased. Mean = 12.6 ± 2.8 compared to normal 0.93 ± 0.28 U/L. *1201*

189.00 **Malignant Neoplasm of Kidney** Markedly increased. Mean = 12.6 ± 2.8 compared to normal 0.93 ± 0.28 U/L. *1201*

201.90 **Hodgkin's Disease** Markedly increased in malignant lymphomas. Mean = 14.6 ± 2.0 compared to normal 0.93 ± 0.28 U/L. *1201*

202.80 **Non-Hodgkins Lymphoma** Markedly increased in malignant lymphomas. Mean = 14.6 ± 2.0 compared to normal 0.93 ± 0.28 U/L. *1201*

Red Blood Cells Absent

282.31 **Hereditary Nonspherocytic Hemolytic Anemia** Deficient in erythrocytes in congenital nonspherocytic hemolytic anemia. *0619*

Hexosamine

Serum Increase

710.00 **Systemic Lupus Erythematosus** Hexosamine and other acute-phase reactants are elevated and remain so to some degree during period of apparent remission. *0999* Have been found to be elevated but are nonspecific. *0962*

714.00 **Rheumatoid Arthritis** Usually parallel the activity of the ESR. *0962*

Serum Normal

277.30 **Amyloidosis** *0120 2246*

Hexosaminidase

Serum Decrease

330.11 **Tay-Sach's Disease** Hexosaminidase A (possessing both acetylglucosaminidase and acetylgalactosaminidase activities) is nearly absent in fetal Tay-Sach's serum. Heterozygotes have intermediate reductions in serum, leukocytes, and cultured fibroblasts. *2246 1716*

Serum Increase

45.90 **Acute Poliomyelitis** Increase in total concentration (hexosaminidase A and B). *1716*

70.00 **Viral Hepatitis** Increase in total concentration (hexosaminidase A and B). *1716*

151.90 **Malignant Neoplasm of Stomach** *1443*

199.00 **Secondary Malignant Neoplasm (Disseminated)** Elevated. *2356*

203.00 **Multiple Myeloma** Elevated. *2356*

211.10 **Benign Neoplasm of Stomach** Elevated. *2356*

250.00 **Diabetes Mellitus** Increase in total concentration (hexosaminidase A and B). *1716*

277.15 **Porphyria Variegata** *1443*

277.16 **Porphyria Cutanea Tarda** *1443*

303.00 **Acute Alcoholic Intoxication** Elevated in 94% of cases. *1166*

410.90 **Acute Myocardial Infarction** Increase in total concentration (hexosaminidase A and B). *1716*

570.00 **Acute and Subacute Necrosis of Liver** Increase in total concentration (hexosaminidase A and B). *1716*

571.90 **Cirrhosis of Liver** Increase in total concentration (hexosaminidase A and B). *1716*

650.00 **Pregnancy** Increase in total concentration (hexosaminidase A and B). *1716*

Urine Increase

580.00 **Acute Poststreptococcal Glomerulonephritis** Decreased levels in urine. *2356*

580.01 **Glomerulonephritis (Focal)** Decreased levels in urine. *2356*

580.02 **Glomerulonephritis (Minimal Change)** Decreased levels in urine. *2356*

580.04 **Glomerulonephritis (Membranous)** Decreased levels in urine. *2356*

580.05 **Glomerulonephritis (Membranoproliferative)** Decreased levels in urine. *2356*

580.40 **Glomerulonephritis (Rapidly Progressive)** Decreased levels in urine. *2356*

584.00 **Acute Renal Failure** Extremely high values observed in acute renal failure following hypotensive episodes. *1525*

585.00 **Chronic Renal Failure** Urinary levels often increased in chronic renal disease and are very sensitive to degree of renal damage. *1525*

590.00 **Chronic Pyelonephritis** Decreased levels in urine. *2356*

714.00 **Rheumatoid Arthritis** Decreased levels in urine. *2356*

715.90 **Osteoarthritis** *1443*

948.00 **Burns** Decreased levels in urine. *2356*

Hippuran Retention

Serum Increase

994.50 **Exercise** During infusion (depends on extent of activity. *0763*

Hippuric Acid

Urine Decrease

572.40 **Hepatic Failure** *0503*

650.00 **Pregnancy** Reduced excretion in normal pregnancy. *1350 0387*

Histamine

Serum Increase

30.00 **Leprosy** Both histamine and histaminase levels are significantly elevated, especially in cases of long duration. Patients with leprosy in reaction had highest levels, whereas tuberculoid, borderline and lepromatous cases had moderate rises. *1879*

193.01 **Medullary Carcinoma of Thyroid** Abnormally increased activity found in medullary carcinoma, falling after surgical removal, and increasing if residual tumor present. *0619*

Histamine (continued)

Serum   Increase (continued)

205.10   Myelocytic Leukemia (Chronic)   Histamine and histamine metabolites are raised in plasma and WBC in most patients. *0173*   In a group of patients with no symptoms attributable to histamine, mean plasma concentration was > 3 X normal. Tends to reflect the number of basophils. *2299   2552*

238.40   Polycythemia Vera   Present in the majority of patients with uncontrolled disease. *2538 0840*

346.00   Migraine   Levels are increased during acute attacks. *0996*

Serum   Normal

289.00   Polycythemia, Secondary   *2538*

Urine   Increase

238.40   Polycythemia Vera   Present in the majority of patients with uncontrolled disease. *2538 0840*

259.20   Carcinoid Syndrome   Some patients with gastric carcinoids have been shown to have frequent and consistent elevations of histamine, which is inconsistently elevated in those with ileal tumors. Often seen in patients with gastric and bronchial carcinoids. *2199*   Persistently elevated in gastric carcinoid tumors. *2404*

White Blood Cells   Increase

346.00   Migraine   Mean spontaneous histamine release was increased 33.7% compared to controls. *2112*

Histidine

Serum   Decrease

714.00   Rheumatoid Arthritis   Frequently low. *2104*

Serum   Increase

270.51   Histidinemia   Quantitative amino acid analysis demonstrate plasma levels of histidine from 5-17 mg/dL (normal = 1-3 mg/dL). *0433*   A marked elevation is the most consistent and characteristic finding. *2246*

Urine   Increase

270.02   Hartnup Disease   5-20 X normal values. *2246   0995*

270.03   Cystinosis   Nonspecific pattern of aminoaciduria. Fanconi's syndrome. *0995*

270.51   Histidinemia   Quantitative amino acid analysis will demonstrate urinary excretion which usually exceeds 300 mg/24h. *0433* Characteristic, but not as specific an indicator as the serum concentration. *2246*

CSF   Increase

270.51   Histidinemia   Frequently elevated. Values of 2-10 X normal have been noted. *2246 0831 2448*

HLA Antigens

Blood   Present

99.30   Reiter's Disease   HLA-B$_2$7 present in 80% of patients versus 9% of controls. *2539*   HLA-B$_2$7 found in 65% of cases. *1503*

242.90   Hyperthyroidism   HLA-DR3 present in 53% of patients with Graves' Disease versus 18% of controls. *2539*

250.00   Diabetes Mellitus   HLA-DR4 present in 38% of patients with insulin dependent disease versus 13% of controls. HLA-DR3 present in 50% of insulin dependent disease versus 21% of controls. *2539*   HLA-B8 and HLA-Bw15 also associated with this disease. *2191*

255.40   Adrenal Cortical Hypofunction   HLA-DR3 present in 70% of patients versus 21% of controls. *2539*

275.00   Hemochromatosis   HLA-A3 present in 72% of patients versus 21% of controls. *2539*

340.00   Multiple Sclerosis   HLA antigen Dw2 found in 36% of patients with this disease compared to 0% of controls. *2051* HLA-DR2 present in 55% of patients versus 23% of control *2539* Increased incidence of HLA-DR2 *1503*

358.00   Myasthenia Gravis   HLA-DR3 present in 30% of patients versus 17% of controls. *2539*

446.20   Goodpasture's Syndrome   HLA-DR2 is twenty five times more likely in patients with this disease and caries with it a worse prognosis. *1503*

446.50   Cranial Arteritis and Related Conditions   Association noted with HLA-DR4. *1503*

446.70   Pulseless Disease (Aortic Arch Syndrome)   Frequency of HLA-Bw52 greater in affected Asians. *1503*

555.90   Regional Enteritis or Ileitis   If associated arthritis HLA-B$_2$7 found more frequently than control group. *1503*

556.00   Ulcerative Colitis   If associated arthritis HLA-B$_2$7 found more frequently than control group. *1503*

571.49   Chronic Active Hepatitis   HLA-DR3 present in 68% of patients versus 24% of controls. *2539*

579.00   Celiac Sprue Disease   HLA-B8 and DRw3 are found. *0793*   HLA-DR3 found in 96% of patients versus 27% of controls. *2539*

694.00   Dermatitis Herpetiformis   HLA antigen DR2 found in 97% of patients with this disease compared to 25% of controls. *2051* HLA-DR3 found in 77% of patients versus 20% of controls. *2539* HLA-B8 and HLA-Bw15 associated with this disease. *2191*

696.10   Psoriasis   HLA-Cw6 present in 50% of caucasian patients versus 23% of controls. *2539*   HLA-B$_2$7 associated with psoriatic spondylitis. *2191*

710.00   Systemic Lupus Erythematosus   HLA-DR3 present in 70% of patients versus 28% of controls. *2539*   HLA-DR2 and HLA-DR3 frequently associated with whites with this disease. *1503* HLA-A17, HLA-B8, HLA-DR2 and HLA-DR3 associated with this disease. *2191*

710.20   Sjögren's Syndrome   HLA-DR3 present in 75% of patients versus 21% of controls. *2539*   HLA-DR3 found in 84% of patients with this disease compared to 24% of controls. *2051* Increased frequency of HLA-DR2 and HLA-DR3 and decrease. HLA-DR4 in primary disease and increased DR4 with normal freq. DR2 and DR3 in secondary. *1503*

714.00   Rheumatoid Arthritis   HLA antigen DR4 found in 54% of patients with this disease compared to 16% of controls. *2051* HLA-B$_2$7 present in 35% of patients versus 11% of controls HLA-DR4 present in 56% of patients versus 15% of controls *2539*

720.00   Rheumatoid (Ankylosing) Spondylitis   HLA antigen B$_2$7 found in 90% of caucasian patients with this disease compared to 8% of controls. *2051*   HLA-B$_2$7 present in 90% of patients versus 8% of controls *2539*

Homocystine

Serum   Increase

270.42   Homocystinuria   Decreased rate of metabolism results in excessive concentration. *2246*

Urine   Increase

270.03   Cystinosis   Nonspecific pattern of aminoaciduria. Fanconi's syndrome. *0995*

270.42   Homocystinuria   Decreased rate of metabolism results in excessive concentration. *2246   0995*

275.10   Hepatolenticular Degeneration   *0503*

CSF   Increase

270.42   Homocystinuria   *2468*

Homogentisic Acid

Urine   Increase

270.21   Alkaptonuria   Excessive amounts are excreted in the urine. The output is proportional to the amount of protein in the diet. *0619*   All diagnostic tests are based on the presence of homogentisic acid in the urine. *2246*

Homovanillic Acid

Urine   Increase

192.50   Neuroblastoma   Urine arylsulfatase and homovanillic acid are inversely related in neuroblastomas. In melanotic tumors, HVA is elevated and arylsulfatase normal or slightly elevated. Amelanotic tumors have low-normal HVA and high arylsulfatase. *1630* Elevated levels receded toward normal after treatment. *1511*

227.91   Pheochromocytoma   Increased in neuroblastomas, benign ganglioneuromas, and pheochromocytomas. *1630*

Urine   Normal

227.91   Pheochromocytoma   Patients with pheochromocytoma excrete normal amounts. *1806*

CSF   Decrease

331.00   Alzheimer's Disease   Lower than in an aged matched control group. *1765*

333.40   Huntington's Chorea   *0878*

335.20   Amyotrophic Lateral Sclerosis   *1495*

CSF   Increase

53.00   Herpes Zoster   Has been reported. *1167*

CSF   Normal

331.00   Alzheimer's Disease   Level was unchanged from normal controls. *2615*

Hyaline Casts

Urine   Increase

124.00   Trichinosis   In severe cases. *2468*

250.00   Diabetes Mellitus   With diabetic nephropathy. *0186*

428.00   Congestive Heart Failure   There are isolated RBC and WBC, hyaline and sometimes granular casts. *2467*

446.00   Polyarteritis-Nodosa   Hyaline and granular casts indicate renal involvement. *0151*

482.90   Bacterial Pneumonia   Protein, WBC, hyaline and granular casts in small amounts are common. *2467*

572.40   Hepatic Failure   WBC, RBC, and hyaline casts were found in 26% of patients with hepatic failure due to decompensated cirrhosis or attacks of acute viral hepatitis. *0379*

580.02   Glomerulonephritis (Minimal Change)   Hyaline, granular, and fatty casts are found. *0151   0433*

580.04   Glomerulonephritis (Membranous)   Usually present. *0433*

710.00   Systemic Lupus Erythematosus   *0433*

Hydrochloric Acid

Gastric Material   Decrease

151.90   Malignant Neoplasm of Stomach   Achlorhydria following histamine or betazole stimulation found in 50% of patients and hypochlorhydria in another 25% of patients. *2467   0962*

211.41   Adenomatous Polyp   Gastric analysis - achlorhydria in 85% of patients. Polyps occur in 5% of patients with pernicious anemia and 2% of patients with achlorhydria. *2467*

280.90   Iron Deficiency Anemia   The augmented histamine test has shown true achlorhydria in 16% of cases. *0995*

281.00   Pernicious Anemia   Gastric parietal cells lose ability to secrete HCl as well as intrinsic factor. Achlorhydria is therefore characteristic of intrinsic factor deficiency but not diagnostic. *0962*

535.00   Gastritis   Most patients with Ménétrier's disease have achlorhydria. However, some patients may have hypersecretion. *2238*   Transient hypochlorhydria or achlorhydria may be observed during episodes of acute gastritis. *2199*

650.00   Pregnancy   Gastric HCl may be decreased. *2468*

Gastric Material   Increase

151.90   Malignant Neoplasm of Stomach   Although rare, does not rule out carcinoma. *2467*

537.00   Pyloric Stenosis, Acquired   Due to excess circulating gastrin. *0587*

Gastric Material   Normal

151.90   Malignant Neoplasm of Stomach   Normal in 25% of patients. *2467*

Hydroxyproline

Serum   Increase

135.00   Sarcoidosis   *0062*

201.90   Hodgkin's Disease   *0592*

242.90   Hyperthyroidism   *0151*

270.82   Hydroxyprolinemia   Elevated > 15-fold above normal concentration. *2246*

Urine   Decrease

242.90   Hyperthyroidism   Reduced excretion in 22 of 33 patients. *2435*

244.90   Hypothyroidism   *0962*

252.10   Hypoparathyroidism   May occur. *2540   0962*

275.32   Hypophosphatasia   Extremely low. *0663*   May be extremely low, reflecting bone destruction. *2341 2246*

359.11   Progressive Muscular Dystrophy   In boys with Duchenne type. *0878*

Urine   Increase

135.00   Sarcoidosis   Considerably increased in acute disease, returning to normal as the chest x-ray abnormality resolves. Chronic disease has normal levels. *0151*

170.90   Malignant Neoplasm of Bone   Marked elevation. *1693*

201.90   Hodgkin's Disease   *0151*

242.90   Hyperthyroidism   Because of excess bone resorption. *0962*   Elevated in 107 of 111 patients, aged 18-61 y and 10 of 14 patients over 65. *2435*

252.00   Hyperparathyroidism   Normal or increased. Increased with significant bone involvement. *2540*   Tends to parallel the extent and severity of bone involvement. Also seen in the secondary hyperparathyroidism of chronic renal disease. *0962*

253.00   Acromegaly   Indicates secretory activity of tumor. *2467*   Increased bone turnover found in this condition may result in elevation. *0962   0151*

268.00   Vitamin D Deficiency Rickets   Increased formation of osteoid tissue results in hydroxyprolinuria, values will decrease with adequate therapy with vitamin D. *0962*

268.20   Osteomalacia   Increased formation of osteoid tissue results in hydroxyprolinuria, values will decrease with adequate therapy with vitamin D. *0962   0999*

270.03   Cystinosis   Nonspecific pattern of aminoaciduria. Fanconi's syndrome. *0995*

270.81   Hyperprolinemia   Hyperaminoaciduria of proline, glycine and hydroxyproline is specific. *2246*

270.82   Hydroxyprolinemia   Greatly increased. Excretion rates of 285-550 mg/24h have been reported in patients aged 12-31 y. *1797 0629*

275.35   Vitamin D Resistant Rickets   Some patients. *0962 2246*

710.10   Progressive Systemic Sclerosis   Increased in some patients, especially those with active disease. *0151*

731.00   Osteitis Deformans   Increase as evidence of enhanced remodeling activity. *0999*

733.00   Osteoporosis   In hypermetabolic osteopenia. *0999*

Urine   Normal

571.60   Biliary Cirrhosis   Not different from age matched controls. *1057*

CSF   Normal

270.82   Hydroxyprolinemia   *2246*

Hypoxanthine

Serum   Increase

410.90   Acute Myocardial Infarction   Myocardial ischemia in 18 patients resulted in an increase of coronary sinus hypoxanthine levels from 1.20 ± 0.52 mg/dL during pain. *1911*

Hypoxanthine (continued)

Serum   Increase (continued)

414.00   Chronic Ischemic Heart Disease   Myocardial ischemia in 18 patients resulted in an increase of coronary sinus hypoxanthine levels from 1.20 ± 0.52 mg/dL during pain. *1911*

Urine   Increase

277.21   Xanthinuria   Characterized by the replacement of uric acid by xanthine and hypoxanthine in urine. *2246*

Imidazolepyruvic Acid

Urine   Increase

270.51   Histidinemia   Chromatography of the urinary metabolites of histidine will reveal the presence of imidazole pyruvic acid. *0433* Excreted in substantial quantities in the urine but no significant concentration was found in the blood. *2246   0151*

Immunoglobulin IgA

Serum   Decrease

127.00   Ascariasis   Immunoglobulin levels, especially IgA, may be depressed owing to enteric protein loss. *2199*

128.00   Larva Migrans (Visceralis)   Immunoglobulin levels, especially IgA, may be depressed owing to enteric protein loss. *2199*

203.00   Multiple Myeloma   May occur in IgG form. *2538*

204.00   Lymphocytic Leukemia (Acute)   *2467*

204.10   Lymphocytic Leukemia (Chronic)   *2467*

205.10   Myelocytic Leukemia (Chronic)   *2467*

245.10   Subacute Thyroiditis   In 40 patients, levels were decreased in those who were BW-35 negative but were normal in the patients who were BW-35 positive. *1715*

260.00   Protein Malnutrition   *0503*

273.23   Heavy Chain Disease (Gamma)   Marked decrease. *2468*

273.30   Waldenström's Macroglobulinemia   *2467*

275.10   Hepatolenticular Degeneration   Decreased in 6 and elevated in 2 of 16 patients. *2278*

277.30   Amyloidosis   Mean concentration (.61 g/L) was significantly decreased in patients with Bence-Jones proteinuria. *0124*

279.01   IgA Deficiency (Selective)   Less than 5 mg/dL. *0793*

279.04   Agammaglobulinemia (Congenital Sex-linked)   Usually < 1% of normal adult values. *2035*   Undetectable. *2538*

279.06   Immunodeficiency (Common Variable)   *0619 2539*

279.07   Dysgammaglobulinemia (Selective Immunoglobulin Deficiency)   Types I, II, and IV; 1 in 500 of the population have IgA deficiency. *0619*   One of the common partial immunoglobulin defects is characterized by a deficiency of IgA and IgG and increased amounts of IgM in the serum. *2035*   In type III. *2468 0881 0433*

279.13   Nezeloff's Syndrome   50% of patients. *2344*

279.20   Severe Combined Immunodeficiency   *0793*

334.80   Ataxia-Telangiectasia   About 80% of patients lack both serum and secretory IgA. *2035*   Deficient in 66% of patients. *1836 2538*

580.02   Glomerulonephritis (Minimal Change)   Usually normal or modestly decreased. *0419*

581.90   Nephrotic Syndrome   *2467*

Serum   Increase

2.00   Typhoid Fever   Moderate hypergammaglobulinemia, especially IgA. *0880*

30.00   Leprosy   High levels have been described but appear to be more variable than IgG. *2035 2387*

38.00   Septicemia   Perinatal infections. *0619*

47.00   Aseptic Meningitis   IgA and IgG increased. *0619*

70.00   Viral Hepatitis   *2467*

75.00   Infectious Mononucleosis   A modest increase may occur. *0961 2538*

86.90   Trypanosomiasis   *1058*

99.10   Lymphogranuloma Venereum   Up to 75% of the patients will experience an elevation. *0433*

115.00   Histoplasmosis   In patients with chronic cavitary disease, IgM and IgG levels were normal although increased IgA was found. *2035   2476*

117.30   Aspergillosis   Elevated in 10 of 15 patients with a mean of 314.6 mg/dL. *1983*

135.00   Sarcoidosis   Elevated in 25% of cases. *0151*   Immunoglobulins are frequently elevated and tend to reflect the overall resolution of disease. Falls to normal with resolution. *1608*

185.00   Malignant Neoplasm of Prostate   22% had elevated levels ranging from 365-550 mg/dL. *0008*

202.10   Mycosis Fungoides   No prognostic significance. *2539* May be elevated *2539*

203.00   Multiple Myeloma   Peak of > 5 g/dL indicates high tumor mass. A peak of < 3 g/dL indicates low tumor mass. *2467*   The abnormal serum M component was IgG in 20 of 35 patients and IgA in 7. There was no correlation between type of M component and presence of renal failure. *0518*

273.22   Heavy Chain Disease (Alpha)   Distinctive increase in IgA heavy chains (alpha chains). *2035*

275.10   Hepatolenticular Degeneration   Decreased in 6 and elevated in 2 of 16 patients. *2278*

277.00   Cystic Fibrosis   Rises with progressive pulmonary disease. *2467   0619*

279.12   Wiskott-Aldrich Syndrome   Elevated levels. *2344 2539*

279.31   Acquired Immunodeficiency Syndrome (AIDS)   Frequently a polyclonal hypergammaglobulinemia is present, usually of IgG and IgA. *2539*   Elevated levels of at least one immunoglobulin was found in 78% of patients. *0646*

287.00   Allergic Purpura   Found in 50% of patients. *2552*

340.00   Multiple Sclerosis   Levels > 388 mg/dL in 13.8% of 64 patients. *1295*

390.00   Rheumatic Fever   Increase in the globulin fraction of the serum proteins is frequent and mainly due to an increase in IgG and IgA. *1108*   Increased immunoglobulins, particularly of IgG and IgA, and elevated immune responses to streptococcal cellular and extracellular products. *2035*

555.90   Regional Enteritis or Ileitis   *0619*

570.00   Acute and Subacute Necrosis of Liver   Slightly increased or normal. *0992*

571.20   Laennec's or Alcoholic Cirrhosis   Moderate hypergammaglobulinemia, especially IgA. *0880   2035*

571.49   Chronic Active Hepatitis   In 50 patients, mean levels of all three major classes of immunoglobulin, IgG, IgM and IgA, were increased but only IgG was markedly raised. *1467   2035*

571.60   Biliary Cirrhosis   Hypergammaglobulinemia is common, involving all classes of immunoglobulins (IgG, IgA, IgM), although IgM may be selectively increased. *0151*

571.90   Cirrhosis of Liver   Hypergammaglobulinemia is common, involving all classes of immunoglobulins. *0151   0433*

579.00   Celiac Sprue Disease   May be increased. *2238*

581.90   Nephrotic Syndrome   Usually normal or elevated. *0419*

710.00   Systemic Lupus Erythematosus   Mean concentrations were within the normal range at diagnosis (271 ± 171 mg/dL) but increased significantly to 349 ± 210 mg/dL during follow-up (P < 0.05) in 39 patients. *2081*   Level decreased progressively after the first trimester *0517*   Slightly elevated except in the presence of protein-losing nephropathy. *0962*

710.10   Progressive Systemic Sclerosis   Usually slightly elevated. *0962   1995*

710.20   Sjögren's Syndrome   Hypergammaglobulinemia characterized by a diffuse increase in IgG, IgA, and IgM is found especially in those patients with the sicca complex not accompanied by a connective tissue disease. *0934   2035*

714.00   Rheumatoid Arthritis   *2467*

720.00   Rheumatoid (Ankylosing) Spondylitis   Mean levels of C4 and IgA were significantly elevated in patients with sporadic disease. *1273*

994.50   Exercise   Approximately 14% increase immediately after. *1837*

Serum   Normal

11.00   Pulmonary Tuberculosis   *2467*

155.00   Malignant Neoplasm of Liver   *2467*

201.90   Hodgkin's Disease   *2467*

205.00   Myelocytic Leukemia (Acute)   *2467*

279.11   DiGeorge's Syndrome   Frequently normal. *0996*

279.12 **Wiskott-Aldrich Syndrome** Normal 0996
335.20 **Amyotrophic Lateral Sclerosis** 0665
994.50 **Exercise** No observed effect 15 min or 1 day after. 0985

Urine   Increase

153.90 **Malignant Neoplasm of Large Intestine** 24 h excretion and renal clearance were significantly increased in localized tumor patients compared to normals and disseminated cancer cases. Increased high molecular weight protein excretion implies glomerular injury in these patients. 1025

162.90 **Malignant Neoplasm of Bronchus and Lung** 24 h excretion and renal clearance were significantly increased in localized tumor patients compared to normals and disseminated cancer cases. Increased high molecular weight protein excretion implies glomerular injury in these patients. 1025

174.90 **Malignant Neoplasm of Breast** 24 h excretion and renal clearance were significantly increased in localized tumor patients compared to normals and disseminated cancer cases. Increased high molecular weight protein excretion implies glomerular injury in these patients. 1025

182.00 **Malignant Neoplasm of Corpus Uteri** 24 h excretion and renal clearance were significantly increased in localized tumor patients compared to normals and disseminated cancer cases. Increased high molecular weight protein excretion implies glomerular injury in these patients. 1025

599.00 **Urinary Tract Infection** Mean concentration = 3.3 mg/24h. Secretory IgA locally produced in the bladder. 1237

CSF   Decrease

345.90 **Epilepsy** Slightly decreased in grand mal epilepsy. 1625

CSF   Increase

47.00 **Aseptic Meningitis** 0619
340.00 **Multiple Sclerosis** 35.9% of patients had CSF values > 0.6 mg/dL. 1295 Found in 5 of 45 patients. 1933
357.00 **Guillain-Barré Syndrome** Early in disease. 0878
357.90 **Polyneuritis** Increased amounts of immunoglobulins particularly IgA and IgM have been demonstrated. 0433
710.00 **Systemic Lupus Erythematosus** Elevation of IgG index was noted in 70% of patients, IgA index in 77% and IgM index in 100% of 13 patients when compared with 20 controls with other neurological disorders. 1887

Saliva   Increase

714.00 **Rheumatoid Arthritis** Significantly elevated in 24% of patients. 80% of the patients with elevated IgA concentrations had keratoconjunctivitis sicca as well. 0162

Semen   Positive

606.90 **Infertility in Males** 20 Patients tested and 50% were positive for sperm-bound IgA. 0408

Immunoglobulin IgD

Serum   Decrease

172.90 **Malignant Melanoma of Skin** Malignant melanoma patients with metastases presented significant decreases in IgD and IgM subpopulations. 0185

279.04 **Agammaglobulinemia (Congenital Sex-linked)** Undetectable. 2538

642.40 **Pre-Eclampsia** Significantly lower than in normal late pregnancy. 2285

Serum   Increase

38.00 **Septicemia** Moderately increased. 2467
135.00 **Sarcoidosis** 0619
203.00 **Multiple Myeloma** Rare. 0992
245.10 **Subacute Thyroiditis** 0619
340.00 **Multiple Sclerosis** 6.4% of patients had concentrations > 29 mg/dL. 1295
446.00 **Polyarteritis-Nodosa** 0619
710.00 **Systemic Lupus Erythematosus** 0619
710.40 **Dermatomyositis/Polymyositis** 0619
714.00 **Rheumatoid Arthritis** 0619

773.00 **Hemolytic Disease of Newborn (Erythroblastosis Fetalis)** 0619

Serum   Normal

277.00 **Cystic Fibrosis** Not appreciably increased. 2467
279.01 **IgA Deficiency (Selective)** 0793

Immunoglobulin IgE

Serum   Decrease

279.04 **Agammaglobulinemia (Congenital Sex-linked)** Undetectable. 2538

279.06 **Immunodeficiency (Common Variable)** 2035

334.80 **Ataxia-Telangiectasia** Decreased or absent serum IgA and IgE causing recurrent pulmonary infections. 2467 Deficient in 80% of patients. 1836 0151

340.00 **Multiple Sclerosis** Median level was slightly lower than in controls. All other serum immunoglobulins were normal. 0068

Serum   Increase

65.00 **Arthropod-Borne Hemorrhagic Fever** 88.2% of patients with dengue hemorrhagic fever had measurable serum IgE, compared to 57.1% of controls. Patient range was 50-5025 U/mL and control was 50-2250 U/mL. 1786

75.00 **Infectious Mononucleosis** 2035

117.30 **Aspergillosis** Markedly elevated in all patients with allergic bronchopulmonary aspergillosis. 1983 High values are found during the episodes of pulmonary eosinophilia. 2035

120.00 **Schistosomiasis** Increased in bilharziasis. 0619 44% in Egypt and 20% in Brazil were above 24 µg/mL in S. Mansoni infestations. 2035

122.90 **Hydatidosis** Increased in parasitic diseases. 2467 Has been reported. 0992

124.00 **Trichinosis** The only correlation between trichinosis and an increase in serum IgE was found in patients with a prior history of allergic disease. 0119 2035

126.90 **Ancylostomiasis (Hookworm Infestation)** Increased in parasitic diseases. 2467 0619

127.00 **Ascariasis** The extent and persistence of elevation is dependent upon several genetically controlled factors. 1738 Parasitic disorders may be associated with elevated IgE levels, especially Ascariasis. 2199 2035

127.20 **Strongyloidiasis** Increased in parasitic diseases. 2467

127.30 **Trichuriasis** Increased in parasitic diseases. 2467

128.00 **Larva Migrans (Visceralis)** The extent and persistence of elevation is dependent upon several genetically controlled factors. 1738 Parasitic disorders may be associated with elevated IgE levels, especially Ascariasis, and visceral larva migrans. 2199 2035

135.00 **Sarcoidosis** 0062
202.10 **Mycosis Fungoides** May be elevated. 2539
203.00 **Multiple Myeloma** Only 5 cases of IgE myeloma have been reported. 0992
279.12 **Wiskott-Aldrich Syndrome** Frequently elevated. 0996

340.00 **Multiple Sclerosis** Serum IgE and measles antibodies were increased more frequently in hypocomplementemic patients than in normal populations. 2375

477.90 **Hay Fever** Increased in atopic diseases. Occurs in about 30% of patients. 2467 During the pollen season. 0619 Allergic persons usually have values 2-6 X normal. 0999

580.02 **Glomerulonephritis (Minimal Change)** May be increased. 0419

581.90 **Nephrotic Syndrome** Usually normal or elevated. 0419

691.80 **Atopic Eczema** Atopic subjects tend to have moderate increases. 0619 Total serum concentration was elevated in 75-81% of the children with asthma, nasal allergy and atopic dermatitis and an elevated serum concentration or blood eosinophilia, or both, was noted in 85% of the patients. 0405 Some patients. 2035 0642

694.40 **Pemphigus** Significant increase in 70% of bullous pemphigoid patients. 2035

Serum   Normal

279.01 **IgA Deficiency (Selective)** 0793
279.11 **DiGeorge's Syndrome** Frequently normal. 0996

Immunoglobulin IgE *(continued)*

Serum   Normal *(continued)*

493.10   Asthma (Intrinsic)   Elevated in most patients with allergic asthma but not in most patients with intrinsic asthma. At this time, however, the IgE level should not be used by itself to differentiate intrinsic from extrinsic asthma. Elevated in 75-81% of the children with asthma, nasal allergy, and atopic dermatitis. Elevated serum IgE concentration or blood eosinophilia, or both, was noted in 85% of the patients. *0405*   Usually found in patients with allergic asthma but not with other forms. *1170   0642*

Pleural Effusion   Increase

482.90   Bacterial Pneumonia   Immunoglobulins are present in large amount. *1913*

Immunoglobulin IgG

Serum   Decrease

203.00   Multiple Myeloma   May occur in IgA form. *2538*

204.10   Lymphocytic Leukemia (Chronic)   *2467*

273.23   Heavy Chain Disease (Gamma)   Marked decrease in IgG. *2468*   Excessive quantities of the Fe fragment of the heavy chain of IgG. *2035*

273.30   Waldenström's Macroglobulinemia   *2467*

277.30   Amyloidosis   Decreased in 50% of primary and 66% of secondary disease. *1334*   Mean concentration (540 mg/dL) was significantly decreased in patients with Bence-Jones proteinuria. *0124*

279.04   Agammaglobulinemia (Congenital Sex-linked)   Minute amounts of IgG and sometimes IgM are identifiable by sensitive methods, functional levels of antibody are absent. *0999*   100 mg/dL. *2035*   In primary acquired form, the serum levels may be as high as 500 mg/dL. *1069*

279.06   Immunodeficiency (Common Variable)   Usually < 500 mg/dL. *2035*   Usually under 500 mg/dL but may not exhibit normal heterogeneity *2539*

279.07   Dysgammaglobulinemia (Selective Immunoglobulin Deficiency)   One of the common partial immunoglobulin defects is characterized by a deficiency of IgA and IgG and increased amounts of IgM in the serum. *2035*   Type I, II, III, IV. *0619   0881*

279.13   Nezeloff's Syndrome   50% of patients. *2344*

279.20   Severe Combined Immunodeficiency   *0793*

287.30   Idiopathic Thrombocytopenic Purpura   Mean IgG levels were subnormal. *1259   2538*

334.80   Ataxia-Telangiectasia   *0999*

359.21   Myotonia Atrophica   In 4 of 8 cases studied. *1158   2246*

579.01   Protein-Losing Enteropathy   *0503*

580.01   Glomerulonephritis (Focal)   May be significantly reduced. *0419*

580.02   Glomerulonephritis (Minimal Change)   May be profoundly depressed during relapse. *0419*

581.90   Nephrotic Syndrome   Higher IgM and lower IgG serum concentrations were found in nephrotic patients than in normal controls (929 ± 537 mg/dL). *2594*   May be significantly reduced. *0419*

642.40   Pre-Eclampsia   Significantly lower than in normal late pregnancy. *0170 1073 2285*

Serum   Increase

11.00   Pulmonary Tuberculosis   *2467*

23.00   Brucellosis   Antibodies elicited early in natural infection are predominantly IgM, with lesser quantities of IgG. As the disease progresses, IgM declines, and IgG increases, reaching its height at the period of maximum resistance to reinfection. *2035*

30.00   Leprosy   High levels are consistently found in the sera of untreated lepromatous patients. *2035   2387*

47.00   Aseptic Meningitis   IgA and IgG increased. *0619*

55.00   Measles   Maternal antibody may be differentiated from that actively produced by the infant by a steadily declining titer, since these tests primarily measure IgG. *0433*

70.00   Viral Hepatitis   Slightly elevated gamma globulins, usually < 2.0 g/dL. IgG rises as illness progresses. *0433*   Frequently transiently elevated. *0962*

75.00   Infectious Mononucleosis   Mean values 50% higher than normal. *0961   2538*

84.00   Malaria   Marked elevation. *0151*   Mean IgG and IgM were significantly increased. Mean IgG = 179 U/mL, range = 119-284 U/mL. *0834*   Despite the considerably increased concentration of immunoglobulins in infected individuals, only 5% of the immune adult IgG combines specifically with P. falciparum antigens. *0426 2035*

85.00   Leishmaniasis   Serum protein increases to values > 10 g/dL, almost entirely due to raised IgG levels. *0151*   Increased intravascular pools of albumin, IgG, and IgM in tropical splenomegaly. IgM and IgG accounting for 42% of the total and albumin for 28%. *0466*   Marked IgG increase in Kala-Azar patients. Mean = 591 U/mL, range = 305-941 U/mL. *0834*

86.90   Trypanosomiasis   *1058*

87.00   Relapsing Fever   Occurs initially after infection, followed by a rise in IgM. *0151*

117.30   Aspergillosis   Elevated in 8 of 15 cases with a mean of 1485 mg/dL. *1983*

135.00   Sarcoidosis   Consistent increase in 1 or more serum immunoglobulins, noted in 79% of 129 cases studied. IgM and/or IgG are the most frequently increased. *0433*   Elevated in 50% of cases. *0151*   Frequently elevated and tends to reflect the overall resolution of disease. With resolution, falls but tends to remain raised for up to 4 y. *1608*

202.80   Non-Hodgkins Lymphoma   In a recent survey, 15 of 348 patients (4.6%) with lymphosarcoma and reticulum cell sarcoma had monoclonal serum components. In 10 instances the component was IgM and in 5 IgG. *1618*

203.00   Multiple Myeloma   Most common. *0992*   The abnormal serum M component was IgG in 20 of 35 patients and IgA in 7. There was no correlation between type of M component and presence of renal failure. *0518*

238.40   Polycythemia Vera   Significant diffuse increases in IgG and IgM have been noted. *2538*

245.20   Hashimoto's Thyroiditis   Often slightly raised. *2035*

250.00   Diabetes Mellitus   The levels of glycosylated IgG were significantly higher. *2644*

273.21   Cryoglobulinemia (Essential Mixed)   Monoclonal spike may occur. *2035*

275.10   Hepatolenticular Degeneration   Elevated in over 50% of patients. *2278*

277.00   Cystic Fibrosis   Rises with progressive pulmonary disease. *2467*

279.07   Dysgammaglobulinemia (Selective Immunoglobulin Deficiency)   *0619*

279.12   Wiskott-Aldrich Syndrome   Elevated levels. *2539*

279.31   Acquired Immunodeficiency Syndrome (AIDS)   Frequently a polyclonal hypergammaglobulinemia is present, usually of IgG and IgA. *2539*   Elevated levels of at least 1 immunoglobulin found in 78% of patients *0646*   27 of 29 children tested. *1760*

282.60   Sickle Cell Anemia   Markedly elevated in both Black and Caucasian patients. *2110*

287.30   Idiopathic Thrombocytopenic Purpura   Children with both acute and chronic disease had significantly greater levels than normal or thrombocytopenic controls. Acute cases were elevated more than chronic. *1407*

340.00   Multiple Sclerosis   Levels > 1871 mg/dL in 12.3% of 64 patients. *1295*

390.00   Rheumatic Fever   Increase in the globulin fraction of the serum proteins is frequent and mainly due to an increase in IgG and IgA. *1108*   Increased immunoglobulins, particularly of IgG and IgA, and elevated immune responses to streptococcal cellular and extracellular products. *2035*

571.20   Laennec's or Alcoholic Cirrhosis   Elevated in about 50% of the patients. *1847*

571.49   Chronic Active Hepatitis   Elevated levels were present in about 50% of the patients. *1847*   In 50 patients, mean levels of all 3 major classes of immunoglobulin, IgG, IgM, and IgA, were increased but only IgG was markedly raised. *1467   2035*

571.60   Biliary Cirrhosis   IgG is more likely to be elevated in chronic hepatitis and cryptogenic cirrhosis, whereas IgM is high in biliary cirrhosis. *1829*   Hypergammaglobulinemia is common, involving all classes of immunoglobulins (IgG, IgA, IgM), although IgM may be selectively increased. *0151*

571.90 Cirrhosis of Liver In about 50% of the patients with cryptogenic cirrhosis, alcoholic cirrhosis, and chronic active hepatitis. *1847* The increase in gamma fraction is polyclonal in nature and is due first to increase in IgM fraction followed by an increase in IgG fraction. *2339 1829*

650.00 Pregnancy Progressive increase. *2286 2287*

710.00 Systemic Lupus Erythematosus The IgG dynamics differed from those of IgA and IgM by high mean IgG concentrations at diagnosis (1492 ± 835 mg/dL) and a significant decrease to 1195 ± 748 mg/dL during follow-up. The pattern was characterized by an inverse relation of IgA and IgG; while IgA concentrations increased significantly during follow-up, a parallel decrease in IgG occurred. *2081* Marked increase in untreated patients, 18.7 ± 5.1 g/L, with only a moderate correlation with disease activity. *1047* Slightly elevated except in the presence of protein-losing nephropathy. *0962*

710.10 Progressive Systemic Sclerosis In most cases and in greatest measure, the increase involves IgG; less often the levels of IgA and IgM are elevated. *2035* Usually slightly elevated. *0962 1995*

710.20 Sjögren's Syndrome The elevated globulin is usually 7S gamma globulin IgG and is not monoclonal. *0433* Hypergammaglobulinemia characterized by a diffuse increase in IgG, IgA, and IgM is found especially in those patients with the sicca complex not accompanied by a connective tissue disease. *0934 2035*

714.00 Rheumatoid Arthritis *2467*

714.30 Juvenile Rheumatoid Arthritis Polyclonal increase. *0793*

994.50 Exercise Approximately 10% increase immediately after. *1837*

Serum Normal

155.00 Malignant Neoplasm of Liver *2467*

201.90 Hodgkin's Disease *2467*

204.00 Lymphocytic Leukemia (Acute) *2467*

205.00 Myelocytic Leukemia (Acute) *2467*

205.10 Myelocytic Leukemia (Chronic) *2467*

279.01 IgA Deficiency (Selective) *0793*

279.07 Dysgammaglobulinemia (Selective Immunoglobulin Deficiency) In type I and II. *2468*

279.11 DiGeorge's Syndrome Frequently normal. *0996 2344*

279.12 Wiskott-Aldrich Syndrome Normal *0996*

334.80 Ataxia-Telangiectasia *2467*

335.20 Amyotrophic Lateral Sclerosis *0665*

994.50 Exercise No observed effect 15 min or 1 day after. *0985*

Urine Increase

153.90 Malignant Neoplasm of Large Intestine 24 h excretion and renal clearance were significantly increased in localized tumor patients compared to normals and disseminated cancer cases. Increased high molecular weight protein excretion implies glomerular injury in these patients. *1025*

162.90 Malignant Neoplasm of Bronchus and Lung 24 h excretion and renal clearance were significantly increased in localized tumor patients compared to normals and disseminated cancer cases. Increased high molecular weight protein excretion implies glomerular injury in these patients. *1025*

174.90 Malignant Neoplasm of Breast 24 h excretion and renal clearance were significantly increased in localized tumor patients compared to normals and disseminated cancer cases. Increased high molecular weight protein excretion implies glomerular injury in these patients. *1025*

182.00 Malignant Neoplasm of Corpus Uteri 24 h excretion and renal clearance were significantly increased in localized tumor patients compared to normals and disseminated cancer cases. Increased high molecular weight protein excretion implies glomerular injury in these patients. *1025*

CSF Decrease

345.90 Epilepsy Slightly decreased in grand mal epilepsy. *1625* Absolute concentration and percent of total CSF protein were low. *2321*

CSF Increase

45.90 Acute Poliomyelitis *0186*

47.00 Aseptic Meningitis *0619*

97.90 Syphilis Increased with obstruction of the spinal canal, especially in neurosyphilis and tuberculous meningitis. *2321*

191.90 Malignant Neoplasm of Brain No consistent CSF IgG pattern was found in brain tumors, but highly vascularized tumors had increased concentrations. *2321*

225.90 Benign Neoplasm of Brain and CNS No consistent CSF IgG pattern was found in brain tumors, but highly vascularized tumors had increased concentrations. *2321*

320.90 Meningitis (Bacterial) Characteristic of brucella meningitis. Increased in acute meningitis due to impairment of blood:CSF barrier. Increases in absolute not relative amount of individual proteins are found in CSF. Little or no IgG was found to be synthesized intrathecally. A high correlation (R = 0.95) was found between plasma and CSF IgG and albumin concentrations. *0809* Increased with obstruction of the spinal canal, especially in neurosyphilis and tuberculous meningitis. *2321 0555*

323.92 Encephalomyelitis Total protein and IgG concentration were increased. *2321*

340.00 Multiple Sclerosis Total IgG is often increased > 15 mg/dL in CSF in all forms of multiple sclerosis. *0999* Concentrations > 4 mg/dL in 77.7% of patients. *1295* Increased due to intrathecal synthesis not blood:CSF barrier damage. *1099* In 62% of cases. *1933 2321*

357.00 Guillain-Barré Syndrome Oligoclonal IgG bands, specific elevation of IgM and complement activation products have been reported during the acute phase of the disease. *1307* IgG and Albumin increased, probably resulting from blood: CSF barrier damage *1099*

710.00 Systemic Lupus Erythematosus Elevation of IgG index was noted in 70% of patients, IgA index in 77% and IgM index in 100% of 13 patients when compared with 20 controls with other neurological disorders. *1887*

CSF Normal

331.00 Alzheimer's Disease No significant difference in levels compared with controls. *0372*

331.90 Cerebral and Cortical Atrophy Within the normal range. *2321*

Pleural Effusion Increase

482.90 Bacterial Pneumonia Predominant immunoglobulin found in effusions. *1913*

Red Blood Cells Increase

283.00 Acquired Hemolytic Anemia (Autoimmune) May be detected on the red cell surface in up to 80% of patients. *0485 2538*

Semen Positive

606.90 Infertility in Males 20 Patients tested and 100% were positive for sperm-bound IgG. *0408*

Immunoglobulin IgM

Serum Decrease

155.00 Malignant Neoplasm of Liver *2467*

172.90 Malignant Melanoma of Skin Malignant melanoma patients with metastases presented significant decreases in IgD and IgM subpopulations. *0185*

203.00 Multiple Myeloma May occur. *2538*

204.10 Lymphocytic Leukemia (Chronic) *2467*

260.00 Protein Malnutrition *2467*

273.23 Heavy Chain Disease (Gamma) Marked decrease. *2467*

277.30 Amyloidosis The most significant finding. All 14 patients without macroglobulinemia had reduced concentration, mean = 0.5 g/L, only 34% of the control value. *0124* Mean concentration (0.46 g/L) was significantly decreased in patients with Bence-Jones proteinuria. *0124*

279.04 Agammaglobulinemia (Congenital Sex-linked) Usually < 1% of normal adult values. *2035* Undetectable. *2538*

279.06 Immunodeficiency (Common Variable) *2539 2468 0619*

279.07 Dysgammaglobulinemia (Selective Immunoglobulin Deficiency) Types I, V, VII. *0619* In type II. *2468*

279.12 Wiskott-Aldrich Syndrome Low levels. *2539* Usually decreased. *0996 2344*

279.20 Severe Combined Immunodeficiency *0793*

Immunoglobulin IgM (continued)

Serum   Decrease (continued)

334.80 Ataxia-Telangiectasia   Low levels have been reported. *0151*

579.00 Celiac Sprue Disease   Reported low in 37% of patients. *2238*

Serum   Increase

23.00 Brucellosis   Antibodies elicited early in natural infection are predominantly IgM, with lesser quantities of IgG. As the disease progresses, IgM declines, and IgG increases, reaching its height at the period of maximum resistance to reinfection. *2035*

30.00 Leprosy   High levels have been described but appear to be more variable than IgG. *2035   2387*

70.00 Viral Hepatitis   Usually increased above 400 mg/dL during acute phase. *2467*   Initial rise in IgM, followed by IgG. *0433*

75.00 Infectious Mononucleosis   Increase up to 100% over control values in almost all cases, then decline over a period of 2-3 months toward normal. *0961   2538*

84.00 Malaria   Marked elevation. *0151*   Especially when particulate antigenic material is present in the blood stream. *0619*   Mean IgG and IgM were significantly increased in malaria patients. Mean IgM = 191 U/mL, range = 87-369. *0834   0426*

85.00 Leishmaniasis   In tropical splenomegaly; increased intravascular pools of albumin, IgG, and IgM. Variance in plasma volume was attributable to increases in these 3 pools, IgM and IgG accounting for 42% of the total and albumin for 28%. *0466*   Marked IgM increase in Kala-Azar patients. Mean = 226 U/mL range = 74-509 U/mL. *0834*

86.90 Trypanosomiasis   Marked increase of immunoglobulins, particularly IgM, may be explained by the continuous production of antibodies against new variants. *2105*   Markedly increased and remains elevated throughout the course of the infection. *1058   2035*

87.00 Relapsing Fever   IgG hyperglobulinemia occurs initially after infection, followed by a rise in IgM. *0151*

88.00 Bartonellosis   Especially when particulate antigenic material is present in the blood stream. *0619*

104.10 Lyme Disease   May be elevated in Lyme Disease. *2639*

117.30 Aspergillosis   Elevated in 10 of 15 cases; mean = 191.6 mg/dL. *1983*

124.00 Trichinosis   In parasitic diseases. *0503*

126.90 Ancylostomiasis (Hookworm Infestation)   In parasitic diseases. *0503*

127.00 Ascariasis   In parasitic diseases. *0503*

127.20 Strongyloidiasis   In parasitic diseases. *0503*

127.30 Trichuriasis   In parasitic diseases. *0503*

128.00 Larva Migrans (Visceralis)   In parasitic diseases. *0503*

130.00 Toxoplasmosis   Acute infections are characterized by an early and relatively transient IgM and complement-fixing antibody response. *2035   0776*

135.00 Sarcoidosis   Frequently elevated and tends to reflect the overall resolution of disease. Falls with resolution but remains significantly above normal. *1608*   Consistent increase in 1 or more serum immunoglobulins, noted in 79% of 129 cases studied. IgG and/or IgM are most frequently increased. *0433*   Serum IgG is elevated in 50%, IgA in 25%, and IgM in 12.5% of cases. *0151*

202.80 Non-Hodgkins Lymphoma   In a recent survey, 15 of 348 patients (4.6%) with lymphosarcoma and reticulum cell sarcoma had monoclonal serum components. In 10 instances the component was IgM and in 5 IgG. *1618*

238.40 Polycythemia Vera   Significant diffuse increases in IgG and IgM have been noted. *2538*

245.10 Subacute Thyroiditis   In 40 patients, there was an increase in serum C3, IgM, alpha$_1$-acid glycoprotein and alpha$_1$-antitrypsin levels. *1715*

245.20 Hashimoto's Thyroiditis   There was an increase in serum C3, IgM, alpha$_1$-acid glycoprotein and alpha$_1$-antitrypsin levels found in 40 patients. *1715*

273.21 Cryoglobulinemia (Essential Mixed)   Monoclonal spike may occur. *2035*

273.30 Waldenström's Macroglobulinemia   IgM > 15% of total serum protein and/or 1,000 mg/dL. *0999*   Immunoelectrophoresis identified IgM as a component of increased globulin. *2468*

275.10 Hepatolenticular Degeneration   Found to be increased in 5 out of 16 patients. *2278*

279.07 Dysgammaglobulinemia (Selective Immunoglobulin Deficiency)   Type I. *2467*   One of the common partial immunoglobulin defects is characterized by a deficiency of IgA and IgG and increased amounts of IgM in the serum. *2035   0433 0881*

340.00 Multiple Sclerosis   Levels > 161 mg/dL in 7.8% of cases; 3.1% had values 34 mg/dL. *1295*

421.91 Loeffler's Endocarditis   Especially when particulate antigenic material is present in the blood stream. *0619*

446.70 Pulseless Disease (Aortic Arch Syndrome)   Serum proteins abnormal with increased gamma globulins, mostly composed of IgM. *2467*   May be present. *2086*

570.00 Acute and Subacute Necrosis of Liver   *0619*

571.49 Chronic Active Hepatitis   In 50 patients, mean levels of all 3 major classes of immunoglobulin, IgG, IgM and IgA, were increased but only IgG was markedly raised. *1467   2035*

571.60 Biliary Cirrhosis   Elevated in about 80% of patients. *0992*   Hypergammaglobulinemia is common, involving all classes of immunoglobulins, although IgM may be selectively increased. *0151*   Hypergammaglobulinemia is mainly due to an elevation of IgM. *0716   2035 0962*

571.90 Cirrhosis of Liver   The increase in gamma fraction is polyclonal in nature and is due first to increase in IgM fraction followed by an increase in IgG fraction. *2339   1829*

580.02 Glomerulonephritis (Minimal Change)   May be increased. *0419*

581.90 Nephrotic Syndrome   Higher IgM and lower IgG serum concentrations were found in nephrotic patients than in normal controls (157 ± 108 mg/dL vs 127 ± 38 mg/dL). *2594   0419*

694.40 Pemphigus   About 70% of patients with this condition have elevated levels. *2373*

710.00 Systemic Lupus Erythematosus   Increased from a mean value of 88 ± 52 mg/dL at diagnosis to 113 ± 181 mg/dL during follow-up. *2081*   Slightly elevated except in the presence of protein-losing nephropathy. *0962   0354*

710.10 Progressive Systemic Sclerosis   Usually slightly elevated. *0962   1995*

710.20 Sjögren's Syndrome   Hypergammaglobulinemia characterized by a diffuse increase in IgG, IgA, and IgM is found especially in those patients with the sicca complex not accompanied by a connective tissue disease. *0934   2035*

714.00 Rheumatoid Arthritis   *2467*

771.00 Congenital Rubella   Frequently increased levels in the first 4 months of life (immunoglobulin > 20 mg/dL). Detection of rubella-specific IgM indicates congenital disease. *0433*   Presence in cord blood indicates congenital rubella infection. *2508*

Serum   Normal

11.00 Pulmonary Tuberculosis   *2467*

201.90 Hodgkin's Disease   *2467*

203.00 Multiple Myeloma   *0992*

204.00 Lymphocytic Leukemia (Acute)   *2467*

205.00 Myelocytic Leukemia (Acute)   *2467*

205.10 Myelocytic Leukemia (Chronic)   *2467*

277.00 Cystic Fibrosis   Not appreciably increased. *2467*

279.01 IgA Deficiency (Selective)   *0793*

279.07 Dysgammaglobulinemia (Selective Immunoglobulin Deficiency)   Normal or increased. *2467*

279.11 DiGeorge's Syndrome   Frequently normal. *0996*

334.80 Ataxia-Telangiectasia   *2467*

335.20 Amyotrophic Lateral Sclerosis   *0665*

571.20 Laennec's or Alcoholic Cirrhosis   *2467*

581.90 Nephrotic Syndrome   *2467*

994.50 Exercise   No observed effect 15 min or 1 day after. *0985*   No effect of exercise observed. *1837*

Urine   Increase

153.90 Malignant Neoplasm of Large Intestine   24 h excretion and renal clearance were significantly increased in localized tumor patients compared to normals and disseminated cancer cases. Increased high molecular weight protein excretion implies glomerular injury in these patients. *1025*

162.90 Malignant Neoplasm of Bronchus and Lung   24 h excretion and renal clearance were significantly increased in localized tumor patients compared to normals and disseminated cancer cases. Increased high molecular weight protein excretion implies glomerular injury in these patients. *1025*

174.90 Malignant Neoplasm of Breast 24 h excretion and renal clearance were significantly increased in localized tumor patients compared to normals and disseminated cancer cases. Increased high molecular weight protein excretion implies glomerular injury in these patients. *1025*

182.00 Malignant Neoplasm of Corpus Uteri 24 h excretion and renal clearance were significantly increased in localized tumor patients compared to normals and disseminated cancer cases. Increased high molecular weight protein excretion implies glomerular injury in these patients. *1025*

CSF Increase

340.00 Multiple Sclerosis Detected in CSF samples from 26.9% of patients. *1295*

357.00 Guillain-Barré Syndrome Oligoclonal IgG bands, specific elevation of IgM and complement activation products have been reported during the acute phase of the disease. *1307*

357.90 Polyneuritis Increased amounts of immunoglobulins particularly IgA and IgM have been demonstrated. *0433*

710.00 Systemic Lupus Erythematosus Elevation of IgG index was noted in 70% of patients, IgA index in 77% and IgM index in 100% of 13 patients when compared with 20 controls with other neurological disorders. *1887*

Synovial Fluid Increase

714.00 Rheumatoid Arthritis Very suggestive of this disease. *0139*

Pleural Effusion Increase

482.90 Bacterial Pneumonia Immunoglobulins are present in large amounts forming a series declining from the IgG (70% of serum concentration) to the IgM (50% of serum concentration). *1913*

Platelet Increase

279.12 Wiskott-Aldrich Syndrome Platelet associated immunoglobulins were increased presplenectomy. *0455*

Semen Negative

606.90 Infertility in Males 20 Patients tested and 0% positive for sperm-bound IgM. *0408*

Immunoglobulins

Serum Decrease

202.80 Non-Hodgkins Lymphoma Low levels were present in several patients in one family who developed malignant lymphoma of the small intestine. *0073*

203.00 Multiple Myeloma The amount of normal immunoglobulin is usually low, but does not correlate with the increased concentration of anomalous protein. *2538*

204.10 Lymphocytic Leukemia (Chronic) All classes of immunoglobulins tend to be reduced either early in the course or later as marrow, spleen, and liver infiltration develops. *2006 2538 2552*

242.90 Hyperthyroidism Possibly due to LATS effect. *2104*

273.23 Heavy Chain Disease (Gamma) Marked decrease in IgG, IgA, and IgM. *2468*

277.30 Amyloidosis Mean serum concentration of all 3 classes of immunoglobulins, IgA, IgM and IgG, were significantly reduced in patients with increased Bence-Jones protein excretion. *0124*

279.04 Agammaglobulinemia (Congenital Sex-linked) All classes are deficient, including the secretory immunoglobulins. *2552*

279.06 Immunodeficiency (Common Variable) IgG primarily deficient, but other immunoglobulins may also be low. *2552 2539*

283.00 Acquired Hemolytic Anemia (Autoimmune) Immunoglobulin deficiency, in the form of generalized hypogammaglobulinemia or selective deficiency of one immunoglobulin, has been observed in a minority of patients, with or without associated lymphoproliferative disease. *2035*

334.80 Ataxia-Telangiectasia Deficiency appears to contribute to the frequent severe infections associated with the syndrome. *2104*

581.90 Nephrotic Syndrome Usually more pronounced in children, averaging about 0.2 g/dL, which explains the high susceptibility to infection. *2104*

642.40 Pre-Eclampsia Decreased; may predispose to infection, especially urinary tract infections. *2286 2287 0387*

642.60 Eclampsia Predisposes patients to infections, especially urinary tract infections. *2286 2287 0387*

650.00 Pregnancy Diminish during gestation and reach lowest levels in early postpartum period. *2104*

Serum Increase

23.00 Brucellosis Antibodies elicited early in natural infection are predominantly IgM, with lesser quantities of IgG. As the disease progresses, IgM declines, and IgG increases, reaching its height at the period of maximum resistance to reinfection. *2035*

78.50 Cytomegalic Inclusion Disease Normal to increased. *1676*

84.00 Malaria Despite the considerably increased concentration of immunoglobulins in infected individuals, only 5% of the immune adult IgG combines specifically with P. falciparum antigens. *0426 2035*

86.90 Trypanosomiasis Marked increase of immunoglobulins, particularly IgM, may be explained by the continuous production of antibodies against new variants. *2105 2035*

87.00 Relapsing Fever IgG hyperglobulinemia occurs initially after infection, followed by a rise in IgM. *0151*

99.10 Lymphogranuloma Venereum Often associated with striking elevations. *2104*

128.00 Larva Migrans (Visceralis) Striking elevations often found with Toxocara cati infection. *2104*

135.00 Sarcoidosis Serum IgG is elevated in 50%, IgA in 25%, and IgM in 12.5% of cases. *0151* Consistent increase in 1 or more serum immunoglobulins, noted in 79% of 129 cases studied. IgG and/or IgM are most frequently increased. *0433*

202.80 Non-Hodgkins Lymphoma In a recent survey, 15 of 348 patients (4.6%) with lymphosarcoma and reticulum cell sarcoma had monoclonal serum components. In 10 instances the component was IgM and in 5 IgG. *1618*

260.00 Protein Malnutrition Usually normal or increased despite protein deficiency in kwashiorkor. *2104*

390.00 Rheumatic Fever Increased immunoglobulins, particularly of IgG and IgA, and elevated immune responses to streptococcal cellular and extracellular products. *2035*

571.49 Chronic Active Hepatitis Pronounced reflecting the immunological aberrations. *2035*

Serum Normal

287.00 Allergic Purpura Except for IgA, the immunoglobulins remain normal. *0962*

335.20 Amyotrophic Lateral Sclerosis *0665*

446.00 Polyarteritis-Nodosa Usually within normal limits. *2035*

493.10 Asthma (Intrinsic) In the absence of any immunoglobulin deficiency, the levels of the other immunoglobulins as well as complement are within normal limits. *2035*

555.90 Regional Enteritis or Ileitis Patterns vary widely within a given patient, and most workers report no consistent deviations in the mean levels of the major Ig classes (including IgE) in sera of patients compared with healthy controls. *1313 2035*

556.00 Ulcerative Colitis Patterns vary widely within a given patient, and most workers report no consistent deviations in the mean levels of the major Ig classes (including IgE) in sera of patients compared with healthy controls. *1313 2035*

Urine Increase

199.00 Secondary Malignant Neoplasm (Disseminated) 24 h excretion and renal clearance of free lambda and kappa light chains of immunoglobulins were significantly increased in disseminated carcinoma compared with localized. *1025*

581.90 Nephrotic Syndrome Severe urinary loss. *2104*

CSF Decrease

345.90 Epilepsy *0619 1625*

CSF Increase

47.00 Aseptic Meningitis IgA and IgG increased. *0619*

55.00 Measles *0619*

97.90 Syphilis *0619*

244.90 Hypothyroidism Disproportionate rise in immunoglobulin fraction of CSF protein in myxedema. Rise is not seen in plasma. *2104*

320.90 Meningitis (Bacterial) Early rise in CSF. *0619*

340.00 Multiple Sclerosis *0619*

Immunoglobulins *(continued)*

CSF Increase *(continued)*
710.00 **Systemic Lupus Erythematosus** *2104*

Pleural Effusion Increase
482.90 **Bacterial Pneumonia** Immunoglobulins are present in large amounts forming a series declining from the IgG (70% of serum concentration) to the IgM (50% of serum concentration). *1913*

Indican

Urine Increase
270.02 **Hartnup Disease** Large, but variable amounts excreted, almost entirely as indoxyl sulfate. *2246*

579.00 **Celiac Sprue Disease** *0995*

579.90 **Malabsorption, Cause Unspecified** Found in several malabsorptive states as well as bacterial overgrowth. *0995*

Indirect Fluorescent Antibodies

Serum Increase
6.00 **Amebiasis** *0151*

84.00 **Malaria** Antibody to malarial parasites may be detected by the indirect fluorescent antibody test and by hemagglutination tests. Interpretation of antibody titers in a variety of situations has not been clarified. *0962*

116.00 **Blastomycosis** May be the most useful serodiagnostic technique. *2508*

130.00 **Toxoplasmosis** Detects predominantly IgG toxoplasma antibody. *2035* Marked elevations of antibody to toxoplasmosis. *2538* Titers of 1:256 or higher indicate recent infection, and titers of 1:1024 or higher accompany active disease. *0962* Found to be as reliable as the Sabin-Feldman dye test. *2368*

694.40 **Pemphigus** Numerous studies have confirmed the presence of autoantibodies specific for an intercellular substance of skin and mucosa in serum from patients with active pemphigus. *0642*

Sputum Increase
483.01 **Mycoplasma Pneumoniae** Detects antibodies in the bronchial secretions of patients with mycoplasma infection; sensitive and specific test. *0202*

Indolamine

Urine Decrease
300.40 **Depressive Neurosis** Documented decrease in urinary excretion of catecholamine and indolamine metabolites reported in depressed patients. Not used as a clinical tool at this time. *0433*

Indoleacetic Acid

Urine Increase
270.02 **Hartnup Disease** Urine chromatography shows greatly increased amounts. *2468* Almost all patients have an elevated excretion of indolic acids on some occasion. *2246*

270.10 **Phenylketonuria** *2246*

270.31 **Maple Syrup Urine Disease** *2246*

Insulin

Serum Decrease
227.91 **Pheochromocytoma** Plasma levels are inappropriately low for the simultaneous blood glucose. *0433* May be a decreased glucose tolerance because of suppressed insulin release and catecholamine-induced insulin resistance. *0962*

250.00 **Diabetes Mellitus** A critical amount of insulin secretory reserve distinguishes between 2 qualitatively distinct clinical syndromes: true diabetes mellitus (the development of signs and symptoms of insulin deficiency) and the syndrome of pure resistance to insulin (signs and symptoms of hyperglycemia in the setting of adequate or excessive insulin secretion, frequently with obesity, but without diabetic complication). *2388* Absent in severe diabetes mellitus with ketosis and weight loss. In less severe cases, insulin is frequently present but only at lower glucose concentrations. *2467*

260.00 **Protein Malnutrition** Decreased fasting plasma levels found in both marasmus and kwashiorkor but no significant difference was found between types of severe protein-energy malnutrition. *1955*

271.01 **Von Gierke's Disease** Basal plasma concentrations were found to be 50-60% of normal in 5 older patients with type I. *1418* *2246*

277.00 **Cystic Fibrosis** Both alpha and beta cell function is disrupted resulting in low insulin and glucagon concentration in contrast to diabetes mellitus. *1633*

642.40 **Pre-Eclampsia** Both the fasting plasma insulin and insulin response following glucose injection were lower in patients with severe pre-eclampsia than in those with mild pre-eclampsia or a normal pregnancy. The differences however were not statistically significant. *2183*

994.50 **Exercise** If exercise strenuous. *0763*

Serum Increase
21.00 **Tularemia** *1889 2123*

66.00 **Phlebotomus Fever** Relative hyperinsulinemia was observed in sandfly fever. *2479*

211.60 **Benign Neoplasm of Pancreas** Fasting blood insulin level over 50 μU/mL in presence of low or normal blood glucose level. Intravenous tolbutamide or administration of leucine causes rapid rise to very high levels within a few minutes with rapid return to normal. *2467* Elevated levels of plasma insulin following an overnight fast, as well as increased concentrations of C-peptide or proinsulin, strongly suggest the presence of insulinoma. *0999 0098*

242.90 **Hyperthyroidism** Significantly elevated in 42 untreated patients, mean concentration was 23 ± 13 μU/mL. *0056*

250.00 **Diabetes Mellitus** Increased in mild cases of untreated obese diabetics; fasting level is often increased. *2467*

251.20 **Hypoglycemia, Unspecified** Increased in reactive hypoglycemia after glucose ingestion, particularly when a diabetic type of glucose tolerance curve is present. *2467*

252.00 **Hyperparathyroidism** Fasting concentrations and response were significantly increased in primary disease. *1265*

253.00 **Acromegaly** Large amounts of growth hormone have a diabetogenic effect. As a result, the basal plasma insulin values may be higher than normal, and their insulin response to a glucose load may be increased. *0962*

255.00 **Adrenal Cortical Hyperfunction (Glucocorticoid Excess)** *0619*

272.10 **Type IV Hyperlipoproteinemia** Occurs in most patients but not with sufficient constancy to indicate a role in causing the disorder. *2246*

278.00 **Obesity** Degree of obesity correlates with the level of insulin elevation. *0996*

359.21 **Myotonia Atrophica** Found in 7 of 7 patients. *1029* 80% of patients had insulin values > 2 S.D. above the normal mean during oral glucose tolerance test and 42% had high fasting plasma values. *0114* In response to glucose load, in myotonic dystrophy. *2246*

401.10 **Essential Benign Hypertension** Significant increase in glucose and insulin response to a 75 gram oral glucose *2017*

571.20 **Laennec's or Alcoholic Cirrhosis** The majority of cirrhotics demonstrated increased levels of circulating insulin due to decreased hormonal catabolism. *1178*

571.90 **Cirrhosis of Liver** The majority of cirrhotics demonstrated increased levels of circulating insulin due to decreased hormonal catabolism. *1178*

585.00 **Chronic Renal Failure** Increased basal immunoreactive insulin levels in chronic uremia may be due to prolonged half-life. *0098 1108*

650.00 **Pregnancy** Excess of circulating insulin in the fasting state. *0811*

Serum   Normal

251.20 Hypoglycemia, Unspecified   Normal in hypoglycemia associated with nonpancreatic tumors. Normal in idiopathic hypoglycemia of childhood except after administration of leucine. *2467*

994.50 Exercise   No effect if of short or moderate duration. *0763*

Blood   Increase

38.00 Septicemia   Fasting hyperglycemia, impaired glucose tolerance, and relative hyperinsulinemia are found. *1889 2123*

Urine   Increase

585.00 Chronic Renal Failure   Markedly elevated. *1445*

Insulin Tolerance

Serum   Decrease

211.60 Benign Neoplasm of Pancreas   An excessive fall in the blood sugar may occur in pancreatic islet cell hyperplasia. *0619*

253.00 Acromegaly   The blood sugar falls by < 25% of its initial value and rapidly returns to the fasting level. *0619*

271.01 Von Gierke's Disease   Increased insulin sensitivity may result in an excessive fall in the blood sugar in some cases. *0619*

Serum   Increase

255.00 Adrenal Cortical Hyperfunction (Glucocorticoid Excess)   The blood sugar falls by < 25% of its initial value and rapidly returns to the fasting level. *0619   2468*

Inulin Clearance

Urine   Decrease

274.00 Gout   Below 90 mL/min in 33% of patients. *0447*   The lowest values are found in older patients or those with hypertension. *0943*

275.10 Hepatolenticular Degeneration   Reduced clearance in 8 of 9 patients; although none had elevated BUN. *0143*

405.91 Renovascular Hypertension   Renal functional impairment. *0962*

710.00 Systemic Lupus Erythematosus   A mean decrease of 14% was observed in 7 female patients. *1269*

Urine   Increase

1013.01 Diet (High Sodium)   There was a tendency for body weight, serum sodium, exchangeable sodium, and inulin clearance to increase with increase in dietary salt. *1274*

Iodide

Serum   Decrease

244.90 Hypothyroidism   The degree of iodine deficiency dictates the severity of the hypothyroidism. *0999*

Urine   Decrease

240.00 Simple Goiter   *0151*

Iron

Serum   Decrease

2.00 Typhoid Fever   Both serum iron and zinc concentrations became significantly depressed in experimentally infected volunteers. *1795*

38.00 Septicemia   Decreased with acute and chronic infection. Frequently develops within of onset. *0619*

40.20 Whipple's Disease   Microcytic, hypochromic red cells and a low serum iron accompany the anemia. *2199   0995*

84.00 Malaria   Decreased cellular iron incorporation found in all cases during parasitemia. *2240*

115.00 Histoplasmosis   Usually an iron deficient normochromic normocytic anemia. *2199*

126.90 Ancylostomiasis (Hookworm Infestation)   Anemia occurring in hookworm disease is a classic iron deficiency anemia. *2199   0151*

127.20 Strongyloidiasis   Anemia, when it occurs, is usually iron deficiency in type. *2199*

151.90 Malignant Neoplasm of Stomach   Repeated small blood losses and consequent iron deficiency fully explain the anemia in most cases of gastric carcinoma. The anemia is of the hypochromic, microcytic type with other features of chronic iron deficiency. *0962*   Chronic occult blood loss. *2199*

152.90 Malignant Neoplasm of Small Intestine   Anemia is common iron deficiency type, due to chronic blood loss. *2199*

153.90 Malignant Neoplasm of Large Intestine   Iron deficiency anemia is common, because of either gross or occult bleeding. *2199*   In 57% of 19 patients at initial hospitalization for this disorder. *0781*

154.10 Malignant Neoplasm of Rectum   Iron deficiency anemia is common, because of either gross or occult bleeding. *2199*

174.90 Malignant Neoplasm of Breast   In 37% of 13 patients at initial hospitalization for this disorder. *0781*

189.00 Malignant Neoplasm of Kidney   Found in 30% of patients. *0836*

197.00 Secondary Malignant Neoplasm of Respiratory System   In 55% of 43 patients at initial hospitalization for this disorder. *0781*

201.90 Hodgkin's Disease   In 77% of 18 patients at initial hospitalization for this disorder. *0781*   Hypoferremia is characteristic and may be associated with excessive uptake of iron by the liver and spleen. *2538   0151 0592*

202.80 Non-Hodgkins Lymphoma   In 58% of 22 patients at initial hospitalization for this disorder. *0781*

211.10 Benign Neoplasm of Stomach   With occult bleeding, iron deficiency anemia may be present. *2199*

238.40 Polycythemia Vera   Frequently decreased, reflecting therapeutic or spontaneous blood loss. *2538*

244.90 Hypothyroidism   The most frequent type of anemia observed is a microcytic, hypochromic anemia caused by iron deficiency. *2538 1351*   Of 202 patients, anemia was present on diagnosis in 39 of 172 women and 14 of 30 men. *1078*   Concentration was < 50 μg/dL. *0532*   Low in 50% of patients. *1078 0582*

260.00 Protein Malnutrition   With kwashiorkor. *2468*   Usually low because of decreased transferrin concentration or actual iron deficiency. *2538*

267.00 Vitamin C Deficiency   Dietary iron deficiency is common. *2538*

272.72 Gaucher's Disease   Iron is diverted from the plasma and stored within Gaucher cells. *1434*

280.90 Iron Deficiency Anemia   Nearly all patients will have serum values < 50 μg/dL. *0433*   As deficiency intensifies, serum concentration falls. *0999*   Usually < 80 μg/dL, associated with a total plasma iron-binding capacity of > 400 μg/dL. *0151*   In well-developed deficiency often below 30 μg/dL. *0962*   Reduced to an average of 28 μg/dL in adults. *0117   2538*

283.21 Paroxysmal Nocturnal Hemoglobinuria   A remarkable amount is often lost in the urine, even in the absence of observable hemoglobinuria. *2538*

289.00 Polycythemia, Secondary   *0151*

410.90 Acute Myocardial Infarction   *2538 0975*

421.00 Bacterial Endocarditis   *2467*

425.40 Cardiomyopathies   Occasionally low. *1108*

446.20 Goodpasture's Syndrome   Secondary to prolonged pulmonary bleeding. *0062*

516.10 Idiopathic Pulmonary Hemosiderosis   Peripheral blood displays the classic changes of severe iron depletion: anisocytosis, poikilocytosis, microcytosis, and hypochromia. *2538*

533.90 Peptic Ulcer, Site Unspecified   An ulcer that bleeds chronically will cause a varying degree of iron deficiency anemia. *0962*

555.90 Regional Enteritis or Ileitis   Iron deficiency is common. *0962*   As a result of chronic blood loss. *2199*   Iron deficiency anemia was found in 36% of 41 patients with ulcerative colitis, and 22% of 64 patients with Crohn's disease. An additional 32% and 2%, respectively, had iron deficiency with normal erythropoiesis. *2351*

556.00 Ulcerative Colitis   Iron deficiency defined by the absence of marrow hemosiderin was found with anemia in 36% of 41 patients. An additional 32% had iron deficiency with normal erythropoiesis. *2351*   Commonly iron deficient. *2199*

562.00 Diverticular Disease of Intestine   Some cases. *2199*

562.11 Diverticulitis of Colon   Some cases. *2199*

Iron (continued)

Serum Decrease (continued)

564.20 Postgastrectomy (Dumping) Syndrome Iron deficiency and vitamin B_{12} deficiency are common following subtotal gastrectomy. *0962*

571.90 Cirrhosis of Liver In 28% of 21 patients at initial hospitalization for this disorder. *0781*

579.00 Celiac Sprue Disease Characteristic iron-deficiency anemia. In some cases, may be the predominant abnormality indicative of malabsorption. *0433* Very common, because the duodenal lesion usually impairs iron absorption in the untreated patient. *2199*

579.90 Malabsorption, Cause Unspecified *0151*

581.90 Nephrotic Syndrome Probably related to loss of specific iron binding serum globulin in the urine. *0619*

585.00 Chronic Renal Failure Normal in mild cases, but with severe failure, both hypo- and hyperferremia have been observed. *0643 0732 2552*

650.00 Pregnancy Progressive fall from midterm onwards, with rising total iron binding capacity. *0619* Anemia is most often caused or aggravated by a concomitant iron deficiency. *2538 0165* Reduced at term to about 35% below the mean in nonpregnant women. *1629*

706.10 Acne Found in 75% of patients with severe nodulocystic disease. *1387*

714.00 Rheumatoid Arthritis Serum iron < 50 $\mu g/dL$. *0532* Seen frequently, often as a result of gastrointestinal blood loss. *0999*

714.30 Juvenile Rheumatoid Arthritis *0136*

994.50 Exercise Response to stress of exercise. *0342*

Serum Increase

70.00 Viral Hepatitis Increase becomes evident only after liver disease has been present for 2-3 weeks. *0153*

204.00 Lymphocytic Leukemia (Acute) Increased in acute leukemias. *0619*

205.00 Myelocytic Leukemia (Acute) Increased in acute leukemias. *0619*

206.00 Monocytic Leukemia Increased in acute leukemias. *0619*

275.00 Hemochromatosis Diagnosis established when concentration > 220 $\mu g/dL$. *0999* Increased serum and hepatic iron concentration. *1850* Average level is 250 $\mu g/dL$, with a range of from 225-325 $\mu g/dL$. *2538* In the absence of infection, inflammation, neoplasia, or recent blood loss, concentrations usually range from 175-275 $\mu g/dL$. *2246 2612*

277.00 Cystic Fibrosis Intestinal absorption. *0338*

277.14 Acute Intermittent Porphyria Frequently markedly elevated. *0433*

277.15 Porphyria Variegata Frequently markedly elevated. *0433*

277.16 Porphyria Cutanea Tarda Often increased. *2552 2389*

277.17 Hereditary Coproporphyria Frequently markedly elevated. *0433*

281.00 Pernicious Anemia Moderately increased unless there is associated iron deficiency. *0366*

281.20 Folic Acid Deficiency Anemia Slightly to moderately increased. *2538* Moderately increased unless there is associated iron deficiency. *0366*

281.30 Vitamin B_6 Deficiency Anemia Increased with pyridoxine-responsive anemia. *2467* Increased serum iron and reduced iron-binding capacity in $> 50\%$ of cases. *0532*

282.00 Hereditary (Congenital) Spherocytosis May occur. *2552* Due to increased rate of blood destruction. *0619*

282.20 Anemias Due To Disorders of Glutathione Metabolism Elevated serum iron and transferrin saturation. Indirect laboratory evidence that hemolysis is present. *0433*

282.41 Thalassemia Major Serum concentration is elevated with increased saturation of iron-binding protein. *0151* In 42 patients (age 3 mo. to 22 y.) with homozygous beta-thalassemia and thalassemia intermedia, serum zinc was significantly decreased while Cu and Fe were increased. *0072* In contrast to the thin cells of iron deficiency, the serum iron is normal or increased. *0962 0349*

282.42 Thalassemia Minor Hypochromic microcytic anemia in these patients can be distinguished from iron deficiency anemia by a normal or even elevated serum iron concentration and by the failure of the anemia to respond to iron. *0999* In 42 patients (age 3 mo-22 y) with homozygous beta-thalassemia and thalassemia intermedia serum zinc was significantly decreased while Cu and Fe were increased. *0072 0995*

284.90 Aplastic Anemia Often > 200 $\mu g/dL$ with 100% saturation of the iron-binding capacity. Decreased number of normal marrow cells. *0433* Increased with an almost complete saturation of iron-binding capacity. May be the first sign of erythroid suppression and is of considerable screening value in patients receiving potentially toxic drugs. *2538*

285.00 Sideroblastic Anemia Characteristically normal to elevated. *0433* Increased with primary inherited sex-linked sideroblastic anemia. *0619* Increased serum iron and reduced iron-binding capacity in $> 50\%$ of cases. *0532 0151*

446.00 Polyarteritis-Nodosa Anemia may be due to chronic blood loss. *0642 0962*

570.00 Acute and Subacute Necrosis of Liver The degree of increase parallels the amount of hepatic necrosis. *2467* In acute hepatitis the serum iron level is increased, presumably due to the liberation of stored iron from necrosing liver cells. *0619* High serum concentrations, more than can be explained by high ferritin levels are found in acute hepatitis. *2624*

571.20 Laennec's or Alcoholic Cirrhosis Presumably due to the liberation of stored iron from necrosing liver cells. *0619*

581.90 Nephrotic Syndrome *0619*

585.00 Chronic Renal Failure Normal in mild cases, but with severe failure, both hypo- and hyperferremia have been observed. *0643 0732 2552*

758.00 Down's Syndrome Patients with anicteric hepatitis whose serum contained hepatitis-B surface antigen, had lower levels than controls. *0153*

984.00 Toxic Effects of Lead and Its Compounds (including Fumes) With hemolysis. *0618*

Serum Normal

272.52 Abetalipoproteinemia *2501*

277.12 Erythropoietic Protoporphyria *2538*

280.90 Iron Deficiency Anemia Usually low in untreated anemia; however, it may be normal. *0656* Mild deficiency is often accompanied by a normal level, and sometimes the deficiency may be symptomatic without measurably depressing the level. *0962 2538*

281.30 Vitamin B_6 Deficiency Anemia Characteristically normal to elevated. *0433*

282.42 Thalassemia Minor *0995*

285.00 Sideroblastic Anemia Characteristically normal to elevated. *0433*

289.00 Polycythemia, Secondary Usually. *1917*

516.10 Idiopathic Pulmonary Hemosiderosis Hypochromic microcytic anemia due to pulmonary hemorrhages with normal serum iron and iron-binding capacity. *2467*

Urine Increase

283.00 Acquired Hemolytic Anemia (Autoimmune) Hemosiderinuria and increased urinary iron excretion indicate recent hemoglobinemia. May occur several days after an acute intravascular hemolytic episode and persist for some time. *0964 2552*

283.21 Paroxysmal Nocturnal Hemoglobinuria The excretion of iron in the urine continues between hemolytic episodes and is a simple and valuable indication of chronic hemoglobinuria. *0433* A remarkable amount is often lost in the urine, even in the absence of observable hemoglobinuria. *2538*

CSF Normal

332.00 Parkinsons's Disease *1763*

Bone Marrow Decrease

211.10 Benign Neoplasm of Stomach With occult bleeding, iron deficiency anemia may be present, in which case the bone marrow will not contain iron. *2199*

238.40 Polycythemia Vera Decreased or absent bone marrow iron stores that are characteristic of this disease. *2538 0657*

280.90 **Iron Deficiency Anemia** Depleted of stainable iron. *2538* Reticuloendothelial stores are severely reduced or absent in marrow and liver. *0117 2552* The amount is not as important diagnostically as presence or absence. The presence is strong evidence against the diagnosis of clinically significant iron deficiency. *0962*

283.21 **Paroxysmal Nocturnal Hemoglobinuria** Often absent. *2538*

555.90 **Regional Enteritis or Ileitis** Iron deficiency defined by the absence of marrow hemosiderin was found with anemia in 36% of 41 patients with ulcerative colitis, and 22% of 64 with Crohn's disease. An additional 32% and 2%, respectively, had iron deficiency with normal erythropoiesis. *2351* As a result of chronic blood loss. *2199*

556.00 **Ulcerative Colitis** Iron deficiency defined by the absence of marrow hemosiderin was found with anemia in 36% of 41 patients. An additional 32% had iron deficiency with normal erythropoiesis. *2351*

Bone Marrow   Increase

277.16 **Porphyria Cutanea Tarda** General increase in body iron stores, in liver, marrow and plasma. *2389*

281.00 **Pernicious Anemia** Marrow sideroblasts and reticuloendothelial stores tend to be increased. *2552*

281.20 **Folic Acid Deficiency Anemia** Marrow sideroblasts and reticuloendothelial stores tend to be increased. *2552*

281.30 **Vitamin B$_6$ Deficiency Anemia** Bone marrow is hyperplastic and contains increased amounts of normoblastic iron, often forming ringed sideroblasts. *2538* Increased in the marrow fragments and in the developing erythroblasts. *0151*

282.31 **Hereditary Nonspherocytic Hemolytic Anemia** Marrow iron content is normal to increased. *0433*

282.41 **Thalassemia Major** Abundance of iron in the reticuloendothelial cells. *2552*

285.00 **Sideroblastic Anemia** Increased in the marrow fragments and in the developing erythroblasts. *0151* Bone marrow is hyperplastic and contains increased amounts of normoblastic iron, often forming ringed sideroblasts. *2538*

303.00 **Acute Alcoholic Intoxication** Iron overload shown by plasma cells containing iron in bone marrow may occur. *1594*

303.90 **Alcoholism** Iron overload shown by plasma cells containing iron in bone marrow may occur. *1594*

Liver   Decrease

280.90 **Iron Deficiency Anemia** Reticuloendothelial stores are severely reduced or absent in marrow and liver. *0117 2552*

Liver   Increase

275.00 **Hemochromatosis** Increased serum and hepatic iron concentrations. *1850* Increased iron deposition principally in the parenchymal cells of the liver. *0962* Large amounts of stainable iron, predominantly within the parenchymal cells. *2612*

277.16 **Porphyria Cutanea Tarda** General increase in body iron stores, in liver, marrow and plasma. *2389*

571.20 **Laennec's or Alcoholic Cirrhosis** Iron deposition in the liver is common. *0962*

Iron-Binding Capacity, Total (TIBC)

Serum   Decrease

38.00 **Septicemia** Acute and chronic infections. The serum iron falls proportionately more than the transferrin content. *0619*

84.00 **Malaria** Decreased significantly in 11 patients with untreated malaria for more than 4 days. *2066*

153.90 **Malignant Neoplasm of Large Intestine** Significantly reduced (median = 2.6 mg/L) compared to controls (3.4 mg/L). 24 h excretion and renal clearance of transferrin were significantly increased in localized tumor patients compared to normals and disseminated cancer cases. Increased high molecular weight protein excretion implies glomerular injury in these patients. *1025* In 10% of 19 patients at initial hospitalization for this disorder. *0781*

162.90 **Malignant Neoplasm of Bronchus and Lung** Significantly reduced (median = 2.6 mg/L), compared to controls (3.4 mg/L). 24 h excretion and renal clearance were significantly increased in localized tumor patients compared to normals and disseminated cancer cases. Increased high molecular weight protein excretion implies glomerular injury in these patients. *1025*

174.90 **Malignant Neoplasm of Breast** Significantly reduced (median = 2.6 mg/L) compared to controls (3.4 mg/L). 24 h excretion and renal clearance were significantly increased in localized tumor patients compared to normal and disseminated cancer cases. Increased high molecular weight protein excretion implies glomerular injury in these patients. *1025* In 21% of 14 patients at initial hospitalization for this disorder. *0781*

182.00 **Malignant Neoplasm of Corpus Uteri** Significantly reduced (median = 2.6 mg/L) compared to controls (3.4 mg/L). Significantly increased in localized tumor patients compared to normals and disseminated cancer cases. Increased high molecular weight protein excretion implies glomerular injury in these patients. *1025*

189.00 **Malignant Neoplasm of Kidney** Found in 30% of patients. *0836*

197.00 **Secondary Malignant Neoplasm of Respiratory System** In 39% of 43 patients at initial hospitalization for this disorder. *0781*

199.00 **Secondary Malignant Neoplasm (Disseminated)** Low serum iron binding capacity (total) due to carcinomatosis. *0619*

201.90 **Hodgkin's Disease** In 32% of 18 patients at initial hospitalization for this disorder. *0781   0151 0592*

202.80 **Non-Hodgkins Lymphoma** In 36% of 22 patients at initial hospitalization for this disorder. *0781*

244.90 **Hypothyroidism** Total IBC < 200-300 μg/dL. *0532*

260.00 **Protein Malnutrition** Albumin, prealbumin and transferrin concentrations were found to be low in cases of protein-energy malnutrition associated with preschool children. *2065*

267.00 **Vitamin C Deficiency** In scurvy. *0619*

275.00 **Hemochromatosis** Reduced transferrin as shown by a low TIBC. *2612* Occurs early in the course of the disease. *1850* Usually < 300 μg/dL. *2246*

280.90 **Iron Deficiency Anemia** Often increased, but may be normal or low. *2552* Mean = 346 μg/dL, ranging from 170-460. Patients with reduced capacity also have hypoalbuminemia. *0117*

281.00 **Pernicious Anemia** In relapse. *0619* Total plasma capacity tends to be slightly reduced. *2552*

281.20 **Folic Acid Deficiency Anemia** Total plasma capacity tends to be slightly reduced. *2552*

281.30 **Vitamin B$_6$ Deficiency Anemia** Somewhat decreased with pyridoxine-responsive anemia. *2467* Normal to low. *0433* Associated increased serum iron and reduced iron-binding capacity in > 50% of cases. *0532*

284.90 **Aplastic Anemia** Serum iron concentration is elevated and total capacity is reduced. *0151*

285.00 **Sideroblastic Anemia** Normal to low. *0433* Associated increased serum iron and reduced iron-binding capacity in > 50% of cases. *0532* Somewhat decreased with pyridoxine-responsive anemia. *2467*

287.30 **Idiopathic Thrombocytopenic Purpura** Anemia from blood loss may be present. *2538*

345.90 **Epilepsy** Mean concentration was 123.66 ± 8.31 μg/dL in grand mal epileptic patients. *1625*

446.60 **Thrombotic Thrombocytopenic Purpura** Anemia from blood loss may be present. *2538*

571.20 **Laennec's or Alcoholic Cirrhosis** Significantly reduced. *1654   2612*

571.60 **Biliary Cirrhosis** In hepatic cirrhosis. *2612*

571.90 **Cirrhosis of Liver** The only protein to be significantly reduced. *1654* In 51% of 21 patients at initial hospitalization for this disorder. *0781   2612*

580.02 **Glomerulonephritis (Minimal Change)** Decreased as a result of heavy protein loss to the urine, especially low molecular weight proteins, such as albumin and transferrin. *0151*

581.90 **Nephrotic Syndrome** Excessive loss of protein-bound iron with low total IBC. *0619   0995*

585.00 **Chronic Renal Failure** Low in both mild and severe renal failure, with the lowest levels found in patients with poor nutritional state. *1734* In 64% of 17 patients at initial hospitalization for this disorder. *0781*

714.00 **Rheumatoid Arthritis** Low; rises with successful steroid therapy. *0619* Total IBC < 200-300 μg/dL. *0532*

714.30 **Juvenile Rheumatoid Arthritis** *0136*

758.00 **Down's Syndrome** Patients with anicteric hepatitis whose serum contained HBsAg, had lower levels than controls. *0153*

Iron-Binding Capacity, Total (TIBC)
(continued)

Serum   Increase

40.20   Whipple's Disease   Iron deficiency anemia is common. *2199*

70.00   Viral Hepatitis   Increases are rare other than in iron deficiency, but they may occur in viral hepatitis. *0962*   May be increased with hepatitis. *2467*

126.90   Ancylostomiasis (Hookworm Infestation)   Classic iron deficiency anemia. *2199*

127.20   Strongyloidiasis   Classic iron deficiency anemia. *2199*

151.90   Malignant Neoplasm of Stomach   Anemia is commonly iron deficient type, due to chronic blood loss. *2199*

152.90   Malignant Neoplasm of Small Intestine   Anemia is common iron deficiency type, due to chronic blood loss. *2199*

154.10   Malignant Neoplasm of Rectum   Anemia is commonly iron deficient, due to chronic blood loss. *2199*

188.90   Malignant Neoplasm of Bladder   Secondary iron deficiency anemia may develop. *0433*

189.00   Malignant Neoplasm of Kidney   Anemia due mainly to urinary blood loss. *0894 1391*

211.10   Benign Neoplasm of Stomach   Anemia is commonly iron deficient type, due to chronic blood loss. *2199*

244.90   Hypothyroidism   The serum iron concentration was < 12 μmol/L (units) in 60 out of 118 patients. The TIBC was increased in only 21 of these 60 patients. *1078*

280.90   Iron Deficiency Anemia   In well-developed iron deficiency, the percentage of saturation of transferrin is usually very low, 16%. Low saturation from other causes is rare. *0962*   Often increased, but may be normal or low. *2552*   Mean = 346 μg/dL, ranging from 170-460. Patients with reduced capacity also have hypoalbuminemia. *0117   2538*

282.00   Hereditary (Congenital) Spherocytosis   Hemolytic anemia, with raised serum iron concentration (i.e., the total transferrin concentration is increased, but the unsaturated iron binding capacity is reduced). *0619*

282.41   Thalassemia Major   Total capacity is increased. *2468*

282.42   Thalassemia Minor   Total capacity is increased. *2468*

286.01   Hemophilia   Depending upon the severity and frequency of bleeding. *2552*

287.00   Allergic Purpura   Anemia from blood loss may be present. *2538*

446.00   Polyarteritis-Nodosa   Anemia may be due to chronic blood loss. *0642 0962*

446.20   Goodpasture's Syndrome   Secondary to prolonged pulmonary bleeding. *0062*

516.10   Idiopathic Pulmonary Hemosiderosis   *2538*

533.90   Peptic Ulcer, Site Unspecified   An ulcer that bleeds chronically will cause a varying degree of iron deficiency anemia. *0962*

535.00   Gastritis   Anemia may be due to chronic blood loss. *0642 0962*

555.90   Regional Enteritis or Ileitis   Frequent iron deficiency anemia. Severity depends upon rate and duration of bleeding. *2199*

556.00   Ulcerative Colitis   Frequent iron deficiency anemia. Severity depends upon rate and duration of bleeding. *2199*

562.00   Diverticular Disease of Intestine   Some cases. *2199*

562.11   Diverticulitis of Colon   Some cases. *2199*

570.00   Acute and Subacute Necrosis of Liver   May be increased with hepatitis. *2467*

571.49   Chronic Active Hepatitis   Alpha$_2$ glycoproteins, ceruloplasmin and transferrin were elevated. *1654*

579.00   Celiac Sprue Disease   Characteristic iron deficiency anemia. *0433*

579.90   Malabsorption, Cause Unspecified   *0151*

650.00   Pregnancy   In late pregnancy. *2612*   In normal pregnancy, the total IBC rises to about 450 μg/dL, while the serum iron falls. *0619*

Serum   Normal

273.30   Waldenström's Macroglobulinemia   *2467*

273.80   Analbuminemia   *2467*

275.00   Hemochromatosis   *0995*

279.04   Agammaglobulinemia (Congenital Sex-linked)   *2467*

281.30   Vitamin B$_6$ Deficiency Anemia   Normal to low. *0433*

285.00   Sideroblastic Anemia   Normal to low. *0433*

289.00   Polycythemia, Secondary   Usually. *1917*

496.01   Alpha$_1$-Antitrypsin Deficiency   *2467*

516.10   Idiopathic Pulmonary Hemosiderosis   Hypochromic microcytic anemia due to pulmonary hemorrhages with normal serum iron and iron-binding capacity. *2467*

706.10   Acne   Normal levels in 29 patients with severe nodulocystic disease. *1387*

Iron Crystals

Urine   Increase

280.90   Iron Deficiency Anemia   If the spun sediment of the morning's first-voided specimen is stained for iron, it may frequently be seen to contain hemosiderin crystals. *0433*

Iron Saturation

Serum   Decrease

40.20   Whipple's Disease   Iron deficiency anemia is common. *2199*

126.90   Ancylostomiasis (Hookworm Infestation)   Classic iron deficiency anemia. *2199*

127.20   Strongyloidiasis   Classic iron deficiency anemia. *2199*

151.90   Malignant Neoplasm of Stomach   Anemia is commonly iron deficiency type, due to chronic blood loss. *2199*

152.90   Malignant Neoplasm of Small Intestine   Anemia is commonly iron deficient type, due to chronic blood loss. *2199*

153.90   Malignant Neoplasm of Large Intestine   In 67% of 19 patients at initial hospitalization for this disorder. *0781*

154.10   Malignant Neoplasm of Rectum   Anemia is commonly iron deficient type, due to chronic blood loss. *2199*

174.90   Malignant Neoplasm of Breast   In 35% of 14 patients at initial hospitalization for this disorder. *0781*

188.90   Malignant Neoplasm of Bladder   Secondary iron deficiency anemia may develop. *0433*

189.00   Malignant Neoplasm of Kidney   Anemia due mainly to urinary blood loss. *0894 1391*

197.00   Secondary Malignant Neoplasm of Respiratory System   In 59% of 43 patients at initial hospitalization for this disorder. *0781*

199.00   Secondary Malignant Neoplasm (Disseminated)   Serum concentration of albumin and transferrin were significantly reduced while haptoglobin was increased in disseminated carcinoma compared with localized. *1025*

201.90   Hodgkin's Disease   In 94% of 18 patients at initial hospitalization for this disorder. *0781*

202.80   Non-Hodgkins Lymphoma   Anemia due to blood loss may occur. *2538*   In 67% of 22 patients at initial hospitalization for this disorder. *0781*

211.10   Benign Neoplasm of Stomach   Anemia is commonly iron deficient type, due to chronic blood loss. *2199*

244.90   Hypothyroidism   Transferrin saturation < 20%. *0532*

280.90   Iron Deficiency Anemia   Transferrin saturation is almost always under 15% and, in severe deficiency, under 10%. *0999*   Saturation of 15% or less is often found. *2538*   16% and averages 7%. *2552*   In well-developed iron deficiency, the percentage of saturation of transferrin is usually very low, < 16. Low saturation from other causes is rare. *0962*   In 92% of 15 patients at initial hospitalization for this disorder. *0781*

286.01   Hemophilia   Depending upon the severity and frequency of bleeding. *2552*

287.00   Allergic Purpura   Anemia from blood loss may be present. *2538*

446.00   Polyarteritis-Nodosa   Anemia may be due to chronic blood loss. *0642 0962*

446.20   Goodpasture's Syndrome   Secondary to prolonged pulmonary bleeding. *0062*

533.90   Peptic Ulcer, Site Unspecified   An ulcer that bleeds chronically will cause a varying degree of iron deficiency anemia. *0962*

535.00   Gastritis   Anemia may be due to chronic blood loss. *0642 0962*

555.90 **Regional Enteritis or Ileitis** Frequent iron deficiency anemia. Severity depends upon rate and duration of bleeding. *2199*

556.00 **Ulcerative Colitis** Frequent iron deficiency anemia. Severity depends upon rate and duration of bleeding. *2199*

579.00 **Celiac Sprue Disease** Characteristic iron deficiency anemia. *0433*

642.40 **Pre-Eclampsia** Found to be significantly lower than in normal pregnant women. *2286*

706.10 **Acne** 11 of 24 patients with severe nodulocystic disease had decreased levels. *1387*

710.00 **Systemic Lupus Erythematosus** *2467*

714.00 **Rheumatoid Arthritis** Transferrin saturation < 20%. *0532 2467*

Serum Increase

275.00 **Hemochromatosis** Usually > 80% and often 100%. *2612* Usually 75%. *2246 2538*

277.16 **Porphyria Cutanea Tarda** Over 70% saturation in 4 of 20 patients. *0670*

281.30 **Vitamin B$_6$ Deficiency Anemia** Invariably increased saturation. *2552*

282.20 **Anemias Due To Disorders of Glutathione Metabolism** Elevated serum iron and transferrin saturation. Indirect laboratory evidence that hemolysis is present. *0433* May be completely saturated. *2552*

282.41 **Thalassemia Major** Serum concentration is elevated with increased saturation of iron-binding protein. *0151* Often totally saturated. *2208*

282.42 **Thalassemia Minor** *0186*

284.90 **Aplastic Anemia** Percent saturation of transferrin is increased. *0999* Almost 100% saturation. *2538*

285.00 **Sideroblastic Anemia** High degree of saturation. *2538*

287.30 **Idiopathic Thrombocytopenic Purpura** Anemia from blood loss may be present. *2538*

446.60 **Thrombotic Thrombocytopenic Purpura** Anemia from blood loss may be present. *2538*

571.20 **Laennec's or Alcoholic Cirrhosis** Moderate to marked rise in percent saturation in hepatic cirrhosis. *2612*

571.60 **Biliary Cirrhosis** Moderate to marked rise in percent saturation in hepatic cirrhosis. *2612*

571.90 **Cirrhosis of Liver** Moderate to marked rise in percent saturation in hepatic cirrhosis. *2612*

650.00 **Pregnancy** Increased in 49% in late normal pregnancy. *2286 2287* Increased saturation in early pregnancy. *2612*

994.50 **Exercise** Raised at 15 min, normal within 1 day. *0985* Approximately 10% increase immediately after exercise. *1837*

Serum Normal

642.40 **Pre-Eclampsia** No change was found compared to normal late pregnancy. *0409*

Isocitrate Dehydrogenase

Serum Increase

70.00 **Viral Hepatitis** Usually elevated in the early stage (5-10 X normal) but returns to normal in 2-3 weeks. *2467* 40 X normal. *0503* Invariably elevated when measured within 10 days of onset of jaundice. *2260*

75.00 **Infectious Mononucleosis** More than 25 U/L, becomes normal in 2-3 weeks. *2467*

157.90 **Malignant Neoplasm of Pancreas** *0619*

197.70 **Secondary Malignant Neoplasm of Liver** Raised in 57% of patients. *2093* Approximately 50% of patients with liver metastases exhibited relatively small elevations. Only those patients with secondary liver involvement had increased concentrations. *2260*

198.30 **Secondary Malignant Neoplasm of Brain** Increased in CSF with secondary cerebral tumors. *0619*

205.00 **Myelocytic Leukemia (Acute)** *0619*

205.10 **Myelocytic Leukemia (Chronic)** *0619*

250.10 **Diabetic Acidosis** In some instances, mostly in severe cases, especially with severe circulatory failure and liver enlargement. *0155*

260.00 **Protein Malnutrition** *0619*

270.42 **Homocystinuria** *0619*

281.00 **Pernicious Anemia** Increased less consistently and to a lesser degree than LD. *2552 0652*

281.20 **Folic Acid Deficiency Anemia** Serum levels 5 X the normal. *0619* In 5 of 9 patients, the plasma level was elevated above the maximum normal limit. *1023* Increased less consistently and to a lesser degree than LD. *0652 2552*

282.60 **Sickle Cell Anemia** Elevated in 15 patients. Values ranged from 1.5-13.0 and the mean was 5.2 (normal = 2.5). *1023*

570.00 **Acute and Subacute Necrosis of Liver** *2467*

571.90 **Cirrhosis of Liver** Normal or slightly increased in 20% of patients. A large increase suggests a poorer prognosis. *2467*

572.00 **Liver Abscess (Pyogenic)** 500-2000 U/L in 1st week; < 800 U/L after 2 weeks; slightly elevated in 3rd week. *2467*

573.30 **Toxic Hepatitis** Hepatitis of liver poisons, normal in 2-3 weeks. *2467*

576.20 **Extrahepatic Biliary Obstruction** 100-500 U/L. *2467*

642.40 **Pre-Eclampsia** Frequently increased indicating placental degeneration within previous 48 h. *0619*

650.00 **Pregnancy** Increased in 3rd trimester. *2468 0491*

985.00 **Toxic Effects of Non-medicinal Metals** Hepatotoxicity may occur with arsenicals. *1446*

Serum Normal

11.00 **Pulmonary Tuberculosis** *2260*

227.91 **Pheochromocytoma** *2260*

242.90 **Hyperthyroidism** *2260*

250.00 **Diabetes Mellitus** *2260*

255.00 **Adrenal Cortical Hyperfunction (Glucocorticoid Excess)** *2260*

277.14 **Acute Intermittent Porphyria** *2260*

279.06 **Immunodeficiency (Common Variable)** *2260*

281.00 **Pernicious Anemia** *2260*

333.40 **Huntington's Chorea** No abnormalities in 8 patients. *0534*

410.90 **Acute Myocardial Infarction** Concentrations were within normal limits in assays performed within 24 h after onset of symptoms. *2260*

480.90 **Viral Pneumonia** *2260*

556.00 **Ulcerative Colitis** *2260*

571.20 **Laennec's or Alcoholic Cirrhosis** Mean serum concentration was normal with portal cirrhosis. *2260*

576.20 **Extrahepatic Biliary Obstruction** Within the normal range in patients with obstruction due to benign or malignant disease. *2260*

577.10 **Chronic Pancreatitis** *2260*

590.10 **Acute Pyelonephritis** *2260*

601.00 **Prostatitis** *2260*

650.00 **Pregnancy** Well within the normal range in term pregnancies. *2559 1561*

714.00 **Rheumatoid Arthritis** *2260*

CSF Increase

191.90 **Malignant Neoplasm of Brain** Increased with primary cerebral tumors. *0619*

320.90 **Meningitis (Bacterial)** *0619*

Red Blood Cells Increase

281.20 **Folic Acid Deficiency Anemia** 6 out of 8 patients had elevated concentration. The highest elevation was 7.3 U/L and the normal upper limit was 2.5 U/L. *1023*

282.60 **Sickle Cell Anemia** Mean RBC concentration was elevated to 2.8 U/L in 15 patients. *1023*

Isoleucine

Serum Decrease

66.00 **Phlebotomus Fever** Most free serum amino acids are depressed in sandfly fever and other mild-moderate infections. *0122*

259.20 **Carcinoid Syndrome** Decreased plasma concentration, but normal urinary excretion was found. *0718*

Isoleucine *(continued)*

Serum   Decrease *(continued)*

333.40   Huntington's Chorea   Reduced fasting plasma concentrations of leucine, isoleucine and valine. *1816*   19 patients showed a significantly lower concentration of proline, aminolevulinic acid, valine, leucine, isoleucine, and tyrosine compared to 38 normal controls. *0534*

572.20   Hepatic Encephalopathy   Branched chain amino acids are generally reduced. *1473*

Serum   Increase

70.00   Viral Hepatitis   A close relationship was found between the onset of encephalopathy and amino acid equilibrium disturbance, characterized by a fall in the molar ratio between valine leucine and isoleucine and phenylalanine and tyrosine. All showed absolute elevations with onset of encephalopathy. *0531*

270.31   Maple Syrup Urine Disease   Excessively high. *1797 2246*

Urine   Increase

270.02   Hartnup Disease   5-20 X normal values. *2246*

270.03   Cystinosis   Nonspecific pattern of aminoaciduria. Fanconi's syndrome. *0995*

270.31   Maple Syrup Urine Disease   Greatly increased. *2468*

275.10   Hepatolenticular Degeneration   *0503*

Ketones

Serum   Increase

71.00   Rabies   Acetone may be present. *0433*

242.90   Hyperthyroidism   Due to increased carbohydrate requirement in thyrotoxicosis. *0619*

250.00   Diabetes Mellitus   Up to 300-400 mg/dL or more. *0619* Increased as a result of disturbed fat and carbohydrate metabolism. *1854*

250.10   Diabetic Acidosis   Initial values range from 11.3-15 mmol/L in several studies. Target ketone concentration was reached in 4-7 h. *1316*   Beta-hydroxybutyrate accumulates and is one of the major causes of acidosis as a result of disturbed carbohydrate and fat metabolism. *1854   0962 0999*

255.00   Adrenal Cortical Hyperfunction (Glucocorticoid Excess) *0619*

260.00   Protein Malnutrition   *0619*

271.01   Von Gierke's Disease   Ketosis is characteristic. *1086* Increased, especially after fasting. *0619*

272.22   Type III Hyperlipoproteinemia   Fasting hyperglycemia and ketosis are uncommon. *2246*

275.34   Familial Periodic Paralysis   Occasional patients. *2246*

787.00   Vomiting   *0619*

992.00   Heat stroke   Increased ketones in blood. Carbohydrate requirement increased with fever. *0619*

994.50   Exercise   Effect marked in untrained individuals only. *1176* Following exercise there is no increase in ketones in trained athletes, whereas there is an increase in untrained subjects. *0619*

Serum   Normal

253.00   Acromegaly   The overt diabetes associated with acromegaly is frequently insulin-resistant and not associated with elevated ketones in the blood or urine. *0962*

Urine   Increase

71.00   Rabies   Acetone may be present. *0433*

242.90   Hyperthyroidism   Children are more liable to develop ketosis than adults with thyrotoxicosis. *0619*

250.00   Diabetes Mellitus   Children are more liable to develop ketosis than adults. *0619*

250.10   Diabetic Acidosis   Accumulates and is one of the major causes of acidosis as a result of disturbed carbohydrate and fat metabolism. *1854   0999 0962*

260.00   Protein Malnutrition   50 mg/dL; more common in children than adults. *0619 2467*

271.01   Von Gierke's Disease   Children are more liable to develop ketosis than adults, especially after fasting. *0619*

482.90   Bacterial Pneumonia   Ketones may occur with severe infection. *2467*

650.00   Pregnancy   *2467*

787.00   Vomiting   Children are more liable to develop ketosis than adults with persistent vomiting. *0619*

992.00   Heat stroke   Children are more liable to develop ketosis than adults with fever. *0619   2467*

1013.00   Diet   High fat diets. *2467*

Kynurenic Acid

Urine   Increase

991.60   Hypothermia   Possibly due to activation of tryptophan oxygenase. *0762*

Lactate Dehydrogenase

Serum   Decrease

990.00   Effects of X-Ray Irradiation   *2467*

Serum   Increase

2.00   Typhoid Fever   Due to complications. *2468*

6.00   Amebiasis   Normal levels returned after complete cure in 92% of cases. Appears to be more useful than antibodies to detect cure or new infection. *1480*

37.00   Tetanus   Elevated above the upper limit of normal in 3 of 5 cases. *1677*

38.00   Septicemia   In 72% of 11 patients at initial hospitalization for this disorder. *0781*

39.90   Actinomycosis   Liver involvement. *1058*

45.90   Acute Poliomyelitis   Mild elevation was recorded in all 8 cases. *1677*

53.00   Herpes Zoster   In 37% of 18 patients at initial hospitalization for this disorder. *0781*

70.00   Viral Hepatitis   Slightly elevated (1-2 fold) values. *0503* 8 of 10 cases showed mild elevation. *1480*   Slight increase. *0962* In 80% of 25 patients at initial hospitalization in this disorder. *0781* Moderate elevation in most cases. *2260*

73.90   Psittacosis   With severe liver involvement. *0433*

75.00   Infectious Mononucleosis   2-4 X normal values. *0503* All 36 patients showed elevated values, which persisted in 50% of the cases for over 4 months after onset of disease. *1658*   Elevations occur in 80-100% during acute illness and return to normal in 3-5 weeks. *2538*   In 80% of 10 patients at initial hospitalization for this disorder. *0781   1089 0962*

78.50   Cytomegalic Inclusion Disease   Slight increase which becomes more marked with clinical hepatitis in some cases. *2468*

99.10   Lymphogranuloma Venereum   May indicate severe liver impairment. *0433*

120.00   Schistosomiasis   Not significantly increased in patients upon the admission, but did increase with nitridazole treatment. LD_4 was the only isoenzyme to elevate and had returned to normal at follow-up 1 month later. *2026*

122.90   Hydatidosis   With liver involvement. *1058*

124.00   Trichinosis   Moderate to marked elevations. *0503*   A consequence of muscular necrosis. *0433*

135.00   Sarcoidosis   In 24% of 25 patients at initial hospitalization for this disorder. *0781*

151.90   Malignant Neoplasm of Stomach   Marked elevation in 20 patients with tumors of the gastrointestinal tract. Mean = 162.0 ± 23.1 U/L compared to 85.4 ± 1.0 U/L. *1201*

152.90   Malignant Neoplasm of Small Intestine   Marked elevation in 20 patients, mean = 162.0 - 23.1 U/L compared to 85.4 ± 1.0 U/L. *1201*

153.90   Malignant Neoplasm of Large Intestine   Marked elevation in 20 patients, mean = 162.0 U/L (compared to 85.4 ± 1.0 U/L). *1201   0992*

155.00   Malignant Neoplasm of Liver   Useful in detecting metastatic or primary liver cancer due to marked sensitivity to carcinomatosis and insensitivity to noncancerous parenchymal hepatic damage. *0503*   Significant elevation occurred in 66% of patients. *0029*   70-85% incidence of elevation. *0364*   In 83% of 13 patients at initial hospitalization for this disorder. *0781*

157.90   Malignant Neoplasm of Pancreas   In 24% of 46 patients at initial hospitalization for this disorder. *0781*

162.90 Malignant Neoplasm of Bronchus and Lung Activity was frequently elevated in 30 patients with primary and 4 with secondary neoplasms. Activity increased with tumor extension and often in relation to chemotherapy, but provided little diagnostic or prognostic value, except to indicate metastases. *0819* Twice the normal mean in 53 patients with bronchogenic carcinomas. Mean = 175.1 ± 10.4 U/L compared to normals, 85.4 ± 1.0 U/L. *1201*

170.90 Malignant Neoplasm of Bone In 36 patients with Ewing's sarcoma, pretreatment levels proved an extremely good indicator of which patients would ultimately develop metastases. 3 of 18 patients with levels below the total group median (201-214 U/L) developed metastases, while 16 of 18 patients with levels above the median developed metastatic spread (P < 0.001). *0279* In 25% of 26 patients at initial hospitalization for this disorder. *0781*

172.90 Malignant Melanoma of Skin Marked elevation in 38 patients with melanoblastomas. Mean = 179.7 ± 20.0 U/L compared to normals, 85.4 ± 1.0 U/L. *1201*

174.90 Malignant Neoplasm of Breast Highly elevated values (> 300 U/L) may be obtained with or without liver involvement in the presence of bone metastases. *1025* Marked elevation in 110 patients. Mean = 207.2 ± 12.4 U/L, compared to normals, 85.4 ± 1.0 U/L. *1201 2575 1157*

180.90 Malignant Neoplasm of Cervix Marked elevation in 26 patients with uterine, cervix and corpus carcinomas. Mean = 142.5 ± 18.2 U/L compared to normals 85.4 ± 1.0 U/L. *1201*

183.00 Malignant Neoplasm of Ovary All 6 cases showed elevation ranging from 150-350 with the upper limit of normal at 120. Marked elevation in 18 patients. *0090* Mean = 158.7 ± 14.9 U/L compared to normals, 85.4 ± 1.0 U/L. *1201*

185.00 Malignant Neoplasm of Prostate In advanced carcinoma following successful stilbestrol therapy and/or orchiectomy. *0619* Borderline or elevated in 32 patients, regardless of the status of the disease. *0543* In 27% of 83 patients at initial hospitalization for this disorder. *0781 0433*

186.90 Malignant Neoplasm of Testis Marked elevation in 47 patients with tumors of the testicle and kidney. Mean = 168.8 ± 19.5 U/L compared to normals, 85.4 ± 1.0 U/L. *1201* In 38% of 23 patients at initial hospitalization for this disorder. *0781*

189.00 Malignant Neoplasm of Kidney Marked elevation in 47 patients with tumors of the testicle and kidney. Mean = 168.8 ± 19.5 U/L compared to normals, 85.4 ± 10.0 U/L. *1201*

197.00 Secondary Malignant Neoplasm of Respiratory System From a study of 50 patients, a semiquantitative relationship appeared with LD, rapidity of tumor growth, and degree of dissemination of the neoplastic process. *2575* In 50% of 574 patients at initial hospitalization for this disorder. *0781*

197.50 Secondary Malignant Neoplasm of Digestive System From a study of 50 patients, a semiquantitative relation appeared between serum LD, rapidity of tumor growth, and degree of dissemination of the neoplastic process. *2575*

197.70 Secondary Malignant Neoplasm of Liver From a study of 50 patients, a semiquantitative relation appeared between serum LD, rapidity of tumor growth, and degree of dissemination of the neoplastic process. *2575* Distinctly elevated in most cases. *2260*

198.30 Secondary Malignant Neoplasm of Brain From a study of 50 patients, a semiquantitative relation appeared between LD, rapidity of tumor growth, and degree of dissemination of the neoplastic process. *2575* Depending on location, growth rate, etc. *2467*

198.50 Secondary Malignant Neoplasm of Bone From a study of 50 patients, a semiquantitative relation appeared between LD, rapidity of tumor growth, and degree of dissemination of the neoplastic process. *2575*

199.00 Secondary Malignant Neoplasm (Disseminated) From a study of 50 patients, a semiquantitative relation appeared between serum LD, rapidity of tumor growth, and degree of dissemination of the neoplastic process. *2575*

201.90 Hodgkin's Disease Normal or relatively increased; depends on the total mass of the tumor and presence of hemolysis. *0503* May be a sign of active disease or may indicate involvement of liver or bone. *0433* Marked elevation in 138 patients with malignant lymphomas. Mean = 177.7 ± 13.8 U/L compared to normals, 85.4 ± 1.0 U/L. *1201* In 37% of 72 patients at initial hospitalization for this disorder. *0781 0206 1089*

202.10 Mycosis Fungoides *2539*

202.80 Non-Hodgkins Lymphoma Increased in about 60% of the patients. *2467 0812* May be a sign of active disease or may indicate involvement of liver or bone. *0433* Marked elevation in 138 patients with malignant lymphomas. Mean = 177.7 ± 13.8 U/L compared to normals, 85.4 ± 1.0 U/L. *1201* In 55% of 73 patients at initial hospitalization for this disorder. *0781 0151 0962*

204.00 Lymphocytic Leukemia (Acute) Increased in acute, but not in chronic lymphocytic leukemia. Usually reflected changes in the course of the disease-falling during remission and rising during relapses, occasionally indicating the onset before the WBC had begun to change. *0221* Frequently elevated when the disease is in relapse. The absolute levels vary considerably from individual to individual. *0936* In 91% of 39 patients at initial hospitalization for this disorder. *0781* Mean value of 54 patients was 2 X normal adult value. 47 of 54 patients had significantly increased activities. *0206 0962*

204.10 Lymphocytic Leukemia (Chronic) Elevated in all 15 patients, mean = 104.3 U/L. *1521* In 64% of 27 patients at initial hospitalization for this disorder. *0781* 84 of 91 patients with leukemias had values elevated above the normal upper limit. *0206*

205.00 Myelocytic Leukemia (Acute) Markedly elevated levels in untreated acute leukemia. *0812* 2-4 X normal values. *0503* Increased in about 90% of the patients. The degree of increase is not correlated with the level of WBC. *2467* In 87% of 34 patients at initial hospitalization for this disorder. *0781* 84 of 91 patients with leukemias had values elevated above the normal upper limit. *0206 0221 0962*

205.10 Myelocytic Leukemia (Chronic) Usually reflects changes in the course of the disease--falling during remission and rising during relapses, occasionally indicating the onset before the WBC had begun to change. *2468* Elevated in all 20 patients, mean = 197.5 U/L. *1521* Considerably elevated, but appears to be a nonspecific abnormality. *1476* In 95% of 20 patients at initial hospitalization for this disorder. *0781* Elevated above the normal upper limit in 84 of 91 patients with leukemias. *0206 0221 2538 0962*

206.00 Monocytic Leukemia In 80% of 22 patients at initial hospitalization for this disorder. *0781*

207.00 Erythroleukemia Normal or high levels. *2538*

212.70 Benign Neoplasm of Cardiovascular Tissue Reflects hemolysis. *2467*

244.90 Hypothyroidism Regularly elevated. *0503* The muscle involvement of this disease appears to be responsible for the elevated levels seen in this condition. *0503* LD and CK activity are elevated, while AST, ALT, and alkaline phos were within normal limits. *1320* In 60% of 13 patients at initial hospitalization for this disorder. *0781 0433 0962*

245.10 Subacute Thyroiditis *0151*

250.00 Diabetes Mellitus Of 200 untreated diabetics, 21% had an unexplainable elevation. *0873*

250.10 Diabetic Acidosis In some instances, mostly severe cases, especially with severe circulatory failure and liver enlargement. *0155*

271.02 McArdle's Disease Slight to moderate increase. *0503* Increases dramatically within h after strenuous exercise. *0970 2246*

272.72 Gaucher's Disease May be abnormal with liver involvement. *0995*

275.00 Hemochromatosis With liver involvement. *0962*

275.10 Hepatolenticular Degeneration With liver involvement. *0995*

275.31 Hyperphosphatasia Pronounced increase. *2259*

276.20 Metabolic Acidosis Increased in type II-B, with lactic acidosis. *2468*

277.41 Dubin-Johnson Syndrome May be normal or moderately increased. *0602*

281.00 Pernicious Anemia Total LD (chiefly LD_1) is markedly increased especially with hemoglobin < 8 g/dL. *2467* In 5 cases, levels ranged from 310 U/L (in relapse) - 4820 U/L (normal = 50-220 U/L). *2253* Mean value in 16 patients was 2335 U/L (normal 116). *0060* Magnitude of increase is related to the degree of anemia. *2552*

Lactate Dehydrogenase *(continued)*

Serum Increase *(continued)*

281.20 Folic Acid Deficiency Anemia In some cases; LD activity and red cell count inversely related in folic acid and/or vitamin B_{12} deficiency. *0619* More sensitive reflection of this disease state than other tests. 2-40 fold elevations. Almost all patients have increased concentrations, often marked. *0812 0503* In 13 patients ranged from normal to 40 fold elevation. *2253* Mean value in 16 patients was 2335 U/L (normal = 116). *0060* Magnitude of increase is related to the degree of anemia. *2552 1023 0962*

282.00 Hereditary (Congenital) Spherocytosis In hemolytic anemia. *0619 0962*

282.10 Hereditary Elliptocytosis In severe cases. *0433*

282.20 Anemias Due To Disorders of Glutathione Metabolism Especially if intravascular; derived from RBCs. *0619* 2-4 X normal values. *0503*

282.31 Hereditary Nonspherocytic Hemolytic Anemia In hemolytic anemias. *2612*

282.41 Thalassemia Major May be markedly elevated in the serum presumably due to marrow hyperplasia and ineffective erythropoiesis. *0433* Usually elevated. *2552*

282.60 Sickle Cell Anemia Usually elevated to about twice normal in the steady state. *1682 0962*

282.71 Hemoglobin C Disease Due to slight hemolysis. *0186*

283.00 Acquired Hemolytic Anemia (Autoimmune) Often increased, although not as high as in megaloblastic anemia. *2552 0962*

283.21 Paroxysmal Nocturnal Hemoglobinuria Very high during active hemolysis. *2552*

284.90 Aplastic Anemia In 42% of 21 patients hospitalized for this disorder. *0781*

289.80 Myelofibrosis May be elevated usually correlating with the degree of myelofibrosis or WBC elevation. *0433* Increased in every patient irrespective of the disease. The maximum rise was observed in cases of myelosclerosis, the smallest in lymphatic leukemia. *1521 2538*

291.00 Delirium Tremens Relatively slight elevations found in almost all patients. Perhaps of skeletal muscle origin since, like the elevated LD values of progressive muscular dystrophy, they are accompanied by increased CK. High elevations irrespective of associated hepatic disease and may arise in muscle. *0503*

303.90 Alcoholism In 42% of 14 patients hospitalized for this disorder. *0781*

304.90 Drug Dependence (Opium and Derivatives) Markedly elevated in 4 heroin addicts after admission. Acute skeletal muscle necrosis in all 4 cases, and acute renal failure in 2 of the 4 occurred as a result of intravenous use of heroin-adulterant mixtures. *1929*

320.90 Meningitis (Bacterial) LD and its isoenzymes are elevated, mostly due to a rise in the leukocyte fraction. Patients with increased brain LD isoenzyme usually develop neurologic sequelae or die. *0151* In 64% of 12 patients hospitalized for this disorder. *0781*

331.81 Reye's Syndrome Markedly elevated reflecting hepatic injury. *0435*

335.11 Familial Progressive Spinal Muscular Atrophy Elevations of serum enzymes are frequently encountered but never reach the magnitude seen in Duchenne muscular dystrophy. *0433*

335.20 Amyotrophic Lateral Sclerosis Especially in the early stages. *0619* Slight elevations of LD are common in adults, but it is unclear whether muscular atrophy or hepatic disease is the cause. *2418*

359.11 Progressive Muscular Dystrophy Particularly during the early and middle stages of the disease. In the late stage of the disease when the muscle mass has been severely reduced, may be only minimally elevated. *0433 1677*

359.21 Myotonia Atrophica Slightly or moderately increased. *0503* In about 10% of the patients. *2467 0433*

359.22 Myotonia Congenita Slightly or moderately increased. *0503*

390.00 Rheumatic Fever In some cases of acute rheumatic carditis. *0619*

410.90 Acute Myocardial Infarction Rises 2-10 fold after the first 12 h and reaches a peak by 24-48 h. The increase is roughly parallel to the degree of cardiac damage and also to the serum AST. *0619* May remain elevated up to 10-14 days after onset; therefore is particularly useful when patient is first seen after sufficient time has elapsed for CK and AST to become normal. *2467* Moderate elevations in almost all patients (92-98%) with proven infarction. The complication by shock leads to higher values of AST and LD and to abnormal levels of enzymes that reflect hepatic injury (ALT, ICD). *0503* Concentrations 2,000 U/L suggest a poor prognosis. *2467 0088 0812 0191*

415.10 Pulmonary Embolism and Infarction 2-4 X normal values. Increased within 24 h of onset of pain. *0503* Combination of increased LD and a normal AST present in 60-75% of patients. *0999* Characteristically a rise of activity and in about 50% of cases no rise of AST activity. Initially considered to be diagnostic, has been shown repeatedly to be not the case. *1108* Frequently elevated within 5 days after the embolic event. Too nonspecific to be diagnostic. *0962 2445 0781*

422.00 Acute Myocarditis Elevated cardiac enzymes may be the earliest evidence of myocarditis. *1108*

425.40 Cardiomyopathies Increased, often to extremely high levels; may rise even further after recovery from shock in cobalt beer cardiomyopathy. *2467*

428.00 Congestive Heart Failure Increased in about 40% of patients. *2467 0433*

431.00 Cerebral Hemorrhage In 40% of 10 patients hospitalized for this disorder. *0781 2560*

434.00 Cerebral Thrombosis Serum elevations were less frequent and independent of those in the CSF. *2560*

444.90 Arterial Embolism and Thrombosis In 32% of 37 patients hospitalized for this disorder. *0781 2079 0992*

480.90 Viral Pneumonia In 60% of 10 patients at initial hospitalization for this disorder. *0781* The increases that did occur were in cases of viral pneumonia. *1126*

482.90 Bacterial Pneumonia In some cases. *2368* In 32% of 17 patients at initial hospitalization for this disorder. *0781*

483.01 Mycoplasma Pneumoniae May be elevated. *2368*

486.01 Resolving Pneumonia In 33% of 62 patients at initial hospitalization for this disorder. *0781*

496.00 Alpha₁-Antitrypsin Deficiency Related to liver disease. *1636*

502.00 Silicosis *0962*

516.00 Pulmonary Alveolar Proteinosis Increases when protein accumulates in lungs and drops to normal when infiltrate resolves. *2467* Values for all 12 patients were above the normal upper limit. *1518*

555.90 Regional Enteritis or Ileitis Liver abnormalities are common. *0995*

556.00 Ulcerative Colitis With liver involvement. *0433*

557.01 Mesenteric Artery Embolism *0433*

560.90 Intestinal Obstruction Increase may indicate strangulation (infarction) of small intestine. *2467* In 32% of 42 patients at initial hospitalization for this disorder. *0781*

570.00 Acute and Subacute Necrosis of Liver Total LD is increased in 50% the cases. Relatively slight elevations or not at all. *0812 0503* Occasionally increased. *0995 1089*

571.20 Laennec's or Alcoholic Cirrhosis Slight increase. *0962* High in 6 of 20 patients with portal cirrhosis. *2260*

571.90 Cirrhosis of Liver Slight increase. *0962* In 32% of 69 patients at initial hospitalization for this disorder. *0781 2575 1089*

572.40 Hepatic Failure May be increased or normal. *0503*

573.30 Toxic Hepatitis LD 4 and 5 due to chemical poisoning. *0812*

576.20 Extrahepatic Biliary Obstruction Slight increase. *0962* In obstruction due to benign or malignant disease. *2260*

577.00 Acute Pancreatitis In some cases. *0619* Nonspecific serum enzymes may also be increased. *2467* In 45% of 21 patients at initial hospitalization for this disorder. *0781*

581.90 Nephrotic Syndrome In 44% of 25 patients at initial hospitalization for this disorder. *0781 0503*

584.00 Acute Renal Failure In 72% of 11 patients at initial hospitalization for this disorder. *0781*

585.00 Chronic Renal Failure Occasional increase but to no clinically useful degree. *2467* Patients with chronic renal disease, especially those with nephrotic syndrome or hemolytic anemia, also have increased values. *0503*

593.81 **Renal Infarction** Occasional increase but to no clinically useful degree. May be increased markedly with arterial infarction of kidneys. Peak on 3rd day; return to normal by 10th day. *2468 0503 0962*

633.90 **Ectopic Pregnancy** In 4 of 10 patients at initial hospitalization for this disorder. *0781*

642.40 **Pre-Eclampsia** Rose to a mean value of 384.1 ± 31.8 U/L in severe pre-eclampsia, over the normal value in pregnancy of 154.5 - 12.2 U/L. *2034* Usually not elevated. When transaminases are found to be elevated, either pronounced hepatic or marked myocardial alterations have occurred. *0433*

650.00 **Pregnancy** Increases variably in normal pregnancy. *0387 0491*

694.00 **Dermatitis Herpetiformis** In 25% of 12 patients at initial hospitalization for this disorder. *0781*

710.00 **Systemic Lupus Erythematosus** Significantly higher in patients with diffuse proliferative lupus nephritis. *1124*

710.10 **Progressive Systemic Sclerosis** Moderate to marked increase with associated myositis. *0503*

710.40 **Dermatomyositis/Polymyositis** Moderate to marked increase. *0503* Elevated at some time in nearly every patient. *0244* Increased but less sensitive indicator of muscle injury. *0962* Elevation in both acute and chronic polymyositis. *1071 2575*

714.00 **Rheumatoid Arthritis** Characteristically abnormal when the arthritis is active. *0433 1089*

773.00 **Hemolytic Disease of Newborn (Erythroblastosis Fetalis)** Derived from red blood cells. *0619*

785.40 **Gangrene** In 24% of 32 patients hospitalized for this disorder. *0781* Slight elevation. *0992*

785.50 **Shock** 2-40 X normal values. *0503*

989.50 **Toxic Effects of Venom** Analysis of 17 patients admitted for wasp stings showed elevated LD in 8/14 cases, elevated AST and CK in 9/17 and 14/17, respectively. *1822*

990.00 **Effects of X-Ray Irradiation** May be increased in cases of radiation injury, indicating major cell and tissue damage. *0151*

991.60 **Hypothermia** Due to hypoxia, acid-base imbalance hypotension. *1471* 20 of 24 patients with hypothermia had elevated concentrations. *1472*

992.00 **Heat stroke** Increases to a mean value 5 X normal by the 3rd day and returns to normal in 2 weeks. Very high levels are often associated with lethal outcome. *2468*

994.50 **Exercise** After a 100 km race, 3 well-trained men, showed normal EKG and good clinical states, but significant elevations in LD, AST and CK were recorded. *2076* Maximum effect observed following day. Marked increase with exercise. *2550* Exercise. *1930 0985*

994.80 **Effects of Electric Current** *0995*

Serum Normal

205.10 **Myelocytic Leukemia (Chronic)** Frequently normal. *2468*

238.40 **Polycythemia Vera** Normal in uncomplicated cases. *2538*

272.31 **Type I Hyperlipoproteinemia** *2246*

275.00 **Hemochromatosis** Over 50% of patients have no laboratory evidence of liver dysfunction. *0995*

277.42 **Gilbert's Disease** *0995*

277.44 **Crigler-Najjar Syndrome** *0469*

280.90 **Iron Deficiency Anemia** Normal, even in severe iron-deficiency. *2468*

333.40 **Huntington's Chorea** No abnormalities in 8 patients. *0534*

358.00 **Myasthenia Gravis** *2057*

359.21 **Myotonia Atrophica** Usually normal. *2246*

413.90 **Angina Pectoris** In 89% of 75 patients hospitalized for this disorder. *0781 2467*

415.10 **Pulmonary Embolism and Infarction** Values may be normal in the presence of embolism. *1108*

441.00 **Dissecting Aortic Aneurysm** Unless complications occur. *2467*

446.50 **Cranial Arteritis and Related Conditions** *0186*

482.90 **Bacterial Pneumonia** Normal in 45 of 50 cases of uncomplicated pneumonia. The increases that did occur were in cases of viral pneumonia. Unreliable screening methods were suggested to account for the increase in LD in pneumonia in a previous study. *1126 0619*

486.01 **Resolving Pneumonia** Levels were normal in 45/50 cases of. uncomplicated pneumonia. Increases that did occur were in cases of viral pneumonia. Unreliable screening methods were suggested to account for the increases in a previous study. *1126*

650.00 **Pregnancy** *1561*

992.00 **Heat stroke** Normal in children. *0548*

Urine Increase

185.00 **Malignant Neoplasm of Prostate** Increased in a high proportion of cases; useful for detection of asymptomatic lesions or screening of susceptible population groups. Increased values usually precede clinical symptoms. *2467 0817 0818*

188.00 **Malignant Neoplasm of Bladder** Increased in a high proportion of cases; useful for detection of asymptomatic lesions or screening of susceptible population groups, and differential diagnosis of renal cysts. This test is chiefly useful in screening for malignancy of kidney, renal pelvis, and bladder; increased values usually precede clinical symptoms. *2467* 60.7% (17 of 28) patients with transitional cell carcinoma showed elevations. *1843 0817 0818*

189.00 **Malignant Neoplasm of Kidney** Mild elevation occurred in 33% of cases. *0818* Elevated in 40% of patients. *0817* In all 16 cases, urinary activity was increased 10 fold but with no rise in tumor tissue level. *1005*

410.90 **Acute Myocardial Infarction** *2467*

580.00 **Acute Poststreptococcal Glomerulonephritis** *2468*

581.90 **Nephrotic Syndrome** *2467*

584.00 **Acute Renal Failure** In acute tubular necrosis. *2467*

585.00 **Chronic Renal Failure** 38% of cases showed elevation. *0817*

590.00 **Chronic Pyelonephritis** Urinary activity was almost invariably elevated. *0817*

590.10 **Acute Pyelonephritis** Increased in 25% of patients. *2467*

593.81 **Renal Infarction** May be increased markedly with arterial infarction of kidney. LD peaks on 3rd day; return to normal by 10th day. *2468 0962*

710.00 **Systemic Lupus Erythematosus** With nephritis. *2467*

Urine Normal

592.00 **Kidney Calculus** *2467*

753.10 **Polycystic Kidney Disease** *2467*

CSF Increase

13.00 **Tuberculosis Meningitis** Increased in all cases in the range of 80-265 U/L (normal = 0-35 U/L), higher in those who were seriously ill and having acute onset of the disease. *1263*

47.00 **Aseptic Meningitis** Invariably slightly elevated, with LD-1 and 2 the elevated isoenzymes. *1684*

191.90 **Malignant Neoplasm of Brain** In primary and metastatic tumors depending on location, growth rate, etc. *2467*

198.30 **Secondary Malignant Neoplasm of Brain** In group of patients with metastatic tumors of the nervous system showed a highly significant difference in the mean CSF LD activity of 67 U/L. All but 2 patients had significantly elevated individual results. *0507 2574*

320.90 **Meningitis (Bacterial)** Elevations varied from 2-100 X the normal values in 23 cases. Significantly lower levels were found in patients with viral meningitis and in CNS infection. *0720* 234 specimens from 183 different children were analyzed. Activity was elevated in patients with meningitis, especially bacterial infections, and CNS leukemia. The isoenzyme pattern generally reflected the number and distribution of lymphocytes and granulocytes in the CSF. *1684*

330.00 **Metachromatic Leukodystrophy** Increases initially, then diminishes. *0078*

331.40 **Acquired Hydrocephalus** Range of LD activity in 9 patients with hydrocephalus for shunt insertion or revision was 17-53 U/L, with normal CSF values from 3-17 U/L. *1684*

431.00 **Cerebral Hemorrhage** In the acute stage of the disease. The increase seems to be the result of blood and plasma reaching the CSF in hemorrhage. *2575* Elevated in all 27 determinations of CSF in 17 patients with hemorrhagic vascular lesions and 13 of 30 patients with nonhemorrhagic lesions. *2560*

434.00 **Cerebral Thrombosis** All of the 17 patients with hemorrhagic lesions showed elevations. 13 of 30 patients with nonhemorrhagic lesions showed similar but smaller elevations in the CSF. Serum elevations were less frequent and independent of those in the CSF. *2560*

Lactate Dehydrogenase *(continued)*

Pleural Effusion   Decrease

423.10 **Constrictive Pericarditis**   Transudate. *0062*

571.90 **Cirrhosis of Liver**   Transudate. *0062*

581.90 **Nephrotic Syndrome**   Transudate. *0062*

585.00 **Chronic Renal Failure**   Transudate. *0062*

Pleural Effusion   Increase

11.00 **Pulmonary Tuberculosis**   Moderate elevation occurred in 50% of cases, especially in active tuberculosis. *0490*

162.90 **Malignant Neoplasm of Bronchus and Lung**   Elevation in pleural fluid without concurrent rise in protein indicates malignancy. *1403*   A markedly elevated pleural LD is consistent with neoplastic involvement of the pleura. Not specific for the diagnosis. *0962*

197.00 **Secondary Malignant Neoplasm of Respiratory System**   A markedly elevated pleural LD is consistent with neoplastic involvement of the pleura. Not specific for the diagnosis. *0962*

415.10 **Pulmonary Embolism and Infarction**   Exudate. *0062*

480.90 **Viral Pneumonia**   Usually higher than in serum; commonly found in chronic pleural effusions and is not useful in differential diagnosis. *2467*

482.90 **Bacterial Pneumonia**   Usually higher than in serum; commonly found in chronic pleural effusions and is not useful in differential diagnosis. *2467*

577.00 **Acute Pancreatitis**   Exudate. *0062*

577.10 **Chronic Pancreatitis**   Exudate. *0062*

Ascitic Fluid   Increase

155.00 **Malignant Neoplasm of Liver**   In malignant effusions. *2199*

157.90 **Malignant Neoplasm of Pancreas**   In malignant effusions. *2199*

189.00 **Malignant Neoplasm of Kidney**   In malignant effusions. *2199*

Pericardial Fluid   Decrease

420.00 **Acute Pericarditis**   Less than 60% of serum levels. *0758*

Pericardial Fluid   Increase

714.00 **Rheumatoid Arthritis**   With rheumatoid pericarditis markedly elevated. *0764*

Gastric Material   Increase

151.90 **Malignant Neoplasm of Stomach**   Increase in activity is found in carcinoma, measured as U/mL or U secreted/h. *0619*   Elevated in gastric cancer. Overlap between noncancer and cancer patients limits usefulness and specificity. *2199*

533.90 **Peptic Ulcer, Site Unspecified**   Moderately increased activity. *0619*

535.00 **Gastritis**   Moderately increased activity. *0619*

Red Blood Cells   Increase

281.20 **Folic Acid Deficiency Anemia**   5 of 15 patients had RBC concentrations above the normal upper limit of 96. *1023*

282.60 **Sickle Cell Anemia**   Mean concentration elevated to 180 U/L (3 X the normal mean) in 15 patients. Values ranged from 83-388 U/L. *1023*

Red Blood Cells   Normal

585.00 **Chronic Renal Failure**   Within normal limits. *1566*

Lactate Dehydrogenase Isoenzyme 5 (LD$_5$)

Serum   Decrease

205.10 **Myelocytic Leukemia (Chronic)**   Isoenzyme 2 and 3 were the most intense and 5 was decreased. *1521* *2253*

359.11 **Progressive Muscular Dystrophy**   In 76 cases of Duchenne MD, was markedly depressed and remained low until the final stages of the disease. Abnormal isoenzyme patterns persisted over time even though the total LD value fell to normal with increasing age of patient. *1070*

Serum   Increase

70.00 **Viral Hepatitis**   Markedly elevated in 7 cases. Comprised 35.4% of the total serum LD (normal = 0-6%). *0852*

75.00 **Infectious Mononucleosis**   Elevated in 35% of the 36 patients with elevated serum LD. *1658*   Mean level in 5 cases was 8.2% of total serum LD. Normal mean = 3.0%. *1658* *0852*

155.00 **Malignant Neoplasm of Liver**   Elevated to a mean of 13% of total LD values (normal = 0-6%). *0852*

157.90 **Malignant Neoplasm of Pancreas**   Mild elevation to a mean of 13% of total LD in patients with carcinoma of the liver, gallbladder and pancreas (normal = 0-6%). *0852*

185.00 **Malignant Neoplasm of Prostate**   Consistently elevated in patients with advanced progressive prostatic carcinoma. In patients in remission, at trace levels as found in the control group. *0543*

281.00 **Pernicious Anemia**   Increased to about the same extent as LD. *0652* *2552*

281.20 **Folic Acid Deficiency Anemia**   Increased to about the same extent as LD. *0652* *2552*

335.11 **Familial Progressive Spinal Muscular Atrophy**   In rapidly destructive neurogenic atrophies such as Werdnig-Hoffmann disease a rise was noted, reflecting a temporary leakage of cytoplasmic LD$_5$ from muscle to peripheral blood. *1070*

335.20 **Amyotrophic Lateral Sclerosis**   In rapidly destructive progressive muscular atrophies, such as amyotrophic lateral sclerosis and Werdnig-Hoffmann disease, a rise was noted reflecting leakage of cytoplasmic LD$_5$ from muscle to peripheral blood. *1070*

359.21 **Myotonia Atrophica**   Elevation of fast moving LD in serum. *2467*

410.90 **Acute Myocardial Infarction**   Almost invariably increased, beginning 12 h after infarction and peaking after 48 h. *1390*   Parallels increase of fast moving LD with peak (3-4 X normal) in 48 h and persistent elevation for up to 2 weeks. *2467*

415.10 **Pulmonary Embolism and Infarction**   Elevated to 8.4% of the total LD value of 736 U/L in 5 cases of pulmonary embolism. *0852*

428.00 **Congestive Heart Failure**   Elevated to 14.5% of total LD in 12 patients with passive congestion. *0852*   LD$_1$ and 5 are elevated. *2467*

480.90 **Viral Pneumonia**   Abnormally elevated to 6.3% of the total LD value of 774 U/mL in 6 cases of lobar pneumonia. *0852*

493.10 **Asthma (Intrinsic)**   Raised activities of LD$_3$ and LD$_5$ comprised the bulk of the increase in total activity. The increment in LD$_3$ activity arose from lung involvement whereas the major portion of the increment in LD$_5$ activity was derived from the liver. *2405*

570.00 **Acute and Subacute Necrosis of Liver**   Present in increased amounts. *0619*   Most marked increase, which occurs during prodromal stage and is greatest at time of onset of jaundice. *2467*

571.20 **Laennec's or Alcoholic Cirrhosis**   LD 4 and 5 are elevated. *0503*

571.90 **Cirrhosis of Liver**   LD 4 and 5 are moderately elevated. *0503*

573.30 **Toxic Hepatitis**   Due to chemical poisoning. *2467*

576.20 **Extrahepatic Biliary Obstruction**   Was markedly elevated in 3 cases. Mean elevation = 11.0% of total LD value. *0852*

577.00 **Acute Pancreatitis**   Elevated to 8.3% of the total value of 861 U/L in 3 cases. Increases occurred in LD isoenzymes 4 and 5. *0852*

581.90 **Nephrotic Syndrome**   May be slightly increased. *2467*

650.00 **Pregnancy**   Mother carrying erythroblastotic child. LD$_4$ and LD$_5$. *2467* *0491*

710.40 **Dermatomyositis/Polymyositis**   In cases of chronic polymyositis, a relative but mild rise was noted. *1071*   May be increased, paralleling the increased LD. *2467*

991.60 **Hypothermia**   Due to hypoxia, acid-base imbalance hypotension. *1471*   20 of 24 patients with hypothermia had elevated concentrations. *1472*

994.50 **Exercise**   *1978*

Serum   Normal

413.90 **Angina Pectoris**   *2467*

441.00 **Dissecting Aortic Aneurysm**   Unless complications occur. *2467*

650.00 **Pregnancy**   *0491*

600.00 Benign Prostatic Hypertrophy The urinalysis may be completely normal or may reveal albuminuria, pyuria, and hematuria as a result of obstruction with infection or stone formation. *0433*

601.00 Prostatitis Following prostatic massage the last portion of voided urine shows an increased WBC compared with the first portion. *0186*

710.00 Systemic Lupus Erythematosus *0433*

Urine   Normal

590.10 Acute Pyelonephritis Acute pyelonephritis may exist in the absence of pyuria and bacteriuria. This may occur in the patient with hematogenous dissemination of infection to the renal parenchyma without communication to urinary drainage, as in renal carbuncle or perinephric abscess. *0433   0277*

591.00 Hydronephrosis In uninfected cases the urine is negative. If infection supervenes, WBC and albumin are noted. *0433*

592.10 Ureter Calculus Children usually have no WBC in their unspun microscopic urine examination. WBC aren't always present in these lower tract obstructions even with moderate symptoms unless infection is present. *0433* Urinalysis often shows no significant alteration from normal. *0433*

600.00 Benign Prostatic Hypertrophy The urinalysis may be completely normal or may reveal albuminuria, pyuria, and hematuria as a result of obstruction with infection or stone formation. *0433*

CSF   Increase

13.00 Tuberculosis Meningitis Up to 1,000/μL, the cells being 30-100% lymphocytes. *0999* Cell count usually varies between 10-500/μL and consists mainly of lymphocytes, except in the early stage when neutrophils predominate. *0962   0151*

36.00 Meningococcal Meningitis Markedly increased (2500-10,000/μL), almost all polymorphonuclear leukocytes. *2468   2400*

45.90 Acute Poliomyelitis Usually 25-500/μL at first. Most are polymorphonuclear leukocytes; after several days most are lymphocytes. *2468   0433*

47.00 Aseptic Meningitis May increase from a few to > 1,000/μL, mostly polymorphonuclears, in acute hemorrhagic encephalitis. *0151* Count ranges from 50-300/μL and rarely 2,000. Marked predominance of lymphocytes except in the earliest stage. *0962*

62.10 Western Equine Encephalitis Up to 1,000/μL. *1058*

62.20 Eastern Equine Encephalitis Up to 1,000/μL. *1058*

72.00 Mumps In meningitis and meningoencephalitis, CSF usually contains fewer than 500/μL with only occasional counts > 2,000/μL. In most cases the cells are almost exclusively mononuclear from the onset; polymorphonuclear leukocytes predominate for the first few days in only a small percentage of patients. Pleocytosis may continue for as long as 5 weeks. *0433*

87.00 Relapsing Fever Pleocytosis can occur. *0433*

97.90 Syphilis Average 500/μL, usually lymphocytes. *0151*

99.10 Lymphogranuloma Venereum Pleocytosis as high as 4,000/μL may occur. *0433*

112.90 Moniliasis Mean count = 600/μL in 28 cases of Candida meningitis. *0138*

114.90 Coccidioidomycosis Fewer than 500/μL with CNS involvement. *1058*

117.50 Cryptococcosis 40-400/μL with meningoencephalitis. *1058*

130.00 Toxoplasmosis In congenital, both RBC and WBC with a predominance of mononuclear elements. In acquired predominantly mononuclear cells, 30-2,000/μL. *1319*

135.00 Sarcoidosis In granulomatous basilar meningitis affecting cranial nerves. *0992*

320.90 Meningitis (Bacterial) Several hundred to 60,000/μL with predominantly polymorphonuclear cells present. *0151* Ranges between 500-20,000/μL, with about 90% polymorphonuclears. Counts > 25,000 suggest a ruptured brain abscess. *0962   0999   2400*

323.91 Myelitis Spinal fluid may be normal or may show increased protein and cells (20-1,000/μL--lymphocytes and mononuclear cells). *2467* Increased WBCs, mononuclear, and polymorphonuclear cells are found. *0999*

323.92 Encephalomyelitis Pleocytosis ranges from 10-500/μL. In most infections, and these are predominantly lymphocytes; however, granulocytes may prevail for 1-2 days after onset. Counts may exceed 100/μL especially in lymphocytic choriomeningitis and eastern equine encephalomyelitis. *0433*

324.00 Intracranial Abscess Counts may be < 100 to several thousand in subdural empyema. *0151* Usually ranges from 50-300/μL and consists predominantly of lymphocytes. With intraventricular rupture, counts may exceed 50,000. *0962* In the range of 50-1,000/μL. *0995*

324.10 Intraspinal Abscess Usually 10-100 WBC/μL with predominantly lymphocytes present in spinal epidural abscess. *0151*

340.00 Multiple Sclerosis A pleocytosis of usually not more than 25 mononuclear cells/μL can be found. *0433*

421.00 Bacterial Endocarditis May reach 100/μL, mostly polymorphonuclears and lymphocytes in bacterial endocarditis with embolism. *0151*

431.00 Cerebral Hemorrhage Count will be commensurate with the amount of bleeding, 1 WBC/1,000 RBC. Increase is caused by the inflammatory reaction in the meninges and may reach levels of 500/μL. *0151*

434.00 Cerebral Thrombosis A slight increase is common in the 1st few days. Rarely, and for unexplained reasons, a brisk transient pleocytosis (400-2,000 polymorphonuclears/μL) occurs on the 3rd day. *0992*

434.10 Cerebral Embolism Septic embolism (e.g., bacterial endocarditis) may cause increased WBC, up to 200/μL with variable lymphocytes and polymorphonuclear leukocytes. *2467*

510.00 Empyema In subdural empyema. (50-1000/μl, 20-80% neutrophils) *0186*

CSF   Normal

71.00 Rabies Usually normal. *0433   1319*

331.40 Acquired Hydrocephalus *1684*

357.00 Guillain-Barré Syndrome Normal cell count; usually below 10 monocytes per mL. The presence of more than 50 mononuclear cells per mL or the presence of any polymorphonuclear cells should suggest another disease. *1307*

Synovial Fluid   Increase

99.30 Reiter's Disease Synovial fluid is typically inflammatory, with cell counts up to 60,000/μL. *0999*

274.00 Gout The synovial fluid is typical of inflammatory reactions showing polymorphonuclear leukocytosis (5,000-5,000/μL). *0999* Counts between 750-45,000/μL in acute attacks. *0962*

282.60 Sickle Cell Anemia Ranged from 600-270,000/μL in 13 patients. Polymorphonuclear cells predominated. *0676*

390.00 Rheumatic Fever Increased number of white cells in synovial fluid, ranging from 300-98,000/μL. *2467   10,000-15,000/μL. 0962*

710.00 Systemic Lupus Erythematosus 5,000/μL. *0962* Usually low (< 5,000/μL) with a low percentage of neutrophils. *0433* Usually does not not exceed 3,000/μL. *1700*

711.00 Acute Arthritis (Pyogenic) May vary from 10,000-300,000/μL, depending upon the stage of infection and inflammatory response. The cells are predominantly polymorphonuclear. *0433* Infected fluid is characteristically turbid or purulent, with a count of 100,000/μL or more, with a differential of 90% polymorphonuclears. *2481   2482*

714.00 Rheumatoid Arthritis Elevated (3,000 to 60,000/μL, with an average of around 10,000/μL), with predominantly polymorphonuclear response at times of active disease. *0999* Less than 15,000/μL. *0962*

714.30 Juvenile Rheumatoid Arthritis *2467*

715.90 Osteoarthritis Counts range from 200-2000/μL. *0151* Synovial fluid is viscid and has few white cells in degenerative joint disease. *0999*

Pleural Effusion   Decrease

428.00 Congestive Heart Failure < 1000/μL. *2017*

571.90 Cirrhosis of Liver < 500/μL. *2017*

Pleural Effusion   Increase

482.90 Bacterial Pneumonia A markedly elevated leukocyte count 10,000/μL), especially with a preponderance of neutrophils, is highly suggestive of a pyogenic infection. *0962*

510.00 Empyema 25,000-100,000/μL. *2017*

577.00 Acute Pancreatitis 5000-20,000/μL. *2017*

577.10 Chronic Pancreatitis 5000-20,000/μL. *2017*

577.20 Pancreatic Cyst and Pseudocyst 5000-20,000/μL. *2017*

714.00 Rheumatoid Arthritis 1000-20,000/μL. *2017*

Leukocytes *(continued)*

Ascitic Fluid Increase

18.00 Disseminated Tuberculosis > 1000 µL usually over 70% lymphocytes. *2626*

151.90 Malignant Neoplasm of Stomach > 1000 µL. *2626*

152.90 Malignant Neoplasm of Small Intestine > 1000 WBC/µL. *2626*

153.90 Malignant Neoplasm of Large Intestine > 1000 µL. *2626*

155.00 Malignant Neoplasm of Liver > 1000/µL. *2626*

197.70 Secondary Malignant Neoplasm of Liver > 1000 WBC/µL. *2626*

425.40 Cardiomyopathies Ascitic fluid and pericardial fluid are usually blood-stained or serous and contain leukocytes in obliterative cardiomyopathies. *1108*

428.00 Congestive Heart Failure Less than 1000 µL. *2626*

567.90 Peritonitis Mean total count = 5,500/µL. *1187* Elevated counts (> 250/µL) indicate peritoneal irritation. *0151* > 1000 µL predominantly polymorphonuclear cells. *2626*

571.20 Laennec's or Alcoholic Cirrhosis In 58 culture-negative patients the ascitic fluid count range was 28-1,800 and 50% of counts were > 300 WBC/µL. The percentage of polymorphonuclear leukocytes ranged from 2-98%. *1872* In 57 uncomplicated alcoholic liver disease patients, total ascitic WBC counts were often markedly elevated. Mean = 360/µL. *1187 1282*

571.90 Cirrhosis of Liver A total WBC exceeding 300/µL with predominantly polymorphonuclear leukocytes indicates associated peritonitis. *0433* Less than 250 cells/µL. {*2626*}

581.90 Nephrotic Syndrome Less than 250 cells per µL. *2626*

Ascitic Fluid Normal

157.90 Malignant Neoplasm of Pancreas Variable *2626*

577.00 Acute Pancreatitis Variable *2626*

577.10 Chronic Pancreatitis Variable *2626*

Pericardial Fluid Increase

425.40 Cardiomyopathies Ascitic fluid and pericardial fluid are usually blood-stained or serous and contain leukocytes in obliterative cardiomyopathies. *1108*

Bone Marrow Decrease

202.80 Non-Hodgkins Lymphoma In histiocytic medullary reticulosis, severe cytopenias may be associated with the abnormal phagocytosis of erythrocytes, platelets or leukocytes seen in the bone marrow. *2538*

Feces Increase

4.90 Bacillary Dysentery During the acute phase, examination of the stool will reveal clumps of polymorphonuclear leukocytes and RBCs, and the stool culture will be positive. *0962*

555.90 Regional Enteritis or Ileitis Large numbers. *2199*

Prostatic Fluid Increase

99.30 Reiter's Disease Reflects urethritis. *0186*

601.00 Prostatitis Since the presence of increased number of leukocytes and oval fat bodies are seen equally in cases of chronic bacterial prostatitis and nonbacterial prostatitis, the microscopic appearance of the expressed prostatic secretions is not specifically diagnostic. *0433* In the chronic form, prostatic fluid usually shows 10-15 WBCs (pus cells) with prostatitis. *2468*

Sputum Increase

482.90 Bacterial Pneumonia Sputum contains very many leukocytes with intracellular gram-positive cocci in staphylococcal pneumonia. *2468*

492.80 Pulmonary Emphysema Often infected on smear; increased WBC and epithelial debris. *0433*

Lipase

Serum Decrease

70.00 Viral Hepatitis Lack of bile salts result in the failure to activate pancreatic lipase in the intestinal lumen. *2104*

157.90 Malignant Neoplasm of Pancreas May be slightly increased in early stages (< 10% of cases); with later destruction, they are normal or decreased. *2467*

260.00 Protein Malnutrition Decreased with protein malnutrition. In kwashiorkor. *0151* Circulating concentration appears consistent with the amount of structural damage to the pancreas, characteristic of kwashiorkor. *2104*

277.00 Cystic Fibrosis *1901*

570.00 Acute and Subacute Necrosis of Liver Lack of bile salts result in the failure to activate pancreatic lipase in the intestinal lumen. *2104*

576.20 Extrahepatic Biliary Obstruction Lack of bile salts result in the failure to activate pancreatic lipase in the intestinal lumen. *2104*

650.00 Pregnancy Less than 50% of nonpregnant level. *0686*

Serum Increase

72.00 Mumps 11.5% of patients had slightly elevated values. *0336*

157.90 Malignant Neoplasm of Pancreas May be slightly increased in early stages (< 10% of cases); with later destruction, they are normal or decreased. *2467* Early obstruction of the pancreatic duct will occasionally elevate. *0151* Increased in 38% of 100 histologically proven cases. *0932*

272.31 Type I Hyperlipoproteinemia During bouts of abdominal pain. *2246*

272.32 Type V Hyperlipoproteinemia During bouts of abdominal pain. *2246*

533.90 Peptic Ulcer, Site Unspecified Perforated or penetrating peptic ulcer especially with involvement of the pancreas. *2467*

575.00 Acute Cholecystitis In some cases. *2467* In 25% of cases. *2238*

576.00 Postcholecystectomy Syndrome If tests are performed repeatedly, immediately after attacks, some abnormalities will appear if there is an organic cause of the syndrome. *0995*

576.20 Extrahepatic Biliary Obstruction Marked elevations should point to the diagnosis of acute pancreatitis of primary nature or secondary to calculus biliary tract disease. *0433*

576.50 Spasm of Sphincter of Oddi Obstruction of the pancreatic duct by drug-induced spasm of the sphincter (e.g.,by opiates, codeine, methyl choline). *2467*

577.00 Acute Pancreatitis Increases in 50% of patients and may remain elevated as long as 14 days after amylase returns to normal. *2467* Usually rises in parallel with the amylase activity, reaching its peak in 72 or 96 h with a gradual fall; values > 2.0 mL of N/100 NaOH are significant. *0151* Elevated in 63%, amylase in 70%, and 83% had parallel elevation of both enzymes. *0080* Elevated in 90% of cases. *2228 0433*

577.10 Chronic Pancreatitis As functioning tissue is destroyed, it is not uncommon to find only normal levels. *2238*

577.20 Pancreatic Cyst and Pseudocyst Laboratory findings preceding acute pancreatitis are present (this is mild and unrecognized in 33% of the cases). Persistent increase of serum amylase and lipase after an acute episode may indicate formation of a pseudocyst. *2467* May be elevated after recent attack of pancreatitis in pseudocyst. *0433*

584.00 Acute Renal Failure May be increased without evidence of pancreatitis in early stage. *2468*

829.00 Fracture of Bone In 30-50% of cases. *2468*

929.00 Crush Injury (Trauma) Activity increases in some patients sustaining severe injury to adipose tissue. *2104*

958.10 Fat Embolism Increased in 30-50% of cases. *2467*

Serum Normal

250.10 Diabetic Acidosis Normal levels. *1887*

577.10 Chronic Pancreatitis As functioning tissue is destroyed, it is not uncommon to find only normal levels. *2238*

633.90 Ectopic Pregnancy Normal levels. *1887*

Pleural Effusion Increase

577.00 Acute Pancreatitis May contain very high concentration, even with normal serum level. If the concentration are lower than the serum, pancreatitis is virtually excluded as the cause. *2199*

Ascitic Fluid Increase

577.00 Acute Pancreatitis May be elevated. *0080*

Duodenal Contents   Normal

577.20   Pancreatic Cyst and Pseudocyst   Duodenal contents after secretin-pancreozymin stimulation usually show decreased bicarbonate content (< 80 mmol/L) but normal volume and normal content of amylase, lipase, and trypsin. *2467*

Gastric Material   Decrease

260.00   Protein Malnutrition   In kwashiorkor. *0151*

Lipids

Serum   Decrease

38.00   Septicemia   Sepsis causes the concentration to decrease. *0049*

242.90   Hyperthyroidism   Total lipids are usually decreased. *2467*

272.52   Abetalipoproteinemia   Concentration of all major lipids reduced to 50% of normal. *2246*

281.00   Pernicious Anemia   Decreased in serum and the red cell membrane. *0619*

282.00   Hereditary (Congenital) Spherocytosis   Generalized hypolipidemia; with reduced phospholipids and total lipids occurs in children as well as adults with uncomplicated cases. *2109*

282.41   Thalassemia Major   Serum total lipid levels were found to be low in children with beta-thalassemia. The difference between the mean total lipid level in patients (365 mg/dL ± 75) as compared to that of the controls (581 mg/dL ± 94) was highly significant. *2607*   In 20 cases of thalassemia, there was reduction in red cell lipids and their fractions, plasma lipids and their fraction, and derangement of liver functions compared to controls. *1260*

282.60   Sickle Cell Anemia   Plasma lipids are significantly reduced and RBC cholesterol is higher in patients than in normal subjects. *0028*

434.90   Brain Infarction   In all patients a significant reduction in total lipids, cholesterol, triglyceride and all lipoproteins was demonstrated after the acute cerebrovascular accident presumedly due to the stress situation. *1192*

496.00   Chronic Obstructive Lung Disease   Decreased in decompensated patients. Amount of decrease correlates with degree of hypoxemia. *2044*

710.00   Systemic Lupus Erythematosus   Total lipid concentration was found to be low but HDL fraction was normal. *1435*

714.00   Rheumatoid Arthritis   In 54 female patients plasma lipid levels were low. *1435*

720.00   Rheumatoid (Ankylosing) Spondylitis   Total lipid concentration was found to be low. *1435*

Serum   Increase

155.00   Malignant Neoplasm of Liver   Sometimes present. Occasionally antedates the discovery of the tumor. *0962*

244.90   Hypothyroidism   Thyroid hormone insufficiency results in abnormal lipid metabolism with minimal to marked increases in circulating levels of cholesterol and triglycerides *0999*

250.10   Diabetic Acidosis   Level of serum sodium depends on degree of increased plasma lipids. *0999*   Often found. *0962*

271.01   Von Gierke's Disease   Rarely is there an increase, which is associated with impaired carbohydrate metabolism and associated ketosis. *0619*   Hyperlipidemia is a dominant feature. *1086*   Total lipids are significantly elevated. *2104*

271.02   McArdle's Disease   Total lipids are significantly elevated. *2104*

271.03   Forbes Disease   Total lipids are significantly elevated. *2104*

272.22   Type III Hyperlipoproteinemia   Diagnosis of abnormal lipoproteins can be done when the lipids are at normal concentration, but most patients are hyperlipidemic before they are diagnosed. *2246*

272.71   Anderson's Disease   Total lipids are significantly elevated. *2104*

303.90   Alcoholism   Rise after ingestion of moderate amounts of alcohol due to increased hepatic production and release of lipoproteins. *0962*

414.00   Chronic Ischemic Heart Disease   The severity of atherosclerosis was slightly positively correlated with triglyceride concentration, especially in the younger patients and (not significantly) with plasma cholesterol concentration. Hyperlipidemia was present in 58.8% of patients. *0508*   Studies of patients with coronary atherosclerotic heart disease and of their families have indicated a significantly higher incidence (16-44%) of elevated plasma cholesterol and/or triglyceride levels, usually classified as type II or type IV. *1108*

440.00   Arteriosclerosis   Hyperlipidemia was present in 43.9% of patients with atherosclerosis of the legs. Hyperlipidemia was frequently found in 219 male and 63 female patients. No significant relationship was found between uric acid and cholesterol or triglyceride. *0108*   *0508*

570.00   Acute and Subacute Necrosis of Liver   Increased in acute hepatitis. *0619*

571.20   Laennec's or Alcoholic Cirrhosis   In 28 patients, 13 showed hypercholesterolemia, 16 increased serum triglyceride and 8 increased serum phospholipid. *1045*   In fatty infiltration of the liver the serum cholesterol, triglyceride and total lipid concentrations were significantly increased, as compared with the normal values and with the figures obtained in the cases of chronic inflammatory liver disease. *0710*

571.60   Biliary Cirrhosis   Common. *0992*

571.90   Cirrhosis of Liver   Gross elevation noted in acute alcoholic liver injury and primary biliary cirrhosis. *0433*

576.20   Extrahepatic Biliary Obstruction   In cholestasis, the increase in alpha$_2$ and beta globulin components correlates with the height of serum lipid values and is a useful point in distinguishing between biliary obstructive lesions and other nonobstructive types of jaundice. *2339*

577.00   Acute Pancreatitis   Transient; subsides shortly after the onset of the disease and reappears with recurrences. These features differentiate the hyperlipidemia of acute pancreatitis from pancreatitis secondarily associated with primary abnormalities of lipid metabolism. *0433*   Patients with disease caused by alcohol may exhibit milky serum as a result of marked elevation of lipids. *2199*

577.10   Chronic Pancreatitis   *0619*

581.90   Nephrotic Syndrome   Characteristic hyperlipidemia occurs with elevations in cholesterol, phospholipids, and triglycerides. *0151*   Characterized by a great increase of all lipid constituents with both quantitative and qualitative alterations in lipoproteins. *0962*

585.00   Chronic Renal Failure   Raised in late renal failure, mainly due to a rise in triglycerides; phospholipids and cholesterol are normal or slightly elevated. *0151*

650.00   Pregnancy   Total serum lipids rise to a maximum by the 30th week, and regain prepregnancy levels by the 8th week postpartum. The increase is due to equal rises in cholesterol and phospholipids. *0619*   *1891*

758.70   Klinefelter's Syndrome (XXY)   Hyperlipidemia found in 8 of 24 patients; in 6, only cholesterol was elevated. *1454*

770.80   Respiratory Distress Syndrome   Plasma lipids, particularly triglycerides complexed with fibrins, were elevated severalfold in patients with adult respiratory distress. Plasma triglycerides complexed with fibrins were significantly higher in patients who died than in those who survived. *1324*

Serum   Normal

335.20   Amyotrophic Lateral Sclerosis   *0665*

Urine   Increase

250.00   Diabetes Mellitus   Lipids in the urine include all fractions. Double refractile (cholesterol) bodies can be seen. *2467*

580.00   Acute Poststreptococcal Glomerulonephritis   Lipid droplets may appear within the first few weeks. *0995*

581.90   Nephrotic Syndrome   All fractions increased. *2467*   Lipiduria is a regular feature of the nephrotic syndrome. It is recognized in the fatty casts present in great numbers as well as in the cells which appear to be shed by the kidney. *0999*

642.60   Eclampsia   Lipids in the urine include all fractions. Double refractile (cholesterol) bodies can be seen. There is a high protein content. *2467*

986.00   Toxic Effects of Carbon Monoxide   Lipids in the urine include all fractions. Double refractile (cholesterol) bodies can be seen. There is a high protein content. *2467*

Lipids *(continued)*

CSF   Decrease

331.90   Cerebral and Cortical Atrophy   Significantly low CSF values for cholesterol and total lipids were found in a group of patients with brain atrophy in comparison with a control group. It is possible that these changes are a function of reduced brain mass or of defect in brain lipid metabolism. *1035*

Feces   Increase

157.90   Malignant Neoplasm of Pancreas   Reduced intraluminal pancreatic enzyme activity with maldigestion of lipid and protein. *0962*

251.50   Zollinger-Ellison Syndrome   Hyperacidity in duodenum inactivates pancreatic enzymes. *0962*

277.00   Cystic Fibrosis   Reduced intraluminal pancreatic enzyme activity with maldigestion of lipid and protein. *0962*

577.10   Chronic Pancreatitis   Reduced intraluminal pancreatic enzyme activity with maldigestion of lipid and protein. *0962*

Red Blood Cells   Decrease

281.00   Pernicious Anemia   Decreased in serum and the red cell membrane. *0619*

282.41   Thalassemia Major   In 20 cases of thalassemia there was reduction in red cell lipids and their fractions, plasma lipids and their fractions, and derangement of liver functions compared to controls. *1260*

Lipoproteins

Serum   Decrease

272.31   Type I Hyperlipoproteinemia   Heavy chylomicronemia and subnormal concentrations of all other lipoproteins. (Type I hyperlipoproteinemia) is a qualitative abnormality which is not a specific marker for a single genetic disease. Occurs in familial lipoprotein lipase deficiency. *2246*

272.52   Abetalipoproteinemia   Only alpha lipoproteins are present. *0151*

282.00   Hereditary (Congenital) Spherocytosis   All classes of lipoproteins were reduced in children as well as adults with uncomplicated cases of congenital hemolytic anemia and spherocytosis. *2109*

334.00   Friedreich's Ataxia   Their total amount of high density lipoprotein was reduced and the composition was abnormal in both Friedreich's and familial spastic ataxia. *1091*

434.90   Brain Infarction   In all patients a significant reduction in total lipids, cholesterol, triglyceride and all lipoproteins was demonstrated after the acute cerebrovascular accident presumedly due to the stress situation. *1192*

Serum   Increase

277.30   Amyloidosis   May be present. *1108*   Has been observed. No correlation with severity or duration of the disease. *0120 2246*

405.91   Renovascular Hypertension   More than 50% of the patients showed obviously abnormal profiles of serum lipoproteins, which returned to normal or near-normal when the disease was ameliorated or corrected surgically. *2446*

440.00   Arteriosclerosis   Hyperuricemia and hyperlipidemia were frequently found in 219 male and 63 female patients. No significant relationship was found between uric acid and cholesterol or triglyceride, when the males were divided into lipoprotein types it was found that those who were normolipoproteinemic or who had type IV hyperlipoproteinemia had a significantly higher mean uric acid level. *0108*

496.01   Alpha$_1$-Antitrypsin Deficiency   Lipoprotein X was increased to an average of 855 mg/dL. *0563*

576.20   Extrahepatic Biliary Obstruction   Alpha$_2$ and beta globulins contain lipoproteins which may be markedly increased in cholestatic lesions of the liver. *2339*

577.00   Acute Pancreatitis   May be present. *2199*

580.00   Acute Poststreptococcal Glomerulonephritis   More than 50% of the patients with glomerulonephritis, nephrotic syndrome and renovascular hypertension showed obviously abnormal lipoprotein profiles, which returned to normal or near-normal when the disease was ameliorated or corrected surgically. *2446*

581.90   Nephrotic Syndrome   More than 50% of the patients with glomerulonephritis, nephrotic syndrome and renovascular hypertension showed obviously abnormal lipoprotein profiles, returning to normal or near-normal when the disease was ameliorated or corrected surgically. *2446   0833*

585.00   Chronic Renal Failure   Characteristically increased. Type IV hyperlipoproteinemia occurs commonly secondary to renal failure. *1038*   42 of 100 patients had type IV hyperlipoproteinemia, which did not correlate with degree of disease, or age, sex, weight or diet of patient. *2557*

Serum   Normal

335.20   Amyotrophic Lateral Sclerosis   *0665*

Pleural Effusion   Increase

482.90   Bacterial Pneumonia   Pleural effusions in patients with bacterial pleurisy contain low density lipoproteins (33% of the serum LDL concentration on average) but almost no very low density lipoproteins (about 1% of the serum VLDL concentration on average). *1913*

Lipoproteins, Beta

Serum   Decrease

256.30   Ovarian Hypofunction   Estrogen effect. *0995*

272.22   Type III Hyperlipoproteinemia   There is generally a decrease in alpha and beta lipoproteins. *0774*   Slight to moderately decreased. *2246   0772 1631*

272.31   Type I Hyperlipoproteinemia   There is generally a decrease in alpha and beta lipoproteins. *0774   0772 1631*

272.32   Type V Hyperlipoproteinemia   In severely affected patients. *2246*   Chylomicronemia and hyperprebeta-lipoproteinemia were accompanied by reduction in pools of beta and alpha lipoproteins. *2177*

272.51   Tangier Disease   Levels tend to be reduced. *0151*

272.52   Abetalipoproteinemia   Complete absence of LDL. *0151*   None present. *0878*

334.00   Friedreich's Ataxia   Total amount of high density lipoprotein reduced in Friedreich's and familial spastic ataxia. *1091*

496.00   Chronic Obstructive Lung Disease   Decreased in decompensated patients. Amount of decrease correlates with degree of hypoxemia. *2044*

Serum   Increase

203.00   Multiple Myeloma   *0774 0772 0773*

244.90   Hypothyroidism   *0774 0772 0773*

250.00   Diabetes Mellitus   *0774 0772 0773*

256.00   Ovarian Hyperfunction   Estrogen effect. *0995*

272.00   Type IIA Hyperlipoproteinemia   Characterized by an increase in beta-lipoproteins clearly visible on electrophoresis. *1108*   Marked increase. *2467   0151*

272.21   Type IIB Hyperlipoproteinemia   Serum cholesterol level is elevated, equal to or > triglyceride level, both LDL and VLDL are increased. *0151*   Characterized by an increase in beta-lipoproteins clearly visible on electrophoresis. *1108*   Marked increase. *2467*

277.14   Acute Intermittent Porphyria   *0151*

277.15   Porphyria Variegata   *0151*

277.17   Hereditary Coproporphyria   *0151*

571.20   Laennec's or Alcoholic Cirrhosis   In fatty infiltration of the liver the serum total lipid concentrations were significantly increased, as compared with the normal values and with the figures obtained in the cases of chronic inflammatory liver disease. Beta and prebeta lipoprotein were increased. *0710*

576.20   Extrahepatic Biliary Obstruction   *0774 0772 0773*

581.90   Nephrotic Syndrome   Untreated uncomplicated nephrotic syndrome is characterized by increased low (beta) and very low (prebeta) density lipoproteins and a diminution of high density (alpha) lipoprotein. Changes correlated strictly with albumin concentrat were more pronounced with albumin concentration < 20 g/L. *0833*   In severe, fully developed cases, increase in low density lipoproteins with normal or decreased alpha lipoproteins has been described. *0962*

585.00   Chronic Renal Failure   Increased mean plasma concentration in chronic failure. *1243*

592.00 Kidney Calculus With corresponding increase in beta:alpha ratio. *2416*

642.40 Pre-Eclampsia Significantly elevated. *0433* Higher than in normal late pregnancy. *1073 2286 0409 0387 2287*

642.60 Eclampsia Significantly elevated. *0433*

1013.00 Diet With high saturated fat and/or cholesterol diet. *0774 0772 0773*

Serum Normal

994.50 Exercise No change was observed after exercise. *1837*

CSF Decrease

346.00 Migraine Significantly lower (P < 0.005). *0825*

Pleural Effusion Present

482.90 Bacterial Pneumonia Pleural effusions in patients with bacterial pleurisy contain low density lipoproteins (33% of the serum LDL concentration on average) but almost no very low density lipoproteins (about 1% of the serum VLDL concentration on average). *1913*

Lipoproteins, Prebeta

Serum Decrease

272.31 Type I Hyperlipoproteinemia Normal or decreased. *0503*

272.52 Abetalipoproteinemia Absent or below standard measuring capabilities. *2246* None present. *0878*

Serum Increase

272.10 Type IV Hyperlipoproteinemia Type IV hyperlipemia is manifested as hyper-prebeta-lipoproteinemia. This is associated with an increase in triglycerides above normal limits and is commonly accompanied by a rise in cholesterol of about 1 mg/dL for each 5 mg/dL increase in triglyceride concentration. *0773* Characteristic lipid abnormality is an increase in plasma triglyceride and VLDL cholesterol levels. *1108* Prebeta-lipoproteins alone are generally increased. *0151*

272.21 Type IIB Hyperlipoproteinemia May be elevated. *0992*

272.22 Type III Hyperlipoproteinemia An increase in very low density lipoproteins of abnormal composition is the basis for type III diagnosis. *1631* VLDL defined as including all lipoproteins of density < 1.006. *2246*

272.31 Type I Hyperlipoproteinemia May be raised. *0995*

272.32 Type V Hyperlipoproteinemia In severely affected patients. *2246* Hyperprebeta-lipoproteinemia accompanied by low alpha and beta lipoproteinemia. *2177*

282.41 Thalassemia Major Mean concentration in 50 children was significantly elevated. *0547*

434.00 Cerebral Thrombosis Significant rise was noticed in all patients. *0112*

581.90 Nephrotic Syndrome Untreated uncomplicated nephrotic syndrome is characterized by increased low (beta) and very low (prebeta) density lipoproteins and a diminution of high density (alpha) lipoprotein. Changes correlated strictly with albumin concentration and were more pronounced with albumin concentration < 20 g/L. *0833*

585.00 Chronic Renal Failure Consistent rise in late renal failure. *0151* Increased mean plasma concentration in chronic failure. *1243*

Serum Normal

272.00 Type IIA Hyperlipoproteinemia *0503*

Pleural Effusion Decrease

482.90 Bacterial Pneumonia Pleural effusions in patients with bacterial pleurisy contain low density lipoproteins (33% of the serum LDL concentration on average) but almost no very low density lipoproteins (about 1% of the serum VLDL concentration on average). *1913*

Lithocholic Acid

Feces Decrease

211.40 Benign Neoplasm of Rectum and Anus Increased cholesterol and decreased lithocholic acid is excreted in patients with familial polyposis. *1895*

Feces Increase

153.90 Malignant Neoplasm of Large Intestine The fecal excretion of cholesterol, coprostanol, coprostanone, total bile acids, deoxycholic acid, lithocholic acid was higher in colonic cancer and adenomatous polyps compared to normal controls as well as in patients with other digestive diseases. *1896*

211.40 Benign Neoplasm of Rectum and Anus The fecal excretion of cholesterol, coprostanol, coprostanone, total bile acids, deoxycholic acid, lithocholic acid was higher in patients with colon cancer and patients with adenomatous polyps compared to normal American and Japanese controls as well as in patients with other digestive diseases. *1896*

Long Acting Thyroid Stimulating Hormone (LATS)

Serum Increase

242.90 Hyperthyroidism Present in most patients with Graves' disease. *2145* Found in at most 80% of patients with Graves' disease, and its presence or level does not correlate uniformly with thyroid hyperactivity. *0151* Detected in about 50% of patients with hyperthyroidism of Graves' disease and in many patients who are euthyroid or hypothyroid. *1415 2035*

245.20 Hashimoto's Thyroiditis Occasionally. *2540*

Luteinizing Hormone (LH)

Serum Decrease

185.00 Malignant Neoplasm of Prostate Patients with prostatic carcinoma and benign prostatic hypertrophy showed lower levels of LH when compared with age-matched controls. *0971*

253.40 Anterior Pituitary Hypofunction Decreased to values seen during follicular phase rather than luteal phase of menstrual cycle with galactorrhea amenorrhea syndromes. *2468* Characterized by absent or reduced production and release. *1108* Compatible with stage of sexual development, not with age. *0399*

275.00 Hemochromatosis Hypogonadism frequently occurs in idiopathic hemochromatosis. *2473* Depressed in 44% of 32 patients; generalized depression of pituitary function. *2266*

282.60 Sickle Cell Anemia Serum LH and FSH before and after stimulation with gonadotropin releasing hormone were consistent with primary testicular failure in all 14 adult male patients tested. *0005*

600.00 Benign Prostatic Hypertrophy Patients with both malignant and benign prostatic disease showed lower concentrations when compared with age-matched controls. *0971*

Serum Increase

242.90 Hyperthyroidism *1731*

256.40 Polycystic Ovaries Elevated in polycystic ovary disease. *0879*

256.41 Stein-Leventhal Syndrome Slightly elevated levels. *0151*

303.90 Alcoholism The basal level of LH was significantly elevated in alcoholics with and without clinically evident sexual disorders. *2169*

627.90 Menopausal and Postmenopausal Symptoms *0433*

758.70 Klinefelter's Syndrome (XXY) Commonly elevated; result of deficient testicular function. *1090* May either be high or normal. *0151*

758.80 Syndromes Due to Sex Chromosome Abnormalities Usually doesn't increase until puberty. *0186*

Urine Increase

758.70 Klinefelter's Syndrome (XXY) *0186*

Luteinizing Hormone (LH) *(continued)*

CSF Increase

194.30 Malignant Neoplasm of Pituitary 21 of 22 patients with suprasellar extension of a pituitary tumor had elevations of one or more CSF adenohypophyseal hormones. *1189*

Lymphocyte B-Cell

Blood Decrease

279.04 Agammaglobulinemia (Congenital Sex-linked) Complete absence. *2539*

279.06 Immunodeficiency (Common Variable) Normal or decreased. *2539*

279.20 Severe Combined Immunodeficiency Absent or markedly reduced. *0793*

Blood Normal

279.01 IgA Deficiency (Selective) *0793*

279.11 DiGeorge's Syndrome *0793*

279.12 Wiskott-Aldrich Syndrome *2539*

279.13 Nezeloff's Syndrome *0793*

Lymphocytes

Blood Decrease

9.00 Gastroenteritis and Colitis In viral gastroenteritis, during acute illness, a transient lymphopenia was noted which involved all lymphocyte subpopulations. *0577*

13.00 Tuberculosis Meningitis *0532*

37.00 Tetanus Lymphopenia is more usual than lymphocytosis. *0433*

38.00 Septicemia In 78% of 14 patients at initial hospitalization for this disorder. *0781*

40.20 Whipple's Disease An absolute lymphopenia due to loss of lymphocytes into the small intestine. *0962*

45.90 Acute Poliomyelitis The numbers of circulating lymphocytes are sharply and regularly reduced. *0783*

52.00 Chickenpox The numbers of circulating lymphocytes are sharply and regularly reduced. *2521*

55.00 Measles The numbers of circulating lymphocytes are sharply and regularly reduced. *2521* *2035*

60.00 Yellow Fever The numbers of circulating lymphocytes are sharply and regularly reduced. *2521* *2035*

70.00 Viral Hepatitis Impaired T-cell reactivity is due to a disturbed function of T-cell and not to a decrease in their number. In cases associated with significant hepatocellular damage, a reduction in the number of circulating B-cells was observed. *1709*

104.10 Lyme Disease Lymphopenia occurs in Lyme Disease. *2639*

130.00 Toxoplasmosis *0532*

135.00 Sarcoidosis Absolute lymphopenia occurs in pulmonary sarcoidosis and correlates very closely with prognosis. A steady increase in absolute number indicates good prognosis (with or without treatment). No increase or a very low and unchanged number indicates very poor prognosis. *0260* In 52% of 25 patients at initial hospitalization for this disorder. *0781*

150.90 Malignant Neoplasm of Esophagus In 55% of 36 patients at initial hospitalization for this disorder. *0781*

151.90 Malignant Neoplasm of Stomach In 60% of 44 patients at initial hospitalization for this disorder. *0781* Relative lymphocytopenia may occur as a result of absolute increase in monocytes and polymorphonuclear cells in inflammatory bowel disease. *2345*

172.90 Malignant Melanoma of Skin Active rosettes (T-EA) were decreased only in metastatic patients, while the total T population (T-ET) was decreased in all stages. Patients whose values were constant remained cancer free, while a reduction heralded the appearance of clinical and/or radiological signs of metastases. *0185*

191.90 Malignant Neoplasm of Brain In 19 different groups of neurological diseases, absolute and relative T-lymphocyte populations were significantly decreased only in patients with acute Guillian-Barre Syndrome, active multiple sclerosis, and malignant cerebral tumor. *2540* In 38% of 23 patients at initial hospitalization for this disorder. *0781*

197.00 Secondary Malignant Neoplasm of Respiratory System In 59% of 581 patients at initial hospitalization for this disorder. *0781*

199.00 Secondary Malignant Neoplasm (Disseminated) Active rosettes (T-EA) were decreased only in metastatic patients, while the total T population (T-ET) was decreased in all stages. Patients whose values were constant remained cancer free, while a reduction heralded the appearance of clinical and/or radiological signs of metastases. *0185*

201.90 Hodgkin's Disease Lymphopenia is common late in the disease. *0999* Absolute counts tend to be at the lower end of the normal range or slightly below the lower limit. Frequently more severe in the presence of disseminated disease. *2035* In 66% of 76 patients at initial hospitalization for this disorder. *0781* *0532*

205.10 Myelocytic Leukemia (Chronic) In 85% of 21 patients at initial hospitalization for this disorder. *0781*

250.00 Diabetes Mellitus The percentage and absolute number of peripheral T-lymphocytes were significantly lower (38.1% and 833/μL) in juvenile-onset diabetics than in normal subjects or maternity-onset diabetics. There was no significant difference between normals and maternity-onset cases. *0360*

250.10 Diabetic Acidosis Often a polymorphonucleocytosis with a lymphopenia and eosinopenia. *0962*

251.50 Zollinger-Ellison Syndrome Often an absolute lymphopenia due to loss of lymphocytes into the small intestine. *0962*

255.00 Adrenal Cortical Hyperfunction (Glucocorticoid Excess) Relative lymphopenia is frequent (differential is usually < 15%). *2468* Patients with hypercortisolism often have neutrophilia, lymphopenia, and eosinopenia. *0962* *0433*

260.00 Protein Malnutrition Decreased total count < 1,500/μL. *0186*

271.30 Lactosuria Often an absolute lymphopenia due to loss of lymphocytes into the small intestine. *0962*

279.04 Agammaglobulinemia (Congenital Sex-linked) There is a decreased number of lymphocytes in the congenital forms. *0433*

279.06 Immunodeficiency (Common Variable) Significant deficiency of T and B Lymphocytes. Clinical findings are usually associated with abnormal T-Lymphocyte function. *2539* *0996* *2468*

279.11 DiGeorge's Syndrome Profound lymphopenia and T_5+/T_8+ cells are relatively more deficient than T_4+ cells. *2539*

279.12 Wiskott-Aldrich Syndrome Diminished T-Lymphocytes in some patients. *0996* *2344*

279.20 Severe Combined Immunodeficiency *0793*

279.31 Acquired Immunodeficiency Syndrome (AIDS) Lymphopenia less than 1500 cells/mL is often present and the absolute number of cells in the T helper/inducer subset is depressed. *2539* < 1500 cells/μL in 26 of 35 patients. 91.6% of patients had decreased concentration of T-Helper cells. *0646* Absolute lymphopenia in 1 of 29 children tested. *1760*

284.90 Aplastic Anemia The absolute count is often decreased. *2538*

288.00 Agranulocytosis The lymphocytes number below about 1,400/μL in children or 1,000/μL in adults. *0151* Variable. *0992*

334.80 Ataxia-Telangiectasia T-lymphocytes and T-cell functions are regularly grossly deficient. *0151* Variable; below 1,000/μL in 33% of patients. *2552*

340.00 Multiple Sclerosis In 19 different groups of neurological diseases, absolute and relative T-lymphocyte populations were significantly decreased only in patients with acute Guillain-Barré Syndrome, active multiple sclerosis and malignant cerebral tumor. *2540*

357.00 Guillain-Barré Syndrome In 19 different groups of neurological diseases, absolute and relative T-lymphocyte populations were significantly decreased only in patients with acute Guillain-Barré Syndrome, active multiple sclerosis and malignant cerebral tumor. *2540* During active phase of disease. *0878*

358.00 Myasthenia Gravis 17 of 32 patients had counts < 1,500/μL and 18 of the 32 did not develop sensitivity to dinitrochlorobenzene. *0003* *2035*

423.10 Constrictive Pericarditis *0999*

480.90 Viral Pneumonia In 52% of 15 patients at initial hospitalization for this disorder. *0781*

487.10 Influenza Leukopenia and lymphopenia are often seen early in influenza but mild leukocytosis is more common. *0999* The numbers of circulating lymphocytes are sharply and regularly reduced. *2521*

540.90 Acute Appendicitis In 80% of 105 patients at initial hospitalization for this disorder. *0781*

570.00 Acute and Subacute Necrosis of Liver Transient. *0992*

579.00 Celiac Sprue Disease Often an absolute lymphopenia due to loss of lymphocytes into the small intestine. *0962* Uncommon but may occur if severe folate or vitamin B_{12} deficiency is present. *2199*

581.90 Nephrotic Syndrome In 41% of 26 patients at initial hospitalization for this disorder. *0781*

584.00 Acute Renal Failure *0277*

585.00 Chronic Renal Failure In 66% of 141 patients at initial hospitalization for this disorder. *0781*

710.00 Systemic Lupus Erythematosus Overall depression of peripheral blood leukocytes frequently with a lymphopenia and a slight shift to the left in the granulocytic series. *0433* In 158 patients with active, untreated disease, lymphopenia was present in 75%, and another 18% of those patients developed lymphopenia subsequent to disease reactivation. Lymphopenia of < 1,500 occurred more frequently than any of the preliminary criteria and it was the most prevalent initial laboratory abnormality. *1949*

756.52 Osteopetrosis Relative lymphocytosis or lymphocytopenia may occur. *2468*

990.00 Effects of X-Ray Irradiation The earliest laboratory finding is lymphopenia, reaching absolute lymphocyte levels below 1,000/μL within the first 48 postexposure h in cases of radiation injury. *0151* Lymphopenia commences immediately becoming maximal within 24-36 h. *0995 0532*

Blood Increase

2.00 Typhoid Fever A low WBC count with a relative lymphocytosis is commonly seen. *0433*

11.00 Pulmonary Tuberculosis *2467*

13.00 Tuberculosis Meningitis *0532*

23.00 Brucellosis Relative lymphocytosis in some cases. *0962 0433*

33.00 Whooping Cough Though the WBC count and the differential counts may be quite variable, > 20,000/μL with more than 70% small lymphocytes indicates this disease. *0433* Moderate to severe leukocytosis, ranging from 15,000-40,000/μL with a differential of 60-90% lymphocytes. *0962* Begins late in the catarrhal stage and rises steeply. *2368*

38.00 Septicemia In convalescence from acute infection. *2467*

49.00 Lymphocytic Choriomeningitis Relative lymphocytosis. *2368*

50.00 Smallpox Leukopenia is found in the first days of illness followed by leukocytosis with lymphocytosis and a high percentage of metamyelocytes. *0433*

56.00 Rubella Increased during the rash. *2468*

66.10 Tick-Borne Fever Relative. *1058*

70.00 Viral Hepatitis A relative lymphocytosis may result with some atypical lymphocytes. *0962 0433 0532*

72.00 Mumps Usually there is a slight predominance of lymphocytes but at times the reverse is true. *1319 2467*

75.00 Infectious Mononucleosis Absolute and relative lymphocytosis are characteristic and requisite for diagnosis. *0433* An absolute increase in the number of atypical lymphocytes is a characteristic finding during all stages of the disease. *1319* Marked lymphocytosis, both relative and absolute. At least 50-60% of the WBCs are lymphocytes or monocytes; and at least 10% are atypical lymphocytes. *0962 2538 2368*

78.50 Cytomegalic Inclusion Disease Increase in WBC to 15,000-20,000/μL with 60-80% lymphocytes, many of which are Downey cell type. *2468*

83.20 Rickettsialpox Typify the acute phase. *0433*

84.00 Malaria Depletion of T cells was found associated with an increased proportion of null cells. K cell activity was also increased and it is likely that some of the increased number of null cells were K cells. *0917*

86.90 Trypanosomiasis Relative lymphocytosis. *1058*

97.90 Syphilis Absolute increase. *1058*

99.10 Lymphogranuloma Venereum Mild leukocytosis with a relative lymphocytosis or monocytosis. *2199*

115.00 Histoplasmosis Leukopenia with lymphocytosis is frequently present. *2368*

130.00 Toxoplasmosis Slight. *0151 0532*

174.90 Malignant Neoplasm of Breast 6 patients with advanced cancer had significantly higher numbers of B lymphocytes than patients with benign breast disease. *1370*

180.90 Malignant Neoplasm of Cervix In 44% of 146 patients at initial hospitalization for this disorder. *0781*

201.90 Hodgkin's Disease Relative lymphocytosis when there is marked neutropenia but not absolute increase. *2246 0532*

202.80 Non-Hodgkins Lymphoma *0433 0532*

203.00 Multiple Myeloma 40-55% lymphocytosis frequently present on differential count, with variable number of immature lymphocytic and plasmacytic forms. *2468* Relative lymphocytosis of 40-55% with a variable proportion of immature lymphocytic and plasmacytic forms. *2035*

204.10 Lymphocytic Leukemia (Chronic) Generally, lymphocytosis consisting of mature lymphocytes with counts > 100,000/μL in a patient over 50 y of age is diagnostic. *0433* In 24 treated patients, the origin of malignant cells was found to be the B lymphocyte population. On the basis of a reactive T lymphocyte proliferation in patients with chronic lymphatic leukemia, a coefficient of active T lymphocytes has been deduced which proved to be a rapid indicator of a short-term prognosis. *0999 0992 1910 0685 0805 0612*

242.90 Hyperthyroidism Although a peripheral blood lymphocytosis has been noted in the past, a recent study of the distribution of T and B lymphocytes showed a slightly decreased number of T cells, and consequently of total lymphocytes. *2403* Relative lymphocytosis. *2540*

253.40 Anterior Pituitary Hypofunction Marked. *0433* Relative lymphocytosis. *0995*

255.40 Adrenal Cortical Hypofunction WBC may be normal or increased with a tendency to lymphocytosis and eosinophilia. *0433* May be a relative lymphocytosis and moderate eosinophilia. *0962*

273.23 Heavy Chain Disease (Gamma) Atypical lymphocytes *0186* Relative lymphocytosis. *2468*

273.30 Waldenström's Macroglobulinemia Absolute lymphocytosis with atypical, immature, and plasmacytic forms in many cases, and occasionally reaching leukemic proportions. *2035* Relative lymphocytosis. *2468*

282.00 Hereditary (Congenital) Spherocytosis During the chronic stage of anemia. *0810 2552*

282.41 Thalassemia Major Especially in infants. *2552*

287.30 Idiopathic Thrombocytopenic Purpura In chronic cases. *0995* Lymphocytosis with abnormal cells resembling those found in infectious mononucleosis. *2552*

288.00 Agranulocytosis Variable and may be decreased, normal or increased. *0992*

304.90 Drug Dependence (Opium and Derivatives) Persistent absolute and relative lymphocytosis occurs with often bizarre and atypical cells that may resemble Downey cells. *2468*

381.00 Otitis Media In 66% of 70 patients hospitalized for this disorder. *0781*

446.60 Thrombotic Thrombocytopenic Purpura Often with a relative lymphocytosis, atypical lymphocytes (particularly in children), and eosinophilia. *2035 2552*

480.90 Viral Pneumonia Normal or low WBC with a relative lymphocytosis. *1905* In 39% of 15 patients at initial hospitalization for this disorder *0781*

483.01 Mycoplasma Pneumoniae May occur during the period of acute illness. *0151*

487.10 Influenza The percentage of T-lymphocytes was decreased but a relative and absolute increase of non-T-lymphocytes occurred. *1152*

570.00 Acute and Subacute Necrosis of Liver Relative lymphocytosis. *0992* Atypical lymphocytes varying between 2-20% is common during the acute phase. *0992*

756.52 Osteopetrosis Relative lymphocytosis or lymphocytopenia may occur. *2468*

990.00 Effects of X-Ray Irradiation *0532*

992.00 Heat stroke *2467*

Blood Normal

205.10 Myelocytic Leukemia (Chronic) Absolute count is usually within normal limits. *2552*

245.10 Subacute Thyroiditis T-lymphocytes may increase with a concomitant decrease in B-lymphocytes. *0151* Usually normal. *2540*

279.04 Agammaglobulinemia (Congenital Sex-linked) Counts are normal (> 2,000/μL). *2035*

Lymphocytes (continued)

Blood Normal (continued)

279.11 DiGeorge's Syndrome Patients have partial or complete T cell immunodeficiency with normal or near normal B cell immune function. *2539* May be normal but virtually all are B-cells. *0996*

284.90 Aplastic Anemia Production is not considered impaired. *2538*

288.00 Agranulocytosis Variable and may be decreased, normal or increased. *0992*

Urine Increase

580.01 Glomerulonephritis (Focal) May be found. *0951*

CSF Increase

13.00 Tuberculosis Meningitis 30-100% of CSF cells are lymphocytes. *0999* Count usually varies between 10-500/μL and consists mainly of lymphocytes, except in the early stage when neutrophils predominate. *0962*

18.00 Disseminated Tuberculosis Predominantly mononuclear pleocytosis (up to several hundred cells/μL). *0999*

45.90 Acute Poliomyelitis Cell count is usually 25-500/μL at first most are polymorphonuclear leukocytes; after several days most are lymphocytes. *2468* *0433*

47.00 Aseptic Meningitis After first day or two differential shifts to predominantly lymphocytes. *0999* Increased in 50% of the patients. *0790* Count ranges from 50-300/μL and rarely > 2,000. Marked predominance of lymphocytes except in the earliest stage. *0962*

49.00 Lymphocytic Choriomeningitis 100-3,000/μL, occasionally up to 30,000. *2468* Cell count is between 50-3,500/μL, 80-95% lymphocytes. *2368*

52.00 Chickenpox With CNS involvement the cells in the CSF number from normal to < 100/μL and are almost exclusively lymphocytes. *1058*

53.00 Herpes Zoster Lymphocytes pleocytosis. *1058* CSF commonly shows a pleocytosis and elevation of protein, even when clinical signs of meningeal irritation or encephalomyelitis are absent. *0151*

62.10 Western Equine Encephalitis Usually predominate. *1058*

62.20 Eastern Equine Encephalitis Usually predominate. *1058*

72.00 Mumps Cell counts range from 500 to several thousand/μL, and are predominantly lymphocytes. *0151* Increased T-cells and decreased B-cells in CSF were found in mumps meningitis. *1214* *0790*

86.90 Trypanosomiasis Up to 2,000/μL with CNS involvement. *1058*

97.90 Syphilis CSF count may be elevated, with 5-10 or more lymphocytes/μL. *0962* Majority of cells are lymphocytes with CNS involvement. *2368* *0151*

100.00 Leptospirosis Lymphocytic pleocytosis is common with counts from 100-300/μL. *2368*

114.90 Coccidioidomycosis Fewer than 500 leukocytes/μL, as many as 50% neutrophils initially with lymphocytes predominating later. *1058*

117.50 Cryptococcosis Characteristically outnumber neutrophils. *1058*

130.00 Toxoplasmosis In congenital and acquired. *1319*

320.90 Meningitis (Bacterial) Lymphocytes will be more prevalent in the CSF if the disease moves into the subacute or chronic stage. Polymorphonuclear neutrophils may predominate in the early phase of an aseptic or viral meningitis. *0433*

323.91 Myelitis Spinal fluid may be normal or may show increased protein and cells (20-1,000/μL -- lymphocytes and mononuclear cells). *2467* *0999*

323.92 Encephalomyelitis Approximately 66% of the patients show a lymphocytic pleocytosis in the spinal fluid, but in the remaining 33%, the CSF is normal. *0433*

324.00 Intracranial Abscess Count usually ranges from 50-300/μL and consists predominantly of lymphocytes. *0962* In the range of 50-1,000/μL. *0995*

324.10 Intraspinal Abscess Usually 1-100 WBC/μL with predominantly lymphocytes present in spinal epidural abscess. *0151*

340.00 Multiple Sclerosis Significant increase in T-lymphocytes. *1214*

357.00 Guillain-Barré Syndrome While it is true most cases show few, if any, lymphocytes, a few show up to 20-30 cells/μL. *0878*

357.90 Polyneuritis CSF shows increased protein and up to several hundred mononuclear cells in polyneuritis due to infectious mononucleosis. *2467*

363.20 Inflammation of Optic Nerve and Retina CSF is normal or may show increased protein and up to 200 lymphocytes/μL. *2467*

CSF Normal

9.00 Gastroenteritis and Colitis Normal except when aseptic meningoencephalitis is part of the overall syndrome. Then lymphocytic pleocytosis is found. *0433*

Synovial Fluid Increase

714.30 Juvenile Rheumatoid Arthritis Abundant lymphocytes (sometimes > 50%) and immature lymphocytes and monocytes present in the synovial fluid. *2467* *2468*

Pleural Effusion Decrease

11.00 Pulmonary Tuberculosis In patients with pulmonary tuberculosis, pulmonary malignancy or nonspecific pleuritis, the percentages and absolute numbers of B lymphocytes were significantly lower in pleural fluid than in peripheral blood. *1809*

197.00 Secondary Malignant Neoplasm of Respiratory System In patients with pulmonary tuberculosis, pulmonary malignancy or nonspecific pleuritis, the percentages and absolute number of B lymphocytes were significantly lower in pleural fluid than in peripheral blood. *1809*

Pleural Effusion Increase

11.00 Pulmonary Tuberculosis Both the percentage and absolute numbers in pleural fluid were significantly higher than in peripheral blood. *1809* 43 of 46 patients had effusions with > 50% small lymphocytes. *1403* The percentage and absolute numbers of B lymphocytes were significantly lower in pleural fluid than in peripheral blood. *1809* Characterized by a protein content of 3 g/dL and the presence of lymphocytes. *0962* A preponderance of lymphocytes is consistent with tuberculosis, carcinoma, or lymphoma. *0962*

162.90 Malignant Neoplasm of Bronchus and Lung Pleural effusion with > 50% of the WBC as small lymphocytes are highly indicative of malignancy or tuberculosis. Of 96 such effusions, 43 were TB and 47 were cancerous. 47 of 90 patients with lung cancer had predominantly small lymphocytes in effusions. *1403* In patients with pulmonary tuberculosis, pulmonary malignancy or nonspecific pleuritis, the percentages and absolute numbers of B lymphocytes were significantly lower in pleural fluid than in peripheral blood. *1809*

201.90 Hodgkin's Disease A preponderance of lymphocytes is consistent with tuberculosis, carcinoma, or lymphoma. *0962*

202.80 Non-Hodgkins Lymphoma A preponderance of lymphocytes is consistent with tuberculosis, carcinoma or lymphoma. *0962*

Ascitic Fluid Increase

11.00 Pulmonary Tuberculosis Characteristic of chronic inflammatory disease, especially tuberculosis. *2199*

18.00 Disseminated Tuberculosis Characteristic of chronic inflammatory disease, especially tuberculosis. *2199*

567.90 Peritonitis A high percentage suggests tuberculous peritonitis. *0151*

Bone Marrow Increase

273.23 Heavy Chain Disease (Gamma) Bone marrow aspirations and lymph node biopsies have demonstrated a proliferation of plasmacytic and lymphocytic forms, along with eosinophils and large reticulum or reticuloendothelial cells, (the pattern of a pleomorphic reticular neoplasm). *2035* Bone marrow may be normal, but usually there is an increased proportion of plasma cells or lymphocytes or both, often accompanied by eosinophilia. *2538*

273.30 Waldenström's Macroglobulinemia Proliferation of lymphocytic and plasmacytic forms with many intermediate and apparently transitional cell types. *2035* *0188*

284.90 Aplastic Anemia 60-100% of the nucleated cells are lymphocytes. *2552*

733.00 Osteoporosis The iliac bone marrow specimens showed infiltrates consisting of elongated mast cells, eosinophils, plasma cells, and varying numbers of lymphocytes. *2334*

Lung Tissue Increase

486.01 Resolving Pneumonia In 13 patients with lymphocytic interstitial pneumonitis, lung biopsies in all cases showed diffuse interstitial infiltrations consisting of mature lymphocytes and plasma cells. *2283*

Peritoneal Fluid Increase

11.00 Pulmonary Tuberculosis Cell count in the peritoneal fluid varies from 2,000-10,000/μL and shows a marked predominance of lymphocytes. *0962*

Sputum Increase

491.00 Chronic Bronchitis *0433*

494.00 Bronchiectasis Microscopic examination reveals polymorphonuclear and lymphocytic, as well as bronchial epithelial cells with varying degrees of metaplasia. *0433*

Lymphocyte T-Cell

Blood Decrease

11.00 Pulmonary Tuberculosis *0793*

18.00 Disseminated Tuberculosis *0793*

30.00 Leprosy *0793*

56.00 Rubella *0793*

199.00 Secondary Malignant Neoplasm (Disseminated) *0793*

201.90 Hodgkin's Disease *0793*

260.00 Protein Malnutrition *0793*

279.06 Immunodeficiency (Common Variable) Normal or decreased. *2539*

279.11 DiGeorge's Syndrome Usually low but may be normal or increased. *0793*

279.12 Wiskott-Aldrich Syndrome Normal immunity initially but may decline with advancing years. *2539*

279.13 Nezeloff's Syndrome Studies of T cell immunity are abnormal but the degree of deficiency may vary. *0793*

279.20 Severe Combined Immunodeficiency Deficient immunity. *0793*

279.31 Acquired Immunodeficiency Syndrome (AIDS) The risk of AIDS is clearly predicted by the total number of circulating OKTA positive lymphocytes (T_4). *0860*

480.90 Viral Pneumonia *0793*

571.49 Chronic Active Hepatitis *0793*

710.00 Systemic Lupus Erythematosus *0793*

Blood Normal

279.01 IgA Deficiency (Selective) *0793*

279.04 Agammaglobulinemia (Congenital Sex-linked) Normal to increased. *2539*

714.00 Rheumatoid Arthritis Increased T_4/T_8 ratio. *0062*

Lysine

Serum Decrease

259.20 Carcinoid Syndrome Decreased plasma concentration, but normal urinary excretion was found. *0718*

Urine Increase

270.01 Cystinuria Characteristic. *2246 2468*

270.03 Cystinosis Nonspecific pattern of aminoaciduria. Fanconi's syndrome. *0995*

Lysolecithin

Gastric Material Increase

533.90 Peptic Ulcer, Site Unspecified Found to be high. *1174*

Lysozyme

Serum Decrease

202.40 Leukemic Reticuloendotheliosis Low, normal or high. *0798*

204.00 Lymphocytic Leukemia (Acute) Low or normal. *0798*

204.10 Lymphocytic Leukemia (Chronic) Low or normal. *0798*

205.00 Myelocytic Leukemia (Acute) Low, normal or moderately increased. *0798*

Serum Increase

11.00 Pulmonary Tuberculosis Isolated cases. *0981*

18.00 Disseminated Tuberculosis Isolated cases. *0981*

135.00 Sarcoidosis Highest in patients with the most extensive disease and falls progressively in stage II to I. All patients with disease involving the spleen showed increased activity. *1777* Most frequently elevated in patients with pulmonary parenchymal involvement. *1968*

201.90 Hodgkin's Disease Significantly higher compared to controls and independent of stage. *0258* Isolated cases *0981*

202.40 Leukemic Reticuloendotheliosis Low, normal or high. *0798*

203.00 Multiple Myeloma Isolated cases. *0981*

205.00 Myelocytic Leukemia (Acute) During the transition from a variety of myeloproliferative disorders to acute myeloblastic or acute myelomonocytic leukemia, there is a striking elevation in serum and urine muramidase activity. *2093* Low, normal, or moderately increased. *0798 0151*

205.10 Myelocytic Leukemia (Chronic) Elevated only in patients who do not have the Philadelphia chromosome. No correlation is apparent between urine and serum levels. *2093*

206.00 Monocytic Leukemia Elevated in serum and urine in some patients with acute monocytic and myelomonocytic leukemia. *0433* During the transition from a variety of myeloproliferative disorders to acute myeloblastic or acute myelomonocytic leukemia, there is a striking elevation in serum and urine muramidase activity. *2093* Markedly increased. *0798*

238.40 Polycythemia Vera Significantly elevated, reflecting participation of the granulocyte in the proliferative process. *2538 0209*

272.72 Gaucher's Disease Increased (15.6 ± 3.37 g/L) in 80% of adult chronic non-neuropathic type I Gaucher's Disease. *2163*

281.20 Folic Acid Deficiency Anemia *2538 1802*

289.80 Myelofibrosis During the transition from a variety of myeloproliferative disorders to acute myeloblastic or acute myelomonocytic leukemia, there is a striking elevation in serum and urine muramidase activity. *2093*

555.90 Regional Enteritis or Ileitis Particularly when the inflammatory process is active. *0693 2199   2035 0694*

556.00 Ulcerative Colitis Increased in severely affected cases. *1297   2035*

994.50 Exercise After protracted exertion. *0985*

Serum Normal

202.40 Leukemic Reticuloendotheliosis Low, normal or high. *0798*

204.00 Lymphocytic Leukemia (Acute) Low or normal. *0798*

204.10 Lymphocytic Leukemia (Chronic) Low or normal. *0798*

205.00 Myelocytic Leukemia (Acute) Low, normal, or moderately increased. *0798*

279.04 Agammaglobulinemia (Congenital Sex-linked) Other serum constituents involved in resistance to infection are normal. *2246   2539*

994.50 Exercise No effect even with strenuous exercise. *1838*

Urine Increase

199.00 Secondary Malignant Neoplasm (Disseminated) 24 h excretion and renal clearance were significantly increased in disseminated carcinoma compared with localized. *1025*

201.90 Hodgkin's Disease *0151*

205.00 Myelocytic Leukemia (Acute) Elevated only in patients who do not have the Philadelphia chromosome. No correlation is apparent between urine and serum levels. *2093* During the transition from a variety of myeloproliferative disorders to acute myeloblastic or acute myelomonocytic leukemia, there is a striking elevation in serum and urine muramidase activity. *2093*

Lysozyme *(continued)*

Urine Increase *(continued)*

206.00 Monocytic Leukemia Elevated in serum and urine in some patients with acute monocytic and myelomonocytic leukemia. *0433* Patients with heavy lysozymuria develop an apparently unique type of glomerular-tubular dysfunction, with hypokalemia, hyperkaluria, and azotemia. *1641* During the transition from a variety of myeloproliferative disorders to acute myeloblastic or acute myelomonocytic leukemia, there is a striking elevation in serum and urine muramidase activity. *2093*

250.00 Diabetes Mellitus Lysozymuria. *0701*

289.80 Myelofibrosis During the transition from a variety of myeloproliferative disorders to acute myeloblastic or acute myelomonocytic leukemia, there is a striking elevation in serum and urine muramidase activity. *2093*

585.00 Chronic Renal Failure Marked increase. *1860*

990.00 Effects of X-Ray Irradiation Often seen for over 45 days following therapy. *2360*

994.50 Exercise Very high clearance: proximal tubular function affected. *1838*

CSF Increase

320.90 Meningitis (Bacterial) May be increased but clinical significance is unknown. *0995*

Magnesium

Serum Decrease

9.00 Gastroenteritis and Colitis Mean serum level of 2.06 ± 0.62 mg/dL in 54 patients with noncholeric gastroenteritis. 7 (13%) had values below the lower normal limit. *0606*

30.00 Leprosy Decrease was highly significant in tuberculoid, lepromatous and borderline lepromatous cases. *2187*

40.20 Whipple's Disease In patients with severe diarrhea and malabsorption. *2199*

70.00 Viral Hepatitis Before treatment, plasma concentration was 0.96 - 0.2. Normal = 1.73 ± 0.13 mmol/L. *0246*

198.50 Secondary Malignant Neoplasm of Bone *2467*

242.90 Hyperthyroidism *1180 0962*

250.00 Diabetes Mellitus Osmotic diuresis secondary to hyperglycemia. *2540*

250.10 Diabetic Acidosis *0962*

252.00 Hyperparathyroidism May occur. *2444* Normal or low. *2540* Found in 14%. *1492 0022*

252.10 Hypoparathyroidism Hypomagnesemia may occur. *2444*

255.10 Adrenal Cortical Hyperfunction (Mineralocorticoid Excess) In many cases. *1108* If hypokalemia is severe. *0995*

260.00 Protein Malnutrition Hypomagnesemia may occur. *2444*

275.21 Hypomagnesemia *0062*

277.14 Acute Intermittent Porphyria Electrolyte depletion and alkalosis associated with azotemia of variable degree are often present on admission but may also develop acutely during the course of the attack. The electrolyte disorders are attributable in many patients to electrolyte depletion with inappropriate and injudicious overhydration. *0433*

303.00 Acute Alcoholic Intoxication *2467*

303.90 Alcoholism *0619*

345.90 Epilepsy In idiopathic grand mal epilepsy the concentrations both in serum and CSF were significantly low just after the seizure. During interseizure period (more than 24 h) the levels increased both in the serum and CSF but in serum it still remained significantly low. *0093*

414.00 Chronic Ischemic Heart Disease May occur in the course of the disease. *2107*

555.90 Regional Enteritis or Ileitis Common feature of severe colitis. *2035*

556.00 Ulcerative Colitis Common feature of severe colitis. *2035*

571.20 Laennec's or Alcoholic Cirrhosis 4 of 11 patients had abnormally low concentration. Mean concentration (1.85 mmol/L) was significantly lower than the normal mean. *2469* May occur. *2444*

571.49 Chronic Active Hepatitis Mean = 1.28 ± 0.18. Normal = 1.73 ± 0.13 mmol/L. *0246*

571.90 Cirrhosis of Liver 4 of 11 patients had abnormally low concentrations. The mean concentration for the cirrhotic patients, 1.85 mmol/L, was significantly lower than the normal mean. *2469* In 35% of 14 patients at initial hospitalization for this disorder. *0781*

572.40 Hepatic Failure Hypomagnesemia is common in hepatic failure. *1775*

577.00 Acute Pancreatitis Low or in the low normal range. *2509* Observed in a few patients and could partly account for the failure of hypocalcemia to respond to exogenous calcium. *2199*

577.10 Chronic Pancreatitis May occur. *2444*

579.00 Celiac Sprue Disease May occur. *2444* Often low. 10% of untreated patients may have levels < 1 mmol/L and may have symptoms from the deficiency. *2238 2199*

579.90 Malabsorption, Cause Unspecified Hypomagnesemia may occur. *2444 0151*

580.00 Acute Poststreptococcal Glomerulonephritis Majority of cases showed a fall in both serum and urinary levels, associated with hypoproteinemia and hypoalbuminemia. *1772* Hypomagnesemia may occur in some cases. *2444*

581.90 Nephrotic Syndrome In a majority of cases, serum levels were low with concomitant increase in urinary concentration due to massive albuminuria, as 35% of Mg is bound to albumin. *1772*

585.00 Chronic Renal Failure Depletion occurs in rare instances. *1570*

590.00 Chronic Pyelonephritis Hypomagnesemia may occur. *2444*

590.10 Acute Pyelonephritis May occur. *2444*

591.00 Hydronephrosis Hypomagnesemia may occur. *2444*

642.60 Eclampsia Both serum and CSF concentrations were found to be low. *0093*

650.00 Pregnancy Decreased progressively from early pregnancy to term. *0517*

733.00 Osteoporosis In severe cases. *0999*

948.00 Burns Moderate and short-lived decrease in serum and erythrocytes occurs immediately after burn. *1335*

Serum Increase

204.00 Lymphocytic Leukemia (Acute) *2538*

205.00 Myelocytic Leukemia (Acute) *2538*

244.90 Hypothyroidism *2467*

250.00 Diabetes Mellitus In diabetic coma before treatment and in controlled diabetes in older age groups. *2467 2290*

250.10 Diabetic Acidosis In the early phase. *0962*

255.40 Adrenal Cortical Hypofunction *2467*

570.00 Acute and Subacute Necrosis of Liver Pathological increase in serum with liver disease. *0619 2026*

584.00 Acute Renal Failure Pathological increase with renal failure. *0619*

585.00 Chronic Renal Failure Increases when GFR falls to < 30 mL/min. *2468* In 43% of 60 patients at initial hospitalization for this disorder. *0781*

Serum Normal

252.10 Hypoparathyroidism Initial diuresis without significant change in serum concentrations. *2540*

333.40 Huntington's Chorea *1252*

994.50 Exercise Observed effect with 12 min cycle-ergometer. *0804*

Urine Decrease

244.90 Hypothyroidism *0837*

252.10 Hypoparathyroidism Initial diuresis without significant change in serum concentrations. *2540*

580.00 Acute Poststreptococcal Glomerulonephritis Majority of cases showed a fall in both serum and urinary levels, associated with hypoproteinemia and hypoalbuminemia. *1772*

Urine Increase

242.90 Hyperthyroidism *1180*

250.00 Diabetes Mellitus Osmotic diuresis secondary to hyperglycemia. *2540*

581.90 Nephrotic Syndrome In a majority of cases, serum levels were low with concomitant increase in urinary concentration due to massive albuminuria, as 35% of Mg is bound to albumin. *1772*

CSF   Decrease

13.00   Tuberculosis Meningitis   Low levels associated with convulsions. *0093*

345.90   Epilepsy   In idiopathic grand mal epilepsy the concentrations both in serum and CSF were significantly low just after the seizure. *0093*

642.60   Eclampsia   Both serum and CSF concentrations were found to be low. *0093*

Red Blood Cells   Decrease

70.00   Viral Hepatitis   2 of 5 patients had abnormally low concentrations. The mean concentration for the entire group, 4.3 mmol/L packed cells, was significantly (P < 0.001) decreased below normal. *2469*   RBC concentration was 3.18 ± 0.78 mmol/L before treatment. Normal = 5.08 ± 0.25 mmol/L. *0246*

260.00   Protein Malnutrition   RBC concentration was decreased in 2 of 4 patients with prolonged malnutrition. *2469*

571.20   Laennec's or Alcoholic Cirrhosis   The mean concentration (4.7 mmol/L packed cells) was significantly below normal values. *2469*

571.49   Chronic Active Hepatitis   Mean RBC concentration = 3.99 ± 0.61 compared to 5.08 ± 0.25 mmol/L. *0246*

571.90   Cirrhosis of Liver   The mean concentration in cirrhotic patients (4.7 mmol/L packed cells) was significantly below normal values. *2469*

948.00   Burns   Moderate and short-lived decrease in serum and erythrocytes occurs immediately after burn. *1335*

Red Blood Cells   Increase

252.10   Hypoparathyroidism   In 5 of 8 patients, the RBC concentration was at or above the normal upper limit. For the group the mean was 6.3 μmol/L packed cells, significantly over the normal (P < 0.001). *2469*

585.00   Chronic Renal Failure   Of 15 patients with a variety of renal lesions and a wide range of BUN, 9 had elevated erythrocyte magnesium levels. Mean concentration for the whole group was significantly raised, 6.7 mmol/L packed cells. *2469*

Red Blood Cells   Normal

333.40   Huntington's Chorea   *0745*

Sweat   Increase

585.00   Chronic Renal Failure   Concentrations of Ca, Mg and phosphate in sweat were significantly elevated due to an increase in the secretion of these electrolytes in the secretory portion of the sweat gland, while that in the reabsorptive duct is normal. *1861*

Malate Dehydrogenase

Serum   Increase

2.00   Typhoid Fever   Slight increase. *0619*

70.00   Viral Hepatitis   *0619*

155.00   Malignant Neoplasm of Liver   In neoplastic disease. *0503*

197.70   Secondary Malignant Neoplasm of Liver   Elevated in 62% of patients. *2093*

205.10   Myelocytic Leukemia (Chronic)   Less elevation than in acute leukemia. *2468*

250.10   Diabetic Acidosis   In some instances, mostly severe cases, especially with severe circulatory failure and liver enlargement. *0155*

281.00   Pernicious Anemia   Increased to about the same extent as LD. *0652 2552*

281.20   Folic Acid Deficiency Anemia   In 17 patients, the plasma content was consistently and markedly elevated. *1023*   Serum levels rise to up to 40 X normal value. *0619*   Increased to about the same extent as LD. *0652 2552 2538*

282.60   Sickle Cell Anemia   Elevated to a median of 193 U/L (normal = 52 U/L) with a range of 87-337 U/L in 15 patients. *1023*

359.11   Progressive Muscular Dystrophy   In Duchenne type. *0878*

410.90   Acute Myocardial Infarction   Elevated 2-10 X above normal in all cases of clinically proved infarction. *2443*   Level rises after 6-24 h to a peak at 24-48 h (2-15 X normal), falling to normal by 5 days. The peak precedes AST and LD, and degree is similar to rise in AST. *0619*   Always elevated, sometimes strikingly. *0210*

577.00   Acute Pancreatitis   Slight increase. *0619*   Nonspecific serum enzymes may be increased. *2467*

650.00   Pregnancy   Variable increase in normal pregnancy. *0387*

710.40   Dermatomyositis/Polymyositis   May be increased but offers no additional diagnostic value. *2467*

994.50   Exercise   Significant effect with exercise. *0804*   Significant effect after 2 h march. *2092*

Serum   Normal

333.40   Huntington's Chorea   No abnormalities in 8 patients. *0534*

Urine   Increase

189.00   Malignant Neoplasm of Kidney   Increased in 75% of patients. *1005*

Red Blood Cells   Increase

281.20   Folic Acid Deficiency Anemia   10 of 16 patients had red cell activity elevated significantly above the normal upper limit of 96. *1023*

282.60   Sickle Cell Anemia   Mean RBC concentration was elevated to 245 ± 93 U/L in 15 patients. Levels ranged from 80-460 U/L (normal = 160 U/L). *1023*

Manganese

Serum   Increase

70.00   Viral Hepatitis   Increase becomes evident only after liver disease has been present for 2-3 weeks. *0153*   During acute phase increase up to four times that seen in normal subjects. *2429*   Significant increase (P < 0.01). *2429*

571.49   Chronic Active Hepatitis   Significant P < 0.001. *2429*

571.90   Cirrhosis of Liver   Significant P < 0.001. *2429*

573.30   Toxic Hepatitis   During acute phase increase up to four times that seen in normal subjects. *2429*

Serum   Normal

650.00   Pregnancy   *0966*

CSF   Normal

332.00   Parkinsons's Disease   *1763*

MCH

Blood   Decrease

40.20   Whipple's Disease   Anemia is common and is usually associated with iron deficiency. *2199*

115.00   Histoplasmosis   A marked to moderate hypochromic anemia occurs in most cases. *0962*

126.90   Ancylostomiasis (Hookworm Infestation)   Anemia occurring in hookworm disease is a classic iron deficiency anemia. *2199*   Development of hypochromic, microcytic anemia depends on the number of worms, recency of infection, and host nutrition. *2368*

127.20   Strongyloidiasis   Anemia, when it occurs, is usually iron deficiency in type. *2199*

127.30   Trichuriasis   In children can be accompanied by a microcytic hypochromic anemia. *0433*

151.90   Malignant Neoplasm of Stomach   The amount of bleeding and the degree of anemia will vary widely. Anemia of more than moderate degree is a late consequence of gastric malignancy. *0962*   Anemia may be of several types. The most common is iron deficiency anemia caused by chronic occult blood loss. *2199 2467*

152.90   Malignant Neoplasm of Small Intestine   Iron deficiency anemia is common because of either gross or occult bleeding. *2199*

153.90   Malignant Neoplasm of Large Intestine   Anemia; may be the only symptom of carcinoma of the right side of the colon (present in > 50% of these patients, usually hypochromic). *2467*   Iron deficiency anemia is common because of either gross or occult bleeding. *2199*

154.10   Malignant Neoplasm of Rectum   Iron deficiency anemia is common because of either gross or occult bleeding. *2199*

MCH (continued)

Blood Decrease (continued)

188.90 Malignant Neoplasm of Bladder May show anemia secondary to iron deficiency or secondary to a diffuse metastatic disease. *0433*

189.00 Malignant Neoplasm of Kidney Anemia occurs in approximately 30% of patients, secondary to bone marrow depression. *0836* 30 of 34 patients with hypernephroma were anemic, due mainly to urinary blood loss. Hemoglobin values varied from 7-12 g/dL. *0894*

202.80 Non-Hodgkins Lymphoma Anemia occurs frequently and may be due to blood loss, bone marrow infiltration, or hemolysis. *2538*

211.10 Benign Neoplasm of Stomach With occult bleeding, iron deficiency anemia may be present. *2199*

238.40 Polycythemia Vera *2468*

242.90 Hyperthyroidism Patients occasionally develop a mild hypochromic anemia. *2540*

244.90 Hypothyroidism Microcytic hypochromic anemia may occur due to blood loss, increased demand or dietary inadequacy. MCH < 27 pg, MCV < 80 fL. *0532*

267.00 Vitamin C Deficiency Associated with anemia of normocytic, macrocytic, or hypochromic variety in about 80% of cases. *2538*

277.11 Congenital Erythropoietic Porphyria (Günther's Disease) Microcytic hypochromic anemia may occur due to blood loss or increased demand. MCH < 27 pg. *0532*

277.12 Erythropoietic Protoporphyria Microcytic hypochromic anemia may occur due to blood loss or increased demand. MCH < 27 pg. *0532* A moderate hypochromic or normochromic anemia is frequently observed. *2538*

277.13 Erythropoietic Coproporphyria Microcytic hypochromic anemia may occur due to blood loss or increased demand. MCH < 27 pg. *0532*

277.14 Acute Intermittent Porphyria Microcytic hypochromic anemia may occur due to blood loss or increased demand. MCH < 27 pg. *0532*

277.15 Porphyria Variegata Microcytic hypochromic anemia may occur due to blood loss or increased demand. MCH < 27 pg. *0532*

277.16 Porphyria Cutanea Tarda Microcytic hypochromic anemia may occur due to blood loss or increased demand. MCH < 27 pg. *0532*

277.17 Hereditary Coproporphyria Microcytic hypochromic anemia may occur due to blood loss or increased demand. MCH < 27 pg. *0532*

280.81 Plummer-Vinson Syndrome Microcytic anemia. *0995*

280.90 Iron Deficiency Anemia Microcytic hypochromic anemia may occur due to blood loss, increased demand or dietary inadequacy. MCH < 27 pg, MCV < 80 fL. *0532* Morphologic changes are paralleled by decreases in the MCV, MCH, and MCHC. The decline in MCHC is the more consistent. *0962* Average is 20 pg, range = 14-29. *0117*

281.30 Vitamin B$_6$ Deficiency Anemia Microcytic hypochromic anemia may occur due to blood loss, increased demand or dietary inadequacy. MCH < 27 pg, MCV < 80 fL. *0532*

282.41 Thalassemia Major Microcytic hypochromic anemia may occur due to blood loss, increased demand or dietary inadequacy. MCH < 27 pg, MCV < 80 fL. *0532* Defective globin synthesis. *0962* *2468*

282.42 Thalassemia Minor The most striking and consistent finding is that of small, poorly hemoglobinized red cells, MCH values of 20-22 pg and MCV values of 50-70 fL. *2538* Mean in 45 cases was 20.26 ± 2.23 pg. *1793*

285.00 Sideroblastic Anemia Microcytic hypochromic anemia may occur due to blood loss, increased demand or dietary inadequacy. MCH < 27 pg, MCV < 80 fL. *0532* Reduced hemoglobin synthesis. Microcytic hypochromic anemia. *2552*

286.01 Hemophilia Presence or absence of anemia depends on the severity and frequency of bleeding. *2552*

287.00 Allergic Purpura Anemia is not usually present unless the hemorrhagic manifestations have been severe. *2538*

289.00 Polycythemia, Secondary *0151*

446.00 Polyarteritis-Nodosa Microcytic hypochromic anemia may occur due to blood loss, increased demand or dietary inadequacy. MCH < 27 pg, MCV < 80 fL. *0532* Mild anemia is frequently present due either to blood loss or to chronic renal failure. *0642* Anemia is found chiefly in cases complicated by renal insufficiency or blood loss. *0962* *0433*

533.90 Peptic Ulcer, Site Unspecified A few patients will have anemia because of chronic blood loss. *0433* An ulcer that bleeds chronically will cause a varying degree of iron deficiency anemia. *0962*

535.00 Gastritis May be low in patients with bleeding. *0433*

553.30 Hernia Diaphragmatic Microcytic anemia (due to loss of blood) may be present. *2467*

555.90 Regional Enteritis or Ileitis Frequently moderate anemia, most often iron deficiency, but occasionally macrocytic caused by poor diet or failure to absorb vitamin B$_{12}$ normally. *2199*

556.00 Ulcerative Colitis Anemia in approximately 70% of cases. *2035* Anemia secondary to colonic blood loss. Severity varies, depending on the rate and duration of bleeding. *2199*

562.00 Diverticular Disease of Intestine Some cases. *2199*

562.11 Diverticulitis of Colon Some cases. *2199*

564.20 Postgastrectomy (Dumping) Syndrome Iron deficiency and vitamin B$_{12}$ deficiency are common following subtotal gastrectomy. *0962*

579.00 Celiac Sprue Disease Characteristic iron deficiency anemia. The peripheral blood smear may show hypochromia. In some cases iron deficiency anemia may be the predominant abnormality indicative of malabsorption. *0433*

579.90 Malabsorption, Cause Unspecified Microcytic hypochromic anemia may occur due to blood loss, increased demand or dietary inadequacy. MCH < 27 pg, MCV < 80 fL. *0532*

710.10 Progressive Systemic Sclerosis A mild hypochromic microcytic anemia may be present. *0433* Found in up to 25% of patients. *0962*

714.00 Rheumatoid Arthritis Microcytic hypochromic anemia may occur due to blood loss, increased demand or dietary inadequacy. MCH < 27 pg, MCV < 80 fL. *0532*

984.00 Toxic Effects of Lead and Its Compounds (including Fumes) Microcytic hypochromic anemia may occur due to blood loss, increased demand or dietary inadequacy. MCH < 27 pg, MCV < 80 fL. *0532*

Blood Increase

123.40 Diphyllobothriasis (Intestinal) When present, anemia is macrocytic. *2199*

205.00 Myelocytic Leukemia (Acute) Often severe anemia, may be macrocytic. *2552*

244.90 Hypothyroidism Mild to moderate normochromic, normocytic, or slightly macrocytic anemia with normal leukocyte and platelet counts. *0433*

281.00 Pernicious Anemia Generally 33-38 pg in moderate anemia, and 33-56 pg, with severe cases (normal = 27-31 pg). *2552* *0995*

281.20 Folic Acid Deficiency Anemia Erythrocytes are increased in diameter and thickness. Abnormalities are reflected in the increased MCV and MCH. *0962* Generally 33-38 pg in moderate anemia, and 33-56 pg, with severe cases (normal = 27-31 pg). *2552*

282.00 Hereditary (Congenital) Spherocytosis Variations usually correspond to changes in volume. *2552*

284.01 Congenital Aplastic Anemia The anemia is normochromic or slightly macrocytic, and macrocytes and target cells may be seen in the blood. *2552*

285.00 Sideroblastic Anemia The anemia is normocytic or slightly macrocytic. *2538*

358.00 Myasthenia Gravis Occasional cases of macrocytic anemia. *2467*

773.00 Hemolytic Disease of Newborn (Erythroblastosis Fetalis) *2468*

Blood Normal

280.90 Iron Deficiency Anemia Red cell indices are related to the duration and severity of anemia. Mild cases or those of short duration may have normal values. *0194*

287.30 Idiopathic Thrombocytopenic Purpura An anemia from blood loss may be present, but the RBC morphology is normal. *0433*

650.00 Pregnancy *1113*

MCHC

Blood   Decrease

40.20   Whipple's Disease   Anemia is common and is usually associated with iron deficiency. *2199*

115.00   Histoplasmosis   A marked to moderate hypochromic anemia occurs in most cases. *0962*

126.90   Ancylostomiasis (Hookworm Infestation)   Anemia occurring in hookworm disease is a classic iron deficiency anemia. *2199*   Development of hypochromic, microcytic anemia depends on the number of worms, recency of infection, and host nutrition. *2368   0151*

127.20   Strongyloidiasis   Anemia, when it occurs, is usually iron deficiency in type. *2199*

127.30   Trichuriasis   In children can be accompanied by a microcytic hypochromic anemia. *0433*

151.90   Malignant Neoplasm of Stomach   The amount of bleeding and the degree of anemia will vary widely. Anemia of more than moderate degree is a late consequence of gastric malignancy. *0962*   Anemia may be of several types. The most common is iron deficiency anemia caused by chronic blood loss. *2199*

152.90   Malignant Neoplasm of Small Intestine   Iron deficiency anemia is common because of either gross or occult bleeding. *2199*

153.90   Malignant Neoplasm of Large Intestine   Anemia; may be the only symptom of carcinoma of the right colon (present in > 50% of these patients, usually hypochromic). *2467*   Iron deficiency anemia is common because of either gross or occult bleeding. *2199*

154.10   Malignant Neoplasm of Rectum   Iron deficiency anemia is common because of either gross or occult bleeding. *2199*

188.90   Malignant Neoplasm of Bladder   May show anemia secondary to iron deficiency or secondary to a diffuse metastatic disease. *0433*

189.00   Malignant Neoplasm of Kidney   Anemia occurs in approximately 30% of patients, secondary to bone marrow depression. *0836*   30 of 34 patients with hypernephroma were anemic, due to urinary blood loss. Hemoglobin values varied from 7-12 g/dL. *0894*

202.80   Non-Hodgkins Lymphoma   Anemia occurs frequently and may be due to blood loss, bone marrow infiltration, or hemolysis. *2538*

211.10   Benign Neoplasm of Stomach   With occult bleeding, iron deficiency anemia may be present. *2199*

238.40   Polycythemia Vera   *2468*

242.90   Hyperthyroidism   Patients occasionally develop a mild hypochromic anemia. *2540*

267.00   Vitamin C Deficiency   Associated with anemia of normocytic, macrocytic, or hypochromic variety in about 80% of cases. *2538*

277.12   Erythropoietic Protoporphyria   A moderate hypochromic or normochromic anemia is frequently observed. *2538*

280.81   Plummer-Vinson Syndrome   Hypochromic anemia associated with dysphagia and cardiospasm in women. *2467*

280.90   Iron Deficiency Anemia   Of little diagnostic value except when anemia is severe. *2538*   Morphologic changes are paralleled by decreases in the MCV, MCH, and MCHC. The decline in MCHC is the more consistent. *0962*   Average is 28 g/dL, ranging from 22-31. *0117   2467 0151 0999*

281.30   Vitamin B$_6$ Deficiency Anemia   Degree of anemia may vary but is usually in the range of 7-8 g/dL of hemoglobin, with a lowered MCHC. *0151*

282.41   Thalassemia Major   Normal or slightly decreased. *2468*   Hypochromic anemia with MCHC between 23-32% *2552   0999*

282.42   Thalassemia Minor   Slightly reduced. Mean in 45 cases was 31.22 ± 0.96 %. *1793*

285.00   Sideroblastic Anemia   Degree of anemia may vary but is usually in the range of 7-8 g/dL of hemoglobin, with a lowered MCHC. *0151*   Reduced hemoglobin synthesis. Microcytic hypochromic anemia. *2552   0532*

286.01   Hemophilia   Presence or absence of anemia depends on the severity and frequency of bleeding. *2552*

287.00   Allergic Purpura   Anemia is not usually present unless the hemorrhagic manifestations have been severe. *2538*

289.00   Polycythemia, Secondary   Low MCHC in addition to microcytosis, especially after large hemorrhages or repeated phlebotomies. *0151*

446.00   Polyarteritis-Nodosa   Mild anemia is frequently present due either to blood loss or to chronic renal failure. *0642*   Anemia is found chiefly in cases complicated by renal insufficiency or blood loss. *0962   0433*

446.20   Goodpasture's Syndrome   Secondary to prolonged pulmonary bleeding. *0062*

533.90   Peptic Ulcer, Site Unspecified   A few patients will have anemia because of chronic blood loss. *0433*   An ulcer that bleeds chronically will cause a varying degree of iron deficiency anemia. *0962*

535.00   Gastritis   May be low in patients with bleeding. *0433*

555.90   Regional Enteritis or Ileitis   Frequently moderate anemia, most often iron deficiency, but occasionally macrocytic caused by poor diet or failure to absorb vitamin B$_{12}$ normally. *2199*

556.00   Ulcerative Colitis   Anemia in approximately 70% of cases. *2035*   Anemia secondary to colonic blood loss. Severity varies, depending on the rate and duration of bleeding. *2199*

562.00   Diverticular Disease of Intestine   Some cases. *2199*

562.11   Diverticulitis of Colon   Some cases. *2199*

564.20   Postgastrectomy (Dumping) Syndrome   Iron deficiency and vitamin B$_{12}$ deficiency are common following subtotal gastrectomy. *0962*

579.00   Celiac Sprue Disease   Characteristic iron deficiency anemia. The peripheral blood smear may show hypochromia. In some cases iron deficiency anemia may be the predominant abnormality indicative of malabsorption. *0433*

585.00   Chronic Renal Failure   Slightly reduced, to about 30-31%. *0151*

710.10   Progressive Systemic Sclerosis   A mild hypochromic microcytic anemia may be present. *0433*   Found in up to 25% of patients. *0962*

984.00   Toxic Effects of Lead and Its Compounds (including Fumes)   Hemolytic anemia. *0484*

Blood   Increase

282.00   Hereditary (Congenital) Spherocytosis   The mean MCHC is usually increased (36-39%) reflecting the loss of membrane surface in relation to cell volume. *0433*   Usually elevated, often as high as 37 %. *0674*   Very high. *0999*   Characteristically high, 37-39 g/dL. *2552   2538*

284.01   Congenital Aplastic Anemia   The anemia is normochromic or slightly macrocytic, and macrocytes and target cells may be seen in the blood. *2552*

Blood   Normal

280.90   Iron Deficiency Anemia   Red cell indices are related to the duration and severity of anemia. Mild cases or those of short duration may have normal values. *0194*

281.00   Pernicious Anemia   When not complicated by iron deficiency, anemia is normochromic and macrocytic. *2552   0995*

281.20   Folic Acid Deficiency Anemia   When not complicated by iron deficiency, anemia is normochromic and macrocytic. *2552*

287.30   Idiopathic Thrombocytopenic Purpura   An anemia from blood loss may be present, but the RBC morphology is normal. *0433*

650.00   Pregnancy   *1113*

773.00   Hemolytic Disease of Newborn (Erythroblastosis Fetalis)   *2468*

MCV

Blood   Decrease

40.20   Whipple's Disease   Microcytic, hypochromic red cells and a low serum iron accompany the anemia. *2199*

126.90   Ancylostomiasis (Hookworm Infestation)   Anemia occurring in hookworm disease is a classic iron deficiency anemia. *2199*   Development of hypochromic, microcytic anemia depends on the number of worms, recency of infection, and host nutrition. *2368*

127.20   Strongyloidiasis   Anemia, when it occurs, is usually iron deficiency in type. *2199*

127.30   Trichuriasis   In children can be accompanied by a microcytic hypochromic anemia. *0433*

151.90   Malignant Neoplasm of Stomach   The anemia is of the hypochromic, microcytic type with other features of chronic iron deficiency. *0962*

MCV *(continued)*

Blood Decrease *(continued)*

152.90 Malignant Neoplasm of Small Intestine Iron deficiency anemia is common because of either gross or occult bleeding. *2199*

153.90 Malignant Neoplasm of Large Intestine Many patients have chronic iron deficiency anemia characterized by hypochromic microcytic red cells. *2199*

154.10 Malignant Neoplasm of Rectum Many patients have chronic iron deficiency anemia characterized by hypochromic microcytic red cells. *2199*

188.90 Malignant Neoplasm of Bladder May show anemia secondary to iron deficiency or secondary to a diffuse metastatic disease. *0433*

189.00 Malignant Neoplasm of Kidney Anemia occurs in approximately 30% of patients, secondary to bone marrow depression. *0836* 30 of 34 patients with hypernephroma were anemic, due mainly to urinary blood loss. Hemoglobin values varied from 7-12g/dL. *0894*

202.80 Non-Hodgkins Lymphoma Anemia occurs frequently and may be due to blood loss, bone marrow infiltration, or hemolysis. *2538*

211.10 Benign Neoplasm of Stomach With occult bleeding, iron deficiency anemia may be present. *2199*

238.40 Polycythemia Vera *2468*

242.90 Hyperthyroidism Decreased in hyperthyroid patients with neither anemia nor a reduced transferrin saturation. After treatment, it rose by an average of 6 fL. A diminution even within the normal range, is an invariable concomitant of hyperthyroidism. *1696 1669*

244.90 Hypothyroidism Microcytic hypochromic anemia may occur due to blood loss, increased demand or dietary inadequacy. MCH < 27 pg, MCV < 80 fL. *0532*

277.11 Congenital Erythropoietic Porphyria (Günther's Disease) Microcytic hypochromic anemia may occur due to blood loss or increased demand. MCV < 80 fL. *0532*

277.12 Erythropoietic Protoporphyria Microcytic hypochromic anemia may occur due to blood loss or increased demand. MCV < 80 fL. *0532* A moderate hypo- or normochromic anemia is frequently observed. *2538*

277.13 Erythropoietic Coproporphyria Microcytic hypochromic anemia may occur due to blood loss or increased demand. MCV < 80 fL. *0532*

277.14 Acute Intermittent Porphyria Microcytic hypochromic anemia may occur due to blood loss or increased demand. MCV < 80 fL. *0532*

277.15 Porphyria Variegata Microcytic hypochromic anemia may occur due to blood loss or increased demand. MCV < 80 fL. *0532*

277.16 Porphyria Cutanea Tarda Microcytic hypochromic anemia may occur due to blood loss or increased demand. MCV < 80 fL. *0532*

277.17 Hereditary Coproporphyria Microcytic hypochromic anemia may occur due to blood loss or increased demand. MCV < 80 fL. *0532*

280.81 Plummer-Vinson Syndrome Hypochromic anemia associated with dysphagia and cardiospasm in women. *2467*

280.90 Iron Deficiency Anemia Microcytic hypochromic anemia may occur due to blood loss, increased demand or dietary inadequacy. MCH < 27 pg, MCV < 80 fL. *0532* In severe uncomplicated anemia, erythrocytes are hypochromic and microcytic. *2538* Hypochromic microcytosis parallels severity of anemia with marked variation in size and shape. *0151* Characteristic of well-developed iron deficiency. *0962* Average is 74 fL, range - 53-93. *0117*

281.30 Vitamin B$_6$ Deficiency Anemia Microcytic hypochromic anemia may occur due to blood loss, increased demand or dietary inadequacy. MCH < 27 pg, MCV < 80 fL. *0532*

282.00 Hereditary (Congenital) Spherocytosis Small, dense, round, red cells (microspherocytes) seen in large numbers. *0999* May be normal, high, or very low. *2552* Mean value in 76 affected patients was 83 ± 8.5 fL; ranging from 62-125 fL. *1470*

282.41 Thalassemia Major MCV < 75 fL are most often due to thalassemia trait. *2468* Microcytic, hypochromic anemia may occur due to blood loss, increased demand or dietary inadequacy. MCH < 27 pg, MCV < 80 fL. *0532* Hypochromic microcytic anemia with MCV between 28-43 fL. *2552* In nonsplenectomized patients, large poikilocytes are common, whereas after splenectomy large flat macrocytes and small deformed microcytes are frequently seen. *2538 0962*

282.42 Thalassemia Minor The most striking and consistent finding is that of small, poorly hemoglobinized red cells, MCH values of 20-22 pg and MCV values of 50-70 fL. *2538* In 45 cases, the range was 52-75, with a mean of 64.7 fL. *1793* Unusually low for the mild degree of anemia. *2552 0151*

282.60 Sickle Cell Anemia Red cell indices are usually normal, but the MCV may be increased or decreased. *2552*

282.72 Hemoglobin E Disease Definite microcytosis. *0433* Homozygotes for hemoglobin E have a relatively mild anemia characterized by microcytosis and targeting of the red cells. *0385 2538*

283.21 Paroxysmal Nocturnal Hemoglobinuria Occasional microcytosis, when urinary iron loss has occurred. *2552*

285.00 Sideroblastic Anemia Microcytic hypochromic anemia may occur due to blood loss, increased demand or dietary inadequacy. MCH < 27 pg, MCV < 80 fL. *0532* Reduced hemoglobin synthesis. Microcytic hypochromic anemia. *2552*

286.01 Hemophilia Presence or absence of anemia depends on the severity and frequency of bleeding. *2552*

287.00 Allergic Purpura Anemia is not usually present unless the hemorrhagic manifestations have been severe. *2538*

289.00 Polycythemia, Secondary Decreased resulting in a smaller increase in hemoglobin than usually would occur with the increased RBC count. Low MCHC and MCV, especially after large hemorrhages or repeated phlebotomies. *0151*

446.00 Polyarteritis-Nodosa Microcytic hypochromic anemia may occur due to blood loss, increased demand or dietary inadequacy. MCH < 27 pg, MCV < 80 fL. *0532*

516.10 Idiopathic Pulmonary Hemosiderosis Peripheral blood displays the classic changes of severe iron depletion: anisocytosis, poikilocytosis, microcytosis, and hypochromia. *2538*

533.90 Peptic Ulcer, Site Unspecified A few patients will have anemia because of chronic blood loss. *0433* An ulcer that bleeds chronically will cause a varying degree of iron deficiency anemia. *0962*

535.00 Gastritis May be low in patients with bleeding. *0433*

553.30 Hernia Diaphragmatic Microcytic anemia (due to loss of blood) may be present. *2467*

555.90 Regional Enteritis or Ileitis As a result of chronic blood loss. *2199*

556.00 Ulcerative Colitis Anemia in approximately 70% of cases. *2035* Anemia secondary to colonic blood loss. Severity varies, depending on the rate and duration of bleeding. *2199 0433*

564.20 Postgastrectomy (Dumping) Syndrome Iron deficiency and vitamin B$_{12}$ deficiency are common following subtotal gastrectomy. *0962*

579.00 Celiac Sprue Disease Characteristic of iron-deficiency anemia the peripheral blood smear may show microcytosis. In some cases iron-deficiency anemia may be the predominant abnormality indicative of malabsorption. *0433*

579.90 Malabsorption, Cause Unspecified Microcytic hypochromic anemia may occur due to blood loss, increased demand or dietary inadequacy. MCH < 27 pg, MCV < 80 fL. *0532*

710.10 Progressive Systemic Sclerosis A mild hypochromic microcytic anemia may be present. *0433* Found in up to 25% of patients. *0962*

714.00 Rheumatoid Arthritis Microcytic hypochromic anemia may occur due to blood loss, increased demand or dietary inadequacy. MCH < 27 pg, MCV < 80 fL. *0532*

984.00 Toxic Effects of Lead and Its Compounds (including Fumes) Microcytic hypochromic anemia may occur due to blood loss, increased demand or dietary inadequacy. MCH < 27 pg, MCV < 80 fL. *0532* Hemolytic anemia. *0484*

Blood Increase

40.20 Whipple's Disease In some patients there is macrocytosis caused by folate deficiency. *2199*

123.40 Diphyllobothriasis (Intestinal) When present, anemia is macrocytic. *2199*

151.90 Malignant Neoplasm of Stomach Macrocytic anemia may be seen in patients with gastric carcinoma and untreated pernicious anemia or folate deficiency. *2199*

203.00 Multiple Myeloma Anemia may be macrocytic. *2538*

205.00 Myelocytic Leukemia (Acute) Often severe anemia, may be macrocytic. *2552*

207.00 Erythroleukemia A mild macrocytosis is sometimes present. *2538*

244.90 **Hypothyroidism** Mean MCV exceeded 90 fL in 29 of 53 patients with normal vitamin B_{12}, folic acid and iron levels. MCV invariably fell with T_4 treatment even if initial levels were within the normal range. 9 of 53 patients with normal folic acid, vitamin B_{12} and iron had anemia and increased MCV -- the macrocytic anemia of hypothyroidism. *1078* Mild to moderate normochromic, normocytic, or slightly macrocytic anemia with normal leukocyte platelet counts. *0433 2538 0248*

267.00 **Vitamin C Deficiency** Associated with anemia of normocytic, macrocytic, or hypochromic variety in about 80% of cases. *2538*

269.90 **Deficiency State (Unspecified)** Macrocytic anemia may occur due to vitamin B_{12} or folate deficiency. MCV > 100 fL. *0532*

279.06 **Immunodeficiency (Common Variable)** High incidence of pernicious anemia. *2538*

281.00 **Pernicious Anemia** Macrocytic anemia may occur due to vitamin B_{12} or folate deficiency. MCV > 100 fL. *0532* Usually macrocytic anemia. Rise in MCV is largely proportional to the degree of anemia. Usual values are 95-110 fL, but may be 110-160 with severe anemia. *2552*

281.20 **Folic Acid Deficiency Anemia** Macrocytic anemia may occur due to vitamin B_{12} or folate deficiency. MCV > 100 fL. *0532* Anemia is normochromic (unless iron deficiency coexists) and macrocytic, with MCV ranging from 100 to > 150 fL. *2538* Erythrocytes are increased in diameter and thickness. Abnormalities are reflected in the increased MCV and MCH. *0962* Usually macrocytic anemia. Rise in MCV is largely proportional to the degree of anemia. Usual values are 95-110 fL, but may be 110-160 with severe anemia. *2552*

282.00 **Hereditary (Congenital) Spherocytosis** May be normal, high, or very low. *2552*

282.31 **Hereditary Nonspherocytic Hemolytic Anemia** Mild to moderate macrocytosis. *2538*

282.60 **Sickle Cell Anemia** Red cell indices are usually normal, but the MCV may be increased or decreased. *2552*

283.00 **Acquired Hemolytic Anemia (Autoimmune)** Reflects increased number of reticulocytes. *0186*

283.21 **Paroxysmal Nocturnal Hemoglobinuria** RBC are usually macrocytic but there may be great variation in size. *2552*

284.01 **Congenital Aplastic Anemia** The anemia is normochromic or slightly macrocytic, and macrocytes and target cells may be seen in the blood. *2552*

284.90 **Aplastic Anemia** Occasional macrocytosis. *0433*

285.00 **Sideroblastic Anemia** The anemia is normocytic or slightly macrocytic. *2538*

287.30 **Idiopathic Thrombocytopenic Purpura** Occasional moderate macrocytosis, if there has been a recent severe hemorrhage. *2552 0995*

358.00 **Myasthenia Gravis** Occasional cases of macrocytic anemia. *2467*

428.00 **Congestive Heart Failure** Overall hypervolemia involving both plasma and red cell volume. *1669*

535.00 **Gastritis** Secondary to B_{12} deficiency with atrophic gastritis. *2199*

555.90 **Regional Enteritis or Ileitis** Macrocytic anemia may occur due to vitamin B_{12} or folate deficiency. MCV > 100 fL. *0532* Macrocytic, megaloblastic anemia may indicate folic acid or vitamin B_{12} deficiency. *2199*

571.20 **Laennec's or Alcoholic Cirrhosis** Occasionally mild macrocytosis, but rarely 115 fL in the absence of megaloblastic changes in marrow. Reported incidence varies from 33-65%. *2552*

571.90 **Cirrhosis of Liver** Occasionally mild macrocytosis, but rarely 115 fL in the absence of megaloblastic changes in marrow. Reported incidence varies from 33-65%. *2552*

579.00 **Celiac Sprue Disease** Macrocytic anemia may occur due to vitamin B_{12} or folate deficiency. MCV > 100 fL. *0532*

579.90 **Malabsorption, Cause Unspecified** Macrocytic anemia may occur due to vitamin B_{12} or folate deficiency. MCV > 100 fL. *0532*

585.00 **Chronic Renal Failure** Slight macrocytosis has been observed. *1421*

650.00 **Pregnancy** Macrocytic anemia may occur due to vitamin B_{12} or folate deficiency. MCV > 100 fL. *0532*

714.00 **Rheumatoid Arthritis** Macrocytic anemia may occur due to vitamin B_{12} or folate deficiency. MCV > 100 fL. *0532*

758.00 **Down's Syndrome** As a whole, the group showed an increase. Macrocytosis increased with age. *0828*

773.00 **Hemolytic Disease of Newborn (Erythroblastosis Fetalis)** *2468*

984.00 **Toxic Effects of Lead and Its Compounds (including Fumes)** Rare increase with poisoning. *0618*

Blood   Normal

244.90 **Hypothyroidism** A true increase occurs in < 10% of the patients, and in these cases it is usually caused by a megaloblastic erythropoiesis due to vitamin B_{12} or folic acid deficiency. *2538 2384*

280.90 **Iron Deficiency Anemia** Red cell indices are related to the duration and severity of anemia. Mild cases or those of short duration may have normal values. *0194*

287.30 **Idiopathic Thrombocytopenic Purpura** An anemia from blood loss may be present, but the RBC morphology is normal. *0433*

289.40 **Hypersplenism** Apparent anemia is often due to expansion of plasma volume in the presence of normal RBC volume. *1824*

650.00 **Pregnancy** *1113*

Melanin

Urine   Increase

172.90 **Malignant Melanoma of Skin** In some patients, when the urine is exposed to air for several h, colorless melanogens are oxidized to melanin and urine becomes deep brown and later black. Melanogenuria occurs in 25% of patients; it is said to be more frequent with extensive liver metastasis. It is not useful for judging completeness of removal or early recurrence. *2467*

197.70 **Secondary Malignant Neoplasm of Liver** Melanogenuria occurs in 25% of patients with malignant melanoma; it is said to be more frequent with extensive liver metastasis. It is not useful for judging completeness of removal or early recurrence. Beware of false positive red-brown or purple suspension due to salicylates. *2467*

Metamyelocytes

Blood   Increase

50.00 **Smallpox** Leukopenia is found in the first days of illness followed by leukocytosis with lymphocytosis and a high percentage of metamyelocytes. *0433*

205.10 **Myelocytic Leukemia (Chronic)** In the great majority of patients. *2538*

289.00 **Polycythemia, Secondary** Are seen. *0151*

289.80 **Myelofibrosis** Can generally be found in myelofibrosis. *2538*

Bone Marrow   Decrease

288.00 **Agranulocytosis** Characteristic lack of granulocytes, including polymorphonuclears, metamyelocytes, and myelocytes. *2552*

Metanephrines, Total

Serum   Increase

227.91 **Pheochromocytoma** Values should be twice upper limit of normal. *0999*

Urine   Increase

192.50 **Neuroblastoma** *1752*

192.90 **Malignant Neoplasm of Other Parts of Nervous System** *1752*

199.00 **Secondary Malignant Neoplasm (Disseminated)** *0503*

225.90 **Benign Neoplasm of Brain and CNS** *1752*

227.91 **Pheochromocytoma** Of the 3 different types of catecholamines present in the urine--the metanephrine test is positive in more than 97% of patients with the disease and is rarely falsely positive in hypertensive subjects who do not have the disease. *1223* In almost all patients, analysis of any 24-h urine collection will reveal increased excretion. *0151   0999 1108 0962*

308.00 **Stress** *0503*

785.50 **Shock** *0503*

Metanephrines, Total (continued)

Urine   Normal
585.00 **Chronic Renal Failure**   Normal urinary excretion. *0649*

Methemalbumin

Serum   Increase
283.00 **Acquired Hemolytic Anemia (Autoimmune)**   Low levels of hemoglobinemia and methemalbuminemia are common. *2035*

283.21 **Paroxysmal Nocturnal Hemoglobinuria**   May be detected at times of active hemolysis. *0433   2552*

577.00 **Acute Pancreatitis**   Consistent methemalbuminemia in patients with hemorrhagic pancreatitis, whereas in patients with acute edematous pancreatitis, none could be detected in serum or ascites. *0826*   Appears after 12 h, reaching peak values by 4-5 days. There is a much higher mortality in acute hemorrhagic pancreatitis than in edematous acute pancreatitis. *0619*   May be present in serum in acute hemorrhagic pancreatitis and not in nonhemorrhagic pancreatitis. *2199   0962*

Ascitic Fluid   Increase
577.00 **Acute Pancreatitis**   Ranged from 2.6-35 g/dL in the patients with hemorrhagic pancreatitis. *0827*

Methionine

Serum   Decrease
260.00 **Protein Malnutrition**   *0151*

270.42 **Homocystinuria**   Low or low normal in homocystinuria caused by deficient 5-methyltetrahydrofolate-dependent homocysteine methylation. *2246*

Serum   Increase
38.00 **Septicemia**   Concentrations determined in 10 burned patients with gram-negative sepsis and 9 burned patients without sepsis revealed an increase in the gluconeogenic precursors alanine, glycine, methionine and phenylalanine in those patients with sepsis. *2543*

259.20 **Carcinoid Syndrome**   The only amino acid found to be increased, all others were decreased or normal. *0718*

270.41 **Cystathioninuria**   *2246*

270.42 **Homocystinuria**   In homocystinuria caused by cystathionine beta-synthetase deficiency. *2246*

271.20 **Hereditary Fructose Intolerance**   During acute intoxication, signs of proximal tubular syndrome and of liver failure are common. *0433*

572.20 **Hepatic Encephalopathy**   Frequently increased and is implicated in the pathogenesis of the disorder. *1473*

Urine   Increase
270.01 **Cystinuria**   Has been reported. *1271 2246*

270.03 **Cystinosis**   Nonspecific pattern of aminoaciduria. Fanconi's syndrome. *0995*

270.42 **Homocystinuria**   *0151*

CSF   Increase
270.42 **Homocystinuria**   *2468*

Methylene Blue (Sabin-Feldman) Dye Test

Serum   Increase
130.00 **Toxoplasmosis**   Specific and sensitive. *2368*   Appears within 1-2 weeks, rises not less than 1:256 and can be as high as 1:32,000 or more. May persist at high levels for several y then fall slowly to 1:64 or less and tends to persist indefinitely. *1319*   Detects predominantly IgG but also IgM antibodies which appear within 2-4 weeks after infection and persist for years. Rising titers in paired sera at least 3 weeks apart are most helpful in the diagnosis of recent infection. *2035*   Titers of 1:16 are considered indicative of past infection or exposure. During active disease, titers of 1:1,000-1:65,000 may be attained. *0962*

Methylmalonate

Urine   Increase
281.00 **Pernicious Anemia**   Relatively specific for vitamin B$_{12}$ deficiency. *0433*

Urine   Normal
281.20 **Folic Acid Deficiency Anemia**   *2538*

Monoamine Oxidase

Blood   Increase
346.00 **Migraine**   Platelet levels are increased during acute attacks. *0996*

Monocytes

Blood   Decrease
202.40 **Leukemic Reticuloendotheliosis**   Severe monocytopenia; 299/μL was the highest count and 6 patients had none at all. *2390*

204.00 **Lymphocytic Leukemia (Acute)**   In 64% of 34 patients at initial hospitalization for this disorder. *0781*

204.10 **Lymphocytic Leukemia (Chronic)**   In 66% of 27 patients at initial hospitalization for this disorder. *0781*

284.90 **Aplastic Anemia**   Absolute monocytopenia and reduction in total circulating white cells usually occurs. *0151   2538*

Blood   Increase
11.00 **Pulmonary Tuberculosis**   Frequently elevated in active disease. Monocytosis of 8-15% may be seen in severe or overwhelming tuberculosis. *0151   2538*

13.00 **Tuberculosis Meningitis**   *0532*

18.00 **Disseminated Tuberculosis**   Frequently elevated in active disease. Monocytosis of 8-15% may be seen in severe or overwhelming tuberculosis. *0151*

23.00 **Brucellosis**   Occurs in certain bacterial infections. *2467 0532*

38.00 **Septicemia**   In acute infection. *2467*

53.00 **Herpes Zoster**   In 65% of 18 patients at initial hospitalization for this disorder. *0781*

70.00 **Viral Hepatitis**   In 55% of 23 patients at initial hospitalization for this disorder. *0781   0532*

72.00 **Mumps**   May occur. *2368*

75.00 **Infectious Mononucleosis**   Relative increase. *2538*   In 54% of 11 patients at initial hospitalization for this disorder. *0781 0532*

82.00 **Rocky Mountain Spotted Fever**   Increases in some Rickettsial infections. *2467*

84.00 **Malaria**   Increases in many protozoan infections. *2467 0532*

85.00 **Leishmaniasis**   Increases in many protozoan infections. *2467*

86.90 **Trypanosomiasis**   Increased in many protozoan infections. *2467*

97.90 **Syphilis**   In neonatal, primary and secondary syphilis. *1975 2538*

99.10 **Lymphogranuloma Venereum**   Mild leukocytosis with a relative lymphocytosis or monocytosis. *2199*

130.00 **Toxoplasmosis**   Slight. *0151   0532*

135.00 **Sarcoidosis**   In 72% of 25 patients at initial hospitalization for this disorder. *0781   2467*

150.90 **Malignant Neoplasm of Esophagus**   In 65% of 37 patients at initial hospitalization for this disorder. *0781*

151.90 **Malignant Neoplasm of Stomach**   Relative lymphocytopenia may occur as a result of absolute increase in monocytes and polymorphonuclear cells in inflammatory bowel disease. *2345*   In 69% of 44 patients at initial hospitalization for this disorder. *0781*

153.90 **Malignant Neoplasm of Large Intestine**   In 57% of 150 patients at initial hospitalization for this disorder. *0781*

154.10 **Malignant Neoplasm of Rectum**   In 59% of 74 patients at initial hospitalization for this disorder. *0781*

155.00 **Malignant Neoplasm of Liver** In 73% of 12 patients at initial hospitalization for this disorder. *0781*

157.90 **Malignant Neoplasm of Pancreas** In 68% of 46 patients at initial hospitalization for this disorder. *0781*

170.90 **Malignant Neoplasm of Bone** In 61% of 24 patients at initial hospitalization for this disorder. *0781*

182.00 **Malignant Neoplasm of Corpus Uteri** In 51% of 150 patients at initial hospitalization for this disorder. *0781*

185.00 **Malignant Neoplasm of Prostate** In 63% of 81 patients at initial hospitalization for this disorder. *0781*

188.90 **Malignant Neoplasm of Bladder** In 59% of 42 patients at initial hospitalization for this disorder. *0781*

191.90 **Malignant Neoplasm of Brain** In 63% of 23 patients at initial hospitalization for this disorder. *0781*

197.00 **Secondary Malignant Neoplasm of Respiratory System** In 61% of 584 patients at initial hospitalization for this disorder. *0781*

201.90 **Hodgkin's Disease** 10-40% of cases exhibited a monocytosis that did not correlate with prognosis. *2398* Appearance of abnormal large mononuclear cells in peripheral blood. *0433* All varieties of lymphomas have been reported on occasion in association with a monocytosis, sometimes varying with disease activity. *1107* In 71% of 77 patients at initial hospitalization for this disorder. *0781 0532 2538*

202.52 **Histiocytosis X** Monocytes, sometimes morphologically quite immature, may be noted in increased numbers in the peripheral blood. *0433*

202.80 **Non-Hodgkins Lymphoma** Appearance of abnormal large mononuclear cells in peripheral blood. *0433* All varieties of lymphomas have been reported on occasion in association with a monocytosis, sometimes varying with disease activity. *1107* In 57% of 74 patients at initial hospitalization for this disorder. *0781* Peripheral monocytosis is especially likely to occur in circumstances of histiocytic proliferation and increased phagocytosis as strikingly manifested in histiocytic medullary reticulosis. *1489*

203.00 **Multiple Myeloma** *2538*

204.00 **Lymphocytic Leukemia (Acute)** On occasion associated with a monocytosis of relatively minor proportions. *1489 2538*

205.00 **Myelocytic Leukemia (Acute)** On occasion associated with a monocytosis of relatively minor proportions. *1489 2538*

205.10 **Myelocytic Leukemia (Chronic)** May be normal or increased. *0992* On occasion associated with a monocytosis of relatively minor proportions. *1489* Increase in absolute number in almost all cases. *2552 0151 2538*

206.00 **Monocytic Leukemia** Occurs in monocytic and other leukemias. *2467* In 38% of 23 patients at initial hospitalization for this disorder. *0781*

238.40 **Polycythemia Vera** *2538*

242.90 **Hyperthyroidism** May occur. *2540*

272.72 **Gaucher's Disease** Lipid storage diseases. *2467*

273.30 **Waldenström's Macroglobulinemia** Has been observed. *0128*

281.30 **Vitamin B$_6$ Deficiency Anemia** Morphologically normal, but the proportion may be moderately increased. *2538*

282.41 **Thalassemia Major** May be somewhat increased. *2552*

282.60 **Sickle Cell Anemia** Leukocytosis with monocytosis (5-25%). *2538*

283.00 **Acquired Hemolytic Anemia (Autoimmune)** *2538*

285.00 **Sideroblastic Anemia** Morphologically normal, but the proportion may be moderately increased. *2538*

287.30 **Idiopathic Thrombocytopenic Purpura** *2538*

288.00 **Agranulocytosis** Sometimes occurs. Increases in the recovery. *2467* May be relatively and absolutely increased. *2552*

289.80 **Myelofibrosis** Peripheral monocytosis is especially likely to occur in circumstances of histiocytic proliferation and increased phagocytosis as strikingly manifested in histiocytic medullary reticulosis. *1489 2538*

421.00 **Bacterial Endocarditis** Elevated WBC up to about 15,000/μL in 50%. Monocytosis may be pronounced. *2467* Found in 15-20% of patients but is not correlated with the presence or number of peripheral phagocytic reticuloendothelial cells. *0488 2538*

446.00 **Polyarteritis-Nodosa** Has been reported. *1489 2538*

446.50 **Cranial Arteritis and Related Conditions** Has been reported. *1489 2538*

555.90 **Regional Enteritis or Ileitis** Relative lymphocytopenia may occur as a result of absolute increase in monocytes and polymorphonuclear cells. *2345 2538*

556.00 **Ulcerative Colitis** Relative lymphocytopenia may occur as a result of absolute increase in monocytes and polymorphonuclear cells. *2345 2538*

579.00 **Celiac Sprue Disease** *2538*

600.00 **Benign Prostatic Hypertrophy** In 63% of 73 patients at initial hospitalization for this disorder. *0781*

694.00 **Dermatitis Herpetiformis** In 63% of 11 patients at initial hospitalization for this disorder. *0781*

708.90 **Urticaria** In 50% of 28 patients at initial hospitalization for this disorder. *0781*

710.00 **Systemic Lupus Erythematosus** Was reported. *1489 2538*

714.00 **Rheumatoid Arthritis** Has been reported. *1489* In 41% of 91 patients at initial hospitalization for this disorder. *0781 2538*

715.90 **Osteoarthritis** In 51% of 125 patients at initial hospitalization for this disorder. *0781*

730.00 **Osteomyelitis** In 55% of 26 patients at initial hospitalization for this disorder. *0781*

992.00 **Heat stroke** *2538*

Urine   Increase

99.10 **Lymphogranuloma Venereum** Vaginovesical fistulas may cause changes that reflect in the urine as numerous leukocytes or inclusion-filled mononuclear cells. *0433*

585.00 **Chronic Renal Failure** 29-33% mononuclear cells found in lupus nephritis and endemic benign nephropathy. *1411*

710.00 **Systemic Lupus Erythematosus** 29-33% mononuclear cells were found in lupus nephritis and endemic benign nephropathy. *1411*

CSF   Increase

13.00 **Tuberculosis Meningitis** Usually range from 50-200/μL. *0151 0999*

32.00 **Diphtheria** Following paralysis. *0433*

87.00 **Relapsing Fever** Sometimes increased. *0433*

102.90 **Yaws** Occasionally found but neither symptoms nor signs of neurologic disability have evolved. *1058*

130.00 **Toxoplasmosis** Moderate number. *1058*

323.91 **Myelitis** Spinal fluid may be normal or may show increased protein and cells (20-1,000/μL - lymphocytes and mononuclear cells). *2467*

340.00 **Multiple Sclerosis** CSF shows a slight increase in mononuclear cells and normal or slightly increased protein (50% of cases). *2467*

431.00 **Cerebral Hemorrhage** Mononuclear cells are increased. *0999*

434.90 **Brain Infarction** Mononuclear cells are increased in CSF early in the course of the disease. *0999*

Pleural Effusion   Increase

11.00 **Pulmonary Tuberculosis** Predominant cell type. *2017*

162.90 **Malignant Neoplasm of Bronchus and Lung** Predominant cell type. *2017*

197.00 **Secondary Malignant Neoplasm of Respiratory System** Predominant cell type. *2017*

428.00 **Congestive Heart Failure** Predominant cell type. *2017*

571.90 **Cirrhosis of Liver** Predominant cell type. *2017*

714.00 **Rheumatoid Arthritis** Predominant cell type. *2017*

Ascitic Fluid   Increase

11.00 **Pulmonary Tuberculosis** Characteristic of chronic inflammatory disease, especially tuberculosis. *2199* Seen with tuberculous peritonitis. *0186*

18.00 **Disseminated Tuberculosis** Characteristic of chronic inflammatory disease, especially tuberculosis. *2199*

567.90 **Peritonitis** Seen with tuberculous peritonitis. *0186*

Peritoneal Fluid   Increase

567.90 **Peritonitis** Most patients have > 80% mononuclear forms. Characterize chronic inflammatory disease, especially tuberculosis. *2199*

Monocytes *(continued)*

Sputum   Increase
491.00   **Chronic Bronchitis**   *0433*

Mucopolysaccharides

Serum   Increase
275.31   **Hyperphosphatasia**   Pronounced increase. *2259*

Urine   Increase
120.00   **Schistosomiasis**   Abnormalities of neutral mucopolysaccharides appear in urine in bilharziasis. *1258*
710.00   **Systemic Lupus Erythematosus**   Have been found to be elevated but are nonspecific. *0962*

Mucoprotein

Serum   Decrease
70.00   **Viral Hepatitis**   *0503*
571.90   **Cirrhosis of Liver**   *0503*

Serum   Increase
390.00   **Rheumatic Fever**   *0962*
576.20   **Extrahepatic Biliary Obstruction**   *0503*
710.00   **Systemic Lupus Erythematosus**   Mucoproteins and other acute-phase reactants are elevated and persist to some degree during periods of apparent remission. *0999*

Urine   Increase
994.50   **Exercise**   Concentration of Tamm-Horsfall protein increased with decreased volume. *1118*

Myelocytes

Blood   Increase
205.10   **Myelocytic Leukemia (Chronic)**   In the great majority of patients. *2538*
289.00   **Polycythemia, Secondary**   Occasionally seen. *0151*
289.80   **Myelofibrosis**   Can generally be found in myelofibrosis. *2538*

Myoglobin

Serum   Decrease
308.00   **Stress**   As much as 50% decrease in pilots flying high performance aircraft. *0430*

Serum   Increase
244.90   **Hypothyroidism**   Significantly higher than normal in patients with primary hypothyroidism. *0573*
304.90   **Drug Dependence (Opium and Derivatives)**   Serum concentrations as high as 0.310 g/L were found in heroin addicts. *1929*
410.90   **Acute Myocardial Infarction**   Very common; first appears in serum within a few h after infarction, reaching a peak before the peak of CK activity. Did not correlate with infarct size as estimated by CK. *1208*
948.00   **Burns**   In 8 thermal burn patients there was a significant increase (P < 0.01). *0933*

Urine   Increase
250.00   **Diabetes Mellitus**   Sporadic; metabolic myoglobinuria. *2467*
271.02   **McArdle's Disease**   Transient attacks of myoglobinuria. *0619*   Myoglobinuria appeared in > 50% of patients following episodes of exercise. *2246*
276.80   **Hypokalemia**   Sporadic; metabolic myoglobinuria. *2467*
303.90   **Alcoholism**   Sporadic; metabolic myoglobinuria. *2467*
304.90   **Drug Dependence (Opium and Derivatives)**   Acute myoglobinuria up to 3.25 g/L in heroin addicts. *1929*
359.11   **Progressive Muscular Dystrophy**   Sporadic. *2467*

359.21   **Myotonia Atrophica**   Metabolic defect, hereditary. *2467*
410.90   **Acute Myocardial Infarction**   Sporadic; ischemic. *2467*
444.90   **Arterial Embolism and Thrombosis**   Sporadic; ischemia. *2467*   Sudden muscle damage due to ischemia, e.g., thrombosis of artery supplying a large muscle mass. *0619*
710.40   **Dermatomyositis/Polymyositis**   In severe cases. *2467*
780.30   **Convulsions**   Sporadic; exertional. *2467*
929.00   **Crush Injury (Trauma)**   Sudden muscle damage. *0619*
986.00   **Toxic Effects of Carbon Monoxide**   Sporadic; metabolic myoglobinuria. *2467*   *0016*
989.50   **Toxic Effects of Venom**   Common after bites. *0619*   Sporadic elevation; metabolic myoglobinuria. *2467*
992.00   **Heat stroke**   Sudden muscle damage. *0619*   Sporadic; metabolic myoglobinuria. *2467*
994.50   **Exercise**   Sporadic; exertional. *2467*
994.80   **Effects of Electric Current**   Sporadic; exertional. *2467*   Sudden muscle damage due to high-voltage electric shock. *0619*   *0016*

NBT Test

Blood   Positive
320.90   **Meningitis (Bacterial)**   Mean percentage of positive neutrophils was 21.5% in 30 patients. Useful in differential diagnosis of bacterial and tubercular meningitis (all tubercular meningitis NBT scores were normal). *0391*
482.90   **Bacterial Pneumonia**   Elevated in 29 of 33 lobar pneumonia patients, mean = 33.5% (control mean = 5.4%). Useful in differential diagnosis of pulmonary infection and thromboembolism (3 of 55 with abnormal scores). *1024*
711.00   **Acute Arthritis (Pyogenic)**   NBT positive cells were found in synovial fluid of 7 of 8 patients, while only 4 showed positive peripheral blood tests. *0939*

Synovial Fluid   Positive
711.00   **Acute Arthritis (Pyogenic)**   NBT positive cells were found in synovial fluid of 7 of 8 patients, while only 4 showed positive peripheral blood tests. *0939*

Neutralizing Antibodies

Serum   Increase
33.00   **Whooping Cough**   These antibodies are produced in low titer and appear only after the 2nd week of disease. *0962*
45.90   **Acute Poliomyelitis**   *1058*
49.00   **Lymphocytic Choriomeningitis**   Appear within 6-10 weeks and persist longer than do CF antibodies. *2368 1058*
50.00   **Smallpox**   Only titers above 1:1,000 or a large increase in titer is significant. *0433*   Increased titer in acute-phase and convalescent-phase sera. *2468*   A rising antibody titer is seen in paired sera. *0962*
53.00   **Herpes Zoster**   A significant (4-fold or greater) anamnestic response usually occurs. *1058*
54.00   **Herpes Simplex**   Increased titer of neutralizing antibodies is shown in convalescent-phase compared with acute-phase in primary infections. *2468*
56.00   **Rubella**   Appear within 1-3 days after rash and reach maximum in 2 wk. May remain positive for > 20 y. *0619*
66.10   **Tick-Borne Fever**   Increases are seen in sera taken during acute and convalescent phases. *2468*   Found in all patients with Colorado tick fever upon follow-up 1 month after onset. 92% showed a 4-fold rise in titer within 30 days. Peak titers were reached in the 20th week. *0891   1058*
72.00   **Mumps**   The most reliable index of the immune status of natural disease or administration of the live attenuated virus vaccine. Unfortunately their determination is impractical as a routine diagnostic procedure. *0433*
78.50   **Cytomegalic Inclusion Disease**   Requires use of multiple serologic types and is too time consuming and not very practical. *1319*
422.00   **Acute Myocarditis**   In viral myocarditis. *1108*
487.10   **Influenza**   May become positive during the 2nd week of illness. *0962*   A 4-fold or greater rise in antibody level between paired sera is accepted as evidence of infection. *0433*

Neutral Sterols

Feces   Increase

556.00   Ulcerative Colitis   The fecal excretion of cholesterol, coprostanol, and cholestane-38 beta, 5 alpha, 6 beta-triol was higher in patients with ulcerative colitis than in other control and patient groups. *1897*

Neutrophils

Blood   Decrease

2.00   Typhoid Fever   Significant neutropenia may occur. *1646 0532 2538*

4.90   Bacillary Dysentery   Significant neutropenia may occur. *2433   2538*

11.00   Pulmonary Tuberculosis   *0532*

23.00   Brucellosis   Significant neutropenia may occur. *0356 2538*

38.00   Septicemia   In early onset group B streptococcal disease 39 (87%) had abnormal absolute neutrophil counts, 25 with neutropenia and 14 with neutrophilia. The absolute immature neutrophil count was elevated in 19 infants (42%). *1499*

50.00   Smallpox   Leukopenia frequently associated with infectious diseases. *1077 2538*

52.00   Chickenpox   Leukopenia frequently associated with infectious diseases. *1077   2538*

55.00   Measles   The total WBC count is low with an absolute neutropenia. *0433*   Leukopenia frequently associated with infectious diseases. *1077   2538*

56.00   Rubella   Leukopenia frequently associated with infectious diseases. *1077   2538*

60.00   Yellow Fever   Leukopenia frequently associated with infectious diseases. *1077   2538*

65.00   Arthropod-Borne Hemorrhagic Fever   Leukopenia frequently associated with infectious diseases. *1077   2538*

66.00   Phlebotomus Fever   Leukopenia frequently associated with infectious diseases. *1077   2538*

66.10   Tick-Borne Fever   There is a relative decrease in mature polymorphonuclear leukocytes with an increase in immature forms. *0433*   Absolute neutropenia. *1058*

73.90   Psittacosis   Rarely, profound granulocytopenia occurs. *0433*

80.00   Epidemic Typhus   Leukopenia frequently associated with infectious diseases. *1077   2538*

81.00   Endemic Typhus   Leukopenia frequently associated with infectious diseases. *1077*

82.00   Rocky Mountain Spotted Fever   Leukopenia frequently associated with infectious diseases. *1077   2538*

84.00   Malaria   Significant neutropenia may occur. *1646   2538*

85.00   Leishmaniasis   Absolute neutropenia with total WBC count < 2,000/μL. *0151*   Significant neutropenia may occur. *1646 2538*

198.50   Secondary Malignant Neoplasm of Bone   Depression of all formed elements of the blood is often seen in disseminated neoplastic disease. *0999*

202.40   Leukemic Reticuloendotheliosis   Absolute neutropenia in 78% of 102 cases; frequently severe. *2390*   Severe bone marrow granulocytopenia and poor blood neutrophil response to stimulation are found. *2587*

202.80   Non-Hodgkins Lymphoma   Often present in addition to anemia, and almost any combination of cytopenias may be produced by bone marrow infiltration and replacement, by hypersplenism or as the result of therapy. *2538*

203.00   Multiple Myeloma   About 33% have leukopenia with diminished granulocytes and decreased platelets. *1980*   Total WBC is often reduced to 3,000-4,000/μL, largely because of neutropenia. *2538*

204.00   Lymphocytic Leukemia (Acute)   The absolute number is almost always decreased, and usually to a greater extent than in acute myelogenous leukemia. *2538*   In 92% of 34 patients at initial hospitalization for this disorder. *0781*

204.10   Lymphocytic Leukemia (Chronic)   Neutropenia and thrombocytopenia, ranging in severity from mild to catastrophic, are characteristically present in patients with marrow replacement in the late stages. *2538*   In 95% of 27 patients at initial hospitalization for this disorder. *0781*

206.00   Monocytic Leukemia   In 94% of 24 patients at initial hospitalization for this disorder. *0781*

242.90   Hyperthyroidism   About 10% of patients develop low count due to decreased neutrophils. *2540*

255.40   Adrenal Cortical Hypofunction   Neutropenia and relative lymphocytosis are common. *2467   0433*

273.30   Waldenström's Macroglobulinemia   In some patients, neutropenia, as part of general pancytopenia, has been observed. *2552 0128*

279.07   Dysgammaglobulinemia (Selective Immunoglobulin Deficiency)   Not uncommon. *0433*

280.90   Iron Deficiency Anemia   WBC is usually normal in number, but slight granulocytopenia may occur in long standing cases. *2437*

281.20   Folic Acid Deficiency Anemia   Neutropenia and thrombocytopenia are less frequent but still common. Rarely severe. *0962*

281.30   Vitamin B$_6$ Deficiency Anemia   Leukopenia is accompanied by neutropenia. *2538*

283.00   Acquired Hemolytic Anemia (Autoimmune)   A minority of patients will have persistent leukopenia and neutropenia. *0680 2538*

283.21   Paroxysmal Nocturnal Hemoglobinuria   Common. *0433*   Leukopenia, especially granulocytopenia, is present at some time in about 60% of patients. *0484   2538*

284.01   Congenital Aplastic Anemia   In most patients, leukopenia has been due to neutropenia, but frequently all types of WBC are affected. *2552*

284.90   Aplastic Anemia   Absolute granulocytopenia invariably occurs. Counts 200/μL indicate high risk of infection. *0151*   Absolute granulocytopenia is always present and is responsible for the leukopenic part of pancytopenia. *2538*   Abnormal granulation of the polymorphonuclear cells has been described. Decreased number of normal marrow cells. *0433*

285.00   Sideroblastic Anemia   Leukopenia is accompanied by neutropenia. *2538*

288.00   Agranulocytosis   Marked decrease or complete absence of mature granulocytes. *0433*   0-2%. May show pyknosis or vacuolization with agranulocytosis. *2468*   Counts of 500-1,000/μL have moderately increased risks, whereas below this the invasion of mucous membranes, skin and blood by microorganisms becomes increasingly frequent and severe. *0151*

289.40   Hypersplenism   Count may be low, even in the range of 1%, but the patient can make pus and usually is not subject to septic disease. *2538*   Due to increased destruction and sequestration. *0214 2246*

381.00   Otitis Media   In 53% of 70 patients hospitalized for this disorder. *0781*

422.00   Acute Myocarditis   Crisis is characterized by acute neutropenia and respiratory alkalosis. *1108*

480.90   Viral Pneumonia   In 52% of 15 patients at initial hospitalization for this disorder. *0781*

487.10   Influenza   Leukopenia frequently associated with infectious diseases. *1077*

570.00   Acute and Subacute Necrosis of Liver   Transient. *0992*

710.00   Systemic Lupus Erythematosus   Reduced counts in 7 of 21 cases. 62% had a subnormal response to etiocholanolone challenge, indicating reduced marrow reserves. *1267*   Present in well over 50% of patients. *0454*   There is usually an overall depression of peripheral blood leukocytes, frequently with a lymphopenia and a slight shift to the left in the granulocytic series. *0433   2538*

714.10   Felty's Syndrome   Most patients appear to have increased cell margination probably with splenic sequestration. About 33% have impaired production. *0415*   Leukopenia (usually due to neutropenia) occurs predisposing patients to infection. *2239*

990.00   Effects of X-Ray Irradiation   A gradual fall begins during the first 2 weeks after exposure, reaches a plateau, and may even rise slightly, followed by a steep fall to a low point at 30 days postexposure in cases of radiation injury. *0151*   Within a few h after irradiation a neutrophilic leukocytosis appears. Following this, an oscillation in the neutrophilic count occurs, the rate at which it falls to the minimum being a function of the dose of radiation. *0995*

Blood   Increase

4.90   Bacillary Dysentery   In many cases there is a significant increase in the number of immature neutrophils, so that the ratio of band to segmented neutrophils often is reversed. *0433*

Neutrophils *(continued)*

Blood Increase *(continued)*

6.00 Amebiasis Moderate neutrophilia present in 75% of cases. *1058*

9.00 Gastroenteritis and Colitis *2538*

18.00 Disseminated Tuberculosis Increase was observed in two cases of tuberculosis of the liver. *1312* Active tuberculosis is usually accompanied by a moderate leukocytosis. Extreme leukocytosis occasionally occurs in patients seriously ill with widespread, necrotizing disease. *2553 0532*

32.00 Diphtheria Slight leukocytosis with neutrophilia usually is noted, although in severe cases leukopenia may occur. *0433* WBC is slightly increased (< 15,000/μL). *2468*

36.00 Meningococcal Meningitis Leukocytosis up to 40,000/μL with 80-90% neutrophils is almost always present. *0151*

37.00 Tetanus Granulocytosis and the appearance of less mature forms of neutrophils. *0433*

38.00 Septicemia In 49% of 14 patients at initial hospitalization for this disorder. *0781* Increased WBC (15,000-30,000/μL) and polymorphonuclear leukocytes are found. *2468*

45.90 Acute Poliomyelitis Occasionally a mild leukocytosis is present. *0962*

75.00 Infectious Mononucleosis Transient increase with intercurrent bacterial infection. *0433 1319 2538*

99.30 Reiter's Disease *2468*

100.00 Leptospirosis Neutrophilia of > 70% is often found regardless of the leukocyte count which may be high or low. *0151* In a high proportion of cases. *2368 0962*

112.90 Moniliasis Leukocytosis of 12,000-22,000/μL and neutrophilia of 75-90% in Candida meningitis. *0138*

124.00 Trichinosis Neutrophilic leukocytosis is common. *2368 0433*

151.90 Malignant Neoplasm of Stomach Neutrophilic leukemoid reactions occur most frequently with gastric, bronchogenic, and pancreatic carcinomas. *2538*

155.00 Malignant Neoplasm of Liver *2538*

157.90 Malignant Neoplasm of Pancreas Neutrophilic leukemoid reactions occur most frequently with gastric, bronchogenic, and pancreatic carcinomas. *2538*

162.90 Malignant Neoplasm of Bronchus and Lung Neutrophilic leukemoid reactions occur most frequently with gastric, bronchogenic, and pancreatic carcinomas. *2538*

188.90 Malignant Neoplasm of Bladder A leukoerythroblastic blood picture would indicate marrow metastasis. *0433*

197.00 Secondary Malignant Neoplasm of Respiratory System In 55% of 584 patients at initial hospitalization for this disorder. *0781*

201.90 Hodgkin's Disease Common. *0433* In 54% of 77 patients at initial hospitalization for this disorder. *0781 0151*

204.10 Lymphocytic Leukemia (Chronic) The percentage is often reduced, but the absolute number may be somewhat increased in early stages of the disease. *0242 2538*

205.00 Myelocytic Leukemia (Acute) The number of blasts can range from 0 to 1 million. Not increased in approximately 40% at time of diagnosis. Normal blood leukocytes are almost always decreased. *0992*

205.10 Myelocytic Leukemia (Chronic) 80-90% of the cells are granulocytes. The distribution shows only a slight shift toward immaturity. *0151* Most patients have > 100,000 granulocytes at time of diagnosis and the count may exceed 1 million. *0992* Granulocytes in all stages of development occur in profusion in the peripheral blood and for the most part appear to be normal in morphology. The most mature elements are ordinarily present in greatest number and the less mature in diminishing frequency. *2538 2552*

238.40 Polycythemia Vera An absolute granulocytosis is seen in the majority of patients with a circulatory count of 15,000-30,000/μL. *0433* Occurs in about 66% of cases. Usually of moderate degree but extreme degrees are sometimes observed late in the course. A moderate shift to the left in the granulocyte series frequently accompanies the increase. *2538*

250.10 Diabetic Acidosis May be associated with a moderate to severe neutrophilia. *2538*

255.00 Adrenal Cortical Hyperfunction (Glucocorticoid Excess) Some patients have granulocytosis, lymphopenia, and eosinopenia. *0151* In many cases. *1108* If hypokalemia is severe. *0995*

274.00 Gout May be associated with a moderate to severe neutrophilia. *2538*

275.34 Familial Periodic Paralysis Occasionally during attacks. *2246*

282.60 Sickle Cell Anemia *2552*

283.00 Acquired Hemolytic Anemia (Autoimmune) Most patients have modestly elevated counts. *2538*

287.00 Allergic Purpura A mild leukocytosis, mainly of polymorphonuclear cells, with WBC counts of 10,000-20,000/μL common. *0433* Modest neutrophilia. *2552*

287.30 Idiopathic Thrombocytopenic Purpura Shift to the left. *0995* Usually normal, but moderate neutrophilia may occur due to severe bleeding. *2552*

320.90 Meningitis (Bacterial) In 55% of 20 patients hospitalized for this disorder. *0781 0433*

324.00 Intracranial Abscess In the acute phase WBC may be markedly elevated with an increase in the polymorphonuclear leukocytes. *0433* Slight increase in neutrophils and lymphocytes (20-100/μL). *2467*

357.00 Guillain-Barré Syndrome A moderate polymorphonuclear leukocytosis. *0878*

357.90 Polyneuritis In 53% of 13 patients hospitalized for this disorder. *0781*

381.00 Otitis Media Usually accompanied by a mild leukocytosis with the appearance of less mature forms of neutrophils. *0433*

390.00 Rheumatic Fever *2538*

410.90 Acute Myocardial Infarction Increase of polymorphonuclear leukocytes, with an increase in young forms. *1108* In 58% of 100 patients hospitalized for this disorder. *0781*

415.10 Pulmonary Embolism and Infarction In 40% of 22 patients at initial hospitalization for this disorder. *0781* With pulmonary infarction there may be a relative increase in neutrophils and a leukocytosis. *0962*

421.00 Bacterial Endocarditis Usually increased numbers of immature granulocytes are found in the blood. *0999* Elevated WBC in 50% of patients with 65-85% neutrophils. *2467* Normal or elevated to 15,000 with 65-85% neutrophils *2488*

431.00 Cerebral Hemorrhage In 45% of 13 patients hospitalized for this disorder. *0781*

444.90 Arterial Embolism and Thrombosis In 50% of 40 patients hospitalized for this disorder. *0781*

446.00 Polyarteritis-Nodosa In about 80% of cases, there is mild leukocytosis with a shift to the left. *2035*

446.50 Cranial Arteritis and Related Conditions In 42% of 14 patients hospitalized for this disorder. *0781*

446.60 Thrombotic Thrombocytopenic Purpura Leukocytosis in 50% with a shift to the left and appearance of immature granulocytes. *2552*

451.90 Phlebitis and Thrombophlebitis In 36% of 49 patients at initial hospitalization for this disorder. *0781*

480.90 Viral Pneumonia In 39% of 15 patients at initial hospitalization for this disorder. *0781*

482.90 Bacterial Pneumonia A polymorphonuclear leukocytosis of above 15,000/μL. However, the count may be normal and in some instances of overwhelming infection a leukopenia may be present. *0433* In 55% of 18 patients at initial hospitalization for this disorder. *0781*

483.01 Mycoplasma Pneumoniae Slight neutrophilia occurs with counts of 60-85% neutrophils. *0151*

486.01 Resolving Pneumonia In 37% of 81 patients at initial hospitalization for this disorder. *0781*

487.10 Influenza Secondary bacterial infection commonly leads to a polymorphonuclear leukocytosis in excess of 15,000/μL. *0433*

491.00 Chronic Bronchitis Neutrophilic cells are present only during the course of an infection. *0433*

493.10 Asthma (Intrinsic) Modest changes in the peripheral WBC count occur along with an occasional increase in the percentage of polymorphonuclear WBC. *0433* In 38% of 122 patients at initial hospitalization for this disorder. *0781*

495.90 Allergic Alveolitis During the acute febrile episodes there is a polymorphonuclear leukocytosis of 15,000-25,000/μL. *0433*

496.00 Chronic Obstructive Lung Disease In 42% of 79 patients at initial hospitalization for this disorder. *0781*

513.00 Abscess of Lung In most patients there is a leukocytosis in the range of 20,000-30,000 cells/μL. The debilitated or elderly patients may fail to respond to the infection with a leukocytosis. *0433*

535.00 Gastritis In 40% of 36 patients at initial hospitalization for this disorder. *0781*

540.90 Acute Appendicitis 96% of patients had either an abnormal total or differential WBC count. Leukocytosis > 10,000/μL or a differential in excess of 75% neutrophils supports this clinical diagnosis. *1872* Raised total leukocyte count in 42%, a raised neutrophil percentage in 93% and a raised absolute neutrophil count in 77%. *0588* In 71% of 106 patients at initial hospitalization for this disorder. *0781 2199*

555.90 Regional Enteritis or Ileitis Relative lymphocytopenia may occur as a result of absolute increase in monocytes and polymorphonuclear cells. *2345* Count increases with increasing disease activity. *1216*

556.00 Ulcerative Colitis Count increases with increasing disease activity. *1216* Relative lymphocytopenia may occur as a result of absolute increase in monocytes and polymorphonuclear cells. *2345*

560.90 Intestinal Obstruction In 39% of 44 patients at initial hospitalization for this disorder. *0781*

562.11 Diverticulitis of Colon In 51% of 36 patients at initial hospitalization for this disorder. *0781* Leukocytosis with an increase in polymorphonuclear forms. *2199*

567.90 Peritonitis Secondary; WBC is elevated with a major increase in polymorphonuclear granulocytes. May not be present in the older age group and those on steroids. *0433*

570.00 Acute and Subacute Necrosis of Liver May be associated with a moderate to severe neutrophilia. *2538*

572.00 Liver Abscess (Pyogenic) Polymorphonuclear leukocytosis in > 90% of patients; usually over 20,000/μL. *2467*

575.00 Acute Cholecystitis In 60% of 15 patients at initial hospitalization for this disorder. *0781* Neutrophilic leukocytosis. *2199*

576.10 Cholangitis Marked increase, up to 30,000/μL with increase in granulocytes in suppurative cholangitis. *2467* In 36% of 11 patients at initial hospitalization for this disorder. *0781*

577.00 Acute Pancreatitis Usually elevated. *0433* In 75% of 20 patients at initial hospitalization for this disorder. *0781 2538*

577.10 Chronic Pancreatitis In 36% of 11 patients at initial hospitalization for this disorder. *0781*

580.00 Acute Poststreptococcal Glomerulonephritis *2538*

581.90 Nephrotic Syndrome In 49% of 26 patients at initial hospitalization for this disorder. *0781*

584.00 Acute Renal Failure In 74% of 12 patients at initial hospitalization for this disorder. *0781 0277*

585.00 Chronic Renal Failure Slight neutrophilic leukocytosis may be observed. *2552 0329* In 67% of 141 patients at initial hospitalization for this disorder. *0781*

590.10 Acute Pyelonephritis Most patients exhibit a leukocytosis of 15,000- 20,000/μL with an increase of immature neutrophils in the differential count. *0433* In 63% of 14 patients at initial hospitalization for this disorder. *0781*

600.00 Benign Prostatic Hypertrophy In 44% of 73 patients at initial hospitalization for this disorder. *0781*

601.00 Prostatitis In 30% of 13 patients at initial hospitalization for this disorder. *0781*

642.60 Eclampsia May be associated with a moderate to severe neutrophilia. *2538*

650.00 Pregnancy Occurs almost entirely in the last trimester but is present in only about 20% of patients. *1329 2538*

694.00 Dermatitis Herpetiformis In 45% of 11 patients at initial hospitalization for this disorder. *0781*

708.90 Urticaria In 28% of 28 patients at initial hospitalization for this disorder. *0781 2538*

711.00 Acute Arthritis (Pyogenic) An elevated absolute neutrophil count. *0650*

714.00 Rheumatoid Arthritis About 25% of patients develop a significant neutrophilic leukocytosis. These patients usually have arthritis of short duration with a high degree of activity and fever. *2154* In 60% of 92 patients at initial hospitalization for this disorder. *0781*

730.00 Osteomyelitis In 44% of 26 patients at initial hospitalization for this disorder. *0781*

773.00 Hemolytic Disease of Newborn (Erythroblastosis Fetalis) *2061*

780.30 Convulsions *2538*

785.40 Gangrene In 63% of 33 patients hospitalized for this disorder. *0781*

787.00 Vomiting *2538*

929.00 Crush Injury (Trauma) *0995*

948.00 Burns *2538*

989.50 Toxic Effects of Venom May be caused by poisoning by chemicals, drugs, or venoms. *2467* Polymorphonuclear leukocytosis of 20,000-30,000/μL. *0995*

990.00 Effects of X-Ray Irradiation Within a few h after irradiation a neutrophilic leukocytosis appears. Following this, an oscillation in the neutrophilic count occurs, the rate at which it falls to the minimum being a function of the dose of radiation. *0995* Increased in electric shock. *2538*

994.50 Exercise *2538*

994.80 Effects of Electric Current Leukocytosis with many large immature granulocytes is common after severe shock. *0995*

Blood Normal

204.10 Lymphocytic Leukemia (Chronic) Usually normal, mean = 6,000/μL. *0242*

Urine Increase

580.00 Acute Poststreptococcal Glomerulonephritis In interstitial nephritis and nephrosclerosis patients, the percentage of polymorphonuclear granulocytes was 76-85%. *1411*

599.00 Urinary Tract Infection The median values for polymorphonuclear granulocytes were > 90% in bacterial renal or urinary tract disease and in polycystic kidney disease. *1411*

753.10 Polycystic Kidney Disease The median values were higher than 90% in bacterial, renal, or urinary tract disease and in polycystic kidney disease. *1411*

CSF Increase

36.00 Meningococcal Meningitis Cell count is elevated to thousands/μL, mostly neutrophils. *0151*

45.90 Acute Poliomyelitis Is usually 25-500/μL at first most are polymorphonuclear leukocytes; after several days most are lymphocytes. *2468 0433*

47.00 Aseptic Meningitis May predominate in the early phase but these cells are also found in bacterial meningitis. *0433*

72.00 Mumps In meningitis and meningoencephalitis fewer than 500 cells/μL with only occasional cell counts exceeding 2,000/μL in most cases the cells are almost exclusively mononuclear from the onset: polymorphonuclear leukocytes predominate for the first few days in only a small percentage of patients. Pleocytosis may continue for as long as 5 weeks. *0433*

114.90 Coccidioidomycosis Fewer than 500 leukocytes/μL, as many as 50% neutrophils initially with lymphocytes predominating later. *1058*

320.90 Meningitis (Bacterial) Several hundred to 60,000/μL with predominantly polymorphonuclear cells present. *0151* Ranges between 500-20,000/μL, with about 90% polymorphonuclears. Counts > 25,000 suggest a ruptured brain abscess. *0962 0999 2400*

323.92 Encephalomyelitis Pleocytosis ranges from 10-500/μL. Granulocytes may prevail for 1-2 days after onset. Counts may exceed 100/μL especially in lymphocytic choriomeningitis and eastern equine encephalomyelitis. *0433*

434.10 Cerebral Embolism In septic embolus, the proportion of lymphocytes and polymorphonuclears varies with the acuteness of the septic process. *0992*

Synovial Fluid Decrease

710.00 Systemic Lupus Erythematosus WBC are usually low (< 5,000/μL) with a low percentage of neutrophils. *0433*

Synovial Fluid Increase

99.30 Reiter's Disease Polymorphonuclear leukocytosis in the range of 2,000-10,000/μL. *0433*

274.00 Gout Increase in percentage of neutrophils in acute attacks; range = 48-94% (Normal less than 5%). *2467*

390.00 Rheumatic Fever Increased number neutrophils, ranging from 8-98/μL. *2467*

711.00 Acute Arthritis (Pyogenic) Increase in number, ranging from 75-100/μL. *2467*

714.00 Rheumatoid Arthritis Increased number, ranging from 5-96/μL. *2467*

Neutrophils (continued)

Pleural Effusion   Increase

11.00 **Pulmonary Tuberculosis**   Neutrophils predominate in very early stages. *1403*

415.10 **Pulmonary Embolism and Infarction**   Predominant cell type. *2017*   Neutrophils predominate in pleural fluid *1403*

482.90 **Bacterial Pneumonia**   Predominant cell type. *2017*

486.01 **Resolving Pneumonia**   Neutrophils predominate in pleural fluid. *1403*

510.00 **Empyema**   Very high counts occur; cells tend to degenerate, with blurred nuclei which do not stain in characteristic purple color. *1403*

567.90 **Peritonitis**   Neutrophils predominate in pleural fluid. *1403*

577.00 **Acute Pancreatitis**   Predominant cell type. *2017*

577.10 **Chronic Pancreatitis**   Predominant cell type. *2017*   Neutrophils predominate in pleural fluid *1403*

714.00 **Rheumatoid Arthritis**   Predominant cells neutrophils or monocytes. *2017*

Ascitic Fluid   Increase

567.90 **Peritonitis**   10 of 11 patients with bacterial peritonitis had counts > 250/μL. Very few patients with other diseases had comparable granulocyte counts. *1187*

Bone Marrow   Decrease

202.40 **Leukemic Reticuloendotheliosis**   Severe bone marrow granulocytopenia and poor neutrophil response to stimulation are found. *2587*

710.00 **Systemic Lupus Erythematosus**   Reduced counts in 7 of 21 cases. 62% had a subnormal response to etiocholanolone challenge, indicating reduced marrow reserves. *1267*

Bone Marrow   Increase

205.10 **Myelocytic Leukemia (Chronic)**   Granulocytic and sometimes megakaryocytic hyperplasia in bone marrow. *0337*   Resemble those in the peripheral blood, but on the average they are about 1 stage less mature. *2538*

Bone Marrow   Absent

288.00 **Agranulocytosis**   Bone marrow shows absence of cells in granulocytic series but normal erythroid and megakaryocytic series. *2468* *2552*

Sputum   Increase

494.00 **Bronchiectasis**   Polymorphonuclear and lymphocytic, as well as bronchial epithelial cells with varying degrees of metaplasia. *0433*

Nickel

Serum   Decrease

70.00 **Viral Hepatitis**   Thought to be caused by hypoalbuminemia. *1559*

410.90 **Acute Myocardial Infarction**   Decreases occur soon after infarction (within 24 h for Caucasian males and before the 3rd day in Caucasian females and Black males), followed by a sharp rise to > 2 X normal value. *2502*

571.90 **Cirrhosis of Liver**   Mean 1.6 (n = 18) compared with controls mean 2.6 μg/L (n = 42). *1559*

572.20 **Hepatic Encephalopathy**   Thought to be caused by hypoalbuminemia. *1559*

572.40 **Hepatic Failure**   Thought to be caused by hypoalbuminemia. *1559*

573.30 **Toxic Hepatitis**   Thought to be caused by hypoalbuminemia. *1559*

581.90 **Nephrotic Syndrome**   Thought to be caused by hypoalbuminemia. *1559*

Serum   Increase

410.90 **Acute Myocardial Infarction**   Decrease occurs soon after infarction (within 24 h for Caucasian males and before the 3rd day in Caucasian females and Black males), followed by a sharp rise to > 2 X normal value. *2502*   Mean 5.2 μg/L (N = 33) compared with control mean of 2.6 μg/L (N = 42). *1559*

434.00 **Cerebral Thrombosis**   Mean 5.2 (n = 33) compared with controls mean 2.6 μg/L (n = 42). *1559*   Increased.

948.00 **Burns**   Mean 7.2 (n = 3) compared with controls mean 2.6 μg/L (n = 42). *1559*

Serum   Normal

291.00 **Delirium Tremens**   Mean 2.3 (n = 35) compared with controls mean 2.6 μg/L (n = 42). *1559*

359.11 **Progressive Muscular Dystrophy**   Mean 2.3 (n = 10) compared with controls mean 2.6 μg/L (n = 42). *1559*

Nicotinamide

Serum   Decrease

270.02 **Hartnup Disease**   From loss of precursor tryptophan. *0995*

Nitrogen

Serum   Decrease

570.00 **Acute and Subacute Necrosis of Liver**   *0619*

Serum   Increase

271.20 **Hereditary Fructose Intolerance**   Amino acid nitrogen increases as a result of deranged hepatic function after administration. *2246*

642.60 **Eclampsia**   Blood-urea tends to decrease, but amino acids and unknown substances are increased. *0619*

Urine   Increase

642.40 **Pre-Eclampsia**   Urinary amines are increased in hypertension resulting from pregnancy. *2623*

642.60 **Eclampsia**   Urinary amines are increased in hypertension resulting from pregnancy. *2623*

Feces   Increase

537.40 **Fistula of Stomach and Duodenum**   *0619*

558.90 **Diarrhea**   *0619*

577.10 **Chronic Pancreatitis**   *0619*

579.00 **Celiac Sprue Disease**   *0619*

Liver   Decrease

260.00 **Protein Malnutrition**   The level of nitrogen in the liver of children with kwashiorkor is markedly decreased over that for children of the same age. *0151*

Norepinephrine

Serum   Increase

346.00 **Migraine**   Levels are increased during acute attacks. *0996*

428.00 **Congestive Heart Failure**   Consistently elevated. Typically average 700-800 pg/mL. *2631*

585.00 **Chronic Renal Failure**   Moderate increase. *0649*

Plasma   Decrease

250.00 **Diabetes Mellitus**   Long-term diabetics with neuropathy showed significant reductions. Diabetics without neuropathy had normal concentrations. *0399*

296.80 **Manic Depressive Disorder**   Usually high in patients with a 6 month or longer history of depression and anxiety, but individual patients may have a markedly low value. *1300*

300.40 **Depressive Neurosis**   Usually high in patients with a 6 month or longer history of depression and anxiety, but individual patients may have a markedly low value. *1300*

Plasma   Increase

38.00 **Septicemia**   In patients with septicemic, traumatic or hemorrhagic shock, epinephrine and norepinephrine concentrations were increased above the normal range. In nonsurvivors norepinephrine concentrations remained persistently elevated while in survivors there was a rapid decline towards the normal range. *0164*

227.91 Pheochromocytoma Blood levels of norepinephrine and to a lesser extent, epinephrine are increased, usually even when patient is asymptomatic and normotensive; rarely are increases found only following a paroxysm. *2467*

244.90 Hypothyroidism Circulating levels are elevated and hypertension is not uncommon. *0999*

250.10 Diabetic Acidosis With fasting, profound exercise and orthostatic changes, norepinephrine secretion is enhanced. *2540*

296.80 Manic Depressive Disorder Usually high in patients with a 6 month or longer history of depression and anxiety, but individual patients may have a markedly low value. *1300*

300.40 Depressive Neurosis Usually high in patients with a 6 month or longer history of depression and anxiety, but individual patients may have a markedly low value. *1300*

410.90 Acute Myocardial Infarction Evidence for a sympathoadrenal response is found in the increased blood and urinary concentration or norepinephrine, epinephrine, or their metabolic products. *1108 1163 1451*

431.00 Cerebral Hemorrhage Plasma concentrations were greatly increased compared to normals, cardiac catheterization patients, and patients with other illnesses. Mean for all the hemorrhagic patients was 0.94 ± 0.10 ng/mL. Patients with poor prognosis had initially higher and markedly higher follow-up concentrations than those with good prognosis. *0163*

533.90 Peptic Ulcer, Site Unspecified *0271*

785.50 Shock In patients with septicemic, traumatic or hemorrhagic shock, epinephrine and norepinephrine concentrations were increased above the normal range. In patients who died, plasma norepinephrine concentrations remained persistently elevated above normal while in those who survived, there was a rapid decline towards the normal range. *0164*

994.50 Exercise Significant effect after physical stress. *0768*

Plasma Normal

250.10 Diabetic Acidosis Following insulin-induced hypoglycemia, there is no change. *2425*

Urine Increase

227.91 Pheochromocytoma Urine levels of norepinephrine and, to a lesser extent, epinephrine are increased, usually even when patient is asymptomatic and normotensive; rarely are increases found only following a paroxysm. *2467* In almost all patients with pheochromocytoma, analysis of any 24-h urine collection will reveal increased excretion of norepinephrine. *0151 0962*

308.00 Stress With physical or emotional stress. *2092*

333.40 Huntington's Chorea *0878*

390.00 Rheumatic Fever Epirephrine and norepinephrine increase in proportion to the severity of circulatory failure. Catecholamine excretion, especially norepinephrine, is significantly raised in grades 3 and 4 of hemodynamic disturbance. *2572*

410.90 Acute Myocardial Infarction Evidence for sympathoadrenal response is found in the increased blood and urinary concentration or norepinephrine, epinephrine, or their metabolic products. *1108* In patients developing heart failure or cardiogenic shock, the urinary level of both free catecholamines rose notably in the 1st week after infarction. In uncomplicated cases, a moderate rise in the norepinephrine level in the 1st week was associated with only a transient rise in the epinephrine level. *1163*

414.00 Chronic Ischemic Heart Disease Increased in proportion to the severity of circulatory failure. Catecholamine excretion especially norepinephrine, is significantly raised in grades 3 and 4 of hemodynamic disturbance. *2572*

415.00 Cor Pulmonale Increased in proportion to the severity of circulatory failure. Catecholamine excretion, especially norepinephrine, is significantly raised in grades 3 and 4 of hemodynamic disturbance. *2572*

991.60 Hypothermia With cold exposure. *2092*

994.50 Exercise Excretion may rise up to 200-300 ng/min. *2200* If strenuous, may be increased 10 fold. *0161*

Urine Normal

333.40 Huntington's Chorea *1662*

Occult Blood

Urine Positive

270.01 Cystinuria *0995*

CSF Positive

431.00 Cerebral Hemorrhage In early subarachnoid hemorrhage (< 8 h after onset of symptoms), test may be positive before xanthochromia develops in CSF. *2467*

Feces Positive

2.00 Typhoid Fever May occur and lead to normochromic anemia later in the disease. *0151* Frequent during the 3rd and 4th weeks. *1058*

4.90 Bacillary Dysentery During the acute phase, examination of the stool will reveal clumps of polymorphonuclear leukocytes and RBCs, and the stool culture will be positive. *0962*

40.20 Whipple's Disease 30% of patients have this finding. *0999*

100.00 Leptospirosis Hemorrhagic manifestations may occur in the first few days of fever. *2368*

126.90 Ancylostomiasis (Hookworm Infestation) Occult or frank blood can be demonstrated at all times. *2368*

127.20 Strongyloidiasis Stools frequently contain occult blood, mucus, and larvae. *2199*

127.30 Trichuriasis Bloody diarrhea. *1058*

150.90 Malignant Neoplasm of Esophagus GI bleeding may occur with malignancies. *2199*

151.90 Malignant Neoplasm of Stomach Persistence of occult blood in the stool is strong evidence of malignancy but, does not indicate the location of the lesion. *0962* Anemia may be of several types. The most common is iron deficiency anemia caused by chronic occult blood loss. *2199*

152.90 Malignant Neoplasm of Small Intestine Persistence of occult blood in the stool is strong evidence of malignancy, but does not indicate the location of the lesion. *0962* Anemia may be of several types. The most common is iron deficiency anemia caused by chronic occult blood loss. *2199*

153.90 Malignant Neoplasm of Large Intestine The most important screening test for cancer of the large bowel in asymptomatic persons. *2549* GI bleeding may occur with malignancies. *2199*

154.10 Malignant Neoplasm of Rectum The most important screening test for cancer of the large bowel in asymptomatic persons. *2549* GI bleeding may occur with malignancies. *2199*

155.00 Malignant Neoplasm of Liver GI bleeding may occur with malignancies. *2199*

155.10 Malignant Neoplasm of Intrahepatic Bile Ducts Frequently positive. *2467*

157.90 Malignant Neoplasm of Pancreas Often found. *0992*

211.10 Benign Neoplasm of Stomach Adenomatous and villous polyps may result in GI bleeding. *2199*

211.40 Benign Neoplasm of Rectum and Anus Large amount of mucus tinged with blood; frequent watery diarrhea. *2467* Adenomatous and villous polyps may result in GI bleeding. *2199*

267.00 Vitamin C Deficiency May be positive in scurvy. *2468*

287.00 Allergic Purpura Stool may show blood. *2468 2552*

441.00 Dissecting Aortic Aneurysm *2199*

516.10 Idiopathic Pulmonary Hemosiderosis Stools may contain occult blood as a result of swallowed blood-laden sputum. *2538*

535.00 Gastritis Upper GI bleeding. *2199*

537.40 Fistula of Stomach and Duodenum The most common presentation. False negative and positives occur. *2512*

553.30 Hernia Diaphragmatic May be positive. *2467*

555.90 Regional Enteritis or Ileitis Stools are not grossly bloody, insidious blood loss with guaiac positive stools is the rule. *0962* Chronic blood loss. *2199 0999*

556.00 Ulcerative Colitis Positive for blood (gross and/or occult). *2467* Lower GI bleeding. *2199*

557.01 Mesenteric Artery Embolism Upper GI bleeding. *2199*

560.90 Intestinal Obstruction Gross rectal blood suggests carcinoma of colon or intussusception. *2467*

562.00 Diverticular Disease of Intestine May occur. *2199*

562.11 Diverticulitis of Colon *2199*

576.20 Extrahepatic Biliary Obstruction May be positive or negative in patients with extrahepatic biliary obstruction. *0999*

577.00 Acute Pancreatitis *2199*

577.10 Chronic Pancreatitis *2199*

984.00 Toxic Effects of Lead and Its Compounds (including Fumes) Bloody diarrhea may occur. *0850*

Occult Blood (continued)

Feces   Positive (continued)

985.00   **Toxic Effects of Non-medicinal Metals**   Bloody diarrhea occurs with arsenic and mercury poisoning. *0889*

Gastric Material   Positive

151.90   **Malignant Neoplasm of Stomach**   Tests for the presence of blood in the gastric contents are positive in a high percentage of cases. Gross blood in the gastric content is a more important finding; found in nearly 50% of the cases. *0962*

560.90   **Intestinal Obstruction**   Positive test suggests strangulation; there may be gross blood if strangulated segment is high in jejunum. *2467*

Ornithine

Urine   Increase

270.01   **Cystinuria**   Characteristic. *2246*

270.03   **Cystinosis**   Nonspecific pattern of aminoaciduria. Fanconi's syndrome. *0995*

Ornithine Carbamoyl Transferase (OCT)

Serum   Increase

70.00   **Viral Hepatitis**   Liver cell damage. *2467*

120.00   **Schistosomiasis**   Consistently and markedly elevated in patients upon admission, during treatment (highest elevations), and at follow-up 1 month later. Elevated levels may indicate liver cell defect which was not corrected by treatment or by improving the dietary conditions. *2026*

155.00   **Malignant Neoplasm of Liver**   Liver cell damage. *2467*

197.70   **Secondary Malignant Neoplasm of Liver**   Liver cell damage. *2467*

291.00   **Delirium Tremens**   Liver cell damage. *2467*

303.90   **Alcoholism**   Liver cell damage. *2467*

428.00   **Congestive Heart Failure**   Liver cell damage. *2467*

570.00   **Acute and Subacute Necrosis of Liver**   Liver cell damage. *2467*

571.20   **Laennec's or Alcoholic Cirrhosis**   Liver cell damage. *2467*

571.90   **Cirrhosis of Liver**   Liver cell damage. *2467*

572.00   **Liver Abscess (Pyogenic)**   Liver cell damage. *2467*

575.00   **Acute Cholecystitis**   Liver cell damage. *2467*

576.20   **Extrahepatic Biliary Obstruction**   Liver cell damage. *2467*

990.00   **Effects of X-Ray Irradiation**   Reflects breakdown of tissue proteins. *0290*

994.50   **Exercise**   Observed to increase following exercise. *0804* Maximum effect observed 7 days after exercise. *0985*

Osmolality

Serum   Decrease

162.90   **Malignant Neoplasm of Bronchus and Lung**   Inappropriate secretion of ADH is associated with hyponatremia, decreased serum osmolality, and inappropriately high sodium concentration in the urine. The entire syndrome resolves following resection of the tumor. *0962*

255.40   **Adrenal Cortical Hypofunction**   *0619*

Serum   Increase

253.50   **Diabetes Insipidus**   If the water intake does not keep pace with the urinary output, there may be mild hypernatremia and a tendency toward serum hyperosmolality. *0962*

Urine   Decrease

203.00   **Multiple Myeloma**   Mean for the group following overnight dehydration was 444 ± 26 mOsm/kg; patients with Bence-Jones proteinuria had further reduced concentrating ability. *0518*

253.50   **Diabetes Insipidus**   Usually < 200 mOsm/kg. *0962*

282.60   **Sickle Cell Anemia**   Chronic defect in renal concentrating ability frequently present. *1001   2538*

405.91   **Renovascular Hypertension**   Renal functional impairment. *0962*

580.01   **Glomerulonephritis (Focal)**   Concentrating capacity is impaired, with urine specific gravity around 1.010. *0962*

584.00   **Acute Renal Failure**   Manifested by oliguria, increasing serum-creatinine, a urine osmolality of < 400 mOsm/kg and a urine/plasma osmolality ratio of < 1·5. *1607*   < 350 mOsm in intrarenal acute renal failure *1595*

585.00   **Chronic Renal Failure**   With renal parenchymal disease. *0838*

590.00   **Chronic Pyelonephritis**   With renal parenchymal disease. *0838*

994.50   **Exercise**   Effect most marked with light exercise. *1205*

Urine   Increase

584.00   **Acute Renal Failure**   > 500 mOsm/kg in prerenal acute renal failure. *1595*

Urine   Normal

585.00   **Chronic Renal Failure**   250-400 mOsm/kg; becomes fixed close to plasma level of 280-295 mOsm/kg. *0186*

Osmotic Fragility

Red Blood Cells   Decrease

238.40   **Polycythemia Vera**   *2468*

280.90   **Iron Deficiency Anemia**   Decreased, reflecting the diminished hemoglobin concentration. *0151*   May be within the normal range, but often there is increased resistance to destruction in hypotonic salt solution. Extreme resistance is unusual. *2552*

281.20   **Folic Acid Deficiency Anemia**   *2467*

281.30   **Vitamin B_6 Deficiency Anemia**   Tends to be decreased. *2538*

282.41   **Thalassemia Major**   Osmotic fragility is reduced; the red cells are usually resistant to hemolysis in hypotonic saline. *0999 0962*

282.42   **Thalassemia Minor**   Decreased osmotic fragility is a method for identifying the heterozygote. *0999*

282.60   **Sickle Cell Anemia**   Decreased (more resistant RBCs). *2467*

282.71   **Hemoglobin C Disease**   Osmotic fragility curves are abnormal, indicating the presence of populations of fragile cells (microspherocytes) and resistant In homozygotes. *2468* Biphasic, with both increased and decreased fragility. *0503   2552 2538*

282.72   **Hemoglobin E Disease**   *2538*

285.00   **Sideroblastic Anemia**   Tends to be decreased. *2538*

289.80   **Myelofibrosis**   Red cell osmotic fragility was decreased in 63% of myelofibrosis patients. *2317*

570.00   **Acute and Subacute Necrosis of Liver**   *2467*

576.20   **Extrahepatic Biliary Obstruction**   Thin, flat erythrocytes are more resistant than normal cells and have decreased osmotic fragility. *0962*

984.00   **Toxic Effects of Lead and Its Compounds (including Fumes)**   Osmotic fragility is decreased and mechanic fragility is increased. *0151*

Red Blood Cells   Increase

84.00   **Malaria**   *1058*

201.90   **Hodgkin's Disease**   A higher degree of light transmission, i.e., osmotic fragility, was found in lymphocytes from Hodgkin's disease patients. After 10 min, light transmission = 70.3% - 5.93% compared to 60% ± 7.33% for normals. *1916*

204.10   **Lymphocytic Leukemia (Chronic)**   Degree of light transmission is used as a measure of lysis of lymphocytes, (i.e., as a measure of osmotic fragility). After 10 min, light transmission of lymphocytes was 78.5% ± 4.65%, compared to 60 ± 7.33%. *1916 2538*

282.00   **Hereditary (Congenital) Spherocytosis**   Almost always increased; in cases in which the cell defect is minor, incubation will bring out the abnormal fragility. *0962*   Typically increased. Hemolysis may be complete at the concentration where it normally commences. *2552   2538 0151*

282.10 **Hereditary Elliptocytosis**   Usually normal but may be increased in patients with overt hemolysis. *2538*

282.20 **Anemias Due To Disorders of Glutathione Metabolism** *2467*

282.31 **Hereditary Nonspherocytic Hemolytic Anemia**   *2467*

282.71 **Hemoglobin C Disease**   Biphasic, with both increased and decreased fragility. *0503*

283.00 **Acquired Hemolytic Anemia (Autoimmune)**   May be normal with mild hemolysis. With more rapid rates of hemolysis, the cumulative curve shows increasing populations of fragile cells correlated with the appearance of spherocytosis in the peripheral blood smear. *2601   2538*

283.21 **Paroxysmal Nocturnal Hemoglobinuria**   Increased in symptomatic hemolytic anemia. *2467*

650.00 **Pregnancy**   Cells may have become more spherical due to inhibition of water. *1113*

773.00 **Hemolytic Disease of Newborn (Erythroblastosis Fetalis)**   Increased with ABO erythroblastosis. *2468*

948.00 **Burns**   Increased after thermal injury. *2467*

Red Blood Cells   Normal

277.11 **Congenital Erythropoietic Porphyria (Günther's Disease)**   *0867*

282.10 **Hereditary Elliptocytosis**   Usually normal even after incubation. *2552*

282.31 **Hereditary Nonspherocytic Hemolytic Anemia**   The osmotic fragility of fresh erythrocytes is usually normal. *2538*

283.00 **Acquired Hemolytic Anemia (Autoimmune)**   Increased in some cases of secondary hemolytic anemia but it is usually normal. *2467*

283.21 **Paroxysmal Nocturnal Hemoglobinuria**   *2552*

284.90 **Aplastic Anemia**   RBC fragility is normal. *2552*

585.00 **Chronic Renal Failure**   *1421*

Osteocalcin

Serum   Decrease

571.60 **Biliary Cirrhosis**   In 15 premenopausal females with this disorder. *1057*

Serum   Increase

585.00 **Chronic Renal Failure**   Markedly elevated. *0671*

731.00 **Osteitis Deformans**   Elevated in 53% of patients. *2535*

Oval Fat Bodies

Urine   Increase

250.00 **Diabetes Mellitus**   With diabetic nephropathy. *0186*

581.90 **Nephrotic Syndrome**   The lipoid material is usually degenerative fatty vacuoles, neutral fat droplets, oval fat bodies, and doubly refractile fat bodies. *0962   0433*

Urine   Positive

446.00 **Polyarteritis-Nodosa**   *0186*

Prostatic Fluid   Increase

601.00 **Prostatitis**   Since the presence of increased number of leukocytes and oval fat bodies are seen equally in cases of chronic bacterial prostatitis and nonbacterial prostatitis, the microscopic appearance of the expressed prostatic secretions is not specifically diagnostic. *0433*

Oxalate

Urine   Increase

555.90 **Regional Enteritis or Ileitis**   *0218*

579.00 **Celiac Sprue Disease**   6 of 9 children with untreated disease had hyperoxaluria. *1726*

579.90 **Malabsorption, Cause Unspecified**   *0186*

Oxygen Saturation

Blood   Decrease

11.00 **Pulmonary Tuberculosis**   Empyema or tuberculous effusion. *0797*

135.00 **Sarcoidosis**   Decreased with lung involvement. *2468*

162.90 **Malignant Neoplasm of Bronchus and Lung**   Impaired diffusion. *2104*

197.00 **Secondary Malignant Neoplasm of Respiratory System**   Impaired diffusion. *0422*

238.40 **Polycythemia Vera**   Mild degrees of unsaturation may occur in patients with otherwise well-documented cases, uncomplicated by independent cardiac or pulmonary disease. *1651*   Arterial oxygen saturation is normal in early cases but mild desaturation is not unusual later in the course of the disease due to the complication of pulmonary emboli. *0433   2538*

242.90 **Hyperthyroidism**   Dyspnea. *2199*

244.90 **Hypothyroidism**   Rare dyspnea secondary to pleural effusion. *2540*

265.00 **Thiamine (B$_1$) Deficiency**   *1108*

272.72 **Gaucher's Disease**   With lung involvement. *2246*

277.00 **Cystic Fibrosis**   Pulmonary involvement. *0438*

282.60 **Sickle Cell Anemia**   The partial pressure of oxygen in arterial blood is usually diminished as a result of shunting within the lung. *0433*   Decreased oxygenation and increased acidosis PO$_2$ and lead to further sickling and further vaso-occlusion. *0874*

282.71 **Hemoglobin C Disease**   Low oxygen affinity. *1649*

282.72 **Hemoglobin E Disease**   RBC oxygen affinity has been found to be decreased, possibly accounting for the anemia. *0433*

289.00 **Polycythemia, Secondary**   *2538*

304.90 **Drug Dependence (Opium and Derivatives)**   Overdose. *0995*

358.00 **Myasthenia Gravis**   Associated respiratory insufficiency. *0995*

359.21 **Myotonia Atrophica**   Respiratory muscle weakness may develop. *0361*

410.90 **Acute Myocardial Infarction**   Very frequent complication; occurs in about 60% of uncomplicated cases. The intensity of hypoxemia is greatest after 2-3 days. The most intense and persisting hypoxemia was seen in patients with shock and/or acute left ventricular failure. Present even 6 months after onset in 25%. *2529*   Patients may develop arterial and tissue hypoxia and metabolic acidosis with a decrease in arterial pH and pO$_2$. *1108*   Arterial pO$_2$ falls, but rarely below 70 mm Hg if there is reasonable cardiovascular function. In left ventricular failure with associated pulmonary edema, the arterial pO$_2$ may fall to 50 mm Hg. *0619   0731*

415.00 **Cor Pulmonale**   Acute hypoxia and hypermetabolism associated with fever and infection. *1108*

415.10 **Pulmonary Embolism and Infarction**   pO$_2$ > 80 mm Hg excludes diagnosis of pulmonary embolism in almost all cases. *2126*   pO$_2$ and pCO$_2$ are both low. *1721*   Abnormal alveolar-arterial gradient for oxygen and resting hypoxemia. Arterial pO$_2$ fails to exceed 55 mm Hg following 100% oxygen breathing. *0962*

486.01 **Resolving Pneumonia**   Moderate to severe hypoxia and respiratory alkalosis in pneumocystis pneumonitis. *1096*   Low pO$_2$ with normal or high pCO$_2$. *2612*

491.00 **Chronic Bronchitis**   Tendency to decrease with the increase in dyspnea severity was apparent. *1496   1497 2335 2612*

492.80 **Pulmonary Emphysema**   Arterial tension in 54 patients with chronic nonspecific lung disease, indicated subnormal results to be more frequent among bronchitics (79% with hypoxemia) than among emphysematous patients (63% with hypoxemia). *1497*   66% of nonasthmatic chronic lung disease patients (bronchitis and emphysema) had a mean pO$_2$ of 72.7 mm Hg. Bronchitics, but not emphysemics, showed a positive correlation between pO$_2$ and ventilatory performance. *2335   2612*

493.10 **Asthma (Intrinsic)**   *0433 2035*

495.90 **Allergic Alveolitis**   Arterial blood gases show decreased pO$_2$ with either slight respiratory alkalosis or normal pH and pCO$_2$. *0433*

496.00 **Chronic Obstructive Lung Disease**   Greatest declines in arterial oxygen saturation occurred during sleep, with intermittent decreases as great as 44% saturation (range, 12-44% saturation). *0748*   Decreased pO$_2$ associated with increased pCO$_2$. *2467*

500.00 **Anthracosis**   Arterial oxygen saturation may fall. *0433*

501.00 **Asbestosis**   Arterial oxygen saturation may fall. *0433*

Oxygen Saturation *(continued)*

Blood   Decrease *(continued)*

502.00   Silicosis   Impaired gas exchange and movement of respiratory cage due to noncompliant lungs. *0151*   Arterial oxygen saturation may fall. *0433*

503.01   Berylliosis   Hypoxemia is frequent. *2608*   Arterial oxygen saturation may fall. *0433*

510.00   Empyema   Empyema or tuberculous effusion. *0797*

516.00   Pulmonary Alveolar Proteinosis   May be normal or reduced. *0151*

518.00   Pulmonary Collapse   Acute massive atelectasis produces a picture of an intrapulmonary right-to-left shunt with a drop in pO_2. *0433*

518.40   Pulmonary Edema   Decreased pO_2 associated with normal or decreased pCO_2. *2467*   Mean arterial O_2 tension measured in 71 patients breathing room air was 59 mm Hg. The 14 acidemic patients had markedly lower pO_2, all under 60 mm Hg. *0554*

553.30   Hernia Diaphragmatic   Severe hypoxia may be present. *0433*   11 out of 20 infants with congenital hernia survived. Of the 9 nonsurvivors, arterial pCO_2 levels were markedly higher (61.3 ± 15.4 mm Hg) and pO_2 levels lower (49.8 ± 14.2) than in survivors (44.3 ± 7.9, 307.9 ± 142.3, respectively). *0245*

577.00   Acute Pancreatitis   Blood gases often reveal a moderate lowering of pO_2. *2199*

642.40   Pre-Eclampsia   In 9 patients with severe pre-eclampsia, there was a significant increase in alveolar-to-arterial pO_2 difference and physiological shunt, indicating a degree of pulmonary ventilation/perfusion imbalance. *2340*

737.30   Kyphoscoliosis   Thoracic bellows defects; decreased pO_2 associated with increased pCO_2. *2467*   Mean pCO_2 increased and pO_2 decreased with age in idiopathic scoliosis. *1206*

770.80   Respiratory Distress Syndrome   Impaired ventilation. *2467*

785.50   Shock   Disturbed RBC 2,3-DPG metabolism results in reduced oxygen affinity and delivery to tissues. *0151*

829.00   Fracture of Bone   Decreased arterial pO_2 associated with normal or decreased pCO_2 with associated fat embolism. *2468*

958.10   Fat Embolism   Decreased arterial pO_2 with normal or decreased pCO_2. *2467*   *2532*

986.00   Toxic Effects of Carbon Monoxide   *2468*

991.60   Hypothermia   Due to hypoxia, acid-base imbalance hypotension. *1471*

Blood   Increase

250.00   Diabetes Mellitus   Diabetics with pronounced hyperlipidemia due to accumulation of chylomicrons showed markedly increased hemoglobin-oxygen affinity (p 50:21.1 vs 26.6 mm Hg). *0568*

272.31   Type I Hyperlipoproteinemia   Hemoglobin-oxygen affinity is increased. *0568*

Blood   Normal

238.40   Polycythemia Vera   Nearly all patients with true polycythemia vera have a near normal arterial oxygen saturation. *2492*   *2538*

Oxytocin

CSF   Normal

331.00   Alzheimer's Disease   No difference from controls. *1881*

Parathyroid Hormone

Serum   Decrease

135.00   Sarcoidosis   Immeasurably low in most patients, both normo- and hypercalcemic. *1909*

242.90   Hyperthyroidism   Subnormal levels were found in 28.9% of cases. Parathyroid hormone correlated inversely to serum calcium and degree of hyperthyroidism. *1638*

252.10   Hypoparathyroidism   *2468 0999*

279.11   DiGeorge's Syndrome   *0793*

Serum   Increase

151.90   Malignant Neoplasm of Stomach   Lung cancer, hypernephroma, gastrointestinal cancer, and other neoplasms can synthesize and secrete parathyroid hormone. *0962*

152.90   Malignant Neoplasm of Small Intestine   Lung cancer, hypernephroma, gastrointestinal cancer, and other neoplasms can synthesize and secrete parathyroid hormone. *0962*

153.90   Malignant Neoplasm of Large Intestine   Lung cancer, hypernephroma, gastrointestinal cancer, and other neoplasms can synthesize and secrete parathyroid hormone. *0962*

162.90   Malignant Neoplasm of Bronchus and Lung   Lung cancer, hypernephroma, gastrointestinal cancer, and other neoplasms can synthesize and secrete parathyroid hormone. *0962*

189.00   Malignant Neoplasm of Kidney   Lung cancer, hypernephroma, gastrointestinal cancer, and other neoplasms can synthesize and secrete parathyroid hormone. *0962*

193.01   Medullary Carcinoma of Thyroid   Elevations in about 50% of medullary cancer patients. *0962*

252.00   Hyperparathyroidism   Raised serum calcium levels fail to depress hormone secretion. *0619*   Concentration rises above baseline level after neck massage only on the side of the adenoma, thereby aiding preoperative localization of the adenoma. *2467*   In over 90% of cases. *0062*   *0520 1492*

268.00   Vitamin D Deficiency Rickets   Decreased calcium absorption in the gut leads to overproduction of parathyroid hormone and the resulting phosphaturia and hypophosphatemia. *1287*   Increased in nutritional rickets. *1909*   *2246*

275.35   Vitamin D Resistant Rickets   Normal or only slight elevations. *2246*

275.42   Pseudohypoparathyroidism   Normally high and can be used to distinguish from true hypoparathyroidism. *2540*   Deficient end organ response. *0062*

303.00   Acute Alcoholic Intoxication   Increased following alcoholic binge of several days duration. *1594*

303.90   Alcoholism   Increased following alcoholic binge of several days duration. *1594*

577.00   Acute Pancreatitis   Elevated and inversely correlated with serum ionized calcium. *2509*

579.00   Celiac Sprue Disease   Malabsorption of calcium results in increased parathyroid hormone production and renal tubular reabsorption of phosphate decreases, leading to mild hypophosphatemia. *1287*

579.90   Malabsorption, Cause Unspecified   Malabsorption of calcium results in increased parathyroid hormone production and renal tubular reabsorption of phosphate decreases, leading to mild hypophosphatemia. *1287*

585.00   Chronic Renal Failure   Reaches 10 X normal late in renal failure. *0151*   Elevated in chronic uremia. *1038*   Increased nearly in all patients. May be extremely high. Rough inverse correlation with renal function. *1909*   *1108*

588.00   Renal Dwarfism   *0151*

588.81   Proximal Renal Tubular Acidosis   Secondary to hypocalcemia. *0277*

588.82   Distal Renal Tubular Acidosis   Secondary to reduced calcium. *0417*

650.00   Pregnancy   Decreased during midgestation and increases thereafter to clearly elevated levels. *1909*

Partial Thromboplastin Time

Plasma   Decrease

630.00   Hydatidiform Mole   Mean time was 32.9/37.1 s in patients compared to 33.6/35.9 in normal pregnancy. Associated with prolonged thrombin time and indicates hypercoagulability. *1430*

994.50   Exercise   Observed effect in exercise. *1839*

Plasma   Increase

84.00   Malaria   Consistent with the diagnosis of disseminated intravascular coagulation. *1058*

85.00   Leishmaniasis   Normal early in the disease but later becomes prolonged. *0151*

205.00   Myelocytic Leukemia (Acute)   Intravascular clotting has been documented in occasional patients. *0890*

205.10   Myelocytic Leukemia (Chronic)   Intravascular clotting has been documented for rare patients. *0890*

206.00 Monocytic Leukemia With disseminated intravascular clotting. *1552*

272.51 Tangier Disease Occasionally prolonged PTT, with normal prothrombin time. *2246*

279.31 Acquired Immunodeficiency Syndrome (AIDS) Noted in 24 of 34 patients with this disorder. Felt to be due to Lupus Anticoagulant. *0229* In 10 patients with AIDS all had elevated times. *0423*

286.01 Hemophilia The most sensitive screening test, usually prolonged if AHG levels are < 20% of normal. *0999* Always significantly prolonged in patients with 20% factor VIII. Individuals with levels ranging between 20-30% may have a PTT value either just outside or at the upper end of the normal range. *2538 0962 2246*

286.10 Christmas Disease In contrast to hemophilia A, the abnormality is corrected by serum but not by adsorbed plasma. *2538 0962 2246*

286.20 Factor XI Deficiency PTT or activated PTT test is prolonged and the prothrombin time normal. *2538 2246*

286.31 Congenital Dysfibrinogenemia Variable. Even when abnormal, rarely as prolonged as the prothrombin time or the thrombin time. *2538*

286.32 Factor XII Deficiency Activated partial thromboplastin time is prolonged. *2538 2246*

286.34 Congenital Afibrinogenemia Corrected by the addition of normal plasma or normal fibrinogen to the patient's plasma. *2538* Infinite. *2246*

286.35 Factor V Deficiency Prothrombin time and partial thromboplastin time, activated or unactivated, are all prolonged. *2538 2246*

286.36 Factor X Deficiency Prolonged. *2538 0433 2246*

286.38 Factor II Deficiency Variable. *2246*

286.40 Von Willebrand's Disease May be prolonged and is related to the decreased factor VIII AHF activity. *2538* Variable. *2246 0962*

286.60 Disseminated Intravascular Coagulopathy Prolonged because of consumption of clotting factors and the anticoagulant effects of fibrin degradation products. *2538*

571.90 Cirrhosis of Liver Severe clotting factor deficiencies are common. *0992*

572.00 Liver Abscess (Pyogenic) *0433*

710.00 Systemic Lupus Erythematosus *0962*

774.40 Jaundice Due to Hepatocellular Damage (Newborn) Markedly prolonged. *0433*

Plasma Normal

286.33 Factor XIII Deficiency *2246*

286.37 Factor VII Deficiency *2538 2246*

287.10 Thrombasthenia (Glanzmann's) *2246*

287.30 Idiopathic Thrombocytopenic Purpura *2552 2246*

446.60 Thrombotic Thrombocytopenic Purpura *2246*

pCO$_2$

Blood Decrease

70.00 Viral Hepatitis Reduced in a high percentage of chronic as well as acute hepatitis patients. *2104*

135.00 Sarcoidosis Mild hyperventilation is frequent except in advanced disease when ventilatory obstruction occurs. *0999* Impaired gas diffusion in pulmonary sarcoid may cause hyperventilation and reduced pCO$_2$. In more severe cases, CO$_2$ retention occurs. *2104* In 26% of 15 patients at initial hospitalization for this disorder. *0781* Decreased with lung involvement. *2468*

162.90 Malignant Neoplasm of Bronchus and Lung Impaired gas diffusion and the accompanying hyperventilation results in a low pCO$_2$, unless the defect is severe and CO$_2$ retention occurs in bronchiolar cell carcinoma. *2104*

202.52 Histiocytosis X With lung involvement, impaired gas diffusion. *2104*

242.90 Hyperthyroidism Respiratory alkalosis may occur. *0962*

250.00 Diabetes Mellitus *1854*

250.10 Diabetic Acidosis Hyperventilation. *2540* Metabolic acidosis may occur. *0962*

252.00 Hyperparathyroidism *2540*

259.20 Carcinoid Syndrome Hyperventilation may occur during the flush. *2540*

265.00 Thiamine (B$_1$) Deficiency Respiratory alkalosis may occur. *0962*

276.20 Metabolic Acidosis Tends to fall below normal range as the blood pH and bicarbonate fall. *0619* Ventilation is stimulated and pCO$_2$ falls. *0962*

291.00 Delirium Tremens Respiratory alkalosis may occur. *0962*

303.90 Alcoholism Plasma bicarbonate ranged from 2-10 mmol/L in acidosis following alcoholic binge. *1594*

306.10 Hyperventilation Syndrome Characteristically, the pCO$_2$ is reduced to 20-30 mm Hg. *0433* Respiratory alkalosis. *2103*

331.81 Reye's Syndrome Hypocapnia is common in children with this syndrome. *0151*

415.10 Pulmonary Embolism and Infarction Decreased pO$_2$ associated with normal or decreased pCO$_2$. *2467* pO$_2$ and pCO$_2$ are both low. *1721* In 62% of 19 patients at initial hospitalization for this disorder. *0781*

421.00 Bacterial Endocarditis In 14 narcotic addicts with bacterial endocarditis the arterial CO$_2$ tension, at 27.8 ± 1.7 mm Hg, was significantly lower than a group of narcotics with other disorders, at 40.1 ± 3.7 mm Hg. *1725*

428.00 Congestive Heart Failure Acidosis occurs when renal insufficiency is associated or there is CO$_2$ retention due to pulmonary insufficiency. *2467*

482.90 Bacterial Pneumonia In 63% of 14 patients at initial hospitalization for this disorder. *0781*

486.01 Resolving Pneumonia Moderate to severe hypoxia and respiratory alkalosis in pneumocystis pneumonitis. *1096* Respiratory alkalosis may occur. *0962* In 40% of 43 patients at initial hospitalization for this disorder. *0781* Impaired gas diffusion and the accompanying hyperventilation results in a low pCO$_2$, unless the defect is severe and CO$_2$ retention occurs. *2104*

491.00 Chronic Bronchitis Can occur due to compensatory increase in ventilatory rate. *2220*

493.10 Asthma (Intrinsic) Reduced in a moderate to severe attack, while normal values are obtained for bicarbonate and pH. As the condition worsens the pCO$_2$ while the pH falls. *0433* pH, total plasma CO$_2$ and pCO$_2$ are decreased as a result of metabolic acidosis in status asthmaticus. *1972* In 30% of 91 patients at initial hospitalization for this disorder. *0781*

501.00 Asbestosis Impaired gas diffusion and the accompanying hyperventilation results in a low pCO$_2$, unless the defect is severe and CO$_2$ retention occurs. *2104*

503.01 Berylliosis Impaired gas diffusion and the accompanying hyperventilation results in a low pCO$_2$, unless the defect is severe and CO$_2$ retention occurs. *2104*

514.00 Pulmonary Congestion and Hypostasis Respiratory alkalosis may occur. *0962*

516.00 Pulmonary Alveolar Proteinosis Impaired gas diffusion and the accompanying hyperventilation results in a low pCO$_2$, unless the defect is severe and CO$_2$ retention occurs. *2104*

516.10 Idiopathic Pulmonary Hemosiderosis Impaired gas diffusion and the accompanying hyperventilation results in a low pCO$_2$, unless the defect is severe and CO$_2$ retention occurs in primary pulmonary hemosiderosis. *2104*

518.00 Pulmonary Collapse Acute massive atelectasis produces a picture of an intrapulmonary right-to-left shunt with a drop in pCO$_2$. *0433* Respiratory alkalosis may occur. *0962*

518.40 Pulmonary Edema Decreased pO$_2$ associated with normal or decreased pCO$_2$. *2467*

537.40 Fistula of Stomach and Duodenum Metabolic acidosis may occur. *0962*

560.90 Intestinal Obstruction Metabolic acidosis secondary to lactic acidosis. *0186*

571.49 Chronic Active Hepatitis Reduced in a high percentage of chronic as well as acute hepatitis patients. *2104*

572.20 Hepatic Encephalopathy Respiratory alkalosis may occur. *0962*

572.40 Hepatic Failure Characteristic of liver failure. *2104*

584.00 Acute Renal Failure Metabolic acidosis may occur. *0962*

585.00 Chronic Renal Failure Metabolic acidosis may occur. *0962* In 63% of 31 patients at initial hospitalization for this disorder. *0781*

650.00 Pregnancy May be induced by progesterone. *1512 1460* Begins to fall early in gestation and persists at 5 mm Hg below normal until parturition. *2104*

pCO₂ *(continued)*

Blood Decrease *(continued)*

710.00 Systemic Lupus Erythematosus Impaired gas diffusion and the accompanying hyperventilation results in a low pCO_2, unless the defect is severe and CO_2 retention occurs. *2104*

714.00 Rheumatoid Arthritis Impaired gas diffusion and the accompanying hyperventilation results in a low pCO_2, unless the defect is severe and CO_2 retention occurs. *2104*

785.40 Gangrene In 22% of 13 patients hospitalized for this disorder. *0781*

785.50 Shock Respiratory alkalosis may occur. *0962*

829.00 Fracture of Bone Decreased arterial pO_2 associated with normal or decreased pCO_2 with associated fat embolism. *2468*

958.10 Fat Embolism Decreased arterial PO_2 with normal or decreased PCO_2. *2467*

991.60 Hypothermia pCO_2 falls as the blood pH and bicarbonate rise with falling body temperatures. *0619*

Blood Increase

37.00 Tetanus At the onset of mild forms, blood gases may be within normal values. Later, when spasms appear and high dosages of sedatives are given, hypoxemia, acidosis plus hypercapnia and metabolic acidosis are present. *0433* Metabolic alkalosis may occur with potassium loss. *0962*

45.90 Acute Poliomyelitis Respiratory acidosis may occur. *0962* Neurological impairment of the respiratory drive. *2612*

135.00 Sarcoidosis In more severe cases, CO_2 retention occurs. *2104*

255.00 Adrenal Cortical Hyperfunction (Glucocorticoid Excess) Metabolic alkalosis may occur with potassium loss. *0962*

255.00 Adrenal Cortical Hyperfunction (Mineralocorticoid Excess) Metabolic alkalosis may occur with potassium loss. *0962*

276.30 Metabolic Alkalosis Normal or slightly elevated. *0962*

277.00 Cystic Fibrosis Salt loss may lead to metabolic alkalosis. *1055*

357.00 Guillain-Barré Syndrome Respiratory acidosis may occur. *0962*

358.00 Myasthenia Gravis Associated respiratory insufficiency. *0995*

359.21 Myotonia Atrophica Respiratory muscle weakness may develop. *0361*

401.00 Malignant Hypertension Metabolic alkalosis may occur with potassium loss. *0962*

415.00 Cor Pulmonale The degree of arterial pCO_2 elevation is in direct proportion to the inadequacy of alveolar ventilation in relation to metabolic production of CO_2. *1108* Increased when Cor Pulmonale is secondary to chest deformities or pulmonary emphysema. *2467*

428.00 Congestive Heart Failure Alkalosis occurs in uncomplicated failure; hyperventilation, alveolar-capillary block due to associated pulmonary fibrosis; hypochloremic alkalosis due to potassium depletion. *2467*

480.90 Viral Pneumonia Low pO_2 with normal or high pCO_2. *2612*

492.80 Pulmonary Emphysema Arterial blood oxygen decreased and CO_2 increased. *2467* Respiratory acidosis may occur. *0962*

493.10 Asthma (Intrinsic) Reduced in a moderate to severe attack, while normal values are obtained for bicarbonate and pH. As the condition worsens the pCO_2 will rise while the pH falls. *0433* Reduction in arterial oxygen tension without concomitant elevation of arterial pCO_2 in moderately severe asthma. Elevation of pCO_2 is dependent upon total reduction in ventilation or will be seen when severe mucus plugging is present. *0433* CO_2 retention, indicating alveolar hypoventilation, has a grave prognostic significance. *0999*

496.00 Chronic Obstructive Lung Disease Decreased pO_2 associated with increased pCO_2. *2467* In 10 patients with hypercapnia, mean renal net acid excretion was elevated and correlated with arterial pCO_2, blood pH and urinary pH. *1479* In 33% of 75 patients at initial hospitalization for this disorder. *0781*

500.00 Anthracosis Impaired gas exchange in established cases. *0151*

501.00 Asbestosis Impaired gas exchange in established cases. *0151*

502.00 Silicosis Impaired gas exchange in established cases. *0151*

503.01 Berylliosis Impaired gas exchange in established cases. *0151*

553.30 Hernia Diaphragmatic 11 out of 20 infants with congenital hernia survived. Of the 9 nonsurvivors, arterial pCO_2 levels were markedly higher (61.3 + - 15.4 mm Hg) and pO_2 levels lower (49.8 ± 14.2) than in survivors (44.3 ± 7.9, 307.9 ± 142.3 respectively). *0245* Severe hypercarbia may be present. *0433*

720.00 Rheumatoid (Ankylosing) Spondylitis Impaired movement of the respiratory cage. *2612*

737.30 Kyphoscoliosis Thoracic bellows defects; decreased pO_2 associated with increased pCO_2. *2467* Mean pCO_2 increased and pO_2 decreased with age in idiopathic scoliosis. *1206*

770.80 Respiratory Distress Syndrome Impaired ventilation. *2467*

991.60 Hypothermia Due to hypoxia, acid-base imbalance hypotension. *1471*

Blood Normal

493.10 Asthma (Intrinsic) The finding of a normal pCO_2 in a patient experiencing a severe asthmatic attack should alert the clinician to impending respiratory failure. *0433*

Pepsin

Gastric Material Decrease

535.00 Gastritis In Ménétrier's Disease hyposecretion is usual finding. *0407*

650.00 Pregnancy May be decreased. *2468*

Pepsinogen

Serum Decrease

151.90 Malignant Neoplasm of Stomach A level < 200 U/L is conclusive of gastric atrophy, a precursor of gastric cancer. *0962*

535.00 Gastritis The combination of high serum gastrin and low pepsinogen is commonly found in patients with atrophic gastritis. *2199*

Serum Increase

533.90 Peptic Ulcer, Site Unspecified Serum acid protease activity at pH 1.8 (pepsin) shows slightly higher levels than normal. *1604* An elevated serum concentration appears to be a subclinical marker of the ulcer diathesis in families with the autosomal dominant form of peptic ulcer disease. Elevated immunoreactive pepsinogen I (> 100 ng/mL) segregated as a dominant trait in the affected families. *1997*

pH

Blood Decrease

1.00 Cholera Metabolic acidosis. *0151*

9.00 Gastroenteritis and Colitis May be noted. *0433*

37.00 Tetanus At the onset of mild forms, blood gases may be within the normal values. Later, when spasms appear and high dosages of sedatives are given, hypoxemia, acidosis plus hypercapnia and metabolic acidosis are present. *0433*

45.90 Acute Poliomyelitis Respiratory acidosis may occur. *0962*

250.00 Diabetes Mellitus From an accumulation of acetoacetate and beta-hydroxybutyric acid. *2540* *1854*

250.10 Diabetic Acidosis Metabolic acidosis may occur. *0962* Acidosis with low plasma pH and bicarbonate (usually < 10 mmol/L) is seen. *0999*

255.40 Adrenal Cortical Hypofunction Raised potassium concentration and metabolic acidosis usually occur. *2612*

256.30 Ovarian Hypofunction Progesterone effect. *0995*

256.41 Stein-Leventhal Syndrome *1337*

260.00 Protein Malnutrition The plasma pH tends to fall. *0619*

268.00 Vitamin D Deficiency Rickets Mild acidosis and hyperchloremia may be observed. *2246*

268.20 Osteomalacia In systemic acidosis. *0995*

270.03 Cystinosis Metabolic, hyperchloremic acidosis. *0433* Marked acidosis. *2246*

271.01 Von Gierke's Disease Acidosis. *0962*

271.03 Forbes Disease Acidosis. *0962*

271.10 Galactosemia Hyperchloremic acidosis. May be secondary to GI disturbance, poor food intake, or renal tubular dysfunction. *2246 1797*

276.20 Metabolic Acidosis Low usually 6.98-7.25 in type II-B, with lactic acidosis. *2468*

282.60 Sickle Cell Anemia Decreased oxygenation and increased acidosis develop and lead to further sickling and further vaso-occlusion. *0874*

303.00 Acute Alcoholic Intoxication Severe metabolic acidosis with pH ranging between 6.96-7.28 occurred after alcoholic binge of several days duration. *1594*

303.90 Alcoholism Severe metabolic acidosis with pH ranging between 6.96 - 7.28 occurred after alcoholic binge of several days duration. *1594*

331.81 Reye's Syndrome Due to impaired oxidative metabolism. *0435*

331.81 Reye's Syndrome Later in disease along with decreased pCO_2 reflecting respiratory acidosis. *0435*

357.00 Guillain-Barré Syndrome Respiratory acidosis may occur. *0962*

405.91 Renovascular Hypertension Acidosis which is out of proportion to the degree of azotemia. *0962*

410.90 Acute Myocardial Infarction Slight metabolic acidosis was observed on the first day of the disease in 37% of the cases, while severe metabolic acidosis was found in 50-60% of the cases during 1 year after myocardial infarction. *2529* Patients may develop arterial and tissue hypoxia and metabolic acidosis with an increase in blood lactate concentration. *1108* Following cardiac arrest, acidosis rapidly develops, and, if not corrected, can result in the inability to defibrillate the heart in ventricular fibrillation. *0962 0731*

428.00 Congestive Heart Failure Acidosis occurs when renal insufficiency is associated or there is CO_2 retention due to pulmonary insufficiency, low plasma sodium, or ammonium chloride toxicity. *2467*

491.00 Chronic Bronchitis In 60% of 20 patients at initial hospitalization for this disorder. *0781*

492.80 Pulmonary Emphysema Respiratory acidosis may occur. *0962*

493.10 Asthma (Intrinsic) In a moderate to severe attack; bicarbonate and pH are lowered. As the condition worsens the pCO_2 will rise while bicarbonate and pH fall. *0433* pH, total plasma CO_2 and pCO_2 are decreased as a result of metabolic acidosis in status asthmaticus. *1972*

496.00 Chronic Obstructive Lung Disease Blood pH was significantly lower in 10 patients with chronic obstructive lung disease than in normocapnic controls. Renal net acid excretion was elevated but urinary pH was not significantly raised. *1479* In 48% of 74 patients at initial hospitalization for this disorder. *0781*

518.00 Pulmonary Collapse Active massive atelectasis produces a picture of intrapulmonary right-to-left shunt with a decrease in pH. *0433*

518.40 Pulmonary Edema Of 71 patients breathing room air, 14 were acidemic; 35 alkalemic and 33 had a pH in the normal range. *0554*

537.40 Fistula of Stomach and Duodenum With high output proximal small bowel or pancreatic fistulas, the patients may be acidotic, because the lost pancreatic and biliary secretions are alkaline. *2199* Metabolic acidosis may occur. *0962*

553.30 Hernia Diaphragmatic Severe acidosis may be present. *0433*

557.01 Mesenteric Artery Embolism Serum electrolytes usually show a depressed CO_2-combining power from the induced severe metabolic acidosis. *0433*

558.90 Diarrhea Tends to fall. *0619*

560.90 Intestinal Obstruction Metabolic acidosis secondary to lactic acidosis. *0186* Reflects the course of the patient and therapy *2467*

584.00 Acute Renal Failure Metabolic acidosis increases within 2nd week. *2468* Mild acidosis is common. *0787 0962*

585.00 Chronic Renal Failure Mild acidosis is common in renal failure. *0787* Metabolic acidosis is an invariable concomitant of chronic failure. *1108* In 31% of 31 patients at initial hospitalization for this disorder. *0781*

588.81 Proximal Renal Tubular Acidosis Tends to fall. *0619 2246*

588.82 Distal Renal Tubular Acidosis *0614*

753.12 Medullary Cystic Disease Characteristic acidosis. *0277*

770.80 Respiratory Distress Syndrome Decreased to 7.3 or less. *2467* Acidosis is first respiratory, later also metabolic. *2061 0702*

780.30 Convulsions In 10 patients with idiopathic seizures studied 3 h after the seizure, arterial and CSF lactate were elevated in association with a mild arterial metabolic acidosis. *0293*

986.00 Toxic Effects of Carbon Monoxide Markedly decreased (metabolic acidosis due to tissue hypoxia). *2468*

991.60 Hypothermia Low blood pH in the form of metabolic acidosis is found in cases of hypothermia, especially if preceded by prolonged shivering and exhaustion. *0151* Due to hypoxia, acid-base imbalance hypotension. *1471*

994.80 Effects of Electric Current Profound metabolic acidosis. *0995*

Blood Increase

9.00 Gastroenteritis and Colitis Increased progressively with increased severity. The lesions became more widespread. Statistically significant differences were observed in pH values between the mild/moderate and severe forms and between the severe and complicated forms. *0340*

37.00 Tetanus Metabolic alkalosis may occur with potassium loss. *0962*

135.00 Sarcoidosis In 72% of 15 patients at initial hospitalization for this disorder. *0781*

242.90 Hyperthyroidism Respiratory alkalosis may occur. *0962*

252.10 Hypoparathyroidism *1337*

255.00 Adrenal Cortical Hyperfunction (Glucocorticoid Excess) Metabolic alkalosis may occur with potassium loss. *0962*

255.10 Adrenal Cortical Hyperfunction (Mineralocorticoid Excess) Metabolic alkalosis may occur with potassium loss. *0962* Metabolic alkalosis. *0995*

256.00 Ovarian Hyperfunction Progesterone effect. *0995*

259.20 Carcinoid Syndrome Hyperventilation may occur during the flush. *2540*

265.00 Thiamine (B_1) Deficiency Respiratory alkalosis may occur. *0962*

275.41 Milk-Alkali Syndrome *0995*

276.30 Metabolic Alkalosis Deficit of hydrogen ion due to loss or alkali administration. *0962*

276.80 Hypokalemia *0995*

277.00 Cystic Fibrosis Salt loss may lead to metabolic alkalosis. *1055*

277.14 Acute Intermittent Porphyria Electrolyte depletion and alkalosis associated with azotemia of variable degree are often present on admission but may also develop acutely during the course of the attack. *0433*

291.00 Delirium Tremens Respiratory alkalosis may occur. *0962*

306.10 Hyperventilation Syndrome The arterial pH is raised to 7.5-7.65. *0433* Respiratory alkalosis. *2103*

401.00 Malignant Hypertension Metabolic alkalosis may occur with potassium loss. *0962*

414.00 Chronic Ischemic Heart Disease In 48% of 184 patients hospitalized for this disorder. *0781*

415.10 Pulmonary Embolism and Infarction May be alkaline in the acute stages. *1721* In 89% of 19 patients at initial hospitalization for this disorder. *0781*

421.00 Bacterial Endocarditis In 14 narcotic addicts with bacterial endocarditis, the blood pH, at 7.47 ± 0.01 was significantly higher than in a group of narcotics with other disorders, at 7.36 ± 0.06. *1725*

422.00 Acute Myocarditis Crisis is characterized by acute neutropenia and respiratory alkalosis. *1108*

428.00 Congestive Heart Failure Occurs in uncomplicated heart failure. *2467*

482.90 Bacterial Pneumonia In 91% of 14 patients at initial hospitalization for this disorder. *0781*

486.01 Resolving Pneumonia Moderate to severe hypoxia and respiratory alkalosis in pneumocystis pneumonitis. *1096* Respiratory alkalosis may occur. *0962* In 79% of 42 patients at initial hospitalization for this disorder. *0781*

pH *(continued)*

Blood   Increase *(continued)*

491.00   Chronic Bronchitis   Can occur due to compensatory increase in ventilatory rate. *2220*

493.10   Asthma (Intrinsic)   In 59% of 92 patients at initial hospitalization for this disorder. *0781*

495.90   Allergic Alveolitis   Arterial blood gases show decreased pO_2 with either slight respiratory alkalosis or normal pH and pCO_2. *0433*

514.00   Pulmonary Congestion and Hypostasis   Respiratory alkalosis may occur. *0962*

518.00   Pulmonary Collapse   Respiratory alkalosis may occur. *0962*

518.40   Pulmonary Edema   Of 71 patients breathing room air, 14 were acidemic; 35 alkalemic and 33 had a pH in the normal range. The acidemic group had markedly lower pO_2, all under 60 mm Hg. *0554*

533.90   Peptic Ulcer, Site Unspecified   May exceed 7.45. Complicated by obstruction. *0433*   Pyloric obstruction with vomiting and loss of gastric secretion results in hypochloremia, hyponatremia, hypokalemia, elevated serum pH and CO_2 content, and azotemia. *0962*

537.40   Fistula of Stomach and Duodenum   In gastric fistula, hypokalemic, hypochloremic alkalosis may result. *2199*

556.00   Ulcerative Colitis   Increased progressively with increased severity of the colitis and as the lesions became more widespread. Significant differences were observed in values between the mild/moderate and severe forms and between the severe and complicated forms (toxic megacolon). *0340*

572.20   Hepatic Encephalopathy   Respiratory alkalosis may occur. *0962*

572.40   Hepatic Failure   Persistent alkalosis in patients with hepatic failure. *1775*

650.00   Pregnancy   Slight rise accompanies reduced alveolar pCO_2. *2104*

785.40   Gangrene   In 74% of 13 patients hospitalized for this disorder. *0781*

785.50   Shock   Respiratory alkalosis may occur. *0962*

787.00   Vomiting   Metabolic alkalosis. *0619*

Blood   Normal

275.35   Vitamin D Resistant Rickets   *2246*

493.10   Asthma (Intrinsic)   In moderate to severe attack. *0433*

Urine   Decrease

250.00   Diabetes Mellitus   From an accumulation of acetoacetate and beta-hydroxybutyric acid. *2540*

260.00   Protein Malnutrition   *2467*

271.30   Lactosuria   Lactose intolerance in children and infants without lactase deficiency:renal acidosis usually exists. *0433*

274.00   Gout   Often low: 5.0-5.5. *0433*   Tends to be low throughout the day, with decreased diurnal variations. *0837*

276.20   Metabolic Acidosis   Urine is strongly acid (pH = 4.5-5.2) if renal function is normal. *2468*

276.50   Dehydration   *2467*

405.91   Renovascular Hypertension   Acidosis which is out of proportion to the degree of azotemia. *0962*

492.80   Pulmonary Emphysema   *2467*

558.90   Diarrhea   *2467*

579.90   Malabsorption, Cause Unspecified   Normal or decreased. *2467*

580.00   Acute Poststreptococcal Glomerulonephritis   May occur early in the course of the illness. *0995*

994.50   Exercise   At all rates of exercise (acid metabolites). *1205*

Urine   Increase

250.00   Diabetes Mellitus   Osmotic diuresis secondary to hyperglycemia. *2540*

252.00   Hyperparathyroidism   *2540*

255.10   Adrenal Cortical Hyperfunction (Mineralocorticoid Excess)   Usually 7.0 or higher. *0999*   Exaggerated ammonia production results in a tendency to a persistently alkaline urine. *1108*   An alkaline urine implies the presence of alkalosis, a characteristic finding in primary aldosteronism. *1108*

255.40   Adrenal Cortical Hypofunction   Normal or increased. *2467*

270.03   Cystinosis   Tends to remain alkaline despite systemic acidosis. *2246*

271.20   Hereditary Fructose Intolerance   Abrupt loss of the ability to acidify urine after ingestion of fructose. *2246*

275.10   Hepatolenticular Degeneration   Value in 50% of patients was > 6.5 with multiple specimens. 9 of 22 patients were unable to adequately acidify their urine during acid loading tests (pH > 5.3). *2278*

276.30   Metabolic Alkalosis   Urine pH > 7.0 (< 7.9) if potassium depletion and concomitant sodium are not severe. *2468*

537.00   Pyloric Stenosis, Acquired   *2467*

584.00   Acute Renal Failure   Normal or increased. *2467*

585.00   Chronic Renal Failure   *2467*

588.81   Proximal Renal Tubular Acidosis   Always relatively high with the gradient defect, no matter how severe the systemic acidosis. *2246*

588.82   Distal Renal Tubular Acidosis   Cardinal clinical finding is a urine pH which is never lower than 6.0, even with severe metabolic acidosis. *0151*   Inappropriately high. *0614*

753.13   Medullary Sponge Kidney   Impaired ability to concentrate or acidify the urine maximally has been reported. *0906 0277*

994.50   Exercise   Effect noted after mild exercise. *1205*

Urine   Normal

253.50   Diabetes Insipidus   *2467*

255.10   Adrenal Cortical Hyperfunction (Mineralocorticoid Excess)   Normal or alkaline. *2467*

255.40   Adrenal Cortical Hypofunction   Normal or increased. *2467*

428.00   Congestive Heart Failure   *2467*

780.80   Hyperhidrosis   *2467*

CSF   Decrease

410.90   Acute Myocardial Infarction   In patients who developed severe anoxia after cardiac arrest, the normal cisternal-lumbar pH gradient was reversed, cisternal fluid was more acid (pH 6.815 vs 6.953), and cisternal potassium concentration was twice that of lumbar (6.7 vs 3.5 mmol/L). During anoxia, potassium and hydrogen ions flow from brain cells into the brain extracellular fluid. Acute changes are reflected more accurately by cisternal than by lumbar fluid. *1213*

Synovial Fluid   Decrease

711.00   Acute Arthritis (Pyogenic)   Close correlation (R = -.92) was found between decreasing pH and increasing WBC in synovial fluid. The high WBC usually found in acute and chronic arthritis results in low pH which may contribute to the poor response to treatment with aminoglycoside antibiotics. *2482*

714.00   Rheumatoid Arthritis   Low pH correlates with increasing WBC count (R = 0.92) in synovial fluid of acute and chronic arthritis. *2482*

Pleural Effusion   Decrease

6.00   Amebiasis   The pleural aspirate from an amebic empyema due to rupture of an amebic liver abscess has an acidic pH. Pleural aspirates of nonamebic etiology were noted to have an alkaline pH. *1875*

11.00   Pulmonary Tuberculosis   May occur in non-neoplastic inflammatory pleural effusion (empyema, rheumatoid disease, tuberculosis). *0797*

162.90   Malignant Neoplasm of Bronchus and Lung   Exudate (pH < 7.3). *0062*

197.00   Secondary Malignant Neoplasm of Respiratory System   Exudate (pH < 7.3). *0062*

244.90   Hypothyroidism   Exudate (pH < 7.3). *0062*

415.10   Pulmonary Embolism and Infarction   Exudate (pH < 7.3). *0062*

480.90   Viral Pneumonia   Pleural fluid pH of < 7.20 or 0.15 below arterial pH frequently occurs in parapneumonic effusions. *1403*

482.90   Bacterial Pneumonia   Exudate (pH < 7.3). *0062*

483.01   Mycoplasma Pneumoniae   Exudate (pH < 7.3). *0062*

510.00 Empyema All 10 patients had a pleural fluid pH of < 7.30. Pleural fluid pH values < 7.30 are likely to result in loculation of the pleural space. *1845* May occur in non-neoplastic inflammatory pleural effusion (empyema, rheumatoid disease, tuberculosis). *0797*

577.00 Acute Pancreatitis Exudate (pH < 7.3). *0062*

577.10 Chronic Pancreatitis Exudate (pH < 7.3). *0062*

577.20 Pancreatic Cyst and Pseudocyst Exudate (pH < 7.3). *0062*

710.00 Systemic Lupus Erythematosus Exudate (pH < 7.3). *0062*

714.00 Rheumatoid Arthritis 7.0-7.2 pH. *0797*

Pleural Effusion Increase

11.00 Pulmonary Tuberculosis pH < 7.3 is rarely encountered in tuberculous effusions. *0962*

162.90 Malignant Neoplasm of Bronchus and Lung pH < 7.40 militates against malignancy, especially in the absence of infection and < 7.30 is rarely encountered in tuberculous pleural disease. *0962*

197.00 Secondary Malignant Neoplasm of Respiratory System pH < 7.40 militates against malignancy, especially in the absence of infection and < 7.30 is rarely encountered in tuberculous pleural disease. *0962*

423.10 Constrictive Pericarditis Transudate (pH > 7.3). *0062*

571.90 Cirrhosis of Liver Transudate (pH > 7.3). *0062*

581.90 Nephrotic Syndrome Transudate (pH > 7.3). *0062*

585.00 Chronic Renal Failure Transudate (pH > 7.3). *0062*

Gastric Material Decrease

151.90 Malignant Neoplasm of Stomach Achlorhydria following histamine or betazole stimulation found in 50% of patients and hypochlorhydria in another 25% of patients. *2467* *0962*

533.90 Peptic Ulcer, Site Unspecified True achlorhydria virtually excludes peptic ulcer disease. In gastric ulcer the average basal gastric secretion is decreased or normal. *0118*

535.00 Gastritis Erosive hemorrhagic gastritis appears to be due to pathologic back diffusion of hydrogen ions caused by a breakdown of the gastric mucosal barrier. *2236* Most patients with Ménétrier's disease have achlorhydria, but some may have hypersecretion. *1115* In Ménétrier's disease hyposecretion of gastric acid is usual finding *0407*

537.00 Pyloric Stenosis, Acquired Due to excess circulating gastrin. *0587*

Gastric Material Increase

151.90 Malignant Neoplasm of Stomach Although rare, does not rule out carcinoma. *2467*

211.41 Adenomatous Polyp Gastric analysis - achlorhydria in 85% of patients. Polyps occur in 5% of patients with pernicious anemia and 2% of patients with achlorhydria. *2467*

244.90 Hypothyroidism True achlorhydria after maximum histamine stimulation occurs in 50% of patients with primary hypothyroidism. *2540* Achlorhydria present in up to 40% of cases *0186*

251.50 Zollinger-Ellison Syndrome Gastric secretion > 100 mmol/12h is strongly indicative of this disorder. *0844* Markedly elevated levels of gastric acid secretion *2540*

533.90 Peptic Ulcer, Site Unspecified No single test of gastric secretion shows abnormal hypersecretion in more than 50% of duodenal ulcer patients. *0118* *0587*

535.00 Gastritis Most patients with Ménétrier's Disease have achlorhydria. However, some patients may have hypersecretion. *2238* Transient hypochlorhydria or achlorhydria may be observed during episodes of acute gastritis. *2199*

650.00 Pregnancy May occur. *2468*

Gastric Material Normal

151.90 Malignant Neoplasm of Stomach Normal in 25% of patients. *2467*

Prostatic Fluid Increase

601.00 Prostatitis The pH of prostatic secretions of males with chronic bacterial prostatitis reached a mean value of 8.1 during inflammation. Values for males without inflammatory prostatic disease was 6.7. *1812*

Phenylalanine

Serum Increase

38.00 Septicemia Concentrations determined in 10 burned patients with gram-negative sepsis and 9 burned patients without sepsis revealed an increase in the gluconeogenic precursors alanine, glycine, methionine and phenylalanine in those patients with sepsis. *2543*

66.00 Phlebotomus Fever Increased during the viral illness in contrast with most other amino acids. *2479*

70.00 Viral Hepatitis A close relationship was found between the onset of encephalopathy and amino acid equilibrium disturbance, characterized by a fall in the molar ratio between valine leucine and isoleucine and phenylalanine and tyrosine. All showed absolute elevations with onset of encephalopathy. *0531*

270.10 Phenylketonuria Patients are clinically normal at birth, distinguishable only by hyperphenylalaninemia, which is established in the 1st postnatal week. *0151* Early diagnosis can only be made by determining the blood concentration. Rises to abnormal levels after the infant has received protein-containing feedings. *2246*

572.20 Hepatic Encephalopathy Consistently elevated. *1473*

Urine Increase

270.02 Hartnup Disease 5-20 X normal values. *2246* *0995*

270.03 Cystinosis Nonspecific pattern of aminoaciduria. Fanconi's syndrome. *0995*

270.10 Phenylketonuria Early diagnosis can only be made by determining the blood concentration. Rises to abnormal levels after the infant has received protein-containing feedings. *2246* *0151*

275.10 Hepatolenticular Degeneration *0503*

Phosphate

Serum Decrease

38.00 Septicemia In 54 patients with gram-negative septicemias; either absolute 2 mg/dL) or relative (P/BUN = 0.04) hypophosphatemia was found in 69% of all determinations. *1934*

40.20 Whipple's Disease An indication of vitamin D and calcium malabsorption. *0962*

172.90 Malignant Melanoma of Skin In 49% of 67 patients at initial hospitalization for this disorder. *0781*

185.00 Malignant Neoplasm of Prostate In 39% of 86 patients at initial hospitalization for this disorder. *0781*

197.00 Secondary Malignant Neoplasm of Respiratory System In 26% of 603 patients at initial hospitalization for this disorder. *0781*

203.00 Multiple Myeloma Common. *0962* Due to renal loss of phosphate. *2468* In 21% of 32 patients at initial hospitalization for this disorder. *0781*

211.60 Benign Neoplasm of Pancreas Hyperinsulinism; during successful treatment of diabetic ketosis, insulin causes phosphate ions to enter the cells with glucose and potassium. *0619 2467*

217.00 Benign Neoplasm of Breast In 43% of 32 patients at initial hospitalization for this disorder. *0781*

227.91 Pheochromocytoma May be caused by ectopic parathyroid hormone production in a few patients but usually results from associated parathyroid hyperplasia in the familial cases. *0433*

250.00 Diabetes Mellitus Osmotic diuresis secondary to hyperglycemia. *2540*

250.10 Diabetic Acidosis During successful treatment of diabetic ketosis insulin causes phosphate ions to enter the cells with glucose and potassium. *0619* Common; usually becomes manifest in 4-12 h of institution of therapy. *1316* Common in patients recovering from severe diabetic ketoacidosis. *1287*

251.50 Zollinger-Ellison Syndrome An indication of vitamin D and calcium malabsorption. *0962*

252.00 Hyperparathyroidism Range of concentration in 34 patients was 1.2-3.4 mg/dL, mean = 4.35 mg/dL. *1904* Occurs in 50% of patients. *0999* In 83% of 19 patients at initial hospitalization for this disorder. *0781* *0151 1957 0962*

252.10 Hypoparathyroidism Initial fall followed by a rise. *2540*

253.40 Anterior Pituitary Hypofunction Hypopituitarism with growth hormone deficiency in children. *0619*

Phosphate *(continued)*

Serum Decrease *(continued)*

255.00 Adrenal Cortical Hyperfunction (Glucocorticoid Excess) Occasional hypophosphatemia as a result of high corticosteroid concentrations. *1287*

255.40 Adrenal Cortical Hypofunction Acute adrenal insufficiency may be accompanied by hypophosphatemia (and hypercalcemia). *0999*

256.30 Ovarian Hypofunction Estrogen effect. *0995*

260.00 Protein Malnutrition Serum concentration generally remains normal but may decline to or slightly below the lower range of normal. *1287*

268.00 Vitamin D Deficiency Rickets Decreased calcium absorption in the gut leads to overproduction of parathyroid hormone and the resulting phosphaturia and hypophosphatemia. *1287* May be low, but usually not as severe as in vitamin D resistant rickets. *2246 0962*

268.20 Osteomalacia Invariably low. May be the only demonstrable abnormality. *0151* Osteomalacia resulting from PO_3 or Ca deficiencies may be associated with moderate hypophosphatemia. *1287 0999*

270.03 Cystinosis Decreased serum concentrations will become normal and then elevated as renal deterioration progress. *2246*

271.01 Von Gierke's Disease Mean fasting inorganic phosphate level was significantly decreased to 3.9 ± 0.3 mg/dL, (normal = 4.8 ± 0.3). Levels were further diminished by fructose and glucagon administration. *1960*

271.20 Hereditary Fructose Intolerance Noted with the chronic syndrome found in young children and after fructose administration in adults. *2246*

271.30 Lactosuria An indication of vitamin D and calcium malabsorption. *0962*

274.00 Gout Hypophosphatemia has been observed in association with acute attacks. *1287*

275.10 Hepatolenticular Degeneration Decreased in 18 of 30 (60%), mean = 3.0 mg/dL. *2278*

275.34 Familial Periodic Paralysis During attacks. *0043*

275.35 Vitamin D Resistant Rickets May be present at birth or develop within the 1st y. *2246* Familial hypophosphatemic rickets; with impaired transport of phosphate ion in both kidney and gut. Usually decreased. *2467*

278.40 Hypervitaminosis D Normal to decreased values. *0503*

282.41 Thalassemia Major 24 h excretion level was higher than net absorption, indicating normal phosphate absorption and high renal phosphaturia, leading to deficiency. *1349*

282.42 Thalassemia Minor 24 h excretion level was higher than net absorption, indicating normal phosphate absorption and high renal phosphaturia, leading to deficiency. *1349*

303.00 Acute Alcoholic Intoxication *0619*

303.90 Alcoholism Occurs in about 50% of hospitalized alcoholics. *1287* An association of hypophosphatemia with chronic alcoholism was found in 11 patients studied. The hypophosphatemia was associated with low levels of RBC ATP, abnormal erythrocyte filtration, and, in at least 1 patient, with hemolytic anemia. *2342*

306.10 Hyperventilation Syndrome Often decreased during prolonged hyperventilation. *0433* Respiratory alkalosis. *2103*

493.10 Asthma (Intrinsic) In 40% of 107 patients at initial hospitalization for this disorder. *0781*

571.90 Cirrhosis of Liver Pronounced hypophosphatemic response in cirrhotic patients after glucose administration. *1287* In 40% of 68 patients at initial hospitalization for this disorder. *0781 1574*

572.40 Hepatic Failure Hypophosphatemia may occur in hepatic failure as a result of intravenous carbohydrate feeding, gram-negative septicemia, endotoxemia, and large dose steroid treatment. *1775*

577.00 Acute Pancreatitis Low or in the low normal range. *2509* In 41% of 21 patients at initial hospitalization for this disorder. *0781*

579.00 Celiac Sprue Disease Low vitamin D absorption from small bowel. *0619* Malabsorption of calcium results in increased parathyroid hormone production and renal tubular reabsorption of phosphate decreases, leading to mild hypophosphatemia. *1287 1115*

579.90 Malabsorption, Cause Unspecified Malabsorption of calcium results in increased parathyroid hormone production and renal tubular reabsorption of phosphate decreases, leading to mild hypophosphatemia. *1287* An indication of vitamin D and calcium malabsorption. *0962*

588.81 Proximal Renal Tubular Acidosis Low in the early stages and increasing to normal values with increasing azotemia. *0503 0433 2246*

588.82 Distal Renal Tubular Acidosis Typical feature of Type I. *0151*

650.00 Pregnancy Levels decreased progressively after the first trimester. *0517* Sometimes a slight decline in serum concentration may occur with no serious complication. *1287*

730.00 Osteomyelitis In 24% of 25 patients at initial hospitalization for this disorder. *0781*

756.52 Osteopetrosis Occasionally in children. *0995*

787.00 Vomiting Of 100 patients with hypophosphatemia, 12% was due to vomiting, 40% to intravenous glucose feeding, and miscellaneous or unexplained in the rest. *0190*

948.00 Burns Patients recovering from burns may remain hypophosphatemic and hypouricemic for months after the initial injury. *1287*

Serum Increase

135.00 Sarcoidosis *2199*

198.50 Secondary Malignant Neoplasm of Bone May be normal or increased (osteolytic metastases (especially from primary tumor of bronchus, breast, kidney, thyroid)). *2467*

203.00 Multiple Myeloma Some cases. *2467* In 27% of 32 patients at initial hospitalization for this disorder. *0781*

204.00 Lymphocytic Leukemia (Acute) Hyperphosphatemia with values of 5.7-9.4 mg/dL was observed within 24-48 h after initiation of chemotherapy. *2622* In 40% of 44 patients at initial hospitalization for this disorder. *0781*

205.00 Myelocytic Leukemia (Acute) *2467*

250.00 Diabetes Mellitus *0619*

250.10 Diabetic Acidosis *0619*

252.10 Hypoparathyroidism Increased (usually 5-6 mg/dL; as high as 12 mg/dL). *2467* Initial fall followed by a rise. May range from 6-16 mg/dL. *2540 0812 0503 0999*

253.00 Acromegaly There may be a mild hyperphosphatemia, a reversal of the diurnal rhythmicity of urinary phosphate excretion, and an increased tubular reabsorption of phosphate. *0962*

255.40 Adrenal Cortical Hypofunction *2467*

256.00 Ovarian Hyperfunction Estrogen effect. *0995*

270.03 Cystinosis Decreased serum concentrations will become normal and then elevated as renal deterioration progress. *2246*

271.20 Hereditary Fructose Intolerance *0151*

275.41 Milk-Alkali Syndrome Normal or elevated. *0503*

275.42 Pseudohypoparathyroidism Normal excretory mechanisms are impaired. *0999 0503*

276.20 Metabolic Acidosis Increased in type II-B, with lactic acidosis. *2468*

278.40 Hypervitaminosis D Usually increased with increased urinary phosphate. *2467 0812 0503*

282.00 Hereditary (Congenital) Spherocytosis *0962*

283.00 Acquired Hemolytic Anemia (Autoimmune) *0962*

303.00 Acute Alcoholic Intoxication Increased following alcoholic binge of several days duration. *1594*

303.90 Alcoholism Increased following alcoholic binge of several days duration. *1594*

331.81 Reye's Syndrome Indicates muscle involvement. *1887*

557.01 Mesenteric Artery Embolism Of 7 patients with massive intestinal infarction, all had elevated concentrations. *1145*

560.90 Intestinal Obstruction *2467*

570.00 Acute and Subacute Necrosis of Liver *2467*

580.05 Glomerulonephritis (Membranoproliferative) As functional loss becomes severe (GFR 50% of normal or less), there is usually a rise in serum phosphate and uric acid. *0962*

580.40 Glomerulonephritis (Rapidly Progressive) As functional loss becomes severe (GFR 50% of normal or less), there is usually a rise in serum phosphate and uric acid. *0962*

581.90 Nephrotic Syndrome In 60% of 25 patients at initial hospitalization for this disorder. *0781*

584.00 Acute Renal Failure Hyperphosphatemia may occur depending on the duration and severity of disease. *0151* In 72% of 11 patients at initial hospitalization for this disorder. *0781 0812*

585.00 Chronic Renal Failure Plasma levels rise late in renal failure and are unrelated to the serum calcium levels. *0151* Increases when creatinine clearance falls to approximately 25 mL/min. *2468* In 75% of 141 patients at initial hospitalization for this disorder. *0781 0962 1393*

588.00 Renal Dwarfism May be normal or elevated. When both phosphate and calcium are high, metastatic calcifications in subcutaneous tissues and conjunctiva may develop. *0999*

597.80 Urethritis Reveals the degree of renal impairment. *0433*

642.60 Eclampsia Slight increase. *0621*

731.00 Osteitis Deformans Usually normal or slightly elevated. *0999 0503*

829.00 Fracture of Bone *0619 2467*

992.00 Heat stroke Concentrations were very high (9.5-15 mg/dL) throughout and later resulted in a fall in serum-calcium in a case of malignant hyperpyrexia. *0541* In children. *0548*

994.50 Exercise Observed effect with 12 min cycle-ergometer. *0804* Effect of muscular exercise. *0161*

Serum Normal

170.90 Malignant Neoplasm of Bone Usually normal in Ewing's Sarcoma and other osteolytic tumors. *2467*

193.01 Medullary Carcinoma of Thyroid Usually normal, in spite of very high titers of plasma calcitonin seen in medullary cancer of the thyroid. *0962*

268.00 Vitamin D Deficiency Rickets In some individuals, serum calcium and phosphate may be normal. *2467* Normal or low. *2246 0433*

275.32 Hypophosphatasia *0619*

277.00 Cystic Fibrosis Normal unless complications occur (e.g., chronic pulmonary disease with accumulation of CO_2, massive salt loss due to sweating). *2467*

588.00 Renal Dwarfism May be normal or elevated. When both phosphate and calcium are high, metastatic calcifications in subcutaneous tissues and conjunctiva may develop. *0999*

714.00 Rheumatoid Arthritis Generally normal. *0962*

730.00 Osteomyelitis Normal in all 39 cases. *2464*

731.00 Osteitis Deformans Normal or slightly increased. *2467*

733.00 Osteoporosis *2467*

756.52 Osteopetrosis *2467*

Urine Decrease

252.10 Hypoparathyroidism Urine phosphate and phosphate clearance is decreased. *2468 0503 0433*

268.20 Osteomalacia *0503*

275.42 Pseudohypoparathyroidism Normal excretory mechanisms are impaired. *0999 0503*

985.00 Toxic Effects of Non-medicinal Metals Highly significant hypercalciuria and decreased serum inorganic phosphate was found in a group of workers with cadmium intoxication. *2098*

Urine Increase

120.00 Schistosomiasis Urinary inorganic phosphate was increased in hepatic bilharziasis despite normal serum levels. *0955*

203.00 Multiple Myeloma Renal loss. *2468*

204.00 Lymphocytic Leukemia (Acute) Marked hyperphosphaturia was observed within 24-48 h after initiation of chemotherapy. *2622*

242.90 Hyperthyroidism Urinary excretion was increased and correlated positively to degree of hyperthyroidism. *1638* Poorly understood. *2540*

250.00 Diabetes Mellitus Osmotic diuresis secondary to hyperglycemia. *2540*

252.00 Hyperparathyroidism Increased unless there is a renal insufficiency or phosphate depletion (especially due to commonly used antacids containing aluminum). *2468* Marked phosphaturia due to parathyroid hormones. *0619 0503*

268.00 Vitamin D Deficiency Rickets Decreased calcium absorption in the gut leads to overproduction of parathyroid hormone and the resulting phosphaturia and hypophosphatemia. *1287*

270.03 Cystinosis Failure of tubular reabsorption. *0995* Usually increased excretion before renal disease is advanced. *0993 2246*

271.20 Hereditary Fructose Intolerance Phosphate reabsorption is impaired. *2246*

275.10 Hepatolenticular Degeneration Marked increase in clearance in 36% (8 of 22). *2278*

275.35 Vitamin D Resistant Rickets High in untreated patients. *2246*

278.40 Hypervitaminosis D In large doses vitamin D causes increased renal excretion of phosphate; to this extent its renal effect resembles parathyroid hormone. *0812 0503*

282.41 Thalassemia Major 24 h excretion level was higher than net absorption, indicating normal phosphate absorption and high renal phosphaturia, leading to deficiency. *1349*

282.42 Thalassemia Minor 24 h excretion level was higher than net absorption, indicating normal phosphate absorption and high renal phosphaturia, leading to deficiency. *1349*

579.00 Celiac Sprue Disease Malabsorption of calcium results in increased parathyroid hormone production and renal tubular reabsorption of phosphate decreases, leading to mild hypophosphatemia. *1287*

579.90 Malabsorption, Cause Unspecified Malabsorption of calcium results in increased parathyroid hormone production and renal tubular reabsorption of phosphate decreases, leading to mild hypophosphatemia. *1287*

588.81 Proximal Renal Tubular Acidosis Excessive loss in urine. *2467 2246 0503*

984.00 Toxic Effects of Lead and Its Compounds (including Fumes) Results from changes in the epithelium in the proximal convoluted tubules. *0151*

Feces Increase

242.90 Hyperthyroidism Poorly understood. *2540*

270.03 Cystinosis Decreased intestinal absorption. *0204 2246*

275.35 Vitamin D Resistant Rickets Diminished intestinal absorption. *2246*

Saliva Increase

252.00 Hyperparathyroidism Increased inorganic phosphate in saliva. *0619*

277.00 Cystic Fibrosis Increased. *1359*

Sweat Increase

585.00 Chronic Renal Failure Concentrations of Ca, Mg and phosphate in sweat were significantly elevated due to an increase in the secretion of these electrolytes in the secretory portion of the sweat gland, while that in the reabsorptive duct is normal. *1861*

Phosphoethanolamine

Serum Increase

275.32 Hypophosphatasia Two X normal. *1882*

Urine Increase

275.32 Hypophosphatasia 3-8 X normal. *1882*

Phosphoglucomutase

Serum Increase

204.00 Lymphocytic Leukemia (Acute) Increases in some cases. *0619*

204.10 Lymphocytic Leukemia (Chronic) Increases in some cases. *0619*

205.00 Myelocytic Leukemia (Acute) In some cases. *0619*

205.10 Myelocytic Leukemia (Chronic) In some cases. *0619*

570.00 Acute and Subacute Necrosis of Liver *0619*

986.00 Toxic Effects of Carbon Monoxide One case with serum level increased 250 X normal reported. *0619*

Phospholipids, Total

Serum Decrease

70.00 Viral Hepatitis Increased in mild but decreased in severe hepatitis. *2467*

Phospholipids, Total *(continued)*

Serum Decrease *(continued)*

242.90 Hyperthyroidism Falls, but not in simple relation to the associated rise in the BMR. Diet has a variable effect on the blood level. *0812*

260.00 Protein Malnutrition *0151*

272.51 Tangier Disease Typically 30-50% below normal. *2246 1292*

272.52 Abetalipoproteinemia Wide range of variation. Reduced by approximately 75%. *1181 2246*

281.00 Pernicious Anemia All phospholipid fractions decreased in relapse. *2471*

282.00 Hereditary (Congenital) Spherocytosis Generalized hypolipidemia; with reduced phospholipids and total lipids occurs in children as well as adults with uncomplicated cases. *2109*

282.60 Sickle Cell Anemia Plasma lipids are significantly reduced and RBC cholesterol is higher in patients than in normal subjects. *0028*

340.00 Multiple Sclerosis Particularly in patients with evidence of recent progression. *0878*

571.60 Biliary Cirrhosis In 4 female patients compared to 6 normal age matched controls. *0127*

770.80 Respiratory Distress Syndrome *2061*

Serum Increase

70.00 Viral Hepatitis Increased in mild but decreased in severe hepatitis. *2467*

242.90 Hyperthyroidism *0619*

244.90 Hypothyroidism *0619*

250.00 Diabetes Mellitus *0619*

271.01 Von Gierke's Disease Striking elevation. *1086 2246*

272.00 Type IIA Hyperlipoproteinemia Moderate elevation in heterozygotes and marked in homozygotes. *2246* Elevated, but not as high as cholesterol. *0992*

272.21 Type IIB Hyperlipoproteinemia Moderate elevation in heterozygotes and marked in homozygotes. *2246* Elevated, but not as high as cholesterol. *0992*

303.90 Alcoholism Fasting serum lipid values were have been analyzed in 85 male and 10 female alcoholics of various ages in connection with an acute drinking bout and compared to control subjects. The most prominent finding was an increase in the mean concentration of triglycerides and phospholipids, most marked in the younger age groups. The elevations were moderate and most alcoholics had the same serum total lipid values as the controls. *0261*

401.00 Malignant Hypertension In 24 male patients, mean concentration was 234.7 - 13.5 mg/dL compared to 204.1 ± 3.5 in normals. *0381*

410.90 Acute Myocardial Infarction Mean concentration was increased to 249.5 ± 7.6 mg/L in 69 male patients, compared to 204.1 ± 3.5 in normals. *0381*

571.20 Laennec's or Alcoholic Cirrhosis 45 patients suffering from steatosis of the liver have been examined with reference to serum lipid abnormalities. 28 of the patients were chronic alcoholics. 13 patients showed hypercholesterolemia, 16 increased serum triglyceride and 8 increased serum phospholipid. *1045*

571.60 Biliary Cirrhosis Marked increase in total cholesterol and phospholipids takes place, with normal triglycerides; serum is not lipemic. The increase is associated with xanthomas and xantholasmas. *2467*

576.20 Extrahepatic Biliary Obstruction In 15 patients (aged 16-78), compared to 23 controls (aged 18-63), there was an increased in cholesterol and phospholipids and increase in phospholipid to cholesterol ratio. *1606*

577.10 Chronic Pancreatitis Increase in cholesterol, phospholipids and neutral fats. *0619*

581.90 Nephrotic Syndrome Elevated cholesterol with lipiduria can be demonstrated; however, phospholipids and triglycerides are even more consistently and strikingly elevated. *0503* Typically elevated. *0962*

Serum Normal

758.00 Down's Syndrome Plasma lipid levels were measured in 20 mongoloid and 16 nonmongoloid mentally retarded subjects. Significant elevations of plasma triglyceride levels were found in patients with Down's syndrome compared with mentally retarded controls. However, no significant difference was found in plasma cholesterol, phospholipid and free fatty acid levels between the mongoloids and control subjects. *1698*

994.50 Exercise But relative reduction of unsaturated acid. *1109*

CSF Increase

340.00 Multiple Sclerosis Raised in patients with high total CSF proteins but lowered in chronic multiple sclerosis. *2371*

Red Blood Cells Decrease

281.00 Pernicious Anemia Decreased concentration in red cells. *0619*

Red Blood Cells Increase

570.00 Acute and Subacute Necrosis of Liver An increase in RBC phospholipid was detected in most patients with hepatocellular disease or cholestatic jaundice but the alteration in RBC lipid content did not correlate with RBC survival. *1848*

576.20 Extrahepatic Biliary Obstruction An increase in RBC phospholipid was detected in most patients with hepatocellular disease or cholestatic jaundice but the alteration in RBC lipid content did not correlate with RBC survival. *1848*

Red Blood Cells Normal

272.51 Tangier Disease *2246*

Phytanic Acid

Plasma Increase

272.52 Abetalipoproteinemia Characteristic. *0995*

Plasma Normal

335.20 Amyotrophic Lateral Sclerosis *0665*

Plasma Cells

Serum Decrease

6.00 Amebiasis Hepatic Amebiasis. *2357 0659 0683*

70.00 Viral Hepatitis Late pregnancy. *2357 0659 0683*

155.00 Malignant Neoplasm of Liver Depressed. *2357 0659 0683*

260.00 Protein Malnutrition Depressed. *2357 0659 0683*

279.06 Immunodeficiency (Common Variable) Decreased in transient hypogammaglobulinemia of infancy. *2468* Ordinarily, sparse in infancy, are absent with disease. *2552*

280.90 Iron Deficiency Anemia Depressed. *2357 0659 0683*

359.11 Progressive Muscular Dystrophy Depressed. *2357 0659 0683*

410.90 Acute Myocardial Infarction *2357 0659 0683*

415.10 Pulmonary Embolism and Infarction Depressed. *2357 0659 0683*

428.00 Congestive Heart Failure Post Surgical. *2357 0659 0683*

571.90 Cirrhosis of Liver Post Surgical. *2357 0659 0683*

585.00 Chronic Renal Failure Depressed. *2357 0659 0683*

650.00 Pregnancy Late pregnancy. *2357 0659 0683*

710.40 Dermatomyositis/Polymyositis Depressed. *2357 0659 0683*

Serum Increase

30.00 Leprosy High levels of precipitating antimycobacterial antibodies in lepromatous leprosy are paralleled by marked plasma cell proliferation. *2035*

49.00 Lymphocytic Choriomeningitis *2468*

52.00 Chickenpox *2468*

55.00 Measles *2468*

56.00 Rubella *2468*

75.00 Infectious Mononucleosis *2468*

203.00 Multiple Myeloma   A small number may be found in the circulating blood of many patients, and if the absolute number of plasma cells exceeds 2,000/μL, the diagnosis of plasma cell leukemia may be made. *2538*

272.10 Type IV Hyperlipoproteinemia   Elevated *2357 0659 0683*

273.23 Heavy Chain Disease (Gamma)   Presence of atypical lymphocytes or plasma cells in the blood. *2538*

282.00 Hereditary (Congenital) Spherocytosis   During the chronic stage of anemia. *0810 2552*

571.49 Chronic Active Hepatitis   Increased plasma cells in bone marrow and may appear in peripheral blood. *2467*

580.02 Glomerulonephritis (Minimal Change)   Elevated *2357 0659 0683*

Synovial Fluid   Increase

714.30 Juvenile Rheumatoid Arthritis   *0793*

Bone Marrow   Decrease

279.04 Agammaglobulinemia (Congenital Sex-linked)   The basic deficiency is an absence of plasma cells from the lymph nodes, spleen, intestine, and bone marrow. *2538 2035 0886*

Bone Marrow   Increase

203.00 Multiple Myeloma   Marked bone marrow plasmacytosis. Many patients had cytoplasmic abnormalities of cells, including size and contour of nucleus, mitochondria and rough ER. *0904* Increased numbers and abnormal forms have been found in all cases, although more than one attempt may be necessary. *2035* Bone marrow infiltrated with over 20% plasma cells in clusters or sheets. *1980*   In average patients with moderately advanced disease, 20-95% of the nucleated cells in the bone marrow are mature or immature plasma cells. The percent varies with the sample and is not a reliable measure of the total amount of disease present. *2538 0992 1744*

273.23 Heavy Chain Disease (Gamma)   Bone marrow aspirations and lymph node biopsies have demonstrated a proliferation of plasmacytic and lymphocytic forms, along with eosinophils and large reticulum or reticuloendothelial cells, (the pattern of a pleomorphic reticular neoplasm). *2035*   Bone marrow may be normal, but usually there is an increased proportion of plasma cells or lymphocytes or both, often accompanied by eosinophilia. *2538*

273.30 Waldenström's Macroglobulinemia   Proliferation of lymphocytic and plasmacytic forms with many intermediate and apparently transitional cell types. *2035   0188*

277.30 Amyloidosis   None of the patients with primary disease had > 15% plasma cells, whereas over 50% of the secondary cases did. Mean percentage of cells was 4 in primary and 23 in secondary. *1334*   A bone marrow plasmacytosis is found in a high proportion of cases. *1108*   Many patients can be shown to have homogeneous immunoglobulins in the serum and/or urine, and plasmacytosis in the marrow, and ultimately to develop morphologic and clinical evidence of a plasma cell dyscrasia. *1127   2538*

284.01 Congenital Aplastic Anemia   There may be many plasma cells and mastocytes. *0695*

288.00 Agranulocytosis   Plasma cells, lymphocytes and reticulum cells may be increased. *2552*

571.49 Chronic Active Hepatitis   Plasmacytosis in the bone marrow is part of the abnormal immunological response. *1151   2035*

733.00 Osteoporosis   The iliac bone marrow specimens showed infiltrates consisting of elongated mast cells, eosinophils, plasma cells, and varying numbers of lymphocytes. *2334*

Lung Tissue   Increase

486.01 Resolving Pneumonia   In 13 patients with lymphocytic interstitial pneumonitis, lung biopsies in all cases showed diffuse interstitial infiltrations consisting of mature lymphocytes and plasma cells. *2283*

Plasminogen

Serum   Decrease

205.10 Myelocytic Leukemia (Chronic)   Below normal in some patients. *2318*

238.40 Polycythemia Vera   Below normal in some patients. *2318*

286.60 Disseminated Intravascular Coagulopathy   Deposition of fibrin usually stimulates local secondary fibrinolysis producing reduced circulating plasminogen level due to consumption and a decrease in systemic fibrinolytic activity. *2538*

570.00 Acute and Subacute Necrosis of Liver   With massive necrosis. *1443*

Serum   Increase

650.00 Pregnancy   *1443*

994.50 Exercise   Observed effect in exercise. *1839*   Vigorous exercise. *1443*

Serum   Normal

286.31 Congenital Dysfibrinogenemia   Invariably normal. *2538*

Platelet Adhesiveness

Blood   Increase

451.90 Phlebitis and Thrombophlebitis   Increased in 7 cases. *2025*

Platelet Aggregation

Blood   Decrease

410.90 Acute Myocardial Infarction   Significantly reduced the first few days. *1289*

Platelet Count

Blood   Decrease

18.00 Disseminated Tuberculosis   Pancytopenia is a common feature. *2538*

38.00 Septicemia   May be associated with defibrination resulting in platelet and coagulation factor consumption in severe gram-positive septicemia. *2538*

50.00 Smallpox   Pronounced thrombocytopenia is commonly found in hemorrhagic smallpox. *0433*

54.00 Herpes Simplex   May be associated with defibrination resulting in platelet and coagulation factor consumption. *2538*

56.00 Rubella   Decrease within 1 week of onset of rash is frequent and may be marked. *2468*   Sometimes very severe in newborn infants infected with rubella. *0451   2538*

65.00 Arthropod-Borne Hemorrhagic Fever   Indicates occurrence of intravascular coagulation in dengue hemorrhagic fever patients experiencing shock. *0247*   May be associated with defibrination resulting in platelet and coagulation factor consumption (Korean Fever, Thai Fever). *2538*

66.10 Tick-Borne Fever   *1058*

70.00 Viral Hepatitis   Patient may show anemia, leukocytosis, thrombocytopenia in fulminant hepatitis with hepatic failure. *2467*

78.50 Cytomegalic Inclusion Disease   Thrombocytopenia usually present in congenital disease. *1319*   Common manifestation; usually transient and rarely associated with significant bleeding. *1676*

81.00 Endemic Typhus   Rarely seen. *0433*

82.00 Rocky Mountain Spotted Fever   Counts below 100,000/μL were seen in 4 of 5 patients. *2589*   May be associated with defibrination resulting in platelet and coagulation factor consumption. *2538*

84.00 Malaria   With disease progression may become apparent. *0433*   Pancytopenia is a common feature. *2538*   May be associated with defibrination resulting in platelet and coagulation factor consumption (overwhelming parasitemia). *2538*

88.00 Bartonellosis   Has been reported. *1058*

100.00 Leptospirosis   Rare. *0992*

115.00 Histoplasmosis   Markedly reduced only in the terminal phases. *2368*

135.00 Sarcoidosis   Pancytopenia is a common feature. *2538*

197.00 Secondary Malignant Neoplasm of Respiratory System   May be associated with defibrination resulting in platelet and coagulation factor consumption. *2538*

197.50 Secondary Malignant Neoplasm of Digestive System   May be associated with defibrination resulting in platelet and coagulation factor consumption. *2538*

Platelet Count (continued)

Blood   Decrease (continued)

198.30   Secondary Malignant Neoplasm of Brain   Platelet count frequently decreased (intracranial hemorrhage). *2467*

198.50   Secondary Malignant Neoplasm of Bone   Depression of all formed elements of the blood is often seen in disseminated neoplastic disease. *0999*

199.00   Secondary Malignant Neoplasm (Disseminated)   May be associated with defibrination resulting in platelet and coagulation factor consumption. *2538*

201.90   Hodgkin's Disease   Pancytopenia is a common feature. May result from hypersplenism. *2538*

202.40   Leukemic Reticuloendotheliosis   Thrombocytopenia found in 84% of patients with counts usually in the 50-150,000 mm^3 range. *2390*

202.52   Histiocytosis X   Thrombocytopenia may occur in patients with the so-called Letterer-Siwe Syndrome and if associated with hemorrhage manifestations constitutes a grave prognostic sign. *0433*   With involvement of the spleen. *2538*

202.80   Non-Hodgkins Lymphoma   Often present in addition to anemia, and almost any combination of cytopenias may be produced by bone marrow infiltration and replacement, by hypersplenism or as the result of therapy. *2538*   Unusual. *2552*

203.00   Multiple Myeloma   Occasionally, moderate to severe leukopenia or thrombocytopenia, or both, may be observed prior to treatment. *2035*   About 33% have leukopenia with diminished granulocytes and decreased platelets. *1980*   Leukopenia and thrombocytopenia were present in 16 and 13% of the patients, respectively. The degree in untreated patients is usually mild. *1333*   In 31% of 31 patients at initial hospitalization for this disorder. *0781*

204.00   Lymphocytic Leukemia (Acute)   Most patients will have thrombocytopenia. *0433*   The absolute number is almost always decreased, and usually to a greater extent than in acute myelogenous leukemia. *2538*   Pronounced at diagnosis. *2552*   In 78% of 29 patients at initial hospitalization for this disorder. *0781*

204.10   Lymphocytic Leukemia (Chronic)   With thrombocytopenia, and associated bleeding diathesis, a microcytic hypochromic picture could be present. *0433*   Anemia and thrombocytopenia develop as the disorder progresses. *0999*   Neutropenia and thrombocytopenia, ranging in severity from mild to catastrophic, are characteristically present in patient with marrow replacement in the late stages. *2538*   Mild thrombocytopenia may occur in < 50% of cases. *2552*   In 47% of 27 patients at initial hospitalization for this disorder. *0781*

205.00   Myelocytic Leukemia (Acute)   Most patients will have thrombocytopenia. *0433*   Common; frequently pronounced at diagnosis. *2552*   In 85% of 35 patients at initial hospitalization for this disorder. *0781*   Intravascular clotting has been documented in occasional patients. *0890*

205.10   Myelocytic Leukemia (Chronic)   Decreased in terminal stages with findings of thrombocytopenic purpura. *2468*   Rarely develops spontaneously in the absence of blastic crisis. *0992*   Severe thrombocytopenia is rare at diagnosis. *2552*   In 56% of 21 patients at initial hospitalization for this disorder. *0781*   Intravascular clotting has been documented in rare patients. *0890*

206.00   Monocytic Leukemia   Usually present. *2538*   In 83% of 24 patients at initial hospitalization for this disorder. *0781*   With disseminated intravascular clotting. *1552*

207.00   Erythroleukemia   In about 50% of the cases. *2538*

212.70   Benign Neoplasm of Cardiovascular Tissue   May be decreased (possibly mechanical) with resultant findings due to thrombocytopenia. *2467*

272.72   Gaucher's Disease   Unexplained splenomegaly with mild-moderate anemia and thrombocytopenia. *1808*   Pancytopenia is a common feature. May become quite severe. *2538*

272.73   Niemann-Pick Disease   Pancytopenia is a common feature. *2538*   May be severe. *0995*

273.23   Heavy Chain Disease (Gamma)   Presumably related to hypersplenism. *2035*   Mild to marked thrombocytopenia. *2538*

273.30   Waldenström's Macroglobulinemia   Leukocytosis and thrombocytopenia are uncommon. *2538*   Found in about 50% of patients suffering from bleeding diathesis. *2552*   *2035*

275.10   Hepatolenticular Degeneration   Frequently decreased; 13 of 32 patients had counts < 100,000/μL. *2278*   *0433*

279.06   Immunodeficiency (Common Variable)   Count is decreased, with bleeding tendency. *2468*   *2035*

279.12   Wiskott-Aldrich Syndrome   Thrombocytopenia. *2539*   *0455*

280.90   Iron Deficiency Anemia   In infants and children, thrombocytopenia occurred almost as frequently (28%) as did thrombocytosis (35%). Associated with more severe anemia. *0927*   *2538*

281.00   Pernicious Anemia   Anemia, leukopenia (primarily granulopenia) and thrombocytopenia. Occasionally, the primary reduction may be in only 1 of these 3 major formed elements of the blood. May present initially with bleeding associated with thrombocytopenia. *0433*   Generally reduced, may be < 100,000/μL. *1756*   *2552*

281.20   Folic Acid Deficiency Anemia   Pancytopenia is a common feature in vitamin B$_{12}$ and folic acid deficiency. *2538*   Neutropenia and thrombocytopenia are less frequent but still common. Rarely severe. *0962*   Generally reduced, may be < 100,000/μL. *1756* *2552*

281.30   Vitamin B$_6$ Deficiency Anemia   Usually normal, but thrombocytopenia and thrombocytosis occurs in a minority of patients. *2538*

282.00   Hereditary (Congenital) Spherocytosis   Rarely moderately reduced. *2552*

282.41   Thalassemia Major   With the gross splenomegaly which may occur, a secondary thrombocytopenia and leukopenia frequently develop, leading to a further tendency to infection and bleeding. *2538*

282.60   Sickle Cell Anemia   Decreased with folate deficiency or during an aplastic crisis. *2552*

282.71   Hemoglobin C Disease   May be low due to hypersplenism. *0433*

283.00   Acquired Hemolytic Anemia (Autoimmune)   Commonly normal or slightly depressed. Severe thrombocytopenia with bleeding is encountered occasionally and has been termed the Evans' Syndrome. *0681*   *2538*

283.21   Paroxysmal Nocturnal Hemoglobinuria   Usually decreased but shows thrombotic rather than hemorrhagic complications. *2468*   Pancytopenia is a common feature. *2538*   Occurs at some stage in the disease in about 66% of patients. *0484*   Moderate thrombocytopenia is common. *0813*

284.90   Aplastic Anemia   Often markedly decreased. *0433*   Peripheral pancytopenia associated with hypocellular bone marrow. *0415*   Invariable finding. Many patients continue to have decreased counts for years after other abnormalities have disappeared. *2538*   *0151*

285.00   Sideroblastic Anemia   Usually normal, but thrombocytopenia and thrombocytosis occurs in a minority of patients. *2538*

286.34   Congenital Afibrinogenemia   Mild to moderate thrombocytopenia occurs occasionally. Count is rarely below 100,000/μL. *2590*

286.40   Von Willebrand's Disease   Usually normal, but thrombocytopenia has been reported in some families. *0456*   *0962*

286.60   Disseminated Intravascular Coagulopathy   Low or falling platelet counts. *0433*   *2538*

287.00   Allergic Purpura   Defect in hemostasis in drug-sensitivity allergic purpura. *0962*

287.10   Thrombasthenia (Glanzmann's)   Count is usually normal, but mild reduction may occur. *0327*

287.30   Idiopathic Thrombocytopenic Purpura   There is a marked decrease with values under 10,000/μL in the acute form. In the chronic form a moderate thrombocytopenia with counts of 30,000-100,000/μL is present. *0433*   Usually severe at the onset; in most cases platelets are < 20,000/μL. *2538*   May be totally absent or only slightly decreased. *2552*   *0962*

288.00   Agranulocytosis   Depending on the underlying process the patient may manifest a reduced platelet count. *0433*

289.40   Hypersplenism   Pancytopenia is a common feature. *2538*   As much as 50-90% of the total plasma mass may be sequestered. *0082*

289.80   Myelofibrosis   Count ranges from 30,000-3,200,000/μL with an average of 400,000/μL. *0433*   Thrombocytopenia occurred in 48% of myelofibrosis patients, mostly in the later stages. Counts > 400,000 occurred in 16% in the early stages. *2317*   Pancytopenia is a common feature. *2538*   In myelofibrosis as the disease progresses, may be aggravated by therapy. *2538*

303.90   Alcoholism   Counts as low as 20,000/μL have been recorded. Recovery to a normal count occurs within 1 week of abstinence. *0962*

421.00   Bacterial Endocarditis   Usually normal but occasionally it is decreased; rarely purpura occurs. *2467*

446.60 Thrombotic Thrombocytopenic Purpura Decreased count--no bleeding until 60,000/μL. *2468* Usually range 10,000-50,000. *2538*

483.01 Mycoplasma Pneumoniae *2368*

487.10 Influenza May be associated with defibrination resulting in platelet and coagulation factor consumption. *2538*

496.01 Alpha₁-Antitrypsin Deficiency With associated hypersplenism. *1636*

570.00 Acute and Subacute Necrosis of Liver Patients with severe acute hepatic necrosis may have findings compatible with intravascular coagulation, thrombocytopenia and increased levels of fibrinogen/fibrin degradation products. *1048 2538*

571.20 Laennec's or Alcoholic Cirrhosis May result from hypersplenism, a direct effect of alcohol or folate deficiency. *0992* Mild; in about 50% of cases. *2137*

571.49 Chronic Active Hepatitis Anemia, leukopenia, and thrombocytopenia occur in 40-60% of patients. *2467* Slight to moderate anemia with leukopenia and thrombocytopenia are seen, particularly in patients with splenomegaly. *2035*

571.90 Cirrhosis of Liver Patients with severe acute hepatic necrosis may have findings compatible with intravascular coagulation, thrombocytopenia and increased levels of fibrinogen/fibrin degradation products. *1048* Mild; in about 50% of cases. *2137* In 38% of 48 patients at initial hospitalization for this disorder. *0781 2538*

572.00 Liver Abscess (Pyogenic) *0433*

572.40 Hepatic Failure As a result of hypersplenism. *0503*

576.10 Cholangitis Characteristic of the acute phase. *2199*

580.40 Glomerulonephritis (Rapidly Progressive) Observed occasionally. *0277*

584.00 Acute Renal Failure As a consequence of peripheral destruction. *0988*

630.00 Hydatidiform Mole May be associated with defibrination resulting in platelet and coagulation factor consumption. *2538*

642.40 Pre-Eclampsia Evidence of intravascular coagulation, as shown by elevated levels of fibrin degradation products and reduced platelet counts, has been found in many women. *0251* An occasional patient is mildly to moderately thrombocytopenic. *0250* Usually thrombocytopenia and high hematocrit values. *0887 2538*

642.60 Eclampsia Marked reduction in some patients with severe toxemia. *1012*

710.00 Systemic Lupus Erythematosus Thrombocytopenia (< 100,000/μL) is common and is most frequently mild without purpura. Severe thrombocytopenia may occur, but purpura is rarely the presenting manifestation. *0433* Mild thrombocytopenia in 32 patients (23%). Purpura or bleeding noted in 5 cases. *0713* May occur, due to increased destruction. *0309*

710.10 Progressive Systemic Sclerosis Has been reported. *0962*

711.10 Mixed Connective Tissue Disease Thrombocytopenia. *0062*

756.52 Osteopetrosis Anemia and pancytopenia. *2468*

773.00 Hemolytic Disease of Newborn (Erythroblastosis Fetalis) Frequently present in the severely affected group. Although partially a result of exchange transfusion, it is predominantly caused by a reduction of marrow megakaryocytes as a result of excess erythropoiesis. Counts < 40,000/μL are not uncommon. *0433* May occur secondary to isoimmune or exchange transfusion. *2538 2061*

774.40 Jaundice Due to Hepatocellular Damage (Newborn) *0433*

829.00 Fracture of Bone *2468*

948.00 Burns Moderate thrombocytopenia is frequently present for 2-4 days following severe thermal injury to more than 10% of the body. Reduction is most pronounced in patients with sepsis. The degree of thrombocytopenia does not correlate closely with prognosis, but rising platelet levels are associated with clinical improvement. *1034 2538*

958.10 Fat Embolism Sometimes quite severe. *2538 2467*

984.00 Toxic Effects of Lead and Its Compounds (including Fumes) Pancytopenia may occur. *1578*

985.00 Toxic Effects of Non-medicinal Metals Pancytopenia may occur in arsenic poisoning. *0484*

989.50 Toxic Effects of Venom *0995*

990.00 Effects of X-Ray Irradiation A gradual fall in the first 2 weeks postexposure and reaches a low point after 30 days in cases of radiation injury. *0151*

992.00 Heat stroke Low in severe cases. *0151 0995*

Blood   Increase

11.00 Pulmonary Tuberculosis In 49% of 12 patients at initial hospitalization for this disorder. *0781*

151.90 Malignant Neoplasm of Stomach In 39% of 35 patients at initial hospitalization for this disorder. *0781*

153.90 Malignant Neoplasm of Large Intestine In 30% of 118 patients at initial hospitalization for this disorder. *0781*

155.00 Malignant Neoplasm of Liver In 46% of 13 patients at initial hospitalization for this disorder. *0781*

162.90 Malignant Neoplasm of Bronchus and Lung In a large proportion of patients. *2168 0532*

186.90 Malignant Neoplasm of Testis In 34% of 23 patients at initial hospitalization for this disorder. *0781*

197.00 Secondary Malignant Neoplasm of Respiratory System May be increased in malignancy especially disseminated, advanced or inoperable. *2468* In 31% of 508 patients at initial hospitalization for this disorder. *0781*

197.50 Secondary Malignant Neoplasm of Digestive System May be increased in malignancy especially disseminated, advanced or inoperable. *2467*

197.70 Secondary Malignant Neoplasm of Liver May be increased in malignancy especially disseminated, advanced or inoperable. *2468*

198.30 Secondary Malignant Neoplasm of Brain May be increased in malignancy especially disseminated, advanced or inoperable. *2468*

198.50 Secondary Malignant Neoplasm of Bone May be increased in malignancy especially disseminated, advanced or inoperable. *2468*

199.00 Secondary Malignant Neoplasm (Disseminated) May be increased in malignancy especially disseminated, advanced or inoperable. *2468*

201.90 Hodgkin's Disease Thrombocytosis (counts > 400,000) encountered at times, and large bizarre forms may be observed. *0999* In 45% of 70 patients at initial hospitalization for this disorder. *0781*

204.00 Lymphocytic Leukemia (Acute) On very rare occasions. *0075*

205.00 Myelocytic Leukemia (Acute) On very rare occasions. *0075*

205.10 Myelocytic Leukemia (Chronic) Elevated in a small percentage of patients, with counts reaching 1-2 million/μL. Occasionally precedes the increase in WBC and a diagnosis of essential or primary thrombocythemia may be made. *0433* A 33% or more of patients have pronounced thrombocytosis. *1520* High in approximately 50% of patients. *1512 2555* In 23% of 21 patients at initial hospitalization for this disorder. *0781 0532 0999 2538*

238.40 Polycythemia Vera Elevated in a majority of cases. *0532* In about 50% of patients at time of diagnosis. Degree is usually modest, with counts in the range of 450,000-800,000/μL. *2538* Usually increased in number and counts as high as 3 million have been reported. *0151 0433 0999*

250.00 Diabetes Mellitus In 23% of 21 patients at initial hospitalization for this disorder. *0781*

259.20 Carcinoid Syndrome In abdominal crises leukocytosis and thrombocytosis are usual. *0433*

277.30 Amyloidosis Mild thrombocytosis in primary disease. *1334*

280.90 Iron Deficiency Anemia In infants and children, thrombocytopenia occurred almost as frequently (28%) as did thrombocytosis (35%). Associated with more severe anemia. *0927* Reported in 50-75% of adults with classic hypochromic anemia due to chronic blood loss. May be found only in those patients who are actively bleeding. *1232* Usually twice the normal level. *2070*

281.30 Vitamin B₆ Deficiency Anemia Usually normal, but thrombocytopenia and thrombocytosis occurs in a minority of patients. *2538*

282.00 Hereditary (Congenital) Spherocytosis Increased during aplastic crises. *0433* Usually within the normal to high range or slight increase. *2552*

282.31 Hereditary Nonspherocytic Hemolytic Anemia Normal or slightly increased. *0433*

282.41 Thalassemia Major The white cell and platelet counts are slightly elevated unless there is secondary hypersplenism. *2538*

Platelet Count (continued)

Blood   Increase (continued)

282.60   Sickle Cell Anemia   Thrombocytosis often accompanies the leukocytosis. *0433*   Increased (300,000-500,000/μL) with abnormal forms. *2467*   Common, but the count may fall during infarctive crisis. *2538*

285.00   Sideroblastic Anemia   Usually normal, but thrombocytopenia and thrombocytosis occurs in a minority of patients. *2538*

286.01   Hemophilia   Usually normal or elevated. *2552*

289.80   Myelofibrosis   Count ranges from 30,000-3,200,000/μL with an average of 400,000/μL. *0433*   May appear large and bizarre with agnogenic myeloid metaplasia. *0151*   In myelofibrosis, occurs in about 33% of cases, especially in the earlier stages, and may at times reach levels of 1,000,000/μL or higher. *2538   0532*

346.00   Migraine   Increased number but depleted of their serotonin concentration. *0996*

415.10   Pulmonary Embolism and Infarction   Implicated as a cause of intravascular thrombosis, but their role is neither clear nor constant. *1108*   In 19% of 15 patients at initial hospitalization for this disorder. *0781*

446.00   Polyarteritis-Nodosa   Counts > 500,000/μL frequently found. *0999   0962*

555.90   Regional Enteritis or Ileitis   May be present. *2199   2035*

556.00   Ulcerative Colitis   Most commonly in those patients having marked leukocytosis. Not associated with coagulation defects. *2199   2035*

571.90   Cirrhosis of Liver   Increased in miscellaneous disease states. *2467*

577.10   Chronic Pancreatitis   *2467*

579.00   Celiac Sprue Disease   May be present and may reflect splenic atrophy. *2199*

581.90   Nephrotic Syndrome   In 43% of 18 patients at initial hospitalization for this disorder. *0781*   Mildly increased. *2322*

585.00   Chronic Renal Failure   Normal or slightly increased. However, platelet function may be severely impaired. *0329 2552*

714.00   Rheumatoid Arthritis   Counts exceeding 400,000/μL are common and correlate best with leukocytosis and highly active disease. *0962*   In 46% of 40 patients at initial hospitalization for this disorder. *0781*

929.00   Crush Injury (Trauma)   Count rises slowly, lasting for 3 weeks in trauma. *2468*

948.00   Burns   Count rises slowly, lasting for 3 weeks in burns and other types of trauma. *2468*

994.50   Exercise   Effect of sudden exercise. *0618*

Blood   Normal

203.00   Multiple Myeloma   Usually within normal limits prior to cytotoxic therapy. *2035*

204.10   Lymphocytic Leukemia (Chronic)   Normal counts in > 50% of patients. *2552*

242.90   Hyperthyroidism   *2540*

273.30   Waldenström's Macroglobulinemia   Count is usually normal, but abnormalities of platelet function appear to be important causes of bleeding in these patients. *2538*

279.20   Severe Combined Immunodeficiency   *2539*

281.30   Vitamin B₆ Deficiency Anemia   Usually normal, but thrombocytopenia and thrombocytosis occurs in a minority of patients. *2538*

282.00   Hereditary (Congenital) Spherocytosis   Normal except during aplastic crises. *0433*

283.21   Paroxysmal Nocturnal Hemoglobinuria   May be normal or reduced. *0433*   Moderate thrombocytopenia, but life span and function are normal. *0813*

285.00   Sideroblastic Anemia   Usually normal, but thrombocytopenia and thrombocytosis occurs in a minority of patients. *2538   0433*

286.31   Congenital Dysfibrinogenemia   *2538*

286.33   Factor XIII Deficiency   *2538*

286.40   Von Willebrand's Disease   Usually normal, but thrombocytopenia has been reported in some families. *0456   2538*

287.00   Allergic Purpura   Count is normal. *2538*   Tourniquet test may be positive but other tests of hemostasis are usually normal. *2552*

287.10   Thrombasthenia (Glanzmann's)   Present in normal numbers and are morphologically normal. Deficient platelet aggregation is the most significant abnormality. *2552   0433 2538*

289.00   Polycythemia, Secondary   *2538*

421.00   Bacterial Endocarditis   Usually normal but occasionally it is decreased; rarely purpura occurs. *2467*

572.00   Liver Abscess (Pyogenic)   *0433*

642.40   Pre-Eclampsia   Usually within the normal range. *2143*

710.00   Systemic Lupus Erythematosus   Most patients have increased production and increased peripheral destruction, with a normal circulating platelet count. *0309*

Bone Marrow   Decrease

202.80   Non-Hodgkins Lymphoma   In histiocytic medullary reticulosis, severe cytopenias may be associated with the abnormal phagocytosis of erythrocytes, platelets or leukocytes seen in the bone marrow. *2538*

Platelet Survival

Blood   Decrease

287.30   Idiopathic Thrombocytopenic Purpura   Markedly shortened. *0433*   The life-span of transfused normal platelets is extremely short, sometimes only a few h. *2538*

446.60   Thrombotic Thrombocytopenic Purpura   Increased platelet destruction results in thrombocytopenia or shortened platelet survival (i.e., compensated thrombocytolytic states). *1230   2035*

pO₂

Blood   Decrease

37.00   Tetanus   At the onset of mild forms, blood gases may be within normal values. Later when spasms appear and high dosages of sedatives are given, hypoxemia, acidosis plus hypercapnia and metabolic acidosis are present, mainly because of inadequate or improper therapeutic management. *0433*

39.90   Actinomycosis   Pulmonary involvement. *1058*

45.90   Acute Poliomyelitis   Neurological impairment of the respiratory drive. *2612*

80.00   Epidemic Typhus   With pulmonary involvement. *0433*

114.90   Coccidioidomycosis   With pulmonary involvement. *1058*

117.50   Cryptococcosis   With pulmonary involvement. *1058*

135.00   Sarcoidosis   In 71% of 14 patients at initial hospitalization for this disorder. *0781*   Decreased with lung involvement. *2468*   Mild hyperventilation is frequent except in advanced disease when ventilatory obstruction occurs. *0999*

162.90   Malignant Neoplasm of Bronchus and Lung   Impaired diffusion. *2104*

197.00   Secondary Malignant Neoplasm of Respiratory System   In 65% of 67 patients at initial hospitalization for this disorder. *0781*

202.52   Histiocytosis X   With lung involvement, impaired gas diffusion. *2104*

242.90   Hyperthyroidism   Dyspnea. *2199*

244.90   Hypothyroidism   Rare dyspnea secondary to pleural effusion. *2540*

272.72   Gaucher's Disease   With lung involvement. *2246*

277.00   Cystic Fibrosis   Pulmonary involvement. *0438*

282.60   Sickle Cell Anemia   The partial pressure of oxygen in arterial blood is usually diminished as a result of shunting within the lung. *0433*   Decreased oxygenation and increased acidosis lead to further sickling and further vaso-occlusion. *0874*

289.00   Polycythemia, Secondary   *2538*

304.90   Drug Dependence (Opium and Derivatives)   Overdose. *0995*

358.00   Myasthenia Gravis   Associated respiratory insufficiency. *0995*

359.21   Myotonia Atrophica   Respiratory muscle weakness may develop. *0361*

410.90 **Acute Myocardial Infarction** Very frequent complication; occurs in 60% of uncomplicated cases. The intensity of hypoxemia is greatest after 2-3 days. The most intense and persisting hypoxemia was seen in patients with shock and/or acute left ventricular failure. Present even 6 months after onset in 25%. *2529* Patients may develop arterial and tissue hypoxia and metabolic acidosis with a decrease in arterial pH and pO_2. *1108* Arterial pO_2 falls, but rarely below 70 mm Hg if there is reasonable cardiovascular function. In left ventricular failure with associated pulmonary edema, the arterial pO_2 may fall to 50 mm Hg. *0619* *0731*

415.00 **Cor Pulmonale** Acute hypoxia and hypermetabolism associated with fever and infection. *1108*

415.10 **Pulmonary Embolism and Infarction** $pO_2 > 80$ mm Hg excludes diagnosis of pulmonary embolism in almost all cases. *2126* pO_2 and pCO_2 are both low. *1721* Abnormal alveolar-arterial gradient for oxygen and resting hypoxemia. Arterial pO_2 fails to exceed 55 mm Hg following 100% oxygen breathing. *0962* In 86% of 17 patients at initial hospitalization for this disorder. *0781*

446.20 **Goodpasture's Syndrome** Secondary to prolonged pulmonary bleeding. *0062*

480.90 **Viral Pneumonia** Low pO_2 with normal or high pCO_2. *2612*

482.90 **Bacterial Pneumonia** Low pO_2 with normal or high pCO_2. *2612* In 98% of 14 patients at initial hospitalization for this disorder. *0781*

486.01 **Resolving Pneumonia** Moderate to severe hypoxia and respiratory alkalosis in pneumocystis pneumonitis. *1096* Low pO_2 with normal or high pCO_2. *2612* In 76% of 41 patients at initial hospitalization for this disorder. *0781*

491.00 **Chronic Bronchitis** Arterial O_2 tension in 54 patients with chronic nonspecific lung disease, indicated subnormal results to be more frequent among bronchitics (79% with hypoxemia) than among emphysematous patients (63% with hypoxemia). *1497* Tendency to decrease witH the increase in dyspnea severity was apparent. *1496* 66% of nonasthmatic chronic lung disease patients (bronchitis and emphysema) had a mean pO_2 of 72.7 mm Hg. Bronchitics but not emphysemics showed a positive correlation between pO_2 and ventilatory performance. *2335* In 61% of 19 patients at initial hospitalization for this disorder. *0781* *2612*

493.10 **Asthma (Intrinsic)** In general, with moderate asthma of whatever type, and even sometimes when there is no obvious distress, a modest reduction of arterial oxygen pressure to 60-70 mm Hg may be found. As an attack becomes more severe, a further reduction may yield values as low as 50-60 mm Hg. *1560* In 74% of 89 patients at initial hospitalization for this disorder. *0781* *2035 2612*

494.00 **Bronchiectasis** Mild to moderate hypoxemia secondary to venous mixture with arterial blood. *2220*

495.90 **Allergic Alveolitis** Arterial blood gases show decreased pO_2 with either slight respiratory alkalosis or normal pH and pCO_2. *0433*

496.00 **Chronic Obstructive Lung Disease** Decreased pO_2 associated with increased pCO_2. *2467* Greatest declines in arterial oxygen saturation occurred during sleep, with intermittent decreases as great as 44% saturation (range = 12-44% saturation). *0748* In 82% of 70 patients at initial hospitalization for this disorder. *0781*

500.00 **Anthracosis** Impaired gas exchange in established cases. *0151* Arterial oxygen saturation may fall. *0433*

501.00 **Asbestosis** Impaired gas exchange in established cases. *0151* Arterial oxygen saturation may fall. *0433*

502.00 **Silicosis** Impaired gas exchange in established cases. *0151* Impaired gas exchange and movement of respiratory cage due to noncompliant lungs. *0151* Arterial oxygen saturation may fall. *0433*

503.01 **Berylliosis** Hypoxemia is frequent. *2608* Impaired gas exchange in established cases. *0151* Arterial oxygen saturation may fall. *0433*

510.00 **Empyema** Empyema or tuberculous effusion. *0797*

514.00 **Pulmonary Congestion and Hypostasis** *0503*

518.00 **Pulmonary Collapse** Acute massive atelectasis produces a picture of an intrapulmonary right-to-left shunt with a drop in pO_2. *0433*

518.40 **Pulmonary Edema** Decreased pO_2 associated with normal or decreased pCO_2. *2467* Mean arterial O_2 tension measured in 71 patients breathing room air was 59 mm Hg. The 14 acidemic patients had markedly lower pO_2, all under 60 mm Hg. *0554*

553.30 **Hernia Diaphragmatic** Severe hypoxia may be present. *0433* 11 out of 20 infants with congenital hernia survived. Of the 9 nonsurvivors, arterial pCO_2 levels were markedly higher (61.3 ± 15.4 mm Hg) and pO_2 levels lower (49.8 ± 14.2) than in survivors (44.3 ± 7.9, 307.9 ± 142.3, respectively). *0245*

577.00 **Acute Pancreatitis** Blood gases often reveal a moderate lowering of pO_2. *2199*

642.40 **Pre-Eclampsia** In 9 patients with severe pre-eclampsia, there was a significant increase in alveolar-to-arterial pO_2 difference and physiological shunt, indicating a degree of pulmonary ventilation/perfusion imbalance. *2340*

720.00 **Rheumatoid (Ankylosing) Spondylitis** Impaired movement of the respiratory cage. *2612*

737.30 **Kyphoscoliosis** Thoracic bellows defects; decreased pO_2 associated with increased pCO_2. *2467* Mean pCO_2 increased and pO_2 decreased with age in idiopathic scoliosis. *1206*

770.80 **Respiratory Distress Syndrome** Impaired ventilation. *2467*

785.40 **Gangrene** In 63% of 11 patients hospitalized for this disorder. *0781*

829.00 **Fracture of Bone** Decreased arterial pO_2 associated with normal or decreased pCO_2 with associated fat embolism. *2468*

958.10 **Fat Embolism** Decreased arterial pO_2 with normal or decreased pCO_2. *2467* *2532*

991.60 **Hypothermia** Due to hypoxia, acid-base imbalance hypotension. *1471*

Blood Normal

289.00 **Polycythemia, Secondary** *2538*

Pleural Effusion Decrease

11.00 **Pulmonary Tuberculosis** Empyema or tuberculous effusion. *0797*

Poikilocytes

Blood Decrease

202.40 **Leukemic Reticuloendotheliosis** Usually normochromic, normocytic anemia; mild anisocytosis and poikilocytosis were common. *2390*

Blood Increase

238.40 **Polycythemia Vera** Mild anisocytosis and poikilocytosis may be seen in the peripheral blood. *2538*

272.52 **Abetalipoproteinemia** Acanthocytosis of 50-70%. *2246*

272.72 **Gaucher's Disease** If splenectomy has been carried out, severe anisocytosis and poikilocytosis occur, with many target cells, some nucleated red cells, and Howell-Jolly bodies usually present. *2538*

280.90 **Iron Deficiency Anemia** Usually there is moderate to marked anisocytosis and poikilocytosis. *0999* Characteristic of well-developed iron deficiency. *0962* A moderate number, especially tailed and elongated forms, are found. *2552* *0151*

281.00 **Pernicious Anemia** Many bizarre-shaped corpuscles are found. *0995*

281.30 **Vitamin B_6 Deficiency Anemia** Blood smear shows poikilocytosis with many bizarre forms, target cells, hypochromia with pyridoxine-responsive anemia. *2467* Prominent findings on blood smear. *2552*

282.00 **Hereditary (Congenital) Spherocytosis** Slight poikilocytosis. *2468*

282.41 **Thalassemia Major** The red cells show marked aniso-poikilocytosis, with hypochromia, target-cell formation, and a variable degree of basophilic stippling. *2538*

282.42 **Thalassemia Minor** Defective globin synthesis. *0962* Aniso- and poikilocytosis may be very striking and far out of proportion to the degree of anemia. *2552*

282.60 **Sickle Cell Anemia** Blood film reveals marked poikilocytosis and anisocytosis, target cells, some macrocytes, and occasional sickled erythrocytes. Nucleated red cells are frequently seen, particularly in children. *0999*

282.73 **Hemoglobin H Disease** Anisopoikilocytosis of RBC. *2246*

285.00 **Sideroblastic Anemia** Blood smear shows poikilocytosis with many bizarre forms, target cells, hypochromia with pyridoxine-responsive anemia. *2467* Prominent findings on blood smear. In hereditary x-linked sideroblastic anemia. *2552*

Poikilocytes *(continued)*

Blood Increase *(continued)*

516.10 Idiopathic Pulmonary Hemosiderosis Peripheral blood displays the classic changes of severe iron depletion: anisocytosis, poikilocytosis, microcytosis, and hypochromia. *2538*

Porphobilinogen

Serum Increase

277.14 Acute Intermittent Porphyria Increased production of the porphyrin precursors. *0145* In patients with severe attacks. *2304*

277.15 Porphyria Variegata Increased production of the porphyrin precursors. *0145*

277.17 Hereditary Coproporphyria Increased production of the porphyrin precursors. *0145*

Urine Increase

199.00 Secondary Malignant Neoplasm (Disseminated) Elevated porphobilinogen occasionally has been observed in carcinomatosis. *0151*

201.90 Hodgkin's Disease Elevated porphobilinogen occasionally has been observed. *0151*

277.13 Erythropoietic Coproporphyria Slight increase. *2246*

277.14 Acute Intermittent Porphyria Occurs fairly specifically in acute idiopathic porphyria. *2499* In 21 symptomatic patients, an average of 83 mg porphobilinogen/24h was excreted. Tends to decrease somewhat during remission. *2254* During relapse the presence of this compound is a constant feature. During remission it is usually present but the absence does not exclude the diagnosis. *2457 2538* Characteristic. *2246 0145 2271 0962 2552*

277.15 Porphyria Variegata May appear during acute attacks. *2552* May be as high as levels in acute intermittent porphyria. *0524 0613*

277.16 Porphyria Cutanea Tarda Rarely occurs. *0613 2246 0995*

277.17 Hereditary Coproporphyria Only during acute attacks. *2552 0995 2246*

571.90 Cirrhosis of Liver Occasionally observed. *0151*

Urine Normal

277.11 Congenital Erythropoietic Porphyria (Günther's Disease) With chromatographic methods, within normal limits. *0867 2426*

277.12 Erythropoietic Protoporphyria *1478*

277.13 Erythropoietic Coproporphyria *0995*

277.16 Porphyria Cutanea Tarda Not present. *1344 2538*

984.00 Toxic Effects of Lead and Its Compounds (including Fumes) *1031*

CSF Increase

277.14 Acute Intermittent Porphyria In patients with severe attacks. *2304*

Liver Increase

277.14 Acute Intermittent Porphyria Large amounts. *0908* Liver and kidney regularly contain large amounts. *2072 2246*

Porphyrins

Urine Increase

70.00 Viral Hepatitis *2467*

277.16 Porphyria Cutanea Tarda Usually enough to produce a pinkish or brown color. *2246*

571.90 Cirrhosis of Liver *2467*

650.00 Pregnancy May be increased. *2468*

984.00 Toxic Effects of Lead and Its Compounds (including Fumes) *2467*

Urine Normal

270.02 Hartnup Disease *2246*

Bone Marrow Normal

277.16 Porphyria Cutanea Tarda *2072*

277.17 Hereditary Coproporphyria No increase demonstrable. *2246 0868*

Feces Increase

277.17 Hereditary Coproporphyria *2246*

Feces Normal

270.02 Hartnup Disease *2246*

277.16 Porphyria Cutanea Tarda Normal or only slightly increased in the stool. *2552* Highly variable. *2246*

Liver Increase

277.16 Porphyria Cutanea Tarda May precede clinical manifestations and persist after remission. *2072*

Potassium

Serum Decrease

1.00 Cholera Marked loss of fluid and electrolytes. *2468* Renal wasting leads to hypokalemic state. *1679*

4.90 Bacillary Dysentery Fluid and electrolyte loss may be quite significant, particularly in pediatric and geriatric populations. *1058*

40.20 Whipple's Disease In patients with severe diarrhea and malabsorption. *2199*

153.90 Malignant Neoplasm of Large Intestine Villous tumor of rectum may cause depletion. *2467*

157.90 Malignant Neoplasm of Pancreas Gastrointestinal wasting as a result of pancreatic islet nonbeta cell tumors. *1679* In 30% of 33 patients at initial hospitalization for this disorder. *0781*

203.00 Multiple Myeloma Common. *0962*

205.00 Myelocytic Leukemia (Acute) Below 3.5 mmol/L in 19 (59%) of 32 patients. *1602*

211.40 Benign Neoplasm of Rectum and Anus Sometimes decreased. *2467*

211.60 Benign Neoplasm of Pancreas Gastrointestinal wasting as a result of pancreatic islet nonbeta cell tumors. *1679*

227.91 Pheochromocytoma High plasma renin activity has been noted and may result in mild hypokalemia. *0433*

250.00 Diabetes Mellitus Osmotic diuresis secondary to hyperglycemia. *2540*

250.10 Diabetic Acidosis Total body deficit. Only 4-10% have decreased plasma concentrations and these patients are at high risk for developing life-threatening hypokalemia during early hours of treatment. *1516* Renal wasting leads to hypokalemic state. *1679* Despite the markedly negative K^+ balance, hyperkalemia is often present because the acidosis causes the K^+ to shift from inside the cells into the extracellular space. *2540*

251.50 Zollinger-Ellison Syndrome Hypokalemia; frequently associated with chronic severe diarrhea. *2468*

252.00 Hyperparathyroidism Related to the hypercalcemia and does not aid in differential diagnosis. *0433* Rare (3%). *0999* Occasionally observed; attributed to decreased distal tubular reabsorption. *0151*

255.00 Adrenal Cortical Hyperfunction (Glucocorticoid Excess) Characterized by low serum concentration and hypertension. *1108* Severe hypokalemia and weakness are best explained by the enormous quantities of cortisol secreted by the hyperplastic adrenals. *0151*

255.10 Adrenal Cortical Hyperfunction (Mineralocorticoid Excess) Progressive weakness and lack of stamina due to potassium depletion are frequent complaints. *0433* Renal wasting leads to hypokalemic state. *1679* Characterized by low serum concentration and hypertension. Mean concentration < 3.0 mmol/L and is usually persistently in this range. *1108 0962*

260.00 Protein Malnutrition Potassium depletion is a major biochemical characteristic of kwashiorkor. *0151*

270.03 Cystinosis Hypokalemia and severe intracellular potassium depletion can be most difficult problems, causing severe muscle weakness. *0433* Due to high urine potassium. *2468* Decreased serum concentrations will become normal and then elevated as renal deterioration progress. *2246*

275.10 Hepatolenticular Degeneration Found in 9 of 31 patients (29%). *2278*

275.34 Familial Periodic Paralysis   Ranges from 2.5-3.5 mmol/L in hypokalemic attacks. May be normal between attacks. *0151* Marked fall. *1172*   Rarely, may shift from extra- to intracellular sites. There is no evidence of GI or renal wasting, volume depletion or total body K depletion. *1679*

276.30 Metabolic Alkalosis   Usually decreased, which is the chief danger in alkalosis. *2468*

276.80 Hypokalemia   *0062*

277.14 Acute Intermittent Porphyria   Electrolyte depletion and alkalosis associated with azotemia of variable degree are often present on admission but may also develop acutely during the course of the attack. The electrolyte disorders are attributable in many patients to electrolyte depletion with inappropriate and injudicious overhydration. *0433*

281.00 Pernicious Anemia   Slightly reduced. *2552*   17 of 34 patients had < 4 mmol/L, the lower limit of normal. *1358*

281.20 Folic Acid Deficiency Anemia   Slightly reduced. *2552* 17 of 34 patients had < 4 mmol/L, the lower limit of normal. *1358*

303.90 Alcoholism   In 26 patients in whom delirium tremens developed, a continuing decrease led to hypokalemia, (mean 2.9 mmol/L) when delirium tremens started. *2449*

331.81 Reye's Syndrome   Hypokalemia and hyponatremia are common. *0151*

401.00 Malignant Hypertension   Many diseases including hyperaldosteronism are characterized by low serum concentration. *1108*

401.10 Essential Benign Hypertension   Characterized by low serum concentration. *1108*   Untreated hypertensive patients frequently presented with low serum concentrations unassociated with acidosis or alkalosis. *2027*

428.00 Congestive Heart Failure   Deficiency is common and excess is occasionally noted in patients under therapy. When failure is severe, an accelerated excretion rate may result from secondary hyperaldosteronism. *1108*   Most often due to the kaliuretic action of diuretics without adequate potassium replacement. *0962*

493.10 Asthma (Intrinsic)   Hypokalemia caused by therapy or gastrointestinal fluid losses in children may intensify or induce respiratory failure by producing muscle weakness. *0433*   May be found in corticosteroid-treated patients. *2035*

496.00 Chronic Obstructive Lung Disease   Suggests a coexisting primary metabolic alkalosis. *0962*

533.90 Peptic Ulcer, Site Unspecified   May be < 3.5 mmol/L when complicated by obstruction. *0433*   Pyloric obstruction with vomiting and loss of gastric secretion results in hypochloremia, hyponatremia, hypokalemia, elevated serum pH and carbon dioxide content, and azotemia. *0962*

537.00 Pyloric Stenosis, Acquired   Secondary to vomiting. *0587*

537.40 Fistula of Stomach and Duodenum   Renal wasting leads to hypokalemic state. *1679*   In gastric fistula, hypokalemic, hypochloremic alkalosis may result. *2199*

555.90 Regional Enteritis or Ileitis   Common feature of severe colitis. *2035*

556.00 Ulcerative Colitis   Serum electrolytes may show losses due to diarrhea, especially hypokalemia, which may contribute to colonic atony and may portend acute toxic dilatation. *0433*   Common feature of severe colitis. *2035*   Portends a worse prognosis, probably because the degree of abnormality parallels clinical severity. *2199*

558.90 Diarrhea   Depletion may develop with any severe diarrhea. *2199*

560.90 Intestinal Obstruction   Metabolic alkalosis secondary to vomiting. *2467*

564.20 Postgastrectomy (Dumping) Syndrome   Jejunal hypersecretion of water and electrolytes, especially potassium. *0995*

567.90 Peritonitis   Secondary to increased aldosterone production. *0995*

571.20 Laennec's or Alcoholic Cirrhosis   Often present in these patients and may represent gastrointestinal losses, decreased oral intake, or increased urinary excretion through acquired renal tubular acidosis. *0999*   *0151*

571.90 Cirrhosis of Liver   Frequent in patients with ascites and edema. *0992*

577.00 Acute Pancreatitis   Usually normal or only slightly depressed. *2199*

579.00 Celiac Sprue Disease   If diarrhea is severe, marked electrolyte depletion. *2199*

579.90 Malabsorption, Cause Unspecified   *0151*

584.00 Acute Renal Failure   Large urinary potassium excretion may cause decreased serum concentration in diuretic stage. *2468* May occur early in renal failure due to diarrhea, vomiting, or spontaneous potassium loss in urine. *0151*

585.00 Chronic Renal Failure   May occur. *0277*

588.81 Proximal Renal Tubular Acidosis   May be a life-threatening complication. *0433*   Hydrogen ion and ammonium ion production by the renal tubule cells is diminished, with excessive loss of potassium in the urine. In any case of severe renal damage, potassium conservation may be impaired. *0619*   Renal wasting leads to hypokalemic state. *1679*   Normal or decreased *2645 2446*

588.82 Distal Renal Tubular Acidosis   Commonly occurs in Type I. *0151*   *0843*

787.00 Vomiting   Deficiency results from decreased intake of potassium, loss in the vomitus, and most important, from renal potassium wasting. *2199*

992.00 Heat stroke   Serum K is low and Cl is high in severe cases. *0151*

994.80 Effects of Electric Current   Unexplained acute hypokalemia leading to respiratory arrest and cardiac arrhythmias has developed in some patients between the 2nd and 4th weeks following injury. *0995*

Serum   Increase

65.00 Arthropod-Borne Hemorrhagic Fever   Occurs in the oliguric phase of epidemic hemorrhagic fever. *0151*

100.00 Leptospirosis   Marked oliguria or anuria develops after the 1st week of disease and is attended by severe azotemia and electrolyte imbalance characteristic of lower nephron nephrosis. *2368*

151.90 Malignant Neoplasm of Stomach   In 30% of 29 patients at initial hospitalization for this disorder. *0781*

205.10 Myelocytic Leukemia (Chronic)   Pseudohyperkalemia due to the release of potassium from white cells during clotting has been reported. *0291*   Artifactual hyperkalemia may occur. *2552*

238.40 Polycythemia Vera   Has been reported in myeloproliferative disorders associated with thrombocytosis. May be spurious and related to K release from the increased number of platelets during the process of blood coagulation. *1656 2538*

250.00 Diabetes Mellitus   hyperkalemia may occur due to low insulin levels, which normally would cause a net influx of K^+ into cells, and low aldosterone levels, which would stimulate K^+ excretion in a normal state. *1854*   In 29% of 107 patients at initial hospitalization for this disorder. *0781*

250.10 Diabetic Acidosis   Usually normal or elevated, despite total body deficit. Only 4-10% have decreased plasma concentrations and these patients are at high risk for developing life-threatening hypokalemia during early hours of treatment. *1516*   Despite the markedly negative K^+ balance, hyperkalemia is often present because the acidosis causes the K^+ to shift from inside the cells into the extracellular space. *2540*   Impaired uptake by the cells secondary to acidosis and increased liberation of cell potassium following protein breakdown and gluconeogenesis. *0619*   *1515*

252.00 Hyperparathyroidism   Incidence of 40% (7 of 17 cases) was reported. Other studies indicate a lower frequency. *2613 1492*

253.00 Acromegaly   *0995*

255.40 Adrenal Cortical Hypofunction   Raised potassium concentration and metabolism acidosis usually occur. *2612*   Normal in mild insufficiency, but in severe insufficiency, particularly of aldosterone, there are hyponatremia and hyperkalemia. *0433* *0999 0962*

259.20 Carcinoid Syndrome   Severe hypokalemia and weakness are common, due to the enormous quantities or cortisol secreted by the hyperplastic adrenals. *0151*

270.03 Cystinosis   Decreased serum concentrations will become normal and then elevated as renal deterioration progress. *2246*

276.20 Metabolic Acidosis   Frequently increased. Often 6-7 mmol/L in type II-B, with lactic acidosis. *2468*

428.00 Congestive Heart Failure   Deficiency is common and excess is occasionally noted in patients under therapy. *1108* Less common than hypokalemia. A common complication in patients on potassium supplements who are not responding to their diuretics. *0962*

492.80 Pulmonary Emphysema   Rises in acidosis but total body potassium is usually depressed. *0433*

496.00 Chronic Obstructive Lung Disease   When acidemia is present, may be falsely high because of potassium ions moving from the extracellular space. *0962*

496.01 Alpha₁-Antitrypsin Deficiency   Seen with Acidosis. *1636*

Potassium (continued)

Serum Increase (continued)

572.20 Hepatic Encephalopathy Decreased concentrations indirectly induce hepatic coma by its effect on ammonia metabolism. Renal production of ammonia increases in the presence of potassium deficiency. *0801*

584.00 Acute Renal Failure During oliguric phase. *0277* May occur depending on the duration and severity of the disease. *0151* Liberated during body cell breakdown, and is not excreted completely in the urine. *0619*

585.00 Chronic Renal Failure Liberated during body cell breakdown, and is not excreted completely in the urine. *0619*

588.82 Distal Renal Tubular Acidosis Some cases. *0186*

597.80 Urethritis Reveals the degree of renal impairment. *0433*

694.40 Pemphigus *0151*

710.00 Systemic Lupus Erythematosus Two patients with long standing disease had persistent hyperkalemia apparently due to defect in renal tubular secretion. *0527*

770.80 Respiratory Distress Syndrome Increased catabolism. *2467* *0702*

929.00 Crush Injury (Trauma) *0995*

992.00 Heat stroke In malignant hyperpyrexia, raised to 9.0 mmol/L (normal = 3.5-5.4 mmol/L) 2 h after the anesthetic was started. *0541*

Serum Normal

250.00 Diabetes Mellitus Normal or increased. *2467*

253.40 Anterior Pituitary Hypofunction Usually. *0995*

275.34 Familial Periodic Paralysis Normal between attacks. *2246*

276.50 Dehydration *2467*

277.00 Cystic Fibrosis Normal unless complications occur (e.g., chronic pulmonary disease with accumulation of CO_2, massive salt loss due to sweating). *2467* *0105*

359.11 Progressive Muscular Dystrophy The differences between the patients and the control group of normal boys for sodium and potassium in serum and urine were not significant. The pathologically elevated sodium:potassium ratio in skeletal muscle is not due to increased aldosterone or other causes of renal wastage of potassium. *0816*

428.00 Congestive Heart Failure Normal or slightly increased (because of shift from hypochloremic alkalosis due to some diuretics. *2467*

492.80 Pulmonary Emphysema *2467*

588.81 Proximal Renal Tubular Acidosis Normal or decreased. *0186*

650.00 Pregnancy Throughout pregnancy. *0517*

780.80 Hyperhidrosis *2467*

Urine Decrease

255.40 Adrenal Cortical Hypofunction Inability of the renal tubules to reabsorb sodium chloride and water and relative inability to excrete potassium. *0619* *0962*

275.34 Familial Periodic Paralysis Excretion decreases at the time of attack. *2467*

558.90 Diarrhea Normal or decreased. *2467*

579.90 Malabsorption, Cause Unspecified *2467*

580.00 Acute Poststreptococcal Glomerulonephritis *0619*

584.00 Acute Renal Failure In acute tubular necrosis the kidney loses it ability to reabsorb sodium, and an increased concentration of urine sodium with a relative decrease in urine potassium will be noted. *0433*

590.00 Chronic Pyelonephritis *0619*

590.10 Acute Pyelonephritis *0619*

Urine Increase

203.00 Multiple Myeloma Due to Myeloma Nephropathy. *0186*

205.00 Myelocytic Leukemia (Acute) Inappropriately large quantities of potassium were excreted in relation to the low serum content. 12 of 32 patients excreted more than the mean potassium intake. *1602*

250.00 Diabetes Mellitus Osmotic diuresis secondary to hyperglycemia. *2540*

252.00 Hyperparathyroidism May occur. *2540*

255.00 Adrenal Cortical Hyperfunction (Glucocorticoid Excess) There is excessive endogenous adrenocortical activity with increased potassium loss in the urine. *0619* *0151*

255.10 Adrenal Cortical Hyperfunction (Mineralocorticoid Excess) Significant urinary potassium loss may be encountered despite hypokalemia. *0999*

260.00 Protein Malnutrition Increased breakdown of the body cells, occurs with release of intracellular potassium. Carbohydrate intake (glucose 100 g/24h) greatly reduces the rate of cell breakdown. *0619*

270.03 Cystinosis *2468*

276.20 Metabolic Acidosis *0619*

276.30 Metabolic Alkalosis *0619*

276.50 Dehydration *2467*

571.20 Laennec's or Alcoholic Cirrhosis *0151*

585.00 Chronic Renal Failure *2467*

588.81 Proximal Renal Tubular Acidosis Renal wasting of potassium. *1679* May result in severe hypokalemic paralysis. *2246*

588.82 Distal Renal Tubular Acidosis Commonly occurs in Type I. *0151* *0843*

787.00 Vomiting *0619*

1013.01 Diet (High Sodium) Urinary K excretion rose progressively as salt intake increased. *1274*

Urine Normal

253.50 Diabetes Insipidus *2467*

255.10 Adrenal Cortical Hyperfunction (Mineralocorticoid Excess) Usually within normal limits in spite of hypokalemia and tissue potassium depletion. *1108*

255.40 Adrenal Cortical Hypofunction Normal or decreased. *2467*

260.00 Protein Malnutrition Increased or normal. *2467*

359.11 Progressive Muscular Dystrophy The differences between the patients and the control group of normal boys for sodium and potassium in serum and urine were not significant. The pathologically elevated sodium:potassium ratio in skeletal muscle is not due to increased aldosterone or other causes of renal wastage of potassium. *0816*

428.00 Congestive Heart Failure *2467*

492.80 Pulmonary Emphysema *2467*

537.00 Pyloric Stenosis, Acquired *2467*

780.80 Hyperhidrosis *2467*

CSF Decrease

275.34 Familial Periodic Paralysis Rarely found to be quite low during attack. *0612*

CSF Increase

410.90 Acute Myocardial Infarction In patients who developed severe anoxia after a cardiac arrest, the cisternal K^+ concentration was twice that of lumbar (6.7 vs 3.5 mmol/L). During anoxia, K^+ and H^+ flow from brain cells into the brain extracellular fluid. Acute changes are reflected more accurately by cisternal than by lumbar fluid. *1213* Of 41 patients with cardiac arrest studied, 20 regained consciousness and 21 did not. In those who did not, was a significant increase in the K^+ concentration found in samples obtained between 40-50 min and between 50-60 min after cardiac arrest. Potassium concentration of cisternal CSF obtained soon after cardiac arrest might give an indication of the degree of cerebral damage. *2159*

CSF Normal

275.34 Familial Periodic Paralysis Only a slight drop during attacks. *1865*

Feces Increase

1.00 Cholera Fecal potassium concentrations are higher than in plasma. *0151*

193.01 Medullary Carcinoma of Thyroid About 33% of patients with medullary carcinoma have watery diarrhea with stools characteristically containing increased sodium and potassium content. *2199*

273.22 Heavy Chain Disease (Alpha) Patients usually present with chronic diarrhea, hypocalcemia, and excessive fecal losses of water and electrolytes. *2538*

273.23 Heavy Chain Disease (Gamma) Patients usually present with chronic diarrhea, hypocalcemia, and excessive fecal losses of water and electrolytes. *2538*

585.00 Chronic Renal Failure May represent an important adaptive response. *1010*

Red Blood Cells   Increase

585.00 Chronic Renal Failure In 36 patients, a normal or high erythrocyte potassium was found. *1162*

Saliva   Increase

428.00 Congestive Heart Failure *2467*

Saliva   Normal

277.00 Cystic Fibrosis Submaxillary saliva has slightly increased chloride and sodium but not potassium. *2467*

Sweat   Increase

277.00 Cystic Fibrosis Striking increase in sweat sodium and chloride and to a lesser extent potassium is present in virtually all homozygous patients. It is present throughout life from time of birth and is not related to severity of disease or organ involvement. *2467*

Prealbumin

Serum   Decrease

70.00 Viral Hepatitis The mean value was 6.0 mg/dL in fatal cases, 7.4 mg/dL in survivors. The difference was not statistically significant. *1291*

84.00 Malaria Decreased significantly in 11 patients untreated for more than 4 days. *2066*

260.00 Protein Malnutrition Albumin, prealbumin and transferrin concentrations, as well as the level of alpha$_2$ macroglobulin were found to be lower in cases of protein-energy malnutrition associated with preschool children. *2065*

555.90 Regional Enteritis or Ileitis Haptoglobin concentrations rise with increasing clinical activity of the disease, while the prealbumin fraction declines. *1510 2035*

556.00 Ulcerative Colitis Haptoglobin concentrations rise with increasing clinical activity of the disease, while the prealbumin fraction declines. *1510 2035*

Serum   Increase

197.50 Secondary Malignant Neoplasm of Digestive System Tends to reflect the nutritional status of patients with primary and metastatic cancer of the large intestine. *2480*

CSF   Increase

345.90 Epilepsy Only protein to increase in CSF of epileptics. Mean concentration was 1.50 ± 0.11 mg/dL. *1625*

Precipitins

Serum   Increase

11.00 Pulmonary Tuberculosis Found in approximately 40% of patients. *2508*

30.00 Leprosy Found in the sera of lepromatous patients and in 50% of the patients with tuberculoid lesions that were bacillary-positive. Not found in the sera of bacillary-negative tuberculoid patients. *2035*

112.90 Moniliasis Serum agglutinin and precipitin titers against Candida are of little value; as many normal individuals harbor the organism without tissue invasion. *2199* A low titer probably makes esophageal candidiasis unlikely. *2199*

114.90 Coccidioidomycosis Highly specific and can be detected in 80% of patients within 2 weeks of onset of symptoms; absent in 90% after 6 months. *2508* Present in approximately 80% of patients with primary nondisseminating infection, preceding the development of CF antibodies, and they appear to represent IgM antibodies. Persisting precipitins have been associated with dissemination, and precipitins may reappear when there is systemic reinfection. *2035* Positive in most patients within a month after onset of symptoms. *0962 2207 2368*

115.00 Histoplasmosis Antibodies are demonstrable, but cross reactions with Blastomyces and Coccidioides are seen in these tests. *0962*

117.30 Aspergillosis Detected in 100% of patients with aspergillomas and 70% with allergic aspergillosis. *2508* 48 and 67% having precipitins to Staphylococcus aureus and hemophilus influenzae. *2035*

124.00 Trichinosis Using bentonite particles, become positive later in the disease and are most helpful when they exhibit a significant change in titer. *0962* Precipitin test appears to be too nonspecific for general use. *1207*

130.00 Toxoplasmosis *2035*

245.20 Hashimoto's Thyroiditis Unusual but, when present, seem to be pathognomonic of Hashimoto's disease. *2035* Precipitin test for thyroglobulin is positive in 60% of chronic thyroiditis cases. The least sensitive test for thyroid antibodies but the most specific. *0999*

495.90 Allergic Alveolitis Found in 17-18%, particularly against the thermophilic actinomycete M. faeni and also, against T. vulgaris and fungi such as the genus Aspergillus and Mucormycosis. *1801 2035*

710.00 Systemic Lupus Erythematosus Found in 15% of patients and 3% of controls. *0344*

CSF   Increase

114.90 Coccidioidomycosis Only rarely found in meningitis. *2035 2207*

Pleural Effusion   Increase

114.90 Coccidioidomycosis May be found in the thoracic fluid in pleural effusions. *2035*

Pregnanediol

Urine   Decrease

217.00 Benign Neoplasm of Breast Average daily values were lower in 109 women with benign disease than normal women. No change was found in plasma estradiol. *1528*

220.00 Benign Neoplasm of Ovary Absent in ovarian tumors. *2468*

220.92 Granulosa Cell Tumor of Ovary Absent in ovarian tumors. *2468*

220.93 Lutein Cell Tumor of Ovary Absent in ovarian tumors. *2468*

220.94 Theca Cell Tumor of Ovary Absent in ovarian tumors. *2468*

256.30 Ovarian Hypofunction Decreased in amenorrhea. *2468*

630.00 Hydatidiform Mole High concentrations of chorionic gonadotropin and reduced pregnanediol suggests diagnosis. *2104*

640.00 Threatened Abortion Sometimes. *2467*

642.40 Pre-Eclampsia Reduced compared to normal pregnant women, but there was considerable overlap in values. *2332* In 58 women with mild pre-eclampsia, mean = 29.5 mg/24h, ranging from 6-63.8. The average decrease of 40% was not found significant because of the wide range of values in both normo- and hypertensive patients. *1218*

642.60 Eclampsia *2467*

656.40 Pregnancy Complicated by Intrauterine Death Fetal death. If < 5 mg/24h then abortion is inevitable. *0619*

780.30 Convulsions The incidence of epileptic seizures was higher in women during the high estrogen period of the menstrual cycle. Number of seizures correlated positively to estrogen:progesterone ratio and negatively to progesterone levels. *0096*

Urine   Increase

181.00 Malignant Neoplasm of Trophoblast (Choriocarcinoma) May be much increased with primary chorionepithelioma of ovary. *2467*

220.95 Arrhenoblastoma In arrhenoblastoma of ovary. *2468*

620.20 Ovarian Cyst Increased in luteal cysts of ovary. *2468*

650.00 Pregnancy Rises progressively as pregnancy progresses, with a slight fall in the last 2 weeks. Range was 26-79.4 mg/24h, with an average of 50. *1218 0850*

Pregnanetriol

Urine Decrease

253.40 Anterior Pituitary Hypofunction Decreased to values seen during follicular phase rather than luteal phase of menstrual cycle with galactorrhea amenorrhea syndromes. *2468*

Urine Increase

194.00 Malignant Neoplasm of Adrenal Gland Virilizing adrenal tumors. *0995*

255.00 Adrenal Cortical Hyperfunction (Glucocorticoid Excess) Increased 17 OH-progesterone in recurring and cancerous patients. *1450*

994.50 Exercise Effect most marked in well trained individuals. *0089*

Progesterone

Plasma Decrease

217.00 Benign Neoplasm of Breast Average daily values were lower in 109 women with benign disease than normal women. No change was found in plasma estradiol. *1528*

220.00 Benign Neoplasm of Ovary Absent in ovarian tumors. *2468*

220.92 Granulosa Cell Tumor of Ovary Absent in ovarian tumors. *2468*

220.93 Lutein Cell Tumor of Ovary Absent in ovarian tumors. *2468*

220.94 Theca Cell Tumor of Ovary Absent in ovarian tumors. *2468*

253.40 Anterior Pituitary Hypofunction Decreased to values seen during follicular phase rather than luteal phase of menstrual cycle with galactorrhea amenorrhea syndromes. *2468*

256.30 Ovarian Hypofunction Decreased in amenorrhea. *2468*

630.00 Hydatidiform Mole High concentrations of chorionic gonadotropin and reduced pregnanediol indicate diagnosis. *2104*

640.00 Threatened Abortion Has been reported to be low, but is often normal prior to spontaneous abortion. *2104*

642.40 Pre-Eclampsia Reduced compared to normal pregnant women, but there was considerable overlap in values. In 58 women with mild pre-eclampsia, mean = 29.5 mg/24h, ranging from 6-63.8. The average decrease of 40% was not found significant because of the wide range of values in both normo- and hypertensive patients. *1218*

642.60 Eclampsia Appears to be unrelated to the severity of the condition. *2104* *2212*

656.40 Pregnancy Complicated by Intrauterine Death Fetal death. If < 5 mg/24h then abortion is inevitable. *0619*

780.30 Convulsions The incidence of epileptic seizures was higher in women during the high estrogen period of the menstrual cycle. Number of seizures correlated positively to estrogen:progesterone ratio and negatively to progesterone levels. *0096*

Plasma Increase

155.00 Malignant Neoplasm of Liver Raised in 36 of 50 men with liver disease compared with 20 healthy male control subjects. Significantly higher in men with nonalcoholic cirrhosis with gynecomastic than those without. *0704*

181.00 Malignant Neoplasm of Trophoblast (Choriocarcinoma) May be much increased with primary chorionepithelioma of ovary. *2467*

220.95 Arrhenoblastoma In arrhenoblastoma of ovary. *2468*

255.00 Adrenal Cortical Hyperfunction (Glucocorticoid Excess) Increased 17 OH-progesterone in recurring and cancerous patients. *1450*

571.90 Cirrhosis of Liver Raised in 36 of 50 men with liver disease compared with 20 healthy male control subjects. Significantly higher in men with nonalcoholic cirrhosis with gynaecomastic than those without. *0704*

600.00 Benign Prostatic Hypertrophy Increased; especially in older patients. *0972*

620.20 Ovarian Cyst Increased in luteal cysts of ovary. *2468*

630.00 Hydatidiform Mole Higher progesterone concentration than found in normal pregnant women in 8 of 13 patients with intact mole, ranging from 17.5-79.2 ng/mL. *1613*

650.00 Pregnancy Among the normotensive subjects, concentrations were elevated as early as the 6t of gestation. While consistent, progressive, further increases were noted in renin substrate, aldosterone and progesterone during pregnancy, renin activity did not continue to rise. *2507* Mean plasma concentrations were 60% higher in twin pregnancies than in normal simplex pregnancies. *0133* *1578*

Proinsulin

Serum Increase

211.60 Benign Neoplasm of Pancreas Elevated levels of plasma insulin following an overnight fast, as well as increased concentrations of C-peptide or proinsulin, strongly suggest the presence of insulinoma. *0999*

250.00 Diabetes Mellitus Increased percentage in 11 of 59 maturity-onset cases and correlated with plasma glucose but not to total insulin. *1485*

Serum Normal

250.00 Diabetes Mellitus No consistent abnormality has been found. Patients with mild diabetes have repeatedly shown normal proportions. Severe cases may have an elevated proinsulin:insulin ratio. *1080*

Prolactin

Serum Decrease

253.40 Anterior Pituitary Hypofunction Patients with pituitary tumors or postpartum pituitary necrosis will be found to have impaired prolactin and growth hormone reserve. *0999* Characterized by absent or reduced production and release. *1108*

297.90 Paranoid States and Other Psychoses Concentrations in 17 drug-free chronic schizophrenic patients correlated inversely with ratings of their psychopathology. *1279*

Serum Increase

84.00 Malaria Slightly increased in falciparum malaria. *2487*

155.00 Malignant Neoplasm of Liver Found in 14% of men with liver disease. Levels unrelated to presence of gynecomastia. *0704*

162.90 Malignant Neoplasm of Bronchus and Lung Elevated. *0918*

174.90 Malignant Neoplasm of Breast Significantly higher concentrations than controls in early breast cancer. In advanced breast cancer elevated levels were only found in postmenopausal patients. *1977* Mean concentration was significantly elevated in 148 breast cancer patients. Incidence of elevation was 22%. *0033*

189.00 Malignant Neoplasm of Kidney Elevated. *0918*

244.90 Hypothyroidism Associated with amenorrhea and pituitary enlargement secondary to primary hypothyroidism. *1256* Over 14.0 ng/mL in 39% of patients with untreated primary disease. Mean = 14.3 ± 1.1, range = 4.7-42.0 ng/mL in 49 subjects. Normal value = 8.2 ± 0.5. Significant differences occurred only between female patients and controls, not with male patients and controls. *1068* Can trigger a mild to moderate increase (20-300 ng/mL) *2637* *2638*

250.10 Diabetic Acidosis Elevated in 8 patients, (24.8 ± 10.2 ng/mL). After correction of the ketoacidosis, levels decreased to 10.9 ± 6.4 ng/mL (normal range men 4.9 ± 0.8, women 5.1 ± 1.6 ng/mL). *0983*

251.20 Hypoglycemia, Unspecified Increased levels. *1887* Can trigger a mild to moderate increase (20-300 ng/mL) *2637*

251.50 Zollinger-Ellison Syndrome Levels were measured in 36 patients with ZES, eight patients had elevated levels. *2245*

253.00 Acromegaly Measured in 73 untreated patients and found to be elevated in 32%. *0521* Can trigger a mild to moderate increase (20-300 ng/mL). *2637*

255.00 Adrenal Cortical Hyperfunction (Glucocorticoid Excess) Can trigger a mild to moderate increase (20-300 ng/mL). *2637*

255.40 Adrenal Cortical Hypofunction Increased levels. *1887*

256.40 Polycystic Ovaries Increased levels. *1887*

308.00 Stress *2113*

359.21 Myotonia Atrophica Basal levels elevated in 3 of 7 patients. *1029*

571.90 Cirrhosis of Liver Found in 14% of men with liver disease. Levels unrelated to presence of gynecomastia. *0704*

585.00 Chronic Renal Failure Significantly decreased in patients with impaired renal function, both in patients on drug therapy and in those not taking any drugs affecting plasma prolactin. No relation was found with age, sex, underlying diagnosis, or duration of uremia. *0460* Increased levels *2638*

606.90 Infertility in Males Four patients with oligospermia were found to have slightly to moderately elevated levels. *2562*

650.00 Pregnancy Increase in a linear pattern, related to supramaximal estrogen augmentation and is a reflection of hypertrophy and hyperplasia of pituitary lactotrophs. *1938* Mean plasma concentrations of human placental lactogen were 60% higher in twin pregnancies than in normal simplex pregnancies. *0133* Can trigger a mild to moderate increase (20-300 ng/mL)

Serum Normal

758.70 Klinefelter's Syndrome (XXY) Usually normal. *1090*

CSF Increase

194.30 Malignant Neoplasm of Pituitary 21 of 22 patients with suprasellar extension of a pituitary tumor had elevations of one or more CSF adenohypophyseal hormones. *1189*

Proline

Serum Decrease

333.40 Huntington's Chorea 19 patients showed a significantly lower concentration of proline, alanine, valine, leucine, isoleucine, and tyrosine compared to 38 normal controls. *0534*

Serum Increase

270.81 Hyperprolinemia Higher in type II than in type I. *2246 0995*

Urine Increase

270.03 Cystinosis Nonspecific pattern of aminoaciduria. Fanconi's syndrome. *0995*

270.81 Hyperprolinemia Hyperaminoaciduria of proline, glycine and hydroxyproline is specific. *2246 0995*

275.10 Hepatolenticular Degeneration *0503*

Proline Hydroxylase

Serum Increase

155.00 Malignant Neoplasm of Liver Markedly elevated in hepatoma, and to a lesser extent lymphosarcoma and pheochromocytoma. *0364*

201.90 Hodgkin's Disease Elevated to a lesser degree than that seen in hepatoma. *0364*

202.80 Non-Hodgkins Lymphoma Elevated to a lesser degree than that seen in hepatoma. *0364*

227.91 Pheochromocytoma Elevated to a lesser degree than that seen in hepatoma. *0364*

Properidin

Serum Decrease

990.00 Effects of X-Ray Irradiation Reflects breakdown of tissue proteins. *0618*

Serum Normal

279.04 Agammaglobulinemia (Congenital Sex-linked) Normal. *2539* Other serum constituents involved in resistance to infection are normal *2246*

Prostaglandin E2

Plasma Decrease

255.00 Adrenal Cortical Hyperfunction (Glucocorticoid Excess) In 4 patients with Cushing's Syndrome values were extremely low in renal venous blood. *1331*

255.10 Adrenal Cortical Hyperfunction (Mineralocorticoid Excess) In 8 patients with primary aldosteronism values were extremely low in renal venous blood. *1331*

Prostaglandins

Serum Decrease

401.10 Essential Benign Hypertension Reduced levels of A_2 in patients with essential hypertension as opposed to normal controls. *1367*

Serum Increase

193.01 Medullary Carcinoma of Thyroid May occur. *0995*

250.00 Diabetes Mellitus Prostaglandin E2 and F2-alpha were significantly elevated in children at all times measured. *0378*

259.20 Carcinoid Syndrome During a flush. *2040*

297.90 Paranoid States and Other Psychoses Increased synthesis in schizophrenia. *1076*

300.40 Depressive Neurosis Increased synthesis in schizophrenia and depression. *1076*

770.80 Respiratory Distress Syndrome During the acute phase, plasma concentrations of the primary prostaglandins E and F were significantly elevated. The ratio of prostaglandin E to F was reversed. *0780*

994.50 Exercise Increase of 340% (mean after exercise). *0909*

1013.00 Diet With ingestion of fats. *0909*

Urine Increase

710.00 Systemic Lupus Erythematosus The mean pretreatment excretion of urinary immunoreactive Prostaglandin E, 42.7 ± 6.4 ng/h, was significantly higher than the value of 29.0 ± 1.9 ng/h for normal subjects. *1269*

Synovial Fluid Increase

714.00 Rheumatoid Arthritis Prostaglandin E2 usually predominates. Concentration does not seem to correlate with clinical course of disease. *0252*

Protein

Serum Decrease

9.00 Gastroenteritis and Colitis Enteric loss of plasma protein. *2199*

11.00 Pulmonary Tuberculosis Hypoproteinemia may be present. There is no specific diagnostic value to patterns of protein distribution in tuberculosis. *0962*

13.00 Tuberculosis Meningitis Hypoproteinemia may be present. There is no specific diagnostic value to patterns of protein distribution in tuberculosis. *0962*

18.00 Disseminated Tuberculosis Hypoproteinemia may be present. There is no specific diagnostic value to patterns of protein distribution in tuberculosis. *0962*

40.20 Whipple's Disease Enteric loss of plasma protein. *2199*

80.00 Epidemic Typhus Hypoproteinemia occurs in severe cases. *2368*

82.00 Rocky Mountain Spotted Fever Hypoproteinemia is common in severe cases. *2368*

84.00 Malaria Significantly lower in patients admitted after 5-10 days to hospital compared with the control group. *2066*

124.00 Trichinosis May be marked. *0433* In severe cases between 2-4 weeks and may last for y. *2468*

151.90 Malignant Neoplasm of Stomach Enteric loss of plasma protein. *2199*

152.90 Malignant Neoplasm of Small Intestine Enteric loss of plasma protein. *2199*

153.90 Malignant Neoplasm of Large Intestine May be lower than normal in carcinoma of colon. *2199* Enteric loss of plasma protein. *2199*

154.10 Malignant Neoplasm of Rectum May be lower than normal in carcinoma of colon. *2199*

201.90 Hodgkin's Disease Enteric loss of plasma protein. *2199* Occurs commonly. *2538* In patients with advanced disease, reduction in serum protein concentration with hypoalbuminemia and hypogammaglobulinemia is frequent. *2462*

202.52 Histiocytosis X May occur in the presence of extensive liver involvement. *0433*

Protein *(continued)*

Serum   Decrease *(continued)*

202.80 Non-Hodgkins Lymphoma   Occurs commonly. *2538* Enteric loss of plasma protein. *2199*   In patients with advanced disease, reduction in serum protein concentration with hypoalbuminemia and hypogammaglobulinemia is frequent. *2462*

204.10 Lymphocytic Leukemia (Chronic)   Reduction in serum protein concentration is a feature of advanced disease and one which carries a poor prognosis. *2538*

242.90 Hyperthyroidism   *2540*

250.00 Diabetes Mellitus   With diabetic nephropathy. *0186*

255.00 Adrenal Cortical Hyperfunction (Glucocorticoid Excess) Cortisol accelerates the catabolism of protein and stimulates the hepatic uptake and deamination of amino acids. *0151*

260.00 Protein Malnutrition   Albumin, prealbumin and transferrin concentrations, as well as the level of $alpha_2$ macroglobulin were found to be lower in cases of protein-energy malnutrition associated with infection than the corresponding values for a group of healthy preschool children. *2065   0151*

265.00 Thiamine (B_1) Deficiency   Characteristic. *1108*

273.80 Analbuminemia   Marked decrease. *2467*

275.10 Hepatolenticular Degeneration   Reduced to 6.0 mg/dL or less in 29% of patients (9 of 31). *2278*

277.30 Amyloidosis   Hypoproteinemia occurs in 15% of cases of cardiac amyloidosis. *0151*

279.06 Immunodeficiency (Common Variable)   *2467*

334.00 Friedreich's Ataxia   In Friedreich's patients, the relative proportion of cholesterol and triglycerides was increased while the relative protein content was greatly reduced. *1091*

401.10 Essential Benign Hypertension   *2467*

423.10 Constrictive Pericarditis   Enteric loss of plasma protein. *2199*

428.00 Congestive Heart Failure   *2467*

533.90 Peptic Ulcer, Site Unspecified   *2467*

535.00 Gastritis   An increased sensitivity of atrophic mucosa to exogenous irritants is suggested by the observation that patients with atrophic gastritis lost excessive amounts of plasma protein when they ingested ethanol. *0397*   In Ménétrier's disease hypoproteinemia is often seen *0407*

537.40 Fistula of Stomach and Duodenum   Anemia and hypoproteinemia reflect malnutrition and chronic disease. *2199*

555.90 Regional Enteritis or Ileitis   Often present; due in some part to diminished intake, but mainly result from excessive enteric protein loss. *2199*

556.00 Ulcerative Colitis   Fever, hypovolemia, tachycardia and hypoproteinemia are major manifestations. *0999*   Malnutrition with protein deficiency. *0433   1161*

557.01 Mesenteric Artery Embolism   *0433*

571.90 Cirrhosis of Liver   Total serum protein is usually normal or decreased. *2467*

573.30 Toxic Hepatitis   Enteric loss of plasma protein. *2199*

575.00 Acute Cholecystitis   *2467*

579.00 Celiac Sprue Disease   Defective amino acid absorption might contribute to the observed reduction in serum protein levels. *2199*   Enteric loss of plasma protein. *2199*

579.90 Malabsorption, Cause Unspecified   *0186*

580.00 Acute Poststreptococcal Glomerulonephritis   Occasionally lowered with reversed A/G ratio. *0999*

580.04 Glomerulonephritis (Membranous)   Proteinuria is non-selective, distinguishing it from minimal change glomerulonephritis. *0151*   Usually occurs, with size of proteins indicating degree of glomerular damage. Albumin is nearly always present. *2545* Onset of disease was marked by proteinuria without nephrotic syndrome in 24.2% of patients. *1701*

585.00 Chronic Renal Failure   Total protein is decreased with chronic renal insufficiency. *2468*

642.40 Pre-Eclampsia   Significantly reduced below the levels for normal pregnancy. *0433*

642.60 Eclampsia   Significantly reduced below the levels for normal pregnancy. *0433*

650.00 Pregnancy   Most plasma proteins decrease with the exception of $alpha_1$ globulins. *0433   1113*

694.40 Pemphigus   Total serum protein may fall as low as 3.6 g/dL with a correspondingly low level of albumin. *0151*   May fall to 50% of normal in untreated patients with advanced disease. *0743*

992.00 Heat stroke   Reduced by 15.7% after 2-11 h heat exposure. *2114*

Serum   Increase

1.00 Cholera   *0151*

85.00 Leishmaniasis   Elevated to values > 10 g/dL, almost entirely due to increased IgG. *0151*

99.10 Lymphogranuloma Venereum   Elevated with a reversal of the A/G ratio. In such cases, the increase occurs in the $alpha_2$ and gamma globulin regions. *0433*

135.00 Sarcoidosis   *2467 0433*

162.90 Malignant Neoplasm of Bronchus and Lung   More than 3 g/L. *2467*

203.00 Multiple Myeloma   Very elevated serum total protein is due to increase in globulins (with decreased A/G ratio) in 50-66% of the patients. *2468*   Over 80 g/L in 18 of 35 patients, all of whom had total globulin concentration > 52 g/L. *0518   0512*

227.91 Pheochromocytoma   Hemoconcentration can cause increased hematocrit and plasma proteins. *0962*

250.10 Diabetic Acidosis   Secondary to dehydration. *0999*

255.40 Adrenal Cortical Hypofunction   Dehydration and hemoconcentration due to severe renal sodium loss. *2612*

259.20 Carcinoid Syndrome   Common and may add to the peripheral manifestations of cardiac failure. *1108*

273.30 Waldenström's Macroglobulinemia   Total serum proteins are increased owing to elevation of gamma globulins. *0433*

276.50 Dehydration   Reduced by 15.7% after 2-11 h heat exposure. *2114*

308.00 Stress   Marked; with psychological stress. *2092*

333.40 Huntington's Chorea   In 23 of 27 patients. *0303*

390.00 Rheumatic Fever   Increase in the globulin fraction of the serum proteins is frequent and mainly due to an increase in IgG and IgA. *1108*

434.10 Cerebral Embolism   In septic embolism. *2467*

571.90 Cirrhosis of Liver   Increased serum globulin may cause increased total protein especially in posthepatic cirrhosis. *2467*

642.60 Eclampsia   Secondary to hemoconcentration. *1012*

770.80 Respiratory Distress Syndrome   *0702*

994.50 Exercise   Significant effect with 12 min on cycle-ergometer. *0804*   9% increase immediately after exercise, normal in 30 min. *1837*

Serum   Normal

60.00 Yellow Fever   No significant variations were found in the total protein concentrations. *1750*

710.00 Systemic Lupus Erythematosus   In 39 patients serum total protein and albumin concentrations were stable throughout the course of disease. *2081*

Urine   Increase

2.00 Typhoid Fever   Proteinuria is seen during febrile periods. *0835   0186*

60.00 Yellow Fever   Occurs in severe cases. *2468*   Occurred in 14 of 21 cases including all 6 of the children who died. *1750*

65.00 Arthropod-Borne Hemorrhagic Fever   Heavy proteinuria progressing to acute renal failure occurs during the hypotensive phase of epidemic hemorrhagic fever. *0151*

71.00 Rabies   Slight. *1058*

72.00 Mumps   Indicates mumps nephritis. *0433*

73.90 Psittacosis   Common during the febrile period. *2368*

81.00 Endemic Typhus   During the febrile period. *0433*

85.00 Leishmaniasis   Frequent. *2468*

87.00 Relapsing Fever   Sometimes; during the febrile period. *0962*

100.00 Leptospirosis   In 75% of patients. *2468*   During the leptospiremic phase. *0962*   Heavy proteinuria during the febrile period. *2368*

126.90 Ancylostomiasis (Hookworm Infestation)   *2199*

203.00 Multiple Myeloma   Unexplained, persistent proteinuria may last for years. *2468*   Minimal elevation (0.15-0.5 g/L) in 7, mild-moderate (0.5-3 g/L) in 17 and heavy (> 3 g/L) in 9 of 35 patients. *0518*

206.00 Monocytic Leukemia A unique type of proteinuria develops in about 50% of patients. In addition to ordinary plasma components, the low molecular weight enzyme lysozyme is excreted in amounts up to 0.6-2.4 g/24h. *1746 2538*

244.90 Hypothyroidism May occur to a mild degree. *0565*

250.00 Diabetes Mellitus With diabetic nephropathy; often > 5g/24h. *0186*

250.10 Diabetic Acidosis *2468*

255.10 Adrenal Cortical Hyperfunction (Mineralocorticoid Excess) In the majority of patients. *0999* Negative to trace amounts. *0995*

270.03 Cystinosis Frequent. *2246*

271.10 Galactosemia *2468*

272.52 Abetalipoproteinemia Proteinuria is an early finding and patients ultimately develop renal failure. *0999*

273.23 Heavy Chain Disease (Gamma) Up to 1 gram/day *0186*

273.30 Waldenström's Macroglobulinemia 5 of 16 patients excreted 2.0 g or more of protein/24 h. *1626 2538*

274.00 Gout Low-grade proteinuria occurs in 20-80% of gouty persons for many y before further evidence of renal disease appears. *2468* Incidence varies from 20-40%. May be intermittent and rarely heavy. *2246*

275.10 Hepatolenticular Degeneration Present in 33% of patients; always minimal and decreases with penicillamine therapy. Probably due to tubular reabsorption than increased GFR of protein. *2278*

275.34 Familial Periodic Paralysis Occasional patients. *2246*

277.30 Amyloidosis Proteinuria is usually the first sign of renal amyloid, may persist for years or temporarily disappear. *0151* Found in 90% of primary and 98% of secondary cases. *1334* Frequently massive, with up to 20 g/24h excreted in patients with renal amyloid. *0125*

279.12 Wiskott-Aldrich Syndrome Increased incidence of renal failure. *0793*

287.00 Allergic Purpura Urine may show hematuria and proteinuria. *2538* Proteinuria is manifest and moderate in quantity. *0962*

390.00 Rheumatic Fever Slight febrile albuminuria. Indicates mild focal nephritis. Concomitant glomerulonephritis appears in up to 2.5% of cases. *2467* Proteinuria may occur. *0151*

401.10 Essential Benign Hypertension May occur with accompanying renal functional impairment. *1108*

421.00 Bacterial Endocarditis Mild to moderate proteinuria is common as a result of joint and muscle inflammation. *0151*

428.00 Congestive Heart Failure Mild to moderate proteinuria varying from 0.5-4 g/24h is not unusual; may be greater in severe failure with a marked decrease in GFR and renal blood flow. *1108 0151*

446.00 Polyarteritis-Nodosa Found in patients with glomerular disease. *0999* With renal involvement. *0962*

446.60 Thrombotic Thrombocytopenic Purpura With kidney involvement. *0962* Proteinuria or hematuria in 90% of patients. *2538*

482.90 Bacterial Pneumonia Protein, WBC, hyaline and granular casts in small amounts are common. *2467*

570.00 Acute and Subacute Necrosis of Liver In a few patients minimal proteinuria. *0992*

580.00 Acute Poststreptococcal Glomerulonephritis Usually occurs, with size of proteins indicating degree of glomerular damage. Albumin is nearly always present. *2545* May reach over 6-8 g/24h, but is more often below 2 g/24h. *2468 0999*

580.01 Glomerulonephritis (Focal) May persist for years, even after other manifestations cease. *0962*

580.02 Glomerulonephritis (Minimal Change) Characterized by heavy proteinuria consisting almost entirely of low molecular weight plasma proteins, especially albumin and transferrin. Values are > 5 g/24h. *0151* Marked proteinuria - usually > 4.5 g/24h; usually exclusively albuminuria in children with lipoid nephrosis, but in glomerulonephritis high- and low-molecular weight proteins are present with nephrotic syndrome. *2468*

580.04 Glomerulonephritis (Membranous) Proteinuria is nonselective, distinguishing it from minimal change glomerulonephritis. *0151* Usually occurs, with size of proteins indicating degree of glomerular damage. Albumin is nearly always present. *2545* Onset of disease was marked by proteinuria without nephrotic syndrome in 24.2% of patients. *1701*

580.05 Glomerulonephritis (Membranoproliferative) *0331*

580.40 Glomerulonephritis (Rapidly Progressive) Usually occurs; with size of proteins indicating degree of glomerular damage. Albumin is nearly always present. *2545* Exceeds 2.5 g/24h in 8 of 29 cases. *1633* Proteinuria is always present. *0962*

581.90 Nephrotic Syndrome Heavy proteinuria must be present for this diagnosis. *0999* High concentrations were observed in 19 patients, including adults and children. *2441*

584.00 Acute Renal Failure In the early stage. *2468*

585.00 Chronic Renal Failure With renal parenchymal disease. *0838*

590.00 Chronic Pyelonephritis With renal parenchymal disease. *0838* Slight, usually < 3 g/24h. *0151*

590.10 Acute Pyelonephritis Usually < 2 g/24h. *0503* Proteinuria is usually mild, rarely exceeding 1.5-2.0 g/24h. *0962* With renal parenchymal disease *0838*

593.81 Renal Infarction Common. *0186*

599.00 Urinary Tract Infection Proteinuria to the extent of +2 (usually < 2 g/24h) occurs. *0962*

600.00 Benign Prostatic Hypertrophy Normal or increased. *0186*

642.40 Pre-Eclampsia Hypertension, edema, and proteinuria characterize toxemia of pregnancy. *0151* This diagnosis is questionable without the presence of proteinuria. Renal leakage of small molecular weight proteins is characteristic. *0387*

642.60 Eclampsia Hypertension, edema, and proteinuria characterize toxemia of pregnancy. *0151* As a result of hemoconcentration. *0621* Constant finding. *0387*

650.00 Pregnancy The presence of proteinuria and pregnancy in the absence of blood pressure elevation increases perinatal mortality to at least twice the rates of patients without proteinuria. *0516*

710.00 Systemic Lupus Erythematosus Levels of hematuria and proteinuria correlate well with severity of morphologic lesions. *1047* Generally precedes hematuria and red cell casts, although small degrees of renal involvement may occur without proteinuria. *0782* Changes in the amount of proteinuria do not reflect histologic changes in the kidneys. *0962*

710.10 Progressive Systemic Sclerosis In urinalysis proteinuria may be the only manifestation. *0962* May be present for extended periods without clinical evidence of progressive renal dysfunction. *0962* Renal involvement. *1700*

753.10 Polycystic Kidney Disease Usually minimal or mild. *0962*

984.00 Toxic Effects of Lead and Its Compounds (including Fumes) Renal damage may occur. *0889*

985.00 Toxic Effects of Non-medicinal Metals With renal damage in arsenic poisoning. *0811* Nephrotoxicity may occur in mercury poisoning. *1514 0651 0889*

986.00 Toxic Effects of Carbon Monoxide Occurs in severe cases. *0151* Nephrotoxicity. *2084*

989.50 Toxic Effects of Venom May cause nephrotoxicity. *2084 0995*

990.00 Effects of X-Ray Irradiation May cause renal damage. *0618*

992.00 Heat stroke *0995*

994.50 Exercise More common with heavy exercise than mild. *1205*

994.80 Effects of Electric Current May cause renal damage. *2084*

Urine   Normal

600.00 Benign Prostatic Hypertrophy Normal or increased. *0186*

CSF   Decrease

331.81 Reye's Syndrome *0416* Low levels of glucose and protein found in the CSF

CSF   Increase

11.00 Pulmonary Tuberculosis *0619*

13.00 Tuberculosis Meningitis Slightly increased in early stages but continues to increase, reaching levels > 300 mg/dL in advanced disease, and much higher levels when block of CSF occurs. *0999 0962 2612*

18.00 Disseminated Tuberculosis *0999*

32.00 Diphtheria With neuritis. *1058* Prolonged elevation following paralysis. *0433*

36.00 Meningococcal Meningitis Values of 80-500 mg/dL. *1058 2400*

Protein (continued)

CSF   Increase (continued)

45.90   Acute Poliomyelitis   Initial values usually fall within range of 25-150 mg/dL. Characteristically modest elevations are found during the first week after onset of CNS symptoms. Levels tend to decrease toward the 10th day, but may increase again in a secondary stage (100-400 mg/dL) in the 3rd and 4th weeks. *0433* Often progressive increase. *0962*   May be high. *2368*

47.00   Aseptic Meningitis   Often increased to 45-200 mg/dL. *0999*   Moderately elevated in acute hemorrhagic encephalitis. *0151*

49.00   Lymphocytic Choriomeningitis   Total concentration may be high. *2368*

52.00   Chickenpox   Normal or slightly increased. *1058*

53.00   Herpes Zoster   CSF commonly shows a pleocytosis and elevation of protein, even when clinical signs of meningeal irritation or encephalomyelitis are absent. *0151*   20-110 mg/dL. *0962*

54.00   Herpes Simplex   Frequently elevated. *0151*

62.10   Western Equine Encephalitis   *0151*

62.20   Eastern Equine Encephalitis   *0151*

71.00   Rabies   A slight increase. *2468*

72.00   Mumps   Normal or slightly elevated. *0433*

78.50   Cytomegalic Inclusion Disease   In congenital disease. *1319*

80.00   Epidemic Typhus   With severe encephalitic manifestations. *0433*

87.00   Relapsing Fever   Sometimes increased in CSF. *2468*

97.90   Syphilis   Usually increased to some degree with CNS involvement. *0962*   Over 45 mg/dL in syphilitic meningitis. *2368* Increased with obstruction of the spinal canal, especially in neurosyphilis and tuberculous meningitis. *2321*   *2612*

99.10   Lymphogranuloma Venereum   High in the early stages of CSF infection, varying from 250-3,750 mg/dL. *0433*

100.00   Leptospirosis   Increased in about 66% of patients, up to 80 mg/dL, indicating meningeal involvement. *2468*   Occasionally observed. *2368*   *0962*

112.90   Moniliasis   Mean = 123 mg/dL in 28 cases of Candida meningitis. *0138*

114.90   Coccidioidomycosis   CSF cell and chemistry are indistinguishable from tuberculous meningitis. *2368*   Moderate increase with CNS involvement. *1058*

117.50   Cryptococcosis   Almost always elevated. *1058*

130.00   Toxoplasmosis   In congenital, as high as 2,000 mg/dL. *1319*

135.00   Sarcoidosis   In granulomatous basilar meningitis affecting cranial nerves. *0992*

191.90   Malignant Neoplasm of Brain   Consistently found with intracranial tumors. Normal value does not exclude the presence of a tumor. *0433*   *1099*

198.30   Secondary Malignant Neoplasm of Brain   Increased protein (meningeal infiltration of leukemic cells). *2467*

203.00   Multiple Myeloma   Usually normal or slightly elevated to values of 50-100 mg/dL. *0151*

204.00   Lymphocytic Leukemia (Acute)   With meningeal infiltration. *2538*

205.00   Myelocytic Leukemia (Acute)   With meningeal infiltration. *2538*

225.90   Benign Neoplasm of Brain and CNS   Protein content > 100 mg/dL is associated with rapidly growing tumors near the ventricles or subarachnoid space. Slowly growing tumors may have only slightly elevated or normal values. *0151*   Total CSF protein is increased. Individual increase of proteins depended on the degree of blood/CSF barrier damage. *1099*   In acoustic neuromas nearly always high (100-500 mg). Cerebellar tumors usually have normal or only moderately increased protein (20-100). *0962*

244.90   Hypothyroidism   Perhaps due to increased capillary permeability. *2540*

250.00   Diabetes Mellitus   Approximately 70% of patients with neuropathy have unusual spinal fluid protein (50-100 mg/dL). *2540*

253.00   Acromegaly   Occasionally seen; reflects the intracranial lesion. *0962*

265.00   Thiamine (B$_1$) Deficiency   *0619*

277.30   Amyloidosis   Usually elevated. *2246*

320.90   Meningitis (Bacterial)   Nearly always elevated above 50 mg/dL. *2400*   Ranges between 50-500 mg/dL, with an average of 200-300. *0962*   Increased with obstruction of the spinal canal, especially in neurosyphilis and tuberculous meningitis. *2321* *0999 0151*

323.91   Myelitis   Increased to 45-200 mg/dL in encephalitis and myelitis. *0999*

323.92   Encephalomyelitis   The protein concentration is elevated but rarely exceeds 150 mg/dL. A slight elevation is common. *0433* Total protein and IgG concentration were increased. *2321*   *2612*

324.00   Intracranial Abscess   Usually elevated, varying between 60-200 mg/dL. *0433*   Raised, particularly if the abscess is near to the surface. 75-300 mg/dL. *0995*   *0962 2368*

324.10   Intraspinal Abscess   Increased (usually 100-400 mg/dL), and WBCs (lymphocytes and neutrophils) are relatively few in number. *2467*

330.00   Metachromatic Leukodystrophy   Common. *0433*

336.00   Syringomyelia and Syringobulbia   In a minority of cases the lumbar CSF protein content is elevated in the range of 40-100 mg/dL. *0433*

340.00   Multiple Sclerosis   A slight increase in mononuclear cells and normal or slightly increased protein (50% of cases). Diagnosis is probable if more than 20% is gamma globulin. *2467*   In all forms of MS approximately 70% of patients have abnormalities of CSF proteins. *0999*   Increased total protein and IgG concentration. *2321*   *2612*

356.30   Refsum's Disease   High CSF protein concentration in the absence of pleocytosis has been found in all cases. *2246*   Elevated in 20 patients, ranging from 55-732 mg/dL. Mean = 275, mode = 165. *0878*

357.00   Guillain-Barré Syndrome   CSF shows albuminocytologic dissociation with normal cell count and increased protein (average, 50-100 mg/dL). Protein increase parallels increasing clinical severity; may be prolonged. *2467*   Increased total protein (1.21 ± 0.274 g/L). *1099*   May reach as high as 2 g/100 mL. *0878*   Usually elevated between 65 and 1000 mg/dL but may not peak until 4 to 6 weeks after onset of neurological sign. Elevation may persist for several months. Primarily Albumin *1307*

357.90   Polyneuritis   From day 3-7 of the illness, over 50% of the patients will have high concentrations, frequently > 100 mg/dL. From the 2-7th week, almost all patients will have high CSF protein values. *0433*   *2612*

363.20   Inflammation of Optic Nerve and Retina   CSF is normal or may show increased protein and up to 200 lymphocytes/µL. *2467*

421.00   Bacterial Endocarditis   Slightly elevated in infection with embolism. *0151*

431.00   Cerebral Hemorrhage   Usually elevated to around 100 mg/dL with maximum levels 8-10 days after bleeding. *0151*

434.00   Cerebral Thrombosis   The total amount may be normal, but frequently it is raised to 50-80 mg/dL. Rarely it is over 100, in which case some other diagnosis should be considered. *0992*

434.10   Cerebral Embolism   Elevated in septic emboli. *0992*

434.90   Brain Infarction   Slight elevations of 60-75 mg/dL are found in 20% of patients. *0151*

446.50   Cranial Arteritis and Related Conditions   May occur due to intracerebral artery involvement. *2468*

510.00   Empyema   In subdural empyema. (75-300 mg/dL) *0186*

710.00   Systemic Lupus Erythematosus   In patients with neurologic symptoms. *1700*

720.00   Rheumatoid (Ankylosing) Spondylitis   Observed in 33% of patients, most often those with severe back pain. *0666*

984.00   Toxic Effects of Lead and Its Compounds (including Fumes)   Increased, with normal cell count in encephalopathy. *2468*   *0850*

CSF   Normal

130.00   Toxoplasmosis   In acquired, usually normal. *1319*

324.00   Intracranial Abscess   Normal or increased. *0995*

336.00   Syringomyelia and Syringobulbia   In a minority of cases the lumbar CSF protein content is elevated in the range of 40-100 mg/dL. *0433*

434.00   Cerebral Thrombosis   The total amount may be normal, but frequently it is raised to 50-80 mg/dL. Rarely it is over 100, in which case some other diagnosis should be considered. *0992*

Synovial Fluid   Decrease

710.00   Systemic Lupus Erythematosus   Synovial fluid may be a transudate with low protein content (< 3 g/dL), especially in patients with asymptomatic joint effusions associated with nephritis and edema. In other patients with inflammatory joint signs, the fluid is an exudate with increased protein content (3-5 g/dL). *0433*

711.00   Acute Arthritis (Pyogenic)   30-40% of the plasma concentration. *1958*

Synovial Fluid   Increase

99.30   Reiter's Disease   *0186*

274.00   Gout   The synovial fluid is typical of inflammatory reactions showing an increase in protein content. *0999*

282.60   Sickle Cell Anemia   Elevated in 6 of 13 patients. *0676*

710.00   Systemic Lupus Erythematosus   Synovial fluid may be a transudate with low protein content (< 3 g/dL), especially in patients with asymptomatic joint effusions associated with nephritis and edema. In other patients with inflammatory joint signs, the fluid is an exudate with increased protein content (3-5 g/dL). *0433*

714.00   Rheumatoid Arthritis   Characteristically turbid with increased protein content. *0999*

Pleural Effusion   Decrease

423.10   Constrictive Pericarditis   Transudate secondary to increased hydrostatic pressure. (< 3 g/dL). *0062*

428.00   Congestive Heart Failure   Consistent with a transudate. *0186*

514.00   Pulmonary Congestion and Hypostasis   Transudate (< 3 g/dL). *0503*

571.90   Cirrhosis of Liver   May cause pleural effusion by several mechanisms; most important of these is transfer of fluid from the peritoneal cavity via either direct diaphragmatic defect or lymphatics. *0216*   Transudate (< 3 g/dL). *2017*

580.00   Acute Poststreptococcal Glomerulonephritis   Pleural effusions are usually transudates (< 3 g/dL). *0062*

580.01   Glomerulonephritis (Focal)   Pleural effusions are usually transudates (< 3 g/dL). *0062*

580.02   Glomerulonephritis (Minimal Change)   Pleural effusions are usually transudates (< 3 g/dL). *0062*

580.04   Glomerulonephritis (Membranous)   Pleural effusions are usually transudates (< 3 g/dL). *0062*

580.05   Glomerulonephritis (Membranoproliferative)   Pleural effusions are usually transudates (< 3 g/dL). *0062*

581.90   Nephrotic Syndrome   Transudate secondary to decreased albumin. (< 3 g/dL). *0062*

585.00   Chronic Renal Failure   Transudate secondary to decreased albumin. (< 3 g/dL). *0062*

Pleural Effusion   Increase

6.00   Amebiasis   Parasitic disease most often associated with an effusion. Exudate *0062*

11.00   Pulmonary Tuberculosis   Concentrations > 6.0 g/dL indicate tuberculosis. *1403*   Characterized by a protein content of 3 g/dL and the presence of lymphocytes. *0962*

162.90   Malignant Neoplasm of Bronchus and Lung   Exudate. *2017*

197.00   Secondary Malignant Neoplasm of Respiratory System   Exudate. *2017*

201.90   Hodgkin's Disease   Pleural effusions are usually exudates. *0062*

202.80   Non-Hodgkins Lymphoma   Pleural effusions are usually exudates. *0062*

203.00   Multiple Myeloma   With pleural involvement increased total protein with a sharp spike in the gamma globulin region. *2021*

204.00   Lymphocytic Leukemia (Acute)   Pleural effusions are usually exudates. *0062*

204.10   Lymphocytic Leukemia (Chronic)   Pleural effusions are usually exudates. *0062*

205.00   Myelocytic Leukemia (Acute)   Pleural effusions are usually exudates. *0062*

205.10   Myelocytic Leukemia (Chronic)   Pleural effusions are usually exudates. *0062*

206.00   Monocytic Leukemia   Pleural effusions are usually exudates. *0062*

244.90   Hypothyroidism   Exudate (> 3 g/dL). *0062*

415.10   Pulmonary Embolism and Infarction   Exudative effusion in about 50% of cases. *0503*

480.90   Viral Pneumonia   Exudate (> 3 g/dL). *0062*

482.90   Bacterial Pneumonia   High total protein concentrations. *0368   1405*

483.01   Mycoplasma Pneumoniae   Rare effusion which is usually small and an exudate (> 3g/dL). *0062*

510.00   Empyema   Exudate. *2017*

577.00   Acute Pancreatitis   Exudate (> 3 g/dL). *0062*

577.10   Chronic Pancreatitis   Exudate (> 3 g/dL). *0062*

577.20   Pancreatic Cyst and Pseudocyst   Exudate. *2017*

714.00   Rheumatoid Arthritis   Tends to produce high total protein concentration. *0368*

Ascitic Fluid   Decrease

571.20   Laennec's or Alcoholic Cirrhosis   Ascitic fluid is usually a transudate with protein < 3.0 g/dL and specific gravity < 1.016. However, protein may exceed 2.5 g/dL in up to 30% of patients. *2199*

571.90   Cirrhosis of Liver   Ascitic fluid is usually a transudate with protein < 3.0 g/dL and specific gravity < 1.016. However, protein may exceed 2.5 g/dL in up to 30% of patients. *2199*   < 2.5 g/dL in ascitic fluid *2626*

581.90   Nephrotic Syndrome   < 2.5 g/dL in ascitic fluid. *2626*

Ascitic Fluid   Increase

18.00   Disseminated Tuberculosis   Often > 2.5 g/dL in ascitic fluid. *2626*

151.90   Malignant Neoplasm of Stomach   > 2.5 g/dL. *2626*

152.90   Malignant Neoplasm of Small Intestine   > 2.5 g/dL. *2626*

153.90   Malignant Neoplasm of Large Intestine   > 2.5 g/dL. *2626*

155.00   Malignant Neoplasm of Liver   > 2.5 g/dL. *2626*

157.90   Malignant Neoplasm of Pancreas   Variable but often > 2.5 g/dL in ascitic fluid. *2626*

197.70   Secondary Malignant Neoplasm of Liver   > 2.5 g/dL in ascitic fluid. *2626*

567.90   Peritonitis   Often > 2.5 g/dL in ascitic fluid. *2626*

577.00   Acute Pancreatitis   Variable but often > 2.5 g/dL in ascitic fluid. *2626*   Total protein varied from 1.2-6.6 g/dL *0827*

577.10   Chronic Pancreatitis   Variable but often > 2.5 g/dL in ascitic fluid. *2626*

Ascitic Fluid   Normal

428.00   Congestive Heart Failure   Variable amounts between 1.5-5.0 g/dL. *2626*

Pericardial Fluid   Decrease

420.00   Acute Pericarditis   Less than 50% of serum levels. *0758*

Pericardial Fluid   Increase

714.00   Rheumatoid Arthritis   With rheumatoid pericarditis a high total protein is common. *0764*

Duodenal Contents   Increase

277.00   Cystic Fibrosis   In excess of that found in the duodenal fluid of controls. *0392*

Feces   Increase

157.90   Malignant Neoplasm of Pancreas   Reduced intraluminal pancreatic enzyme activity with maldigestion of lipid and protein. *0962*

251.50   Zollinger-Ellison Syndrome   Hyperacidity in duodenum inactivates pancreatic enzymes. *0962*

277.00   Cystic Fibrosis   Reduced intraluminal pancreatic enzyme activity with maldigestion of lipid and protein. *0962*

535.00   Gastritis   An increased sensitivity of atrophic mucosa to exogenous irritants is suggested by the observation that patients with atrophic gastritis lost excessive amounts of plasma protein when they ingested ethanol. *0397*

577.10   Chronic Pancreatitis   Reduced intraluminal pancreatic enzyme activity with maldigestion of lipid and protein. *0962*

Protein (continued)

Peritoneal Fluid   Increase

11.00 Pulmonary Tuberculosis   Usually, but not always, over 3 g/dL. *0962*

157.90 Malignant Neoplasm of Pancreas   Greater than 30 g/L in 70% of cases of pancreatic ascites. *0586*

567.90 Peritonitis   Exceeds 2.5 g/dL in 85-100% of patients with tuberculous peritonitis. Exudate with protein concentration > 3.0 g/dL usually found with tuberculous and bacterial peritonitis. *2199*

577.00 Acute Pancreatitis   Greater than 30 g/L in 70% of cases of pancreatic ascites. *0586*

577.10 Chronic Pancreatitis   Greater than 30 g/L in 70% of cases of pancreatic ascites. *0586*

Prostatic Fluid   Decrease

601.00 Prostatitis   Average amount of protein and protein-like substance was low 28.0 g/L, range 15.0-37.7, compared to normal 42.6, range 37.5-64. *0084*

Saliva   Increase

277.00 Cystic Fibrosis   Submaxillary saliva is more turbid, with increased calcium, total protein, and amylase. These changes are not generally found in parotid saliva. *2467*

Protein Bound Iodine (PBI)

Serum   Decrease

240.00 Simple Goiter   Normal or slightly low. *0962*

242.90 Hyperthyroidism   Reduced in 24 of 33 patients. *2435*

244.90 Hypothyroidism   Ranges from 0 to 3 mg/dL. After treatment returns to normal in about 3 weeks. *0619*

245.10 Subacute Thyroiditis   May be subnormal later in the disease. *2540*   Characteristically low. *0151*

245.20 Hashimoto's Thyroiditis   May be decreased and may vary over a period of time (because of thyroid destruction and regeneration). *2468*   May be low owing to butanol-insoluble iodinated albumin in plasma. *0151*   Later in the disease. *2540*

253.00 Acromegaly   *0619*

253.40 Anterior Pituitary Hypofunction   *0151*

255.00 Adrenal Cortical Hyperfunction (Glucocorticoid Excess) *2540*

260.00 Protein Malnutrition   Occasionally. *2104*

269.90 Deficiency State (Unspecified)   Decreased in malnutrition. *0619*

570.00 Acute and Subacute Necrosis of Liver   In severe liver disease. *2104*

571.90 Cirrhosis of Liver   In severe liver disease. *2104*

572.00 Liver Abscess (Pyogenic)   In severe liver disease. *2104*

581.90 Nephrotic Syndrome   Urinary loss of TBG results in lowering of most blood thyroid hormones and increased T_3 uptake. *0962* *2104*

991.60 Hypothermia   Occasionally decreased. *2467*   In accidental hypothermia. *0619*

Serum   Increase

70.00 Viral Hepatitis   Not infrequently. May be due to biliary reflux of conjugated T_4. *2540* *2104*

174.90 Malignant Neoplasm of Breast   Occasionally increased. *2467*

181.00 Malignant Neoplasm of Trophoblast (Choriocarcinoma)   Occasionally increased in metastatic choriocarcinoma. *2467*

186.90 Malignant Neoplasm of Testis   Occasionally increased in embryonal testicular carcinoma. *2467*

220.01 Teratoma (Dermoid)   Occasionally increased in certain tumors. *2467*

242.90 Hyperthyroidism   In thyrotoxicosis, levels may range from 7-20 mg/dL. With treatment, the level falls to normal more rapidly than does the BMR. *0619*   Elevated in 60 of 76 patients over the age of 60 y. *0512*   May be present. *0962*

245.10 Subacute Thyroiditis   Early in the disease. *0992*   Usually elevated even higher than T_4. *1106*   Often disproportionately higher than the T_4 iodine concentration, indicating the presence of abnormal iodinated material. *2540* *0999 0151 2104*

245.20 Hashimoto's Thyroiditis   Slightly elevated early in the disease. *2540*   May be increased and may vary over a period of time (because of thyroid destruction and regeneration). *2468*

277.14 Acute Intermittent Porphyria   Occasionally. *2254*

570.00 Acute and Subacute Necrosis of Liver   *0619*

630.00 Hydatidiform Mole   Occasionally increased. *2467*

650.00 Pregnancy   From about the 4th week until up to 6th week postpartum. *2467*   Most plasma proteins decrease with the exception of alpha₁ globulins which account for elevation of protein-bound iodine and blood cortisol. *0433*   In normal pregnancy the level may rise to 15 mg/dL. The level falls in threatened abortion. *0619* *2104*

Serum   Normal

220.01 Teratoma (Dermoid)   Occasionally increased in certain tumors. *2467*

227.91 Pheochromocytoma   No characteristic changes. *1108*

238.40 Polycythemia Vera   *2467*

240.00 Simple Goiter   Normal or slightly low. *0962*   Usually. *2540*

245.20 Hashimoto's Thyroiditis   May be normal and may vary over a period of time because of thyroid destruction and regeneration. *2468*   PBI may be disproportionately higher than the BEI because of circulating nonfunctioning iodinated proteins. *0962*

250.00 Diabetes Mellitus   *2467*

253.00 Acromegaly   *2467*

255.40 Adrenal Cortical Hypofunction   *2467*

994.50 Exercise   No effect observed. *0511*

Urine   Increase

277.14 Acute Intermittent Porphyria   Occasionally increased. *2467* *0151*

Protein Casts

Urine   Increase

84.00 Malaria   May be demonstrable in severe falciparum infection. *0433*

Prothrombin Consumption

Blood   Decrease

273.30 Waldenström's Macroglobulinemia   Evidence of impaired platelet function. *2538*

286.40 Von Willebrand's Disease   May be present and is related to the decreased factor VIII AHF activity. *2538*

287.30 Idiopathic Thrombocytopenic Purpura   Defect phase I or II blood coagulation. *2467* *2552*

Blood   Increase

38.00 Septicemia   May be associated with defibrination resulting in platelet and coagulation factor consumption in severe gram-positive septicemia. *2538*

54.00 Herpes Simplex   May be associated with defibrination resulting in platelet and coagulation factor consumption. *2538*

65.00 Arthropod-Borne Hemorrhagic Fever   May be associated with defibrination resulting in platelet and coagulation factor consumption (Korean and Thai fever). *2538*

82.00 Rocky Mountain Spotted Fever   May be associated with defibrination resulting in platelet and coagulation factor consumption. *2538*

84.00 Malaria   May be associated with defibrination resulting in platelet and coagulation factor consumption (in overwhelming parasitemia). *2538*

197.00 Secondary Malignant Neoplasm of Respiratory System   May be associated with defibrination resulting in platelet and coagulation factor consumption. *2538*

199.00 Secondary Malignant Neoplasm (Disseminated)   May be associated with defibrination resulting in platelet and coagulation factor consumption. *2538*

286.10 Christmas Disease   In severe cases. *2467*

286.20 Factor XI Deficiency   *2468*

286.32 Factor XII Deficiency   *2468*

286.35 **Factor V Deficiency** Increase in prothrombin consumption is not corrected by administration of vitamin K, with factor V deficiency. *2468*

286.36 **Factor X Deficiency** Abnormal results. *2246*

287.10 **Thrombasthenia (Glanzmann's)** *2552*

487.10 **Influenza** May be associated with defibrination resulting in platelet and coagulation factor consumption. *2538*

630.00 **Hydatidiform Mole** May be associated with defibrination resulting in platelet and coagulation factor consumption. *2538*

Blood Normal

287.10 **Thrombasthenia (Glanzmann's)** *2246*

Prothrombin Time

Plasma Decrease

256.00 **Ovarian Hyperfunction** *0995*

555.90 **Regional Enteritis or Ileitis** *0995*

Plasma Increase

38.00 **Septicemia** May be associated with defibrination resulting in platelet and coagulation factor consumption in severe gram-positive septicemia. *2538*

40.20 **Whipple's Disease** *0999*

54.00 **Herpes Simplex** May be associated with defibrination resulting in platelet and coagulation factor consumption. *2538*

70.00 **Viral Hepatitis** May be slightly prolonged but bleeding problems are uncommon. A greatly prolonged prothrombin time heralds massive hepatic necrosis and is a sign of poor prognosis. *0433* Usually normal, and if prolonged, suggests severe hepatitis. If the prolongation increases, it is indicative of fulminant hepatitis. *0962*

84.00 **Malaria** Consistent with the diagnosis of disseminated intravascular coagulation. *1058*

85.00 **Leishmaniasis** Normal early in the disease but later becomes prolonged. *0151*

100.00 **Leptospirosis** In some patients. *0992* May occur with jaundice. *2368*

155.00 **Malignant Neoplasm of Liver** Prolonged in 26.6% of patients. *1115* Abnormal in 21 of 24 hepatoma patients with cirrhosis and 11 of 16 without cirrhosis in tests done within 1 month of death. *1783*

157.90 **Malignant Neoplasm of Pancreas** May be increased but will be correctable with parenterally administered vitamin K. *0433*

189.00 **Malignant Neoplasm of Kidney** Increased in the absence of hepatic metastases. *0186*

197.70 **Secondary Malignant Neoplasm of Liver** Prolonged in liver disease. *0962*

205.00 **Myelocytic Leukemia (Acute)** Intravascular clotting has been documented in occasional patients. *0890*

205.10 **Myelocytic Leukemia (Chronic)** Intravascular clotting has been documented for rare patients. *0890*

206.00 **Monocytic Leukemia** With disseminated intravascular clotting. *1552*

251.50 **Zollinger-Ellison Syndrome** An indication of vitamin K malabsorption. *0962*

271.30 **Lactosuria** An indication of vitamin K malabsorption. *0962*

272.52 **Abetalipoproteinemia** Frequently prolonged, secondary to vitamin K malabsorption. *0566* Abnormal bleeding is rare. *0095*

275.10 **Hepatolenticular Degeneration** Mean time = 17.3 sec., abnormally prolonged in 79% (26 of 33) patients. *2278*

277.00 **Cystic Fibrosis** Secondary to vitamin K deficiency. *0551*

279.31 **Acquired Immunodeficiency Syndrome (AIDS)** Three of seven patients studied. *0423*

286.31 **Congenital Dysfibrinogenemia** Usually prolonged, but in some cases no clot forms at all. *2538* In many cases. *2246*

286.34 **Congenital Afibrinogenemia** Corrected by the addition of normal plasma or normal fibrinogen to the patient's plasma. *2538* Infinite. *2246*

286.35 **Factor V Deficiency** Deficient factor V (labile). *0433* Not corrected by administration of vitamin K. *2468* Prothrombin time and partial thromboplastin time, activated or unactivated, are all prolonged. *2538* *2246*

286.36 **Factor X Deficiency** Not corrected by administration of vitamin K. Prolonged. *2538* *2246*

286.37 **Factor VII Deficiency** Usually greatly prolonged. *0035* *2538* *2246*

286.38 **Factor II Deficiency** *0433* *2246*

286.60 **Disseminated Intravascular Coagulopathy** Prolonged because of consumption of clotting factors and the anticoagulant effects of fibrin degradation products. *2538* *0433*

289.80 **Myelofibrosis** Prolonged in 75% of patients with agnogenic myeloid metaplasia. *2468*

331.81 **Reye's Syndrome** May be prolonged. *0416* Reflects Hepatic damage *0151*

428.00 **Congestive Heart Failure** Frequently elevated. *0433* May be slightly increased, with increased sensitivity to anticoagulant drugs. *2467*

556.00 **Ulcerative Colitis** Hypoprothrombinemia (prolonged time) is a commonly found defect in moderate or severe disease. *2199*

557.01 **Mesenteric Artery Embolism** *0433*

570.00 **Acute and Subacute Necrosis of Liver** Due to poor fat absorption. *2467* Increased time indicates degree of parenchymal damage; marked prolongation (> 20 sec) is an early reflection of massive necrosis. *0151* *0433*

571.20 **Laennec's or Alcoholic Cirrhosis** Severe clotting factor deficiencies are common. *0992*

571.49 **Chronic Active Hepatitis** Often prolonged. *0992* Patients with marked prolongation, despite vitamin K replacement and a positive LE cell test, have the worst prognosis. *0962*

571.60 **Biliary Cirrhosis** Laboratory findings of steatorrhea but prothrombin time is normal or restored to normal by parenteral vitamin K. *2467*

571.90 **Cirrhosis of Liver** Hypoprothrombinemia unresponsive to parenteral vitamin K is indicative of severe hepatocellular dysfunction. *0433* *0962*

572.00 **Liver Abscess (Pyogenic)** Increased in cases of severe liver damage due to poisons, hepatitis, cirrhosis. *2467* *0433*

572.20 **Hepatic Encephalopathy** Prolonged in liver disease. *0962*

572.40 **Hepatic Failure** *0503*

573.30 **Toxic Hepatitis** Increased in cases of severe liver damage due to poisons. *2467*

576.20 **Extrahepatic Biliary Obstruction** Prolonged, with response to parenteral vitamin K more frequent than in hepatic parenchymal cell disease. *2467*

579.00 **Celiac Sprue Disease** An indication of vitamin K malabsorption. *0962* May be prolonged in celiac sprue owing to malabsorption of vitamin K. *2199*

579.90 **Malabsorption, Cause Unspecified** An indication of vitamin K malabsorption. *0962*

642.60 **Eclampsia** Higher than normal in pregnant patients. *1012*

710.00 **Systemic Lupus Erythematosus** A prolonged time may suggest the possibility of a circulating anticoagulant, which is particularly likely to be found in patients with a chronic false positive serologic test for syphilis. *0433*

773.00 **Hemolytic Disease of Newborn (Erythroblastosis Fetalis)** *2061*

774.40 **Jaundice Due to Hepatocellular Damage (Newborn)** Markedly prolonged. *0433*

989.50 **Toxic Effects of Venom** May be greatly prolonged in severe cases of snake bite. *0151*

990.00 **Effects of X-Ray Irradiation** *0889*

992.00 **Heat stroke** May occur with prolonged hot weather. *1095*

994.50 **Exercise** Observed effect in exercise. *1839*

1013.00 **Diet** Prolonged due to inadequate vitamin K in diet. *2467*

Plasma Normal

238.40 **Polycythemia Vera** *2491*

272.51 **Tangier Disease** Occasionally prolonged PTT, with normal prothrombin time. *2246*

286.01 **Hemophilia** Bleeding time and prothrombin time are not significantly prolonged. *2538* *2246*

286.10 **Christmas Disease** All patients have a normal test using human brain tissue factor (thromboplastin), but when ox-brain tissue factor is used, the prothrombin time is prolonged in approximately 6% of cases. *2538* *2538* *2246*

286.20 **Factor XI Deficiency** PTT or activated PTT test is prolonged and the prothrombin time normal. *2538* *2246*

Prothrombin Time (continued)

Plasma Normal (continued)

286.32 **Factor XII Deficiency** Prothrombin and bleeding times are normal. *2538 2246*

286.33 **Factor XIII Deficiency** *2246*

286.40 **Von Willebrand's Disease** *0962 2246*

287.10 **Thrombasthenia (Glanzmann's)** *2246*

287.30 **Idiopathic Thrombocytopenic Purpura** *0433 2552 2246*

446.60 **Thrombotic Thrombocytopenic Purpura** *2246 0054*

Protoporphyrin

Serum Increase

277.12 **Erythropoietic Protoporphyria** Frequently elevated. *1478* Most striking finding is the elevation in RBC, feces, and plasma. *2246*

Urine Increase

277.12 **Erythropoietic Protoporphyria** *1752*

Feces Increase

277.11 **Congenital Erythropoietic Porphyria (Günther's Disease)** Variable although not significantly elevated. *2246*

277.12 **Erythropoietic Protoporphyria** Usually but not always increased in symptomatic patients, from 30-300 μg/g dry weight and occasionally higher. *1458* Contains only increased protoporphyrin, a unique finding among porphyrias. *2538* In some carriers, elevated even with normal RBC porphyrins. Fluctuates markedly from one time period to another in the same patient. *0579 2552 2246*

277.14 **Acute Intermittent Porphyria** Slight or moderate elevation. *2498* Small increases may be found. *2246*

277.15 **Porphyria Variegata** The most characteristic and consistent abnormality. *2254* Large amounts. *0524* Even when clinical manifestations are minimal. *0928 0962 2246*

277.16 **Porphyria Cutanea Tarda** Large amounts. *0995* Highly variable. *2314 2246*

277.17 **Hereditary Coproporphyria** Increased but not to the same extent as coproporphyrin. *2538 2246*

Feces Normal

277.11 **Congenital Erythropoietic Porphyria (Günther's Disease)** Variable although not significantly elevated. *2246*

277.13 **Erythropoietic Coproporphyria** *0995*

277.17 **Hereditary Coproporphyria** Normal or only slightly increased. *2552*

Red Blood Cells Decrease

285.00 **Sideroblastic Anemia** May be characteristically high or very low, depending upon the type of sideroblastic anemia. Usually high in idiopathic and low in hereditary. *2552 2538*

Red Blood Cells Increase

277.11 **Congenital Erythropoietic Porphyria (Günther's Disease)** As in other hemolytic conditions. *2497 2538*

277.12 **Erythropoietic Protoporphyria** The red cells hemolyze if blood in thin layers is exposed to ultraviolet light. *0990 2538* Increased 5-30 X. *1478* Reported values range from 300-4,500 mg/dL (normal < 50). *2552* Excess does not occur in all cells, from 7-60% were found to contain excess. *1224* May be up to 100-fold. *1477* Marked increase. *2246*

277.13 **Erythropoietic Coproporphyria** Small increase. *2246 0995*

280.90 **Iron Deficiency Anemia** Defective heme synthesis is associated with raised RBC protoporphyrin. *2538 0151*

281.30 **Vitamin B₆ Deficiency Anemia** Almost always moderately increased, and rarely it is markedly so. *1326* Elevated (40-300 mg/dL compared to normal levels of 15-35 mg/dL) reflecting a functional block to hemoglobin synthesis. *0433 2538*

282.41 **Thalassemia Major** *1457*

282.42 **Thalassemia Minor** May be increased on occasion. *0349*

284.90 **Aplastic Anemia** *2552*

285.00 **Sideroblastic Anemia** Almost always moderately increased, and rarely it is markedly so. *1326* Elevated (40-300 mg/dL compared to normal levels of 15-35 mg/dL) reflecting a functional block to hemoglobin synthesis. *0433* May be characteristically high or very low, depending upon the type of sideroblastic anemia. Usually high in idiopathic and low in hereditary. *2552 2538*

585.00 **Chronic Renal Failure** May be moderately increased. *1421 2552*

650.00 **Pregnancy** *0249*

984.00 **Toxic Effects of Lead and Its Compounds (including Fumes)** Accumulates in the erythrocytes as a result of the blocks in the synthetic process. *0151* Free erythrocyte protoporphyrin ranges from 300-3,000 mg/dL (normal = 15-60). *0151* Log of RBC protoporphyrin level closely correlated to blood level (R = 0.72) in lead-exposed workers. Especially useful in the detection of mild increases in blood lead concentrations under conditions of occupational exposure. *2366*

Red Blood Cells Normal

277.14 **Acute Intermittent Porphyria** *0995*

277.15 **Porphyria Variegata** *0995 2246*

277.16 **Porphyria Cutanea Tarda** *0995*

277.17 **Hereditary Coproporphyria** No increase demonstrable. *2246 0868 0995*

Pseudocholinesterase

Serum Decrease

37.00 **Tetanus** Activity may be decreased in severe cases due to inhibition by the tetanus toxin. *0433* Reduced levels correlate with degree of severity of disease. *1841*

38.00 **Septicemia** In conditions which may have decreased serum albumin. *2467*

70.00 **Viral Hepatitis** Tends to be more marked in patients ill with chronic liver disease, such as cirrhosis than in those ill with acute conditions, such as viral hepatitis, ascending cholangitis and acute anoxic hepatomegaly. Peaks and depressions in cholinesterase activity in acute liver disease are related to the extent of hepatic parenchymal damage. *2441 1452*

124.00 **Trichinosis** May last up to 6 months. *2468*

197.70 **Secondary Malignant Neoplasm of Liver** Some patients. *2467*

250.10 **Diabetic Acidosis** Decreases 2-3 days after episodes of ketoacidosis. *0155*

260.00 **Protein Malnutrition** May be decreased in some conditions in which albumin is low. *2467* In Kwashiorkor. *0151*

269.90 **Deficiency State (Unspecified)** Low in malnourished patients (from starvation, anorexia, or debilitating disease) reflecting protein depletion and hepatic function impairment. The rise to normal levels parallels nutritional improvement and weight gain. *2441*

281.20 **Folic Acid Deficiency Anemia** *2538 1573*

410.90 **Acute Myocardial Infarction** May occur with decrease in serum albumin. *2467*

428.00 **Congestive Heart Failure** Some patients. *2467*

570.00 **Acute and Subacute Necrosis of Liver** Depression of enzyme concentration tends to be more marked in patients ill with chronic liver disease, such as cirrhosis, than in those ill with acute conditions, such as viral hepatitis, ascending cholangitis, and acute anoxic hepatomegaly. Peaks and depressions in cholinesterase activity in acute liver disease are related to the extent of hepatic parenchymal damage. *2441*

571.90 **Cirrhosis of Liver** Tends to be more marked in chronic liver disease, such as cirrhosis than in acute disorders. Sixty patients with chronic liver disease showed a serum cholinesterase range of 0.73-0.008. *2441*

572.00 **Liver Abscess (Pyogenic)** Liver diseases, especially hepatitis. Lowest level corresponds to peak of disease and becomes normal with recovery. *2467*

579.00 **Celiac Sprue Disease** May be decreased in some cases of malnutrition in which albumin is decreased. *2467*

579.90 **Malabsorption, Cause Unspecified** May be decreased in some cases of malnutrition in which albumin is decreased. *2467*

710.40 **Dermatomyositis/Polymyositis** With serum albumin. *2467*

Serum   Increase

242.90   **Hyperthyroidism**   In some cases of thyrotoxicosis. Not a useful measure of thyroid activity, because of the wide overlap with normal cases. *0619*

250.00   **Diabetes Mellitus**   Obese type. *0619*

272.10   **Type IV Hyperlipoproteinemia**   Both GGT and pseudocholinesterase were increased in hypertriglyceridemic subjects. Both strongly correlated with the logarithm of serum triglyceride and the prebeta electrophoretic fraction. Increase of GGT was rather characteristic for gross hypertriglyceridemia. *0480*

281.00   **Pernicious Anemia**   *2441*

303.90   **Alcoholism**   *0126 0619*

334.00   **Friedreich's Ataxia**   Altered or increased in 7 of 23 patients. However, the elevation was considered to be significant in only 3. *1956*

401.10   **Essential Benign Hypertension**   *0126*

571.90   **Cirrhosis of Liver**   In active cirrhosis. *0619*

581.90   **Nephrotic Syndrome**   18 of 19 patients had values elevated above 12.5 U/mL. *2441*

Pyridoxine

Serum   Decrease

297.90   **Paranoid States and Other Psychoses**   Has been noted in schizophrenia. *2104*

303.00   **Acute Alcoholic Intoxication**   Has been noted in acute alcoholism. *2104*

345.90   **Epilepsy**   Has been noted in epilepsy. *2104*

556.00   **Ulcerative Colitis**   Anemia may be due to blood loss, simple iron deficiency, deficiencies in folic acid, pyridoxine, or vitamin B_{12}. *0433*

579.00   **Celiac Sprue Disease**   Lack of B_6 results in failure to metabolize tryptophan and high concentrations of tryptophan metabolites. *2104*

592.00   **Kidney Calculus**   A relationship may exist between deficient B_6 and endogenous oxalic acid production and stone formation. *2104*

Urine   Decrease

714.00   **Rheumatoid Arthritis**   Patients with active disease excrete abnormally low B_6 and related metabolites. *2104*

Pyrophosphate

Serum   Increase

265.00   **Thiamine (B_1) Deficiency**   Thiamine pyrophosphate is elevated prior to thiamine administration but falls rapidly after therapy. *1108*

Urine   Increase

268.00   **Vitamin D Deficiency Rickets**   *0151*

Synovial Fluid   Increase

244.90   **Hypothyroidism**   Has been identified. *2088*

252.00   **Hyperparathyroidism**   Has been identified. *2088*

253.00   **Acromegaly**   Has been identified. *2088*

274.00   **Gout**   Moderately elevated levels. *1132*

275.00   **Hemochromatosis**   Has been identified. *2088*

275.10   **Hepatolenticular Degeneration**   Has been identified. *2088*

715.90   **Osteoarthritis**   Moderately elevated levels. *1132*

Synovial Fluid   Normal

714.00   **Rheumatoid Arthritis**   Near normal levels. *1132*

Pyruvate

Blood   Decrease

994.50   **Exercise**   Slight fall within 1 h and then steep drop. *0618*

Blood   Increase

151.90   **Malignant Neoplasm of Stomach**   Elevated in 8 patients with tumors of the gastrointestinal tract, mean = 1.93 ± 0.18 U/L. *1201*

152.90   **Malignant Neoplasm of Small Intestine**   Moderately elevated in 8 patients, mean = 1.93 ± 0.18 U/L. *1201*

153.90   **Malignant Neoplasm of Large Intestine**   Moderately elevated in 8 patients with tumors of the gastrointestinal tract. Mean = 1.93 ± 0.18 U/L. *1201*

162.90   **Malignant Neoplasm of Bronchus and Lung**   Mildly elevated in 5 patients with bronchogenic carcinomas. Mean = 0.88 ± 0.13 U/L. *1201*

174.90   **Malignant Neoplasm of Breast**   Moderately elevated in 6 patients, mean = 1.5 ± 0.35 U/L. *1201*

186.90   **Malignant Neoplasm of Testis**   Mildly elevated in 8 patients with tumors of the testicle. Mean = 0.89 ± 0.18 U/L. *1201*

189.00   **Malignant Neoplasm of Kidney**   Mildly elevated in 8 patients, mean = 0.89 ± 0.18 U/L. *1201*

201.90   **Hodgkin's Disease**   Moderately elevated in 20 patients with malignant lymphomas. Mean = 1.1 ± 0.15 U/L. *1201*

202.80   **Non-Hodgkins Lymphoma**   Moderately elevated in 20 of 20 patients with malignant lymphomas. Mean = 1.1 - 0.15 U/L. *1201*

250.00   **Diabetes Mellitus**   Raised levels have been reported in unstable diabetes (insulin sensitive). *0619*

250.10   **Diabetic Acidosis**   Can be demonstrated after removal of acetoacetic acid. *0619*

265.00   **Thiamine (B_1) Deficiency**   Acute advanced beriberi (vitamin B_1 deficiency). Many cases of alcoholic polyneuritis are due to vitamin B_1 deficiency. *0619*   In 16 of 17 untreated cases. *2350*

270.01   **Cystinuria**   *0995*

270.03   **Cystinosis**   In some but not all patients. *2246*

271.01   **Von Gierke's Disease**   Striking elevation. *1086 2246*

275.10   **Hepatolenticular Degeneration**   Reverts to normal after treatment with copper-chelating agent. *0619*

275.34   **Familial Periodic Paralysis**   *1535*

340.00   **Multiple Sclerosis**   Raised levels have been reported in some cases. The cause for this has not been discovered. *0619* High concentrations noted in these patients imply a defect in carbohydrate metabolism. *2104*

493.10   **Asthma (Intrinsic)**   Lactic acid, pyruvic acid, and the lactic/pyruvic ratio are increased in some patients. *1972*

570.00   **Acute and Subacute Necrosis of Liver**   Very advanced liver stage. *0619*

780.30   **Convulsions**   May occur with febrile convulsions in children. *2178*

985.00   **Toxic Effects of Non-medicinal Metals**   Arsenic, antimony, gold, and mercury inhibit pyruvate oxidation. *0619*

994.50   **Exercise**   After exercise to exhaustion 1.7 X control. *1837*

CSF   Increase

780.30   **Convulsions**   May occur with febrile convulsions in children. *2178*

Pyruvate Kinase

Red Blood Cells   Decrease

282.31   **Hereditary Nonspherocytic Hemolytic Anemia**   PK deficiency is limited to the red cell; the leukocyte does not share the deficiency. *2538*

Recalcification Time

Blood   Increase

286.01   **Hemophilia**   Greatly prolonged. *2552*

286.34   **Congenital Afibrinogenemia**   Corrected by the addition of normal plasma or normal fibrinogen to the patient's plasma. *2538*

Blood   Normal

286.31   **Congenital Dysfibrinogenemia**   The clotting time of whole blood or the recalcification time of platelet-poor plasma has usually been normal. *2538*

Reduced Glutathione

Red Blood Cells   Increase

289.80 **Myelofibrosis**   RBC reduced glutathione occurred in 16 of 17 myelofibrosis patients. *2317*   In myelofibrosis, usually increased. *0900   2538*

Renin Activity

Plasma   Decrease

244.90 **Hypothyroidism**   *2540*

250.00 **Diabetes Mellitus**   Decreased catecholamine levels, which reduce renin secretion, are common. *1854*

253.40 **Anterior Pituitary Hypofunction**   Both plasma renin substrate and angiotensin are low and unresponsive to adequate stimulation *0103*

255.00 **Adrenal Cortical Hyperfunction (Glucocorticoid Excess)**   In 4 patients with Cushing's Syndrome values were extremely low in renal venous blood. *1331*

255.10 **Adrenal Cortical Hyperfunction (Mineralocorticoid Excess)**   Markedly decreased (normal or increased in secondary aldosteronism). It cannot be stimulated by use of salt restriction and upright posture to deplete plasma volume. *0725*   Low value is essential for the diagnosis of primary aldosteronism. *1108*   In 8 patients with primary aldosteronism values were extremely low in renal venous blood *1331*

401.10 **Essential Benign Hypertension**   Decreased in 20% of patients at diagnosis. *2467*   Suppressed plasma renin activity. *0371*   Can be high, low or normal. *1108*

642.40 **Pre-Eclampsia**   In hypertensive groups, plasma renin activity and aldosterone concentration were significantly suppressed during the last trimester despite levels of renin substrate and progesterone that were not significantly different from those observed in normotensive pregnancy. *2507*   During normal pregnancy, plasma levels of renin, angiotensin II, and aldosterone are increased. Paradoxically with pregnancy-induced hypertension they commonly decrease towards the normal. *1859*

642.60 **Eclampsia**   In hypertensive groups, plasma renin activity and aldosterone concentration were significantly suppressed during the last trimester despite levels of renin substrate and progesterone that were not significantly different from those observed in normotensive pregnancy. *2507*   During normal pregnancy, plasma levels of renin, angiotensin II, and aldosterone are increased. Paradoxically with pregnancy-induced hypertension, they commonly decrease towards the normal. *1859*

1013.01 **Diet (High Sodium)**   Increased plasma volume due to high-sodium diet. *2467*   Plasma renin activity increased with decreased dietary sodium. *1274*

Plasma   Increase

84.00 **Malaria**   Increased in acute renal failure due to falciparum malaria. *2190*

189.00 **Malignant Neoplasm of Kidney**   Elevation occurred in 37% of cases of renal adenocarcinoma and was associated with high grade, high stage lesions of mixed histologic cell type and predicted poor prognosis. *2291*   Significantly higher in renal vein from affected side and maintains circadian rhythm despite marked elevation with renin-producing renal tumors. *2468*

242.90 **Hyperthyroidism**   *1004*

255.40 **Adrenal Cortical Hypofunction**   Due to reduced plasma volume. *2467*

296.80 **Manic Depressive Disorder**   High resting renin activity was found in a group of manic depressives, but no relation to mood was observed. Aldosterone production rates were inappropriate for the renin activity found. *1098*

303.00 **Acute Alcoholic Intoxication**   Increased more than 100%, when 1.5-2.3 g ethanol/kg body weight was ingested over a 3-h period. During hangover the increase even exceed 200%. *1412*

401.00 **Malignant Hypertension**   Most patients. *0995   1108   0151*

401.10 **Essential Benign Hypertension**   Mean level, measured after 1 h supine rest, was significantly higher in the hypertensive subjects, while the upright PRA was normal. *1211*   Greater in plasma of hypertensive patients and uremic patients than in plasma of normotensive control subjects. *1310*   Can be high, low or normal. *1108*

405.91 **Renovascular Hypertension**   *0992*

496.00 **Chronic Obstructive Lung Disease**   Plasma renin and aldosterone tended to have higher than normal baseline values, especially in hypercapnic patients. *0698*

571.90 **Cirrhosis of Liver**   Increased levels. *1887*

584.00 **Acute Renal Failure**   Increased in failure due to falciparum malaria. *2190*

642.40 **Pre-Eclampsia**   Greater increase in pre-eclamptic than in normal pregnant women. *2309*   At term, hypertensive, toxemic pregnant women had elevated aldosterone and plasma renin activity, which remained elevated > 1 week after delivery. *0066   0387*

642.60 **Eclampsia**   At term, hypertensive, toxemic pregnant women had elevated aldosterone and plasma renin activity, which remained elevated > 1 week after delivery. *0066*

650.00 **Pregnancy**   Highest in the first trimester and decreases thereafter. Both concentration and activity are increased. *2194*   Among the normotensive subjects, activity was elevated as early as the 6th week of gestation. While consistent, progressive, further increases were noted in renin substrate, aldosterone and progesterone continue to rise. Renin activity did not continue to rise. *2507   0387*

710.10 **Progressive Systemic Sclerosis**   Extremely elevated levels are a frequent accompaniment of renal scleroderma. *0962*

992.00 **Heat stroke**   Plasma activity increased by 174% after 1 week of thermal stress. *0100*

1013.02 **Diet (Low Sodium)**   Reduced plasma volume due to low-sodium diet. *2467*

Plasma   Normal

401.10 **Essential Benign Hypertension**   Can be high, low or normal. *1108*

642.40 **Pre-Eclampsia**   Renin activity was found to be about the same, or less, than in normotensive pregnant women. *2421   0387*

642.60 **Eclampsia**   Average concentration and activity are slightly less than in normotensive pregnancies, but nearly all values in each group are in the same range. *0387   2421*

Urine   Decrease

401.10 **Essential Benign Hypertension**   *1362*

Reptilase Time

Blood   Increase

286.31 **Congenital Dysfibrinogenemia**   Usually prolonged, but in some cases no clot forms at all. *2538*

286.34 **Congenital Afibrinogenemia**   Corrected by the addition of normal plasma or normal fibrinogen to the patient's plasma. *2538   0433*

Reticulocytes

Blood   Decrease

38.00 **Septicemia**   The absolute count is reduced. *0433*

202.80 **Non-Hodgkins Lymphoma**   *2552*

204.00 **Lymphocytic Leukemia (Acute)**   Usually low. *0433*   Reflects decreased cell production. *2552*

205.00 **Myelocytic Leukemia (Acute)**   Usually low, however, if RBC morphology is bizarre, and nucleated RBCs and an increased reticulocyte count are present, erythroleukemia should be suspected. *0433*   Reflects decreased cell production. *2552*

244.90 **Hypothyroidism**   *0433*

253.40 **Anterior Pituitary Hypofunction**   Absolute count is decreased. *0433*

255.40 **Adrenal Cortical Hypofunction**   Absolute count is decreased. *0433*

257.20 **Testicular Hypofunction**   The absolute count is decreased. *0433*

260.00 **Protein Malnutrition**   Normal or slightly decreased. *2538*

280.90 **Iron Deficiency Anemia**   Rarely reduced. *2552*   Usually normal or decreased. *2538*

281.00 **Pernicious Anemia**   Inappropriately low corrected count due to marrow failure. *0999*

281.20 **Folic Acid Deficiency Anemia**   Lower than normal, both in absolute and in percentage terms. *2538*   Tends to be low or at the low extreme of the normal range. *0962*

281.30 Vitamin B₆ Deficiency Anemia   Absolute count is usually reduced. *0151*

284.01 Congenital Aplastic Anemia   May be slightly increased relatively but the absolute count is reduced. *2552*

284.90 Aplastic Anemia   Percentage ranges from 0 to as high as 5%, but the absolute number is usually subnormal. Many are large and immature, possibly reflecting an increased concentration of erythropoietin and a short bone marrow transit time. *1049   0151   2538*

285.00 Sideroblastic Anemia   Absolute count is usually reduced. *0151*   Inappropriately low. *2538*

571.20 Laennec's or Alcoholic Cirrhosis   Reticulocytosis can be suppressed by alcohol. *2552 1147*

571.90 Cirrhosis of Liver   Reticulocytosis can be suppressed by alcohol. *2552 1147*

585.00 Chronic Renal Failure   Anemia is characteristically normocytic and normochromic, and is associated with a normal or slightly decreased number of reticulocytes. *2538*

990.00 Effects of X-Ray Irradiation   May decrease or disappear in the first 48 postexposure h in cases of radiation injury. *0151*

Blood   Increase

70.00 Viral Hepatitis   Mild hemolytic anemia with increase in the reticulocyte count are commonly found. *0962*

84.00 Malaria   Occurs several days after therapy has begun. *0151*

86.90 Trypanosomiasis   *2035*

115.00 Histoplasmosis   25% of patients with disseminated disease. *0999*

198.50 Secondary Malignant Neoplasm of Bone   Possibly increased. *2467*

201.90 Hodgkin's Disease   In patients with advanced disease. *2538*

204.10 Lymphocytic Leukemia (Chronic)   Secondary to hemolysis. *2538*

205.10 Myelocytic Leukemia (Chronic)   Generally normal or slightly increased. *2538   2552*

206.00 Monocytic Leukemia   Usually modest in degree, considering the severity of the anemia. *2538*

207.00 Erythroleukemia   Occasionally. *0936*

212.70 Benign Neoplasm of Cardiovascular Tissue   Hemolytic anemia, mechanical in origin (due to local turbulence of blood) is usual and may be severe. The anemia is recognized in about 50% of patients with this tumor. *2467*

238.40 Polycythemia Vera   Possibly increased. *2467*

267.00 Vitamin C Deficiency   Normocytic, normochromic anemia with a reticulocytosis of 5-10%. *2538*

272.52 Abetalipoproteinemia   Reflects increased RBC turnover. *1583*

272.72 Gaucher's Disease   A modest reticulocytosis is often present in anemic patients. *2538*

277.11 Congenital Erythropoietic Porphyria (Günther's Disease)   With moderate to severe anemia. *2552*   Secondary to increased hemolytic activity. *2073   2246*

280.90 Iron Deficiency Anemia   Both the percentage and absolute number tend to be normal or slightly increased. *0117*   Occasionally a count of 2-3% may be noted. *2538*

281.30 Vitamin B₆ Deficiency Anemia   Count is usually normal but may be slightly increased. *2538*

282.00 Hereditary (Congenital) Spherocytosis   Is increased 5-20%. *0433*   Characteristic increase. *2552*   Common chronic hemolytic findings. *2246   2538*

282.10 Hereditary Elliptocytosis   In patients with more severe forms of this disease there may be a compensated hemolytic anemia with raised reticulocyte count. *0433*   The great majority of these patients manifest only mild hemolysis with hemoglobin > 12 g/dL, reticulocytes < 4%. In 10-15% of patients the rate of hemolysis is increased and reticulocytosis ranging to 20%. *2538*

282.20 Anemias Due To Disorders of Glutathione Metabolism   Laboratory clue that hemolysis may be present. *0433*   As the hemoglobin level falls, reticulocytosis occurs, and polychromasia is seen. *2538*

282.31 Hereditary Nonspherocytic Hemolytic Anemia   Increase in count is marked, even with mild anemia with hereditary nonspherocytic hemolytic anemias. *2468*

282.41 Thalassemia Major   Moderately elevated. *2538*   Only slightly increased. *0962*   Moderate (19,000-25,000/µL). *0995*

282.42 Thalassemia Minor   Count is increased (2-10%) with thalassemias. *2468*   Normal or slightly increased. *1774*

282.60 Sickle Cell Anemia   In 15 cases, mean count was 345,000/µL with a range of 62,-750,000/µL, markedly increased over the normal value of 50,000/µL. *1023*   Reticulocytosis (5-20%) with circulating nucleated red cells. Count is diminished during aplastic crises. *2538*

282.71 Hemoglobin C Disease   Count is increased (2-10%). *2468*   Manifested by a hemolytic state. *0962*

282.73 Hemoglobin H Disease   Usually in the 5% range. *2538   0433 2246*

283.00 Acquired Hemolytic Anemia (Autoimmune)   Increased polychromasia, reflecting reticulocytosis in patients with slightly or moderately increased erythrocyte destruction. *2538*   In cases with more active hemolysis, anemia may be moderate to severe (with hematocrit's in the 10- 25% range) and the reticulocyte count markedly elevated to 50% or more. *2035*

283.21 Paroxysmal Nocturnal Hemoglobinuria   May be greatly increased from 20-24% depending on the severity of the hemolysis and the degree of marrow response. *0433*   Count may be elevated above the level usually seen in iron deficiency. *2538*   There may be relative reticulocytosis but the absolute count is often inappropriately low in relation to the severity of the anemia. *2552*

285.00 Sideroblastic Anemia   Count is usually normal but may be slightly increased. *2538*

287.30 Idiopathic Thrombocytopenic Purpura   Occasionally, if there has been a recent severe hemorrhage. *2552   0995*

289.00 Polycythemia, Secondary   Percentage is usually normal, but the absolute number is increased. *0151*

289.80 Myelofibrosis   Greater than 1% in 75% of myelofibrosis patients; total count > 60,000/µL occurred in 51%. *2317   0151*

446.60 Thrombotic Thrombocytopenic Purpura   In most cases. *2552*   Averaged 20%. *0054*

483.01 Mycoplasma Pneumoniae   Sometimes seen in convalescence. *0726*

570.00 Acute and Subacute Necrosis of Liver   Mild. *0992*

571.20 Laennec's or Alcoholic Cirrhosis   Average = 8.6%, ranging from 2.3-24.6% in 16 patients. *1147*

571.90 Cirrhosis of Liver   Average = 8.6%, ranging from 2.3-24.6% in 16 patients. *1147*

585.00 Chronic Renal Failure   1-4 X normal after correction for reduced RBC. *0151*   May be moderately increased. *1421 2552*   Highest values (6%) observed when the BUN was 300-350 mg/dL. *2130*

773.00 Hemolytic Disease of Newborn (Erythroblastosis Fetalis)   Counts normally 5-10% may be markedly elevated in the erythroblastic infant (up to 25-50% in severe cases). *0433*   Correlates roughly with the level of hemoglobin in the cord blood, although well-compensated hemolysis may occur. *2538*   Percentage is a rough indicator of prognosis. *2061*

984.00 Toxic Effects of Lead and Its Compounds (including Fumes)   Hemolytic anemia. *0889*

985.00 Toxic Effects of Non-medicinal Metals   Values up to 18% have been observed following toxicity with arsenicals. *0977*

Blood   Normal

204.10 Lymphocytic Leukemia (Chronic)   Normal or slightly decreased. *0157*

205.10 Myelocytic Leukemia (Chronic)   Normal or slightly increased. *0157*

277.44 Crigler-Najjar Syndrome   No evidence of hemolytic anemia or splenomegaly. *2246   0469*

280.90 Iron Deficiency Anemia   Usually normal. *0995*   Usually normal or decreased. *2538*

281.00 Pernicious Anemia   Usually within normal limits in untreated patients. *0995*

282.41 Thalassemia Major   Reticulocyte index normal or slightly increased. *0999*

Rheumatoid Factor

Serum   Increase

11.00 Pulmonary Tuberculosis   The incidence of seropositivity exceeds that of a normal population. *2035*   11% positivity. *0123   0422 0962*

Rheumatoid Factor *(continued)*

Serum Increase *(continued)*

13.00 Tuberculosis Meningitis Positive tests may be seen in connective tissue diseases such as tuberculosis. *0999* 11% positivity. *0123 0422*

18.00 Disseminated Tuberculosis 11% positivity. *0422 0123* The incidence of seropositivity exceeds that of a normal population. *2035*

30.00 Leprosy Found in 50%. *2035* The incidence of seropositivity exceeds that of a normal population. *2035* Found in 24% of patients. *0422 0123 0962*

70.00 Viral Hepatitis 24% positivity. *0422 0123 0962*

75.00 Infectious Mononucleosis *0962*

84.00 Malaria High prevalence of IgM rheumatoid factors showed a positive correlation with malaria antibodies. *2438 2035*

85.00 Leishmaniasis Parasitic diseases that involve the liver and reticuloendothelial system have a significant incidence of seropositivity, suggesting that these factors may be produced in the tissues locally. *0962*

86.00 Trypanosomiasis Parasitic diseases that involve the liver and reticuloendothelial system have a significant incidence of seropositivity, suggesting that these factors may be produced in the tissues locally. *0962* 27% positivity. *0422 0123*

97.90 Syphilis The incidence of seropositivity exceeds that of a normal population. *2035* 13% positivity. *0422 0123 0962*

120.00 Schistosomiasis Parasitic diseases that involve the liver and reticuloendothelial system have a significant incidence of seropositivity, suggesting that these factors may be produced in these tissues locally. *0962*

128.00 Larva Migrans (Visceralis) Parasitic diseases that involve the liver and reticuloendothelial system have a significant incidence of seropositivity, suggesting that these factors may be produced in these tissues locally. *0962*

135.00 Sarcoidosis The incidence of seropositivity exceeds that of a normal population. *2035* High incidence of seropositive tests among those who had the disease for 2 y, especially among those who also had arthritis. *0962* 17% positivity. *0422 0123*

174.90 Malignant Neoplasm of Breast Treated patients with no evidence of residual tumor had an 89% rate of positive tests. The incidence of seropositivity was low among untreated patients with similar tumors. *2394*

201.90 Hodgkin's Disease Dysproteinemias and paraproteinemias present significant seropositivity. *0962* Found in 18% of patients. *0422 0123*

202.80 Non-Hodgkins Lymphoma Dysproteinemias and paraproteinemias present significant seropositivity. *0962*

203.00 Multiple Myeloma Dysproteinemias and paraproteinemias may present significant seropositivity. *0962*

204.00 Lymphocytic Leukemia (Acute) Dysproteinemias and paraproteinemias present significant seropositivity. *0962*

205.00 Myelocytic Leukemia (Acute) Dysproteinemias and paraproteinemias present significant seropositivity. *0962*

242.90 Hyperthyroidism Titers > 1:160 are more common in Graves' disease patients than in controls. In patients under 40, titers > 1:80 are more frequent than in control subjects. *2162*

273.21 Cryoglobulinemia (Essential Mixed) High titer when tested at 37 C. *2035*

273.30 Waldenström's Macroglobulinemia Occasionally. *2035* Dysproteinemias and paraproteinemias present significant seropositivity. *0962* In some cases. *0020*

279.07 Dysgammaglobulinemia (Selective Immunoglobulin Deficiency) Dysproteinemias and paraproteinemias present significant seropositivity. *0962*

358.00 Myasthenia Gravis Somewhat elevated compared to the population at large. Demonstrated in a small percentage of patients. *2035*

410.90 Acute Myocardial Infarction Found in 12% of patients. *0422 0123*

421.00 Bacterial Endocarditis Elevated levels of IgG and IgM rheumatoid factor were found in patients with subacute infection. *0348* 13 (24%) of 55 patients were seropositive at some point in their courses. More severe cases were more likely to develop rheumatoid factor. *2132* May be used to confirm the diagnosis. Following remission, titers fall to 0. *0962* Positive in 17 of 36 patients but did not correlate with renal failure. *1798 2035*

446.00 Polyarteritis-Nodosa Present in some patients. *0999 2024*

446.50 Cranial Arteritis and Related Conditions Present in serum in 7.5% of patients with polymyalgia rheumatica. *2468*

482.90 Bacterial Pneumonia Positive latex fixation in 22% of 50 patients. *0448*

491.00 Chronic Bronchitis Found in 62% of patients. *0422 0123*

493.10 Asthma (Intrinsic) Found in 17% of patients. *0422 0123*

500.00 Anthracosis 42% of patients without associated arthritis had a positive sheep cell agglutination test, while 80% with associated rheumatoid arthritis were found to be seropositive. *0962*

501.00 Asbestosis 21% positivity. *0123 0422 0962*

502.00 Silicosis Positive in 15% of patients. *0123 0422 0962*

571.20 Laennec's or Alcoholic Cirrhosis Found in 36% of patients. *0422 0123*

571.90 Cirrhosis of Liver Dysproteinemias and paraproteinemias present significant seropositivity. *0962*

710.00 Systemic Lupus Erythematosus Positive tests (titer of 1:80 or more) were found in 50% (61) of patients. *0713* Rheumatoid factors are present in almost 50% of patients at some time during their course, but intermittently and at low titer. *0999* In 15% of cases. *1700*

710.10 Progressive Systemic Sclerosis Present in 33% of sera from 47 patients with scleroderma. *1995* 25-33% of patients have positive tests. In most cases the titers have been 1:320 or less. *2035* Almost 50% of patients have factor present in serum but it does not correlate with the existence of joint disease. *0999*

710.20 Sjögren's Syndrome Detected in > 70% of cases, regardless of the presence or absence of rheumatoid arthritis. *2134* High incidence even when not associated with a connective disease; the incidence of seropositivity is greatest in definite RA. *0962* 96% positivity. *0422 2035 0123*

710.40 Dermatomyositis/Polymyositis Positive (> 1:40) in 18 of 82 recorded (20%): including 5 patients (6%) with pure polymyositis (Type I), 4 (5%) with pure dermatomyositis (Type II), and 9 (10%) with the overlap type (Type V). *2035* Positive in 10-50% of patients. *0151* Reported to be positive in 40%. Positive only in a few cases of uncomplicated disease. Positive titer in 10% contrary to other reports. Higher titers were found in patients with other complications. *0244*

711.10 Mixed Connective Tissue Disease Found in over 50% of cases. Titer is usually very high. *0062*

714.00 Rheumatoid Arthritis The majority of rheumatoid sera give positive reactions; the incidence varies with different techniques, but at least 70%. A high degree of correlation of rheumatoid factors and subcutaneous nodules, symmetrical deforming arthritis of the hands and wrists, and various visceral manifestations of rheumatoid arthritis. *2035* Correlated with anatomical stage, class and course of disease and ESR. *0550* Low values associated with more severe disease and poorer prognosis. *0313 0999*

714.10 Felty's Syndrome Serologic tests are positive; may be present in high titers. *2467 2468*

714.30 Juvenile Rheumatoid Arthritis No more than 10% of patients have a positive rheumatoid factor in sera. *0151* Found in only 10-20% of children. *1700*

720.00 Rheumatoid (Ankylosing) Spondylitis Serologic tests are positive in 15% of patients with arthritis of the vertebral region in ankylosing spondylitis. *2468*

Serum Normal

99.30 Reiter's Disease *0186*

117.10 Sporotrichosis Normal in all patients with Sporotrichosis arthritis. *0478*

274.00 Gout *2467*

390.00 Rheumatic Fever *2467*

446.00 Polyarteritis-Nodosa Usually absent, and when present should suggest that the arteritis is part of another disorder. *2035*

446.50 Cranial Arteritis and Related Conditions Characteristically absent. *2035*

556.00 Ulcerative Colitis Usually negative even with associated arthritis. *2199*

714.30 Juvenile Rheumatoid Arthritis No more than 10% of patients have a positive rheumatoid factor in sera. *0151* Found in only 10-20% of children. *1700* In acute systemic form. *0136*

715.90 Osteoarthritis *2467*

720.00 Rheumatoid (Ankylosing) Spondylitis Occurs no more frequently than in the general population. *0666*

Urine   Increase

270.02   **Hartnup Disease**   *0995*

CSF   Increase

320.90   **Meningitis (Bacterial)**   In 18 samples of CSF from patients with pneumococcal meningitis, 11 were found to be positive by the latex fixation test. *0448*

Synovial Fluid   Increase

714.00   **Rheumatoid Arthritis**   Low values associated with more severe disease and poorer prognosis. *0313*

Synovial Fluid   Normal

99.30   **Reiter's Disease**   *0999*

714.30   **Juvenile Rheumatoid Arthritis**   Absent in synovial fluid. *2468*

Pleural Effusion   Increase

162.90   **Malignant Neoplasm of Bronchus and Lung**   May be present with rheumatoid disease, but may also be found in other types of pleural effusions (e.g., carcinoma, tuberculosis, bacterial pneumonia). *2467*

197.00   **Secondary Malignant Neoplasm of Respiratory System**   May be present with rheumatoid disease, but may also be found in other types of pleural effusions (e.g., carcinoma, tuberculosis, bacterial pneumonia). *2467*

482.90   **Bacterial Pneumonia**   May be present with rheumatoid disease, but may also be found in other types of pleural effusions (e.g., carcinoma, tuberculosis, bacterial pneumonia). *2467*

Riboflavin

Serum   Decrease

242.90   **Hyperthyroidism**   Secondary to increased metabolic processes. *2540*

Ribose

Urine   Increase

359.11   **Progressive Muscular Dystrophy**   Probably derived from the nucleoprotein of breaking down muscle cells. *0619*

Selenium

Plasma   Decrease

440.00   **Arteriosclerosis**   Low concentrations of selenium in plasma in coronary atherogenesis. *1620*

Serine

Serum   Decrease

274.00   **Gout**   *2604*

Urine   Increase

270.02   **Hartnup Disease**   5-20 X normal values. *2246*   *0995*

270.03   **Cystinosis**   Nonspecific pattern of aminoaciduria. Fanconi's syndrome. *0995*

Sialic Acid

Serum   Increase

590.00   **Chronic Pyelonephritis**   Increased in 84 chronic patients, correlated with activity of pathologic process and distinguished it from glomerulonephritis. *2362*

Sickle Cells

Blood   Increase

282.60   **Sickle Cell Anemia**   Sickled erythrocytes may not be numerous in the blood smear, but in blood deoxygenated with sodium metabisulfite virtually all the red cells are sickled. *0151* Mean number of irreversibly sickled cells was 9 ± 5.06 in 25 patients. Number of cells correlated inversely with RBC life span. *1541*

282.71   **Hemoglobin C Disease**   Sickling produces prominent clinical manifestations. *2538*

Synovial Fluid   Increase

282.60   **Sickle Cell Anemia**   Sickled erythrocytes were found in 7 of 13 joint fluid specimens. *0676*

Sodium

Serum   Decrease

4.90   **Bacillary Dysentery**   Fluid and electrolyte loss may be quite significant, particularly in pediatric and geriatric populations. *1058*

9.00   **Gastroenteritis and Colitis**   Either elevated or diminished may be noted. *0433*

11.00   **Pulmonary Tuberculosis**   Sometimes found in extensive chronic disease. Usually caused by abnormal retention of water. *0151*   May be decreased (110-125 mmol/L) especially in aged or in overwhelming infection. *2468*   Occasionally found, due to inappropriate secretion of ADH with consequent water retention. *0962*

13.00   **Tuberculosis Meningitis**   May be decreased (110-125 mmol/L) especially in aged or in overwhelming infection. *2468* Occasionally found, due to inappropriate secretion of ADH with consequent water retention. *0962*

18.00   **Disseminated Tuberculosis**   Often occurs, frequently caused by inappropriate secretion of antidiuretic hormone. *0151*

80.00   **Epidemic Typhus**   Chronic illness from rickettsial disease result in hyponatremia. *2104*

81.00   **Endemic Typhus**   Chronic illness from rickettsial disease results in hyponatremia. *2104*

81.10   **Brill's Disease**   Chronic illness from Rickettsial disease result in hyponatremia. *2104*

81.20   **Mite-Borne Typhus**   Chronic illness from Rickettsial disease results in hyponatremia. *2104*

82.00   **Rocky Mountain Spotted Fever**   Chronic illness from Rickettsial disease result in hyponatremia. *2104*

83.20   **Rickettsialpox**   Chronic illness from Rickettsial disease result in hyponatremia. *2104*

84.00   **Malaria**   Caused by salt depletion and water retention. *1058 0761 1593*

162.90   **Malignant Neoplasm of Bronchus and Lung**   Inappropriate secretion of ADH is associated with hyponatremia, decreased serum osmolality, and inappropriately high sodium concentration in the urine. The entire syndrome resolves following resection of the tumor. *0962*

191.90   **Malignant Neoplasm of Brain**   Associated with excessive ADH production *2104* . Serum sodium usually less than 130 mEq/L. *0062*

198.30   **Secondary Malignant Neoplasm of Brain**   Associated with excessive ADH production. *2104*   Serum Sodium usually less than 130 mEq/L *0062*

203.00   **Multiple Myeloma**   In 31% of 28 patients at initial hospitalization for this disorder. *0781*

225.90   **Benign Neoplasm of Brain and CNS**   Associated with excessive ADH production. *2104*   Serum Sodium usually less than 130 mEq/L *0062* .

244.90   **Hypothyroidism**   Significant hyponatremia can occur. *0433*

245.10   **Subacute Thyroiditis**   Severe hyponatremia and hypoglycemia may occur as a manifestation of primary or secondary thyroid failure. *0151*

250.00   **Diabetes Mellitus**   Osmotic diuresis secondary to hyperglycemia. *2540*   In 22% of 104 patients at initial hospitalization for this disorder. *0781*

250.10   **Diabetic Acidosis**   Despite the markedly negative sodium balance, the plasma concentration may be hypernormal, normal or subnormal. *2540*   *0962*

Sodium (continued)

Serum Decrease (continued)

253.40 Anterior Pituitary Hypofunction May be 120 mmol/L or lower without symptoms of adrenal insufficiency. *0151 0433*

255.40 Adrenal Cortical Hypofunction Normal in mild insufficiency, but in severe insufficiency, particularly of aldosterone, there are hyponatremia and hyperkalemia. *0433* Often occurs. *0962* Serum concentration may remain normal until a crisis, when sodium loss exceeds water loss. *2612*

256.00 Ovarian Hyperfunction Progesterone effect. *0995*

272.32 Type V Hyperlipoproteinemia Lipemia was associated with significant hyponatremia. *2177*

277.00 Cystic Fibrosis Normal unless complications occur (e.g., chronic pulmonary disease with accumulation of CO_2, massive salt loss due to sweating). *2467 0105*

277.14 Acute Intermittent Porphyria Electrolyte depletion and alkalosis associated with azotemia of variable degree are often present on admission but may also develop acutely during the course of the attack. The severity of the hyponatremia is a particularly striking feature, and although it may by symptomless, it is often associated with the encephalopathic manifestations of the acute attack. Attributable in many patients to electrolyte depletion with inappropriate and injudicious overhydration. *0433 2254*

320.90 Meningitis (Bacterial) Serum concentrations below 135 mmol/L were noted on admission in 72 of 124 (58.1%) of patients. Low initial concentration and prolonged depression despite fluid restriction correlated significantly with the presence of neurologic sequelae of the disease. *0712* Associated with excessive ADH production. *2104 0062*

323.92 Encephalomyelitis Associated with excessive ADH production. *2104* Serum sodium is usually less than 130 mEq/L *0062*

331.81 Reye's Syndrome Hyponatremia is common in children. *0151*

401.10 Essential Benign Hypertension Slight but highly significant depression in circulating concentration. Mean in 130 hypertensives was 137.7 mmol/L and 140.4 mmol/L in 123 normotensives. *2104*

410.90 Acute Myocardial Infarction Frequent hyponatremia, degree of loss seems to correlate with severity of myocardial involvement. *2104*

428.00 Congestive Heart Failure May be the result of over-vigorous use of diuretics in an already dehydrated patient who is on a sodium-restricted diet. A common hyponatremic syndrome is observed in patients who continue to have edema and clinical heart failure. Total body sodium in these patients is increased, but the amount of retained water is even greater. Is true dilutional hyponatremia. *0962*

431.00 Cerebral Hemorrhage Associated with excessive ADH production. *2104* Serum sodium is usually less than 130 mEq/L *0062*

434.00 Cerebral Thrombosis Associated with excessive ADH production. *2104* Serum sodium is usually less than 130 mEq/L. *0062*

434.10 Cerebral Embolism Associated with excessive ADH production. *2104* Serum sodium is usually less than 130 mEq/L *0062*

533.90 Peptic Ulcer, Site Unspecified May be < 135 mmol/L when complicated by obstruction. *0433* Pyloric obstruction with vomiting and loss of gastric secretion results in hypochloremia, hyponatremia, hypokalemia, elevated serum pH and carbon dioxide content, and azotemia. *0962*

537.00 Pyloric Stenosis, Acquired Secondary to vomiting. *0587*

537.40 Fistula of Stomach and Duodenum Small intestinal aspiration or fistula. The loss of sodium/day (430 mmol) is > the loss of chloride (270 mmol). *0619*

555.90 Regional Enteritis or Ileitis Common feature of severe colitis. *2035*

556.00 Ulcerative Colitis Common feature of severe colitis. *2035*

558.90 Diarrhea 60 mmol/day may be lost. *0619* Hyponatremia commonly results. *2199*

571.20 Laennec's or Alcoholic Cirrhosis Frequent in patients with ascites or edema. *0992*

571.60 Biliary Cirrhosis Frequently found, especially in patients with ascites. *2104*

571.90 Cirrhosis of Liver Characteristic. *2537* Especially in patients with ascites. *2104*

572.40 Hepatic Failure In hepatic failure patients, sodium loss in urine may be high if the GFR falls below 24 mL/min. *2536* Frequently depressed in hepatic failure. Severe hyponatremic states are found in end-stage hepatic cirrhosis with uniformly poor prognosis. *1775* Hyponatremia (< 130 mmol/L) occurred in 61% of patients with hepatic failure due to decompensated cirrhosis of liver. *0379*

579.00 Celiac Sprue Disease If diarrhea is severe, marked electrolyte depletion. *2199*

579.90 Malabsorption, Cause Unspecified *2467 0151*

580.00 Acute Poststreptococcal Glomerulonephritis The decreased GFR and increased aldosterone secretion lead to retention of sodium and water with resultant hypervolemia. *1108*

584.00 Acute Renal Failure Often decreased, in the 2nd week. *2468*

585.00 Chronic Renal Failure Decreased because of tubular damage with loss in urine, vomiting, diarrhea, diet restriction, etc. *2468*

588.81 Proximal Renal Tubular Acidosis Normal or decreased. *0186* Hyponatremia may develop *2246*

597.80 Urethritis Reveals the degree of renal impairment. *0433*

642.40 Pre-Eclampsia Rarely. *0387* Serum concentrations tend to decline as severity increases. *2104*

642.60 Eclampsia Rarely. *0387* Reduced concentrations as a result of hemodilution. Averages 4-8 mmol/L lower than in normal nonpregnant women. *2104*

650.00 Pregnancy Average reduction in cations (chiefly sodium) was 4.7 mmol/L during pregnancy. *1690*

694.40 Pemphigus *0151*

753.10 Polycystic Kidney Disease Renal salt wasting. *0277 0433*

753.12 Medullary Cystic Disease Renal salt wasting. *0277 0433*

780.80 Hyperhidrosis *2467*

785.40 Gangrene In 47% of 27 patients hospitalized for this disorder. *0781*

948.00 Burns Reduced concentration in plasma, but an increase in RBC concentration occurs even in minor burns. *2104*

985.00 Toxic Effects of Non-medicinal Metals May occur with established mercury poisoning. *0618*

991.60 Hypothermia Glucose solution acts as a relatively inert extracellular fluid volume expander when the body temperature is lowered. *0619*

Serum Increase

1.00 Cholera Marked loss of fluid and electrolytes occurs. *2468*

4.90 Bacillary Dysentery Fluid and electrolyte loss may be quite significant, particularly in pediatric and geriatric populations. *1058*

9.00 Gastroenteritis and Colitis Reflects the loss of greater volumes of fluid than salt. Either elevated or diminished may be noted. *0433*

202.80 Non-Hodgkins Lymphoma In 88% of 73 patients at initial hospitalization for this disorder. *0781*

204.00 Lymphocytic Leukemia (Acute) In 94% of 39 patients at initial hospitalization for this disorder. *0781*

204.10 Lymphocytic Leukemia (Chronic) In 99% of 27 patients at initial hospitalization for this disorder. *0781*

205.00 Myelocytic Leukemia (Acute) In 98% of 34 patients at initial hospitalization for this disorder. *0781*

205.10 Myelocytic Leukemia (Chronic) In 100% of 20 patients at initial hospitalization for this disorder. *0781*

250.10 Diabetic Acidosis May be normal or elevated depending on the relative losses of sodium and water and the degree of increased plasma lipids. Because of the increase in plasma lipids a sodium concentration of 150 mmol/L of plasma may represent 170 mmol/L of water. *0999* Despite the markedly negative sodium balance, the plasma concentration may be hypernormal, normal or subnormal. *2540*

253.00 Acromegaly *0995*

253.50 Diabetes Insipidus If the water intake does not keep pace with the urinary output, there may be mild hypernatremia and a tendency toward serum hyperosmolality. *0962*

255.00 Adrenal Cortical Hyperfunction (Glucocorticoid Excess) Sodium retention and elevated blood pressure can occur. *0151*

255.10 Adrenal Cortical Hyperfunction (Mineralocorticoid Excess) Frequent, although not constant. *1108* May be seen. *0962*

256.30 Ovarian Hypofunction Estrogen effect. *0995*

275.34 Familial Periodic Paralysis Precedes attack. *2246*

276.50 Dehydration *2467*

428.00 Congestive Heart Failure Sodium retention. *1985*

558.90 Diarrhea In osmotic diarrhea water loss is proportionately greater than that of sodium. Dehydration with hypernatremia may occur. *2199*

560.90 Intestinal Obstruction Secondary to dehydration. *0995*

567.90 Peritonitis Secondary to increased aldosterone production. *0995*

572.40 Hepatic Failure Marked sodium retention (9 mmol/24h) may occur in fulminant hepatic failure when GFR exceeds 40 mL/min. *2536*

585.00 Chronic Renal Failure Much less common. *0277*

787.00 Vomiting Resulting in relative depletion of chloride and hydrogen ions (developing metabolic alkalosis), can lead to an increase in plasma sodium concentration in the presence of gross dehydration. *0619*

1013.01 Diet (High Sodium) There was a tendency for body weight, serum sodium, exchangeable sodium, and inulin clearance to increase as dietary sodium increased. *1274*

Serum Normal

253.50 Diabetes Insipidus Normal or increased. *2467*

255.00 Adrenal Cortical Hyperfunction (Glucocorticoid Excess) Sodium retention leads to increased total body concentration, but serum concentration is normal due to water retention. *2612*

255.40 Adrenal Cortical Hypofunction Normal in mild insufficiency, but in severe insufficiency, particularly of aldosterone, there are hyponatremia and hyperkalemia. *0433*

260.00 Protein Malnutrition *2467*

277.00 Cystic Fibrosis Normal unless complications occur (e.g., chronic pulmonary disease with accumulation of CO_2, massive salt loss due to sweating). *2467 0105*

359.11 Progressive Muscular Dystrophy The differences between the patient group and the group of normal boys for sodium and potassium in serum and urine were not significant. The pathologically elevated sodium:potassium ratio in skeletal muscle is not due to increased aldosterone or other causes of renal wastage of potassium. *0816*

401.10 Essential Benign Hypertension Sodium homeostasis is usually maintained in gradual renal failure. *1985*

492.80 Pulmonary Emphysema *2467*

585.00 Chronic Renal Failure Usually. *0277*

588.81 Proximal Renal Tubular Acidosis Normal or decreased. *0186*

650.00 Pregnancy Throughout pregnancy. *0517*

Urine Decrease

255.10 Adrenal Cortical Hyperfunction (Mineralocorticoid Excess) *2467*

275.34 Familial Periodic Paralysis Precedes attack. *2246*

405.91 Renovascular Hypertension A 50% or greater decrease in volume excreted and a 15% or greater decrease in sodium concentration indicated renal artery obstruction and reversible renovascular hypertension. *1108 2440*

428.00 Congestive Heart Failure As the heart improves, urinary output increases but is low in sodium and has a high specific gravity. *0151* Patients may, when renal function is intact, reduce urinary sodium concentration virtually to zero. They may retain nearly 100% of the sodium offered them. Hypervolemia and edema result. *1108* Sodium retention. *1985 0731*

492.80 Pulmonary Emphysema *2467*

496.00 Chronic Obstructive Lung Disease Hypercapnic patients showed low effective renal plasma flow, impaired water and sodium excretion compared to normocapnic patients and normal controls. *0698*

537.00 Pyloric Stenosis, Acquired *2467*

558.90 Diarrhea *2467*

572.20 Hepatic Encephalopathy Hyponatremia (< 130 mmol/L) occurred in 61% of patients with hepatic failure due to decompensated cirrhosis of liver. *0379*

572.40 Hepatic Failure Marked sodium retention (9 mmol/24 h) may occur in fulminant hepatic failure when GFR exceeds 40 mL/min. *2536* Hyponatremia (< 130 mmol/L) occurred in 61% of patients with hepatic failure due to decompensated cirrhosis of liver. *0379*

579.90 Malabsorption, Cause Unspecified *2467*

580.00 Acute Poststreptococcal Glomerulonephritis Very low (< 15 mmol/L). *0995* Reflects avid salt reabsorption in the distal nephron. *0062*

581.90 Nephrotic Syndrome Results from increased aldosterone secretion and reduced GFR. *0151*

584.00 Acute Renal Failure *0151*

585.00 Chronic Renal Failure *0151*

642.40 Pre-Eclampsia Reduced to a greater extent than that of normal pregnancy. *2104*

642.60 Eclampsia Reduced to a greater extent than that of normal pregnancy. *2104*

780.80 Hyperhidrosis *2467*

Urine Increase

162.90 Malignant Neoplasm of Bronchus and Lung Excessive excretion due to water retention resulting from abnormally regulated secretion of ADH. *0151* Inappropriate secretion of ADH is associated with hyponatremia, decreased serum osmolality, and inappropriately high sodium concentration in the urine. The entire syndrome resolves following resection of the tumor. *0962*

191.90 Malignant Neoplasm of Brain Urine is almost always hypertonic to plasma *0062* .

198.30 Secondary Malignant Neoplasm of Brain Urine is almost always hypertonic to plasma *0062* .

225.90 Benign Neoplasm of Brain and CNS Urine is almost always hypertonic to plasma *0062* .

250.00 Diabetes Mellitus Osmotic diuresis secondary to hyperglycemia. *2540 2467*

252.00 Hyperparathyroidism *2540*

253.40 Anterior Pituitary Hypofunction Increased output in Addison's Disease and hypopituitarism. *0619* There is diminished tubular sodium reabsorption because of adrenal cortical steroid deficiency. The urine volume is increased, with loss of the normal diurnal variation, and an increased sodium and chloride concentration. *0619*

255.40 Adrenal Cortical Hypofunction Inability of the renal tubules to reabsorb sodium and water and relative inability to excrete potassium. *0619 2467*

260.00 Protein Malnutrition Normal or increased. *2467*

276.50 Dehydration *2467*

320.90 Meningitis (Bacterial) Urine is almost always hypertonic to plasma *0062* .

323.92 Encephalomyelitis Urine is almost always hypertonic to plasma *0062* .

401.10 Essential Benign Hypertension Significantly higher excretion in subjects with diastolic blood pressure between 95 and 109 mm Hg than in the group with diastolic blood pressure below 90 mm Hg. *0596*

431.00 Cerebral Hemorrhage Urine is almost always hypertonic to plasma *0062* .

434.00 Cerebral Thrombosis Urine is almost always hypertonic to plasma *0062* .

434.10 Cerebral Embolism Urine is almost always hypertonic to plasma *0062* .

560.90 Intestinal Obstruction Specific gravity increases, with deficit of water and electrolytes unless pre-existing renal disease is present. *2467*

572.40 Hepatic Failure In hepatic failure patients, sodium loss in urine may be high if the GFR falls below 24 mL/min. *2536*

584.00 Acute Renal Failure In acute tubular necrosis the kidney loses its ability to reabsorb sodium, and an increased concentration of urine sodium with a relative decrease in urine potassium will be noted. *0433*

585.00 Chronic Renal Failure *2467*

588.81 Proximal Renal Tubular Acidosis *2467*

588.82 Distal Renal Tubular Acidosis Characteristic complication of metabolic acidosis. *2050*

753.12 Medullary Cystic Disease Characteristic renal salt wasting. *0277*

Sodium (continued)

Urine   Normal

253.50 **Diabetes Insipidus**   *2467*

359.11 **Progressive Muscular Dystrophy**   The differences between the patient group and the control group for sodium and potassium in serum and urine were significant. The pathologically elevated sodium potassium ratio in skeletal muscle is not due to increased aldosterone or other causes of renal wastage of potassium. *0816*

CSF   Increase

242.90 **Hyperthyroidism**   *0619*

Feces   Increase

1.00 **Cholera**   Fecal concentrations are increased above normal, but are consistently lower than the plasma values. *0151*

193.01 **Medullary Carcinoma of Thyroid**   About 33% of patients with medullary carcinoma have watery diarrhea with stools characteristically containing increased sodium and potassium content. *2199*

273.22 **Heavy Chain Disease (Alpha)**   Patients usually present with chronic diarrhea, hypocalcemia, and excessive fecal losses of water and electrolytes. *2538*

273.23 **Heavy Chain Disease (Gamma)**   Patients usually present with chronic diarrhea, hypocalcemia, and excessive fecal losses of water and electrolytes. *2538*

Red Blood Cells   Decrease

585.00 **Chronic Renal Failure**   Erythrocytes sodium values showed a wide range, from very high to very low, and the rate constant for Na+ efflux was found to be higher than normal. *1162*

Red Blood Cells   Increase

84.00 **Malaria**   The content of infected and uninfected erythrocytes is increased as a result of increased permeability. *1058*

242.90 **Hyperthyroidism**   *0902*

585.00 **Chronic Renal Failure**   Erythrocytes sodium values showed a wide range, from very high to very low, and the rate constant for Na efflux was found to be higher than normal. *1162* In 25% of uremic patients. *2515*

948.00 **Burns**   Reduced concentration in plasma, but an increase in RBC concentration occurs even in minor burns. *2104*

Saliva   Decrease

255.10 **Adrenal Cortical Hyperfunction (Mineralocorticoid Excess)**   Low sweat and salivary concentration while total body exchangeable sodium is high. *1108*

428.00 **Congestive Heart Failure**   *2467*

Saliva   Increase

277.00 **Cystic Fibrosis**   Submaxillary saliva has slightly increased chloride and sodium but not potassium; however, considerable overlap with normal individuals prevents diagnostic usage. *2467*

714.00 **Rheumatoid Arthritis**   The concentrations of salivary sodium and IgA were significantly elevated in 24% of patients. 80% of the patients with elevated sodium and IgA concentrations had keratoconjunctivitis sicca as well. *0162*

Sweat   Decrease

255.10 **Adrenal Cortical Hyperfunction (Mineralocorticoid Excess)**   Low sweat and salivary concentration while total body exchangeable sodium is high. *1108*

Sweat   Increase

277.00 **Cystic Fibrosis**   A sweat sodium value of above 70 mmol/L is consistent with the diagnosis. *0433* Striking increase in sweat sodium and chloride is present in virtually all homozygous patients. Present throughout life from time of birth and is not related to severity of disease or organ involvement. *2467* Sweat sodium and T$_3$ normalized after 1 y of oral essential fatty acid therapy. *1987* *0151*

577.10 **Chronic Pancreatitis**   Concentrations exceeded 90 mmol/L in 26% and 120 mmol/L in 6% of noncalcific pancreatitis patients. *0111*

Somatomedin

Serum   Decrease

253.40 **Anterior Pituitary Hypofunction**   Dwarfism. *1443*

260.00 **Protein Malnutrition**   *1443*

570.00 **Acute and Subacute Necrosis of Liver**   *1443*

571.90 **Cirrhosis of Liver**   *1443*

Serum   Increase

253.00 **Acromegaly**   *1443*

Somatomedin-C

Serum   Decrease

244.90 **Hypothyroidism**   *2634*

260.00 **Protein Malnutrition**   Decreased *2634*

571.90 **Cirrhosis of Liver**   *2634*

572.40 **Hepatic Failure**   *2634*

Serum   Increase

253.00 **Acromegaly**   *2634*

255.10 **Adrenal Cortical Hyperfunction (Mineralocorticoid Excess)**   *2634*

Somatostatin

CSF   Decrease

300.40 **Depressive Neurosis**   Low levels appear to be a state marker for episodes of depression. *0023*

331.00 **Alzheimer's Disease**   Significantly lower mean CSF levels than other neurological patients. All 11 patients with Alzheimer's Disease or Parkinsons Disease dementia had levels well below 21.8 ng/ml. *2119* Significant difference from elderly normal subjects but did not differ from normal younger subjects *1881* Significantly decreased compared to other neurological patients (14.6 pg/mL versus 26.7 pg/mL) *2119*

332.00 **Parkinsons's Disease**   Significantly lower mean CSF levels than other neurological patients. All 11 patients with Alzheimer's Disease or Parkinsons Disease dementia had levels well below 21.8 ng/ml. *2119* Significantly decreased in demented Parkinsonian patient *2119*

Sorbitol Dehydrogenase

Serum   Increase

120.00 **Schistosomiasis**   Markedly elevated upon admission, during treatment, and at follow-up. *2026*

250.10 **Diabetic Acidosis**   In some instances, mostly in severe cases, especially with severe circulatory failure and liver enlargement. *0155*

994.50 **Exercise**   Significant effect after 2 h march. *2092*

Specific Gravity

Serum   Increase

1.00 **Cholera**   Due to severe dehydration. *0151*

Urine   Decrease

9.00 **Gastroenteritis and Colitis**   *0433*

70.00 **Viral Hepatitis**   Concentrating ability is sometimes decreased. *2467*

202.52 **Histiocytosis X**   Low, fixed specific gravity of urine is characteristic in patients with hypothalamic involvement. *0433*

244.90 **Hypothyroidism**   May occur to a mild degree. *0565*

252.00 **Hyperparathyroidism**   Polyuria due to the inability to concentrate the urine. Related to the hypercalcemia and does not aid in differential diagnosis. *0433*

253.00 **Acromegaly**   Usually 1.001-1.005. *0151*

253.50 **Diabetes Insipidus**   Always abnormal. *0433* Polyuria and hyposthenuria. *2246* *0962*

255.10 Adrenal Cortical Hyperfunction (Mineralocorticoid Excess) Less than 1.015 due to impaired ability to concentrate urine. *0995*

275.10 Hepatolenticular Degeneration Reduced concentrating ability; 20% had maximum specific gravities of < 1.015 on overnight specimens. *2278*

282.60 Sickle Cell Anemia Despite the relative benignity of sickle cell trait, adults with this condition are unable to concentrate their urine and characteristically have a urine specific gravity around 1.010. *0433* Specific gravity is low reflecting the loss of renal concentrating ability due to repeated microinfarcts in the medulla of the kidneys. *0999*

405.91 Renovascular Hypertension Renal functional impairment. *0962*

428.00 Congestive Heart Failure May be high during the phases of salt and water retention and low during periods of diuresis. *1108*

580.01 Glomerulonephritis (Focal) Concentrating capacity is impaired, with urine specific gravity around 1.010. *0962*

580.40 Glomerulonephritis (Rapidly Progressive) Concentrating capacity is impaired, with urine specific gravity around 1.010. *0962*

584.00 Acute Renal Failure A low, fixed specific gravity indicates tubular damage. *0433*

585.00 Chronic Renal Failure With decreased renal function, specific gravity is 1.020, as renal impairment is more severe, specific gravity approaches 1.010. The test is sensitive for early loss of renal function, but a normal finding does not necessarily rule out active kidney disease. *2467*

590.00 Chronic Pyelonephritis The urine is usually of low specific gravity or at least no more than isosmotic plasma. *0433*

590.10 Acute Pyelonephritis Urine concentrating ability is impaired relatively early. *0962*

753.12 Medullary Cystic Disease Characteristic hyposthenuria. *0277*

753.13 Medullary Sponge Kidney Impaired ability to concentrate or acidify the urine maximally has been reported. *0906 0277*

994.50 Exercise Reduced ability to concentration at all rates. *1205*

Urine Increase

71.00 Rabies The urine is concentrated, particularly when the body temperature is elevated and/or the kidney function is diminished. *0433*

250.10 Diabetic Acidosis *0962*

428.00 Congestive Heart Failure Urine is concentrated, with specific gravity 1.020. Oliguria is a characteristic feature of right-sided failure. *2467* May be high during the phases of salt and water retention and low during periods of diuresis. *1108*

560.90 Intestinal Obstruction Urinalysis may be entirely normal in intestinal obstruction with the exception of relatively high specific gravity. *0433* Increases with deficit of water and electrolytes unless pre-existing renal disease is present. Urinalysis helps rule out renal colic, diabetic acidosis, etc. *2467*

580.00 Acute Poststreptococcal Glomerulonephritis May occur early in the course of the illness. *0995*

584.00 Acute Renal Failure May be high in the early stage. *2468*

Pleural Effusion Decrease

423.10 Constrictive Pericarditis Transudate (< 1.016). *0062*

571.90 Cirrhosis of Liver Transudate (< 1.016). *0062*

581.90 Nephrotic Syndrome Transudate (< 1.016). *0062*

585.00 Chronic Renal Failure Transudate (< 1.016). *0062*

Pleural Effusion Increase

6.00 Amebiasis Exudate (> 1.016). *0062*

11.00 Pulmonary Tuberculosis Exudate (> 1.016). *0062*

162.90 Malignant Neoplasm of Bronchus and Lung Exudate (> 1.016). *0062*

197.00 Secondary Malignant Neoplasm of Respiratory System Exudate (> 1.016). *0062*

244.90 Hypothyroidism Exudate (> 1.016). *0062*

415.10 Pulmonary Embolism and Infarction Exudate (> 1.016). *0062*

480.90 Viral Pneumonia Exudate (> 1.016). *0062*

482.90 Bacterial Pneumonia Exudate (> 1.016). *0062*

483.01 Mycoplasma Pneumoniae Exudate (> 1.016). *0062*

577.00 Acute Pancreatitis Exudate (> 1.016). *0062*

577.10 Chronic Pancreatitis Exudate (> 1.016). *0062*

577.20 Pancreatic Cyst and Pseudocyst Exudate (> 1.016). *0062*

710.00 Systemic Lupus Erythematosus Exudate (> 1.016). *0062*

Ascitic Fluid Decrease

571.20 Laennec's or Alcoholic Cirrhosis Ascitic fluid is usually a transudate with protein < 3.0 g/dL and specific gravity < 1.016. However, protein may exceed 2.5 g/dL in up to 30% of patients. *2199*

571.90 Cirrhosis of Liver Ascitic fluid is usually a transudate with protein < 3.0 g/dL and specific gravity < 1.016. However, protein may exceed 2.5 g/dL in up to 30% of patients. *2199*

Peritoneal Fluid Increase

567.90 Peritonitis Exudate with specific gravity > 1.016 usually found with tuberculous and bacterial peritonitis. *2199*

Sulfate

Serum Increase

584.00 Acute Renal Failure In metabolic acidosis accompanying renal failure. Serves as a reliable index of insufficiency. *2104*

585.00 Chronic Renal Failure In metabolic acidosis accompanying renal failure. Serves as a reliable index of insufficiency. *2104*

Urine Decrease

570.00 Acute and Subacute Necrosis of Liver Patients with liver disease often have reduced urinary sulfate. *2104*

571.90 Cirrhosis of Liver Patients with liver disease often have reduced urinary sulfate. *2104*

572.00 Liver Abscess (Pyogenic) Patients with liver disease often have reduced urinary sulfate. *2104*

T_3 Uptake

Serum Decrease

244.90 Hypothyroidism Mean T_3 was 76.7 ± 76 ng/mL, ranging from 20-600. 72 of 100 patients had subnormal values. No correlation with TSH was found. *1323*

245.20 Hashimoto's Thyroiditis Mean value was 76.7 ± 76 ng/dL, ranging from 20-600. 72 of 100 patients had subnormal values. No correlation was found with TSH. *1323* In the far advanced stage of thyroid destruction, all tests show the results of hypothyroidism. *2035*

650.00 Pregnancy From about the 10th week of pregnancy until up to 12th week postpartum. *2467* Combination of raised T_4 and low resin uptake due to increased TBG concentration occurs in pregnancy, estrogen therapy, and oral contraceptive use. *2612*

Serum Increase

174.90 Malignant Neoplasm of Breast Slight but significant differences were found, with a higher mean value for thyrotropin, reverse-T_3 and T_3-resin uptake and a lower mean value for T_3. *0014*

242.90 Hyperthyroidism Elevated in 57% of 21 patients in an elderly population. 9 of the patients with normal T_3 uptakes had elevated PBI. T_3 uptake was not a useful indicator of metabolic status. *0512* May be present. *0962*

245.10 Subacute Thyroiditis *0962*

260.00 Protein Malnutrition T_3 resin uptake is significantly elevated in the acute stage of kwashiorkor and returns to normal after 2 weeks of appropriate refeeding. *1123*

358.00 Myasthenia Gravis Thyrotoxicosis may occur in conjunction with this disease. *0995*

581.90 Nephrotic Syndrome Urinary loss of TBG results in lowering of most blood thyroid hormones and increased T_3 uptake. *0962* Low T_4 and raised resin uptake due to reduced TBG concentration occurs with protein loss. *2612*

640.00 Threatened Abortion *2467*

Serum Normal

193.01 Medullary Carcinoma of Thyroid *2467*

240.00 Simple Goiter *2467*

T$_3$ Uptake (continued)

Serum   Normal (continued)

250.00   Diabetes Mellitus   *2467*

253.00   Acromegaly   Thyroid functions were all found to be normal in active disease, contrary to several earlier reports. *0458*

255.40   Adrenal Cortical Hypofunction   *2467*

300.00   Anxiety Neurosis   *2467*

Taurine

Plasma   Decrease

296.80   Manic Depressive Disorder   Mean concentration in depressed patients free of any drugs and under drug therapy was 29 ± 2 and 25 ± 3 nmol/mL platelet-free plasma respectively. Normal mean was 45 ± 4 nmol/mL. *2313*

300.40   Depressive Neurosis   Mean concentration in depressed patients free of any drugs and under drug therapy was 29 ± 2 and 25 ± 3 nmol/mL platelet-free plasma respectively. Normal mean was 45 ± 4 nmol/mL. *2313*

Urine   Increase

281.00   Pernicious Anemia   Amino aciduria with an excess excretion of taurine, especially if there is associated subacute combined degeneration of the spinal cord. Amino aciduria does not occur in other megaloblastic anemias. *2468*   May be slight excess of urinary amino acids, especially taurine. *0755 2364*

281.20   Folic Acid Deficiency Anemia   May be slight excess of urinary amino acids, especially taurine. *0755 2364*

990.00   Effects of X-Ray Irradiation   Tissue destruction. *1556*

Testosterone

Serum   Increase

706.10   Acne   Elevated in 38% of 26 females with acne between ages 27 and 42 y. *2074*

Serum   Normal

706.10   Acne   Free and total testosterone were measured in 34 men and 14 women suffering from acne but otherwise healthy. *2294*

Plasma   Decrease

253.00   Acromegaly   Have been reported to be low in the presence of normal gonadotropin levels. *0433*

253.40   Anterior Pituitary Hypofunction   Decreased in hypopituitarism and hypogonadism. *0619*

255.00   Adrenal Cortical Hyperfunction (Glucocorticoid Excess)   Decreased in male patients. *1450*

257.20   Testicular Hypofunction   Decreased in primary and secondary hypogonadism. *2467 2468*

275.00   Hemochromatosis   Found in 12 of 12 patients. *0199*

282.60   Sickle Cell Anemia   Basal serum testosterone, dihydrotestosterone, and androstenedione were lower in 32 adult male patients. Secondary sex characteristics were abnormal in 29 of 32 patients. *0005*

303.90   Alcoholism   After abstaining from alcohol and cigarettes for one week, the testosterone levels in 30 alcoholics allowed alcohol during the second week dropped rapidly and significantly, but did not correlate with amount of alcohol ingested. *1805*

758.70   Klinefelter's Syndrome (XXY)   Reported to be low in most studies, although there is considerable overlap between normal males and Klinefelter males. Generally higher in mosaics than in pure Klinefelter patients. *1090*   Quite variable but often tends to be midway between the normal male and female. *0962*

Plasma   Increase

174.90   Malignant Neoplasm of Breast   Plasma hormone concentrations were measured in sequential samples from 6 women and were compared to concentrations in 6 control women matched for age, years since menopause, and parity. Concentrations in each cancer patient were significantly higher than in each matched control. *1543*

220.00   Benign Neoplasm of Ovary   Plasma testosterone levels are elevated and confirmatory. *0433*

244.90   Hypothyroidism   *1731*

256.41   Stein-Leventhal Syndrome   On occasion. *0995*

600.00   Benign Prostatic Hypertrophy   Increased; especially in older patients. *0972*

650.00   Pregnancy   Mean concentration in pregnant women with female fetuses was 597 ± 167 pg/mL, and in women with male fetuses, mean value was 828 ± 298 pg/mL, significantly higher (p = < 0.01). Increases began in week 7, reaching a maximum by 9-11. *1284   1031*

758.80   Syndromes Due to Sex Chromosome Abnormalities   In XYY males. *0619*

Plasma   Normal

255.40   Adrenal Cortical Hypofunction   Androgen deficiency is not clinically evident because testosterone production is unimpaired. *2612*

Tetrahydroaldosterone

Urine   Increase

255.10   Adrenal Cortical Hyperfunction (Mineralocorticoid Excess)   Patients with primary aldosteronism can be shown at some time to have increased urinary excretion of aldosterone and/or tetrahydroaldosterone. *1108*

Thiamine

Serum   Decrease

242.90   Hyperthyroidism   Secondary to increased metabolic processes. *2540*

265.00   Thiamine (B$_1$) Deficiency   *2468*

Urine   Decrease

265.00   Thiamine (B$_1$) Deficiency   Urinary excretion of thiamine of 0-14 mg in 24 h has been reported in beriberi, and early signs have been observed with excretions of < 40 mg/24 h. *0151*

Threonine

Serum   Decrease

66.00   Phlebotomus Fever   Most free serum amino acids are depressed in sandfly fever and other mild-moderate infections. *0122*

585.00   Chronic Renal Failure   Mean concentration decreased with deteriorating renal function in children. *0192*

Urine   Decrease

714.00   Rheumatoid Arthritis   *2104*

Urine   Increase

270.02   Hartnup Disease   5-20 X normal values. *2246   0995*

270.03   Cystinosis   Nonspecific pattern of aminoaciduria. Fanconi's syndrome. *0995*

275.10   Hepatolenticular Degeneration   *0503*

Thrombin Time

Plasma   Increase

84.00   Malaria   Consistent with the diagnosis of disseminated intravascular coagulation. *1058*

205.00   Myelocytic Leukemia (Acute)   Intravascular clotting has been demonstrated in occasional patients. *0890*

205.10   Myelocytic Leukemia (Chronic)   Intravascular clotting has been documented for rare patients. *0890*

206.00   Monocytic Leukemia   With disseminated intravascular clotting. *1552*

273.30   Waldenström's Macroglobulinemia   Coagulation defect detected most frequently is prolongation of the thrombin time. *2538*

286.31   Congenital Dysfibrinogenemia   Usually prolonged, but in some cases no clot forms at all. *2538*   Abnormally long. *2246*

286.34 **Congenital Afibrinogenemia** Corrected by the addition of normal plasma or normal fibrinogen to the patient's plasma. *2538* Infinite. *2246 0433*

286.60 **Disseminated Intravascular Coagulopathy** Prolonged because of consumption of clotting factors and the anticoagulant effects of fibrin degradation products. *2538*

630.00 **Hydatidiform Mole** Mean time was 21.1/16.6 s in patients compared to 17.6/15.9 in normal pregnancy. Prolonged time and associated reduction of partial thromboplastin time indicates hypercoagulability and high fibrinogen turnover rate. *1430*

Plasma   Normal

286.01 **Hemophilia** *0962 0995 2246*

286.10 **Christmas Disease** *2246*

286.20 **Factor XI Deficiency** *2246*

286.32 **Factor XII Deficiency** *0433 2246*

286.33 **Factor XIII Deficiency** *0433 2246*

286.35 **Factor V Deficiency** *0433 0995 2246*

286.36 **Factor X Deficiency** *0433 0995 2246*

286.37 **Factor VII Deficiency** *0995 2246*

286.38 **Factor II Deficiency** *0433 2246*

286.40 **Von Willebrand's Disease** *0962 2246*

287.10 **Thrombasthenia (Glanzmann's)** *2246*

287.30 **Idiopathic Thrombocytopenic Purpura** *2246*

446.60 **Thrombotic Thrombocytopenic Purpura** *2246*

Thromboglobulin, Beta

Serum   Increase

451.90 **Phlebitis and Thrombophlebitis** Increased in 7 cases. *2025*

Thromboplastin Generation

Blood   Increase

273.30 **Waldenström's Macroglobulinemia** Evidence of impaired platelet function. *2538*

286.01 **Hemophilia** Due to deficient function of the adsorbed plasma reagent. *2552 2538*

286.10 **Christmas Disease** In mild deficiency, may be the only abnormal test. *2467* In contrast to hemophilia A, the abnormality resides in the serum rather than in the adsorbed plasma. *2538*

286.20 **Factor XI Deficiency** The most marked abnormality is found when the patient's adsorbed plasma and serum are incubated together. *2538*

286.35 **Factor V Deficiency** Abnormal when the reaction mixture contains adsorbed plasma from the patient, but is normal when serum from the patient is used. *0995 2538 2246*

286.36 **Factor X Deficiency** *2538*

287.10 **Thrombasthenia (Glanzmann's)** Contact activation is abnormal, resulting in abnormal TGT test. *2552*

571.90 **Cirrhosis of Liver** Reflects various abnormalities. *2467*

581.90 **Nephrotic Syndrome** Has been noted. *1249*

710.00 **Systemic Lupus Erythematosus** The type of anticoagulant most commonly found inhibits the conversion of prothrombin to thrombin and exhibits prolonged thromboplastin and prothrombin times. *0962*

Blood   Normal

238.40 **Polycythemia Vera** Conventional coagulation tests are usually normal. *0009 2538*

286.31 **Congenital Dysfibrinogenemia** *2538*

286.35 **Factor V Deficiency** Abnormal when the reaction mixture contains adsorbed plasma from the patient but is normal when serum from the patient is used. *2538* Abnormal when the reaction mixture includes the serum reagent prepared for the patient. *2538* Abnormal results. *2246*

286.37 **Factor VII Deficiency** *2246*

287.10 **Thrombasthenia (Glanzmann's)** *2246*

CSF   Increase

320.90 **Meningitis (Bacterial)** Increased thromboplastic activity is about 145 fold more common in bacterial meningitis than in viral meningitis. *2392*

Thromboxane B$_2$

Serum   Decrease

346.00 **Migraine** The patients ability to produce Thromboxane B$_2$ was reduced in both children and adults with migraine. *1245*

Thymol Turbidity

Serum   Increase

11.00 **Pulmonary Tuberculosis** *0619*

18.00 **Disseminated Tuberculosis** *0619*

70.00 **Viral Hepatitis** Usually increased during acute phase. *2467* More useful in assessing the rate of recovery, although it may be increased early in the disease. It remains positive in convalescence after the cephalin cholesterol reaction has become normal. *0619*

75.00 **Infectious Mononucleosis** Reflected the presence and extent of hepatic damage, and paralleled the severity of subjective symptoms in 36 patients. *1912* Show abnormal results in most cases. *1319*

78.50 **Cytomegalic Inclusion Disease** Slight increased which becomes more marked with clinical hepatitis in some cases. *2468*

100.00 **Leptospirosis** Jaundice may appear at the end of the 1st week of fever. Liver tests show hepatic decompensation of the intrahepatic type. *2368 0992*

135.00 **Sarcoidosis** Increased due to alteration of serum proteins. *2467*

155.00 **Malignant Neoplasm of Liver** *0503*

157.90 **Malignant Neoplasm of Pancreas** May be slightly elevated, usually normal. *0433*

203.00 **Multiple Myeloma** In both beta- and gamma- types. *0619*

277.41 **Dubin-Johnson Syndrome** May be increased. *2467*

304.90 **Drug Dependence (Opium and Derivatives)** Thymol turbidity and cephalin flocculation are commonly increased in 75% of patients. *2468*

421.00 **Bacterial Endocarditis** Increased due to altered serum proteins and increased gamma globulins. *2467*

423.10 **Constrictive Pericarditis** Increased in some cases. *2467*

570.00 **Acute and Subacute Necrosis of Liver** Active liver disease; in active hepatitis thymol turbidity becomes positive later than transaminase elevation; may remain positive after cephalin flocculation has become negative. In cirrhosis it may be normal. *2467*

571.20 **Laennec's or Alcoholic Cirrhosis** Possibly the bile-cholesterol-phospholipid combination has a stabilizing effect on the serum proteins. *0619*

571.49 **Chronic Active Hepatitis** Usually increased. *2467*

571.60 **Biliary Cirrhosis** Usually increased. *2467*

571.90 **Cirrhosis of Liver** Possibly the bile-cholesterol-phospholipid combination has a stabilizing effect on the serum proteins. *0619*

572.40 **Hepatic Failure** *0503*

573.30 **Toxic Hepatitis** Normal or slight increase. *2467*

576.20 **Extrahepatic Biliary Obstruction** Normal or may later become only slightly increased. *2467*

710.00 **Systemic Lupus Erythematosus** Frequently positive and reflects nonspecific serum protein abnormalities. *0962*

714.00 **Rheumatoid Arthritis** Characteristically abnormal when the arthritis is active. *0433*

985.00 **Toxic Effects of Non-medicinal Metals** Hepatotoxicity may occur with arsenicals. *1446*

Serum   Normal

277.30 **Amyloidosis** Usually normal. *0125*

571.20 **Laennec's or Alcoholic Cirrhosis** May be normal. *2467*

571.90 **Cirrhosis of Liver** May be normal. *2467*

642.40 **Pre-Eclampsia** No abnormal results were found in a study of 20 mild and 20 severe pre-eclamptic patients. *2597* Usually normal. *0429 0387*

Thymol Turbidity (continued)

Serum Normal (continued)

642.60 **Eclampsia** Usually normal. 0429 0387

650.00 **Pregnancy** Found to be normal in a study of 40 normal pregnant women. 2597 Usually normal. 0429 0387

Thyro-Binding Index

Serum Normal

250.00 **Diabetes Mellitus** Serum T_4, T_3RU free T_4 and TSH in patients prior to therapy was not significantly different from normal subjects. 1203

Thyroid Stimulating Hormone (TSH)

Serum Decrease

242.90 **Hyperthyroidism** Plasma TSH levels are actually subnormal in Graves' disease in its hyperthyroid stage, normal in its euthyroid stage, and supranormal if the patient becomes hypothyroid. 2035 Significantly reduced, but may occasionally fall in the normal range. 0960 0962 2612

244.90 **Hypothyroidism** Not increased in pituitary hypothyroidism and does not respond to TRH administration. 2540

253.00 **Acromegaly** The expanding tumor within the pituitary fossa may cause a diminution of secretion of other pituitary hormones. Loss of thyroid-stimulating hormone will cause hypothyroidism. 0960

253.40 **Anterior Pituitary Hypofunction** May be deficient and lead to secondary hypothyroidism. 2612 Characterized by absent or reduced production and release. 1108

650.00 **Pregnancy** 2467

758.70 **Klinefelter's Syndrome (XXY)** Administration of TRH revealed a decreased TSH reserve in the Klinefelter patients. 2203

Serum Increase

84.00 **Malaria** 2487

162.90 **Malignant Neoplasm of Bronchus and Lung** ACTH producing small cell carcinoma. 0536

174.90 **Malignant Neoplasm of Breast** Mean concentrations higher than in normals or other cancers. The difference was statistically significant only in those with advanced disease. 12% of the early cancer and 15% of the advanced had elevated plasma concentrations. 1976 Elevated in 148 patients (38%) with breast cancer. Mean survival and disease free intervals were shorter for patients with elevated TSH, but not significantly. 0033 Slight but significant differences were found with a higher mean value for thyrotropin, reverse-T_3 and T_3-resin uptake. 0014

240.00 **Simple Goiter** Normal or slightly increased. 0962

242.90 **Hyperthyroidism** Plasma TSH levels are actually subnormal in Graves' disease in its hyperthyroid stages, normal in its euthyroid stage, and supranormal if the patient becomes hypothyroid. 2035

244.90 **Hypothyroidism** Elevated in all patients, mean = 76.7 ± 55 µU/mL, range = 11-240. Mean values for patients < 20 y old was significantly higher than for older patients. 1323 Not increased in pituitary hypothyroidism and does not respond to TRH administration. 2540 Raised in all cases due to primary thyroid disease. 0960 2612

245.10 **Subacute Thyroiditis** Defective hormonal synthesis causes increased secretion of TSH. 0999 During recovery the TSH may be transiently elevated while T_4 is depressed, and then over a period of 2-3 months all tests return to normal. 0151

245.20 **Hashimoto's Thyroiditis** Elevated in all patients, mean = 76.7 ± 55 µU/mL, range = 11-240. Mean values for patients < 20 years old was significantly higher than for older patients. 1323 May occur as disease progresses. 2540 Endogenous serum TSH may be normal or moderately elevated. 0962 2035

571.20 **Laennec's or Alcoholic Cirrhosis** The mean serum TSH level was 3.1 µU/mL in the normals and 7.1 µU/mL in the cirrhotic patients. 15% of the hepatic patients had serum TSH values above 10 µU/mL. 1703

571.90 **Cirrhosis of Liver** The mean serum TSH level was 3.1 µU/mL in the normals and 7.1 µU/mL in the cirrhotic patients. 15% of the hepatic patients had serum TSH values above 10 µU/mL. 1703

630.00 **Hydatidiform Mole** 9 of 14 patients were hyperthyroid. Found in high concentrations in 13 preoperative patients. Close correlation with human chorionic gonadotropins suggests that the hCG molecule, when present in large amounts, stimulates thyroid function. 1044

Serum Normal

240.00 **Simple Goiter** Normal or slightly low. 0962 Usually. 2540 Normal in nontoxic goiter without autoimmune thyroiditis. 0960

245.20 **Hashimoto's Thyroiditis** Usually normal at time of diagnosis. 2540

250.00 **Diabetes Mellitus** Serum T_4, T_3RU free T_4 and TSH in patients prior to therapy was not significantly elevated compared to normals. 1203

252.00 **Hyperparathyroidism** 1226

253.00 **Acromegaly** Normal, even with thyroid enlargement. 0960

255.00 **Adrenal Cortical Hyperfunction (Glucocorticoid Excess)** 2467

260.00 **Protein Malnutrition** In frank kwashiorkor, concentrations were within the normal range throughout the entire course of dietary therapy, indicating that the children remained euthyroid. 1122

571.90 **Cirrhosis of Liver** Patients with severe alcoholic hepatitis often are euthyroid sick with low T_3 low T_4 and elevated rT_3 and normal TSH. 0335

585.00 **Chronic Renal Failure** 1617

650.00 **Pregnancy** 1113

758.70 **Klinefelter's Syndrome (XXY)** Usually normal. 1090

991.60 **Hypothermia** No change observed. 1754

Thyroxine Binding Globulin

Serum Decrease

2.00 **Typhoid Fever** Patients with fever had significantly lowered levels. 2327

38.00 **Septicemia** 2540

84.00 **Malaria** In patients with fever. 2327

242.90 **Hyperthyroidism** 2104

253.00 **Acromegaly** 0062

256.30 **Ovarian Hypofunction** Estrogen effect. 0995

260.00 **Protein Malnutrition** Decreased in nephrosis and other causes of marked hypoproteinemia. 2467 In hypoproteinemias. 2104

308.00 **Stress** 0062

571.90 **Cirrhosis of Liver** In chronic liver disease. 0062

579.00 **Celiac Sprue Disease** Decreased in hypoproteinemia. 2467

579.01 **Protein-Losing Enteropathy** Decreased in nephrosis and other causes of marked hypoproteinemia. 2467 2104

579.90 **Malabsorption, Cause Unspecified** Decreased with hypoproteinemia. 2467

581.90 **Nephrotic Syndrome** Urinary loss of TBG results in lowering of most blood thyroid hormones and increased T_3 uptake. 0962 Low T_4 and raised resin uptake due to reduced TBG concentration occurs with protein loss. 2612 2540 2104

Serum Increase

70.00 **Viral Hepatitis** Not infrequently. 2540 Increased level. 1887

193.00 **Malignant Neoplasm of Thyroid Gland** Elevations > 300 ng/mL were found only in patients with thyroid cancer, with or without irradiation, and in all stages. 0529

242.90 **Hyperthyroidism** Elevated in all patients and fell to normal with therapy; patients whose illness recurred after cessation of drug therapy had higher pretreatment thyroglobulin values and no fall during treatment. 0296 1108

244.90 **Hypothyroidism** Marked elevations found in the vast majority of patients with chronic lymphocytic thyroiditis, though an occasional patient will have low or nonmeasurable titers. 0999

245.10 **Subacute Thyroiditis** Serum thyroglobulin was elevated in 92% of 38 patients in the early stage of this disorder. After two months of corticosteroid treatment the levels were significantly decreased in 25 patients who could be rechecked. 1474 Elevated during acute stage 1106

245.20 Hashimoto's Thyroiditis Elevated and fell to normal with therapy; patients whose illness recurred after cessation of drug therapy had higher pretreatment thyroglobulin values and no fall during treatment. *0296*

256.00 Ovarian Hyperfunction Estrogen effect. *0995*

277.14 Acute Intermittent Porphyria *2540 2254*

555.90 Regional Enteritis or Ileitis Mean levels were high in these patients, mainly due to the high levels in female patients. *1150*

556.00 Ulcerative Colitis Mean serum values were high in these patients, mainly due to the high levels in female patients. *1150*

571.60 Biliary Cirrhosis *0062*

571.90 Cirrhosis of Liver Increased. *1887*

573.30 Toxic Hepatitis Increased levels. *1887*

650.00 Pregnancy Due to estrogen stimulation. *0791* Combination of raised T_4 and low resin uptake due to increased resin uptake due to increased TBG concentration occurs in pregnancy, estrogen therapy, and oral contraceptive use. *2612 2540 2104*

Serum   Normal

244.90 Hypothyroidism In some cases. *2467*

Thyroxine Binding Prealbumin

Serum   Decrease

650.00 Pregnancy Decreased 27% in late normal pregnancy. *2287 2286*

Thyroxine, Free

Serum   Decrease

244.90 Hypothyroidism *0186*

Serum   Increase

242.90 Hyperthyroidism *0186*

Serum   Normal

250.00 Diabetes Mellitus Serum T_4, T_3RU free T_4 and TSH in patients prior to therapy was not significantly different from controls. *1203*

252.00 Hyperparathyroidism *1226*

Thyroxine Index, Free (FTI)

Serum   Decrease

244.90 Hypothyroidism *2467*

Serum   Increase

242.90 Hyperthyroidism *2467*

571.90 Cirrhosis of Liver In 11 patients with decompensated cirrhosis, the free T_4 index and free T_4 by dialysis method and its absolute value were significantly raised, due to disturbance in the protein binding capacity. *0823*

Serum   Normal

650.00 Pregnancy Normal even though T_3 and T_4 alone are abnormal. *2467 1446*

Thyroxine (T₄)

Serum   Decrease

174.90 Malignant Neoplasm of Breast Four patients with plasma TSH levels above 85 $\mu U/mL$ had subnormal plasma T_4 levels. *1976*

240.00 Simple Goiter Normal or slightly low. *0962*

244.90 Hypothyroidism Average T_4 was 1.8 ± 1.5 $\mu g/dL$, range = 0.2-7.0. An inverse correlation was found with TSH and T_4, r = 0.73. *1323*

245.10 Subacute Thyroiditis May be subnormal late in the disease. *2540*

245.20 Hashimoto's Thyroiditis In the far advanced stage of thyroid destruction, all tests show the results of hypothyroidism. *2035* May be depressed, depending on the stage of development of the process. *0151* Average T_4 was 1.8 ± 1.5 $\mu g/dL$, range = 0.2-7.0. An inverse correlation was found with TSH and T_4, r = 0.73. *1323* Normal in 25 euthyroid, reduced in 22 hypothyroid and increased in 4 hyperthyroid patients with Hashimoto's thyroiditis. No specific abnormalities in serum concentrations of thyroid hormones were found. *0832 0999 2540*

250.10 Diabetic Acidosis In 19 euthyroid patients with severe ketoacidosis, a 'low T_3 syndrome' was found, with lowered serum concentrations of T_3, increased reverse T_3, slightly low T_4 (T_4) and normal thyrotropin. *1663*

253.40 Anterior Pituitary Hypofunction Low or low normal levels are suggestive but not diagnostic. *2612*

260.00 Protein Malnutrition Decreased T_4 with hypoproteinemia. *2467*

579.00 Celiac Sprue Disease Decreased in hypoproteinemia. *2467 2415*

579.01 Protein-Losing Enteropathy Decreased T_4 with hypoproteinemia. *2467*

579.90 Malabsorption, Cause Unspecified Decreased with hypoproteinemia. *2467*

581.90 Nephrotic Syndrome Urinary loss of TBG results in lowering of most blood thyroid hormones and increased T_3 uptake. *0962* Low T_4 and raised resin uptake due to reduced TBG concentration occurs with protein loss. *2612 2540*

585.00 Chronic Renal Failure Significant decrease in total and free T_4; total T_4 mean = 5.3 ± 1.9 $\mu g/dL$. Levels were even further depleted in terminal failure. *1298* In 56% of 26 patients at initial hospitalization for this disorder. *0781* Normal or decreased *1617*

994.50 Exercise Significant effect with strenuous exercise. *2092*

Serum   Increase

2.00 Typhoid Fever Slightly increased in all patients. *1481* During fever both percentage of free T_4 and absolute free T_4 were elevated. *2327*

36.00 Meningococcal Meningitis Slightly increased in all patients. *1481*

70.00 Viral Hepatitis Not infrequently. *2540*

84.00 Malaria Stable or increasing in falciparum. *2487* Increased free T_4 during fever. *2327*

242.90 Hyperthyroidism May be present. *0962 0999*

245.10 Subacute Thyroiditis Elevated in 50% of patients. *1106* The association of a very low iodine uptake with an elevated T_4 is characteristic of the early phase of disease. *2540 0151*

245.20 Hashimoto's Thyroiditis Normal in 25 euthyroid, reduced in 22 hypothyroid and increased in 4 hyperthyroid patients with Hashimoto's thyroiditis. No specific abnormalities in serum concentrations of thyroid hormones were found. *0832*

304.90 Drug Dependence (Opium and Derivatives) Significantly raised in heroin addiction. *1053*

358.00 Myasthenia Gravis Thyrotoxicosis may occur in conjunction with this disease. *0995*

571.20 Laennec's or Alcoholic Cirrhosis The mean free T_4 value was significantly higher (3.3 ng/dL) than in the normal subjects (2.1 ng/dL). *1703*

571.90 Cirrhosis of Liver In 11 patients with decompensated cirrhosis, the free T_4 index and free T_4 by dialysis method and its absolute value were significantly raised, due to disturbance in the protein binding capacity. *0823*

630.00 Hydatidiform Mole 9 of 14 patients were hyperthyroid. T_4 varied from 18-34 mg/dL. *1044* In patients with gestational trophoblastic disease without signs of hyperthyroidism, the mean serum total and free T_4 concentrations were 43% and 92% higher than those in normal pregnancy. *1740*

642.40 Pre-Eclampsia The mean serum T_4 and free T_4 concentrations were significantly higher than those in normal pregnant women. *1740*

650.00 Pregnancy Elevation thought to be caused by an increase in T_4 binding protein secondary to high circulating-estrogen levels. *0999* Elevated in normal pregnancy, while free T_4 and free T_3 are normal. *1740* Combination of raised T_4 and low resin uptake due to increased TBG concentration occurs in pregnancy, estrogen therapy, and oral contraceptive use. *2612*

Thyroxine (T₄) *(continued)*

Serum   Normal

193.00 Malignant Neoplasm of Thyroid Gland Usually euthyroid. *1200*

240.00 Simple Goiter Normal or slightly low. *0962* Usually. *2540*

245.10 Subacute Thyroiditis May be normal with acute thyroiditis. *0151*

245.20 Hashimoto's Thyroiditis The majority of patients are euthyroid at diagnosis with normal T_3, T_4, free hormones and TSH. *1106* Normal in 25 euthyroid, reduced in 22 hypothyroid and increased in 4 hyperthyroid patients with Hashimoto's thyroiditis. No specific abnormalities in serum concentrations of thyroid hormones were found. *0832   0962*

250.00 Diabetes Mellitus Serum T_4, T_3RU free T_4 and TSH in patients prior to therapy was not significantly different from controls. *1203*

252.00 Hyperparathyroidism *1226*

253.00 Acromegaly Thyroid functions were all found to be normal in active disease, contrary to several earlier reports. *0458*

275.34 Familial Periodic Paralysis *2246*

Urine   Decrease

592.00 Kidney Calculus In male renal calcium stone patients (20-40 y) urinary T_4 is lower than in age-matched controls. *2097*

Urine   Increase

590.00 Chronic Pyelonephritis Urinary loss exceeds the normal mean 10-fold. *0733*

Transcortin

Serum   Decrease

256.30 Ovarian Hypofunction Estrogen effect. *0995*

Serum   Increase

256.00 Ovarian Hyperfunction Estrogen effect. *0995*

Trehalase

Serum   Increase

250.00 Diabetes Mellitus Increased but does not correlate with blood sugar concentration. *0155*

994.50 Exercise Observed to increase with exercise. *0804*

Urine   Increase

994.50 Exercise Observed to increase with exercise. *0804*

Triglycerides

Serum   Decrease

242.90 Hyperthyroidism Falls, but not in simple relation to the associated rise in the BMR. Diet has a variable effect on the blood level. *0812*

252.00 Hyperparathyroidism Levels were about 22% in females and 60% lower in males compared to controls. After operation levels normalized. *0401*

260.00 Protein Malnutrition *2468*

269.90 Deficiency State (Unspecified) *2467*

271.30 Lactosuria Significantly decreased in the lactose malabsorption group (after taking into account the effects of other variables). Other lipids and proteins were not different from the control group. *2022*

272.52 Abetalipoproteinemia Usually below accurate measuring capabilities of conventional lab methods. *2246*

282.00 Hereditary (Congenital) Spherocytosis The majority of values were low (15/18 children) but there was a greater scatter of triglyceride than cholesterol concentrations. *2109*

434.90 Brain Infarction In all patients a significant reduction in total lipids, cholesterol, triglyceride and all lipoproteins was demonstrated after the acute cerebrovascular accident presumedly due to the stress situation. *1192*

496.00 Chronic Obstructive Lung Disease Decreased in decompensated patients. Amount of decrease correlates with degree of hypoxemia. *2044*

994.50 Exercise *2104*

Serum   Increase

38.00 Septicemia Sepsis causes the concentration to increase. *0049*

70.00 Viral Hepatitis In 12 children a relationship was suggested between ALT and triglycerides, in which the triglycerides provide an energy substrate, thereby freeing glucose for alanine synthesis. *0026*

244.90 Hypothyroidism Thyroid hormone insufficiency results in abnormal lipid metabolism with minimal to marked increases in circulating levels of cholesterol and triglycerides. *0999   2540*

250.00 Diabetes Mellitus Higher values correlate with hyperglycemia and poorer control of diabetes; reduced by insulin therapy. *2467* Mean levels for children were elevated 120 ± 63 vs 85 ± 23 μg/dL for controls. 8 had hypercholesterolemia, 5 had hypertriglyceridemia, and 9 had combined hypercholesterolemia and hypertriglyceridemia. *0377* In 228 patients, a significant positive association between GGT and triglyceride concentration was found. May reflect hepatic microsomal *1517*

271.01 Von Gierke's Disease Types I and VI glycogen storage disease. *0619* Striking elevation. *1086 2246*

272.00 Type IIA Hyperlipoproteinemia Usually a marked elevation of plasma cholesterol and a modest elevation of plasma triglyceride. *1108* Normal to elevated at 100-400 mg/dL. *0962* Occasionally. Usually normal in heterozygotes but may at times be > 250 mg/dL. *2246   0433*

272.10 Type IV Hyperlipoproteinemia Seldom exceeds 1000 mg/dL. Cholesterol is usually < half when triglyceride exceeds 500 mg/dL. *0433* Characteristic increase in plasma triglyceride and VLDL cholesterol levels. *1108* Elevated, sometimes to an extreme degree. *0962* Values of 200-500 mg/dL are common. *2246   0999*

272.21 Type IIB Hyperlipoproteinemia Serum cholesterol and triglycerides are usually elevated to a similar extent. Neither generally exceeds 400 mg/dL and triglyceride levels are not more than 100 mg/dL higher than cholesterol levels. *0433*

272.22 Type III Hyperlipoproteinemia Cholesterol and triglycerides are usually elevated to a similar extent; levels often exceed 400 mg/dL. *0433* Increased in all 49 cases of type III. *1631* Usually range from 200-800, and tend to exceed cholesterol. *2246*

272.31 Type I Hyperlipoproteinemia Often exceed 1,000 mg/dL with only moderate elevation of cholesterol. *0433* Grossly elevated, range from 2,500-12,000 mg/dL in lipoprotein lipase deficiency. *2246   0915 2177 0619 0151*

272.32 Type V Hyperlipoproteinemia In 11 patients with type V hyperlipoproteinemia. *2177* Averages 10-20 X normal. *2246*

272.51 Tangier Disease Slight increase in homozygotes. *0151* Range from 150-330 mg/dL. *2246* Unique combination of low cholesterol and high triglycerides is indicative. *2246   0999*

274.00 Gout 75-84% of patients. *0717 0115 2246*

278.00 Obesity Hypertriglyceridemia is frequent. *0996*

281.00 Pernicious Anemia In relapse, increased free fatty acid and triglyceride concentrations but decreased concentrations of total cholesterol, unesterified cholesterol and all examined phospholipid fractions. *2471*

282.41 Thalassemia Major Significantly elevated mean concentrations were found in 50 children. *0547*

303.90 Alcoholism 19 (26%) of these male patients had serum concentrations > 150 mg/dL. *1402* 38% of the patients had a type IV hyperlipoproteinemia with elevated serum triglycerides still after 17 days of abstinence. *2472* Rise after ingestion of moderate amounts of alcohol due to increased hepatic production and release of lipoproteins. *0962*

308.00 Stress Stressful situations evoke catecholamine excretion, producing an increased circulating concentration with surprising speed. *2104*

401.00 Malignant Hypertension In 24 male patients, mean concentration was 93.4 ± 6.3 mg/dL compared to 76.1 ± 3.7 in controls. *0381*

401.10 Essential Benign Hypertension Frequently elevated. *0995*

405.91 Renovascular Hypertension Predisposes to development of arteriosclerosis. *0992*

410.90 Acute Myocardial Infarction Rises to peak in 3 weeks; the increase may persist for 1 year. *2467* Mean concentration was 92.5 ± 3.5 mg/dL in 69 male patients, compared to 76.1 ± 3.7 in controls. *0381* Tends to be moderately elevated for a few weeks following a brief decrease. *1108 0771*

414.00 Chronic Ischemic Heart Disease The severity of atherosclerosis was positively correlated with plasma concentration, especially in the younger patients (R = 0.29, P < 0.05), and (not significantly) with plasma cholesterol concentration. *0508* Studies of patients with coronary atherosclerotic heart disease and of their families have indicated a significantly higher incidence (16-44%) of elevated plasma cholesterol and/or triglyceride levels, usually classified as type II or type IV. *1108*

434.00 Cerebral Thrombosis Significant rise noticed in all patients. *0112*

440.00 Arteriosclerosis The severity of disease showed a slight positive correlation with plasma triglyceride concentrations, especially in the younger patients. *0508* Frequently found in 219 male and 63 female patients. No significant relationship was found between uric acid and triglyceride. *0108*

496.01 Alpha$_1$-Antitrypsin Deficiency Average 336 mg/dL. *0563*

570.00 Acute and Subacute Necrosis of Liver *2467*

571.20 Laennec's or Alcoholic Cirrhosis In fatty infiltration of the liver the serum cholesterol, triglyceride and total lipid concentrations were significantly increased, as compared with the normal values and with the figures obtained in the cases of chronic inflammatory liver disease. *0710* In 28 patients, 13 showed hypercholesterolemia, 16 increased serum triglyceride and 8 increased serum phospholipid. *1045*

571.60 Biliary Cirrhosis With time, all lipids rise, including triglycerides. *2238*

576.20 Extrahepatic Biliary Obstruction A marked and persistent elevation. The increase is of similar magnitude to that for cholesterol and phospholipid. Following relief of obstruction the triglycerides returned to normal. Associated with a clear serum and negative cold aggregation test in contrast to the changes in cases of endogenous (type IV) hypertriglyceridemia. *1606*

577.00 Acute Pancreatitis Often imparts a lactescence to the serum. Elevated because of a transient inhibition to chylomicron removal from the circulation. *0962* May reach 1,000 mg/dL or higher. *2199*

577.10 Chronic Pancreatitis Increase in cholesterol, phospholipids, and neutral fats. *0619*

581.90 Nephrotic Syndrome Elevated cholesterol with lipiduria can be demonstrated; however, phospholipids and triglycerides are even more consistently and strikingly elevated. *0503* Typically elevated. *0962*

585.00 Chronic Renal Failure Endogenous VLDL triglyceride production rate was significantly raised in 13 patients who were not on dialysis treatment. *0465* Characteristically increased. Type IV hyperlipoproteinemia occurs commonly secondary to renal failure. *1038* Hypertriglyceridemia was found in 43% of patients. 20 men had values > 200 mg/dL and 23 women had 150 mg/dL or greater. *2557* Increased mean plasma concentration in chronic failure. *1243* Present in most patients whether or not they are dialyzed. *1108 0151 0099*

650.00 Pregnancy Steep rise. *0930*

758.00 Down's Syndrome Plasma lipid levels were measured in 20 mongoloid and 16 nonmongoloid mentally retarded subjects. Significant elevations of plasma triglyceride levels were found in patients with Down's syndrome compared with mentally retarded controls. However, no significant difference was found in plasma cholesterol, phospholipid and free fatty acid levels between the mongoloids and control subjects. *1698*

770.80 Respiratory Distress Syndrome Plasma lipids, particularly triglycerides complexed with fibrins were elevated several-fold in patients with adult disease. Triglycerides complexed with fibrins were significantly higher in patients who died than in those who survived. *1324*

829.00 Fracture of Bone After traumatic fracture. *2468*

958.10 Fat Embolism *2467*

1013.00 Diet With high carbohydrate diet. *2104*

Serum Normal

272.21 Type IIB Hyperlipoproteinemia Normal to elevated at 100-400 mg/dL. *0962* Occasionally. Usually normal in heterozygotes but may at times be > 250 mg/dL. *2246* Occasionally normal. *0995*

272.51 Tangier Disease Some patients. *2246* May be normal in the postabsorptive state. *2246*

334.00 Friedreich's Ataxia Significantly higher in Friedreich's ataxia, but remained within the normal limit. *1091*

571.60 Biliary Cirrhosis Marked increase in total cholesterol and phospholipids takes place, with normal triglycerides; serum is not lipemic. *2467*

994.50 Exercise With relative reduction of unsaturated acid. *1109*

Tri-iodothyronine, Free

Serum Decrease
244.90 Hypothyroidism *0186*

Serum Increase
242.90 Hyperthyroidism *0186*

Tri-iodothyronine, Reverse

Serum Decrease
244.90 Hypothyroidism *1617*

Serum Increase
250.00 Diabetes Mellitus Prior to Rx. serum rT$_3$ was significantly higher than in normal controls. *1203*

571.20 Cirrhosis of Liver Patients with severe alcoholic hepatitis often are euthyroid sick with low T$_3$ low T$_4$ and elevated rT$_3$ and normal TSH. *0335*

Serum Normal
252.00 Hyperparathyroidism Despite the low serum total T$_3$ levels. *1226*

585.00 Chronic Renal Failure Reverse T$_3$ is normal but free reverse T$_3$ is usually elevated. *1617*

Tri-iodothyronine (T$_3$)

Serum Decrease
2.00 Typhoid Fever Patients with fever had significantly lowered levels. *2327* Significantly low in all patients. Fall in T$_3$ was inversely related to the degree of fever. *1481*

36.00 Meningococcal Meningitis Significantly low in all patients. Fall in T$_3$ is inversely related to the degree of fever. *1481*

84.00 Malaria Abruptly declined during falciparum infection. *2487* Patients with fever of infection had significantly lowered levels. *2327*

174.90 Malignant Neoplasm of Breast Slight but significant differences were found with a higher mean value for thyrotropin reverse T$_3$ and T$_3$ resin uptake and a lower mean value for T$_3$. *0014*

244.90 Hypothyroidism Usually decreased but may be normal in approximately 20% of patients. *2468 2540*

245.20 Hashimoto's Thyroiditis Normal in 25 euthyroid, reduced in 22 hypothyroid and increased in 4 hyperthyroid patients with Hashimoto's thyroiditis. No specific abnormalities in serum concentrations of thyroid hormones were found. *0832*

250.10 Diabetic Acidosis In 19 euthyroid patients with severe ketoacidosis a 'low T$_3$ syndrome' was found, with lowered serum concentrations of T$_3$, increased reverse T$_3$, slightly low T$_4$ (T$_4$), and normal thyrotropin. *1663*

252.00 Hyperparathyroidism Significantly lower in patients with primary hyperparathyroidism (118 ng/dL) than normal controls (147 ng/dL). There was a significant inverse correlation between serum levels of total T$_3$ and PTH. *1226*

260.00 Protein Malnutrition Protein-calorie malnutrition in a group of 43 children aged 18-30 months was characterized by a sharp fall in T$_3$ concentration to 25-30% of the mean value in controls. This decrease was significantly more pronounced in kwashiorkor of recent onset than in long-term. *1122* Mean serum reverse T$_3$ was elevated in patients with severe protein calorie malnutrition to 53 ng/dL. In the same patients after feeing treatment the value dropped to 22 ng/dL. *0394*

410.90 Acute Myocardial Infarction Decreased to 66% at day 9 and then returned to normal within 2 months. *2215*

Tri-iodothyronine (T₃) *(continued)*

Serum   Decrease *(continued)*

556.00 Ulcerative Colitis   The concentration was lower in the severely ill patients than in those who were mildly-moderately ill, while T₄ and TBG were not affected by the severity of the disease. *1150*

571.20 Laennec's or Alcoholic Cirrhosis   The mean serum T₃ value, 85 ng/dL, was significantly reduced in the hepatic patients as compared to a mean serum T₃ value of 126 ng/dL in the normal subjects, while the free T₃ value was 0.28 ng/dL in both groups. The reduction of the serum total and free T₃ values were closely correlated with the degree of liver damage. *1703*

579.00 Celiac Sprue Disease   *2415*

581.90 Nephrotic Syndrome   Urinary loss of TBG results in lowering of most blood thyroid hormones and increased T₃ uptake. *0962*

585.00 Chronic Renal Failure   Although mean serum total T₃ concentration was normal, 43% had low serum T₃ and 54% had low serum free T₃ concentrations. *2233*   Reduced total and free T₃, mean total T₃ = 65.4 ± 17.4 ng/dL. *1298*   Decreased *1617*

770.80 Respiratory Distress Syndrome   In preterm infants with this disorder, cord blood T₃ concentration was significantly lower than that in cord blood of babies without this disease (22 ± 2.6 vs 36 ± 5 ng/dL). There was no significant rise at 24 h of age (22 ± 2.6 vs 34.0 ± 8 ng/dL) and remained low for 3 weeks. *0006*

Serum   Increase

193.00 Malignant Neoplasm of Thyroid Gland   Rarely in follicular cancer. *1200*

240.00 Simple Goiter   Normal or increased. *0962*

242.90 Hyperthyroidism   A small group of patients whose hypermetabolism is due to T₃ excess alone has been identified. These patients are clinically hyperthyroid but have normal levels of total serum T₄ and free T₄. Their radioiodine uptakes are variable, but are usually in the upper normal range. Total serum T₃ values are high. *0999*   Increased before overt hyperthyroidism is apparent and before serum T₄ levels have increased. *0619*   May be present. *0962 2468*

245.10 Subacute Thyroiditis   Invariably elevated at some time during acute stage. *1106*

245.20 Hashimoto's Thyroiditis   May occur as disease progresses. *2540*   Normal in 25 euthyroid, reduced in 22 hypothyroid and increased in 4 hyperthyroid patients with Hashimoto's thyroiditis. No specific abnormalities in serum concentrations of thyroid hormones were found. *0832*

250.00 Diabetes Mellitus   Prior to Rx. serum T₃ was significantly lower than in normal controls. *1203*

358.00 Myasthenia Gravis   Thyrotoxicosis may occur in conjunction with this disease. *0995*

555.90 Regional Enteritis or Ileitis   The concentration was lower in the severely ill patients than in those who were mildly-moderately ill, while T₄ and TBG were not affected by the severity of the disease. *1150*

571.90 Cirrhosis of Liver   Mean serum reverse T₃ and free reverse T₃ (450 pg/dL) were increased in hepatic cirrhosis. *0394*

630.00 Hydatidiform Mole   9 of 14 patients were hyperthyroid. Serum T₃ ranged from 300-800 ng/dL. Correlated closely with chorionic gonadotropins. *1044*   High in 13 of 15 patients with molar pregnancy, paralleling that of T₄. *2487*

650.00 Pregnancy   The total T₃ is elevated, thought to be caused by an increase in T₄ binding protein secondary to high circulating-estrogen levels. *0999*   Elevated in normal pregnancy, while free T₄ and free T₃ are normal. *1740*

Serum   Normal

193.00 Malignant Neoplasm of Thyroid Gland   Usually euthyroid. *1200*

240.00 Simple Goiter   Normal or slightly low. *0962*   Usually. *2540*

245.20 Hashimoto's Thyroiditis   The majority of patients are euthyroid at diagnosis with normal T₃, T₄, free hormones and TSH. *1106*   Normal in 25 euthyroid, reduced in 22 hypothyroid and increased in 4 hyperthyroid patients with Hashimoto's thyroiditis. No specific abnormalities in serum concentrations of thyroid hormones were found. *0832 0962*

253.00 Acromegaly   Thyroid functions were all found to be normal in active disease, contrary to several reports. *0458*

275.34 Familial Periodic Paralysis   *2246*

Urine   Decrease

585.00 Chronic Renal Failure   Reduced excretion, 27 ± 44 ng/24h. *1298*

Triolein ¹³¹I Test

Feces   Positive

40.20 Whipple's Disease   Positive test for lipid droplets in the stool, but results are inconsistent. *0962*

251.50 Zollinger-Ellison Syndrome   Positive test for lipid droplets in the stool, but results are inconsistent. *0962*

271.30 Lactosuria   Positive test for lipid droplets in the stool, but results are inconsistent. *0962*

577.10 Chronic Pancreatitis   Abnormal in 33% of patients. *2467*

579.00 Celiac Sprue Disease   Positive test for lipid droplets in the stool, but results are inconsistent. *0962*

579.90 Malabsorption, Cause Unspecified   Positive test for lipid droplets in the stool, results are inconsistent. *0962*

Trypsin

Serum   Decrease

277.00 Cystic Fibrosis   *1901*

Serum   Increase

157.90 Malignant Neoplasm of Pancreas   Mean serum concentration in 7 patients was 394 U/L. (normal < 100 U) *1678*

250.00 Diabetes Mellitus   High incidence of pancreatic abnormality in patients with no clinical evidence of pancreatic acinar disease. *2406*

571.90 Cirrhosis of Liver   High incidence of pancreatic abnormality in patients with no clinical evidence of pancreatic acinar disease. *2406*

577.00 Acute Pancreatitis   10-40 X higher than normal. *2199*

577.10 Chronic Pancreatitis   Mean circulatory concentration in 16 cases was 433 U/L. Normal < 100 U/L. *1678*

Duodenal Contents   Normal

577.20 Pancreatic Cyst and Pseudocyst   Duodenal contents after secretin-pancreozymin stimulation usually show decreased bicarbonate content (< 80 mmol/L) but normal volume and normal content of amylase, lipase, and trypsin. *2467*

Gastric Material   Decrease

260.00 Protein Malnutrition   In kwashiorkor. *0151*

Trypsin Inhibitor

Serum   Increase

199.00 Secondary Malignant Neoplasm (Disseminated)   Elevated compared to normal controls or patients with non-neoplastic disorders. *1590*

Synovial Fluid   Increase

714.00 Rheumatoid Arthritis   Elevated in 36 patients with involvement of the knee joint. *1953*

Tryptophan

Serum   Decrease

259.20 Carcinoid Syndrome   Due to increased production of serotonin by the tumor; may result in clinical pellagra. *0718*

260.00 Protein Malnutrition   *0151*

270.02 Hartnup Disease   Reduced blood levels of tryptophan metabolites. *0151*

555.90 Regional Enteritis or Ileitis   In 32 patients, 13 fell into a distinct group of low tryptophan sera levels. Patients in this group ate less, had low albumin levels and greater intestinal protein loss than normal tryptophan patients. *0150*

991.60 Hypothermia   Decreased with cold exposure although total amino acids are unaffected. *0762*

Serum   Increase

572.20 **Hepatic Encephalopathy**   The only amino acid with increased CSF concentrations compared to normals and stable cirrhotics, probably attributable to increased plasma free tryptophan in hepatic coma patients. *1733*

580.00 **Acute Poststreptococcal Glomerulonephritis**   Tyrosine and tryptophan usually rise in acute and chronic glomerulonephritis. *2104*

580.01 **Glomerulonephritis (Focal)**   Tyrosine and tryptophan usually rise in acute and chronic glomerulonephritis. *2104*

580.02 **Glomerulonephritis (Minimal Change)**   Tyrosine and tryptophan usually rise in acute and chronic glomerulonephritis. *2104*

580.04 **Glomerulonephritis (Membranous)**   Tyrosine and tryptophan usually rise in acute and chronic glomerulonephritis. *2104*

580.05 **Glomerulonephritis (Membranoproliferative)**   Tyrosine and tryptophan usually rise in acute and chronic glomerulonephritis. *2104*

580.40 **Glomerulonephritis (Rapidly Progressive)**   Tyrosine and tryptophan usually rise in acute and chronic glomerulonephritis. *2104*

Urine   Increase

270.02 **Hartnup Disease**   Urine chromatography shows greatly increased amount. *2468*   5-20 X normal values. *2246*

270.03 **Cystinosis**   Nonspecific pattern of aminoaciduria. Fanconi's syndrome. *0995*

275.10 **Hepatolenticular Degeneration**   *0503*

CSF   Increase

13.00 **Tuberculosis Meningitis**   *2468*

571.90 **Cirrhosis of Liver**   Increased concentrations due to decreased plasma branched chain amino acids. *1733*

572.20 **Hepatic Encephalopathy**   The only amino acid with increased CSF concentrations compared to normals and stable cirrhotics, probably attributable to increased plasma free tryptophan in hepatic coma patients. *1733*

CSF   Normal

333.40 **Huntington's Chorea**   In 7 patients. *2591*

Tryptophan, Free

Serum   Decrease

333.40 **Huntington's Chorea**   Markedly reduced as a result of the increased concentrations of nonesterified fatty acids. In induced hypoglycemia, the difference in free tryptophan between control and diseased groups was much less severe. *1816*

Tyrosine

Serum   Decrease

66.00 **Phlebotomus Fever**   Most free amino acids are depressed in sandfly fever and other mild-moderate infections. *0122*

260.00 **Protein Malnutrition**   *0151*

270.10 **Phenylketonuria**   With normal phenylalanine intake. *0186*

333.40 **Huntington's Chorea**   19 patients showed a significantly lower concentration of proline, alanine, valine, leucine, isoleucine, and tyrosine compared to 38 normal controls. *0534*

580.01 **Glomerulonephritis (Focal)**   Mean concentration of essential amino acids and tyrosine were significantly lower, resulting in a low essential/total ratio. *1545*

580.04 **Glomerulonephritis (Membranous)**   Mean concentration of essential amino acids and tyrosine were significantly lower, resulting in a low essential/total ratio. *1545*

585.00 **Chronic Renal Failure**   Children with mild renal insufficiency showed a significant decrease in tyrosine and arginine and an increase in cystine. Tyrosine showed a linear correlation between decreasing plasma concentration and GFR (R = 0.4). *0192*

714.00 **Rheumatoid Arthritis**   Frequently low. *2104*

753.10 **Polycystic Kidney Disease**   Mean concentration of essential amino acids and tyrosine were significantly lower, resulting in a low essential/total ratio. *1545*

991.60 **Hypothermia**   Decreased with cold exposure although total amino acids are unaffected. *0762*

Serum   Increase

70.00 **Viral Hepatitis**   A close relationship was found between the onset of encephalopathy and amino acid equilibrium disturbance, characterized by a fall in the molar ratio between valine, leucine, and isoleucine, and phenylalanine and tyrosine. All showed absolute elevations with onset of encephalopathy. *0531*

271.20 **Hereditary Fructose Intolerance**   During acute intoxication, signs of proximal tubular syndrome and of liver failure are common. *0433*

571.90 **Cirrhosis of Liver**   In 30 patients with alcoholic liver cirrhosis, portal hypertension and bleeding esophageal varices. *1165*

580.00 **Acute Poststreptococcal Glomerulonephritis**   Tyrosine and tryptophan usually rise in acute and chronic glomerulonephritis. *2104*

580.01 **Glomerulonephritis (Focal)**   Tyrosine and tryptophan usually rise in acute and chronic glomerulonephritis. *2104*

580.02 **Glomerulonephritis (Minimal Change)**   Tyrosine and tryptophan usually rise in acute and chronic glomerulonephritis. *2104*

580.04 **Glomerulonephritis (Membranous)**   Tyrosine and tryptophan usually rise in acute and chronic glomerulonephritis. *2104*

580.05 **Glomerulonephritis (Membranoproliferative)**   Tyrosine and tryptophan usually rise in acute and chronic glomerulonephritis. *2104*

580.40 **Glomerulonephritis (Rapidly Progressive)**   Tyrosine and tryptophan usually rise in acute and chronic glomerulonephritis. *2104*

Urine   Increase

270.02 **Hartnup Disease**   5-20 X normal values. *2246*   *0995*

270.03 **Cystinosis**   Nonspecific pattern of aminoaciduria. Fanconi's syndrome. *0995*

271.10 **Galactosemia**   General aminoaciduria - identified by chromatography. *2468*   Manifestation of a renal toxicity syndrome. *1066*

275.10 **Hepatolenticular Degeneration**   *0503*

572.40 **Hepatic Failure**   *0503*

CSF   Normal

333.40 **Huntington's Chorea**   In 7 patients. *2591*

Tyrosine Crystals

Urine   Increase

570.00 **Acute and Subacute Necrosis of Liver**   Acute yellow atrophy. *2467*

Urea Nitrogen

Serum   Decrease

253.00 **Acromegaly**   In some patients, because of the high uptake of amino acids required for enhanced protein synthesis. *0962*

260.00 **Protein Malnutrition**   Indicates decreased protein metabolism. *0186 0016   0151*

275.10 **Hepatolenticular Degeneration**   Mildly elevated between 20-25 mg/dL in 6 of 35 (17%) and decreased < 10 mg/dL in 4 cases. *2278*

277.00 **Cystic Fibrosis**   In 46% of 13 patients at initial hospitalization for this disorder. *0781*

570.00 **Acute and Subacute Necrosis of Liver**   Abnormally low levels have been attributed to liver failure. This is not a rare finding today and its significance should not be overlooked. Values of 5 mg/dL or less observed in 1% of 16,000 determinations. *0803 0503*

571.20 **Laennec's or Alcoholic Cirrhosis**   With severe cirrhosis. *0992*

571.90 **Cirrhosis of Liver**   Often decreased (< 10 mg/dL). *2467 0376*

572.40 **Hepatic Failure**   Only if hepatic tissue is severely damaged. *2104*

Urea Nitrogen (continued)

Serum Decrease (continued)

573.30 Toxic Hepatitis With severe damage due to hepatotoxic agents. *2104*

579.00 Celiac Sprue Disease Impaired protein absorption. *2467*

581.90 Nephrotic Syndrome Some patients. *2467*

642.40 Pre-Eclampsia Low (9 ± 2 mg/dL) and low creatinine (0.75 ± 0.2 mg/dL) in late pregnancy are indicative of toxemia. *0151*

642.60 Eclampsia Low (9 ± 2 mg/dL) and low creatinine (0.75 ± 0.2 mg/dL) in late pregnancy are indicative of toxemia. *0151* Tends to decrease. *0619*

650.00 Pregnancy Slightly lower than in the nonpregnant state. *0433* 18 mg/dL is definitely abnormal in pregnancy although normal in nonpregnant women. Decreases approximately 25%, especially during first 2 trimesters. *2468* Found to be 8.7 mg ± 1.5 from the 15th week of pregnancy to term compared to 13.1 mg ± 3.0 for nonpregnant subjects. *2179* Decreased markedly throughout pregnancy *0517* *0503*

994.50 Exercise Observed effect with 12 min cycle-ergometer. *1205*

1013.00 Diet With low protein and high carbohydrate diet. *2467*

Serum Increase

1.00 Cholera Due to severe dehydration. *0992*

32.00 Diphtheria Elevation with increase in serum globulins may occur. *0433*

38.00 Septicemia In 49% of 12 patients at initial hospitalization for this disorder. *0781* A condition that may be associated with excessive protein catabolism. *0503*

39.90 Actinomycosis Kidney involvement. *1058*

53.00 Herpes Zoster In 31% of 18 patients at initial hospitalization for this disorder. *0781*

60.00 Yellow Fever With kidney involvement. *1058* Concentrations of 220 mg/dL were recorded in 3 patients, all of whom died. *1179*

73.90 Psittacosis With severe renal involvement. *0433*

80.00 Epidemic Typhus With varying degrees of renal involvement. *0433* Azotemia is common. *2368*

82.00 Rocky Mountain Spotted Fever Azotemia is common in severe cases. *2368* *0433*

100.00 Leptospirosis Usually associated with jaundice. *0992* During leptospiremic phase, azotemia may be present. *0962* Marked oliguria or anuria develops after the 1st week of disease and is attended by severe azotemia and electrolyte imbalance characteristic of lower nephron nephrosis. *2368*

117.30 Aspergillosis Either as a result of underlying disease or the infection. Azotemia develops rapidly. *1058*

188.90 Malignant Neoplasm of Bladder In 40% of 45 patients at initial hospitalization for this disorder. *0781*

202.80 Non-Hodgkins Lymphoma In 26% of 74 patients at initial hospitalization for this disorder. *0781*

203.00 Multiple Myeloma Ranged from 5.0-92.1 mmol/L in 35 patients. *0518* In 51% of 33 patients at initial hospitalization for this disorder. *0781* Impaired renal function in > 50%, decreasing concentrating ability and azotemia. *2468* *0433*

204.00 Lymphocytic Leukemia (Acute) Can be elevated in kidney infiltration and should be followed especially if nephrotoxic antibiotics are used. *0433*

204.10 Lymphocytic Leukemia (Chronic) Can be elevated in kidney infiltration and should be followed especially if nephrotoxic antibiotics are used. *0433* In 54% of 27 patients at initial hospitalization for this disorder. *0781*

205.00 Myelocytic Leukemia (Acute) Can be elevated in kidney infiltration and should be followed especially if nephrotic antibiotics are used. *0433* In 33% of 37 patients at initial hospitalization for this disorder. *0781*

205.10 Myelocytic Leukemia (Chronic) Can be elevated in kidney infiltration and should be followed especially if nephrotoxic antibiotics are used. *0433* In 23% of 21 patients at initial hospitalization for this disorder. *0781*

206.00 Monocytic Leukemia In 36% of 24 patients at initial hospitalization for this disorder. *0781*

242.90 Hyperthyroidism Excessive protein catabolism. *0503*

244.90 Hypothyroidism May be slightly elevated but returns to normal with replacement therapy *0433* . Usually normal. *2540*

250.00 Diabetes Mellitus Uncontrolled diabetes mellitus may be associated with excessive protein catabolism. *0503* In 29% of 117 patients at initial hospitalization for this disorder. *0781*

250.10 Diabetic Acidosis May reflect prerenal azotemia or diabetic nephropathy. *0962*

252.00 Hyperparathyroidism May occur. *2540*

255.00 Adrenal Cortical Hyperfunction (Glucocorticoid Excess) A condition that may be associated with excessive protein catabolism. *0503*

255.40 Adrenal Cortical Hypofunction Dehydration and hypotension lead to prerenal impairment of renal function. *0433* Dehydration may result in hemoconcentration. *0962* Fluid depletion leads to reduced circulating blood volume and renal circulatory insufficiency. *2612*

270.03 Cystinosis Elevated with advanced renal disease as early as 2 y of age in some patients. *2246* *0995*

273.23 Heavy Chain Disease (Gamma) Increased (30-50 mg/dL). *2468*

273.30 Waldenström's Macroglobulinemia Elevated in 5 of 16 patients. *1626* *2538*

274.00 Gout Rises with renal failure, but these changes may be subtle and slow. *0433*

275.10 Hepatolenticular Degeneration Mildly elevated between 20-25 mg/dL in 6 of 35 (17%) and decreased < 10 mg/dL in 4 cases. *2278*

275.41 Milk-Alkali Syndrome *0995*

276.30 Metabolic Alkalosis May be increased. *2468*

276.50 Dehydration Salt and water depletion causes reduced renal blood flow leading to prerenal azotemia. *2467* Dehydration. *0812* *0503*

277.14 Acute Intermittent Porphyria Frequent. *2254* During an attack. *0433* *2538*

277.30 Amyloidosis *0433*

279.12 Wiskott-Aldrich Syndrome Increased incidence of renal failure. *0793*

283.00 Acquired Hemolytic Anemia (Autoimmune) In 82% of 12 patients hospitalized for this disorder. *0781*

287.00 Allergic Purpura Elevated in the presence of renal failure. *2538* Azotemia is a common but transient finding. *2552*

308.00 Stress Increased protein catabolism (serum creatinine remains normal). *2467*

320.90 Meningitis (Bacterial) Dehydration. *0995*

331.81 Reye's Syndrome Markedly elevated reflecting renal injury. *0435*

401.00 Malignant Hypertension *1853*

401.10 Essential Benign Hypertension *1853*

410.90 Acute Myocardial Infarction In 36% of 119 patients hospitalized for this disorder. *0781* 18 of 22 patients showed elevations at some time during the study, usually within 3 days after admission. *2530* *2467*

421.00 Bacterial Endocarditis Increased--usually 25-75 mg/dL. *2468* *0433* *1798*

428.00 Congestive Heart Failure May be as high as 80-100 mg/dL as a result of prerenal azotemia. *0433* Moderate azotemia (BUN usually < 60 mg/dL) is evident with severe oliguria; may increase with vigorous diuresis. *2467* *0812* *0503*

440.00 Arteriosclerosis Several mechanisms are involved. *0503* In 36% of 75 patients hospitalized for this disorder. *0781*

444.90 Arterial Embolism and Thrombosis Progressive azotemia. *1108* In 34% of 42 patients hospitalized for this disorder. *0781*

446.00 Polyarteritis-Nodosa With renal involvement. *0995*

446.20 Goodpasture's Syndrome Progressive renal failure. *0062*

446.60 Thrombotic Thrombocytopenic Purpura Renal function may be impaired. *0962* Elevated initially in 50% of patients and more terminally. *2538*

533.90 Peptic Ulcer, Site Unspecified Pyloric obstruction with vomiting and loss of gastric secretion results in hypochloremia, hyponatremia, hypokalemia, elevated serum pH and carbon dioxide content, and azotemia. *0962*

557.01 Mesenteric Artery Embolism Will reflect the hemoconcentration secondary to fluid loss into the bowel and peritoneal cavity following bowel infarction. *0433*

558.90 Diarrhea Observed in patients with diarrhea and severe dehydration, who were rapidly dehydrated with concomitant fall of BUN to normal or subnormal levels. *0803*

560.90 Intestinal Obstruction Azotemia may be striking; also with massive hemorrhage. *0503* Increase suggests blood in intestine or renal damage. *2467*

567.90 Peritonitis Secondary; may be increased owing to hemoconcentration from extracellular fluid loss into the peritoneal cavity. *0433*

571.90 Cirrhosis of Liver Increased with gastrointestinal hemorrhage. *2467 0812*

572.40 Hepatic Failure Blood levels of urea were raised in 20 cases (40%) of which in 9 cases it was > 60 mg/dL in patients with hepatic failure arising from decompensated cirrhosis or attacks of acute viral hepatitis. *0379*

577.00 Acute Pancreatitis Not uncommon with more severe cases, especially when shock and oliguria are present. *0151* Rarely exceeds 4 mg/dL. *2199*

580.00 Acute Poststreptococcal Glomerulonephritis All fractions of nonprotein nitrogen increase. *0812* Elevated in 50% of patients. *0995*

580.04 Glomerulonephritis (Membranous) Occurs late in course. *0419*

580.05 Glomerulonephritis (Membranoproliferative) BUN and creatinine rise as GFR decreases. *0962*

580.40 Glomerulonephritis (Rapidly Progressive) Usually > 80 mg/dL. *2468* BUN and creatinine rise as GFR decreases. *0962*

581.90 Nephrotic Syndrome In 51% of 26 patients at initial hospitalization for this disorder. *0781*

584.00 Acute Renal Failure Rises < 20 mg/dL/day in transfusion reaction. Rises > 50 mg/dL/day in overwhelming infection or severe crushing injuries in early stage. Continues to rise for several days after onset of diuresis in the 2nd week. *2468* Excessive tubular reabsorption of urea and several other nonprotein nitrogen constituents may play a role in diseases producing this state. *0503* In 99% of 12 patients at initial hospitalization for this disorder. *0781 1853*

585.00 Chronic Renal Failure Damage to the nephrons leads to faulty urine formation and excretion. The blood-urea begins to rise when the equivalent of one kidney lost, or when the GFR falls below 10 mL/min. *0619* In 98% of 148 patients at initial hospitalization for this disorder. *0781 1853*

590.00 Chronic Pyelonephritis May be elevated. *0151 1853*

590.10 Acute Pyelonephritis Uncomplicated disease does not characteristically exhibit evidence of renal insufficiency; however, a nonspecific elevation of BUN may be a reflection of volume contraction and and dehydration. *0433* In 24% of 16 patients at initial hospitalization for this disorder. *0781*

591.00 Hydronephrosis In cases of advanced renal damage elevation of the BUN and secondary anemia may be noted secondary to uremia. *0433* In 20% of 10 patients at initial hospitalization for this disorder. *0781*

597.80 Urethritis Reveals the degree of renal impairment. *0433*

600.00 Benign Prostatic Hypertrophy In 29% of 80 patients at initial hospitalization for this disorder. *0781*

642.40 Pre-Eclampsia If the hypertension has reached relatively severe levels, may be elevated, indicating renal damage. *0433*

710.00 Systemic Lupus Erythematosus Elevated, usually > 100 mg/dL. Indicates uremia. *1269* Correlates well with severity of morphologic lesions. *1047*

710.10 Progressive Systemic Sclerosis Renal function may be impaired. *0962*

714.00 Rheumatoid Arthritis At times increased. Somewhat elevated (30-40 mg/dL) during active phase. *0433*

753.10 Polycystic Kidney Disease Azotemia. *1853*

753.12 Medullary Cystic Disease Characteristic azotemia. *0277*

770.80 Respiratory Distress Syndrome Increased catabolism. *2467*

780.80 Hyperhidrosis Salt and water depletion causes reduced renal blood flow leading to prerenal azotemia. *2467* Dehydration. *0812 0503*

785.50 Shock A decrease in plasma volume secondary to dehydration, blood loss, hypotension or shock is often referred to as prerenal azotemia. *0812 0503*

787.00 Vomiting Salt and water depletion causes reduced renal blood flow leading to prerenal azotemia. *2467* Dehydration. *0812 0503*

984.00 Toxic Effects of Lead and Its Compounds (including Fumes) May cause renal damage. *2084*

985.00 Toxic Effects of Non-medicinal Metals Nephrotoxicity is common with therapeutic doses of arsenicals. *0811*

986.00 Toxic Effects of Carbon Monoxide Occurs in severe cases. *0151* Nephrotoxicity. *2084*

989.50 Toxic Effects of Venom May cause nephrotoxicity. *2084 0995*

990.00 Effects of X-Ray Irradiation May cause renal damage. *2084*

992.00 Heat stroke Elevated in severe cases. *0151*

994.50 Exercise Raised at 15 min, partial return to normal in 24 h. *0985*

994.80 Effects of Electric Current May cause renal damage. *2084*

Serum   Normal

244.90 Hypothyroidism Usually normal. *2540*

252.10 Hypoparathyroidism *2540*

253.40 Anterior Pituitary Hypofunction Usually. *0995*

273.30 Waldenström's Macroglobulinemia Renal insufficiency is reported to be uncommon. *1469 2538*

275.35 Vitamin D Resistant Rickets *2246*

642.60 Eclampsia No significant increase. *0621*

994.50 Exercise Moderate degrees of exercise will not change BUN if sufficient calories to meet the energy demand are provided. *2104*

Saliva   Increase

277.00 Cystic Fibrosis Increased. *1359*

584.00 Acute Renal Failure A near perfect correlation (R = 0.97) was found for saliva, plasma urea nitrogen ratios in 56 pairs of samples from patients with renal failure. The mean serum concentration before dialysis was 81.2 ± 30.9 mg/dL. In unstimulated saliva, the urea nitrogen saliva: plasma ratio remained constant at 1.3. *2125*

585.00 Chronic Renal Failure A near perfect correlation (R = 0.97) was found for saliva: plasma urea nitrogen ratios in 56 pairs of samples from patients with renal failure. The mean serum urea nitrogen level for renal failure patients before dialysis was 81.2 ± 30.9 mg/dL. In unstimulated saliva, the urea nitrogen saliva: plasma ratio remained constant at 1.3. *2125*

Uric Acid

Serum   Decrease

162.90 Malignant Neoplasm of Bronchus and Lung Hypouricemia accompanied hyponatremia (< 130 mmol/L) in 75% of patients with the syndrome of inappropriate antidiuretic hormone and small cell carcinoma of the lung. *1778 0962*

201.90 Hodgkin's Disease Decreased uric acid is seen in occasional cases of neoplasms such as Hodgkin's disease. *2467* Hypouricemia associated with markedly elevated clearance has been reported. *1241* Rarely reported. *0962*

203.00 Multiple Myeloma Occasionally decreased due to altered renal tubular function. *2468* Common. *0962*

253.00 Acromegaly Some patients. *2467*

270.02 Hartnup Disease There is possibly a congenital tubular defect resulting in decreased reabsorption. *0619*

270.03 Cystinosis Failure of reabsorption. *0995*

275.10 Hepatolenticular Degeneration Renal tubular reabsorption of uric acid is reduced, possibly as a result of damage to the tubule cells by excess unbound copper. *0619* Occurs in most patients with untreated disease. *2546* Decreased urate, mean = 2.5 mg/dL in 25 of 32 (78%). One patient had an elevated concentration. *2278 2104*

275.34 Familial Periodic Paralysis *2104*

277.21 Xanthinuria Characterized by the replacement of uric acid by xanthine and hypoxanthine in urine. *2246* Concentrations below level of detection have been documented as well as elevations. *2104 0962*

281.00 Pernicious Anemia Decreased in some patients in relapse. *2467* Rarely reported. *0962*

281.20 Folic Acid Deficiency Anemia Often depressed. *2538*

571.20 Laennec's or Alcoholic Cirrhosis Serum concentration was 4.18 ± 0.25 mg/dL in 22 male patients, significantly lower than in age-matched controls, 6.44 ± 0.19. An inverse correlation (R = 0.70) was found with serum bilirubin. *1580*

571.60 Biliary Cirrhosis May occur. *2467*

Uric Acid *(continued)*

Serum Decrease *(continued)*

571.90 Cirrhosis of Liver *2467*

579.00 Celiac Sprue Disease Slight. *2467*

588.81 Proximal Renal Tubular Acidosis Hypouricemia, secondary to increased renal clearance of uric acid, is present in some patients (children). *0433*

650.00 Pregnancy Averages 3.86 mg/dL in nonpregnant controls compared to 2.72 mg/dL before 16 weeks of pregnancy, 2.6 mg/dL between 17 and 28 weeks and 3.61 mg/dL after 28 weeks. May explain the observation that gout tends to improve in pregnancy. *0266* Decreased in early pregnancy but returned to normal by term. *0517*

948.00 Burns Patients recovering from burns may remain hypophosphatemic and hypouricemic for months after the initial injury. *1287*

Serum Increase

11.00 Pulmonary Tuberculosis In 48% of 26 patients at initial hospitalization for this disorder. *0781*

13.00 Tuberculosis Meningitis Increased in both blood and CSF with a lowered blood:CSF ratio, possibly due to cellular breakdown and nucleoprotein catabolism. *2301*

38.00 Septicemia In 54% of 11 patients at initial hospitalization for this disorder. *0781*

70.00 Viral Hepatitis Mean levels were 8.0 ± 0.6 (normal = 6.5 ± 0.6 mg/dL) in 16 patients. Values for the entire group were not statistically significant, but individual decreases measured upon recovery showed significant individual elevations. *1890*

85.00 Leishmaniasis In tropical splenomegaly syndrome. *1139*

135.00 Sarcoidosis May occur even with normal renal function in up to 50% of patients. *2468* In 52% of 25 patients at initial hospitalization for this disorder. *0781* *1283 0962*

150.90 Malignant Neoplasm of Esophagus In 46% of 40 patients at initial hospitalization for this disorder. *0781*

151.90 Malignant Neoplasm of Stomach In 36% of 47 patients at initial hospitalization for this disorder. *0781*

153.90 Malignant Neoplasm of Large Intestine In 35% of 149 patients at initial hospitalization for this disorder. *0781*

154.10 Malignant Neoplasm of Rectum In 43% of 73 patients at initial hospitalization for this disorder. *0781*

157.90 Malignant Neoplasm of Pancreas In 29% of 46 patients at initial hospitalization for this disorder. *0781*

170.90 Malignant Neoplasm of Bone In 37% of 26 patients at initial hospitalization for this disorder. *0781*

172.90 Malignant Melanoma of Skin In 38% of 67 patients at initial hospitalization for this disorder. *0781*

174.90 Malignant Neoplasm of Breast In 25% of 300 patients at initial hospitalization for this disorder. *0781*

182.00 Malignant Neoplasm of Corpus Uteri In 36% of 151 patients at initial hospitalization for this disorder. *0781*

185.00 Malignant Neoplasm of Prostate In 42% of 86 patients at initial hospitalization for this disorder. *0781*

186.90 Malignant Neoplasm of Testis In 61% of 24 patients at initial hospitalization for this disorder. *0781*

188.90 Malignant Neoplasm of Bladder In 43% of 45 patients at initial hospitalization for this disorder. *0781*

197.00 Secondary Malignant Neoplasm of Respiratory System In 39% of 602 patients at initial hospitalization for this disorder. *0781*

201.90 Hodgkin's Disease Hyperuricemia occurs occasionally. *0999* Especially post x-irradiation. *2467* In 31% of 72 patients at initial hospitalization for this disorder. *0781*

202.80 Non-Hodgkins Lymphoma May occur, but more often is normal. *1639* Especially post x-radiation. *2467* In 39% of 73 patients at initial hospitalization for this disorder. *0781*

203.00 Multiple Myeloma Seen in about 33% of patients. *0433* 10 of 35 patients had hyperuricemia (> 416 mmol/L). 8 of these had only mild elevations, consistent with the severity of renal insufficiency. *0518* May accompany renal failure or may occur in the absence of azotemia. *2538* In 63% of 33 patients at initial hospitalization for this disorder. *0781* *0962*

204.00 Lymphocytic Leukemia (Acute) Frequent biochemical abnormality. Secondary to the increased cell turnover. *0433* Frequently elevated when the disease is in relapse. The absolute levels vary considerably from individual to individual. *0270* In 50% of patients. *1042* In 39% of 46 patients at initial hospitalization for this disorder. *0781* *2538*

204.10 Lymphocytic Leukemia (Chronic) A frequent association of the treated condition. *0433* Not as frequent as in other leukemias. *0992*

205.00 Myelocytic Leukemia (Acute) Frequent biochemical abnormality. Secondary to the increased cell turnover. *0433* In approximately 50% of patients. *1042 2552* In 44% of 35 patients at initial hospitalization for this disorder. *0781* Due to excessive excretion of urate, but no correlation was found between serum and urinary levels in myeloid patients, contrary to normal controls (R = 0.85). Serum levels tends to fall in relapse. *1601* *0962*

205.10 Myelocytic Leukemia (Chronic) Frequent biochemical abnormality. *0433* Especially with high WBC and antileukemic therapy. Urinary obstruction may develop on account of intrarenal and extrarenal crystallization. *2468* Often moderately elevated; increased production. *2552* In 80% of 21 patients at initial hospitalization for this disorder. *0781* *0962*

206.00 Monocytic Leukemia In 55% of 23 patients at initial hospitalization for this disorder. *0781*

207.00 Erythroleukemia Normal or high levels. *2538*

225.90 Benign Neoplasm of Brain and CNS In 31% of 22 patients at initial hospitalization for this disorder. *0781*

238.40 Polycythemia Vera Increased RBC formation produces hyperuricemia and hyperuricosuria in 30-50% of patients at the time of diagnosis. Both tend to increase in frequency and severity as the disease progresses and may remain asymptomatic but approximately 5-10% of patients develop symptoms and signs of gout. *2538 0839 2603* High in a significant proportion of patients. *0999*

244.90 Hypothyroidism May be slightly elevated but returns to normal with replacement therapy. *0433* In 45% of 13 patients at initial hospitalization for this disorder. *0781* *1283 0962 2104*

250.00 Diabetes Mellitus Increased occurrence of hyperuricemia has been reported. *1585* In 28% of 104 patients at initial hospitalization for this disorder. *0781*

250.10 Diabetic Acidosis Elevated in 50% of patients; parallels the degree of ketoacidosis and returns to normal when diabetes is controlled. *1757* Frequently increased. *0999* Often found. *0962 1283*

252.00 Hyperparathyroidism Over 6.8 mg/dL in 62% of patients. *0999* Increased frequency of hyperuricemia and gout. 66% of the patients showed elevations, with no difference of frequency among males or females or with type of disease. *1492* In 54% of 18 patients at initial hospitalization for this disorder. *0781* *1600 1283 0962*

252.10 Hypoparathyroidism In primary cases. *0601* *1283 0962*

253.00 Acromegaly Increased in some patients. *2467*

253.50 Diabetes Insipidus Occasionally. *0893* *0962*

260.00 Protein Malnutrition High in starvation, ketosis, and high fat diets. *1757* *1283 0962*

270.21 Alkaptonuria *2104*

271.01 Von Gierke's Disease Fasting blood levels were > 2 X normal mean; further significant increases occurred after fructose and glucagon administration in children. *1960* Hyperuricemia appears in early infancy, but rarely becomes symptomatic before age 10. May become a major problem in the adult. *2246 1086* Significant elevations generally occur in the glycogen storage diseases. *2104* *1283 0962*

271.02 McArdle's Disease Significant elevations generally occur in the glycogen storage diseases. *2104*

271.03 Forbes Disease Usually but not always. *2246*

272.00 Type IIA Hyperlipoproteinemia Common. *0992*

272.10 Type IV Hyperlipoproteinemia Hyperuricemia is common. *0151* 9 of 22 patients. *2246* Occurs in most patients but not with sufficient constancy to indicate a role in causing the disorder. *2246* *0962*

272.21 Type IIB Hyperlipoproteinemia Common. *0992*

272.22 Type III Hyperlipoproteinemia 15-20% of patients. *0619* In 40% of patients. *2246* *0915*

272.32 Type V Hyperlipoproteinemia Common in type V. *0915* In 40% of patients. *2246*

272.71 Anderson's Disease Significant elevations generally occur in the glycogen storage diseases. *2104*

273.23 Heavy Chain Disease (Gamma) Increased, (> 8.5 mg/dL). *2468*

273.30 Waldenström's Macroglobulinemia May occur. *2552 0962*

274.00 Gout More than 95% of patients eventually have an elevated serum concentration. *0433* May rise above 6.0 mg/dL in men, or 5.5 mg/dL in women. Possibly the rise is due to increased renal tubular reabsorption. 25% of patients' relatives have raised serum concentration also, but without symptoms of gout (possibly the effect of a single autosomal dominant gene). *0619*

277.21 Xanthinuria Concentrations below level of detection have been documented as well as elevations. *2104*

277.22 Lesch-Nyhan Syndrome Ranges from 7-18 mg/dL in the absence of renal insufficiency. Occasionally a normal value may occur. *0182 2246*

277.30 Amyloidosis Increased in 22% of primary and 31% of secondary cases. *1334*

281.00 Pernicious Anemia Especially after treatment. *0619 1283 0962*

282.00 Hereditary (Congenital) Spherocytosis *1283 0962*

282.20 Anemias Due To Disorders of Glutathione Metabolism *2467*

282.41 Thalassemia Major *0962*

282.60 Sickle Cell Anemia May be increased. *2467* *0962*

283.00 Acquired Hemolytic Anemia (Autoimmune) In 63% of 11 patients hospitalized for this disorder. *0781* *0962*

289.00 Polycythemia, Secondary *0151 0962*

289.80 Myelofibrosis May be elevated usually correlating with the degree of myelofibrosis or WBC elevation. *0433* In myelofibrosis, secondary gout and the formation of urinary uric acid calculi are frequent consequences of the hyperuricosuria. *2538* *1283 0962*

296.80 Manic Depressive Disorder Increased in both blood and CSF with a lowered CSF:blood ratio, possibly due to cellular breakdown and nucleoprotein catabolism. *2301*

297.90 Paranoid States and Other Psychoses Increased in both blood and CSF with a lowered CSF:blood ratio, possibly due to cellular breakdown and nucleoprotein catabolism. *2301* In 34% of 36 patients hospitalized for this disorder. *0781*

300.40 Depressive Neurosis Increased in both blood and CSF with a lowered CSF:blood ratio, possibly due to cellular breakdown and nucleoprotein catabolism. *2301*

303.90 Alcoholism Increased lactic acid concentration inhibits uric acid excretion in the distal renal tubule. Usually decreases to normal within 1 week after abstinence. *0962* *1283*

320.90 Meningitis (Bacterial) Increased in both blood and CSF with a lowered blood:CSF ratio, possibly due to cellular breakdown and nucleoprotein catabolism. *2301* In 36% of 11 patients hospitalized for this disorder. *0781*

323.92 Encephalomyelitis Increased in both blood and CSF with a lowered blood:CSF ratio, possibly due to cellular breakdown and nucleoprotein catabolism. *2301*

401.10 Essential Benign Hypertension Found in 58% of 470 patients (27% of 333 untreated patients). Degree or occurrence of hyperuricemia did not correlate with severity of hypertension. *0275* In 54% of 102 patients hospitalized for this disorder. *0781* *0962*

405.91 Renovascular Hypertension Increased incidence of hyperuricemia. *0992*

410.90 Acute Myocardial Infarction In several studies, mean concentration ranged from 5.13 ± 1.10 to 7.32 mg/dL. Males were found to have a higher concentration (8.25 - 1.21) than females (7.16 ± 1.17) compared to normal, 3.59 ± 0.80, 3.01 ± 0.82, respectively. *2184* Frequently occurs. *0599* In 60% of 110 patients hospitalized for this disorder. *0781* *0962*

413.90 Angina Pectoris In 55% of 72 patients hospitalized for this disorder. *0781*

414.00 Chronic Ischemic Heart Disease Occurs frequently. In 92 young adults with coronary heart disease, mean level was 5.13 - 0.12, ranging from 3.0-7.8 mg/dL. *0599* In 59% of 475 patients hospitalized for this disorder. *0781* *2184*

428.00 Congestive Heart Failure Frequently elevated from either prerenal azotemia or, more commonly, the use of diuretics *0433* *1283*

431.00 Cerebral Hemorrhage Increased in both blood and CSF with a lowered CSF:blood ratio, possibly due to cellular breakdown and nucleoprotein catabolism. *2301*

434.00 Cerebral Thrombosis Increased in both blood and CSF with a lowered CSF:blood ratio, possibly due to cellular breakdown and nucleoprotein catabolism. *2301* Found in 25% of patients of both sexes with acute stroke. *1790* In 24% of 12 patients hospitalized for this disorder. *0781*

434.10 Cerebral Embolism Increased in both blood and CSF with a lowered CSF:blood ratio, possibly due to cellular breakdown and nucleoprotein catabolism. *2301* Found in 25% of both sexes with acute stroke. *1790*

434.90 Brain Infarction Increased in both blood and CSF with a lowered CSF:blood ratio, possibly due to cellular breakdown and nucleoprotein catabolism. *2301* In 36% of 115 cases of acute infarction. *1790*

435.90 Transient Cerebral Ischemia In 46% of 50 patients hospitalized for this disorder. *0781*

440.00 Arteriosclerosis Increased in 80% of patients with elevated serum triglycerides. *2467* Frequently found in 219 male and 63 female patients. No significant relationship was found between uric acid and serum lipids. *0108* In 59% of 71 patients hospitalized for this disorder. *0781*

486.01 Resolving Pneumonia *2467*

493.10 Asthma (Intrinsic) Has been observed and is thought to be a consequence of the excessive use of sympathomimetic drugs. *0997* *0642*

503.01 Berylliosis *2467*

555.90 Regional Enteritis or Ileitis *2035*

556.00 Ulcerative Colitis *2035*

571.20 Laennec's or Alcoholic Cirrhosis Hyperuricemia resulting from depressed urinary excretion of uric acid parallels lactic acidosis. *0151*

571.90 Cirrhosis of Liver In 52% of 68 patients at initial hospitalization for this disorder. *0781*

579.00 Celiac Sprue Disease *0962*

580.01 Glomerulonephritis (Focal) As functional loss becomes severe (GFR 50% of normal or less), there is usually a rise in serum phosphate and uric acid. *0962*

580.40 Glomerulonephritis (Rapidly Progressive) As functional loss becomes severe (GFR 50% of normal or less), there is usually a rise in serum phosphate and uric acid. *0962*

581.90 Nephrotic Syndrome In 52% of 25 patients at initial hospitalization for this disorder. *0781*

584.00 Acute Renal Failure In 99% of 11 patients at initial hospitalization for this disorder. *0781*

585.00 Chronic Renal Failure Increase is usually < 10 mg/dL. *2468* Rise begins very early, but is so slight that the level becomes consistently abnormal only when the GFR falls to about 15 mL/min. In late renal failure there is a further increase in fractional urate clearance so that plasma urate rises less steeply than plasma urea or creatinine. *0151* In 91% of 140 patients at initial hospitalization for this disorder. *0781*

600.00 Benign Prostatic Hypertrophy In 48% of 80 patients at initial hospitalization for this disorder. *0781*

642.40 Pre-Eclampsia Elevations of plasma urate is an early feature of pre-eclampsia. *1899* Perinatal mortality was markedly increased when maternal plasma-urate concentration were raised, generally in associated with severe pre-eclampsia of early onset. Maternal hypertension, even severe, without hyperuricemia, was associated with an excellent prognosis for the fetus. When maternal hypertension was mild and hyperuricemia was severe, the prognosis for the fetus was poor. *1898* *1283*

642.60 Eclampsia Serial determinations to follow therapeutic response and estimate prognosis. *2467* Hyperuricemia usually precedes the development of azotemia due to reduced urate clearance. *0151* Consistently observed. *0621*

656.40 Pregnancy Complicated by Intrauterine Death Perinatal mortality was markedly increased when maternal plasma-urate concentrations were raised, generally in association with severe pre-eclampsia of early onset. Maternal hypertension, even severe, without hyperuricemia, was associated with an excellent prognosis for the fetus. When maternal hypertension was mild and hyperuricemia was severe, the prognosis for the fetus was poor. *1898*

696.10 Psoriasis Slight elevation may occur, especially in male patients. *1343* Increased with increased extent and severity of cutaneous lesions. *0743* Found in 30-40% of patients. *2104* Increased nucleic acid turnover. *2612* *1283*

714.00 Rheumatoid Arthritis Slight elevation may occur, especially in male patients. *1343*

Uric Acid (continued)

Serum Increase (continued)

758.00 Down's Syndrome Some cases. *0619 2104*

770.80 Respiratory Distress Syndrome Higher serum concentrations during the first 3 days of life, and the urinary excretion over the period of 12-36 h of age is also higher than in the normal infants. Neonatal hyperuricemia is not due to renal retention but to increased production of uric acid. *1874*

780.30 Convulsions Significant increases were found in 17 patients with 2 or more grand mal seizures within 24 h. In 6 cases, concentrations were reached at which hyperuricemic renal failure may develop. *1449 1784*

984.00 Toxic Effects of Lead and Its Compounds (including Fumes) Moonshine whiskey causing 'saturnine gout'. *0619* Increased in serum due to reduced renal clearance. *0106 1283 0962*

990.00 Effects of X-Ray Irradiation Reflects cellular breakdown. *0865*

992.00 Heat stroke In children. *0548*

994.50 Exercise Marked increase with prolonged exercise. Correlates closely with serum lactic acid concentration. *2104*

1013.00 Diet Increased in a high-protein weight reduction diet and a diet with excess nucleoprotein (sweetbreads and liver). *2467* With high fat diets. *2104*

Serum Normal

202.80 Non-Hodgkins Lymphoma Usually normal. *2552*

204.10 Lymphocytic Leukemia (Chronic) Usually normal. *2039*

255.10 Adrenal Cortical Hyperfunction (Mineralocorticoid Excess) In the absence of azotemia. *0995*

272.00 Type IIA Hyperlipoproteinemia *0962*

272.21 Type IIB Hyperlipoproteinemia *0962*

282.60 Sickle Cell Anemia Patients have normal serum levels as a result of increased clearance. *0553*

320.90 Meningitis (Bacterial) High CSF levels of 0.9-1.3 mg/dL, with normal serum levels. *1338*

323.92 Encephalomyelitis High CSF levels of 0.9-1.3 mg/dL, with normal serum levels are seen in acute encephalitis. *1338*

331.90 Cerebral and Cortical Atrophy In the chronic stage. *1338*

340.00 Multiple Sclerosis Very low CSF levels of 0.02-0.04 mg/dL, with normal serum levels found in the chronic stage of disease. *1338*

642.40 Pre-Eclampsia Values may or may not be elevated in severe cases. When elevated, may represent liver or kidney dysfunction. *0433*

714.00 Rheumatoid Arthritis Generally normal. *0962*

Urine Decrease

277.21 Xanthinuria Characterized by the replacement of uric acid by xanthine and hypoxanthine in urine. *2246*

281.20 Folic Acid Deficiency Anemia Often depressed. *2538*

984.00 Toxic Effects of Lead and Its Compounds (including Fumes) Reduced renal clearance. *0106*

Urine Increase

13.00 Tuberculosis Meningitis Increased excretion in neurological and psychiatric disorders; progressive rise in urinary level following slight rise in blood, due to disturbed purine metabolism. *2301*

70.00 Viral Hepatitis 24 h excretion was markedly elevated in patients (1405 ± 149 mg/day) compared to controls (748 ± 58 mg/day). *1890*

202.80 Non-Hodgkins Lymphoma May occur, but more often is normal. *1639*

204.00 Lymphocytic Leukemia (Acute) Secondary to the increased cell turnover. *0433* Almost invariably. *1042*

204.10 Lymphocytic Leukemia (Chronic) Not as frequent as in other leukemias. *0992*

205.00 Myelocytic Leukemia (Acute) Mean urate excretion was 0.774 ± 0.057 mg/min, significantly higher than normal, 0.595 ± 0.035. *1601* Almost invariable. *1042 2552*

205.10 Myelocytic Leukemia (Chronic) Often 2-3 X normal in patients with active disease, and if aggressive therapy leads to rapid cell lysis, excretion of the additional purine load may produce urinary tract blockage. *1315* Almost invariably increased; gout may occur. *2552*

238.40 Polycythemia Vera Increased formation produces hyperuricemia and hyperuricosuria in 30-50% of patients at the time of diagnosis. Both tend to increase in frequency and severity as the disease progresses and may remain asymptomatic, but approximately 5-10% of patients develop symptoms and signs of gout. *2538 0839 2603*

268.20 Osteomalacia Reflects variable degree of disturbance of proximal tubular function. *0995*

270.03 Cystinosis Failure of reabsorption. *0995*

270.21 Alkaptonuria *2104*

271.01 Von Gierke's Disease Mean excretion was 1.5 ± 0.6 mg/mg creatinine, slightly elevated compared to 0.6 ± 0.1 mg/mg creatinine in normal children. *1960*

271.20 Hereditary Fructose Intolerance *0151*

274.00 Gout May occur during acute attack. *0091*

275.10 Hepatolenticular Degeneration Due to decreased renal tubular reabsorption. *0619*

275.34 Familial Periodic Paralysis Uricosuria accompanies attacks. *2104*

277.22 Lesch-Nyhan Syndrome Markedly increased. Ranges from 25-143 mg/kg/day compared to 18 as the normal upper limit in children. *1581 2246*

282.60 Sickle Cell Anemia Increased tubular secretion of urate; patients have normal serum levels as a result of increased clearance. *0553*

289.00 Polycythemia, Secondary *0619*

289.80 Myelofibrosis In myelofibrosis, secondary and the formation of urinary uric acid calculi are frequent consequences of the hyperuricemia and hyperuricosuria. *2538*

296.80 Manic Depressive Disorder Increased excretion in neurological and psychiatric disorders; progressive rise in urinary level following slight rise in blood, due to disturbed purine metabolism. *2301*

297.90 Paranoid States and Other Psychoses Increased excretion in neurological and psychiatric disorders; progressive rise in urinary level following slight rise in blood, due to disturbed purine metabolism. *2301*

300.40 Depressive Neurosis Increased excretion in neurological and psychiatric disorders; progressive rise in urinary level following slight rise in blood, due to disturbed purine metabolism. *2301*

320.90 Meningitis (Bacterial) Increased excretion in neurological and psychiatric disorders; progressive rise in urinary level following slight rise in blood, due to disturbed purine metabolism. *2301*

323.92 Encephalomyelitis Increased excretion in neurological and psychiatric disorders; progressive rise in urinary level following slight rise in blood, due to disturbed purine metabolism. *2301*

431.00 Cerebral Hemorrhage Increased excretion in neurological and psychiatric disorders; progressive rise in urinary level following slight rise in blood, due to disturbed purine metabolism. *2301*

434.00 Cerebral Thrombosis Increased excretion in neurological and psychiatric disorders; progressive rise in urinary level following slight rise in blood, due to disturbed purine metabolism. *2301*

434.10 Cerebral Embolism Increased excretion in neurological and psychiatric disorders; progressive rise in urinary level following slight rise in blood, due to disturbed purine metabolism. *2301*

434.90 Brain Infarction Increased excretion in neurological and psychiatric disorders; progressive rise in urinary level following slight rise in blood, due to disturbed purine metabolism. *2301*

555.90 Regional Enteritis or Ileitis High levels may be found. *0282 2035*

556.00 Ulcerative Colitis High levels may be found. *0282 2035*

588.81 Proximal Renal Tubular Acidosis Hypouricemia, secondary to increased renal clearance of uric acid, is present in some patients (children). *0433*

770.80 Respiratory Distress Syndrome Higher serum concentrations during the first 3 days of life, and the urinary excretion over the period of 12-36 h of age was also higher than in the normal infants. Neonatal hyperuricemia is not due to renal retention but to increased production of uric acid. *1874*

990.00 Effects of X-Ray Irradiation Reflects cellular breakdown. *0865*

Urine   Normal

202.80   **Non-Hodgkins Lymphoma**   Usually normal. *2552*

204.10   **Lymphocytic Leukemia (Chronic)**   Often normal. *2039*

CSF   Decrease

331.90   **Cerebral and Cortical Atrophy**   Very low CSF levels of 0.02-0.04 mg/dL, with normal serum levels found in the chronic stage of disease. *1338*

340.00   **Multiple Sclerosis**   Very low CSF levels of 0.02-0.04 mg/dL, with normal serum levels found in the chronic stage of disease. *1338*

CSF   Increase

13.00   **Tuberculosis Meningitis**   Markedly increased with decreased CSF:blood ratio, possibly due to cellular breakdown and nucleoprotein catabolism. *2301*

291.00   **Delirium Tremens**   High CSF levels of 0.9-1.3 mg/dL, with normal serum levels. *1338*

296.80   **Manic Depressive Disorder**   Markedly increased with decreased CSF:blood ratio, possibly due to cellular breakdown and nucleoprotein catabolism. *2301*

297.90   **Paranoid States and Other Psychoses**   Markedly increased with decreased CSF:blood ratio, possibly due to cellular breakdown and nucleoprotein catabolism. *2301*

300.40   **Depressive Neurosis**   Markedly increased with decreased CSF:blood ratio, possibly due to cellular breakdown and nucleoprotein catabolism. *2301*

320.90   **Meningitis (Bacterial)**   High CSF levels of 0.9-1.3 mg/dL, with normal serum levels. *1338*   Markedly increased with decreased blood:CSF ratio, possibly due to cellular breakdown and nucleoprotein catabolism. *2301*

323.92   **Encephalomyelitis**   High CSF levels of 0.9-1.3 mg/dL, with normal serum levels are seen in acute encephalitis. *1338*   Markedly increased with decreased blood:CSF ratio, possibly due to cellular breakdown and nucleoprotein catabolism. *2301*

431.00   **Cerebral Hemorrhage**   Markedly increased with decreased CSF:blood ratio, possibly due to cellular breakdown and nucleoprotein catabolism. *2301*

434.00   **Cerebral Thrombosis**   Markedly increased with decreased CSF:blood ratio, possibly due to cellular breakdown and nucleoprotein catabolism. *2301*

434.10   **Cerebral Embolism**   Markedly increased with decreased CSF:blood ratio, possibly due to cellular breakdown and nucleoprotein catabolism. *2301*

434.90   **Brain Infarction**   Markedly increased with decreased CSF:blood ratio, possibly due to cellular breakdown and nucleoprotein catabolism. *2301*

CSF   Normal

274.00   **Gout**   Very low in normal and gouty patients. Probably explains the absence of tophaceous deposits in the CNS. *2582*

Synovial Fluid   Increase

274.00   **Gout**   Many patients have a concentration which is greater than in serum. *1903*

Saliva   Increase

277.00   **Cystic Fibrosis**   Increased. *1359*

Uric Acid Clearance

Urine   Increase

201.90   **Hodgkin's Disease**   Hypouricemia associated with markedly elevated clearance has been reported. *1241*

275.10   **Hepatolenticular Degeneration**   Consistently high renal clearance even though some patients have total excretion values within the normal range. *2546*   Mean clearance = 17.1 mL/min/1.73 m^2. 87% of 24 patients had elevated clearance. *2278 2104*

282.60   **Sickle Cell Anemia**   Increased tubular secretion of urate; patients have normal serum levels as a result of increased clearance. *0553*

585.00   **Chronic Renal Failure**   Increases slightly early in renal failure and again in the late stages, causing plasma urate to rise less steeply than urea or creatinine. *0151*

588.81   **Proximal Renal Tubular Acidosis**   Hypouricemia, secondary to increased renal clearance of uric acid, is present in some patients (children). *0433*

948.00   **Burns**   Significantly increased renal clearance is found. *2506*

1013.00   **Diet**   High protein and carbohydrate diets accelerate renal clearance. *2104*

Urobilin

Feces   Increase

242.90   **Hyperthyroidism**   May be secondary to erythroid hyperplasia. *2540*

289.00   **Polycythemia, Secondary**   Increased slightly. *0151*

Urobilinogen

Urine   Decrease

157.90   **Malignant Neoplasm of Pancreas**   Absent in carcinoma of head of pancreas. *2467*

277.42   **Gilbert's Disease**   Normal or decreased. *2467*

277.44   **Crigler-Najjar Syndrome**   Normal or decreased. *2467*

576.20   **Extrahepatic Biliary Obstruction**   *2467*

Urine   Increase

70.00   **Viral Hepatitis**   At peak of the disease, it disappears for days or weeks. *2467*   Increases during defervescent period. *0433*

100.00   **Leptospirosis**   Jaundice may appear at the end of the 1st week of fever. Liver tests show hepatic decompensation of the intrahepatic type. *2368*

238.40   **Polycythemia Vera**   Rarely. *0995*

277.16   **Porphyria Cutanea Tarda**   May be increased because of liver disease. *2458*

277.41   **Dubin-Johnson Syndrome**   Urine contains bile and urobilinogen. *2467*

277.43   **Rotor's Syndrome**   Normal or increased. *2467*

281.00   **Pernicious Anemia**   Possibly in some cases. *0619*

282.00   **Hereditary (Congenital) Spherocytosis**   *0995 2538*

282.10   **Hereditary Elliptocytosis**   In severe cases. *0433*

282.20   **Anemias Due To Disorders of Glutathione Metabolism**   Increased hemolysis. *2467*

282.41   **Thalassemia Major**   Increased in urine without bile. *2468*

282.60   **Sickle Cell Anemia**   Urine contains increased urobilinogen but is negative for bile. *2467   0999*

283.00   **Acquired Hemolytic Anemia (Autoimmune)**   Commonly increased. *2538   2035*

283.21   **Paroxysmal Nocturnal Hemoglobinuria**   Increased blood destruction. *2552*

289.00   **Polycythemia, Secondary**   Increased slightly. *0151*

415.10   **Pulmonary Embolism and Infarction**   Hemorrhage into tissues. *2467*

428.00   **Congestive Heart Failure**   With hepatic anoxia. *0619 1108*

516.10   **Idiopathic Pulmonary Hemosiderosis**   Occasional findings of hemolytic type of anemia. *2467*   Excretion may be increased by the increased porphyrin catabolism. *2538*

570.00   **Acute and Subacute Necrosis of Liver**   Early hepatitis (usually the first 48 h, but it may persist for 1-2 days longer in some cases). Also in hepatic necrosis. *0619*   May precede the onset of jaundice by several days. *0999*

571.60   **Biliary Cirrhosis**   Urine contains urobilinogen and bilirubin. *2467*

571.90   **Cirrhosis of Liver**   In early and recovery stages. *2467*

573.30   **Toxic Hepatitis**   Normal or increased during preicteric phase. *2467*

575.00   **Acute Cholecystitis**   Usually disappears within 24-48 h after the attack subsides. *2199*

576.10   **Cholangitis**   With parenchymal cell necrosis and malfunction. *2467*   With infection of the biliary tract. In cholangitis very high concentrations are attained. *0619*

Urobilinogen *(continued)*

Urine   Increase *(continued)*

576.20   Extrahepatic Biliary Obstruction   With infection of the biliary tract. In cholangitis very high concentrations of urine urobilinogen are attained. Probably bacteria act in the proximal parts of the bile-ducts, on the bile-pigments. *0619*

773.00   Hemolytic Disease of Newborn (Erythroblastosis Fetalis)   Parallels serum levels. *2468*   Excess consistent with exaggerated hemolysis. *2061*

984.00   Toxic Effects of Lead and Its Compounds (including Fumes)   Possibly in some cases as evidence of increased red cell destruction. *0619   2468*

Urine   Normal

571.20   Laennec's or Alcoholic Cirrhosis   Normal or increased. *2467*

571.90   Cirrhosis of Liver   Normal or increased. *2467*

573.30   Toxic Hepatitis   *2467*

774.40   Jaundice Due to Hepatocellular Damage (Newborn)   *2467*

Feces   Decrease

70.00   Viral Hepatitis   Disappears at peak of disease. *2467*

157.90   Malignant Neoplasm of Pancreas   Absent in cancer of head of pancreas. *2467*

277.41   Dubin-Johnson Syndrome   *0995*

277.42   Gilbert's Disease   Normal or decreased. *2467*

277.43   Rotor's Syndrome   *2467*

277.44   Crigler-Najjar Syndrome   Usually very low but stool is of normal color. *2246*

573.30   Toxic Hepatitis   *2467*

576.20   Extrahepatic Biliary Obstruction   Marked decrease. Clay colored stools. *2467*   When very high serum bilirubin levels are attained, a little bilirubin may diffuse into the bowel, resulting in the appearance of small quantities of urobilinogen in the stools. Otherwise none is detected. *0619*

774.40   Jaundice Due to Hepatocellular Damage (Newborn)   Normal or decreased. *2467*

Feces   Increase

207.00   Erythroleukemia   Evidence of a mild or moderate increase in hemolysis is commonly observed, but the erythrokinetic findings are those of ineffective erythropoiesis. *2538*

277.11   Congenital Erythropoietic Porphyria (Günther's Disease)   *2073 2246*

281.00   Pernicious Anemia   Possibly in some cases. *0619*

282.00   Hereditary (Congenital) Spherocytosis   As much as 5-20 X normal. *2552   2538*

282.10   Hereditary Elliptocytosis   In severe cases. *0433*

282.41   Thalassemia Major   *2468*

282.60   Sickle Cell Anemia   *0999*

283.00   Acquired Hemolytic Anemia (Autoimmune)   Uniformly increased, but seldom necessary or useful for clinical purposes at present. *2538*

570.00   Acute and Subacute Necrosis of Liver   *2467*

773.00   Hemolytic Disease of Newborn (Erythroblastosis Fetalis)   Parallels serum levels of indirect bilirubin. *2468*

Urocanic Acid

Urine   Decrease

270.51   Histidinemia   Chromatography of the urinary metabolites of histidine will reveal an absence of urocanic acid. *0433*   Reported to be absent from urine in several studies, but normal concentrations are low and methods of detection lack specificity. *2246 2570 1065*

Uropepsinogen

Urine   Decrease

280.90   Iron Deficiency Anemia   With achlorhydria. *0619*

281.00   Pernicious Anemia   With achlorhydria. *0619*

535.00   Gastritis   With atrophic gastritis. *0587*

Urine   Increase

650.00   Pregnancy   Moderate increase in output. *0619*

948.00   Burns   *0619*

Uroporphyrin

Serum   Increase

277.11   Congenital Erythropoietic Porphyria (Günther's Disease)   Variable. *2246 2072*

Urine   Increase

277.11   Congenital Erythropoietic Porphyria (Günther's Disease)   Most characteristic metabolic abnormality. *2552*   Large amounts. *2538*   Daily excretion of 500 µg/24h has been reported. *0935*   Up to 500 µg/24h has been reported. *2246*

277.12   Erythropoietic Protoporphyria   Only in patients with hepatic complications. *2246*

277.14   Acute Intermittent Porphyria   Excessive amounts. *0995*   May contain little if any increase. *0443*   May develop in urine on standing. *2246*

277.15   Porphyria Variegata   During acute attacks. *0995*   Characteristic finding in urine and feces. *1940*   Sharp rise in acute attacks. *0613   2538*

277.16   Porphyria Cutanea Tarda   In 66 patients, average was 2,819 µg/L and exceeded 1,000 µg/L in 70% of the group (normal < 40 mg/24h). *0611*   During acute attacks. *0995*   Usually 1-10 mg/24h. *0613*

277.17   Hereditary Coproporphyria   *0995*

984.00   Toxic Effects of Lead and Its Compounds (including Fumes)   *2468*

Urine   Normal

277.12   Erythropoietic Protoporphyria   *1478 2246*

277.13   Erythropoietic Coproporphyria   *1529*

Bone Marrow   Increase

277.11   Congenital Erythropoietic Porphyria (Günther's Disease)   Bone marrow is studded with red cell precursors containing uroporphyrin in the nucleus and showing intense fluorescence when examined under ultraviolet light. *2073   2538 2072*

Feces   Increase

277.11   Congenital Erythropoietic Porphyria (Günther's Disease)   Usually large amounts. *2246*

277.14   Acute Intermittent Porphyria   In some patients. *2498*   Small increases may be found. *2246*

277.15   Porphyria Variegata   May be increased. *2303*   Variable. *0868*

277.16   Porphyria Cutanea Tarda   Highly variable. *2314*

Feces   Normal

277.12   Erythropoietic Protoporphyria   *2246*

277.13   Erythropoietic Coproporphyria   *0995*

Liver   Increase

277.14   Acute Intermittent Porphyria   Has been isolated from hepatic tissue in some cases. *2072 2246*

Red Blood Cells   Increase

277.11   Congenital Erythropoietic Porphyria (Günther's Disease)   High concentrations. *2072*   High RBC concentration of uroporphyrin I. *2072 2246*

277.12   Erythropoietic Protoporphyria   Moderate concentrations. *0995*

277.13   Erythropoietic Coproporphyria   Moderate concentrations. *0995*

Red Blood Cells   Normal

277.14   Acute Intermittent Porphyria   *0995*

277.15   Porphyria Variegata   *0995 2246*

277.16   Porphyria Cutanea Tarda   *0995*

277.17   Hereditary Coproporphyria   No increase demonstrable. *2246 0868   0995*

Valine

Serum   Decrease

66.00   Phlebotomus Fever   Most free serum amino acid are depressed in sandfly fever and other mild-moderate infections. *0122*

259.20   Carcinoid Syndrome   Decreased plasma concentration, but normal urinary excretion was found. *0718*

260.00   Protein Malnutrition   *0151*

333.40   Huntington's Chorea   Reduced fasting plasma concentrations of leucine, isoleucine and valine. *1816*   19 patients showed a significantly lower concentration of proline, aminolevulinic acid, valine, leucine, isoleucine, and tyrosine compared to 38 normal controls. *0534*

572.20   Hepatic Encephalopathy   Branched chain amino acids are generally reduced. *1473*

Serum   Increase

70.00   Viral Hepatitis   A close relationship was found between the onset of encephalopathy and amino acid equilibrium disturbance, characterized by a fall in the molar ratio between valine, leucine and isoleucine, and phenylalanine and tyrosine. All showed absolute elevations with onset of encephalopathy. *0531*

270.31   Maple Syrup Urine Disease   Excessively high. *1797 2246*

Urine   Increase

270.02   Hartnup Disease   5-20 X normal values. *2246   0995*

270.03   Cystinosis   Nonspecific pattern of aminoaciduria. Fanconi's syndrome. *0995*

270.31   Maple Syrup Urine Disease   Greatly increased urinary excretion. *2468*

275.10   Hepatolenticular Degeneration   *0503*

Vanillylamine

Serum   Increase

227.91   Pheochromocytoma   Values should be twice upper limit of normal (normal < 6.8 mg/day) *0999*

Urine   Increase

192.50   Neuroblastoma   False positive results may occur due to certain foods and certain drugs. Detects 75% of neuroblastomas, ganglioneuromas and ganglioblastomas if used alone. In combination with HVA or total catecholamines, 95-100% may be detected. *2467*   Excretion > 2 X normal is diagnostic providing all dietary restrictions have been followed. *2612*

227.91   Pheochromocytoma   False positive results may occur due to certain foods and certain drugs. Monamine oxidase inhibitors may increase metanephrine and decrease VMA. Excretion is considerably increased. *2467*   In almost all patients analysis of any 24 h urine collection will reveal increased excretion. *0151*   Phenolic acids of dietary origin may yield many false positive tests. *1108*   Excretion > 2 X normal is diagnostic providing all dietary restrictions have been followed. *2612   1630 2440 0962*

346.00   Migraine   Levels are increased during acute attacks. *0996*

390.00   Rheumatic Fever   Increased VMA excretion was observed in cases of grade 4 hemodynamic disturbance. *2572*

401.00   Malignant Hypertension   May occur. *0995*

414.00   Chronic Ischemic Heart Disease   Increased excretion was observed in cases of grade 4 hemodynamic disturbance. *2572*

415.00   Cor Pulmonale   Increased excretion observed in cases of grade 4 hemodynamic disturbance. *2572*

994.50   Exercise   Significant effect after physical stress. *0768*

Urine   Normal

335.20   Amyotrophic Lateral Sclerosis   *0665*

585.00   Chronic Renal Failure   Normal urinary excretion. *0649*

Vasopressin

CSF   Decrease

331.00   Alzheimer's Disease   Significant decrease in arginine vasopressin compared to elderly and younger normal control subjects. *1881*

VDRL

Serum   Positive

11.00   Pulmonary Tuberculosis   False positive serologic tests may be seen. *0999*

13.00   Tuberculosis Meningitis   False positive serologic tests for syphilis may be seen. *0999*

18.00   Disseminated Tuberculosis   False positive serologic tests may be seen. *0999*

23.00   Brucellosis   False positive serologic tests are sometimes seen. *0999*

30.00   Leprosy   False positive serologic test occurs in 40% of patients. *2468*   Found in 70%. *2035*   Frequent biological false positive reactions. *2368*

55.00   Measles   False positive tests are sometimes seen. *0999*

75.00   Infectious Mononucleosis   False positive serologic tests for syphilis are sometimes seen. *0999*   Occurs occasionally, usually reverts to negative by the 3rd week. *1319*   The incidence of false positive reactions is 5%. *1108*   Positive tests occur but are unusual. *0502   2538*

80.00   Epidemic Typhus   In 20% of patients. *1058*

84.00   Malaria   False positive may occur. *0151*   Found in 100% of cases. *1058*

86.90   Trypanosomiasis   False positive in 10% of cases. *1058*

87.00   Relapsing Fever   45% false positive. *2230*   30% false positive. *1058   2468*

97.90   Syphilis   Negative at the onset of primary syphilis, but within 7-14 days it becomes positive in the majority of cases. Almost all sera from patients with secondary syphilis are positive. Asymptomatic or latent syphilis can be diagnosed only by a positive serologic test. *0999*   Becomes positive in most patients 2-3 weeks after the appearance of the chancre or 6 weeks after the initial contact. In the secondary stage, especially when generalized eruptions occur, it is positive in virtually 100% of patients. *0962*

99.10   Lymphogranuloma Venereum   Biologic false-positive serologic tests are not infrequent. *2199*   20% false positive. *1058*

100.00   Leptospirosis   10% false positive. *1058*

102.90   Yaws   All serological tests for syphilis are positive. *1058*

114.90   Coccidioidomycosis   Low incidence of false positive results. *1058*

245.20   Hashimoto's Thyroiditis   Persistent false positive reactions are seen. *0999*   A false positive serologic test may occur. *0962*

273.30   Waldenström's Macroglobulinemia   Biologic false positive found in some cases. *0020*

304.90   Drug Dependence (Opium and Derivatives)   Incidence of false positive reactions is 20% in narcotic addicts. *1108*

390.00   Rheumatic Fever   Not uncommon to encounter biologic false-positive reactions. *0151*

446.60   Thrombotic Thrombocytopenic Purpura   In 10% of patients (biological false-positive). *0054*

483.01   Mycoplasma Pneumoniae   False positive reactions in screening tests are common. *2368*

710.00   Systemic Lupus Erythematosus   A persistent biologic false positive serologic test for syphilis may precede overt manifestations by many months or years. *0999*   Biologic false positive results in 14% of patients. *0713*   Incidence of false positive reactions is 15%. *1108*

710.10   Progressive Systemic Sclerosis   Occasionally there are biologic false-positive tests. *1700*

714.00   Rheumatoid Arthritis   Biologic false positive tests reported in 5-10% of patients. Those patients are more likely to have positive LE cell tests. *0962*

CSF   Positive

97.90   Syphilis   In asymptomatic neurosyphilis the blood and spinal fluid VDRL are usually both reactive. *0962*   Positive as a result of serum or blood leaking into the CSF. *0999*

Viscosity

Serum   Increase

84.00   Malaria   Significantly increased in 15 patients with acute renal failure due to falciparum infection. *2190*

Viscosity (continued)

Serum   Increase (continued)

203.00   Multiple Myeloma   An increase of IgM is the most common clinical situation producing hyperviscosity of serum. *0962* Occurs in only 2-4% of patients. *2226*

238.40   Polycythemia Vera   Clinical manifestations may be related to increased blood viscosity. *0999*

273.30   Waldenström's Macroglobulinemia   The relative serum viscosity was elevated above 4 in 41% of patients and 36% of these patients developed symptoms of hyperviscosity sometime in the course of their disease. *1469*   A great increase in serum viscosity. Is usually associated with the presence of macroglobulins. *2538*   Some increase in serum viscosity is found in about 66% of patients tested, but only 50% of these will manifest symptoms of the hyperviscosity syndrome. *2552 0962*

282.60   Sickle Cell Anemia   Increased viscosity of circulating whole blood may contribute to vaso-occlusion. *0874*

282.71   Hemoglobin C Disease   Blood viscosity is increased. *0962*

410.90   Acute Myocardial Infarction   Due to alterations in serum proteins during the acute phase of illness. *1108   1146*

415.00   Cor Pulmonale   An increase in blood viscosity, red blood cell mass, and blood volume is thought to further compromise the pressure-flow relationships of the constricted and restricted pulmonary vascular bed. *1108*

496.00   Chronic Obstructive Lung Disease   An increase in blood viscosity, red blood cell mass, and blood volume is thought to further compromise the pressure-flow relationships of the constricted and restricted pulmonary vascular bed. *1108*

584.00   Acute Renal Failure   Significantly increased in 15 patients with acute failure due to falciparum malaria. *2190*

642.40   Pre-Eclampsia   Apparent blood viscosity rises sharply as the hematocrit increases due to hemoconcentration. *0387*

642.60   Eclampsia   Apparent blood viscosity rises sharply as the hematocrit increases due to hemoconcentration. *0387*

710.00   Systemic Lupus Erythematosus   Modest increases may be seen, but no hyperviscosity syndromes have been reported. *2135*

948.00   Burns   Rises acutely and remains elevated for 4-5 days although hematocrit has returned to normal. *2468*

Synovial Fluid   Decrease

274.00   Gout   *0962*

390.00   Rheumatic Fever   *0962*

710.00   Systemic Lupus Erythematosus   Slightly decreased. *0962*

714.00   Rheumatoid Arthritis   *0962*

720.00   Rheumatoid (Ankylosing) Spondylitis   Lower than blood. *0666*

Synovial Fluid   Normal

715.90   Osteoarthritis   *0666*

Red Blood Cells   Increase

282.71   Hemoglobin C Disease   A tendency to increased intracellular viscosity with decreased cell deformability. *2552*

Vitamin A

Serum   Decrease

18.00   Disseminated Tuberculosis   Impaired absorption. *0619*

70.00   Viral Hepatitis   In severe hepatitis. *2467*

259.20   Carcinoid Syndrome   Secondary to malabsorption or steatorrhea. *2540*

260.00   Protein Malnutrition   Extremely low. *0151*

269.90   Deficiency State (Unspecified)   *0619*

272.51   Tangier Disease   Occasionally low. *0878*

272.52   Abetalipoproteinemia   Very low. *0878   1242*

277.00   Cystic Fibrosis   *0055*

570.00   Acute and Subacute Necrosis of Liver   *0619*

571.90   Cirrhosis of Liver   *0619*

572.40   Hepatic Failure   *0503*

576.20   Extrahepatic Biliary Obstruction   *0619*

577.10   Chronic Pancreatitis   Some cases. *0619*

579.00   Celiac Sprue Disease   Due to faulty fat absorption. *0619   0433*

Serum   Increase

581.90   Nephrotic Syndrome   *0619*

585.00   Chronic Renal Failure   *0619*

Serum   Normal

272.51   Tangier Disease   *2246*

Vitamin B$_{12}$

Serum   Decrease

7.10   Giardiasis   Vitamin B$_{12}$ absorption is decreased. *0996*

123.40   Diphyllobothriasis (Intestinal)   Loss of ingested vitamin B$_{12}$. *2467   2538*

151.90   Malignant Neoplasm of Stomach   Inadequate absorption, lack of intrinsic factor, loss of gastric mucosa. *2467*

242.90   Hyperthyroidism   Secondary to increased metabolic processes. *2540*

244.90   Hypothyroidism   Almost 50% of patients have achlorhydria with intrinsic factor failure and low vitamin B$_{12}$; rarely megaloblastic anemia develops. *2467   1078*

273.22   Heavy Chain Disease (Alpha)   Impaired absorption. *2035*

281.00   Pernicious Anemia   Markedly decreased, mean value in 39 patients was 34 pg/mL compared to 385 pg/mL in normals. *1990   2538*

340.00   Multiple Sclerosis   Malabsorption of vitamin B$_{12}$ was found in 11.9% of 52 patients. *0938*

535.00   Gastritis   With atrophic gastritis. *2199*

555.90   Regional Enteritis or Ileitis   Tests may be abnormal. *0151* Frequently moderate anemia, most often iron deficiency, but occasionally macrocytic caused by poor diet or failure to absorb vitamin B$_{12}$ normally. *2199*

556.00   Ulcerative Colitis   Anemia may be due to blood loss, simple iron deficiency, deficiencies in folic acid, pyridoxine, or vitamin B$_{12}$. *0433*

564.20   Postgastrectomy (Dumping) Syndrome   Iron deficiency and vitamin B$_{12}$ deficiency are common following subtotal gastrectomy. *0962*

579.00   Celiac Sprue Disease   Patients may show a megaloblastic anemia and leukopenia secondary to folic acid or vitamin B$_{12}$ deficiency. Malabsorption. *2467*   If severe ileal disease is present, vitamin B$_{12}$ absorption is abnormally low both with and without added intrinsic factor. *2199   0433 2538*

579.90   Malabsorption, Cause Unspecified   Particularly in tropical sprue and bacterial overgrowth. *0151*

650.00   Pregnancy   Progressive decrease during pregnancy. *2467*

710.10   Progressive Systemic Sclerosis   A selective vitamin B$_{12}$ deficiency only or a decrease in iron stores may be present without other obvious signs of the malabsorption syndrome. *0962*

Serum   Increase

197.70   Secondary Malignant Neoplasm of Liver   *2467*

202.80   Non-Hodgkins Lymphoma   High levels were found in 15 patients with lymphomas, mean = 1,059 compared to normal, 385 pg/mL. *1990*   Usually normal. *2552*

204.10   Lymphocytic Leukemia (Chronic)   About 33% of cases. *2467*   Significant increase in 19 patients, mean = 1223 compared to normal, 385 pg/mL. *1990*

205.00   Myelocytic Leukemia (Acute)   Acute myelocytic leukemic cells may secrete a vitamin B$_{12}$ binding protein in large quantity, accounting for high serum levels of B$_{12}$. *0151*   Usually high, in contrast to acute lymphocytic leukemia. *0142   2538*

205.10   Myelocytic Leukemia (Chronic)   Significant increase found in 27 patients, mean for the group = 675, compared to normal, 385. *1990*   Increased to an average of approximately 15 X the normal mean concentration, generally proportional to the height of the leukocyte count in untreated patients, but still 4 X normal in patients who have normal WBC counts during remissions. *2538   0151*

206.00   Monocytic Leukemia   Increases in some cases. *2467*

207.00   Erythroleukemia   In many, but not all patients. *2538*

238.40 Polycythemia Vera   Usually increased. *0999*   Marked increase; mean was 741 pg/mL in 40 patients (normal = 385). *1990* Above 900 pg/mL found in about 33% of patients before treatment or during relapse. *2538*

260.00 Protein Malnutrition   Usually increased with kwashiorkor. *2468*

280.90 Iron Deficiency Anemia   Slight increase; mean = 466 pg/mL in 118 patients (normal = 385). *1990*

289.80 Myelofibrosis   Normal or elevated in myelofibrosis. *2317* Significantly increased in 7 cases of myelofibrosis, mean = 1,525 compared to normal, 385 pg/mL. *1990*   Serum concentration is generally raised, as is the binding power, but neither of them is as high as in chronic granulocytic leukemia (in myelofibrosis). *0841 2538 0142*

570.00 Acute and Subacute Necrosis of Liver   The blood level may be 3-8 X the normal concentration. Predominantly the free form is increased. *0619*

571.90 Cirrhosis of Liver   May be 3-8 X the normal concentration. The increase is mainly in the alpha-globulin bound fraction. *0619* Markedly increased; mean = 608 pg/mL in 33 patients. *1990*

572.20 Hepatic Encephalopathy   May increase to 30-40 X the normal level. The increase is mainly in the free form. *0619*

Serum   Normal

201.90 Hodgkin's Disease   *2467*

202.80 Non-Hodgkins Lymphoma   Usually normal. *2538*

203.00 Multiple Myeloma   *2467*

204.00 Lymphocytic Leukemia (Acute)   Usually normal, in contrast to acute myelogenous leukemia. *0142*

204.10 Lymphocytic Leukemia (Chronic)   *2468 0142*

272.52 Abetalipoproteinemia   *1583*

281.20 Folic Acid Deficiency Anemia   *2538*

289.00 Polycythemia, Secondary   *2538*

Feces   Increase

340.00 Multiple Sclerosis   Malabsorption of vitamin B$_{12}$ was found in 11.9% of 52 patients. *0938*

Vitamin B$_{12}$ Binding Capacity

Serum   Decrease

579.90 Malabsorption, Cause Unspecified   *0151*

Serum   Increase

201.90 Hodgkin's Disease   Significant elevation; usually correlated with WBC in peripheral blood. *1990*

202.80 Non-Hodgkins Lymphoma   Significant elevation; usually correlated with WBC in peripheral blood. *1990*

203.00 Multiple Myeloma   Significant elevation; usually correlated with WBC in peripheral blood. *1990*

204.00 Lymphocytic Leukemia (Acute)   Significant elevation; usually correlated with WBC in peripheral blood. *1990*

204.10 Lymphocytic Leukemia (Chronic)   Significant elevation; usually correlated with WBC in peripheral blood. *1990*

205.00 Myelocytic Leukemia (Acute)   Significant elevation; usually correlated with WBC in peripheral blood. *1990*

205.10 Myelocytic Leukemia (Chronic)   Increased in the vast majority of patients with myeloproliferative disorders, reflective of the WBC pool size. *0337*   Despite the increased amount of vitamin B$_{12}$, there is considerable additional unsaturated binding capacity. *1825 2538 2552*

238.40 Polycythemia Vera   Significant elevation; usually correlated with WBC in peripheral blood. *1990*   Increased to values > 2,200 pg/mL in about 75% of these patients. Found to be related directly to disease activity. *2538 0841*

281.00 Pernicious Anemia   Increased binding capacity, mean = 1,682 (normal = 1,208 pg/mL) and decreased serum concentration. *1990*

281.20 Folic Acid Deficiency Anemia   Significant elevation; usually correlated with WBC in peripheral blood. *1990*

289.80 Myelofibrosis   Significant elevation; usually correlated with WBC in peripheral blood. *1990*   In myelofibrosis, serum concentration is generally raised as is the binding power, but neither of them is as high as in chronic granulocytic leukemia. *0841 2538*

571.90 Cirrhosis of Liver   Significant elevation; usually correlated with WBC in peripheral blood. *1990*

710.00 Systemic Lupus Erythematosus   Significant elevation; usually correlated with WBC in peripheral blood. *1990*

Serum   Normal

202.80 Non-Hodgkins Lymphoma   Usually normal. *2538*

272.52 Abetalipoproteinemia   *1583*

289.00 Polycythemia, Secondary   *2538*

Vitamin E (Tocopherol)

Serum   Decrease

272.51 Tangier Disease   One subject. *2246*

272.52 Abetalipoproteinemia   Very low concentration. *1215*

277.00 Cystic Fibrosis   *0896*

571.60 Biliary Cirrhosis   Deficiency might be expected in patients with defective fat absorption. *2104*

579.00 Celiac Sprue Disease   Decreased. *2053*

1013.00 Diet   Low concentrations indicate a diet high in unsaturated fats. *2104*

Serum   Increase

650.00 Pregnancy   Average is about 65% higher than normal at term. *2104*

Vitamin K

Serum   Decrease

277.00 Cystic Fibrosis   Occasionally occurs. *0551*

576.20 Extrahepatic Biliary Obstruction   Due to fat malabsorption. *2104*

579.00 Celiac Sprue Disease   Due to malabsorption. *2538*

579.90 Malabsorption, Cause Unspecified   Deficiency and resulting bleeding tendency is to be expected with fat malabsorption. *2104*

Volume

Plasma   Decrease

84.00 Malaria   Initial hypovolemia followed by hypervolemia or normovolemia in acute renal failure due to falciparum. *2190*   A rare and serious complication. *1058*

227.91 Pheochromocytoma   Low in < 33% of patients. *0433*

238.40 Polycythemia Vera   Most often. *0995*

244.90 Hypothyroidism   Total volume is reduced by 25% on the average. *1669*

250.00 Diabetes Mellitus   *2467*

253.50 Diabetes Insipidus   *2467*

255.00 Adrenal Cortical Hyperfunction (Glucocorticoid Excess)   Polycythemia occurs in 10-20% of patients, due either to an increase in red cell volume or decrease in plasma volume. *1669*

255.40 Adrenal Cortical Hypofunction   Fluid depletion leads to reduced circulating blood volume and renal circulatory insufficiency. *2612*

256.00 Ovarian Hyperfunction   Progesterone effect. *0995*

260.00 Protein Malnutrition   Normal or decreased. *2467*

276.50 Dehydration   Reduced 13.6% after 2-11 h heat exposure. *2114*

277.14 Acute Intermittent Porphyria   Frequently observed during attacks. *2254*

410.90 Acute Myocardial Infarction   Probably the result of reflex adrenergic discharge and vasoconstriction, pooling or trapping of blood, sweating, or the development of pulmonary edema. *1108*

537.00 Pyloric Stenosis, Acquired   *2467*

556.00 Ulcerative Colitis   Fever, hypovolemia, tachycardia and hypoproteinemia are major manifestations. *0999*

558.90 Diarrhea   When salt and water are lost in isotonic proportions, a contraction of the extracellular fluid compartment occurs and hemoconcentration develops. *2199 2467*

Volume *(continued)*

Plasma Decrease *(continued)*

564.20 Postgastrectomy (Dumping) Syndrome Jejunal hypersecretion of water and electrolytes, with resultant reduced plasma volume. *0995*

567.90 Peritonitis Exudation of fluid leads to reduction in effective circulating volume. *0995*

579.90 Malabsorption, Cause Unspecified *0151*

581.90 Nephrotic Syndrome In nephrotic syndrome, even with edema, blood volume is normal or decreased. *1669*

584.00 Acute Renal Failure Initial hypovolemia followed by hyper- or normovolemia in acute renal failure due to falciparum malaria. *2190*

585.00 Chronic Renal Failure Hydremia and dehydration are common. Changes will exaggerate or minimize the degree of anemia. *2552*

588.81 Proximal Renal Tubular Acidosis *2467*

642.40 Pre-Eclampsia Hemoconcentration is an index of severity and prognosis. *0387*

642.60 Eclampsia Hemoconcentration is an index of severity and prognosis. *0387* In severe cases. *0621*

787.00 Vomiting *0619*

948.00 Burns Decreased plasma volume and blood volume follows marked drop in cardiac output. Greatest decrease occurs in first 12 h and continues at a slower rate for 6-12 h longer. In a 40% burn, plasma volume falls 25%. *2468*

992.00 Heat stroke Reduced 13.6% after 2-11 h heat exposure. *2114*

994.80 Effects of Electric Current Immediately following major injury. *0995*

Plasma Increase

84.00 Malaria Initial hypovolemia followed by hypervolemia or normovolemia in acute renal failure due to falciparum. *2190* A rare and serious complication. *1058*

85.00 Leishmaniasis In 64 cases of tropical splenomegaly, plasma volumes ranged from 52-129 mL/kg. 70% of the increase was attributable to increased intravascular pools of IgG and IgM (42%) and albumin (28%). *0466*

203.00 Multiple Myeloma Often expands as the amount of myeloma protein increases in the serum, and the resulting hemodilution may be great enough to produce a significant reduction in hemoglobin concentration with little or no change in total red cell mass. *1301* *2538*

238.40 Polycythemia Vera The greatest increase occurs in patients with a significant degree of hepatosplenomegaly. *2538* *1835*

242.90 Hyperthyroidism Corpuscular and total hypervolemia may occur to facilitate oxygen delivery to tissues. *1669* Increase in plasma volume keeps the hemoglobin concentration from reaching polycythemic values. *2538* *1642*

255.10 Adrenal Cortical Hyperfunction (Mineralocorticoid Excess) An increased volume, with slight decrease of the Hct value, is usual. *1108*

256.30 Ovarian Hypofunction Estrogen effect. *0995*

260.00 Protein Malnutrition Plasma volume expressed in mL/kg of body weight was increased. Dilution was a major factor responsible for the reduction in hemoglobin concentration. *2538*

273.30 Waldenström's Macroglobulinemia *0186*

289.00 Polycythemia, Secondary Red cell mass increased. *0619*

289.40 Hypersplenism When the spleen is greatly enlarged, the plasma volume and total blood volume are significantly expanded. *2538* Apparent anemia is often due to expansion of plasma volume in the presence of normal RBC volume. *1824*

410.90 Acute Myocardial Infarction Significant increases in plasma volume, reflected by changes in hct. Average change was 12%. For the patients with accompanying pulmonary edema, the change was 17%. *2554*

415.00 Cor Pulmonale An increase in blood viscosity, red blood cell mass, and blood volume is thought to further compromise the pressure-flow relationships of the constricted and restricted pulmonary vascular bed. *1108*

428.00 Congestive Heart Failure Overall hypervolemia involving both plasma and red cell volume. *1669* May be normal or increased. *1108* *0619*

492.80 Pulmonary Emphysema Normal or increased. *2467*

496.00 Chronic Obstructive Lung Disease An increase in blood viscosity, red blood cell mass, and blood volume is thought to further compromise the pressure-flow relationships of the constricted and restricted pulmonary vascular bed. *1108*

571.20 Laennec's or Alcoholic Cirrhosis With nutritional cirrhosis; usually moderate and occurs in approximately 33% of the patients. *1311* Averages 15% above normal. Hemodilution exaggerates anemia. *1268* In 64% of patients. *1669* *1108*

571.90 Cirrhosis of Liver Averages 15% above normal. Hemodilution exaggerates anemia. *1268* In 64% of patients. *1669*

580.00 Acute Poststreptococcal Glomerulonephritis Plasma volume may be as much as 50% above normal during edematous phase. *1669* The decreased GFR and increased aldosterone secretion lead to retention of sodium and water with resultant hypervolemia. *1108*

584.00 Acute Renal Failure Initial hypovolemia followed by hyper- or normovolemia in acute renal failure due to falciparum malaria. *2190* *2467*

585.00 Chronic Renal Failure Hydremia and dehydration are common. Changes will exaggerate or minimize the degree of anemia. *2552*

650.00 Pregnancy The increment averages 40% above non-pregnant values, its magnitude varying with the parity of the mother and with her body composition. *1108* Begins to increase about the 6th week and reaches a maximum between the 26-36 weeks. *0387* *2538*

694.40 Pemphigus *0151*

Plasma Normal

84.00 Malaria Initial hypovolemia followed by hypervolemia or normovolemia in acute renal failure due to falciparum. *2190* A rare and serious complication. *1058*

238.40 Polycythemia Vera Within the normal range in the majority of patients, reduced in some, and increased in others. *2538* *1100*

492.80 Pulmonary Emphysema Normal or increased. *2467*

780.80 Hyperhidrosis *2467*

Urine Decrease

80.00 Epidemic Typhus Oliguria is common. *2368*

82.00 Rocky Mountain Spotted Fever Oliguria is common. *2368*

255.40 Adrenal Cortical Hypofunction Normal or decreased. *2467*

260.00 Protein Malnutrition In total colonic starvation. *0995*

276.50 Dehydration *2467*

277.14 Acute Intermittent Porphyria Prolonged vomiting may cause dehydration, oliguria, and azotemia. *0151*

428.00 Congestive Heart Failure With edema. *0619*

537.00 Pyloric Stenosis, Acquired *2467*

558.90 Diarrhea *2467*

560.90 Intestinal Obstruction Urinary output diminishes early in the disease. *0151*

571.20 Laennec's or Alcoholic Cirrhosis With ascites and edema. *0619*

571.90 Cirrhosis of Liver With ascites and edema. *0619*

580.00 Acute Poststreptococcal Glomerulonephritis The disease is sometimes ushered in by oliguria which may progress to complete anuria. *0995* *0619*

580.40 Glomerulonephritis (Rapidly Progressive) Oliguria < 500 mL/24h was present in 20 of 29 cases and dialysis was required in 22. *1633*

584.00 Acute Renal Failure Urine is scant in volume (often < 50 mL/day) for 2 weeks, in the early stage. Daily volume of 400 mL indicates onset of tubular recovery. Daily volume of 1,000 mL occurs in several days or < 2 weeks. *2468* Manifested by oliguria, urine osmolality of < 400 mOsm/kg and a urine/plasma osmolality ratio of < 1-5. *1607* *2467*

585.00 Chronic Renal Failure With renal parenchymal disease. *0838* Terminal chronic nephritis *0619*

590.00 Chronic Pyelonephritis With renal parenchymal disease. *0838*

590.10 Acute Pyelonephritis With renal parenchymal disease. *0838 0619*

992.00 Heat stroke Urine volume is low in severe cases. *0151*

994.50 Exercise With heavy exercise. *1205*

Urine Increase

242.90 Hyperthyroidism Mild polyuria. *2199*

250.00 Diabetes Mellitus As the urine sugar content rises, glucose acts as a diuretic, i.e., the renal tubules are reabsorbing glucose at their maximum rate and the excess glucose prevents further water reabsorption. *0619*

250.10 Diabetic Acidosis *2540*

252.00 Hyperparathyroidism Polyuria due to the inability to concentrate the urine. Related to the hypercalcemia and does not aid in differential diagnosis. *0433*

253.40 Anterior Pituitary Hypofunction Diminished tubular sodium reabsorption because of adrenal cortical steroid deficiency. The urine volume is increased, with loss of the normal diurnal variation, and an increased sodium and chloride concentration. *0619*

253.50 Diabetes Insipidus Large volume (4-15 L/24h) is characteristic. *2468* After ingestion of 1,000 mL of 1% sodium chloride the urine volume in normal subjects and in pathological polydipsia is 25% of the ingested fluid. In diabetes insipidus the excretion rate is unchanged. *0619* Usually > 3 L/day. *0962* Polyuria and hyposthenuria. *2246 0151*

255.00 Adrenal Cortical Hyperfunction (Glucocorticoid Excess) Polyuria. *0995*

255.10 Adrenal Cortical Hyperfunction (Mineralocorticoid Excess) *2467*

260.00 Protein Malnutrition In semistarvation, polyuria of 2-3 L/day and nocturia. *0995*

405.91 Renovascular Hypertension A 50% or greater decrease in volume excreted and a 15% or greater decrease in sodium concentration indicated renal artery obstruction and reversible renovascular hypertension. *1108 2440*

588.81 Proximal Renal Tubular Acidosis Characterized by polyuria. *2246 2467*

650.00 Pregnancy May increase up to 25% in last trimester. *2468*

753.10 Polycystic Kidney Disease Common. *0186*

753.12 Medullary Cystic Disease Polyuria. *0995*

994.50 Exercise With mild exercise. *1205*

Urine Normal

255.40 Adrenal Cortical Hypofunction Normal or decreased. *2467*

492.80 Pulmonary Emphysema *2467*

579.90 Malabsorption, Cause Unspecified *2467*

780.80 Hyperhidrosis *2467*

Duodenal Contents Normal

577.20 Pancreatic Cyst and Pseudocyst Duodenal contents after secretin-pancreozymin stimulation usually show decreased bicarbonate content (< 80 mmol/L) but normal volume and normal content of amylase, lipase, and trypsin. *2467*

Feces Increase

579.90 Malabsorption, Cause Unspecified Unabsorbed fats and fatty acids cause stools to be bulky and voluminous. *0151*

Platelet Decrease

279.12 Wiskott-Aldrich Syndrome Mean platelet volume was markedly decreased but returned to normal post- splenectomy. *0455*

Red Blood Cells Decrease

227.91 Pheochromocytoma Decreased in the hypertension resulting from pheochromocytoma. *1669*

285.00 Sideroblastic Anemia Erythrocytes are formed in normal numbers but are reduced in size. *2552*

440.00 Arteriosclerosis RBC volume is decreased in the hypertension resulting from renal artery stenosis. *1669*

571.90 Cirrhosis of Liver 25% of patients. *1669*

Red Blood Cells Increase

189.00 Malignant Neoplasm of Kidney True polycythemia may occur. *1669*

238.40 Polycythemia Vera Unless the RBC volume is > 38 mL/kg for males and 36 mL/kg for females, the diagnosis of polycythemia vera cannot be considered established. *0151*

255.00 Adrenal Cortical Hyperfunction (Glucocorticoid Excess) Polycythemia occurs in 10-20% of patients, due either to an increase in red cell volume or decrease in plasma volume. *1669*

428.00 Congestive Heart Failure Overall hypervolemia involving both plasma and red cell volume. *1669*

440.00 Arteriosclerosis True polycythemia with a considerable increase of red cell volume may occur. *1669*

591.00 Hydronephrosis True polycythemia with a considerable increase of red cell volume may occur. *1669*

650.00 Pregnancy Red cell volume actually increases by about 20%. *2538* Although both plasma volume and RBC mass increase, plasma volume increases earlier and proportionately more, leading to relative hemodilution, the physiologic anemia of pregnancy. *1108* Increases progressively throughout pregnancy but proportionately less than does the plasma volume. *1858*

753.10 Polycystic Kidney Disease True polycythemia with a considerable increase of red cell volume may occur. *1669*

Red Blood Cells Normal

642.40 Pre-Eclampsia In 14 cases in the late stages, mean red cell volume was identical with that of normal pregnant women in the same gestational period. *0224*

642.60 Eclampsia In 14 cases in the late stages of eclampsia and pre-eclampsia, mean red cell volume was identical with that of normal pregnant women in the same gestational period. *0224*

Weil-Felix Reaction

Serum Negative

81.10 Brill's Disease A negative test in the presence of rising complement-fixing antibodies distinguishes Brill-Zinsser from primary louse-borne typhus. *0151* Positive reactions develop in 10-20% of cases that occur 10 or more years after the primary attack. *1058*

83.20 Rickettsialpox With Proteus OX-19, OX-2 and OX-K. *1319* Negative in Rickettsial Pox, Q fever, and trench fever. *2368*

Serum Positive

23.00 Brucellosis *0503*

66.10 Tick-Borne Fever Agglutinins against OX-19 develop during the 2nd week. *0151*

75.00 Infectious Mononucleosis Positive tests occur but are unusual. *0502*

80.00 Epidemic Typhus Serum obtained 5-12 days after onset of symptoms usually shows a positive reaction with agglutinating antibody for Proteus Ox 19 and rarely Proteus Ox 2. *0433*

81.00 Endemic Typhus With Proteus OX-9 and OX-2. *0503* Antibodies to Proteus OX-19 are present in significant titers by the third week. *0433* May be superior to complement-fixation procedure in typhus and Rocky Mountain spotted fever. *1813*

81.20 Mite-Borne Typhus Four fold or greater rises in Weil-Felix OX-K titers are found in almost all untreated patients and 75% of those treated with antimicrobial therapy. *0151* The only rickettsial disease in which OX-K antibody is present. *0962* Agglutinins for Proteus OX-K but not for OX-19 or OX-2 are present. *2368*

82.00 Rocky Mountain Spotted Fever Agglutinins against Proteus OX-19 and OX-2 develop by the 2nd or 3rd week. *1319* Antibodies first appear between the 8th and 12th day of illness. *2508 0151*

83.20 Rickettsialpox Appears in 2nd-3rd week of illness. Agglutinins for Proteus OX-19, OX-2, and OX-K do not rise in titer. *2368*

87.00 Relapsing Fever Reactive in titers of 1:80 or higher. *0151* Proteus OX K > 90% positive (> / = 1:40). *2230*

Xanthine

Urine Increase

277.21 Xanthinuria Characterized by the replacement of uric acid by xanthine and hypoxanthine in urine. *2246*

Xanthurenic Acid

Urine   Increase

281.30 Vitamin B₆ Deficiency Anemia   Abnormal tryptophan metabolism indicated by excessive excretion of xanthurenic acid following TRP load has been found in 33% of cases. *2552* Detects pyridoxine (B₆) deficiency. *2538*

285.00 Sideroblastic Anemia   Abnormal tryptophan metabolism indicated by excessive excretion in response to loading dose of L-tryptophan has been found in pyridoxine responsive cases. *2552*

297.90 Paranoid States and Other Psychoses   Has been noted in schizophrenia. *2104*

303.00 Acute Alcoholic Intoxication   Has been noted in acute alcoholism. *2104*

345.90 Epilepsy   Has been noted in epilepsy. *2104*

991.60 Hypothermia   Possibly due to activation of tryptophan oxygenase. *0762*

Xylose Tolerance Test

Urine   Abnormal

38.00 Septicemia   An inverse association between amount of xylose excreted and serum gamma globulin and IgG concentrations was significant. *0440*

40.20 Whipple's Disease   *0999*

250.00 Diabetes Mellitus   Defects of multiple stages of digestion-absorption. *2199*

277.00 Cystic Fibrosis   48 children had 1-h blood xylose levels within the normal range, but the means at 90, 120, and 180 min after load exceeded significantly those of controls. *0325*

570.00 Acute and Subacute Necrosis of Liver   In patients with ascites, the urine level is low. *2467*

577.10 Chronic Pancreatitis   With malabsorption. *2238*

579.00 Celiac Sprue Disease   The 1 h value was found to be more reliable than was fecal fat analysis in screening children for celiac disease. *0325*   One h after 5 g xylose, the blood-xylose is 20 mg/dL or more in treated disease or in cases other than celiac disease. In untreated disease, the 1 h blood-xylose is < 20 mg/dL. *0619*   Usually found at the time of initial diagnosis. *0999 2199*

579.90 Malabsorption, Cause Unspecified   *0995*

Urine   Normal

260.00 Protein Malnutrition   *2467*

269.90 Deficiency State (Unspecified)   *2467*

555.90 Regional Enteritis or Ileitis   *2467*

556.00 Ulcerative Colitis   *2467*

571.90 Cirrhosis of Liver   *2467*

Zinc

Serum   Decrease

2.00 Typhoid Fever   Both serum iron and zinc were significantly depressed in experimentally infected volunteers. *1795*

11.00 Pulmonary Tuberculosis   Decreased levels are characteristic. *0239*

70.00 Viral Hepatitis   Generally declines to values comparable to those found in other acute infections. Serum Zn exists almost entirely in a diffusible state with very little protein-bound. *0153*

151.90 Malignant Neoplasm of Stomach   Increased in 35 cases of primary malignant tumors, (1.24 ± 0.34 ppm) and plasma zinc decreased (8.83 ± 0.18 ppm). *1125*

153.90 Malignant Neoplasm of Large Intestine   In 35 cases of primary malignant tumors of the digestive organs, plasma concentrations were decreased 0.83 ± 0.18 ppm. *1125*

183.00 Malignant Neoplasm of Ovary   Does not result from a shift of zinc into or release of copper out of malignant tumor tissue. *1406*

197.70 Secondary Malignant Neoplasm of Liver   Low in advanced carcinoma with liver metastases. *1125*

199.00 Secondary Malignant Neoplasm (Disseminated)   Decreased. *2297*

201.90 Hodgkin's Disease   *1087*

202.80 Non-Hodgkins Lymphoma   Decreased. *2297*

204.00 Lymphocytic Leukemia (Acute)   Decreased. *2297*

204.10 Lymphocytic Leukemia (Chronic)   Decreased. *2297*

205.00 Myelocytic Leukemia (Acute)   Decreased. *2297*

205.10 Myelocytic Leukemia (Chronic)   Decreased. *2297*

206.00 Monocytic Leukemia   Decreased. *2297*

253.00 Acromegaly   Decreased. *2297 1308*

255.00 Adrenal Cortical Hyperfunction (Glucocorticoid Excess)   *0794*

260.00 Protein Malnutrition   Decreased. *2297 2043*

277.00 Cystic Fibrosis   Decreased. *2297*

281.00 Pernicious Anemia   Decreased. *2297 2000*

282.41 Thalassemia Major   In 42 patients aging from 3 months to 22 years with homozygous beta-thalassemia and thalassemia intermedia. Mean serum concentration was significantly decreased. *0072*

282.60 Sickle Cell Anemia   Decreased. *2297 2120*

303.90 Alcoholism   Elevated in alcoholics with normal or fatty liver and low in those with alcoholic hepatitis or cirrhosis. *0998* Statistically significant *2188   0126*

308.00 Stress   *1443*

401.10 Essential Benign Hypertension   *0126*

410.90 Acute Myocardial Infarction   A significant decrease was observed. *2428*   Falls immediately to low levels following a myocardial infarction, rising to the original normal level over the next 10-14 days. *0962*

482.90 Bacterial Pneumonia   Statistically significant. *2188*

491.00 Chronic Bronchitis   Statistically significant. *2188*

570.00 Acute and Subacute Necrosis of Liver   Found to be low in patients with hepatitis. *0998*

571.20 Laennec's or Alcoholic Cirrhosis   Found to be low in patients with alcoholic cirrhosis or hepatitis, and elevated in alcoholics with normal or fatty liver. *0998*

571.49 Chronic Active Hepatitis   Significant P < 0.001. *2429*

571.90 Cirrhosis of Liver   Patients had serum levels < 70 μg/dL with a mean of 53.4 ± 11 μg/dL (normal mean = 85 ± 11 μg/dL). *2567* Lower concentrations of total serum zinc (540 ± 111 mg/L), and of albumin-bound serum zinc (295 ± 113 mg/L) and a higher concentration of alpha₂ macroglobulin-bound zinc (245 ± 69 mg/L) were found in 28 healthy patients with decompensated hepatic cirrhosis, compared to 28 healthy subjects (835 ± 91; 679 ± 83; 156 ± 27 mg/1 respectively). *0802*   Significant P < 0.001 *2429 2188   2064*

579.00 Celiac Sprue Disease   Depression of plasma zinc and lowered taste discrimination were observed in untreated patients. With confirmation of plasma copper depression indicates that trace metal deficiency is a common nutritional complication of adult celiac disease. *2225*

579.90 Malabsorption, Cause Unspecified   Decreased. *2297*

581.90 Nephrotic Syndrome   Decreased. *2297*   Associated protein loss *1893*

650.00 Pregnancy   In 84 women with complications such as abnormal labor or atonic bleeding, serum concentrations were significantly reduced during early pregnancy. Women who gave birth to immature infants delivered in the 37th week or earlier or in the 43rd week or later showed significantly lower serum zinc during early pregnancy compared to women delivered in the 40th week. *1143*   Lower in early and late pregnancy *0969*

696.10 Psoriasis   Decreased. *2297 0910*

758.00 Down's Syndrome   Decreased. *2297*

Serum   Increase

170.90 Malignant Neoplasm of Bone   Patients with primary osteosarcoma had elevated levels, those with metastases had depressed levels. The ratio of serum copper/serum zinc in metastatic osteosarcoma patients is higher than in patients with primary osteosarcoma. Determination of serum copper and serum zinc in osteosarcoma patients may be of value in prognoses and therapy evaluation. Their ratio may be useful in discriminating between patients with primary and metastatic osteosarcoma. *0735*

198.50 Secondary Malignant Neoplasm of Bone   Serum Cu:Zn concentrations were evaluated in 19 patients with sarcomas, 12 of which were osteosarcomas at various stages. Patients with primary or metastatic osteosarcoma had elevated Cu. Patients with primary osteosarcoma had elevated Zn, those with metastases had depressed Zn. The ratio of Cu:Zn in osteosarcoma. patients may be of value in prognosis and therapy evaluation. The ratio of Cu:Zn may be useful in discriminating between patients with primary and metastatic osteosarcoma. *0735*

201.90 **Hodgkin's Disease** *0151*

303.90 **Alcoholism** Elevated in alcoholics with normal or fatty liver and low in those with alcoholic hepatitis or cirrhosis. *0998*

414.00 **Chronic Ischemic Heart Disease** Epidemiologic and metabolic data are consistent with the hypothesis that a metabolic imbalance in regard to zinc and copper is a major factor in the etiology of coronary heart disease. A metabolic imbalance is either a relative or an absolute deficiency of copper characterized by a high ratio of zinc to copper. The imbalance results in hypercholesterolemia and an increased mortality due to coronary heart disease. *1280*

440.00 **Arteriosclerosis** High serum concentrations were found in 13 patients when compared with controls. The Zn:Cu ratio is much higher in arteriosclerotic patients than in healthy subjects. *0324*

Serum   Normal

606.90 **Infertility in Males** No significant difference from fertile male controls. *2247*

Urine   Increase

252.00 **Hyperparathyroidism** Mean 24 h excretion was above normal in 17 patients with untreated primary disease. *1490*

CSF   Decrease

191.90 **Malignant Neoplasm of Brain** Significantly less. *0648*

225.90 **Benign Neoplasm of Brain and CNS** Significantly less. *0648*

571.90 **Cirrhosis of Liver** Mean CSF concentrations of 2.8 ± 1.8 μg/dL. Normal mean for control group was 4.0 ± 2.6 μg/dL. *2567*

Red Blood Cells   Decrease

282.60 **Sickle Cell Anemia** RBC and hair zinc concentration were decreased in adult male patients. RBC zinc correlated ($R = 0.61$) with serum testosterone, which was low (primary testicular failure) in all patients tested. *0005*

Red Blood Cells   Normal

606.90 **Infertility in Males** No significant difference between fertile and infertile males. *2247*

4 DISEASE LISTINGS BY ICD-9-CM CLASSIFICATION

INFECTIOUS AND PARASITIC DISEASES

Intestinal Infectious Diseases

1.00 Cholera

Antistreptolysin O *Serum Increase* Above normal titers may occur. *1752*

Bicarbonate *Feces Increase* Fecal carbonate concentration is higher than in plasma. *0151*

Chloride *Serum Increase* Due to marked loss of fluid and electrolytes. *2468*

Feces Increase Fecal concentrations are above normal, but are consistently lower than the plasma values. *0151*

Erythrocytes *Blood Increase* Due to severe dehydration. *0992*

Hemagglutination Inhibition *Serum Increase* *1058*

Hematocrit *Blood Increase* Due to severe dehydration. *0151*

Hemoglobin *Blood Increase* Due to severe dehydration. *0992*

Leukocytes *Blood Increase* Acute infections cause leukocytosis. *2467* Due to severe dehydration. *0151*

pH *Blood Decrease* Metabolic acidosis. *0151*

Potassium *Serum Decrease* Marked loss of fluid and electrolytes. *2468* Renal wasting leads to hypokalemic state. *1679*

Feces Increase Fecal potassium concentrations are higher than in plasma. *0151*

Protein *Serum Increase* *0151*

Sodium *Serum Increase* Marked loss of fluid and electrolytes occurs. *2468*

Feces Increase Fecal concentrations are increased above normal, but are consistently lower than the plasma values. *0151*

Specific Gravity *Serum Increase* Due to severe dehydration. *0151*

Urea Nitrogen *Serum Increase* Due to severe dehydration. *0992*

2.00 Typhoid Fever

Adenosine Deaminase *Serum Increase* Found to be significantly elevated in children. *1873*

Agglutination Tests *Serum Positive* The diagnostic value of the Widal reaction has been diminished by the widespread use of TAB vaccination. In an unimmunized patient, it does not become positive until after 7-10 days of illness. *0433*

Albumin *Urine Increase* Common during the febrile period. *0151* *0433*

Alkaline Phosphatase *Serum Increase* Increased due to complications. *2468*

Alkaline Phosphatase Isoenzymes *Serum Increase* Increased incidence of the Regan (placental) isoenzyme. *0740*

Aspartate Aminotransferase *Serum Increase* Frequently seen due to complications. *2468*

Copper *Serum Increase* Before the onset of overt clinical illness. *1795*

Creatine Kinase *Serum Increase* Occurs in some patients. *2468*

Eosinophils *Blood Decrease* *0151*

Erythrocyte Sedimentation Rate *Blood Decrease* *2468*

Blood Normal *0186*

Globulin *Serum Increase* Moderate hypergammaglobulinemia, especially IgA. *0880* *2035*

Hematocrit *Blood Decrease* Normochromic anemia usually develops and may be aggravated by blood loss in stools. *0151* Normochromic anemia is common present late in illness and during convalescence. *0962* *1058*

Hemoglobin *Blood Decrease* Normochromic anemia usually develops and may be aggravated by blood loss in the stools. *0151* Commonly present late in illness and during convalescence. *0962* *1058*

Immunoglobulin IgA *Serum Increase* Moderate hypergammaglobulinemia, especially IgA. *0880*

Iron *Serum Decrease* Both serum iron and zinc concentrations became significantly depressed in experimentally infected volunteers. *1795*

Lactate Dehydrogenase *Serum Increase* Due to complications. *2468*

Leukocytes *Blood Decrease* A low count with a relative lymphocytosis commonly seen. *0433* Counts range from 4,000-6,000/μL during the first 2 weeks and 3,000-5,000/μL during the 3rd and 4th week. Leukopenia is generally moderate, rarely falling below 2,500/μL. *1058* Frequent, with a decrease in neutrophilic granulocytes. *0962*

Blood Increase Moderate leukocytosis to 12,000/μL may be observed in some patients. *1058*

Lymphocytes *Blood Increase* A low WBC count with a relative lymphocytosis is commonly seen. *0433*

Malate Dehydrogenase *Serum Increase* Slight increase. *0619*

Neutrophils *Blood Decrease* Significant neutropenia may occur. *1646* *0532 2538*

Occult Blood *Feces Positive* May occur and lead to normochromic anemia later in the disease. *0151* Frequent during the 3rd and 4th weeks. *1058*

Protein *Urine Increase* Proteinuria is seen during febrile periods. *0835* *0186*

Thyroxine Binding Globulin *Serum Decrease* Patients with fever had significantly lowered levels. *2327*

Thyroxine (T$_4$) *Serum Increase* Slightly increased in all patients. *1481* During fever both percentage of free T$_4$ and absolute free T$_4$ were elevated. *2327*

Tri-iodothyronine (T$_3$) *Serum Decrease* Patients with fever had significantly lowered levels. *2327* Significantly low in all patients. Fall in T$_3$ was inversely related to the degree of fever. *1481*

Zinc *Serum Decrease* Both serum iron and zinc were significantly depressed in experimentally infected volunteers. *1795*

4.90 Bacillary Dysentery

Chloride *Serum Decrease* Fluid and electrolyte loss may be quite significant, particularly in pediatric and geriatric populations. *1058*

Erythrocytes *Blood Normal* Anemia is uncommon. *0992*

Hemagglutination Inhibition *Serum Increase* Generally demonstrable. *1058*

Hematocrit *Blood Normal* Anemia is uncommon. *0992*

Hemoglobin *Blood Normal* Anemia is uncommon. *0992*

Leukocytes *Blood Decrease* The total peripheral WBC count is not characteristic in this disease; a leukopenia, leukocytosis, or a normal count may be seen. *0433*

Blood Increase The total peripheral WBC count is not characteristic in this disease; a leukopenia, leukocytosis, or a normal count may be seen. *0433*

Feces Increase During the acute phase, examination of the stool will reveal clumps of polymorphonuclear leukocytes and RBCs, and the stool culture will be positive. *0962*

Neutrophils *Blood Decrease* Significant neutropenia may occur. *2433 2538*

Blood Increase In many cases there is a significant increase in the number of immature neutrophils, so that the ratio of band to segmented neutrophils often is reversed. *0433*

Occult Blood *Feces Positive* During the acute phase, examination of the stool will reveal clumps of polymorphonuclear leukocytes and RBCs, and the stool culture will be positive. *0962*

Potassium *Serum Decrease* Fluid and electrolyte loss may be quite significant, particularly in pediatric and geriatric populations. *1058*

Sodium *Serum Decrease* Fluid and electrolyte loss may be quite significant, particularly in pediatric and geriatric populations. *1058*

Serum Increase Fluid and electrolyte loss may be quite significant, particularly in pediatric and geriatric populations. *1058*

6.00 Amebiasis

5'-Nucleotidase *Serum Increase* With liver involvement. *1058*

Alanine Aminotransferase *Serum Increase* With liver involvement. *1058*

Alkaline Phosphatase *Serum Increase* Becomes elevated earliest with liver abscess. *0433*

Aspartate Aminotransferase *Serum Increase* With liver involvement. *1058*

Bilirubin *Serum Normal* With liver involvement, jaundice is uncommon and bilirubin is usually normal. *1058*

Complement Fixation *Serum Increase* Usually positive during active (especially hepatic) disease. Significant positive titer is > 1:16. *2468*

Eosinophils *Blood Increase* *2538*

Erythrocyte Sedimentation Rate *Blood Increase* The general rule. *1058* Increased with liver abscess. *2468*

Gamma Glutamyl Transferase (GGT) *Serum Increase* With liver involvement. *1058*

Hemagglutination Inhibition *Serum Increase* Positive test is > 1:128. *2468* Usually positive in the presence of tissue invasion and approach 100% with extracolonic disease such as liver abscess. *0999* Test for E. histolytica has been found to be positive in over 90% of patients with proven amebic liver abscess. *0962*

Hematocrit *Blood Decrease* Normochromic or hypochromic anemia is found in 75% of cases. *1058* Mild degree of anemia is common, either normochromic or hypochromic. Severity is related to duration of symptoms. *0015*

Hemoglobin *Blood Decrease* Normochromic or hypochromic anemia is found in 75% of cases. *1058* Mild degree of anemia is common, either normochromic or hypochromic. Severity is related to duration of symptoms. *0015*

Indirect Fluorescent Antibodies *Serum Increase* *0151*

Lactate Dehydrogenase *Serum Increase* Normal levels returned after complete cure in 92% of cases. Appears to be more useful than antibodies to detect cure or new infection. *1480*

Leukocytes *Blood Increase* A leukocytosis with a predominance of immature forms is common. *0433* Increased in the majority of cases. *0015*

Neutrophils *Blood Increase* Moderate neutrophilia present in 75% of cases. *1058*

pH *Pleural Effusion Decrease* The pleural aspirate from an amebic empyema due to rupture of an amebic liver abscess has an acidic pH. Pleural aspirates of nonamebic etiology were noted to have an alkaline pH. *1875*

Plasma Cells *Serum Decrease* Hepatic Amebiasis. *2357 0659 0683*

Protein *Pleural Effusion Increase* Parasitic disease most often associated with an effusion. Exudate *0062*

Specific Gravity *Pleural Effusion Increase* Exudate (> 1.016). *0062*

7.10 Giardiasis

Antibody Titer *Serum Increase* Anti-Giardia IgM and IgG by ELISA was found. Specificity and Sensitivity was 96%. *0862*

Vitamin B$_{12}$ *Serum Decrease* Vitamin B$_{12}$ absorption is decreased. *0996*

9.00 Gastroenteritis and Colitis

Albumin *Serum Decrease* Hypoalbuminemia and persistent diarrhea in cytomegalovirus enteritis. *2401*

Bicarbonate *Serum Decrease* May be noted. *0433*

Chloride *Serum Decrease* Either elevated or diminished may be noted. *0433*

Serum Increase Reflects the loss of greater volumes of fluid than salt. Either elevated or diminished may be noted. *0433*

Glucose *Serum Decrease* Of 868 infants with dehydration from gastroenteritis, 7.9% of cases had blood sugar levels of 0-50 mg/dL. A high mortality rate was found in patients with hypoglycemia. *0857*

Serum Increase Of 868 infants with dehydration from gastroenteritis, blood sugar levels in 10.2% were > 200 mg/dL. High mortality rate was found in patients with hyperglycemia. *0857*

CSF Decrease In children with severe dehydration. *0433*

Hematocrit *Blood Increase* Normal to elevated, depending on the amount of dehydration. *0433*

Hemoglobin *Blood Increase* Hemoglobin and Hct are normal to elevated, depending on the amount of dehydration. *0433*

Leukocytes *Blood Normal* Usually within the normal limits of 5,000-10,000/μL. *0433*

Lymphocytes *Blood Decrease* In viral gastroenteritis, during acute illness, a transient lymphopenia was noted which involved all lymphocyte subpopulations. *0577*

CSF Normal Normal except when aseptic meningoencephalitis is part of the overall syndrome. Then lymphocytic pleocytosis is found. *0433*

Magnesium *Serum Decrease* Mean serum level of 2.06 ± 0.62 mg/dL in 54 patients with noncholeric gastroenteritis. 7 (13%) had values below the lower normal limit. *0606*

Neutrophils *Blood Increase* *2538*

pH *Blood Decrease* May be noted. *0433*

Blood Increase Increased progressively with increased severity. The lesions became more widespread. Statistically significant differences were observed in pH values between the mild/moderate and severe forms and between the severe and complicated forms. *0340*

Protein *Serum Decrease* Enteric loss of plasma protein. *2199*

Sodium *Serum Decrease* Either elevated or diminished may be noted. *0433*

Serum Increase Reflects the loss of greater volumes of fluid than salt. Either elevated or diminished may be noted. *0433*

Specific Gravity *Urine Decrease* *0433*

Tuberculosis

11.00 Pulmonary Tuberculosis

1,25-Dihydroxy-Vitamin D$_3$ *Serum Increase* *0062*

Albumin *Serum Decrease* Tends to be reduced to a degree proportional to the severity of the lesions. *1821 2104* In 36% of 26 patients at initial hospitalization for this disorder. *0781*

Alkaline Phosphatase *Serum Increase* Isolated elevation suggests liver involvement in the absence of other causes. *0433* Elevated in 50% of cases, ranging from 25-270 U/L, with only 10% of cases having values > 100. *0503* In 25% of 26 patients at initial hospitalization for this disorder. *0781*

Amylase   *Pleural Effusion   Increase*   Pleural fluid levels may be high. *1584*

Angiotensin-Converting Enzyme (ACE)   *Serum   Normal*   No difference in levels found between control group of 108 and TB group of 100. *0907*

Antibody Titer   *Serum   Increase*   Used to differentiate pulmonary sarcoidosis from tuberculosis. Antituberculous antibodies were found in TB in 83%; in sarcoidosis in 22%. *1309*

Antidiuretic Hormone   *Serum   Increase*   Inappropriate secretion of ADH with consequent water retention can occur. *0962*

Antistreptolysin O   *Serum   Increase*   Above normal titers may occur. *1752*

Arylsulfatase   *Urine   Increase*   Considerable increase. *0610*

Aspartate Aminotransferase   *Serum   Increase*   In 35% of 26 patients at initial hospitalization for this disorder. *0781*

Basophils   *Blood   Increase*   *2538*

Bicarbonate   *Serum   Increase*   In 64% of 23 patients at initial hospitalization for this disorder. *0781*

Carcinoembryonic Antigen   *Serum   Increase*   37% of patients had values > 2.5 ng/mL. *2199*

Pleural Effusion   Increase   Benign inflammatory effusions (tuberculosis, empyema, pneumonia) had mean CEA activity of 6.2 ± 3.4 ng/mL, higher than effusions caused by congestive heart failure (2.9 ± 1.5) and other noninflammatory effusions. *1945*

Cells   *Peritoneal Fluid   Increase*   Cell count in the peritoneal fluid varies from 2,000-10,000/µL and shows a marked predominance of lymphocytes. *0962*

Cholesterol   *Serum   Decrease*   In 34% of 26 patients at initial hospitalization for this disorder. *0781*

Pleural Effusion   Increase   Rarely. *0418*

Complement Fixation   *Serum   Increase*   Used to differentiate pulmonary sarcoidosis from tuberculosis. Antituberculous antibodies were found in TB is 83%; in sarcoidosis 22%. *1309*

Copper   *Serum   Increase*   Characteristically elevated in whole blood, plasma, and erythrocytes. *0239*

Red Blood Cells   Increase   Characteristically elevated levels. *0239*

C-Reactive Protein   *Serum   Increase*   Increased inconsistently. *2467*

Erythrocytes   *Pleural Effusion   Increase*   < 10,0000/µL. *2017 0962*

Erythrocyte Sedimentation Rate   *Blood   Increase*   Usually elevated. *0433*   Normal rates may be seen on occasion in patients with active tuberculosis. *0962*

Globulin   *Serum   Increase*   Advanced pulmonary and extrapulmonary tuberculosis. *2104*

Glucose   *Pleural Effusion   Decrease*   Levels less than 3.3 mmol/L (60 mg/dL). *1444*

Ascitic Fluid   Decrease   Seen with tuberculous peritonitis. *0186*

Hematocrit   *Blood   Decrease*   Anemia is common because of the effects of the infection on RBC production and survival and because of coexistent iron and nutritional deficiencies. *0433*

Hemoglobin   *Blood   Decrease*   Anemia is common because of the effects of the infection on RBC production and survival and because of coexistent iron and nutritional deficiencies. *0433*

Immunoglobulin IgA   *Serum   Normal*   *2467*

Immunoglobulin IgG   *Serum   Increase*   *2467*

Immunoglobulin IgM   *Serum   Normal*   *2467*

Isocitrate Dehydrogenase   *Serum   Normal*   *2260*

Lactate Dehydrogenase   *Pleural Effusion   Increase*   Moderate elevation occurred in 50% of cases, especially in active tuberculosis. *0490*

Leukocytes   *Blood   Increase*   Leukocytosis and rarely a leukemoid reaction may occur; however, the WBC is frequently normal. In more acute forms of the disease, the ratio of leukocytes may be increased with decreased lymphocytes. *0433*

Blood   Normal   Leukocytosis and rarely a leukemoid reaction may occur; however, the WBC is frequently normal. In more acute forms of the disease, the ratio of leukocytes may be increased with decreased lymphocytes. *0433*   Usually not elevated. Leukocytosis suggests the presence of secondary infection but may occur in acute tuberculous pneumonia. *0962*

Lymphocytes   *Blood   Increase*   *2467*

Pleural Effusion   Decrease   In patients with pulmonary tuberculosis, pulmonary malignancy or nonspecific pleuritis, the percentages and absolute numbers of B lymphocytes were significantly lower in pleural fluid than in peripheral blood. *1809*

Pleural Effusion   Increase   Both the percentage and absolute numbers in pleural fluid were significantly higher than in peripheral blood. *1809*   43 of 46 patients had effusions with > 50% small lymphocytes. *1403*   The percentage and absolute numbers of B lymphocytes were significantly lower in pleural fluid than in peripheral blood. *1809*   Characterized by a protein content of 3 g/dL and the presence of lymphocytes. *0962*   A preponderance of lymphocytes is consistent with tuberculosis, carcinoma, or lymphoma. *0962*

Ascitic Fluid   Increase   Characteristic of chronic inflammatory disease, especially tuberculosis. *2199*

Peritoneal Fluid   Increase   Cell count in the peritoneal fluid varies from 2,000-10,000/µL and shows a marked predominance of lymphocytes. *0962*

Lymphocyte T-Cell   *Blood   Decrease*   *0793*

Lysozyme   *Serum   Increase*   Isolated cases. *0981*

Monocytes   *Blood   Increase*   Frequently elevated in active disease. Monocytosis of 8-15% may be seen in severe or overwhelming tuberculosis. *0151   2538*

Pleural Effusion   Increase   Predominant cell type. *2017*

Ascitic Fluid   Increase   Characteristic of chronic inflammatory disease, especially tuberculosis. *2199*   Seen with tuberculous peritonitis. *0186*

Neutrophils   *Blood   Decrease*   *0532*

Pleural Effusion   Increase   Neutrophils predominate in very early stages. *1403*

Oxygen Saturation   *Blood   Decrease*   Empyema or tuberculous effusion. *0797*

pH   *Pleural Effusion   Decrease*   May occur in non-neoplastic inflammatory pleural effusion (empyema, rheumatoid disease, tuberculosis). *0797*

Pleural Effusion   Increase   pH < 7.3 is rarely encountered in tuberculous effusions. *0962*

Platelet Count   *Blood   Increase*   In 49% of 12 patients at initial hospitalization for this disorder. *0781*

pO₂   *Pleural Effusion   Decrease*   Empyema or tuberculous effusion. *0797*

Precipitins   *Serum   Increase*   Found in approximately 40% of patients. *2508*

Protein   *Serum   Decrease*   Hypoproteinemia may be present. There is no specific diagnostic value to patterns of protein distribution in tuberculosis. *0962*

CSF   Increase   *0619*

Pleural Effusion   Increase   Concentrations > 6.0 g/dL indicate tuberculosis. *1403*   Characterized by a protein content of 3 g/dL and the presence of lymphocytes. *0962*

Peritoneal Fluid   Increase   Usually, but not always, over 3 g/dL. *0962*

Rheumatoid Factor   *Serum   Increase*   The incidence of seropositivity exceeds that of a normal population. *2035*   11% positivity. *0123 0422 0962*

Sodium   *Serum   Decrease*   Sometimes found in extensive chronic disease. Usually caused by abnormal retention of water. *0151*   May be decreased (110-125 mmol/L) especially in aged or in overwhelming infection. *2468*   Occasionally found, due to inappropriate secretion of ADH with consequent water retention. *0962*

Specific Gravity   *Pleural Effusion   Increase*   Exudate (> 1.016). *0062*

Thymol Turbidity   *Serum   Increase*   *0619*

Uric Acid   *Serum   Increase*   In 48% of 26 patients at initial hospitalization for this disorder. *0781*

VDRL   *Serum   Positive*   False positive serologic tests may be seen. *0999*

Zinc   *Serum   Decrease*   Decreased levels are characteristic. *0239*

13.00   Tuberculosis Meningitis

Antidiuretic Hormone   *Serum   Increase*   Inappropriate secretion of ADH with consequent water retention. *0962*

Cells   *CSF   Increase*   25-500/µL; chiefly lymphocytes. *0962*

Chloride   *Serum   Decrease*   Fall may be due to vomiting. *0619*

CSF   Decrease   May be due mainly to the associated fall in the plasma level following vomiting, but may be associated with alteration in the plasma/CSF barrier. *0619*   525-675 mg/dL. *0962*

Erythrocyte Sedimentation Rate   *Blood   Increase*   Over 100 mm/h indicate serious disease. *0532*

13.00 Tuberculosis Meningitis (continued)

Globulin *Serum Increase* Advanced pulmonary and extrapulmonary tuberculosis. *2104*

Glucose *CSF Decrease* Falls to < 50% of blood glucose. *2468* 40 mg/dL. *0999* Normal or moderately decreased. *0962 1894*

Lactate Dehydrogenase *CSF Increase* Increased in all cases in the range of 80-265 U/L (normal = 0-35 U/L), higher in those who were seriously ill and having acute onset of the disease. *1263*

Leukocytes *CSF Increase* Up to 1,000/μL, the cells being 30-100% lymphocytes. *0999* Cell count usually varies between 10-500/μL and consists mainly of lymphocytes, except in the early stage when neutrophils predominate. *0962 0151*

Lymphocytes *Blood Decrease* 0532

Blood Increase 0532

CSF Increase 30-100% of CSF cells are lymphocytes. *0999* Count usually varies between 10-500/μL and consists mainly of lymphocytes, except in the early stage when neutrophils predominate. *0962*

Magnesium *CSF Decrease* Low levels associated with convulsions. *0093*

Monocytes *Blood Increase* 0532

CSF Increase Usually range from 50-200/μL. *0151 0999*

Protein *Serum Decrease* Hypoproteinemia may be present. There is no specific diagnostic value to patterns of protein distribution in tuberculosis. *0962*

CSF Increase Slightly increased in early stages but continues to increase, reaching levels > 300 mg/dL in advanced disease, and much higher levels when block of CSF occurs. *0999 0962 2612*

Rheumatoid Factor *Serum Increase* Positive tests may be seen in connective tissue diseases such as tuberculosis. *0999* 11% positivity. *0123 0422*

Sodium *Serum Decrease* May be decreased (110-125 mmol/L) especially in aged or in overwhelming infection. *2468* Occasionally found, due to inappropriate secretion of ADH with consequent water retention. *0962*

Tryptophan *CSF Increase* 2468

Uric Acid *Serum Increase* Increased in both blood and CSF with a lowered blood:CSF ratio, possibly due to cellular breakdown and nucleoprotein catabolism. *2301*

Urine Increase Increased excretion in neurological and psychiatric disorders; progressive rise in urinary level following slight rise in blood, due to disturbed purine metabolism. *2301*

CSF Increase Markedly increased with decreased CSF:blood ratio, possibly due to cellular breakdown and nucleoprotein catabolism. *2301*

VDRL *Serum Positive* False positive serologic tests for syphilis may be seen. *0999*

18.00 Disseminated Tuberculosis

1,25-Dihydroxy-Vitamin D$_3$ *Serum Increase* 0062

5'-Nucleotidase *Serum Increase* 2 cases were reported in which the tests were 25 and 118 U/L (Normal = 2-11 U/L). *1312* Serum 5'-nucleotidase was significantly elevated in 2 of 3 patients with liver granulomata. *1312*

Alanine Aminotransferase *Serum Increase* In 5 cases of hepatic granuloma, ALT was 70 U/L with a range of 50-115 U/L. *1452*

Alkaline Phosphatase *Serum Increase* Constant chemical finding due to diffuse involvement of the liver with granulomas. *0962* Marked elevation in all 5 cases of granuloma of liver. Maximum upper limit of normal = 85 U/L. Average elevated value = 425 U/L. Range = 191-700 U/L. *1452 0999*

Antistreptolysin O *Serum Increase* Above normal titers may occur. *1752*

Arylsulfatase *Urine Increase* Considerable increase in urinary activity in pulmonary and renal tuberculosis. *1890 0610*

Aspartate Aminotransferase *Serum Increase* In 5 cases of granuloma of liver, 100% were mildly elevated, showing a mean elevation of 36 U/L over the normal maximum limit of 24 U/L. *1452*

Bilirubin *Serum Increase* Bilirubin usually only minimally elevated. *0999 2538 0486*

Cells *CSF Increase* Spinal fluid shows predominantly mononuclear pleocytosis (up to several hundred cells/μL). *0999*

Cholesterol *Pericardial Fluid Increase* High levels (2.6-5.2 mmol/L; 100 to 200 mg/dL). *0274*

Erythrocytes *Blood Decrease* Pancytopenia is a common feature. *2538*

Ascitic Fluid Increase > 10,000 cells/μL seen in about 5% of patients. *2626*

Erythrocyte Sedimentation Rate *Blood Increase* Increased in disseminated or advanced tuberculosis but is not used as an index of activity. *2468*

Gamma Glutamyl Transferase (GGT) *Serum Increase* In 5 patients with liver granulomas, including miliary tuberculosis and sarcoidosis, serum GGT levels were all elevated, mean = 303, range = 116-740 U/L. *1452*

Globulin *Serum Increase* 0999

Glucose *CSF Decrease* 0999

Peritoneal Fluid Decrease Usually < 1.7 mmol/L. *0298*

Hematocrit *Blood Decrease* 2538 0486

Hemoglobin, Free *Serum Increase* 2538 0486

Leucine Aminopeptidase *Serum Increase* In 12 patients with granulomatous hepatitis, all showed elevated LAP levels, varying from 380-1,000 U/L, with a mean of 622 (normal = 322). *0281*

Leukocytes *Blood Decrease* Leukopenia, sometimes as low as 3,500-4,000/μL, with a large number of immature forms. *0151* Pancytopenia is a common feature. *2538* May be low or normal to markedly elevated with the leukemoid reaction. *0962 2467 0999*

Blood Increase Leukocytosis up to 20,000/μL (leukemoid reaction). *0999* Active tuberculosis is usually accompanied by a moderate leukocytosis. Extreme leukocytosis occasionally occurs in patients seriously ill with widespread, necrotizing disease. *2553* May be low or normal to markedly elevated with the leukemoid reaction. *0962 2538*

Ascitic Fluid Increase > 1000 μL usually over 70% lymphocytes. *2626*

Lymphocytes *CSF Increase* Predominantly mononuclear pleocytosis (up to several hundred cells/μL). *0999*

Ascitic Fluid Increase Characteristic of chronic inflammatory disease, especially tuberculosis. *2199*

Lymphocyte T-Cell *Blood Decrease* 0793

Lysozyme *Serum Increase* Isolated cases. *0981*

Monocytes *Blood Increase* Frequently elevated in active disease. Monocytosis of 8-15% may be seen in severe or overwhelming tuberculosis. *0151*

Ascitic Fluid Increase Characteristic of chronic inflammatory disease, especially tuberculosis. *2199*

Neutrophils *Blood Increase* Increase was observed in two cases of tuberculosis of the liver. *1312* Active tuberculosis is usually accompanied by a moderate leukocytosis. Extreme leukocytosis occasionally occurs in patients seriously ill with widespread, necrotizing disease. *2553 0532*

Platelet Count *Blood Decrease* Pancytopenia is a common feature. *2538*

Protein *Serum Decrease* Hypoproteinemia may be present. There is no specific diagnostic value to patterns of protein distribution in tuberculosis. *0962*

CSF Increase 0999

Ascitic Fluid Increase Often > 2.5 g/dL in ascitic fluid. *2626*

Rheumatoid Factor *Serum Increase* 11% positivity. *0422 0123* The incidence of seropositivity exceeds that of a normal population. *2035*

Sodium *Serum Decrease* Often occurs, frequently caused by inappropriate secretion of antidiuretic hormone. *0151*

Thymol Turbidity *Serum Increase* 0619

VDRL *Serum Positive* False positive serologic tests may be seen. *0999*

Vitamin A *Serum Decrease* Impaired absorption. *0619*

Bacterial Diseases

20.00 Plague

Erythrocytes *Blood Normal* Usually normal. *0996*

Leukocytes *Blood Increase* Greater than 20,000/μL and there is a predominance of polymorphonuclear leukocytes. *0996* Significantly higher. *0864*

21.00   Tularemia

Agglutination Tests   *Serum Positive*   Positive between the 1st and 3rd weeks, and a rising titer is usually demonstrable between acute and convalescent sera. *0962*   Agglutination reaction becomes positive in 2nd week of infection. Significant titer is 1:40; usually it becomes > 1:320 by 3rd week. Peaks at 4-7 weeks 1:100), then gradually decreases during next year. *2468*

Albumin   *Urine Increase*   Mild albuminuria may occur at the height of illness. *0151*

C-Reactive Protein   *Serum Increase*   Elevated in proportion to the activity of the disease. *0433   1058*

Erythrocyte Sedimentation Rate   *Blood Increase*   Elevated in proportion to the activity of the disease. *0433*   During the active stages. *0151   1058*

Glucose   *Serum Increase*   *2123 1889*

Glucose Tolerance   *Serum Decrease*   *2123 1889*

Insulin   *Serum Increase*   *1889 2123*

Leukocytes   *Blood Decrease*   Usually normal or low. *0151 2467*

    Blood Increase   Usually normal or slightly increased. *0962*

    Blood Normal   Usually normal, may be low or slightly increased. *0962 0151*

23.00   Brucellosis

5'-Nucleotidase   *Serum Increase*   Significantly elevated in 2 of 3 patients with liver granulomata. *1312*

Agglutination Tests   *Serum Positive*   Of 200 cases of symptomatic brucella infection, 198 had titers of 160 or > in the standard tube agglutination test. *0307*   Agglutinins appear 1-2 weeks after onset of infection. *0962*   Becomes positive during 2nd to 3rd week of illness; 90% of patients have titers of > 1:320, and may remain positive long after infection has been cured. *2468*

Alanine Aminotransferase   *Serum Increase*   In 5 cases of hepatic granuloma, ALT was elevated to a mean value of 70 U/L (normal = 50 U/L) and a range of 50-115 U/L. *1452*

Alkaline Phosphatase   *Serum Increase*   Marked elevation in all 5 cases of granuloma of liver. Maximum upper limit of normal = 85 U/L. Average elevated value = 425 U/L. Range = 191-700 U/L. *1452*

Antibody Titer   *Serum Increase*   Antibodies elicited early in natural infection are predominantly IgM, with lesser quantities of IgG. As the disease progresses, IgM declines, and IgG increases, reaching its height at the period of maximum resistance to reinfection. *2035*

Aspartate Aminotransferase   *Serum Increase*   In 5 cases of granuloma of liver, 100% were mildly elevated, showing a mean elevation of 36 U/L over the normal maximum limit of 24 U/L. *1452*

Complement Fixation   *Serum Increase*   In late active disease, usually 1:16 or higher. *1058*

Coombs' Test   *Blood Positive*   The modified Coombs' test overcomes the blocking antibody and prozone phenomenon. *2035*

Erythrocyte Sedimentation Rate   *Blood Increase*   Occurs in < 25% of patients and usually in nonlocalized type. *2468*

Hemagglutination Inhibition   *Serum Increase*   When a series of known positive sera were submitted to 6 recognized laboratories highly variable reports were received, ranging from negative to titers as high as 1:640 for the same serum. In view of many variables there can hardly be a titer considered to be diagnostic. In general a titer of 1:320 or higher in the presence of significant symptoms and a reasonable exposure history may be considered presumptive evidence of the disease. *0433   2035*

Immunoglobulin IgG   *Serum Increase*   Antibodies elicited early in natural infection are predominantly IgM, with lesser quantities of IgG. As the disease progresses, IgM declines, and IgG increases, reaching its height at the period of maximum resistance to reinfection. *2035*

Immunoglobulin IgM   *Serum Increase*   Antibodies elicited early in natural infection are predominantly IgM, with lesser quantities of IgG. As the disease progresses, IgM declines, and IgG increases, reaching its height at the period of maximum resistance to reinfection. *2035*

Immunoglobulins   *Serum Increase*   Antibodies elicited early in natural infection are predominantly IgM, with lesser quantities of IgG. As the disease progresses, IgM declines, and IgG increases, reaching its height at the period of maximum resistance to reinfection. *2035*

Leucine Aminopeptidase   *Serum Increase*   In 12 patients with granulomatous hepatitis, all showed elevated LAP levels, varying from 380-1,000 U/L, with a mean of 622 (normal = 322). *0281*

Leukocytes   *Blood Decrease*   May be normal or slightly elevated in the acute disease but a moderate leukopenia with a relative lymphocytosis is commonly observed. *0433*   Leukopenia is seen in infections especially bacterial infections. Usually < 10,000/μL with significant decreases occurring in 33% of patients. *2468*

    Blood Increase   May be normal or slightly elevated in the acute disease but a moderate leukopenia with a relative lymphocytosis is commonly observed. *0433*

Lymphocytes   *Blood Increase*   Relative lymphocytosis in some cases. *0962   0433*

Monocytes   *Blood Increase*   Occurs in certain bacterial infections. *2467   0532*

Neutrophils   *Blood Decrease*   Significant neutropenia may occur. *0356   2538*

VDRL   *Serum Positive*   False positive serologic tests are sometimes seen. *0999*

Weil-Felix Reaction   *Serum Positive*   *0503*

30.00   Leprosy

Albumin   *Serum Decrease*   Markedly decreased in lepromatous leprosy and lepra reaction. *2045*

Alpha₁-Globulin   *Serum Decrease*   Decreased in dimorphic leprosy. *2045*

Angiotensin-Converting Enzyme (ACE)   *Serum Increase*   *1398 2014*

Antinuclear Antibodies   *Serum Increase*   Found in 30%. *2035*

Calcium   *Serum Decrease*   Significantly decreased in all types of leprosy except tuberculoid. *2187*

Cholesterol   *Serum Decrease*   Slightly decreased. *2468*

Complement C3   *Serum Increase*   High levels of both C2 and C3 have been recorded. *2035   2387*

Complement, Total   *Serum Increase*   Sarcoidosis, leprosy, and Wegener's granulomatosis have elevated levels. *1699*

Cryoglobulins   *Serum Increase*   Found in 95%. *2035*

Erythrocyte Sedimentation Rate   *Blood Increase*   ESR directly correlates with the increase in plasma fibrinogen in lepromatous leprosy. *1878*

Fibrinogen   *Plasma Increase*   Significant increases were noted in cases with lepra reaction, particularly those manifesting necrotizing skin, kidney, and sclerodermic lesions. *1878*

Fibrin Split Products (FSP)   *Plasma Decrease*   In lepromatous leprosy. *1878*

Globulin   *Serum Increase*   In 50 cases of leprosy, (10 tuberculoid, 25 lepromatous leprosy, 10 lepra reaction, 5 dimorphic leprosy, all showed a rise). *2045*   Lepromatous leprosy. *2104*   Often present *0962*

Hematocrit   *Blood Decrease*   Anemia, when present, is usually mild. *0962*

Hemoglobin   *Blood Decrease*   Anemia, when present, is usually mild. *0962*

Histamine   *Serum Increase*   Both histamine and histaminase levels are significantly elevated, especially in cases of long duration. Patients with leprosy in reaction had highest levels, whereas tuberculoid, borderline and lepromatous cases had moderate rises. *1879*

Immunoglobulin IgA   *Serum Increase*   High levels have been described but appear to be more variable than IgG. *2035   2387*

Immunoglobulin IgG   *Serum Increase*   High levels are consistently found in the sera of untreated lepromatous patients. *2035 2387*

Immunoglobulin IgM   *Serum Increase*   High levels have been described but appear to be more variable than IgG. *2035   2387*

LE Cells   *Blood Increase*   Found in 8%. *2035*

Leukocytes   *Blood Increase*   Moderate leukocytosis may occur during exacerbations. *0962*

Lymphocyte T-Cell   *Blood Decrease*   *0793*

Magnesium   *Serum Decrease*   Decrease was highly significant in tuberculoid, lepromatous and borderline lepromatous cases. *2187*

Plasma Cells   *Serum Increase*   High levels of precipitating antimycobacterial antibodies in lepromatous leprosy are paralleled by marked plasma cell proliferation. *2035*

Precipitins   *Serum Increase*   Found in the sera of lepromatous patients and in 50% of the patients with tuberculoid lesions that were bacillary-positive. Not found in the sera of bacillary-negative tuberculoid patients. *2035*

30.00 Leprosy (continued)

Rheumatoid Factor *Serum Increase* Found in 50%. *2035* The incidence of seropositivity exceeds that of a normal population. *2035* Found in 24% of patients. *0422 0123 0962*

VDRL *Serum Positive* False positive serologic test occurs in 40% of patients. *2468* Found in 70%. *2035* Frequent biological false positive reactions. *2368*

32.00 Diphtheria

Albumin *Urine Increase* Common, particularly in severe forms of the disease. *0433*

Casts *Urine Increase* Frequently present. *2468*

Cells *CSF Increase* With neuritis, a pleocytosis can occur. *1058*

Erythrocyte Sedimentation Rate *Blood Increase* *0962*

Globulin *Serum Increase* May occur *0433* .

Glucose *Serum Decrease* Occurs frequently. *2468*

Hemagglutination Inhibition *Serum Increase* Assays antitoxin titer of patient's serum. 4-fold increase between titer in acute and convalescent sera confirms diagnosis. *2468*

Hematocrit *Blood Decrease* Moderate anemia persisting into convalescence is common. *0433*

Hemoglobin *Blood Decrease* Moderate anemia persisting into convalescence is common. *0433*

Leukocytes *Blood Decrease* In severe cases. *0433*

Blood Increase Slight leukocytosis with neutrophilia usually is noted, although in severe cases leukopenia may occur. *0433* WBC is slightly increased (< 15,000/μL). *2468* Mild to moderate leukocytosis of about 15,000/μL with increase in immature neutrophils. *0962*

Monocytes *CSF Increase* Following paralysis. *0433*

Neutrophils *Blood Increase* Slight leukocytosis with neutrophilia usually is noted, although in severe cases leukopenia may occur. *0433* WBC is slightly increased (< 15,000/μL). *2468*

Protein *CSF Increase* With neuritis. *1058* Prolonged elevation following paralysis. *0433*

Urea Nitrogen *Serum Increase* Elevation with increase in serum globulins may occur. *0433*

33.00 Whooping Cough

Agglutination Tests *Serum Positive* These antibodies are produced in low titer and appear only after the second week of disease. *0962*

Complement Fixation *Serum Increase* These antibodies are produced in low titer and appear only after the second week of disease. *0962*

Leukocytes *Blood Increase* Leukemoid reactions (> 50,000/μL) are frequently associated with severe complications. *0433* WBC > 20,000/μL with > 70% small lymphocytes indicates this disease. *0433* Moderate to severe leukocytosis, ranging from 15,000- 40,000/μL with a differential of 60-90% lymphocytes. *0962* Begins late in the catarrhal stage and rises steeply. *2368*

Lymphocytes *Blood Increase* Though the WBC count and the differential counts may be quite variable, > 20,000/μL with more than 70% small lymphocytes indicates this disease. *0433* Moderate to severe leukocytosis, ranging from 15,000-40,000/μL with a differential of 60-90% lymphocytes. *0962* Begins late in the catarrhal stage and rises steeply. *2368*

Neutralizing Antibodies *Serum Increase* These antibodies are produced in low titer and appear only after the 2nd week of disease. *0962*

34.10 Scarlet Fever

Eosinophils *Blood Increase* *0779*

36.00 Meningococcal Meningitis

Albumin *Urine Increase* May occur. *2468*

Cells *CSF Increase* Cell count is elevated to thousands/μL, mostly neutrophils. *0151*

Erythrocytes *Urine Increase* May show increase. *2468*

Glucose *CSF Decrease* Usually < 35 mg/dL. *1058 2400*

Leukocytes *Blood Increase* Up to 40,000/μL with 80-90% neutrophils almost always occurs. *0151 1058*

CSF Increase Markedly increased (2500-10,000/μL), almost all polymorphonuclear leukocytes. *2468 2400*

Neutrophils *Blood Increase* Leukocytosis up to 40,000/μL with 80-90% neutrophils is almost always present. *0151*

CSF Increase Cell count is elevated to thousands/μL, mostly neutrophils. *0151*

Protein *CSF Increase* Values of 80-500 mg/dL. *1058 2400*

Thyroxine (T₄) *Serum Increase* Slightly increased in all patients. *1481*

Tri-iodothyronine (T₃) *Serum Decrease* Significantly low in all patients. Fall in T_3 is inversely related to the degree of fever. *1481*

37.00 Tetanus

Alanine Aminotransferase *Serum Increase* Mainly in the more severe cases. *0433*

Albumin *Urine Increase* Some patients show proteinuria. *0433*

Aldolase *Serum Increase* Very high serum levels are found in severe cases. *0619 1643*

Aspartate Aminotransferase *Serum Increase* Mainly in the more severe cases. *0433* Elevation occurred in 2 of 5 cases. *1677*

Bicarbonate *Serum Decrease* The lowest values are found in the more severe cases. *0433*

Serum Increase Metabolic alkalosis may occur with potassium loss. *0962*

Catecholamines *Plasma Increase* Found in patients with severe disease. It is believed that this increase is caused by autonomic nervous system overactivity. *0433*

Urine Increase Usually found in patients with severe disease. It is believed that this increase is caused by autonomic nervous system overactivity. *0433*

Creatine Kinase *Serum Increase* Levels were found to be elevated in 75 cases and related to the clinical severity of disease. Values higher than 2.97 mU/mL were found to be highly suggestive of disease. *2407 1643*

Erythrocyte Sedimentation Rate *Blood Increase* Is often increased. *0433*

Lactate Dehydrogenase *Serum Increase* Elevated above the upper limit of normal in 3 of 5 cases. *1677*

Leukocytes *Blood Increase* Probably caused by bacterial superimposed infections in the respiratory tract or in the injured tissues responsible for the infection (focus). *0433*

Urine Increase Some patients show degenerate leukocytes. *0433*

Lymphocytes *Blood Decrease* Lymphopenia is more usual than lymphocytosis. *0433*

Neutrophils *Blood Increase* Granulocytosis and the appearance of less mature forms of neutrophils. *0433*

pCO₂ *Blood Increase* At the onset of mild forms, blood gases may be within normal values. Later, when spasms appear and high dosages of sedatives are given, hypoxemia, acidosis plus hypercapnia and metabolic acidosis are present. *0433* Metabolic alkalosis may occur with potassium loss. *0962*

pH *Blood Decrease* At the onset of mild forms, blood gases may be within the normal values. Later, when spasms appear and high dosages of sedatives are given, hypoxemia, acidosis plus hypercapnia and metabolic acidosis are present. *0433*

Blood Increase Metabolic alkalosis may occur with potassium loss. *0962*

pO₂ *Blood Decrease* At the onset of mild forms, blood gases may be within normal values. Later when spasms appear and high dosages of sedatives are given, hypoxemia, acidosis plus hypercapnia and metabolic acidosis are present, mainly because of inadequate or improper therapeutic management. *0433*

Pseudocholinesterase *Serum Decrease* Activity may be decreased in severe cases due to inhibition by the tetanus toxin. *0433* Reduced levels correlate with degree of severity of disease. *1841*

38.00 Septicemia

5'-Nucleotidase *Serum Increase* 4 patients with extrahepatic infection showed elevated levels, ranging from 21-75 U/L (Normal = 3-17). *1681*

17-Hydroxycorticosteroids *Urine Increase* Increased due to severe stress. *2467*

17-Ketogenic Steroids *Urine Increase* Increased due to severe stress. *2467*

Alanine *Serum Increase* Concentrations determined in 10 burned patients with gram-negative sepsis and 9 burned patients without sepsis revealed an increase in the gluconeogenic precursors alanine, glycine, methionine and phenylalanine in those patients with sepsis. *2543*

Alanine Aminotransferase *Serum Increase* Elevations observed in 6 cases of extrahepatic sepsis. *1681*

Albumin *Serum Decrease* Decreased in 6 cases of extrahepatic sepsis. *1681* In 54% of 11 patients at initial hospitalization for this disorder. *0781*

Urine Increase Transient slight increase. *2468*

Alkaline Phosphatase *Serum Increase* Elevated in 5 of 6 cases of extrahepatic sepsis, with levels as high as 460 U/L recorded. *1681* In 27% of 11 patients at initial hospitalization for this disorder. *0781*

Leukocyte Increase Usually increased in untreated disease. *2467 0619*

Antistreptolysin O *Serum Increase* Appear in the serum 10-21 days after onset of acute streptococcal infection. *0962*

Apolipoprotein AI *Serum Decrease* Sepsis causes the concentration to decrease. *0049*

Apolipoprotein B *Serum Decrease* Sepsis causes the concentration to decrease. *0049*

Aspartate Aminotransferase *Serum Increase* Elevations observed in 6 cases of extrahepatic sepsis. *1681* In 27% of 11 patients at initial hospitalization for this disorder. *0781*

Catecholamines *Plasma Increase* Severe stress resulting from sepsis, hypovolemia or hypercapnia causes hypersecretion. *2236*

Urine Increase Increased due to severe stress. *2467* Severe stress resulting from sepsis, hypovolemia or hypocapnia causes hypersecretion. *2236*

Cholesterol *Serum Decrease* May fall, during convalescence the level rises, sometimes above the normal range. *0619* May fall. *0049* In 54% of 11 patients at initial hospitalization for this disorder. *0781*

Cholesterol, High Density Lipoprotein *Serum Decrease* Sepsis causes the concentration to decrease. *0049*

Complement C1q *Serum Normal* Normal concentrations of C1, C3, and C4. *2522*

Complement C2 *Serum Normal* Normal concentrations of C1, C2, and C4. *2522*

Complement C3 *Serum Decrease* In severe gram-negative infection associated with shock, depression of C3, C5, C6, and C9 may occur, with normal concentrations of C1, C2, and C4. Abnormalities develop early, before shock. C3 concentration correlates with mortality. *2522 0452 1275 0375*

Complement C4 *Serum Normal* In severe gram-negative infection associated with shock, depression of C3, C5, C6, and C9 may occur, with normal concentrations of C1, C2, and C4. Abnormalities develop early, before shock. C3 concentration correlates with mortality. *2522*

Complement, Total *Serum Decrease* In severe gram-negative infection associated with shock, depression of C3, C5, C6, and C9 may occur, with normal concentrations of C1, C2, and C4. Abnormalities develop early, before shock. C3 concentration correlates with mortality. *2522* In 51 patients, 24% had decreased values. *2223*

Serum Increase In 51 patients, 27% had increased values. *2223*

Copper *Serum Increase* Increased in acute and chronic infections. *2467*

C-Reactive Protein *Serum Increase* Increased inconsistently. *2467*

Creatine *Urine Increase* Increased breakdown of muscle. *2467*

Creatinine *Serum Increase* In 49% of 12 patients at initial hospitalization for this disorder. *0781*

Epinephrine *Plasma Increase* In patients with septicemic, traumatic or hemorrhagic shock, plasma epinephrine and norepinephrine concentrations were increased above the normal range. *0164*

Erythrocyte Casts *Urine Increase* Transient slight increase. *2468*

Erythrocyte Sedimentation Rate *Blood Increase* Increased in most bacterial infections; reflects the activity of the infectious process. *0962*

Factor II *Plasma Decrease* May be associated with defibrination resulting in platelet and coagulation factor consumption in severe gram-positive septicemia. *2538*

Factor IV *Plasma Decrease* May be associated with defibrination resulting in platelet and coagulation factor consumption in severe gram-positive septicemia. *2538*

Fibrinogen *Plasma Decrease* May be associated with defibrination resulting in platelet and coagulation factor consumption in severe gram-positive septicemia. *2538*

Fibrin Split Products (FSP) *Plasma Increase* Raised levels are common with other evidence of enhanced fibrinolysis. *1253* Elevation is much more common in fatal cases than in survivors. *2193*

Globulin *Serum Increase* Increased in 6 cases of extrahepatic sepsis. *1681*

Glucose *Serum Increase* Fasting hyperglycemia, impaired glucose tolerance and relative hyperinsulinemia are found. *1889 2123* In 56% of 12 patients at initial hospitalization for this disorder. *0781*

Urine Increase *0619*

Glucose Tolerance *Serum Decrease* Fasting hyperglycemia, impaired glucose tolerance and relative hyperinsulinemia are found. *2123 1889*

Glycine *Serum Increase* Concentrations determined in 10 burned patients with gram-negative sepsis and 9 burned patients without sepsis revealed an increase in the gluconeogenic precursors alanine, glycine, methionine and phenylalanine in those patients with sepsis. *2543*

Hematocrit *Blood Decrease* Mild to moderate anemia may occur during the course of chronic infections. *0433*

Hemoglobin *Blood Decrease* Mild to moderate anemia may occur during the course of chronic infections. *0433*

Immunoglobulin IgA *Serum Increase* Perinatal infections. *0619*

Immunoglobulin IgD *Serum Increase* Moderately increased. *2467*

Insulin *Blood Increase* Fasting hyperglycemia, impaired glucose tolerance, and relative hyperinsulinemia are found. *1889 2123*

Iron *Serum Decrease* Decreased with acute and chronic infection. Frequently develops within of onset. *0619*

Iron-Binding Capacity, Total (TIBC) *Serum Decrease* Acute and chronic infections. The serum iron falls proportionately more than the transferrin content. *0619*

Lactate Dehydrogenase *Serum Increase* In 72% of 11 patients at initial hospitalization for this disorder. *0781*

Leukocytes *Blood Decrease* Although leukocytosis generally accompanies acute bacterial infection, leukopenia may be found, and in general, the WBC is not diagnostic. *0433 2467*

Blood Increase Although leukocytosis generally accompanies acute bacterial infection, leukopenia may be found, and in general, the WBC is not diagnostic. *0433* Total counts may become extremely high. *2538* Moderate to marked leukocytosis with a shift to left generally occurs. *0962* In 63% of 14 patients at initial hospitalization for this disorder. *0781 2467*

Lipids *Serum Decrease* Sepsis causes the concentration to decrease. *0049*

Lymphocytes *Blood Decrease* In 78% of 14 patients at initial hospitalization for this disorder. *0781*

Blood Increase In convalescence from acute infection. *2467*

Methionine *Serum Increase* Concentrations determined in 10 burned patients with gram-negative sepsis and 9 burned patients without sepsis revealed an increase in the gluconeogenic precursors alanine, glycine, methionine and phenylalanine in those patients with sepsis. *2543*

Monocytes *Blood Increase* In acute infection. *2467*

Neutrophils *Blood Decrease* In early onset group B streptococcal disease 39 (87%) had abnormal absolute neutrophil counts, 25 with neutropenia and 14 with neutrophilia. The absolute immature neutrophil count was elevated in 19 infants (42%). *1499*

Blood Increase In 49% of 14 patients at initial hospitalization for this disorder. *0781* Increased WBC (15,000-30,000/μL) and polymorphonuclear leukocytes are found. *2468*

Norepinephrine *Plasma Increase* In patients with septicemic, traumatic or hemorrhagic shock, epinephrine and norepinephrine concentrations were increased above the normal range. In non-survivors norepinephrine concentrations remained persistently elevated while in survivors there was a rapid decline towards the normal range. *0164*

Phenylalanine *Serum Increase* Concentrations determined in 10 burned patients with gram-negative sepsis and 9 burned patients without sepsis revealed an increase in the gluconeogenic precursors alanine, glycine, methionine and phenylalanine in those patients with sepsis. *2543*

Phosphate *Serum Decrease* In 54 patients with gram-negative septicemias; either absolute 2 mg/dL or relative (P/BUN = 0.04) hypophosphatemia was found in 69% of all determinations. *1934*

38.00   Septicemia   *(continued)*

Platelet Count   *Blood   Decrease*   May be associated with defibrination resulting in platelet and coagulation factor consumption in severe gram-positive septicemia. *2538*

Prothrombin Consumption   *Blood   Increase*   May be associated with defibrination resulting in platelet and coagulation factor consumption in severe gram-positive septicemia. *2538*

Prothrombin Time   *Plasma   Increase*   May be associated with defibrination resulting in platelet and coagulation factor consumption in severe gram-positive septicemia. *2538*

Pseudocholinesterase   *Serum   Decrease*   In conditions which may have decreased serum albumin. *2467*

Reticulocytes   *Blood   Decrease*   The absolute count is reduced. *0433*

Thyroxine Binding Globulin   *Serum   Decrease*   *2540*

Triglycerides   *Serum   Increase*   Sepsis causes the concentration to increase. *0049*

Urea Nitrogen   *Serum   Increase*   In 49% of 12 patients at initial hospitalization for this disorder. *0781*   A condition that may be associated with excessive protein catabolism. *0503*

Uric Acid   *Serum   Increase*   In 54% of 11 patients at initial hospitalization for this disorder. *0781*

Xylose Tolerance Test   *Urine   Abnormal*   An inverse association between amount of xylose excreted and serum gamma globulin and IgG concentrations was significant. *0440*

39.90   Actinomycosis

Alanine Aminotransferase   *Serum   Increase*   Liver involvement. *1058*

Alkaline Phosphatase   *Serum   Increase*   May be elevated in cases with osteomyelitis. *0433*

Erythrocyte Sedimentation Rate   *Blood   Increase*   Almost always elevated. *0433*

Gamma Glutamyl Transferase (GGT)   *Serum   Increase*   Liver involvement. *1058*

Hematocrit   *Blood   Decrease*   A mild to moderate normocytic, normochromic anemia frequently accompanies this disease. *0433*

Hemoglobin   *Blood   Decrease*   A mild to moderate normocytic, normochromic anemia frequently accompanies this disease. *0433*

Lactate Dehydrogenase   *Serum   Increase*   Liver involvement. *1058*

Leukocytes   *Blood   Increase*   In uncomplicated disease the peripheral WBC usually ranges between 8,000-14,000/μL. Counts over 15,000/μL are unusual except in cases with secondary superinfection. *0433*   May occur when destructive tissue lesions are present. *0962*

pO₂   *Blood   Decrease*   Pulmonary involvement. *1058*

Urea Nitrogen   *Serum   Increase*   Kidney involvement. *1058*

40.20   Whipple's Disease

17-Hydroxycorticosteroids   *Urine   Decrease*   Reduced 24-h excretion of 17-hydroxycorticosteroids and 17-ketosteroids has been found in debilitated patients. *2199*

17-Ketogenic Steroids   *Urine   Decrease*   Reduced 24 h excretion of 17-hydroxycorticosteroids and 17-ketosteroids has been found in debilitated patients. *2199*

17-Ketosteroids   *Urine   Decrease*   Reduced 24-h excretion of 17-hydroxycorticosteroids and 17-ketosteroids has been found in debilitated patients. *2199*

Albumin   *Serum   Decrease*   Excessive loss into GI tract and decreased production. *0995*   A low serum albumin will reflect possible malabsorption of protein or protein-losing enteropathy. *0962*   In patients with severe diarrhea and malabsorption. *2199   0999*

Alkaline Phosphatase   *Serum   Decrease*   An indication of vitamin D and calcium malabsorption. *0962*

Serum   Increase   An indication of vitamin K malabsorption. *0962*

Calcium   *Serum   Decrease*   An indication of vitamin D and calcium malabsorption. *0962*   In patients with severe diarrhea and malabsorption. *2199   0995*

Carotene   *Serum   Decrease*   A useful indication of fat malabsorption low levels are found in as many 80% of patients with steatorrhea. *0962*   Common. *2199*

Cholesterol   *Serum   Decrease*   Common. *2199   0999*

Erythrocyte Sedimentation Rate   *Blood   Increase*   *0999*

Fat   *Feces   Increase*   In small intestinal disease. *2199*

Folate   *Serum   Decrease*   In some cases. *2199*

Glucose Tolerance   *Serum   Increase*   Flat peak. Poor absorption from the GI tract (normal IV GTT curve). *2467*

Hematocrit   *Blood   Decrease*   Anemia is common and is usually associated with iron deficiency. *2199*

Hemoglobin   *Blood   Decrease*   Anemia is common and is usually associated with iron deficiency. *2199*

Iron   *Serum   Decrease*   Microcytic, hypochromic red cells and a low serum iron accompany the anemia. *2199   0995*

Iron-Binding Capacity, Total (TIBC)   *Serum   Increase*   Iron deficiency anemia is common. *2199*

Iron Saturation   *Serum   Decrease*   Iron deficiency anemia is common. *2199*

Leukocytes   *Blood   Increase*   Seen in the period of clinical activity. *0999*   Mild to moderate leukocytosis may be present, especially in febrile patients. *2199*

Lymphocytes   *Blood   Decrease*   An absolute lymphopenia due to loss of lymphocytes into the small intestine. *0962*

Magnesium   *Serum   Decrease*   In patients with severe diarrhea and malabsorption. *2199*

MCH   *Blood   Decrease*   Anemia is common and is usually associated with iron deficiency. *2199*

MCHC   *Blood   Decrease*   Anemia is common and is usually associated with iron deficiency. *2199*

MCV   *Blood   Decrease*   Microcytic, hypochromic red cells and a low serum iron accompany the anemia. *2199*

Blood   Increase   In some patients there is macrocytosis caused by folate deficiency. *2199*

Occult Blood   *Feces   Positive*   30% of patients have this finding. *0999*

Phosphate   *Serum   Decrease*   An indication of vitamin D and calcium malabsorption. *0962*

Potassium   *Serum   Decrease*   In patients with severe diarrhea and malabsorption. *2199*

Protein   *Serum   Decrease*   Enteric loss of plasma protein. *2199*

Prothrombin Time   *Plasma   Increase*   *0999*

Triolein ¹³¹I Test   *Feces   Positive*   Positive test for lipid droplets in the stool, but results are inconsistent. *0962*

Xylose Tolerance Test   *Urine   Abnormal*   *0999*

Viral Diseases of the CNS

45.90   Acute Poliomyelitis

Aspartate Aminotransferase   *Serum   Increase*   A mild rise was reported in all 8 cases. *1677*

CSF   Increase   Always increased but does not correlate with serum level or with severity of paralysis; reaches peak in 1 week and returns to normal by 4 weeks. *2468*

Bicarbonate   *Serum   Increase*   Respiratory acidosis may occur. *0962*

Cells   *CSF   Increase*   Is usually 25-500/μL. At first most are polymorphonuclear leukocytes; after several days most are lymphocytes. *2468*   Chiefly lymphocytes. *0962*

Chloride   *CSF   Decrease*   670-750 mg/dL. *0962*

CSF   Normal   *2368*

Complement Fixation   *Serum   Increase*   *1058*

Coproporphyrin   *Urine   Increase*   Possibly derived from nervous system. *0619*

Creatine   *Serum   Increase*   *0619*

Urine   Increase   Increased formation; myopathy. *2467*

Creatine Kinase   *Serum   Increase*   Mild elevation was reported in 50% of 8 cases. *1677*

Gamma Globulin   *CSF   Increase*   Especially IgG. *0186*

Glucose   *CSF   Normal*   *0962 2368*

Hexosaminidase   *Serum   Increase*   Increase in total concentration (hexosaminidase A and B). *1716*

Immunoglobulin IgG   *CSF   Increase*   *0186*

Lactate Dehydrogenase   *Serum   Increase*   Mild elevation was recorded in all 8 cases. *1677*

Leukocytes   *Blood   Increase*   Blood shows early moderate increase 15,000/μL. *2468*   Occasionally a mild leukocytosis is present. *0962*

CSF Increase Usually 25-500/µL at first. Most are polymorphonuclear leukocytes; after several days most are lymphocytes. *2468 0433*

Lymphocytes *Blood Decrease* The numbers of circulating lymphocytes are sharply and regularly reduced. *0783*

CSF Increase Cell count is usually 25-500/µL at first most are polymorphonuclear leukocytes; after several days most are lymphocytes. *2468 0433*

Neutralizing Antibodies *Serum Increase 1058*

Neutrophils *Blood Increase* Occasionally a mild leukocytosis is present. *0962*

CSF Increase Is usually 25-500/µL at first most are polymorphonuclear leukocytes; after several days most are lymphocytes. *2468 0433*

pCO₂ *Blood Increase* Respiratory acidosis may occur. *0962* Neurological impairment of the respiratory drive. *2612*

pH *Blood Decrease* Respiratory acidosis may occur. *0962*

pO₂ *Blood Decrease* Neurological impairment of the respiratory drive. *2612*

Protein *CSF Increase* Initial values usually fall within range of 25-150 mg/dL. Characteristically modest elevations are found during the first week after onset of CNS symptoms. Levels tend to decrease toward the 10th day, but may increase again in a secondary stage (100-400 mg/dL) in the 3rd and 4th weeks. *0433* Often progressive increase. *0962* May be high. *2368*

47.00 Aseptic Meningitis

Cells *CSF Increase* A pleocytosis of up to 3,000/µL may occur. In the first day or two of illness, polymorphonuclears may predominate, but the cell differential then shifts to one predominantly of lymphocytes. *0999*

Fibrin Split Products (FSP) *Plasma Increase* Elevation is much more common in fatal cases than in survivors. *2193*

Glucose *CSF Normal* Normal but may be depressed in mumps meningitis. *0962*

Immunoglobulin IgA *Serum Increase* IgA and IgG increased. *0619*

CSF Increase 0619

Immunoglobulin IgG *Serum Increase* IgA and IgG increased. *0619*

CSF Increase 0619

Immunoglobulins *CSF Increase* IgA and IgG increased. *0619*

Lactate Dehydrogenase *CSF Increase* Invariably slightly elevated, with LD-1 and 2 the elevated isoenzymes. *1684*

Lactate Dehydrogenase Isoenzymes *CSF Increase* Slight elevation of isoenzymes 1 and 2 invariably occurs. *1684*

Leukocytes *Blood Normal* Peripheral WBC is generally within normal limits. *0962*

CSF Increase May increase from a few to > 1,000/µL, mostly polymorphonuclears, in acute hemorrhagic encephalitis. *0151* Count ranges from 50-300/µL and rarely 2,000. Marked predominance of lymphocytes except in the earliest stage. *0962*

Lymphocytes *CSF Increase* After first day or two differential shifts to predominantly lymphocytes. *0999* Increased in 50% of the patients. *0790* Count ranges from 50-300/µL and rarely > 2,000. Marked predominance of lymphocytes except in the earliest stage. *0962*

Neutrophils *CSF Increase* May predominate in the early phase but these cells are also found in bacterial meningitis. *0433*

Protein *CSF Increase* Often increased to 45-200 mg/dL. *0999* Moderately elevated in acute hemorrhagic encephalitis. *0151*

49.00 Lymphocytic Choriomeningitis

Complement Fixation *Serum Increase* Develops within 2-4 weeks. *2368 1058*

Globulin *CSF Increase* May be found in the 2nd week. *2368*

Glucose *CSF Normal* Normal or low normal. *2368*

Leukocytes *Blood Decrease* Moderate leukopenia. *2368*

Blood Normal Usually within normal limits in all types. *2368*

Lymphocytes *Blood Increase* Relative lymphocytosis. *2368*

CSF Increase 100-3,000/µL, occasionally up to 30,000. *2468* Cell count is between 50-3,500/µL, 80-95% lymphocytes. *2368*

Neutralizing Antibodies *Serum Increase* Appear within 6-10 weeks and persist longer than do CF antibodies. *2368 1058*

Plasma Cells *Serum Increase 2468*

Protein *CSF Increase* Total concentration may be high. *2368*

Viral Diseases

50.00 Smallpox

Albumin *Urine Increase* With the elimination of toxic material. *0433*

Basophils *Blood Increase 2467*

Coagulation Time *Blood Increase* Commonly found in hemorrhagic smallpox. *0433*

Complement Fixation *Serum Increase* Highly significant in an unvaccinated patient or when vaccination was performed years previously. *0433* A rising antibody titer is seen in paired sera. *0962*

Hemagglutination Inhibition *Serum Increase* Only titers above 1,:1000 or a great increase in titer is significant. *0433* A rising antibody titer is seen in paired sera. *0962*

Leukocytes *Blood Decrease* Leukopenia is found in the first days of illness followed by leukocytosis with lymphocytosis and a high percentage of metamyelocytes. *0433* Leukopenia. *1077 2538*

Blood Increase Leukopenia is found in the first days of illness followed by leukocytosis with lymphocytosis and a high percentage of metamyelocytes. *0433* Increased during pustular rash. *2468*

Lymphocytes *Blood Increase* Leukopenia is found in the first days of illness followed by leukocytosis with lymphocytosis and a high percentage of metamyelocytes. *0433*

Metamyelocytes *Blood Increase* Leukopenia is found in the first days of illness followed by leukocytosis with lymphocytosis and a high percentage of metamyelocytes. *0433*

Neutralizing Antibodies *Serum Increase* Only titers above 1:1,000 or a large increase in titer is significant. *0433* Increased titer in acute-phase and convalescent-phase sera. *2468* A rising antibody titer is seen in paired sera. *0962*

Neutrophils *Blood Decrease* Leukopenia frequently associated with infectious diseases. *1077 2538*

Platelet Count *Blood Decrease* Pronounced thrombocytopenia is commonly found in hemorrhagic smallpox. *0433*

52.00 Chickenpox

Albumin *Serum Decrease* May be decreased with increased beta and gamma globulins. *2468*

Basophils *Blood Increase 2467*

Beta-Globulin *Serum Increase* May be increased. *2468*

Bilirubin *Serum Increase 2538 1857*

Cells *CSF Increase* Encephalitis. *2467*

Globulin *Serum Increase* May be increased. *2468*

Glucose *CSF Normal 1058*

Hematocrit *Blood Decrease 2538 1857*

Hemoglobin, Free *Serum Increase 2538 1857*

Leukocytes *Blood Decrease* Leukopenia frequently associated with infectious diseases. *1077 2538*

Lymphocytes *Blood Decrease* The numbers of circulating lymphocytes are sharply and regularly reduced. *2521*

CSF Increase With CNS involvement the cells in the CSF number from normal to < 100/µL and are almost exclusively lymphocytes. *1058*

Neutrophils *Blood Decrease* Leukopenia frequently associated with infectious diseases. *1077 2538*

Plasma Cells *Serum Increase 2468*

Protein *CSF Increase* Normal or slightly increased. *1058*

53.00 Herpes Zoster

5-Hydroxyindoleacetic Acid (5-HIAA) *CSF Increase* Has been reported. *1167*

Albumin *Serum Decrease* In 32% of 18 patients at initial hospitalization for this disorder. *0781*

Alkaline Phosphatase *Serum Increase* In 31% of 18 patients at initial hospitalization for this disorder. *0781*

Aspartate Aminotransferase *Serum Increase* In 36% of 18 patients at initial hospitalization for this disorder. *0781*

53.00   Herpes Zoster   *(continued)*

Cells   *CSF   Increase*   40% of patients show increased cells (< 300 mononuclear cells/μL). *2468   0962*

Cholesterol   *Serum   Decrease*   In 21% of 18 patients at initial hospitalization for this disorder. *0781*

Complement Fixation   *Serum   Increase*   A significant (4-fold or greater) anamnestic response usually occurs. *1058*   11 of 12 children showed a rise in CF antibody during convalescence. *0302*

Creatinine   *Serum   Increase*   In 15% of 17 patients at initial hospitalization for this disorder. *0781*

Glucose   *CSF   Normal*   *0962*

Hematocrit   *Blood   Decrease*   In 37% of 18 patients at initial hospitalization for this disorder. *0781*

Hemoglobin   *Blood   Decrease*   In 38% of 18 patients at initial hospitalization for this disorder. *0781*

Homovanillic Acid   *CSF   Increase*   Has been reported. *1167*

Lactate Dehydrogenase   *Serum   Increase*   In 37% of 18 patients at initial hospitalization for this disorder. *0781*

Lymphocytes   *CSF   Increase*   Lymphocytes pleocytosis. *1058* CSF commonly shows a pleocytosis and elevation of protein, even when clinical signs of meningeal irritation or encephalomyelitis are absent. *0151*

Monocytes   *Blood   Increase*   In 65% of 18 patients at initial hospitalization for this disorder. *0781*

Neutralizing Antibodies   *Serum   Increase*   A significant (4-fold or greater) anamnestic response usually occurs. *1058*

Protein   *CSF   Increase*   CSF commonly shows a pleocytosis and elevation of protein, even when clinical signs of meningeal irritation or encephalomyelitis are absent. *0151*   20-110 mg/dL. *0962*

Urea Nitrogen   *Serum   Increase*   In 31% of 18 patients at initial hospitalization for this disorder. *0781*

54.00   Herpes Simplex

Bilirubin   *Serum   Increase*   *2538 1857*

Cells   *CSF   Increase*   Up to 500/μL, with lymphocytes or mononuclear cells predominating. *0151*

Complement Fixation   *Serum   Increase*   Increased titer of complement-fixation and neutralizing antibodies is shown in convalescent-phase compared with acute-phase sera in primary infections. *2468*

Erythrocytes   *CSF   Increase*   RBC or xanthochromia frequently found, reflecting hemorrhagic nature of the lesions. *0151*

Erythrocyte Sedimentation Rate   *Blood   Increase*   26 patients with vulval and cervical herpetic lesions showed highly significant elevations compared to normals. *1272*

Factor II   *Plasma   Decrease*   May be associated with defibrination resulting in platelet and coagulation factor consumption. *2538*

Factor IV   *Plasma   Decrease*   May be associated with defibrination resulting in platelet and coagulation factor consumption. *2538*

Fibrinogen   *Plasma   Decrease*   May be associated with defibrination resulting in platelet and coagulation factor consumption. *2538*

Hematocrit   *Blood   Decrease*   *2538 1857*

Hemoglobin, Free   *Serum   Increase*   *2538 1857*

Neutralizing Antibodies   *Serum   Increase*   Increased titer of neutralizing antibodies is shown in convalescent-phase compared with acute-phase in primary infections. *2468*

Platelet Count   *Blood   Decrease*   May be associated with defibrination resulting in platelet and coagulation factor consumption. *2538*

Protein   *CSF   Increase*   Frequently elevated. *0151*

Prothrombin Consumption   *Blood   Increase*   May be associated with defibrination resulting in platelet and coagulation factor consumption. *2538*

Prothrombin Time   *Plasma   Increase*   May be associated with defibrination resulting in platelet and coagulation factor consumption. *2538*

55.00   Measles

Bilirubin   *Serum   Increase*   *2538 1857*

Cells   *CSF   Increase*   *2467*

Sputum   Increase   Wright's stain of sputum shows measles multinucleated giant cells, especially during prodrome and early rash. *2468*

Complement Fixation   *Serum   Increase*   Antibodies tend to decrease with time but may be used for diagnosing recent infection. *0433*   Becomes positive 1 week after onset. *2468*   CF antibody appeared at the same time as the rash and rose to a maximum titer of 1:512 between the 5th and 16th days after the axanthem. *2368*

Hemagglutination Inhibition   *Serum   Increase*   Circulating antibody is present by the time the rash develops. HI antibodies and neutralizing antibodies remain indefinitely. *0433*

Hematocrit   *Blood   Decrease*   *2538 1857*

Hemoglobin, Free   *Serum   Increase*   *2538 1857*

Immunoglobulin IgG   *Serum   Increase*   Maternal antibody may be differentiated from that actively produced by the infant by a steadily declining titer, since these tests primarily measure IgG. *0433*

Immunoglobulins   *CSF   Increase*   *0619*

Leukocytes   *Blood   Decrease*   Total WBC count is low with an absolute neutropenia. *0433*   Leukopenia frequently associated with infectious diseases. *1077   2538*

Blood   Increase   Slight increase at onset, then falls to 5000/μL with increased lymphocyte count. Increased WBC with shift to left suggests bacterial complication. *2468*

Lymphocytes   *Blood   Decrease*   The numbers of circulating lymphocytes are sharply and regularly reduced. *2521   2035*

Neutrophils   *Blood   Decrease*   The total WBC count is low with an absolute neutropenia. *0433*   Leukopenia frequently associated with infectious diseases. *1077   2538*

Plasma Cells   *Serum   Increase*   *2468*

VDRL   *Serum   Positive*   False positive tests are sometimes seen. *0999*

56.00   Rubella

Cells   *CSF   Increase*   *2467*

Complement Fixation   *Serum   Increase*   Antibodies appear within 1 week after rash; therefore acute-phase serum must be collected promptly or the rise in titer may not be detected. They may last for 8 months to years. *2468*

Hemagglutination Inhibition   *Serum   Increase*   Change in titer from acute-phase to convalescent-phase sera is the most useful technique to demonstrate a rise in antibody titer. With rubella rash, diagnosis is established if acute sample titer is > 1:10 or if convalescent-phase serum taken 7 days after rash shows a 4-fold increase in titer. *2468*   Does not distinguish between IgM and IgG antibodies but absence of HI antibodies in cord blood makes diagnosis unlikely. *2508*

Leukocytes   *Blood   Decrease*   Decreased before the rash appears. *2468*   Leukopenia frequently associated with infectious diseases. *1077   2538*

Lymphocytes   *Blood   Increase*   Increased during the rash. *2468*

Lymphocyte T-Cell   *Blood   Decrease*   *0793*

Neutralizing Antibodies   *Serum   Increase*   Appear within 1-3 days after rash and reach maximum in 2 wk. May remain positive for > 20 y. *0619*

Neutrophils   *Blood   Decrease*   Leukopenia frequently associated with infectious diseases. *1077   2538*

Plasma Cells   *Serum   Increase*   *2468*

Platelet Count   *Blood   Decrease*   Decrease within 1 week of onset of rash is frequent and may be marked. *2468*   Sometimes very severe in newborn infants infected with rubella. *0451   2538*

60.00   Yellow Fever

Alanine Aminotransferase   *Serum   Increase*   Activity was above normal in all sera tested, the degree of increase approximately proportional to the severity of disease. *1179*

Albumin   *Urine   Increase*   Sudden development of intense albuminuria about day 3-4 is characteristic, often reaching levels of 3-5 g/L or higher. *0151*   Most marked on the 3rd-4th day of illness and declined thereafter. *1179*

Amino Acids   *Plasma   Increase*   Increased in severe cases. *0619*

Antismooth Muscle Antibodies   *Serum   Increase*   Occasionally positive in low titer. *1829*

Aspartate Aminotransferase   *Serum   Increase*   Activity was above normal in all sera tested, the degree of increase approximately proportional to the severity of disease. *1179*

Bilirubin   *Serum   Increase*   Slightly increased. *2468*   Has been reported. *1179*

Cholesterol   *Serum   Decrease*   Infections associated with liver damage. *0619*

Complement Fixation   *Serum   Increase*   Can be confirmed by CF antibody rises in paired sera. *1179*

Globulin   *Serum   Decrease*   Decreased percentage during the course of the disease. *1750*

Glucose   *Serum   Decrease*   Deficiency in available glycogen. *0619*

Leukocytes   *Blood   Decrease*   Most marked by 6th day, associated with decreased lymphocytes. *2468*   Leukopenia frequently associated with infectious diseases. *1077*   In 23 cases, no consistent WBC picture was found. Leukopenia was present in a few cases, especially during the first few days of illness. *1179   2538*

Lymphocytes   *Blood   Decrease*   The numbers of circulating lymphocytes are sharply and regularly reduced. *2521   2035*

Neutrophils   *Blood   Decrease*   Leukopenia frequently associated with infectious diseases. *1077   2538*

Protein   *Serum   Normal*   No significant variations were found in the total protein concentrations. *1750*

Urine   Increase   Occurs in severe cases. *2468*   Occurred in 14 of 21 cases including all 6 of the children who died. *1750*

Urea Nitrogen   *Serum   Increase*   With kidney involvement. *1058* Concentrations of 220 mg/dL were recorded in 3 patients, all of whom died. *1179*

62.10   Western Equine Encephalitis

Chloride   *CSF   Normal*   *1058*

Glucose   *CSF   Normal*   *1058*

Leukocytes   *Blood   Decrease*   May be present early in the disease. *0151*

Blood   Increase   Mild leukocytosis with polymorphonuclear cells predominating is common. Leukopenia may be present early in the disease. *0151*

CSF   Increase   Up to 1,000/μL. *1058*

Lymphocytes   *CSF   Increase*   Usually predominate. *1058*

Protein   *CSF   Increase*   *0151*

62.20   Eastern Equine Encephalitis

Chloride   *CSF   Normal*   *1058*

Glucose   *CSF   Normal*   *1058*

Leukocytes   *Blood   Decrease*   Marked decrease occurs with relative lymphocytosis. *2468*

Blood   Increase   May occur. *0433*   Polymorphonuclear leukocytosis may reach 50,000/μL. *0151*

CSF   Increase   Up to 1,000/μL. *1058*

Lymphocytes   *CSF   Increase*   Usually predominate. *1058*

Protein   *CSF   Increase*   *0151*

65.00   Arthropod-Borne Hemorrhagic Fever

Bleeding Time   *Blood   Increase*   Prolonged in hemorrhagic fever caused by dengue viruses. *0151*

Factor II   *Plasma   Decrease*   May be associated with defibrination resulting in platelet and coagulation factor consumption (Korean and Thai fever). *2538*

Factor IV   *Plasma   Decrease*   May be associated with defibrination resulting in platelet and coagulation factor consumption (Korean and Thai fever). *2538*

Fibrinogen   *Plasma   Decrease*   Indicates occurrence of intravascular coagulation in dengue hemorrhagic fever patients experiencing shock. *0247*   May be associated with defibrination resulting in platelet and coagulation factor consumption (Korean and Thai fever). *2538*

Fibrin Split Products (FSP)   *Plasma   Increase*   Indicates occurrence of intravascular coagulation in Dengue hemorrhagic fever patients experiencing shock. *0247*

Hematocrit   *Blood   Increase*   Values may reach 70% in the hypotensive phase of epidemic hemorrhagic fever. *0151*

Immunoglobulin IgE   *Serum   Increase*   88.2% of patients with dengue hemorrhagic fever had measurable serum IgE, compared to 57.1% of controls. Patient range was 50-5025 U/mL and control was 50-2250 U/mL. *1786*

Leukocytes   *Blood   Decrease*   Almost invariably decreased reaching levels of 1,000/μL by the 4th day in hemorrhagic fever caused by arenaviruses (Argentine, Bolivian, and Lassa fever). *0151 1077 2538*

Blood   Normal   Usually normal but may be elevated in severe cases of Dengue fever. *0151*

Neutrophils   *Blood   Decrease*   Leukopenia frequently associated with infectious diseases. *1077   2538*

Platelet Count   *Blood   Decrease*   Indicates occurrence of intravascular coagulation in dengue hemorrhagic fever patients experiencing shock. *0247*   May be associated with defibrination resulting in platelet and coagulation factor consumption (Korean Fever, Thai Fever). *2538*

Potassium   *Serum   Increase*   Occurs in the oliguric phase of epidemic hemorrhagic fever. *0151*

Protein   *Urine   Increase*   Heavy proteinuria progressing to acute renal failure occurs during the hypotensive phase of epidemic hemorrhagic fever. *0151*

Prothrombin Consumption   *Blood   Increase*   May be associated with defibrination resulting in platelet and coagulation factor consumption (Korean and Thai fever). *2538*

66.00   Phlebotomus Fever

Amino Acids   *Plasma   Decrease*   Basal hypoaminoacidemia. After intravenous glucose administration the total amino acid concentration rapidly decreased as much as or more than the original decline. *2479*

Glucose   *Serum   Increase*   Impaired glucose tolerance with relative hyperinsulinemia was observed in sandfly fever. *2479*

Glucose Tolerance   *Serum   Decrease*   Impaired glucose tolerance with relative hyperinsulinemia was observed in sandfly fever. *2479*

Glutamine   *Serum   Decrease*   Most free serum amino acids are depressed in sandfly fever and other mild-moderate infections. *0122*

Insulin   *Serum   Increase*   Relative hyperinsulinemia was observed in sandfly fever. *2479*

Isoleucine   *Serum   Decrease*   Most free serum amino acids are depressed in sandfly fever and other mild-moderate infections. *0122*

Leukocytes   *Blood   Decrease*   Leukopenia frequently associated with infectious diseases. *1077   2538*

Neutrophils   *Blood   Decrease*   Leukopenia frequently associated with infectious diseases. *1077   2538*

Phenylalanine   *Serum   Increase*   Increased during the viral illness in contrast with most other amino acids. *2479*

Threonine   *Serum   Decrease*   Most free serum amino acids are depressed in sandfly fever and other mild-moderate infections. *0122*

Tyrosine   *Serum   Decrease*   Most free amino acids are depressed in sandfly fever and other mild-moderate infections. *0122*

Valine   *Serum   Decrease*   Most free serum amino acid are depressed in sandfly fever and other mild-moderate infections. *0122*

66.10   Tick-Borne Fever

Complement Fixation   *Serum   Increase*   Increased in sera taken during acute and convalescent phases. *2468*

Hematocrit   *Blood   Decrease*   Anemia develops in some patients. *1058*

Hemoglobin   *Blood   Decrease*   Anemia develops in some patients. *1058*

Leukocytes   *Blood   Decrease*   Invariably decreased. Noted by the 2nd or 3rd day of illness. Often drops to 2,000/μL. *0433*   Characterized by a profound leukopenia and occasional thrombocytopenia which is usually greatest during the second febrile episode. *0151* Initial mean count from confirmed cases of Colorado tick fever was 3,900/μL. 67% had counts < 4,500 and the mean for the leukopenic group was 2,400. No relation was found between leukopenia and age, sex, or recovery. *0891*

Lymphocytes   *Blood   Increase*   Relative. *1058*

Neutralizing Antibodies   *Serum   Increase*   Increases are seen in sera taken during acute and convalescent phases. *2468*   Found in all patients with Colorado tick fever upon follow-up 1 month after onset. 92% showed a 4-fold rise in titer within 30 days. Peak titers were reached in the 20th week. *0891   1058*

Neutrophils   *Blood   Decrease*   There is a relative decrease in mature polymorphonuclear leukocytes with an increase in immature forms. *0433*   Absolute neutropenia. *1058*

66.10   Tick-Borne Fever *(continued)*

Platelet Count   *Blood   Decrease*   1058

Weil-Felix Reaction   *Serum   Positive*   Agglutinins against OX-19 develop during the 2nd week. *0151*

70.00   Viral Hepatitis

5'-Nucleotidase   *Serum   Increase*   Elevations ranging from 8-103 U/L (normal = 2-11) were observed in 24 patients. *1312   0151*

Acid Phosphatase   *Serum   Increase*   Closely parallels serum bilirubin. *2104*

Adenosine Deaminase   *Serum   Increase*   Found to be significantly elevated in children. *1873*

Alanine Aminopeptidase   *Serum   Increase*   1443

Alanine Aminotransferase   *Serum   Increase*   Appears to reflect acute hepatic disease somewhat more specifically than is true of AST. Striking elevations of 220-1,800 U/L. *0503*   May be elevated 2-4 weeks before the onset of jaundice and may reach peak levels after 1-2 weeks. Reflects organelle injury rather than necrosis or alteration of the permeability of the plasma membranes. Elevations as high as 2,000-3,000 U/L may be seen. *0433*   Increases provide early indication of impending relapse, before clinically apparent. *2368*   Marked elevation in nearly all patients. *2260   2576 0962 0781*

Albumin   *Serum   Decrease*   Levels may be normal in the early stages of the disease process and may gradually decrease only after parenchymal damage has occurred. In severe and prolonged cases, levels bear a close relation to the clinical state and are helpful prognostically and in following results of treatment. *2339*   In 32% of 24 patients at initial hospitalization for this disorder. *0781   0724*

Serum   Normal   Normal in acute hepatitis; a decrease suggests chronic liver disease. *0962*

Urine   Increase   A few RBC or mild proteinuria. *0433*

Aldolase   *Serum   Increase*   Increased in 90% of patients up to 10 X normal. It parallels transaminase with a sharp rise before serum bilirubin rises and a return to normal 2-3 weeks after jaundice begins (acute icteric period). *2467   0962*

Alkaline Phosphatase   *Serum   Increase*   Approximately 90% of patients have elevated values. *0503*   40% of cases have values > 210 U/L. *2104*   In 72% of 25 patients at initial hospitalization for this disorder. *0781   2576 1312*

Leukocyte   Increase   2467

Alkaline Phosphatase Isoenzymes   *Serum   Increase*   Isoenzyme I was elevated in 12 of 12 patients. Isoenzyme IV was elevated in only 5 cases. *1221*

Alpha₁-Antitrypsin   *Serum   Increase*   Increased. *1866 0042 1946 1947 2129*

Alpha₁-Globulin   *Serum   Decrease*   Indicates acute hepatocellular damage. *2467*

Alpha₁-Glycoprotein   *Serum   Increase*   It was found to have a sensitivity of 65% and a specificity of 80% with severe liver disease. *0709*

Alpha₂-Globulin   *Serum   Decrease*   Indicates acute hepatocellular damage. *2467*

Serum   Increase   Slight to moderate increase (related to the increase in alpha-lipoprotein). *0619*

Alpha₂-Macroglobulin   *Serum   Increase*   2640

Alpha-Fetoprotein   *Serum   Increase*   Levels > 30 ng/mL were found in 87% of patients with acute hepatitis and in 58% with chronic active hepatitis. *0036*   Among 51 patients with fulminant hepatitis and coma, AFP was detected in 17 (85%) of 20 who survived and in only 12 (38.7%) of 31 fatal cases, (p = 0.002). Positivity was related to the severity of the disease and its appearance was followed by recovery. High values in severe forms are a favorable prognostic sign. *1231*   In some cases. *1255*

Amino Acids   *Urine   Increase*   Amount of urinary loss reflects degree of hepatic involvement. *2104*

Aminolevulinic Acid   *Urine   Increase*   May occur. *0503*

Amylase   *Serum   Increase*   Mild pancreatitis may occur and is a contributing factor in mortality. Morphological evidence of pancreatitis found in 44% of 19 hepatitis patients at autopsy. *2031*   Moderate elevation found in some patients. *2104*

Antimitochondrial Antibodies   *Serum   Normal*   1840

Antinuclear Antibodies   *Serum   Increase*   Found in 23% of patients and 2% of controls. *1840*

Antismooth Muscle Antibodies   *Serum   Increase*   IgM smooth muscle antibody may appear as opposed to the IgG antibody found in chronic hepatitis. *1829*   Transiently positive. *0703*   11% of patients were positive (6% of controls). *1840 2251   2035*

Antistreptolysin O   *Serum   Increase*   Above normal titers may occur. *1752*

Aspartate Aminotransferase   *Serum   Increase*   Striking elevations (145-200 U/L) are seen in patients with acute hepatic necrosis. *0503*   May be elevated 2-4 weeks before the onset of jaundice and may reach peak levels after 1-2 weeks. Reflects organelle injury rather than necrosis or alteration of the permeability of the plasma membrane. *0433*   In 92% of 25 patients at initial hospitalization for this disorder. *0781   0999 0962*

Beta₂-Macroglobulin   *Serum   Increase*   An increased serum concentration is characteristic. *1236*

Beta-Globulin   *Serum   Increase*   Increased in cholangiolitis. May reach very high levels in chronic progressive disease. *2339*   Associated with intrahepatic biliary obstruction. *0619*

Bile Acids   *Serum   Increase*   In one study with viral hepatitis type B, bile acids and transaminase were of equal sensitivity. *2199*

Bilirubin   *Serum   Increase*   Jaundice becomes apparent when concentration exceeds 2 mg/dL. Usually rises for 10-14 days to an average peak of about 10 mg/dL. But much higher levels are encountered especially when hemolysis is present. The rate of decline from the peak level is more gradual and often requires 2-6 weeks. The level has no prognostic significance. *0433*   On occasion there is severe hemolytic anemia resulting in a marked rise in the serum bilirubin, this frequently occurs in patients with glucose-6-phosphate dehydrogenase deficiency. *0962*   In 78% of 24 patients at initial hospitalization for this disorder. *0781   2156 2576*

Urine   Increase   Appears a few days before the onset of jaundice. *0433*   Seen in anicteric hepatitis. *0151   0999*

Feces   Decrease   2467

Bilirubin, Direct   *Serum   Increase*   Serum bilirubin is 50-75% direct in the early stage; later, indirect bilirubin is proportionately more in acute icteric period. *2467*   Direct and indirect bilirubin are equally elevated in the icteric phase. *0151*   In 93% of 19 patients at initial hospitalization for this disorder. *0781   0999*

Bilirubin, Indirect   *Serum   Increase*   Serum bilirubin is 50-75% direct in the early stage; later, indirect bilirubin is proportionately more. *2467*   In 75% of 18 patients at initial hospitalization for this disorder. *0781*

BSP Retention   *Serum   Increase*   Useful in screening for anicteric disease and during convalescence. *0433*   The earliest abnormality, followed by bilirubinuria, before serum bilirubin increases. *2467*

Carcinoembryonic Antigen   *Serum   Increase*   30% of patients had values > 2.5 ng/mL. *2199*

Cephalin Flocculation   *Serum   Increase*   Occurs frequently; concurrent with increase in direct bilirubin. *2467*

Chenodeoxycholic Acid   *Serum   Increase*   Increased serum bile acids in anicteric viral hepatitis from either A or B virus. Elevated postprandial levels may persist even after transaminase and BSP retention have returned to normal. *1154*

Cholesterol   *Serum   Decrease*   Magnitude of depression is directly related to degree of hepatic damage. A progressive fall is a grave prognostic sign. *2104*   In 25% of 19 patients at initial hospitalization for this disorder. *0781*   Normal or mildly depressed in hepatitis; but markedly depressed in severe hepatitis. *0503*

Red Blood Cells   Increase   25-50% increase in the membrane concentration, resulting in the characteristic target cell. *2552*

Cholesterol Esters   *Serum   Decrease*   Striking decrease as liver involvement progresses. *2104*

Cholesterol, Very Low Density Lipoprotein   *Serum   Increase*   Marked elevation. *0062*

Cholic Acid   *Serum   Increase*   Increased serum bile acids in anicteric viral hepatitis from either A or B virus. Elevated postprandial levels may persist even after transaminase and BSP retention have returned to normal. *1154*

Cold Agglutinins   *Serum   Increase*   Elevated titers may persist for weeks or months. *2035*

Copper   *Serum   Increase*   Significant P < 0.001. *2429*

Coproporphyrin   *Urine   Increase*   0619

Creatine Kinase   *Serum   Normal*   0962

Cryomacroglobulins   *Serum   Increase*   0863

Erythrocyte Sedimentation Rate   *Blood   Increase*   High (mean = 24.1 ± 10.7 mm/h) in cases of uncomplicated HBsAg-negative hepatitis and normal (mean < 10 mm/h) in HBsAG positive cases. *1575*   Nonspecific. *1900*

Fat *Feces Increase* May be excessive amounts of fecal fat. *2104*

Folate *Serum Increase* Increased. *0741 0866*

Gamma Glutamyl Transferase (GGT) *Serum Increase* The mean elevation (152 U/L) in 17 patients was 5.2 X the upper limit of normal. *1452* In 77% of 14 patients at initial hospitalization for this disorder. *0781*

Saliva Normal Infectious Hepatitis. *1164*

Globulin *Serum Increase* Mean total serum values were highest in acute viral hepatitis, primary hepatocellular carcinoma and cirrhosis, in that order. *0724* Frequent transiently elevated *0962*

Glucaric Acid *Urine Increase* A 3 fold increase of D-glucaric acid was found in the early stages of disease (37.13 μmol/24h ± 3.08 vs. 9.91 ± 1.18 in controls) when serum transaminases and bilirubin were very high. A lower but significantly raised level was found during recovery when the transaminases and bilirubin were greatly reduced. *0346*

Glucose *Serum Decrease* Can occur with various types of liver disease. Hepatic hypoglycemia is a fasting hypoglycemia and often only transiently relieved by food. *0962 2104*

Glucose Tolerance *Serum Decrease* Subnormal insulin response to oral glucose tolerance test was found in 5 of 14 patients in the icteric phase. *1548*

Glycoproteins *Serum Decrease* In acute fulminant hepatitis, the values showed a statistically significant difference between fatal (21.9 mg/dL) and surviving cases (37.4 mg/dL). *1291*

Granular Casts *Urine Increase* During the early icteric phase may reflect renal abnormalities. *0151*

Hematocrit *Blood Decrease* May develop late in the course of the disease. *0151* A mild degree of transient anemia. *0962*

Hemoglobin *Blood Decrease* Mild anemia may appear late in the course of acute disease. *0151* A mild degree of transient anemia. *0962*

Hepatitis B Surface Antigen *Serum Increase* Can be present during incubation period and acute phase; occasionally may persist. *2467* About 80% of patients with clinical signs of viral hepatitis type B have been found to have the antigen in their blood when multiple timed sample were taken. *0962*

Hexosaminidase *Serum Increase* Increase in total concentration (hexosaminidase A and B). *1716*

Immunoglobulin IgA *Serum Increase* *2467*

Immunoglobulin IgG *Serum Increase* Slightly elevated gamma globulins, usually < 2.0 g/dL. IgG rises as illness progresses. *0433* Frequently transiently elevated. *0962*

Immunoglobulin IgM *Serum Increase* Usually increased above 400 mg/dL during acute phase. *2467* Initial rise in IgM, followed by IgG. *0433*

Iron *Serum Increase* Increase becomes evident only after liver disease has been present for 2-3 weeks. *0153*

Iron-Binding Capacity, Total (TIBC) *Serum Increase* Increases are rare other than in iron deficiency, but they may occur in viral hepatitis. *0962* May be increased with hepatitis. *2467*

Isocitrate Dehydrogenase *Serum Increase* Usually elevated in the early stage (5-10 X normal) but returns to normal in 2-3 weeks. *2467* 40 X normal. *0503* Invariably elevated when measured within 10 days of onset of jaundice. *2260*

Isoleucine *Serum Increase* A close relationship was found between the onset of encephalopathy and amino acid equilibrium disturbance, characterized by a fall in the molar ratio between valine leucine and isoleucine and phenylalanine and tyrosine. All showed absolute elevations with onset of encephalopathy. *0531*

Lactate Dehydrogenase *Serum Increase* Slightly elevated (1-2 fold) values. *0503* 8 of 10 cases showed mild elevation. *1480* Slight increase. *0962* In 80% of 25 patients at initial hospitalization in this disorder. *0781* Moderate elevation in most cases. *2260*

Lactate Dehydrogenase Isoenzyme 5 (LD$_5$) *Serum Increase* Markedly elevated in 7 cases. Comprised 35.4% of the total serum LD (normal = 0-6%). *0852*

Lactate Dehydrogenase Isoenzymes *Serum Decrease* In 7 cases, LD$_1$ and LD$_2$ were markedly decreased (13.0% and 19.3% respectively). *0852*

Serum Increase In 7 cases, LD$_4$ was markedly increased (11.0%). Total LD was elevated to a mean level of 2057 U/L. *0852*

Lecithin *Red Blood Cells Increase* 25-50% increase in the membrane concentration, resulting in the characteristic target cell. *2552*

Leucine *Serum Increase* A close relationship was found between the onset of encephalopathy and amino acid equilibrium disturbance, characterized by a fall in the molar ratio between valine, leucine, and isoleucine, and phenylalanine and tyrosine. All showed absolute elevations with onset of encephalopathy. *0531*

Leucine Aminopeptidase *Serum Increase* In 12 patients, 92% showed elevated values, ranging from 320-900 U/L and a mean of 592 U/L. *0281*

Leukocytes *Blood Decrease* There may be a slight transient drop but rarely to leukopenic levels. *0433* Leukopenia (lymphopenia and neutropenia) is noted with onset of fever, followed by relative lymphocytosis and monocytosis. *2467 0999 0962*

Lipase *Serum Decrease* Lack of bile salts result in the failure to activate pancreatic lipase in the intestinal lumen. *2104*

Lymphocytes *Blood Decrease* Impaired T-cell reactivity is due to a disturbed function of T-cell and not to a decrease in their number. In cases associated with significant hepatocellular damage, a reduction in the number of circulating B-cells was observed. *1709*

Blood Increase A relative lymphocytosis may result with some atypical lymphocytes. *0962 0433 0532*

Magnesium *Serum Decrease* Before treatment, plasma concentration was 0.96 - 0.2. Normal = 1.73 ± 0.13 mmol/L. *0246*

Red Blood Cells Decrease 2 of 5 patients had abnormally low concentrations. The mean concentration for the entire group, 4.3 mmol/L packed cells, was significantly (P < 0.001) decreased below normal. *2469* RBC concentration was 3.18 ± 0.78 mmol/L before treatment. Normal = 5.08 ± 0.25 mmol/L. *0246*

Malate Dehydrogenase *Serum Increase* *0619*

Manganese *Serum Increase* Increase becomes evident only after liver disease has been present for 2-3 weeks. *0153* During acute phase increase up to four times that seen in normal subjects. *2429* Significant increase (P < 0.01). *2429*

Monocytes *Blood Increase* In 55% of 23 patients at initial hospitalization for this disorder. *0781 0532*

Mucoprotein *Serum Decrease* *0503*

Nickel *Serum Decrease* Thought to be caused by hypoalbuminemia. *1559*

Ornithine Carbamoyl Transferase (OCT) *Serum Increase* Liver cell damage. *2467*

pCO$_2$ *Blood Decrease* Reduced in a high percentage of chronic as well as acute hepatitis patients. *2104*

Phenylalanine *Serum Increase* A close relationship was found between the onset of encephalopathy and amino acid equilibrium disturbance, characterized by a fall in the molar ratio between valine leucine and isoleucine and phenylalanine and tyrosine. All showed absolute elevations with onset of encephalopathy. *0531*

Phospholipids, Total *Serum Decrease* Increased in mild but decreased in severe hepatitis. *2467*

Serum Increase Increased in mild but decreased in severe hepatitis. *2467*

Plasma Cells *Serum Decrease* Late pregnancy. *2357 0659 0683*

Platelet Count *Blood Decrease* Patient may show anemia, leukocytosis, thrombocytopenia in fulminant hepatitis with hepatic failure. *2467*

Porphyrins *Urine Increase* *2467*

Prealbumin *Serum Decrease* The mean value was 6.0 mg/dL in fatal cases. 7.4 mg/dL in survivors. The difference was not statistically significant. *1291*

Protein Bound Iodine (PBI) *Serum Increase* Not infrequently. May be due to biliary reflux of conjugated T$_4$. *2540 2104*

Prothrombin Time *Plasma Increase* May be slightly prolonged but bleeding problems are uncommon. A greatly prolonged prothrombin time heralds massive hepatic necrosis and is a sign of poor prognosis. *0433* Usually normal, and if prolonged, suggests severe hepatitis. If the prolongation increases, it is indicative of fulminant hepatitis. *0962*

Pseudocholinesterase *Serum Decrease* Tends to be more marked in patients ill with chronic liver disease, such as cirrhosis than in those ill with acute conditions, such as viral hepatitis, ascending cholangitis and acute anoxic hepatomegaly. Peaks and depressions in cholinesterase activity in acute liver disease are related to the extent of hepatic parenchymal damage. *2441 1452*

Reticulocytes *Blood Increase* Mild hemolytic anemia with increase in the reticulocyte count are commonly found. *0962*

Rheumatoid Factor *Serum Increase* 24% positivity. *0422 0123 0962*

70.00 Viral Hepatitis *(continued)*

Specific Gravity *Urine Decrease* Concentrating ability is sometimes decreased. *2467*

Thymol Turbidity *Serum Increase* Usually increased during acute phase. *2467* More useful in assessing the rate of recovery, although it may be increased early in the disease. It remains positive in convalescence after the cephalin cholesterol reaction has become normal. *0619*

Thyroxine Binding Globulin *Serum Increase* Not infrequently. *2540* Increased level. *1887*

Thyroxine (T$_4$) *Serum Increase* Not infrequently. *2540*

Triglycerides *Serum Increase* In 12 children a relationship was suggested between ALT and triglycerides, in which the triglycerides provide an energy substrate, thereby freeing glucose for alanine synthesis. *0026*

Tyrosine *Serum Increase* A close relationship was found between the onset of encephalopathy and amino acid equilibrium disturbance, characterized by a fall in the molar ratio between valine, leucine, and isoleucine, and phenylalanine and tyrosine. All showed absolute elevations with onset of encephalopathy. *0531*

Uric Acid *Serum Increase* Mean levels were 8.0 ± 0.6 (normal = 6.5 ± 0.6 mg/dL) in 16 patients. Values for the entire group were not statistically significant, but individual decreases measured upon recovery showed significant individual elevations. *1890*

Urine Increase 24 h excretion was markedly elevated in patients (1405 ± 149 mg/day) compared to controls (748 ± 58 mg/day). *1890*

Urobilinogen *Urine Increase* At peak of the disease, it disappears for days or weeks. *2467* Increases during defervescent period. *0433*

Feces Decrease Disappears at peak of disease. *2467*

Valine *Serum Increase* A close relationship was found between the onset of encephalopathy and amino acid equilibrium disturbance, characterized by a fall in the molar ratio between valine, leucine and isoleucine, and phenylalanine and tyrosine. All showed absolute elevations with onset of encephalopathy. *0531*

Vitamin A *Serum Decrease* In severe hepatitis. *2467*

Zinc *Serum Decrease* Generally declines to values comparable to those found in other acute infections. Serum Zn exists almost entirely in a diffusible state with very little protein-bound. *0153*

71.00 Rabies

Albumin *Urine Increase* May be present. *2468*

Cells *CSF Increase* Usually < 1,000/μL but counts between 1,500-4,000/μL have been observed. *1319*

Erythrocytes *Saliva Increase* May be bloody. *2368*

Glucose *Serum Decrease* May be somewhat below normal. *0433*

Ketones *Serum Increase* Acetone may be present. *0433*

Urine Increase Acetone may be present. *0433*

Leukocytes *Blood Increase* Leukocytosis with a relative increase of neutrophils is the rule. May be moderate but high values are not unusual. The maximum count observed was 32,000/μL. *0433 1319*

CSF Normal Usually normal. *0433 1319*

Protein *Urine Increase* Slight. *1058*

CSF Increase A slight increase. *2468*

Specific Gravity *Urine Increase* The urine is concentrated, particularly when the body temperature is elevated and/or the kidney function is diminished. *0433*

72.00 Mumps

Albumin *Urine Increase* Proteinuria should suggest a diagnosis of mumps nephritis. *0433*

Amylase *Serum Increase* Increased during the period of swelling and for about 10 days thereafter in 90% of patients. *0433* 96.2% of 224 patients showed elevations during the course of the disease. In 83.77% of patients the elevations occurred in the first week and fell progressively. *0336 1319*

Urine Increase Increased during first week. *2468*

Cells *CSF Increase* In meningitis and meningoencephalitis fewer than 500/μL with only occasional cell counts exceeding 2,000/μL. In most cases the cells are almost exclusively mononuclear from the onset: polymorphonuclear leukocytes predominate for the first few days in only a small percentage of patients. Pleocytosis may continue for as long as 5 weeks. *0433*

Cold Agglutinins *Serum Increase* Increased titer. *0186*

Complement Fixation *Serum Increase* Antibodies against the S and V antigens are the most widely used serologic test. The S antibodies usually rise within the first week of illness, the V antibodies appearing 1-2 weeks later. A presumptive diagnosis can therefore be made when elevated S antibodies are found in the absence of V antibodies. *0433* Positive during 2nd week and remains elevated > 6 weeks; paired sera showing a 4-fold increase in titer confirm recent infection. *2368 1319*

Erythrocyte Casts *Urine Increase* Suggests a diagnosis of mumps nephritis. *0433*

Erythrocytes *Urine Increase* Suggests a diagnosis of mumps nephritis. *0433*

Erythrocyte Sedimentation Rate *Blood Increase* May occur with mumps arthritis and orchitis. *0433*

Gamma Glutamyl Transferase (GGT) *Saliva Normal* *1164*

Glucose *Serum Decrease* *0619*

CSF Decrease Usually normal, however, recent reports have emphasized that depressed CSF concentrations (< 40 mg/dL) may be present initially and persist for several days. *0433 1319*

Hemagglutination Inhibition *Serum Increase* Develops later and persists longer by several months than complement-fixation test. *2468* A 4-fold difference in titer between the 1st and 3rd week is diagnostic. *2368*

Leukocytes *Blood Decrease* May be depressed, normal or elevated, with or without a relative lymphocytosis; they are of little value in establishing a diagnosis. *0433*

Blood Increase Total count often reaches 15,000-20,000/μL, with a high percentage of polymorphonuclear cells. *0151* May be depressed, normal or elevated, with or without a relative lymphocytosis; they are of little value in establishing a diagnosis. *0433*

Blood Normal Usually within normal limits. *2368*

CSF Increase In meningitis and meningoencephalitis, CSF usually contains fewer than 500/μL with only occasional counts > 2,000/μL. In most cases the cells are almost exclusively mononuclear from the onset: polymorphonuclear leukocytes predominate for the first few days in only a small percentage of patients. Pleocytosis may continue for as long as 5 weeks. *0433*

Lipase *Serum Increase* 11.5% of patients had slightly elevated values. *0336*

Lymphocytes *Blood Increase* Usually there is a slight predominance of lymphocytes but at times the reverse is true. *1319 2467*

CSF Increase Cell counts range from 500 to several thousand/μL, and are predominantly lymphocytes. *0151* Increased T-cells and decreased B-cells in CSF were found in mumps meningitis. *1214 0790*

Monocytes *Blood Increase* May occur. *2368*

Neutralizing Antibodies *Serum Increase* The most reliable index of the immune status of natural disease or administration of the live attenuated virus vaccine. Unfortunately their determination is impractical as a routine diagnostic procedure. *0433*

Neutrophils *CSF Increase* In meningitis and meningoencephalitis fewer than 500 cells/μL with only occasional cell counts exceeding 2,000/μL in most cases the cells are almost exclusively mononuclear from the onset: polymorphonuclear leukocytes predominate for the first few days in only a small percentage of patients. Pleocytosis may continue for as long as 5 weeks. *0433*

Protein *Urine Increase* Indicates mumps nephritis. *0433*

CSF Increase Normal or slightly elevated. *0433*

73.90 Psittacosis

Alanine Aminotransferase *Serum Increase* With severe liver involvement. *0433*

Albumin *Urine Increase* Frequently seen. *0433*

Alkaline Phosphatase *Serum Increase* With severe liver involvement. *0433*

Angiotensin-Converting Enzyme (ACE) *Serum Normal* Not elevated in active hypersensitivity pneumonitis. *1539*

Aspartate Aminotransferase *Serum Increase* With severe liver involvement. *0433*

Cold Agglutinins *Serum Normal* *2468*

Complement Fixation *Serum Increase* Positive but not conclusive tests are presumptive in diagnosis because of false positives with other infections and cross reactions with lymphogranuloma venereum. *2468* A low titer is highly suspicious during the acute phase of the illness, and the diagnosis is confirmed by a 4-fold increase in titer. *0962 2368*

Creatinine *Serum Increase* With severe renal involvement. *0433*

Erythrocytes *Sputum Increase* Occasionally bloody. *2368*

Erythrocyte Sedimentation Rate *Blood Increase* Usually is increased but may be normal. *2468*

Blood Normal Frequently normal. *2368*

Gamma Glutamyl Transferase (GGT) *Serum Increase* With severe liver involvement. *0433*

Globulin *Serum Increase* Often associated with hypergammaglobulinemia. *2104*

Lactate Dehydrogenase *Serum Increase* With severe liver involvement. *0433*

Leukocytes *Blood Decrease* Normal or decreased in acute phase, then increases in convalescence. *2368* During the early stage of the illness. *0962 2467 0433 2468*

Blood Increase May occur during the late or convalescent stage. *0962 2368*

Neutrophils *Blood Decrease* Rarely, profound granulocytopenia occurs. *0433*

Protein *Urine Increase* Common during the febrile period. *2368*

Urea Nitrogen *Serum Increase* With severe renal involvement. *0433*

75.00   Infectious Mononucleosis

Acid Phosphatase *Leukocyte Increase* *1388*

Alanine Aminotransferase *Serum Increase* Reflected the presence and extent of hepatic damage, and the severity of subjective symptoms in 36 patients. *1912* Show abnormal results in most cases. *1319* Elevations occur in 80-100% during acute illness and return to normal in 3-5 weeks. *2538 0619 2467 0962*

Aldolase *Serum Increase* *0962*

Alkaline Phosphatase *Serum Increase* Increased in many cases, with maximum values during the 3rd week of the disease. 60-70% of cases are elevated ranging from 25-215 U/L. Only 20% of cases had values > 107 U/L. *0619* 30 (65%) had dissociation with serum bilirubin concentration. Occasionally high levels, even with normal bilirubin concentration. *2156* May occur; hepatic involvement is usually mild. *2538 1687 0962*

Alkaline Phosphatase Isoenzymes *Serum Increase* An electrophoretically distinct isoenzyme (phosphatase N) was found in the serum of all 22 patients. Values ranged from 13-100% of the total activity, with 6 cases having > 80% phos-N activity. *1687*

Amylase *Serum Increase* May be associated with hyperamylasemia. *1386*

Antibody Titer *Serum Increase* The presence of EB virus antibody is essential for diagnosis in heterophil-negative cases. Antibody to early antigen and EB virus-specific IgM antibody occurs in 75-85% of acute cases. *1028 2538*

Antinuclear Antibodies *Serum Increase* 65% of patients were positive. *1799* May be present without positive LE cell test. *0619*

Antismooth Muscle Antibodies *Serum Increase* IgM smooth muscle antibody may appear as opposed to the IgG antibody found in chronic hepatitis. *1829* Transiently positive. *1062 2035*

Aspartate Aminotransferase *Serum Increase* In 80% of patients moderate (50-300 U/L) increases are observed. Usual values 25-400 U/L. *0503* Elevations occur in 80-100% during acute illness and return to normal in 3-5 weeks. *2538* In 90% of 11 patients at initial hospitalization for this disorder. *0781 0812 1912 0962*

Bilirubin *Serum Increase* Over 1 mg/dL in 37% of patients. *0433* May occur; hepatic involvement is usually mild. *2538 0962*

BSP Retention *Serum Increase* May occur; hepatic involvement is usually mild. *2538*

Cephalin Flocculation *Serum Increase* Maximal by 2nd week and normal by 5th week. *0619* Reflected the presence and extent of hepatic damage, and paralleled the severity of subjective symptoms in 36 patients. *1912* In most cases. *1319 2368*

Cholesterol *Serum Decrease* In 60% of 10 patients at initial hospitalization for this disorder. *0781*

Cold Agglutinins *Serum Increase* Occur frequently; they are present mostly in the IgM fraction and have anti-I specificity. *0502* Elevated titers may persists for weeks or months. *2035 0330 2538*

Coproporphyrin *Urine Increase* *0151*

Cryomacroglobulins *Serum Increase* *0863*

Erythrocyte Sedimentation Rate *Blood Decrease* Low readings may reflect the intracellular nature of the offending organism or liver involvement that causes decreased synthesis of fibrinogen. *0962*

Gamma Glutamyl Transferase (GGT) *Serum Increase* Levels correlate with serum alkaline phosphatase and 5'-nucleotidase levels. *0619*

Globulin *Serum Increase* Often associated with hypergammaglobulinemia. *2104*

Hematocrit *Blood Decrease* Anemia is rare. *1319*

Blood Increase In 27% of 11 patients at initial hospitalization for this disorder. *0781*

Hemoglobin *Blood Decrease* Anemia is rare. *1319*

Blood Increase In 45% of 11 patients at initial hospitalization for this disorder. *0781*

Heterophil Antibody *Serum Increase* Elevated titers which agglutinate sheep RBCs; 40% have positive tests during 1st week of illness and 80% by the 3rd week. *2508* Elevated titers may persist longer than a year in 75% of patients. Over 95% of typical cases are heterophil antibody positive if followed long enough. *0679* Develop in the 1st week of illness in most patients and ultimately appear in 80-90% of patients and persist for 3-6 months. *0962 2538 0151*

Immunoglobulin IgA *Serum Increase* A modest increase may occur. *0961 2035*

Immunoglobulin IgE *Serum Increase* *2035*

Immunoglobulin IgG *Serum Increase* Mean values 50% higher than normal. *0961 2538*

Immunoglobulin IgM *Serum Increase* Increase up to 100% over control values in almost all cases, then decline over a period of 2-3 months toward normal. *0961 2538*

Isocitrate Dehydrogenase *Serum Increase* More than 25 U/L, becomes normal in 2-3 weeks. *2467*

Lactate Dehydrogenase *Serum Increase* 2-4 X normal values. *0503* All 36 patients showed elevated values, which persisted in 50% of the cases for over 4 months after onset of disease. *1658* Elevations occur in 80-100% during acute illness and return to normal in 3-5 weeks. *2538* In 80% of 10 patients at initial hospitalization for this disorder. *0781 1089 0962*

Lactate Dehydrogenase Isoenzyme 5 (LD$_5$) *Serum Increase* Elevated in 35% of the 36 patients with elevated serum LD. *1658* Mean level in 5 cases was 8.2% of total serum LD. Normal mean = 3.0%. *1658 0852*

Lactate Dehydrogenase Isoenzymes *Serum Increase* Elevated in all 36 patients. Isoenzymes 1, 2, and 3 were most often elevated and remained so for 4 months after onset. *1658*

Leucine Aminopeptidase *Serum Increase* In 4 patients all had serum levels above the upper limit of normal, ranging from 330-740 U/L. *1682*

Leukocytes *Blood Decrease* During the first week of illness the count and distribution may be normal; infrequently there is moderate leukopenia. *0433 2467 1319*

Blood Increase During the 1st week, WBC count and distribution may be normal; infrequently there is moderate leukopenia. In the 2nd week, total count rises and persists into the 3rd week; then it declines. *0433* Leukopenia is toward the end of the 1st week or the start of the 2nd week; with counts rising to between 10,000-20,000/μL. Rarely, counts from 30,000-80,000 are seen. *1794 1319 2538 0781 2368*

Blood Normal During the first week of illness the leukocyte count and distribution may be normal; infrequently there is moderate leukopenia. *0433* Usually within normal limits during the first week or two of disease, but progressively rises. *0962 1319*

Lymphocytes *Blood Increase* Absolute and relative lymphocytosis are characteristic and requisite for diagnosis. *0433* An absolute increase in the number of atypical lymphocytes is a characteristic finding during all stages of the disease. *1319* Marked lymphocytosis, both relative and absolute. At least 50-60% of the WBCs are lymphocytes or monocytes; and at least 10% are atypical lymphocytes. *0962 2538 2368*

Monocytes *Blood Increase* Relative increase. *2538* In 54% of 11 patients at initial hospitalization for this disorder. *0781 0532*

Neutrophils *Blood Increase* Transient increase with intercurrent bacterial infection. *0433 1319 2538*

Plasma Cells *Serum Increase* *2468*

Rheumatoid Factor *Serum Increase* *0962*

75.00   Infectious Mononucleosis   (continued)

Thymol Turbidity   *Serum   Increase*   Reflected the presence and extent of hepatic damage, and paralleled the severity of subjective symptoms in 36 patients. *1912*   Show abnormal results in most cases. *1319*

VDRL   *Serum   Positive*   False positive serologic tests for syphilis are sometimes seen. *0999*   Occurs occasionally, usually reverts to negative by the 3rd week. *1319*   The incidence of false positive reactions is 5%. *1108*   Positive tests occur but are unusual. *0502 2538*

Weil-Felix Reaction   *Serum   Positive*   Positive tests occur but are unusual. *0502*

78.50   Cytomegalic Inclusion Disease

Alanine Aminotransferase   *Serum   Increase*   Slight increase which becomes more marked with clinical hepatitis in some cases. *2468*

Alkaline Phosphatase   *Serum   Increase*   Increased in infants. *0619*

Alpha-Fetoprotein   *Serum   Increase*   Among 54 patients with verified infection, 8 (15%) had raised levels in sera taken after the onset of infection. *0802*   In the newborn, the level was abnormal but disappeared by the end of the 1st month. *1598*

Aspartate Aminotransferase   *Serum   Increase*   Slight increase which becomes more marked with clinical hepatitis in some cases. *2468*

Bilirubin   *Serum   Increase*   Hemolytic anemia. *2538 0767*

Bilirubin, Direct   *Serum   Increase*   Usually > 5% of total concentration and may be 50%. *2368*

Bilirubin, Indirect   *Serum   Increase*   In hemolytic anemia. *1058*

Cells   *CSF   Increase*   Pleocytosis in congenital disease. *1319*

Cephalin Flocculation   *Serum   Increase*   Slight increase which becomes more marked with clinical hepatitis in some cases. *2468*

Cold Agglutinins   *Serum   Increase*   *2468*

Complement Fixation   *Serum   Increase*   Requires use of multiple serologic types and is too time consuming and not very practical. *1319*

Erythrocyte Sedimentation Rate   *Blood   Increase*   Slightly increased. *2468*

Haptoglobin   *Serum   Decrease*   Hemolytic anemia. *1058*

Hematocrit   *Blood   Decrease*   Anemia usually present in congenital disease. *1319*   Hemolytic anemia. *0767 2538*

Hemoglobin   *Blood   Decrease*   Anemia usually present in congenital disease. *1319*   Hemolytic anemia. *0767 2538*

Hemoglobin, Free   *Serum   Increase*   Hemolytic anemia. *0767 2538*

Immunoglobulins   *Serum   Increase*   Normal to increased. *1676*

Lactate Dehydrogenase   *Serum   Increase*   Slight increase which becomes more marked with clinical hepatitis in some cases. *2468*

Leukocytes   *Blood   Increase*   Increase to 15,000-20,000/μL with 60-80% lymphocytes, many of which are Downey cell type. *2468*

Lymphocytes   *Blood   Increase*   Increase in WBC to 15,000-20,000/μL with 60-80% lymphocytes, many of which are Downey cell type. *2468*

Neutralizing Antibodies   *Serum   Increase*   Requires use of multiple serologic types and is too time consuming and not very practical. *1319*

Platelet Count   *Blood   Decrease*   Thrombocytopenia usually present in congenital disease. *1319*   Common manifestation; usually transient and rarely associated with significant bleeding. *1676*

Protein   *CSF   Increase*   In congenital disease. *1319*

Thymol Turbidity   *Serum   Increase*   Slight increased which becomes more marked with clinical hepatitis in some cases. *2468*

80.00   Epidemic Typhus

Albumin   *Urine   Increase*   During the febrile period. *0433*

Antibody Titer   *Serum   Increase*   Antibodies are demonstrable in significant titers by the 3rd week. *0433*   Acute phase antibodies are of the IgM type. *0151*

Cells   *CSF   Increase*   With severe encephalitis manifestations. *0433*

Complement Fixation   *Serum   Increase*   Antibodies first appear in the serum between the 7-12 days. *0151*   A demonstration of a 4-fold increase is considered significant. *1319*   Antibodies develop which are both group- and species- specific. *0962   0433*

Creatinine   *Serum   Increase*   With varying degrees of renal involvement. *0433*

Eosinophils   *Blood   Decrease*   Absent or rare in the early stages. *2368*

Erythrocytes   *Urine   Increase*   Microscopic hematuria can be expected. *0433*

Globulin   *Serum   Increase*   Often associated with hypergammaglobulinemia. *2104*

Hematocrit   *Blood   Decrease*   Normal early, falls significantly during the illness. *0433*   May develop in the 2nd or 3rd week. *2368*

Hemoglobin   *Blood   Decrease*   Normal early, falls significantly during the illness. *0433*   May develop in the 2nd or 3rd week. *2368*

Leukocytes   *Blood   Decrease*   Leukopenia frequently associated with infectious diseases. *1077*   In first few days of illness. *2368 2538*

 Blood   Increase   May signal secondary bacterial infection. *0433*   Only slightly elevated unless complications ensue. *2368*

Neutrophils   *Blood   Decrease*   Leukopenia frequently associated with infectious diseases. *1077   2538*

pO₂   *Blood   Decrease*   With pulmonary involvement. *0433*

Protein   *Serum   Decrease*   Hypoproteinemia occurs in severe cases. *2368*

 CSF   Increase   With severe encephalitic manifestations. *0433*

Sodium   *Serum   Decrease*   Chronic illness from rickettsial disease result in hyponatremia. *2104*

Urea Nitrogen   *Serum   Increase*   With varying degrees of renal involvement. *0433*   Azotemia is common. *2368*

VDRL   *Serum   Positive*   In 20% of patients. *1058*

Volume   *Urine   Decrease*   Oliguria is common. *2368*

Weil-Felix Reaction   *Serum   Positive*   Serum obtained 5-12 days after onset of symptoms usually shows a positive reaction with agglutinating antibody for Proteus Ox 19 and rarely Proteus Ox 2. *0433*

81.00   Endemic Typhus

Complement Fixation   *Serum   Increase*   Antibodies develop which are both group- and species- specific. Appear during the 2nd week of illness and reach a peak during the 4th week. *0962*

Hematocrit   *Blood   Normal*   *0433*

Leukocytes   *Blood   Decrease*   Leukopenia frequently associated with infectious diseases. *1077*   Normal or slightly low. *0433*

Neutrophils   *Blood   Decrease*   Leukopenia frequently associated with infectious diseases. *1077*

Platelet Count   *Blood   Decrease*   Rarely seen. *0433*

Protein   *Urine   Increase*   During the febrile period. *0433*

Sodium   *Serum   Decrease*   Chronic illness from rickettsial disease results in hyponatremia. *2104*

Weil-Felix Reaction   *Serum   Positive*   With Proteus OX-9 and OX-2. *0503*   Antibodies to Proteus OX-19 are present in significant titers by the third week. *0433*   May be superior to complement-fixation procedure in typhus and Rocky Mountain spotted fever. *1813*

81.10   Brill's Disease

Albumin   *Urine   Increase*   Transient albuminuria may occur. *0433*

Antibody Titer   *Serum   Increase*   Acute-phase antibodies are of the IgG class. *0151*

Complement Fixation   *Serum   Increase*   The diagnosis can be made by demonstrating a rising titer of antibodies which fix complement in the presence of epidemic typhus antigen or agglutinate suspensions of washed Rickettsia prowazekii. The antibody occurs earlier (4-6th day) and peaks between the 8-10th day. *0433   2368*

Sodium   *Serum   Decrease*   Chronic illness from Rickettsial disease result in hyponatremia. *2104*

Weil-Felix Reaction   *Serum   Negative*   A negative test in the presence of rising complement-fixing antibodies distinguishes Brill-Zinsser from primary louse-borne typhus. *0151*   Positive reactions develop in 10-20% of cases that occur 10 or more years after the primary attack. *1058*

81.20　Mite-Borne Typhus

Complement Fixation　*Serum　Increase*　Available antigens detect complement fixing antibody in only about 50% of the cases. *0962*　Irregular results. *2368*

Leukocytes　*Blood　Decrease*　Leukopenia is seen in Rickettsial diseases. *2467*

Blood　Normal　Usually. *1058*

Sodium　*Serum　Decrease*　Chronic illness from Rickettsial disease results in hyponatremia. *2104*

Weil-Felix Reaction　*Serum　Positive*　Four fold or greater rises in Weil-Felix OX-K titers are found in almost all untreated patients and 75% of those treated with antimicrobial therapy. *0151*　The only rickettsial disease in which OX-K antibody is present. *0962*　Agglutinins for Proteus OX-K but not for OX-19 or OX-2 are present. *2368*

82.00　Rocky Mountain Spotted Fever

Albumin　*Serum　Decrease*　Common. *0433*

Urine　Increase　Varying degrees. *0433*

Aspartate Aminotransferase　*Serum　Increase*　Common. *0433*

Casts　*Urine　Increase*　Varying degrees. *0433*

Complement Fixation　*Serum　Increase*　Antibodies develop which are both group- and species- specific. Appear during the 2nd week of illness and reach a peak during the 4th week. *0962*　A 4-fold or greater rise is considered confirmatory. *0151*　Significant rise in titer occurs by the 3rd week. *1319*

Factor II　*Plasma　Decrease*　May be associated with defibrination resulting in platelet and coagulation factor consumption. *2538*

Factor IV　*Plasma　Decrease*　May be associated with defibrination resulting in platelet and coagulation factor consumption. *2538*

Factor XII　*Plasma　Decrease*　May be associated with defibrination resulting in platelet and coagulation factor consumption. *2538*　Hypofibrinogenemia in 2 of 5 cases with marked reduction of factor XII. *2589*

Fibrinogen　*Plasma　Decrease*　May be associated with defibrination resulting in platelet and coagulation factor consumption. *2538*　Hypofibrinogenemia in 2 of 5 cases with marked reduction of factor XII. *2589*

Hemagglutination Inhibition　*Serum　Increase*　May be superior to complement-fixation procedure in typhus and Rocky Mountain spotted fever. *1813*

Hematocrit　*Blood　Decrease*　Anemia may develop in the 2nd-3rd weeks. *2368*

Hemoglobin　*Blood　Decrease*　Anemia may develop in the 2nd-3rd weeks. *2368*

Leukocytes　*Blood　Decrease*　Leukopenia frequently associated with infectious diseases. *1077　2538*

Blood　Increase　Common. *0433*

Monocytes　*Blood　Increase*　Increases in some Rickettsial infections. *2467*

Neutrophils　*Blood　Decrease*　Leukopenia frequently associated with infectious diseases. *1077　2538*

Platelet Count　*Blood　Decrease*　Counts below 100,000/μL were seen in 4 of 5 patients. *2589*　May be associated with defibrination resulting in platelet and coagulation factor consumption. *2538*

Protein　*Serum　Decrease*　Hypoproteinemia is common in severe cases. *2368*

Prothrombin Consumption　*Blood　Increase*　May be associated with defibrination resulting in platelet and coagulation factor consumption. *2538*

Sodium　*Serum　Decrease*　Chronic illness from Rickettsial disease result in hyponatremia. *2104*

Urea Nitrogen　*Serum　Increase*　Azotemia is common in severe cases. *2368　0433*

Volume　*Urine　Decrease*　Oliguria is common. *2368*

Weil-Felix Reaction　*Serum　Positive*　Agglutinins against Proteus OX-19 and OX-2 develop by the 2nd or 3rd week. *1319*　Antibodies first appear between the 8th and 12th day of illness. *2508　0151*

83.20　Rickettsialpox

Complement Fixation　*Serum　Increase*　A 4-fold or greater rise in antibody titer in paired sera. Because of cross reactions, the Rocky Mountain spotted fever test will also be positive. *1319*

Leukocytes　*Blood　Decrease*　Typify the acute phase. *0433*　Usual. *1058*

Lymphocytes　*Blood　Increase*　Typify the acute phase. *0433*

Sodium　*Serum　Decrease*　Chronic illness from Rickettsial disease result in hyponatremia. *2104*

Weil-Felix Reaction　*Serum　Negative*　With Proteus OX-19, OX-2 and OX-K. *1319*　Negative in Rickettsial Pox, Q fever, and trench fever. *2368*

Serum　Positive　Appears in 2nd-3rd week of illness. Agglutinins for Proteus OX-19, OX-2, and OX-K do not rise in titer. *2368*

84.00　Malaria

Alanine Aminotransferase　*Serum　Increase*　Moderate increase. *2468*

Albumin　*Serum　Decrease*　*2468*

Urine　Increase　In uncomplicated infection, mild. *0433*

Alkaline Phosphatase　*Serum　Increase*　Moderate increase. *2468*

Antinuclear Antibodies　*Serum　Increase*　An unusually high incidence was observed during chronic infection. *0916　2035*

Aspartate Aminotransferase　*Serum　Decrease*　Activity was increased in 11 patients untreated for more than 4 days. *2066*　May be elevated. *0962*

Serum　Increase　Moderate increase. *2468*

Bilirubin　*Serum　Increase*　Evidence of hemolysis. *2468*

Bilirubin, Indirect　*Serum　Increase*　Evidence of hemolysis. *2468*

Cold Agglutinins　*Serum　Increase*　An unusually high incidence was observed during chronic infection. *0916　2035 1826*

Complement C3　*Serum　Decrease*　Only in patients with defective hemoglobin synthesis. *2240*

Complement Fixation　*Serum　Increase*　In natural infections, the complement-fixation and indirect hemagglutination tests detect malarial antibodies equally efficiently for the first 2 months after onset, but titers obtained by complement-fixation rapidly decline within a year, while the indirect hemagglutination titers remain elevated. *2547*

Coombs' Test　*Blood　Positive*　Patients occasionally have a Coombs'-positive hemolytic anemia. *0151*

Creatinine　*Serum　Increase*　In all patients, independent of the duration of the acute infection, levels were significantly raised. *2066*

Eosinophils　*Blood　Decrease*　During acute infections. *0433*

Blood　Increase　Depressed during acute infections but may become elevated during convalescence. *0433　2538*

Erythrocytes　*Blood　Decrease*　Anemia with an average 2.5 million/μL is usually hypochromic; may be macrocytic in severe chronic cases. *2468*　Pancytopenia is a common feature. *2538　0151*

Erythrocyte Sedimentation Rate　*Blood　Increase*　*2468*

Factor II　*Plasma　Decrease*　May be associated with defibrination resulting in platelet and coagulation factor consumption (in overwhelming parasitemia). *2538*

Factor IV　*Plasma　Decrease*　May be associated with defibrination resulting in platelet and coagulation factor consumption (in overwhelming parasitemia). *2538*

Fibrinogen　*Plasma　Decrease*　May be associated with defibrination resulting in platelet and coagulation factor consumption (overwhelming parasitemia). *2538*

Plasma　Increase　In 25 patients with acute renal failure due to falciparum malaria, marked increase in fibrinogen and fibrin degradation products were observed. The other coagulation parameters were within the normal limits. *2190*

Fibrin Split Products (FSP)　*Plasma　Increase*　In 25 patients with acute renal failure due to falciparum malaria, marked increase in plasma fibrinogen and elevation of serum fibrin degradation products were observed. The other coagulation parameters were within the normal limits. *2190*

Globulin　*Serum　Increase*　Often associated with hypergammaglobulinemia. *2104*　Especially euglobulin fraction *2468　1058*

Glomerular Filtration Rate (GFR)　*Urine　Decrease*　In acute renal failure due to falciparum malaria. *2190*

Glycoproteins　*Serum　Increase*　Serum alpha$_1$ glycoproteins are increased and alpha$_2$ glycoproteins are decreased. *0151*

Haptoglobin　*Serum　Decrease*　Intravascular hemolysis due to parasites. *2467*

84.00 Malaria (continued)

Hemagglutination Inhibition *Serum Increase* Antibody to malarial parasites may be detected by the indirect fluorescent antibody test and by hemagglutination tests. *0962* In natural infections, the complement-fixation and indirect hemagglutination tests detect malarial antibodies equally efficiently for the first 2 months after onset, but titers obtained by complement-fixation rapidly decline within a year, while the indirect hemagglutination titers remain elevated. *2547*

Hematocrit *Blood Decrease* With disease progression a normocytic, normochromic anemia may become apparent. *0433* Marked anemia was found only in the patients with defective hemoglobin synthesis. *2240* Anemia is present in proportion to the severity of the infection. *0962*

Hemoglobin *Blood Decrease* With disease progression, a normocytic, normochromic anemia may become apparent. *0433* Marked anemia was found in patients with defective hemoglobin synthesis. *2240* Anemia is present in proportion to the severity of the infection. *0962*

Hemoglobin, Free *Serum Increase* Intravascular hemolysis due to parasites. *2467*

Urine Increase In severe falciparum infection may be demonstrable. *0433* Intravascular hemolysis due to parasites. *2467*

Immunoglobulin IgG *Serum Increase* Marked elevation. *0151* Mean IgG and IgM were significantly increased. Mean IgG = 179 U/mL, range = 119-284 U/mL. *0834* Despite the considerably increased concentration of immunoglobulins in infected individuals, only 5% of the immune adult IgG combines specifically with P. falciparum antigens. *0426 2035*

Immunoglobulin IgM *Serum Increase* Marked elevation. *0151* Especially when particulate antigenic material is present in the blood stream. *0619* Mean IgG and IgM were significantly increased in malaria patients. Mean IgM = 191 U/mL, range = 87-369. *0834 0426*

Immunoglobulins *Serum Increase* Despite the considerably increased concentration of immunoglobulins in infected individuals, only 5% of the immune adult IgG combines specifically with P. falciparum antigens. *0426 2035*

Indirect Fluorescent Antibodies *Serum Increase* Antibody to malarial parasites may be detected by the indirect fluorescent antibody test and by hemagglutination tests. Interpretation of antibody titers in a variety of situations has not been clarified. *0962*

Iron *Serum Decrease* Decreased cellular iron incorporation found in all cases during parasitemia. *2240*

Iron-Binding Capacity, Total (TIBC) *Serum Decrease* Decreased significantly in 11 patients with untreated malaria for more than 4 days. *2066*

Leukocytes *Blood Decrease* Pancytopenia is a common feature. *2538* Occasionally leukopenia is present. *0962*

Lymphocytes *Blood Increase* Depletion of T cells was found associated with an increased proportion of null cells. K cell activity was also increased and it is likely that some of the increased number of null cells were K cells. *0917*

Monocytes *Blood Increase* Increases in many protozoan infections. *2467 0532*

Neutrophils *Blood Decrease* Significant neutropenia may occur. *1646 2538*

Osmotic Fragility *Red Blood Cells Increase* *1058*

Partial Thromboplastin Time *Plasma Increase* Consistent with the diagnosis of disseminated intravascular coagulation. *1058*

Platelet Count *Blood Decrease* With disease progression may become apparent. *0433* Pancytopenia is a common feature. *2538* May be associated with defibrination resulting in platelet and coagulation factor consumption (overwhelming parasitemia). *2538*

Prealbumin *Serum Decrease* Decreased significantly in 11 patients untreated for more than 4 days. *2066*

Prolactin *Serum Increase* Slightly increased in falciparum malaria. *2487*

Protein *Serum Decrease* Significantly lower in patients admitted after 5-10 days to hospital compared with the control group. *2066*

Protein Casts *Urine Increase* May be demonstrable in severe falciparum infection. *0433*

Prothrombin Consumption *Blood Increase* May be associated with defibrination resulting in platelet and coagulation factor consumption (in overwhelming parasitemia). *2538*

Prothrombin Time *Plasma Increase* Consistent with the diagnosis of disseminated intravascular coagulation. *1058*

Renin Activity *Plasma Increase* Increased in acute renal failure due to falciparum malaria. *2190*

Reticulocytes *Blood Increase* Occurs several days after therapy has begun. *0151*

Rheumatoid Factor *Serum Increase* High prevalence of IgM rheumatoid factors showed a positive correlation with malaria antibodies. *2438 2035*

Sodium *Serum Decrease* Caused by salt depletion and water retention. *1058 0761 1593*

Red Blood Cells Increase The content of infected and uninfected erythrocytes is increased as a result of increased permeability. *1058*

Thrombin Time *Plasma Increase* Consistent with the diagnosis of disseminated intravascular coagulation. *1058*

Thyroid Stimulating Hormone (TSH) *Serum Increase* *2487*

Thyroxine Binding Globulin *Serum Decrease* In patients with fever. *2327*

Thyroxine (T$_4$) *Serum Increase* Stable or increasing in falciparum. *2487* Increased free T$_4$ during fever. *2327*

Tri-iodothyronine (T$_3$) *Serum Decrease* Abruptly declined during falciparum infection. *2487* Patients with fever of infection had significantly lowered levels. *2327*

VDRL *Serum Positive* False positive may occur. *0151* Found in 100% of cases. *1058*

Viscosity *Serum Increase* Significantly increased in 15 patients with acute renal failure due to falciparum infection. *2190*

Volume *Plasma Decrease* Initial hypovolemia followed by hypervolemia or normovolemia in acute renal failure due to falciparum. *2190* A rare and serious complication. *1058*

Plasma Increase Initial hypovolemia followed by hypervolemia or normovolemia in acute renal failure due to falciparum. *2190* A rare and serious complication. *1058*

Plasma Normal Initial hypovolemia followed by hypervolemia or normovolemia in acute renal failure due to falciparum. *2190* A rare and serious complication. *1058*

85.00 Leishmaniasis

Albumin *Serum Decrease* Decreased with reversed A/G ratio. *2468*

Serum Increase In tropical splenomegaly, increased plasma volume occurs mainly due to raised intravascular pools of albumin IgG and IgM. The variance in plasma volume was attributable to increases in these 3 pools, IgM and IgG accounting for 42% of the total and albumin for 28%. *0466*

Bilirubin *Serum Increase* Hemolytic anemia. *2538 2568*

Bilirubin, Indirect *Serum Increase* Hemolytic anemia. *2538 2568*

Clotting Time *Blood Increase* Normal early in the disease but later becomes prolonged. *0151*

Complement Fixation *Serum Increase* Positive but is also positive in tuberculosis. *2468*

Erythrocytes *Urine Increase* Frequent. *2468*

Erythrocyte Sedimentation Rate *Blood Increase* Increased due to increased serum globulin. *2468*

Globulin *Serum Increase* Increased with reversed A/G ratio. *2468* Often associated with hypergammaglobulinemia *2104*

Haptoglobin *Serum Decrease* Intravascular hemolysis due to parasites. *2467* Hemolytic anemia. *2568*

Hemagglutination Inhibition *Serum Increase* Used for diagnosis but requires fuller development for routine use. *0503*

Hematocrit *Blood Decrease* Normochromic, normocytic anemia develops slowly but becomes severe later in the disease. *0151* Hemolytic anemia. *2568 2538*

Hemoglobin *Blood Decrease* Hemolytic anemia. *2568* Normocytic, normochromic anemia develops slowly but becomes severe later in the disease. *0151*

Hemoglobin, Free *Serum Increase* Hemolytic anemia. *2568 2538*

Immunoglobulin IgG *Serum Increase* Serum protein increases to values > 10 g/dL, almost entirely due to raised IgG levels. *0151* Increased intravascular pools of albumin, IgG, and IgM in tropical splenomegaly. IgM and IgG accounting for 42% of the total and albumin for 28%. *0466* Marked IgG increase in Kala-Azar patients. Mean = 591 U/mL, range = 305-941 U/mL. *0834*

Immunoglobulin IgM *Serum Increase* In tropical splenomegaly; increased intravascular pools of albumin, IgG, and IgM. Variance in plasma volume was attributable to increases in these 3 pools, IgM and IgG accounting for 42% of the total and albumin for 28%. *0466* Marked IgM increase in Kala-Azar patients. Mean = 226 U/mL range = 74-509 U/mL. *0834*

Leukocytes *Blood Decrease* Characteristic, with counts < 2,000/μL in 75% of cases. *0151*

Monocytes *Blood Increase* Increases in many protozoan infections. *2467*

Neutrophils *Blood Decrease* Absolute neutropenia with total WBC count < 2,000/μL. *0151* Significant neutropenia may occur. *1646 2538*

Partial Thromboplastin Time *Plasma Increase* Normal early in the disease but later becomes prolonged. *0151*

Protein *Serum Increase* Elevated to values > 10 g/dL, almost entirely due to increased IgG. *0151*

Urine Increase Frequent. *2468*

Prothrombin Time *Plasma Increase* Normal early in the disease but later becomes prolonged. *0151*

Rheumatoid Factor *Serum Increase* Parasitic diseases that involve the liver and reticuloendothelial system have a significant incidence of seropositivity, suggesting that these factors may be produced in the tissues locally. *0962*

Uric Acid *Serum Increase* In tropical splenomegaly syndrome. *1139*

Volume *Plasma Increase* In 64 cases of tropical splenomegaly, plasma volumes ranged from 52-129 mL/kg. 70% of the increase was attributable to increased intravascular pools of IgG and IgM (42%) and albumin (28%). *0466*

86.90 Trypanosomiasis

Albumin *Serum Decrease* *1058*

Cold Agglutinins *Serum Increase* *2035 1826*

Complement Fixation *Serum Increase* *1058*

CSF Increase *1058*

Erythrocyte Survival *Red Blood Cells Decrease* Hematological studies indicate the presence of a hemolytic process. *2569 2035*

Globulin *Serum Increase* *1058*

CSF Increase In 22% of cases. *0846*

Haptoglobin *Serum Decrease* Intravascular hemolysis due to parasites. *2467*

Hematocrit *Blood Decrease* Anemia is a characteristic feature. *2569* Mild normocytic normochromic anemia associated with reduced marrow activity. *1058 2035*

Hemoglobin *Blood Decrease* Anemia is a characteristic feature. Hematological studies indicate the presence of a hemolytic process. *2569* Mild normocytic normochromic anemia associated with reduced marrow activity. *1058*

Hemoglobin, Free *Serum Increase* Intravascular hemolysis due to parasites. *2467*

Immunoglobulin IgA *Serum Increase* *1058*

Immunoglobulin IgG *Serum Increase* *1058*

Immunoglobulin IgM *Serum Increase* Marked increase of immunoglobulins, particularly IgM, may be explained by the continuous production of antibodies against new variants. *2105* Markedly increased and remains elevated throughout the course of the infection. *1058 2035*

Immunoglobulins *Serum Increase* Marked increase of immunoglobulins, particularly IgM, may be explained by the continuous production of antibodies against new variants. *2105 2035*

Leukocytes *Blood Normal* Usually. *1058*

Lymphocytes *Blood Increase* Relative lymphocytosis. *1058*

CSF Increase Up to 2,000/μL with CNS involvement. *1058*

Monocytes *Blood Increase* Increased in many protozoan infections. *2467*

Reticulocytes *Blood Increase* *2035*

Rheumatoid Factor *Serum Increase* Parasitic diseases that involve the liver and reticuloendothelial system have a significant incidence of seropositivity, suggesting that these factors may be produced in the tissues locally. *0962* 27% positivity. *0422 0123*

VDRL *Serum Positive* False positive in 10% of cases. *1058*

87.00 Relapsing Fever

Albumin *Urine Increase* Noted occasionally. *0433*

Bilirubin *Serum Increase* Occurs late in the course of the disease. *0962*

Urine Increase Noted occasionally. *0433*

Cells *CSF Increase* Mononuclear cells sometimes increased. *2468*

Complement Fixation *Serum Increase* Antibodies develop but antigens are not sufficiently well standardized to be useful. *0962*

Erythrocytes *Urine Increase* There may be blood in urine during the febrile period. *0962*

Erythrocyte Sedimentation Rate *Blood Increase* Common. *0433*

Haptoglobin *Serum Decrease* Intravascular hemolysis due to parasites. *2467*

Hematocrit *Blood Decrease* Moderate anemia may occur later in the disease. *0962* Intravascular hemolysis due to parasites. *2467*

Hemoglobin *Blood Decrease* Moderate anemia may occur later in the disease. *0962*

Hemoglobin, Free *Serum Increase* Intravascular hemolysis due to parasites. *2467*

Immunoglobulin IgG *Serum Increase* Occurs initially after infection, followed by a rise in IgM. *0151*

Immunoglobulin IgM *Serum Increase* IgG hyperglobulinemia occurs initially after infection, followed by a rise in IgM. *0151*

Immunoglobulins *Serum Increase* IgG hyperglobulinemia occurs initially after infection, followed by a rise in IgM. *0151*

Leukocytes *Blood Decrease* May be elevated or decreased but is usually normal. *0433*

Blood Increase From the onset, there is marked polymorphonuclear leukocytosis, of 15,000-25,000/μL, with increase in immature forms. *0151* During the febrile period, with a shift to the left. *0962*

Blood Normal May be elevated or decreased but is usually normal. *0433*

CSF Increase Pleocytosis can occur. *0433*

Monocytes *CSF Increase* Sometimes increased. *0433*

Protein *Urine Increase* Sometimes; during the febrile period. *0962*

CSF Increase Sometimes increased in CSF. *2468*

VDRL *Serum Positive* 45% false positive. *2230* 30% false positive. *1058 2468*

Weil-Felix Reaction *Serum Positive* Reactive in titers of 1:80 or higher. *0151* Proteus OX K > 90% positive (> / = 1:40). *2230*

88.00 Bartonellosis

Bilirubin *Serum Increase* *2538 1918*

Bilirubin, Indirect *Serum Increase* *2538 1918*

Haptoglobin *Serum Decrease* Intravascular hemolysis due to parasites. *2467*

Hematocrit *Blood Decrease* Intravascular hemolysis due to parasites. *2467 2538 1918*

Hemoglobin *Urine Increase* Intravascular hemolysis parasites (Oroya fever); due to Bartonella bacilliformis. *2467*

Hemoglobin, Free *Serum Increase* Intravascular hemolysis due to parasites. *2467 2538 1918*

Immunoglobulin IgM *Serum Increase* Especially when particulate antigenic material is present in the blood stream. *0619*

Leukocytes *Blood Decrease* Normal, increased or decreased. *1058*

Blood Increase Normal, increased or decreased. *1058*

Blood Normal Normal, increased or decreased. *1058*

Platelet Count *Blood Decrease* Has been reported. *1058*

97.90 Syphilis

Alpha$_2$-Macroglobulin *CSF Normal* Neurosyphilis. *2069*

Cells *CSF Increase* Increased in meningovascular syphilis. *0999* First sign of asymptomatic syphilis arising from latency is pleocytosis of > 4 cells/μL, followed by increase in protein. With progress to parenchymatous neurosyphilis, 150 cells/μL and marked increase in protein (globulin) is found. *0151 0962*

Chloride *CSF Decrease* Usually slightly decreased. *0962*

97.90   Syphilis   (continued)

Complement Fixation   *Serum   Increase*   Kolmer test. *1058*

Cryomacroglobulins   *Serum   Increase*   *0863*

Erythrocyte Sedimentation Rate   *Blood   Increase*   Raised in 66.6% of seronegative primary cases, 80% of seropositive cases, 100% secondary cases, 80% early latent cases, and 73.9% of late latent cases. Also raised in 16/17 cases of neurosyphilis and 11/11 cases of cardiovascular syphilis. *0759*

Gamma Globulin   *CSF   Increase*   In active disease. *2174*

Globulin   *Serum   Increase*   All 3 stages. *2104*

CSF   Increase   Reflected in an abnormal Lange curve. *0151*

Glucose   *Serum   Increase*   *0619*

CSF   Decrease   Decreased in 50% of the patients. *0962*   10-45 mg/dL. *2368*

Hematocrit   *Blood   Decrease*   Secondary anemia. *1058*

Hemoglobin   *Blood   Decrease*   Secondary anemia. *1058*

Immunoglobulin IgG   *CSF   Increase*   Increased with obstruction of the spinal canal, especially in neurosyphilis and tuberculous meningitis. *2321*

Immunoglobulins   *CSF   Increase*   *0619*

Leukocytes   *Blood   Increase*   In secondary syphilis. *1058*

CSF   Increase   Average 500/μL, usually lymphocytes. *0151*

Lymphocytes   *Blood   Increase*   Absolute increase. *1058*

CSF   Increase   CSF count may be elevated, with 5-10 or more lymphocytes/μL. *0962*   Majority of cells are lymphocytes with CNS involvement. *2368   0151*

Monocytes   *Blood   Increase*   In neonatal, primary and secondary syphilis. *1975   2538*

Protein   *CSF   Increase*   Usually increased to some degree with CNS involvement. *0962*   Over 45 mg/dL in syphilitic meningitis. *2368*   Increased with obstruction of the spinal canal, especially in neurosyphilis and tuberculous meningitis. *2321   2612*

Rheumatoid Factor   *Serum   Increase*   The incidence of seropositivity exceeds that of a normal population. *2035*   13% positivity. *0422 0123   0962*

VDRL   *Serum   Positive*   Negative at the onset of primary syphilis, but within 7-14 days it becomes positive in the majority of cases. Almost all sera from patients with secondary syphilis are positive. Asymptomatic or latent syphilis can be diagnosed only by a positive serologic test. *0999*   Becomes positive in most patients 2-3 weeks after the appearance of the chancre or 6 weeks after the initial contact. In the secondary stage, especially when generalized eruptions occur, it is positive in virtually 100% of patients. *0962*

CSF   Positive   In asymptomatic neurosyphilis the blood and spinal fluid VDRL are usually both reactive. *0962*   Positive as a result of serum or blood leaking into the CSF. *0999*

99.10   Lymphogranuloma Venereum

Alanine Aminotransferase   *Serum   Increase*   May indicate severe liver impairment. *0433*

Albumin   *Serum   Decrease*   A common finding during active infection. Often reversal of the A/G ratio. *0962   2199*

Alpha$_2$-Globulin   *Serum   Increase*   Elevated with a reversal of the A/G ratio. In such cases, the increase occurs in the alpha$_2$ and gamma globulin regions. *0433*

Aspartate Aminotransferase   *Serum   Increase*   May indicate severe liver impairment. *0433*

Bilirubin   *Serum   Increase*   May indicate severe liver impairment. *0433*

Complement Fixation   *Serum   Increase*   Early in the course of the disease, in symptomatic and asymptomatic patients, titers of 1:40-1:160 will occur. Later stages may produce titers as high as 1:640 in most patients. *0433*   This test is nonspecific and may be positive following infections with other chlamydiae. *0962*   A rising titer strongly indicates acute disease. May remain positive after antimicrobial therapy and an apparent clinical remission. *2199*   Much more sensitive than the Frei test, but cross reacts with other chlamydiae infections, such as psittacosis. *2060 2368   2468*

Erythrocyte Sedimentation Rate   *Blood   Increase*   Is often increased. *0433   0962 2199*

Frei Test   *Skin   Positive*   Diagnostic skin test. A 6 mm nodule with surrounding erythema 48 h after intradermal injection is positive reaction. *2368*   May be up to 60% false-negative reactions even in established cases. *2060*

Globulin   *Serum   Increase*   Are increased with reversed A/G ratio. A common finding during active infection. Often reversal of the albumin:globulin ratio. *0962*   Elevated with a reversal of the A/G ratio. In such cases, the increase occurs in the alpha$_2$ and gamma globulin regions. *0433*   Often associated with hypergammaglobulinemia *2104   2199*

Glucose   *CSF   Decrease*   In the early stages of infection. *0433*   Characteristically low. *1319*

Hematocrit   *Blood   Decrease*   Anemia and leukopenia are most common when enlargement of the liver and spleen and generalized lymphadenopathy occur. *0433   2199*

Hemoglobin   *Blood   Decrease*   Anemia and leukopenia are most common when enlargement of the liver and spleen and generalized lymphadenopathy occur. *0433   2199*

Immunoglobulin IgA   *Serum   Increase*   Up to 75% of the patients will experience an elevation. *0433*

Immunoglobulins   *Serum   Increase*   Often associated with striking elevations. *2104*

Lactate Dehydrogenase   *Serum   Increase*   May indicate severe liver impairment. *0433*

Leukocytes   *Blood   Decrease*   Anemia and leukopenia are most common when enlargement of the liver and spleen and generalized lymphadenopathy occur. *0433*

Blood   Increase   When the nodes suppurate, a leukocytosis of 7,000-19,000/μL and a slight monocytosis may occur. *0433*   Mild leukocytosis with a relative lymphocytosis or monocytosis. *2199*

Urine   Increase   Vaginovesical fistulas may cause changes that reflect in the urine as numerous leukocytes or inclusion-filled mononuclear cells. *0433*

CSF   Increase   Pleocytosis as high as 4,000/μL may occur. *0433*

Lymphocytes   *Blood   Increase*   Mild leukocytosis with a relative lymphocytosis or monocytosis. *2199*

Monocytes   *Blood   Increase*   Mild leukocytosis with a relative lymphocytosis or monocytosis. *2199*

Urine   Increase   Vaginovesical fistulas may cause changes that reflect in the urine as numerous leukocytes or inclusion-filled mononuclear cells. *0433*

Protein   *Serum   Increase*   Elevated with a reversal of the A/G ratio. In such cases, the increase occurs in the alpha$_2$ and gamma globulin regions. *0433*

CSF   Increase   High in the early stages of CSF infection, varying from 250-3,750 mg/dL. *0433*

VDRL   *Serum   Positive*   Biologic false-positive serologic tests are not infrequent. *2199*   20% false positive. *1058*

99.30   Reiter's Disease

Alpha$_2$-Globulin   *Serum   Increase*   Evidence of nonspecific inflammation. *0433*

Antinuclear Antibodies   *Serum   Normal*   *0999*

Cells   *Synovial Fluid   Present*   Reiter's Cells (macrophages with partially digested neutrophils). *0186*

Complement, Total   *Serum   Increase*   Elevated during active inflammation and subsides with remission. *2090*   In 14 patients, 64% had increased values. *2223*

Synovial Fluid   Increase   Usually higher than in most other types of effusions in contrast to the very low levels in rheumatoid arthritis. *0433*   Elevated levels appear to be directly related to the severity and duration of joint inflammation. *2090*

Erythrocyte Sedimentation Rate   *Blood   Increase*   The increased ESR parallels clinical course. *2468*   Common. *0999*

Globulin   *Serum   Increase*   Increased in long-standing disease. *2468*

Glucose   *Synovial Fluid   Decrease*   Usually normal but may be decreased when leukocyte count is increased. *0186*

Synovial Fluid   Normal   Usually normal but may be decreased when leukocyte count is increased. *0186*

Hematocrit   *Blood   Decrease*   There may be a mild anemia. *0433*

Hemoglobin   *Blood   Decrease*   There may be a mild anemia. *0433*

HLA Antigens   *Blood   Present*   HLA-B$_2$7 present in 80% of patients versus 9% of controls. *2539*   HLA-B$_2$7 found in 65% of cases. *1503*

Leukocytes   *Blood   Increase*   A range of 10,000-18,000/μL. *0433*   Common. *0999*

Urine   Increase   Reflects urethritis. *0186*

Synovial Fluid Increase Synovial fluid is typically inflammatory, with cell counts up to 60,000/μL. *0999*

Prostatic Fluid Increase Reflects urethritis. *0186*

Neutrophils *Blood Increase* *2468*

Synovial Fluid Increase Polymorphonuclear leukocytosis in the range of 2,000-10,000/μL. *0433*

Protein *Synovial Fluid Increase* *0186*

Rheumatoid Factor *Serum Normal* *0186*

Synovial Fluid Normal *0999*

100.00 Leptospirosis

Agglutination Tests *Serum Positive* Antibodies appear during 2nd week of illness. *0962* Tests reach peaks in 4-7 weeks and may last for many years. An individual titer of 1:300 is suggestive of this disease. *2468*

Alanine Aminotransferase *Serum Increase* Increased in 50% of the patients but average levels are not as high as in hepatitis. *2468*

Albumin *Serum Decrease* May occur with jaundice after the 1st week of fever. *2368*

Alkaline Phosphatase *Serum Increase* Increased in 50% of the patients. *2468* Jaundice may appear at the end of the 1st week of fever. Liver tests show hepatic decompensation of the intrahepatic type. *2368*

Alpha₂-Globulin *Serum Increase* May occur with jaundice after the 1st week of fever. *2368*

Antibody Titer *Serum Increase* The contrast between negative acute-phase and positive convalescent phase sera is diagnostic. *2368*

Aspartate Aminotransferase *Serum Increase* Increased in 50% of the patients but average levels are not as high as in hepatitis. *2468* Values are rarely increased more than 2-3 X normal regardless of the degree of hyperbilirubinemia. *0151* Elevated in patients without clinically evident liver disease. *0962*

Bilirubin *Serum Increase* Increased in 50% of the patients. *2468* May reach 65 mg/dL but is < 20 mg/dL in 66% of patients. *0151* Elevated values found in patients without clinically evident liver disease. *0962* Jaundice may appear at the end of the 1st week of fever. Liver tests show hepatic decompensation of the intrahepatic type. *2368* *0992*

Bilirubin, Direct *Serum Increase* Hyperbilirubinemia, which is predominantly conjugated (direct) may reach 65 mg/dL but is < 20 mg/dL in 66% of patients. *0151*

Casts *Urine Increase* Urine is abnormal in 75% of patients. *2468* During the leptospiremic phase. *0962*

Cells *CSF Increase* Increased up to 500/μL in about 66% of patients. Indicates meningeal involvement. *2468* Pleocytosis of 25-500 cells/μL in > 75% of cases. *0962*

Cholesterol *Serum Decrease* May occur with jaundice. *2368*

Complement Fixation *Serum Increase* Antibodies appear during second week of illness. *0962*

Creatine Kinase *Serum Increase* Increased in 33% of patients during the 1st week. Differentiates the condition from hepatitis. *2468*

Creatinine *Serum Increase* Marked oliguria or anuria develops after the 1st week of disease and is attended by severe azotemia and electrolyte imbalance characteristic of lower nephron nephrosis. *2368*

Erythrocytes *Urine Increase* In 75% of patients. *2468* During the leptospiremic phase. *0962* Hemorrhagic manifestations may occur in the first few days of fever. *2368* Hematuria, pyuria, and cylindruria in most cases. *2368*

Erythrocyte Sedimentation Rate *Blood Increase* Increased in > 50% of the patients but is usually < 50 mm/h. *0151*

Globulin *Serum Increase* May occur with jaundice after the 1st week of fever. *2368*

Glucose *CSF Normal* *0992* *0962*

Hematocrit *Blood Decrease* With jaundice, anemia may be severe due to intravascular hemolysis. Anemia is unusual in anicteric patients. *0992*

Hemoglobin *Blood Decrease* With jaundice, anemia may be severe due to intravascular hemolysis. Anemia is unusual in anicteric patients. *0992*

Lactic Acid *Blood Increase* *0619*

Leukocytes *Blood Decrease* May occur. *0151*

Blood Increase Mild elevations in anicteric patients. *0151* As high as 50,000/μL in patients with jaundice. *0992* Often normal in mild cases and ranges up to 40,000/μL in severe cases. *0962* With a preponderance of polymorphonuclears and immature forms. *2368*

Urine Increase In 75% of patients. *2468* During the leptospiremic phase. *0962*

Lymphocytes *CSF Increase* Lymphocytic pleocytosis is common with counts from 100-300/μL. *2368*

Neutrophils *Blood Increase* Neutrophilia of > 70% is often found regardless of the leukocyte count which may be high or low. *0151* In a high proportion of cases. *2368* *0962*

Occult Blood *Feces Positive* Hemorrhagic manifestations may occur in the first few days of fever. *2368*

Platelet Count *Blood Decrease* Rare. *0992*

Potassium *Serum Increase* Marked oliguria or anuria develops after the 1st week of disease and is attended by severe azotemia and electrolyte imbalance characteristic of lower nephron nephrosis. *2368*

Protein *Urine Increase* In 75% of patients. *2468* During the leptospiremic phase. *0962* Heavy proteinuria during the febrile period. *2368*

CSF Increase Increased in about 66% of patients, up to 80 mg/dL, indicating meningeal involvement. *2468* Occasionally observed. *2368* *0962*

Prothrombin Time *Plasma Increase* In some patients. *0992* May occur with jaundice. *2368*

Thymol Turbidity *Serum Increase* Jaundice may appear at the end of the 1st week of fever. Liver tests show hepatic decompensation of the intrahepatic type. *2368* *0992*

Urea Nitrogen *Serum Increase* Usually associated with jaundice. *0992* During leptospiremic phase, azotemia may be present. *0962* Marked oliguria or anuria develops after the 1st week of disease and is attended by severe azotemia and electrolyte imbalance characteristic of lower nephron nephrosis. *2368*

Urobilinogen *Urine Increase* Jaundice may appear at the end of the 1st week of fever. Liver tests show hepatic decompensation of the intrahepatic type. *2368*

VDRL *Serum Positive* 10% false positive. *1058*

102.90 Yaws

Monocytes *CSF Increase* Occasionally found but neither symptoms nor signs of neurologic disability have evolved. *1058*

VDRL *Serum Positive* All serological tests for syphilis are positive. *1058*

104.10 Lyme Disease

Aspartate Aminotransferase *Serum Increase* May be elevated in Lyme Disease if mild hepatic involvement persists. *2639*

Cryoglobulins *Serum Increase* May be detected in Lyme Disease. *2639*

Erythrocyte Sedimentation Rate *Blood Increase* Often mildly elevated in Lyme Disease. *2639*

Gamma Glutamyl Transferase (GGT) *Serum Increase* With liver involvement. *1503*

Immunoglobulin IgM *Serum Increase* May be elevated in Lyme Disease. *2639*

Lymphocytes *Blood Decrease* Lymphopenia occurs in Lyme Disease. *2639*

112.90 Moniliasis

Agglutination Tests *Serum Positive* Serum agglutinin and precipitin titers against Candida are of little value, as many normal individuals harbor the organism without tissue invasion. A low titer probably makes esophageal candidiasis unlikely. *2199*

Cells *CSF Increase* Pleocytosis in all patients with Candida meningitis, predominantly lymphocytic. *0138*

Leukocytes *Blood Increase* Leukocytosis of 12,000-22,000/μL and neutrophilia of 75-90% in Candida meningitis. *0138*

CSF Increase Mean count = 600/μL in 28 cases of Candida meningitis. *0138*

Neutrophils *Blood Increase* Leukocytosis of 12,000-22,000/μL and neutrophilia of 75-90% in Candida meningitis. *0138*

112.90 Moniliasis *(continued)*

Precipitins *Serum Increase* Serum agglutinin and precipitin titers against Candida are of little value, as many normal individuals harbor the organism without tissue invasion. *2199* A low titer probably makes esophageal candidiasis unlikely. *2199*

Protein *CSF Increase* Mean = 123 mg/dL in 28 cases of Candida meningitis. *0138*

114.90 Coccidioidomycosis

Angiotensin-Converting Enzyme (ACE) *Serum Increase* Decreased. *1398*

Cells *CSF Increase* CSF cell and chemistry are indistinguishable from tuberculous meningitis. *2368*

Complement Fixation *Serum Increase* Highly specific and has prognostic significance. Positive in about 60% of cases with chronic coccidioidal cavities, but often negative in patients with asymptomatic coccidioidomas. *0151* Positive 4-6 weeks following onset of symptoms with maximum response at 2-3 months. Titers > 1:2 may indicate active disease and 80% with disseminated infection have titers > 1:16. *2508* Titer correlates with increasing severity of the disease. A rising titer may indicate spread of the disease to extrapulmonary sites. *0433 2207 0962 2368*

CSF Increase Generally the titer is lower than in the serum. *2207* Pleural, joint, and CSF fluids contain complement-fixing antibody but in lower titer than in serum. *0151* In 75% of patients with coccidioidal meningitis. *2368 2035*

Synovial Fluid Increase Pleural, joint, and CSF fluids contain complement-fixing antibody but in lower titer than in serum. *0151*

Pleural Effusion Increase Generally the titer is lower than in the serum. *2207* Pleural, joint, and CSF fluids contain complement-fixing antibody but in lower titer than in serum. *0151 2035*

Peritoneal Fluid Increase Generally the titer is lower than in the serum. *2207 2035*

Eosinophils *Blood Increase* Occasional eosinophilia during either the primary or the disseminated stages. *0433* In the initial infection. *2368*

Erythrocyte Sedimentation Rate *Blood Increase* In active infection. *2368*

Glucose *CSF Decrease* Often an early significant change with CNS involvement. *0151*

CSF Increase CSF cell and chemistry are indistinguishable from tuberculous meningitis. *2368*

Leukocytes *Blood Increase* Moderate leukocytosis sometimes with eosinophilia. *0151* Frequently slightly elevated with a shift to the left. *2368 2468*

CSF Increase Fewer than 500/μL with CNS involvement. *1058*

Lymphocytes *CSF Increase* Fewer than 500 leukocytes/μL, as many as 50% neutrophils initially with lymphocytes predominating later. *1058*

Neutrophils *CSF Increase* Fewer than 500 leukocytes/μL, as many as 50% neutrophils initially with lymphocytes predominating later. *1058*

pO₂ *Blood Decrease* With pulmonary involvement. *1058*

Precipitins *Serum Increase* Highly specific and can be detected in 80% of patients within 2 weeks of onset of symptoms; absent in 90% after 6 months. *2508* Present in approximately 80% of patients with primary nondisseminating infection, preceding the development of CF antibodies, and they appear to represent IgM antibodies. Persisting precipitins have been associated with dissemination, and precipitins may reappear when there is systemic reinfection. *2035* Positive in most patients within a month after onset of symptoms. *0962 2207 2368*

CSF Increase Only rarely found in meningitis. *2035 2207*

Pleural Effusion Increase May be found in the thoracic fluid in pleural effusions. *2035*

Protein *CSF Increase* CSF cell and chemistry are indistinguishable from tuberculous meningitis. *2368* Moderate increase with CNS involvement. *1058*

VDRL *Serum Positive* Low incidence of false positive results. *1058*

115.00 Histoplasmosis

5'-Nucleotidase *Serum Increase* Significantly elevated in 2 of 3 patients with liver granulomata. *1312*

Agglutination Tests *Serum Positive* Antibodies are demonstrable, but cross reactions with Blastomyces and Coccidioides are seen in these tests. *0962*

Alanine Aminotransferase *Serum Increase* In 5 cases of hepatic granuloma, ALT was elevated to a mean value of 70 U/L (normal = 50 U/L) and a range of 50-115 U/L. *1452*

Albumin *Serum Decrease* Concentrations of < 3.0 g/dL occur in 60% of patients with disseminated disease. *0999*

Alkaline Phosphatase *Serum Increase* Present in 50% of patients with disseminated disease. *0999* Marked elevation in all 5 cases of granuloma of liver. Maximum upper limit of normal = 85 U/L. Average elevated value = 425 U/L. Range = 191-700 U/L. *1452*

Angiotensin-Converting Enzyme (ACE) *Serum Increase* Elevated in 25% of 86 patients. *2015* Rises acutely in all patients with Histo and then falls gradually towards baseline (n = 44). *0506*

Antibody Titer *Serum Increase* Elevated convalescent phase titer may be the result of skin testing or of active disease. *2508*

Aspartate Aminotransferase *Serum Increase* Present in 70% of patients with disseminated disease. *0999* In 5 cases of granuloma of liver, 100% were mildly elevated, showing a mean elevation of 36 U/L over the normal maximum limit of 24 U/L. *1452*

Bilirubin *Serum Increase* Greater than 1.0 mg/dL in 25% of patients with disseminated disease. *0999*

BSP Retention *Serum Increase* Elevated in 70% of patients with disseminated disease. *0999*

Cells *Bone Marrow Normal* Marrow smears reveal no cellular abnormalities. *2368*

Complement Fixation *Serum Increase* Of 79 consecutive patients with positive test 28 (35%) were false-positive results. 12 patients (15%) had titers of > 1:32, without cultural or histological evidence of active infection. Using histoplasmin as antigen detected antibodies in the sera of 72.8% of the 70 proven cases, while yeast antigen detected antibodies in 94%. *2343* Initially positive in 74% of 228 cases (titers > 1:64). *0892* In primary pulmonary infection, antibodies to yeast antigen appear 10-21 days following fungus exposure. Histoplasmin antibodies are of greater importance in chronic infection, in which antibodies to yeast antigen may be decreased or absent. Titer of > 1:8 is presumed to indicate active infection, most patients have titers > 1:16. *2508* CF antibodies are produced in a high percentage of patients in the acute phase, and fade out as the infection becomes asymptomatic or inactive. *2368 0962*

Gamma Glutamyl Transferase (GGT) *Serum Increase* In 5 patients with liver granulomas, including miliary tuberculosis and sarcoidosis, serum GGT levels were all elevated, mean = 303, range = 116-740 U/L. *1452*

Globulin *Serum Increase* Levels > 3.0 g/dL occur in 50% of patients with disseminated disease. *0999* Often associated with Hypergammaglobulinemia *2104*

Hematocrit *Blood Decrease* 50% of the patients with disseminated disease may have anemia. *0999* A marked to moderate hypochromic anemia occurs in most cases. *0962* Usually an iron deficient normochromic normocytic anemia. *2199* Normochromic anemia. *2368*

Blood Normal The anemia of chronic disease is conspicuously absent. Normal values found in 91% of patients. Differentiates chronic pulmonary histoplasmosis from pulmonary tuberculosis. *0892*

Hemoglobin *Blood Decrease* 50% of the patients may have anemia in disseminated disease. *0999* A marked to moderate hypochromic anemia occurs in most cases. *0962* Usually an iron deficient normochromic normocytic anemia. *2199* Normochromic anemia. *2368*

Blood Normal The anemia of chronic disease is conspicuously absent. Normal values found in 91% of patients. differentiate chronic pulmonary histoplasmosis from pulmonary tuberculosis. *0892*

Immunoglobulin IgA *Serum Increase* In patients with chronic cavitary disease, IgM and IgG levels were normal although increased IgA was found. *2035 2476*

Iron *Serum Decrease* Usually an iron deficient normochromic normocytic anemia. *2199*

Leucine Aminopeptidase *Serum Increase* In 12 patients with granulomatous hepatitis, all showed elevated LAP levels, varying from 380-1,000 U/L, with a mean of 622 (normal = 322). *0281*

Leukocytes *Blood Decrease* In 25% of patients with disseminated disease. *0999* Characteristic. *0962* Leukopenia with lymphocytosis is frequently present. *2368 2199*

Blood Increase Occurs in 12% of patients with disseminated disease. *0999*

Lymphocytes *Blood Increase* Leukopenia with lymphocytosis is frequently present. *2368*

MCH *Blood Decrease* A marked to moderate hypochromic anemia occurs in most cases. *0962*

MCHC *Blood Decrease* A marked to moderate hypochromic anemia occurs in most cases. *0962*

Platelet Count *Blood Decrease* Markedly reduced only in the terminal phases. *2368*

Precipitins *Serum Increase* Antibodies are demonstrable, but cross reactions with Blastomyces and Coccidioides are seen in these tests. *0962*

Reticulocytes *Blood Increase* 25% of patients with disseminated disease. *0999*

116.00   Blastomycosis

Alkaline Phosphatase *Serum Increase* May be increased with bone lesions. *2468*

Complement Fixation *Serum Increase* Titers of 1:8 or greater may be present in 33-50% of the patients. Positive titers of 1:32 or higher are highly suggestive of active disease. *0433* High titer is correlated with poor prognosis. *2468* Reactions are transient and inconsistent with poor sensitivity and high incidence of cross-reactivity. *2508*

Erythrocyte Sedimentation Rate *Blood Increase* Most common hematologic abnormality. *0433*

Globulin *Serum Increase* Slightly increased. *2468*

Hematocrit *Blood Decrease* Present in < 50% of patients. *0433*

Hemoglobin *Blood Decrease* Present in < 50% of patients. *0433*

Indirect Fluorescent Antibodies *Serum Increase* May be the most useful serodiagnostic technique. *2508*

Leukocytes *Blood Increase* Appears in < 50% of patients. *0433*

117.10   Sporotrichosis

Antinuclear Antibodies *Serum Normal* Normal in all patients with Sporotrichosis arthritis. *0478*

Complement, Total *Serum Normal* Normal in all patients with Sporotrichosis arthritis. *0478*

Erythrocyte Sedimentation Rate *Blood Increase* Elevated in all 4 patients studied. *1459* Elevated in all patients with Sporotrichosis arthritis (average 55 mm/h). *0478*

LE Cells *Blood Negative* Normal in all patients with Sporotrichosis arthritis. *0478*

Leukocytes *Blood Normal* Near normal (2000-6150/μL). *1459*

Rheumatoid Factor *Serum Normal* Normal in all patients with Sporotrichosis arthritis. *0478*

117.30   Aspergillosis

Bilirubin *Serum Increase* Hemolytic anemia. *2538 1950*

Bilirubin, Indirect *Serum Increase* Hemolytic anemia. *2538 1950*

Eosinophils *Blood Increase* Mean percentage was 16.2, ranging from 8-29% in 20 cases of allergic bronchopulmonary aspergillosis. *1983*

Erythrocytes *Urine Increase* With urinary tract obstruction. *1058*

Erythrocyte Survival *Red Blood Cells Decrease* Hemolytic anemia. *1950 2538*

Hematocrit *Blood Decrease* Hemolytic anemia. *2538 1950*

Hemoglobin *Blood Decrease* Hemolytic anemia. *2538 1950*

Hemoglobin, Free *Serum Increase* Hemolytic anemia. *2538 1950*

Immunoglobulin IgA *Serum Increase* Elevated in 10 of 15 patients with a mean of 314.6 mg/dL. *1983*

Immunoglobulin IgE *Serum Increase* Markedly elevated in all patients with allergic bronchopulmonary aspergillosis. *1983* High values are found during the episodes of pulmonary eosinophilia. *2035*

Immunoglobulin IgG *Serum Increase* Elevated in 8 of 15 cases with a mean of 1485 mg/dL. *1983*

Immunoglobulin IgM *Serum Increase* Elevated in 10 of 15 cases; mean = 191.6 mg/dL. *1983*

Precipitins *Serum Increase* Detected in 100% of patients with aspergillomas and 70% with allergic aspergillosis. *2508* 48 and 67% having precipitins to Staphylococcus aureus and hemophilus influenzae. *2035*

Urea Nitrogen *Serum Increase* Either as a result of underlying disease or the infection. Azotemia develops rapidly. *1058*

117.50   Cryptococcosis

Agglutination Tests *Serum Positive* With CNS involvement about 66% of patients have antigen in their serum, CSF or both. *1058*

CSF Positive With CNS involvement about 66% of patients have antigen in their serum, CSF or both. *1058*

Antibody Titer *Serum Increase* Several serologic tests for anticryptococcal antibody are in use. Although sometimes of value, false positive reactions limit the utility of these tests. *1058*

Complement Fixation *Serum Increase* With CNS involvement about 66% of patients have antigen in their serum, CSF or both. *1058*

CSF Increase With CNS involvement about 66% of patients have antigen in their serum, CSF or both. *1058*

Erythrocyte Sedimentation Rate *Blood Normal* Even in extensive infection, the blood WBC, hct, and ESR remain normal. *1058*

Glucose *CSF Decrease* In about 50% of cases of symptomatic meningoencephalitis. *1058*

Hematocrit *Blood Normal* Even in extensive infection, the blood WBC, hct, and ESR remain normal. *1058*

Leukocytes *Blood Normal* Even in extensive infection, the blood WBC, hct, and ESR remain normal. *1058*

CSF Increase 40-400/μL with meningoencephalitis. *1058*

Lymphocytes *CSF Increase* Characteristically outnumber neutrophils. *1058*

pO₂ *Blood Decrease* With pulmonary involvement. *1058*

Protein *CSF Increase* Almost always elevated. *1058*

120.00   Schistosomiasis

5'-Nucleotidase *Serum Increase* Elevated above normal upon admission and rose to 2 X normal during treatment. *2026* Significantly elevated in 2 of 3 patients with live granulomata. *1312*

Alanine Aminotransferase *Serum Increase* May be mild elevations, but jaundice is uncommon. *0962* In 5 cases of hepatic granuloma, ALT was elevated to a mean value of 70 U/L (normal = 50 U/L) and a range of 50-115 U/L. *1452*

Albumin *Serum Decrease* A significant decrease associated with a compensatory increase in globulin throughout the course of the disease. The drop may be due to decreased anabolism or increased catabolism. *2026*

Alkaline Phosphatase *Serum Increase* Found in 50% of adult patients but is not useful in children. *2468* Consistently elevated and remains high for 1 month after treatment. *2026* Marked elevation in all 5 cases of granuloma of liver. Maximum upper limit of normal = 85 U/L. Average elevated value = 425 U/L. Range = 191-700 U/L. *1452 0151 0962*

Aspartate Aminotransferase *Serum Increase* Markedly increased without concomitant elevation of ALT. Remains elevated from admission, through nitridazole treatment, and at follow-up 1 month later. *2026* May be mild elevations, but jaundice is uncommon. *0962* In 5 cases of granuloma of liver, 100% were mildly elevated, showing a mean elevation of 36 U/L over the normal maximum limit of 24 U/L. *1452*

Bilirubin *Serum Increase* May be mild elevations, but jaundice is uncommon. *0962*

BSP Retention *Serum Increase* 5% retention upon admission. *2026* Common. *0962*

Calcium *Urine Increase* Increased despite normal serum levels. *0955*

Cephalin Flocculation *Serum Increase* Positive in acute disease. *2468*

Complement Fixation *Serum Increase* The best serologic procedure to diagnose chronic disease (100% specific and 95% sensitive). *2468*

Creatinine Clearance *Urine Decrease* Significantly decreased in 35 children with hepatic bilharziasis. *0955*

Eosinophils *Blood Increase* Eosinophilia occurs and may be 20-60%. *2468* In 64 patients (22%) showed eosinophil counts > 1,000/μL. *2028* Tends to decrease with chronicity. *2199*

Erythrocyte Sedimentation Rate *Blood Increase* Increased in acute disease. *2468*

120.00 Schistosomiasis (continued)

Gamma Glutamyl Transferase (GGT) *Serum Increase* In 5 patients with liver granulomas, including miliary tuberculosis and sarcoidosis, serum GGT levels were all elevated, mean = 303, range = 116-740 U/L. *1452*

Globulin *Serum Increase* Significant increase throughout the course of the disease. The increase in gamma globulin, the main isoenzyme causing the total elevation, may be due to the parasite's presence. The increase in gamma globulin, the main isoenzyme causing the total elevation may be due to the parasite's presence *2026* May be Present *2199*

Hemagglutination Inhibition *Serum Increase* Indirect hemagglutination. *1058*

Immunoglobulin IgE *Serum Increase* Increased in bilharziasis. *0619* 44% in Egypt and 20% in Brazil were above 24 μg/mL in S. Mansoni infestations. *2035*

Lactate Dehydrogenase *Serum Increase* Not significantly increased in patients upon the admission, but did increase with nitridazole treatment. LD_4 was the only isoenzyme to elevate and had returned to normal at follow-up 1 month later. *2026*

Lactate Dehydrogenase Isoenzymes *Serum Increase* Total LD was not significantly increased in patients upon admission, but did increase with nitridazole treatment LD_4 was the only isoenzyme to elevate and had returned to normal at follow-up 1 month later. *2026*

Leucine Aminopeptidase *Serum Increase* In 12 patients with granulomatous hepatitis, all showed elevated LAP levels, varying from 380-1,000 U/L, with a mean of 622 (normal = 322). *0281*

Leukocytes *Blood Increase* Tends to decrease with chronicity. *2199*

Mucopolysaccharides *Urine Increase* Abnormalities of neutral mucopolysaccharides appear in urine in bilharziasis. *1258*

Ornithine Carbamoyl Transferase (OCT) *Serum Increase* Consistently and markedly elevated in patients upon admission, during treatment (highest elevations), and at follow-up 1 month later. Elevated levels may indicate liver cell defect which was not corrected by treatment or by improving the dietary conditions. *2026*

Phosphate *Urine Increase* Urinary inorganic phosphate was increased in hepatic bilharziasis despite normal serum levels. *0955*

Rheumatoid Factor *Serum Increase* Parasitic diseases that involve the liver and reticuloendothelial system have a significant incidence of seropositivity, suggesting that these factors may be produced in these tissues locally. *0962*

Sorbitol Dehydrogenase *Serum Increase* Markedly elevated upon admission, during treatment, and at follow-up. *2026*

122.90 Hydatidosis

Alanine Aminotransferase *Serum Increase* With liver involvement. *1058*

Alkaline Phosphatase *Serum Increase* May increase with obstruction of biliary system. *0812* With bone involvement. *1058*

Aspartate Aminotransferase *Serum Increase* With liver involvement. *1058*

Bilirubin *Serum Increase* With liver involvement. *1058*

Complement Fixation *Serum Increase* *1058*

Creatine Kinase *Serum Increase* With bone involvement. *1058*

Eosinophils *Blood Increase* Occurs in parasitic infestation especially with tissue invasion. *2467* *2538*

Gamma Glutamyl Transferase (GGT) *Serum Increase* With liver involvement. *1058*

Hemagglutination Inhibition *Serum Increase* *1058*

Immunoglobulin IgE *Serum Increase* Increased in parasitic diseases. *2467* Has been reported. *0992*

Lactate Dehydrogenase *Serum Increase* With liver involvement. *1058*

123.40 Diphyllobothriasis (Intestinal)

Eosinophils *Blood Increase* May be a mild eosinophilia, between 5-10%. *2199*

Hematocrit *Blood Decrease* When present, anemia is macrocytic. *2199*

Hemoglobin *Blood Decrease* When present, anemia is macrocytic. *2199*

MCH *Blood Increase* When present, anemia is macrocytic. *2199*

MCV *Blood Increase* When present, anemia is macrocytic. *2199*

Vitamin B₁₂ *Serum Decrease* Loss of ingested vitamin B₁₂. *2467* *2538*

124.00 Trichinosis

Alanine Aminotransferase *Serum Increase* May show a moderate rise. *0433* *0962*

Albumin *Serum Decrease* Decrease occurs in severe cases between 2-4 weeks and may last for years. *2468* In severe cases there may be hypoalbuminemia. *0962* *0433*

Urine Increase In severe cases. *2468* Possibly due to capillary leakage. *0992*

Aldolase *Serum Increase* Moderate rise probably related to myositis. *0992* *0962*

Alpha₂-Globulin *Serum Increase* *0433*

Aspartate Aminotransferase *Serum Increase* Moderate to marked. *0503* During the acute stage. *0962*

Complement Fixation *Serum Increase* Becomes positive about 2 weeks after occurrence of eosinophilia and may remain positive for 6 months. *2468* Using bentonite particles, become positive later in the disease and are most helpful when they exhibit a significant change in titer. *0962*

Creatine *Urine Increase* Constant finding. *0433*

Creatine Kinase *Serum Increase* Moderate to marked increase. *0503* Is observed as the consequence of muscular necrosis. *0433* During the acute stage. *0962*

Eosinophils *Blood Increase* May reach 8,000/μL and persists for several weeks. In fatal cases, it is the only sign of disease. *0433* The most constant finding and one of significance early in the course of disease. Generally appears before the end of the 2nd week. *0992* Characteristic. *2508* Marked; ranging from 15-50% of the total WBC. Highest during the active stage of the disease. *0962* *2199*

Erythrocyte Sedimentation Rate *Blood Decrease* Characteristically slow. *0992*

Blood Increase Normal or moderately increased in some patients. *0433*

Globulin *Serum Increase* Increase in relative and absolute concentrations parallels titer of serologic tests and of thymol turbidity. The increase occurs between 5-8 weeks and may last 6 months or more. *2468* Often associated with hypergammaglobulinemia. *2104*

Hemagglutination Inhibition *Serum Increase* Tannic acid hemagglutination proved to be very sensitive; antibodies were detected in 6 days. *1207*

Hematocrit *Blood Decrease* Prolonged infection may result in secondary anemia. *2368*

Hemoglobin *Blood Decrease* Prolonged infection may result in secondary anemia. *2368*

Hyaline Casts *Urine Increase* In severe cases. *2468*

Immunoglobulin IgE *Serum Increase* The only correlation between trichinosis and an increase in serum IgE was found in patients with a prior history of allergic disease. *0119* *2035*

Immunoglobulin IgM *Serum Increase* In parasitic diseases. *0503*

Lactate Dehydrogenase *Serum Increase* Moderate to marked elevations. *0503* A consequence of muscular necrosis. *0433*

Leukocytes *Blood Increase* Typically, a leukocytosis with a marked hypereosinophilia ranging between 20-75% or more. *2199* Counts as high as 20,000-50,000/μL are found. *2368*

Neutrophils *Blood Increase* Neutrophilic leukocytosis is common. *2368* *0433*

Precipitins *Serum Increase* Using bentonite particles, become positive later in the disease and are most helpful when they exhibit a significant change in titer. *0962* Precipitin test appears to be too nonspecific for general use. *1207*

Protein *Serum Decrease* May be marked. *0433* In severe cases between 2-4 weeks and may last for y. *2468*

Pseudocholinesterase *Serum Decrease* May last up to 6 months. *2468*

126.90 Ancylostomiasis (Hookworm Infestation)

Albumin *Serum Decrease* *2199*

Basophils *Blood Increase* *2538*

Cholesterol *Serum Increase* *2199*

Eosinophils *Blood Increase* Very characteristic. *0433* Generally an eosinophilia of 7-15%, and it may exceed 50% in severe cases. *2199* Common in hookworm anemia. *1924* *2538*

Erythrocytes *Blood Decrease* May be reduced. *2368*

Hematocrit *Blood Decrease* A microcytic, hypochromic anemia attributed directly to blood loss; when the patient has severe malnutrition, however, the anemia may be macrocytic hypochromic anemia. *0433* Anemia occurring in hookworm disease is a classic iron deficiency anemia. *2199* Development of hypochromic, microcytic anemia depends on the number of worms, recency of infection, and host nutrition. *2368*

Hemoglobin *Blood Decrease* A microcytic, hypochromic anemia attributed directly to blood loss; when the patient has severe malnutrition, however, the anemia may be macrocytic hypochromic anemia. *0433* Anemia occurring in hookworm disease is a classic iron deficiency anemia. *2199* Development of hypochromic, microcytic anemia depends on the numbers of worms, recency of infection, and host nutrition. *2368* *0151*

Immunoglobulin IgE *Serum Increase* Increased in parasitic diseases. *2467* *0619*

Immunoglobulin IgM *Serum Increase* In parasitic diseases. *0503*

Iron *Serum Decrease* Anemia occurring in hookworm disease is a classic iron deficiency anemia. *2199* *0151*

Iron-Binding Capacity, Total (TIBC) *Serum Increase* Classic iron deficiency anemia. *2199*

Iron Saturation *Serum Decrease* Classic iron deficiency anemia. *2199*

Leukocytes *Blood Increase* In some early cases may be marked. *0992*

MCH *Blood Decrease* Anemia occurring in hookworm disease is a classic iron deficiency anemia. *2199* Development of hypochromic, microcytic anemia depends on the number of worms, recency of infection, and host nutrition. *2368*

MCHC *Blood Decrease* Anemia occurring in hookworm disease is a classic iron deficiency anemia. *2199* Development of hypochromic, microcytic anemia depends on the number of worms, recency of infection, and host nutrition. *2368* *0151*

MCV *Blood Decrease* Anemia occurring in hookworm disease is a classic iron deficiency anemia. *2199* Development of hypochromic, microcytic anemia depends on the number of worms, recency of infection, and host nutrition. *2368*

Occult Blood *Feces Positive* Occult or frank blood can be demonstrated at all times. *2368*

Protein *Urine Increase* *2199*

127.00 Ascariasis

Eosinophils *Blood Increase* May occur, but this finding is more characteristic of hookworm infection and strongyloidiasis. *0433* Increased during symptomatic phase, especially pulmonary phase. *2468* May be a mild eosinophilia ranging between 5-10%. *1105* *2199* *0151* *2538*

Sputum Increase *0151*

Hemagglutination Inhibition *Serum Increase* *0503*

Immunoglobulin IgA *Serum Decrease* Immunoglobulin levels, especially IgA, may be depressed owing to enteric protein loss. *2199*

Immunoglobulin IgE *Serum Increase* The extent and persistence of elevation is dependent upon several genetically controlled factors. *1738* Parasitic disorders may be associated with elevated IgE levels, especially Ascariasis. *2199* *2035*

Immunoglobulin IgM *Serum Increase* In parasitic diseases. *0503*

127.20 Strongyloidiasis

Albumin *Serum Decrease* Has been observed. *2199*

Eosinophils *Blood Increase* 10% eosinophilia is usual and counts of 50% or even higher are occasionally found. *0433* Increase is almost always present, but the number usually decreased with chronicity. *2468* Typically, an eosinophilia between 8-10% and in very severe infections, up to 50%. *2199* *2538*

Globulin *Serum Increase* Has been observed. *2199*

Hematocrit *Blood Decrease* Anemia, when it occurs, is usually iron deficiency in type. *2199*

Hemoglobin *Blood Decrease* Anemia, when it occurs, is usually iron deficiency in type. *2199*

Immunoglobulin IgE *Serum Increase* Increased in parasitic diseases. *2467*

Immunoglobulin IgM *Serum Increase* In parasitic diseases. *0503*

Iron *Serum Decrease* Anemia, when it occurs, is usually iron deficiency in type. *2199*

Iron-Binding Capacity, Total (TIBC) *Serum Increase* Classic iron deficiency anemia. *2199*

Iron Saturation *Serum Decrease* Classic iron deficiency anemia. *2199*

Leukocytes *Blood Increase* In some patients, there may be a very marked leukocytosis. *2199*

MCH *Blood Decrease* Anemia, when it occurs, is usually iron deficiency in type. *2199*

MCHC *Blood Decrease* Anemia, when it occurs, is usually iron deficiency in type. *2199*

MCV *Blood Decrease* Anemia, when it occurs, is usually iron deficiency in type. *2199*

Occult Blood *Feces Positive* Stools frequently contain occult blood, mucus, and larvae. *2199*

127.30 Trichuriasis

Eosinophils *Blood Increase* May be > 25%. *2468* *0433*

Erythrocytes *Blood Decrease* In children can be accompanied by a microcytic hypochromic anemia. *0433*

Hematocrit *Blood Decrease* In children can be accompanied by a microcytic hypochromic anemia. *0433*

Hemoglobin *Blood Decrease* In children can be accompanied by a microcytic hypochromic anemia. *0433*

Immunoglobulin IgE *Serum Increase* Increased in parasitic diseases. *2467*

Immunoglobulin IgM *Serum Increase* In parasitic diseases. *0503*

Leukocytes *Blood Increase* May be present. *2468*

MCH *Blood Decrease* In children can be accompanied by a microcytic hypochromic anemia. *0433*

MCHC *Blood Decrease* In children can be accompanied by a microcytic hypochromic anemia. *0433*

MCV *Blood Decrease* In children can be accompanied by a microcytic hypochromic anemia. *0433*

Occult Blood *Feces Positive* Bloody diarrhea. *1058*

128.00 Larva Migrans (Visceralis)

Complement Fixation *Serum Increase* Positive in 75% of patients. *0992*

Eosinophils *Blood Increase* Highest level of eosinophilia has been described due to Toxocara canis or catis infection in children. *2035* Severe eosinophilia, splenomegaly, and lymphadenopathy in several members of the same family were infected from a common environmental source. *0585* Characteristic feature. *2368* *2538*

Globulin *Serum Increase* Often increased. *2104* Characteristic feature. *2368*

Hemagglutination Inhibition *Serum Increase* Tests with Ascaris and Toxocara antigen are helpful, but are rarely diagnostic because cross reactions with other helminths are common. *1058*

Immunoglobulin IgA *Serum Decrease* Immunoglobulin levels, especially IgA, may be depressed owing to enteric protein loss. *2199*

Immunoglobulin IgE *Serum Increase* The extent and persistence of elevation is dependent upon several genetically controlled factors. *1738* Parasitic disorders may be associated with elevated IgE levels, especially Ascariasis, and visceral larva migrans. *2199* *2035*

Immunoglobulin IgM *Serum Increase* In parasitic diseases. *0503*

Immunoglobulins *Serum Increase* Striking elevations often found with Toxocara cati infection. *2104*

Leukocytes *Blood Increase* *2468*

Rheumatoid Factor *Serum Increase* Parasitic diseases that involve the liver and reticuloendothelial system have a significant incidence of seropositivity, suggesting that these factors may be produced in these tissues locally. *0962*

130.00   Toxoplasmosis

Alpha-Fetoprotein   *Serum   Increase*   In newborn but disappeared by the end of the 1st month. *1598*

Antibody Titer   *CSF   Increase*   Congenital infection is indicated when CSF antibody concentration is higher for toxoplasmosis than for rubeola. *1360*

Bilirubin   *Serum   Increase*   *2538 0486*

Cells   *CSF   Increase*   In congenital, both RBC and WBC with a predominance of mononuclear elements. In acquired predominantly mononuclear cells, 30-2000/μL. *1319*

Complement Fixation   *Serum   Increase*   Antibody is present within 1-2 months of infection and is usually negative within 2 y. *2035* Becomes positive later than the other serologic tests, and its titer declines earlier. *0962*   In 26 patients with congenital infection and in 22 of their mothers, tests results were positive on all specimens from the patients younger than 2 y of age and on 69% of specimens collected from older patients. *1244*   CF antibodies appear later than Sabin-Feldman or hemagglutinating antibodies and diminish more rapidly. *2368   1319*

Eosinophils   *Blood   Increase*   *2538*

Erythrocytes   *Blood   Decrease*   Anemia is present. *2468*

Globulin   *Serum   Increase*   *2468*

Glucose   *CSF   Normal*   In acquired, usually normal. *1319*

Hemagglutination Inhibition   *Serum   Increase*   Specific and sensitive. *0433*   Hemagglutinating antibody appears later and rises more slowly than IFA antibody. *2035*   Marked elevations of antibody to toxoplasmosis. *2538   2571*

Hematocrit   *Blood   Decrease*   Anemia is present. *2468   2538 0486*

Hemoglobin   *Blood   Decrease*   Anemia is present. *2468*

Hemoglobin, Free   *Serum   Increase*   *2538 0486*

Immunoglobulin IgM   *Serum   Increase*   Acute infections are characterized by an early and relatively transient IgM and complement-fixing antibody response. *2035   0776*

Indirect Fluorescent Antibodies   *Serum   Increase*   Detects predominantly IgG toxoplasma antibody. *2035*   Marked elevations of antibody to toxoplasmosis. *2538*   Titers of 1:256 or higher indicate recent infection, and titers of 1:1024 or higher accompany active disease. *0962*   Found to be as reliable as the Sabin-Feldman dye test. *2368*

Leukocytes   *Blood   Decrease*   WBC varies from leukopenia to leukemoid reaction; atypical lymphocytes may be found. *2468*

Blood   Increase   WBC varies from leukopenia to leukemoid reaction; atypical lymphocytes may be found. *2468*

CSF   Increase   In congenital, both RBC and WBC with a predominance of mononuclear elements. In acquired predominantly mononuclear cells, 30-2,000/μL. *1319*

Lymphocytes   *Blood   Decrease*   *0532*

Blood   Increase   Slight. *0151   0532*

CSF   Increase   In congenital and acquired. *1319*

Methylene Blue (Sabin-Feldman) Dye Test   *Serum   Increase*   Specific and sensitive. *2368*   Appears within 1-2 weeks, rises not less than 1:256 and can be as high as 1:32,000 or more. May persist at high levels for several y then fall slowly to 1:64 or less and tends to persist indefinitely. *1319*   Detects predominantly IgG but also IgM antibodies which appear within 2-4 weeks after infection and persist for years. Rising titers in paired sera at least 3 weeks apart are most helpful in the diagnosis of recent infection. *2035*   Titers of 1:16 are considered indicative of past infection or exposure. During active disease, titers of 1:1,000-1:65,000 may be attained. *0962*

Monocytes   *Blood   Increase*   Slight. *0151   0532*

CSF   Increase   Moderate number. *1058*

Precipitins   *Serum   Increase*   *2035*

Protein   *CSF   Increase*   In congenital, as high as 2,000 mg/dL. *1319*

CSF   Normal   In acquired, usually normal. *1319*

135.00   Sarcoidosis

1,25-Dihydroxy-Vitamin D₃   *Serum   Increase*   *0062*

5'-Nucleotidase   *Serum   Increase*   Levels ranging from 14.5-91.3 U/L were observed in 5 cases. *1312*   Significantly elevated in 2 of 3 patients with liver granulomata. *1312*

Alanine Aminotransferase   *Serum   Increase*   In 5 cases of hepatic granuloma, ALT was elevated to a mean value of 70 U/L (normal = 50 U/L) and a range of 50-115 U/L. *1452*

Albumin   *Serum   Decrease*   Associated with increased globulin in 'sarcoid step' characteristic patterns. *2468*

Serum   Increase   Some cases when active. *0619*

Alkaline Phosphatase   *Serum   Increase*   Elevated in 40% of cases involving the liver, usually ranging from 25-97 U/L, with < 15% presenting values > 107 U/L. *0503*   Marked elevation in all 5 cases of granuloma of liver. Maximum upper limit of normal = 85 U/L. Average elevated value = 425 U/L. Range = 191-700 U/L. *1452 1312 0999*

Alkaline Phosphatase Isoenzymes   *Serum   Increase*   Elevated hepatic isoenzyme is characteristically present. *0999*

Alpha₂-Globulin   *Serum   Increase*   Stepwise increase of alpha₂, beta, and gamma globulin 'sarcoid steps' helps differentiate from other lung disease *2467*   Marked increase is frequent. *0619*

Angiotensin-Converting Enzyme (ACE)   *Serum   Increase*   Most frequently elevated in patients with pulmonary parenchymal involvement. *1968*   Elevated in 33% of patients with Sarcoidosis. *0941* Elevated in 60-80% of cases. *0560*   Increased levels in 67.2% of 100 patients. *2041*   Elevated in 75% of patients. *2118   1400*

Antibody Titer   *Serum   Increase*   Used to differentiate pulmonary sarcoidosis from tuberculosis. Antituberculous antibodies were found in TB in 83%; in sarcoidosis 22%. *1309*

Aspartate Aminotransferase   *Serum   Increase*   In 36% of 24 patients at initial hospitalization for this disorder. *0781*   In 5 cases of granuloma of liver, 100% were mildly elevated, showing a mean elevation of 36 U/L over the normal maximum limit of 24 U/L. *1452*

Beta₂-Macroglobulin   *Serum   Increase*   Elevated in 63% of patients. *1773*

Beta-Globulin   *Serum   Increase*   Stepwise increase of alpha₂, beta, and gamma globulin. 'sarcoid steps' help differentiate from other lung disease. *2467*

Bicarbonate   *Serum   Increase*   In 55% of 20 patients at initial hospitalization for this disorder. *0781*

Calcium   *Serum   Increase*   Much less frequent than hypercalciuria. Found in 6-13% of cases. *0433*   Occurs in approximately 33% of patients at some stage of disease. *1083   0962 2199*

Urine   Increase   30-60% of the patients. *0503*   Solitary hypercalciuria without hyperparathyroidism indicates sarcoidosis. *0503 0433* Occurs in approximately 33% of patients at some stage. Urinary levels are high, stool content low, and serum phosphate normal or low. *1083   0999 1361 2199*

Feces   Decrease   At some stage of disease. *1083*

Cells   *CSF   Increase*   In granulomatous basilar meningitis affecting cranial nerves. *0992*

Chloride   *Serum   Decrease*   Suggests the presence of sarcoidosis or malignancy in conjunction with other tests. *0433*

Complement Fixation   *Serum   Increase*   Used to differentiate pulmonary sarcoidosis from tuberculosis. Antituberculous antibodies were found in TB in 83%; in sarcoidosis 22%. *1309*

Complement, Total   *Serum   Increase*   *0151 1699*

Copper   *Liver   Increase*   Increased in hepatocytes in 5 patients. *2004*

Creatinine   *Serum   Increase*   In 38% of 13 patients at initial hospitalization for this disorder. *0781*

Cyclic Adenosine Monophosphate   *Urine   Decrease*   *0575*

Eosinophils   *Blood   Increase*   Occurs in 15% of patients. *2468* In 44% of 25 patients at initial hospitalization for this disorder. *0781 2538*

Erythrocytes   *Blood   Decrease*   Pancytopenia is a common feature. *2538*

Erythrocyte Sedimentation Rate   *Blood   Increase*   May reflect raised immunoglobulin levels, or associated erythema nodosum or secondary infection. *0151   0433*

Fibrinogen   *Plasma   Increase*   Indicates active disease. *1964*

Gamma Glutamyl Transferase (GGT)   *Serum   Increase*   In 5 patients with liver granulomas, including miliary tuberculosis and sarcoidosis, serum GGT levels were all elevated, mean = 303, range = 116-740 U/L. *1452*

Globulin   *Serum   Increase*   Has been observed in 23.5-61% of cases. *0433*   Increased in 75% of patients, producing reduced A/G ratio and increased total protein in 30% of patients. *2468*   Increase of Alpha 2, and gamma globulins help differentiate from other lung disease *2467*

Glucose   *CSF   Decrease*   Due to multiple tumors in the meninges, in rare cases, involving the central nervous system. *0619*

Hydroxyproline   *Serum   Increase*   *0062*

Urine Increase Considerably increased in acute disease, returning to normal as the chest x-ray abnormality resolves. Chronic disease has normal levels. *0151*

Immunoglobulin IgA *Serum Increase* Elevated in 25% of cases. *0151* Immunoglobulins are frequently elevated and tend to reflect the overall resolution of disease. Falls to normal with resolution. *1608*

Immunoglobulin IgD *Serum Increase* *0619*

Immunoglobulin IgE *Serum Increase* *0062*

Immunoglobulin IgG *Serum Increase* Consistent increase in 1 or more serum immunoglobulins, noted in 79% of 129 cases studied. IgM and/or IgG are the most frequently increased. *0433* Elevated in 50% of cases. *0151* Frequently elevated and tends to reflect the overall resolution of disease. With resolution, falls but tends to remain raised for up to 4 y. *1608*

Immunoglobulin IgM *Serum Increase* Frequently elevated and tends to reflect the overall resolution of disease. Falls with resolution but remains significantly above normal. *1608* Consistent increase in 1 or more serum immunoglobulins, noted in 79% of 129 cases studied. IgG and/or IgM are most frequently increased. *0433* Serum IgG is elevated in 50%, IgA in 25%, and IgM in 12.5% of cases. *0151*

Immunoglobulins *Serum Increase* Serum IgG is elevated in 50%, IgA in 25%, and IgM in 12.5% of cases. *0151* Consistent increase in 1 or more serum immunoglobulins, noted in 79% of 129 cases studied. IgG and/or IgM are most frequently increased. *0433*

Lactate Dehydrogenase *Serum Increase* In 24% of 25 patients at initial hospitalization for this disorder. *0781*

Leucine Aminopeptidase *Serum Increase* In 12 patients with granulomatous hepatitis, all showed elevated LAP levels, varying from 380-1,000 U/L, with a mean of 622 (normal = 322). *0281*

Leukocytes *Blood Decrease* In 30% of patients. *2468* Pancytopenia is a common feature. *2538*

CSF Increase In granulomatous basilar meningitis affecting cranial nerves. *0992*

Lymphocytes *Blood Decrease* Absolute lymphopenia occurs in pulmonary sarcoidosis and correlates very closely with prognosis. A steady increase in absolute number indicates good prognosis (with or without treatment). No increase or a very low and unchanged number indicates very poor prognosis. *0260* In 52% of 25 patients at initial hospitalization for this disorder. *0781*

Lysozyme *Serum Increase* Highest in patients with the most extensive disease and falls progressively in stage II to I. All patients with disease involving the spleen showed increased activity. *1777* Most frequently elevated in patients with pulmonary parenchymal involvement. *1968*

Monocytes *Blood Increase* In 72% of 25 patients at initial hospitalization for this disorder. *0781 2467*

Oxygen Saturation *Blood Decrease* Decreased with lung involvement. *2468*

Parathyroid Hormone *Serum Decrease* Immeasurably low in most patients, both normo- and hypercalcemic. *1909*

pCO₂ *Blood Decrease* Mild hyperventilation is frequent except in advanced disease when ventilatory obstruction occurs. *0999* Impaired gas diffusion in pulmonary sarcoid may cause hyperventilation and reduced pCO_2. In more severe cases, CO_2 retention occurs. *2104* In 26% of 15 patients at initial hospitalization for this disorder. *0781* Decreased with lung involvement. *2468*

Blood Increase In more severe cases, CO_2 retention occurs. *2104*

pH *Blood Increase* In 72% of 15 patients at initial hospitalization for this disorder. *0781*

Phosphate *Serum Increase* *2199*

Platelet Count *Blood Decrease* Pancytopenia is a common feature. *2538*

pO₂ *Blood Decrease* In 71% of 14 patients at initial hospitalization for this disorder. *0781* Decreased with lung involvement. *2468* Mild hyperventilation is frequent except in advanced disease when ventilatory obstruction occurs. *0999*

Protein *Serum Increase* *2467 0433*

CSF Increase In granulomatous basilar meningitis affecting cranial nerves. *0992*

Rheumatoid Factor *Serum Increase* The incidence of seropositivity exceeds that of a normal population. *2035* High incidence of seropositive tests among those who had the disease for 2 y, especially among those who also had arthritis. *0962* 17% positivity. *0422 0123*

Thymol Turbidity *Serum Increase* Increased due to alteration of serum proteins. *2467*

Uric Acid *Serum Increase* May occur even with normal renal function in up to 50% of patients. *2468* In 52% of 25 patients at initial hospitalization for this disorder. *0781 1283 0962*

NEOPLASMS

Primary Malignant Neoplasms

150.90 Malignant Neoplasm of Esophagus

Albumin *Serum Decrease* In 35% of 40 patients at initial hospitalization for this disorder. *0781*

Aldolase *Serum Increase* Significantly elevated in tumors of the gastrointestinal tract. Mean = 4.9 ± 0.8 U/L compared to normal, 1.6 ± 0.21. *1201*

Alkaline Phosphatase *Serum Increase* In 29% of 40 patients at initial hospitalization for this disorder. *0781*

Amylase *Serum Increase* *0062*

Aspartate Aminotransferase *Serum Increase* In 41% of 40 patients at initial hospitalization for this disorder. *0781*

Calcium *Serum Increase* Neoplasm without evidence of direct bone involvement. Parathyroid hormone-secreting tumors. *0503*

Carcinoembryonic Antigen *Serum Increase* In 66% of patients with localized upper GI tract malignancy, mean = 4.9 ng/mL. *1817 2467 2035 0795*

Pleural Effusion Increase The highest levels (> 1,000 ng/mL) were found in samples from patients with gastrointestinal carcinomas. *0622* 24 (34%) of 70 malignant effusions had levels 12 ng/mL. *1945*

Ascitic Fluid Increase CEA > 10 ng/mL ascites indicating cancerous effusion. *1420*

Peritoneal Fluid Increase The highest levels (> 1,000 ng/mL) were found in samples from patients with gastrointestinal carcinomas. *0622*

Complement C3 *Serum Increase* Increased in patients with local disease. Very closely linked to the stage of the disease. Patients in remission had normal levels, but further increases were noted in distant metastases. Levels dropped significantly in the terminal phase of the disease. *2427*

Complement C4 *Serum Increase* Increased in patients with local disease. Very closely linked to the stage of the disease. Patients in remission had normal levels, but further increases were noted in distant metastases. Levels dropped significantly in the terminal phase of disease. *2427*

Complement, Total *Serum Increase* Found to be very closely linked to the stage of the disease. Patients in remission had normal levels, but further increases were noted in distant metastases. Levels dropped significantly in the terminal phase of the disease. *2427*

Hematocrit *Blood Decrease* In 24% of 40 patients at initial hospitalization for this disorder. *0781*

Hemoglobin *Blood Decrease* In 27% of 39 patients at initial hospitalization for this disorder. *0781*

Hexokinase *Serum Increase* Increased in gastrointestinal tumors. Mean 15.3 ± 3.5 compared to normal, 0.93 ± 0.28 U/L. *1201*

Leukocytes *Blood Increase* In 37% of 40 patients at initial hospitalization for this disorder. *0781*

Lymphocytes *Blood Decrease* In 55% of 36 patients at initial hospitalization for this disorder. *0781*

Monocytes *Blood Increase* In 65% of 37 patients at initial hospitalization for this disorder. *0781*

Occult Blood *Feces Positive* GI bleeding may occur with malignancies. *2199*

Uric Acid *Serum Increase* In 46% of 40 patients at initial hospitalization for this disorder. *0781*

151.90 Malignant Neoplasm of Stomach

Albumin *Serum Decrease* Found occasionally, due to leakage into stomach. *0992* In 38% of 47 patients at initial hospitalization for this disorder. *0781*

Aldolase *Serum Increase* Significantly elevated in tumors of the gastrointestinal tract. Mean = 4.9 ± 0.8 U/L compared to normal, 1.6 ± 0.21. *1201*

Alkaline Phosphatase *Serum Increase* In 38% of 45 patients at initial hospitalization for this disorder. *0781*

151.90 Malignant Neoplasm of Stomach *(continued)*

Alkaline Phosphatase *(continued)*

Leukocyte Decrease Low activity is present irrespective of tumor category, activity of disease, or type of therapy. In 11 patients, median activity was 5 U/L (normal = 55). *1423*

Alkaline Phosphatase Isoenzymes *Serum Increase* Concentration of Regan isoenzyme was 12.5-34.2 U/L. *0549*

Alpha-Fetoprotein *Serum Increase* Elevated in 18% of cases. *1348*

Androgens *Urine Decrease* Both androsterone and etiocholanolone were significantly lower in 18 male patients than in controls and patients with rectal cancer. *2333*

Androsterone *Urine Decrease* Both androsterone and etiocholanolone were significantly lower in 18 male patients than in controls and patients with rectal cancer. *2333*

Aspartate Aminotransferase *Serum Increase* In 28% of 47 patients at initial hospitalization for this disorder. *0781*

Beta-Glucuronidase *Gastric Material Increase* Greater than 1 U/mg protein in 90% of subjects with cancer or gastric atrophy. *0992* Elevated in gastric cancer. Overlap between noncancer and cancer patients limits usefulness and specificity. *2199 1266*

Carcinoembryonic Antigen *Serum Increase* In 66% of patients with localized upper GI tract malignancy, mean = 4.9 ng/mL. *1817 2035 0795*

Pleural Effusion Increase The highest levels (> 1,000 ng/mL) were found in samples from patients with gastrointestinal carcinomas. *0622* 24 (34%) of 70 malignant effusions had levels 12 ng/mL. *1945*

Ascitic Fluid Increase CEA > 10 ng/mL ascites indicating cancerous effusion. *1420*

Peritoneal Fluid Increase The highest levels (> 1,000 ng/mL) were found in samples from patients with gastrointestinal carcinomas. *0622*

Ceruloplasmin *Serum Increase* High only in gastric and pulmonary cancer. In 58 cases there was a correlation between copper and ceruloplasmin levels in the same subject; significant only in gastric forms. *2058*

Chloride *Serum Increase* In 34% of 29 patients at initial hospitalization for this disorder. *0781*

Complement C3 *Serum Increase* Increased in patients with local disease. Very closely linked to the stage of the disease. Patients in remission had normal levels, but further increases were noted in distant metastases. Levels dropped significantly in the terminal phase of disease. *2427*

Complement C4 *Serum Increase* Increased in patients with local disease. Very closely linked to the stage of the disease. Patients in remission had normal levels, but further increases were noted in distant metastases. Levels dropped significantly in the terminal phase of disease. *2427*

Complement, Total *Serum Increase* CH50, C1q, C3, and C4 were significantly higher in cancer patients than in matched controls. The increase was dependent upon the stage of disease and the therapy. *2427*

Copper *Serum Increase* A correlation between copper and ceruloplasmin was reported in 58 cases of gastric neoplasm. *2058* In 35 cases of primary malignant tumors of the digestive organs, plasma copper was increased (1.24 ± 0.34 ppm). *1125*

Cryofibrinogen *Serum Increase* *2035 1551*

Erythrocytes *Ascitic Fluid Increase* > 10,000 cells/µL seen in 20% of cases. *2626*

Erythrocyte Sedimentation Rate *Blood Increase* Normal in peptic ulcer, but accelerated in carcinoma of the stomach. *0962*

Etiocholanolone *Urine Decrease* Both androsterone and etiocholanolone were significantly lower in 18 male patients than in controls and patients with rectal cancer. *2333*

Fucose *Serum Increase* Total concentration was increased in patients with both malignant and benign tumors of breast, lung and stomach. The glycoprotein-bound fraction was markedly elevated in cases of malignancy and not in benign disease. Mucoprotein fraction was raised in both diseases. *2331* Mean value = 13.52 ± 0.65 in 35 patients. (normal = 6.84 ± 0.13 mg/dL). *1342*

Gastrin *Serum Increase* Found to be normal in 26 patients with gastric cancer. Elevated levels may occur in some patients, due to the accompanying atrophy of the oxyntic glands. *1130*

Serum Normal Found to be normal in 26 patients with gastric cancer. Elevated levels may occur in some patients, due to the accompanying atrophy of the oxyntic glands. *1130*

Glucose *Serum Decrease* *2467*

Gonadotropin, Chorionic *Serum Increase* Ectopic production. *0001 0265 0299 1691*

Gonadotropin, Pituitary *Serum Increase* Can cause the syndrome of ectopic gonadotropin production. *0962*

Growth Hormone *Serum Increase* Elevated. *0918*

Haptoglobin *Serum Increase* *0992*

Hematocrit *Blood Decrease* The amount of bleeding and the degree of anemia will vary widely. Anemia of more than moderate degree is a late consequence of gastric malignancy. *0962* Anemia may be of several types. The most common is iron deficiency anemia caused by chronic occult blood loss. *2199* In 43% of 47 patients at initial hospitalization for this disorder. *0781*

Hemoglobin *Blood Decrease* The amount of bleeding and the degree of anemia will vary widely. Anemia of more than moderate degree is a late consequence of gastric malignancy. *0962* Anemia may be of several types. The most common is iron deficiency anemia caused by chronic occult blood loss. *2199* In 46% of 46 patients at initial hospitalization for this disorder. *0781*

Hexokinase *Serum Increase* Increased in gastrointestinal tumors. Mean = 15.3 ± 3.5 compared to normal, 0.93 ± 0.28 U/L. *1201*

Hexosaminidase *Serum Increase* *1443*

Hydrochloric Acid *Gastric Material Decrease* Achlorhydria following histamine or betazole stimulation found in 50% of patients and hypochlorhydria in another 25% of patients. *2467 0962*

Gastric Material Increase Although rare, does not rule out carcinoma. *2467*

Gastric Material Normal Normal in 25% of patients. *2467*

Iron *Serum Decrease* Repeated small blood losses and consequent iron deficiency fully explain the anemia in most cases of gastric carcinoma. The anemia is of the hypochromic, microcytic type with other features of chronic iron deficiency. *0962* Chronic occult blood loss. *2199*

Iron-Binding Capacity, Total (TIBC) *Serum Increase* Anemia is commonly iron deficient type, due to chronic blood loss. *2199*

Iron Saturation *Serum Decrease* Anemia is commonly iron deficiency type, due to chronic blood loss. *2199*

Lactate Dehydrogenase *Serum Increase* Marked elevation in 20 patients with tumors of the gastrointestinal tract. Mean = 162.0 ± 23.1 U/L compared to 85.4 ± 1.0 U/L. *1201*

Gastric Material Increase Increase in activity is found in carcinoma, measured as U/mL or U secreted/h. *0619* Elevated in gastric cancer. Overlap between noncancer and cancer patients limits usefulness and specificity. *2199*

Lactic Acid *Blood Increase* In 8 patients with localized tumors, mean concentration was 21.5 ± 5.7 mg/dL compared to normal, 11.7 ± 0.72 mg/dL. *1201*

Gastric Material Increase Greater than 100 g/L in 50% of patients with carcinoma, but in only 2% of patients with gastric ulcer. *0992* Elevated in gastric cancer. Overlap between noncancer and cancer patients limits usefulness and specificity. *2199 1823*

Leukocytes *Blood Increase* Complicated by degeneration, infection, or metastasis, there may be an elevation of the count and proportionate increase in the percentage of neutrophils. A marked leukocytosis is rare usually associated with malignant invasion of the bone marrow or large infected tumor tissues. *0962* In 26% of 47 patients at initial hospitalization for this disorder. *0781*

Blood Normal There are no characteristic early changes in the leukocyte count in large malignant tumors of the stomach. *0962*

Ascitic Fluid Increase > 1000 µL. *2626*

Lymphocytes *Blood Decrease* In 60% of 44 patients at initial hospitalization for this disorder. *0781* Relative lymphocytopenia may occur as a result of absolute increase in monocytes and polymorphonuclear cells in inflammatory bowel disease. *2345*

MCH *Blood Decrease* The amount of bleeding and the degree of anemia will vary widely. Anemia of more than moderate degree is a late consequence of gastric malignancy. *0962* Anemia may be of several types. The most common is iron deficiency anemia caused by chronic occult blood loss. *2199 2467*

MCHC *Blood Decrease* The amount of bleeding and the degree of anemia will vary widely. Anemia of more than moderate degree is a late consequence of gastric malignancy. *0962* Anemia may be of several types. The most common is iron deficiency anemia caused by chronic blood loss. *2199*

MCV *Blood Decrease* The anemia is of the hypochromic, microcytic type with other features of chronic iron deficiency. *0962*

Blood Increase Macrocytic anemia may be seen in patients with gastric carcinoma and untreated pernicious anemia or folate deficiency. *2199*

Monocytes *Blood Increase* Relative lymphocytopenia may occur as a result of absolute increase in monocytes and polymorphonuclear cells in inflammatory bowel disease. *2345* In 69% of 44 patients at initial hospitalization for this disorder. *0781*

Neutrophils *Blood Increase* Neutrophilic leukemoid reactions occur most frequently with gastric, bronchogenic, and pancreatic carcinomas. *2538*

Occult Blood *Feces Positive* Persistence of occult blood in the stool is strong evidence of malignancy but, does not indicate the location of the lesion. *0962* Anemia may be of several types. The most common is iron deficiency anemia caused by chronic occult blood loss. *2199*

Gastric Material Positive Tests for the presence of blood in the gastric contents are positive in a high percentage of cases. Gross blood in the gastric content is a more important finding; found in nearly 50% of the cases. *0962*

Parathyroid Hormone *Serum Increase* Lung cancer, hypernephroma, gastrointestinal cancer, and other neoplasms can synthesize and secrete parathyroid hormone. *0962*

Pepsinogen *Serum Decrease* A level < 200 U/L is conclusive of gastric atrophy, a precursor of gastric cancer. *0962*

pH *Gastric Material Decrease* Achlorhydria following histamine or betazole stimulation found in 50% of patients and hypochlorhydria in another 25% of patients. *2467* *0962*

Gastric Material Increase Although rare, does not rule out carcinoma. *2467*

Gastric Material Normal Normal in 25% of patients. *2467*

Platelet Count *Blood Increase* In 39% of 35 patients at initial hospitalization for this disorder. *0781*

Potassium *Serum Increase* In 30% of 29 patients at initial hospitalization for this disorder. *0781*

Protein *Serum Decrease* Enteric loss of plasma protein. *2199*

Ascitic Fluid Increase > 2.5 g/dL. *2626*

Pyruvate *Blood Increase* Elevated in 8 patients with tumors of the gastrointestinal tract, mean = 1.93 ± 0.18 U/L. *1201*

Uric Acid *Serum Increase* In 36% of 47 patients at initial hospitalization for this disorder. *0781*

Vitamin B$_{12}$ *Serum Decrease* Inadequate absorption, lack of intrinsic factor, loss of gastric mucosa. *2467*

Zinc *Serum Decrease* Increased in 35 cases of primary malignant tumors, (1.24 ± 0.34 ppm) and plasma zinc decreased (8.83 ± 0.18 ppm). *1125*

152.90 Malignant Neoplasm of Small Intestine

Aldolase *Serum Increase* Significantly elevated in tumors of the gastrointestinal tract. Mean = 4.9 ± 0.8 U/L compared to normal, 1.6 ± 0.21. *1201*

Carcinoembryonic Antigen *Serum Increase* In 66% of patients with localized upper GI tract malignancy, mean = 4.9 ng/mL. *1817 2035 0795*

Pleural Effusion Increase The highest levels (> 1,000 ng/mL) were found in samples from patients with gastrointestinal carcinomas. *0622* 24 (34%) of 70 malignant effusions had levels > 12 ng/mL. *1945*

Ascitic Fluid Increase CEA > 10 ng/mL ascites indicating cancerous effusion. *1420*

Peritoneal Fluid Increase The highest levels (> 1,000 ng/mL) were found in samples from patients with gastrointestinal carcinomas. *0622*

Complement C3 *Serum Increase* Increased in patients with local disease. Very closely linked to the stage of the disease. Patients in remission had normal levels, but further increases were noted in distant metastases. Levels dropped significantly in the terminal phase of the disease. *2427*

Complement C4 *Serum Increase* Increased in patients with local disease. Very closely linked to the stage of the disease. Patients in remission had normal levels, but further increases were noted in distant metastases. Levels dropped significantly in the terminal phase of disease. *2427*

Cryofibrinogen *Serum Increase* *2035 1551*

Erythrocytes *Ascitic Fluid Increase* > 10,000 cells/µL seen in 20% of cases. *2626*

Hematocrit *Blood Decrease* Anemia may be of several types. The most common is iron deficiency anemia caused by chronic occult blood loss. *2199*

Hemoglobin *Blood Decrease* Anemia may be of several types. The most common is iron deficiency anemia caused by chronic occult blood loss. *2199*

Hexokinase *Serum Increase* Increased in gastrointestinal tumors. Mean = 15.3 ± 3.5 compared to normal, 0.93 ± 0.28 U/L. *1201*

Iron *Serum Decrease* Anemia is common iron deficiency type, due to chronic blood loss. *2199*

Iron-Binding Capacity, Total (TIBC) *Serum Increase* Anemia is common iron deficiency type, due to chronic blood loss. *2199*

Iron Saturation *Serum Decrease* Anemia is commonly iron deficient type, due to chronic blood loss. *2199*

Lactate Dehydrogenase *Serum Increase* Marked elevation in 20 patients, mean = 162.0 - 23.1 U/L compared to 85.4 ± 1.0 U/L. *1201*

Lactic Acid *Blood Increase* In 8 patients with tumors of the gastrointestinal tract, mean concentration was 21.5 ± 5.7 mg/dL compared to normal, 11.7 ± 0.72 mg/dL. *1201*

Leukocytes *Ascitic Fluid Increase* > 1000 WBC/µL. *2626*

MCH *Blood Decrease* Iron deficiency anemia is common because of either gross or occult bleeding. *2199*

MCHC *Blood Decrease* Iron deficiency anemia is common because of either gross or occult bleeding. *2199*

MCV *Blood Decrease* Iron deficiency anemia is common because of either gross or occult bleeding. *2199*

Occult Blood *Feces Positive* Persistence of occult blood in the stool is strong evidence of malignancy, but does not indicate the location of the lesion. *0962* Anemia may be of several types. The most common is iron deficiency anemia caused by chronic occult blood loss. *2199*

Parathyroid Hormone *Serum Increase* Lung cancer, hypernephroma, gastrointestinal cancer, and other neoplasms can synthesize and secrete parathyroid hormone. *0962*

Protein *Serum Decrease* Enteric loss of plasma protein. *2199*

Ascitic Fluid Increase > 2.5 g/dL. *2626*

Pyruvate *Blood Increase* Moderately elevated in 8 patients, mean = 1.93 ± 0.18 U/L. *1201*

153.90 Malignant Neoplasm of Large Intestine

Albumin *Serum Decrease* Significantly reduced (median = 35.7 g/L compared to controls (44.0 g/L). *1025* In 28% of 149 patients at initial hospitalization for this disorder. *0781*

Urine Increase 24 h excretion and renal clearance were significantly increased in localized tumor patients compared to normals and disseminated cancer cases. Increased high molecular weight protein excretion implies glomerular injury in these patients. *1025*

Aldolase *Serum Increase* Significantly elevated in tumors of the gastrointestinal tract. Mean = 4.9 ± 0.8 U/L compared to normal, 1.6 ± 0.21. *1201*

Alkaline Phosphatase *Serum Increase* In 24% of 150 patients at initial hospitalization for this disorder. *0781 0992*

Leukocyte Decrease Low activity is present irrespective of tumor category, activity of disease, or type of therapy. In 11 patients median value was 18 U/L (normal = 55). *1423*

Alkaline Phosphatase Isoenzymes *Serum Increase* Increased incidence of the Regan (placental) isoenzyme. *0740* 13.25% had increased concentration of the Regan isoenzyme, ranging from 7.17-24.3 U/L. *0549*

Alpha$_2$-Globulin *Serum Increase* Increased plasma concentrations in primary cancer. Haptoglobin values were especially useful to indicate tumor activity. *0450*

Alpha-Fetoprotein *Serum Increase* Elevated in 5% of cases. *1348*

Arylsulfatase *Urine Increase* Urinary arylsulfatase B was observed in high concentrations in patients with colon carcinoma. Increased activity correlated with the extent of disease. Elevations were observed in only 28% of patients with Dukes' A disease. 55% of those with Dukes' B, and in more than 75% of patients with Dukes' C and D lesions. *2093*

Beta-Glucuronidase *Serum Increase* Increased. *0741 0866*

153.90 Malignant Neoplasm of Large Intestine
(continued)

Carcinoembryonic Antigen *Serum Increase* Increased in about 80% of the patients. *2467* 55% of patients had elevated concentrations (mean = 6.3 ng/mL). 91% of patients had positive plasma assays. *0830* In 73% of cases. *2199* In 66% of patients with localized upper GI tract malignancy, mean = 4.9 ng/mL. *1817 2035 0795*

Pleural Effusion *Increase* The highest levels (> 1,000 ng/mL) were found in patients with gastrointestinal carcinomas. *0622* 24 (34%) of 70 malignant effusions had levels > 12 ng/mL. *1945*

Ascitic Fluid *Increase* Ascitic fluid assays detected 11 of 13 cases; (CEA > 10 ng/mL ascites indicating cancerous effusion). *1420*

Peritoneal Fluid *Increase* The highest levels (> 1,000 ng/mL) were found in patients with gastrointestinal carcinomas. *0622*

Cholesterol *Serum Decrease* The mean levels were lower (202.2 mg/dL) than controls (219.5). Patients with Duke B stage cancer accounted for most of the difference. *1686*

Feces *Increase* Fecal excretion of cholesterol, coprostanol, coprostanone, total bile acids, deoxycholic acid, lithocholic acid was higher in colonic cancer and adenomatous polyps compared to normal controls as well as in patients with other digestive diseases. *1896*

Complement C3 *Serum Increase* Increased in patients with local disease. Found to be very closely linked to the stage of the disease. Patients in remission had normal levels, but further increases were noted in distant metastases. Dropped significantly in the terminal phase of disease. *2427*

Complement C4 *Serum Increase* Increased in patients with local disease. Very closely linked to the stage of the disease. Patients in remission had normal levels, but further increases were noted in distant metastases. Levels dropped significantly in the terminal phase of disease. *2427*

Complement, Total *Serum Increase* Found to be very closely linked to stage of disease. Patients in remission had normal levels, but further increases were noted in distant metastases. Levels dropped significantly in the terminal phase of disease. *2427*

Copper *Serum Increase* Increased in 35 cases of primary malignant tumors of the digestive organs, (mean = 1.24 ± 0.34 ppm). *1125*

Creatine Kinase *Serum Increase* Highest activity of CK-BB in brain and smooth muscle. *1347*

Creatinine *Serum Increase* In 34% of 63 patients at initial hospitalization for this disorder. *0781*

Cryofibrinogen *Serum Increase* *2035 1551*

Deoxycholic Acid *Feces Increase* The fecal excretion of cholesterol, coprostanol, coprostanone, total bile acids, deoxycholic acid, lithocholic acid was higher in colonic cancer and adenomatous polyps compared to normal controls as well as in patients with other digestive diseases. *1896*

Erythrocytes *Ascitic Fluid Increase* > 10,000 cells/μL seen in 20% of cases. *2626*

Erythrocyte Sedimentation Rate *Blood Increase* Increased in significant tissue necrosis. Extreme elevation frequently occurs. Indicates inflammation. *2467 0962*

Fucose *Serum Increase* In 17 patients, mean value was 11.79 ± 0.72 (normal = 6.84 ± 0.13 mg/dL). *1342*

Gonadotropin, Chorionic *Serum Increase* Ectopic production. *0001 0265 0299 1691*

Haptoglobin *Serum Increase* Increased in primary cancer, and rises in metastatic cancer especially involving the liver. Values are useful to indicate tumor activity. *0450* Increased in patients (2.2 g/L) compared to normals (1.1 g/L). *1025*

Urine Increase 24 h excretion and renal clearance were significantly increased in localized tumor patients compared to normals and disseminated cancer cases. Increased high molecular weight protein excretion implies glomerular injury in these patients. *1025*

Hematocrit *Blood Decrease* Anemia; may be the only symptom of carcinoma of the right side of colon (present in > 50% of these patients, usually hypochromic). *2467* Iron deficiency anemia is common, because of either gross or occult bleeding. *2199* In 35% of 154 patients at initial hospitalization for this disorder. *0781* Incidence of anemia between 22-74.6%. *2199*

Hemoglobin *Blood Decrease* Anemia; may be the only symptom of carcinoma of the right side of colon (present in > 50% of these patients; usually hypochromic. *2467* Incidence of anemia between 22-74.6%. Iron deficiency anemia is common, because of either gross or occult bleeding. *2199* In 45% of 153 patients at initial hospitalization for this disorder. *0781*

Hexokinase *Serum Increase* Increased in gastrointestinal tumors. Mean = 15.3 ± 3.5 compared to normal, 0.93 ± 0.28 U/L. *1201*

Immunoglobulin IgA *Urine Increase* 24 h excretion and renal clearance were significantly increased in localized tumor patients compared to normals and disseminated cancer cases. Increased high molecular weight protein excretion implies glomerular injury in these patients. *1025*

Immunoglobulin IgG *Urine Increase* 24 h excretion and renal clearance were significantly increased in localized tumor patients compared to normals and disseminated cancer cases. Increased high molecular weight protein excretion implies glomerular injury in these patients. *1025*

Immunoglobulin IgM *Urine Increase* 24 h excretion and renal clearance were significantly increased in localized tumor patients compared to normals and disseminated cancer cases. Increased high molecular weight protein excretion implies glomerular injury in these patients. *1025*

Iron *Serum Decrease* Iron deficiency anemia is common, because of either gross or occult bleeding. *2199* In 57% of 19 patients at initial hospitalization for this disorder. *0781*

Iron-Binding Capacity, Total (TIBC) *Serum Decrease* Significantly reduced (median = 2.6 mg/L) compared to controls (3.4 mg/L). 24 h excretion and renal clearance of transferrin were significantly increased in localized tumor patients compared to normals and disseminated cancer cases. Increased high molecular weight protein excretion implies glomerular injury in these patients. *1025* In 10% of 19 patients at initial hospitalization for this disorder. *0781*

Iron Saturation *Serum Decrease* In 67% of 19 patients at initial hospitalization for this disorder. *0781*

Lactate Dehydrogenase *Serum Increase* Marked elevation in 20 patients, mean = 162.0 U/L (compared to 85.4 ± 1.0 U/L). *1201 0992*

Lactic Acid *Blood Increase* In patients with tumors of the gastrointestinal tract, mean concentration was 21.5 ± 5.7 mg/dL compared to normal, 11.7 ± 0.72 mg/dL. *1201*

Leukocytes *Blood Increase* May be noted in patients with inflammatory complications, such as necrosis of tumor, or local colonic perforation. *2199* In 25% of 154 patients at initial hospitalization for this disorder. *0781*

Ascitic Fluid Increase > 1000 μL. *2626*

Lithocholic Acid *Feces Increase* The fecal excretion of cholesterol, coprostanol, coprostanone, total bile acids, deoxycholic acid, lithocholic acid was higher in colonic cancer and adenomatous polyps compared to normal controls as well as in patients with other digestive diseases. *1896*

MCH *Blood Decrease* Anemia; may be the only symptom of carcinoma of the right side of the colon (present in > 50% of these patients, usually hypochromic). *2467* Iron deficiency anemia is common because of either gross or occult bleeding. *2199*

MCHC *Blood Decrease* Anemia; may be the only symptom of carcinoma of the right colon (present in > 50% of these patients, usually hypochromic). *2467* Iron deficiency anemia is common because of either gross or occult bleeding. *2199*

MCV *Blood Decrease* Many patients have chronic iron deficiency anemia characterized by hypochromic microcytic red cells. *2199*

Monocytes *Blood Increase* In 57% of 150 patients at initial hospitalization for this disorder. *0781*

Occult Blood *Feces Positive* The most important screening test for cancer of the large bowel in asymptomatic persons. *2549* GI bleeding may occur with malignancies. *2199*

Parathyroid Hormone *Serum Increase* Lung cancer, hypernephroma, gastrointestinal cancer, and other neoplasms can synthesize and secrete parathyroid hormone. *0962*

Platelet Count *Blood Increase* In 30% of 118 patients at initial hospitalization for this disorder. *0781*

Potassium *Serum Decrease* Villous tumor of rectum may cause depletion. *2467*

Protein *Serum Decrease* May be lower than normal in carcinoma of colon. *2199* Enteric loss of plasma protein. *2199*

Ascitic Fluid Increase > 2.5 g/dL. *2626*

Pyruvate *Blood Increase* Moderately elevated in 8 patients with tumors of the gastrointestinal tract. Mean = 1.93 ± 0.18 U/L. *1201*

Uric Acid *Serum Increase* In 35% of 149 patients at initial hospitalization for this disorder. *0781*

Zinc *Serum Decrease* In 35 cases of primary malignant tumors of the digestive organs, plasma concentrations were decreased 0.83 ± 0.18 ppm. *1125*

154.10 Malignant Neoplasm of Rectum

Aldolase *Serum Increase* Significantly elevated in tumors of the gastrointestinal tract. Mean = 4.9 ± 0.8 U/L compared to normal, 1.6 ± 0.21. *1201*

Alpha$_2$-Globulin *Serum Increase* alpha$_2$-globulins, especially haptoglobins, were generally increased in primary colorectal cancer, and the liver. Haptoglobin values were useful to indicate tumor activity. *0450*

Androgens *Urine Decrease* Significantly decreased, 1.86 ± 0.20 mg/g creatinine in 16 male patients. *2333*

Androsterone *Urine Decrease* Significantly decreased, 1.86 ± 0.20 mg/g creatinine in 16 male patients. *2333*

Carcinoembryonic Antigen *Serum Increase* In 73% of cases. *2199* In 66% of patients with localized upper GI tract malignancy, mean = 4.9 ng/mL. *1817 2035 0795*

Pleural Effusion Increase The highest levels (> 1,000 ng/mL) were found in samples from patients with gastrointestinal carcinomas. *0622* 24 (34%) of 70 malignant effusions had levels > 12 ng/mL. *1945*

Ascitic Fluid Increase CEA > 10 ng/mL ascites indicating cancerous effusion. *1420*

Peritoneal Fluid Increase The highest levels (> 1,000 ng/mL were found in patients with gastrointestinal carcinomas. *0622*

Complement C3 *Serum Increase* Increased in patients with local disease. Found to be very closely linked to the stage of the disease. Patients in remission had normal levels, but further increases were noted in distant metastases. Dropped significantly in the terminal phase of disease. *2427*

Complement C4 *Serum Increase* Increased in patients with local disease. Very closely linked to the stage of the disease. Patients in remission had normal levels, but further increases were noted in distant metastases. Levels dropped significantly in the terminal phase of disease. *2427*

Hematocrit *Blood Decrease* Iron deficiency anemia is common, because of either gross or occult bleeding. *2199*

Hemoglobin *Blood Decrease* Iron deficiency anemia is common, because of either gross or occult bleeding. *2199*

Hexokinase *Serum Increase* Increased in gastrointestinal tumors. Mean = 15.3 ± 3.5 compared to normal, 0.93 ± 0.28 U/L. *1201*

Iron *Serum Decrease* Iron deficiency anemia is common, because of either gross or occult bleeding. *2199*

Iron-Binding Capacity, Total (TIBC) *Serum Increase* Anemia is commonly iron deficient, due to chronic blood loss. *2199*

Iron Saturation *Serum Decrease* Anemia is commonly iron deficient type, due to chronic blood loss. *2199*

Leukocytes *Blood Increase* May be noted in patients with inflammatory complications of their carcinoma, such as necrosis of tumor, or local colonic perforation. *2199*

MCH *Blood Decrease* Iron deficiency anemia is common because of either gross or occult bleeding. *2199*

MCHC *Blood Decrease* Iron deficiency anemia is common because of either gross or occult bleeding. *2199*

MCV *Blood Decrease* Many patients have chronic iron deficiency anemia characterized by hypochromic microcytic red cells. *2199*

Monocytes *Blood Increase* In 59% of 74 patients at initial hospitalization for this disorder. *0781*

Occult Blood *Feces Positive* The most important screening test for cancer of the large bowel in asymptomatic persons. *2549* GI bleeding may occur with malignancies. *2199*

Protein *Serum Decrease* May be lower than normal in carcinoma of colon. *2199*

Uric Acid *Serum Increase* In 43% of 73 patients at initial hospitalization for this disorder. *0781*

155.00 Malignant Neoplasm of Liver

^{131}I Uptake *Serum Increase* In hepatic disease. *2104*

5'-Nucleotidase *Serum Increase* 88.4% of 51 hepatoma patients had values > 10% above the normal upper limit. *1115 0503*

Adenosine Deaminase *Serum Increase* Increased in obstructive jaundice seen with neoplastic disease. *0655 1737 2235*

Alanine Aminotransferase *Serum Increase* In all cases of intrahepatic malignant disease, values were above normal, and all but 1 showed higher AST than ALT. ALT values ranged from 31-43 U/L. *2576* Elevated in only 34% of 32 patients with primary hepatoma (normal = 2.4-17 U/L). *0029*

Albumin *Serum Decrease* Mean values were found to be highest in the healthy subjects followed by acute viral hepatitis, primary hepatocellular carcinoma and cirrhosis, in that order. Both the mean albumin and mean total globulin of each group of subjects were significantly different from the respective means of the other 3 groups. *0724* Reversed A/G ratio in 54% of 51 hepatoma patients. *1115* In 42% of 14 patients at initial hospitalization for this disorder. *0781*

Aldolase *Serum Increase* *0962*

Alkaline Phosphatase *Serum Increase* Due to obstruction, elevated in 88% of patients with primary cancer. *0029* Elevated in 95-100% of primary cancers, usually ranging from 80-215 U/L, with only 80% having values 107 U/L. *0503* Usually moderately elevated; 40-50% of patients have concentration between 20-75 U/L and 15-30% are above 81 U/L. *0364* Elevated in 80.5% of 62 patients with hepatoma. *1115* In about 80% of cases. *0962* In 90% of 12 patients at initial hospitalization for this disorder. *0781 0151*

Alkaline Phosphatase Isoenzymes *Serum Increase* Of 15 cases all had increased values of isoenzyme-I and 6 had increased isoenzyme-IV as well. *1221*

Alpha$_1$-Antitrypsin *Serum Increase* Significant elevation compared with controls (n = 58). *0700*

Alpha$_1$-Glycoprotein *Serum Increase* It was found to have a sensitivity of 65% and a specificity of 80% with severe liver disease. *0709*

Alpha$_2$-Globulin *Serum Increase* alpha$_2$-globulins, especially haptoglobins, were generally increased in primary colorectal cancer, and the liver. Haptoglobin values were useful to indicate tumor activity. *0450*

Alpha$_2$-Macroglobulin *Serum Increase* Moderate elevation. *1082*

Alpha-Fetoprotein *Serum Increase* Detectable in 14 of 19 (76%) patients. *0029* Incidence of positivity varies with geographical area from 50-90%; in this country 50% is a more accurate estimate. Serum concentration > 500 ng/mL indicates hepatoma 97% of the time. Postoperative serial determinations show an exponential fall to normal when the tumor has been completely excised. Recurrence of elevated levels indicates tumor recurrence. *2583* Above 30 ng/mL in 69%. Levels declined as age increased. Appeared to be related to the tumor cell type: the relatively immature *0036 0383 2116*

Pleural Effusion Increase Positive results were most frequently found in samples derived from patients with liver tumors. The highest levels (6 and 30 ng/mL), were determined in samples of two hepatoma patients. *0622*

Aminolevulinic Acid *Urine Increase* May occur. *0503*

Antithrombin III *Plasma Decrease* Decreased in parenchymatous liver disease. *2353 1482*

Antithyroglobulin Antibodies *Serum Increase* Rare. *1736*

Aspartate Aminotransferase *Serum Increase* Levels may be 10-100 X normal and remain elevated for long periods. *0812* Elevated from 2-5 X the normal level in 66-70% of patients with primary carcinoma. *0029* Elevated in 80%. *0364* Over 10% above normal upper limit in 83.3% of 66 hepatoma patients. *1115* In 98% of 12 patients at initial hospitalization for this disorder. *0781*

Beta-Glucuronidase *Serum Increase* Increased. *0741 0866*

Bilirubin *Serum Increase* In patients with primary tumors, values ranged from 3.5-5.2 mg/dL (normal < 1.0). *2576* Commonly found (60-70%), but concentration > 85 mmol/L were found in only 10-25% of patients. *0364* Over 10% above upper limit of normal in 43.2% in 67 cases of hepatoma. *1115* In 38% of 13 patients at initial hospitalization for this disorder. *0781*

BSP Retention *Serum Increase* Increased retention in 90% of cases. *0364*

Calcium *Serum Increase* A serious complication in many cases of hepatoma. *1246 1507* Sometimes present. Occasionally antedate the discovery of the tumor. *0962*

Carcinoembryonic Antigen *Serum Increase* In 67% of cases. *2199 0795 2035*

Ascitic Fluid Increase In malignant effusions. *2199*

155.00 Malignant Neoplasm of Liver (continued)

Cholesterol *Serum Decrease* The close relationship between serum levels of cholesterol and bile acids has been confirmed in 46 patients with primary hepatoma, serum levels of cholesterol and bile acids are roughly correlated with serum AFP. Because the relationship between serum cholesterol and bile acids did not exist in common hepatocellular diseases, the results suggest a peculiar sterol metabolism occurring in human hepatoma. *1050* 20-30% incidence. *0364*

Cholesterol, Low Density Lipoprotein *Serum Increase* Moderate increase secondary to lack of feedback inhibition of hepatic cholesterol synthesis by dietary cholesterol. *0062*

Cryofibrinogen *Serum Increase* *2035 1551*

Erythrocytes *Blood Increase* In the absence of systemic hypoxia, erythrocytosis may develop in hepatocellular carcinoma as a compensatory response to local liver hypoxia. *2377* Erythrocytosis occurs in about 11% of hepatoma patients with increased red cell mass and bone marrow erythroid hyperplasia. *0300 1507* Occasional erythrocytosis. *0962*

Ascitic Fluid Increase Strongly suggests neoplasm, especially hepatoma. *0151* A large number of RBC, especially grossly bloody ascites, suggests a neoplasm, particularly hepatoma or ovarian cancer. *2199* > 10,000 cells/μL seen in 20% of cases *0696*

Erythrocyte Sedimentation Rate *Blood Increase* Sometimes increased. *2467*

Erythropoietin *Serum Increase* Increased plasma concentrations are found in patients with erythrocytosis associated with several types of tumor, especially lung, kidney and liver. *0263 1416 1507*

Fibrin Split Products (FSP) *Ascitic Fluid Increase* In malignant effusions. *2199*

Fucose *Serum Increase* Markedly increased. *1342*

Gamma Glutamyl Transferase (GGT) *Serum Increase* *0503*

Saliva Increase Significantly higher (10.4 units/L) versus controls (5.12 U/L). *1164*

Globulin *Serum Increase* Mean values were found to be lowest in controls followed by acute viral hepatitis, primary hepatocellular carcinoma, and cirrhosis, in that order. *0724* Reversed A/G ratio in 54% of 51 hepatoma patients. *1115*

Glucose *Serum Decrease* 5-25% incidence. *0364* Hypoglycemia noted in about 30% of hepatoma patients in some studies. *1507* Sometimes present. Occasionally antedates the discovery of the tumor. *0962* Can occur with various types of liver disease. Hepatic hypoglycemia is a fasting hypoglycemia and often only transiently relieved by food. *0962 2104*

Gonadotropin, Chorionic *Serum Increase* Ectopic production. *0001 0265 0299 1691*

Hematocrit *Blood Decrease* In 35% of 14 patients at initial hospitalization for this disorder. *0781*

Hemoglobin *Blood Decrease* In 49% of 14 patients at initial hospitalization for this disorder. *0781*

Hepatitis B Surface Antigen *Serum Increase* Reported incidence varies from 5-80%. *0364* Prevalence of antigen in sera varies with geographic location; 40% incidence was found in an African study and 80% in a study in Taiwan. *1507*

Immunoglobulin IgA *Serum Normal* *2467*

Immunoglobulin IgG *Serum Normal* *2467*

Immunoglobulin IgM *Serum Decrease* *2467*

Lactate Dehydrogenase *Serum Increase* Useful in detecting metastatic or primary liver cancer due to marked sensitivity to carcinomatosis and insensitivity to noncancerous parenchymal hepatic damage. *0503* Significant elevation occurred in 66% of patients. *0029* 70-85% incidence of elevation. *0364* In 83% of 13 patients at initial hospitalization for this disorder. *0781*

Ascitic Fluid Increase In malignant effusions. *2199*

Lactate Dehydrogenase Isoenzyme 5 (LD$_5$) *Serum Increase* Elevated to a mean of 13% of total LD values (normal = 0-6%). *0852*

Leucine Aminopeptidase *Serum Increase* *0503*

Leukocytes *Blood Increase* Sometimes increased. *2467* In 45% of 13 patients at initial hospitalization for this disorder. *0781*

Ascitic Fluid Increase > 1000/μL. *2626*

Lipids *Serum Increase* Sometimes present. Occasionally antedates the discovery of the tumor. *0962*

Malate Dehydrogenase *Serum Increase* In neoplastic disease. *0503*

Monocytes *Blood Increase* In 73% of 12 patients at initial hospitalization for this disorder. *0781*

Neutrophils *Blood Increase* *2538*

Occult Blood *Feces Positive* GI bleeding may occur with malignancies. *2199*

Ornithine Carbamoyl Transferase (OCT) *Serum Increase* Liver cell damage. *2467*

Plasma Cells *Serum Decrease* Depressed. *2357 0659 0683*

Platelet Count *Blood Increase* In 46% of 13 patients at initial hospitalization for this disorder. *0781*

Progesterone *Plasma Increase* Raised in 36 of 50 men with liver disease compared with 20 healthy male control subjects. Significantly higher in men with nonalcoholic cirrhosis with gynecomastic than those without. *0704*

Prolactin *Serum Increase* Found in 14% of men with liver disease. Levels unrelated to presence of gynecomastia. *0704*

Proline Hydroxylase *Serum Increase* Markedly elevated in hepatoma, and to a lesser extent lymphosarcoma and pheochromocytoma. *0364*

Protein *Ascitic Fluid Increase* > 2.5 g/dL. *2626*

Prothrombin Time *Plasma Increase* Prolonged in 26.6% of patients. *1115* Abnormal in 21 of 24 hepatoma patients with cirrhosis and 11 of 16 without cirrhosis in tests done within 1 month of death. *1783*

Thymol Turbidity *Serum Increase* *0503*

155.10 Malignant Neoplasm of Intrahepatic Bile Ducts

Alanine Aminotransferase *Serum Increase* Found in all cases of malignant disease of biliary tract; ranging from 65.5-87 U/L. *2576*

Alkaline Phosphatase *Serum Increase* In all cases; elevated from 94-263 U/L (normal = 25 U/L) due to common duct obstruction. *2576*

Alkaline Phosphatase Isoenzymes *Serum Increase* Regan isoenzyme concentration was 27.6 U/L. *0549*

Aspartate Aminotransferase *Serum Increase* May be slightly elevated, but rarely higher than 200 U/L. *0151*

Bilirubin *Serum Increase* Markedly elevated levels, ranging from 16.0-23.2 mg/dL. *2576* Values exceed 10 mg/dL in most cases, with a mean value of about 18 mg/dL. *0151*

Carcinoembryonic Antigen *Ascitic Fluid Increase* In malignant effusions. *2199*

Cholesterol *Serum Increase* Averages about 400 mg/dL. *0151*

Cryofibrinogen *Serum Increase* *2035 1551*

Fibrin Split Products (FSP) *Ascitic Fluid Increase* In malignant effusions. *2199*

Occult Blood *Feces Positive* Frequently positive. *2467*

156.00 Malignant Neoplasm of Gallbladder

Alkaloids *Serum Increase* Increased. *0655 1737*

157.90 Malignant Neoplasm of Pancreas

5'-Nucleotidase *Serum Increase* Due to biliary tract obstruction, values range from 28.0-40.0 U/L (normal = 4.0). *2576* Values are elevated when there is an element of obstruction of the common bile duct or metastases to the liver. *0151 1312*

Alanine Aminotransferase *Serum Increase* Elevated due to extrahepatic biliary tract obstruction. *2576* In 40% of 10 patients at initial hospitalization for this disorder. *0781*

Albumin *Serum Decrease* In 44% of 46 patients at initial hospitalization for this disorder. *0781*

Alkaline Phosphatase *Serum Increase* Due to biliary tract obstruction values range from 150-215 U/L (normal = 21 U/L). *2576* Elevated without marked abnormalities in all liver function tests. *0267* Elevated in 85 of 100 patients with histologically proven disease. *0932* In 82% of 46 patients at initial hospitalization for this disorder. *0781 0151*

Leukocyte Decrease Low activity is present irrespective of tumor category, activity of disease, or type of therapy. In 11 patients, median activity was 5 U/L (normal = 55). *1423*

Alkaline Phosphatase Isoenzymes *Serum Increase* Highest concentrations were found in sera of patients with cancer of the pancreas. Ranges were 11.8-81.4 U/L. *0549*

Alpha$_1$-Antitrypsin *Serum Increase* Significantly higher than controls. Pancreatic Ca. patients average 487 mg/dL, Controls average 434 mg/dL. *2370* Only 3 of 16 patients had elevated levels. *1856*

Alpha-Fetoprotein *Serum Increase* Over 50 ng/mL in 10-15% of cases. *2116*

Amylase *Serum Decrease* Slightly increased in early stages (< 10% of cases). With later destruction of pancreas, normal or decreased. *2467*

Serum Increase May be slightly increased in early stages (< 10% of cases). With later destruction of pancreas, normal or decreased. *2467* Early obstruction of the pancreatic duct. *0151* Elevated serum and urinary S-amylase has been reported. *2151* Hyperamylasemia found in only 9% of 100 histologically proven cases. *0932* May be mildly elevated in a few patients as a result of pancreatitis secondary to an obstructing tumor. *2199* In 35% of 14 patients at initial hospitalization for this disorder. *0781*

Serum Normal May be slightly increased in early stages (< 10% of cases). With later destruction of pancreas, normal or decreased. *2467*

Urine Increase 1 h excretion is increased in up to 30% of patients. *0992* Elevated serum and urinary S-amylase has been reported. *2151* May be mildly elevated in a few patients as a result of pancreatitis secondary to an obstructing tumor. *2199*

Pleural Effusion Increase Carcinoma of the pancreas and other organs. *1405*

Aspartate Aminotransferase *Serum Increase* Slight elevation occurred in 2 of 4 cases. Range of values was 12.5-45, while the maximum upper limit of normal is 24 U/L. *1452* 63% of patients showed elevated values. *0932* In 74% of 46 patients at initial hospitalization for this disorder. *0781*

Beta-Glucuronidase *Serum Increase* Increased. *0741 0866*

Bicarbonate *Duodenal Contents Decrease* Acinar destruction (as in pancreatitis) shows normal volume (20-30 mL/10 min collection period) but bicarbonate and enzyme levels may be decreased. In carcinoma, the test result depends on the relative extent and combination of acinar destruction and of duct obstruction. *2467*

Duodenal Contents Normal Secretin-pancreozymin stimulation evidences duct obstruction when duodenal intubation shows decreased volume of duodenal contents (< 10 mL/10 min collection period) with usually normal bicarbonate and enzyme levels in duodenal contents. *2467*

Bilirubin *Serum Increase* Markedly elevated with values ranging from 4.0-17.9 mg/dL. *2576* May become significantly elevated with direct fraction greater than the indirect fraction. *0433* Increased (12-25 mg/dL), mostly direct. Increase is persistent and nonfluctuating. *2467* Elevated without marked abnormalities in liver all function tests. *0267* In 39% of 46 patients at initial hospitalization for this disorder. *0781*

Bilirubin, Direct *Serum Increase* In 91% of 14 patients at initial hospitalization for this disorder. *0781*

Bilirubin, Indirect *Serum Increase* In 56% of 14 patients at initial hospitalization for this disorder. *0781*

Calcium *Serum Increase* Without evidence of direct bone involvement. Parathyroid hormone-secreting tumors. *0503 1509*

Urine Decrease No evidence of direct bone involvement. Parathyroid hormone-secreting tumors. *0503*

Carcinoembryonic Antigen *Serum Increase* Elevated levels were noted in 33% of the patients with tumors localized to the pancreas. When the carcinoma had extended beyond the pancreas or distant metastases were present, 78% of patients had elevated levels. *1767* In 92% of cases. *2199 2035 0795*

Ascitic Fluid Increase In malignant effusions. *2199*

Carotene *Serum Decrease* Secondary to malabsorption. *2199*

Cephalin Flocculation *Serum Normal* Usually normal. *2467*

Cholesterol *Serum Decrease* In 27% of 43 patients at initial hospitalization for this disorder. *0781*

Serum Increase May remain normal until late in the disease. *0433* Increased (usually > 300 mg/dL) with esters not decreased. *2467*

Complement C3 *Serum Increase* Increased in patients with local disease. Very closely linked to the stage of the disease, patients in remission had normal levels, but further increases were noted in distant metastases. Dropped significantly in the terminal phase of disease. *2427*

Complement C4 *Serum Increase* Increased in patients with local disease. Very closely linked to the stage of the disease. Patients in remission had normal levels, but further increases were noted in distant metastases. Levels dropped significantly in the terminal phase of disease. *2427*

Complement, Total *Serum Increase* Very closely linked to the stage of the disease. Patients in remission had normal levels, but further increases were noted in distant metastases. Dropped significantly in the terminal phase of disease. *2427*

Corticotropin *Plasma Increase* Uncommon. *1562*

Cryofibrinogen *Serum Increase* *2035 1551*

Erythrocytes *Ascitic Fluid Increase* Grossly bloody ascites suggests neoplasm. *2199*

Fat *Feces Increase* Steatorrhea is found in approximately 10% of the cases as judged by abnormal chemical fat excretion. *0151* Deficient intraluminal pancreatic enzymes. *2199*

Fibrin Split Products (FSP) *Plasma Increase* *1253*

Ascitic Fluid Increase In malignant effusions. *2199*

Fucose *Serum Increase* Markedly increased. *1342*

Gamma Glutamyl Transferase (GGT) *Serum Increase* Greatest in cases of primary carcinoma of the head of the pancreas and adenocarcinoma of bile duct. In 4 patients range was 264-1,040 U/L, mean = 590. *1452* In 100% of 10 patients at initial hospitalization for this disorder. *0781*

Glucagon *Plasma Decrease* Decreased. *0306 0620 0513*

Glucose *Serum Decrease* In children. Decreased due to excess insulin. *0619 0812*

Serum Increase 59% of 100 patients had fasting hyperglycemia. *0932* Diabetes mellitus occurs in 25-50% of cases and is manifest most frequently as an abnormal glucose tolerance test rather than overt glucosuria or fasting hyperglycemia. *2199* In 46% of 46 patients at initial hospitalization for this disorder. *0781*

Urine Increase Diabetes mellitus occurs in 25-50% of cases and is manifest most frequently as an abnormal glucose tolerance test rather than overt glucosuria or fasting hyperglycemia. *2199*

Glucose Tolerance *Serum Decrease* Test is abnormal in 25-50% of patients and is a more frequent abnormality than frank glycosuria or fasting hyperglycemia. *0151* Abnormal in 25-50% of patients. More frequently than frank glucosuria or fasting hyperglycemia. *2199*

Glutamic Acid *Serum Increase* High levels of glutamic acid and normal glutamine levels were found in 9 of 10 patients. Mean value = 3.40 ± 2.22 mg/dL. *0359*

Glutamine *Serum Normal* High levels of glutamic acid and normal glutamine levels were found in 9 of 10 patients. Mean value = 3.40 ± 2.22 mg/dL. *0359*

Gonadotropin, Chorionic *Serum Increase* Elevated immunoreactive hCG was found in 33% of patients. *0740*

Hematocrit *Blood Decrease* 34% of patients were anemic. *0932* In 33% of 46 patients at initial hospitalization for this disorder. *0781*

Hemoglobin *Blood Decrease* In 41% of 45 patients at initial hospitalization for this disorder. *0781*

Isocitrate Dehydrogenase *Serum Increase* *0619*

Lactate Dehydrogenase *Serum Increase* In 24% of 46 patients at initial hospitalization for this disorder. *0781*

Ascitic Fluid Increase In malignant effusions. *2199*

Lactate Dehydrogenase Isoenzyme 5 (LD$_5$) *Serum Increase* Mild elevation to a mean of 13% of total LD in patients with carcinoma of the liver, gallbladder and pancreas (normal = 0-6%). *0852*

Lactate Dehydrogenase Isoenzymes *Serum Increase* Elevated LD$_2$ and LD$_3$. *0503*

Leucine Aminopeptidase *Serum Increase* In 3 cases without hepatic metastases, all had markedly elevated values ranging from 430-730 U/L. *0281* Consistently elevated. *0341* Variable, especially if there is no associated increase in either serum alkaline phosphatase or serum AST. *0619* When there is an element of obstruction of the common bile duct or metastasis to the liver. *0151*

Urine Increase Marked increase. *0619* Over 300 U/L in 60% of patients due to liver metastases or biliary tract obstruction. May also be increased in chronic liver disease. *2467*

Leukocytes *Blood Increase* Over 12,000/μL in 12% of histologically proven cases. *0932* In 32% of 46 patients at initial hospitalization for this disorder. *0781*

Ascitic Fluid Normal Variable *2626*

Lipase *Serum Decrease* May be slightly increased in early stages (< 10% of cases); with later destruction, they are normal or decreased. *2467*

Serum Increase May be slightly increased in early stages (< 10% of cases); with later destruction, they are normal or decreased. *2467* Early obstruction of the pancreatic duct will occasionally elevate. *0151* Increased in 38% of 100 histologically proven cases. *0932*

Lipids *Feces Increase* Reduced intraluminal pancreatic enzyme activity with maldigestion of lipid and protein. *0962*

Monocytes *Blood Increase* In 68% of 46 patients at initial hospitalization for this disorder. *0781*

157.90   Malignant Neoplasm of Pancreas   *(continued)*

Neutrophils   *Blood   Increase*   Neutrophilic leukemoid reactions occur most frequently with gastric, bronchogenic, and pancreatic carcinomas. *2538*

Occult Blood   *Feces   Positive*   Often found. *0992*

Potassium   *Serum   Decrease*   Gastrointestinal wasting as a result of pancreatic islet nonbeta cell tumors. *1679*   In 30% of 33 patients at initial hospitalization for this disorder. *0781*

Protein   *Ascitic Fluid   Increase*   Variable but often > 2.5 g/dL in ascitic fluid. *2626*

Feces   Increase   Reduced intraluminal pancreatic enzyme activity with maldigestion of lipid and protein. *0962*

Peritoneal Fluid   Increase   Greater than 30 g/L in 70% of cases of pancreatic ascites. *0586*

Prothrombin Time   *Plasma   Increase*   May be increased but will be correctable with parenterally administered vitamin K. *0433*

Thymol Turbidity   *Serum   Increase*   May be slightly elevated, usually normal. *0433*

Trypsin   *Serum   Increase*   Mean serum concentration in 7 patients was 394 U/L (normal < 100 U). *1678*

Uric Acid   *Serum   Increase*   In 29% of 46 patients at initial hospitalization for this disorder. *0781*

Urobilinogen   *Urine   Decrease*   Absent in carcinoma of head of pancreas. *2467*

Feces   Decrease   Absent in cancer of head of pancreas. *2467*

162.90   Malignant Neoplasm of Bronchus and Lung

2,3-Diphosphoglycerate   *Red Blood Cells   Increase*   Synthesis is increased in response to hypoxia. *0159*

5-Hydroxyindoleacetic Acid (5-HIAA)   *Urine   Increase*   Oat-cell carcinoma of the bronchus and bronchial adenoma of carcinoid type may cause excess secretion. *0619*   Rarely a carcinoid syndrome is associated with bronchogenic carcinoma with the laboratory manifestation of abnormal urinary levels of 5-HIAA. *0962*

5-Hydroxytryptamine (Serotonin)   *Blood   Increase*   Oat-cell carcinoma of the bronchus and bronchial adenoma of carcinoid type may cause excessive secretion. *0619*   Rarely a carcinoid syndrome is associated with bronchogenic carcinoma with the laboratory manifestation of abnormal urinary levels of 5-HIAA. *0962*

17-Hydroxycorticosteroids   *Urine   Increase*   Ectopic ACTH production. *0536*

17-Ketogenic Steroids   *Urine   Increase*   Ectopic ACTH production. *0536*

Acid Phosphatase   *Serum   Increase*   In a series of 25 cases of lung cancer 36% had elevated levels. Acid phosphatase is of no value as a marker for lung cancer. *1637*

Albumin   *Serum   Decrease*   Significantly reduced (median = 35.7 g/L) in patients with carcinoma compared to controls (44.0 g/L). *1025*

Urine   Increase   24 h excretion and renal clearance were significantly increased in localized tumor patients compared to normals and disseminated cancer cases. Increased high molecular weight protein excretion implies glomerular injury in these patients. *1025*

Aldolase   *Serum   Increase*   Slightly elevated in bronchogenic carcinomas. Mean = 2.8 ± 0.6 U/L compared to normal, 1.6 ± 0.21. *1201*

Alkaline Phosphatase   *Serum   Increase*   Elevated shortly before death or with tumor extension. Little diagnostic use but helpful in detecting metastases to bone. *0819*   In 9 patients, initial values ranged from 43-263 U/L (normal < 105 U/L). *2267*

Leukocyte   Decrease   Low activity is present irrespective of tumor category, activity of disease, or type of therapy. In 12 patients median activity was 8 U/L (normal = 55). *1423*

Alpha₁-Globulin   *Serum   Increase*   Increased in squamous, large and small cell carcinoma and adenocarcinoma of lung. A 2-fold decrease in trypsin inhibitory capacity was also found in association. *0989*

Alpha₁-Glycoprotein   *Pleural Effusion   Increase*   Highest levels found in malignant exudates. *1239 1672 1866   1947 2096 2170*

Amylase   *Serum   Increase*   May occur. *0178*   Markedly increased in serum, urine and tumor tissue. *2598*

Urine   Increase   Markedly increased in serum, urine and tumor tissue. *2598*

Pleural Effusion   Increase   High pleural fluid concentrations may occur. *0662*   Elevated in primary or metastatic lung cancer, pancreatitis, or esophageal perforation. *2031*

Pleural Effusion   Normal   Usually less than or equal to serum level. *2017*

Angiotensin-Converting Enzyme (ACE)   *Serum   Decrease*   In 141 patients with newly diagnosed primary lung cancer it was found to be lower than in the control group. This suggests that low levels may be associated with a poor prognosis in this condition. *1967 1501*

Antidiuretic Hormone   *Serum   Increase*   Inappropriate secretion of ADH is associated with hyponatremia, decreased serum osmolality, and inappropriately high sodium concentration in the urine. The entire syndrome resolves following resection of the tumor. *0962*

Aspartate Aminotransferase   *Serum   Increase*   Becomes elevated only shortly before death. In most cases, elevated values indicate the presence of metastases. *0819*

Calcitonin   *Serum   Increase*   Elevated in 75% of patients with oat cell carcinoma. *1553*   8 of 11 patients with oat cell carcinoma (including 4 with skeletal metastases) had concentrations > 0.1 ng/mL, ranging up to 5 ng/mL. *0445*   Elevated in 54 (68%) of 79 patients with small cell carcinoma. 20 patients (25%) had levels usually associated with medullary carcinoma of the thyroid. *0980*   Increase found in both thyroid and bronchogenic carcinomas. Medullary thyroid cancer is characterized by the presence of at least 7 different fractions, ranging from fraction I (> 30,000 molecular weight) to V (2,500 molecular weight). Bronchogenic cancers had a predominance of high molecular weight fractions (I and IIa). *0146*   High levels can also be produced ectopically by small cell cancer of the lung. *0962 1589*

Calcium   *Serum   Increase*   In squamous cell neoplasm without evidence of direct bone involvement. Parathyroid hormone-secreting tumors. *0503*   Frequent hypercalcemia in advanced cases. *0393*

Carcinoembryonic Antigen   *Serum   Increase*   Very high titers have been found in 76% of patients. *0431*   88 of 115 (or 77%) of patients had an initial concentration > 2.5 ng/mL. Of 28 patients with concentration 15 ng/mL at the time of initial examination, 27 were found to have locally extensive or disseminated disease. *2432*   Found in > 50 % of the patients *0925*   Concentrations > 40 µg/L were found in 40.6% of patients with oat cell carcinoma. *1553*   In 72% of cases. *2199   0795 2035*

Pleural Effusion   Increase   24 (34%) of 70 malignant effusions had levels > 12 ng/mL. *1945*

Ceruloplasmin   *Serum   Increase*   High in gastric and pulmonary cancer. *2058*

Complement C3   *Serum   Increase*   Increased in patients with local disease. Very closely linked to the stage of the disease. Patients in remission had normal levels, but further increases were noted in distant metastases. Levels dropped significantly in the terminal phase of the disease. *2427*

Complement C4   *Serum   Increase*   Increased in patients with local disease. Very closely linked to the stage of the disease. Patients in remission had normal levels, but further increases were noted in distant metastases. Levels dropped significantly in the terminal phase of disease. *2427*

Complement, Total   *Serum   Increase*   Closely linked to the stage of the disease. Patients in remission had normal levels, but further increases were noted in distant metastases. Levels dropped significantly in the terminal phase of disease. *2427*

Copper   *Serum   Increase*   Extremely high in 82% of the 34 patients. *1296*   Increased in stomach, lung and large intestine neoplasm. Serum ceruloplasmin was high in gastric and lung cancer but not in the large intestine. *2058*

Creatine Kinase   *Serum   Increase*   Highest activity of CK-BB in brain and smooth muscle. *1347*

Cryofibrinogen   *Serum   Increase*   *2035 1551*

Erythrocytes   *Pleural Effusion   Increase*   1000-> 100,000/µL. *2017 0962*

Erythropoietin   *Serum   Increase*   Increased plasma concentrations are found in patients with erythrocytosis associated with several types of tumor, especially lung, kidney and liver. *0263 1416 1507*

Ferritin   *Serum   Increase*   Increased levels were found in more than 50% of patients. *0925*

Fucose   *Serum   Increase*   Increased in patients with both malignant and benign tumors of breast, lung and stomach. The glycoprotein-bound fraction was very markedly elevated in cases of malignancy and not in benign disease. Mucoprotein fraction was raised in both diseases. *2331*   In 15 patients, mean = 15.98 ± 1.43. Normal value = 6.84 ± 0.13 mg/dL. *1342*

Globulin   *Serum   Increase*   Good correlation between hypergammaglobulinemia and neoplastic disease, especially bronchogenic carcinoma. *2104*

Glucose *Serum Decrease* Occasionally, bronchogenic carcinoma is associated with insulin-like activity which may be reflected by hypoglycemia. *0962*

Pleural Effusion Decrease Approximately 15% of malignancies have low concentrations in pleural fluids. *1403* Markedly reduced, 20 mg/dL or less, is very suggestive and virtually diagnostic of rheumatoid disease. A low level in the range of 40 mg/dL can be found in infectious processes and in malignant pleural effusions. *0962 0174*

Glycoproteins *Serum Increase* Increased levels found in > 50% of patients. *0925*

Gonadotropin, Chorionic *Serum Increase* Ectopic production. *0001 0265 0299 1691 0536*

Gonadotropin, Pituitary *Serum Increase* Gonadotropin activity is clinically manifested by gynecomastia and by elevated gonadotropin blood levels. *0962* All cell types of bronchogenic cancer can cause the syndrome of ectopic gonadotropin production. *0962* Anaplastic large cell carcinoma. *0799*

Growth Hormone *Serum Increase* Elevated. *0918*

Haptoglobin *Serum Increase* Increased to 2.2 g/L, compared to normals, 1.1 g/L. *1025*

Urine Increase 24 h excretion and renal clearance were significantly increased in localized tumor patients compared to normals and disseminated cancer cases. Increased high molecular weight protein excretion implies glomerular injury in these patients. *1025*

Hexokinase *Serum Increase* Significantly increased. Mean = 20.4 ± 5.4 compared to normal, 0.93 ± 0.28 U/L. *1201*

Immunoglobulin IgA *Urine Increase* 24 h excretion and renal clearance were significantly increased in localized tumor patients compared to normals and disseminated cancer cases. Increased high molecular weight protein excretion implies glomerular injury in these patients. *1025*

Immunoglobulin IgG *Urine Increase* 24 h excretion and renal clearance were significantly increased in localized tumor patients compared to normals and disseminated cancer cases. Increased high molecular weight protein excretion implies glomerular injury in these patients. *1025*

Immunoglobulin IgM *Urine Increase* 24 h excretion and renal clearance were significantly increased in localized tumor patients compared to normals and disseminated cancer cases. Increased high molecular weight protein excretion implies glomerular injury in these patients. *1025*

Iron-Binding Capacity, Total (TIBC) *Serum Decrease* Significantly reduced (median = 2.6 mg/L), compared to controls (3.4 mg/L). 24 h excretion and renal clearance were significantly increased in localized tumor patients compared to normals and disseminated cancer cases. Increased high molecular weight protein excretion implies glomerular injury in these patients. *1025*

Lactate Dehydrogenase *Serum Increase* Activity was frequently elevated in 30 patients with primary and 4 with secondary neoplasms. Activity increased with tumor extension and often in relation to chemotherapy, but provided little diagnostic or prognostic value, except to indicate metastases. *0819* Twice the normal mean in 53 patients with bronchogenic carcinomas. Mean = 175.1 ± 10.4 U/L compared to normals, 85.4 ± 1.0 U/L. *1201*

Pleural Effusion Increase Elevation in pleural fluid without concurrent rise in protein indicates malignancy. *1403* A markedly elevated pleural LD is consistent with neoplastic involvement of the pleura. Not specific for the diagnosis. *0962*

Lactate Dehydrogenase Isoenzymes *Pleural Effusion Increase* Pleural effusions with a predominant LD_2 are highly indicative of malignancy. *1403*

Lactic Acid *Blood Increase* In 5 patients with bronchogenic tumors, mean concentration was 13.7 ± 3.6 mg/dL compared to normal, 11.7 ± 0.72 mg/dL. *1201*

Lymphocytes *Pleural Effusion Increase* Pleural effusion with > 50% of the WBC as small lymphocytes are highly indicative of malignancy or tuberculosis. Of 96 such effusions, 43 were TB and 47 were cancerous. 47 of 90 patients with lung cancer had predominantly small lymphocytes in effusions. *1403* In patients with pulmonary tuberculosis, pulmonary malignancy or nonspecific pleuritis, the percentages and absolute numbers of B lymphocytes were significantly lower in pleural fluid than in peripheral blood. *1809*

Monocytes *Pleural Effusion Increase* Predominant cell type. *2017*

Neutrophils *Blood Increase* Neutrophilic leukemoid reactions occur most frequently with gastric, bronchogenic, and pancreatic carcinomas. *2538*

Osmolality *Serum Decrease* Inappropriate secretion of ADH is associated with hyponatremia, decreased serum osmolality, and inappropriately high sodium concentration in the urine. The entire syndrome resolves following resection of the tumor. *0962*

Oxygen Saturation *Blood Decrease* Impaired diffusion. *2104*

Parathyroid Hormone *Serum Increase* Lung cancer, hypernephroma, gastrointestinal cancer, and other neoplasms can synthesize and secrete parathyroid hormone. *0962*

pCO_2 *Blood Decrease* Impaired gas diffusion and the accompanying hyperventilation results in a low pCO_2, unless the defect is severe and CO_2 retention occurs in bronchiolar cell carcinoma. *2104*

pH *Pleural Effusion Decrease* Exudate (pH < 7.3). *0062*

Pleural Effusion Increase pH < 7.40 militates against malignancy, especially in the absence of infection and < 7.30 is rarely encountered in tuberculous pleural disease. *0962*

Platelet Count *Blood Increase* In a large proportion of patients. *2168 0532*

pO_2 *Blood Decrease* Impaired diffusion. *2104*

Prolactin *Serum Increase* Elevated. *0918*

Protein *Serum Increase* More than 3 g/L. *2467*

Pleural Effusion Increase Exudate. *2017*

Pyruvate *Blood Increase* Mildly elevated in 5 patients with bronchogenic carcinomas. Mean = 0.88 ± 0.13 U/L. *1201*

Rheumatoid Factor *Pleural Effusion Increase* May be present with rheumatoid disease, but may also be found in other types of pleural effusions (e.g., carcinoma, tuberculosis, bacterial pneumonia). *2467*

Sodium *Serum Decrease* Inappropriate secretion of ADH is associated with hyponatremia, decreased serum osmolality, and inappropriately high sodium concentration in the urine. The entire syndrome resolves following resection of the tumor. *0962*

Urine Increase Excessive excretion due to water retention resulting from abnormally regulated secretion of ADH. *0151* Inappropriate secretion of ADH is associated with hyponatremia, decreased serum osmolality, and inappropriately high sodium concentration in the urine. The entire syndrome resolves following resection of the tumor. *0962*

Specific Gravity *Pleural Effusion Increase* Exudate (> 1.016). *0062*

Thyroid Stimulating Hormone (TSH) *Serum Increase* ACTH producing small cell carcinoma. *0536*

Uric Acid *Serum Decrease* Hypouricemia accompanied hyponatremia (< 130 mmol/L) in 75% of patients with the syndrome of inappropriate antidiuretic hormone and small cell carcinoma of the lung. *1778 0962*

170.90 Malignant Neoplasm of Bone

Acid Phosphatase *Serum Increase* The multinucleated giant cells of giant cell tumors are rich in acid phosphatase yet only rarely is this enzyme elevated in the patient's serum. *0536*

Alkaline Phosphatase *Serum Increase* Marked increase up to 40 X normal in osteogenic forms, parallels clinical course. *2467* In predominantly osteolytic forms remains normal or only moderately increased. *0619* All groups of bone tumors showed a significant increase when compared to the norm. Maximum values were found in the group of osteosarcomas and minimum in that of fibrosarcomas. *0301* In 39% of 26 patients at initial hospitalization for this disorder. *0781 0503*

Serum Normal Usually normal in Ewing's sarcoma and other osteolytic tumors. *2467*

Aspartate Aminotransferase *Serum Increase* In 32% of 25 patients at initial hospitalization for this disorder. *0781*

Bence-Jones Protein *Urine Present* Uncommon in osteogenic sarcoma. *0619*

Calcium *Serum Increase* Lytic tumors involving bone can lead to nephrocalcinosis and renal failure. The most frequent cause of hypercalcemia. *0619 2467 0503*

Serum Normal Usually normal in Ewing's sarcoma and other osteolytic tumors. *2467*

Urine Increase Lytic tumors. *0503 0619*

Ceruloplasmin *Serum Increase* A highly significant increase over normal levels in sera from patients with osteosarcoma. *2155*

Complement, Total *Serum Increase* Levels from sera of 21 bone tumors showed normal or slightly elevated titers. *0369*

170.90   Malignant Neoplasm of Bone   (continued)

Copper   *Serum   Increase*   12 cases of osteosarcoma at various stages were analyzed. Elevations occurred in primary and metastatic cases. Patients with advanced cases had the highest levels. *0735* Significantly elevated in 18 patients with primary untreated osteogenic sarcoma (173 ± 30 μg/dL). *0276*

Cyclic Adenosine Monophosphate   *Urine   Decrease   0575*

Eosinophils   *Blood   Increase*   Increases in tumors involving the bone. *2467*

Hematocrit   *Blood   Decrease*   In 24% of 24 patients at initial hospitalization for this disorder. *0781*

Hemoglobin   *Blood   Decrease*   In 36% of 24 patients at initial hospitalization for this disorder. *0781*

Hydroxyproline   *Urine   Increase*   Marked elevation. *1693*

Lactate Dehydrogenase   *Serum   Increase*   In 36 patients with Ewing's sarcoma, pretreatment levels proved an extremely good indicator of which patients would ultimately develop metastases. 3 of 18 patients with levels below the total group median (201-214 U/L) developed metastases, while 16 of 18 patients with levels above the median developed metastatic spread (P < 0.001). *0279*   In 25% of 26 patients at initial hospitalization for this disorder. *0781*

Monocytes   *Blood   Increase*   In 61% of 24 patients at initial hospitalization for this disorder. *0781*

Phosphate   *Serum   Normal*   Usually normal in Ewing's Sarcoma and other osteolytic tumors. *2467*

Uric Acid   *Serum   Increase*   In 37% of 26 patients at initial hospitalization for this disorder. *0781*

Zinc   *Serum   Increase*   Patients with primary osteosarcoma had elevated levels, those with metastases had depressed levels. The ratio of serum copper/serum zinc in metastatic osteosarcoma patients is higher than in patients with primary osteosarcoma. Determination of serum copper and serum zinc in osteosarcoma patients may be of value in prognoses and therapy evaluation. Their ratio may be useful in discriminating between patients with primary and metastatic osteosarcoma. *0735*

172.90   Malignant Melanoma of Skin

Aldolase   *Serum   Increase*   Markedly elevated in melanoblastomas. Mean = 9.0 ± 2.9 compared to 1.6 ± 0.21 U/L. *1201*

Alkaline Phosphatase   *Leukocyte   Decrease*   Low activity is present irrespective of tumor category, activity of disease, or type of therapy. In 11 patients, median activity was 5 U/L (normal = 55). *1423*

Dopa (3,4-Dihydroxyphenylalanine)   *Serum   Increase*   Significantly increased (P < 0.001) in plasma of all 65 patients with active disease (stage II), 2.08 μg/L compared with 32 normal control values of 1.23 μg/L. *0696*

Eosinophils   *Blood   Increase*   *2538*

Hexokinase   *Serum   Increase*   Significantly increased in melanoblastomas. Mean 17.4 ± 3.5 compared to normal 0.93 ± 0.28 U/L. *1201*

Immunoglobulin IgD   *Serum   Decrease*   Malignant melanoma patients with metastases presented significant decreases in IgD and IgM subpopulations. *0185*

Immunoglobulin IgM   *Serum   Decrease*   Malignant melanoma patients with metastases presented significant decreases in IgD and IgM subpopulations. *0185*

Lactate Dehydrogenase   *Serum   Increase*   Marked elevation in 38 patients with melanoblastomas. Mean = 179.7 ± 20.0 U/L compared to normals, 85.4 ± 1.0 U/L. *1201*

Lymphocytes   *Blood   Decrease*   Active rosettes (T-EA) were decreased only in metastatic patients, while the total T population (T-ET) was decreased in all stages. Patients whose values were constant remained cancer free, while a reduction heralded the appearance of clinical and/or radiological signs of metastases. *0185*

Melanin   *Urine   Increase*   In some patients, when the urine is exposed to air for several h, colorless melanogens are oxidized to melanin and urine becomes deep brown and later black. Melanogenuria occurs in 25% of patients; it is said to be more frequent with extensive liver metastasis. It is not useful for judging completeness of removal or early recurrence. *2467*

Phosphate   *Serum   Decrease*   In 49% of 67 patients at initial hospitalization for this disorder. *0781*

Uric Acid   *Serum   Increase*   In 38% of 67 patients at initial hospitalization for this disorder. *0781*

174.90   Malignant Neoplasm of Breast

17-Ketosteroids   *Urine   Decrease*   Total 17-ketosteroids and the sum of the fractions were significantly decreased in comparison with controls. *0390*

Acid Phosphatase   *Serum   Increase*   Female patients with metastatic breast cancer, selected at random and including both treated and untreated cases, had a mean serum activity which was significantly (P < 0.001) above that seen in females with benign disease. *1921   0812 1157*

Albumin   *Serum   Decrease*   Significantly reduced (median = 35.7 g/L) in patients with carcinoma compared to controls (44.0 g/L). *1025*

Urine   Increase   24 h excretion and renal clearance were significantly increased in localized tumor patients compared to normals and disseminated cancer cases. Increased high molecular weight protein excretion implies glomerular injury in these patients. *1025*

Aldolase   *Serum   Increase*   Significantly elevated; mean = 4.8 ± 0.7 U/L compared to normal, 1.6 ± 0.21. *1201*

Alkaline Phosphatase   *Serum   Increase*   Mean level in patients without bone metastases was above the normal range. The mean levels with metastases to bone was even higher, with 56% of all cases above the normal range. *2566*

Serum   Normal   No significant elevation was found in patients without bone metastases. *1312*

Leukocyte   Decrease   Low activity is present irrespective of tumor category, activity of disease, or type of therapy. In 21 patients, median value = 25 U/L (normal = 55). *1423*

Alkaline Phosphatase Isoenzymes   *Serum   Increase*   Cancer of the ovary, endometrium, cervix and breast as a group exhibited the highest frequency of Regan isoenzyme (placental). *0326*

Alpha-Fetoprotein   *Serum   Increase*   Elevated *1348*

Alpha-Glucosidase   *Serum   Increase*   The elevations were observed when the disease was in an early clinical stage. *0808*

Androgens   *Plasma   Increase*   Plasma testosterone concentrations were measured in sequential samples from 6 women and were compared to concentrations in 6 control women matched for age, y since menopause, and parity. Concentrations in each cancer patient were significantly higher than in each matched control. *1543*

Urine   Decrease   Significantly decreased in comparison with controls. *0390*

Androsterone   *Urine   Decrease*   Significantly decreased in comparison with controls. *0390*

Aspartate Aminotransferase   *Serum   Increase*   In 25% of 296 patients at initial hospitalization for this disorder. *0781*

Beta-Glucuronidase   *Serum   Increase*   Increased. *0741 0866*

Calcitonin   *Serum   Normal*   In 107 patients with breast cancer; CEA, ferritin and calcitonin levels were measured. CEA and ferritin but not calcitonin levels were statistically higher in those patients with metastases. *0200*

Calcium   *Serum   Increase*   Neoplasm without evidence of direct bone involvement. Parathyroid hormone-secreting tumors. Metastatic or lytic tumors involving bone. *0503*   Frequent hypercalcemia in advanced cases. *0393*

Urine   Increase   *0503*

Carcinoembryonic Antigen   *Serum   Increase*   12 of 17 patients had initially elevated values. Levels in later stages of the disease were usually higher than those in earlier stages. Referring to the international TNM classification, values were particularly elevated in both the T_3 and T_4 stages, with axillary node involvement and with the presence of bone metastases. *2374*   In 52% of cases. *2199 0200   0795 2035*

Pleural Effusion   Increase   24 (34%) of 70 malignant effusions had levels > 12 ng/mL. *1945*

Ascitic Fluid   Increase   4 of 6 breast cancer patients were detected by CEA estimations in ascitic fluid. Values > 10 ng/mL were considered cancerous effusions. *1420*

Complement C3   *Serum   Increase*   Increased in patients with local disease. Very closely linked to the stage of the disease. Patients in remission had normal levels, but further increases were noted in distant metastases. Dropped significantly in the terminal phase of the disease. *2427*

Complement C4   *Serum   Increase*   Increased in patients with local disease. Very closely linked to the stage of the disease. Patients in remission had normal levels, but further increases were noted in distant metastases. Levels dropped significantly in the terminal phase of the disease. *2427*

Complement, Total *Serum Increase* Very closely linked to the stage of the disease. Patients in remission had normal levels, but further increases were noted in distant metastases. Levels dropped significantly in the terminal phase of disease. *2427*

Copper *Serum Increase* All 23 patients demonstrated elevations (299 ± 34 mg/dL) compared to normal (108 ± 10 mg/dL). *0519 2094*

C-Reactive Protein *Serum Increase* 14 of 16 patients with overt metastases had elevated C-reactive proteins (> 10 mg/L). *0446*

Erythrocyte Sedimentation Rate *Blood Increase* Extreme elevation frequently occurs. *2467* In 385 patients, the frequency distribution curve was found to be distorted when compared to controls. *1939 0962*

Ferritin *Serum Increase* In 107 patients with breast cancer; CEA, ferritin and calcitonin levels were measured. CEA and ferritin but not calcitonin levels were statistically higher in those patients with metastases. *0200*

Fucose *Serum Increase* Increased in patients with both malignant and benign tumors of breast, lung and stomach. The glycoprotein-bound fraction was very markedly elevated in cases of malignancy and not in benign disease. Mucoprotein fraction was raised in both diseases. *2331* Mean elevation in 15 cases was 11.12 ± 0.68 (normal = 6.84 ± 0.13 mg/dL). Elevation was less significant in early and locally restricted breast cancer. *1342*

Gamma Glutamyl Transferase (GGT) *Serum Increase* In 49% of 41 patients at initial hospitalization for this disorder. *0781*

Glycoproteins *Serum Increase* Significant preoperative elevation of beta$_2$ glycoprotein in cancer patients compared to patients with benign breast tumors. *1810*

Haptoglobin *Serum Increase* Increased to 2.2 g/L compared to normals (1.1 g/L). *1025*

Urine Increase 24 h excretion and renal clearance were significantly increased in localized tumor patients compared to normals and disseminated cancer cases. Increased high molecular weight protein excretion implies glomerular injury in these patients. *1025*

Hexokinase *Serum Increase* Markedly increased. Mean = 22.8 ± 3.7 U/L compared to 0.93 ± 0.28 U/L in normals. *1201*

Immunoglobulin IgA *Urine Increase* 24 h excretion and renal clearance were significantly increased in localized tumor patients compared to normals and disseminated cancer cases. Increased high molecular weight protein excretion implies glomerular injury in these patients. *1025*

Immunoglobulin IgG *Urine Increase* 24 h excretion and renal clearance were significantly increased in localized tumor patients compared to normals and disseminated cancer cases. Increased high molecular weight protein excretion implies glomerular injury in these patients. *1025*

Immunoglobulin IgM *Urine Increase* 24 h excretion and renal clearance were significantly increased in localized tumor patients compared to normals and disseminated cancer cases. Increased high molecular weight protein excretion implies glomerular injury in these patients. *1025*

Iron *Serum Decrease* In 37% of 13 patients at initial hospitalization for this disorder. *0781*

Iron-Binding Capacity, Total (TIBC) *Serum Decrease* Significantly reduced (median = 2.6 mg/L) compared to controls (3.4 mg/L). 24 h excretion and renal clearance were significantly increased in localized tumor patients compared to normal and disseminated cancer cases. Increased high molecular weight protein excretion implies glomerular injury in these patients. *1025* In 21% of 14 patients at initial hospitalization for this disorder. *0781*

Iron Saturation *Serum Decrease* In 35% of 14 patients at initial hospitalization for this disorder. *0781*

Lactate Dehydrogenase *Serum Increase* Highly elevated values (> 300 U/L) may be obtained with or without liver involvement in the presence of bone metastases. *1025* Marked elevation in 110 patients. Mean = 207.2 ± 12.4 U/L, compared to normals, 85.4 ± 1.0 U/L. *1201 2575 1157*

Lactic Acid *Blood Increase* In 5 cases, mean concentration was 25.8 ± 4.0 mg/dL compared to normal, 11.7 ± 0.72 mg/dL. *1201*

Lymphocytes *Blood Increase* 6 patients with advanced cancer had significantly higher numbers of B lymphocytes than patients with benign breast disease. *1370*

Prolactin *Serum Increase* Significantly higher concentrations than controls in early breast cancer. In advanced breast cancer elevated levels were only found in postmenopausal patients. *1977* Mean concentration was significantly elevated in 148 breast cancer patients. Incidence of elevation was 22%. *0033*

Protein Bound Iodine (PBI) *Serum Increase* Occasionally increased. *2467*

Pyruvate *Blood Increase* Moderately elevated in 6 patients, mean = 1.5 ± 0.35 U/L. *1201*

Rheumatoid Factor *Serum Increase* Treated patients with no evidence of residual tumor had an 89% rate of positive tests. The incidence of seropositivity was low among untreated patients with similar tumors. *2394*

T$_3$ Uptake *Serum Increase* Slight but significant differences were found, with a higher mean value for thyrotropin, reverse-T$_3$ and T$_3$-resin uptake and a lower mean value for T$_3$. *0014*

Testosterone *Plasma Increase* Plasma hormone concentrations were measured in sequential samples from 6 women and were compared to concentrations in 6 control women matched for age, years since menopause, and parity. Concentrations in each cancer patient were significantly higher than in each matched control. *1543*

Thyroid Stimulating Hormone (TSH) *Serum Increase* Mean concentrations higher than in normals or other cancers. The difference was statistically significant only in those with advanced disease. 12% of the early cancer and 15% of the advanced had elevated plasma concentrations. *1976* Elevated in 148 patients (38%) with breast cancer. Mean survival and disease free intervals were shorter for patients with elevated TSH, but not significantly. *0033* Slight but significant differences were found with a higher mean value for thyrotropin, reverse-T$_3$ and T$_3$-resin uptake. *0014*

Thyroxine (T$_4$) *Serum Decrease* Four patients with plasma TSH levels above 85 µU/mL had subnormal plasma T$_4$ levels. *1976*

Tri-iodothyronine (T$_3$) *Serum Decrease* Slight but significant differences were found with a higher mean value for thyrotropin reverse T$_3$ and T$_3$ resin uptake and a lower mean value for T$_3$. *0014*

Uric Acid *Serum Increase* In 25% of 300 patients at initial hospitalization for this disorder. *0781*

180.90 Malignant Neoplasm of Cervix

Aldolase *Serum Increase* Mildly elevated in uterine cervix and corpus carcinomas. Mean = 2.9 ± 1.1 U/L compared to normal, 1.6 ± 0.21 U/L. *1201*

Alkaline Phosphatase Isoenzymes *Serum Increase* Cancer of the ovary, endometrium, cervix and breast as a group exhibited the highest frequency of Regan isoenzyme (placental). *0326*

Alpha$_1$-Antitrypsin *Serum Increase* Increased. *1866 0042 1946 1947 2129*

Alpha-Fetoprotein *Serum Increase* CEA, AFP and hCG were measured in 253 patients with gynecologic malignancies and in 317 patients with benign gynecologic diseases. Concentrations of each of these antigens were elevated in a significantly greater number of patients with invasive cancer. *0580*

Beta-Glucuronidase *Serum Increase* Increased. *0741 0866*

Carcinoembryonic Antigen *Serum Increase* Of the 156 patients with carcinoma in situ, 14 (9%) were positive. Progressive increase in the percentage of positive patients as stage increases, from 26% in stage I to 88% in stage IV. 52 of 61 (85%) with recurrent squamous cell carcinoma showed a positive value. *0564* 59% positivity reported. In advanced disease 84% had elevated values. *0740* Elevations found in cervical adenocarcinoma (19%) and squamous cell carcinoma of the uterine cervix (10%). *2386* Elevated (> 2.5 ng/mL) in 48% of 300 patients, and varied directly with stage of disease and histologic differentiation of the tumor. Rising of concentration indicated recurrence in 29 patients. *2413* In 42% of cases. *2199 0580*

Cholesterol *Urine Increase* Nonesterified cholesterol hyperexcretion (values > 1.5 mg/24h) occurred in 65 of 68 women with active carcinoma including 13 with carcinoma in situ. *0012*

Complement C3 *Serum Increase* Increased in patients with local disease. Closely linked to the stage of the disease. Patients in remission had normal levels, but further increases were noted in distant metastases. Dropped significantly in the terminal phase of the disease. *2427*

Complement C4 *Serum Increase* Increased in patients with local disease. Very closely linked to the stage of the disease. Patients in remission had normal levels, but further increases were noted in distant metastases. Levels dropped significantly in the terminal phase of disease. *2427*

Complement, Total *Serum Increase* Closely linked to the stage of the disease, patients in remission had normal levels, but further increases were noted in distant metastases. Levels dropped significantly in the terminal phase of the disease. *2427*

180.90   Malignant Neoplasm of Cervix   (continued)

Copper   *Serum   Increase*   Elevations are related to the stage of the disease and decrease in response to treatment. *1719   2094*

Ferritin   *Serum   Increase*   In 98 patients with untreated disease 51% had elevated serum levels. *1129*

Fucose   *Serum   Increase*   Markedly elevated and correlated with clinical stage of disease. Values ranged from 12.2-32.2 mg/dL. *0607*

Gonadotropin, Chorionic   *Serum   Increase*   CEA, AFP and hCG were measured in 253 patients with gynecologic malignancies and in 317 patients with benign gynecologic diseases. Concentrations of each of these antigens were elevated in a significantly greater number of patients with invasive cancer. *0580*

Hexokinase   *Serum   Increase*   Markedly increased. Mean = 32.0 ± 4.7 U/L. *1201*

Lactate Dehydrogenase   *Serum   Increase*   Marked elevation in 26 patients with uterine, cervix and corpus carcinomas. Mean = 142.5 ± 18.2 U/L compared to normals 85.4 ± 1.0 U/L. *1201*

Lymphocytes   *Blood   Increase*   In 44% of 146 patients at initial hospitalization for this disorder. *0781*

181.00   Malignant Neoplasm of Trophoblast (Choriocarcinoma)

Alpha-Fetoprotein   *Serum   Normal*   In pure choriocarcinomas, human chorionic gonadotropins are always elevated and AFP is absent. *2583*

Estrogens   *Serum   Increase*   May be much increased with primary chorionepithelioma of ovary. *2467*

Gonadotropin, Chorionic   *Serum   Increase*   In pure choriocarcinomas, human chorionic gonadotropins are always elevated and AFP is absent. *2583*

Urine   Increase   Markedly increased with primary chorionepithelioma of ovary. *2467*

Gonadotropin, Pituitary   *Serum   Increase*   *0962*

Pregnanediol   *Urine   Increase*   May be much increased with primary chorionepithelioma of ovary. *2467*

Progesterone   *Plasma   Increase*   May be much increased with primary chorionepithelioma of ovary. *2467*

Protein Bound Iodine (PBI)   *Serum   Increase*   Occasionally increased in metastatic choriocarcinoma. *2467*

182.00   Malignant Neoplasm of Corpus Uteri

Albumin   *Serum   Decrease*   Significantly reduced (median = 35.7 g/L ± 2.6 g/L) compared to controls (44.0 g/L ± 3.4 g/L). *1025*

Urine   Increase   24 h excretion and renal clearance were significantly increased in localized tumor patients compared to normals and disseminated cancer cases. Increased high molecular weight protein excretion implies glomerular injury in these patients. *1025*

Carcinoembryonic Antigen   *Serum   Increase*   Positive in 25 of 47 patients with adenocarcinoma of the endometrium. A tendency toward higher values in the advanced stages evidenced by 24% incidence in stage I in contrast to a 57% incidence in stage III. *0564*   67% positivity; incidence rose to 84% in advanced cases. *0740*   In 27% of the cases. *2199*

Cholesterol   *Urine   Increase*   Hyperexcretion in 42 of 45 women with active carcinoma, sequential studies demonstrated an almost perfect correlation between excretion and the clinical status of the patient following surgical and/or radiation therapy. *0012*

Creatinine   *Serum   Increase*   In 35% of 35 patients at initial hospitalization for this disorder. *0781*

Estrogens   *Serum   Increase*   Mean value was 76.65 ng/dL in 28 patients with endometrial carcinoma. Highest elevations were found in obese patients. *0034*

Haptoglobin   *Serum   Increase*   Increased (2.2 g/L) compared to normals (1.1 g/L). *1025*

Urine   Increase   24 h excretion and renal clearance were significantly increased in localized tumor patients compared to normals and disseminated cancer cases. Increased high molecular weight protein excretion implies glomerular injury in these patients. *1025*

Hematocrit   *Blood   Decrease*   In 25% of 155 patients at initial hospitalization for this disorder. *0781*

Hemoglobin   *Blood   Decrease*   In 30% of 154 patients at initial hospitalization for this disorder. *0781*

Immunoglobulin IgA   *Urine   Increase*   24 h excretion and renal clearance were significantly increased in localized tumor patients compared to normals and disseminated cancer cases. Increased high molecular weight protein excretion implies glomerular injury in these patients. *1025*

Immunoglobulin IgG   *Urine   Increase*   24 h excretion and renal clearance were significantly increased in localized tumor patients compared to normals and disseminated cancer cases. Increased high molecular weight protein excretion implies glomerular injury in these patients. *1025*

Immunoglobulin IgM   *Urine   Increase*   24 h excretion and renal clearance were significantly increased in localized tumor patients compared to normals and disseminated cancer cases. Increased high molecular weight protein excretion implies glomerular injury in these patients. *1025*

Iron-Binding Capacity, Total (TIBC)   *Serum   Decrease*   Significantly reduced (median = 2.6 mg/L) compared to controls (3.4 mg/L). Significantly increased in localized tumor patients compared to normals and disseminated cancer cases. Increased high molecular weight protein excretion implies glomerular injury in these patients. *1025*

Monocytes   *Blood   Increase*   In 51% of 150 patients at initial hospitalization for this disorder. *0781*

Uric Acid   *Serum   Increase*   In 36% of 151 patients at initial hospitalization for this disorder. *0781*

183.00   Malignant Neoplasm of Ovary

Aldolase   *Serum   Increase*   Mildly elevated. Mean = 3.8 ± 1.0 U/L compared to normal, 1.6 ± 0.21. *1201*

Alkaline Phosphatase   *Serum   Increase*   In 5 cases, the initial value was 45-190 U/L (normal < 107 U/L). *0326*

Alkaline Phosphatase Isoenzymes   *Serum   Increase*   In 5 cases, the initial value was 44.7-191 (normal 106.5 U/L). The Regan isoenzyme was found in all cases and ranged from 99-264 U/L placental isoenzyme units. *2267*   Cancer of the ovary, endometrium, cervix and breast as a group exhibited the highest frequency of Regan isoenzyme (placental) in malignancies. *0326*

Pleural Effusion   Increase   59% (13 of 22) patients had detectable regan isoenzyme in malignant effusions. *2268*

Ascitic Fluid   Increase   59% (13 of 22) patients had detectable regan isoenzyme. *2268*

Alpha-Fetoprotein   *Serum   Increase*   Present in embryonal carcinoma (in 27% of cases) or malignant teratoma (60% of cases) of ovary and testis. *2467*   15 out of 20 cases of teratoblastoma of testis and ovary showed raised levels. *0007*   Over 50 ng/mL in 33% of cases of gonadal teratoblastoma. *2116 0580*

Serum   Normal   No elevations are seen in conjunction with pure dysgerminomas of the ovary. *2583*

Amylase   *Serum   Increase*   Hyperamylasemia may occur in ovarian papillary cystadenocarcinoma. *1373*

Pleural Effusion   Increase   Rare occurrence of ovarian carcinoma producing amylase-rich ascites and pleural effusions. Salivary type amylase has been identified in tumor tissue. *0457*

Ascitic Fluid   Increase   Rare occurrence of ovarian carcinoma producing amylase-rich ascites and pleural effusions was reported; salivary type amylase was identified in tumor tissue. *0457*

Carcinoembryonic Antigen   *Serum   Increase*   Of the 132 patients with adenocarcinoma, 73 had positive values. The largest number of patients were in the stage III category where 45 of 77 patients (58%) were positive. *0564*   77% positivity. *0740*   Most commonly found in ovarian cancer. Elevated levels occurred in 6 of 30 cases, all at advanced stages III or IV. *2386*   In 35% of cases. *2199 0580*

Ascitic Fluid   Increase   In malignant effusions. *2199*

Cholesterol   *Urine   Increase*   Hyperexcretion in 18 of 19 cystadenocarcinomas of the serous and/or mucinous types; 1 of 1 endometrial carcinoma; 4 of 4 malignant granulosa cell tumors; two of two mixed malignant germ cell tumors; and one of one malignant mixed Müllerian tumor. A normal excretion was characteristic of 19 of 21 surviving patients treated by surgery and adjunctive therapy. The 94% correlation between the presence of proven active ovarian carcinomas and urinary hyperexcretion is significant. *0013*

Peritoneal Fluid   Increase   Markedly increased in active cases. *1547*

Complement C3 *Serum Increase* Increased in patients with local disease. Closely linked to the stage of the disease. Patients in remission had normal levels, but further increases were noted in distant metastases. Levels dropped significantly in the terminal phase of disease. *2427*

Complement C4 *Serum Increase* Increased in patients with local disease. Very closely linked to the stage of the disease. Patients in remission had normal levels, but further increases were noted in distant metastases. Levels dropped significantly in the terminal phase of the disease. *2427*

Complement, Total *Serum Increase* Closely linked to the stage of the disease. Patients in remission had normal levels, but further increases were noted in distant metastases. Dropped significantly in the terminal phase of disease. *2427*

Copper *Serum Increase* Does not result from a shift of zinc into or release of copper out of malignant tumor tissue. *1406*

Cryofibrinogen *Serum Increase* *2035 1551*

Eosinophils *Blood Increase* *2467*

Erythrocytes *Ascitic Fluid Increase* A large number of RBC, especially grossly bloody ascites, suggests a neoplasm, particularly hepatoma or ovarian cancer. *2199*

Estradiol *Plasma Increase* In estrogen producing tumors estradiol is the most active estrogen. *0002 1720 0046*

Fibrin Split Products (FSP) *Ascitic Fluid Increase* In malignant effusions. *2199*

Follicle Stimulating Hormone (FSH) *Urine Decrease* *0211*

Gonadotropin, Chorionic *Serum Increase* The highest incidence was found in patients with carcinoma of testis (61%), adenocarcinoma of ovary (42%), and pancreas (33%). *0740* In 22 patients, 30% had hCG positive serum. *2268* Elevated with invasive carcinoma. *0580*

Pleural Effusion Increase In 22 patients, 30% had positive serum while 68% had positive pleural and ascites effusions. *2268*

Ascitic Fluid Increase In 22 patients, 30% had positive serum while 68% had positive pleural and ascites effusions. *2268*

Hexokinase *Serum Increase* Markedly increased. Mean = 22.8 ± 4.0 U/L compared to normal, 0.93 ± 0.28 U/L. *1201*

Lactate Dehydrogenase *Serum Increase* All 6 cases showed elevation ranging from 150-350 with the upper limit of normal at 120. Marked elevation in 18 patients. *0090* Mean = 158.7 ± 14.9 U/L compared to normals, 85.4 ± 1.0 U/L. *1201*

Zinc *Serum Decrease* Does not result from a shift of zinc into or release of copper out of malignant tumor tissue. *1406*

185.00 Malignant Neoplasm of Prostate

Acid Phosphatase *Serum Increase* May be raised, especially if the tumor has extended outside the gland. Anaplastic tumors secrete minimal enzyme. *0619* Useful in detecting metastases but is of no value in detecting the presence of resectable carcinoma. 50-75% of patients with carcinoma extended beyond the capsule have elevated levels. Patients with carcinoma still confined within the capsule usually have normal serum levels. *0812 0503* Normal levels do not exclude possibility of carcinoma. 26% of proved cases *0944 1175 0433*

Serum Normal Percentage of patients with normal levels varied from 14-96% depending upon the stage of disease. *1052* Normal levels do not exclude possibility of this cancer. *1175* Some patients with known metastatic carcinoma have low values, possibly due to a recent episode of hyper- or hypothermia, as the enzyme is subject to common serum inhibitors. *0433 1426*

Bone Marrow Increase Significant in detecting unsuspected metastases before they become radiologically apparent. Bone marrow levels elevate at an earlier stage in the disease than serum levels. *1513* Of the 25 patients with histologically confirmed malignancy, 18 had an elevation in bone marrow while only 11 had serum elevations. *1261 0404 2422*

Adenosine Deaminase *Serum Increase* Increased. *0655 1737 2235*

Albumin *Serum Decrease* In 31% of 86 patients at initial hospitalization for this disorder. *0781*

Aldolase *Serum Increase* Cell destruction. *2467 0962*

Alkaline Phosphatase *Serum Increase* Levels were elevated above the normal range in cases without bone metastases. With bone metastases, levels were much higher and 90% of patients showed marked elevations. *2566* In 54% of 83 patients at initial hospitalization for this disorder. *0781 0870 1863*

Leukocyte *Decrease* Low activity is present irrespective of tumor category, activity of disease, or type of therapy. In 11 patients, median activity was 5 U/L (normal = 55). *1423*

Amylase *Serum Increase* Reported in 95% of patients with benign hypertrophy and 70% of carcinomas. Similar results have not been reported elsewhere. *0973*

Aspartate Aminotransferase *Serum Increase* In 25% of 86 patients at initial hospitalization for this disorder. *0781*

Carcinoembryonic Antigen *Serum Increase* 30% of patients with advanced urologic tumors have elevated plasma levels. There is a good correlation between the stage of carcinoma and the degree of elevation. In general, with advanced active disease positive results exceed the normal level of 2.5 ng., whereas levels in inactive disease have been negative or at least below normal. *0433* In 40% of cases. *2199* 35% of patients. *2503 0795 2035*

Cholesterol *Serum Decrease* Pretreatment levels (196 ± 1.3 mg/dL) (normal = 1093) were significantly lower than those reported for age-matched controls. *2102*

Serum Increase Nonesterified cholesterol hyperexcretion occurred in 44.8% of stage A and B and in 52.6% of stage C and D. Total cholesterol was elevated in 52.2% and 63.2% respectively. *1196*

Urine Increase In 42 patients, 62% were found to have levels 2.6 mg/24h. *0403*

Complement C3 *Serum Increase* 26% had raised levels ranging from 208-440 mg/dL. *0008* Levels were found to be very closely linked to the stage of the disease. Patients in remission had normal levels, but further increases were noted in distant metastases. Levels dropped significantly in the terminal phase of disease. *2427*

Complement C4 *Serum Increase* Increased in patients with local disease. Very closely linked to the stage of the disease. Patients in remission had normal levels, but further increases were noted in distant metastases. Levels dropped significantly in the terminal phase of disease. *2427*

Complement, Total *Serum Increase* Closely linked to the stage of the disease. Patients in remission had normal levels, but further increases were noted in distant metastases. Dropped significantly in the terminal phase of the disease. *2427*

Creatine Kinase *Serum Increase* *1347*

Creatinine *Serum Increase* In 59% of 59 patients at initial hospitalization for this disorder. *0781*

Cryofibrinogen *Serum Increase* *2035 1551*

Fibrin Split Products (FSP) *Plasma Increase* Especially with metastases. *1253* Fibrinolysins are found in 12% of patients. *2468*

Gamma Glutamyl Transferase (GGT) *Serum Increase* In 48% of 12 patients at initial hospitalization for this disorder. *0781*

Glucose *Serum Increase* In 36% of 86 patients at initial hospitalization for this disorder. *0781*

Gonadotropin, Chorionic *Serum Decrease* Patients with seminomas and teratomas should have a low titer. *0536*

Gonadotropin, Pituitary *Serum Decrease* Patients with prostatic carcinoma and benign prostatic hypertrophy showed lower levels of LH when compared with age-matched controls. *0971*

Hematocrit *Blood Decrease* In 43% of 87 patients at initial hospitalization for this disorder. *0781*

Hemoglobin *Blood Decrease* In 43% of 87 patients at initial hospitalization for this disorder. *0781*

Immunoglobulin IgA *Serum Increase* 22% had elevated levels ranging from 365-550 mg/dL. *0008*

Lactate Dehydrogenase *Serum Increase* In advanced carcinoma following successful stilbestrol therapy and/or orchiectomy. *0619* Borderline or elevated in 32 patients, regardless of the status of the disease. *0543* In 27% of 83 patients at initial hospitalization for this disorder. *0781 0433*

Urine Increase Increased in a high proportion of cases; useful for detection of asymptomatic lesions or screening of susceptible population groups. Increased values usually precede clinical symptoms. *2467 0817 0818*

Lactate Dehydrogenase Isoenzyme 5 (LD₅) *Serum Increase* Consistently elevated in patients with advanced progressive prostatic carcinoma. In patients in remission, at trace levels as found in the control group. *0543*

Lactate Dehydrogenase Isoenzymes *Serum Increase* Some correlation between the LD 5:1 ratio, and the degree of differentiation and the stage of the disease in the patient. *0433* LD₄ and LD₅ were consistently elevated in patients with advanced progressive carcinomas. In patients in remission, LD₄ and LD₅ were at trace levels as found in the control group. *0543* Rise in LD₄. *1863*

Leucine Aminopeptidase *Serum Decrease* *0950*

185.00 Malignant Neoplasm of Prostate *(continued)*

Luteinizing Hormone (LH) *Serum Decrease* Patients with prostatic carcinoma and benign prostatic hypertrophy showed lower levels of LH when compared with age-matched controls. *0971*

Monocytes *Blood Increase* In 63% of 81 patients at initial hospitalization for this disorder. *0781*

Phosphate *Serum Decrease* In 39% of 86 patients at initial hospitalization for this disorder. *0781*

Uric Acid *Serum Increase* In 42% of 86 patients at initial hospitalization for this disorder. *0781*

186.90 Malignant Neoplasm of Testis

17-Hydroxycorticosteroids *Urine Increase* *2467*

17-Ketogenic Steroids *Urine Increase* *2467*

Aldolase *Serum Increase* Mildly elevated in tumors of the testicle and kidney. Mean = 4.1 ± 0.5 U/L compared to normal, 1.6 ± 0.21. *1201*

Alkaline Phosphatase Isoenzymes *Serum Increase* Gonadal neoplasms (ovary and testis) showed the greatest frequency of Regan isoenzymes (placental) in cancers. *0740*

Alpha-Fetoprotein *Serum Increase* Present in embryonal carcinoma (in 27% of cases) or malignant teratoma (in 60% of cases). Concentrations > 40 g/L are found in 75% of patients with teratocarcinoma *2467* Elevated in 60% of stage A and B cases and all patients with stage 3 disease *0756* In patients with nonseminomatous testicular germ cell malignant growths during and after therapeutic interventions, an elevated marker assay indicated the presence of active disease. A normal marker assay does not exclude active disease. *1621* 15 out of 20 cases of teratoblastoma of testis and ovary showed raised levels. *0007* Over 50 ng/mL in 33% of cases of gonadal teratoblastoma. *2116 2337*

Serum Normal No elevations are found in conjunction with pure seminomas of the testis. In teratoblastoma, both AFP and hCG are usually absent, but may be increased in tumors with small areas of extra-embryonic tumor tissue. *2583*

Carcinoembryonic Antigen *Serum Increase* In 57% of cases. *2199*

Creatinine *Serum Increase* In 53% of 13 patients at initial hospitalization for this disorder. *0781*

Eosinophils *Blood Increase* In 46% of 27 patients at initial hospitalization for this disorder. *0781*

Estrogens *Urine Increase* *2467*

Follicle Stimulating Hormone (FSH) *Urine Increase* Increased with seminoma. *0619*

Gonadotropin, Chorionic *Serum Increase* Elevated marker assay indicates active disease in nonseminomatous testicular germ cell tumors, during and after therapeutic interventions. Normal does not exclude active disease being present. *1621* The highest incidence of immunoreactive hCG (61%) found in cancers. *0740* This is an effective tumor marker in the staging and management of testicular cancer and potentially of nontrophoblastic cancers *1111* Elevated in 60% of stage A and B cases and all patients with stage C disease *0756*

Urine Increase 90% of patients with testicular tumors are positive; useful in gauging efficacy of chemotherapy. *2467* An elevation of the gonadotropins usually indicates the presence of a tumor containing chorionic tissue and indicates poor prognosis. *0433*

Gonadotropin, Pituitary *Urine Increase* Increased with seminoma. *0619*

Hexokinase *Serum Increase* Markedly increased. Mean = 12.6 ± 2.8 compared to normal 0.93 ± 0.28 U/L. *1201*

Lactate Dehydrogenase *Serum Increase* Marked elevation in 47 patients with tumors of the testicle and kidney. Mean = 168.8 ± 19.5 U/L compared to normals, 85.4 ± 1.0 U/L. *1201* In 38% of 23 patients at initial hospitalization for this disorder. *0781*

Lactic Acid *Blood Increase* Mildly elevated in 8 patients with tumors of the testicle mean concentration was 21.5 ± 5.7 mg/dL compared to normal, 11.7 ± 0.72 mg/dL. *1201*

Platelet Count *Blood Increase* In 34% of 23 patients at initial hospitalization for this disorder. *0781*

Protein Bound Iodine (PBI) *Serum Increase* Occasionally increased in embryonal testicular carcinoma. *2467*

Pyruvate *Blood Increase* Mildly elevated in 8 patients with tumors of the testicle. Mean = 0.89 ± 0.18 U/L. *1201*

Uric Acid *Serum Increase* In 61% of 24 patients at initial hospitalization for this disorder. *0781*

188.90 Malignant Neoplasm of Bladder

Adenosine Deaminase *Serum Increase* Increased. *0655 1737 2235*

Lymphocytes Increase Lymphocyte concentrations were elevated in all patients with transitional cell bladder carcinoma and correlated with stage, activity, clinical course and tumor resection but not with grade. Erythrocyte levels were also elevated in all cases but showed no correlation to disease parameters. *2293*

Red Blood Cells Increase Lymphocyte concentrations were elevated in all patients with transitional cell bladder carcinoma and correlated with stage, activity, clinical course and tumor resection but not with grade. Erythrocyte levels were also elevated in all cases but showed no correlation to disease parameters. *2293*

Albumin *Serum Decrease* In 27% of 45 patients at initial hospitalization for this disorder. *0781*

Urine Increase May be completely negative or may show microscopic evidence of hematuria, pyuria, albumin, and threads of mucus. *0433*

Alkaline Phosphatase *Urine Increase* Elevated in 43% of 35 patients. *0817* Elevated in 10 of 26 (38.5%) of active transitional cell carcinomas. *1843 0818*

Alpha-Fetoprotein *Serum Increase* Of 112 cases, 59 (52.8%) showed positive results, and no false positive results occurred. *0045*

Arylsulfatase *Urine Increase* Up to 40-fold increase in urinary activity. *0610* Arylsulfatase A (100%) and B (82.8%) were elevated in 29 cases of active disease. *1843*

Calcium *Serum Increase* Neoplasm without evidence of direct bone involvement. Parathyroid hormone-secreting tumors. *0503*

Urine Increase No evidence of bone involvement. Parathyroid hormone-secreting tumors. *0503*

Carcinoembryonic Antigen *Serum Increase* Increased in 53% of the patients (without urinary infection). No false positive results. *1304* In 33% of cases. *2199* *0795 2035*

Ascitic Fluid Increase In malignant effusions. *2199*

Complement C3 *Serum Increase* Increased in patients with local disease. Closely linked to the stage of the disease. Patients in remission had normal levels, but further increases were noted in distant metastases. Dropped significantly in the terminal phase of disease. *2427*

Complement C4 *Serum Increase* Increased in patients with local disease. Very closely linked to the stage of the disease. Patients in remission had normal levels, but further increases were noted in distant metastases. Levels dropped significantly in the terminal phase of the disease. *2427*

Complement, Total *Serum Increase* Closely linked to the stage of the disease. Patients in remission had normal levels, but further increases were noted in distant metastases. Dropped significantly in the terminal phase of disease. *2427*

Creatinine *Serum Increase* In 70% of 37 patients at initial hospitalization for this disorder. *0781*

Cryofibrinogen *Serum Increase* *2035 1551*

Erythrocytes *Urine Increase* By far the most common symptom; may be intermittent or persistent, gross or microscopic. The urine can be completely negative or may show microscopic evidence of hematuria, pyuria, albumin, and threads of mucus. *0433*

Fibrin Split Products (FSP) *Urine Increase* A high degree of accuracy (90%) was found in correlating cytology and urinary fibrinogen degradation products with the activity of the disease. *2455*

Hematocrit *Blood Decrease* May show anemia secondary to iron deficiency or secondary to a diffuse metastatic disease. *0433* In 22% of 46 patients at initial hospitalization for this disorder. *0781*

Hemoglobin *Blood Decrease* May show anemia secondary to iron deficiency or secondary to a diffuse metastatic disease. *0433* In 26% of 45 patients at initial hospitalization for this disorder. *0781*

Iron-Binding Capacity, Total (TIBC) *Serum Increase* Secondary iron deficiency anemia may develop. *0433*

Iron Saturation *Serum Decrease* Secondary iron deficiency anemia may develop. *0433*

Lactate Dehydrogenase *Urine Increase* Increased in a high proportion of cases; useful for detection of asymptomatic lesions or screening of susceptible population groups, and differential diagnosis of renal cysts. This test is chiefly useful in screening for malignancy of kidney, renal pelvis, and bladder; increased values usually precede clinical symptoms. *2467* 60.7% (17 of 28) patients with transitional cell carcinoma showed elevations. *1843* *0817 0818*

Leukocytes *Urine Increase* Pyuria without hematuria is occasionally the only finding associated with widespread epidermoid carcinoma. Urine can be completely negative or may show microscopic evidence of hematuria, pyuria, albumin and threads of mucus. *0433*

MCH *Blood Decrease* May show anemia secondary to iron deficiency or secondary to a diffuse metastatic disease. *0433*

MCHC *Blood Decrease* May show anemia secondary to iron deficiency or secondary to a diffuse metastatic disease. *0433*

MCV *Blood Decrease* May show anemia secondary to iron deficiency or secondary to a diffuse metastatic disease. *0433*

Monocytes *Blood Increase* In 59% of 42 patients at initial hospitalization for this disorder. *0781*

Neutrophils *Blood Increase* A leukoerythroblastic blood picture would indicate marrow metastasis. *0433*

Urea Nitrogen *Serum Increase* In 40% of 45 patients at initial hospitalization for this disorder. *0781*

Uric Acid *Serum Increase* In 43% of 45 patients at initial hospitalization for this disorder. *0781*

189.00   Malignant Neoplasm of Kidney

Adenosine Deaminase *Lymphocytes Decrease* Decreased concentration in lymphocyte adenosine deaminase is found in renal cell carcinoma. Progression of disease is associated with a fall in lymphocyte values in all patients. RBC concentrations are low only in blood types B and O. *2292*

Albumin *Serum Decrease* *0151*

Urine Increase Albuminuria often accompanies hematuria but may occur alone in metastatic renal tumors, especially those of lymphatic or leukemic origin. *0433*

Aldolase *Serum Increase* Mildly elevated in tumors of the testicle and kidney. Mean = 4.1 ± 0.5 U/L compared to normal, 1.6 ± 0.21. *1201*

Alkaline Phosphatase *Urine Increase* Occurs mainly when a tumor has extended beyond the renal parenchyma or into bladder muscle. *0818* Elevated in 55% of patients. *0817*

Alkaline Phosphatase Isoenzymes *Serum Increase* Increased incidence of the Regan (placental) isoenzyme. *0740*

Alpha₂-Globulin *Serum Increase* *0151*

Alpha-Fetoprotein *Serum Normal* Not elevated. *1348*

Beta-Glucuronidase *Urine Increase* All 17 patients with renal adenocarcinoma had slightly elevated activity with values ranging from 32-55 U/L (mean 42.8 ± 6.1 U). Uncomplicated renal cysts revealed normal urinary enzyme activities (mean = 17.9 ± 12.8). *1525*

Calcium *Serum Increase* 5-15% of patients with hypernephroma develop hypercalcemia usually secondary to metastases. *0836*

Carcinoembryonic Antigen *Serum Increase* In 35% of cases. *2199*

Ascitic Fluid Increase In malignant effusions. *2199*

Cryofibrinogen *Serum Increase* *2035 1551*

Erythrocytes *Blood Increase* Erythrocytosis is common; disappears after nephrectomy if no metastases are present. *1391* Erythrocytosis has been associated with hypernephromas. *1982 1992*

Urine Increase 95% of patients with this disease will have either gross or microscopic hematuria at some time. *0433* Intermittent hematuria found in 60%, occasionally causes colic. *1391* Urinalysis in malignant tumors usually reveals only painless hematuria. *0962*

Ascitic Fluid Increase Grossly bloody ascites suggests neoplasm. *2199*

Erythrocyte Sedimentation Rate *Blood Increase* Unusually high rates of up to 150 mm/h are characteristic. *0151* Common. *0836* Values over 100 mm/h found in 16 of 34 patients. *0894*

Erythropoietin *Serum Increase* Increased in 49 of 92 patients with renal cell carcinoma or renal cysts. Highest values were found in patients developing metastases after removal of renal carcinoma. *1609* Elevated in 63% of patients but did not correlate with tumor grade, type, stage, prognosis. *2291* Increased plasma concentrations are found in patients with erythrocytosis associated with several types of tumor, especially lung, kidney, and liver. *0263 1416 1507*

Fibrin Split Products (FSP) *Ascitic Fluid Increase* In malignant effusions. *2199*

Gamma Glutamyl Transferase (GGT) *Serum Increase* *1739*

Urine Decrease The only renal disorder to demonstrate a decreased value in urine. *1005*

Gonadotropin, Pituitary *Serum Increase* Can cause the syndrome of ectopic gonadotropin production. *0962*

Haptoglobin *Serum Increase* May be elevated without metastases. *0836*

Hematocrit *Blood Decrease* Anemia occurs in approximately 30% of patients, secondary to bone marrow depression. *0836* 30 of 34 patients with hypernephroma were anemic, due mainly to urinary blood loss. Hemoglobin values varied from 7-12%. *0894* Anemia is a frequent presenting symptom. *1391*

Blood Increase Occurs occasionally due to erythropoietin formation by the tumor. *0186*

Hemoglobin *Blood Decrease* Anemia occurs in approximately 30% of patients with renal cell carcinoma, secondary to bone marrow depression by tumor. *0836* 30 of 34 patients with hypernephroma were anemic. Due mainly to urinary blood loss. Values varied from 7-12%. *0894* A frequent presenting symptom. *1391*

Blood Increase Occurs occasionally due to erythropoietin formation by the tumor. *0186*

Hexokinase *Serum Increase* Markedly increased. Mean = 12.6 ± 2.8 U/L compared to 0.93 ± 0.28 U/L. *1201*

Iron *Serum Decrease* Found in 30% of patients. *0836*

Iron-Binding Capacity, Total (TIBC) *Serum Decrease* Found in 30% of patients. *0836*

Serum Increase Anemia due mainly to urinary blood loss. *0894 1391*

Iron Saturation *Serum Decrease* Anemia due mainly to urinary blood loss. *0894 1391*

Lactate Dehydrogenase *Serum Increase* Marked elevation in 47 patients with tumors of the testicle and kidney. Mean = 168.8 ± 19.5 U/L compared to normals, 85.4 ± 10.0 U/L. *1201*

Urine Increase Mild elevation occurred in 33% of cases. *0818* Elevated in 40% of patients. *0817* In all 16 cases, urinary activity was increased 10 fold but with no rise in tumor tissue level. *1005*

Ascitic Fluid Increase In malignant effusions. *2199*

Lactic Acid *Blood Increase* Mild elevation in 8 patients, mean = 13.6 - 2.8 mg/dL compared to normal, 11.7 ± 0.72 mg/dL. *1201*

Leukocytes *Blood Increase* Leukocytosis ranging up to 100,000/μL may occur. *0151*

Malate Dehydrogenase *Urine Increase* Increased in 75% of patients. *1005*

MCH *Blood Decrease* Anemia occurs in approximately 30% of patients, secondary to bone marrow depression. *0836* 30 of 34 patients with hypernephroma were anemic, due mainly to urinary blood loss. Hemoglobin values varied from 7-12 g/dL. *0894*

MCHC *Blood Decrease* Anemia occurs in approximately 30% of patients, secondary to bone marrow depression. *0836* 30 of 34 patients with hypernephroma were anemic, due to urinary blood loss. Hemoglobin values varied from 7-12 g/dL. *0894*

MCV *Blood Decrease* Anemia occurs in approximately 30% of patients, secondary to bone marrow depression. *0836* 30 of 34 patients with hypernephroma were anemic, due mainly to urinary blood loss. Hemoglobin values varied from 7-12g/dL. *0894*

Parathyroid Hormone *Serum Increase* Lung cancer, hypernephroma, gastrointestinal cancer, and other neoplasms can synthesize and secrete parathyroid hormone. *0962*

Prolactin *Serum Increase* Elevated. *0918*

Prothrombin Time *Plasma Increase* Increased in the absence of hepatic metastases. *0186*

Pyruvate *Blood Increase* Mildly elevated in 8 patients, mean = 0.89 ± 0.18 U/L. *1201*

Renin Activity *Plasma Increase* Elevation occurred in 37% of cases of renal adenocarcinoma and was associated with high grade, high stage lesions of mixed histologic cell type and predicted poor prognosis. *2291* Significantly higher in renal vein from affected side and maintains circadian rhythm despite marked elevation with renin-producing renal tumors. *2468*

Volume *Red Blood Cells Increase* True polycythemia may occur. *1669*

191.90   Malignant Neoplasm of Brain

Aldolase *Serum Increase* The serum of cancer patients contains a greater proportion of aldolase A (muscle-type) than serum from normal persons. Gliomas and normal brain tissue contain aldolase C (nerve and brain variant), but in meningiomas or tumor metastatic to brain, only aldolase A (liver and fetal form) is detected. *2093*

Alpha₂-Macroglobulin *CSF Normal* Neurotumors. *2069*

Antidiuretic Hormone *Serum Increase* Associated with excessive ADH production resulting in sodium loss. *2104*

191.90 Malignant Neoplasm of Brain *(continued)*

Aspartate Aminotransferase *Serum Increase* In occasional cases. *2467* In 33% of 24 patients at initial hospitalization for this disorder. *0781*

Beta-Galactosidase *Serum Decrease* Mean serum concentration in patients with tumors (both benign and malignant) were depressed to 0.065 ± 0.009 mmol/min/L, compared with 0.243 ± 0.038 in controls. *1099*

Bicarbonate *Serum Increase* In 74% of 21 patients at initial hospitalization for this disorder. *0781*

Cells *CSF Increase* Mononuclear cells are increased. *0999*

Creatine Kinase *Serum Increase* Highest activity of CK-BB in brain and smooth muscle. *1347* In necrotic glioma *0619*

Eosinophils *Blood Increase* In 41% of 23 patients at initial hospitalization for this disorder. *0781*

Erythrocytes *Blood Increase* Erythrocytosis seen in association with cerebellar hemangioblastomas appears to be due to the secretion of erythropoietin by these lesions. *1992*

Erythropoietin *Serum Increase* Erythrocytosis seen in association with cerebellar hemangioblastomas appears to be due to the secretion of erythropoietin by these lesions. *1992*

Gamma Glutamyl Transferase (GGT) *Serum Increase* Elevated preoperatively in 13 of 23 patients. Those showing elevations included 7 of 13 patients with astrocytomas, grades I-IV, 4 of 6 patients with metastatic brain tumors, and 2 of 4 patients with cerebral meningiomas. *0684*

Glomerular Filtration Rate (GFR) *Urine Increase* Associated excess ADH may tend to accelerate GFR. *2104*

Immunoglobulin IgG *CSF Increase* No consistent CSF IgG pattern was found in brain tumors, but highly vascularized tumors had increased concentrations. *2321*

Isocitrate Dehydrogenase *CSF Increase* Increased with primary cerebral tumors. *0619*

Lactate Dehydrogenase *CSF Increase* In primary and metastatic tumors depending on location, growth rate, etc. *2467*

Lead *CSF Increase* Markedly increased (ratio 2.11: tumor patients/control patients). *0647*

Lymphocytes *Blood Decrease* In 19 different groups of neurological diseases, absolute and relative T-lymphocyte populations were significantly decreased only in patients with acute Guillian-Barre Syndrome, active multiple sclerosis, and malignant cerebral tumor. *2540* In 38% of 23 patients at initial hospitalization for this disorder. *0781*

Monocytes *Blood Increase* In 63% of 23 patients at initial hospitalization for this disorder. *0781*

Protein *CSF Increase* Consistently found with intracranial tumors. Normal value does not exclude the presence of a tumor. *0433 1099*

Sodium *Serum Decrease* Associated with excessive ADH production *2104* . Serum sodium usually less than 130 mEq/L. *0062*

Urine Increase Urine is almost always hypertonic to plasma *0062*

Zinc *CSF Decrease* Significantly less. *0648*

192.50 Neuroblastoma

Arylsulfatase *Urine Increase* Urine arylsulfatase and homovanillic acid are inversely related in neuroblastomas. In melanotic tumors, HVA is elevated and arylsulfatase normal or slightly elevated. Amelanotic tumors have low-normal HVA and high arylsulfatase. *1630*

Carcinoembryonic Antigen *Serum Increase* In 100% of cases. *2199*

Catecholamines *Plasma Increase* Catecholamine secretion is as high or higher than in pheochromocytoma. *2612*

Dopa (3,4-Dihydroxyphenylalanine) *Serum Increase* Increased production by neuroblastoma cell system. *1630*

Urine Increase Elevated levels receded toward normal after treatment. *1511*

Dopamine *Serum Increase* Excess secretion in some tumors. *2612*

Urine Increase Elevated levels receded toward normal after treatment. *1511*

Homovanillic Acid *Urine Increase* Urine arylsulfatase and homovanillic acid are inversely related in neuroblastomas. In melanotic tumors, HVA is elevated and arylsulfatase normal or slightly elevated. Amelanotic tumors have low-normal HVA and high arylsulfatase. *1630* Elevated levels receded toward normal after treatment. *1511*

Metanephrines, Total *Urine Increase* *1752*

Vanillylamine *Urine Increase* False positive results may occur due to certain foods and certain drugs. Detects 75% of neuroblastomas, ganglioneuromas and ganglioblastomas if used alone. In combination with HVA or total catecholamines, 95-100% may be detected. *2467* Excretion > 2 X normal is diagnostic providing all dietary restrictions have been followed. *2612*

192.90 Malignant Neoplasm of Other Parts of Nervous System

Glucose *CSF Decrease* Due to multiple tumors in the meninges, but these are rare causes. *0619*

Metanephrines, Total *Urine Increase* *1752*

193.00 Malignant Neoplasm of Thyroid Gland

Antithyroglobulin Antibodies *Serum Increase* In 20% of cases. *0058*

Thyroxine Binding Globulin *Serum Increase* Elevations > 300 ng/mL were found only in patients with thyroid cancer, with or without irradiation, and in all stages. *0529*

Thyroxine (T$_4$) *Serum Normal* Usually euthyroid. *1200*

Tri-iodothyronine (T$_3$) *Serum Increase* Rarely in follicular cancer. *1200*

Serum Normal Usually euthyroid. *1200*

193.01 Medullary Carcinoma of Thyroid

5-Hydroxytryptamine (Serotonin) *Blood Increase* In medullary cancer. *0962*

Aspartate Aminotransferase *Serum Increase* In 31% of 22 patients at initial hospitalization for this disorder. *0781*

Calcitonin *Serum Increase* Increased baseline levels or increased level after calcium infusion indicates medullary carcinoma. May be found even in absence of palpable mass in the thyroid. *2468* Observed in 2 patients with medullary cancer of the thyroid. *1587* Increased in both thyroid and bronchogenic carcinomas. Medullary thyroid cancer is characterized by the presence of at least 7 different fractions, ranging from fraction I to V. Bronchogenic cancers had a predominance of high molecular weight fractions (I and IIa). *0146 0962*

Urine Increase Urinary calcitonin is high in medullary cancer patients. *0962*

Calcium *Serum Normal* Usually normal, in spite of very high titers of plasma calcitonin seen in medullary cancer of the thyroid. *0962*

Carcinoembryonic Antigen *Serum Increase* Over 5 ng/mL in 20% of patients. All patients with medullary carcinoma had considerably elevated levels (> 25 ng/mL). *0624*

Corticotropin *Plasma Increase* May occur. *0995*

Fucose *Serum Increase* Elevation was less significant in early and locally restricted disease. Mean value was 10.36 ± 0.41 (normal = 6.48 ± 0.13 mg/dL). *1342*

Histamine *Serum Increase* Abnormally increased activity found in medullary carcinoma, falling after surgical removal, and increasing if residual tumor present. *0619*

Parathyroid Hormone *Serum Increase* Elevations in about 50% of medullary cancer patients. *0962*

Phosphate *Serum Normal* Usually normal, in spite of very high titers of plasma calcitonin seen in medullary cancer of the thyroid. *0962*

Potassium *Feces Increase* About 33% of patients with medullary carcinoma have watery diarrhea with stools characteristically containing increased sodium and potassium content. *2199*

Prostaglandins *Serum Increase* May occur. *0995*

Sodium *Feces Increase* About 33% of patients with medullary carcinoma have watery diarrhea with stools characteristically containing increased sodium and potassium content. *2199*

T$_3$ Uptake *Serum Normal* *2467*

194.00 Malignant Neoplasm of Adrenal Gland

11-Hydroxycorticosteroids *Urine Increase* Usually very high. *2612*

17-Hydroxycorticosteroids *Urine Increase* *0503*

Urine Normal Can be normal to moderately elevated in masculinizing or feminizing tumors. *0995*

17-Ketogenic Steroids *Urine Increase* Very high values in Cushing's suggests ectopic ACTH production or adrenocortical carcinoma. *2612*

Urine Normal Can be normal to moderately elevated in masculinizing or feminizing tumors. *0995*

17-Ketosteroids *Urine Increase* Usually very high. *2612 2467 0619*

Aldosterone *Plasma Increase* In tumors of the zona glomerulosa. *0536*

Urine Increase In tumors of the zona glomerulosa. *0536*

Androgens *Plasma Increase* Excessive androgen secretion in adrenocortical carcinoma. *2612*

Corticosterone *Plasma Increase* In tumors of the zona glomerulosa or zona fasciculata. *0536*

Corticotropin *Plasma Decrease* Very low or undetectable in Cushing's patients with adrenocortical tumors. *2612*

Cortisol *Plasma Increase* Both 9 h and 23 h basal plasma concentrations are very high. *2612* In tumors of the zona fasciculata. *0536*

Dehydroepiandrosterone (DHEA) *Serum Increase* Virilizing adrenal tumors. *0995*

Dehydroepiandrosterone Sulfate (DHEA-S) *Serum Increase* *0046 1692*

Dehydroisoandrosterone *Urine Increase* *2467*

Estrogens *Urine Increase* Principally due to increments in estriol and also to increments in estradiol and estrone. *0995*

Follicle Stimulating Hormone (FSH) *Urine Decrease* *0211*

Gonadotropin, Pituitary *Serum Increase* Feminizing adrenal tumor can cause the syndrome of ectopic gonadotropin production. *0962*

Pregnanetriol *Urine Increase* Virilizing adrenal tumors. *0995*

194.30 Malignant Neoplasm of Pituitary

Corticotropin *CSF Increase* 21 of 22 patients with suprasellar extension of a pituitary tumor had elevations of one or more CSF adenohypophyseal hormones. *1189*

Follicle Stimulating Hormone (FSH) *CSF Increase* 21 of 22 patients with suprasellar extension of a pituitary tumor had elevations of one or more CSF adenohypophyseal hormones. *1189*

Growth Hormone *CSF Increase* 21 of 22 patients with suprasellar extension of a pituitary tumor had elevations of one or more CSF adenohypophyseal hormones. *1189*

Luteinizing Hormone (LH) *CSF Increase* 21 of 22 patients with suprasellar extension of a pituitary tumor had elevations of one or more CSF adenohypophyseal hormones. *1189*

Prolactin *CSF Increase* 21 of 22 patients with suprasellar extension of a pituitary tumor had elevations of one or more CSF adenohypophyseal hormones. *1189*

197.00 Secondary Malignant Neoplasm of Respiratory System

Alanine Aminotransferase *Serum Increase* In 24% of 33 patients at initial hospitalization for this disorder. *0781*

Albumin *Serum Decrease* In 30% of 601 patients at initial hospitalization for this disorder. *0781*

Alkaline Phosphatase *Serum Increase* In 49% of 588 patients at initial hospitalization for this disorder. *0781*

Leukocyte Decrease Patients with metastases of the lung, bone and skin all showed decreased activity, with median values of 6.4 20.5, and 10.0 U/L respectively (normal = 55 U). *1423*

Alpha₁-Glycoprotein *Serum Increase* Elevated with metastases and larger tumor mass. *1239 1672 1866 1947 2096 2170*

Pleural Effusion Increase Highest levels found in malignant exudates. *1239 1672 1866 1947 2096 2170*

Amylase *Pleural Effusion Normal* Usually less than or equal to serum level. *2017*

Aspartate Aminotransferase *Serum Increase* In 48% of 592 patients at initial hospitalization for this disorder. *0781*

Bicarbonate *Serum Increase* In 41% of 280 patients at initial hospitalization for this disorder. *0781*

Calcium *Serum Increase* In 7 cases of bronchogenic metastases, hypercalcemia was recorded (range 10.6-16.4 mg/dL). *1904*

Carcinoembryonic Antigen *Ascitic Fluid Increase* In malignant effusions. *2199*

Erythrocytes *Pleural Effusion Increase* 1000-> 100,000/μL. *2017 0962*

Factor II *Plasma Decrease* May be associated with defibrination resulting in platelet and coagulation factor consumption. *2538*

Factor IV *Plasma Decrease* May be associated with defibrination resulting in platelet and coagulation factor consumption. *2538*

Fibrinogen *Plasma Decrease* May be associated with defibrination resulting in platelet and coagulation factor consumption. *2538*

Gamma Glutamyl Transferase (GGT) *Serum Increase* In 62% of 106 patients at initial hospitalization for this disorder. *0781*

Glucose *Pleural Effusion Decrease* Markedly reduced, 20 mg/dL or less, is very suggestive and virtually diagnostic of rheumatoid disease. A low level in the range of 40 mg/dL can be found in infectious processes and in malignant pleural effusions. *0962*

Hematocrit *Blood Decrease* In 28% of 603 patients at initial hospitalization for this disorder. *0781*

Hemoglobin *Blood Decrease* In 37% of 597 patients at initial hospitalization for this disorder. *0781*

Iron *Serum Decrease* In 55% of 43 patients at initial hospitalization for this disorder. *0781*

Iron-Binding Capacity, Total (TIBC) *Serum Decrease* In 39% of 43 patients at initial hospitalization for this disorder. *0781*

Iron Saturation *Serum Decrease* In 59% of 43 patients at initial hospitalization for this disorder. *0781*

Lactate Dehydrogenase *Serum Increase* From a study of 50 patients, a semiquantitative relationship appeared with LD, rapidity of tumor growth, and degree of dissemination of the neoplastic process. *2575* In 50% of 574 patients at initial hospitalization for this disorder. *0781*

Pleural Effusion Increase A markedly elevated pleural LD is consistent with neoplastic involvement of the pleura. Not specific for the diagnosis. *0962*

Leukocytes *Blood Increase* In 25% of 604 patients at initial hospitalization for this disorder. *0781*

Lymphocytes *Blood Decrease* In 59% of 581 patients at initial hospitalization for this disorder. *0781*

Pleural Effusion Decrease In patients with pulmonary tuberculosis, pulmonary malignancy or nonspecific pleuritis, the percentages and absolute number of B lymphocytes were significantly lower in pleural fluid than in peripheral blood. *1809*

Monocytes *Blood Increase* In 61% of 584 patients at initial hospitalization for this disorder. *0781*

Pleural Effusion Increase Predominant cell type. *2017*

Neutrophils *Blood Increase* In 55% of 584 patients at initial hospitalization for this disorder. *0781*

Oxygen Saturation *Blood Decrease* Impaired diffusion. *0422*

pH *Pleural Effusion Decrease* Exudate (pH < 7.3). *0062*

Pleural Effusion Increase pH < 7.40 militates against malignancy, especially in the absence of infection and < 7.30 is rarely encountered in tuberculous pleural disease. *0962*

Phosphate *Serum Decrease* In 26% of 603 patients at initial hospitalization for this disorder. *0781*

Platelet Count *Blood Decrease* May be associated with defibrination resulting in platelet and coagulation factor consumption. *2538*

Blood Increase May be increased in malignancy especially disseminated, advanced or inoperable. *2468* In 31% of 508 patients at initial hospitalization for this disorder. *0781*

pO₂ *Blood Decrease* In 65% of 67 patients at initial hospitalization for this disorder. *0781*

Protein *Pleural Effusion Increase* Exudate. *2017*

Prothrombin Consumption *Blood Increase* May be associated with defibrination resulting in platelet and coagulation factor consumption. *2538*

Rheumatoid Factor *Pleural Effusion Increase* May be present with rheumatoid disease, but may also be found in other types of pleural effusions (e.g., carcinoma, tuberculosis, bacterial pneumonia). *2467*

Specific Gravity *Pleural Effusion Increase* Exudate (> 1.016). *0062*

197.00   Secondary Malignant Neoplasm of Respiratory System *(continued)*

Uric Acid   *Serum   Increase*   In 39% of 602 patients at initial hospitalization for this disorder. *0781*

197.50   Secondary Malignant Neoplasm of Digestive System

Alpha₁-Antitrypsin   *Serum   Decrease*   Increased levels of alpha₁ antitrypsin and alpha₁ acid glycoprotein are associated with metastases to the large bowel. *2480*

Serum   Increase   Increased levels of alpha₁ antitrypsin and alpha₁ acid glycoprotein are associated with metastases to the large bowel. *2480*

Alpha₁-Glycoprotein   *Serum   Increase*   Elevated with metastases and larger tumor mass. *1239 1672 1866   1947 2096 2170*

Carcinoembryonic Antigen   *Serum   Increase*   All but 1 of the patients with metastatic disease of the GI tract had elevated concentrations of CEA. Mean value for upper GI tract disease was 21.8 ± 22.7 ng/mL, and 285.2 ± 441 ng/mL for lower GI tract disease. *1817*

Factor II   *Plasma   Decrease*   May be associated with defibrination resulting in platelet and coagulation factor consumption. *2538*

Factor IV   *Plasma   Decrease*   May be associated with defibrination resulting in platelet and coagulation factor consumption. *2538*

Fibrinogen   *Plasma   Decrease*   May be associated with defibrination resulting in platelet and coagulation factor consumption. *2538*

Glycoproteins   *Serum   Increase*   Metastases are indicated when levels increase in patients with large intestinal cancer. *2480*

Haptoglobin   *Serum   Increase*   High levels of haptoglobin may suggest involvement of the bowel wall by recurrent cancer. *2480*

Lactate Dehydrogenase   *Serum   Increase*   From a study of 50 patients, a semiquantitative relation appeared between serum LD, rapidity of tumor growth, and degree of dissemination of the neoplastic process. *2575*

Platelet Count   *Blood   Decrease*   May be associated with defibrination resulting in platelet and coagulation factor consumption. *2538*

Blood   Increase   May be increased in malignancy especially disseminated, advanced or inoperable. *2467*

Prealbumin   *Serum   Increase*   Tends to reflect the nutritional status of patients with primary and metastatic cancer of the large intestine. *2480*

197.70   Secondary Malignant Neoplasm of Liver

5'-Nucleotidase   *Serum   Increase*   Five patients with carcinoma of head of pancreas metastatic to liver showed elevations ranging from 20-118 U/L (normal = 2-11). *1312*

Acid Phosphatase   *Serum   Increase*   Closely parallels serum bilirubin. *2104*

Alanine Aminotransferase   *Serum   Increase*   Generally parallels AST but the increase is less marked. *2467*   Modestly elevated (145 U/L). All cases of intrahepatic disease showed elevations. Values ranged from 12.5-116 U/L. *2576*   83% of 12 patients showed increase. Mean elevation 72 U/L (normal = 24). *1452*   Raised in 33% of cases of liver metastases. *2093*   Occasional elevation. *2260 0503 0962*

Aldolase   *Serum   Increase*   Elevated in 75% of cases of liver metastases. *2093*

Alkaline Phosphatase   *Serum   Increase*   Degree of elevation may at times be striking with little or no rise in bilirubin. Occurs in 80% of cases, usually ranging from 25-375 U/L with 20% of cases showing values > 107 U/L. *0503*   Useful index of partial obstruction of the biliary tree when serum bilirubin is usually normal and urine bilirubin is increased. Increased in 80% of patients with metastatic carcinoma. *2467*   Consistent elevation with metastases. *1312*

Leukocyte   Increase   Parallel alkaline phosphatase but is not affected by bone disease. *2467*   Liver metastases appear to be the only metastatic site which tends to increase activity. Patients with liver metastases had a median value of 65 U/L (normal = 55). Other primary and secondary malignancies usually present significantly low levels. *1423*

Alkaline Phosphatase Isoenzymes   *Serum   Increase*   23 of 24 patients with metastatic carcinoma of liver had markedly elevated liver alpha₁ and alpha₂ alkaline phosphatase isoenzyme levels. Mean values were 19 ± 18 U/L and 45 ± 28 U/L respectively. *1926*

Alpha₁-Glycoprotein   *Serum   Increase*   It was found to have a sensitivity of 65% and a specificity of 80% with severe liver disease. *0709*

Alpha-Fetoprotein   *Serum   Increase*   Present in some patients with liver metastases from carcinoma of the stomach or pancreas. *2467*

Pleural Effusion   Increase   Positive results were most frequently found in samples derived from patients with secondary or primary liver tumors. The highest levels (6 and 30 ng/mL) were determined in samples of 2 hepatoma patients. *0622*

Aminolevulinic Acid   *Urine   Increase*   May occur. *0503*

Aspartate Aminotransferase   *Serum   Increase*   Approximately 50% of patients with metastatic carcinoma have elevated values, usually in the same range as patients with cirrhosis and posthepatic jaundice. Usual values < 145 U/L. *0503*   All 12 cases of liver metastases showed a moderate elevation (mean = 106). Normal upper limit 24 U/L. *1452   0962*

Beta-Glucuronidase   *Serum   Increase*   Increased. *0741 0866*

Bilirubin   *Serum   Increase*   Elevated serum bilirubin values of 2.6-12.2 mg/dL were reported in patients with carcinoma metastatic to liver. *2576*

Serum   Normal   Common finding. *0186*

Urine   Increase   Increased serum alkaline phosphatase is the most useful index of partial obstruction of the biliary tree when serum bilirubin is usually normal and urine bilirubin is increased. *2467*

BSP Retention   *Serum   Increase*   Increased serum alkaline phosphatase and increased BSP retention is 65% reliable to establish this diagnosis. *2467*

Carcinoembryonic Antigen   *Serum   Increase*   Markedly increased (> 25 ng/mL) values are highly suggestive of metastatic cancer, particularly hepatic metastasis. *0859*

Ascitic Fluid   Increase   In malignant effusions. *2199*

Cholesterol   *Serum   Decrease*   *0503*

Copper   *Serum   Increase*   High in advanced carcinoma with liver metastases. *1125*

Creatine   *Urine   Increase*   Increased formation. *0619*

Dopa (3,4-Dihydroxyphenylalanine)   *Urine   Increase*   Found to be elevated in the urine of patients with metastatic disease. Excretion appears to be proportional to the tumor burden. *1511*

Erythrocytes   *Ascitic Fluid   Increase*   > 10,000 cells/μL seen in 20% of cases. *2626*

Fibrin Split Products (FSP)   *Ascitic Fluid   Increase*   In malignant effusions. *2199*

Gamma Glutamyl Transferase (GGT)   *Serum   Increase*   Parallels alkaline phosphatase; elevation precedes positive liver scans. *2467*   Marked elevations were observed in 12 patients. Mean 396 U/L was 13.2 X the normal upper limit (range = 208-820). *1452*

Glucose   *Serum   Decrease*   Can occur with various types of liver disease. Hepatic hypoglycemia is a fasting hypoglycemia and often only transiently relieved by food. *0962   2104*

Glutathione Reductase   *Serum   Increase*   Raised in 47% of cases. *2093*

Haptoglobin   *Serum   Increase*   alpha₂-globulins, especially haptoglobins were generally increased in primary colorectal cancer, and rose in metastatic cancer especially when it involved the liver. Haptoglobin values were useful to indicate tumor activity. *0450*

Isocitrate Dehydrogenase   *Serum   Increase*   Raised in 57% of patients. *2093*   Approximately 50% of patients with liver metastases exhibited relatively small elevations. Only those patients with secondary liver involvement had increased concentrations. *2260*

Lactate Dehydrogenase   *Serum   Increase*   From a study of 50 patients, a semiquantitative relation appeared between serum LD, rapidity of tumor growth, and degree of dissemination of the neoplastic process. *2575*   Distinctly elevated in most cases. *2260*

Leucine Aminopeptidase   *Serum   Increase*   Of 30 patients with hepatic metastases, 93% had elevated levels, ranging from 305-1,000 U/L with a mean of 572 U/L. *0281*   Moderate increase in serum, which occurs even in the absence of jaundice (especially if steroids given). *0619*

Leukocytes   *Ascitic Fluid   Increase*   > 1000 WBC/μL. *2626*

Malate Dehydrogenase   *Serum   Increase*   Elevated in 62% of patients. *2093*

Melanin   *Urine   Increase*   Melanogenuria occurs in 25% of patients with malignant melanoma; it is said to be more frequent with extensive liver metastasis. It is not useful for judging completeness of removal or early recurrence. Beware of false positive red-brown or purple suspension due to salicylates. *2467*

Ornithine Carbamoyl Transferase (OCT)   *Serum   Increase*   Liver cell damage. *2467*

Platelet Count   *Blood   Increase*   May be increased in malignancy especially disseminated, advanced or inoperable. *2468*

Protein *Ascitic Fluid Increase* > 2.5 g/dL in ascitic fluid. *2626*

Prothrombin Time *Plasma Increase* Prolonged in liver disease. *0962*

Pseudocholinesterase *Serum Decrease* Some patients. *2467*

Vitamin B$_{12}$ *Serum Increase* *2467*

Zinc *Serum Decrease* Low in advanced carcinoma with liver metastases. *1125*

198.30 Secondary Malignant Neoplasm of Brain

Aldolase *Serum Increase* The serum of cancer patients contains a greater proportion of aldolase A (muscle-type) than serum from normal persons. Gliomas and normal brain tissue contain aldolase C (nerve and brain variant), but in meningiomas or tissue metastatic to brain, only aldolase A (liver and fetal form) is detected. *2093*

Antidiuretic Hormone *Serum Increase* Associated with excessive ADH production resulting in sodium loss. *2104*

Aspartate Aminotransferase *CSF Increase* Elevated activities were associated with metastatic carcinoma of CNS. Patients with primary tumors generally showed normal levels. *0507* In all but 2 patients with metastatic tumors of the CNS, the activity was significantly raised. The mean for the group was 20.4 U/L. *0507*

Cells *CSF Increase* Increased cells which are not usually recognized as blast cells because of poor preservation (meningeal infiltration of leukemic cells). *2467*

Glomerular Filtration Rate (GFR) *Urine Increase* Associated excess ADH may tend to accelerate GFR. *2104*

Glucose *CSF Decrease* Less than 50% of blood level (meningeal infiltration of leukemic cells). *2467*

Isocitrate Dehydrogenase *Serum Increase* Increased in CSF with secondary cerebral tumors. *0619*

Lactate Dehydrogenase *Serum Increase* From a study of 50 patients, a semiquantitative relation appeared between LD, rapidity of tumor growth, and degree of dissemination of the neoplastic process. *2575* Depending on location, growth rate, etc. *2467*

CSF Increase In group of patients with metastatic tumors of the nervous system showed a highly significant difference in the mean CSF LD activity of 67 U/L. All but 2 patients had significantly elevated individual results. *0507* *2574*

Leukocytes *Blood Increase* More frequent when WBC is > 100,000/μL and with rapid increase in WBC, especially in blastic crises (intracranial hemorrhage). *2467*

Platelet Count *Blood Decrease* Platelet count frequently decreased (intracranial hemorrhage). *2467*

Blood Increase May be increased in malignancy especially disseminated, advanced or inoperable. *2468*

Protein *CSF Increase* Increased protein (meningeal infiltration of leukemic cells). *2467*

Sodium *Serum Decrease* Associated with excessive ADH production. *2104* Serum Sodium usually less than 130 mEq/L *0062*

Urine Increase Urine is almost always hypertonic to plasma *0062*

198.50 Secondary Malignant Neoplasm of Bone

Acid Phosphatase *Serum Increase* Especially from breast carcinoma; concentrations > 9 U/L indicate active invasion. *0619* Often slightly increased, especially in prostatic metastases (osteolytic metastases), and especially in primary tumor of bronchus, breast, kidney, and thyroid. *2467* Occurred in 61% of cases. Normal levels were found in 39% of cases when bone metastases were present. *1954*

Bone Marrow Increase Early bone metastases were detected by an increased activity in the bone marrow before any serum elevation or discernible radiographic changes occurred. Bone marrow activity was consistently much higher than in the serum in patients with histologically confirmed bone metastases. *0404* *1261*

Alkaline Phosphatase *Serum Increase* Rises in proportion to the formation of new bone cells. *0812* Usually increased in osteoblastic metastases (especially from primary tumor in prostate). *2467* Especially secondary to prostate *1954* and breast carcinoma. *2566* 23% of patients with bone metastasis showed normal concentrations. *2062* *0503*

Leukocyte Decrease Patients with metastases of the lung, bone and skin all showed decreased activity, with median values of 6.4, 20.5, and 10.0 U/L respectively (Normal = 55 U). *1423*

Alkaline Phosphatase Isoenzymes *Serum Increase* 5 of 7 patients with metastatic lesions of bone had elevated isoenzyme-II. Isoenzymes I and IV were elevated in 2 of the 7 cases. *1221*

Calcitonin *Serum Increase* 8 patients with skeletal metastases had increased concentrations, ranging from 0.15 ng/mL - 9.0 ng/mL. *0445*

Calcium *Serum Increase* May be normal or increased in osteolytic metastases (especially from primary tumor of bronchus, breast, kidney, thyroid). *2467* Elevations in patients with carcinoma of prostate metastatic to bone were negligible at first but mild hypercalcemia developed at some time in 9% of patients. *2566* *1904*

Urine Decrease Low in osteoblastic metastases (especially from primary tumor in prostate). *2467*

Urine Increase Patients with osteolytic metastatic neoplasms (especially with active or extensive lesions) may display hypercalcemia and hypercalciuria which can be further complicated by nephrocalcinosis and renal failure. *0503* Often increased; marked increase may reflect increased rate of tumor growth. *2467* *0151*

Copper *Serum Increase* 12 cases of osteosarcoma at various stages were analyzed for Cu and Zn serum levels. Elevated Cu occurred in primary and metastatic cases, while elevated Zn occurred only in primary osteosarcoma and depressed serum Zn in metastases. Patients with advanced cases had the highest serum Cu:Zn ratios. *0735*

Erythrocytes *Blood Decrease* Depression of all formed elements of the blood is often seen in disseminated neoplastic disease. *0999*

Erythrocyte Sedimentation Rate *Blood Increase* *0962*

Gamma Glutamyl Transferase (GGT) *Serum Increase* In 4 patients with carcinoma metastatic to bone, 25% (1) had a slightly elevated concentration (54 U/L). *1452*

Hematocrit *Blood Decrease* Depression of all formed elements of the blood is often seen in disseminated neoplastic disease. *0999*

Hemoglobin *Blood Decrease* Depression of all formed elements of the blood is often seen in disseminated neoplastic disease. *0999*

Lactate Dehydrogenase *Serum Increase* From a study of 50 patients, a semiquantitative relation appeared between LD, rapidity of tumor growth, and degree of dissemination of the neoplastic process. *2575*

Leukocytes *Blood Decrease* Depression of all formed elements of the blood is often seen in disseminated neoplastic disease. *0999*

Magnesium *Serum Decrease* *2467*

Neutrophils *Blood Decrease* Depression of all formed elements of the blood is often seen in disseminated neoplastic disease. *0999*

Phosphate *Serum Increase* May be normal or increased (osteolytic metastases (especially from primary tumor of bronchus, breast, kidney, thyroid)). *2467*

Platelet Count *Blood Decrease* Depression of all formed elements of the blood is often seen in disseminated neoplastic disease. *0999*

Blood Increase May be increased in malignancy especially disseminated, advanced or inoperable. *2468*

Reticulocytes *Blood Increase* Possibly increased. *2467*

Zinc *Serum Increase* Serum Cu:Zn concentrations were evaluated in 19 patients with sarcomas, 12 of which were osteosarcomas at various stages. Patients with primary or metastatic osteosarcoma had elevated Cu. Patients with primary osteosarcoma had elevated Zn, those with metastases had depressed Zn. The ratio of Cu:Zn in osteosarcoma. patients may be of value in prognosis and therapy evaluation. The ratio of Cu:Zn may be useful in discriminating between patients with primary and metastatic osteosarcoma. *0735*

199.00 Secondary Malignant Neoplasm (Disseminated)

Albumin *Serum Decrease* Serum concentration of albumin and transferrin were significantly reduced while haptoglobin was increased in disseminated carcinoma compared with localized. *1025*

Aldolase *Serum Increase* Variable rises in serum levels may be found in carcinomatosis. Serum aldolase and phosphohexose isomerase are roughly parallel. *0619*

Alkaline Phosphatase *Leukocyte Decrease* Patients with metastases of the lung, bone, and skin all showed decreased activity, with median values of 6.4, 20.5, and 10.0 U/L respectively (Normal = 55 U). *1423*

Alpha$_1$-Antichymotrypsin *Serum Increase* Increased with any kind of invasive tumor. *1262* *1248*

Alpha$_1$-Antitrypsin *Serum Increase* Increased. *1866* *0042* *1946* *1947* *2129*

199.00   Secondary Malignant Neoplasm (Disseminated)
(continued)

Alpha₁-Globulin   *Serum   Increase*   2467

Alpha₁-Glycoprotein   *Serum   Increase*   Elevated with metastases and larger tumor mass. *1239 1672 1866   1947 2096 2170*

Alpha₂-Globulin   *Serum   Increase*   2467

Alpha₂-Macroglobulin   *Serum   Increase*   1438

Amylase   *Ascitic Fluid   Increase*   With carcinomatous peritonitis 91% of the increased amylase activity was of salivary type and the remainder of pancreatic type. *1364*   Parallels the degree of metastatic involvement of the peritoneum. *2104*

Angiotensin-Converting Enzyme (ACE)   *Serum   Decrease*   Most cancer patients present with normal to low levels. *1501*

Serum   Normal   Most cancer patients present with normal to low levels. *1501*

Antithrombin III   *Plasma   Decrease*   Seen with carcinoma. *2353 1482*

Beta₂-Macroglobulin   *Urine   Increase*   24 h excretion and renal clearance were significantly increased in disseminated carcinoma compared with localized. *1025*

Beta-Globulin   *Serum   Decrease*   2467

Calcitonin   *Serum   Increase*   Elevated. *0918*

Carcinoembryonic Antigen   *Serum   Increase*   High preoperative values had been shown to be associated with an increased risk of metastases or recurrence in patients who apparently had a successful resection of a carcinoma of the large bowel. Measurements after surgery provide an earlier warning of metastases and recurrence often with a lead time of many months. *0450*

Cholesterol   *Serum   Decrease*   Among 150 men who died of cancer, cholesterol level fell 22.7 mg/dL more than in survivors over the equivalent period. *2148*

Pericardial Fluid   Increase   High levels (2.6-5.2 mmol/L; 100 to 200 mg/dL). *0274*

Cryofibrinogen   *Serum   Increase*   2035 1551

Dopa (3,4-Dihydroxyphenylalanine)   *Urine   Increase*   Found to be elevated in the urine of patients with metastatic disease. Excretion appears to be proportional to the tumor burden. *1511*

Eosinophils   *Blood   Increase*   2538

Erythrocyte Sedimentation Rate   *Blood   Increase*   ESR > 100 mm in the 1st h indicates serious disease, as in tuberculosis and carcinomatosis. *0532*

Factor II   *Plasma   Decrease*   May be associated with defibrination resulting in platelet and coagulation factor consumption. *2538*

Factor IV   *Plasma   Decrease*   May be associated with defibrination resulting in platelet and coagulation factor consumption. *2538*

Fibrinogen   *Plasma   Decrease*   May be associated with defibrination resulting in platelet and coagulation factor consumption. *2538*

Folate   *Serum   Decrease*   Decreased with extensive skin disease. *0299 2357 0367*

Fucose   *Serum   Increase*   Markedly increased. *1342*

Glycoproteins   *Serum   Increase*   Metastases are indicated when levels increase in patients with large intestinal cancer. *2480*

Haptoglobin   *Serum   Increase*   Serum concentration of albumin and transferrin were significantly reduced while haptoglobin was increased in disseminated carcinoma compared with localized. *1025*

Hexosaminidase   *Serum   Increase*   Elevated. *2356*

Immunoglobulins   *Urine   Increase*   24 h excretion and renal clearance of free lambda and kappa light chains of immunoglobulins were significantly increased in disseminated carcinoma compared with localized. *1025*

Iron-Binding Capacity, Total (TIBC)   *Serum   Decrease*   Low serum iron binding capacity (total) due to carcinomatosis. *0619*

Iron Saturation   *Serum   Decrease*   Serum concentration of albumin and transferrin were significantly reduced while haptoglobin was increased in disseminated carcinoma compared with localized. *1025*

Lactate Dehydrogenase   *Serum   Increase*   From a study of 50 patients, a semiquantitative relation appeared between serum LD, rapidity of tumor growth, and degree of dissemination of the neoplastic process. *2575*

Leucine Aminopeptidase   *Serum   Increase*   Elevated in disseminated malignant disease. *1814*

Lymphocytes   *Blood   Decrease*   Active rosettes (T-EA) were decreased only in metastatic patients, while the total T population (T-ET) was decreased in all stages. Patients whose values were constant remained cancer free, while a reduction heralded the appearance of clinical and/or radiological signs of metastases. *0185*

Lymphocyte T-Cell   *Blood   Decrease*   0793

Lysozyme   *Urine   Increase*   24 h excretion and renal clearance were significantly increased in disseminated carcinoma compared with localized. *1025*

Metanephrines, Total   *Urine   Increase*   0503

Platelet Count   *Blood   Decrease*   May be associated with defibrination resulting in platelet and coagulation factor consumption. *2538*

Blood   Increase   May be increased in malignancy especially disseminated, advanced or inoperable. *2468*

Porphobilinogen   *Urine   Increase*   Elevated porphobilinogen occasionally has been observed in carcinomatosis. *0151*

Prothrombin Consumption   *Blood   Increase*   May be associated with defibrination resulting in platelet and coagulation factor consumption. *2538*

Trypsin Inhibitor   *Serum   Increase*   Elevated compared to normal controls or patients with non-neoplastic disorders. *1590*

Zinc   *Serum   Decrease*   Decreased. *2297*

201.90   Hodgkin's Disease

5'-Nucleotidase   *Serum   Increase*   Six patients showed elevations varying from 18.8-126.2 U/L (normal = 2-11). *1312*

Alanine Aminotransferase   *Serum   Increase*   May be a systemic sign of active disease or may indicate involvement of liver or bone. *0433*   In 30% of 10 patients at initial hospitalization for this disorder. *0781*

Albumin   *Serum   Decrease*   With active disease. *2538 0073*   In 22% of 72 patients at initial hospitalization for this disorder. *0781 2552*

Aldolase   *Serum   Increase*   Markedly elevated in malignant lymphomas. Mean = 5.0 ± 0.4 U/L compared to normal, 1.6 - 0.21. *1201*

Alkaline Phosphatase   *Serum   Increase*   Progressive increase in patients over 20 y of age with elevated concentrations found with advancing clinical stage. Patients < 20 had frequent (50%) occurrence of elevations but this did not correlate with stage of disease. More sensitive than GGT in following the clinical course. *0160*   May be a systemic sign of active disease or may indicate involvement of liver or bone. *2538 1204*   Lymphoma associated with hyperbilirubinemia is accompanied by elevations from 43-331 U/L. In some cases, reflects osteoblastic lesions as well as metastases. *2576   0433 0781*

Leukocyte   Decrease   Activity is low irrespective of tumor category, activity of disease, or type of therapy. In 17 cases of malignant lymphoma, median LAP was 17 U/L (Normal = 55). *1423*

Leukocyte   Increase   In 4 cases, mean value was 135, ranging from 92-182. Activities were elevated in patients in spite of good remission with no clinical and radiological sign of disease. *1563*   22 of 23 patients with active disease had significant LAP elevations, mean score of 164 ± 51. Of 19 patients with inactive disease, 15 had normal scores, 63 ± 17, and the 4 with elevated scores soon redeveloped symptoms of activity. *0167*   Elevated during active phases. Normal during remission. *2538   0151*

Alpha₁-Globulin   *Serum   Increase*   In the presence of fever. *2552*   Increased alpha₁ and alpha₂-globulins suggest disease activity. *2468*

Alpha₂-Globulin   *Serum   Increase*   Frequently increased in later stages of disease. *2450*   With active disease. *2538 0073*   Often quite high. *2552*

Angiotensin-Converting Enzyme (ACE)   *Serum   Decrease*   No relationship was found between enzyme activity and stage, activity, histo- pathology, etc. Levels were lower than healthy controls but not significantly *0258   1969*

Aspartate Aminotransferase   *Serum   Increase*   Minimal elevation was observed in 5 of 11 patients. *0160*   May be a systemic sign of active disease or may indicate involvement of liver or bone. *0433*

Basophils   *Blood   Increase*   2467

Beta₂-Macroglobulin   *Serum   Increase*   May be increased. *1236 0388*

CSF   Increase   May be increased in lymphomas involving the central nervous system. *1236*   With Involvement of the CNS *0388*

Beta-Globulin   *Serum   Decrease*   2467

Serum   Increase   Active disease. *0073*

Bicarbonate   *Serum   Increase*   In 60% of 45 patients at initial hospitalization for this disorder. *0781*

Bilirubin   *Serum   Increase*   May be a systemic sign of active disease or may indicate involvement of liver or bone. *0433*

Bleeding Time *Blood Decrease* Has been reported. *2538 1087* Thrombocytopenia. *2246*

BSP Retention *Serum Increase* May be a systemic sign of active disease or may indicate involvement of liver or bone. *0433*

Calcium *Serum Increase* Observed in 6 cases (range 10.6 - 16.4 mg/dL). *1904* In patients with bone and liver disease. *2538 1204* Metastatic or lytic tumor involving bone. *0503* Indicates bone involvement. *0433*

Urine Increase *0503*

Carcinoembryonic Antigen *Serum Increase* In 22% of cases. *2199*

Serum Normal Levels are low in this malignancy, remaining within the normal range or just above it. *2374*

Ceruloplasmin *Serum Increase* *0151*

Cholesterol *Serum Decrease* In 27% of 72 patients at initial hospitalization for this disorder. *0781*

Cholesterol, Very Low Density Lipoprotein *Serum Increase* Moderate increase due to presence of IgG or IgM that forms complexes with chylomicron remnants and/or VLDL thereby decreasing catabolism. *0062*

Chylomicrons *Serum Increase* Moderate increase due to presence of IgG or IgM that forms complexes with chylomicron remnants and/or VLDL thereby decreasing catabolism. *0062*

Clot Retraction *Blood Poor* With thrombocytopenia. *2246*

Complement, Total *Serum Increase* 58 of 72 patients had elevated total complement levels which were associated with C-reactive protein, ESR and beta globulin levels. *1998* A highly significant increase of the mean total serum hemolytic complement activity was found in stages III-A and IV-A and all stages with systemic symptoms in Hodgkin's disease. *2450*

Coombs' Test *Blood Positive* Usually negative, but on occasion it is positive. *0641 2538*

Copper *Serum Increase* Correlates significantly to stage of disease and amount of tumor tissue. Varies with activity of the disease-- increases with progression and decreases with improvement. *2354* Has been reported. *2538 1087* In all 50 patients with lymphoma, invariably found to be raised. After radiotherapy, the level was significantly lowered. *1888*

C-Reactive Protein *Serum Increase* Increased during active stages; may be normal during remission. *2468*

Creatinine *Serum Increase* In 36% of 37 patients at initial hospitalization for this disorder. *0781*

Cryofibrinogen *Serum Increase* *2035 1551*

Cryoglobulins *Serum Increase* May be associated with cryoglobulinemia. *2468*

Eosinophils *Blood Increase* Occasionally seen. *0433* Eosinophilia, usually < 10%, may be seen in 10-20% of cases. *0999* Tends to occur in patients with severe and longstanding pruritus. *0151* A striking eosinophilia is the outstanding characteristic. *1484* In 29% of 77 patients at initial hospitalization for this disorder. *0781* *0532 2538*

Liver Increase Eosinophilic predominance occurs mainly in the fibrotic types of Hodgkin's disease. The survival time of patients with eosinophilic predominance was significantly shorter than that of the controls. *2369*

Erythrocytes *Blood Decrease* Pancytopenia is a common feature. *2538*

Erythrocyte Sedimentation Rate *Blood Increase* Commonly elevated in patients with active disease. *0151* Increases with stage of disease. *2450* Increased in significant tissue necrosis, especially neoplasms - most frequently malignant lymphoma, cancer of the colon and breast. *2468*

Erythrocyte Survival *Red Blood Cells Decrease* Mild or moderate hemolytic anemia, with a negative Coombs' test, is common in disseminated lymphoma. *0433*

Erythropoietin *Serum Decrease* The most frequent finding is a normochromic anemia, most often a result of decreased erythropoiesis *0999*

Ferritin *Serum Increase* Serum levels are raised due to increased production by splenic tumor tissue. *2047* A high circulating concentration is characteristic. *2538 1185* Significant elevation *2244*

Fibrinogen *Plasma Increase* Increases with stage of disease. *2450*

Fucose *Serum Increase* Markedly elevated and correlated with clinical stage of disease. Values ranged from 13 mg/dL in stage 1 to 29.5 mg/dL in stage 4. *0607*

Gamma Glutamyl Transferase (GGT) *Serum Increase* Elevated in 36% (4 of 11) patients. *0160* In 73% of 12 patients at initial hospitalization for this disorder. *0781*

Globulin *Serum Decrease* Infrequent. Concentrations < 200 mg/dL are rarely documented. *1061* Rare occasions. *1060*

Serum Increase May be increased with macroglobulins present and evidence of autoimmune process. *2468* With active disease. *2538 0073* Electrophoretic studies of serum proteins are often normal early in the course of the disease but may show a hyperglobulinemia (commonly alpha$_2$) *0999*

Haptoglobin *Serum Increase* Increased in disseminated neoplasms; conditions associated with increased ESR and alpha$_2$-globulin. *2467* *0151*

Hematocrit *Blood Decrease* Mild or moderate hemolytic anemia, with a negative Coombs' test, is common in disseminated lymphoma. *0433* Present in 33% of all patients at diagnosis. Develops in nearly every patient who has fever, sweats, or other systemic manifestations. Becomes worse as the disease advances and improves with remission. *2538 0414* In 38% of 76 patients at initial hospitalization for this disorder. *0781*

Hemoglobin *Blood Decrease* Mild to moderate hemolytic anemia, with a negative Coombs' test, is common in disseminated lymphoma. *0433* Present in 33% of all patients at diagnosis. Develops in nearly every patient who has fever, sweats, or other systemic manifestations. Becomes worse as the disease advances and improves with remission. *2538 0414* In 44% of 76 patients at initial hospitalization for this disorder. *0781*

Heterophil Antibody *Serum Increase* Very rare. *0503*

Hexokinase *Serum Increase* Markedly increased in malignant lymphomas. Mean = 14.6 $\pm$ 2.0 compared to normal 0.93 $\pm$ 0.28 U/L. *1201*

Hydroxyproline *Serum Increase* *0592*

Urine Increase *0151*

Immunoglobulin IgA *Serum Normal* *2467*

Immunoglobulin IgG *Serum Normal* *2467*

Immunoglobulin IgM *Serum Normal* *2467*

Iron *Serum Decrease* In 77% of 18 patients at initial hospitalization for this disorder. *0781* Hypoferremia is characteristic and may be associated with excessive uptake of iron by the liver and spleen. *2538* *0151 0592*

Iron-Binding Capacity, Total (TIBC) *Serum Decrease* In 32% of 18 patients at initial hospitalization for this disorder. *0781* *0151 0592*

Iron Saturation *Serum Decrease* In 94% of 18 patients at initial hospitalization for this disorder. *0781*

Lactate Dehydrogenase *Serum Increase* Normal or relatively increased; depends on the total mass of the tumor and presence of hemolysis. *0503* May be a sign of active disease or may indicate involvement of liver or bone. *0433* Marked elevation in 138 patients with malignant lymphomas. Mean = 177.7 $\pm$ 13.8 U/L compared to normals, 85.4 $\pm$ 1.0 U/L. *1201* In 37% of 72 patients at initial hospitalization for this disorder. *0781* *0206 1089*

Lactate Dehydrogenase Isoenzymes *Serum Increase* LD$_3$ and LD$_4$ (may even increase LD$_2$); also useful for following effect of chemotherapy. *0812*

Lactic Acid *Blood Increase* In 20 patients with malignant lymphomas, mean concentration = 23.2 $\pm$ 2.9 mg/dL compared to normal, 11.7 $\pm$ 0.72 mg/dL. *1201*

Leukocytes *Blood Decrease* Variable, maybe normal, decreased, or markedly increased. *2468* Pancytopenia is a common feature. *2538*

Blood Increase Variable, maybe normal, decreased, or markedly increased. *2468* Moderately increased and a granulocytosis and monocytosis may be observed. *0999* In the untreated patient, or if therapy has been minimal, moderate to marked neutrophilic leukocytosis and thrombocytosis are characteristic of active, symptomatic Hodgkin's disease. *0151* In 56% of 77 patients at initial hospitalization for this disorder. *0781*

Lymphocytes *Blood Decrease* Lymphopenia is common late in the disease. *0999* Absolute counts tend to be at the lower end of the normal range or slightly below the lower limit. Frequently more severe in the presence of disseminated disease. *2035* In 66% of 76 patients at initial hospitalization for this disorder. *0781 0532*

Blood Increase Relative lymphocytosis when there is marked neutropenia but not absolute increase. *2246 0532*

Pleural Effusion Increase A preponderance of lymphocytes is consistent with tuberculosis, carcinoma, or lymphoma. *0962*

Lymphocyte T-Cell *Blood Decrease* *0793*

201.90   Hodgkin's Disease   (continued)

Lysozyme   *Serum   Increase*   Significantly higher compared to controls and independent of stage. *0258*   Isolated cases *0981*

Urine   Increase   *0151*

Monocytes   *Blood   Increase*   10-40% of cases exhibited a monocytosis that did not correlate with prognosis. *2398*   Appearance of abnormal large mononuclear cells in peripheral blood. *0433*   All varieties of lymphomas have been reported on occasion in association with a monocytosis, sometimes varying with disease activity. *1107*   In 71% of 77 patients at initial hospitalization for this disorder. *0781*   *0532 2538*

Neutrophils   *Blood   Increase*   Common. *0433*   In 54% of 77 patients at initial hospitalization for this disorder. *0781*   *0151*

Osmotic Fragility   *Red Blood Cells   Increase*   A higher degree of light transmission, i.e., osmotic fragility, was found in lymphocytes from Hodgkin's disease patients. After 10 min, light transmission = 70.3% - 5.93% compared to 60% ± 7.33% for normals. *1916*

Platelet Count   *Blood   Decrease*   Pancytopenia is a common feature. May result from hypersplenism. *2538*

Blood   Increase   Thrombocytosis (counts > 400,000) encountered at times, and large bizarre forms may be observed. *0999*   In 45% of 70 patients at initial hospitalization for this disorder. *0781*

Porphobilinogen   *Urine   Increase*   Elevated porphobilinogen occasionally has been observed. *0151*

Proline Hydroxylase   *Serum   Increase*   Elevated to a lesser degree than that seen in hepatoma. *0364*

Protein   *Serum   Decrease*   Enteric loss of plasma protein. *2199*   Occurs commonly. *2538*   In patients with advanced disease, reduction in serum protein concentration with hypoalbuminemia and hypogammaglobulinemia is frequent. *2462*

Pleural Effusion   Increase   Pleural effusions are usually exudates. *0062*

Pyruvate   *Blood   Increase*   Moderately elevated in 20 patients with malignant lymphomas. Mean = 1.1 ± 0.15 U/L. *1201*

Reticulocytes   *Blood   Increase*   In patients with advanced disease. *2538*

Rheumatoid Factor   *Serum   Increase*   Dysproteinemias and paraproteinemias present significant seropositivity. *0962*   Found in 18% of patients. *0422*   *0123*

Uric Acid   *Serum   Decrease*   Decreased uric acid is seen in occasional cases of neoplasms such as Hodgkin's disease. *2467*   Hypouricemia associated with markedly elevated clearance has been reported. *1241*   Rarely reported. *0962*

Serum   Increase   Hyperuricemia occurs occasionally. *0999*   Especially post x-irradiation. *2467*   In 31% of 72 patients at initial hospitalization for this disorder. *0781*

Uric Acid Clearance   *Urine   Increase*   Hypouricemia associated with markedly elevated clearance has been reported. *1241*

Vitamin B$_{12}$ *Serum   Normal*   *2467*

Vitamin B$_{12}$ Binding Capacity   *Serum   Increase*   Significant elevation; usually correlated with WBC in peripheral blood. *1990*

Zinc   *Serum   Decrease*   *1087*

Serum   Increase   *0151*

202.10   Mycosis Fungoides

Beta$_2$-Macroglobulin   *Serum   Increase*   Compared with healthy controls. *1354*   Elevated compared to normal controls *1353*

Eosinophils   *Blood   Increase*   Eosinophilia. *2539*

Immunoglobulin IgA   *Serum   Increase*   No prognostic significance. *2539*   May be elevated *2539*

Immunoglobulin IgE   *Serum   Increase*   May be elevated. *2539*

Lactate Dehydrogenase   *Serum   Increase*   *2539*

202.40   Leukemic Reticuloendotheliosis

Acid Phosphatase   *Leukocyte   Increase*   *1388*

Anisocytes   *Blood   Increase*   Usually normochromic, normocytic anemia; mild anisocytosis and poikilocytosis were common. *2390*

Erythrocytes   *Blood   Decrease*   Pancytopenia was found in almost 50% of all patients (102). *2390*

Hematocrit   *Blood   Decrease*   Usually normochromic, normocytic anemia; mild anisocytosis and poikilocytosis were common. *2390*

Hemoglobin   *Blood   Decrease*   Usually normochromic, normocytic anemia; mild anisocytosis and poikilocytosis were common. *2390*

Leukocytes   *Blood   Decrease*   Leukopenia in 63 of 102 patients, while mild leukocytosis was found in 15. *2390*

Blood   Increase   Leukopenia in 63 of 102 patients, while mild leukocytosis was found in 15. *2390*

Lysozyme   *Serum   Decrease*   Low, normal or high. *0798*

Serum   Increase   Low, normal or high. *0798*

Serum   Normal   Low, normal or high. *0798*

Monocytes   *Blood   Decrease*   Severe monocytopenia; 299/μL was the highest count and 6 patients had none at all. *2390*

Neutrophils   *Blood   Decrease*   Absolute neutropenia in 78% of 102 cases; frequently severe. *2390*   Severe bone marrow granulocytopenia and poor blood neutrophil response to stimulation are found. *2587*

Bone Marrow   Decrease   Severe bone marrow granulocytopenia and poor neutrophil response to stimulation are found. *2587*

Platelet Count   *Blood   Decrease*   Thrombocytopenia found in 84% of patients with counts usually in the 50-150,000 mm^3 range. *2390*

Poikilocytes   *Blood   Decrease*   Usually normochromic, normocytic anemia; mild anisocytosis and poikilocytosis were common. *2390*

202.52   Histiocytosis X

Bilirubin   *Serum   Increase*   May occur in the presence of extensive liver involvement. *0433*

Eosinophils   *Blood   Normal*   No associated eosinophilia. *2552*

Erythrocyte Sedimentation Rate   *Blood   Increase*   Correlates with the prognosis and extent of disease. *2348*

Hematocrit   *Blood   Decrease*   A normocytic, normochromic anemia, sometimes severe and sometimes hemolytic in nature, may be present, especially in patients with disseminated disease. Aplastic anemia has also been described. *0433*

Hemoglobin   *Blood   Decrease*   A normocytic, normochromic anemia, sometimes severe and sometimes hemolytic in nature, may be present, especially in patients with disseminated disease. Aplastic anemia has also been described. *0433*

Leukocytes   *Blood   Decrease*   May be normal, decreased, or increased. *0433*

Blood   Increase   May be normal, decreased, or increased. *0433*

Monocytes   *Blood   Increase*   Monocytes, sometimes morphologically quite immature, may be noted in increased numbers in the peripheral blood. *0433*

pCO$_2$ *Blood   Decrease*   With lung involvement, impaired gas diffusion. *2104*

Platelet Count   *Blood   Decrease*   Thrombocytopenia may occur in patients with the so-called Letterer-Siwe Syndrome and if associated with hemorrhage manifestations constitutes a grave prognostic sign. *0433*   With involvement of the spleen. *2538*

pO$_2$ *Blood   Decrease*   With lung involvement, impaired gas diffusion. *2104*

Protein   *Serum   Decrease*   May occur in the presence of extensive liver involvement. *0433*

Specific Gravity   *Urine   Decrease*   Low, fixed specific gravity of urine is characteristic in patients with hypothalamic involvement. *0433*

202.80   Non-Hodgkins Lymphoma

1,25-Dihydroxy-Vitamin D$_3$ *Serum   Decrease*   In five patients with adult T-Cell Lymphoma. All had levels at or below the normal range. These data show that calcitriol levels are not uniformly elevated in this order and may not be the usual cause of hypercalcemia. *0574*

Serum   Increase   Three patients had elevated levels (56,72,77 pg/mL) compared to normal (< 50). *0280*

Serum   Normal   In five patients with adult T-Cell Lymphoma. All had levels at or below the normal range. These data show that calcitriol levels are not uniformly elevated in this order and may not be the usual cause of hypercalcemia. *0574*

5-Hydroxyindoleacetic Acid (5-HIAA)   *Urine   Decrease*   Absent from urine. *0619*

5'-Nucleotidase   *Serum   Increase*   Ten patients with lymphosarcoma, showed 5'-nucleotidase activities ranging from 16-59 U/L (normal = 2-11). *1312*

Acid Phosphatase *Serum Increase* In a few patients, a striking increase has been noted. *2523* A patient with histiocytic medullary reticulosis was found to have up to 60 X the normal upper limit, which then paralleled the activity of disease during temporary responses to therapy. *2523*

Leukocyte Decrease *1388*

Alanine Aminotransferase *Serum Increase* May be a systemic sign of active disease or may indicate involvement of liver or bone. *0433* In 30% of 10 patients at initial hospitalization for this disorder. *0781*

Albumin *Serum Decrease* In patients with advanced disease, reduction in serum protein concentration with hypoalbuminemia and hypogammaglobulinemia is frequent. *2462* In 40% of 74 patients at initial hospitalization for this disorder. *0781* *2538*

Aldolase *Serum Increase* Markedly elevated in malignant lymphomas. Mean = 5.0 ± 0.4 U/L compared to normal, 1.6 ± 0.21. *1201*

Alkaline Phosphatase *Serum Increase* In 10 patients with lymphosarcoma involving the liver, value was 69 ± 28 U/L. *1312* May be increased as a result of liver and less frequently bone disease. *0025* May be a systemic sign of active disease or may indicate involvement of liver or bone. *0433* Lymphoma associated with hyperbilirubinemia is accompanied by elevations from 43-331 U/L. In some cases, reflects osteoblastic lesions as well as metastases. *2576*

Leukocyte Decrease Activity is low irrespective of tumor category, activity of disease, or type of therapy. In 17 cases of malignant lymphoma, median LAP was 17 U/L (Normal = 55). *1423*

Leukocyte Increase Usually increased in untreated diseases. Increased in lymphoma (including Hodgkin's disease and reticulum cell sarcoma). *2467*

Leukocyte Normal In 10 cases, mean activity was found to be in the normal range or slightly below, irrespective of treatment. *1563* *2467*

Alpha₁-Antitrypsin *Serum Increase* Increased. *1866 0042 1946 1947 2129*

Alpha₂-Globulin *Serum Increase* Moderate increase. *0619*

Angiotensin-Converting Enzyme (ACE) *Serum Decrease* Patients with low values had a poorer prognosis. *1969*

Aspartate Aminotransferase *Serum Increase* May be a systemic sign of active disease or may indicate involvement of liver or bone. *0433* In 24% of 72 patients at initial hospitalization for this disorder. *0781*

Bence-Jones Protein *Urine Present* 30-40% of patients. *2478*

Beta₂-Macroglobulin *CSF Increase* With involvement of the CNS. *0388* May be increased in lymphomas involving the central nervous system *1236*

Beta-Globulin *Serum Decrease* *2467*

Bilirubin *Serum Increase* May be a systemic sign of active disease or may indicate involvement of liver or bone. *0433*

BSP Retention *Serum Increase* May be a systemic sign of active disease or may indicate involvement of liver or bone. *0433*

Calcium *Serum Increase* Has been observed in the absence of hyperparathyroidism or of skeletal metastases. *2180* Metastatic or lytic tumor involving bone. *0503* *2538*

Urine Increase Neoplasm. Metastatic tumors involving the bone. *0503*

Carcinoembryonic Antigen *Serum Increase* In 22% of cases. *2199*

Cells *Bone Marrow Increase* Erythrocytic and granulocytic hyperplasia may develop in the bone marrow. *2538*

Cholesterol *Serum Decrease* In 24% of 74 patients at initial hospitalization for this disorder. *0781*

Cholesterol, Very Low Density Lipoprotein *Serum Increase* Moderate increase due to presence of IgG or IgM that forms complexes with chylomicron remnants and/or VLDL thereby decreasing catabolism. *0062*

Chylomicrons *Serum Increase* Moderate increase due to presence of IgG or IgM that forms complexes with chylomicron remnants and/or VLDL thereby decreasing catabolism. *0062*

Cold Agglutinins *Serum Increase* *2035*

Coombs' Test *Blood Positive* Autoimmune hemolytic anemia, with a positive Coombs' test, occurs in a few patients. *1186* May occur. *2552* *2538*

Copper *Serum Increase* Invariably raised in all 50 patients with lymphoma. Significantly lowered after radiotherapy. *1888*

Creatinine *Serum Increase* In 42% of 47 patients at initial hospitalization for this disorder. *0781*

Cryoglobulins *Serum Increase* May be associated with cryoglobulinemia. *2468*

Erythrocytes *Bone Marrow Decrease* In histiocytic medullary reticulosis, severe cytopenias may be associated with the abnormal phagocytosis of erythrocytes, platelets or leukocytes seen in the bone marrow. *2538*

Erythrocyte Sedimentation Rate *Blood Increase* Increased in significant tissue necrosis, especially neoplasms - most frequently malignant lymphoma, cancer of the colon and breast. *2467*

Erythrocyte Survival *Red Blood Cells Decrease* Characteristically short in patients with bulky lymph nodes or with enlargement of the liver and spleen. *1186* *2538*

Ferritin *Serum Increase* Significant elevation. *2244*

Fucose *Serum Increase* Markedly elevated and correlated with clinical stage of disease. Values ranged from 13 mg/dL in stage 1 to 29.5 mg/dL in stage 4. *0607*

Gamma Glutamyl Transferase (GGT) *Serum Increase* In 67% of 16 patients at initial hospitalization for this disorder. *0781*

Globulin *Serum Decrease* In patients with advanced disease, reduction in serum protein concentration with hypoalbuminemia and hypogammaglobulinemia is frequent. *2462* *2538*

Haptoglobin *Serum Increase* Conditions associated with increased ESR and alpha₂-globulin. *2467*

Hematocrit *Blood Decrease* Anemia may result from blood loss, hemolysis, or bone marrow infiltration. *2538* Present in < 50% of cases and is rarely severe at time of diagnosis. *2552* In 22% of 74 patients at initial hospitalization for this disorder. *0781*

Blood Normal Anemia is often conspicuously lacking, especially early in the disease. *1984*

Hemoglobin *Blood Decrease* Anemia occurs frequently and may be due to blood loss, bone marrow infiltration, or hemolysis. *2538* Present in < 50% of patients and is rarely severe at the time of diagnosis. *2552* In 51% of 73 patients at initial hospitalization for this disorder. *0781*

Blood Normal Anemia is often conspicuously lacking, especially early in the disease. Hemoglobin above 12 g/dL found in 90% of 1269 cases. *1984*

Hexokinase *Serum Increase* Markedly increased in malignant lymphomas. Mean = 14.6 ± 2.0 compared to normal 0.93 ± 0.28 U/L. *1201*

Immunoglobulin IgG *Serum Increase* In a recent survey, 15 of 348 patients (4.6%) with lymphosarcoma and reticulum cell sarcoma had monoclonal serum components. In 10 instances the component was IgM and in 5 IgG. *1618*

Immunoglobulin IgM *Serum Increase* In a recent survey, 15 of 348 patients (4.6%) with lymphosarcoma and reticulum cell sarcoma had monoclonal serum components. In 10 instances the component was IgM and in 5 IgG. *1618*

Immunoglobulins *Serum Decrease* Low levels were present in several patients in one family who developed malignant lymphoma of the small intestine. *0073*

Serum Increase In a recent survey, 15 of 348 patients (4.6%) with lymphosarcoma and reticulum cell sarcoma had monoclonal serum components. In 10 instances the component was IgM and in 5 IgG. *1618*

Iron *Serum Decrease* In 58% of 22 patients at initial hospitalization for this disorder. *0781*

Iron-Binding Capacity, Total (TIBC) *Serum Decrease* In 36% of 22 patients at initial hospitalization for this disorder. *0781*

Iron Saturation *Serum Decrease* Anemia due to blood loss may occur. *2538* In 67% of 22 patients at initial hospitalization for this disorder. *0781*

Lactate Dehydrogenase *Serum Increase* Increased in about 60% of the patients. *2467 0812* May be a sign of active disease or may indicate involvement of liver or bone. *0433* Marked elevation in 138 patients with malignant lymphomas. Mean = 177.7 ± 13.8 U/L compared to normals, 85.4 ± 1.0 U/L. *1201* In 55% of 73 patients at initial hospitalization for this disorder. *0781* *0151 0962*

Lactic Acid *Blood Increase* In 20 patients with malignant lymphomas, mean concentration = 23.2 ± 2.9 mg/dL compared to normal, 11.7 ± 0.72 mg/dL. *1201*

Leukocytes *Blood Decrease* Uncommon. *2552* In 8% of 73 patients at initial hospitalization for this disorder. *0781*

Blood Increase Uncommon. *2552* In 13% of 73 patients at initial hospitalization for this disorder. *0781*

202.80   Non-Hodgkins Lymphoma *(continued)*

Leukocytes *(continued)*

Bone Marrow   Decrease   In histiocytic medullary reticulosis, severe cytopenias may be associated with the abnormal phagocytosis of erythrocytes, platelets or leukocytes seen in the bone marrow. *2538*

Lymphocytes   *Blood   Increase*   *0433 0532*

Pleural Effusion   Increase   A preponderance of lymphocytes is consistent with tuberculosis, carcinoma or lymphoma. *0962*

MCH   *Blood   Decrease*   Anemia occurs frequently and may be due to blood loss, bone marrow infiltration, or hemolysis. *2538*

MCHC   *Blood   Decrease*   Anemia occurs frequently and may be due to blood loss, bone marrow infiltration, or hemolysis. *2538*

MCV   *Blood   Decrease*   Anemia occurs frequently and may be due to blood loss, bone marrow infiltration, or hemolysis. *2538*

Monocytes   *Blood   Increase*   Appearance of abnormal large mononuclear cells in peripheral blood. *0433*   All varieties of lymphomas have been reported on occasion in association with a monocytosis, sometimes varying with disease activity. *1107*   In 57% of 74 patients at initial hospitalization for this disorder. *0781*   Peripheral monocytosis is especially likely to occur in circumstances of histiocytic proliferation and increased phagocytosis as strikingly manifested in histiocytic medullary reticulosis. *1489*

Neutrophils   *Blood   Decrease*   Often present in addition to anemia, and almost any combination of cytopenias may be produced by bone marrow infiltration and replacement, by hypersplenism or as the result of therapy. *2538*

Platelet Count   *Blood   Decrease*   Often present in addition to anemia, and almost any combination of cytopenias may be produced by bone marrow infiltration and replacement, by hypersplenism or as the result of therapy. *2538*   Unusual. *2552*

Bone Marrow   Decrease   In histiocytic medullary reticulosis, severe cytopenias may be associated with the abnormal phagocytosis of erythrocytes, platelets or leukocytes seen in the bone marrow. *2538*

Proline Hydroxylase   *Serum   Increase*   Elevated to a lesser degree than that seen in hepatoma. *0364*

Protein   *Serum   Decrease*   Occurs commonly. *2538*   Enteric loss of plasma protein. *2199*   In patients with advanced disease, reduction in serum protein concentration with hypoalbuminemia and hypogammaglobulinemia is frequent. *2462*

Pleural Effusion   Increase   Pleural effusions are usually exudates. *0062*

Pyruvate   *Blood   Increase*   Moderately elevated in 20 of 20 patients with malignant lymphomas. Mean = 1.1 - 0.15 U/L. *1201*

Reticulocytes   *Blood   Decrease*   *2552*

Rheumatoid Factor   *Serum   Increase*   Dysproteinemias and paraproteinemias present significant seropositivity. *0962*

Sodium   *Serum   Increase*   In 88% of 73 patients at initial hospitalization for this disorder. *0781*

Urea Nitrogen   *Serum   Increase*   In 26% of 74 patients at initial hospitalization for this disorder. *0781*

Uric Acid   *Serum   Increase*   May occur, but more often is normal. *1639*   Especially post x-radiation. *2467*   In 39% of 73 patients at initial hospitalization for this disorder. *0781*

Serum   Normal   Usually normal. *2552*

Urine   Increase   May occur, but more often is normal. *1639*

Urine   Normal   Usually normal. *2552*

Vitamin B$_{12}$ *Serum   Increase*   High levels were found in 15 patients with lymphomas, mean = 1,059 compared to normal, 385 pg/mL. *1990*   Usually normal. *2552*

Serum   Normal   Usually normal. *2538*

Vitamin B$_{12}$ Binding Capacity   *Serum   Increase*   Significant elevation; usually correlated with WBC in peripheral blood. *1990*

Serum   Normal   Usually normal. *2538*

Zinc   *Serum   Decrease*   Decreased. *2297*

203.00   Multiple Myeloma

Acid Phosphatase   *Serum   Increase*   May be elevated even in the absence of prostatic carcinoma. *0433*   2 patients showed elevated levels of both total and prostatic fraction of the serum acid phos. *0775*   *0812 0948 1375*

Leukocyte   Normal   *1388*

Albumin   *Serum   Decrease*   In 57% of 33 patients at initial hospitalization for this disorder. *0781 2467*

Urine   Increase   Occurs in 90% of patients. *0433*   Frequent proteinuria due to albumin and globulins. *2468*   Greater than 1.0 g/day. *0518*

Alkaline Phosphatase   *Serum   Increase*   In the absence of fracture with callus formation, the level is usually normal, although elevated levels have been reported. *0433*   Normal or slightly elevated, even in patients with extensive bone lesions. *2538*   In 27% of 31 patients at initial hospitalization for this disorder. *0781*

Serum   Normal   Usually normal. *0433   0992*

Leukocyte   Increase   Over a 13 y period, 60 of 62 patients had consistently elevated levels. One patient had a normal level, and one had an initially normal level which later increased. Elevations could not be correlated with age, hemoglobin, WBC, or BUN. *0292*

Alpha$_2$-Globulin   *Serum   Increase*   Marked increase. *0619*   Homogeneous component seen in some patients. *0992*

Alpha$_2$-Macroglobulin   *Serum   Decrease*   Mild. *1141*

Amino Acids   *Urine   Increase*   Aminoaciduria may be nonselective and associated with renal glycosuria and mild renal acidosis. *0962*

Angiotensin-Converting Enzyme (ACE)   *Serum   Decrease*   Depression of activity. Significant decrease *1969*

Aspartate Aminotransferase   *Serum   Increase*   In 45% of 33 patients at initial hospitalization for this disorder. *0781*

Bence-Jones Protein   *Serum   Present*   Demonstrable in the serum or urine, or both, of over 90% of cases of overt, symptomatic myeloma, it is only the rare case in which there is not an abnormal serum or urinary protein. *2035*   Electrophoresis of sera reveals a double spike. *2436*

Urine   Present   Kappa or lambda light chains with no heavy chains attached found in 26 of 35 patients. 11 excreted large amounts (> 1 g/day). *0518*   Demonstrable in the serum or urine, or both, of over 90% of cases of overt, symptomatic myeloma, it is only the rare case in which there is not an abnormal serum or urinary protein. *2035*   The amount excreted varies from a few mg to 25-40 g/24h. Found in the urine of 70-80% of patients. *1333*   Highly indicative. *2218 2538*

Beta$_2$-Macroglobulin   *Serum   Increase*   Showed the best correlation with survival. May be increased. *1236*

Beta-Globulin   *Serum   Increase*   Markedly increased. *0619*

Calcium   *Serum   Increase*   Found in about 21% of patients. *2566*   If the renal excretory capacity for calcium is exceeded. *2035*   Frequent hypercalcemia in advanced cases. *0393*   Elevated above 11.0 mg/dL in about 30% of patients at the time of diagnosis, and rises above this level in an additional 30% during the course of the disease. *0176   1904 0962*

Urine   Increase   Skeletal destruction results in hypercalciuria in virtually all cases. *2035*

Chloride   *Serum   Increase*   Typical hyperchloremic acidosis with respiratory compensation in 9 of 35 patients. *0518*

Cholesterol   *Serum   Decrease*   150 mg/dL in 25% of patients while only 5% have a level > 300 mg/dL. *0433*   In 27% of 31 patients at initial hospitalization for this disorder. *0781*

Serum   Increase   150 mg/dL in 25% of patients while only 5% have a level > 300 mg/dL. *0433*

Cholesterol, Very Low Density Lipoprotein   *Serum   Increase*   Moderate increase due to presence of IgG or IgM that forms complexes with chylomicron remnants and/or VLDL thereby decreasing catabolism. *0062*

Chylomicrons   *Serum   Increase*   Moderate increase due to presence of IgG or IgM that forms complexes with chylomicron remnants and/or VLDL thereby decreasing catabolism. *0062*

Cold Agglutinins   *Serum   Increase*   Cold agglutinin or cryoglobulins with lymphocytes. *2468*

Coombs' Test   *Blood   Negative*   Usually. *2538*

Creatinine   *Serum   Increase*   Not uncommon. *0433*   Ranged from 53.0-981 µmol/L in 35 patients. *0518*   In 68% of 28 patients at initial hospitalization for this disorder. *0781*

Creatinine Clearance   *Urine   Decrease*   Clearance ranged from 0.03-2.02 mL/s (2-121 mL/min) in 35 cases. 19 had rates > 0.83 mL/s. Mean clearance was significantly lower in the patients with Bence-Jones proteinuria. *0518*

Cryofibrinogen   *Serum   Increase*   *2035 1551*

Cryoglobulins   *Serum   Increase*   Associated cryoglobulinemia. *2468*

Erythrocytes   *Blood   Decrease*   Overgrowth of plasma cells may produce pancytopenia, or may evoke a leukoerythroblastic reaction. *2538*

Blood *Increase* Has been found in a small number of patients. *1357*

Erythrocyte Sedimentation Rate *Blood Increase* Typically increased but a normal or modestly elevated rate does not exclude the diagnosis. Approximately 25% of patients have a ESR > 50 mm/h (Westergren). *0433* Over 100 mm/h in almost 50% of patients. *1980* A result of hyperglobulinemia. *2538* *0962*

Ferritin *Serum Increase* Significant elevation. *2244*

Globulin *Serum Decrease* *0615*

Serum Increase Very elevated serum total protein is due to increase in globulins (with decreased A/G ratio) in 50-66% of the patients. *2468* Plasma cell dyscrasias are among the most common causes of serum elevations, which may exceed 5 g/dL. *0999* Greater than 32 g/L in 27 of 35 patients and reduced 20 g/L) in 1 case. *0518* Over 80 g/L in 60% of patients. *1980* A Homogeneous protein component ranging from slow gamma to alpha₂-globulin is seen in 60% of patients *0992*

Urine Increase *2468*

CSF Increase Increased in about 66% of patients, with corresponding colloidal gold curve. *0151*

Glomerular Filtration Rate (GFR) *Urine Decrease* Renal function is decreased. There is no correlation between the degree of Bence-Jones proteinuria and renal functional impairment. *0962* Marked reduction in PAH clearance in patients with Bence-Jones proteinuria 3.22 ± 0.65 mL/s. Diminished out of proportion to the GFR. *0518*

Glucose *Urine Increase* Aminoaciduria may be nonselective and associated with renal glycosuria and mild renal acidosis. *0962*

Hematocrit *Blood Decrease* A normocytic, normochromic anemia is present in 66% of patients at the time of diagnosis. *0433* Virtually all patients exhibit anemia of varying severity, either at the time of diagnosis or subsequently with disease progression. *2035* In 69% of 33 patients at initial hospitalization for this disorder. *0781*

Hemoglobin *Blood Decrease* A normocytic, normochromic anemia is present in 66% of patients at the time of diagnosis. *0433* High tumor mass is indicated if hemoglobin < 8.5 g/dL, low tumor mass is present in hemoglobin > 10.5 g/dL. *2467* Virtually all patients exhibit anemia of varying severity, either at the time of diagnosis or subsequently with disease progression. *2035* Reduced to < 12.0 g/dL in 62% of the patients. *1333* In 78% of 33 patients at initial hospitalization for this disorder. *0781* *2468* *2538*

Hemoglobin, Fetal *Blood Increase* *2467*

Hexosaminidase *Serum Increase* Elevated. *2356*

Immunoglobulin IgA *Serum Decrease* May occur in IgG form. *2538*

Serum Increase Peak of > 5 g/dL indicates high tumor mass. A peak of < 3 g/dL indicates low tumor mass. *2467* The abnormal serum M component was IgG in 20 of 35 patients and IgA in 7. There was no correlation between type of M component and presence of renal failure. *0518*

Immunoglobulin IgD *Serum Increase* Rare. *0992*

Immunoglobulin IgE *Serum Increase* Only 5 cases of IgE myeloma have been reported. *0992*

Immunoglobulin IgG *Serum Decrease* May occur in IgA form. *2538*

Serum Increase Most common. *0992* The abnormal serum M component was IgG in 20 of 35 patients and IgA in 7. There was no correlation between type of M component and presence of renal failure. *0518*

Immunoglobulin IgM *Serum Decrease* May occur. *2538*

Serum Normal *0992*

Immunoglobulins *Serum Decrease* The amount of normal immunoglobulin is usually low, but does not correlate with the increased concentration of anomalous protein. *2538*

Leukocytes *Blood Decrease* Progressive plasma cell proliferation in the marrow may result in leukopenia. *0999* Occasionally, moderate to severe leukopenia or thrombocytopenia, or both, may be observed prior to treatment. *2035* About 33% have leukopenia with diminished granulocytes and decreased platelets. *1980* Leukopenia and thrombocytopenia were present in 16 and 13% of the patients, respectively. The degree of disease in untreated patients is usually mild. *1333*

Blood Normal Usually within normal limits prior to cytotoxic therapy. *2035*

Lipoproteins, Beta *Serum Increase* *0774 0772 0773*

Lymphocytes *Blood Increase* 40-55% lymphocytosis frequently present on differential count, with variable number of immature lymphocytic and plasmacytic forms. *2468* Relative lymphocytosis of 40-55% with a variable proportion of immature lymphocytic and plasmacytic forms. *2035*

Lysozyme *Serum Increase* Isolated cases. *0981*

MCV *Blood Increase* Anemia may be macrocytic. *2538*

Monocytes *Blood Increase* *2538*

Neutrophils *Blood Decrease* About 33% have leukopenia with diminished granulocytes and decreased platelets. *1980* Total WBC is often reduced to 3,000-4,000/μL, largely because of neutropenia. *2538*

Osmolality *Urine Decrease* Mean for the group following overnight dehydration was 444 ± 26 mOsm/kg; patients with Bence-Jones proteinuria had further reduced concentrating ability. *0518*

Phosphate *Serum Decrease* Common. *0962* Due to renal loss of phosphate. *2468* In 21% of 32 patients at initial hospitalization for this disorder. *0781*

Serum Increase Some cases. *2467* In 27% of 32 patients at initial hospitalization for this disorder. *0781*

Urine Increase Renal loss. *2468*

Plasma Cells *Serum Increase* A small number may be found in the circulating blood of many patients, and if the absolute number of plasma cells exceeds 2,000/μL, the diagnosis of plasma cell leukemia may be made. *2538*

Bone Marrow Increase Marked bone marrow plasmacytosis. Many patients had cytoplasmic abnormalities of cells, including size and contour of nucleus, mitochondria and rough ER. *0904* Increased numbers and abnormal forms have been found in all cases, although more than one attempt may be necessary. *2035* Bone marrow infiltrated with over 20% plasma cells in clusters or sheets. *1980* In average patients with moderately advanced disease, 20-95% of the nucleated cells in the bone marrow are mature or immature plasma cells. The percent varies with the sample and is not a reliable measure of the total amount of disease present. *2538* *0992* *1744*

Platelet Count *Blood Decrease* Occasionally, moderate to severe leukopenia or thrombocytopenia, or both, may be observed prior to treatment. *2035* About 33% have leukopenia with diminished granulocytes and decreased platelets. *1980* Leukopenia and thrombocytopenia were present in 16 and 13% of the patients, respectively. The degree in untreated patients is usually mild. *1333* In 31% of 31 patients at initial hospitalization for this disorder. *0781*

Blood Normal Usually within normal limits prior to cytotoxic therapy. *2035*

Potassium *Serum Decrease* Common. *0962*

Urine Increase Due to Myeloma Nephropathy. *0186*

Protein *Serum Increase* Very elevated serum total protein is due to increase in globulins (with decreased A/G ratio) in 50-66% of the patients. *2468* Over 80 g/L in 18 of 35 patients, all of whom had total globulin concentration > 52 g/L. *0518* *0512*

Urine Increase Unexplained, persistent proteinuria may last for years. *2468* Minimal elevation (0.15-0.5 g/L) in 7, mild-moderate (0.5-3 g/L) in 17 and heavy (> 3 g/L) in 9 of 35 patients. *0518*

CSF Increase Usually normal or slightly elevated to values of 50-100 mg/dL. *0151*

Pleural Effusion Increase With pleural involvement increased total protein with a sharp spike in the gamma globulin region. *2021*

Rheumatoid Factor *Serum Increase* Dysproteinemias and paraproteinemias may present significant seropositivity. *0962*

Sodium *Serum Decrease* In 31% of 28 patients at initial hospitalization for this disorder. *0781*

Thymol Turbidity *Serum Increase* In both beta- and gamma-types. *0619*

Urea Nitrogen *Serum Increase* Ranged from 5.0-92.1 mmol/L in 35 patients. *0518* In 51% of 33 patients at initial hospitalization for this disorder. *0781* Impaired renal function in > 50%, decreasing concentrating ability and azotemia. *2468* *0433*

Uric Acid *Serum Decrease* Occasionally decreased due to altered renal tubular function. *2468* Common. *0962*

Serum Increase Seen in about 33% of patients. *0433* 10 of 35 patients had hyperuricemia (> 416 mmol/L). 8 of these had only mild elevations, consistent with the severity of renal insufficiency. *0518* May accompany renal failure or may occur in the absence of azotemia. *2538* In 63% of 33 patients at initial hospitalization for this disorder. *0781* *0962*

203.00   Multiple Myeloma *(continued)*

Viscosity   *Serum   Increase*   An increase of IgM is the most common clinical situation producing hyperviscosity of serum. *0962* Occurs in only 2-4% of patients. *2226*

Vitamin B₁₂   *Serum   Normal   2467*

Vitamin B₁₂ Binding Capacity   *Serum   Increase*   Significant elevation; usually correlated with WBC in peripheral blood. *1990*

Volume   *Plasma   Increase*   Often expands as the amount of myeloma protein increases in the serum, and the resulting hemodilution may be great enough to produce a significant reduction in hemoglobin concentration with little or no change in total red cell mass. *1301   2538*

204.00   Lymphocytic Leukemia (Acute)

Albumin   *Serum   Decrease*   Normal at diagnosis and declines as disease advances. *0689 2552*   In 30% of 44 patients at initial hospitalization for this disorder. *0781*

Alkaline Phosphatase   *Serum   Increase*   Infiltration of the liver may result in obstruction of biliary system. *2468*   Elevations > 95 U/L. *1322*   In 56% of 42 patients at initial hospitalization for this disorder. *0781*

Leukocyte   Increase   The mean activity score was 159.4 ranging from 83-308 (12 cases). *1563*   Tend to be high, in contrast to acute myelogenous leukemia. *1011*

Alkaline Phosphatase Isoenzymes   *Serum   Increase*   In all 6 patients, an electrophoretically distinct isoenzyme (phosphatase N) was present in the serum. The range of phosphatase N was 26-100% of the total alkaline phosphatase activity. *1687*

Alpha₁-Globulin   *Serum   Increase*   Often reflects the presence of fever or infection. *0689 2552*

Alpha₁-Glycoprotein   *Serum   Increase*   Elevated levels in states associated with cell proliferation. *1239 1672*   *1947 2096 2170 1866*

Alpha₂-Globulin   *Serum   Increase*   Often reflects the presence of fever or infection. *0689 2552*

Antinuclear Antibodies   *Serum   Increase*   Positive in 25% of patients. *1799*

Aspartate Aminotransferase   *Serum   Increase*   Infiltration of the liver. *0619*   Moderately elevated levels are observed in lymphomas and leukemia but less frequently than in other hepatic disease. *0503* In 71% of 43 patients at initial hospitalization for this disorder. *0781*

Bence-Jones Protein   *Urine   Present   0619*

Beta₂-Macroglobulin   *Serum   Increase*   May be increased in leukemia of B-lymphocyte lineage. *1236*

Beta-Globulin   *Serum   Decrease*   Common. *0689 2552*

Calcium   *Serum   Decrease*   Hypocalcemia with values of 6.6-8.3 mg/dL was observed within 24-48 h after initiation of chemotherapy. *2622*

Serum   Increase   May be increased in some cases. *0503*   Elevated levels (> 11.0 mg/dL) may occur with leukemic infiltration of bone. *1322*   Has been observed but is uncommon. *2552*

Urine   Increase   May be increased in some cases. *0503*

Carcinoembryonic Antigen   *Serum   Increase*   Above 2.5 ng/mL in 38% of patients with acute and chronic leukemia. *0211*

Cells   *CSF   Increase*   Pleocytosis with meningeal infiltration. *2538*

Bone Marrow   Increase   Almost always hypercellular and heavily infiltrated or replaced by abnormal lymphoid elements. *2538*

Cholesterol   *Serum   Decrease*   In 37% of 42 patients at initial hospitalization for this disorder. *0781*

Cold Agglutinins   *Serum   Increase*   Tends to rise. *1752*

Copper   *Serum   Increase*   Significant increase observed in 16 children with acute leukemias. Drop in concentration occurs in cases who respond to quadruple chemotherapy while those who failed to respond showed persistently high serum levels. *0645*

Creatine   *Serum   Increase*   Increased formation. *0619*

Urine   Increase   Pronounced increase in children and adult males with acute leukemias. *2104*   Extremely variable. *2453*

Creatinine   *Serum   Increase*   In 49% of 16 patients at initial hospitalization for this disorder. *0781*

Erythropoietin   *Serum   Increase*   Found to be increased and negatively correlated with hemoglobin concentration. *1785*

Urine   Increase   Urine levels are usually increased in lymphoblastic but not myeloblastic leukemia. *1785*

Ferritin   *Serum   Increase*   Significant elevation. *2244*

Fibrinogen   *Plasma   Increase*   Frequently elevated when the disease is in relapse. The absolute levels vary considerably from individual to individual. *0270   2538*

Globulin   *Serum   Decrease   2467*

Serum   Normal   Most often normal in contrast to acute myelogenous leukemia. *0689 2552*

Glucose   *CSF   Decrease*   With meningeal infiltration. *2538*

Hematocrit   *Blood   Decrease*   Most patients will have anemia. *0433*   Often severe, usually normochromic, normocytic. *2552*   In 81% of 36 patients at initial hospitalization for this disorder. *0781*

Hemoglobin   *Blood   Decrease*   Most patients will have anemia. *0433*   Often severe, usually normochromic, normocytic. *2552*   In 82% of 37 patients at initial hospitalization for this disorder. *0781*

Heterophil Antibody   *Serum   Decrease*   Positive presumptive test but negative differential test if Forsman antigen is used. *1752*

Serum   Increase   Positive presumptive test but negative differential test if Forsman antigen is used. *1752*

Immunoglobulin IgA   *Serum   Decrease   2467*

Immunoglobulin IgG   *Serum   Normal   2467*

Immunoglobulin IgM   *Serum   Normal   2467*

Iron   *Serum   Increase*   Increased in acute leukemias. *0619*

Lactate Dehydrogenase   *Serum   Increase*   Increased in acute, but not in chronic lymphocytic leukemia. Usually reflected changes in the course of the disease-falling during remission and rising during relapses, occasionally indicating the onset before the WBC had begun to change. *0221*   Frequently elevated when the disease is in relapse. The absolute levels vary considerably from individual to individual. *0936*   In 91% of 39 patients at initial hospitalization for this disorder. *0781*   Mean value of 54 patients was 2 X normal adult value. 47 of 54 patients had significantly increased activities. *0206 0962*

Leukocytes   *Blood   Decrease*   Variable and can be very high (> 100,000/μL), moderately elevated (20,000-100,000), normal or low. *0433*

Blood   Increase   Initial counts above 100,000/μL significantly indicate poor prognosis. *2176*   Elevated in slightly over 50% of patients. *2552*

Blood   Normal   Variable and can be very high (> 100,000/μL), moderately elevated (20,000-100,000/μL), normal, or low. *0433*

Lysozyme   *Serum   Decrease*   Low or normal. *0798*

Serum   Normal   Low or normal. *0798*

Magnesium   *Serum   Increase   2538*

Monocytes   *Blood   Decrease*   In 64% of 34 patients at initial hospitalization for this disorder. *0781*

Blood   Increase   On occasion associated with a monocytosis of relatively minor proportions. *1489   2538*

Neutrophils   *Blood   Decrease*   The absolute number is almost always decreased, and usually to a greater extent than in acute myelogenous leukemia. *2538*   In 92% of 34 patients at initial hospitalization for this disorder. *0781*

Phosphate   *Serum   Increase*   Hyperphosphatemia with values of 5.7-9.4 mg/dL was observed within 24-48 h after initiation of chemotherapy. *2622*   In 40% of 44 patients at initial hospitalization for this disorder. *0781*

Urine   Increase   Marked hyperphosphaturia was observed within 24-48 h after initiation of chemotherapy. *2622*

Phosphoglucomutase   *Serum   Increase*   Increases in some cases. *0619*

Platelet Count   *Blood   Decrease*   Most patients will have thrombocytopenia. *0433*   The absolute number is almost always decreased, and usually to a greater extent than in acute myelogenous leukemia. *2538*   Pronounced at diagnosis. *2552*   In 78% of 29 patients at initial hospitalization for this disorder. *0781*

Blood   Increase   On very rare occasions. *0075*

Protein   *CSF   Increase*   With meningeal infiltration. *2538*

Pleural Effusion   Increase   Pleural effusions are usually exudates. *0062*

Reticulocytes   *Blood   Decrease*   Usually low. *0433*   Reflects decreased cell production. *2552*

Rheumatoid Factor   *Serum   Increase*   Dysproteinemias and paraproteinemias present significant seropositivity. *0962*

Sodium   *Serum   Increase*   In 94% of 39 patients at initial hospitalization for this disorder. *0781*

Urea Nitrogen   *Serum   Increase*   Can be elevated in kidney infiltration and should be followed especially if nephrotoxic antibiotics are used. *0433*

Uric Acid   *Serum Increase*   Frequent biochemical abnormality. Secondary to the increased cell turnover. *0433*   Frequently elevated when the disease is in relapse. The absolute levels vary considerably from individual to individual. *0270*   In 50% of patients. *1042*   In 39% of 46 patients at initial hospitalization for this disorder. *0781 2538*

Urine Increase   Secondary to the increased cell turnover. *0433*   Almost invariably. *1042*

Vitamin B$_{12}$ *Serum Normal*   Usually normal, in contrast to acute myelogenous leukemia. *0142*

Vitamin B$_{12}$ Binding Capacity   *Serum Increase*   Significant elevation; usually correlated with WBC in peripheral blood. *1990*

Zinc   *Serum Decrease*   Decreased. *2297*

204.10   Lymphocytic Leukemia (Chronic)

5'-Nucleotidase   *Lymphocytes Decrease*   Reduced or absent in the lymphocytes of most patients. *1429 2538*

Acid Phosphatase   *Leukocyte Decrease*   *1388*

Albumin   *Serum Decrease*   In 47% of 27 patients at initial hospitalization for this disorder. *0781 2467*

Serum Normal   Usually within normal limits. *0241 2552*

Alkaline Phosphatase   *Serum Increase*   Infiltration of the liver may result in obstruction of the biliary system. *2468*   Elevations > 95 U/L. *1322*   In 42% of 27 patients at initial hospitalization for this disorder. *0781*

Leukocyte Increase   Mean score of 139.4 with a range of 73-180. *1563*   The range of actual enzyme levels per 10^{10} leukocytes was 2.5-68.2 with a mean of 20.8. Only 3 determinations were higher than 26.5. Normal = 25.8, ranging from 13.4-58.0. *0144*

Alkaline Phosphatase Isoenzymes   *Serum Increase*   A distinct isoenzyme (phosphatase N) was found in the serum of 5 patients. Values ranged from 35-39% of the total activity. *1687*

Alpha$_1$-Globulin   *Serum Normal*   Usually within normal limits. *0241*

Alpha$_1$-Glycoprotein   *Serum Increase*   Elevated levels in states associated with cell proliferation. *1239 1672   1947 2096 2170 1866*

Alpha$_2$-Globulin   *Serum Normal*   Usually within normal limits. *0241 2552*

Angiotensin-Converting Enzyme (ACE)   *Serum Decrease*   Significant decrease. Depression of Activity *1969*

Antinuclear Antibodies   *Serum Increase*   Positive in 20% of patients. *1799*

Aspartate Aminotransferase   *Serum Increase*   Moderately elevated levels are observed in lymphomas and leukemia but less frequently than in other hepatic disease. *0503*   In 27% of 27 patients at initial hospitalization for this disorder. *0781*

Bence-Jones Protein   *Urine Present*   *0619*

Beta$_2$-Macroglobulin   *Serum Increase*   May be increased in leukemia of B-lymphocyte lineage. *1236*   With leukemia of B-lymphocyte lineage *2232*

Beta-Globulin   *Serum Decrease*   *2467*

Serum Normal   Usually within normal limits. *0241 2552*

Bilirubin   *Serum Increase*   20% of patients develop severe hemolysis. *0992*

Bilirubin, Indirect   *Serum Increase*   20% of patients develop severe hemolysis. *0992*

Calcium   *Serum Increase*   Elevations > 11 mg/dL may occur with leukemic infiltration of bone. *1322   0503*

Urine Increase   *0503*

Carcinoembryonic Antigen   *Serum Increase*   Above 2.5 ng/mL in 38% of patients with acute and chronic leukemia. *0211*

Cholesterol   *Serum Decrease*   In 43% of 27 patients at initial hospitalization for this disorder. *0781*

Cold Agglutinins   *Serum Increase*   Tends to rise. *1752*

Coombs' Test   *Blood Positive*   20% of patients develop severe hemolysis. *0992*

Copper   *Serum Increase*   In acute and chronic leukemias. *2468*

Creatine   *Urine Increase*   Increased breakdown. *2468*

Creatinine   *Serum Increase*   In 49% of 24 patients at initial hospitalization for this disorder. *0781*

Cryofibrinogen   *Serum Increase*   *2035 1551*

Cryoglobulins   *Serum Increase*   May be associated with cryoglobulinemia. *2468*

Erythrocytes   *Blood Decrease*   Reduced production plus shortened survival. *2538*

Erythrocyte Survival   *Red Blood Cells Decrease*   Characteristically short even when there is no evidence of autoimmunity. *2489 2538*

Globulin   *Serum Decrease*   Concentration of 0.7-0.8 g/dL are common in early and uncomplicated disease. As disease advances, may fall to 0.3-0.4 g/dL, at which time patients become vulnerable to infections. *2399   2538 0692*

Haptoglobin   *Serum Decrease*   20% of patients develop severe hemolysis. *0992*

Hematocrit   *Blood Decrease*   Characteristically normochromic normocytic anemia. *0433*   Anemia is not a feature of early disease; it may begin to develop when 50% or more of the bone marrow is usurped by lymphoid tissue. *2489*   Anemia, usually mild, was present at diagnosis in 50% of patients. *2552*   In 76% of 27 patients at initial hospitalization for this disorder. *0781   2538*

Hemoglobin   *Blood Decrease*   Characteristically normochromic normocytic anemia. *0433*   Anemia is not a feature of early disease; it may begin to develop when 50% or more of the bone marrow is usurped by lymphoid tissue. *2489*   Anemia, usually mild, was present at diagnosis in 50% of patients. *2552*   In 76% of 27 patients at initial hospitalization for this disorder. *0781   2538*

Hemoglobin, Free   *Serum Increase*   On occasion, severe hemolytic anemia is present at diagnosis. *0092 2258   2552*

Immunoglobulin IgA   *Serum Decrease*   *2467*

Immunoglobulin IgG   *Serum Decrease*   *2467*

Immunoglobulin IgM   *Serum Decrease*   *2467*

Immunoglobulins   *Serum Decrease*   All classes of immunoglobulins tend to be reduced either early in the course or later as marrow, spleen, and liver infiltration develops. *2006   2538 2552*

Lactate Dehydrogenase   *Serum Increase*   Elevated in all 15 patients, mean = 104.3 U/L. *1521*   In 64% of 27 patients at initial hospitalization for this disorder. *0781*   84 of 91 patients with leukemias had values elevated above the normal upper limit. *0206*

Lactate Dehydrogenase Isoenzymes   *Serum Increase*   Isoenzyme 2 was usually the most intensive, LD$_1$ was also increased, and LD$_5$ was only detectable in a few cases. *1521*

Leukocytes   *Blood Increase*   Usually 50,000-250,000/µL with 90% lymphocytes. *2468   0433*

Lymphocytes   *Blood Increase*   Generally, lymphocytosis consisting of mature lymphocytes with counts > 100,000/µL in a patient over 50 y of age is diagnostic. *0433*   In 24 treated patients, the origin of malignant cells was found to be the B lymphocyte population. On the basis of a reactive T lymphocyte proliferation in patients with chronic lymphatic leukemia, a coefficient of active T lymphocytes has been deduced which proved to be a rapid indicator of a short-term prognosis. *0999 0992 1910 0685 0805 0612*

Lysozyme   *Serum Decrease*   Low or normal. *0798*

Serum Normal   Low or normal. *0798*

Monocytes   *Blood Decrease*   In 66% of 27 patients at initial hospitalization for this disorder. *0781*

Neutrophils   *Blood Decrease*   Neutropenia and thrombocytopenia, ranging in severity from mild to catastrophic, are characteristically present in patients with marrow replacement in the late stages. *2538*   In 95% of 27 patients at initial hospitalization for this disorder. *0781*

Blood Increase   The percentage is often reduced, but the absolute number may be somewhat increased in early stages of the disease. *0242   2538*

Blood Normal   Usually normal, mean = 6,000/µL. *0242*

Osmotic Fragility   *Red Blood Cells Increase*   Degree of light transmission is used as a measure of lysis of lymphocytes, (i.e., as a measure of osmotic fragility). After 10 min, light transmission of lymphocytes was 78.5% ± 4.65%, compared to 60 ± 7.33%. *1916 2538*

Phosphoglucomutase   *Serum Increase*   Increases in some cases. *0619*

Platelet Count   *Blood Decrease*   With thrombocytopenia, and associated bleeding diathesis, a microcytic hypochromic picture could be present. *0433*   Anemia and thrombocytopenia develop as the disorder progresses. *0999*   Neutropenia and thrombocytopenia, ranging in severity from mild to catastrophic, are characteristically present in patient with marrow replacement in the late stages. *2538*   Mild thrombocytopenia may occur in < 50% of cases. *2552*   In 47% of 27 patients at initial hospitalization for this disorder. *0781*

Blood Normal   Normal counts in > 50% of patients. *2552*

Protein   *Serum Decrease*   Reduction in serum protein concentration is a feature of advanced disease and one which carries a poor prognosis. *2538*

204.10   Lymphocytic Leukemia (Chronic)   (continued)

Protein   (continued)

Pleural Effusion   Increase   Pleural effusions are usually exudates. *0062*

Reticulocytes   *Blood   Increase*   Secondary to hemolysis. *2538*

Blood   Normal   Normal or slightly decreased. *0157*

Sodium   *Serum   Increase*   In 99% of 27 patients at initial hospitalization for this disorder. *0781*

Urea Nitrogen   *Serum   Increase*   Can be elevated in kidney infiltration and should be followed especially if nephrotoxic antibiotics are used. *0433*   In 54% of 27 patients at initial hospitalization for this disorder. *0781*

Uric Acid   *Serum   Increase*   A frequent association of the treated condition. *0433*   Not as frequent as in other leukemias. *0992*

Serum   Normal   Usually normal. *2039*

Urine   Increase   Not as frequent as in other leukemias. *0992*

Urine   Normal   Often normal. *2039*

Vitamin B$_{12}$ *Serum   Increase*   About 33% of cases. *2467*   Significant increase in 19 patients, mean = 1223 compared to normal, 385 pg/mL. *1990*

Serum   Normal   *2468 0142*

Vitamin B$_{12}$ Binding Capacity   *Serum   Increase*   Significant elevation; usually correlated with WBC in peripheral blood. *1990*

Zinc   *Serum   Decrease*   Decreased. *2297*

205.00   Myelocytic Leukemia (Acute)

Alanine Aminotransferase   *Serum   Increase*   Infiltration of the liver. *0619*   Moderate elevation observed in lymphomas and leukemia but less frequently than in other hepatic disease. *0503*

Albumin   *Serum   Decrease*   Normal at diagnosis, but falls as disease progresses. *0689 2552*   In 34% of 36 patients at initial hospitalization for this disorder. *0781*

Aldolase   *Serum   Increase*   Slight elevation in 50% of patients. *2468*

Alkaline Phosphatase   *Serum   Increase*   Infiltration of the liver may result in obstruction of the biliary system. *2468*   Elevations > 95 U/L. *1322*

Leukocyte   Decrease   The range of activity per 10^{10} leukocytes was 0.0-6.2 U/L, the mean being 1.6 U/L. The tendency toward low levels for both alkaline and acid phosphatase activity suggests that the blast form is poor in phosphatase; the activity being attributable chiefly to the more mature cells in acute leukemia. *0144*   leukemia. *1949 1563   2552*

Leukocyte   Increase   Slightly elevated in > 50% of cases. *2552*

Alpha$_1$-Antichymotrypsin   *Serum   Increase*   Increased 24-48 hours after chemotherapy in patients with or without DIC. *1262 0807*

Alpha$_1$-Globulin   *Serum   Increase*   Often reflects the presence of fever or infection. *0689 2552*

Alpha$_1$-Glycoprotein   *Serum   Increase*   Elevated levels in states associated with cell proliferation. *1239 1672   1947 2096 2170 1866*

Alpha$_2$-Globulin   *Serum   Increase*   Often reflects the presence of fever or infection. *0689 2552*

Angiotensin-Converting Enzyme (ACE)   *Serum   Decrease*   Mean value for group 19.9 U/L compared with 24.4 U/L for control group. *1969*

Antinuclear Antibodies   *Serum   Increase*   Positive in 25% of patients. *1799*

Arylsulfatase   *Serum   Increase*   30-50% increase in serum activity. *0610*

Aspartate Aminotransferase   *Serum   Increase*   Moderately elevated levels are observed in lymphomas and leukemia but less frequently than in other hepatic disease. *0503*   In 37% of 36 patients at initial hospitalization for this disorder. *0781*

Basophils   *Blood   Increase*   Occasionally. *0992*

Bence-Jones Protein   *Serum   Present*   *0619*

Beta-Globulin   *Serum   Increase*   Common. *0689 2552*

Calcium   *Serum   Increase*   Elevation (> 11 mg/dL) may occur with leukemic infiltration of bone. *1322*   Has been observed, but is uncommon. *2552 0503*

Urine   Increase   *0503*

Carcinoembryonic Antigen   *Serum   Increase*   Above 2.5 ng/mL in 38% of patients with acute and chronic leukemia. *0211*

Cells   *CSF   Increase*   Pleocytosis with meningeal infiltration. *2538*

Bone Marrow   Increase   Marked occurrence of either sea-blue histiocytes or Gaucher like cells, or of both, was observed in bone marrow smears and the hematopoietic tissues of 23 patients with chronic disease and in acute, but with lower frequency and degree. *2319*   Blast cells are present even when none are found in the peripheral blood. *2468*

Cholesterol   *Serum   Decrease*   In 51% of 36 patients at initial hospitalization for this disorder. *0781*

Copper   *Serum   Increase*   Significant increase observed in 16 cases of acute leukemia. Drop occurs in cases who respond to quadruple chemotherapy while those who failed to respond showed persistently high levels. *0645*

Creatine   *Urine   Increase*   Pronounced increase in children and adult males with acute leukemias. *2104*   Extremely variable. *2453*

Creatinine   *Serum   Increase*   In 55% of 27 patients at initial hospitalization for this disorder. *0781*

Eosinophils   *Blood   Increase*   Occasionally. *0992*

Erythropoietin   *Serum   Increase*   Increased and negatively correlated with hemoglobin concentration. *1785*

Factor V   *Plasma   Decrease*   Intravascular clotting has been documented in occasional patients. *0890*

Factor VIII   *Plasma   Decrease*   Intravascular clotting has been documented in occasional patients. *0890*

Ferritin   *Serum   Increase*   Significant elevation. *2244*

Fibrinogen   *Plasma   Decrease*   Moderate depression occurs. *0619*   Intravascular clotting has been documented in occasional patients. *0890*

Fibrin Split Products (FSP)   *Plasma   Increase*   Intravascular clotting has been documented in occasional patients. *0890*

Globulin   *Serum   Increase*   Diffuse hypergammaglobulinemia is common. *0689 2552*

Glucose   *CSF   Decrease*   With meningeal infiltration. *2538*

Hematocrit   *Blood   Decrease*   Most patients will have anemia. *0433*   Often severe, may be macrocytic. *2552*   In 90% of 35 patients at initial hospitalization for this disorder. *0781*

Hemoglobin   *Blood   Decrease*   Most patients will have anemia. *0433*   Often severe, may be macrocytic. *2552*   In 90% of 35 patients at initial hospitalization for this disorder. *0781*

Hemoglobin, Fetal   *Blood   Increase*   Increased in some leukemias (especially juvenile myeloid leukemia); with HbF of 30-60%, absence of Philadelphia chromosome, rapid fatal course, more pronounced thrombocytopenia, and lower total WBC count. *2468*

Heterophil Antibody   *Serum   Decrease*   Positive presumptive test but negative differential test if Forsman antigen is used. *1752*

Serum   Increase   Positive presumptive test but negative differential test if Forsman antigen is used. *1752*

Immunoglobulin IgA   *Serum   Normal*   *2467*

Immunoglobulin IgG   *Serum   Normal*   *2467*

Immunoglobulin IgM   *Serum   Normal*   *2467*

Iron   *Serum   Increase*   Increased in acute leukemias. *0619*

Isocitrate Dehydrogenase   *Serum   Increase*   *0619*

Lactate Dehydrogenase   *Serum   Increase*   Markedly elevated levels in untreated acute leukemia. *0812*   2-4 X normal values. *0503*   Increased in about 90% of the patients. The degree of increase is not correlated with the level of WBC. *2467*   In 87% of 34 patients at initial hospitalization for this disorder. *0781*   84 of 91 patients with leukemias had values elevated above the normal upper limit. *0206 0221 0962*

Leukocytes   *Blood   Decrease*   Variable and can be very high (> 100,000/μL), moderately elevated (20,000-100,000), normal or low. *0433*   In 26% of 34 patients at initial hospitalization for this disorder. *0781*

Blood   Increase   Variable and can be very high (> 100,000/μL), moderately elevated (20,000-10,000/μL), normal or low. *0433*   Number of blasts can range from 0 to 1 million. Not increased in approximately 40% at time of diagnosis. Normal blood leukocytes are almost always decreased. *0992*   Slightly elevated in > 50% of cases. *2552*   In 46% of 34 patients at initial hospitalization for this disorder. *0781*

Blood   Normal   Variable and can be very high, moderately elevated, normal or low. *0433*

Lysozyme   *Serum   Decrease*   Low, normal or moderately increased. *0798*

Serum   Increase   During the transition from a variety of myeloproliferative disorders to acute myeloblastic or acute myelomonocytic leukemia, there is a striking elevation in serum and urine muramidase activity. *2093*   Low, normal, or moderately increased. *0798   0151*

Serum Normal Low, normal, or moderately increased. *0798*

Urine Increase Elevated only in patients who do not have the Philadelphia chromosome. No correlation is apparent between urine and serum levels. *2093* During the transition from a variety of myeloproliferative disorders to acute myeloblastic or acute myelomonocytic leukemia, there is a striking elevation in serum and urine muramidase activity. *2093*

Magnesium *Serum Increase 2538*

MCH *Blood Increase* Often severe anemia, may be macrocytic. *2552*

MCV *Blood Increase* Often severe anemia, may be macrocytic. *2552*

Monocytes *Blood Increase* On occasion associated with a monocytosis of relatively minor proportions. *1489 2538*

Neutrophils *Blood Increase* The number of blasts can range from 0 to 1 million. Not increased in approximately 40% at time of diagnosis. Normal blood leukocytes are almost always decreased. *0992*

Partial Thromboplastin Time *Plasma Increase* Intravascular clotting has been documented in occasional patients. *0890*

Phosphate *Serum Increase 2467*

Phosphoglucomutase *Serum Increase* In some cases. *0619*

Platelet Count *Blood Decrease* Most patients will have thrombocytopenia. *0433* Common; frequently pronounced at diagnosis. *2552* In 85% of 35 patients at initial hospitalization for this disorder. *0781* Intravascular clotting has been documented in occasional patients. *0890*

Blood Increase On very rare occasions. *0075*

Potassium *Serum Decrease* Below 3.5 mmol/L in 19 (59%) of 32 patients. *1602*

Urine Increase Inappropriately large quantities of potassium were excreted in relation to the low serum content. 12 of 32 patients excreted more than the mean potassium intake. *1602*

Protein *CSF Increase* With meningeal infiltration. *2538*

Pleural Effusion Increase Pleural effusions are usually exudates. *0062*

Prothrombin Time *Plasma Increase* Intravascular clotting has been documented in occasional patients. *0890*

Reticulocytes *Blood Decrease* Usually low, however, if RBC morphology is bizarre, and nucleated RBCs and an increased reticulocyte count are present, erythroleukemia should be suspected. *0433* Reflects decreased cell production. *2552*

Rheumatoid Factor *Serum Increase* Dysproteinemias and paraproteinemias present significant seropositivity. *0962*

Sodium *Serum Increase* In 98% of 34 patients at initial hospitalization for this disorder. *0781*

Thrombin Time *Plasma Increase* Intravascular clotting has been demonstrated in occasional patients. *0890*

Urea Nitrogen *Serum Increase* Can be elevated in kidney infiltration and should be followed especially if nephrotic antibiotics are used. *0433* In 33% of 37 patients at initial hospitalization for this disorder. *0781*

Uric Acid *Serum Increase* Frequent biochemical abnormality. Secondary to the increased cell turnover. *0433* In approximately 50% of patients. *1042 2552* In 44% of 35 patients at initial hospitalization for this disorder. *0781* Due to excessive excretion of urate, but no correlation was found between serum and urinary levels in myeloid patients, contrary to normal controls (R = 0.85). Serum levels tends to fall in relapse. *1601 0962*

Urine Increase Mean urate excretion was 0.774 ± 0.057 mg/min, significantly higher than normal, 0.595 ± 0.035. *1601* Almost invariable. *1042 2552*

Vitamin B$_{12}$ *Serum Increase* Acute myelocytic leukemic cells may secrete a vitamin B$_{12}$ binding protein in large quantity, accounting for high serum levels of B$_{12}$. *0151* Usually high, in contrast to acute lymphocytic leukemia. *0142 2538*

Vitamin B$_{12}$ Binding Capacity *Serum Increase* Significant elevation; usually correlated with WBC in peripheral blood. *1990*

Zinc *Serum Decrease* Decreased. *2297*

205.10 Myelocytic Leukemia (Chronic)

Acid Phosphatase *Serum Increase* 9 of 16 patients with myeloid metaplasia or chronic granulocytic leukemia were found to have slight but significant elevations. *0129*

Alanine Aminotransferase *Serum Increase* Less elevation than in acute leukemia. *2468*

Albumin *Serum Decrease* Electrophoresis shows decrease. *2468* In 46% of 21 patients at initial hospitalization for this disorder. *0781*

Serum Normal Usually normal. *2552*

Aldolase *Serum Increase* Less elevation than in acute leukemia. *2468*

Alkaline Phosphatase *Serum Increase* Infiltration of the liver may result in obstruction of the biliary system. *2468* 21 of 54 patients had levels > 95 U/L. *1322* In 54% of 21 patients at initial hospitalization for this disorder. *0781*

Leukocyte Decrease In 60 patients, mean = 33 U/L, ranging from 0-294 U/L. In untreated cases, the mean score was 6.6 U/L, ranging from 0-28 U/L. Mean in 19 treated cases was 45.15 U/L with a range of 3-294 U/L. Leukopenic cases showed the average score as 104 U/L, ranging from 52-208 U/L. *1563* 25% of 38 patients who achieved remission had normal activity. *1991* A striking decrease can be demonstrated; about 20% of normal mature granulocytes give a positive reaction. *2538* Abnormally low and may actually be absent *0525 2552*

Leukocyte Increase Occasionally can be elevated if some complicating condition (ulcerative colitis, a second neoplasm, or an acute infection) is present. *0433*

Alpha$_1$-Globulin *Serum Increase* Increased alpha and gamma globulins. *2468*

Alpha$_2$-Globulin *Serum Increase* Increased alpha and gamma globulins. *2468*

Alpha-Ketoglutarate *Serum Increase* Increased in the vast majority of patients with myeloproliferative disorders, reflective of the WBC pool size. *0337*

Antithrombin III *Plasma Decrease* Below normal in some patients. *2318*

Arylsulfatase *Serum Increase* 30-50% increase in serum activity. *0610*

Aspartate Aminotransferase *Serum Increase* Infiltration of the liver. *0619* Moderately elevated levels are observed in lymphomas and leukemia but less frequently than in other hepatic disease. *0503* Less elevation than in acute leukemia. *2468* In 54% of 21 patients at initial hospitalization for this disorder. *0781*

Basophils *Blood Increase* Particularly in the stage preceding acute blastic crisis. *0433* Slight to moderate persistent basophilia may occur. Often regarded as a poor prognostic sign. *2538* High absolute number in almost all patients. *2552 0992*

Bone Marrow Increase May be considerably increased; usually in proportion to their number in the circulating blood. *2538*

Bence-Jones Protein *Serum Present 0619*

Calcium *Serum Increase* Elevation > 11 mg/dL may occur with leukemic infiltration of bone. *1322* Has been described occasionally. *0109 1392*

Urine Increase 0503

Carcinoembryonic Antigen *Serum Increase* Above 2.5 ng/mL in 38% of patients with acute and chronic leukemia. *0211*

Cells *Bone Marrow Increase* Occurrence of either sea-blue histiocytes or Gaucher like cells, or of both, was observed in bone marrow smears of 23 patients and in the hematopoietic tissues of 44 of the examined cases; particularly marked in chronic disease and in acute forms, though less in frequency or degree. *2319* Bone marrow aspirated from almost any site usually yields a grossly hypercellular specimen in which the fat is practically absent. *2538*

Cholesterol *Serum Increase* In 65% of 21 patients at initial hospitalization for this disorder. *0781*

Complement C4 *Serum Decrease* Occasionally occurs. *1120*

Complement, Total *Serum Decrease* Occasionally occurs. *1120*

Coombs' Test *Blood Positive* Positive in 33% of patients. *2468*

Creatine *Urine Increase* Increased breakdown. *2467 2468*

Creatinine *Serum Increase* In 83% of 13 patients at initial hospitalization for this disorder. *0781*

Eosinophils *Blood Increase* Increased in percentage, which means a striking absolute increase. *0151* Characteristic shift toward immaturity of the granulocytes and the increase in eosinophils and basophils. *0151* Often regarded as a poor prognostic sign. *2538* Absolute increase in almost all cases. *2552 0992*

Bone Marrow Increase Particularly in the stage preceding acute blastic crisis. *0433* May be considerably increased; usually in proportion to their number in the circulating blood. *2538*

Erythrocyte Survival *Red Blood Cells Decrease* Some shortening of survival occurs in the presence of gross splenomegaly and hepatomegaly. *2538*

205.10 Myelocytic Leukemia (Chronic) *(continued)*

Factor II *Plasma Decrease* Low levels found. *2318*

Factor V *Plasma Decrease* Low levels found. *2318* Intravascular clotting has been documented for rare patients. *0890*

Factor VIII *Plasma Decrease* Intravascular clotting has been documented for rare patients. *0890*

Fat *Bone Marrow Decrease* Bone marrow aspirated from almost any site usually yields a grossly hypercellular specimen in which the fat is practically absent. *2538*

Ferritin *Serum Increase* Significant elevation. *2244*

Fibrinogen *Plasma Decrease* Moderate depression. *0619* Intravascular clotting has been documented for rare patients. *0890*

Plasma Increase Either elevated or normal. *2318*

Fibrin Split Products (FSP) *Plasma Increase* Intravascular clotting has been documented for rare patients. *0890*

Globulin *Serum Increase* Increased alpha and gamma globulins. *2468* Often moderately elevated. *2552*

Glucose *Serum Decrease* Artifactual hypoglycemia may be due to leukocyte glucose utilization in vitro. *0730* *2552*

Serum Increase In 49% of 21 patients at initial hospitalization for this disorder. *0781*

Hematocrit *Blood Decrease* Anemia, when present, is characteristically normochromic normocytic. *0433* Anemia is almost always a feature of active disease, and generally increases in severity as the disease advances. Usually normocytic and normochromic with little evidence of iron deficiency, accelerated RBC hemolysis, or erythrocyte abnormality. *2538* In 75% of 20 patients at initial hospitalization for this disorder. *0781* *2552*

Blood Increase In a small percentage of patients there may be a mild elevation. *0433*

Hemoglobin *Blood Decrease* Anemia, when present, is characteristically normochromic normocytic. *0433* Anemia is almost always a feature of active disease, and generally increases in severity as the disease advances. Usually normocytic and normochromic with little evidence of iron deficiency, accelerated RBC hemolysis, or erythrocyte abnormality. *2538* In 85% of 22 patients at initial hospitalization for this disorder. *0781* *2552*

Blood Increase In a small percentage of patients there may be a mild elevation. *0433*

Histamine *Serum Increase* Histamine and histamine metabolites are raised in plasma and WBC in most patients. *0173* In a group of patients with no symptoms attributable to histamine, mean plasma concentration was > 3 X normal. Tends to reflect the number of basophils. *2299* *2552*

Immunoglobulin IgA *Serum Decrease* *2467*

Immunoglobulin IgG *Serum Normal* *2467*

Immunoglobulin IgM *Serum Normal* *2467*

Isocitrate Dehydrogenase *Serum Increase* *0619*

Lactate Dehydrogenase *Serum Increase* Usually reflects changes in the course of the disease--falling during remission and rising during relapses, occasionally indicating the onset before the WBC had begun to change. *2468* Elevated in all 20 patients, mean = 197.5 U/L. *1521* Considerably elevated, but appears to be a nonspecific abnormality. *1476* In 95% of 20 patients at initial hospitalization for this disorder. *0781* Elevated above the normal upper limit in 84 of 91 patients with leukemias. *0206* *0221 2538 0962*

Serum Normal Frequently normal. *2468*

Lactate Dehydrogenase Isoenzyme 5 (LD₅) *Serum Decrease* Isoenzyme 2 and 3 were the most intense and 5 was decreased. *1521* *2253*

Red Blood Cells Increase Increase observed in hemolysates. In 5 cases values ranged from 5-16% activity while normal = 2%. *2249*

Lactate Dehydrogenase Isoenzymes *Serum Increase* Fractions 2 and 3 were increased and fraction 5 was decreased. *2253*

Leukocytes *Blood Increase* Increase due to increase in myeloid series is earliest change. In earlier stages the more mature forms predominate with sequentially fewer cells of the younger forms; in the later, more advanced stages the younger cells become predominant. *2468* Characteristically > 75,000/µL, and may exceed 500,000/µL. *0999* Over 100,000/µL in 62-90% at diagnosis. *1512 2555* In 94% of 22 patients at initial hospitalization for this disorder. *0781* *2552*

Lymphocytes *Blood Decrease* In 85% of 21 patients at initial hospitalization for this disorder. *0781*

Blood Normal Absolute count is usually within normal limits. *2552*

Lysozyme *Serum Increase* Elevated only in patients who do not have the Philadelphia chromosome. No correlation is apparent between urine and serum levels. *2093*

Malate Dehydrogenase *Serum Increase* Less elevation than in acute leukemia. *2468*

Metamyelocytes *Blood Increase* In the great majority of patients. *2538*

Monocytes *Blood Increase* May be normal or increased. *0992* On occasion associated with a monocytosis of relatively minor proportions. *1489* Increase in absolute number in almost all cases. *2552* *0151 2538*

Myelocytes *Blood Increase* In the great majority of patients. *2538*

Neutrophils *Blood Increase* 80-90% of the cells are granulocytes. The distribution shows only a slight shift toward immaturity. *0151* Most patients have > 100,000 granulocytes at time of diagnosis and the count may exceed 1 million. *0992* Granulocytes in all stages of development occur in profusion in the peripheral blood and for the most part appear to be normal in morphology. The most mature elements are ordinarily present in greatest number and the less mature in diminishing frequency. *2538* *2552*

Bone Marrow Increase Granulocytic and sometimes megakaryocytic hyperplasia in bone marrow. *0337* Resemble those in the peripheral blood, but on the average they are about 1 stage less mature. *2538*

Partial Thromboplastin Time *Plasma Increase* Intravascular clotting has been documented for rare patients. *0890*

Phosphoglucomutase *Serum Increase* In some cases. *0619*

Plasminogen *Serum Decrease* Below normal in some patients. *2318*

Platelet Count *Blood Decrease* Decreased in terminal stages with findings of thrombocytopenic purpura. *2468* Rarely develops spontaneously in the absence of blastic crisis. *0992* Severe thrombocytopenia is rare at diagnosis. *2552* In 56% of 21 patients at initial hospitalization for this disorder. *0781* Intravascular clotting has been documented in rare patients. *0890*

Blood Increase Elevated in a small percentage of patients, with counts reaching 1-2 million/µL. Occasionally precedes the increase in WBC and a diagnosis of essential or primary thrombocythemia may be made. *0433* A 33% or more of patients have pronounced thrombocytosis. *1520* High in approximately 50% of patients. *1512 2555* In 23% of 21 patients at initial hospitalization for this disorder. *0781* *0532 0999 2538*

Potassium *Serum Increase* Pseudohyperkalemia due to the release of potassium from white cells during clotting has been reported. *0291* Artifactual hyperkalemia may occur. *2552*

Protein *Pleural Effusion Increase* Pleural effusions are usually exudates. *0062*

Prothrombin Time *Plasma Increase* Intravascular clotting has been documented for rare patients. *0890*

Reticulocytes *Blood Increase* Generally normal or slightly increased. *2538 2552*

Blood Normal Normal or slightly increased. *0157*

Sodium *Serum Increase* In 100% of 20 patients at initial hospitalization for this disorder. *0781*

Thrombin Time *Plasma Increase* Intravascular clotting has been documented for rare patients. *0890*

Urea Nitrogen *Serum Increase* Can be elevated in kidney infiltration and should be followed especially if nephrotoxic antibiotics are used. *0433* In 23% of 21 patients at initial hospitalization for this disorder. *0781*

Uric Acid *Serum Increase* Frequent biochemical abnormality. *0433* Especially with high WBC and antileukemic therapy. Urinary obstruction may develop on account of intrarenal and extrarenal crystallization. *2468* Often moderately elevated; increased production. *2552* In 80% of 21 patients at initial hospitalization for this disorder. *0781 0962*

Urine Increase Often 2-3 X normal in patients with active disease, and if aggressive therapy leads to rapid cell lysis, excretion of the additional purine load may produce urinary tract blockage. *1315* Almost invariably increased; gout may occur. *2552*

Vitamin B₁₂ *Serum Increase* Significant increase found in 27 patients, mean for the group = 675, compared to normal, 385. *1990* Increased to an average of approximately 15 X the normal mean concentration, generally proportional to the height of the leukocyte count in untreated patients, but still 4 X normal in patients who have normal WBC counts during remissions. *2538 0151*

Vitamin B₁₂ Binding Capacity *Serum Increase* Increased in the vast majority of patients with myeloproliferative disorders, reflective of the WBC pool size. *0337* Despite the increased amount of vitamin B₁₂, there is considerable additional unsaturated binding capacity. *1825 2538 2552*

Zinc *Serum Decrease* Decreased. *2297*

206.00 Monocytic Leukemia

Albumin *Serum Decrease* In 33% of 23 patients at initial hospitalization for this disorder. *0781*

Alkaline Phosphatase *Serum Increase* In 34% of 21 patients at initial hospitalization for this disorder. *0781*

Leukocyte Increase Mean value in 13 cases of acute monomyelocytic leukemia was 103.4 with a range of 12-208. *1563*

Aspartate Aminotransferase *Serum Increase* In 63% of 23 patients at initial hospitalization for this disorder. *0781*

Beta-Globulin *Serum Decrease* *2467*

Cholesterol *Serum Decrease* In 51% of 23 patients at initial hospitalization for this disorder. *0781*

Creatinine *Serum Increase* In 49% of 22 patients at initial hospitalization for this disorder. *0781*

Factor V *Plasma Decrease* With disseminated intravascular clotting. *1552*

Factor VIII *Plasma Decrease* With disseminated intravascular clotting. *1552*

Fibrinogen *Plasma Decrease* With disseminated intravascular clotting. *1552*

Fibrin Split Products (FSP) *Plasma Increase* With disseminated intravascular clotting. *1552*

Globulin *Serum Increase* An increased concentration of heterogeneous or polyclonal gamma globulin in the plasma occurs frequently. *2538 2467*

Hematocrit *Blood Decrease* Anemia is often quite severe, usually normochromic and normocytic. *2552* In 90% of 24 patients at initial hospitalization for this disorder. *0781*

Hemoglobin *Blood Decrease* Anemia is often quite severe, usually normochromic and normocytic. *2552* In 91% of 24 patients at initial hospitalization for this disorder. *0781*

Iron *Serum Increase* Increased in acute leukemias. *0619*

Lactate Dehydrogenase *Serum Increase* In 80% of 22 patients at initial hospitalization for this disorder. *0781*

Leukocytes *Blood Decrease* Variable percentage of abnormal monocytes in about 33% of all patients initially. Usually present. *2538* Patients are usually leukopenic. *2552*

Blood Increase The majority have a moderate to pronounced leukocytosis, with some 50-75% of the WBC being monocytes, promonocytes, or monoblasts. *2538* In 58% of 24 patients at initial hospitalization for this disorder. *0781*

Lysozyme *Serum Increase* Elevated in serum and urine in some patients with acute monocytic and myelomonocytic leukemia. *0433* During the transition from a variety of myeloproliferative disorders to acute myeloblastic or acute myelomonocytic leukemia, there is a striking elevation in serum and urine muramidase activity. *2093* Markedly increased. *0798*

Urine Increase Elevated in serum and urine in some patients with acute monocytic and myelomonocytic leukemia. *0433* Patients with heavy lysozymuria develop an apparently unique type of glomerular-tubular dysfunction, with hypokalemia, hyperkaluria, and azotemia. *1641* During the transition from a variety of myeloproliferative disorders to acute myeloblastic or acute myelomonocytic leukemia, there is a striking elevation in serum and urine muramidase activity. *2093*

Monocytes *Blood Increase* Occurs in monocytic and other leukemias. *2467* In 38% of 23 patients at initial hospitalization for this disorder. *0781*

Neutrophils *Blood Decrease* In 94% of 24 patients at initial hospitalization for this disorder. *0781*

Partial Thromboplastin Time *Plasma Increase* With disseminated intravascular clotting. *1552*

Platelet Count *Blood Decrease* Usually present. *2538* In 83% of 24 patients at initial hospitalization for this disorder. *0781* With disseminated intravascular clotting. *1552*

Protein *Urine Increase* A unique type of proteinuria develops in about 50% of patients. In addition to ordinary plasma components, the low molecular weight enzyme lysozyme is excreted in amounts up to 0.6-2.4 g/24h. *1746 2538*

Pleural Effusion Increase Pleural effusions are usually exudates. *0062*

Prothrombin Time *Plasma Increase* With disseminated intravascular clotting. *1552*

Reticulocytes *Blood Increase* Usually modest in degree, considering the severity of the anemia. *2538*

Thrombin Time *Plasma Increase* With disseminated intravascular clotting. *1552*

Urea Nitrogen *Serum Increase* In 36% of 24 patients at initial hospitalization for this disorder. *0781*

Uric Acid *Serum Increase* In 55% of 23 patients at initial hospitalization for this disorder. *0781*

Vitamin B$_{12}$ *Serum Increase* Increases in some cases. *2467*

Zinc *Serum Decrease* Decreased. *2297*

207.00 Erythroleukemia

Alkaline Phosphatase *Leukocyte Increase* In 2 cases of erythroleukemia, the scores from polymorphonuclears were 24 and 78. Normal mean = 61.9. *1563 2538*

Bilirubin *Serum Increase* Evidence of a mild or moderate increase in hemolysis is commonly observed, but the erythrokinetic findings are those of ineffective erythropoiesis. *2538*

Cells *Bone Marrow Increase* Marrow is nearly always hypercellular and characteristically shows a selective hyperplasia of the erythroid cells, with a myeloid/erythroid ratio of 1.0 or even lower. *2538*

Coombs' Test *Blood Negative* *2538*

Erythrocyte Survival *Red Blood Cells Decrease* Evidence of a mild or moderate increase in hemolysis is commonly observed, but the erythrokinetic findings are those of ineffective erythropoiesis. *2538*

Haptoglobin *Serum Decrease* Evidence of a mild or moderate increase in hemolysis is commonly observed, but the erythrokinetic findings are those of ineffective erythropoiesis. *2538*

Hematocrit *Blood Decrease* Anemia is nearly always present, but its severity is variable. Usually normocytic and normochromic. *2538*

Hemoglobin *Blood Decrease* Anemia is nearly always present, but its severity is variable. Usually normocytic and normochromic. *2538*

Lactate Dehydrogenase *Serum Increase* Normal or high levels. *2538*

Leukocytes *Blood Increase* Count varies from subnormal to frankly leukemic levels but tends to rise as the disease progresses. *2538*

MCV *Blood Increase* A mild macrocytosis is sometimes present. *2538*

Platelet Count *Blood Decrease* In about 50% of the cases. *2538*

Reticulocytes *Blood Increase* Occasionally. *0936*

Uric Acid *Serum Increase* Normal or high levels. *2538*

Urobilinogen *Feces Increase* Evidence of a mild or moderate increase in hemolysis is commonly observed, but the erythrokinetic findings are those of ineffective erythropoiesis. *2538*

Vitamin B$_{12}$ *Serum Increase* In many, but not all patients. *2538*

211.10 Benign Neoplasm of Stomach

Albumin *Serum Decrease* Secondary to protein-losing enteropathy in adenocarcinoma. *2104*

Fucose *Serum Increase* Total concentration was increased in patients with both malignant and benign tumors. The glycoprotein-bound fraction was very markedly elevated in cases of malignancy and not in benign disease. Mucoprotein fraction was raised in both diseases. *2331*

Hematocrit *Blood Decrease* With occult bleeding, iron deficiency anemia may be present, in which case the bone marrow will not contain iron. *2199*

Hemoglobin *Blood Decrease* With occult bleeding, iron deficiency anemia may be present, in which case the bone marrow will not contain iron. *2199*

Hexosaminidase *Serum Increase* Elevated. *2356*

Iron *Serum Decrease* With occult bleeding, iron deficiency anemia may be present. *2199*

Bone Marrow Decrease With occult bleeding, iron deficiency anemia may be present, in which case the bone marrow will not contain iron. *2199*

Iron-Binding Capacity, Total (TIBC) *Serum Increase* Anemia is commonly iron deficient type, due to chronic blood loss. *2199*

Iron Saturation *Serum Decrease* Anemia is commonly iron deficient type, due to chronic blood loss. *2199*

MCH *Blood Decrease* With occult bleeding, iron deficiency anemia may be present. *2199*

211.10   Benign Neoplasm of Stomach (continued)

MCHC   *Blood   Decrease*   With occult bleeding, iron deficiency anemia may be present. *2199*

MCV   *Blood   Decrease*   With occult bleeding, iron deficiency anemia may be present. *2199*

Occult Blood   *Feces   Positive*   Adenomatous and villous polyps may result in GI bleeding. *2199*

211.40   Benign Neoplasm of Rectum and Anus

Carcinoembryonic Antigen   *Serum   Increase*   14 (15%) of 93 adult patients with sporadic colorectal adenomata had concentration > 2.5 ng/mL. No associations were found with age, polyp volume, or villous histology. *0587*   19% of patients had values > 2.5 ng/mL. *2199*

Cholesterol   *Feces   Increase*   The fecal excretion of cholesterol, coprostanol, coprostanone, total bile acids, deoxycholic acid, lithocholic acid was higher in patients with colon cancer and patients with adenomatous polyps compared to normal American and Japanese controls as well as in patients with other digestive diseases. *1896*   Although the total fecal neutral sterol concentrations were not different between the groups, the patients with familial polyposis excreted a high amount of cholesterol and low levels of coprostanol and coprostanone compared with other groups. Increased cholesterol and decreased lithocholic acid is excreted in patients with familial polyposis. *1895*

Deoxycholic Acid   *Feces   Increase*   The fecal excretion was higher in patients with colon cancer and patients with adenomatous polyps compared to normal American and Japanese controls as well as patients with other digestive diseases. *1896*

Lithocholic Acid   *Feces   Decrease*   Increased cholesterol and decreased lithocholic acid is excreted in patients with familial polyposis. *1895*

Feces   Increase   The fecal excretion of cholesterol, coprostanol, coprostanone, total bile acids, deoxycholic acid, lithocholic acid was higher in patients with colon cancer and patients with adenomatous polyps compared to normal American and Japanese controls as well as in patients with other digestive diseases. *1896*

Occult Blood   *Feces   Positive*   Large amount of mucus tinged with blood; frequent watery diarrhea. *2467*   Adenomatous and villous polyps may result in GI bleeding. *2199*

Potassium   *Serum   Decrease*   Sometimes decreased. *2467*

211.41   Adenomatous Polyp

Hydrochloric Acid   *Gastric Material   Decrease*   Gastric analysis - achlorhydria in 85% of patients. Polyps occur in 5% of patients with pernicious anemia and 2% of patients with achlorhydria. *2467*

pH   *Gastric Material   Increase*   Gastric analysis - achlorhydria in 85% of patients. Polyps occur in 5% of patients with pernicious anemia and 2% of patients with achlorhydria. *2467*

211.60   Benign Neoplasm of Pancreas

Glucose   *Serum   Decrease*   Decreased glucose due to excess insulin in pancreatic islet cell. *0619   0812*

Glucose Tolerance   *Serum   Increase*   Flat peak. Late hypoglycemia. *2467*

Insulin   *Serum   Increase*   Fasting blood insulin level over 50 μU/mL in presence of low or normal blood glucose level. Intravenous tolbutamide or administration of leucine causes rapid rise to very high levels within a few minutes with rapid return to normal. *2467*   Elevated levels of plasma insulin following an overnight fast, as well as increased concentrations of C-peptide or proinsulin, strongly suggest the presence of insulinoma. *0999   0098*

Insulin Tolerance   *Serum   Decrease*   An excessive fall in the blood sugar may occur in pancreatic islet cell hyperplasia. *0619*

Phosphate   *Serum   Decrease*   Hyperinsulinism; during successful treatment of diabetic ketosis, insulin causes phosphate ions to enter the cells with glucose and potassium. *0619 2467*

Potassium   *Serum   Decrease*   Gastrointestinal wasting as a result of pancreatic islet nonbeta cell tumors. *1679*

Proinsulin   *Serum   Increase*   Elevated levels of plasma insulin following an overnight fast, as well as increased concentrations of C-peptide or proinsulin, strongly suggest the presence of insulinoma. *0999*

212.70   Benign Neoplasm of Cardiovascular Tissue

Aspartate Aminotransferase   *Serum   Increase*   May reflect many small emboli to striated muscle. *2467*

C-Reactive Protein   *Serum   Increase*   May be increased in myxoma of left atrium. *2467*

Erythrocyte Sedimentation Rate   *Blood   Increase*   Reflection of abnormal serum proteins. *2467*   Occurs with myxoma, possibly reflecting tumor emboli or tumor breakdown products. *1108*

Erythrocyte Survival   *Red Blood Cells   Decrease*   Hemolytic anemia and mechanical in origin (due to local turbulence of blood) may occur and may be severe. The anemia is recognized in about 50% of the patients. *2467*   Occurs with myxoma, possibly reflecting tumor emboli or tumor breakdown products. *1108*

Globulin   *Serum   Increase*   Occurs with myxoma, possibly reflecting tumor emboli or tumor breakdown products. *1108*   Recognized to be increased in about 50% of patients *2467*

Hematocrit   *Blood   Decrease*   Hemolytic anemia, and mechanical in origin (due to local turbulence of blood) may occur and may be severe. The anemia is recognized in about 50% of patients. *2467*   Occurs with myxoma, possibly reflecting tumor emboli or tumor breakdown products. *1108*

Hemoglobin   *Blood   Decrease*   Hemolytic anemia, mechanical in origin (due to local turbulence of blood) is usual and may be severe. The anemia is recognized in about 50% of patients with this tumor. *2467*   Occurs with myxoma, possibly reflecting tumor emboli or tumor breakdown products. *1108*

Blood   Increase   Often elevated without arterial hypoxemia in right atrial myxoma. *1108*

Lactate Dehydrogenase   *Serum   Increase*   Reflects hemolysis. *2467*

Leukocytes   *Blood   Increase*   Occurs with myxoma, possibly reflecting tumor emboli or tumor breakdown products. *1108*

Urine   Increase   Occasionally. *2467*

Platelet Count   *Blood   Decrease*   May be decreased (possibly mechanical) with resultant findings due to thrombocytopenia. *2467*

Reticulocytes   *Blood   Increase*   Hemolytic anemia, mechanical in origin (due to local turbulence of blood) is usual and may be severe. The anemia is recognized in about 50% of patients with this tumor. *2467*

217.00   Benign Neoplasm of Breast

Bicarbonate   *Serum   Increase*   In 42% of 14 patients at initial hospitalization for this disorder. *0781*

Carcinoembryonic Antigen   *Serum   Increase*   15% of patients had values > 2.5 ng/mL. *2199*

Fucose   *Serum   Increase*   Total concentration was increased in patients with both malignant and benign tumors. The glycoprotein-bound fraction was very markedly elevated in cases of malignancy and not in benign disease. Mucoprotein fraction was raised in both diseases. *2331*

Growth Hormone   *Serum   Increase*   Elevated. *0918*

Phosphate   *Serum   Decrease*   In 43% of 32 patients at initial hospitalization for this disorder. *0781*

Pregnanediol   *Urine   Decrease*   Average daily values were lower in 109 women with benign disease than normal women. No change was found in plasma estradiol. *1528*

Progesterone   *Plasma   Decrease*   Average daily values were lower in 109 women with benign disease than normal women. No change was found in plasma estradiol. *1528*

220.00   Benign Neoplasm of Ovary

17-Ketosteroids   *Urine   Increase*   May be slightly increased in arrhenoblastoma. May be moderately increased in Leydig cell tumors in masculinizing ovarian tumors. *2467*

Androgens   *Plasma   Increase*   *0433*

Estradiol   *Plasma   Increase*   In estrogen producing tumors estradiol is the most active estrogen. *0002   1720 0046*

Estrogens   *Urine   Increase*   *2467*

Follicle Stimulating Hormone (FSH)   *Urine   Decrease*   Inhibited by increased estrogen. *2467*

Gonadotropin, Pituitary   *Urine   Decrease*   Inhibited by increased estrogen. *2467*

Pregnanediol   *Urine   Decrease*   Absent in ovarian tumors. *2468*

Progesterone   *Plasma   Decrease*   Absent in ovarian tumors. *2468*

Testosterone *Plasma Increase* Plasma testosterone levels are elevated and confirmatory. *0433*

220.01 Teratoma (Dermoid)

17-Hydroxycorticosteroids *Urine Increase* *0503*

17-Ketogenic Steroids *Urine Increase* *0503*

Alpha-Fetoprotein *Serum Normal* *2468*

Protein Bound Iodine (PBI) *Serum Increase* Occasionally increased in certain tumors. *2467*

Serum Normal Occasionally increased in certain tumors. *2467*

220.92 Granulosa Cell Tumor of Ovary

17-Ketosteroids *Serum Increase* Ketosteroids are increased in virilizing ovarian tumors (e.g., adrenal rest tumor, granulosa cell tumor, hilar cell tumor, Brenner tumor, and most frequently, arrhenoblastoma) increased in 50% of patients and normal in 50% of the patients. *2467*

Urine Increase Urine 17-KS may be slightly increased in arrhenoblastoma. May be markedly increased in adrenal tumors of ovary. May be moderately increased in Leydig cell tumors in masculinizing ovarian tumors. *2467*

Estrogens *Serum Increase* Estrogens are increased in granulosa cell tumor of ovary. *2468*

Urine Increase Normal urinary excretion of total estrogens will be below 10 µg/24h. Values > 20 µg/24h are suggestive of a granulosa cell tumor. *0433*

Follicle Stimulating Hormone (FSH) *Urine Decrease* Inhibited by increased estrogen. *2467*

Pregnanediol *Urine Decrease* Absent in ovarian tumors. *2468*

Progesterone *Plasma Decrease* Absent in ovarian tumors. *2468*

220.93 Lutein Cell Tumor of Ovary

17-Ketogenic Steroids *Urine Increase* Increased in lutein cell tumor of the ovary if androgenic *2467*

17-Ketosteroids *Serum Increase* Ketosteroids are increased in virilizing ovarian tumors (e.g., adrenal rest tumor, granulosa cell tumor, hilar cell tumor, Brenner tumor, and most frequently, arrhenoblastoma) increased in 50% of the patients and normal in 50% of the patients. *2467*

Urine Increase Urine 17-KS may be slightly increased in arrhenoblastoma. May be markedly increased in adrenal tumors of ovary. May be moderately increased in Leydig cell tumors in masculinizing ovarian tumors. *2467*

Estrogens *Serum Increase* Estrogens are increased in luteoma of ovary. *2467* *2468*

Urine Increase *2467*

Follicle Stimulating Hormone (FSH) *Urine Decrease* Inhibited by increased estrogen. *2467*

Pregnanediol *Urine Decrease* Absent in ovarian tumors. *2468*

Progesterone *Plasma Decrease* Absent in ovarian tumors. *2468*

220.94 Theca Cell Tumor of Ovary

17-Ketosteroids *Serum Increase* Ketosteroids are increased in virilizing ovarian tumors (e.g., adrenal rest tumor, granulosa cell tumor, hilar cell tumor, Brenner tumor, and most frequently, arrhenoblastoma) increased in 50% of patients and normal in 50% of the patients. *2467*

Urine Increase Urinary 17-KS may be slightly increased in arrhenoblastoma. May be markedly increased in adrenal tumors of ovary. May be moderately increased in Leydig cell tumors in masculinizing ovarian tumors. *2467*

Estrogens *Serum Increase* Estrogens are increased in theca-cell tumor of ovary. *2467* *2468*

Urine Increase *0619*

Follicle Stimulating Hormone (FSH) *Urine Decrease* Inhibited by increased estrogen. *2467*

Pregnanediol *Urine Decrease* Absent in ovarian tumors. *2468*

Progesterone *Plasma Decrease* Absent in ovarian tumors. *2468*

220.95 Arrhenoblastoma

17-Hydroxycorticosteroids *Urine Increase* *0503*

17-Ketogenic Steroids *Urine Increase* *0503*

17-Ketosteroids *Urine Increase* May be slightly increased in arrhenoblastoma. May be moderately increased in Leydig cell tumors in masculinizing ovarian tumors. *2467*

Pregnanediol *Urine Increase* In arrhenoblastoma of ovary. *2468*

Progesterone *Plasma Increase* In arrhenoblastoma of ovary. *2468*

222.00 Benign Neoplasm of Testis

17-Ketogenic Steroids *Urine Increase* The 17-ketosteroids occasionally are elevated when a Leydig cell tumor is present. *0433*

17-Ketosteroids *Urine Increase* *0619*

Estrogens *Urine Increase* *0619*

225.90 Benign Neoplasm of Brain and CNS

Aldolase *Serum Increase* The serum of cancer patients contains a greater proportion of aldolase A (muscle-type) than serum from normal persons. Gliomas and normal brain tissue contain aldolase C (nerve and brain variant), but in meningiomas or tissue metastatic to brain, only aldolase A (liver and fetal form) is detected. *2093*

Antidiuretic Hormone *Serum Increase* Associated with excessive ADH production resulting in sodium loss. *2104*

Aspartate Aminotransferase *Serum Increase* In 31% of 22 patients at initial hospitalization for this disorder. *0781*

Beta-Galactosidase *Serum Decrease* Mean serum concentration in patients with tumors (both benign and malignant) were depressed to 0.065 ± 0.009 mmol/min/L, compared to 0.243 ± 0.038 in normals. *1099*

Bicarbonate *Serum Increase* In 74% of 16 patients at initial hospitalization for this disorder. *0781*

Cells *CSF Increase* Elevated from 5-100/µL in 33% of cases. May exceed 1,000, particularly if the tumor involves the ventricular wall and has undergone necrosis. *0151* *0962*

Chloride *CSF Decrease* *0962*

Glomerular Filtration Rate (GFR) *Urine Increase* Associated excess ADH may tend to accelerate GFR. *2104*

Glucose *CSF Decrease* Values are characteristically < 40 mg/dL in patients with diffuse neoplastic involvement of the meninges, but are normal in other tumors of the brain. *0151*

Hematocrit *Blood Increase* In 22% of 22 patients at initial hospitalization for this disorder. *0781*

Hemoglobin *Blood Increase* In 31% of 22 patients at initial hospitalization for this disorder. *0781*

Immunoglobulin IgG *CSF Increase* No consistent CSF IgG pattern was found in brain tumors, but highly vascularized tumors had increased concentrations. *2321*

Metanephrines, Total *Urine Increase* *1752*

Protein *CSF Increase* Protein content > 100 mg/dL is associated with rapidly growing tumors near the ventricles or subarachnoid space. Slowly growing tumors may have only slightly elevated or normal values. *0151* Total CSF protein is increased. Individual increase of proteins depended on the degree of blood/CSF barrier damage. *1099* In acoustic neuromas nearly always high (100-500 mg). Cerebellar tumors usually have normal or only moderately increased protein (20-100). *0962*

Sodium *Serum Decrease* Associated with excessive ADH production. *2104* Serum Sodium usually less than 130 mEq/L *0062*

Urine Increase Urine is almost always hypertonic to plasma *0062*

Uric Acid *Serum Increase* In 31% of 22 patients at initial hospitalization for this disorder. *0781*

Zinc *CSF Decrease* Significantly less. *0648*

227.00 Benign Neoplasm of Adrenal Cortex

11-Hydroxycorticosteroids *Urine Increase* In Cushingoid patients. *2612*

17-Ketogenic Steroids *Urine Increase* May be normal or raised. *2612*

17-Ketosteroids *Urine Increase* In Cushing patients with adrenocortical adenoma. *2612*

227.00 Benign Neoplasm of Adrenal Cortex (continued)

Corticotropin *Plasma Decrease* Very low or undetectable in Cushing's patients with adrenocortical tumor. 2612

Cortisol *Plasma Increase* Basal plasma concentrations may be normal or raised at 9 h and raised at 23 h. 2612

Dehydroepiandrosterone Sulfate (DHEA-S) *Serum Increase* 0046 1692

227.91 Pheochromocytoma

Calcitonin *Serum Increase* 1589

Calcium *Serum Increase* May be caused by ectopic parathyroid hormone production in a few patients but usually results from associated parathyroid hyperplasia in the familial cases. 0433 Hypercalcemia can occur independently or in association with coexistent hyperparathyroidism. 0962 Can occur, disappearing after removal of the tumor. 0962

Catecholamines *Plasma Increase* In pediatric cases, venous catheterization showed a great increase in catecholamine efflux from the left adrenal vein, while dopamine-beta-hydroxylase (DBH) was only slightly elevated. Circulating catecholamines fluctuated greatly during removal of tumors, but DBH decreased gradually. 1021 Twice upper limit of normal. 0999 Usually very high, there is significant overlap with values that may be obtained with excitement, emotional disturbance, essential hypertension and depression. 0151

Urine Increase Of the 3 different types of catecholamines present in the urine - the metanephrine test is positive in more than 97% of patients with the disease and is rarely falsely positive in hypertensive subjects who do not have the disease. 1223 Most excrete > 300 µg/24h. 1108 0999 0962

Cholesterol *Serum Normal* No characteristic changes. 1108

Dopamine Hydroxylase *Serum Increase* In pediatric cases, venous catheterization showed a great increase in catecholamine efflux from the left adrenal vein, while dopamine-beta-hydroxylase (DBH) was only slightly elevated. Circulating catecholamines fluctuated greatly during removal of tumors, but DBH decreased gradually. 1021

Epinephrine *Urine Increase* In almost all patients, analysis of any 24 h urine collection will reveal increased excretion. 0151 0962

Erythrocytes *Blood Increase* Erythrocytosis associated with pheochromocytoma. 2461

Urine Increase Gross or microscopic hematuria may occur early. 0433

Erythropoietin *Serum Increase* Large amounts. 1992

Fatty Acids, Free (FFA) *Serum Increase* Plasma insulin levels are inappropriately low and free fatty acids are correspondingly high. 0433 May be elevated. 0962

Gastrin *Serum Increase* In a few patients, elevated concentrations have become normal after tumor resection. 2199

Glucose *Serum Increase* Fasting level is elevated in about 50% the patients, usually only slightly above normal values. 1108 May be elevated. 0962 Attacks may be accompanied by hyperglycemia and glucosuria. 2612

Urine Increase Usually intermittent. 1108 Attacks may be accompanied by hyperglycemia and glucosuria. 2612 0999

Glucose Tolerance *Serum Decrease* Impaired glucose tolerance which may be misdiagnosed as diabetes mellitus. 0151 May be decreased because of suppressed insulin release and catecholamine-induced insulin resistance. 0962

Hematocrit *Blood Increase* Occasionally found and may be due to a decreased plasma volume, a true increase in RBC mass, or both. 0433 Hemoconcentration is not uncommon. 0962 Hemoconcentration can cause increased hematocrit and plasma proteins. 0962

Hemoglobin *Blood Increase* Hemoconcentration is not uncommon. 0962

Homovanillic Acid *Urine Increase* Increased in neuroblastomas, benign ganglioneuromas, and pheochromocytomas. 1630

Urine Normal Patients with pheochromocytoma excrete normal amounts. 1806

Insulin *Serum Decrease* Plasma levels are inappropriately low for the simultaneous blood glucose. 0433 May be a decreased glucose tolerance because of suppressed insulin release and catecholamine-induced insulin resistance. 0962

Isocitrate Dehydrogenase *Serum Normal* 2260

Metanephrines, Total *Serum Increase* Values should be twice upper limit of normal. 0999

Urine Increase Of the 3 different types of catecholamines present in the urine--the metanephrine test is positive in more than 97% of patients with the disease and is rarely falsely positive in hypertensive subjects who do not have the disease. 1223 In almost all patients, analysis of any 24-h urine collection will reveal increased excretion. 0151 0999 1108 0962

Norepinephrine *Plasma Increase* Blood levels of norepinephrine and to a lesser extent, epinephrine are increased, usually even when patient is asymptomatic and normotensive; rarely are increases found only following a paroxysm. 2467

Urine Increase Urine levels of norepinephrine and, to a lesser extent, epinephrine are increased, usually even when patient is asymptomatic and normotensive; rarely are increases found only following a paroxysm. 2467 In almost all patients with pheochromocytoma, analysis of any 24-h urine collection will reveal increased excretion of norepinephrine. 0151 0962

Phosphate *Serum Decrease* May be caused by ectopic parathyroid hormone production in a few patients but usually results from associated parathyroid hyperplasia in the familial cases. 0433

Potassium *Serum Decrease* High plasma renin activity has been noted and may result in mild hypokalemia. 0433

Proline Hydroxylase *Serum Increase* Elevated to a lesser degree than that seen in hepatoma. 0364

Protein *Serum Increase* Hemoconcentration can cause increased hematocrit and plasma proteins. 0962

Protein Bound Iodine (PBI) *Serum Normal* No characteristic changes. 1108

Vanillylamine *Serum Increase* Values should be twice upper limit of normal (normal < 6.8 mg/day) 0999

Urine Increase False positive results may occur due to certain foods and certain drugs. Monamine oxidase inhibitors may increase metanephrine and decrease VMA. Excretion is considerably increased. 2467 In almost all patients analysis of any 24 h urine collection will reveal increased excretion. 0151 Phenolic acids of dietary origin may yield many false positive tests. 1108 Excretion > 2 X normal is diagnostic providing all dietary restrictions have been followed. 2612 1630 2440 0962

Volume *Plasma Decrease* Low in < 33% of patients. 0433

Red Blood Cells Decrease Decreased in the hypertension resulting from pheochromocytoma. 1669

238.40 Polycythemia Vera

Alanine Aminotransferase *Serum Normal* Normal in uncomplicated cases. 1379 2538

Albumin *Urine Increase* Occasionally. 2552

Alkaline Phosphatase *Leukocyte Increase* Three polycythemic patients showed elevations the mean = 82, compared with the mean of the normal group (25.8) and that of the group with chronic myelocytic leukemia (4.0). 0144 70-90% of patients have above the upper limits of normal, while a small number of patients have normal values. No clinical or hematologic differences are apparent in patients with normal activity as compared with those with increased activity. 0069 Strikingly increased. 1610 2468 1563 2538

Anisocytes *Blood Increase* Mild anisocytosis and poikilocytosis may be seen in the peripheral blood. 2538

Antithrombin III *Plasma Decrease* Below normal in some patients. 2318

Aspartate Aminotransferase *Serum Normal* Normal in uncomplicated cases. 1379 2538

Basophilic Stippling *Blood Increase* May be found. 2552

Basophils *Blood Increase* Usually a mild basophilia. 0433 Increase in the absolute count (above 65/µL) is observed in about 66% of cases. 0840 Slight to moderate persistent basophilia may occur. 2538

Bone Marrow Increase An unusually high number may be found. 2552

Bence-Jones Protein *Urine Present* Appears in the urine uncommonly. 0619

Bilirubin *Serum Increase* Slightly elevated. 0181 Rarely. 0995

Bleeding Time *Blood Normal* 2468

Calcium *Serum Increase* Slight rise, cause unknown. 0619

Casts *Urine Increase* Occasionally. 2552

Cells *Bone Marrow Increase* Hyperplasia of erythroid, myeloid and megakaryocytic elements within those areas of the skeleton that normally contain active marrow. Marrow differential count may be normal or may reveal a reduction in the myeloid/erythroid ratio, reflecting a predominant normoblastic hyperplasia. 2538

Clot Retraction *Blood Poor* A common defect has been the excessive number of untrapped RBCs after clot retraction (the escape phenomenon of excessive red cell fallout). An increased rate of retraction has also been observed. *2538 1883 1989* Bleeding time and coagulation time are normal but clot retraction may be poor *2468*

Coagulation Time *Blood Normal 2468*

Cold Agglutinins *Serum Increase 2035*

Cryoglobulins *Serum Increase* Variable elevation of cryoglobulins. *2104*

Cryomacroglobulins *Serum Increase 0863*

Eosinophils *Blood Increase* Sometimes eosinophilia. *0433*

Bone Marrow Increase An unusually high number may be found. *2552*

Erythrocytes *Blood Increase* RBC is 7-12 million; may increase to > 15 million/µL. *2468* RBC > 6.5 million/µL in men and 5.6 million in women. *0532*

Erythrocyte Sedimentation Rate *Blood Decrease* Characteristically decreased and may be 0. *2538*

Erythrocyte Survival *Red Blood Cells Decrease* As the disease progresses, there are increasing degrees of extramedullary ineffective hematopoiesis with progressive shortening of the red cell lifespan secondary to increasing splenic sequestration. *2538 1835*

Red Blood Cells Normal Red cell life span is normal as is arterial oxygen saturation. *0999*

Erythropoietin *Serum Decrease* Usually lower than normal or undetectable. *0999* In 21 proved cases, concentrations were all < 5 mU/mL (the limit of sensitivity) whereas 35 control subjects had a mean of 7.8 mU/mL. *0673*

Urine Decrease Poor sensitivity of the assay techniques prevents a reliable method to differentiate secondary polycythemia from polycythemia vera. *0433 0999*

Factor V *Plasma Decrease* Low levels found. *2318*

Fibrinogen *Plasma Decrease* Usually normal although a moderate decrease (115-200 mg/dL) was found in one study. *2491 2538*

Glomerular Filtration Rate (GFR) *Urine Normal* GFR is kept to almost normal levels by an increased renal blood flow. *2483 2552*

Hematocrit *Blood Increase* Over 60% in males and 55% in females. *0433* Before treatment, Hct values range between 55-80. *0999*

Heterophil Antibody *Serum Decrease* Positive presumptive test but negative differential test if Forsman antigen is used. *1752*

Serum Increase Positive presumptive test but negative differential test if Forsman antigen is used. *1752*

Histamine *Serum Increase* Present in the majority of patients with uncontrolled disease. *2538 0840*

Urine Increase Present in the majority of patients with uncontrolled disease. *2538 0840*

Immunoglobulin IgG *Serum Increase* Significant diffuse increases in IgG and IgM have been noted. *2538*

Immunoglobulin IgM *Serum Increase* Significant diffuse increases in IgG and IgM have been noted. *2538*

Iron *Serum Decrease* Frequently decreased, reflecting therapeutic or spontaneous blood loss. *2538*

Bone Marrow Decrease Decreased or absent bone marrow iron stores that are characteristic of this disease. *2538 0657*

Lactate Dehydrogenase *Serum Normal* Normal in uncomplicated cases. *2538*

Leukocytes *Blood Increase* Elevated in a majority of cases. *0532* A peripheral leukocytosis, with an absolute granulocytosis, occurs in about 66% of cases. *2538 0999*

Lysozyme *Serum Increase* Significantly elevated, reflecting participation of the granulocyte in the proliferative process. *2538 0209*

MCH *Blood Decrease 2468*

MCHC *Blood Decrease 2468*

MCV *Blood Decrease 2468*

Monocytes *Blood Increase 2538*

Neutrophils *Blood Increase* An absolute granulocytosis is seen in the majority of patients with a circulatory count of 15,000-30,000/µL. *0433* Occurs in about 66% of cases. Usually of moderate degree but extreme degrees are sometimes observed late in the course. A moderate shift to the left in the granulocyte series frequently accompanies the increase. *2538*

Osmotic Fragility *Red Blood Cells Decrease 2468*

Oxygen Saturation *Blood Decrease* Mild degrees of unsaturation may occur in patients with otherwise well-documented cases, uncomplicated by independent cardiac or pulmonary disease. *1651* Arterial oxygen saturation is normal in early cases but mild desaturation is not unusual later in the course of the disease due to the complication of pulmonary emboli. *0433 2538*

Blood Normal Nearly all patients with true polycythemia vera have a near normal arterial oxygen saturation. *2492 2538*

Plasminogen *Serum Decrease* Below normal in some patients. *2318*

Platelet Count *Blood Increase* Elevated in a majority of cases. *0532* In about 50% of patients at time of diagnosis. Degree is usually modest, with counts in the range of 450,000-800,000/µL. *2538* Usually increased in number and counts as high as 3 million have been reported. *0151 0433 0999*

Poikilocytes *Blood Increase* Mild anisocytosis and poikilocytosis may be seen in the peripheral blood. *2538*

Potassium *Serum Increase* Has been reported in myeloproliferative disorders associated with thrombocytosis. May be spurious and related to K release from the increased number of platelets during the process of blood coagulation. *1656 2538*

Protein Bound Iodine (PBI) *Serum Normal 2467*

Prothrombin Time *Plasma Normal 2491*

Reticulocytes *Blood Increase* Possibly increased. *2467*

Thromboplastin Generation *Blood Normal* Conventional coagulation tests are usually normal. *0009 2538*

Uric Acid *Serum Increase* Increased RBC formation produces hyperuricemia and hyperuricosuria in 30-50% of patients at the time of diagnosis. Both tend to increase in frequency and severity as the disease progresses and may remain asymptomatic but approximately 5-10% of patients develop symptoms and signs of gout. *2538 0839 2603* High in a significant proportion of patients. *0999*

Urine Increase Increased formation produces hyperuricemia and hyperuricosuria in 30-50% of patients at the time of diagnosis. Both tend to increase in frequency and severity as the disease progresses and may remain asymptomatic, but approximately 5-10% of patients develop symptoms and signs of gout. *2538 0839 2603*

Urobilinogen *Urine Increase* Rarely. *0995*

Viscosity *Serum Increase* Clinical manifestations may be related to increased blood viscosity. *0999*

Vitamin B$_{12}$ *Serum Increase* Usually increased. *0999* Marked increase; mean was 741 pg/mL in 40 patients (normal = 385). *1990* Above 900 pg/mL found in about 33% of patients before treatment or during relapse. *2538*

Vitamin B$_{12}$ Binding Capacity *Serum Increase* Significant elevation; usually correlated with WBC in peripheral blood. *1990* Increased to values > 2,200 pg/mL in about 75% of these patients. Found to be related directly to disease activity. *2538 0841*

Volume *Plasma Decrease* Most often. *0995*

Plasma Increase The greatest increase occurs in patients with a significant degree of hepatosplenomegaly. *2538 1835*

Plasma Normal Within the normal range in the majority of patients, reduced in some, and increased in others. *2538 1100*

Red Blood Cells Increase Unless the RBC volume is > 38 mL/kg for males and 36 mL/kg for females, the diagnosis of polycythemia vera cannot be considered established. *0151*

ENDOCRINE, NUTRITIONAL AND METABOLIC DISEASES, AND IMMUNITY DISORDERS

Diseases of the Endocrine Glands

240.00 Simple Goiter

^{131}I Uptake *Serum Increase* In some patients, elevated to the 70-95% range. *0151 0962*

Serum Normal Usually normal. *2540*

Butanol Extractable Iodine (BEI) *Serum Decrease* Normal or slightly low. *0962*

Serum Normal Normal or slightly low. *0962*

Eosinophils *Blood Increase* In 50% of 19 patients at initial hospitalization for this disorder. *0781*

Iodide *Urine Decrease 0151*

240.00 Simple Goiter (continued)

Protein Bound Iodine (PBI) *Serum Decrease* Normal or slightly low. *0962*

Serum Normal Normal or slightly low. *0962* Usually. *2540*

T$_3$ Uptake *Serum Normal* *2467*

Thyroid Stimulating Hormone (TSH) *Serum Increase* Normal or slightly increased. *0962*

Serum Normal Normal or slightly low. *0962* Usually. *2540* Normal in nontoxic goiter without autoimmune thyroiditis. *0960*

Thyroxine (T$_4$) *Serum Decrease* Normal or slightly low. *0962*

Serum Normal Normal or slightly low. *0962* Usually. *2540*

Tri-iodothyronine (T$_3$) *Serum Increase* Normal or increased. *0962*

Serum Normal Normal or slightly low. *0962* Usually. *2540*

242.90 Hyperthyroidism

^{131}I Uptake *Serum Increase* Thyroid uptake is increased. It is relatively more affected at 1, 2, or 6 h than at 24 h. It may be normal in presence of recent iodine ingestion. *2467* Uptake is > 30% in 6 h, > 40% in 12 h, and > 55% in 24 h, with rapid release. *0619* Mean uptake = 63.6% in patients over 60 y of age. *0512* May be present. *0962*

2,3-Diphosphoglycerate *Red Blood Cells Increase* Results in reduced oxygen affinity. *1596*

11-Hydroxycorticosteroids *Urine Normal* *2540*

17-Hydroxycorticosteroids *Urine Decrease* *0503*

Urine Increase Normal or slightly increased. *2540*

17-Ketogenic Steroids *Urine Decrease* May be moderately reduced. *2540*

Urine Increase Normal or slightly increased. *2540*

Alanine Aminotransferase *Serum Increase* Slight rise (mean = 12.1 U/L, normal = 8.1). The differences between hyper- and euthyroid groups were statistically significant but individually, minor changes would be of little positive diagnostic significance. *1320*

Albumin *Serum Decrease* Possibly due to rapid turnover in severe thyrotoxicosis. *0619 2467*

Aldosterone *Plasma Normal* *1448*

Alkaline Phosphatase *Serum Increase* Mean level was 42.5 U/L or 55% higher in the hyperthyroid than in the euthyroid group. *1320 0999*

Amino Acids *Plasma Increase* Slight increase. *0619*

Amylase *Serum Decrease* Severe thyrotoxicosis. *0619* When accompanied by severe liver damage. *2467*

Angiotensin-Converting Enzyme (ACE) *Serum Increase* Significantly elevated in 21 patients with hyperthyroidism (mean 65 U/mL) compared with healthy control subjects (mean 30 U/mL). *2600* Consistently elevated in untreated patients compared with controls. *1673 2165 0278* Significantly higher than hypothyroid or normal subjects. Higher than all other groups but fell from 30.8 to 17.4 U/mL with therapy in 35 patients studied *0901 2202*

Antithyroglobulin Antibodies *Serum Increase* High incidence reflects focal toxicity in the gland and correlates with the development of postoperative hypothyroidism. *2612* Patients with Graves' disease often have some or all of the thyroid autoantibodies of Hashimoto's disease. *2035*

Ascorbic Acid *Serum Decrease* Secondary to increased metabolic processes. *2540*

Aspartate Aminotransferase *Serum Increase* A slight rise in mean activity over the normal with hepatic dysfunction (mean 13.5, normal = 11.1). *1320*

Basophils *Blood Decrease* *0532*

Bicarbonate *Serum Decrease* Respiratory alkalosis may occur. *0962*

Bilirubin *Serum Increase* Due to hemolysis. *0151*

BSP Retention *Serum Increase* Mild retention. *2540*

Butanol Extractable Iodine (BEI) *Serum Increase* May be present. *0962*

Calcium *Serum Increase* An incidental finding and an uncommon complication. *0999* Ionized and total calcium levels were elevated in 21 of 45 (47%) and in 12 of 45 (27%) thyrotoxic patients, respectively. Mean ionized and total calcium levels were higher in these 45 patients than in normal persons. *0319* Usually normal but may occur in as many as 20% of patients. *2540* Found in rare occasions with severe thyrotoxicosis due to increased turnover of bone. *2612 0962*

Serum Normal Significant hypercalcemia did not occur in patients over 60 years of age. *0512*

Urine Increase Urinary excretion was increased and correlated positively to degree of hyperthyroidism. *1638 0999 1083*

Feces Increase Excess of thyroid hormone induces a marked increase in fecal and urinary excretion. *1083*

Catecholamines *Plasma Decrease* Decreased plasma levels correlate inversely with total T$_4$. *2139*

Plasma Normal *2540*

Urine Normal *2540*

Cholesterol *Serum Decrease* Direct stimulation of synthesis and metabolism. *2540* Falls, but not in simple relation to the associated rise in the BMR. Diet has a variable effect on the blood level. *0812*

Cholesterol Esters *Serum Increase* *1336*

Copper *Serum Increase* *2467 0619*

Creatine *Serum Increase* Excess T$_4$ or TSH stimulates creatinuria. *2104*

Urine Increase Increased excretion when the muscle mass is reduced, or is unable to take up creatine due to muscle catabolism. *0619*

Creatine Kinase *Serum Decrease* Below normal but increased after treatment. *0573*

Creatinine *Serum Increase* *0503*

Urine Decrease With associated rise in urine creatine. *0619*

Eosinophils *Blood Increase* Often occurs. *2540*

Erythrocyte Sedimentation Rate *Blood Increase* Raised in 12% of patients over 60. *0512*

Erythrocyte Survival *Red Blood Cells Decrease* In patients with thyrotoxicosis, a moderate shortening. *2538 1537*

Estrogens *Serum Normal* Estradiol is normal. *1731*

Factor VIII *Plasma Increase* May reflect increased adrenergic activity. *2540* Increased activity in hyperthyroid states. *0636*

Fatty Acids, Free (FFA) *Serum Increase* Increased lipid degradation. *2540*

Gastrin *Serum Increase* Mean fasting levels in untreated hyperthyroid patients was 356 ± 26 pg/mL, (normal = 89 ± 4 pg/mL). No correlation was apparent between gastrin level and any parameter of thyroid function. *2108*

Globulin *Serum Normal* *2467*

Glucose *Serum Increase* Possibly due to increased circulating epinephrine in thyrotoxicosis. Increased rate of absorption from intestine. *0619* Significantly elevated in 42 untreated patients, mean concentration was 92 ± 8 mg/dL. *0056*

Urine Increase *2468*

Glucose Tolerance *Serum Decrease* Early high peak due to increased intestinal absorption (normal IV curve) with normal return to fasting level. Decreased formation of glycogen with low fasting levels and subsequent hypoglycemia. *2467* Oral test resulted in significantly increased responses in 20 untreated patients. *0056*

Glycerol *Serum Increase* Increased lipid degradation. *2540*

Gonadotropin, Pituitary *Serum Decrease* *2035*

Hematocrit *Blood Decrease* Patients occasionally develop a mild hypochromic anemia. *2540*

Hemoglobin *Blood Decrease* In 239 patients with uncomplicated disease, the concentration was < 12.0 g/dL in 37 of 207 women and < 13.0 g/dL in 9 of 32 men. A small fall is usual and it may sometimes be sufficient to cause a mild degree of anemia. *1696* Often patients develop a normochromic and normocytic anemia with 9-11 g/dL. *0151 2540*

HLA Antigens *Blood Present* HLA-DR3 present in 53% of patients with Graves' Disease versus 18% of controls. *2539*

Hydroxyproline *Serum Increase* *0151*

Urine Decrease Reduced excretion in 22 of 33 patients. *2435*

Urine Increase Because of excess bone resorption. *0962* Elevated in 107 of 111 patients, aged 18-61 y and 10 of 14 patients over 65. *2435*

Immunoglobulins *Serum Decrease* Possibly due to LATS effect. *2104*

Insulin *Serum Increase* Significantly elevated in 42 untreated patients, mean concentration was 23 ± 13 µU/mL. *0056*

Isocitrate Dehydrogenase *Serum Normal* *2260*

Ketones *Serum Increase* Due to increased carbohydrate requirement in thyrotoxicosis. *0619*

Urine Increase Children are more liable to develop ketosis than adults with thyrotoxicosis. *0619*

Leukocytes *Blood Decrease* About 10% of patients develop low count due to decreased neutrophils. *2540*

Lipids *Serum Decrease* Total lipids are usually decreased. *2467*

Long Acting Thyroid Stimulating Hormone (LATS) *Serum Increase* Present in most patients with Graves' disease. *2145* Found in at most 80% of patients with Graves' disease, and its presence or level does not correlate uniformly with thyroid hyperactivity. *0151* Detected in about 50% of patients with hyperthyroidism of Graves' disease and in many patients who are euthyroid or hypothyroid. *1415 2035*

Luteinizing Hormone (LH) *Serum Increase 1731*

Lymphocytes *Blood Increase* Although a peripheral blood lymphocytosis has been noted in the past, a recent study of the distribution of T and B lymphocytes showed a slightly decreased number of T cells, and consequently of total lymphocytes. *2403* Relative lymphocytosis. *2540*

Magnesium *Serum Decrease 1180 0962*

Urine Increase 1180

MCH *Blood Decrease* Patients occasionally develop a mild hypochromic anemia. *2540*

MCHC *Blood Decrease* Patients occasionally develop a mild hypochromic anemia. *2540*

MCV *Blood Decrease* Decreased in hyperthyroid patients with neither anemia nor a reduced transferrin saturation. After treatment, it rose by an average of 6 fL. A diminution even within the normal range, is an invariable concomitant of hyperthyroidism. *1696 1669*

Monocytes *Blood Increase* May occur. *2540*

Neutrophils *Blood Decrease* About 10% of patients develop low count due to decreased neutrophils. *2540*

Oxygen Saturation *Blood Decrease* Dyspnea. *2199*

Parathyroid Hormone *Serum Decrease* Subnormal levels were found in 28.9% of cases. Parathyroid hormone correlated inversely to serum calcium and degree of hyperthyroidism. *1638*

pCO₂ *Blood Decrease* Respiratory alkalosis may occur. *0962*

pH *Blood Increase* Respiratory alkalosis may occur. *0962*

Phosphate *Urine Increase* Urinary excretion was increased and correlated positively to degree of hyperthyroidism. *1638* Poorly understood. *2540*

Feces Increase Poorly understood. *2540*

Phospholipids, Total *Serum Decrease* Falls, but not in simple relation to the associated rise in the BMR. Diet has a variable effect on the blood level. *0812*

Serum Increase 0619

Platelet Count *Blood Normal 2540*

pO₂ *Blood Decrease* Dyspnea. *2199*

Protein *Serum Decrease 2540*

Protein Bound Iodine (PBI) *Serum Decrease* Reduced in 24 of 33 patients. *2435*

Serum Increase In thyrotoxicosis, levels may range from 7-20 mg/dL. With treatment, the level falls to normal more rapidly than does the BMR. *0619* Elevated in 60 of 76 patients over the age of 60 y. *0512* May be present. *0962*

Pseudocholinesterase *Serum Increase* In some cases of thyrotoxicosis. Not a useful measure of thyroid activity, because of the wide overlap with normal cases. *0619*

Renin Activity *Plasma Increase 1004*

Rheumatoid Factor *Serum Increase* Titers > 1:160 are more common in Graves' disease patients than in controls. In patients under 40, titers > 1:80 are more frequent than in control subjects. *2162*

Riboflavin *Serum Decrease* Secondary to increased metabolic processes. *2540*

Sodium *CSF Increase 0619*

Red Blood Cells Increase 0902

T₃ Uptake *Serum Increase* Elevated in 57% of 21 patients in an elderly population. 9 of the patients with normal T₃ uptakes had elevated PBI. T₃ uptake was not a useful indicator of metabolic status. *0512* May be present. *0962*

Thiamine *Serum Decrease* Secondary to increased metabolic processes. *2540*

Thyroid Stimulating Hormone (TSH) *Serum Decrease* Plasma TSH levels are actually subnormal in Graves' disease in its hyperthyroid stage, normal in its euthyroid stage, and supranormal if the patient becomes hypothyroid. *2035* Significantly reduced, but may occasionally fall in the normal range. *0960 0962 2612*

Serum Increase Plasma TSH levels are actually subnormal in Graves' disease in its hyperthyroid stages, normal in its euthyroid stage, and supranormal if the patient becomes hypothyroid. *2035*

Thyroxine Binding Globulin *Serum Decrease 2104*

Serum Increase Elevated in all patients and fell to normal with therapy; patients whose illness recurred after cessation of drug therapy had higher pretreatment thyroglobulin values and no fall during treatment. *0296 2540*

Thyroxine, Free *Serum Increase 0186*

Thyroxine Index, Free (FTI) *Serum Increase 2467*

Thyroxine (T₄) *Serum Increase* May be present. *0962 0999*

Triglycerides *Serum Decrease* Falls, but not in simple relation to the associated rise in the BMR. Diet has a variable effect on the blood level. *0812*

Tri-iodothyronine, Free *Serum Increase 0186*

Tri-iodothyronine (T₃) *Serum Increase* A small group of patients whose hypermetabolism is due to T₃ excess alone has been identified. These patients are clinically hyperthyroid but have normal levels of total serum T₄ and free T₄. Their radioiodine uptakes are variable, but are usually in the upper normal range. Total serum T₃ values are high. *0999* Increased before overt hyperthyroidism is apparent and before serum T₄ levels have increased. *0619* May be present. *0962 2468*

Urea Nitrogen *Serum Increase* Excessive protein catabolism. *0503*

Urobilin *Feces Increase* May be secondary to erythroid hyperplasia. *0619*

Vitamin B₁₂ *Serum Decrease* Secondary to increased metabolic processes. *2540*

Volume *Plasma Increase* Corpuscular and total hypervolemia may occur to facilitate oxygen delivery to tissues. *1669* Increase in plasma volume keeps the hemoglobin concentration from reaching polycythemic values. *2538 1642*

Urine Increase Mild polyuria. *2199*

244.90 Hypothyroidism

¹³¹I Uptake *Serum Decrease* Usually low but may be normal or in a rare patient slightly elevated at 2 or 4 h. *0999*

11-Hydroxycorticosteroids *Plasma Increase* Due to slow disposal of circulating cortisol. *0619*

17-Hydroxycorticosteroids *Urine Decrease* As a result of decreased rate of turnover of cortisol. *2540* Low in untreated disease. Does not necessarily indicate pituitary origin. *2612*

17-Ketogenic Steroids *Urine Decrease* As a result of decreased rate of turnover of cortisol. *2540* Low in untreated disease. Does not necessarily indicate pituitary origin. *2612*

17-Ketosteroids *Urine Decrease* Low in untreated disease. Does not necessarily indicate pituitary origin. *2612*

Albumin *Serum Increase* Increase in total pool may occur. *2540* In 37% of 13 patients at initial hospitalization for this disorder. *0781*

Urine Increase Urinalysis commonly demonstrates mild proteinuria without significant formed elements, and there is preservation of normal concentrating ability. *0433*

Aldolase *Serum Increase* May be elevated. *0433*

Aldosterone *Plasma Normal 1448*

Alkaline Phosphatase *Serum Decrease* Characteristically low in infantile and juvenile cases. *2540 2468*

Serum Increase Excess enzyme originates from the bone. *2468* In 24% of 12 patients at initial hospitalization for this disorder. *0781*

Angiotensin-Converting Enzyme (ACE) *Serum Decrease* Levels 13.9 U/mL in hypothyroid patients versus 17.0 U/mL in controls. In 12 hypothyroid patients levels rose from 11.6 to 15.8 U/mL after thyroid replacement therapy. Patients with thyroxine index less than 5.0 had significantly lower levels than normal controls *0278 2202*

Serum Normal Patients had levels within the normal range. *0309 1673*

Anisocytes *Blood Increase* A minor degree of anisocytosis and also acanthocytosis (32 of 172) was demonstrated. *1078*

Antibody Titer *Serum Increase* Antiparietal cell antibodies present in up to 40% of cases. *0186*

244.90   Hypothyroidism (continued)

Antithyroglobulin Antibodies   Serum   Increase   May be detected in high titer if due to thyroiditis. 2612   Found in 50% of cases of myxedema. 0058

Aspartate Aminotransferase   Serum   Increase   The muscle involvement of this disease appears to be responsible for the elevation. 0503   May be elevated. 0433   In 58% of 13 patients at initial hospitalization for this disorder. 0781

Basophils   Blood   Increase   2467

Bicarbonate   Serum   Increase   Significant CO_2 retention can occur. 0433   In 60% of 13 patients at initial hospitalization for this disorder. 0781

Butanol Extractable Iodine (BEI)   Serum   Decrease   2468

Calcium   Serum   Increase   Sometimes increased. 2468

Serum   Normal   Usually. 2540

Urine   Decrease   In general. 2540

Carcinoembryonic Antigen   Serum   Increase   32% of patients had values > 2.5 ng/mL. 0979

Carotene   Serum   Increase   2468

Catecholamines   Plasma   Increase   2139

Plasma   Normal   2540

Urine   Increase   2139

Cholesterol   Serum   Increase   A moderate elevation that may reflect depression in overall metabolism is almost always demonstrable. 0503   In true myxedema, level is usually > 200 mg/dL, but may be normal if there is also associated malnutrition. 0619   Values ranged from 143-556 in 10 patients. 0905   In pituitary hypothyroidism, may be normal or low. 2540   In 58% of 12 patients at initial hospitalization for this disorder. 0781

Pericardial Fluid   Increase   High levels (2.6-5.2 mmol/L; 100 to 200 mg/dL). 0274

Cholesterol Esters   Serum   Decrease   No significant difference in rate of esterification between hypo-, hyper- and euthyroid subjects. The fractional rates were highly significant, decreased in hypo- and increased in hyperthyroid patients. 1336

Cholesterol, Low Density Lipoprotein   Serum   Increase   Marked elevation secondary to decreased catabolism. 0062 2614

Cholesterol, Very Low Density Lipoprotein   Serum   Increase   2614

Chylomicrons   Serum   Increase   Increased. 1380 1936 1948

Copper   Serum   Increase   2467

Cortisol   Plasma   Normal   2540

Creatine   Urine   Decrease   2467

Creatine Kinase   Serum   Increase   Abnormally high serum levels found. 0619   Muscle involvement appears to be responsible for the elevation. 0503   Significantly higher than in normal controls in patients with primary hypothyroidism. 0573   Found in 66% of 15 patients. Values returned to normal after restoration of thyroid function. 0905   Slight increase. 0962   Often raised, but of no diagnostic value. 2612   0642

Creatinine   Urine   Increase   Occasionally increased. 0619   Usually normal. 2540

Urine   Normal   Usually normal. 2540

Cryofibrinogen   Serum   Increase   2035 0856 1551 2046

Cyclic Adenosine Monophosphate   Urine   Decrease   Lack of primary messenger necessary to activate adenyl cyclase system resulting in decreased levels. No hormonal effect noted. 2356

Erythrocyte Sedimentation Rate   Blood   Increase   2467

Estrogens   Serum   Increase   Increased estradiol. 1731

Factor VIII   Plasma   Decrease   May occur. 2175

Factor IX   Plasma   Decrease   May occur. 2175

Folate   Serum   Decrease   May occur. 2540

Gastrin   Serum   Decrease   Mean fasting plasma level was 64 ± 5 pg/mL compared to normal, 89 ± 4 pg/mL. No correlation was found between gastrin and any other parameters of thyroid function. 2121

Glomerular Filtration Rate (GFR)   Urine   Decrease   2540

Glucose   Serum   Decrease   Fasting blood sugar is decreased. 2468

Serum   Increase   In 35% of 14 patients at initial hospitalization for this disorder. 0781

Glucose Tolerance   Serum   Increase   Curve may be flat. 2612

Gonadotropin, Pituitary   Serum   Increase   0962

Hematocrit   Blood   Decrease   Seldom < 30%. 0433   Mild to moderate normochromic, normocytic, or slightly macrocytic anemia with normal leukocyte and platelet counts. 0433   Of 202 patients, anemia was present on diagnosis in 39 of 172 women and 14 of 30 men. Microcytic anemia was present in only 9 patients in the entire series. 1078   Many patients have a hypoplastic anemia which is unresponsive to therapy with iron, vitamin B_{12}, or folic acid. The degree is mild to moderate. 2538   Anemia observed in 21-60% of patients. 2552   0532 0781

Hemoglobin   Blood   Decrease   Seldom < 9 g/dL. Of 202 patients, anemia was present on diagnosis in 39 of 172 women and 14 of 30 men. Microcytic anemia was present in only 9 patients in the entire series. 1078   Anemia may occur, hemoglobin < 13 g/dL. 0532   Many patients have a hypoplastic anemia which is unresponsive to therapy with iron, vitamin B_{12}, or folic acid. The degree is mild to moderate, with concentration rarely < 8-9 g/dL. 2538   Anemia observed in 21-60% of patients. 2552   In 42% of 14 patients at initial hospitalization for this disorder. 0781

Hydroxyproline   Urine   Decrease   0962

Immunoglobulins   CSF   Increase   Disproportionate rise in immunoglobulin fraction of CSF protein in myxedema. Rise is not seen in plasma. 2104

Iodide   Serum   Decrease   The degree of iodine deficiency dictates the severity of the hypothyroidism. 0999

Iron   Serum   Decrease   The most frequent type of anemia observed is a microcytic, hypochromic anemia caused by iron deficiency. 2538 1351   Of 202 patients, anemia was present on diagnosis in 39 of 172 women and 14 of 30 men. 1078   Concentration was < 50 µg/dL. 0532   Low in 50% of patients. 1078   0582

Iron-Binding Capacity, Total (TIBC)   Serum   Decrease   Total IBC < 200-300 µg/dL. 0532

Serum   Increase   The serum iron concentration was < 12 µmol/L (units) in 60 out of 118 patients. The TIBC was increased in only 21 of these 60 patients. 1078

Iron Saturation   Serum   Decrease   Transferrin saturation < 20%. 0532

Lactate Dehydrogenase   Serum   Increase   Regularly elevated. 0503   The muscle involvement of this disease appears to be responsible for the elevated levels seen in this condition. 0503   LD and CK activity are elevated, while AST, ALT, and alkaline phos were within normal limits. 1320   In 60% of 13 patients at initial hospitalization for this disorder. 0781   0433 0962

Lipids   Serum   Increase   Thyroid hormone insufficiency results in abnormal lipid metabolism with minimal to marked increases in circulating levels of cholesterol and triglycerides 0999

Lipoproteins, Beta   Serum   Increase   0774 0772 0773

Magnesium   Serum   Increase   2467

Urine   Decrease   0837

MCH   Blood   Decrease   Microcytic hypochromic anemia may occur due to blood loss, increased demand or dietary inadequacy. MCH < 27 pg, MCV < 80 fL. 0532

Blood   Increase   Mild to moderate normochromic, normocytic, or slightly macrocytic anemia with normal leukocyte and platelet counts. 0433

MCV   Blood   Decrease   Microcytic hypochromic anemia may occur due to blood loss, increased demand or dietary inadequacy. MCH < 27 pg, MCV < 80 fL. 0532

Blood   Increase   Mean MCV exceeded 90 fL in 29 of 53 patients with normal vitamin B_{12}, folic acid and iron levels. MCV invariably fell with T_4 treatment even if initial levels were within the normal range. 9 of 53 patients with normal folic acid, vitamin B_{12} and iron had anemia and increased MCV -- the macrocytic anemia of hypothyroidism. 1078   Mild to moderate normochromic, normocytic, or slightly macrocytic anemia with normal leukocyte platelet counts. 0433   2538 0248

Blood   Normal   A true increase occurs in < 10% of the patients, and in these cases it is usually caused by a megaloblastic erythropoiesis due to vitamin B_{12} or folic acid deficiency. 2538 2384

Myoglobin   Serum   Increase   Significantly higher than normal in patients with primary hypothyroidism. 0573

Norepinephrine   Plasma   Increase   Circulating levels are elevated and hypertension is not uncommon. 0999

Oxygen Saturation   Blood   Decrease   Rare dyspnea secondary to pleural effusion. 2540

pH   Pleural Effusion   Decrease   Exudate (pH < 7.3). 0062

Gastric Material   Increase   True achlorhydria after maximum histamine stimulation occurs in 50% of patients with primary hypothyroidism. 2540   Achlorhydria present in up to 40% of cases 0186

Phospholipids, Total   Serum   Increase   0619

pO$_2$ *Blood Decrease* Rare dyspnea secondary to pleural effusion. *2540*

Prolactin *Serum Increase* Associated with amenorrhea and pituitary enlargement secondary to primary hypothyroidism. *1256* Over 14.0 ng/mL in 39% of patients with untreated primary disease. Mean = 14.3 ± 1.1, range = 4.7-42.0 ng/mL in 49 subjects. Normal value = 8.2 ± 0.5. Significant differences occurred only between female patients and controls, not with male patients and controls. *1068* Can trigger a mild to moderate increase (20-300 ng/mL) *2637 2638*

Protein *Urine Increase* May occur to a mild degree. *0565*

CSF Increase Perhaps due to increased capillary permeability. *2540*

Pleural Effusion Increase Exudate (> 3 g/dL). *0062*

Protein Bound Iodine (PBI) *Serum Decrease* Ranges from 0 to 3 mg/dL. After treatment returns to normal in about 3 weeks. *0619*

Pyrophosphate *Synovial Fluid Increase* Has been identified. *2088*

Renin Activity *Plasma Decrease 2540*

Reticulocytes *Blood Decrease 0433*

Sodium *Serum Decrease* Significant hyponatremia can occur. *0433*

Somatomedin-C *Serum Decrease 2634*

Specific Gravity *Urine Decrease* May occur to a mild degree. *0565*

Pleural Effusion Increase Exudate (> 1.016). *0062*

T$_3$ Uptake *Serum Decrease* Mean T$_3$ was 76.7 ± 76 ng/mL, ranging from 20-600. 72 of 100 patients had subnormal values. No correlation with TSH was found. *1323*

Testosterone *Plasma Increase 1731*

Thyroid Stimulating Hormone (TSH) *Serum Decrease* Not increased in pituitary hypothyroidism and does not respond to TRH administration. *2540*

Serum Increase Elevated in all patients, mean = 76.7 ± 55 µU/mL, range = 11-240. Mean values for patients < 20 y old was significantly higher than for older patients. *1323* Not increased in pituitary hypothyroidism and does not respond to TRH administration. *2540* Raised in all cases due to primary thyroid disease. *0960 2612*

Thyroxine Binding Globulin *Serum Increase* Marked elevations found in the vast majority of patients with chronic lymphocytic thyroiditis, though an occasional patient will have low or nonmeasurable titers. *0999*

Serum Normal In some cases. *2467*

Thyroxine, Free *Serum Decrease 0186*

Thyroxine Index, Free (FTI) *Serum Decrease 2467*

Thyroxine (T$_4$) *Serum Decrease* Average T$_4$ was 1.8 ± 1.5 µg/dL, range = 0.2-7.0. An inverse correlation was found with TSH and T$_4$, r = 0.73. *1323*

Triglycerides *Serum Increase* Thyroid hormone insufficiency results in abnormal lipid metabolism with minimal to marked increases in circulating levels of cholesterol and triglycerides. *0999 2540*

Tri-iodothyronine, Free *Serum Decrease 0186*

Tri-iodothyronine, Reverse *Serum Decrease 1617*

Tri-iodothyronine (T$_3$) *Serum Decrease* Usually decreased but may be normal in approximately 20% of patients. *2468 2540*

Urea Nitrogen *Serum Increase* May be slightly elevated but returns to normal with replacement therapy *0433* . Usually normal. *2540*

Serum Normal Usually normal. *2540*

Uric Acid *Serum Increase* May be slightly elevated but returns to normal with replacement therapy. *0433* In 45% of 13 patients at initial hospitalization for this disorder. *0781 1283 0962 2104*

Vitamin B$_{12}$ *Serum Decrease* Almost 50% of patients have achlorhydria with intrinsic factor failure and low vitamin B$_{12}$; rarely megaloblastic anemia develops. *2467 1078*

Volume *Plasma Decrease* Total volume is reduced by 25% on the average. *1669*

245.10 Subacute Thyroiditis

^{131}I Uptake *Serum Decrease* The association of a very low uptake with a normal or high serum T$_4$ concentration is characteristic of the early phase of disease. Subnormal values for thyroid ^{131}I uptake are usually found. *2540* Extremely low. *0962 2104*

Alkaline Phosphatase *Serum Increase* Elevated in 3 of 10 patients; no apparent relation to degree of T$_4$ elevation and of unknown origin. *0489*

Alpha$_1$-Antitrypsin *Serum Decrease* These conditions reduce activity. *2633*

Antithyroglobulin Antibodies *Serum Increase* Circulating thyroid antibodies are present in low titer in a minority of cases and disappear when disease subsides. *2540*

Aspartate Aminotransferase *Serum Increase 0151*

Carotene *Serum Increase 0151*

Cholesterol *Serum Increase* If hypothyroid. *0151*

Complement C3 *Serum Increase* Increased serum C3, IgM, alpha$_1$-acid glycoprotein and alpha$_1$-antitrypsin levels in 40 patients. *1715*

Creatine Kinase *Serum Increase* If hypothyroid. *0151*

Erythrocyte Sedimentation Rate *Blood Increase* Consistently increased, normal rate mitigates against the diagnosis. *0433* Invariably elevated in the 1st month, reaching very high levels that appear out of proportion to the degree of inflammation and remain so long after symptoms disappear. *1106* Frequently greatly elevated. *0962*

Gamma Glutamyl Transferase (GGT) *Serum Increase* Elevated in 3 patients, suggesting hepatic origin of the enzymes. *0489*

Glucose *Serum Decrease* Severe hyponatremia and hypoglycemia may occur as a manifestation of primary or secondary thyroid failure. *0151*

Glycoproteins *Serum Increase* Increased serum C3, alpha$_1$-acid glycoprotein and alpha$_1$-antitrypsin levels found in 40 patients. *1715*

Immunoglobulin IgA *Serum Decrease* In 40 patients, levels were decreased in those who were BW-35 negative but were normal in the patients who were BW-35 positive. *1715*

Immunoglobulin IgD *Serum Increase 0619*

Immunoglobulin IgM *Serum Increase* In 40 patients, there was an increase in serum C3, IgM, alpha$_1$-acid glycoprotein and alpha$_1$-antitrypsin levels. *1715*

Lactate Dehydrogenase *Serum Increase 0151*

Leukocytes *Blood Increase* A slight leukocytosis may or may not be present. *0433* May be moderately elevated to 15,000-20,000. *1106 0151*

Lymphocytes *Blood Normal* T-lymphocytes may increase with a concomitant decrease in B-lymphocytes. *0151* Usually normal. *2540*

Protein Bound Iodine (PBI) *Serum Decrease* May be subnormal later in the disease. *2540* Characteristically low. *0151*

Serum Increase Early in the disease. *0992* Usually elevated even higher than T$_4$. *1106* Often disproportionately higher than the T$_4$ iodine concentration, indicating the presence of abnormal iodinated material. *2540 0999 0151 2104*

Sodium *Serum Decrease* Severe hyponatremia and hypoglycemia may occur as a manifestation of primary or secondary thyroid failure. *0151*

T$_3$ Uptake *Serum Increase 0962*

Thyroid Stimulating Hormone (TSH) *Serum Increase* Defective hormonal synthesis causes increased secretion of TSH. *0999* During recovery the TSH may be transiently elevated while T$_4$ is depressed, and then over a period of 2-3 months all tests return to normal. *0151*

Thyroxine Binding Globulin *Serum Increase* Serum thyroglobulin was elevated in 92% of 38 patients in the early stage of this disorder. After two months of corticosteroid treatment the levels were significantly decreased in 25 patients who could be rechecked. *1474* Elevated during acute stage *1106*

Thyroxine (T$_4$) *Serum Decrease* May be subnormal late in the disease. *2540*

Serum Increase Elevated in 50% of patients. *1106* The association of a very low iodine uptake with an elevated T$_4$ is characteristic of the early phase of disease. *2540 0151*

Serum Normal May be normal with acute thyroiditis. *0151*

Tri-iodothyronine (T$_3$) *Serum Increase* Invariably elevated at some time during acute stage. *1106*

245.20   Hashimoto's Thyroiditis

[131]I Uptake   *Serum Decrease*   Markedly depressed. *0992*   Subnormal values are usually found early in the disease. *2540*   In the far advanced stage of thyroid destruction, all tests show the results of hypothyroidism: radioiodide uptake is low normal to low. *2035*   May be normal, elevated, or low. *0962*

Serum Increase   An early abnormality is a relative impairment of the process of organification of iodide trapped by the thyroid cell. Radioiodide uptake studies from 20 min to 6 h after administration may be relatively high, compared to the 24 h uptake. *2035*   May be normal or elevated in euthyroid patients. *1106*   May be slightly elevated in chronic patients. *0999*   May be normal, elevated, or low. *0962*

Serum Normal 0962

Alkaline Phosphatase   *Serum Increase*   Elevated in 3 patients, suggesting hepatic origin of the enzymes. *0489*

Alpha$_1$-Antitrypsin   *Serum Decrease*   Reduced activity. *2633*

Serum Increase   There was an increase in serum C3, IgM, alpha$_1$-acid glycoprotein and alpha$_1$-antitrypsin levels found in 40 patients. *1715*   Increased *1866   0042 1946 1947 2129*

Antibody Titer   *Serum Increase*   Characteristically present in high titer during the active phase of chronic thyroiditis. *0999*   Virtually all patients with this disease have circulating autoantibodies. *2540*   Antimicrosomal antibodies present in 78% of patients. *0992*   Almost all patients have thyroid autoantibodies in their serum, and extremely high titers of any of the autoantibodies are inconsistent with most other diagnoses. *2035*

Antimitochondrial Antibodies   *Serum Increase*   Presence correlates with degree of lymphocytic infiltration of the gland. *0186*

Antinuclear Antibodies   *Serum Increase*   Present in 1-8% of cases. *0995*

Antithyroglobulin Antibodies   *Serum Increase*   May be detected in high titer. *2612*   Characteristically present in high titer during the active phase of chronic thyroiditis. *0999*   Almost all patients have thyroid autoantibodies in their serum, and extremely high titers of any of the autoantibodies are inconsistent with most other diagnoses. *2035*   In over 80% of cases. *0058*   In most patients present in high titers (> 1:25,000 in tanned red cell test). Young patients may have low titers of autoantibodies. *2540*

Butanol Extractable Iodine (BEI)   *Serum Decrease*   Depressed in chronic thyroiditis patients. *0999*

Serum Normal 0962

Complement C3   *Serum Increase*   There was an increase in serum C3, IgM, alpha$_1$-acid glycoprotein and alpha$_1$-antitrypsin levels found in 40 patients. *1715*

Complement Fixation   *Serum Increase*   Virtually all patients with this disease have circulating autoantibodies. *2540*   Antimicrosomal antibodies present in 78% of patients. *0992*   Positive for cytoplasmic microsomal antigen in > 80% of cases. High titers of 1:256 usually occur in chronic thyroiditis. *0999*

Erythrocyte Sedimentation Rate   *Blood Increase*   In 50% of chronic thyroiditis patients. *0999*   May be mildly elevated. *0962*

Globulin   *Serum Increase*   Occurs in approximately 50% of chronic patients, and may reflect the degree of thyroiditis or autoantibody production. *0999*   May be present *0962*

Gonadotropin, Pituitary   *Serum Increase*   In the far advanced stage of thyroid destruction, all tests show the results of hypothyroidism. *2035*

Immunoglobulin IgG   *Serum Increase*   Often slightly raised. *2035*

Immunoglobulin IgM   *Serum Increase*   There was an increase in serum C3, IgM, alpha$_1$-acid glycoprotein and alpha$_1$-antitrypsin levels found in 40 patients. *1715*

Long Acting Thyroid Stimulating Hormone (LATS)   *Serum Increase*   Occasionally. *2540*

Precipitins   *Serum Increase*   Unusual but, when present, seem to be pathognomonic of Hashimoto's disease. *2035*   Precipitin test for thyroglobulin is positive in 60% of chronic thyroiditis cases. The least sensitive test for thyroid antibodies but the most specific. *0999*

Protein Bound Iodine (PBI)   *Serum Decrease*   May be decreased and may vary over a period of time (because of thyroid destruction and regeneration). *2468*   May be low owing to butanol-insoluble iodinated albumin in plasma. *0151*   Later in the disease. *2540*

Serum Increase   Slightly elevated early in the disease. *2540*   May be increased and may vary over a period of time (because of thyroid destruction and regeneration). *2468*

Serum Normal   May be normal and may vary over a period of time because of thyroid destruction and regeneration. *2468*   PBI may be disproportionately higher than the BEI because of circulating nonfunctioning iodinated proteins. *0962*

T$_3$ Uptake   *Serum Decrease*   Mean value was 76.7 ± 76 ng/dL, ranging from 20-600. 72 of 100 patients had subnormal values. No correlation was found with TSH. *1323*   In the far advanced stage of thyroid destruction, all tests show the results of hypothyroidism. *2035*

Thyroid Stimulating Hormone (TSH)   *Serum Increase*   Elevated in all patients, mean = 76.7 ± 55 μU/mL, range = 11-240. Mean values for patients < 20 years old was significantly higher than for older patients. *1323*   May occur as disease progresses. *2540*   Endogenous serum TSH may be normal or moderately elevated. *0962 2035*

Serum Normal   Usually normal at time of diagnosis. *2540*

Thyroxine Binding Globulin   *Serum Increase*   Elevated and fell to normal with therapy; patients whose illness recurred after cessation of drug therapy had higher pretreatment thyroglobulin values and no fall during treatment. *0296*

Thyroxine (T$_4$)   *Serum Decrease*   In the far advanced stage of thyroid destruction, all tests show the results of hypothyroidism. *2035*   May be depressed, depending on the stage of development of the process. *0151*   Average T$_4$ was 1.8 ± 1.5 μg/dL, range = 0.2-7.0. An inverse correlation was found with TSH and T$_4$, r = 0.73. *1323*   Normal in 25 euthyroid, reduced in 22 hypothyroid and increased in 4 hyperthyroid patients with Hashimoto's thyroiditis. No specific abnormalities in serum concentrations of thyroid hormones were found. *0832   0999 2540*

Serum Increase   Normal in 25 euthyroid, reduced in 22 hypothyroid and increased in 4 hyperthyroid patients with Hashimoto's thyroiditis. No specific abnormalities in serum concentrations of thyroid hormones were found. *0832*

Serum Normal   The majority of patients are euthyroid at diagnosis with normal T$_3$, T$_4$, free hormones and TSH. *1106*   Normal in 25 euthyroid, reduced in 22 hypothyroid and increased in 4 hyperthyroid patients with Hashimoto's thyroiditis. No specific abnormalities in serum concentrations of thyroid hormones were found. *0832   0962*

Tri-iodothyronine (T$_3$)   *Serum Decrease*   Normal in 25 euthyroid, reduced in 22 hypothyroid and increased in 4 hyperthyroid patients with Hashimoto's thyroiditis. No specific abnormalities in serum concentrations of thyroid hormones were found. *0832*

Serum Increase   May occur as disease progresses. *2540*   Normal in 25 euthyroid, reduced in 22 hypothyroid and increased in 4 hyperthyroid patients with Hashimoto's thyroiditis. No specific abnormalities in serum concentrations of thyroid hormones were found. *0832*

Serum Normal   The majority of patients are euthyroid at diagnosis with normal T$_3$, T$_4$, free hormones and TSH. *1106*   Normal in 25 euthyroid, reduced in 22 hypothyroid and increased in 4 hyperthyroid patients with Hashimoto's thyroiditis. No specific abnormalities in serum concentrations of thyroid hormones were found. *0832   0962*

VDRL   *Serum Positive*   Persistent false positive reactions are seen. *0999*   A false positive serologic test may occur. *0962*

250.00   Diabetes Mellitus

2,3-Diphosphoglycerate   *Urine Increase   0503*

Red Blood Cells Increase   Increased to 15.0 μmol/g (normal = 13.7). Concentrations vary in response to plasma inorganic phosphate levels. *0567*

17-Hydroxycorticosteroids   *Urine Decrease   0503*

17-Ketogenic Steroids   *Urine Decrease   0503*

Acid Phosphatase   *Serum Increase*   In 90 diabetics, an increased activity 137%, P < 0.001) was found. The increase was moderate (55%) in uncomplicated diabetics with slightly elevated glycemia (148 ± 24 mg/dL), and about twice normal levels in diabetics with either vasculopathies or marked hyperglycemia (343 ± 108 mg/dL). *0154*   Increased activity correlated with blood sugar concentration. *0155*

Alanine   *Serum Decrease*   Decreased. *0094 0269 2149*

Albumin   *Serum Decrease*   Tends to be low with increased alpha$_2$-globulins, particularly with vascular complications. *2104*   In 29% of 105 patients at initial hospitalization for this disorder. *0781*

Urine Increase   An early sign of diabetic nephropathy. *2104*

Aldosterone   *Plasma Decrease*   Commonly found, a result of reduced renin secretion or a specific defect in synthesis are common. *1854*

Urine Decrease   Commonly found, a result of reduced renin secretion or a specific defect in synthesis are common. *1854*

Alkaline Phosphatase *Serum Increase* Occurred in 11-17% of the patients. Ketoacidosis and death occurred more often among patients with elevated serum enzymes than those with normal levels. *0873* In 24% of 105 patients at initial hospitalization for this disorder. *0781* Elevated by 40% in 44% of 166 untreated patients. Activity did not correlate with blood sugar concentration. *0155*

Alpha₂-Antiplasmin *Serum Increase* High fast-antiplasmin levels and low or missing slow-antiplasmin levels. *0051*

Alpha₂-Globulin *Serum Increase* *2467*

Alpha₂-Macroglobulin *Serum Increase* All age groups. *1142* Extent of elevation is usually found to directly correlate with duration of disease and presence of vascular complications. *2630 1203 0107*

Amino Acids *Plasma Increase* Found with ketosis, probably associated with gluconeogenesis. *0619*

Urine Increase In severe diabetic ketosis. *0619*

Ammonia *Urine Increase* Reflects severity of acidosis and parallels the degree of ketonuria. *0619*

Amylase *Serum Decrease* Both abnormally high and low values have been observed. *2104*

Serum Increase High incidence of pancreatic abnormality in patients with no clinical evidence of pancreatic acinar disease. *2406* Increased activity correlated with blood sugar concentration. *0155*

Urine Increase High incidence of pancreatic abnormality in patients with no clinical evidence of pancreatic acinar disease. *2406*

Angiotensin-Converting Enzyme (ACE) *Serum Increase* Elevated levels were detected in 24% of 265 patients with this disease. *1399* Elevated in 32% of 81 patients. *2068*

Antibody Titer *Serum Increase* Antibodies to Islet cells. Present in 60% of juvenile onset diabetics of less than 1 years duration. Such antibodies tend to disappear rapidly after the disease is recognized clinically. *1670*

Antithrombin III *Plasma Decrease* Reports of increased and decreased levels. *2353 1482*

Plasma Increase Reports of increased and decreased levels. *2353 1482*

Plasma Normal Normal levels seen with diabetic nephropathy. *0365*

Aspartate Aminotransferase *Serum Increase* Of 200 untreated diabetics, 12% had unexplainable elevations. *0873*

Basophils *Blood Increase* *2538*

Beta-Globulin *Serum Increase* *2467*

Beta-Glucuronidase *Serum Increase* Increased activity correlated with blood sugar concentration. *0155*

Beta-Glusosaminidase *Serum Increase* Increased activity correlated with blood sugar concentration. *0155*

Bicarbonate *Serum Decrease* *2467*

Calcium *Serum Decrease* Osmotic diuresis secondary to hyperglycemia. *2540*

Urine Increase Osmotic diuresis secondary to hyperglycemia. *2540*

Carcinoembryonic Antigen *Serum Increase* 38% of patients had values > 2.5 ng/mL. *2199*

Carotene *Serum Increase* *2467*

Catecholamines *Plasma Decrease* Common. *1854* Long-term diabetics with neuropathy showed significant reductions. Diabetics without neuropathy had normal concentrations. *0399*

Urine Decrease Common. *1854* Long-term diabetics with neuropathy showed significant reductions. Diabetics without neuropathy had normal concentrations. *0399*

Chloride *Serum Decrease* Osmotic diuresis secondary to hyperglycemia. *2540*

Urine Increase Osmotic diuresis secondary to hyperglycemia. *2540*

Cholesterol *Serum Increase* Moderate increase. *0503* Mean levels in children (205 ± 78 mg/dL) were significantly higher than for controls (155 ± 27 mg/dL), as were mean triglyceride levels. 8 with diabetes had hypercholesterolemia, 5 had hypertriglyceridemia, and 9 had combined hypercholesterolemia and hypertriglyceridemia. *0377*

Cholesterol, High Density Lipoprotein *Serum Decrease* Decreased. *0131 1519 2556*

Cholesterol, Very Low Density Lipoprotein *Serum Increase* Marled elevation due to increased secretion and decreased catabolism secondary to reduced lipoprotein lipase activity. *0062 2614*

Chylomicrons *Serum Increase* Increased. *1380 1936 1948* Minimal elevation secondary to decreased catabolism due to reduced lipoprotein lipase activity. *0062*

Creatine *Serum Increase* Increased formation and decreased renal absorption. *0619*

Urine Increase Creatinuria occurs with gonadal dysfunction in males and females. *2104*

Creatinine *Serum Increase* High levels may be the result of interference by the high levels of glucose and acetone present. *1003* In 49% of 102 patients at initial hospitalization for this disorder. *0781*

Cryofibrinogen *Serum Increase* *2035 0856 1551 2046*

Factor VIII *Plasma Increase* Increased activity has been reported. *0635*

Fat *Feces Increase* Defects of multiple stages of digestion-absorption. *2199*

Fatty Acids, Free (FFA) *Serum Increase* Marked elevation in circulating concentration due to release of fatty acids from fat stores. *2104*

Fibrinogen *Plasma Increase* Significantly higher in both juvenile and maturity onset diabetics. *0149*

Fibrin Split Products (FSP) *Urine Increase* With diabetic nephropathy the greater the degree of proteinuria the greater the loss of fibrinogen degradation product in the urine. *0365*

Gamma Glutamyl Transferase (GGT) *Serum Increase* A study of 228 patients has shown a significant positive association between serum GGT and triglyceride levels. Both fall with treatment, the most marked reduction occurring in patients on insulin. This association may reflect hepatic triglyceride levels in new diabetics may reflect hepatic microsomal enzyme induction of the rate-limiting enzymes of triglyceride synthesis. Serum GGT does not seem to correlate with hepatomegaly in diabetes mellitus. *1517* In 50% of 20 patients at initial hospitalization for this disorder. *0781 0876*

Glucose *Serum Increase* Diagnosis can be readily made when there is an unequivocal and persistent elevation of the fasting plasma glucose. For venous plasma, the fasting glucose is normally between 60-100 mg/100 mL and values consistently > 120 should be considered diagnostic of diabetes. *0999 0812 0433*

Serum Normal May be normal in mild diabetes. *0812* A large percentage of patients with early diabetes have perfectly normal fasting blood glucose levels. When elevated this test is very helpful, but when normal it is of little consequence. This is a poor screening test for diabetes. *0433*

Urine Increase Urine testing as a preliminary screening procedure for diabetes is the cheapest method available, however, it is not very productive. *0433* Glycosuria is characteristic of the diabetic state, but its presence is neither necessary nor sufficient for the diagnosis. *1919*

Glucose Tolerance *Serum Decrease* Decreased tolerance; decreased utilization with slow fall to fasting level. *2467* The responses in nondiabetic and diabetic population do not describe a bimodal distribution, but constitute a single curve skewed in the direction of higher blood sugar values. *0999*

Granular Casts *Urine Increase* With diabetic nephropathy. *0186*

Growth Hormone *Serum Increase* In insulin-dependent diabetics high values are usually observed. *0858* Often abnormally high. *2104*

Hemoglobin A₁C *Blood Increase* All patients classified as diabetic were found to have values greater than 9.9%. *1171* 2-3 fold increase in the red cells of diabetic patients. By providing an integrated measurement of blood glucose, Hb A₁C is useful in assessing the degree of diabetic control. *0315*

Hexosaminidase *Serum Increase* Increase in total concentration (hexosaminidase A and B). *1716*

HLA Antigens *Blood Present* HLA-DR4 present in 38% of patients with insulin dependent disease versus 13% of controls. HLA-DR3 present in 50% of insulin dependent disease versus 21% of controls. *2539* HLA-B8 and HLA-Bw15 also associated with this disease. *2191*

Hyaline Casts *Urine Increase* With diabetic nephropathy. *0186*

Immunoglobulin IgG *Serum Increase* The levels of glycosylated IgG were significantly higher. *2644*

Insulin *Serum Decrease* A critical amount of insulin secretory reserve distinguishes between 2 qualitatively distinct clinical syndromes: true diabetes mellitus (the development of signs and symptoms of insulin deficiency) and the syndrome of pure resistance to insulin (signs and symptoms of hyperglycemia in the setting of adequate or excessive insulin secretion, frequently with obesity, but without diabetic complication. *2388* Absent in severe diabetes mellitus with ketosis and weight loss. In less severe cases, insulin is frequently present but only at lower glucose concentrations. *2467*

250.00   Diabetes Mellitus *(continued)*

Insulin *(continued)*
Serum   Increase   Increased in mild cases of untreated obese diabetics; fasting level is often increased. *2467*

Isocitrate Dehydrogenase   *Serum   Normal   2260*

Ketones   *Serum   Increase*   Up to 300-400 mg/dL or more. *0619* Increased as a result of disturbed fat and carbohydrate metabolism. *1854*

Urine   Increase   Children are more liable to develop ketosis than adults. *0619*

Lactate Dehydrogenase   *Serum   Increase*   Of 200 untreated diabetics, 21% had an unexplainable elevation. *0873*

Lactic Acid   *Blood   Increase*   Moderately elevated in 11 of 28 diabetics. *0796*

Lipids   *Urine   Increase*   Lipids in the urine include all fractions. Double refractile (cholesterol) bodies can be seen. *2467*

Lipoproteins, Beta   *Serum   Increase*   *0774 0772 0773*

Lymphocytes   *Blood   Decrease*   The percentage and absolute number of peripheral T-lymphocytes were significantly lower (38.1% and 833/μL) in juvenile-onset diabetics than in normal subjects or maternity-onset diabetics. There was no significant difference between normals and maternity-onset cases. *0360*

Lysozyme   *Urine   Increase*   Lysozymuria. *0701*

Magnesium   *Serum   Decrease*   Osmotic diuresis secondary to hyperglycemia. *2540*

Serum   Increase   In diabetic coma before treatment and in controlled diabetes in older age groups. *2467   2290*

Urine   Increase   Osmotic diuresis secondary to hyperglycemia. *2540*

Myoglobin   *Urine   Increase*   Sporadic; metabolic myoglobinuria. *2467*

Norepinephrine   *Plasma   Decrease*   Long-term diabetics with neuropathy showed significant reductions. Diabetics without neuropathy had normal concentrations. *0399*

Oval Fat Bodies   *Urine   Increase*   With diabetic nephropathy. *0186*

Oxygen Saturation   *Blood   Increase*   Diabetics with pronounced hyperlipidemia due to accumulation of chylomicrons showed markedly increased hemoglobin-oxygen affinity (p 50:21.1 vs 26.6 mm Hg). *0568*

pCO$_2$ *Blood   Decrease*   *1854*

pH   *Blood   Decrease*   From an accumulation of acetoacetate and beta-hydroxybutyric acid. *2540   1854*

Urine   Decrease   From an accumulation of acetoacetate and beta-hydroxybutyric acid. *2540*

Urine   Increase   Osmotic diuresis secondary to hyperglycemia. *2540*

Phosphate   *Serum   Decrease*   Osmotic diuresis secondary to hyperglycemia. *2540*

Serum   Increase   *0619*

Urine   Increase   Osmotic diuresis secondary to hyperglycemia. *2540*

Phospholipids, Total   *Serum   Increase*   *0619*

Platelet Count   *Blood   Increase*   In 23% of 21 patients at initial hospitalization for this disorder. *0781*

Potassium   *Serum   Decrease*   Osmotic diuresis secondary to hyperglycemia. *2540*

Serum   Increase   hyperkalemia may occur due to low insulin levels, which normally would cause a net influx of K$^+$ into cells, and low aldosterone levels, which would stimulate K$^+$ excretion in a normal state. *1854*   In 29% of 107 patients at initial hospitalization for this disorder. *0781*

Serum   Normal   Normal or increased. *2467*

Urine   Increase   Osmotic diuresis secondary to hyperglycemia. *2540*

Proinsulin   *Serum   Increase*   Increased percentage in 11 of 59 maturity-onset cases and correlated with plasma glucose but not to total insulin. *1485*

Serum   Normal   No consistent abnormality has been found. Patients with mild diabetes have repeatedly shown normal proportions. Severe cases may have an elevated proinsulin:insulin ratio. *1080*

Prostaglandins   *Serum   Increase*   Prostaglandin E2 and F2-alpha were significantly elevated in children at all times measured. *0378*

Protein   *Serum   Decrease*   With diabetic nephropathy. *0186*

Urine   Increase   With diabetic nephropathy; often > 5g/24h. *0186*

CSF   Increase   Approximately 70% of patients with neuropathy have unusual spinal fluid protein (50-100 mg/dL). *2540*

Protein Bound Iodine (PBI)   *Serum   Normal   2467*

Pseudocholinesterase   *Serum   Increase*   Obese type. *0619*

Pyruvate   *Blood   Increase*   Raised levels have been reported in unstable diabetes (insulin sensitive). *0619*

Renin Activity   *Plasma   Decrease*   Decreased catecholamine levels, which reduce renin secretion, are common. *1854*

Sodium   *Serum   Decrease*   Osmotic diuresis secondary to hyperglycemia. *2540*   In 22% of 104 patients at initial hospitalization for this disorder. *0781*

Urine   Increase   Osmotic diuresis secondary to hyperglycemia. *2540   2467*

T$_3$ Uptake   *Serum   Normal   2467*

Thyro-Binding Index   *Serum   Normal*   Serum T$_4$, T$_3$RU free T$_4$ and TSH in patients prior to therapy was not significantly different from normal subjects. *1203*

Thyroid Stimulating Hormone (TSH)   *Serum   Normal*   Serum T$_4$, T$_3$RU free T$_4$ and TSH in patients prior to therapy was not significantly elevated compared to normals. *1203*

Thyroxine, Free   *Serum   Normal*   Serum T$_4$, T$_3$RU free T$_4$ and TSH in patients prior to therapy was not significantly different from controls. *1203*

Thyroxine (T$_4$)   *Serum   Normal*   Serum T$_4$, T$_3$RU free T$_4$ and TSH in patients prior to therapy was not significantly different from controls. *1203*

Trehalase   *Serum   Increase*   Increased but does not correlate with blood sugar concentration. *0155*

Triglycerides   *Serum   Increase*   Higher values correlate with hyperglycemia and poorer control of diabetes; reduced by insulin therapy. *2467*   Mean levels for children were elevated 120 ± 63 vs 85 ± 23 μg/dL for controls. 8 had hypercholesterolemia, 5 had hypertriglyceridemia, and 9 had combined hypercholesterolemia and hypertriglyceridemia. *0377*   In 228 patients, a significant positive association between GGT and triglyceride concentration was found. May reflect hepatic microsomal *1517*

Tri-iodothyronine, Reverse   *Serum   Increase*   Prior to Rx. serum rT$_3$ was significantly higher than in normal controls. *1203*

Tri-iodothyronine (T$_3$)   *Serum   Increase*   Prior to Rx. serum T$_3$ was significantly lower than in normal controls. *1203*

Trypsin   *Serum   Increase*   High incidence of pancreatic abnormality in patients with no clinical evidence of pancreatic acinar disease. *2406*

Urea Nitrogen   *Serum   Increase*   Uncontrolled diabetes mellitus may be associated with excessive protein catabolism. *0503*   In 29% of 117 patients at initial hospitalization for this disorder. *0781*

Uric Acid   *Serum   Increase*   Increased occurrence of hyperuricemia has been reported. *1585*   In 28% of 104 patients at initial hospitalization for this disorder. *0781*

Volume   *Plasma   Decrease   2467*

Urine   Increase   As the urine sugar content rises, glucose acts as a diuretic, i.e., the renal tubules are reabsorbing glucose at their maximum rate and the excess glucose prevents further water reabsorption. *0619*

Xylose Tolerance Test   *Urine   Abnormal*   Defects of multiple stages of digestion-absorption. *2199*

250.10   Diabetic Acidosis

Alanine Aminotransferase   *Serum   Increase*   In some instances, mostly in severe cases, especially with severe circulatory failure and liver enlargement. *0155*

Albumin   *Serum   Decrease   0619*

Urine   Increase   0962

Amylase   *Serum   Increase*   Raised in ketoacidosis. *2485* Occurs frequently; 21 of 35 patients (60%) had elevated concentrations. Occurs most often when blood sugar > 500 mg/dL. *0869*   21 of 35 patients were hyperamylasemic, with 6 showing values > 1,000 Somogyi U. No relation was found between degree of elevation and morbidity and mortality or acidosis or azotemia. Relation was found with degrees of hyperglycemia. *1286*   Elevated levels *2646*

Aspartate Aminotransferase   *Serum   Increase*   Mild-moderate abnormalities may occur in 20-65% of patients but bears no relation to degree of abdominal pain or prognosis. *1316*   In some instances, mostly in severe cases, especially with severe circulatory failure and liver enlargement. *0155*

Bicarbonate *Serum Decrease* May be < 2 mmol/L in profound cases and 15 mmol/L in severe cases. *2540* Metabolic acidosis may occur. *0962*

Casts *Urine Increase 2468*

Catecholamines *Plasma Increase 2540*

Chloride *Serum Decrease 0962*

Cortisol *Plasma Increase 2425*

Creatine Kinase *Serum Increase* Mild-moderate abnormalities may occur in 20-65% of patients but bears no relation to degree of abdominal pain or prognosis. *1316*

Eosinophils *Blood Decrease* Often a polymorphonucleocytosis with a lymphopenia and eosinopenia. *0962*

Epinephrine *Plasma Increase 2425*

Gamma Glutamyl Transferase (GGT) *Saliva Increase* Significantly higher (11.6 U/L) versus controls (5.12 U/L). *1164*

Glucagon *Plasma Increase* Frequently observed. *1644*

Glucose *Serum Increase* Increased, usually > 300 mg/dL. *2467* Seldom in excess of 800 mg/dL. *1316 0999*

Urine Increase 0999 0962

Glutamate Dehydrogenase *Serum Increase* In some instances, mostly in severe cases, especially with severe circulatory failure and liver enlargement. *0155*

Growth Hormone *Serum Increase 2540*

Hematocrit *Blood Increase* Secondary to dehydration. *0999* May be moderately increased because of hemoconcentration. *0962*

Isocitrate Dehydrogenase *Serum Increase* In some instances, mostly in severe cases, especially with severe circulatory failure and liver enlargement. *0155*

Ketones *Serum Increase* Initial values range from 11.3-15 mmol/L in several studies. Target ketone concentration was reached in 4-7 h. *1316* Beta-hydroxybutyrate accumulates and is one of the major causes of acidosis as a result of disturbed carbohydrate and fat metabolism. *1854 0962 0999*

Urine Increase Accumulates and is one of the major causes of acidosis as a result of disturbed carbohydrate and fat metabolism. *1854 0999 0962*

Lactate Dehydrogenase *Serum Increase* In some instances, mostly severe cases, especially with severe circulatory failure and liver enlargement. *0155*

Lactic Acid *Blood Increase* Accumulates and is one of the major causes of acidosis as a result of disturbed carbohydrate and fat metabolism. *1854* Coexistent and biochemically significant lactic acidosis is a relatively infrequent complication of ketoacidosis; usually due to underlying disorders associated with poor tissue perfusion. *1316*

Leukocytes *Blood Increase* Leukocytosis is common (15,000-30,000/μL). *2540* Often a polymorphonucleocytosis with a lymphopenia and eosinopenia. *0962*

Lipase *Serum Normal* Normal levels. *1887*

Lipids *Serum Increase* Level of serum sodium depends on degree of increased plasma lipids. *0999* Often found. *0962*

Lymphocytes *Blood Decrease* Often a polymorphonucleocytosis with a lymphopenia and eosinopenia. *0962*

Magnesium *Serum Decrease 0962*

Serum Increase In the early phase. *0962*

Malate Dehydrogenase *Serum Increase* In some instances, mostly severe cases, especially with severe circulatory failure and liver enlargement. *0155*

Neutrophils *Blood Increase* May be associated with a moderate to severe neutrophilia. *2538*

Norepinephrine *Plasma Increase* With fasting, profound exercise and orthostatic changes, norepinephrine secretion is enhanced. *2540*

Plasma Normal Following insulin-induced hypoglycemia, there is no change. *2425*

pCO$_2$ *Blood Decrease* Hyperventilation. *2540* Metabolic acidosis may occur. *0962*

pH *Blood Decrease* Metabolic acidosis may occur. *0962* Acidosis with low plasma pH and bicarbonate (usually < 10 mmol/L) is seen. *0999*

Phosphate *Serum Decrease* During successful treatment of diabetic ketosis insulin causes phosphate ions to enter the cells with glucose and potassium. *0619* Common; usually becomes manifest in 4-12 h of institution of therapy. *1316* Common in patients recovering from severe diabetic ketoacidosis. *1287*

Serum Increase 0619

Potassium *Serum Decrease* Total body deficit. Only 4-10% have decreased plasma concentrations and these patients are at high risk for developing life-threatening hypokalemia during early hours of treatment. *1516* Renal wasting leads to hypokalemic state. *1679* Despite the markedly negative K$^+$ balance, hyperkalemia is often present because the acidosis causes the K$^+$ to shift from inside the cells into the extracellular space. *2540*

Serum Increase Usually normal or elevated, despite total body deficit. Only 4-10% have decreased plasma concentrations and these patients are at high risk for developing life-threatening hypokalemia during early hours of treatment. *1516* Despite the markedly negative K$^+$ balance, hyperkalemia is often present because the acidosis causes the K$^+$ to shift from inside the cells into the extracellular space. *2540* Impaired uptake by the cells secondary to acidosis and increased liberation of cell potassium following protein breakdown and gluconeogenesis. *0619 1515*

Prolactin *Serum Increase* Elevated in 8 patients, (24.8 ± 10.2 ng/mL). After correction of the ketoacidosis, levels decreased to 10.9 ± 6.4 ng/mL (normal range men 4.9 ± 0.8, women 5.1 ± 1.6 ng/mL). *0983*

Protein *Serum Increase* Secondary to dehydration. *0999*

Urine Increase 2468

Pseudocholinesterase *Serum Decrease* Decreases 2-3 days after episodes of ketoacidosis. *0155*

Pyruvate *Blood Increase* Can be demonstrated after removal of acetoacetic acid. *0619*

Sodium *Serum Decrease* Despite the markedly negative sodium balance, the plasma concentration may be hypernormal, normal or subnormal. *2540 0962*

Serum Increase May be normal or elevated depending on the relative losses of sodium and water and the degree of increased plasma lipids. Because of the increase in plasma lipids a sodium concentration of 150 mmol/L of plasma may represent 170 mmol/L of water. *0999* Despite the markedly negative sodium balance, the plasma concentration may be hypernormal, normal or subnormal. *2540*

Sorbitol Dehydrogenase *Serum Increase* In some instances, mostly in severe cases, especially with severe circulatory failure and liver enlargement. *0155*

Specific Gravity *Urine Increase 0962*

Thyroxine (T$_4$) *Serum Decrease* In 19 euthyroid patients with severe ketoacidosis, a 'low T$_3$ syndrome' was found, with lowered serum concentrations of T$_3$, increased reverse T$_3$, slightly low T$_4$ (T$_4$) and normal thyrotropin. *1663*

Tri-iodothyronine (T$_3$) *Serum Decrease* In 19 euthyroid patients with severe ketoacidosis a 'low T$_3$ syndrome' was found, with lowered serum concentrations of T$_3$, increased reverse T$_3$, slightly low T$_4$ (T$_4$), and normal thyrotropin. *1663*

Urea Nitrogen *Serum Increase* May reflect prerenal azotemia or diabetic nephropathy. *0962*

Uric Acid *Serum Increase* Elevated in 50% of patients; parallels the degree of ketoacidosis and returns to normal when diabetes is controlled. *1757* Frequently increased. *0999* Often found. *0962 1283*

Volume *Urine Increase 2540*

251.20 Hypoglycemia, Unspecified

Glucagon *Plasma Increase 0619*

Glucose *Serum Decrease* Insulin excess probably due to excessively rapid absorption as in postgastrectomy. This may occur particularly in: underweight, poorly nourished babies; twins; premature infants. A low birth-weight baby with a proportionally large head is very prone to hypoglycemia. Infants of diabetic mothers (fetal blood glucose is controlled by the maternal blood glucose level, but at term the newborn infant's pancreas may respond to maternal hyperglycemia by secretion of insulin and hence hypoglycemia). *0619*

CSF Decrease 0619

Glycine *Serum Increase* Persistently elevated and is generally higher than in secondary hyperglycinemias. *0433*

Urine Increase Persistently elevated and are generally higher than in secondary hyperglycinemias. *0433*

Growth Hormone *Serum Increase 0619*

Insulin *Serum Increase* Increased in reactive hypoglycemia after glucose ingestion, particularly when a diabetic type of glucose tolerance curve is present. *2467*

251.20   Hypoglycemia, Unspecified *(continued)*

Insulin *(continued)*

Serum   Normal   Normal in hypoglycemia associated with nonpancreatic tumors. Normal in idiopathic hypoglycemia of childhood except after administration of leucine. *2467*

Prolactin   *Serum   Increase*   Increased levels. *1887*   Can trigger a mild to moderate increase (20-300 ng/mL) *2637*

251.50   Zollinger-Ellison Syndrome

Albumin   *Serum   Decrease*   Serum concentration in 20 patients with proved or presumed ZE syndrome (4.1 ± 0.8 g/dL) were significantly lower than observed in 40 normal controls (5.1 ± 0.3). 40 duodenal ulcer patients (5.1 ± 0.4 g/dL). Total gastrectomy induced a rise in serum albumin in 8 patients studied. *1345*   A low serum albumin will reflect possible malabsorption of protein or protein-losing enteropathy. *0962*

Alkaline Phosphatase   *Serum   Decrease*   An indication of vitamin D and calcium malabsorption. *0962*

Calcitonin   *Serum   Increase*   In some cases. *1041*

Calcium   *Serum   Decrease*   An indication of vitamin D and calcium malabsorption. *0962*

Carotene   *Serum   Decrease*   A useful indication of fat malabsorption, low levels are found in as many as 80% of patients with steatorrhea. *0962*

Fat   *Feces   Increase*   Hyperacidity in duodenum inactivates pancreatic enzymes. *0962*

Gastrin   *Serum   Increase*   Significant correlation between basal levels and malignant gastrinoma but not with benign tumors. *2244*   Concentrations reach 2,800-300,000 pg/mL associated with non-insulin producing pancreatic tumors *0619*

Gonadotropin, Chorionic   *Serum   Increase*   Significant correlation between basal levels and malignant gastrinoma but not with benign tumors. *2244*

Lipids   *Feces   Increase*   Hyperacidity in duodenum inactivates pancreatic enzymes. *0962*

Lymphocytes   *Blood   Decrease*   Often an absolute lymphopenia due to loss of lymphocytes into the small intestine. *0962*

pH   *Gastric Material   Increase*   Gastric secretion > 100 mmol/12h is strongly indicative of this disorder. *0844*   Markedly elevated levels of gastric acid secretion *2540*

Phosphate   *Serum   Decrease*   An indication of vitamin D and calcium malabsorption. *0962*

Potassium   *Serum   Decrease*   Hypokalemia; frequently associated with chronic severe diarrhea. *2468*

Prolactin   *Serum   Increase*   Levels were measured in 36 patients with ZES, eight patients had elevated levels. *2245*

Protein   *Feces   Increase*   Hyperacidity in duodenum inactivates pancreatic enzymes. *0962*

Prothrombin Time   *Plasma   Increase*   An indication of vitamin K malabsorption. *0962*

Triolein ^{131}I Test   *Feces   Positive*   Positive test for lipid droplets in the stool, but results are inconsistent. *0962*

252.00   Hyperparathyroidism

1,25-Dihydroxy-Vitamin D$_3$ *Serum   Increase*   *0062*

Acid Phosphatase   *Serum   Increase*   Found in 28 cases with definite skeletal changes. Activity was increased in every instance from 1.4-16 X the normal maximum. *0948   0812*

Alkaline Phosphatase   *Serum   Increase*   Found to be elevated in only 30%, and each of these showed normal results for other liver function tests. Correlated well with serum calcium, but only significant in female patients. *1492*   Following the removal of the parathyroid tumor, the increased serum concentration persists and may even rise temporarily, falling gradually over a period of months as bone repair is completed. *0619*

Alpha$_2$-Globulin   *Serum   Increase*   Slightly increased but return to normal after parathyroidectomy. *2467*

Amino Acids   *Urine   Increase*   Quite common. *2540*

Antibody Titer   *Serum   Increase*   Parathyroid antibodies. *1670*

Bicarbonate   *Serum   Decrease*   Decreased bicarbonate in 24% of cases. *1492*

Calcitonin   *Serum   Decrease*   *0619 0520*

Calcium   *Serum   Increase*   Of 50 primary cases, 47 had increased concentration (> 10.3 mg/dL). *1957*   In 149 samples, 0.7% of serum ionized calcium and 7.5% of total calcium determinations were within the normal range. All patients exhibited abnormally elevated values upon repeated testing. *0626*   Hyperparathyroidism associated with pathologic lesions, shows hypercalcemia 10.5 mg/dL. Probably the single most important diagnostic aid. *0503   2595 1083 0812 1492 0781 0589*

Urine   Decrease   Although they may have hypercalciuria, compared with normal controls, they have very low rates for their serum calcium. *2540*

Urine   Increase   24 h excretion is high because of significant hypercalcemia, even though the renal clearance of calcium is relatively reduced. *0151*   39 of 54 patients had elevations above the normal upper limit (250-300 mg/24h). *2161*   Found in about 50% of primary cases. *1957*   Most patients are hypercalcemic and hypercalciuric. *1492   0433*

Chloride   *Serum   Increase*   The chloride values were higher (mean = 107 mmol/L) and phosphate, lower (mean = 2.6 mg/dL mL) in the 25 hyperparathyroid patients, whereas the chloride concentrations were lower (mean = 98 mmol/L) and phosphate, higher (mean = 4.5 mg/dL) in the 27 patients with hypercalcemia from other causes. The chloride to phosphate ratio ranged from 31.8-80 in hyperparathyroidism, with 96% more than 33, and from 17.1-32.3 in those with hypercalcemia from other causes, with 92% < 30. *1766*   Increases and phosphate decreases resulting in a Cl/PO$_3$ ratio > 33. *1957*   Hyperchloremic acidosis occurs as a result of renal effects *2541 0781*

Serum   Normal   Appears to be more reliable than inorganic phosphate for differentiating hyperparathyroidism from other causes of hypercalcemia. *2542*

Cholesterol   *Serum   Decrease*   Hypercalcemia due to hyperparathyroidism is linked with low cholesterol levels and high parathyroid hormone and calcitonin production. An average increase of 41 μg/dL occurred after corrective surgery. *0520*   About 8-10% lower in both females and males compared with corresponding control cases. *0401*

Citrate   *Serum   Increase*   Elevated in the high normal range. *2540*

Urine   Increase   High or in high normal range. *2540*   Often elevated. *0992*

Copper   *Serum   Increase*   Slightly > normal mean. *1490*

Urine   Increase   Mean 24 h urinary excretion was greater than normal in 17 patients with untreated disease. *1490*

Creatinine   *Serum   Increase*   Mean concentration was 4.8 ± 1.8 mg/dL. *1475*   In 45% of 11 patients at initial hospitalization for this disorder. *0781*

Creatinine Clearance   *Urine   Decrease*   Strong negative correlation between creatinine clearance and serum calcium. *1492*

Cyclic Adenosine Monophosphate   *Urine   Increase*   Parathyroid hormone action on the kidney leads to increased cAMP excretion. Mean urinary concentration was almost twice that of normals. *1492*

Urine   Normal   In 21 patients, mean urinary excretion of cAMP/24h was 5.0 ± 1.9 μmol uncorrected. When correlated to albumin-corrected serum calcium, this overlap between hyperparathyroidism and normality disappears completely. Excretion is influenced to a considerable degree by the biological activity of circulating parathyroid hormone. *1475   1492*

Erythrocyte Sedimentation Rate   *Blood   Increase*   Raised in 48%, without apparent explanation. *1492   0999*

Gastrin   *Serum   Increase*   Elevated in patients without ulcer and fell to normal after parathyroidectomy. *2277*   Mean preoperative concentration in 18 uncomplicated patients was 122 ± 39 pg/mL. *0545*   Patients may be hypergastrinemic. Some of these patients also have gastric hypersecretion. In these the hypergastrinemia can be consider pathologic. *2199*   Gastrin levels above normal occurred in 22% of patients with primary hyperparathyroidism *2606*

Hematocrit   *Blood   Decrease*   Unexplained anemia found in 21% of 57 patients. *1492*

Hemoglobin   *Blood   Decrease*   Unexplained anemia found in 21% of 57 patients. *1492*

Hydroxyproline   *Urine   Increase*   Normal or increased. Increased with significant bone involvement. *2540*   Tends to parallel the extent and severity of bone involvement. Also seen in the secondary hyperparathyroidism of chronic renal disease. *0962*

Insulin   *Serum   Increase*   Fasting concentrations and response were significantly increased in primary disease. *1265*

Leukocytes   *Blood   Decrease*   Frequently found. *2467*

Magnesium   *Serum   Decrease*   May occur. *2444*   Normal or low. *2540*   Found in 14%. *1492   0022*

Parathyroid Hormone *Serum Increase* Raised serum calcium levels fail to depress hormone secretion. *0619* Concentration rises above baseline level after neck massage only on the side of the adenoma, thereby aiding preoperative localization of the adenoma. *2467* In over 90% of cases. *0062 0520 1492*

pCO₂ *Blood Decrease* 2540

pH *Urine Increase* 2540

Phosphate *Serum Decrease* Range of concentration in 34 patients was 1.2-3.4 mg/dL, mean = 4.35 mg/dL. *1904* Occurs in 50% of patients. *0999* In 83% of 19 patients at initial hospitalization for this disorder. *0781 0151 1957 0962*

Urine Increase Increased unless there is a renal insufficiency or phosphate depletion (especially due to commonly used antacids containing aluminum). *2468* Marked phosphaturia due to parathyroid hormones. *0619 0503*

Saliva Increase Increased inorganic phosphate in saliva. *0619*

Potassium *Serum Decrease* Related to the hypercalcemia and does not aid in differential diagnosis. *0433* Rare (3%). *0999* Occasionally observed; attributed to decreased distal tubular reabsorption. *0151*

Serum Increase Incidence of 40% (7 of 17 cases) was reported. Other studies indicate a lower frequency. *2613 1492*

Urine Increase May occur. *2540*

Pyrophosphate *Synovial Fluid Increase* Has been identified. *2088*

Sodium *Urine Increase* 2540

Specific Gravity *Urine Decrease* Polyuria due to the inability to concentrate the urine. Related to the hypercalcemia and does not aid in differential diagnosis. *0433*

Thyroid Stimulating Hormone (TSH) *Serum Normal* 1226

Thyroxine, Free *Serum Normal* 1226

Thyroxine (T₄) *Serum Normal* 1226

Triglycerides *Serum Decrease* Levels were about 22% in females and 60% lower in males compared to controls. After operation levels normalized. *0401*

Tri-iodothyronine, Reverse *Serum Normal* Despite the low serum total T₃ levels. *1226*

Tri-iodothyronine (T₃) *Serum Decrease* Significantly lower in patients with primary hyperparathyroidism (118 ng/dL) than normal controls (147 ng/dL). There was a significant inverse correlation between serum levels of total T₃ and PTH. *1226*

Urea Nitrogen *Serum Increase* May occur. *2540*

Uric Acid *Serum Increase* Over 6.8 mg/dL in 62% of patients. *0999* Increased frequency of hyperuricemia and gout. 66% of the patients showed elevations, with no difference of frequency among males or females or with type of disease. *1492* In 54% of 18 patients at initial hospitalization for this disorder. *0781 1600 1283 0962*

Volume *Urine Increase* Polyuria due to the inability to concentrate the urine. Related to the hypercalcemia and does not aid in differential diagnosis. *0433*

Zinc *Urine Increase* Mean 24 h excretion was above normal in 17 patients with untreated primary disease. *1490*

252.10 Hypoparathyroidism

1,25-Dihydroxy-Vitamin D₃ *Serum Decrease* 0062

Alkaline Phosphatase *Serum Decrease* Normal or slightly low. *2540*

Serum Normal Normal or slightly low. *2540*

Bicarbonate *Serum Increase* 1337

Calcium *Serum Decrease* Rapidly reduced to a stable low level following removal of gland. *2104* Decreased PTH causes increased serum phosphate and reduced serum calcium. *0503*

Urine Decrease Rises acutely, then falls to low levels as plasma calcium falls. *2540*

Urine Increase Rises acutely, then falls to low levels as plasma calcium falls. *2540*

Chloride *Urine Decrease* May occur. *2540*

Urine Normal Usually. *2540*

Citrate *Serum Decrease* 2540

Glucose Tolerance *Serum Increase* Flat peak. Poor absorption from the GI tract (normal IV GTT curve). *2467*

Hydroxyproline *Urine Decrease* May occur. *2540 0962*

Magnesium *Serum Decrease* Hypomagnesemia may occur. *2444*

Serum Normal Initial diuresis without significant change in serum concentrations. *2540*

Urine Decrease Initial diuresis without significant change in serum concentrations. *2540*

Red Blood Cells Increase In 5 of 8 patients, the RBC concentration was at or above the normal upper limit. For the group the mean was 6.3 μmol/L packed cells, significantly over the normal (P < 0.001). *2469*

Parathyroid Hormone *Serum Decrease* 2468 0999

pH *Blood Increase* 1337

Phosphate *Serum Decrease* Initial fall followed by a rise. *2540*

Serum Increase Increased (usually 5-6 mg/dL; as high as 12 mg/dL). *2467* Initial fall followed by a rise. May range from 6-16 mg/dL. *2540 0812 0503 0999*

Urine Decrease Urine phosphate and phosphate clearance is decreased. *2468 0503 0433*

Urea Nitrogen *Serum Normal* 2540

Uric Acid *Serum Increase* In primary cases. *0601 1283 0962*

253.00 Acromegaly

17-Hydroxycorticosteroids *Urine Increase* 0503

17-Ketogenic Steroids *Urine Increase* 0433

17-Ketosteroids *Urine Decrease* Varies from low, normal to high. *0503*

Urine Increase Varies from low, normal to high. *0503 0151*

Urine Normal Varies from low, normal to high. *0503*

Acetoacetate *Serum Increase* Elevated levels. *2356*

Alkaline Phosphatase *Serum Increase* May indicate secretory activity of tumor. *2467* Increased bone turnover found in this condition may result in elevation. *0962*

Androgens *Plasma Decrease* Testosterone has been reported to be low in the presence of normal gonadotropin levels. *0433*

Calcium *Serum Increase* In 20 patients with active disease, gut absorption was greater than normal and positively correlated with both the elevated serum and urine concentration. *2161* Often noted, because of increase GI absorption. *0962*

Urine Increase In 20 patients with active disease, gut absorption was greater than normal and positively correlated with both the elevated serum and urine concentrations. *2161 0151*

Cholesterol, Very Low Density Lipoprotein *Serum Increase* Minimal elevation due to increased secretion. *0062*

Creatine *Serum Increase* Accelerated rate of synthesis may result in high serum and urine concentrations. *2104*

Urine Increase Accelerated rate of synthesis may result in high serum and urine concentrations. *2104*

Creatinine *Serum Increase* Increased rate of formation. *2467*

Urine Increase 0619

Fatty Acids, Free (FFA) *Serum Increase* May be elevated because of decreased lipogenesis. *0962*

Glomerular Filtration Rate (GFR) *Urine Increase* May be abnormally high. *0962 0433*

Glucocorticoids *Urine Increase* 0151

Glucose *Serum Increase* Overt diabetes is found manifested by fasting hyperglycemia. *0962*

Urine Increase Increase in glucose tolerance because of glycosuria. *0619*

Glucose Tolerance *Serum Decrease* Impaired in most patients with acromegaly and gigantism. *2468* In 50% of these patients, the oral administration of glucose will demonstrate decreased tolerance. *0962*

Gonadotropin, Pituitary *Serum Decrease* Serum and urinary gonadotropins may be diminished; azoospermia and amenorrhea may ensue. *0962*

Urine Decrease Serum and urinary gonadotropins may be diminished; azoospermia and amenorrhea may ensue. *0962*

Growth Hormone *Serum Increase* The definitive test for diagnosis an increase of 10 ng/mL, which is not suppressible by glucose. *0433* Usually basal levels > 20 ng/mL. High basal growth hormone levels and failure of suppression by glucose at 1 or 2 h are the definitive criteria for the diagnosis. *0962 0151*

Hydroxyproline *Urine Increase* Indicates secretory activity of tumor. *2467* Increased bone turnover found in this condition may result in elevation. *0962 0151*

253.00 Acromegaly *(continued)*

Insulin *Serum Increase* Large amounts of growth hormone have a diabetogenic effect. As a result, the basal plasma insulin values may be higher than normal, and their insulin response to a glucose load may be increased. *0962*

Insulin Tolerance *Serum Decrease* The blood sugar falls by < 25% of its initial value and rapidly returns to the fasting level. *0619*

Ketones *Serum Normal* The overt diabetes associated with acromegaly is frequently insulin-resistant and not associated with elevated ketones in the blood or urine. *0962*

Phosphate *Serum Increase* There may be a mild hyperphosphatemia, a reversal of the diurnal rhythmicity of urinary phosphate excretion, and an increased tubular reabsorption of phosphate. *0962*

Potassium *Serum Increase* *0995*

Prolactin *Serum Increase* Measured in 73 untreated patients and found to be elevated in 32%. *0521* Can trigger a mild to moderate increase (20-300 ng/mL). *2637*

Protein *CSF Increase* Occasionally seen; reflects the intracranial lesion. *0962*

Protein Bound Iodine (PBI) *Serum Decrease* *0619*

Serum Normal *2467*

Pyrophosphate *Synovial Fluid Increase* Has been identified. *2088*

Sodium *Serum Increase* *0995*

Somatomedin *Serum Increase* *1443*

Somatomedin-C *Serum Increase* *2634*

Specific Gravity *Urine Decrease* Usually 1.001-1.005. *0151*

T₃ Uptake *Serum Normal* Thyroid functions were all found to be normal in active disease, contrary to several earlier reports. *0458*

Testosterone *Plasma Decrease* Have been reported to be low in the presence of normal gonadotropin levels. *0433*

Thyroid Stimulating Hormone (TSH) *Serum Decrease* The expanding tumor within the pituitary fossa may cause a diminution of secretion of other pituitary hormones. Loss of thyroid-stimulating hormone will cause hypothyroidism. *0962*

Serum Normal Normal, even with thyroid enlargement. *0960*

Thyroxine Binding Globulin *Serum Decrease* *0062*

Thyroxine (T₄) *Serum Normal* Thyroid functions were all found to be normal in active disease, contrary to several earlier reports. *0458*

Tri-iodothyronine (T₃) *Serum Normal* Thyroid functions were all found to be normal in active disease, contrary to several reports. *0458*

Urea Nitrogen *Serum Decrease* In some patients, because of the high uptake of amino acids required for enhanced protein synthesis. *0962*

Uric Acid *Serum Decrease* Some patients. *2467*

Serum Increase Increased in some patients. *2467*

Zinc *Serum Decrease* Decreased. *2297 1308*

253.40 Anterior Pituitary Hypofunction

¹³¹I Uptake *Serum Decrease* *0995*

Serum Normal The thyroidal uptake is often inexplicably normal even when the patient is clinically hypothyroid. *0151*

17-Hydroxycorticosteroids *Urine Decrease* *0999*

Urine Normal *2467*

17-Ketogenic Steroids *Urine Decrease* Low or low normal levels are suggestive but not diagnostic. *2612*

Urine Normal *2467*

17-Ketosteroids *Urine Decrease* Low or low normal levels are suggestive but not diagnostic. *2612 0151*

Aldosterone *Plasma Decrease* *2467*

Urine Decrease *2467*

Androgens *Plasma Decrease* Decreased testosterone in hypopituitarism and hypogonadism. *0619*

Angiotensin *Plasma Decrease* Both plasma renin substrate and angiotensin are low and unresponsive to adequate stimulation *0103*

Calcium *Serum Decrease* *0503*

Serum Increase *0433*

Chloride *Urine Increase* Diminished tubular sodium reabsorption because of adrenal cortical steroid deficiency. The urine volume is increased, with loss of the normal diurnal variation, and an increased sodium and chloride concentration. *0619*

Cholesterol *Serum Increase* In some cases due to secondary hypothyroidism. *0433*

Chylomicrons *Serum Increase* Increased. *1380 1936 1948*

Corticotropin *Plasma Decrease* May be deficient and lead to secondary adrenocortical hypofunction. *2612 0995*

Cortisol *Plasma Decrease* Low or low normal levels are suggestive but not diagnostic. *2612*

Eosinophils *Blood Increase* With reduced adrenal cortical or pituitary function eosinophilia may be seen. *0433*

Follicle Stimulating Hormone (FSH) *Serum Decrease* Characterized by absent or reduced production and release. *1108* Compatible with stage of sexual development, not with age. *0399*

Glucocorticoids *Urine Decrease* *0151*

Glucose *Serum Decrease* May result from growth hormone and cortisol deficiency. *2612 0433 0151*

Glucose Tolerance *Serum Increase* Late hypoglycemia. *2467*

Gonadotropin, Pituitary *Serum Decrease* Decreased in secondary hypogonadism. *2467*

Urine Decrease Deficiency leads to amenorrhea and genital atrophy. *2612 0995*

Growth Hormone *Serum Decrease* Characterized by absent or reduced production and release. *1108* Deficiency may lead to dwarfism in children and contribute to hypoglycemia in children and adults. *2612 0995*

Hematocrit *Blood Decrease* In some cases slight anemia is seen. *0433* Reduced thyroid, adrenal cortical, pituitary or testicular function can produce anemia. The hematocrit is seldom < 30%. The RBC is normochromic and normocytic. *0433*

Hemoglobin *Blood Decrease* In some cases slight anemia is seen. *0433* Reduced thyroid, adrenal cortical, pituitary or testicular function can produce anemia. The hemoglobin is seldom < 9 g/dL. The RBC is normochromic and normocytic. *0433*

Leukocytes *Blood Decrease* With reduced adrenal cortical or pituitary function leukopenia may be seen. *0433*

Luteinizing Hormone (LH) *Serum Decrease* Decreased to values seen during follicular phase rather than luteal phase of menstrual cycle with galactorrhea amenorrhea syndromes. *2468* Characterized by absent or reduced production and release. *1108* Compatible with stage of sexual development, not with age. *0399*

Lymphocytes *Blood Increase* Marked. *0433* Relative lymphocytosis. *0995*

Phosphate *Serum Decrease* Hypopituitarism with growth hormone deficiency in children. *0619*

Potassium *Serum Normal* Usually. *0995*

Pregnanetriol *Urine Decrease* Decreased to values seen during follicular phase rather than luteal phase of menstrual cycle with galactorrhea amenorrhea syndromes. *2468*

Progesterone *Plasma Decrease* Decreased to values seen during follicular phase rather than luteal phase of menstrual cycle with galactorrhea amenorrhea syndromes. *2468*

Prolactin *Serum Decrease* Patients with pituitary tumors or postpartum pituitary necrosis will be found to have impaired prolactin and growth hormone reserve. *0999* Characterized by absent or reduced production and release. *1108*

Protein Bound Iodine (PBI) *Serum Decrease* *0151*

Renin Activity *Plasma Decrease* Both plasma renin substrate and angiotensin are low and unresponsive to adequate stimulation *0103*

Reticulocytes *Blood Decrease* Absolute count is decreased. *0433*

Sodium *Serum Decrease* May be 120 mmol/L or lower without symptoms of adrenal insufficiency. *0151 0433*

Urine Increase Increased output in Addison's Disease and hypopituitarism. *0619* There is diminished tubular sodium reabsorption because of adrenal cortical steroid deficiency. The urine volume is increased, with loss of the normal diurnal variation, and an increased sodium and chloride concentration. *0619*

Somatomedin *Serum Decrease* Dwarfism. *1443*

Testosterone *Plasma Decrease* Decreased in hypopituitarism and hypogonadism. *0619*

Thyroid Stimulating Hormone (TSH) *Serum Decrease* May be deficient and lead to secondary hypothyroidism. *2612* Characterized by absent or reduced production and release. *1108*

Thyroxine (T₄) *Serum Decrease* Low or low normal levels are suggestive but not diagnostic. *2612*

Urea Nitrogen *Serum Normal* Usually. *0995*

Volume *Urine Increase* Diminished tubular sodium reabsorption because of adrenal cortical steroid deficiency. The urine volume is increased, with loss of the normal diurnal variation, and an increased sodium and chloride concentration. *0619*

253.50 Diabetes Insipidus

Antidiuretic Hormone *Serum Decrease* Posterior pituitary insufficiency is signaled by the deficiency of ADH. *1108*

Bicarbonate *Serum Normal* *2467*

Chloride *Serum Increase* *2467*

Urine Decrease Urine chloride concentration is very low, but because of the large urine volume, the daily output is normal. *0619*

Osmolality *Serum Increase* If the water intake does not keep pace with the urinary output, there may be mild hypernatremia and a tendency toward serum hyperosmolality. *0962*

Urine Decrease Usually < 200 mOsm/kg. *0962*

pH *Urine Normal* *2467*

Potassium *Urine Normal* *2467*

Sodium *Serum Increase* If the water intake does not keep pace with the urinary output, there may be mild hypernatremia and a tendency toward serum hyperosmolality. *0962*

Serum Normal Normal or increased. *2467*

Urine Normal *2467*

Specific Gravity *Urine Decrease* Always abnormal. *0433* Polyuria and hyposthenuria. *2246* *0962*

Uric Acid *Serum Increase* Occasionally. *0893* *0962*

Volume *Plasma Decrease* *2467*

Urine Increase Large volume (4-15 L/24h) is characteristic. *2468* After ingestion of 1,000 mL of 1% sodium chloride the urine volume in normal subjects and in pathological polydipsia is 25% of the ingested fluid. In diabetes insipidus the excretion rate is unchanged. *0619* Usually > 3 L/day. *0962* Polyuria and hyposthenuria. *2246* *0151*

255.00 Adrenal Cortical Hyperfunction (Glucocorticoid Excess)

11-Hydroxycorticosteroids *Plasma Increase* Cortisol-binding globulin becomes saturated at the upper limit of normal for plasma cortisol, resulting in a disproportionately high unbound cortisol concentration. *0999* Increased free plasma concentration and failure to reduce secretion with dexamethasone. *2612*

Urine Increase Raised and relatively constant urinary excretions usually occur, but values may fluctuate from normal to elevated over a period of days. *0978* Increased in all forms of the syndrome. *2612* *0999*

17-Hydroxycorticosteroids *Urine Increase* Increased excretion of 17-OHCS and 17-KS is characteristic. *0842* Elevated values at a time when the patient is not under acute exogenous stress strongly favor the diagnosis. Confirmed by demonstrating nonsuppressibility of urinary 17-OHCS to low-dose dexamethasone. *1108*

17-Ketogenic Steroids *Urine Increase* Over 4 X normal in 50% of adrenal carcinomas, 15% of extrapituitary tumors that secrete ACTH, 3% of adrenal hyperplasias without tumors with Cushing's Syndrome. *2467* Diagnosis is confirmed by demonstrating nonsuppressibility of 17-KS to low-dose dexamethasone. *1108* Very high values suggest ectopic ACTH production or adrenocortical carcinoma. *2612* *0151*

Urine Normal May be normal in pituitary-dependent Cushing's syndrome. *2612*

17-Ketosteroids *Urine Increase* Characteristic. *0842* May be very high in Cushing's syndrome with adrenocortical carcinoma. *2612*

Urine Normal Usually normal in hyperplasia and adenoma of adrenal cortex. *2612*

Alanine *Serum Increase* Increased. *0094* *0269* *2149*

Alkaline Phosphatase *Serum Increase* Presumably due to excess ACTH. *0619*

Alpha₂-Globulin *Serum Increase* May be moderately increased. *2467*

Amino Acids *Plasma Decrease* Cortisol accelerates the catabolism of protein and stimulates the hepatic uptake and deamination of amino acids. *0151*

Androgens *Plasma Increase* Secretion may be increased and may be a factor in hirsutism, but virilization is rare. *2612*

Angiotensin II *Plasma Decrease* In 4 patients with Cushing's Syndrome values were extremely low in renal venous blood. *1331*

Bicarbonate *Serum Increase* Metabolic alkalosis may occur with potassium loss. *0962*

Calcium *Serum Increase* Some cases with osteoporosis. *0619*

Urine Increase *0503*

Chloride *Serum Decrease* *0995*

Cholesterol *Serum Increase* Slight elevations. *0503*

Cholesterol, Low Density Lipoprotein *Serum Increase* Moderate elevation secondary to increased conversion of VLDL to LDL. *0062*

Cholesterol, Very Low Density Lipoprotein *Serum Increase* Minimal elevation due to increased secretion. *0062*

Corticotropin *Plasma Decrease* Very low or undetectable in Cushing's patients with primary adrenocortical tumor. *2612*

Plasma Increase Loss of the diurnal rhythm, with 6 P.M. levels abnormally raised in spite of increased cortisol concentration. Secondary disease (pituitary) *0619*

Cortisol *Plasma Increase* Untreated patients almost always have concentrations in excess of 15 µg/dL at all times. *0151* All forms demonstrate some degree of autonomous secretion of excessive amounts of cortisol. *0999* Increased due to adrenal hyperplasia and adrenal neoplasia. *1450* Elevated night values or the lack of significant day-night variation is a consistent feature. *0978* *2612*

Creatine *Serum Increase* Increased formation. *0619*

Urine Increase Increased formation. *2468*

Dehydroepiandrosterone Sulfate (DHEA-S) *Serum Increase* *0046* *1692*

Eosinophils *Blood Decrease* Eosinopenia is frequent (usually < 100/µL). *2468* Patients with hypercortisolism often have neutrophilia, lymphopenia, and eosinophilia. *0962* Below 100/µL in 90% of cases. *0995* *0433*

Erythrocytes *Blood Increase* Mild erythrocytosis in some patients. *2538* *0151*

Erythrocyte Survival *Red Blood Cells Increase* *0999*

Globulin *Serum Decrease* May be decreased. *2468*

Glucocorticoids *Plasma Increase* In most cases of hypercortisolism, the baseline plasma and urinary corticosteroids are elevated. Loss of the normal diurnal rhythm is usually noted. *0962* Diagnosed by demonstrating an excessive secretion of glucocorticoid hormone. *1108*

Urine Increase In most cases of hypercortisolism, the baseline plasma and urinary corticosteroids are elevated. Loss of the normal diurnal rhythm is usually noted. *0962*

Glucose *Serum Increase* Frequently complicated by an insulin resistant diabetes. *2467* Abnormally high amounts of cortisol tend to raise the blood glucose. *0151*

Urine Increase Glycosuria appears in 50% of patients. *2468* *0433*

Glucose Tolerance *Serum Decrease* Decreased in < 50% of patients. *2467* Frequently abnormal. *0962*

Growth Hormone *Serum Decrease* Basal levels are often low and respond poorly to stimuli. *0962*

Hematocrit *Blood Decrease* Normal or occasionally slightly elevated unless a malignancy is present in which case it may be depressed. *0433* Patients with ectopic ACTH syndrome may be anemic. *0962*

Blood Increase Normal or occasionally slightly elevated unless a malignancy is present in which case it may be depressed. *0433*

Blood Normal Normal or occasionally slightly elevated unless a malignancy is present in which case it may be depressed. *0433*

Hemoglobin *Blood Decrease* Normal or occasionally slightly elevated unless a malignancy is present in which case it may be depressed. *0433* Patients with ectopic ACTH syndrome may be anemic. *0962*

Blood Increase Normal or occasionally slightly elevated unless a malignancy is present in which case it may be depressed. *0433*

Blood Normal Normal or occasionally slightly elevated unless a malignancy is present in which case it may be depressed. *0433*

Insulin *Serum Increase* *0619*

Insulin Tolerance *Serum Increase* The blood sugar falls by < 25% of its initial value and rapidly returns to the fasting level. *0619* *2468*

Isocitrate Dehydrogenase *Serum Normal* *2260*

Ketones *Serum Increase* *0619*

255.00 Adrenal Cortical Hyperfunction (Glucocorticoid Excess) *(continued)*

Leukocytes *Blood Increase* May be elevated as a result of the ability of glucocorticoids to increase circulating polymorphonuclear neutrophils. *0433* Mild neutrophilic leukocytosis. *0995 2467*

Lymphocytes *Blood Decrease* Relative lymphopenia is frequent (differential is usually < 15%). *2468* Patients with hypercortisolism often have neutrophilia, lymphopenia, and eosinopenia. *0962 0433*

Neutrophils *Blood Increase* Some patients have granulocytosis, lymphopenia, and eosinopenia. *0151* In many cases. *1108* If hypokalemia is severe. *0995*

pCO₂ *Blood Increase* Metabolic alkalosis may occur with potassium loss. *0962*

pH *Blood Increase* Metabolic alkalosis may occur with potassium loss. *0962*

Phosphate *Serum Decrease* Occasional hypophosphatemia as a result of high corticosteroid concentrations. *1287*

Potassium *Serum Decrease* Characterized by low serum concentration and hypertension. *1108* Severe hypokalemia and weakness are best explained by the enormous quantities of cortisol secreted by the hyperplastic adrenals. *0151*

Urine Increase There is excessive endogenous adrenocortical activity with increased potassium loss in the urine. *0619 0151*

Pregnanetriol *Urine Increase* Increased 17 OH-progesterone in recurring and cancerous patients. *1450*

Progesterone *Plasma Increase* Increased 17 OH-progesterone in recurring and cancerous patients. *1450*

Prolactin *Serum Increase* Can trigger a mild to moderate increase (20-300 ng/mL). *2637*

Prostaglandin E2 *Plasma Decrease* In 4 patients with Cushing's Syndrome values were extremely low in renal venous blood. *1331*

Protein *Serum Decrease* Cortisol accelerates the catabolism of protein and stimulates the hepatic uptake and deamination of amino acids. *0151*

Protein Bound Iodine (PBI) *Serum Decrease 2540*

Renin Activity *Plasma Decrease* In 4 patients with Cushing's Syndrome values were extremely low in renal venous blood. *1331*

Sodium *Serum Increase* Sodium retention and elevated blood pressure can occur. *0151*

Serum Normal Sodium retention leads to increased total body concentration, but serum concentration is normal due to water retention. *2612*

Testosterone *Plasma Decrease* Decreased in male patients. *1450*

Thyroid Stimulating Hormone (TSH) *Serum Normal 2467*

Urea Nitrogen *Serum Increase* A condition that may be associated with excessive protein catabolism. *0503*

Volume *Plasma Decrease* Polycythemia occurs in 10-20% of patients, due either to an increase in red cell volume or decrease in plasma volume. *1669*

Urine Increase Polyuria. *0995*

Red Blood Cells Increase Polycythemia occurs in 10-20% of patients, due either to an increase in red cell volume or decrease in plasma volume. *1669*

Zinc *Serum Decrease 0794*

255.10 Adrenal Cortical Hyperfunction (Mineralocorticoid Excess)

17-Hydroxycorticosteroids *Urine Increase* May cause high excretion with feminization and no Cushing's syndrome involved. *0999* Urine 17-hydroxycorticosteroids and 17-KS excretion levels are always within normal range in patients with aldosteronomas but may occasionally be elevated in more rare instances of primary aldosteronism due to adrenal carcinoma. *0995*

Urine Normal Urine 17-hydroxycorticosteroids and 17-KS excretion levels are always within normal range in patients with aldosteronomas but may occasionally be elevated in more rare instances of primary aldosteronism due to adrenal carcinoma. *0995*

17-Hydroxyprogesterone *Plasma Increase* Congenital Adrenal Hyperplasia. *2596*

17-Ketosteroids *Urine Increase* Urine 17-hydroxycorticosteroids and 17-KS excretion levels are always within normal range in patients with aldosteronomas but may occasionally be elevated in more rare instances of primary aldosteronism due to adrenal carcinoma. *0995 0999*

Aldosterone *Plasma Increase* If the secretion rate is elevated, it may be assumed that the patient has either primary or secondary aldosteronism. *0151 0433*

Urine Increase Increased on normal salt diet (not detectable on all days); cannot be reduced by high sodium intake and DOCA administration. Increased in primary and secondary hyperaldosteronism due to adrenal adenoma and adrenal carcinoma. *2468*

Ammonia *Urine Increase* In primary hyperaldosteronism, possibly due to hormone action on the renal tubule cells or to the associated potassium depletion. *0619* Exaggerated ammonia production results in a tendency to a persistently alkaline urine. *1108*

Angiotensin II *Plasma Decrease* In 8 patients with primary aldosteronism values were extremely low in renal venous blood. *1331*

Bicarbonate *Serum Increase* Most patients exhibit a CO₂ content in the range of 32-38 mmol/L. *1108* Metabolic alkalosis may occur with potassium loss. *0962 2467*

Chloride *Serum Decrease* May be seen. *0962* Depressed reciprocally with the bicarbonate elevation. *1108*

Serum Increase The electrolyte pumps respond to mineralocorticoids by conserving sodium and chloride and by wasting bodily potassium. *2540*

Chylomicrons *Serum Increase* Increased. *1380 1936 1948*

Cortisol *Plasma Increase* Untreated patients almost always have concentration in excess of 15 µg/dL at all times. *0151* All forms demonstrate some degree of autonomous secretion of excessive amounts of cortisol. *0999* Increased due to adrenal hyperplasia and adrenal carcinoma. *1450* Elevated night values or the lack of significant day-night variation is a consistent feature. *0978*

Dehydroepiandrosterone Sulfate (DHEA-S) *Serum Increase 0046 1692*

Hematocrit *Blood Decrease* An increased volume, with slight decrease of the Hct value, is usual. *1108 0962*

Hemoglobin *Blood Decrease* An increased volume, with slight decrease of the Hct value, is usual. *1108 0962*

Leukocytes *Urine Increase* Pyuria due to the predilection of potassium depleted kidneys for infection. *0995*

Magnesium *Serum Decrease* In many cases. *1108* If hypokalemia is severe. *0995*

pCO₂ *Blood Increase* Metabolic alkalosis may occur with potassium loss. *0962*

pH *Blood Increase* Metabolic alkalosis may occur with potassium loss. *0962* Metabolic alkalosis. *0995*

Urine Increase Usually 7.0 or higher. *0999* Exaggerated ammonia production results in a tendency to a persistently alkaline urine. *1108* An alkaline urine implies the presence of alkalosis, a characteristic finding in primary aldosteronism. *1108*

Urine Normal Normal or alkaline. *2467*

Potassium *Serum Decrease* Progressive weakness and lack of stamina due to potassium depletion are frequent complaints. *0433* Renal wasting leads to hypokalemic state. *1679* Characterized by low serum concentration and hypertension. Mean concentration < 3.0 mmol/L and is usually persistently in this range. *1108 0962*

Urine Increase Significant urinary potassium loss may be encountered despite hypokalemia. *0999*

Urine Normal Usually within normal limits in spite of hypokalemia and tissue potassium depletion. *1108*

Prostaglandin E2 *Plasma Decrease* In 8 patients with primary aldosteronism values were extremely low in renal venous blood. *1331*

Protein *Urine Increase* In the majority of patients. *0999* Negative to trace amounts. *0995*

Renin Activity *Plasma Decrease* Markedly decreased (normal or increased in secondary aldosteronism). It cannot be stimulated by use of salt restriction and upright posture to deplete plasma volume. *0725* Low value is essential for the diagnosis of primary aldosteronism. *1108* In 8 patients with primary aldosteronism values were extremely low in renal venous blood *1331*

Sodium *Serum Increase* Frequent, although not constant. *1108* May be seen. *0962*

Urine Decrease 2467

Saliva Decrease Low sweat and salivary concentration while total body exchangeable sodium is high. *1108*

Sweat Decrease Low sweat and salivary concentration while total body exchangeable sodium is high. *1108*

Somatomedin-C *Serum Increase* 2634

Specific Gravity *Urine Decrease* Less than 1.015 due to impaired ability to concentrate urine. 0995

Tetrahydroaldosterone *Urine Increase* Patients with primary aldosteronism can be shown at some time to have increased urinary excretion of aldosterone and/or tetrahydroaldosterone. 1108

Uric Acid *Serum Normal* In the absence of azotemia. 0995

Volume *Plasma Increase* An increased volume, with slight decrease of the Hct value, is usual. 1108

Urine Increase 2467

255.40   Adrenal Cortical Hypofunction

11-Hydroxycorticosteroids *Plasma Decrease* 0619

17-Hydroxycorticosteroids *Urine Decrease* Low for males in the diagnosis of Addison's Disease. 0999

Urine Normal 2467

17-Ketogenic Steroids *Urine Decrease* Markedly decreased. 2468

17-Ketosteroids *Urine Decrease* Markedly decreased. 2467 0999

Aldosterone *Plasma Decrease* Adrenal cortex destruction results in deficiency of glucocorticoids, androgens, and mineralocorticoids. 2612

Urine Decrease Decreased as a result of the progressive destruction of the adrenal cortex. 0619

Ammonia *Urine Decrease* 0619

Androgens *Plasma Decrease* Adrenal cortex destruction results in deficiency of glucocorticoids, androgens, and mineralocorticoids. 2612

Plasma Normal 2612

Antibody Titer *Serum Increase* Antibodies to adrenocortical cell in primary Addison's Disease. 1670

Bicarbonate *Serum Decrease* Dehydration and hypotension lead to prerenal impairment of renal function. 0433   Normal or decreased. 2467 0999

Serum Normal Normal or decreased. 2467

Calcium *Serum Increase* In most instances the clinical picture is not altered by the hypercalcemia. It is not clear in all cases that the hypercalcemia reflects an increase in ionized calcium since hemoconcentration may contribute to the elevation if nausea, vomiting, and dehydration are prominent. Hypercalcemia may appear, however, with acute withdrawal of exogenous corticosteroids. It usually vanishes promptly with small doses of steroids. 0999   0503

Chloride *Serum Decrease* 2467

Serum Increase 2468

Urine Decrease Inability of the renal tubules to reabsorb sodium chloride and water and relative inability to excrete potassium. 0619

Corticosterone *Plasma Decrease* Adrenal cortex destruction results in deficiency of glucocorticoids, androgens, and mineralocorticoids. 2612

Corticotropin *Plasma Increase* Results from the lack of cortisol-suppression feedback mechanism. 2612

Cortisol *Plasma Decrease* Markedly decreased (< 5 μg/dL) and fails to rise to more than twice this level 1 h after injection of ACTH. This is a reliable easy screening test to establish primary adrenocortical insufficiency. 2467   Adrenal cortex destruction results in deficiency of glucocorticoids, androgens, and mineralocorticoids. 2612 0433

Creatinine *Serum Increase* Dehydration and hypotension lead to prerenal impairment of renal function. 0433

Dehydroepiandrosterone Sulfate (DHEA-S) *Serum Decrease* 0046 1692

Eosinophils *Blood Increase* A total count of 50/μL is evidence against severe adrenocortical hypofunction. 2468   With reduced adrenal cortical or pituitary function. 0433   May be a relative lymphocytosis and moderate eosinophilia. 0962

Glomerular Filtration Rate (GFR) *Urine Decrease* Dehydration may result in hemoconcentration. 0962   Fluid depletion leads to reduced circulating blood volume and renal circulatory insufficiency. 2612

Glucocorticoids *Plasma Decrease* Baseline plasma and urinary corticosteroids will be low in Addison's disease. 0962   Adrenal cortex destruction results in deficiency of glucocorticoids, androgens, and mineralocorticoids. 2612

Urine Decrease Baseline plasma and urinary corticosteroids will be low in Addison's disease. 0962

Glucose *Serum Decrease* Patients with diminished glucocorticoid secretion commonly manifest low levels of blood glucose, and symptomatic hypoglycemia may follow a period of fasting. Occasionally, patients with glucocorticoid deficiency exhibit hypoglycemic symptoms late in the postprandial period. 0999   Fasting blood sugar may be low, and the glucose tolerance test may be flat. 0962   May occur due to insulin hypersensitivity in the hypoadrenal state. 2612

Glucose Tolerance *Serum Increase* Flat peak. Poor absorption from the GI tract (normal IV GTT curve). 2467   Fasting blood sugar may be low, and the glucose tolerance test may be flat. 0962   Curve is flat in adrenal hypofunction. 2612

Hematocrit *Blood Decrease* Reduced thyroid, adrenal cortical, pituitary or testicular function can produce anemia. Hematocrit is seldom < 30%. The RBC is normochromic and normocytic. 0433

Blood Increase Dehydration and hemoconcentration due to severe renal sodium loss. 2612   0433 0962

Hemoglobin *Blood Decrease* Reduced thyroid, adrenal cortical, pituitary or testicular function can produce anemia. Hemoglobin is seldom < 9 g/dL. 0433

HLA Antigens *Blood Present* HLA-DR3 present in 70% of patients versus 21% of controls. 2539

Leukocytes *Blood Decrease* With reduced adrenal cortical or pituitary function leukopenia may be seen. 0433

Blood Increase May be normal or increased with a tendency to lymphocytosis and eosinophilia. 0433   With relative or absolute lymphocytosis and eosinophilia in Addison's disease. 0999

Lymphocytes *Blood Increase* WBC may be normal or increased with a tendency to lymphocytosis and eosinophilia. 0433   May be a relative lymphocytosis and moderate eosinophilia. 0962

Magnesium *Serum Increase* 2467

Neutrophils *Blood Decrease* Neutropenia and relative lymphocytosis are common. 2467   0433

Osmolality *Serum Decrease* 0619

pH *Blood Decrease* Raised potassium concentration and metabolic acidosis usually occur. 2612

Urine Increase Normal or increased. 2467

Urine Normal Normal or increased. 2467

Phosphate *Serum Decrease* Acute adrenal insufficiency may be accompanied by hypophosphatemia (and hypercalcemia). 0999

Serum Increase 2467

Potassium *Serum Increase* Raised potassium concentration and metabolism acidosis usually occur. 2612   Normal in mild insufficiency, but in severe insufficiency, particularly of aldosterone, there are hyponatremia and hyperkalemia. 0433   0999 0962

Urine Decrease Inability of the renal tubules to reabsorb sodium chloride and water and relative inability to excrete potassium. 0619 0962

Urine Normal Normal or decreased. 2467

Prolactin *Serum Increase* Increased levels. 1887

Protein *Serum Increase* Dehydration and hemoconcentration due to severe renal sodium loss. 2612

Protein Bound Iodine (PBI) *Serum Normal* 2467

Renin Activity *Plasma Increase* Due to reduced plasma volume. 2467

Reticulocytes *Blood Decrease* Absolute count is decreased. 0433

Sodium *Serum Decrease* Normal in mild insufficiency, but in severe insufficiency, particularly of aldosterone, there are hyponatremia and hyperkalemia. 0433   Often occurs. 0962   Serum concentration may remain normal until a crisis, when sodium loss exceeds water loss. 2612

Serum Normal Normal in mild insufficiency, but in severe insufficiency, particularly of aldosterone, there are hyponatremia and hyperkalemia. 0433

Urine Increase Inability of the renal tubules to reabsorb sodium and water and relative inability to excrete potassium. 0619   2467

T₃ Uptake *Serum Normal* 2467

Testosterone *Plasma Normal* Androgen deficiency is not clinically evident because testosterone production is unimpaired. 2612

Urea Nitrogen *Serum Increase* Dehydration and hypotension lead to prerenal impairment of renal function. 0433   Dehydration may result in hemoconcentration. 0962   Fluid depletion leads to reduced circulating blood volume and renal circulatory insufficiency. 2612

255.40 Adrenal Cortical Hypofunction *(continued)*

Volume *Plasma Decrease* Fluid depletion leads to reduced circulating blood volume and renal circulatory insufficiency. *2612*

Urine Decrease Normal or decreased. *2467*

Urine Normal Normal or decreased. *2467*

256.00 Ovarian Hyperfunction

Apolipoprotein AI *Serum Increase* Estrogen effect. *0995*

Calcium *Serum Increase* Estrogen effect. *0995*

Ceruloplasmin *Serum Increase* Estrogen effect. *0995*

Chloride *Serum Decrease* Progesterone effect. *0995*

Cholesterol *Serum Decrease* Estrogen effect. *0995*

Copper *Serum Increase* Estrogen effect. *0995*

Factor II *Plasma Increase* Estrogen effect. *0995*

Lipoproteins, Beta *Serum Increase* Estrogen effect. *0995*

pH *Blood Increase* Progesterone effect. *0995*

Phosphate *Serum Increase* Estrogen effect. *0995*

Prothrombin Time *Plasma Decrease* *0995*

Sodium *Serum Decrease* Progesterone effect. *0995*

Thyroxine Binding Globulin *Serum Increase* Estrogen effect. *0995*

Transcortin *Serum Increase* Estrogen effect. *0995*

Volume *Plasma Decrease* Progesterone effect. *0995*

256.30 Ovarian Hypofunction

Apolipoprotein AI *Serum Decrease* Estrogen effect. *0995*

Calcium *Serum Decrease* Estrogen effect. *0995*

Ceruloplasmin *Serum Decrease* Estrogen effect. *0995*

Chloride *Serum Increase* Estrogen effect. *0995*

Cholesterol *Serum Increase* Estrogen effect. *0995*

Copper *Serum Decrease* Estrogen effect. *0995*

Creatine *Urine Increase* Creatinuria occurs with gonadal dysfunction in males and females. *2104*

Estrogens *Serum Decrease* Decreased in primary and secondary hypofunction of ovary. *2467*

Urine Decrease *2467 0619*

Factor II *Plasma Decrease* Estrogen effect. *0995*

Gonadotropin, Pituitary *Urine Decrease* Increased or decreased depending on whether it is primary or secondary failure. *2540*

Urine Increase Increased or decreased depending on whether it is primary or secondary failure. *2540 2467*

Lipoproteins, Beta *Serum Decrease* Estrogen effect. *0995*

pH *Blood Decrease* Progesterone effect. *0995*

Phosphate *Serum Decrease* Estrogen effect. *0995*

Pregnanediol *Urine Decrease* Decreased in amenorrhea. *2468*

Progesterone *Plasma Decrease* Decreased in amenorrhea. *2468*

Sodium *Serum Increase* Estrogen effect. *0995*

Thyroxine Binding Globulin *Serum Decrease* Estrogen effect. *0995*

Transcortin *Serum Decrease* Estrogen effect. *0995*

Volume *Plasma Increase* Estrogen effect. *0995*

256.40 Polycystic Ovaries

Androgens *Plasma Increase* Women with polycystic ovary had significantly higher plasma androgen levels than women with 'simple' amenorrhea both before treatment and during induction of ovulation. *1356*

Gonadotropin, Pituitary *Serum Increase* Elevated in polycystic ovary disease. *0879*

Luteinizing Hormone (LH) *Serum Increase* Elevated in polycystic ovary disease. *0879*

Prolactin *Serum Increase* Increased levels. *1887*

256.41 Stein-Leventhal Syndrome

17-Hydroxycorticosteroids *Urine Increase* *0503*

17-Ketosteroids *Urine Increase* *2540*

Androgens *Plasma Increase* Plasma levels of androstenedione and dehydroepiandosterone are elevated. *0995*

Androstenedione *Serum Increase* Plasma levels of androstenedione and dehydroepiandosterone are elevated. *0995*

Dehydroepiandrosterone (DHEA) *Serum Increase* Plasma levels of androstenedione and dehydroepiandosterone are elevated. *0995*

Dehydroepiandrosterone Sulfate (DHEA-S) *Serum Increase* *0046 1692*

Follicle Stimulating Hormone (FSH) *Serum Decrease* *0151*

Gonadotropin, Pituitary *Serum Decrease* *0151*

Serum Increase Slightly elevated levels of LH in Stein-Leventhal syndrome. *0151*

Luteinizing Hormone (LH) *Serum Increase* Slightly elevated levels. *0151*

pH *Blood Decrease* *1337*

Testosterone *Plasma Increase* On occasion. *0995*

257.20 Testicular Hypofunction

17-Hydroxycorticosteroids *Urine Decrease* Decreased with castration in men. *2467*

17-Ketogenic Steroids *Urine Decrease* Decreased with castration in men. *2467*

17-Ketosteroids *Urine Decrease* Decreased in primary and secondary hypogonadism. *2467*

Androgens *Plasma Decrease* Decreased testosterone in primary and secondary hypogonadism. *2467*

Creatine *Urine Increase* Increased formation. *2467*

Estrogens *Serum Increase* The average daily production of estrogen is increased and the circulating levels of estrogen are relatively constant. *0151*

Gonadotropin, Pituitary *Urine Decrease* Decreased in secondary hypogonadism. *2468*

Urine Increase Increased in primary hypogonadism. *2468*

Hematocrit *Blood Decrease* Reduced testicular function can produce anemia. Hematocrit is seldom < 30%. The RBC is normochromic and normocytic. *0433*

Hemoglobin *Blood Decrease* Reduced testicular function can produce anemia. The hemoglobin is seldom < 9 g/dL. The RBC is normocytic and normochromic. *0433*

Reticulocytes *Blood Decrease* The absolute count is decreased. *0433*

Testosterone *Plasma Decrease* Decreased in primary and secondary hypogonadism. *2467 2468*

259.20 Carcinoid Syndrome

5-Hydroxyindoleacetic Acid (5-HIAA) *Urine Increase* Diagnostic of a carcinoid tumor. *1108* Normally there are 2-9 mg/24h while levels up to 1 g/24h may occur in the carcinoid syndrome. *0962* 75% of 75 patients with this disorder had elevated levels *0719* Excretions > 130 mmol/24h is diagnostic provided walnuts and bananas have been excluded from the diet for 24 h. *2612* Usually associated with 5-HIAA urinary concentrations 25 mg/24h. *2404* Increased, usually when tumor is far advanced, but may not be increased despite massive metastases. Useful in confirming diagnosis in only 5-7% *2468*

Urine Normal Hyperserotoninemia with normal urinary 5-HIAA in ileal carcinoid tumors. *2404*

5-Hydroxytryptamine (Serotonin) *Blood Increase* Systemic symptoms appear only after metastasis to the liver; the serotonin released from the metastasis passes directly to the systemic circulation, avoiding hepatic metabolism. *0962* Carcinoid tumors differ widely in their ability to produce or store 5-HT. Excessive production remains their most characteristic chemical abnormality. *2199* Usually associated with an excess of circulating 5-HT. *2612* Serotonin and related products are the biochemical markers of this disorder. *2404*

Urine Increase Systemic symptoms appear only after metastasis to the liver; the serotonin released from the metastasis passes directly to the systemic circulation, avoiding hepatic metabolism. *0962* Carcinoid tumors differ widely in their ability to produce or store 5-HT. Excessive production remains their most characteristic chemical abnormality. *2199* Usually associated with an excess of circulating 5-HT. *2612*

17-Hydroxycorticosteroids *Urine Increase* May be 10 X normal. *0151*

17-Ketogenic Steroids *Urine Increase* *0151*

Albumin *Serum Decrease* Commonly observed in patients with carcinoid tumor. *1508*

Amino Acids *Plasma Decrease* Decreased tryptophan, valine, isoleucine, lysine and ornithine were found. All others were normal except methionine, which was elevated. The low plasma levels were not due to hyperexcretion, as urinary levels were normal. *0718*

Bilirubin *Serum Increase* Rare until extensive hepatic metastases occur. *2540*

BSP Retention *Serum Increase* May be seen in later course of disease. *2540*

Calcitonin *Serum Increase* Secreted in bronchial and intestinal carcinoid tumors. *1589*

Carotene *Serum Decrease* Secondary to malabsorption or steatorrhea. *2540*

Catecholamines *Urine Increase* Catecholamines and their metabolites have been elevated in the urine of some patients. This abnormality is unusual and to date has not been correlated with specific symptoms or origins of the tumors. *2199 1568*

Cholesterol *Serum Decrease* Secondary to malabsorption or steatorrhea. *2540*

Cortisol *Plasma Increase* *0151*

Fat *Feces Increase* Secondary to malabsorption or steatorrhea. *2540*

Glucose *Serum Decrease* *2540*

Glucose Tolerance *Serum Normal* *2540*

Growth Hormone *Serum Increase* Elevated. *0918*

Histamine *Urine Increase* Some patients with gastric carcinoids have been shown to have frequent and consistent elevations of histamine, which is inconsistently elevated in those with ileal tumors. Often seen in patients with gastric and bronchial carcinoids. *2199* Persistently elevated in gastric carcinoid tumors. *2404*

Isoleucine *Serum Decrease* Decreased plasma concentration, but normal urinary excretion was found. *0718*

Leukocytes *Blood Increase* In abdominal crises leukocytosis and thrombocytosis are usual. *0433*

Lysine *Serum Decrease* Decreased plasma concentration, but normal urinary excretion was found. *0718*

Methionine *Serum Increase* The only amino acid found to be increased, all others were decreased or normal. *0718*

pCO$_2$ *Blood Decrease* Hyperventilation may occur during the flush. *2540*

pH *Blood Increase* Hyperventilation may occur during the flush. *2540*

Platelet Count *Blood Increase* In abdominal crises leukocytosis and thrombocytosis are usual. *0433*

Potassium *Serum Increase* Severe hypokalemia and weakness are common, due to the enormous quantities or cortisol secreted by the hyperplastic adrenals. *0151*

Prostaglandins *Serum Increase* During a flush. *2040*

Protein *Serum Increase* Common and may add to the peripheral manifestations of cardiac failure. *1108*

Tryptophan *Serum Decrease* Due to increased production of serotonin by the tumor; may result in clinical pellagra. *0718*

Valine *Serum Decrease* Decreased plasma concentration, but normal urinary excretion was found. *0718*

Vitamin A *Serum Decrease* Secondary to malabsorption or steatorrhea. *2540*

260.00   Protein Malnutrition

17-Hydroxycorticosteroids *Urine Decrease* *2467*

17-Ketogenic Steroids *Urine Decrease* *2467*

Albumin *Serum Decrease* Usually 1.5-2.5 g/dL but may be < l g/dL. Correlates with the degree of fatty liver and of edema; becomes normal after 3 weeks of normal diet; standard test for diagnosis of kwashiorkor and to monitor response to treatment. *2468* Albumin, prealbumin and transferrin concentrations were found to be lower in cases of protein-energy malnutrition associated with infection than the corresponding values for a group of healthy preschool children. *2065*

Alkaline Phosphatase *Serum Decrease* Marked reductions are recognized characteristics. *0151* Decreased unless dehydration is present with marasmus. *2468*

Alpha$_1$-Antichymotrypsin *Serum Increase* Elevated in children with clinical protein malnutrition. *2067*

Alpha$_1$-Antitrypsin *Serum Decrease* Decreased. *1866 0042 1946 1947 2129* These conditions reduce activity *2633*

Alpha$_2$-Macroglobulin *Serum Decrease* Found to be lower in cases of protein-energy malnutrition associated with preschool children. *2065*

Alpha-Amino-Nitrogen *Plasma Decrease* Abnormally low. *0151*

Amino Acids *Plasma Normal* In starvation, the amino acid level in the blood does not usually fall below the normal fasting level. Protein level is maintained at the expense of body protein. *0619* Severe protein deficiency alters the qualitative pattern, not the total amount. *2104*

Ammonia *Urine Increase* *0619*

Amylase *Serum Decrease* Marked reductions are recognized characteristics. *0151* Circulating concentration appears consistent with the amount of structural damage to the pancreas, characteristic of kwashiorkor. *2104*

Gastric Material Decrease Activity is lowered almost to zero in kwashiorkor. *0151*

Beta-Amino-Isobutyric-Acid *Plasma Increase* In Kwashiorkor, there is an increase in beta-aminoisobutyric acid. During recovery ethanolamine is elevated. *0619*

Urine Increase Increased beta-aminoisobutyric acid and ethanolamine in urine of patients with kwashiorkor. *0619*

Beta-Globulin *Serum Decrease* Tends to be both relatively and absolutely decreased. *0151*

Calcium *Serum Decrease* Decreased in hypoproteinemia. *0503*

Carotene *Serum Decrease* Extremely low in children with kwashiorkor. *0151*

Cells *Bone Marrow Decrease* Normally cellular or slightly hypocellular, and the erythroid/myeloid ratio was decreased. *2538*

Ceruloplasmin *Serum Decrease* Moderate transient deficiencies in patients with nephrosis. *2467*

Chloride *Serum Normal* *2467*

Cholesterol *Serum Decrease* With protein malnutrition. *2468* In kwashiorkor. *0151*

Complement C1q *Serum Decrease* *1732*

Complement C1s *Serum Decrease* *1732*

Complement C2 *Serum Decrease* {793} {2522}

Complement C3 *Serum Decrease* All complement components except C4 and C5 were significantly lower in children with protein-calorie malnutrition: C3 and C9 were the most severely depressed. C5 was the only complement that was significantly higher in malnourished children than in normal children. *1732* C3 was the only fraction which is significantly diminished in marasmic infants. *0956*

Complement C4 *Serum Normal* All complement components except C4 and C5 were significantly lower in children with protein-calorie malnutrition: C3 and C9 were the most severely depressed. C5 was the only complement that was significantly higher in malnourished children than in normal children. *1732*

Complement, Total *Serum Decrease* Individual components of the complement system were significantly lower in kwashiorkor than in normal controls. *0956* All complement components except C4 and C5 were significantly lower in children with protein-calorie malnutrition: C3 and C9 were the most severely depressed. C5 was the only complement that was significantly higher in malnourished children than in normal children. *1732* Mean activity in children with kwashiorkor was significantly less on hospital days 1 and 4 than in control subjects. On day 8 it rose to normal, and by day 50 it was significantly higher than the controls. 11 (40%) evidence anticomplementary activity in their serum on either day 1 or day 4. *2298*

Copper *Serum Decrease* Serum, erythrocyte and urinary copper levels showed decline in marasmic malnutrition and kwashiorkor. Marked fall of serum and erythrocyte copper level in children suffering from kwashiorkor. *1140*

Urine Decrease Serum, erythrocyte, and urinary copper levels showed decline in marasmic malnutrition and kwashiorkor. *1140*

Red Blood Cells Decrease Serum, erythrocyte, and urinary copper levels showed decline in marasmic malnutrition and kwashiorkor. Marked fall of serum and erythrocyte copper level in children suffering from kwashiorkor. *1140*

Creatinine *Urine Decrease* Decreased 24 hour urinary creatinine. *0186*

Cystine *Serum Decrease* *0151*

260.00   Protein Malnutrition   *(continued)*

Epinephrine   *Plasma Increase*   Marasmic and normal weight infants excreted proportionally 3-4 X less epinephrine than norepinephrine (ratio: 0.20-0.38). Children with kwashiorkor excreted nearly similar amounts of epinephrine and norepinephrine (ratio: 0.88). In marasmus, norepinephrine may predominate and in kwashiorkor epinephrine may predominate, in the regulation of the metabolic adaptations to assure survival. *1877*

Erythrocyte Sedimentation Rate   *Blood Decrease*   With cachexia. *2231*

Factor VIII   *Plasma Decrease*   During 10 days of total fasting in healthy normal weight males, a reduction of plasma activity with a concomitant decrease in factor VIII antigen was found, without other laboratory evidence for a disseminated intravascular coagulation. *0632*

Factor B   *Plasma Decrease*   *1979 2356*

Fatty Acids, Free (FFA)   *Serum Increase*   *0619*

FIGLU (N-Formiminoglutamic Acid)   *Urine Increase*   Increased in some cases of marasmus. *2467*

Folate   *Serum Decrease*   *2468*

Globulin   *Serum Decrease*   Minimal reduction. *0995*

Serum Increase   Relatively high as a result of concurrent infectious process. *0151*   Slightly increased with marasmus. *2468*

Glucose   *Serum Decrease*   In kwashiorkor. *0151*   Decreased due to excess insulin resulting from deficiency in available glycogen. *0619*

Glucose Tolerance   *Serum Increase*   In kwashiorkor. *0151*

Growth Hormone   *Serum Increase*   Elevated fasting plasma concentrations in all groups of malnourished children. *1955*

Hematocrit   *Blood Decrease*   There may be moderate anemia. *0433*   Mild or moderate normocytic normochromic anemia occurs after 24 weeks of controlled semistarvation. *2538*

Hemoglobin   *Blood Decrease*   Mild anemia. *0433*   In infants and children, may fall to 8-10 g/dL of blood, but some children are admitted with normal levels, probably due to a shrunken plasma volume. *2538*   Mild or moderate normocytic normochromic anemia occurs after 24 weeks of controlled semistarvation. Fall was 11 g/dL in males and 9.5 g/dL in females. *2538*

Immunoglobulin IgA   *Serum Decrease*   *0503*

Immunoglobulin IgM   *Serum Decrease*   *2467*

Immunoglobulins   *Serum Increase*   Usually normal or increased despite protein deficiency in kwashiorkor. *2104*

Insulin   *Serum Decrease*   Decreased fasting plasma levels found in both marasmus and kwashiorkor but no significant difference was found between types of severe protein-energy malnutrition. *1955*

Iron   *Serum Decrease*   With kwashiorkor. *2468*   Usually low because of decreased transferrin concentration or actual iron deficiency. *2538*

Iron-Binding Capacity, Total (TIBC)   *Serum Decrease*   Albumin, prealbumin and transferrin concentrations were found to be low in cases of protein-energy malnutrition associated with preschool children. *2065*

Isocitrate Dehydrogenase   *Serum Increase*   *0619*

Ketones   *Serum Increase*   *0619*

Urine Increase   50 mg/dL; more common in children than adults. *0619 2467*

Leukocytes   *Blood Decrease*   Leukopenia with a mean count diminishing from 6,346 to 4,129/μL. *0995*

Lipase   *Serum Decrease*   Decreased with protein malnutrition. In kwashiorkor. *0151*   Circulating concentration appears consistent with the amount of structural damage to the pancreas, characteristic of kwashiorkor. *2104*

Gastric Material Decrease   In kwashiorkor. *0151*

Lymphocytes   *Blood Decrease*   Decreased total count < 1,500/μL. *0186*

Lymphocyte T-Cell   *Blood Decrease*   *0793*

Magnesium   *Serum Decrease*   Hypomagnesemia may occur. *2444*

Red Blood Cells Decrease   RBC concentration was decreased in 2 of 4 patients with prolonged malnutrition. *2469*

Methionine   *Serum Decrease*   *0151*

Nitrogen   *Liver Decrease*   The level of nitrogen in the liver of children with kwashiorkor is markedly decreased over that for children of the same age. *0151*

pH   *Blood Decrease*   The plasma pH tends to fall. *0619*

Urine Decrease   *2467*

Phosphate   *Serum Decrease*   Serum concentration generally remains normal but may decline to or slightly below the lower range of normal. *1287*

Phospholipids, Total   *Serum Decrease*   *0151*

Plasma Cells   *Serum Decrease*   Depressed. *2357 0659 0683*

Potassium   *Serum Decrease*   Potassium depletion is a major biochemical characteristic of kwashiorkor. *0151*

Urine Increase   Increased breakdown of the body cells, occurs with release of intracellular potassium. Carbohydrate intake (glucose 100 g/24h) greatly reduces the rate of cell breakdown. *0619*

Urine Normal   Increased or normal. *2467*

Prealbumin   *Serum Decrease*   Albumin, prealbumin and transferrin concentrations, as well as the level of alpha$_2$ macroglobulin were found to be lower in cases of protein-energy malnutrition associated with preschool children. *2065*

Protein   *Serum Decrease*   Albumin, prealbumin and transferrin concentrations, as well as the level of alpha$_2$ macroglobulin were found to be lower in cases of protein-energy malnutrition associated with infection than the corresponding values for a group of healthy preschool children. *2065   0151*

Protein Bound Iodine (PBI)   *Serum Decrease*   Occasionally. *2104*

Pseudocholinesterase   *Serum Decrease*   May be decreased in some conditions in which albumin is low. *2467*   In Kwashiorkor. *0151*

Reticulocytes   *Blood Decrease*   Normal or slightly decreased. *2538*

Sodium   *Serum Normal*   *2467*

Urine Increase   Normal or increased. *2467*

Somatomedin   *Serum Decrease*   *1443*

Somatomedin-C   *Serum Decrease*   Decreased *2634*

T$_3$ Uptake   *Serum Increase*   T$_3$ resin uptake is significantly elevated in the acute stage of kwashiorkor and returns to normal after 2 weeks of appropriate refeeding. *1123*

Thyroid Stimulating Hormone (TSH)   *Serum Normal*   In frank kwashiorkor, concentrations were within the normal range throughout the entire course of dietary therapy, indicating that the children remained euthyroid. *1122*

Thyroxine Binding Globulin   *Serum Decrease*   Decreased in nephrosis and other causes of marked hypoproteinemia. *2467*   In hypoproteinemias. *2104*

Thyroxine (T$_4$)   *Serum Decrease*   Decreased T$_4$ with hypoproteinemia. *2467*

Triglycerides   *Serum Decrease*   *2468*

Tri-iodothyronine (T$_3$)   *Serum Decrease*   Protein-calorie malnutrition in a group of 43 children aged 18-30 months was characterized by a sharp fall in T$_3$ concentration to 25-30% of the mean value in controls. This decrease was significantly more pronounced in kwashiorkor of recent onset than in long-term. *1122*   Mean serum reverse T$_3$ was elevated in patients with severe protein calorie malnutrition to 53 ng/dL. In the same patients after feeing treatment the value dropped to 22 ng/dL. *0394*

Trypsin   *Gastric Material Decrease*   In kwashiorkor. *0151*

Tryptophan   *Serum Decrease*   *0151*

Tyrosine   *Serum Decrease*   *0151*

Urea Nitrogen   *Serum Decrease*   Indicates decreased protein metabolism. *0186 0016   0151*

Uric Acid   *Serum Increase*   High in starvation, ketosis, and high fat diets. *1757   1283 0962*

Valine   *Serum Decrease*   *0151*

Vitamin A   *Serum Decrease*   Extremely low. *0151*

Vitamin B$_{12}$ *Serum Increase*   Usually increased with kwashiorkor. *2468*

Volume   *Plasma Decrease*   Normal or decreased. *2467*

Plasma Increase   Plasma volume expressed in mL/kg of body weight was increased. Dilution was a major factor responsible for the reduction in hemoglobin concentration. *2538*

Urine Decrease   In total colonic starvation. *0995*

Urine Increase   In semistarvation, polyuria of 2-3 L/day and nocturia. *0995*

Xylose Tolerance Test   *Urine Normal*   *2467*

Zinc   *Serum Decrease*   Decreased. *2297 2043*

265.00   Thiamine (B₁) Deficiency

Bicarbonate   *Serum   Decrease*   Respiratory alkalosis may occur. *0962*

Glucose   *Serum   Increase*   *0619*

Hematocrit   *Blood   Decrease*   Characteristic. *1108*

Hemoglobin   *Blood   Decrease*   Characteristic. *1108*

Oxygen Saturation   *Blood   Decrease*   *1108*

pCO₂   *Blood   Decrease*   Respiratory alkalosis may occur. *0962*

pH   *Blood   Increase*   Respiratory alkalosis may occur. *0962*

Protein   *Serum   Decrease*   Characteristic. *1108*

  CSF   Increase   *0619*

Pyrophosphate   *Serum   Increase*   Thiamine pyrophosphate is elevated prior to thiamine administration but falls rapidly after therapy. *1108*

Pyruvate   *Blood   Increase*   Acute advanced beriberi (vitamin B₁ deficiency). Many cases of alcoholic polyneuritis are due to vitamin B₁ deficiency. *0619*   In 16 of 17 untreated cases. *2350*

Thiamine   *Serum   Decrease*   *2468*

  Urine   Decrease   Urinary excretion of thiamine of 0-14 mg in 24 h has been reported in beriberi, and early signs have been observed with excretions of < 40 mg/24 h. *0151*

267.00   Vitamin C Deficiency

Albumin   *Serum   Decrease*   Decreased in scurvy. *0619*

Alkaline Phosphatase   *Serum   Decrease*   *0619*

Ascorbic Acid   *Serum   Decrease*   Plasma level of ascorbic acid is decreased--usually 0 in frank scurvy. Normal is 0.5-1.5 mg/dL but lower level does not prove diagnosis. *2468*   Not reliable for diagnostic purposes because tissue levels vary widely. Ascorbic acid assay of the buffy coat for the WBC and platelet count of this vitamin is more helpful, the normal level being 20-30 mg/dL. In latent or overt deficiency, this level falls to 0-2 mg/dL. *0433*

Bleeding Time   *Blood   Normal*   *2467*

Cells   *Bone Marrow   Increase*   Normoblastic hyperplasia in the bone marrow. *2538*

Erythrocytes   *Urine   Present*   Microscopic hematuria is present is 33% of patients with scurvy. *2468*

Fibrinogen   *Plasma   Decrease*   Moderate depression occurs in scurvy. *0619*

Folate   *Serum   Decrease*   Decreased. *0299 2357 0367*

Haptoglobin   *Serum   Increase*   Conditions associated with increased ESR and alpha 2 globulin; increases in collagen diseases. *2467*

Hematocrit   *Blood   Decrease*   Associated with anemia of normocytic, macrocytic, or hypochromic variety in about 80% of cases. *2538*

Hemoglobin   *Blood   Decrease*   Associated with anemia of normocytic, macrocytic, or hypochromic variety in about 80% of cases. *2538*

Iron   *Serum   Decrease*   Dietary iron deficiency is common. *2538*

Iron-Binding Capacity, Total (TIBC)   *Serum   Decrease*   In scurvy. *0619*

MCH   *Blood   Decrease*   Associated with anemia of normocytic, macrocytic, or hypochromic variety in about 80% of cases. *2538*

MCHC   *Blood   Decrease*   Associated with anemia of normocytic, macrocytic, or hypochromic variety in about 80% of cases. *2538*

MCV   *Blood   Increase*   Associated with anemia of normocytic, macrocytic, or hypochromic variety in about 80% of cases. *2538*

Occult Blood   *Feces   Positive*   May be positive in scurvy. *2468*

Reticulocytes   *Blood   Increase*   Normocytic, normochromic anemia with a reticulocytosis of 5-10%. *2538*

268.00   Vitamin D Deficiency Rickets

Alkaline Phosphatase   *Serum   Increase*   The earliest and most reliable biochemical abnormality; until bone healing is complete. *2467* Increased in active rickets, the degree of elevation corresponding to the severity of the disease. The average phosphatase in 9 cases of uncomplicated rickets was 0.75, with a range of 0.3-1.4. *2213*   Consistently elevated. *2246   0503 0441 0442*

  Leukocyte   Decrease   *0151*

Amino Acids   *Urine   Increase*   Decreased net reabsorption, probably due to increased circulating parathyroid hormone. *2246*

Calcium   *Serum   Decrease*   Decreased absorption in the gut leads to overproduction of parathyroid hormone and the resulting phosphaturia and hypophosphatemia. *1287*   Concentrations < 8 mg/dL are common. *2246   0999*

  Serum   Normal   Usually normal or slightly decreased. *2467   0433*

  Urine   Decrease   Low in the untreated state. *2246*

  Urine   Increase   In young persons. *0151   0503*

  Feces   Increase   Urine and serum concentration is low with high stool content. *2246*

Chloride   *Serum   Increase*   Mild acidosis and hyperchloremia may be observed. *2246*

Hydroxyproline   *Urine   Increase*   Increased formation of osteoid tissue results in hydroxyprolinuria, values will decrease with adequate therapy with vitamin D. *0962*

Parathyroid Hormone   *Serum   Increase*   Decreased calcium absorption in the gut leads to overproduction of parathyroid hormone and the resulting phosphaturia and hypophosphatemia. *1287* Increased in nutritional rickets. *1909   2246*

pH   *Blood   Decrease*   Mild acidosis and hyperchloremia may be observed. *2246*

Phosphate   *Serum   Decrease*   Decreased calcium absorption in the gut leads to overproduction of parathyroid hormone and the resulting phosphaturia and hypophosphatemia. *1287*   May be low, but usually not as severe as in vitamin D resistant rickets. *2246 0962*

  Serum   Normal   In some individuals, serum calcium and phosphate may be normal. *2467*   Normal or low. *2246   0433*

  Urine   Increase   Decreased calcium absorption in the gut leads to overproduction of parathyroid hormone and the resulting phosphaturia and hypophosphatemia. *1287*

Pyrophosphate   *Urine   Increase*   *0151*

268.20   Osteomalacia

25-Hydroxy Vitamin D₃   *Serum   Decrease*   Vitamin D deficiency. *0995*

Alkaline Phosphatase   *Serum   Increase*   In adults this test represents the single most sensitive indicator of active disease. The earliest biochemical alteration. *2467*   Persistently raised concentration despite evident relief of symptoms. *0441*   Typically. *2199   0503 0999*

Amino Acids   *Urine   Increase*   Aminoaciduria secondary to PTH excess is seen. *0999*

Bence-Jones Protein   *Urine   Present*   *0619*

Calcium   *Serum   Decrease*   Advanced and sustained vitamin D deficiency. Renal tubular acidosis, hypophosphatasia, and dietary deficiency or a failure of absorption of calcium and vitamin D as well as other causes of increased loss of calcium must be considered in patients with osteomalacia. *2467 0503*   Advanced disease. *2199 0999*

  Serum   Normal   In early stages, stimulation of skeletal mobilization of calcium compensates for the high renal loss or the low intestinal absorption. Serum concentration is therefore normal or low normal. *2199*

  Urine   Decrease   *0503 2467*

  Urine   Increase   Other factors than vitamin D in adults. *0503*

Glucose   *Urine   Increase*   Reflects variable degree of disturbance of proximal tubular function. *0995*

Hydroxyproline   *Urine   Increase*   Increased formation of osteoid tissue results in hydroxyprolinuria, values will decrease with adequate therapy with vitamin D. *0962   0999*

pH   *Blood   Decrease*   In systemic acidosis. *0995*

Phosphate   *Serum   Decrease*   Invariably low. May be the only demonstrable abnormality. *0151*   Osteomalacia resulting from PO₃ or Ca deficiencies may be associated with moderate hypophosphatemia. *1287   0999*

  Urine   Decrease   *0503*

Uric Acid   *Urine   Increase*   Reflects variable degree of disturbance of proximal tubular function. *0995*

269.00   Vitamin K Deficiency

Factor VII   *Plasma   Decrease*   Synthesized in the liver by a process that requires vitamin K. *0992*

Factor IX   *Plasma   Decrease*   Synthesized in the liver by a process that requires vitamin K. *0992*

269.00   Vitamin K Deficiency *(continued)*

Factor X   *Plasma   Decrease*   Synthesized in the liver by a process that requires vitamin K. *0992*

269.90   Deficiency State (Unspecified)

Albumin   *Serum   Decrease*   Serum concentration falls before other indicators change. *0619*

Alkaline Phosphatase   *Serum   Decrease*   Decreased in malnutrition. *2467   0503*

FIGLU (N-Formiminoglutamic Acid)   *Urine   Increase*   Some patients. *2467*

Glucose   *Serum   Decrease*   *2467*

MCV   *Blood   Increase*   Macrocytic anemia may occur due to vitamin B_{12} or folate deficiency. MCV > 100 fL. *0532*

Protein Bound Iodine (PBI)   *Serum   Decrease*   Decreased in malnutrition. *0619*

Pseudocholinesterase   *Serum   Decrease*   Low in malnourished patients (from starvation, anorexia, or debilitating disease) reflecting protein depletion and hepatic function impairment. The rise to normal levels parallels nutritional improvement and weight gain. *2441*

Triglycerides   *Serum   Decrease*   *2467*

Vitamin A   *Serum   Decrease*   *0619*

Xylose Tolerance Test   *Urine   Normal*   *2467*

270.01   Cystinuria

Amino Acids   *Urine   Increase*   Cystine, lysine, arginine, and ornithine are increased in urine. *0619*

Arginine   *Urine   Increase*   Characteristic. *2246*

Cystathionine   *Urine   Increase*   Has been reported. *0785 2246*

Cystine   *Urine   Increase*   Increased (20-30 X normal) with cystinuria. *2468*   Characteristic. *2246*

Glycine   *Urine   Increase*   *0786*

Lysine   *Urine   Increase*   Characteristic. *2246   2468*

Methionine   *Urine   Increase*   Has been reported. *1271 2246*

Occult Blood   *Urine   Positive*   *0995*

Ornithine   *Urine   Increase*   Characteristic. *2246*

Pyruvate   *Blood   Increase*   *0995*

270.02   Hartnup Disease

5-Hydroxyindoleacetic Acid (5-HIAA)   *Urine   Decrease*   Low; may represent a slight diversion of tryptophan from serotonin formation. *2246*

5-Hydroxytryptamine (Serotonin)   *Blood   Decrease*   Low; may represent a slight diversion of tryptophan from serotonin formation. *2246*

Alanine   *Urine   Increase*   5-20 X normal values. *2246   0995*

Amino Acids   *Plasma   Decrease*   Reduced about 30% due to increased excretion and reduced absorption. *2246*

Urine   Increase   Aminoaciduria is the single most important diagnostic finding; it is constantly present, even between episodes of symptoms. An increased urinary excretion of the monoamino-monocarboxylic amino acids with neutral or aromatic side chains, i.e., alanine, serine, threonine, valine, leucine, isoleucine, phenylalanine, tyrosine, histidine, asparagine, glutamine, and tryptophan is characteristic. *0433*   Usually at least a 10-fold increase. *2246   0995*

Feces   Increase   Closely mirrors the pattern in urine. *2246*

Saliva   Normal   *2246*

Sweat   Normal   *2246*

Ammonia   *Blood   Decrease*   *0433*

Asparagine   *Urine   Increase*   5-20 X normal values. *2246   0995*

Calcium   *Urine   Increase*   *2467*

Citrulline   *Urine   Increase*   5-20 X normal values. *2246*

Glutamine   *Urine   Increase*   Urine chromatography shows greatly increased amount of glutamine. *2468*   5-20 X normal values. *2246*

Glycine   *Urine   Increase*   5-20 X normal values. *2246*

Urine   Normal   *0631*

Histidine   *Urine   Increase*   5-20 X normal values. *2246   0995*

Indican   *Urine   Increase*   Large, but variable amounts excreted, almost entirely as indoxyl sulfate. *2246*

Indoleacetic Acid   *Urine   Increase*   Urine chromatography shows greatly increased amounts. *2468*   Almost all patients have an elevated excretion of indolic acids on some occasion. *2246*

Isoleucine   *Urine   Increase*   5-20 X normal values. *2246*

Leucine   *Urine   Increase*   5-20 X normal values. *2246   0995*

Nicotinamide   *Serum   Decrease*   From loss of precursor tryptophan. *0995*

Phenylalanine   *Urine   Increase*   5-20 X normal values. *2246   0995*

Porphyrins   *Urine   Normal*   *2246*

Feces   Normal   *2246*

Rheumatoid Factor   *Urine   Increase*   *0995*

Serine   *Urine   Increase*   5-20 X normal values. *2246   0995*

Threonine   *Urine   Increase*   5-20 X normal values. *2246   0995*

Tryptophan   *Serum   Decrease*   Reduced blood levels of tryptophan metabolites. *0151*

Urine   Increase   Urine chromatography shows greatly increased amount. *2468*   5-20 X normal values. *2246*

Tyrosine   *Urine   Increase*   5-20 X normal values. *2246   0995*

Uric Acid   *Serum   Decrease*   There is possibly a congenital tubular defect resulting in decreased reabsorption. *0619*

Valine   *Urine   Increase*   5-20 X normal values. *2246   0995*

270.03   Cystinosis

Alanine   *Urine   Increase*   Nonspecific pattern of aminoaciduria. Fanconi's syndrome. *0995*

Alkaline Phosphatase   *Serum   Increase*   With the appearance of rickets. *2246*

Amino Acids   *Urine   Increase*   Aminoaciduria with increased cystine. *0619*   May be masked by severely reduced GFR, so that total urinary amino acids are in the normal range. *2246*

Urine   Normal   Aminoaciduria with increased cystine. *0619*   May be masked by severely reduced GFR, so that total urinary amino acids are in the normal range. *2246*

Ammonia   *Urine   Increase*   Increased ammonium ion. *2246*

Arginine   *Urine   Increase*   Nonspecific pattern of aminoaciduria. Fanconi's syndrome. *0995*

Asparagine   *Urine   Increase*   Nonspecific pattern of aminoaciduria. Fanconi's syndrome. *0995*

Bicarbonate   *Serum   Decrease*   Metabolic, hyperchloremic acidosis. *0433*   Reflects renal bicarbonate loss. *2246*

Calcium   *Serum   Decrease*   Hypocalcemic, hypophosphatemic rickets resistant to the usual doses of vitamin D. *0433*

Urine   Increase   Secondary from acidosis. *0995*

Chloride   *Serum   Increase*   Metabolic, hyperchloremic acidosis. *0433*

Creatinine   *Serum   Increase*   Elevated with advanced renal disease as early as 2 y of age in some patients. *2246*

Cystathionine   *Urine   Increase*   Nonspecific pattern of aminoaciduria. Fanconi's syndrome. *0995*

Cysteine   *Urine   Increase*   Nonspecific pattern of aminoaciduria. Fanconi's syndrome. *0995*

Cystine   *Urine   Increase*   Generally increased in the same proportion as other amino acids. *2246*   Nonspecific pattern of aminoaciduria. Fanconi's syndrome. *0995*

Erythrocytes   *Urine   Increase*   As glomerular damage progresses. *2246*

Erythrocyte Sedimentation Rate   *Blood   Increase*   Usually. *2246*

Globulin   *Urine   Increase*   Over 50 X the normal excretion of light chain gamma globulin. *2460*

Glomerular Filtration Rate (GFR)   *Urine   Decrease*   Diminishes with advancing renal disease. *2246*

Glucose   *Serum   Normal*   *0995*

Urine   Increase   May be scanty and intermittent or profuse and constant. *0995*   Up to 5 g/dL. *2246*

Glutamic Acid   *Urine   Increase*   Nonspecific pattern of aminoaciduria. Fanconi's syndrome. *0995*

Granular Casts   *Urine   Increase*   As glomerular damage progresses. *2246*

Growth Hormone   *Serum   Normal*   Growth failure is characteristic even though growth hormone concentrations are normal. *2246*

Hematocrit   *Blood   Decrease*   Often significant anemia before renal failure is substantial. *2246*

Hemoglobin *Blood Decrease* Often significant anemia before renal failure is substantial. *2246*

Histidine *Urine Increase* Nonspecific pattern of aminoaciduria. Fanconi's syndrome. *0995*

Homocystine *Urine Increase* Nonspecific pattern of aminoaciduria. Fanconi's syndrome. *0995*

Hydroxyproline *Urine Increase* Nonspecific pattern of aminoaciduria. Fanconi's syndrome. *0995*

Isoleucine *Urine Increase* Nonspecific pattern of aminoaciduria. Fanconi's syndrome. *0995*

Leucine *Urine Increase* Nonspecific pattern of aminoaciduria. Fanconi's syndrome. *0995*

Lysine *Urine Increase* Nonspecific pattern of aminoaciduria. Fanconi's syndrome. *0995*

Methionine *Urine Increase* Nonspecific pattern of aminoaciduria. Fanconi's syndrome. *0995*

Ornithine *Urine Increase* Nonspecific pattern of aminoaciduria. Fanconi's syndrome. *0995*

pH *Blood Decrease* Metabolic, hyperchloremic acidosis. *0433* Marked acidosis. *2246*

Urine Increase Tends to remain alkaline despite systemic acidosis. *2246*

Phenylalanine *Urine Increase* Nonspecific pattern of aminoaciduria. Fanconi's syndrome. *0995*

Phosphate *Serum Decrease* Decreased serum concentrations will become normal and then elevated as renal deterioration progress. *2246*

Serum Increase Decreased serum concentrations will become normal and then elevated as renal deterioration progress. *2246*

Urine Increase Failure of tubular reabsorption. *0995* Usually increased excretion before renal disease is advanced. *0993* *2246*

Feces Increase Decreased intestinal absorption. *0204* *2246*

Potassium *Serum Decrease* Hypokalemia and severe intracellular potassium depletion can be most difficult problems, causing severe muscle weakness. *0433* Due to high urine potassium. *2468* Decreased serum concentrations will become normal and then elevated as renal deterioration progress. *2246*

Serum Increase Decreased serum concentrations will become normal and then elevated as renal deterioration progress. *2246*

Urine Increase *2468*

Proline *Urine Increase* Nonspecific pattern of aminoaciduria. Fanconi's syndrome. *0995*

Protein *Urine Increase* Frequent. *2246*

Pyruvate *Blood Increase* In some but not all patients. *2246*

Serine *Urine Increase* Nonspecific pattern of aminoaciduria. Fanconi's syndrome. *0995*

Threonine *Urine Increase* Nonspecific pattern of aminoaciduria. Fanconi's syndrome. *0995*

Tryptophan *Urine Increase* Nonspecific pattern of aminoaciduria. Fanconi's syndrome. *0995*

Tyrosine *Urine Increase* Nonspecific pattern of aminoaciduria. Fanconi's syndrome. *0995*

Urea Nitrogen *Serum Increase* Elevated with advanced renal disease as early as 2 y of age in some patients. *2246* *0995*

Uric Acid *Serum Decrease* Failure of reabsorption. *0995*

Urine Increase Failure of reabsorption. *0995*

Valine *Urine Increase* Nonspecific pattern of aminoaciduria. Fanconi's syndrome. *0995*

270.10 Phenylketonuria

5-Hydroxyindoleacetic Acid (5-HIAA) *Urine Decrease* *2468*

Amino Acids *Plasma Increase* Phenylalanine is increased. *0619*

Urine Increase Phenylalanine and ketoderivatives are increased. *0619*

Indoleacetic Acid *Urine Increase* *2246*

Phenylalanine *Serum Increase* Patients are clinically normal at birth, distinguishable only by hyperphenylalaninemia, which is established in the 1st postnatal week. *0151* Early diagnosis can only be made by determining the blood concentration. Rises to abnormal levels after the infant has received protein-containing feedings. *2246*

Urine Increase Early diagnosis can only be made by determining the blood concentration. Rises to abnormal levels after the infant has received protein-containing feedings. *2246* *0151*

Tyrosine *Serum Decrease* With normal phenylalanine intake. *0186*

270.21 Alkaptonuria

Homogentisic Acid *Urine Increase* Excessive amounts are excreted in the urine. The output is proportional to the amount of protein in the diet. *0619* All diagnostic tests are based on the presence of homogentisic acid in the urine. *2246*

Uric Acid *Serum Increase* *2104*

Urine Increase *2104*

270.31 Maple Syrup Urine Disease

Alloisoleucine *Serum Increase* Alloisoleucine, an amino acid not normally present in plasma, is elevated. *0433*

Amino Acids *Plasma Increase* The branched-chain amino acids valine, leucine, and isoleucine, are increased to 10-30 X above normal levels. *0433* Large excess of branched-chain amino acids and keto acids in blood and urine in the untreated patient. *2246*

Urine Increase Valine, leucine, and isoleucine are present in the urine. *0619* Large excess of branched-chain amino acids and keto acids in blood and urine in the untreated patient. *2246*

Glucose *Serum Decrease* Hypoglycemic episodes are probably caused by the high concentrations of leucine. *1797* *2246*

Indoleacetic Acid *Urine Increase* *2246*

Isoleucine *Serum Increase* Excessively high. *1797* *2246*

Urine Increase Greatly increased. *2468*

Leucine *Serum Increase* Excessively high. *1797* *2246*

Urine Increase Greatly increased. *2468*

Valine *Serum Increase* Excessively high. *1797* *2246*

Urine Increase Greatly increased urinary excretion. *2468*

270.41 Cystathioninuria

Amino Acids *Urine Increase* Elevated cystathionine. *0631* *2246*

Cystathionine *Serum Increase* *0151*

Urine Increase *0151* *2246*

Glycine *Urine Increase* *2468*

Methionine *Serum Increase* *2246*

270.42 Homocystinuria

Amino Acids *Urine Increase* Increased homocystine. *0631*

Homocystine *Serum Increase* Decreased rate of metabolism results in excessive concentration. *2246*

Urine Increase Decreased rate of metabolism results in excessive concentration. *2246* *0995*

CSF Increase *2468*

Isocitrate Dehydrogenase *Serum Increase* *0619*

Methionine *Serum Decrease* Low or low normal in homocystinuria caused by deficient 5-methyltetrahydrofolate-dependent homocysteine methylation. *2246*

Serum Increase In homocystinuria caused by cystathionine beta-synthetase deficiency. *2246*

Urine Increase *0151*

CSF Increase *2468*

270.51 Histidinemia

5-Hydroxytryptamine (Serotonin) *Blood Decrease* In the 3 cases in which serotonin concentration has been determined, values were found to be 50% of the normal concentration. *2246*

Alanine *Serum Decrease* *0995*

Urine Increase Moderate increase. *0831* *2246*

Amino Acids *Urine Increase* Slight increase in several amino acids other than histidine. *0831* *2246*

Ammonia *Blood Increase* Postprandial elevation. *0995*

Glutamic Acid *Serum Decrease* *0995*

CSF Decrease In some reports. *0831* *1065* *2246*

Glutamine *CSF Increase* In some reports. *0831* *1065* *2246*

270.51 Histidinemia (continued)

Histidine *Serum Increase* Quantitative amino acid analysis demonstrate plasma levels of histidine from 5-17 mg/dL (normal = 1-3 mg/dL). *0433* A marked elevation is the most consistent and characteristic finding. *2246*

Urine Increase Quantitative amino acid analysis will demonstrate urinary excretion which usually exceeds 300 mg/24h. *0433* Characteristic, but not as specific an indicator as the serum concentration. *2246*

CSF Increase Frequently elevated. Values of 2-10 X normal have been noted. *2246 0831 2448*

Imidazolepyruvic Acid *Urine Increase* Chromatography of the urinary metabolites of histidine will reveal the presence of imidazole pyruvic acid. *0433* Excreted in substantial quantities in the urine but no significant concentration was found in the blood. *2246 0151*

Urocanic Acid *Urine Decrease* Chromatography of the urinary metabolites of histidine will reveal an absence of urocanic acid. *0433* Reported to be absent from urine in several studies, but normal concentrations are low and methods of detection lack specificity. *2246 2570 1065*

270.61 Citrullinemia

Alanine *Serum Increase* Mild elevations have been found. *2246*

Amino Acids *Urine Increase* Generalized hyperaminoaciduria may be found in severely affected infants. *2246*

Ammonia *Blood Increase* Characteristic elevation. May rise to 400-1,000 mg/dL postprandial. *2246*

Citrulline *Serum Increase* Marked accumulation. Increased to 1-4.5 μmol/L, at least 40 X normal. Concentration does not correlate with severity of symptoms. *2246*

Urine Increase Ranges from several hundred mg/24h in infants to several g/24h in adults. *2246 2468*

CSF Increase Greatly increased. Ranges between 0.1-0.3 μmol/L (normal < 0.003). CSF concentrations are lower than in blood. *2246*

Glutamine *Serum Increase* Mild elevations have been found. *2246*

270.81 Hyperprolinemia

Amino Acids *Urine Increase* Hyperaminoaciduria of proline, glycine and hydroxyproline is specific. *2246*

Glycine *Urine Increase* Hyperaminoaciduria of proline, glycine and hydroxyproline is specific. *2246 2468*

Hydroxyproline *Urine Increase* Hyperaminoaciduria of proline, glycine and hydroxyproline is specific. *2246*

Proline *Serum Increase* Higher in type II than in type I. *2246 0995*

Urine Increase Hyperaminoaciduria of proline, glycine and hydroxyproline is specific. *2246 0995*

270.82 Hydroxyprolinemia

Amino Acids *Plasma Increase* Other amino acids (excluding hydroxyproline) are normal. *2246*

Hydroxyproline *Serum Increase* Elevated > 15-fold above normal concentration. *2246*

Urine Increase Greatly increased. Excretion rates of 285-550 mg/24h have been reported in patients aged 12-31 y. *1797 0629*

CSF Normal 2246

271.01 Von Gierke's Disease

Alanine Aminotransferase *Serum Normal* Liver may be massively enlarged but liver function tests are normal. *2246*

Aspartate Aminotransferase *Serum Normal* Liver may be massively enlarged but liver function tests are normal. *2246*

Bleeding Time *Blood Increase* Prolonged bleeding is a major clinical problem, probably due to impaired platelet function. *2246*

BSP Retention *Serum Normal* Liver may be massively enlarged but liver function tests are normal. *2246*

Cholesterol *Serum Increase* Striking elevation. *1086 2246* Significant elevations generally occur in the glycogen storage diseases. *2104*

Cholesterol, Very Low Density Lipoprotein *Serum Increase* Marked elevation due to increased secretion and decreased catabolism due to reduced lipoprotein lipase activity. *0062*

Chylomicrons *Serum Increase* Minimal elevation secondary to decreased catabolism due to reduced lipoprotein lipase activity. *0062*

Fatty Acids, Free (FFA) *Serum Increase* Due to hypoglycemia. *1086 2246*

Glucose *Serum Decrease* Decreased glucose due to excess insulin as a result of deficiency in available glycogen. *0619* Degree of hypoglycemia is variable. *2246* Usually low. *2104 0812*

Glucose-6-Phosphatase *Liver Decrease* Deficient enzyme in the liver. *2246*

Glucose Tolerance *Serum Decrease* Decreased tolerance:excessive peak decreased formation of glycogen with low fasting levels and subsequent hypoglycemia. *2467* Decreased because of inability to form glycogen from administered glucose. *0619* Characteristically diabetic. *1086*

Glycerol *Serum Increase* Has been observed. *1722*

Haptoglobin *Serum Decrease* Reflects chronic hemolysis. *0186*

Hematocrit *Blood Decrease* *0995*

Hemoglobin *Blood Decrease* *0995*

Insulin *Serum Decrease* Basal plasma concentrations were found to be 50-60% of normal in 5 older patients with type I. *1418 2246*

Insulin Tolerance *Serum Decrease* Increased insulin sensitivity may result in an excessive fall in the blood sugar in some cases. *0619*

Ketones *Serum Increase* Ketosis is characteristic. *1086* Increased, especially after fasting. *0619*

Urine Increase Children are more liable to develop ketosis than adults, especially after fasting. *0619*

Lactic Acid *Blood Increase* Striking elevation. *1086 2246* Significant elevations generally occur in the glycogen storage diseases. *2104*

Lipids *Serum Increase* Rarely is there an increase, which is associated with impaired carbohydrate metabolism and associated ketosis. *0619* Hyperlipidemia is a dominant feature. *1086* Total lipids are significantly elevated. *2104*

pH *Blood Decrease* Acidosis. *0962*

Phosphate *Serum Decrease* Mean fasting inorganic phosphate level was significantly decreased to 3.9 ± 0.3 mg/dL, (normal = 4.8 ± 0.3). Levels were further diminished by fructose and glucagon administration. *1960*

Phospholipids, Total *Serum Increase* Striking elevation. *1086 2246*

Pyruvate *Blood Increase* Striking elevation. *1086 2246*

Triglycerides *Serum Increase* Types I and VI glycogen storage disease. *0619* Striking elevation. *1086 2246*

Uric Acid *Serum Increase* Fasting blood levels were > 2 X normal mean; further significant increases occurred after fructose and glucagon administration in children. *1960* Hyperuricemia appears in early infancy, but rarely becomes symptomatic before age 10. May become a major problem in the adult. *2246 1086* Significant elevations generally occur in the glycogen storage diseases. *2104 1283 0962*

Urine Increase Mean excretion was 1.5 ± 0.6 mg/mg creatinine, slightly elevated compared to 0.6 ± 0.1 mg/mg creatinine in normal children. *1960*

271.02 McArdle's Disease

Aldolase *Serum Increase* Increases dramatically within h after strenuous exercise. *0970 2246*

Alpha-Glucosidase *Serum Decrease* Absence of activity in skeletal muscle or liver biopsy tissue or in the blood leukocytes. *1108 1097*

Aspartate Aminotransferase *Serum Increase* Slight to moderate increase. *0503*

Cholesterol *Serum Increase* Significant elevations generally occur in the glycogen storage diseases. *2104*

Creatine Kinase *Serum Increase* During myoglobinuric attacks. *0619* Increases dramatically within h after strenuous exercise. *0970 2246 0503*

Glucose *Serum Decrease* Usually low. *2104*

Serum Normal The blood sugar level, glucose tolerance, and galactose tolerance are normal, as is the response to injected glucagon and epinephrine. *1108* Type V patients are not hypoglycemic. *2246*

Glucose Tolerance *Serum Normal* The blood sugar level, glucose tolerance, and galactose tolerance are normal, as is the response to injected glucagon and epinephrine. *1108*

Lactate Dehydrogenase *Serum Increase* Slight to moderate increase. *0503* Increases dramatically within h after strenuous exercise. *0970 2246*

Lactic Acid *Blood Increase* Significant elevations generally occur in the glycogen storage diseases. *2104*

Lipids *Serum Increase* Total lipids are significantly elevated. *2104*

Myoglobin *Urine Increase* Transient attacks of myoglobinuria. *0619* Myoglobinuria appeared in > 50% of patients following episodes of exercise. *2246*

Uric Acid *Serum Increase* Significant elevations generally occur in the glycogen storage diseases. *2104*

271.03   Forbes Disease

Alanine Aminotransferase *Serum Increase* There may be some mild abnormalities of liver function. Elevations of AST and ALT are common, especially in Type III. *0433*

Aspartate Aminotransferase *Serum Increase* There may be some mild abnormalities of liver function. Elevations of AST and ALT are common, especially in Type III. *0433*

Cholesterol *Serum Increase* Concentrations vary from 200 to > 1,400 mg/dL. Extreme variability of cholesterol and triglyceride concentration is a diagnostic feature and in distinct contrast to the steady elevations in Type II. *0772* Increased in all 49 cases. *1631* Significant elevations generally occur in the glycogen storage diseases. *2104*

Glucose *Serum Decrease* Usually low. *2104*

Lactic Acid *Blood Increase* Significant elevations generally occur in the glycogen storage diseases. *2104*

Lipids *Serum Increase* Total lipids are significantly elevated. *2104*

pH *Blood Decrease* Acidosis. *0962*

Uric Acid *Serum Increase* Usually but not always. *2246*

271.10   Galactosemia

Alanine Aminotransferase *Serum Increase* Deranged liver function. *2246*

Albumin *Urine Increase* Manifestation of a renal toxicity syndrome. *1067*

Amino Acids *Plasma Increase* Frequent in patients receiving a milk diet. *2104*

Urine Increase General aminoaciduria - identified by chromatography. *2468* Manifestation of a renal toxicity syndrome. *1066*

Aspartate Aminotransferase *Serum Increase* Deranged liver function. *2246*

BSP Retention *Serum Increase* Deranged liver function. *2246*

Chloride *Serum Increase* Hyperchloremic acidosis. May be secondary to GI disturbance, poor food intake, or renal tubular dysfunction. *2246 1797*

Galactose *Serum Increase* Galactosemia (equal to total reducing sugar minus glucose oxidase sugar) with galactosemia. *2468 1067 2246*

Urine Increase Galactosuria--detected by nonspecific reducing tests; identified by chromatography with galactosemia. *2468* May be intermittent. *1067 2246*

Glucose *Serum Decrease* In children; following ingestion of galactose blood glucose falls (as blood galactose rises) to dangerously low levels. *0619 2467* On rare occasions. *2246* Replacement or destruction of functioning hepatic tissue may evoke hypoglycemia. *2104*

pH *Blood Decrease* Hyperchloremic acidosis. May be secondary to GI disturbance, poor food intake, or renal tubular dysfunction. *2246 1797*

Protein *Urine Increase* *2468*

Tyrosine *Urine Increase* General aminoaciduria - identified by chromatography. *2468* Manifestation of a renal toxicity syndrome. *1066*

271.20   Hereditary Fructose Intolerance

Alanine Aminotransferase *Serum Increase* Marked rise was noted within 1.5 h after a single large dose of fructose. *2246*

Albumin *Urine Increase* Characteristic symptom in small children. *0177* Develops rapidly after ingestion. *2246*

Aldolase *Serum Increase* Marked rise was noted within 1.5 h after a single large dose of fructose. *2246*

Amino Acids *Plasma Increase* Excess amino acids in serum and urine. *0151*

Urine Increase During acute intoxication, signs of a proximal tubular syndrome and of liver failure are common. *0433* Characteristic symptom in small children. *0177* Develops rapidly after ingestion. *2246*

Aspartate Aminotransferase *Serum Increase* Marked rise was noted within 1.5 h after a single large dose of fructose. *2246*

Bilirubin *Serum Increase* Noted with the chronic syndrome found in young children and after fructose administration in adults. *2246*

Fructose *Serum Increase* Noted with the chronic syndrome found in young children and after fructose administration in adults. *2246*

Urine Increase Noted with the chronic syndrome found in young children and after fructose administration in adults. *2246*

Glucose *Serum Decrease* The causes of hypoglycemia are complex and include impairment of glycogenolysis. *0433* Frequent severe attacks of hypoglycemia. *2246*

Urine Increase During acute intoxication, signs of a proximal tubular syndrome and of liver failure are common. *0433*

Methionine *Serum Increase* During acute intoxication, signs of proximal tubular syndrome and of liver failure are common. *0433*

Nitrogen *Serum Increase* Amino acid nitrogen increases as a result of deranged hepatic function after administration. *2246*

pH *Urine Increase* Abrupt loss of the ability to acidify urine after ingestion of fructose. *2246*

Phosphate *Serum Decrease* Noted with the chronic syndrome found in young children and after fructose administration in adults. *2246*

Serum Increase *0151*

Urine Increase Phosphate reabsorption is impaired. *2246*

Tyrosine *Serum Increase* During acute intoxication, signs of proximal tubular syndrome and of liver failure are common. *0433*

Uric Acid *Urine Increase* *0151*

271.30   Lactosuria

Albumin *Serum Decrease* A low serum albumin will reflect possible malabsorption of protein or protein-losing enteropathy. *0962*

Alkaline Phosphatase *Serum Decrease* An indication of vitamin D and calcium malabsorption. *0962*

Calcium *Serum Decrease* An indication of vitamin D and calcium malabsorption. *0962*

Carotene *Serum Decrease* A useful indication of fat malabsorption, low levels are found in as many as 80% of patients with steatorrhea. *0962*

Lactose *Urine Increase* Lactose intolerance in children and infants without lactase deficiency:lactosuria usually exists. *0433*

Intestinal Contents Increase Deficiency of intestinal lactase results in high concentration of intraluminal lactose with osmotic diarrhea. *0962*

Lymphocytes *Blood Decrease* Often an absolute lymphopenia due to loss of lymphocytes into the small intestine. *0962*

pH *Urine Decrease* Lactose intolerance in children and infants without lactase deficiency:renal acidosis usually exists. *0433*

Phosphate *Serum Decrease* An indication of vitamin D and calcium malabsorption. *0962*

Prothrombin Time *Plasma Increase* An indication of vitamin K malabsorption. *0962*

Triglycerides *Serum Decrease* Significantly decreased in the lactose malabsorption group (after taking into account the effects of other variables). Other lipids and proteins were not different from the control group. *2022*

Triolein ¹³¹**I Test** *Feces Positive* Positive test for lipid droplets in the stool, but results are inconsistent. *0962*

272.00   Type IIA Hyperlipoproteinemia

Albumin *Serum Decrease* Reduced, while the serum gamma globulin fraction is increased. *0619 2467*

Apolipoprotein AI *Serum Increase* *2246*

272.00 Type IIA Hyperlipoproteinemia *(continued)*

Beta-Globulin *Serum Increase* Marked increase due to primary xanthomatosis. *0619*

Calcium *Serum Increase* The greatest increment being in the protein-bound calcium form. *0503*

Carotene *Serum Increase* Increased concentration carried in beta lipoproteins are easily visible. *0992*

Cholesterol *Serum Increase* The plasma is clear even with extremely elevated cholesterol. *0962* Manifested by high cholesterol concentration in low density lipoproteins. Generally 2 X normal mean for heterozygotes and 6 X normal in homozygotes. *2246 1108*

Cholesterol, High Density Lipoprotein *Serum Normal 2614*

Cholesterol, Low Density Lipoprotein *Serum Increase 2614*

Cholesterol, Very Low Density Lipoprotein *Serum Normal 2614*

Dehydroepiandrosterone (DHEA) *Serum Decrease 0299 2356 2540*

Globulin *Serum Increase* Serum albumin is reduced, while the serum gamma globulin fraction is increased. *0619 2467*

Glucose Tolerance *Serum Normal 0962 0992*

Lipoproteins, Beta *Serum Increase* Characterized by an increase in beta-lipoproteins clearly visible on electrophoresis. *1108* Marked increase. *2467 0151*

Lipoproteins, Prebeta *Serum Normal 0503*

Phospholipids, Total *Serum Increase* Moderate elevation in heterozygotes and marked in homozygotes. *2246* Elevated, but not as high as cholesterol. *0992*

Triglycerides *Serum Increase* Usually a marked elevation of plasma cholesterol and a modest elevation of plasma triglyceride. *1108* Normal to elevated at 100-400 mg/dL. *0962* Occasionally. Usually normal in heterozygotes but may at times be > 250 mg/dL. *2246 0433*

Uric Acid *Serum Increase* Common. *0992*

Serum Normal 0962

272.10 Type IV Hyperlipoproteinemia

Cholesterol *Serum Increase* An increase in cholesterol of about 1 mg/dL for each 5 mg/dL increase in triglyceride concentration. *0773* The percentage of esterified cholesterol in plasma and the esterification rate were always reduced when the triglyceride concentration exceeded 600 mg/dL and the rate of esterification rose significantly with appropriate triglyceride-lowering therapy in patients with hypertriglyceridemia. *0897 0151 0962*

Serum Normal Usually found to be normal or only moderately elevated. *1108 0151*

Cholesterol, High Density Lipoprotein *Serum Decrease* Decreased. {0131,1519,2556}

Cholesterol, Low Density Lipoprotein *Serum Normal 2614*

Cholesterol, Very Low Density Lipoprotein *Serum Increase 2614*

Dehydroepiandrosterone (DHEA) *Serum Decrease 0299 2356 2540*

Gamma Glutamyl Transferase (GGT) *Serum Increase* Both GGT and pseudocholinesterase were increased in hypertriglyceridemic subjects. Both strongly correlated with the logarithm of serum triglyceride and the prebeta electrophoretic fraction. Increase of GGT was rather characteristic for gross hypertriglyceridemia. *0480*

Glucagon *Plasma Increase 0619*

Glucose *Serum Increase* Hyperglycemia is only occasionally severe enough to produce symptoms of diabetes. *0151*

Glucose Tolerance *Serum Decrease* Present in 19 of 36 patients (52%). *0855* Occurs in most patients but not with sufficient constancy to indicate a role in causing the disorder. *2246 0995*

Hemoglobin A$_{1C}$ *Blood Increase* Triglyceride concentrations greater than 1750 mg/dL would falsely raise the HbA1 levels. *1498*

Insulin *Serum Increase* Occurs in most patients but not with sufficient constancy to indicate a role in causing the disorder. *2246*

Lipoproteins, Prebeta *Serum Increase* Type IV hyperlipemia is manifested as hyper-prebeta-lipoproteinemia. This is associated with an increase in triglycerides above normal limits and is commonly accompanied by a rise in cholesterol of about 1 mg/dL for each 5 mg/dL increase in triglyceride concentration. *0773* Characteristic lipid abnormality is an increase in plasma triglyceride and VLDL cholesterol levels. *1108* Prebeta-lipoproteins alone are generally increased. *0151*

Plasma Cells *Serum Increase* Elevated *2357 0659 0683*

Pseudocholinesterase *Serum Increase* Both GGT and pseudocholinesterase were increased in hypertriglyceridemic subjects. Both strongly correlated with the logarithm of serum triglyceride and the prebeta electrophoretic fraction. Increase of GGT was rather characteristic for gross hypertriglyceridemia. *0480*

Triglycerides *Serum Increase* Seldom exceeds 1000 mg/dL. Cholesterol is usually < half when triglyceride exceeds 500 mg/dL. *0433* Characteristic increase in plasma triglyceride and VLDL cholesterol levels. *1108* Elevated, sometimes to an extreme degree. *0962* Values of 200-500 mg/dL are common. *2246 0999*

Uric Acid *Serum Increase* Hyperuricemia is common. *0151* 9 of 22 patients. *2246* Occurs in most patients but not with sufficient constancy to indicate a role in causing the disorder. *2246 0962*

272.21 Type IIB Hyperlipoproteinemia

Albumin *Serum Decrease* Reduced, while the serum gamma globulin fraction is increased. *0619 2467*

Alpha$_1$-Antitrypsin *Serum Increase 2246*

Beta-Globulin *Serum Increase* Marked increase due to primary xanthomatosis. *0619*

Calcium *Serum Increase* The greatest increment being in the protein-bound calcium form. *0503*

Carotene *Serum Increase* Increased concentration carried in beta lipoproteins are easily visible. *0992*

Cholesterol *Serum Increase* The plasma is clear even with extremely elevated cholesterol. *0962* Manifested by high cholesterol concentration in low density lipoproteins. Generally 2 X normal mean for heterozygotes and 6 X normal in homozygotes. *2246 1108*

Cholesterol, High Density Lipoprotein *Serum Normal 2614*

Cholesterol, Low Density Lipoprotein *Serum Increase* Serum cholesterol level is elevated, equal to, or greater than the triglyceride level; both LDL and VLDL are increased. *0151 2614*

Cholesterol, Very Low Density Lipoprotein *Serum Increase* Serum cholesterol level is elevated, equal to,or greater than triglyceride level Both LDL and VLDL are increased. *0151 2614*

Dehydroepiandrosterone (DHEA) *Serum Decrease 0299 2356 2540*

Globulin *Serum Increase* Serum albumin is reduced, while the serum gamma globulin fraction is increased. *0619 2467 0088*

Glucose Tolerance *Serum Normal 0962 0992*

Lipoproteins, Beta *Serum Increase* Serum cholesterol level is elevated, equal to or > triglyceride level, both LDL and VLDL are increased. *0151* Characterized by an increase in beta-lipoproteins clearly visible on electrophoresis. *1108* Marked increase. *2467*

Lipoproteins, Prebeta *Serum Increase* May be elevated. *0992*

Phospholipids, Total *Serum Increase* Moderate elevation in heterozygotes and marked in homozygotes. *2246* Elevated, but not as high as cholesterol. *0992*

Triglycerides *Serum Increase* Serum cholesterol and triglycerides are usually elevated to a similar extent. Neither generally exceeds 400 mg/dL and triglyceride levels are not more than 100 mg/dL higher than cholesterol levels. *0433*

Serum Normal Normal to elevated at 100-400 mg/dL. *0962* Occasionally. Usually normal in heterozygotes but may at times be > 250 mg/dL. *2246* Occasionally normal. *0995*

Uric Acid *Serum Increase* Common. *0992*

Serum Normal 0962

272.22 Type III Hyperlipoproteinemia

Alpha$_1$-Lipoprotein *Serum Decrease* There is generally a decrease in alpha and beta lipoproteins. *0774*

Apolipoprotein AI *Serum Decrease* There is generally a decrease in alpha and beta lipoproteins. *0774* An excess of lipoproteins with beta mobility but abnormally low density. *0772* Decreased concentration of both low and high density lipoproteins. *1631* Slight to moderately decreased. *2246*

Beta-Globulin *Serum Increase* Marked increase due to essential hyperlipemia. *0619*

Cholesterol *Serum Increase* Usually > 300 mg/dL. *2246*

Cholesterol, High Density Lipoprotein *Serum Normal 2614*

Cholesterol, Low Density Lipoprotein *Serum Increase 2614*

Cholesterol, Very Low Density Lipoprotein *Serum Increase 2614*

Dehydroepiandrosterone (DHEA) *Serum Decrease 0299 2356 2540*

Glucagon *Plasma Increase 0619*

Glucose *Serum Increase* Fasting hyperglycemia and ketosis are uncommon. *2246*

Glucose Tolerance *Serum Decrease* In roughly 55% of cases. *2246*

Ketones *Serum Increase* Fasting hyperglycemia and ketosis are uncommon. *2246*

Lipids *Serum Increase* Diagnosis of abnormal lipoproteins can be done when the lipids are at normal concentration, but most patients are hyperlipidemic before they are diagnosed. *2246*

Lipoproteins, Beta *Serum Decrease* There is generally a decrease in alpha and beta lipoproteins. *0774* Slight to moderately decreased. *2246 0772 1631*

Lipoproteins, Prebeta *Serum Increase* An increase in very low density lipoproteins of abnormal composition is the basis for type III diagnosis. *1631* VLDL defined as including all lipoproteins of density < 1.006. *2246*

Triglycerides *Serum Increase* Cholesterol and triglycerides are usually elevated to a similar extent; levels often exceed 400 mg/dL. *0433* Increased in all 49 cases of type III. *1631* Usually range from 200-800, and tend to exceed cholesterol. *2246*

Uric Acid *Serum Increase* 15-20% of patients. *0619* In 40% of patients. *2246 0915*

272.31   Type I Hyperlipoproteinemia

Alanine Aminotransferase *Serum Normal 2246*

Alpha₁-Lipoprotein *Serum Decrease* There is generally a decrease in alpha and beta lipoproteins. *0774*

Amylase *Serum Increase* During bouts of abdominal pain. *2246*

Apolipoprotein AI *Serum Decrease* There is generally a decrease in alpha and beta lipoproteins in hyperlipoproteinemia. *0774* Decreased concentration of both low and high density lipoproteins. *1631 0772*

Aspartate Aminotransferase *Serum Normal 2246*

Beta-Globulin *Serum Increase* Marked increase due to essential hyperlipemia. *0619*

Carotene *Serum Increase 2467*

Cholesterol *Serum Increase* Moderate elevation. *0433*

Cholesterol, Free *Serum Increase* The proportion of free cholesterol is elevated to about 50% instead of 30%. *0774* The unesterified cholesterol proportion may be as high as 50%. *2246*

Cholesterol, High Density Lipoprotein *Serum Decrease 2614*

Cholesterol, Low Density Lipoprotein *Serum Normal 2614*

Cholesterol, Very Low Density Lipoprotein *Serum Normal 2614*

Chylomicrons *Serum Increase* Chylomicronemia develops as soon as fat is ingested, and the disorder has been diagnosed during the 1st week of life. *0151* Characterized by the presence of chylomicrons in high concentration in plasma 14 h or more after the last meal of normal diet. *0774* Heavy chylomicronemia and subnormal concentrations of all other lipoproteins. A qualitative abnormality which is not a specific marker for a single genetic disease. Occurs in familial lipoprotein lipase deficiency. *2246*

Dehydroepiandrosterone (DHEA) *Serum Decrease 0299 2356 2540*

Glucose Tolerance *Serum Decrease* May follow pancreatitis, but is not a feature of uncomplicated disease. *2246*

Hematocrit *Blood Normal 2246*

Hemoglobin *Blood Normal 2246*

Hemoglobin A₁c *Blood Increase* Triglyceride concentrations greater than 1750 mg/dL would falsely raise the HbA1 levels. *1498*

Lactate Dehydrogenase *Serum Normal 2246*

Lipase *Serum Increase* During bouts of abdominal pain. *2246*

Lipoproteins *Serum Decrease* Heavy chylomicronemia and subnormal concentrations of all other lipoproteins. (Type I hyperlipoproteinemia) is a qualitative abnormality which is not a specific marker for a single genetic disease. Occurs in familial lipoprotein lipase deficiency. *2246*

Lipoproteins, Beta *Serum Decrease* There is generally a decrease in alpha and beta lipoproteins. *0774 0772 1631*

Lipoproteins, Prebeta *Serum Decrease* Normal or decreased. *0503*

Serum Increase May be raised. *0995*

Oxygen Saturation *Blood Increase* Hemoglobin-oxygen affinity is increased. *0568*

Triglycerides *Serum Increase* Often exceed 1,000 mg/dL with only moderate elevation of cholesterol. *0433* Grossly elevated, range from 2,500-12,000 mg/dL in lipoprotein lipase deficiency. *2246 0915 2177 0619 0151*

272.32   Type V Hyperlipoproteinemia

Alpha₁-Lipoprotein *Serum Decrease* Hyperprebeta-lipoproteinemia accompanied by low alpha and beta lipoproteins. *2177*

Amylase *Serum Increase* During bouts of abdominal pain. *2246*

Apolipoprotein AI *Serum Decrease* Reduced pools of alpha and beta lipoproteins. *2177* In severe affected patients. *2246*

Cholesterol *Serum Increase* In 11 patients with Type V hyperlipoproteinemia, concentration ranged from 212-1,512 mg/dL. *2177* Usually abnormally high, although initial normal values are frequently found. *2246*

Cholesterol, High Density Lipoprotein *Serum Decrease 2614*

Cholesterol, Low Density Lipoprotein *Serum Normal 2614*

Cholesterol, Very Low Density Lipoprotein *Serum Increase 2614*

Chylomicrons *Serum Increase* In severely affected patients. *2246* Chylomicronemia and hyperprebeta-lipoproteinemia. *2177*

Dehydroepiandrosterone (DHEA) *Serum Decrease 0299 2356 2540*

Glucose *Serum Increase 0995*

Glucose Tolerance *Serum Decrease* More than 75% of patients. *0855* Abnormal in 80%. *2246*

Hemoglobin A₁c *Blood Increase* Triglyceride concentrations greater than 1750 mg/dL would falsely raise the HbA1 levels. *1498*

Lipase *Serum Increase* During bouts of abdominal pain. *2246*

Lipoproteins, Beta *Serum Decrease* In severely affected patients. *2246* Chylomicronemia and hyperprebeta-lipoproteinemia were accompanied by reduction in pools of beta and alpha lipoproteins. *2177*

Lipoproteins, Prebeta *Serum Increase* In severely affected patients. *2246* Hyperprebeta-lipoproteinemia accompanied by low alpha and beta lipoproteinemia. *2177*

Sodium *Serum Decrease* Lipemia was associated with significant hyponatremia. *2177*

Triglycerides *Serum Increase* In 11 patients with type V hyperlipoproteinemia. *2177* Averages 10-20 X normal. *2246*

Uric Acid *Serum Increase* Common in type V. *0915* In 40% of patients. *2246*

272.51   Tangier Disease

Apolipoprotein AI *Serum Decrease* Almost none. *0151* Congenital absence or gross reduction. *0619 2467* Electrophoretically absent, irrespective of the medium used. *2246*

Carotene *Serum Decrease* Tends to be low, probably due to the absence of high and low density lipoproteins, not malabsorption. *2246* Occasionally low. *0878*

Cholesterol *Serum Decrease* Ranges from 30-125 mg/dL. *2246* Unique combination of low cholesterol and high triglycerides is indicative. Ranges from 40-125 mg/dL.

Red Blood Cells Normal 2246

Chylomicrons *Serum Increase* Frequently. *2246*

Lipoproteins, Beta *Serum Decrease* Levels tend to be reduced. *0151*

Partial Thromboplastin Time *Plasma Increase* Occasionally prolonged PTT, with normal prothrombin time. *2246*

Phospholipids, Total *Serum Decrease* Typically 30-50% below normal. *2246 1292*

272.51 Tangier Disease *(continued)*

Phospholipids, Total *(continued)*
Red Blood Cells Normal 2246

Prothrombin Time *Plasma Normal* Occasionally prolonged PTT, with normal prothrombin time. *2246*

Triglycerides *Serum Increase* Slight increase in homozygotes. *0151* Range from 150-330 mg/dL. *2246* Unique combination of low cholesterol and high triglycerides is indicative. *2246 0999*

Serum Normal Some patients. *2246* May be normal in the postabsorptive state. *2246*

Vitamin A *Serum Decrease* Occasionally low. *0878*
Serum Normal 2246

Vitamin E (Tocopherol) *Serum Decrease* One subject. *2246*

272.52 Abetalipoproteinemia

Alanine Aminotransferase *Serum Increase* Two subjects. *2246*

Apolipoprotein AI *Serum Increase* Highly variable. *2246*
Serum Normal 0878

Apolipoprotein B *Serum Decrease 0062*

Bilirubin *Serum Increase* Reflects increased RBC turnover. *1583*

Carotene *Serum Decrease* Very low. *0878*

Cholesterol *Serum Decrease* Diagnosis is established by finding very low cholesterol concentration (about 50 mg/dL). The lowest serum cholesterol level in any disease. *0619* Markedly reduced. Averages < 50 mg/dL. *0172 2246 0999*

Cholesterol, Low Density Lipoprotein *Serum Decrease* Absent. *0062*

Cholesterol, Very Low Density Lipoprotein *Serum Decrease* Absent. *0062*

Chylomicrons *Serum Decrease* Complete absence of chylomicrons. *0151* Totally absent. *2246* None present. *0878*

Coombs' Test *Blood Negative 0130*

Erythrocyte Sedimentation Rate *Blood Decrease* High percentage of acanthocytes results in low ESR. *2246*

Erythrocyte Survival *Red Blood Cells Decrease* Usually shortened, but may be normal. *2501 2091 2246 1583*

Fat *Feces Increase* Marked impairment of GI fat absorption. *2467* By 4th or 5th year of life, steatorrhea becomes less marked. *2246*

Fatty Acids, Free (FFA) *Serum Decrease* Slightly diminished or at low normal concentrations. *1583 0095*

Folate *Serum Decrease* Secondary to malabsorption of fat. *2030*

Haptoglobin *Serum Decrease* Reflects increased red cell turnover. *2171*

Hematocrit *Blood Decrease* Anemia has been described. *2246* Severe anemia with hemoglobin as low as 4-8 g/dL is common in children. Most adult patients do not have significant anemia. *2246 1583*

Hemoglobin *Blood Decrease* Severe anemia with hemoglobin as low as 4-8 g/dL is common in children. Most adult patients do not have significant anemia. *2246 1583*

Iron *Serum Normal 2501*

Lipids *Serum Decrease* Concentration of all major lipids reduced to 50% of normal. *2246*

Lipoproteins *Serum Decrease* Only alpha lipoproteins are present. *0151*

Lipoproteins, Beta *Serum Decrease* Complete absence of LDL. *0151* None present. *0878*

Lipoproteins, Prebeta *Serum Decrease* Absent or below standard measuring capabilities. *2246* None present. *0878*

Phospholipids, Total *Serum Decrease* Wide range of variation. Reduced by approximately 75%. *1181 2246*

Phytanic Acid *Plasma Increase* Characteristic. *0995*

Poikilocytes *Blood Increase* Acanthocytosis of 50-70%. *2246*

Protein *Urine Increase* Proteinuria is an early finding and patients ultimately develop renal failure. *0999*

Prothrombin Time *Plasma Increase* Frequently prolonged, secondary to vitamin K malabsorption. *0566* Abnormal bleeding is rare. *0095*

Reticulocytes *Blood Increase* Reflects increased RBC turnover. *1583*

Triglycerides *Serum Decrease* Usually below accurate measuring capabilities of conventional lab methods. *2246*

Vitamin A *Serum Decrease* Very low. *0878 1242*

Vitamin B$_{12}$ *Serum Normal 1583*

Vitamin B$_{12}$ Binding Capacity *Serum Normal 1583*

Vitamin E (Tocopherol) *Serum Decrease* Very low concentration. *1215*

272.71 Anderson's Disease

Alanine Aminotransferase *Serum Increase* Liver involvement. *2246*

Aspartate Aminotransferase *Serum Increase* Liver involvement. *2246*

Cholesterol *Serum Increase* Significant elevations generally occur in the glycogen storage diseases. *2104*

Glucose *Serum Decrease* Usually low. *2104*

Lactic Acid *Blood Increase* Significant elevations generally occur in the glycogen storage diseases. *2104*

Lipids *Serum Increase* Total lipids are significantly elevated. *2104*

Uric Acid *Serum Increase* Significant elevations generally occur in the glycogen storage diseases. *2104*

272.72 Gaucher's Disease

5'-Nucleotidase *Serum Increase* May be abnormal with liver involvement. *0995*

Acid Phosphatase *Serum Increase* Commonly elevated or high normal serum concentrations, irrespective of the patient's clinical status. The excess is caused by spillage from tissue accumulations, primarily from the spleen. *0474* In 12 proved cases, there was a range of 12-25 U/L , with a mean of 16.8 U/L, (normal range = 7-9 U/L). *2382* A 5-50 fold elevation in serum activity in 8 patients with the adult, non-neuropathic form of Gaucher's Disease was found. *0363 1571*

Alanine Aminotransferase *Serum Increase* May be abnormal with liver involvement. *0995*

Alkaline Phosphatase *Serum Increase* With bone resorption. *0619 0812*

Angiotensin-Converting Enzyme (ACE) *Serum Increase* Elevated. *1398*

Anisocytes *Blood Increase* If splenectomy has been carried out, severe anisocytosis and poikilocytosis occur, with many target cells, some nucleated red cells, and Howell-Jolly bodies usually present. *2538*

Beta-Glucosidase *Serum Decrease* At pH 4.0, individuals demonstrate a marked reduction. However, little or no reduction is found at the optimum pH, 5.5. *1808*

Beta-Glucuronidase *Serum Increase 1723 2538*

Erythrocytes *Blood Decrease* Pancytopenia is a common feature. *2538*

Factor IX *Plasma Decrease* Clotting factor abnormalities may be present. Factor IX deficiency seems to be particularly common, and it does not appear to be related to liver disease. *2538*

Gamma Glutamyl Transferase (GGT) *Serum Increase* May be abnormal with liver involvement. *0995*

Glucocerebroside Beta-Glucosidase *Serum Increase* Frequently increased, with highly variable range of values. *2246*

Liver Increase Many times the normal concentration. *2246*

Red Blood Cells Increase Frequently increased, with highly variable range of values. *2246*

Hematocrit *Blood Decrease* Unexplained splenomegaly with mild-moderate anemia and thrombocytopenia. *1808* A normocytic, normochromic anemia is frequently present, but Hb levels rarely fall below 8 g/dL. *2538*

Hemoglobin *Blood Decrease* Unexplained splenomegaly with mild-moderate anemia and thrombocytopenia. *1808* A normocytic, normochromic anemia is frequently present, but concentrations rarely fall below 8 g/dL. *2538*

Iron *Serum Decrease* Iron is diverted from the plasma and stored within Gaucher cells. *1434*

Lactate Dehydrogenase *Serum Increase* May be abnormal with liver involvement. *0995*

Leukocytes *Blood Decrease* Pancytopenia is a common feature. May be decreased to levels as low as 1,000/μL, although milder degrees of leukopenia are much more common. *2538*

Lysozyme *Serum Increase* Increased (15.6 ± 3.37 g/L) in 80% of adult chronic non-neuropathic type I Gaucher's Disease. *2163*

Monocytes *Blood Increase* Lipid storage diseases. *2467*

Oxygen Saturation *Blood Decrease* With lung involvement. *2246*

Platelet Count *Blood Decrease* Unexplained splenomegaly with mild-moderate anemia and thrombocytopenia. *1808* Pancytopenia is a common feature. May become quite severe. *2538*

pO2 *Blood Decrease* With lung involvement. *2246*

Poikilocytes *Blood Increase* If splenectomy has been carried out, severe anisocytosis and poikilocytosis occur, with many target cells, some nucleated red cells, and Howell-Jolly bodies usually present. *2538*

Reticulocytes *Blood Increase* A modest reticulocytosis is often present in anemic patients. *2538*

272.73   Niemann-Pick Disease

Acid Phosphatase *Serum Increase* Ranging from 35-45 U/L over a 4 month period in a patient with this disease. *1000* Increased levels have been documented in only a few cases. *0473 0474*

Serum Normal Eleven measurements on 6 different patients all fell within the normal range for their respective age groups. Observations of increased concentration have not been able to be confirmed. *0473 0474 1000*

Alanine Aminotransferase *Serum Increase* Seen in type B disease. *2246*

Aldolase *CSF Increase* *0619*

Alkaline Phosphatase *Serum Increase* Seen in type B disease. *2246*

Aspartate Aminotransferase *Serum Increase* Seen in type B disease. *2246*

Cells *Bone Marrow Increase* Bone marrow contains typical foam cells, containing small droplets throughout the cytoplasm. *2538*

Cholesterol *Liver Increase* Usually elevated, may be more prominent than sphingomyelin in type D. *2246*

Erythrocytes *Blood Decrease* Pancytopenia is a common feature. *2538*

Hematocrit *Blood Decrease* May be normal or mild anemia may be present. *2538*

Hemoglobin *Blood Decrease* May be normal, or mild anemia may be present. *2538*

Leukocytes *Blood Decrease* Pancytopenia is a common feature. *2538*

Platelet Count *Blood Decrease* Pancytopenia is a common feature. *2538* May be severe. *0995*

273.21   Cryoglobulinemia (Essential Mixed)

Albumin *Urine Increase* Common. *0433*

Cold Agglutinins *Serum Increase* *2035*

Complement C1q *Serum Decrease* Low levels of early components (C1q, C1s, and C4). *2329*

Complement C3 *Serum Normal* In 26 patients affected by essential cryoglobulinemia, a peculiar pattern was observed which was characterized by: low levels of early components (C1q, C1s and C4), normal levels of C3 and high concentrations of late components (C5,C9) and CH50 values significantly lower than normal. *2329* May be normal in mixed cryoglobulinemia. *2522*

Complement C4 *Serum Decrease* In 26 patients affected by essential cryoglobulinemia, a peculiar pattern was observed which was characterized by: low levels of early components (C1q, C1s and C4), normal levels of C3 and high concentrations of late components (C5, C9) and CH50 values significantly lower than normal. *2329* C1q, C2, and C4 are especially decreased whereas C3 may be normal in mixed cryoglobulinemia. *2522*

Complement, Total *Serum Decrease* In 26 patients affected by essential cryoglobulinemia, peculiar pattern was observed which was characterized by: low levels of early components (C1q, C1s and C4), normal levels of C3 and high concentrations of late components (C5,C9) and CH50 values significantly lower than normal. *2329*

Serum Increase In 26 patients affected by essential cryoglobulinemia, a peculiar pattern was observed which was characterized by: low levels of early components (C1q, C1s and C4), normal levels of C3 and high concentrations of late components (C5,C9) and CH50 values significantly lower than normal. *2329*

Erythrocytes *Urine Increase* Urinary sediment contains erythrocytes and finely granular casts. *0433*

Erythrocyte Sedimentation Rate *Blood Decrease* Rare finding of a rate approaching 0 mm/h (in the absence of marked hypofibrinogenemia). *2035*

Blood Increase May be increased at 37 C. *2468*

Blood Normal Normal at room temperature. *2468*

Granular Casts *Urine Increase* Urinary sediment contains erythrocytes and finely granular casts. *0433*

Immunoglobulin IgG *Serum Increase* Monoclonal spike may occur. *2035*

Immunoglobulin IgM *Serum Increase* Monoclonal spike may occur. *2035*

Rheumatoid Factor *Serum Increase* High titer when tested at 37 C. *2035*

273.22   Heavy Chain Disease (Alpha)

Albumin *Serum Decrease* Usually reduced with reversed A/G ratio. *2538*

Alpha2-Globulin *Serum Increase* Markedly elevated broad peak. *2035*

Bence-Jones Protein *Urine Absent* *2468*

Beta-Globulin *Serum Increase* Markedly elevated broad peak. *2035*

Calcium *Serum Decrease* Patients usually present with chronic diarrhea, hypocalcemia, and excessive fecal losses of water and electrolytes. *2538*

Chloride *Feces Increase* Patients usually present with chronic diarrhea, hypocalcemia, and excessive fecal losses of water and electrolytes. *2538*

Immunoglobulin IgA *Serum Increase* Distinctive increase in IgA heavy chains (alpha chains). *2035*

Potassium *Feces Increase* Patients usually present with chronic diarrhea, hypocalcemia, and excessive fecal losses of water and electrolytes. *2538*

Sodium *Feces Increase* Patients usually present with chronic diarrhea, hypocalcemia, and excessive fecal losses of water and electrolytes. *2538*

Vitamin B12 *Serum Decrease* Impaired absorption. *2035*

273.23   Heavy Chain Disease (Gamma)

Albumin *Serum Decrease* Usually reduced with reversed A/G ratio. *2538*

Bence-Jones Protein *Urine Absent* *2468*

Calcium *Serum Decrease* Patients usually present with chronic diarrhea, hypocalcemia, and excessive fecal losses of water and electrolytes. *2538*

Cephalin Flocculation *Serum Increase* *2468*

Chloride *Feces Increase* Patients usually present with chronic diarrhea, hypocalcemia, and excessive fecal losses of water and electrolytes. *2538*

Eosinophils *Blood Increase* Eosinophilia sometimes marked with relative lymphocytosis. *2468* Often associated with mild to marked leukopenia and eosinophilia. *2035*

Bone Marrow Increase Bone marrow aspirations and lymph node biopsies have demonstrated a proliferation of plasmacytic and lymphocytic forms, along with eosinophils and large reticulum or reticuloendothelial cells, (the pattern of a pleomorphic reticular neoplasm). *2035* Bone marrow may be normal, but usually there is an increased proportion of plasma cells or lymphocytes or both, often accompanied by eosinophilia. *2538*

Erythrocyte Sedimentation Rate *Blood Increase* *0186*

Globulin *Serum Decrease* Almost absent on electrophoresis. *2467* In 50% of patients the concentration of the anomalous protein is > 2.0 g/dL and marked hypogammaglobulinemia is present. *2538*

Hematocrit *Blood Decrease* Normochromic, normocytic anemia present in all cases. *0999* Presumably related to hypersplenism. *2035* All patients have mild to moderate anemia. *2538*

273.23 Heavy Chain Disease (Gamma) *(continued)*

Hemoglobin *Blood Decrease* Normochromic, normocytic anemia present in all cases of gamma heavy chain disease. *0999* Presumably related to hypersplenism. *2035* All patients have mild to moderate anemia. *2538*

Immunoglobulin IgA *Serum Decrease* Marked decrease. *2468*

Immunoglobulin IgG *Serum Decrease* Marked decrease in IgG. *2468* Excessive quantities of the Fe fragment of the heavy chain of IgG. *2035*

Immunoglobulin IgM *Serum Decrease* Marked decrease. *2467*

Immunoglobulins *Serum Decrease* Marked decrease in IgG, IgA, and IgM. *2468*

Leukocytes *Blood Decrease* Presumably related to hypersplenism. *2035* Often associated with mild to marked leukopenia and eosinophilia. *2538* *0999*

Lymphocytes *Blood Increase* Atypical lymphocytes *0186* Relative lymphocytosis. *2468*

Bone Marrow Increase Bone marrow aspirations and lymph node biopsies have demonstrated a proliferation of plasmacytic and lymphocytic forms, along with eosinophils and large reticulum or reticuloendothelial cells, (the pattern of a pleomorphic reticular neoplasm). *2035* Bone marrow may be normal, but usually there is an increased proportion of plasma cells or lymphocytes or both, often accompanied by eosinophilia. *2538*

Plasma Cells *Serum Increase* Presence of atypical lymphocytes or plasma cells in the blood. *2035*

Bone Marrow Increase Bone marrow aspirations and lymph node biopsies have demonstrated a proliferation of plasmacytic and lymphocytic forms, along with eosinophils and large reticulum or reticuloendothelial cells, (the pattern of a pleomorphic reticular neoplasm). *2035* Bone marrow may be normal, but usually there is an increased proportion of plasma cells or lymphocytes or both, often accompanied by eosinophilia. *2538*

Platelet Count *Blood Decrease* Presumably related to hypersplenism. *2035* Mild to marked thrombocytopenia. *2538*

Potassium *Feces Increase* Patients usually present with chronic diarrhea, hypocalcemia, and excessive fecal losses of water and electrolytes. *2538*

Protein *Urine Increase* Up to 1 gram/day *0186*

Sodium *Feces Increase* Patients usually present with chronic diarrhea, hypocalcemia, and excessive fecal losses of water and electrolytes. *2538*

Urea Nitrogen *Serum Increase* Increased (30-50 mg/dL). *2468*

Uric Acid *Serum Increase* Increased, (> 8.5 mg/dL). *2468*

273.30 Waldenström's Macroglobulinemia

Acid Phosphatase *Leukocyte Increase* *1388*

Albumin *Serum Decrease* *2467*

Alpha₁-Antitrypsin *Serum Normal* *2467*

Antinuclear Antibodies *Serum Increase* Positive in 16%. *1799*

Antithyroglobulin Antibodies *Serum Increase* Rare. *2373*

Basophils *Bone Marrow Increase* Characteristic presence of large numbers of basophils and tissue mast cells interspersed among the other cells. *2552*

Bence-Jones Protein *Urine Present* Present in approximately 10% of cases, but renal functional impairment is much less common than in myeloma. *2035* Reported to occur in 25% of patients. *2538*

Beta₂-Macroglobulin *Serum Increase* Marked increase. *2467*

Bleeding Time *Blood Increase* Evidence of impaired platelet function. *2538*

Cells *Bone Marrow Increase* Bone marrow sections are always hypercellular and show extensive infiltration with atypical lymphocytes and also plasma cells, with macroglobulinemia. *2468* Bone marrow punctures may result in dry tap due to great cellularity of the marrow combined with increased viscosity of the tissue fluid. *1225*

Cephalin Flocculation *Serum Increase* In some cases. *1225* *0020* *2035*

Cholesterol, Very Low Density Lipoprotein *Serum Increase* Moderate increase due to presence of IgG or IgM that forms complexes with chylomicron remnants and/or VLDL thereby decreasing catabolism. *0062*

Chylomicrons *Serum Increase* Moderate increase due to presence of IgG or IgM that forms complexes with chylomicron remnants and/or VLDL thereby decreasing catabolism. *0062*

Clot Retraction *Blood Poor* Evidence of impaired platelet function. *2538*

Cold Agglutinins *Serum Increase* *2035*

Complement C3 *Serum Normal* *2467*

Complement, Total *Serum Decrease* In some cases. *0020*

Coombs' Test *Blood Negative* Almost always negative. *2538*

Creatinine *Serum Normal* *0062*

Cryofibrinogen *Serum Increase* *0186*

Cryoglobulins *Serum Increase* Demonstrated in the sera of 37% of the tested patients. *2538* Marked elevation of cryoglobulins. *2104*

Eosinophils *Blood Increase* *2035* *0128*

Erythrocyte Sedimentation Rate *Blood Increase* Markedly increased. *2552* The presence of cryomacroglobulins may give the appearance of a normal ESR. *0433* *2035*

Blood Normal The presence of cryomacroglobulins may give the appearance of a normal ESR. *2467*

Erythrocyte Survival *Red Blood Cells Decrease* Found in 6 of 8 patients. *0413* *2538*

Factor II *Plasma Decrease* A number of patients have reduced activity of one or more coagulation factors. *2538*

Factor V *Plasma Decrease* A number of patients have reduced activity of one or more coagulation factors. *2538*

Factor VII *Plasma Decrease* A number of patients have reduced activity of 1 or more coagulation factors. *2538*

Factor VIII *Plasma Decrease* A number of patients have reduced activity of one or more coagulation factors. *2538*

Factor X *Plasma Decrease* A number of patients have reduced activity of one or more coagulation factors. *2538*

Fibrinogen *Plasma Decrease* A number of patients have reduced activity of one or more coagulation factors. *2538*

Globulin *Serum Increase* Electrophoresis shows an intense sharp peak in globulin fraction, usually in the gamma zone, and takes PAS stain. Total serum protein and globulin are markedly increased. Immunoelectrophoresis identifies IgM as a component of increased globulin *2468*

Haptoglobin *Serum Normal* *2467*

Hematocrit *Blood Decrease* Anemia is the most common presenting manifestation and is frequently profound. Usually due to a combination of factors including accelerated RBC destruction, blood loss, and especially decreased erythropoiesis. *2035* A normochromic, normocytic anemia is usually present. *2538*

Hemoglobin *Blood Decrease* Anemia is the most common presenting manifestation and is frequently profound, with Hb levels in the range of 6-9 g/dL. Usually due to a combination of factors including accelerated RBC destruction, blood loss, and especially decreased erythropoiesis. *2035* A normochromic, normocytic anemia is usually present. *2538*

Immunoglobulin IgA *Serum Decrease* *2467*

Immunoglobulin IgG *Serum Decrease* *2467*

Immunoglobulin IgM *Serum Increase* IgM > 15% of total serum protein and/or 1,000 mg/dL. *0999* Immunoelectrophoresis identified IgM as a component of increased globulin. *2468*

Iron-Binding Capacity, Total (TIBC) *Serum Normal* *2467*

Leukocytes *Blood Decrease* WBC is decreased with relative lymphocytosis. *2468* *2035*

Blood Normal Leukocytosis and thrombocytopenia are uncommon. *2538*

Lymphocytes *Blood Increase* Absolute lymphocytosis with atypical, immature, and plasmacytic forms in many cases, and occasionally reaching leukemic proportions. *2035* Relative lymphocytosis. *2468*

Bone Marrow Increase Proliferation of lymphocytic and plasmacytic forms with many intermediate and apparently transitional cell types. *2035* *0188*

Monocytes *Blood Increase* Has been observed. *0128*

Neutrophils *Blood Decrease* In some patients, neutropenia, as part of general pancytopenia, has been observed. *2552* *0128*

Plasma Cells *Bone Marrow Increase* Proliferation of lymphocytic and plasmacytic forms with many intermediate and apparently transitional cell types. *2035* *0188*

Platelet Count *Blood Decrease* Leukocytosis and thrombocytopenia are uncommon. *2538* Found in about 50% of patients suffering from bleeding diathesis. *2552* *2035*

Blood Normal Count is usually normal, but abnormalities of platelet function appear to be important causes of bleeding in these patients. *2538*

Protein *Serum Increase* Total serum proteins are increased owing to elevation of gamma globulins. *0433*

Urine Increase 5 of 16 patients excreted 2.0 g or more of protein/24 h. *1626 2538*

Prothrombin Consumption *Blood Decrease* Evidence of impaired platelet function. *2538*

Rheumatoid Factor *Serum Increase* Occasionally. *2035* Dysproteinemias and paraproteinemias present significant seropositivity. *0962* In some cases. *0020*

Thrombin Time *Plasma Increase* Coagulation defect detected most frequently is prolongation of the thrombin time. *2538*

Thromboplastin Generation *Blood Increase* Evidence of impaired platelet function. *2538*

Urea Nitrogen *Serum Increase* Elevated in 5 of 16 patients. *1626 2538*

Serum Normal Renal insufficiency is reported to be uncommon. *1469 2538*

Uric Acid *Serum Increase* May occur. *2552 0962*

VDRL *Serum Positive* Biologic false positive found in some cases. *0020*

Viscosity *Serum Increase* The relative serum viscosity was elevated above 4 in 41% of patients and 36% of these patients developed symptoms of hyperviscosity sometime in the course of their disease. *1469* A great increase in serum viscosity. Is usually associated with the presence of macroglobulins. *2538* Some increase in serum viscosity is found in about 66% of patients tested, but only 50% of these will manifest symptoms of the hyperviscosity syndrome. *2552 0962*

Volume *Plasma Increase* *0186*

273.80 Analbuminemia

Albumin *Serum Decrease* Marked decrease due to impaired synthesis. *2104* Cannot be detected by routine lab methods. *0433*

Alpha$_1$-Antitrypsin *Serum Normal* *2467*

Alpha$_1$-Globulin *Serum Normal* *2467*

Alpha$_2$-Globulin *Serum Increase* *2467*

Beta-Globulin *Serum Increase* *2467*

Calcium *Serum Decrease* Lower limits of normal. *0433*

Cholesterol *Serum Increase* Often elevated. *0433*

Complement C3 *Serum Normal* *2467*

Erythrocyte Sedimentation Rate *Blood Increase* Usually elevated owing to the increased globulin level. *0433*

Globulin *Serum Increase* Usually present in increased concentration *0433 2467*

Haptoglobin *Serum Normal* *2467*

Iron-Binding Capacity, Total (TIBC) *Serum Normal* *2467*

Protein *Serum Decrease* Marked decrease. *2467*

274.00 Gout

17-Hydroxycorticosteroids *Urine Decrease* *0503*

17-Ketogenic Steroids *Urine Decrease* *0503*

17-Ketosteroids *Urine Decrease* Moderate decrease. *0503*

Adenosine Deaminase *Serum Increase* Increased. *0655 1737 2235*

Alanine *Serum Increase* Increased. *0094 0269 2149*

Alkaline Phosphatase *Synovial Fluid Decrease* *0619*

Alpha$_1$-Globulin *Serum Decrease* alpha$_1$ and alpha$_2$-globulins reduced in many gouty patients. *0050*

Alpha$_2$-Globulin *Serum Decrease* alpha$_1$ and alpha$_2$-globulins reduced in many gouty patients. *0050*

Aspartate Aminotransferase *Serum Increase* Increased levels have been reported in acute stages. *0619*

Cholesterol *Serum Increase* Many patients. *0991* Frequently elevated in individual patients; no correlation has been shown between urate and cholesterol. *2246*

Complement, Total *Serum Decrease* Depleted in serum by urate crystals. *1664*

Serum Increase Elevated during active inflammation and subsides with remission. *2090*

Synovial Fluid Increase Frequently occurs. *2090*

Creatinine *Serum Increase* Rises with renal failure, but these changes may be subtle and slow. *0433*

Erythrocyte Sedimentation Rate *Blood Increase* Frequently elevated with acute gout. *0433* Increased in gouty arthritis. *0962 0999*

Glomerular Filtration Rate (GFR) *Urine Decrease* Moderate but significant reduction in all age groups. *0943*

Glucose *Synovial Fluid Decrease* Typical of inflammatory reactions sometimes showing a slight reduction in glucose. *0999*

Glutamic Acid *Serum Increase* Remains elevated even after casein loading. Fasting values range from 68-72 μmol (45-51 in controls). *1758*

Red Blood Cells Increase Average values range from 214-243 μmol compared to 216 in controls. *1758*

Glutamine *Serum Normal* *2246*

Glycine *Serum Decrease* Distinct reduction. *2604*

Inulin Clearance *Urine Decrease* Below 90 mL/min in 33% of patients. *0447* The lowest values are found in older patients or those with hypertension. *0943*

Leukocytes *Blood Increase* Occurs during acute attacks. *2467* Usually accompanied by leukocytosis. *0999 0433*

Synovial Fluid Increase The synovial fluid is typical of inflammatory reactions showing polymorphonuclear leukocytosis (5,000-5,000/μL). *0999* Counts between 750-45,000/μL in acute attacks. *0962*

Neutrophils *Blood Increase* May be associated with a moderate to severe neutrophilia. *2538*

Synovial Fluid Increase Increase in percentage of neutrophils in acute attacks; range = 48-94% (Normal less than 5%). *2467*

pH *Urine Decrease* Often low: 5.0-5.5. *0433* Tends to be low throughout the day, with decreased diurnal variations. *0837*

Phosphate *Serum Decrease* Hypophosphatemia has been observed in association with acute attacks. *1287*

Protein *Urine Increase* Low-grade proteinuria occurs in 20-80% of gouty persons for many y before further evidence of renal disease appears. *2468* Incidence varies from 20-40%. May be intermittent and rarely heavy. *2246*

Synovial Fluid Increase The synovial fluid is typical of inflammatory reactions showing an increase in protein content. *0999*

Pyrophosphate *Synovial Fluid Increase* Moderately elevated levels. *1132*

Rheumatoid Factor *Serum Normal* *2467*

Serine *Serum Decrease* *2604*

Triglycerides *Serum Increase* 75-84% of patients. *0717 0115 2246*

Urea Nitrogen *Serum Increase* Rises with renal failure, but these changes may be subtle and slow. *0433*

Uric Acid *Serum Increase* More than 95% of patients eventually have an elevated serum concentration. *0433* May rise above 6.0 mg/dL in men, or 5.5 mg/dL in women. Possibly the rise is due to increased renal tubular reabsorption. 25% of patients' relatives have raised serum concentration also, but without symptoms of gout (possibly the effect of a single autosomal dominant gene). *0619*

Urine Increase May occur during acute attack. *0091*

CSF Normal Very low in normal and gouty patients. Probably explains the absence of tophaceous deposits in the CNS. *2582*

Synovial Fluid Increase Many patients have a concentration which is greater than in serum. *1903*

Viscosity *Synovial Fluid Decrease* *0962*

275.00 Hemochromatosis

5'-Nucleotidase *Serum Increase* With liver involvement. *0962*

Serum Normal Over 50% of patients have no laboratory evidence of liver dysfunction. *0995*

Adenosine Deaminase *Serum Increase* Increased. *0655 1737 2235*

Alkaline Phosphatase *Serum Increase* With liver involvement. *0962*

Serum Normal Over 50% of patients have no laboratory evidence of liver dysfunction. *0995*

Androgens *Plasma Decrease* Decreased testosterone found in 12 of 12 patients. *0199*

Aspartate Aminotransferase *Serum Increase* With liver involvement. *0962*

275.00   Hemochromatosis *(continued)*

Aspartate Aminotransferase *(continued)*
Serum   Normal   Over 50% of patients have no laboratory evidence of liver dysfunction. *0995*

Bilirubin   *Serum   Increase*   With liver involvement. *0962*

Serum   Normal   Over 50% of patients have no laboratory evidence of liver dysfunction. *0995*

BSP Retention   *Serum   Increase*   With liver involvement. *0962*

Serum   Normal   Over 50% of patients have no laboratory evidence of liver dysfunction. *0995*

Copper   *Serum   Increase*   *0999*

Corticotropin   *Plasma   Decrease*   9 of 15 patients had pituitary dysfunction. *2265*   A frequent complication. *2246*

Ferritin   *Serum   Increase*   Concentration was grossly raised in all 41 patients, ranging from 670-4,100 µg/L. *1850*   Markedly increased due to gross increase in iron stores. *0141*   Plasma concentration of > 1,000 ng/mL is indicative of increased body iron stores, although it does not differentiate between reticuloendothelial and parenchymal storage. Correlates well with iron stores in cirrhotic patients with primary disease. *2246   2538*

Serum   Normal   Normal or marginal elevation in the precirrhotic stage. *2246*

Follicle Stimulating Hormone (FSH)   *Serum   Decrease*   Frequently occurs in idiopathic hemochromatosis. *2473*

Gamma Glutamyl Transferase (GGT)   *Serum   Increase*   With liver involvement. *0962*

Serum   Normal   Over 50% of patients have no laboratory evidence of liver dysfunction. *0995*

Glucose   *Serum   Increase*   About 82% of all patients with this disorder develop diabetes mellitus. *0995*

Glucose Tolerance   *Serum   Decrease*   Decreased tolerance:excessive peak decreased utilization with slow fall to fasting level. *2467*

Gonadotropin, Pituitary   *Serum   Decrease*   Basal gonadotropin levels and/or their response to LHRH were low in 9 of 12 patients. *0199*

Urine   Decrease   9 of 15 patients had pituitary dysfunction. *2265*   A frequent complication. *2246*

Growth Hormone   *Serum   Decrease*   9 of 15 patients had pituitary dysfunction. *2265*   A frequent complication. *2246*

Urine   Increase   Marked elevation. *1445*

Hematocrit   *Blood   Normal*   Anemia is not usually present with primary hemochromatosis; when present, anemia suggests secondary causes such as alcoholic cirrhosis, transfusion-induced iron overload, sideroblastic anemia, or thalassemia. *0433*

Hemoglobin   *Blood   Normal*   Anemia is not usually present with primary hemochromatosis; when present, anemia suggests secondary causes such as alcoholic cirrhosis, transfusion-induced iron overload, sideroblastic anemia, or thalassemia. *0433*

HLA Antigens   *Blood   Present*   HLA-A3 present in 72% of patients versus 21% of controls. *2539*

Iron   *Serum   Increase*   Diagnosis established when concentration > 220 µg/dL. *0999*   Increased serum and hepatic iron concentration. *1850*   Average level is 250 µg/dL, with a range of from 225-325 µg/dL. *2538*   In the absence of infection, inflammation, neoplasia, or recent blood loss, concentrations usually range from 175-275 µg/dL. *2246   2612*

Liver   Increase   Increased serum and hepatic iron concentrations. *1850*   Increased iron deposition principally in the parenchymal cells of the liver. *0962*   Large amounts of stainable iron, predominantly within the parenchymal cells. *2612*

Iron-Binding Capacity, Total (TIBC)   *Serum   Decrease*   Reduced transferrin as shown by a low TIBC. *2612*   Occurs early in the course of the disease. *1850*   Usually < 300 µg/dL. *2246*

Serum   Normal   *0995*

Iron Saturation   *Serum   Increase*   Usually > 80% and often 100%. *2612*   Usually 75%. *2246   2538*

Lactate Dehydrogenase   *Serum   Increase*   With liver involvement. *0962*

Serum   Normal   Over 50% of patients have no laboratory evidence of liver dysfunction. *0995*

Leucine Aminopeptidase   *Serum   Increase*   With liver involvement. *0962*

Serum   Normal   Over 50% of patients have no laboratory evidence of liver dysfunction. *0995*

Luteinizing Hormone (LH)   *Serum   Decrease*   Hypogonadism frequently occurs in idiopathic hemochromatosis. *2473*   Depressed in 44% of 32 patients; generalized depression of pituitary function. *2266*

Pyrophosphate   *Synovial Fluid   Increase*   Has been identified. *2088*

Testosterone   *Plasma   Decrease*   Found in 12 of 12 patients. *0199*

275.10   Hepatolenticular Degeneration

5'-Nucleotidase   *Serum   Increase*   With liver involvement. *0995*

Alanine   *Urine   Increase*   *0503*

Alanine Aminotransferase   *Serum   Increase*   Minimal elevation in 14% (5 of 37 patients). Mean = 30 U/L. *2278*

Albumin   *Serum   Decrease*   Reduced in 27% or 10 of 37 patients. *2278*

Alkaline Phosphatase   *Serum   Increase*   With liver involvement. *0995*

Alpha-Amino-Nitrogen   *Urine   Increase*   Increased in 79% of patients. *2278*

Amino Acids   *Urine   Increase*   77% of patients tested before penicillamine therapy had hyperaminoaciduria. Urinary excretion of amino acids decreased after therapy. *2278*

Aspartate Aminotransferase   *Serum   Increase*   Minimally elevated in 36% (14 of 39 patients). Mean = 30 U/L. *2278*

Bicarbonate   *Serum   Decrease*   Decreased serum CO_2 in 12 of 27 patients (44%). *2278*

Bilirubin   *Serum   Increase*   Elevated in 13 of 38 (34%) patients; mean = 1.45 mg/dL. Direct bilirubin was increased in 9 of 36 (25%) patients. *2278*

Bilirubin, Direct   *Serum   Increase*   Increased in 9 of 36 (25%) patients. *2278*

BSP Retention   *Serum   Increase*   Excretion was delayed in 76% of cases. Mean retention in 29 patients tested was 15%, and 9 patients had values > 20%. *2278*

Calcium   *Serum   Decrease*   Related to decreased albumin. *2280*

Urine   Increase   Slightly increased clearance in 19% of patients. *2278*

Ceruloplasmin   *Serum   Decrease*   Most patients are deficient; concentration is usually 15 mg/dL, but patients are seen with concentration within the normal range (25-45 mg/dL). This is particularly likely to be the case when liver damage predominates. *0433*   Low ceruloplasmin and elevated copper are characteristic. This is the result of an impaired ability to incorporate copper into protein, particularly ceruloplasmin, which causes unbound copper to be deposited in tissues and fluids throughout the body. *0999*

Serum   Normal   Normal in 5% of patients with overt disease. *2467*

Chloride   *Serum   Increase*   Frequent hyperchloremia; occurred in 13 of 31 patients (42%). *2278*

Cholesterol   *Serum   Decrease*   Related to liver disease. *2280*

Copper   *Serum   Decrease*   The serum concentration is directly related to that of the ceruloplasmin, for the protein binds the majority of the metal. Estimation of the serum copper seldom gives additional diagnostic information unless there is a discrepancy indicating a higher level of serum copper than can be accounted for by that present in ceruloplasmin. The normal serum concentration is between 90-140 µg/dL; in untreated disease it is commonly between 40-60 µg/dL but the range of variation is enormous. *0433   2467*

Urine   Increase   In untreated disease the amount is usually > 200 µg/24h but occasionally much lower, particularly in young presymptomatic siblings. *0433*   A good indirect indicator of the copper concentration in the liver. *1506*   The ceruloplasmin fraction is defective. Copper is excreted in the urine, bound to amino acids which act as chelating agents. *0619*

Liver   Increase   Liver biopsy shows high copper concentration 250 µg/g of dry liver). *2467*   Hepatic copper concentration is the most exact criterion in the diagnosis. In the course of the penicillamine therapy the copper content in the liver decreases, but normal values are achieved only after 5 or more y of treatment. The urinary copper excretion is a good indicator of the copper concentration in the liver. *1506*

Copper, Nonceruloplasmin *Serum Increase* Heterozygotes and treated homozygotes had nonceruloplasmin copper concentration ± 5.9 and 9.8 ± µg/dL, respectively) which did not differ significantly from normal (10.1 ± 1.6 µg/dL). Untreated patients had very significantly raised free copper concentration (22.9 ± 4.5 µg/dL). *1296* There is a complete absence of ceruloplasmin in this condition, and copper is deposited in the liver, brain, and renal tubules. The copper-carrying protein present is abnormal. *0619*

Creatine Kinase *Serum Normal* Normal. *2280*

Creatinine *Serum Decrease* Definitely elevated in 4 of 30 (13%) but decreased in 3 others. *2278*

Serum Increase Definitely elevated in 4 of 30 (13%) but decreased in 3 others. *2278*

Creatinine Clearance *Urine Decrease* Reduced in 7 of 24 patients (29%). *2278*

Erythrocytes *Urine Increase* Microscopic hematuria may occur. *2278*

Erythrocyte Sedimentation Rate *Blood Increase* May be increased, particularly if liver damage is present. *0433*

Erythrocyte Survival *Red Blood Cells Decrease* Reduced and found to correlate with splenic enlargement. *2279*

Gamma Glutamyl Transferase (GGT) *Serum Increase* With liver involvement. *0995*

Glomerular Filtration Rate (GFR) *Urine Decrease* Significantly reduced. *0143*

Glucose *Serum Decrease* In 5% of patients related to malnutrition. *2280*

Serum Increase Fasting glucose consistently elevated. *2278*

Urine Increase Tubular reabsorption of glucose is frequently impaired. *0143*

Glucose Tolerance *Serum Decrease* Abnormal in some patients. Fasting blood sugar levels are consistently increased. *2278*

Haptoglobin *Serum Decrease* Hemolytic anemia. *0995*

Hematocrit *Blood Decrease* Mild normochromic anemia with anisocytosis and poikilocytosis. *0433* Pancytopenia occurred frequently; hematocrit, platelets, WBC were often decreased. *2278*

Hemoglobin *Blood Decrease* Mild normochromic anemia with anisocytosis and poikilocytosis. *0433* *0530*

Hemoglobin, Free *Serum Increase* Hemolytic episodes frequently occur several years prior to onset of other symptoms; due to increased oxidative stress on RBC from excess copper. *0530*

Homocystine *Urine Increase* *0503*

Immunoglobulin IgA *Serum Decrease* Decreased in 6 and elevated in 2 of 16 patients. *2278*

Serum Increase Decreased in 6 and elevated in 2 of 16 patients. *2278*

Immunoglobulin IgG *Serum Increase* Elevated in over 50% of patients. *2278*

Immunoglobulin IgM *Serum Increase* Found to be increased in 5 out of 16 patients. *2278*

Inulin Clearance *Urine Decrease* Reduced clearance in 8 of 9 patients; although none had elevated BUN. *0143*

Isoleucine *Urine Increase* *0503*

Lactate Dehydrogenase *Serum Increase* With liver involvement. *0995*

Leucine *Urine Increase* *0503*

Leucine Aminopeptidase *Serum Increase* With liver involvement. *0995*

Leukocytes *Blood Decrease* Pancytopenia occurred frequently; Hct, platelets, WBC were often decreased. *2278* *0433*

pH *Urine Increase* Value in 50% of patients was > 6.5 with multiple specimens. 9 of 22 patients were unable to adequately acidify their urine during acid loading tests (pH > 5.3). *2278*

Phenylalanine *Urine Increase* *0503*

Phosphate *Serum Decrease* Decreased in 18 of 30 (60%), mean = 3.0 mg/dL. *2278*

Urine Increase Marked increase in clearance in 36% (8 of 22). *2278*

Platelet Count *Blood Decrease* Frequently decreased; 13 of 32 patients had counts < 100,000/µL. *2278* *0433*

Potassium *Serum Decrease* Found in 9 of 31 patients (29%). *2278*

Proline *Urine Increase* *0503*

Protein *Serum Decrease* Reduced to 6.0 mg/dL or less in 29% of patients (9 of 31). *2278*

Urine Increase Present in 33% of patients; always minimal and decreases with penicillamine therapy. Probably due to tubular reabsorption than increased GFR of protein. *2278*

Prothrombin Time *Plasma Increase* Mean time = 17.3 sec., abnormally prolonged in 79% (26 of 33) patients. *2278*

Pyrophosphate *Synovial Fluid Increase* Has been identified. *2088*

Pyruvate *Blood Increase* Reverts to normal after treatment with copper-chelating agent. *0619*

Specific Gravity *Urine Decrease* Reduced concentrating ability; 20% had maximum specific gravities of < 1.015 on overnight specimens. *2278*

Threonine *Urine Increase* *0503*

Tryptophan *Urine Increase* *0503*

Tyrosine *Urine Increase* *0503*

Urea Nitrogen *Serum Decrease* Mildly elevated between 20-25 mg/dL in 6 of 35 (17%) and decreased < 10 mg/dL in 4 cases. *2278*

Serum Increase Mildly elevated between 20-25 mg/dL in 6 of 35 (17%) and decreased < 10 mg/dL in 4 cases. *2278*

Uric Acid *Serum Decrease* Renal tubular reabsorption of uric acid is reduced, possibly as a result of damage to the tubule cells by excess unbound copper. *0619* Occurs in most patients with untreated disease. *2546* Decreased urate, mean = 2.5 mg/dL in 25 of 32 (78%). One patient had an elevated concentration. *2278* *2104*

Urine Increase Due to decreased renal tubular reabsorption. *0619*

Uric Acid Clearance *Urine Increase* Consistently high renal clearance even though some patients have total excretion values within the normal range. *2546* Mean clearance = 17.1 mL/min/1.73 m². 87% of 24 patients had elevated clearance. *2278* *2104*

Valine *Urine Increase* *0503*

275.21 Hypomagnesemia

Calcium *Serum Decrease* Plasma ionized calcium is reduced. *0619*

Magnesium *Serum Decrease* *0062*

275.31 Hyperphosphatasia

Acid Phosphatase *Serum Increase* Increased in this uncommon inherited disorder showing painful swelling of the periosteal soft tissue and spontaneous fractures. *2467* The lesions show pronounced increases in the amount of alkaline and acid phosphatase, aminopeptidase and lactic dehydrogenase, acid mucopolysaccharides and reticulin. *2259*

Alanine Aminopeptidase *Serum Increase* Increased in the uncommon inherited disorder showing painful swelling of the periosteal soft tissue and spontaneous fractures. *2467* Pronounced increase. *2259*

Alkaline Phosphatase *Serum Increase* Pronounced increase. *2259*

Lactate Dehydrogenase *Serum Increase* Pronounced increase. *2259*

Mucopolysaccharides *Serum Increase* Pronounced increase. *2259*

275.32 Hypophosphatasia

Alkaline Phosphatase *Serum Decrease* Marked reduction in activity is one of the cardinal features of hypophosphatasia. Reduced to 25% of the lower limit of normal, the mean levels varying widely with individual cases between almost no activity to 40% activity. There is no correlation between the degree of serum depression and the severity of the clinical manifestations. *0769* *0503*

Leukocyte Decrease In untreated hereditary hypophosphatasia. *2467*

Calcium *Serum Increase* Intermittent hypercalcemia may be observed in these patients, who also demonstrate an increase in phosphoethanolamine in their blood and urine. *0503* Total serum concentration was elevated in 10 patients and normal or undetermined in 6. Individual readings tended to vary widely and hypercalcemic patients had normal readings occasionally. *0769*

Urine Increase *2246*

Hydroxyproline *Urine Decrease* Extremely low. *0663* May be extremely low, reflecting bone destruction. *2341* *2246*

Phosphate *Serum Normal* *0619*

Phosphoethanolamine *Serum Increase* Two X normal. *1882*

275.32 Hypophosphatasia *(continued)*

Phosphoethanolamine *(continued)*
Urine Increase 3-8 X normal. *1882*

275.34 Familial Periodic Paralysis

17-Ketosteroids *Urine Increase* In the most severe attacks. *0903 2246*

Aldolase *Serum Increase* Occasional patients with paramyotonia congenita. *0760*

Aldosterone *Urine Increase* Striking change noted prior to attack. *2246*

Aspartate Aminotransferase *Serum Increase* Occasional patients with paramyotonia congenita. *0760*

Chloride *Urine Decrease* Precedes attack. *2246*

Eosinophils *Blood Decrease* Occasionally during attacks. *2246*

Follicle Stimulating Hormone (FSH) *Urine Increase* During attack. *0362*

Glucose *Urine Increase* Occasional patients. *2246*

Gonadotropin, Pituitary *Urine Increase* During attack. *0362*

Ketones *Serum Increase* Occasional patients. *2246*

Lactic Acid *Blood Increase* *1535*

Leukocytes *Blood Increase* Occasionally during attacks. *2246*

Neutrophils *Blood Increase* Occasionally during attacks. *2246*

Phosphate *Serum Decrease* During attacks. *0043*

Potassium *Serum Decrease* Ranges from 2.5-3.5 mmol/L in hypokalemic attacks. May be normal between attacks. *0151* Marked fall. *1172* Rarely, may shift from extra- to intracellular sites. There is no evidence of GI or renal wasting, volume depletion or total body K depletion. *1679*

Serum Normal Normal between attacks. *2246*

Urine Decrease Excretion decreases at the time of attack. *2467*

CSF Decrease Rarely found to be quite low during attack. *0612*

CSF Normal Only a slight drop during attacks. *1865*

Protein *Urine Increase* Occasional patients. *2246*

Pyruvate *Blood Increase* *1535*

Sodium *Serum Increase* Precedes attack. *2246*

Urine Decrease Precedes attack. *2246*

Thyroxine (T₄) *Serum Normal* *2246*

Tri-iodothyronine (T₃) *Serum Normal* *2246*

Uric Acid *Serum Decrease* *2104*

Urine Increase Uricosuria accompanies attacks. *2104*

275.35 Vitamin D Resistant Rickets

1,25-Dihydroxy-Vitamin D₃ *Serum Decrease* *0062*

Alkaline Phosphatase *Serum Increase* In older infants or children. *0503* Many children and patients continued to show persistently raised concentration, despite evident relief of symptoms in those with rickets or osteomalacia and increased growth rate in the school children. *0441* As skeletal changes develop. *2246*

Serum Normal Normal in most patients without radiologic signs of rickets. *2246*

Amino Acids *Urine Increase* Generalized aminoaciduria is present. *0433*

Urine Normal Normal, in contrast to Vitamin D deficient rickets. *2246*

Bicarbonate *Serum Normal* *2246*

Calcium *Serum Normal* Usually normal. *2246*

Urine Decrease In children, urinary excretion is 10-20 mg/24h whereas in adults urinary excretion ranges between 50-120 mg/24h. *0151* Usually low in untreated cases. *2246*

Feces Increase Diminished intestinal absorption. *2246*

Cyclic Adenosine Monophosphate *Urine Normal* Reported to be normal in untreated heterozygotes and homozygotes, with normal response to PTH infusion. *0853 2246*

Glomerular Filtration Rate (GFR) *Urine Decrease* Characteristic of the 1st few months of life. May result in a normal phosphate concentration even if the tubular defect is already present. *0994*

Glucose *Serum Normal* Found in excess quantities in the urine but not in the plasma. *0433*

Urine Increase Found in excess quantities in the urine but not in the plasma. *0433* Mild renal glycosuria has been reported in a few cases. *2246*

Glycine *Serum Normal* Found in excess quantities in the urine but not in the plasma. *0433*

Urine Increase Found in excess quantities in the urine but not in the plasma. *0433*

Hydroxyproline *Urine Increase* Some patients. *0962 2246*

Parathyroid Hormone *Serum Increase* Normal or only slight elevations. *2246*

pH *Blood Normal* *2246*

Phosphate *Serum Decrease* May be present at birth or develop within the 1st y. *2246* Familial hypophosphatemic rickets; with impaired transport of phosphate ion in both kidney and gut. Usually decreased. *2467*

Urine Increase High in untreated patients. *2246*

Feces Increase Diminished intestinal absorption. *2246*

Urea Nitrogen *Serum Normal* *2246*

275.41 Milk-Alkali Syndrome

Alkaline Phosphatase *Serum Decrease* *2467*

Calcium *Serum Increase* An unusual complication of intensive peptic ulcer therapy is the evolution of hypercalcemia from excessive intake of milk and absorbable alkali. *0999*

Urine Increase *0503*

pH *Blood Increase* *0995*

Phosphate *Serum Increase* Normal or elevated. *0503*

Urea Nitrogen *Serum Increase* *0995*

275.42 Pseudohypoparathyroidism

1,25-Dihydroxy-Vitamin D₃ *Serum Decrease* *0062*

Calcitonin *Serum Increase* *0619*

Calcium *Serum Decrease* End-organ failure. A rare cause of hypocalcemia. Must be considered in osteomalacia. *0503 0999*

Urine Decrease *0503*

Parathyroid Hormone *Serum Increase* Normally high and can be used to distinguish from true hypoparathyroidism. *2540* Deficient end organ response. *0062*

Phosphate *Serum Increase* Normal excretory mechanisms are impaired. *0999 0503*

Urine Decrease Normal excretory mechanisms are impaired. *0999 0503*

276.20 Metabolic Acidosis

2,3-Diphosphoglycerate *Red Blood Cells Decrease* Concentration will be low. *0158*

Aspartate Aminotransferase *Serum Increase* In type II-B, with lactic acidosis. *2468*

Bicarbonate *Serum Decrease* Total plasma CO_2 content is decreased; < 15 mmol/L almost certainly rules out respiratory alkalosis. *2468* Serum bicarbonate falls as hydrogen ions accumulate. *0962*

Calcium *Serum Increase* Increase in ionized calcium. *0791*

Urine Increase *0503*

Lactate Dehydrogenase *Serum Increase* Increased in type II-B, with lactic acidosis. *2468*

Lactic Acid *Blood Increase* Increased blood lactate with lactate-pyruvate ratio greater than 10:1 in type II-B, with lactic acidosis. *2468*

Leukocytes *Blood Increase* Intoxications due to metabolic causes can cause leukocytosis. *2467* Increased WBC in Type II-B, with lactic acidosis. *2468*

pCO₂ *Blood Decrease* Tends to fall below normal range as the blood pH and bicarbonate fall. *0619* Ventilation is stimulated and pCO₂ falls. *0962*

pH *Blood Decrease* Low usually 6.98-7.25 in type II-B, with lactic acidosis. *2468*

Urine Decrease Urine is strongly acid (pH = 4.5-5.2) if renal function is normal. *2468*

Phosphate *Serum Increase* Increased in type II-B, with lactic acidosis. *2468*

Potassium *Serum Increase* Frequently increased. Often 6-7 mmol/L in type II-B, with lactic acidosis. *2468*

Urine Increase 0619

276.30 Metabolic Alkalosis

Bicarbonate *Serum Increase* Total plasma CO_2 is increased (bicarbonate > 30 mmol/L). *2468*

Calcium *Serum Decrease* Decrease in ionized calcium. *0791*

Urine Decrease 0503

Chloride *Serum Decrease* Is relatively lower than sodium. *2468*

pCO$_2$ *Blood Increase* Normal or slightly elevated. *0962*

pH *Blood Increase* Deficit of hydrogen ion due to loss or alkali administration. *0962*

Urine Increase Urine pH > 7.0 (< 7.9) if potassium depletion and concomitant sodium are not severe. *2468*

Potassium *Serum Decrease* Usually decreased, which is the chief danger in alkalosis. *2468*

Urine Increase 0619

Urea Nitrogen *Serum Increase* May be increased. *2468*

276.50 Dehydration

Albumin *Serum Increase* By approximately 11.6% after heat exposure for 2-11 h. *2114*

Bicarbonate *Serum Decrease* Normal or decreased. *2467*

Serum Normal Normal or decreased. *2467*

Chloride *Serum Increase 2467*

Creatinine *Serum Increase* Leading to reduced renal blood flow (prerenal azotemia). *2467*

Creatinine Clearance *Urine Decrease* Following overnight dehydration. *2114*

Hematocrit *Blood Increase 2467*

Hemoglobin *Blood Increase 2467*

pH *Urine Decrease 2467*

Potassium *Serum Normal 2467*

Urine Increase 2467

Protein *Serum Increase* Reduced by 15.7% after 2-11 h heat exposure. *2114*

Sodium *Serum Increase 2467*

Urine Increase 2467

Urea Nitrogen *Serum Increase* Salt and water depletion causes reduced renal blood flow leading to prerenal azotemia. *2467* Dehydration. *0812 0503*

Volume *Plasma Decrease* Reduced 13.6% after 2-11 h heat exposure. *2114*

Urine Decrease 2467

276.80 Hypokalemia

Creatine Kinase *Serum Increase* Patients with severe hypokalemia such as that occurring in hyperaldosteronism with muscle weakness may have elevated CK directly related to their hypokalemia. In other patients with hypokalemia, 10% may have increased CK but this is related to other disease processes. *0467*

Myoglobin *Urine Increase* Sporadic; metabolic myoglobinuria. *2467*

pH *Blood Increase 0995*

Potassium *Serum Decrease 0062*

277.00 Cystic Fibrosis

2,3-Diphosphoglycerate *Red Blood Cells Increase* A study of 35 patients demonstrated that increasing severity of pulmonary involvement was associated with a mild but definite increase in erythrocyte 2,3-DPG and a decrease in hemoglobin affinity for oxygen. *1988*

25-Hydroxy Vitamin D$_3$ *Serum Decrease* Patients supplemented with multivitamins still presented a 36% decrease in 25-OH vitamin D concentration. *0959*

Albumin *Serum Decrease* With advanced lung disease the development of hypoalbuminemia suggests expansion of plasma volume secondary to Cor Pulmonale. *0433* May be found before cardiac involvement is clinically apparent. *2467* In 56% of 12 patients at initial hospitalization for this disorder. *0781 2284*

Duodenal Contents Increase In excess of that found in the duodenal fluid of controls. *0392*

Alkaline Phosphatase *Serum Increase* Noted in 40% of 36 children. Serum activity as a whole is fairly insensitive to occurrence and degree of disease because of high upper limits for normal children. *0578* In 65% of 12 patients at initial hospitalization for this disorder. *0781*

Alkaline Phosphatase Isoenzymes *Serum Increase* Liver fraction. *2246*

Alpha$_1$-Antichymotrypsin *Serum Increase* Increase compared to matched controls. *2504*

Alpha-Fetoprotein *Serum Normal* In 30 patients, the highest value obtained was 10.2 ng/mL and in a control 10.8 ng/mL. These are within published normal limits. Previously reported large increases in CF patients and in heterozygote carriers have not been confirmed. *0285* In CF patients 97.5% and in normal children 95% of the values were within the normal range for healthy adults (1-9 ng/mL). *1288*

Alpha-Glucosidase *Serum Increase* Acutely ill patients with cystic fibrosis demonstrated significant increases compared with cystic fibrosis outpatients. *1842*

Amylase *Saliva Increase* In healthy adults and children the value for pancreatic:salivary amylase is > 1. In 80% of gene carriers, the P:S is < 1 with a mean of 0.68 ± 0.13. In addition to the higher total amylase activity, in homozygotes P:S is < 0.1, and even 0.001. The phenomenon is explained by a compensatory enhancement of salivary activity. *2316* Submaxillary saliva is turbid, with increased calcium, total protein, and amylase. These changes are not generally found in parotid saliva. *2467*

Aspartate Aminotransferase *Serum Increase* In 56% of 12 patients at initial hospitalization for this disorder. *0781* With liver involvement. *1235*

Bile Acids *Serum Increase* Serum bile acid determination seems to be of no value in evaluating the extent of liver disease in cystic fibrosis. Chenodeoxycholic acids are more frequent and more elevated than cholic acid. *2274*

Bleeding Time *Blood Increase* Secondary to vitamin K deficiency. *0551*

Calcium *Serum Decrease* Hypoalbuminemia. *2467*

Serum Normal Normal unless complications occur (e.g., chronic pulmonary disease with accumulation of CO_2, massive salt loss due to sweating). *2467*

Saliva Increase Submaxillary saliva is turbid, with increased calcium, total protein, and amylase. These changes are not generally found in parotid saliva. *2467*

Chenodeoxycholic Acid *Serum Increase* Fifteen patients had elevated levels not correlated to liver morphology.

Chloride *Serum Increase 0619*

Serum Normal Serum electrolytes are normal unless complications occur (e.g., chronic pulmonary disease with accumulation of CO_2, massive salt loss due to sweating). *2467*

Saliva Increase Submaxillary saliva has slightly increased chloride and sodium but not potassium; however, considerable overlap with normal individuals prevents diagnostic usage. *2467*

Sweat Increase A value > 60 mmol/L is consistent with the diagnosis. *0433* Striking increase in sweat sodium and chloride 60 mmol/L) and to a lesser extent potassium is present in virtually all homozygous patients. It is present throughout life from time of birth and is not related to severity of disease or organ involvement. *2467 0151*

Cholesterol *Serum Increase* In 91% of 12 patients at initial hospitalization for this disorder. *0781*

Cholic Acid *Serum Increase* Of cystic fibrosis patients with steatorrhea, 38% had fasting levels greater than 3 standard deviation above mean fasting control levels. *0505* Eight patients had elevated levels not correlated with liver pathology.

Chymotrypsin *Serum Decrease 1901*

Feces Decrease Fecal concentrations may be related to the severity of pancreatic insufficiency. *0113*

Complement C3 *Serum Increase* Found in 13 patients. *1834*

Serum Normal 1397

Erythrocytes *Blood Increase* Slight, in older children. *0338*

277.00 Cystic Fibrosis (continued)

Fat *Feces Increase* Deficient intraluminal pancreatic enzymes. *2199* In this study of 12 patients, average was 41 g/day, compared to < 7 g/day for controls. *2246*

Fatty Acids, Free (FFA) *Serum Decrease* Analyses of children with this disease have indicated a deficiency in essential fatty acids. Arachidonic acid was found only in trace amounts or was absent. *1987* The oleate fatty acids increase while the linoleatic portion decreases. The basis for this seems to be that oleic and linoleic acid differ in changes in oxygen pressure. The oxygen complex of linoleic acid dissociates at relatively high pressures, whereas that of oleic dissociates only at low pressures. *0334*

Globulin *Serum Increase* Rises with progressive pulmonary disease, mainly due to IgG and IgA; IgM and IgD are not appreciably increased. *2467*

Duodenal Contents Increase In excess of that found in the duodenal fluid of controls. *0392*

Glucagon *Plasma Decrease* Both alpha and beta cell function is disrupted resulting in low insulin and glucagon concentration in contrast to diabetes mellitus. *1633*

Glucose *Serum Increase* Fasting hyperglycemia and glycosuria occurred in only 8% of patients. *1633* In 45% of 13 patients at initial hospitalization for this disorder. *0781*

Urine Increase Urinalysis reveals glycosuria due to chemical diabetes. *0433* Fasting hyperglycemia and glycosuria occurred in only 8% of patients. *1633*

Glucose Tolerance *Serum Decrease* Up to 40% of patients are known to have varying degrees of intolerance. Probably secondary to strangulation of the islets by fibrosis. More common with advancing age. *1633* Found in 36% of 31 patients. *0976*

Growth Hormone *Serum Decrease* *0914*

Hematocrit *Blood Decrease* In late stages of chronic lung disease, decreased serum electrolytes, hemoglobin, hematocrit, etc. may reflect hemodilution. *2467*

Hemoglobin *Blood Decrease* In late stages of chronic lung disease, decreased serum electrolytes, hemoglobin, hematocrit, etc., may reflect hemodilution. *2467*

Immunoglobulin IgA *Serum Increase* Rises with progressive pulmonary disease. *2467* *0619*

Immunoglobulin IgD *Serum Normal* Not appreciably increased. *2467*

Immunoglobulin IgG *Serum Increase* Rises with progressive pulmonary disease. *2467*

Immunoglobulin IgM *Serum Normal* Not appreciably increased. *2467*

Insulin *Serum Decrease* Both alpha and beta cell function is disrupted resulting in low insulin and glucagon concentration in contrast to diabetes mellitus. *1633*

Iron *Serum Increase* Intestinal absorption. *0338*

Leukocytes *Blood Increase* In 79% of 16 patients at initial hospitalization for this disorder. *0781*

Lipase *Serum Decrease* *1901*

Lipids *Feces Increase* Reduced intraluminal pancreatic enzyme activity with maldigestion of lipid and protein. *0962*

Oxygen Saturation *Blood Decrease* Pulmonary involvement. *0438*

pCO$_2$ *Blood Increase* Salt loss may lead to metabolic alkalosis. *1055*

pH *Blood Increase* Salt loss may lead to metabolic alkalosis. *1055*

Phosphate *Serum Normal* Normal unless complications occur (e.g., chronic pulmonary disease with accumulation of CO_2, massive salt loss due to sweating). *2467*

Saliva Increase Increased. *1359*

pO$_2$ *Blood Decrease* Pulmonary involvement. *0438*

Potassium *Serum Normal* Normal unless complications occur (e.g., chronic pulmonary disease with accumulation of CO_2, massive salt loss due to sweating). *2467* *0105*

Saliva Normal Submaxillary saliva has slightly increased chloride and sodium but not potassium. *2467*

Sweat Increase Striking increase in sweat sodium and chloride and to a lesser extent potassium is present in virtually all homozygous patients. It is present throughout life from time of birth and is not related to severity of disease or organ involvement. *2467*

Protein *Duodenal Contents Increase* In excess of that found in the duodenal fluid of controls. *0392*

Feces Increase Reduced intraluminal pancreatic enzyme activity with maldigestion of lipid and protein. *0962*

Saliva Increase Submaxillary saliva is more turbid, with increased calcium, total protein, and amylase. These changes are not generally found in parotid saliva. *2467*

Prothrombin Time *Plasma Increase* Secondary to vitamin K deficiency. *0551*

Sodium *Serum Decrease* Normal unless complications occur (e.g., chronic pulmonary disease with accumulation of CO_2, massive salt loss due to sweating). *2467* *0105*

Serum Normal Normal unless complications occur (e.g., chronic pulmonary disease with accumulation of CO_2, massive salt loss due to sweating). *2467* *0105*

Saliva Increase Submaxillary saliva has slightly increased chloride and sodium but not potassium; however, considerable overlap with normal individuals prevents diagnostic usage. *2467*

Sweat Increase A sweat sodium value of above 70 mmol/L is consistent with the diagnosis. *0433* Striking increase in sweat sodium and chloride is present in virtually all homozygous patients. Present throughout life from time of birth and is not related to severity of disease or organ involvement. *2467* Sweat sodium and T_3 normalized after 1 y of oral essential fatty acid therapy. *1987* *0151*

Trypsin *Serum Decrease* *1901*

Urea Nitrogen *Serum Decrease* In 46% of 13 patients at initial hospitalization for this disorder. *0781*

Saliva Increase Increased. *1359*

Uric Acid *Saliva Increase* Increased. *1359*

Vitamin A *Serum Decrease* *0055*

Vitamin E (Tocopherol) *Serum Decrease* *0896*

Vitamin K *Serum Decrease* Occasionally occurs. *0551*

Xylose Tolerance Test *Urine Abnormal* 48 children had 1-h blood xylose levels within the normal range, but the means at 90, 120, and 180 min after load exceeded significantly those of controls. *0325*

Zinc *Serum Decrease* Decreased. *2297*

277.11 Congenital Erythropoietic Porphyria (Günther's Disease)

Aminolevulinic Acid *Urine Normal* With chromatographic methods, within normal limits. *0867* *0995 2426*

Coproporphyrin *Urine Increase* Large amounts but less than the uroporphyrin. *2072*

Bone Marrow Increase *2072*

Feces Increase Large amounts. *2073* *2538 2246*

Red Blood Cells Increase Elevated, but lower than uroporphyrins. *2246* Variable. *2246 2072*

Erythrocyte Survival *Red Blood Cells Decrease* With moderate to severe anemia. *2552* Hemolysis occurs in most patients. *2073 2246*

Hematocrit *Blood Decrease* Anemia is normohromic and normocytic and tends to be mild in degree. *2552* Normochromic anemia, only rarely severe. *2073*

Hemoglobin *Blood Decrease* Anemia is normochromic and normocytic and tends to be mild in degree. *2552* In most patients, reduction was only slight and hemolysis was compensated by increased RBC production. *2073 2246*

MCH *Blood Decrease* Microcytic hypochromic anemia may occur due to blood loss or increased demand. MCH < 27 pg. *0532*

MCV *Blood Decrease* Microcytic hypochromic anemia may occur due to blood loss or increased demand. MCV < 80 fL. *0532*

Osmotic Fragility *Red Blood Cells Normal* *0867*

Porphobilinogen *Urine Normal* With chromatographic methods, within normal limits. *0867* *2426*

Protoporphyrin *Feces Increase* Variable although not significantly elevated. *2246*

Feces Normal Variable although not significantly elevated. *2246*

Red Blood Cells Increase As in other hemolytic conditions. *2497 2538*

Reticulocytes *Blood Increase* With moderate to severe anemia. *2552* Secondary to increased hemolytic activity. *2073* *2246*

Urobilinogen *Feces Increase* *2073 2246*

Uroporphyrin *Serum Increase* Variable. *2246 2072*

Urine Increase Most characteristic metabolic abnormality. *2552* Large amounts. *2538* Daily excretion of 500 µg/24h has been reported. *0935* Up to 500 µg/24h has been reported. *2246*

Bone Marrow Increase Bone marrow is studded with red cell precursors containing uroporphyrin in the nucleus and showing intense fluorescence when examined under ultraviolet light. *2073 2538 2072*

Feces Increase Usually large amounts. *2246*

Red Blood Cells Increase High concentrations. *2072* High RBC concentration of uroporphyrin I. *2072 2246*

277.12 Erythropoietic Protoporphyria

Aminolevulinic Acid *Urine Normal 0995 1478*

Coproporphyrin *Urine Normal 1478*

Feces Increase At times. *2538* In some carriers, elevated even with normal RBC porphyrins. Fluctuates markedly from one time period to another in the same patient. *0579 2246*

Feces Normal 2538

Red Blood Cells Increase 0619

Hematocrit *Blood Decrease* A moderate hypochromic or normochromic anemia is frequently observed. *2538*

Blood Normal In most reported patients, there have been no quantitative blood abnormalities. *2552*

Hemoglobin *Blood Decrease* A moderate hypochromic or normochromic anemia is frequently observed. *2538*

Blood Normal In most reported patients, there have been no quantitative blood abnormalities. *2552*

Iron *Serum Normal 2538*

MCH *Blood Decrease* Microcytic hypochromic anemia may occur due to blood loss or increased demand. MCH < 27 pg. *0532* A moderate hypochromic or normochromic anemia is frequently observed. *2538*

MCHC *Blood Decrease* A moderate hypochromic or normochromic anemia is frequently observed. *2538*

MCV *Blood Decrease* Microcytic hypochromic anemia may occur due to blood loss or increased demand. MCV < 80 fL. *0532* A moderate hypo- or normochromic anemia is frequently observed. *2538*

Porphobilinogen *Urine Normal 1478*

Protoporphyrin *Serum Increase* Frequently elevated. *1478* Most striking finding is the elevation in RBC, feces, and plasma. *2246*

Urine Increase 1752

Feces Increase Usually but not always increased in symptomatic patients, from 30-300 μg/g dry weight and occasionally higher. *1458* Contains only increased protoporphyrin, a unique finding among porphyrias. *2538* In some carriers, elevated even with normal RBC porphyrins. Fluctuates markedly from one time period to another in the same patient. *0579 2552 2246*

Red Blood Cells Increase The red cells hemolyze if blood in thin layers is exposed to ultraviolet light. *0990 2538* Increased 5-30 X. *1478* Reported values range from 300-4,500 mg/dL (normal < 50). *2552* Excess does not occur in all cells, from 7-60% were found to contain excess. *1224* May be up to 100-fold. *1477* Marked increase. *2246*

Uroporphyrin *Urine Increase* Only in patients with hepatic complications. *2246*

Urine Normal 1478 2246

Feces Normal 2246

Red Blood Cells Increase Moderate concentrations. *0995*

277.13 Erythropoietic Coproporphyria

Aminolevulinic Acid *Urine Normal 0995 1478*

Coproporphyrin *Urine Normal 0619*

Feces Normal 2538

Red Blood Cells Increase Large amounts. *0619*

Hematocrit *Blood Decrease* Microcytic hypochromic anemia may occur due to blood loss or increased demand. *0532*

Hemoglobin *Blood Decrease* Microcytic hypochromic anemia may occur due to blood loss or increased demand. *0532*

MCH *Blood Decrease* Microcytic hypochromic anemia may occur due to blood loss or increased demand. MCH < 27 pg. *0532*

MCV *Blood Decrease* Microcytic hypochromic anemia may occur due to blood loss or increased demand. MCV < 80 fL. *0532*

Porphobilinogen *Urine Increase* Slight increase. *2246*

Urine Normal 0995

Protoporphyrin *Feces Normal 0995*

Red Blood Cells Increase Small increase. *2246 0995*

Uroporphyrin *Urine Normal 1529*

Feces Normal 0995

Red Blood Cells Increase Moderate concentrations. *0995*

277.14 Acute Intermittent Porphyria

17-Hydroxycorticosteroids *Urine Increase* In acute attacks. *2246*

17-Ketogenic Steroids *Urine Increase* In acute attacks. *2246*

Amino Acids *Urine Increase 1565*

Aminolevulinic Acid *Serum Increase* Severe attacks. *2246*

Urine Increase In the hereditary hepatic porphyrias. *0145* A reduction in the activity of the enzyme uroporphyrinogen I synthetase appears to explain the accumulation in body fluids and increased amounts in the urine. Excessive accumulation is further aggravated by an increased ALA synthetase activity. *2271* May contain as much as 180 mg/24h. *1529* In 21 symptomatic patients, an average of 43 mg ALA/24h was excreted. Tends to decrease somewhat during remission. *2254 0962 2552*

Antidiuretic Hormone *Serum Increase* Syndrome of inappropriate ADH secretion has been documented in a number of cases. *2552*

BSP Retention *Serum Increase* Normal liver function tests except for BSP. Over 10% BSP retained in 79% of symptomatic patients and in 55% of those in remission. *2254*

Chloride *Serum Decrease* Hyponatremia, hypochloremia, hypokalemia, hypomagnesemia, and alkalosis associated with azotemia of variable degree are often present on admission but may also develop acutely during the course of the attack. The electrolyte disorders are attributable in many patients to electrolyte depletion with inappropriate and injudicious overhydration. *0433 2538*

Cholesterol *Urine Increase 0151*

Cholesterol, Low Density Lipoprotein *Serum Increase* Moderate elevation. *0062*

Coproporphyrin *Urine Increase* Excessive amounts. *0995*

Feces Increase Slight to moderate increase. *2498* Small increases may be found. *2246*

Liver Increase Has been isolated from hepatic tissue in some cases. *2072 2246*

Red Blood Cells Normal 0995

Erythrocyte Survival *Red Blood Cells Normal* Suggests that the decreased RBC mass results from reduced effective erythropoiesis. *0230*

Globulin *Serum Increase* Constant finding. *0433*

Hematocrit *Blood Decrease* Microcytic hypochromic anemia may occur due to blood loss or increased demand. *0532*

Hemoglobin *Blood Decrease* Microcytic hypochromic anemia may occur due to blood loss or increased demand. *0532*

Iron *Serum Increase* Frequently markedly elevated. *0433*

Isocitrate Dehydrogenase *Serum Normal 2260*

Leukocytes *Blood Increase* Occasionally during acute attacks. *2254 0151*

Lipoproteins, Beta *Serum Increase 0151*

Magnesium *Serum Decrease* Electrolyte depletion and alkalosis associated with azotemia of variable degree are often present on admission but may also develop acutely during the course of the attack. The electrolyte disorders are attributable in many patients to electrolyte depletion with inappropriate and injudicious overhydration. *0433*

MCH *Blood Decrease* Microcytic hypochromic anemia may occur due to blood loss or increased demand. MCH < 27 pg. *0532*

MCV *Blood Decrease* Microcytic hypochromic anemia may occur due to blood loss or increased demand. MCV < 80 fL. *0532*

pH *Blood Increase* Electrolyte depletion and alkalosis associated with azotemia of variable degree are often present on admission but may also develop acutely during the course of the attack. *0433*

Porphobilinogen *Serum Increase* Increased production of the porphyrin precursors. *0145* In patients with severe attacks. *2304*

Urine Increase Occurs fairly specifically in acute idiopathic porphyria. *2499* In 21 symptomatic patients, an average of 83 mg porphobilinogen/24h was excreted. Tends to decrease somewhat during remission. *2254* During relapse the presence of this compound is a constant feature. During remission it is usually present but the absence does not exclude the diagnosis. *2457 2538* Characteristic. *2246 0145 2271 0962 2552*

CSF Increase In patients with severe attacks. *2304*

277.14 Acute Intermittent Porphyria *(continued)*

Porphobilinogen *(continued)*

Liver Increase Large amounts. *0908* Liver and kidney regularly contain large amounts. *2072 2246*

Potassium *Serum Decrease* Electrolyte depletion and alkalosis associated with azotemia of variable degree are often present on admission but may also develop acutely during the course of the attack. The electrolyte disorders are attributable in many patients to electrolyte depletion with inappropriate and injudicious overhydration. *0433*

Protein Bound Iodine (PBI) *Serum Increase* Occasionally. *2254*

Urine Increase Occasionally increased. *2467 0151*

Protoporphyrin *Feces Increase* Slight or moderate elevation. *2498* Small increases may be found. *2246*

Red Blood Cells Normal 0995

Sodium *Serum Decrease* Electrolyte depletion and alkalosis associated with azotemia of variable degree are often present on admission but may also develop acutely during the course of the attack. The severity of the hyponatremia is a particularly striking feature, and although it may by symptomless, it is often associated with the encephalopathic manifestations of the acute attack. Attributable in many patients to electrolyte depletion with inappropriate and injudicious overhydration. *0433 2254*

Thyroxine Binding Globulin *Serum Increase 2540 2254*

Urea Nitrogen *Serum Increase* Frequent. *2254* During an attack. *0433 2538*

Uroporphyrin *Urine Increase* Excessive amounts. *0995* May contain little if any increase. *0443* May develop in urine on standing. *2246*

Feces Increase In some patients. *2498* Small increases may be found. *2246*

Liver Increase Has been isolated from hepatic tissue in some cases. *2072 2246*

Red Blood Cells Normal 0995

Volume *Plasma Decrease* Frequently observed during attacks. *2254*

Urine Decrease Prolonged vomiting may cause dehydration, oliguria, and azotemia. *0151*

277.15 Porphyria Variegata

Aminolevulinic Acid *Urine Increase* May appear during acute attacks. *2552* Normal or moderate increase in asymptomatic patients. Sharp rise with acute attacks. *0613 0995*

Cholesterol *Urine Increase 0151*

Coproporphyrin *Urine Increase* Characteristic finding in urine and feces. *1940* Sharp rise in acute attacks. *0613* During acute attacks. *2246 2538*

Feces Increase The most characteristic and consistent abnormality. *2254* Ranges from 70 - > 1,000 μg/g dry weight (normal < 100 μg/g). *2552* Large amounts. *0524* Even when clinical manifestations are minimal. *0928*

Red Blood Cells Normal 0995 2246

Globulin *Serum Increase* Constant finding. *0433*

Hexosaminidase *Serum Increase 1443*

Iron *Serum Increase* Frequently markedly elevated. *0433*

Leukocytes *Blood Increase 0151*

Lipoproteins, Beta *Serum Increase 0151*

MCH *Blood Decrease* Microcytic hypochromic anemia may occur due to blood loss or increased demand. MCH < 27 pg. *0532*

MCV *Blood Decrease* Microcytic hypochromic anemia may occur due to blood loss or increased demand. MCV < 80 fL. *0532*

Porphobilinogen *Serum Increase* Increased production of the porphyrin precursors. *0145*

Urine Increase May appear during acute attacks. *2552* May be as high as levels in acute intermittent porphyria. *0524 0613*

Protoporphyrin *Feces Increase* The most characteristic and consistent abnormality. *2254* Large amounts. *0524* Even when clinical manifestations are minimal. *0928 0962 2246*

Red Blood Cells Normal 0995 2246

Uroporphyrin *Urine Increase* During acute attacks. *0995* Characteristic finding in urine and feces. *1940* Sharp rise in acute attacks. *0613 2538*

Feces Increase May be increased. *2303* Variable. *0868*

Red Blood Cells Normal 0995 2246

277.16 Porphyria Cutanea Tarda

Alanine Aminotransferase *Serum Increase* Liver function is highly variable. May be mildly elevated. *2552*

Aminolevulinic Acid *Urine Increase* During acute stage. *0995* Rarely occurs. *0613 2246*

Urine Normal 1344

Aspartate Aminotransferase *Serum Increase* Liver function is highly variable. May be mildly elevated. *2552*

BSP Retention *Serum Increase* Usually abnormal. *2458*

Coproporphyrin *Urine Increase* Average in 66 patients was 560 μg/24h (normal < 200 μg/24h). *0611 2552*

Feces Increase Large amounts. *0995* Highly variable, but never as high as in variegata porphyria. *2314 2246*

Red Blood Cells Normal 0995

Hematocrit *Blood Decrease* Microcytic hypochromic anemia may occur due to blood low or increased demand. *0532*

Hemoglobin *Blood Decrease* Microcytic hypochromic anemia may occur due to blood low or increased demand. *0532*

Hexosaminidase *Serum Increase 1443*

Iron *Serum Increase* Often increased. *2552 2389*

Bone Marrow Increase General increase in body iron stores, in liver, marrow and plasma. *2389*

Liver Increase General increase in body iron stores, in liver, marrow and plasma. *2389*

Iron Saturation *Serum Increase* Over 70% saturation in 4 of 20 patients. *0670*

MCH *Blood Decrease* Microcytic hypochromic anemia may occur due to blood loss or increased demand. MCH < 27 pg. *0532*

MCV *Blood Decrease* Microcytic hypochromic anemia may occur due to blood loss or increased demand. MCV < 80 fL. *0532*

Porphobilinogen *Urine Increase* Rarely occurs. *0613 2246 0995*

Urine Normal Not present. *1344 2538*

Porphyrins *Urine Increase* Usually enough to produce a pinkish or brown color. *2246*

Bone Marrow Normal 2072

Feces Normal Normal or only slightly increased in the stool. *2552* Highly variable. *2246*

Liver Increase May precede clinical manifestations and persist after remission. *2072*

Protoporphyrin *Feces Increase* Large amounts. *0995* Highly variable. *2314 2246*

Red Blood Cells Normal 0995

Urobilinogen *Urine Increase* May be increased because of liver disease. *2458*

Uroporphyrin *Urine Increase* In 66 patients, average was 2,819 μg/L and exceeded 1,000 μg/L in 70% of the group (normal < 40 mg/24h). *0611* During acute attacks. *0995* Usually 1-10 mg/24h. *0613*

Feces Increase Highly variable. *2314*

Red Blood Cells Normal 0995

277.17 Hereditary Coproporphyria

17-Hydroxycorticosteroids *Urine Increase* In acute attacks. *2246*

17-Ketogenic Steroids *Urine Increase* In acute attacks. *2246*

Aminolevulinic Acid *Urine Increase* Mild increase during latent and acute stage. *0995* Only during acute attacks. *2552 2246*

Cholesterol *Urine Increase 0151*

Coproporphyrin *Urine Increase* May occur during symptomatic periods but is usually normal during remission. *2552 2538 2246*

Feces Increase Between 100-3,000 μg/g dry weight (normal < 40). *2552* Unremitting excretion of large amounts. *2538* Striking abnormality, large excess of coproporphyrin III. *2246*

Red Blood Cells Normal No increase demonstrable. *2246 0868 0995*

Globulin *Serum Increase* Constant finding. *0433*

Hematocrit *Blood Decrease* Microcytic hypochromic anemia may occur due to blood loss or increased demand. *0532*

Hemoglobin *Blood Decrease* Microcytic hypochromic anemia may occur due to blood loss or increased demand. *0532*

Iron *Serum Increase* Frequently markedly elevated. *0433*

Leukocytes *Blood Increase 0151*

Lipoproteins, Beta *Serum Increase* 0151

MCH *Blood Decrease* Microcytic hypochromic anemia may occur due to blood loss or increased demand. MCH < 27 pg. 0532

MCV *Blood Decrease* Microcytic hypochromic anemia may occur due to blood loss or increased demand. MCV < 80 fL. 0532

Porphobilinogen *Serum Increase* Increased production of the porphyrin precursors. 0145

Urine Increase Only during acute attacks. 2552 0995 2246

Porphyrins *Bone Marrow Normal* No increase demonstrable. 2246 0868

Feces Increase 2246

Protoporphyrin *Feces Increase* Increased but not to the same extent as coproporphyrin. 2538 2246

Feces Normal Normal or only slightly increased. 2552

Red Blood Cells Normal No increase demonstrable. 2246 0868 0995

Uroporphyrin *Urine Increase* 0995

Red Blood Cells Normal No increase demonstrable. 2246 0868 0995

277.21 Xanthinuria

Hypoxanthine *Urine Increase* Characterized by the replacement of uric acid by xanthine and hypoxanthine in urine. 2246

Uric Acid *Serum Decrease* Characterized by the replacement of uric acid by xanthine and hypoxanthine in urine. 2246 Concentrations below level of detection have been documented as well as elevations. 2104 0962

Serum Increase Concentrations below level of detection have been documented as well as elevations. 2104

Urine Decrease Characterized by the replacement of uric acid by xanthine and hypoxanthine in urine. 2246

Xanthine *Urine Increase* Characterized by the replacement of uric acid by xanthine and hypoxanthine in urine. 2246

277.22 Lesch-Nyhan Syndrome

Dopamine Hydroxylase *Serum Decrease* Decreased although norepinephrine is normal. 1300

Erythrocytes *Urine Increase* Hematuria often occurs. 2246

Folate *Serum Decrease* Decreased. 0299 2357 0367

Hematocrit *Blood Decrease* Many patients are anemia prior to the occurrence of renal insufficiency. 2246

Hemoglobin *Blood Decrease* Many patients are anemic prior to the occurrence of renal insufficiency. 2246

Uric Acid *Serum Increase* Ranges from 7-18 mg/dL in the absence of renal insufficiency. Occasionally a normal value may occur. 0182 2246

Urine Increase Markedly increased. Ranges from 25-143 mg/kg/day compared to 18 as the normal upper limit in children. 1581 2246

277.30 Amyloidosis

Acid Phosphatase *Serum Increase* Increased in 66% of 14 patients tested. The tartrate inhibition (< 20%) was within normal limits. 1334

Alanine Aminotransferase *Serum Normal* Usually normal. 0125

Albumin *Serum Decrease* Found to be < 3.0 g/dL in 76% of patients. 1334 Frequently found with liver involvement. 0962 Has been observed. No correlation with severity or duration of disease. 0120 2246

Urine Increase Frequently seen. Massive proteinuria (over 10 g/24h) and other manifestations of the nephrotic syndrome may also be present. 0433

Alkaline Phosphatase *Serum Increase* Frequently elevated, usually ranging from 25-535 U/L. No jaundice. In patients with space-occupying lesions such as amyloidosis the degree of elevation at times may be striking with little or no rise in the serum bilirubin values. 2467 0138 0140 Increased in almost 50% of patients with primary disease, mean value = 108 U/L. 1334 Frequently found with liver involvement. 0962 With hepatic involvement. 0125 0503

Alpha₁-Antitrypsin *Serum Increase* In patients with rheumatoid arthritis complicated by amyloidosis. 1526

Alpha₂-Globulin *Serum Increase* Hyperglobulinemia occurs in 15% of cases of cardiac amyloidosis; alpha₂ and gamma fractions moderately increased. 0151

Alpha₂-Macroglobulin *Serum Increase* Has been observed. No correlation with severity or duration of disease. 0120 2246

Amino Acids *Plasma Normal* 2246

Aspartate Aminotransferase *Serum Increase* Elevated in > 33% of patients with primary disease. 1334

Serum Normal Usually normal. 0125

Bence-Jones Protein *Serum Present* May occur. 0999 Found in 21 of 22 patients with primary disease. 1745

Urine Present Found in 57% of secondary and only 8% of primary cases. 1334 Detected in 6 of 15 cases; excretion was < 1 g/24h in all patients. 0125

Bilirubin *Serum Increase* 10% of patients had increased direct bilirubin and 5% had high indirect bilirubin. 1334

Bilirubin, Direct *Serum Increase* 10% of patients had increased direct bilirubin and 5% had high indirect bilirubin. 1334

Bilirubin, Indirect *Serum Increase* 10% of patients had increased direct bilirubin and 5% had high indirect bilirubin. 1334

BSP Retention *Serum Increase* Retention is increased in 75% of patients with liver involvement. 2468 Found to be elevated in over 50% of patients 5% in 1 h), contrary to the suggestion that hepatomegaly with normal or only slightly abnormal liver function is characteristic. 1334 With hepatic involvement. 0125 0962

Calcium *Serum Normal* Rarely elevated in primary disease. 1334

Cholesterol *Serum Increase* High concentrations found in 33% of primary cases and < 20% of secondary cases. 1334

Complement C3 *Serum Increase* Found mostly in the recovery phase. 0793 0452 1275 0509 0375

Congo Red Test *Blood Positive* Of 20 patients with amyloidosis, only 9 had > 60% disappearance of congo red from blood in 1 h. False-negative tests may be expected in > 50% of cases. 0341 Positive in 33% of patients with primary and in 66% of patients with secondary amyloidosis. 2468 Positive in up to 50% of patients with cardiac amyloidosis. 0151

Creatinine *Serum Increase* Increased in > 50% of patients at time of diagnosis due to renal insufficiency. 1334

Erythrocytes *Urine Increase* Microscopic hematuria is frequently seen. 0433

Erythrocyte Sedimentation Rate *Blood Increase* Over 55 mm/h (Westergren) in 50% of patients. 1334

Fat *Feces Increase* In small intestinal disease. 2199

Globulin *Serum Decrease* In 25% of patients. 1334 Hypogammaglobulinemia was found in patients with Bence-Jones proteinuria but not in any other patients. 0125 A low Albumin and globulin profile 0433

Serum Increase Increased concentration with reversed A/G ratio is frequent. 2468 Hyperglobulinemia occurs in 15% of cases of cardiac amyloidosis; alpha₂ and gamma fractions moderately increased. 0151 Has been observed. No correlation with severity or duration of disease 0120 2246

Glomerular Filtration Rate (GFR) *Urine Decrease* Decreased due to reduced filtration surface (fewer functioning glomeruli). 0619

Haptoglobin *Serum Increase* Conditions associated with increased ESR and alpha₂-globulin. 2467

Hematocrit *Blood Decrease* Mild anemia present in < 50% of patients. 1334

Hemoglobin *Blood Decrease* Mild anemia present in < 50% of patients. 1334

Hexosamine *Serum Normal* 0120 2246

Immunoglobulin IgA *Serum Decrease* Mean concentration (.61 g/L) was significantly decreased in patients with Bence-Jones proteinuria. 0124

Immunoglobulin IgG *Serum Decrease* Decreased in 50% of primary and 66% of secondary disease. 1334 Mean concentration (540 mg/dL) was significantly decreased in patients with Bence-Jones proteinuria. 0124

Immunoglobulin IgM *Serum Decrease* The most significant finding. All 14 patients without macroglobulinemia had reduced concentration, mean = 0.5 g/L, only 34% of the control value. 0124 Mean concentration (0.46 g/L) was significantly decreased in patients with Bence-Jones proteinuria. 0124

277.30   Amyloidosis   (continued)

Immunoglobulins   *Serum   Decrease*   Mean serum concentration of all 3 classes of immunoglobulins, IgA, IgM and IgG, were significantly reduced in patients with increased Bence-Jones protein excretion. *0124*

Leukocytes   *Blood   Decrease*   Leukopenia, if present, suggests multiple myeloma as the cause for amyloidosis. *0433*

Blood   Increase   Frequently increased (> 12,000/μL). *2468   0433*

Lipoproteins   *Serum   Increase*   May be present. *1108*   Has been observed. No correlation with severity or duration of the disease. *0120 2246*

Plasma Cells   *Bone Marrow   Increase*   None of the patients with primary disease had > 15% plasma cells, whereas over 50% of the secondary cases did. Mean percentage of cells was 4 in primary and 23 in secondary. *1334*   A bone marrow plasmacytosis is found in a high proportion of cases. *1108*   Many patients can be shown to have homogeneous immunoglobulins in the serum and/or urine, and plasmacytosis in the marrow, and ultimately to develop morphologic and clinical evidence of a plasma cell dyscrasia. *1127   2538*

Platelet Count   *Blood   Increase*   Mild thrombocytosis in primary disease. *1334*

Protein   *Serum   Decrease*   Hypoproteinemia occurs in 15% of cases of cardiac amyloidosis. *0151*

Urine   Increase   Proteinuria is usually the first sign of renal amyloid, may persist for years or temporarily disappear. *0151*   Found in 90% of primary and 98% of secondary cases. *1334*   Frequently massive, with up to 20 g/24h excreted in patients with renal amyloid. *0125*

CSF   Increase   Usually elevated. *2246*

Thymol Turbidity   *Serum   Normal*   Usually normal. *0125*

Urea Nitrogen   *Serum   Increase*   *0433*

Uric Acid   *Serum   Increase*   Increased in 22% of primary and 31% of secondary cases. *1334*

277.41   Dubin-Johnson Syndrome

Alanine Aminotransferase   *Serum   Increase*   May be normal or moderately increased. *0602*

Serum   Normal   Routine liver function tests are normal. *0962*

Alkaline Phosphatase   *Serum   Increase*   May be normal or moderately increased. *0602*

Serum   Normal   Routine liver function tests are normal. *0962*

Aspartate Aminotransferase   *Serum   Increase*   May be normal or moderately increased. *0602*

Serum   Normal   Routine liver function tests are normal. *0962*

Bilirubin   *Serum   Increase*   Characterized by chronic nonhemolytic, predominantly conjugated hyperbilirubinemia. *0180*   The total serum bilirubin ranges between 2-10 mg/24h. *0962*   Slight to marked in degree with marked fluctuations in intensity. *0602 2246*

Urine   Increase   May be seen. *0180*   Patient presents with intermittent jaundice and bilirubinuria. *0962   0999*

Bilirubin, Direct   *Serum   Increase*   Characterized by chronic nonhemolytic, predominantly conjugated hyperbilirubinemia associated with jaundice. *0180*   Familial, conjugated hyperbilirubinemia due to a defect in the excretion of bilirubin from the liver. *0962   0999   2246*

Bilirubin, Indirect   *Serum   Increase*   *0995*

BSP Retention   *Serum   Increase*   Higher at 90 min than at 45 min after IV administration. *0180*   Normal or slightly impaired excretion. *2246*   Normal decrease in serum concentration 45 min after injection, followed by a rise at 2 h, due to difficulty in its excretion from the liver with leakage back into the bloodstream. *0962*

Cephalin Flocculation   *Serum   Increase*   May be positive. *2467*

Coproporphyrin   *Urine   Increase*   Increases in the urinary excretion of coproporphyrin I have been found not only in patients with this syndrome but also in close relatives. *0962*   Mean excretion is 3-4 X that of normal subjects. *2561*   Total excretion is normal or slightly increased, but 84-90% in type I isomer, strikingly different from normal. *2246*

Urine   Normal   Total excretion is normal or slightly increased, but 84-90% in type I isomer, strikingly different from normal. *2246*

Red Blood Cells   Normal   Total concentration is normal but the isomer percentages are reversed. Normally, coproporphyrin III constitutes 75%, while in homozygous patients it is over 80% of the total. *0180*

Lactate Dehydrogenase   *Serum   Increase*   May be normal or moderately increased. *0602*

Thymol Turbidity   *Serum   Increase*   May be increased. *2467*

Urobilinogen   *Urine   Increase*   Urine contains bile and urobilinogen. *2467*

Feces   Decrease   *0995*

277.42   Gilbert's Disease

Alanine Aminotransferase   *Serum   Normal*   *0995*

Alkaline Phosphatase   *Serum   Normal*   *0995*

Aspartate Aminotransferase   *Serum   Normal*   *0995*

Bile Acids   *Serum   Normal*   An elevated bilirubin coexisting with a normal bile acid level suggests Gilbert's Disease. *2199*   Fasting and post prandial levels were normal with reduced and normal caloric loads. *0283*

Bilirubin   *Serum   Increase*   Mild increase in unconjugated serum bilirubin reduced by phenobarbital and increased within 24 h of a reduced calorie diet. *0619*   Degree of elevation does not correlate with symptoms. *0180*   Highest after fasting and rarely exceeds 3 mg/dL. *0962*   Usually in range of 1.2-3 mg/dL, rarely > 5 mg/dL. *0995*

Urine   Normal   *2246*

Feces   Decrease   *2467*

Bilirubin, Direct   *Serum   Normal*   20% of total bilirubin. *0995*

Bilirubin, Indirect   *Serum   Increase*   Mild asymptomatic increase of indirect serum bilirubin, usually discovered on routine lab exam. May rise to 18 mg/dL but usually is < 4 mg/dL. *2467*   Unexplained, mild, chronic elevation. *2246   0962*

BSP Retention   *Serum   Increase*   Mild 45 min retention has been observed in 20% of patients. *0180*   In a significant number of patients. *0179*

Chenodeoxycholic Acid   *Serum   Normal*   Normal levels in hyperbilirubinemic patients. *2642 0751*

Cholic Acid   *Serum   Decrease*   Significantly reduced in hyperbilirubinemic patients. *2642*

Serum   Normal   Fasting levels were normal in all 24 patients studied. *2642*

Erythrocyte Survival   *Red Blood Cells   Decrease*   Mild, but fully compensated hemolysis in a significant number of patients. *0754*

Hemoglobin, Free   *Serum   Increase*   Mild, but fully compensated hemolysis in a significant number of patients. *0754*

Lactate Dehydrogenase   *Serum   Normal*   *0995*

Urobilinogen   *Urine   Decrease*   Normal or decreased. *2467*

Feces   Decrease   Normal or decreased. *2467*

277.43   Rotor's Syndrome

Alanine Aminotransferase   *Serum   Normal*   Routine liver function tests are normal. *0962*

Alkaline Phosphatase   *Serum   Normal*   Routine liver function tests are normal. *0962*

Aspartate Aminotransferase   *Serum   Normal*   Routine liver function tests are normal. *0962*

Bilirubin   *Serum   Increase*   The total serum bilirubin ranges between 2-10 mg/24h. *0962*   Slight to moderate direct bilirubinemia. *2246*

Urine   Increase   Patient presents with intermittent jaundice and bilirubinuria. *0962   2467*

Urine   Normal   *2246*

Feces   Decrease   *0503*

Bilirubin, Direct   *Serum   Increase*   Familial, conjugated hyperbilirubinemia due to a defect in the excretion of bilirubin from the liver. *0962*

Bilirubin, Indirect   *Serum   Increase*   *2467*

BSP Retention   *Serum   Increase*   Marked retention. *2246*   Defects in the excretion of BSP and of gallbladder dye may reveal a normal decrease in its serum concentration 45 min after injection, followed by a rise at 2 h, due to difficulty in its excretion from the live with leakage back into the bloodstream. *0962*

Coproporphyrin   *Urine   Increase*   Increases in the urinary excretion of coproporphyrin I have been found not only in patients with this syndrome but also in close relatives. *0962*   Marked increase in some patients. *2465*

Urobilinogen   *Urine   Increase*   Normal or increased. *2467*

Feces   Decrease   *2467*

277.44   Crigler-Najjar Syndrome

Alanine Aminotransferase   *Serum   Normal*   Liver function tests were uniformly normal. *2246   0469*

Alkaline Phosphatase   *Serum   Normal   0469*

Aspartate Aminotransferase   *Serum   Normal*   Liver function tests were uniformly normal. *2246   0469*

Bilirubin   *Serum   Increase*   Patients with apparent autosomal recessive pattern of inheritance with severe hyperbilirubinemia (20-31 mg/dL). *0999*   Almost invariably in the range of 15-48 mg/dL with virtually all giving an indirect van den Bergh reaction. Fluctuations are frequent, with higher values in winter and incidental illness. *2071 2246*

Urine   Normal   None detectable. *2246*

Feces   Decrease   2467 0503

Bilirubin, Direct   *Serum   Decrease   2246*

Bilirubin, Indirect   *Serum   Increase*   Increased; it appears on 1st or 2nd day of life, rises to 12-45 mg/dL, and persists for life. *2467* Familial unconjugated hyperbilirubinemia due to low or absent hepatic glucuronyl-transferase activity. *0962*

BSP Retention   *Serum   Normal*   Liver function tests were uniformly normal. *2246*

Hematocrit   *Blood   Normal*   No evidence of hemolytic anemia or splenomegaly. *2246   0469*

Hemoglobin   *Blood   Normal*   No evidence of hemolytic anemia or splenomegaly. *2246   0469*

Lactate Dehydrogenase   *Serum   Normal   0469*

Reticulocytes   *Blood   Normal*   No evidence of hemolytic anemia or splenomegaly. *2246   0469*

Urobilinogen   *Urine   Decrease*   Normal or decreased. *2467*

Feces   Decrease   Usually very low but stool is of normal color. *2246*

278.00   Obesity

17-Hydroxycorticosteroids   *Urine   Increase*   Increased 24 hour hydroxycorticoid excretion. *0062*

Cholesterol   *Serum   Increase*   Hyperlipidemia. *0996 2641*

Cortisol   *Plasma   Increase   0062*

Endorphin, Beta   *Plasma   Increase*   Baseline concentrations were two times higher than in nonobese adolescents and children. *0824*

Fatty Acids, Free (FFA)   *Serum   Increase*   Increased turnover. *0996*   Significantly higher *0864*

Glucagon   *Plasma   Normal*   Similar levels were obtained in 10 nonobese patients. *0864*

Growth Hormone   *Serum   Increase*   Secretory response to a variety of stimuli is attenuated. *0062*

Serum   Normal   Similar levels were obtained in 10 nonobese patients. *0864*

Insulin   *Serum   Increase*   Degree of obesity correlates with the level of insulin elevation. *0996*

Triglycerides   *Serum   Increase*   Hypertriglyceridemia is frequent. *0996*

278.40   Hypervitaminosis D

Alkaline Phosphatase   *Serum   Decrease   0503*

Calcium   *Serum   Increase*   Especially with added calcium in the diet; hypercalcemia corrected by steroids. *0619*   4 cases with hypercalcemia (range 10.6-16.4 mg/dL). *1904   2199*

Urine   Increase   2199

Feces   Decrease   Decreased in stool. More calcium is absorbed from the diet than normal. *0619*

Phosphate   *Serum   Decrease*   Normal to decreased values. *0503*

Serum   Increase   Usually increased with increased urinary phosphate. *2467   0812 0503*

Urine   Increase   In large doses vitamin D causes increased renal excretion of phosphate; to this extent its renal effect resembles parathyroid hormone. *0812 0503*

279.01   IgA Deficiency (Selective)

Alpha$_1$-Antitrypsin   *Serum   Normal*   No deficiency was found in children with this disorder. *1747*

Immunoglobulin IgA   *Serum   Decrease*   Less than 5 mg/dL. *0793*

Immunoglobulin IgD   *Serum   Normal   0793*

Immunoglobulin IgE   *Serum   Normal   0793*

Immunoglobulin IgG   *Serum   Normal   0793*

Immunoglobulin IgM   *Serum   Normal   0793*

Lymphocyte B-Cell   *Blood   Normal   0793*

Lymphocyte T-Cell   *Blood   Normal   0793*

279.04   Agammaglobulinemia (Congenital Sex-linked)

Albumin   *Serum   Normal   2467*

Alpha$_1$-Antitrypsin   *Serum   Normal   2467*

Alpha$_1$-Globulin   *Serum   Normal   2538*

Alpha$_2$-Globulin   *Serum   Normal   2538*

Antibody Titer   *Serum   Decrease*   Very low levels of antibody to certain animal viruses can be demonstrated. *2035*

Beta-Globulin   *Serum   Normal   2538*

Complement C3   *Serum   Normal   2467*

Complement, Total   *Serum   Normal*   Other serum constituents involved in resistance to infection are normal. *2246*   Normal *2539 2035*

Erythrocyte Survival   *Red Blood Cells   Decrease*   Hemolytic anemia. *2035*

Globulin   *Serum   Decrease*   The total serum globulins are decreased (100-200 mg/dL). Paper electrophoresis of serum shows complete absence of gamma globulins. *0433*   Serum contains < 100 mg gamma G globulin/dL. Gamma A & M globulins are present in concentrations < 1% of normal *2246*

Haptoglobin   *Serum   Normal   2467*

Hematocrit   *Blood   Decrease*   Hemolytic anemia. *2035*   Hemolytic anemia frequently occurs. *2246*

Hemoglobin   *Blood   Decrease*   Hemolytic anemia. *2035*   Hemolytic anemia frequently occurs. *2246*

Hemoglobin, Free   *Serum   Increase*   Hemolytic anemia frequently occurs. *2246*

Immunoglobulin IgA   *Serum   Decrease*   Usually < 1% of normal adult values. *2035*   Undetectable. *2538*

Immunoglobulin IgD   *Serum   Decrease*   Undetectable. *2538*

Immunoglobulin IgE   *Serum   Decrease*   Undetectable. *2538*

Immunoglobulin IgG   *Serum   Decrease*   Minute amounts of IgG and sometimes IgM are identifiable by sensitive methods, functional levels of antibody are absent. *0999*   100 mg/dL. *2035*   In primary acquired form, the serum levels may be as high as 500 mg/dL. *1069*

Immunoglobulin IgM   *Serum   Decrease*   Usually < 1% of normal adult values. *2035*   Undetectable. *2538*

Immunoglobulins   *Serum   Decrease*   All classes are deficient, including the secretory immunoglobulins. *2552*

Iron-Binding Capacity, Total (TIBC)   *Serum   Normal   2467*

Leukocytes   *Blood   Decrease*   Not uncommon to observe either leukopenia or striking leukocytosis in these patients at the time of severe pyogenic infections. *2035*

Blood   Increase   Not uncommon to observe either leukopenia or striking leukocytosis in these patients at the time of severe pyogenic infections. *2035*

Lymphocyte B-Cell   *Blood   Decrease*   Complete absence. *2539*

Lymphocytes   *Blood   Decrease*   There is a decreased number of lymphocytes in the congenital forms. *0433*

Blood   Normal   Counts are normal (> 2,000/μL). *2035*

Lymphocyte T-Cell   *Blood   Normal*   Normal to increased. *2539*

Lysozyme   *Serum   Normal*   Other serum constituents involved in resistance to infection are normal. *2246   2539*

Plasma Cells   *Bone Marrow   Decrease*   The basic deficiency is an absence of plasma cells from the lymph nodes, spleen, intestine, and bone marrow. *2538   2035 0886*

Properidin   *Serum   Normal*   Normal. *2539*   Other serum constituents involved in resistance to infection are normal *2246*

279.06   Immunodeficiency (Common Variable)

Adenosine Deaminase   *Serum   Decrease*   Decreased in Severe Combined Immunodeficiency Disease. *0655 1737 2235*

Albumin   *Serum   Normal   2467*

Alpha$_1$-Globulin   *Serum   Normal   2467*

Alpha$_2$-Globulin   *Serum   Normal   2467*

279.06   Immunodeficiency (Common Variable)
(continued)

Antibody Titer   *Serum   Decrease*   Antibody responses to most antigens are low or absent. *2552*

Beta-Globulin   *Serum   Normal*   *2467*

Fat   *Feces   Increase*   In small intestinal disease. *2199*

Globulin   *Serum   Decrease*   *2467*

Hematocrit   *Blood   Decrease*   High incidence of pernicious anemia. *2538*

Hemoglobin   *Blood   Decrease*   High incidence of pernicious anemia. *2538*

Immunoglobulin IgA   *Serum   Decrease*   *0619 2539*

Immunoglobulin IgE   *Serum   Decrease*   *2035*

Immunoglobulin IgG   *Serum   Decrease*   Usually < 500 mg/dL. *2035*   Usually under 500 mg/dL but may not exhibit normal heterogeneity *2539*

Immunoglobulin IgM   *Serum   Decrease*   *2539 2468 0619*

Immunoglobulins   *Serum   Decrease*   IgG primarily deficient, but other immunoglobulins may also be low. *2552*   *2539*

Isocitrate Dehydrogenase   *Serum   Normal*   *2260*

Lymphocyte B-Cell   *Blood   Decrease*   Normal or decreased. *2539*

Lymphocytes   *Blood   Decrease*   Significant deficiency of T and B Lymphocytes. Clinical findings are usually associated with abnormal T-Lymphocyte function. *2539*   *0996 2468*

Lymphocyte T-Cell   *Blood   Decrease*   Normal or decreased. *2539*

MCV   *Blood   Increase*   High incidence of pernicious anemia. *2538*

Plasma Cells   *Serum   Decrease*   Decreased in transient hypogammaglobulinemia of infancy. *2468*   Ordinarily, sparse in infancy, are absent with disease. *2552*

Platelet Count   *Blood   Decrease*   Count is decreased, with bleeding tendency. *2468*   *2035*

Protein   *Serum   Decrease*   *2467*

279.07   Dysgammaglobulinemia (Selective Immunoglobulin Deficiency)

Hematocrit   *Blood   Decrease*   Not uncommon. *0433*

Hemoglobin   *Blood   Decrease*   Not uncommon. *0433*

Immunoglobulin IgA   *Serum   Decrease*   Types I, II, and IV; 1 in 500 of the population have IgA deficiency. *0619*   One of the common partial immunoglobulin defects is characterized by a deficiency of IgA and IgG and increased amounts of IgM in the serum. *2035*   In type III. *2468*   *0881 0433*

Immunoglobulin IgG   *Serum   Decrease*   One of the common partial immunoglobulin defects is characterized by a deficiency of IgA and IgG and increased amounts of IgM in the serum. *2035*   Type I, II, III, IV. *0619*   *0881*

Serum   Increase   *0619*

Serum   Normal   In type I and II. *2468*

Immunoglobulin IgM   *Serum   Decrease*   Types I, V, VII. *0619*   In type II. *2468*

Serum   Increase   Type I. *2467*   One of the common partial immunoglobulin defects is characterized by a deficiency of IgA and IgG and increased amounts of IgM in the serum. *2035*   *0433 0881*

Serum   Normal   Normal or increased. *2467*

Neutrophils   *Blood   Decrease*   Not uncommon. *0433*

Rheumatoid Factor   *Serum   Increase*   Dysproteinemias and paraproteinemias present significant seropositivity. *0962*

279.11   DiGeorge's Syndrome

Calcium   *Serum   Decrease*   *2344*

Immunoglobulin IgA   *Serum   Normal*   Frequently normal. *0996*

Immunoglobulin IgE   *Serum   Normal*   Frequently normal. *0996*

Immunoglobulin IgG   *Serum   Normal*   Frequently normal. *0996 2344*

Immunoglobulin IgM   *Serum   Normal*   Frequently normal. *0996*

Lymphocyte B-Cell   *Blood   Normal*   *0793*

Lymphocytes   *Blood   Decrease*   Profound lymphopenia and T_5+/T_8+ cells are relatively more deficient than T_4+ cells. *2539*

Blood   Normal   Patients have partial or complete T cell immunodeficiency with normal or near normal B cell immune function. *2539*   May be normal but virtually all are B-cells. *0996*

Lymphocyte T-Cell   *Blood   Decrease*   Usually low but may be normal or increased. *0793*

Parathyroid Hormone   *Serum   Decrease*   *0793*

279.12   Wiskott-Aldrich Syndrome

Creatinine   *Serum   Increase*   Increased incidence of renal failure. *0793*

Immunoglobulin IgA   *Serum   Increase*   Elevated levels. *2344 2539*

Serum   Normal   Normal *0996*

Immunoglobulin IgE   *Serum   Increase*   Frequently elevated. *0996*

Immunoglobulin IgG   *Serum   Increase*   Elevated levels. *2539*

Serum   Normal   Normal *0996*

Immunoglobulin IgM   *Serum   Decrease*   Low levels. *2539*   Usually decreased. *0996 2344*

Platelet   Increase   Platelet associated immunoglobulins were increased presplenectomy. *0455*

Lymphocyte B-Cell   *Blood   Normal*   *2539*

Lymphocytes   *Blood   Decrease*   Diminished T-Lymphocytes in some patients. *0996 2344*

Lymphocyte T-Cell   *Blood   Decrease*   Normal immunity initially but may decline with advancing years. *2539*

Platelet Count   *Blood   Decrease*   Thrombocytopenia. *2539 0455*

Protein   *Urine   Increase*   Increased incidence of renal failure. *0793*

Urea Nitrogen   *Serum   Increase*   Increased incidence of renal failure. *0793*

Volume   *Platelet   Decrease*   Mean platelet volume was markedly decreased but returned to normal post-splenectomy. *0455*

279.13   Nezeloff's Syndrome

Granulocytes   *Blood   Decrease*   *2344*

Immunoglobulin IgA   *Serum   Decrease*   50% of patients. *2344*

Immunoglobulin IgG   *Serum   Decrease*   50% of patients. *2344*

Lymphocyte B-Cell   *Blood   Normal*   *0793*

Lymphocyte T-Cell   *Blood   Decrease*   Studies of T cell immunity are abnormal but the degree of deficiency may vary. *0793*

279.20   Severe Combined Immunodeficiency

Adenosine Deaminase   *Serum   Normal*   Normal levels. *0793*

Eosinophils   *Blood   Increase*   Commonly elevated. *2539*

Immunoglobulin IgA   *Serum   Decrease*   *0793*

Immunoglobulin IgG   *Serum   Decrease*   *0793*

Immunoglobulin IgM   *Serum   Decrease*   *0793*

Leukocytes   *Blood   Decrease*   *2539*

Lymphocyte B-Cell   *Blood   Decrease*   Absent or markedly reduced. *0793*

Lymphocytes   *Blood   Decrease*   *0793*

Lymphocyte T-Cell   *Blood   Decrease*   Deficient immunity. *0793*

Platelet Count   *Blood   Normal*   *2539*

279.31   Acquired Immunodeficiency Syndrome (AIDS)

Antibody Titer   *Serum   Increase*   Using the enzyme-linked immunosorbent assay (ELISA) for HTLV-III antibodies, 82% of 88 patients with AIDS were positive, 16% borderline and 2% negative. Only 1% of 297 volunteer controls were positive, 6% borderline and 93% negative for a specificity of 98.6% and sensitivity of 97.3%. *2511*

Beta$_2$-Macroglobulin   *Serum   Increase*   Elevated > 2.5 mg/L in 29 or 37 patients. *0646*   Found frequently. *1318*

Immunoglobulin IgA   *Serum   Increase*   Frequently a polyclonal hypergammaglobulinemia is present, usually of IgG and IgA. *2539*   Elevated levels of at least one immunoglobulin was found in 78% of patients. *0646*

Immunoglobulin IgG   *Serum   Increase*   Frequently a polyclonal hypergammaglobulinemia is present, usually of IgG and IgA. *2539*   Elevated levels of at least 1 immunoglobulin found in 78% of patients *0646*   27 of 29 children tested. *1760*

Leukocytes *Blood Decrease* Less than 4500 cells/μL in 25 of 37 patients. *0646*

Lymphocytes *Blood Decrease* Lymphopenia less than 1500 cells/mL is often present and the absolute number of cells in the T helper/inducer subset is depressed. *2539* < 1500 cells/μL in 26 of 35 patients. 91.6% of patients had decreased concentration of T-Helper cells. *0646* Absolute lymphopenia in 1 of 29 children tested. *1760*

Lymphocyte T-Cell *Blood Decrease* The risk of AIDS is clearly predicted by the total number of circulating OKTA positive lymphocytes (T$_4$). *0860*

Partial Thromboplastin Time *Plasma Increase* Noted in 24 of 34 patients with this disorder. Felt to be due to Lupus Anticoagulant. *0229* In 10 patients with AIDS all had elevated times. *0423*

Prothrombin Time *Plasma Increase* Three of seven patients studied. *0423*

DISEASES OF THE BLOOD

Deficiency Anemias

280.81 Plummer-Vinson Syndrome

Hematocrit *Blood Decrease* Hypochromic anemia associated with dysphagia and cardiospasm in women. *2467*

Hemoglobin *Blood Decrease* Hypochromic anemia associated with dysphagia and cardiospasm in women. *2467*

MCH *Blood Decrease* Microcytic anemia. *0995*

MCHC *Blood Decrease* Hypochromic anemia associated with dysphagia and cardiospasm in women. *2467*

MCV *Blood Decrease* Hypochromic anemia associated with dysphagia and cardiospasm in women. *2467*

280.90 Iron Deficiency Anemia

2,3-Diphosphoglycerate *Red Blood Cells Increase* Synthesis is increased in response to hypoxia. *0159*

Albumin *Serum Normal* 2467

Alpha$_1$-Antitrypsin *Serum Normal* 2467

Anisocytes *Blood Increase* Usually there is moderate to marked anisocytosis and poikilocytosis. *0999* Characteristic of well-developed iron deficiency. *0962 0151*

Bilirubin *Serum Decrease* A test of minor or incidental importance. *0433 0151*

Catalase *Red Blood Cells Decrease* Has been demonstrated to be decreased in RBCs. *0104*

Cells *Bone Marrow Increase* Characterized by erythroid hyperplasia of mild-moderate degree. *2552*

Cholesterol *Serum Decrease* 0812

Chylomicrons *Serum Increase* Increased. *1380 1936 1948*

Complement C3 *Serum Normal* 2467

Copper *Serum Decrease* Decreases in some iron-deficiency anemias of childhood (that require copper as well as iron therapy). *2467* Ceruloplasmin lost in urine *2467*

Serum Increase 0433 0619

Coproporphyrin *Urine Increase* 0619

Erythrocytes *Blood Decrease* 2467

Blood Increase In infants and children, hypochromia may occur earlier in the course of iron deficiency and counts > 5.5 million/μL are sometimes encountered. *2538*

Erythrocyte Survival *Red Blood Cells Decrease* Slight to moderate shortening. *2538 1436* Somewhat shortened. High correlation with the number of morphologically abnormal cells. Only severe changes can be detected by the ^{53}Cr method. *0561 2552*

Ferritin *Serum Decrease* Invariably reduced. *0999* Concentration < 10 ng/mL is characteristic. The usefulness of the assay is limited by the fact that when iron deficiency and inflammatory disease coexist, concentration may be within the normal range. *2538*

Serum Normal Concentration < 10 ng/mL is characteristic. The usefulness of the assay is limited by the fact that when iron deficiency and inflammatory disease coexist, concentration may be within the normal range. *2538*

Bone Marrow *Absent* The amount is not as important diagnostically as presence or absence. The presence is strong evidence against the diagnosis of clinically significant iron deficiency. *0962*

Glutamic Acid *Red Blood Cells Increase* Raised RBC L-glutamate levels occur in iron deficiency anemias in the presence of a large population of young cells. *2411*

Haptoglobin *Serum Normal* 2467

Hematocrit *Blood Decrease* 0999 0151

Hemoglobin *Blood Decrease* Reduced to a mean of 7.6 g/dL in 371 patients. *0198 0999 0151*

Hemoglobin A$_{1C}$ *Blood Increase* 2539

Hydrochloric Acid *Gastric Material Decrease* The augmented histamine test has shown true achlorhydria in 16% of cases. *0995*

Iron *Serum Decrease* Nearly all patients will have serum values < 50 μg/dL. *0433* As deficiency intensifies, serum concentration falls. *0999* Usually < 80 μg/dL, associated with a total plasma iron-binding capacity of > 400 μg/dL. *0151* In well-developed deficiency often below 30 μg/dL. *0962* Reduced to an average of 28 μg/dL in adults. *0117 2538*

Serum Normal Usually low in untreated anemia; however, it may be normal. *0656* Mild deficiency is often accompanied by a normal level, and sometimes the deficiency may be symptomatic without measurably depressing the level. *0962 2538*

Bone Marrow Decrease Depleted of stainable iron. *2538* Reticuloendothelial stores are severely reduced or absent in marrow and liver. *0117 2552* The amount is not as important diagnostically as presence or absence. The presence is strong evidence against the diagnosis of clinically significant iron deficiency. *0962*

Liver Decrease Reticuloendothelial stores are severely reduced or absent in marrow and liver. *0117 2552*

Iron-Binding Capacity, Total (TIBC) *Serum Decrease* Often increased, but may be normal or low. *2552* Mean = 346 μg/dL, ranging from 170-460. Patients with reduced capacity also have hypoalbuminemia. *0117*

Serum Increase In well-developed iron deficiency, the percentage of saturation of transferrin is usually very low, 16%. Low saturation from other causes is rare. *0962* Often increased, but may be normal or low. *2552* Mean = 346 μg/dL, ranging from 170-460. Patients with reduced capacity also have hypoalbuminemia. *0117 2538*

Iron Crystals *Urine Increase* If the spun sediment of the morning's first-voided specimen is stained for iron, it may frequently be seen to contain hemosiderin crystals. *0433*

Iron Saturation *Serum Decrease* Transferrin saturation is almost always under 15% and, in severe deficiency, under 10%. *0999* Saturation of 15% or less is often found. *2538* 16% and averages 7%. *2552* In well-developed iron deficiency, the percentage of saturation of transferrin is usually very low, < 16. Low saturation from other causes is rare. *0962* In 92% of 15 patients at initial hospitalization for this disorder. *0781*

Lactate Dehydrogenase *Serum Normal* Normal, even in severe iron-deficiency. *2468*

Lactate Dehydrogenase Isoenzymes *Serum Increase* LD$_3$ was elevated to 31% in serum of patients with hypochromic microcytic anemia. *0852*

Leukocytes *Blood Decrease* 14% were found to have counts between 3,000-4,000/μL. Leukopenia was unrelated to severity of anemia and could not be ascribed to any other condition. Differential counts were normal. *1232 2538*

MCH *Blood Decrease* Microcytic hypochromic anemia may occur due to blood loss, increased demand or dietary inadequacy. MCH < 27 pg, MCV < 80 fL. *0532* Morphologic changes are paralleled by decreases in the MCV, MCH, and MCHC. The decline in MCHC is the more consistent. *0962* Average is 20 pg, range = 14-29. *0117*

Blood Normal Red cell indices are related to the duration and severity of anemia. Mild cases or those of short duration may have normal values. *0194*

MCHC *Blood Decrease* Of little diagnostic value except when anemia is severe. *2538* Morphologic changes are paralleled by decreases in the MCV, MCH, and MCHC. The decline in MCHC is the more consistent. *0962* Average is 28 g/dL, ranging from 22-31. *0117 2467 0151 0999*

Blood Normal Red cell indices are related to the duration and severity of anemia. Mild cases or those of short duration may have normal values. *0194*

280.90   Iron Deficiency Anemia *(continued)*

MCV *Blood Decrease* Microcytic hypochromic anemia may occur due to blood loss, increased demand or dietary inadequacy. MCH < 27 pg, MCV < 80 fL. *0532* In severe uncomplicated anemia, erythrocytes are hypochromic and microcytic. *2538* Hypochromic microcytosis parallels severity of anemia with marked variation in size and shape. *0151* Characteristic of well-developed iron deficiency. *0962* Average is 74 fL, range - 53-93. *0117*

Blood Normal Red cell indices are related to the duration and severity of anemia. Mild cases or those of short duration may have normal values. *0194*

Neutrophils *Blood Decrease* WBC is usually normal in number, but slight granulocytopenia may occur in long standing cases. *2437*

Osmotic Fragility *Red Blood Cells Decrease* Decreased, reflecting the diminished hemoglobin concentration. *0151* May be within the normal range, but often there is increased resistance to destruction in hypotonic salt solution. Extreme resistance is unusual. *2552*

Plasma Cells *Serum Decrease* Depressed. *2357 0659 0683*

Platelet Count *Blood Decrease* In infants and children, thrombocytopenia occurred almost as frequently (28%) as did thrombocytosis (35%). Associated with more severe anemia. *0927 2538*

Blood Increase In infants and children, thrombocytopenia occurred almost as frequently (28%) as did thrombocytosis (35%). Associated with more severe anemia. *0927* Reported in 50-75% of adults with classic hypochromic anemia due to chronic blood loss. May be found only in those patients who are actively bleeding. *1232* Usually twice the normal level. *2070*

Poikilocytes *Blood Increase* Usually there is moderate to marked anisocytosis and poikilocytosis. *0999* Characteristic of well-developed iron deficiency. *0962* A moderate number, especially tailed and elongated forms, are found. *2552   0151*

Protoporphyrin *Red Blood Cells Increase* Defective heme synthesis is associated with raised RBC protoporphyrin. *2538   0151*

Reticulocytes *Blood Decrease* Rarely reduced. *2552* Usually normal or decreased. *2538*

Blood Increase Both the percentage and absolute number tend to be normal or slightly increased. *0117* Occasionally a count of 2-3% may be noted. *2538*

Blood Normal Usually normal. *0995* Usually normal or decreased. *2538*

Uropepsinogen *Urine Decrease* With achlorhydria. *0619*

Vitamin B$_{12}$ *Serum Increase* Slight increase; mean = 466 pg/mL in 118 patients (normal = 385). *1990*

281.00   Pernicious Anemia

2,3-Diphosphoglycerate *Red Blood Cells Increase* Synthesis is increased in response to hypoxia. *0159*

Albumin *Serum Decrease 0619*

Aldolase *Serum Increase* Increased less consistently and to a lesser degree than LD. *0652 2552*

Alkaline Phosphatase *Serum Decrease* 33% of patients. *2467* Decreased activity. *2410*

Amino Acids *Urine Increase* Amino aciduria with an excess excretion of taurine, especially if there is associated subacute combined degeneration of the spinal cord. Amino aciduria does not occur in other megaloblastic anemias. *2468* May be slight excess of urinary amino acids, especially taurine. *0755 2364*

Antibody Titer *Serum Increase* Antibodies against parietal cells are found in 75% of all patients. Antibodies against intrinsic factor are seen in 50% of these patients. *0962*

Antithyroglobulin Antibodies *Serum Increase* In 25% of cases. *0058*

Bilirubin *Serum Increase* Mild due to increase in indirect fraction. *0995*

Bilirubin, Indirect *Serum Increase* Mild unconjugated hyperbilirubinemia. *0151* Slight indirect hyperbilirubinemia as a result of increased production of bile pigment. Normal values are common and values > 2 mg/dL are unusual. *2552*

Bleeding Time *Blood Increase* May be prolonged. *2552*

Calcitonin *Serum Increase* In some cases. *1041*

Cholesterol *Serum Decrease* Decreases in relapse; during remission, or following treatment the serum cholesterol increases as the reticulocyte count rises. *0812* In relapse, increased fatty acid and triglyceride concentrations but decreased concentrations of total cholesterol, unesterified cholesterol and all examined phospholipid fractions. *2471*

Cholesterol, Free *Serum Decrease* In relapse, increased free fatty acid and triglyceride concentrations but decreased concentrations of total cholesterol, unesterified cholesterol and all examined phospholipid fractions. *2471*

Clot Retraction *Blood Poor* May be poor. *2552*

Complement C3 *Serum Decrease* Significantly reduced in patients with vitamin B$_{12}$ deficiency. Levels correlate with the degree of anemia but not with serum vitamin B$_{12}$ levels at diagnosis. *1079*

Copper *Serum Increase* *2467 0619*

Creatine Kinase *Serum Normal* *2467*

Eosinophils *Blood Increase* Occurs in some hematopoietic diseases. *2467*

Erythrocyte Survival *Red Blood Cells Decrease* Moderately reduced. *2552* Ranged from 27-75 days in 5 patients (normal 120 days). *1442 2181*

Fatty Acids, Free (FFA) *Serum Increase* In relapse, increased free fatty acid and triglyceride concentrations but decreased concentrations of total cholesterol, unesterified cholesterol and all examined phospholipid fractions. *2471*

Fibrinogen *Plasma Increase* Moderate depression of fibrinogen formation occurs. *0619*

FIGLU (N-Formiminoglutamic Acid) *Urine Increase* Increased urinary formiminoglutamate after an oral histidine load. *0433*

Folate *Serum Increase* Normal or high. *0999*

Gastrin *Serum Increase* High level may approach that in the Zollinger-Ellison Syndrome. *2467* Concentration in the serum is high, probably because of the high pH within the lumen of the stomach. *0999* May be due to G cell hyperplasia in the pyloric antral mucosa. *1382   1534*

Glucose-6-Phosphate Dehydrogenase *Red Blood Cells Increase* Increased to about the same extent as LD. *0652 2552*

Haptoglobin *Serum Decrease* Probably due at least partly to impaired formation. *0619   0433*

Hematocrit *Blood Decrease* Classical anemia, leukopenia (primarily granulopenia) and thrombocytopenia. Occasionally, the primary reduction may be in only 1 of these 3 major formed elements of the blood. Although patients usually present primarily with anemia they may occasionally present initially with infection associated with granulocytopenia or with bleeding associated with thrombocytopenia. *0433* In 5 cases, hematocrit varied from 12-20% (normal = 37-54%). *2253* Anemia may be very severe or very mild. *2552*

Hemoglobin *Blood Decrease* Classical anemia, leukopenia (primarily granulocytopenia) and thrombocytopenia. Occasionally, the primary reduction may be in only 1 of these 3 major formed elements of the blood. Although patients usually present primarily with anemia they may occasionally present initially with infection associated with granulocytopenia or with bleeding associated with thrombocytopenia. *0433* Concentration ranges from very severe to near normal. Usually 7-8 g/dL at presentation. *2552*

Hemoglobin, Fetal *Blood Increase* In 50% of untreated patients; increases after treatment and then gradually decreases during next 6 months; some patients still have slight elevation thereafter. *2467*

Hydrochloric Acid *Gastric Material Decrease* Gastric parietal cells lose ability to secrete HCl as well as intrinsic factor. Achlorhydria is therefore characteristic of intrinsic factor deficiency but not diagnostic. *0962*

Iron *Serum Increase* Moderately increased unless there is associated iron deficiency. *0366*

Bone Marrow Increase Marrow sideroblasts and reticuloendothelial stores tend to be increased. *2552*

Iron-Binding Capacity, Total (TIBC) *Serum Decrease* In relapse. *0619* Total plasma capacity tends to be slightly reduced. *2552*

Isocitrate Dehydrogenase *Serum Increase* Increased less consistently and to a lesser degree than LD. *2552 0652*

Serum Normal *2260*

Lactate Dehydrogenase *Serum Increase* Total LD (chiefly LD₁) is markedly increased especially with hemoglobin < 8 g/dL. *2467* In 5 cases, levels ranged from 310 U/L (in relapse) - 4820 U/L (normal = 50-220 U/L). *2253* Mean value in 16 patients was 2335 U/L (normal 116). *0060* Magnitude of increase is related to the degree of anemia. *2552*

Lactate Dehydrogenase Isoenzyme 5 (LD₅) *Serum Increase* Increased to about the same extent as LD. *0652 2552*

Lactate Dehydrogenase Isoenzymes *Serum Increase* Predominantly LD₁, in untreated cases. *2467* LD₁ and LD₂ account for the increase in total LD. *2552*

Leukocytes *Blood Decrease* Anemia, leukopenia (primarily granulopenia) and thrombocytopenia. Occasionally, the primary reduction may be in only 1 of these 3 major formed elements of the blood. *0433* Hematopoietic diseases. *2467* Varies with degree of anemia from normal to very low. Usually due to absolute neutropenia. *2552*

Lipids *Serum Decrease* Decreased in serum and the red cell membrane. *0619*

Red Blood Cells Decrease Decreased in serum and the red cell membrane. *0619*

Malate Dehydrogenase *Serum Increase* Increased to about the same extent as LD. *0652 2552*

MCH *Blood Increase* Generally 33-38 pg in moderate anemia, and 33-56 pg, with severe cases (normal = 27-31 pg). *2552 0995*

MCHC *Blood Normal* When not complicated by iron deficiency, anemia is normochromic and macrocytic. *2552 0995*

MCV *Blood Increase* Macrocytic anemia may occur due to vitamin B₁₂ or folate deficiency. MCV > 100 fL. *0532* Usually macrocytic anemia. Rise in MCV is largely proportional to the degree of anemia. Usual values are 95-110 fL, but may be 110-160 with severe anemia. *2552*

Methylmalonate *Urine Increase* Relatively specific for vitamin B₁₂ deficiency. *0433*

Phospholipids, Total *Serum Decrease* All phospholipid fractions decreased in relapse. *2471*

Red Blood Cells Decrease Decreased concentration in red cells. *0619*

Platelet Count *Blood Decrease* Anemia, leukopenia (primarily granulopenia) and thrombocytopenia. Occasionally, the primary reduction may be in only 1 of these 3 major formed elements of the blood. May present initially with bleeding associated with thrombocytopenia. *0433* Generally reduced, may be < 100,000/μL. *1756 2552*

Poikilocytes *Blood Increase* Many bizarre-shaped corpuscles are found. *0995*

Potassium *Serum Decrease* Slightly reduced. *2552* 17 of 34 patients had < 4 mmol/L, the lower limit of normal. *1358*

Pseudocholinesterase *Serum Increase* *2441*

Reticulocytes *Blood Decrease* Inappropriately low corrected count due to marrow failure. *0999*

Blood Normal Usually within normal limits in untreated patients. *0995*

Taurine *Urine Increase* Amino aciduria with an excess excretion of taurine, especially if there is associated subacute combined degeneration of the spinal cord. Amino aciduria does not occur in other megaloblastic anemias. *2468* May be slight excess of urinary amino acids, especially taurine. *0755 2364*

Triglycerides *Serum Increase* In relapse, increased free fatty acid and triglyceride concentrations but decreased concentrations of total cholesterol, unesterified cholesterol and all examined phospholipid fractions. *2471*

Uric Acid *Serum Decrease* Decreased in some patients in relapse. *2467* Rarely reported. *0962*

Serum Increase Especially after treatment. *0619 1283 0962*

Urobilinogen *Urine Increase* Possibly in some cases. *0619*

Feces Increase Possibly in some cases. *0619*

Uropepsinogen *Urine Decrease* With achlorhydria. *0619*

Vitamin B₁₂ *Serum Decrease* Markedly decreased, mean value in 39 patients was 34 pg/mL compared to 385 pg/mL in normals. *1990 2538*

Vitamin B₁₂ Binding Capacity *Serum Increase* Increased binding capacity, mean = 1,682 (normal = 1,208 pg/mL) and decreased serum concentration. *1990*

Zinc *Serum Decrease* Decreased. *2297 2000*

281.20 Folic Acid Deficiency Anemia

Acetylcholinesterase *Red Blood Cells Decrease* Megaloblastic Anemia during relapse. *1443*

Aldolase *Serum Increase* 12 of 16 patients had levels elevated from 2-20 X the normal mean. *1023* Increased less consistently and to a lesser degree than LD. *2552 0652*

Alkaline Phosphatase *Serum Decrease* *2538 2410*

Amino Acids *Urine Increase* Aminoaciduria reportedly occurs, but observers differ on its frequency and significance. *2538* May be slight excess of urinary amino acids, especially taurine. *0755 2364*

Bilirubin *Serum Increase* Slightly to moderately increased. *2538 0151*

Bilirubin, Indirect *Serum Increase* Slight indirect hyperbilirubinemia as a result of increased production of bile pigment. Normal values are common and values 2 mg/dL are unusual. *2552*

Bleeding Time *Blood Increase* May be prolonged. *2552*

Cells *Bone Marrow Increase* Bone marrow shows megaloblastic dysplasia that varies from mild to marked in megaloblastic anemia of infancy. *2467* Aspirated bone marrow is cellular and often hyperplastic. *2538*

Cholesterol *Serum Decrease* Hypocholesterolemia occurred consistently in 10 patients with anemia. Values ranged from 80-180 mg/dL. *2519 0140*

Clot Retraction *Blood Poor* May be poor. *2552*

Complement C3 *Serum Decrease* Significantly reduced in patients with vitamin B₁₂ deficiency. Levels correlate with the degree of anemia but not with serum vitamin B₁₂ levels at diagnosis. *1079*

Copper *Serum Increase* A secondary finding. *0151* Due to intramedullary hemolysis found in megaloblastic anemias. *2467*

Erythrocytes *Blood Decrease* Pancytopenia is a common feature in vitamin B₁₂ and folic acid deficiency. *2538* Depressed to a greater degree than other parameters. *0962*

Erythrocyte Survival *Red Blood Cells Decrease* Moderately reduced. *2552* Ranged from 27-75 days in 5 patients (normal = 120 days). *1442 2181*

FIGLU (N-Formiminoglutamic Acid) *Urine Increase* Urine FIGLU is increased; disappears after folic acid treatment in megaloblastic anemia of infancy. *2467* Less specific than the serum folate assay. It becomes abnormal later and thus gives a better measure of tissue coenzyme levels. *2538* Increased excretion is a consistent feature of folate deficiency but is not confined to that situation. *0962*

Folate *Serum Decrease* Low; < 4 ng/mL. *0999* When intake is reduced, the serum level falls promptly and precedes evidence of tissue deficiency. *0962*

Red Blood Cells Decrease A better measure of tissue folate and is less dependent on recent intake than serum. *0962*

Glucose-6-Phosphate Dehydrogenase *Serum Increase* Elevated in 12 of 12 patients from 2.5-20 X the normal mean. *1023* Increased to about the same extent as LD. *0652 2552 2538 1022*

Red Blood Cells Increase Elevated in 5 of 9 patients. Upper limit of normal = 4.6. *1023*

Hematocrit *Blood Decrease* Hematocrit levels ranged from 12-25% in 10 patients. *2519* Anemia is normochromic (unless iron deficiency coexists) and macrocytic, with MCV ranging from 100 to 150 fL. *2538* Anemia ranges from absent to severe. *0962* Anemia may be very severe or very mild. *2552*

Hemoglobin *Blood Decrease* Anemia is normochromic (unless iron deficiency coexists) and macrocytic, with MCV ranging from 100 to > 150 fL. *2538* Anemia ranges from absent to severe. *0962* Concentration ranges from very severe to near normal. Usually < 7-8 g/dL at presentation. *2552*

Hemoglobin, Fetal *Blood Increase* Minimal elevation occurs in about 15% of patients with megaloblastic anemia. *2467*

Iron *Serum Increase* Slightly to moderately increased. *2538* Moderately increased unless there is associated iron deficiency. *0366*

Bone Marrow Increase Marrow sideroblasts and reticuloendothelial stores tend to be increased. *2552*

Iron-Binding Capacity, Total (TIBC) *Serum Decrease* Total plasma capacity tends to be slightly reduced. *2552*

Isocitrate Dehydrogenase *Serum Increase* Serum levels 5 X the normal. *0619* In 5 of 9 patients, the plasma level was elevated above the maximum normal limit. *1023* Increased less consistently and to a lesser degree than LD. *0652 2552*

Red Blood Cells Increase 6 out of 8 patients had elevated concentration. The highest elevation was 7.3 U/L and the normal upper limit was 2.5 U/L. *1023*

281.20　Folic Acid Deficiency Anemia *(continued)*

Lactate Dehydrogenase *Serum Increase* In some cases; LD activity and red cell count inversely related in folic acid and/or vitamin B_{12} deficiency. *0619* More sensitive reflection of this disease state than other tests. 2-40 fold elevations. Almost all patients have increased concentrations, often marked. *0812 0503* In 13 patients ranged from normal to 40 fold elevation. *2253* Mean value in 16 patients was 2335 U/L (normal = 116). *0060* Magnitude of increase is related to the degree of anemia. *2552 1023 0962*

Red Blood Cells Increase 5 of 15 patients had RBC concentrations above the normal upper limit of 96. *1023*

Lactate Dehydrogenase Isoenzyme 5 (LD₅) *Serum Increase* Increased to about the same extent as LD. *0652 2552*

Lactate Dehydrogenase Isoenzymes *Serum Increase* Isozymes 1 and 2 are markedly elevated in rough proportion to the severity of the anemia. *0660* LD_1 and LD_2 account for the increase in total LD. *2552 2538*

Red Blood Cells Increase In normal erythrocytes, LD_2 activity exceeds that of LD_1. In megaloblastic anemia, LD_1 exceeds LD_2. *2551 2538*

Lactic Acid *Blood Increase* *0151*

Leukocytes *Blood Decrease* Pancytopenia is a common feature in vitamin B_{12} and folic acid deficiency. *2538* Varies with degree of anemia from normal to very low. Usually due to absolute neutropenia. *2552*

Lysozyme *Serum Increase* *2538 1802*

Malate Dehydrogenase *Serum Increase* In 17 patients, the plasma content was consistently and markedly elevated. *1023* Serum levels rise to up to 40 X normal value. *0619* Increased to about the same extent as LD. *0652 2552 2538*

Red Blood Cells Increase 10 of 16 patients had red cell activity elevated significantly above the normal upper limit of 96. *1023*

MCH *Blood Increase* Erythrocytes are increased in diameter and thickness. Abnormalities are reflected in the increased MCV and MCH. *0962* Generally 33-38 pg in moderate anemia, and 33-56 pg, with severe cases (normal = 27-31 pg). *2552*

MCHC *Blood Normal* When not complicated by iron deficiency, anemia is normochromic and macrocytic. *2552*

MCV *Blood Increase* Macrocytic anemia may occur due to vitamin B_{12} or folate deficiency. MCV > 100 fL. *0532* Anemia is normochromic (unless iron deficiency coexists) and macrocytic, with MCV ranging from 100 to > 150 fL. *2538* Erythrocytes are increased in diameter and thickness. Abnormalities are reflected in the increased MCV and MCH. *0962* Usually macrocytic anemia. Rise in MCV is largely proportional to the degree of anemia. Usual values are 95-110 fL, but may be 110-160 with severe anemia. *2552*

Methylmalonate *Urine Normal* *2538*

Neutrophils *Blood Decrease* Neutropenia and thrombocytopenia are less frequent but still common. Rarely severe. *0962*

Osmotic Fragility *Red Blood Cells Decrease* *2467*

Platelet Count *Blood Decrease* Pancytopenia is a common feature in vitamin B_{12} and folic acid deficiency. *2538* Neutropenia and thrombocytopenia are less frequent but still common. Rarely severe. *0962* Generally reduced, may be < 100,000/μL. *1756 2552*

Potassium *Serum Decrease* Slightly reduced. *2552* 17 of 34 patients had < 4 mmol/L, the lower limit of normal. *1358*

Pseudocholinesterase *Serum Decrease* *2538 1573*

Reticulocytes *Blood Decrease* Lower than normal, both in absolute and in percentage terms. *2538* Tends to be low or at the low extreme of the normal range. *0962*

Taurine *Urine Increase* May be slight excess of urinary amino acids, especially taurine. *0755 2364*

Uric Acid *Serum Decrease* Often depressed. *2538*

Urine Decrease Often depressed. *2538*

Vitamin B_{12} *Serum Normal* *2538*

Vitamin B_{12} Binding Capacity *Serum Increase* Significant elevation; usually correlated with WBC in peripheral blood. *1990*

281.30　Vitamin B₆ Deficiency Anemia

Acetylcholinesterase *Red Blood Cells Decrease* Megaloblastic Anemia during relapse. *1443*

Alkaline Phosphatase *Leukocyte Decrease* Score is reduced in about 50% of the patients. *1327*

Anisocytes *Blood Increase* Blood smear shows anisocytosis with many bizarre forms, target cells, hypochromia with pyridoxine-responsive anemia. *2467* Prominent findings on blood smear. *2552*

Basophilic Stippling *Blood Increase* Prominent findings on blood smear. *2552*

Bilirubin *Serum Normal* Rarely elevated despite the mild hemolytic anemia. *0433*

Cells *Bone Marrow Increase* Bone marrow is characterized by intense erythroid hyperplasia, often associated with a shift to younger forms, particularly polychromatophilic normoblasts, some of which show megaloblastic nuclear changes. *2538*

Erythrocytes *Blood Decrease* Reported to be low in about 80% of patients. *0433*

Folate *Serum Decrease* Reported to be low in about 80% of patients. *1462 2538*

Haptoglobin *Serum Decrease* Decreased in hemoglobinemias (related to the duration and severity of hemolysis) due to extravascular hemolysis. *2467*

Hematocrit *Blood Decrease* The anemia is normocytic or slightly macrocytic. *2538*

Hemoglobin *Blood Increase* The degree of anemia is variable, ranging from concentrations as low as 5 g/dL, severely affected boys with sex-linked sideroblastic anemia to almost normal levels in the milder cases. Older people with idiopathic or secondary forms of this disease usually have moderate anemias with concentration ranging from 7-10 g/dL. *0433* Normocytic or slightly macrocytic. *2538 0151*

Iron *Serum Increase* Increased with pyridoxine-responsive anemia. *2467* Increased serum iron and reduced iron-binding capacity in > 50% of cases. *0532*

Serum Normal Characteristically normal to elevated. *0433*

Bone Marrow Increase Bone marrow is hyperplastic and contains increased amounts of normoblastic iron, often forming ringed sideroblasts. *2538* Increased in the marrow fragments and in the developing erythroblasts. *0151*

Iron-Binding Capacity, Total (TIBC) *Serum Decrease* Somewhat decreased with pyridoxine-responsive anemia. *2467* Normal to low. *0433* Associated increased serum iron and reduced iron-binding capacity in > 50% of cases. *0532*

Serum Normal Normal to low. *0433*

Iron Saturation *Serum Increase* Invariably increased saturation. *2552*

Leukocytes *Blood Decrease* Count varies from normal to leukopenic levels; when present, leukopenia is accompanied by neutropenia. *2538*

MCH *Blood Decrease* Microcytic hypochromic anemia may occur due to blood loss, increased demand or dietary inadequacy. MCH < 27 pg, MCV < 80 fL. *0532*

MCHC *Blood Decrease* Degree of anemia may vary but is usually in the range of 7-8 g/dL of hemoglobin, with a lowered MCHC. *0151*

MCV *Blood Decrease* Microcytic hypochromic anemia may occur due to blood loss, increased demand or dietary inadequacy. MCH < 27 pg, MCV < 80 fL. *0532*

Monocytes *Blood Increase* Morphologically normal, but the proportion may be moderately increased. *2538*

Neutrophils *Blood Decrease* Leukopenia is accompanied by neutropenia. *2538*

Osmotic Fragility *Red Blood Cells Decrease* Tends to be decreased. *2538*

Platelet Count *Blood Decrease* Usually normal, but thrombocytopenia and thrombocytosis occurs in a minority of patients. *2538*

Blood Increase Usually normal, but thrombocytopenia and thrombocytosis occurs in a minority of patients. *2538*

Blood Normal Usually normal, but thrombocytopenia and thrombocytosis occurs in a minority of patients. *2538*

Poikilocytes *Blood Increase* Blood smear shows poikilocytosis with many bizarre forms, target cells, hypochromia with pyridoxine-responsive anemia. *2467* Prominent findings on blood smear. *2552*

Protoporphyrin *Red Blood Cells Increase* Almost always moderately increased, and rarely it is markedly so. *1326* Elevated (40-300 mg/dL compared to normal levels of 15-35 mg/dL) reflecting a functional block to hemoglobin synthesis. *0433 2538*

Reticulocytes *Blood Decrease* Absolute count is usually reduced. *0151*

Blood Increase Count is usually normal but may be slightly increased. *2538*

Xanthurenic Acid *Urine Increase* Abnormal tryptophan metabolism indicated by excessive excretion of xanthurenic acid following TRP load has been found in 33% of cases. *2552* Detects pyridoxine (B₆) deficiency. *2538*

282.00 Hereditary (Congenital) Spherocytosis

Alanine Aminotransferase *Serum Increase 0962*

Aldolase *Serum Increase 0962*

Anisocytes *Blood Increase* Anisocytosis is marked. *2468*

Aspartate Aminotransferase *Serum Increase 0962*

Basophils *Blood Increase* During the chronic stage of anemia. *0810 2552*

Bilirubin *Serum Increase* Primarily indirect. *2538*

Bilirubin, Indirect *Serum Increase* Mean = 1.6 ± 1.1 mg/dL. *1470 2538*

Calcium *Red Blood Cells Increase* RBC content of Ca++ is increased. *0711* In 18 cases of congenital hemolytic anemias, increased erythrocytic Ca++ level was observed in 10 cases. *0184* A marked increase in calcium uptake was observed in the ATP depleted red cells of the unsplenectomized patients *2643*

Cholesterol *Serum Decrease* Observed in 8 patients. Values ranged from 110-170 mg/dL. *1942* Low serum values correlated well with hemoglobin concentration. *2109*

Coombs' Test *Blood Negative* Usually negative. *2552*

Coproporphyrin *Urine Increase* Increased hemopoiesis. *0619 0151*

Creatine Kinase *Serum Decrease 2538*

Serum Normal 0962

Erythrocytes *Blood Decrease* Anemia may be absent, moderate or severe. The RBC is reduced proportionately to the hemoglobin concentration. *0433* Reductions in RBC may not be proportional to hemoglobin. *2552*

Erythrocyte Sedimentation Rate *Blood Decrease* Very low rate. *2231*

FIGLU (N-Formiminoglutamic Acid) *Urine Increase 2467*

Haptoglobin *Serum Decrease* Decreased in hemoglobinemia (related to the duration and severity of hemolysis) due to extravascular hemolysis. Seen in hereditary spherocytosis with marked hemolysis. Becomes normal in 4-6 days after treatment with splenectomy. *2467*

Hematocrit *Blood Decrease* Anemia may be absent, moderate or severe. RBC is reduced proportionately to the hemoglobin concentration. *0433* Hct values ranged from 21-36% in 8 patients. *2519* In 91% of 12 patients at initial hospitalization for this disorder. *1404 2538 0781*

Hemoglobin *Blood Decrease* The mean value of the hemoglobin concentration in a large series is usually 11.5 g/dL rarely 7 g/dL. *0433* Concentrations between 9-12 g/dL are most common. Rapid fall to 3-4 g/dL may occur during a crisis. *2552* In 91% of 12 patients at initial hospitalization for this disorder. *0781 2538*

Blood Normal In approximately 10-20% of patients, particularly young men. *2246*

Hemoglobin, Free *Serum Normal* Very little or none. Hemoglobin released during hemolysis is catabolized at the site of destruction. *2246*

Iron *Serum Increase* May occur. *2552* Due to increased rate of blood destruction. *0619*

Iron-Binding Capacity, Total (TIBC) *Serum Increase* Hemolytic anemia, with raised serum iron concentration (i.e., the total transferrin concentration is increased, but the unsaturated iron binding capacity is reduced). *0619*

Lactate Dehydrogenase *Serum Increase* In hemolytic anemia. *0619 0962*

Leukocytes *Blood Decrease* Normal except during aplastic crises. *0433*

Blood Increase Generally slightly increased. Marked increase and shift to the left after a crisis. *2552* In 40% of 12 patients at initial hospitalization for this disorder. *0781*

Blood Normal Normal except during aplastic crises. *0433*

Lipids *Serum Decrease* Generalized hypolipidemia; with reduced phospholipids and total lipids occurs in children as well as adults with uncomplicated cases. *2109*

Lipoproteins *Serum Decrease* All classes of lipoproteins were reduced in children as well as adults with uncomplicated cases of congenital hemolytic anemia and spherocytosis. *2109*

Lymphocytes *Blood Increase* During the chronic stage of anemia. *0810 2552*

MCH *Blood Increase* Variations usually correspond to changes in volume. *2552*

MCHC *Blood Increase* The mean MCHC is usually increased (36-39%) reflecting the loss of membrane surface in relation to cell volume. *0433* Usually elevated, often as high as 37 %. *0674* Very high. *0999* Characteristically high, 37-39 g/dL. *2552 2538*

MCV *Blood Decrease* Small, dense, round, red cells (microspherocytes) seen in large numbers. *0999* May be normal, high, or very low. *2552* Mean value in 76 affected patients was 83 ± 8.5 fL; ranging from 62-125 fL. *1470*

Blood Increase May be normal, high, or very low. *2552*

Osmotic Fragility *Red Blood Cells Increase* Almost always increased; in cases in which the cell defect is minor, incubation will bring out the abnormal fragility. *0962* Typically increased. Hemolysis may be complete at the concentration where it normally commences. *2552 2538 0151*

Phosphate *Serum Increase 0962*

Phospholipids, Total *Serum Decrease* Generalized hypolipidemia; with reduced phospholipids and total lipids occurs in children as well as adults with uncomplicated cases. *2109*

Plasma Cells *Serum Increase* During the chronic stage of anemia. *0810 2552*

Platelet Count *Blood Decrease* Rarely moderately reduced. *2552*

Blood Increase Increased during aplastic crises. *0433* Usually within the normal to high range or slight increase. *2552*

Blood Normal Normal except during aplastic crises. *0433*

Poikilocytes *Blood Increase* Slight poikilocytosis. *2468*

Reticulocytes *Blood Increase* Is increased 5-20%. *0433* Characteristic increase. *2552* Common chronic hemolytic findings. *2246 2538*

Triglycerides *Serum Decrease* The majority of values were low (15/18 children) but there was a greater scatter of triglyceride than cholesterol concentrations. *2109*

Uric Acid *Serum Increase 1283 0962*

Urobilinogen *Urine Increase 0995 2538*

Feces Increase As much as 5-20 X normal. *2552 2538*

282.10 Hereditary Elliptocytosis

Bilirubin *Serum Increase* In patients with more severe forms of this disease there may be a compensated hemolytic anemia with raised serum bilirubin. *0433* Primarily indirect. *0995* Hemolysis and hyperbilirubinemia have been observed in the newborn period. *0087*

Bilirubin, Indirect *Serum Increase 2538*

Coombs' Test *Blood Negative* In uncomplicated cases. *2552*

Erythrocyte Survival *Red Blood Cells Decrease 2538*

Haptoglobin *Serum Decrease* In patients with more severe forms of this disease there may be a compensated hemolytic anemia with reduced serum haptoglobin. *0433 2538*

Hematocrit *Blood Decrease* In severe cases. *2538*

Hemoglobin *Blood Decrease* In severe cases, levels rarely fall below 9-10 g/dL. *2538*

Hemoglobin A$_{1C}$ *Blood Decrease* Significantly lower (P < 0.0005) in patients with hemolytic anemia (n = 20) compared to patients with nonhemolytic anemia and normal controls. *1769*

Hemoglobin, Free *Serum Increase* In 10-15% of patients the rate of hemolysis is substantially increased with red cell half-life times as short as 5 days. *2538* Hemolysis and hyperbilirubinemia have been observed in the newborn period. *0087*

Lactate Dehydrogenase *Serum Increase* In severe cases. *0433*

Osmotic Fragility *Red Blood Cells Increase* Usually normal but may be increased in patients with overt hemolysis. *2538*

Red Blood Cells Normal Usually normal even after incubation. *2552*

Reticulocytes *Blood Increase* In patients with more severe forms of this disease there may be a compensated hemolytic anemia with raised reticulocyte count. *0433* The great majority of these patients manifest only mild hemolysis with hemoglobin > 12 g/dL and reticulocytes < 4%. In 10-15% of patients the rate of hemolysis is increased and reticulocytosis ranging to 20%. *2538*

Urobilinogen *Urine Increase* In severe cases. *0433*

Feces Increase In severe cases. *0433*

282.20 Anemias Due To Disorders of Glutathione Metabolism

Albumin *Serum Normal* 2467

Alkaline Phosphatase *Leukocyte Normal* 2467

Alpha₁-Antitrypsin *Serum Normal* 2467

Bilirubin *Serum Increase* Varying degrees may be evident. 2538

Bilirubin, Indirect *Serum Increase* Indirect laboratory evidence that hemolysis is present. 0433

Cholesterol *Serum Decrease* 0812

Complement C3 *Serum Normal* 2467

Erythrocyte Survival *Red Blood Cells Decrease* 2538

Folate *Serum Decrease* Excessive utilization due to marked cellular proliferation. 2467

Haptoglobin *Serum Decrease* 2467

Hemoglobin *Blood Decrease* As the hemoglobin level falls, reticulocytosis occurs and polychromasia is seen. 2538

Hemoglobin A₁c *Blood Decrease* Significantly lower (P < 0.0005) in patients with hemolytic anemia (n = 20) compared to patients with nonhemolytic anemia and normal controls. 1769

Hemoglobin, Free *Serum Increase* Indirect laboratory evidence that hemolysis is present. 0433

Urine Increase Indirect laboratory evidence that hemolysis is present. 0433 Intravascular hemolysis due to antibodies. 2467

Iron *Serum Increase* Elevated serum iron and transferrin saturation. Indirect laboratory evidence that hemolysis is present. 0433

Iron Saturation *Serum Increase* Elevated serum iron and transferrin saturation. Indirect laboratory evidence that hemolysis is present. 0433 May be completely saturated. 2552

Lactate Dehydrogenase *Serum Increase* Especially if intravascular; derived from RBCs. 0619 2-4 X normal values. 0503

Lactate Dehydrogenase Isoenzymes *Serum Increase* Indirect laboratory evidence that hemolysis is present. 0433

Osmotic Fragility *Red Blood Cells Increase* 2467

Reticulocytes *Blood Increase* Laboratory clue that hemolysis may be present. 0433 As the hemoglobin level falls, reticulocytosis occurs, and polychromasia is seen. 2538

Uric Acid *Serum Increase* 2467

Urobilinogen *Urine Increase* Increased hemolysis. 2467

282.31 Hereditary Nonspherocytic Hemolytic Anemia

Bilirubin, Indirect *Serum Increase* In some cases. 2538

Cells *Bone Marrow Increase* Erythroid hyperplasia. 2538

Haptoglobin *Serum Decrease* Reflects chronic hemolysis. 0186

Hematocrit *Blood Decrease* Anemia. 2538

Hemoglobin *Blood Decrease* In most subjects, the range is 5-11.5 g/dL. 2538

Hemoglobin, Free *Serum Increase* During acute hemolysis. 0433

Urine Increase During acute hemolysis. 0433 Hemosiderinuria and hemoglobinuria, particularly when oxidative stresses have been induced by drugs or other environmental factors. 2538

Hexokinase *Red Blood Cells Absent* Deficient in erythrocytes in congenital nonspherocytic hemolytic anemia. 0619

Iron *Bone Marrow Increase* Marrow iron content is normal to increased. 0433

Lactate Dehydrogenase *Serum Increase* In hemolytic anemias. 2612

Leukocytes *Blood Increase* Tends to be normal or elevated with some increase in the immature granulocytes. 0433

Blood Normal Tends to be normal or elevated with some increase in the immature granulocytes. 0433

MCV *Blood Increase* Mild to moderate macrocytosis. 2538

Osmotic Fragility *Red Blood Cells Increase* 2467

Red Blood Cells Normal The osmotic fragility of fresh erythrocytes is usually normal. 2538

Platelet Count *Blood Increase* Normal or slightly increased. 0433

Pyruvate Kinase *Red Blood Cells Decrease* PK deficiency is limited to the red cell; the leukocyte does not share the deficiency. 2538

Reticulocytes *Blood Increase* Increase in count is marked, even with mild anemia with hereditary nonspherocytic hemolytic anemias. 2468

282.41 Thalassemia Major

Adenosine Deaminase *Serum Increase* Significantly elevated and related to the transfusion schedule of the patient. 1873

Amino Acids *Urine Increase* Found to be markedly increased in children. 0395

Anisocytes *Blood Increase* The red cells show marked aniso-poikilocytosis, with hypochromia, target-cell formation, and a variable degree of basophilic stippling. 2538 2246

Aspartate Aminotransferase *Serum Increase* Usually elevated. 2552

Basophilic Stippling *Blood Increase* The red cells show marked anisopoikilocytosiss, with hypochromia, target-cell formation, and a variable degree of basophilic stippling. 2538

Bilirubin *Serum Increase* Usually increased. 0999

Bilirubin, Indirect *Serum Increase* Unconjugated bilirubinemia (1-3 mg/dL) and slightly increased icterus index. 2552

Cells *Bone Marrow Increase* Bone marrow is cellular and shows erythroid hyperplasia. 2468

Copper *Serum Increase* In 42 patients (age 3 mo. to 22 y.) with homozygous beta-thalassemia and thalassemia intermedia, serum zinc was significantly decreased while Cu and Fe were increased. 0072 May be increased. 2552

Erythrocytes *Blood Decrease* With the more severe expression of the disease, homozygote or heterozygote, all parameters of erythrocyte numbers are depressed. 0962 Count is often between 2-3 million/μL, with great variation in size and shape of cells. 2552

Erythrocyte Survival *Red Blood Cells Decrease* Usually shortened. 2538 Generally ranges from 7-22 days as measured by [51] Chromium-labeling. 2289

Glucose Tolerance *Serum Decrease* 50% of patients had some abnormality in their oral test, 5 falling into the diabetic category. Intolerance correlated with number of transfusions received and age. 2054

Gonadotropin, Pituitary *Serum Decrease* Markedly impaired gonadotropin response to LH releasing hormones in beta thalassemia. 1346

Haptoglobin *Serum Decrease* Decreased in hemoglobinemias (related to the duration and severity of hemolysis) due to extravascular hemolysis. 2467

Hematocrit *Blood Decrease* Anemia is severe, microcytic and hypochromic. 0995

Hemoglobin *Blood Decrease* Common very low in untransfused patients usually below 7 g/dL. 0433 Severe hemolytic anemia, hypochromic and microcytic in type, is found. 0999 May be in the 2-3 g/dL range or even lower. 2538

Hemoglobin A₁c *Blood Decrease* 2539

Hemoglobin, Fetal *Blood Increase* The proportion is usually between 20-60%, but values as high as 90% may occur. 0151 Increased, ranging from 10-90% is characteristic and there may be a total deficiency of hemoglobin A synthesis. 2538

Hemoglobin, Free *Serum Increase* Moderate increase. 2467

Iron *Serum Increase* Serum concentration is elevated with increased saturation of iron-binding protein. 0151 In 42 patients (age 3 mo. to 22 y.) with homozygous beta-thalassemia and thalassemia intermedia, serum zinc was significantly decreased while Cu and Fe were increased. 0072 In contrast to the thin cells of iron deficiency, the serum iron is normal or increased. 0962 0349

Bone Marrow Increase Abundance of iron in the reticuloendothelial cells. 2552

Iron-Binding Capacity, Total (TIBC) *Serum Increase* Total capacity is increased. 2468

Iron Saturation *Serum Increase* Serum concentration is elevated with increased saturation of iron-binding protein. 0151 Often totally saturated. 2208

Lactate Dehydrogenase *Serum Increase* May be markedly elevated in the serum presumably due to marrow hyperplasia and ineffective erythropoiesis. 0433 Usually elevated. 2552

Leukocytes *Blood Decrease* With the gross splenomegaly which may occur, a secondary thrombocytopenia and leukopenia frequently develop, leading to a further tendency to infection and bleeding. 2538

Blood Increase Normoblasts, reticulocytes, and leukocytosis (about 20,000/μL) with a shift to the left in the peripheral blood reflect the bone marrow hyperplasia. 0999 Leukocytosis may be marked and persistent. 0151 Slightly elevated unless there is secondary hypersplenism. 2538

Lipids *Serum Decrease* Serum total lipid levels were found to be low in children with beta-thalassemia. The difference between the mean total lipid level in patients (365 mg/dL ± 75) as compared to that of the controls (581 mg/dL ± 94) was highly significant. *2607* In 20 cases of thalassemia, there was reduction in red cell lipids and their fractions, plasma lipids and their fraction, and derangement of liver functions compared to controls. *1260*

Red Blood Cells Decrease In 20 cases of thalassemia there was reduction in red cell lipids and their fractions, plasma lipids and their fractions, and derangement of liver functions compared to controls. *1260*

Lipoproteins, Prebeta *Serum Increase* Mean concentration in 50 children was significantly elevated. *0547*

Lymphocytes *Blood Increase* Especially in infants. *2552*

MCH *Blood Decrease* Microcytic hypochromic anemia may occur due to blood loss, increased demand or dietary inadequacy. MCH < 27 pg, MCV < 80 fL. *0532* Defective globin synthesis. *0962 2468*

MCHC *Blood Decrease* Normal or slightly decreased. *2468* Hypochromic anemia with MCHC between 23-32% *2552 0999*

MCV *Blood Decrease* MCV < 75 fL are most often due to thalassemia trait. *2468* Microcytic, hypochromic anemia may occur due to blood loss, increased demand or dietary inadequacy. MCH < 27 pg, MCV < 80 fL. *0532* Hypochromic microcytic anemia with MCV between 28-43 fL. *2552* In nonsplenectomized patients, large poikilocytes are common, whereas after splenectomy large flat macrocytes and small deformed microcytes are frequently seen. *2538 0962*

Monocytes *Blood Increase* May be somewhat increased. *2552*

Osmotic Fragility *Red Blood Cells Decrease* Osmotic fragility is reduced; the red cells are usually resistant to hemolysis in hypotonic saline. *0999 0962*

Phosphate *Serum Decrease* 24 h excretion level was higher than net absorption, indicating normal phosphate absorption and high renal phosphaturia, leading to deficiency. *1349*

Urine Increase 24 h excretion level was higher than net absorption, indicating normal phosphate absorption and high renal phosphaturia, leading to deficiency. *1349*

Platelet Count *Blood Decrease* With the gross splenomegaly which may occur, a secondary thrombocytopenia and leukopenia frequently develop, leading to a further tendency to infection and bleeding. *2538*

Blood Increase The white cell and platelet counts are slightly elevated unless there is secondary hypersplenism. *2538*

Poikilocytes *Blood Increase* The red cells show marked anisopoikilocytosis, with hypochromia, target-cell formation, and a variable degree of basophilic stippling. *2538*

Protoporphyrin *Red Blood Cells Increase* *1457*

Reticulocytes *Blood Increase* Moderately elevated. *2538* Only slightly increased. *0962* Moderate (19,000-25,000/μL). *0995*

Blood Normal Reticulocyte index normal or slightly increased. *0999*

Triglycerides *Serum Increase* Significantly elevated mean concentrations were found in 50 children. *0547*

Uric Acid *Serum Increase* *0962*

Urobilinogen *Urine Increase* Increased in urine without bile. *2468*

Feces Increase *2468*

Zinc *Serum Decrease* In 42 patients aging from 3 months to 22 years with homozygous beta-thalassemia and thalassemia intermedia. Mean serum concentration was significantly decreased. *0072*

282.42 Thalassemia Minor

Anisocytes *Blood Increase* Defective globin synthesis. *0962* Aniso- and poikilocytosis may be very striking and far out of proportion to the degree of anemia. *2552*

Basophilic Stippling *Blood Increase* Mild anemia, usually with microcytosis, hypochromia, stippling, and target cells usually occurs in heterozygous beta thalassemia. *0151*

Cells *Bone Marrow Increase* Bone marrow is cellular and shows erythroid hyperplasia and contains stainable iron with thalassemias. *2468*

Copper *Serum Increase* In 42 patients (age 3 mo-22 y) with homozygous beta-thalassemia and thalassemia intermedia, serum zinc was significantly decreased while Cu and Fe were increased. *0072* May be increased on occasion. *0349*

Erythrocytes *Blood Decrease* With the more severe expression of the disease, homozygote or heterozygote, all parameters of erythrocyte numbers are depressed. *0962*

Blood Increase Typically, the RBC are increased in number but are microcytic hypochromic and show prominent poikilocytosis and targeting. *0433* Over 5.7 million/μL and MCV is < 75 fL are most often due to thalassemia trait. *2468* In many heterozygotes the hematocrit and hemoglobin are slightly depressed but the erythrocyte number is normal or increased. *0962*

Blood Normal In many heterozygotes the hematocrit and hemoglobin are slightly depressed but the erythrocyte number is normal or increased. *0962*

Erythrocyte Survival *Red Blood Cells Decrease* Normal or slightly shortened. *1792*

Ferritin *Serum Normal* *0186*

Folate *Serum Decrease* Reflects increased marrow utilization of folate. *0186*

Hematocrit *Blood Decrease* Mild anemia, usually with microcytosis, hypochromia, stippling, and target cells usually occurs in heterozygous beta thalassemia. *0151* In periods of stress such as pregnancy or during severe infection, a moderate degree of anemia may be present. *2538*

Hemoglobin *Blood Decrease* Tends to be 1-2 g/dL lower than in normal subjects. *0433* Mild anemia, usually with microcytosis, hypochromia, stippling, and target cells usually occurs. *0151* In periods of stress such as pregnancy or during severe infection, a moderate degree of anemia may be present in these patients. *2538* Hypochromic microcytic anemia in thalassemia minor can be distinguished from iron deficiency by a normal or even elevated serum iron concentration and by the failure of the anemia to respond to iron. *0999*

Hemoglobin, Fetal *Blood Increase* Elevated in about 50% of patients, usually to 1-3% and rarely to more than 5%. *2538*

Iron *Serum Increase* Hypochromic microcytic anemia in these patients can be distinguished from iron deficiency anemia by a normal or even elevated serum iron concentration and by the failure of the anemia to respond to iron. *0999* In 42 patients (age 3 mo-22 y) with homozygous beta-thalassemia and thalassemia intermedia serum zinc was significantly decreased while Cu and Fe were increased. *0072 0995*

Serum Normal *0995*

Iron-Binding Capacity, Total (TIBC) *Serum Increase* Total capacity is increased. *2468*

Iron Saturation *Serum Increase* *0186*

MCH *Blood Decrease* The most striking and consistent finding is that of small, poorly hemoglobinized red cells, MCH values of 20-22 pg and MCV values of 50-70 fL. *2538* Mean in 45 cases was 20.26 ± 2.23 pg. *1793*

MCHC *Blood Decrease* Slightly reduced. Mean in 45 cases was 31.22 ± 0.96 %. *1793*

MCV *Blood Decrease* The most striking and consistent finding is that of small, poorly hemoglobinized red cells, MCH values of 20-22 pg and MCV values of 50-70 fL. *2538* In 45 cases, the range was 52-75, with a mean of 64.7 fL. *1793* Unusually low for the mild degree of anemia. *2552 0151*

Osmotic Fragility *Red Blood Cells Decrease* Decreased osmotic fragility is a method for identifying the heterozygote. *0999*

Phosphate *Serum Decrease* 24 h excretion level was higher than net absorption, indicating normal phosphate absorption and high renal phosphaturia, leading to deficiency. *1349*

Urine Increase 24 h excretion level was higher than net absorption, indicating normal phosphate absorption and high renal phosphaturia, leading to deficiency. *1349*

Poikilocytes *Blood Increase* Defective globin synthesis. *0962* Aniso- and poikilocytosis may be very striking and far out of proportion to the degree of anemia. *2552*

Protoporphyrin *Red Blood Cells Increase* May be increased on occasion. *0349*

Reticulocytes *Blood Increase* Count is increased (2-10%) with thalassemias. *2468* Normal or slightly increased. *1774*

282.60 Sickle Cell Anemia

Acid Phosphatase *Serum Increase* Marked rise may occur during a severe hemolytic episode. *2104*

Albumin *Urine Increase* May develop. *0433*

282.60 Sickle Cell Anemia (continued)

Aldolase *Serum Increase* Slightly elevated in a group of 15 patients. The range was 1.0-7.3 U/L with a mean of 2.7 U/L (normal = 1.8 U/L). *1023*

Red Blood Cells Increase Mean red cell concentrations were slightly elevated in 15 patients. Mean = 2.2 U/L (normal = 1.2 U/L) and range = 0.9-3.9 U/L. *1023*

Alkaline Phosphatase *Serum Increase* Serum concentration and the isoenzyme pattern appear to be in concordance with severity of sickle cell crisis. Bone isoenzyme is the principal enzyme fraction that increases during symptomatic crises. Serum concentration may be an additional indicator of degree, frequency, and persistence of tissue i injuries. Increased during crisis, representing vaso-occlusive bone injury as well as liver damage with sickle cell disease. *2467 0288*

Leukocyte Decrease Decreased activity. *2468* Low levels found. *2454*

Alkaline Phosphatase Isoenzymes *Serum Increase* Serum concentration and the isoenzyme pattern appear to be in concordance with severity of sickle cell crisis. Bone isoenzyme is the principal enzyme fraction that increases during symptomatic crises. *2467*

Androgens *Plasma Decrease* Deficient as a result of primary rather than secondary hypogonadism in 29 of 32 adult male patients. *0005*

Androstenedione *Serum Decrease* Basal serum testosterone, dihydrotestosterone, and androstenedione were lower in 32 adult male patients. Secondary sex characteristics were abnormal in 29 of 32 patients. *0005*

Anisocytes *Blood Increase* Blood film reveals marked poikilocytosis and anisocytosis, target cells, some macrocytes, and occasional sickled erythrocytes. Nucleated red cells are frequently seen, particularly in children. *0999*

Bilirubin *Serum Increase* Intrahepatic cholestasis with extremely high circulating levels also appears to be characteristic. *2538*

Bilirubin, Indirect *Serum Increase* Elevation is always seen but late in the course true liver function abnormalities also develop. *0433* Laboratory signs of hemolysis with increased indirect-reacting serum bilirubin. *2538*

Cholesterol *Serum Decrease* Hypocholesterolemia was found in 8 cases. Values ranged from 2.6-4.3 mmol/L. *2519* Plasma lipids are significantly reduced. *0028*

Red Blood Cells Increase Plasma lipids are significantly reduced and RBC cholesterol is higher in sickle cell patients than in normal subjects. *0028*

Complement, Total *Synovial Fluid Normal* Total hemolytic complement ranged from 22-80 U/L, usually at the upper limit of normal. *0676*

Copper *Serum Increase* Significantly increased in patients with SS compared to controls P < 0.001 Increased. *2052 1729*

Erythrocytes *Blood Decrease* Usually between 2.0-3.5 million/µL. *2538 0999*

Urine Increase Hematuria is frequent. *2467 2538 1001*

Erythrocyte Sedimentation Rate *Blood Decrease* Decreased ESR becomes normal after blood is aerated. *2467* Consistently decreased. *2552*

Blood Increase Elevated in 6 of 18 patients. *0676*

Erythrocyte Survival *Red Blood Cells Decrease* Mean red cell life span was 17.32 ± 4.51 days and half-life was 10.11 ± 2.82 days. Mean life span was inversely correlated with number of sickled cells. *1541* Shortened in all the varieties of sickle cell disease. *2538*

Factor VIII *Plasma Increase* May be increased. *1931 2552*

Factor IX *Plasma Normal* *1931 2552*

Factor XI *Plasma Normal* *1931 2552*

Factor XII *Plasma Normal* *1931 2552*

Factor B *Plasma Decrease* *1979 2356*

Follicle Stimulating Hormone (FSH) *Serum Decrease* Consistent with primary testicular failure in all 14 adult male patients tested. *0005*

Glucose-6-Phosphate Dehydrogenase *Serum Increase* Elevated in 15 cases. Values ranged from 10-14 with a mean of 4.8 (normal = 1.6). *1023*

Red Blood Cells Increase Mean concentrations in red cells were slightly increased to a mean of 5.4 (range = 1.5-9.8). *1023*

Gonadotropin, Pituitary *Serum Decrease* Serum LH and FSH before and after stimulation with gonadotropin releasing hormone were consistent with primary testicular failure in all 14 adult male patients tested. *0005*

Haptoglobin *Serum Decrease* RBC destruction is partially intravascular, producing elevated plasma heme proteins and decreased haptoglobin concentration. *0476 2552 2538*

Hematocrit *Blood Decrease* Decreased in 7 cases, ranging from 17-24%. *2519*

Hemoglobin *Blood Decrease* Mild anemia. *0433* Steady-state is usually between 5-11 g/dL. The anemia is normochromic. *2538*

Hemoglobin A$_{1c}$ *Blood Decrease* Due to increased RBC turnover.

Blood Increase Significantly elevated in children with this disease (13.1% n = 36) compared with normal children (6.25% n = 27). *1197*

Hemoglobin, Fetal *Blood Increase* Increased in various hemoglobinopathies; HBF over 30% protects the cell from sickling; therefore, infants with homozygous S have few problems before age of 3 months. *2467* Electrophoresis of the hemoglobin confirms the diagnosis by showing the typical pattern of homozygous sickle inheritance: Hb S with variable amounts of Hb F and no Hb A. *0999*

Hemoglobin, Free *Serum Increase* Seen between as well as during crises, and no consistent increase in this value occurs in crises. *0433*

Immunoglobulin IgG *Serum Increase* Markedly elevated in both Black and Caucasian patients. *2110*

Isocitrate Dehydrogenase *Serum Increase* Elevated in 15 patients. Values ranged from 1.5-13.0 and the mean was 5.2 (normal = 2.5). *1023*

Red Blood Cells Increase Mean RBC concentration was elevated to 2.8 U/L in 15 patients. *1023*

Lactate Dehydrogenase *Serum Increase* Usually elevated to about twice normal in the steady state. *1682 0962*

Red Blood Cells Increase Mean concentration elevated to 180 U/L (3 X the normal mean) in 15 patients. Values ranged from 83-388 U/L. *1023*

Lactate Dehydrogenase Isoenzymes *Serum Increase* LD$_1$ and LD$_2$. *2467 0812*

Leukocytes *Blood Increase* Leukocytosis, even after correction for nucleated red blood cells, is the rule. *0433* Tends to persist and increase during crises, when counts > 20,000/µL are common. *0151* Polymorphonuclear leukocytosis with a left shift is common even in the steady state and may be due in part to redistribution of leukocytes from the marginal to the circulating granulocyte pool. *0243 2538*

Synovial Fluid Increase Ranged from 600-270,000/µL in 13 patients. Polymorphonuclear cells predominated. *0676*

Lipids *Serum Decrease* Plasma lipids are significantly reduced and RBC cholesterol is higher in patients than in normal subjects. *0028*

Luteinizing Hormone (LH) *Serum Decrease* Serum LH and FSH before and after stimulation with gonadotropin releasing hormone were consistent with primary testicular failure in all 14 adult male patients tested. *0005*

Malate Dehydrogenase *Serum Increase* Elevated to a median of 193 U/L (normal = 52 U/L) with a range of 87-337 U/L in 15 patients. *1023*

Red Blood Cells Increase Mean RBC concentration was elevated to 245 ± 93 U/L in 15 patients. Levels ranged from 80-460 U/L (normal = 160 U/L). *1023*

MCV *Blood Decrease* Red cell indices are usually normal, but the MCV may be increased or decreased. *2552*

Blood Increase Red cell indices are usually normal, but the MCV may be increased or decreased. *2552*

Monocytes *Blood Increase* Leukocytosis with monocytosis (5-25%). *2538*

Neutrophils *Blood Increase* *2552*

Osmolality *Urine Decrease* Chronic defect in renal concentrating ability frequently present. *1001 2538*

Osmotic Fragility *Red Blood Cells Decrease* Decreased (more resistant RBCs). *2467*

Oxygen Saturation *Blood Decrease* The partial pressure of oxygen in arterial blood is usually diminished as a result of shunting within the lung. *0433* Decreased oxygenation and increased acidosis PO$_2$ and lead to further sickling and further vaso-occlusion. *0874*

pH *Blood Decrease* Decreased oxygenation and increased acidosis develop and lead to further sickling and further vaso-occlusion. *0874*

Phospholipids, Total *Serum Decrease* Plasma lipids are significantly reduced and RBC cholesterol is higher in patients than in normal subjects. *0028*

Platelet Count *Blood Decrease* Decreased with folate deficiency or during an aplastic crisis. *2552*

Blood Increase Thrombocytosis often accompanies the leukocytosis. *0433* Increased (300,000-500,000/μL) with abnormal forms. *2467* Common, but the count may fall during infarctive crisis. *2538*

pO₂ *Blood Decrease* The partial pressure of oxygen in arterial blood is usually diminished as a result of shunting within the lung. *0433* Decreased oxygenation and increased acidosis lead to further sickling and further vaso-occlusion. *0874*

Poikilocytes *Blood Increase* Blood film reveals marked poikilocytosis and anisocytosis, target cells, some macrocytes, and occasional sickled erythrocytes. Nucleated red cells are frequently seen, particularly in children. *0999*

Protein *Synovial Fluid Increase* Elevated in 6 of 13 patients. *0676*

Reticulocytes *Blood Increase* In 15 cases, mean count was 345,000/μL with a range of 62,-750,000/μL, markedly increased over the normal value of 50,000/μL. *1023* Reticulocytosis (5-20%) with circulating nucleated red cells. Count is diminished during aplastic crises. *2538*

Sickle Cells *Blood Increase* Sickled erythrocytes may not be numerous in the blood smear, but in blood deoxygenated with sodium metabisulfite virtually all the red cells are sickled. *0151* Mean number of irreversibly sickled cells was 9 ± 5.06 in 25 patients. Number of cells correlated inversely with RBC life span. *1541*

Synovial Fluid Increase Sickled erythrocytes were found in 7 of 13 joint fluid specimens. *0676*

Specific Gravity *Urine Decrease* Despite the relative benignity of sickle cell trait, adults with this condition are unable to concentrate their urine and characteristically have a urine specific gravity around 1.010. *0433* Specific gravity is low reflecting the loss of renal concentrating ability due to repeated microinfarcts in the medulla of the kidneys. *0999*

Testosterone *Plasma Decrease* Basal serum testosterone, dihydrotestosterone, and androstenedione were lower in 32 adult male patients. Secondary sex characteristics were abnormal in 29 of 32 patients. *0005*

Uric Acid *Serum Increase* May be increased. *2467 0962*

Serum Normal Patients have normal serum levels as a result of increased clearance. *0553*

Urine Increase Increased tubular secretion of urate; patients have normal serum levels as a result of increased clearance. *0553*

Uric Acid Clearance *Urine Increase* Increased tubular secretion of urate; patients have normal serum levels as a result of increased clearance. *0553*

Urobilinogen *Urine Increase* Urine contains increased urobilinogen but is negative for bile. *2467 0999*

Feces Increase *0999*

Viscosity *Serum Increase* Increased viscosity of circulating whole blood may contribute to vaso-occlusion. *0874*

Zinc *Serum Decrease* Decreased. *2297 2120*

Red Blood Cells Decrease RBC and hair zinc concentration were decreased in adult male patients. RBC zinc correlated (R = 0.61) with serum testosterone, which was low (primary testicular failure) in all patients tested. *0005*

282.71 Hemoglobin C Disease

Bilirubin *Serum Increase* Increase is minimal. *2468*

Bilirubin, Indirect *Serum Increase* Manifested by a hemolytic state. *0962*

Cells *Blood Increase* One of the most striking features of homozygous disease is the marked increase in the number of target cells in the peripheral blood. *2538*

Erythrocytes *Blood Increase* Seen in large numbers in Hemoglobin C disease. *0999*

Erythrocyte Survival *Red Blood Cells Decrease* Mean life span 30-55 days. *2347*

Haptoglobin *Serum Decrease* Substantially reduced or even absent. *2538*

Hematocrit *Blood Decrease* Mild anemia, Hct usually between 30-35. *0433*

Hemoglobin *Blood Decrease* Mild anemia. *0433* Hemoglobin concentration of 8-12 g/dL. *2538*

Hemoglobin, Fetal *Blood Increase* Slightly increased. *2468*

Hemoglobin, Free *Serum Increase* Slight to moderate increase. *2467* Manifested by a hemolytic state. *0962*

Lactate Dehydrogenase *Serum Increase* Due to slight hemolysis. *0186*

Leukocytes *Blood Decrease* May be low due to hypersplenism. *0433*

Osmotic Fragility *Red Blood Cells Decrease* Osmotic fragility curves are abnormal, indicating the presence of populations of fragile cells (microspherocytes) and resistant In homozygotes. *2468* Biphasic, with both increased and decreased fragility. *0503 2552 2538*

Red Blood Cells Increase Biphasic, with both increased and decreased fragility. *0503*

Oxygen Saturation *Blood Decrease* Low oxygen affinity. *1649*

Platelet Count *Blood Decrease* May be low due to hypersplenism. *0433*

Reticulocytes *Blood Increase* Count is increased (2-10%). *2468* Manifested by a hemolytic state. *0962*

Sickle Cells *Blood Increase* Sickling produces prominent clinical manifestations. *2538*

Viscosity *Serum Increase* Blood viscosity is increased. *0962*

Red Blood Cells Increase A tendency to increased intracellular viscosity with decreased cell deformability. *2552*

282.72 Hemoglobin E Disease

Haptoglobin *Serum Decrease* Substantially reduced or even absent. *2538*

Hematocrit *Blood Decrease* Exhibits mild or no anemia. *0433* Homozygotes for hemoglobin E have a relatively mild anemia characterized by microcytosis and targeting of the red cells. *0385 2538*

Hemoglobin *Blood Decrease* Exhibits mild or no anemia. *0433* Homozygotes for hemoglobin E have a relatively mild anemia characterized by microcytosis and targeting of the red cells. *0385 2538*

Hemoglobin, Fetal *Blood Increase* Sometimes slightly increased. *2468*

MCV *Blood Decrease* Definite microcytosis. *0433* Homozygotes for hemoglobin E have a relatively mild anemia characterized by microcytosis and targeting of the red cells. *0385 2538*

Osmotic Fragility *Red Blood Cells Decrease* *2538*

Oxygen Saturation *Blood Decrease* RBC oxygen affinity has been found to be decreased, possibly accounting for the anemia. *0433*

282.73 Hemoglobin H Disease

Anisocytes *Blood Increase* Anisopoikilocytosis of RBC. *2246*

Haptoglobin *Serum Decrease* Substantially reduced or even absent. *2538*

Hematocrit *Blood Decrease* Life-long anemia with variable splenomegaly and bone changes. *2538* Variable degree of anemia. *2246*

Hemoglobin *Blood Decrease* Concentration in these patients usually range from about 7-10 g/dL. Both higher and lower levels have been observed. *0433* Life-long anemia with variable splenomegaly and bone changes. *2538* Variable degree of anemia. Hb A constitutes the majority and Hb H varies from 5-30%. *2246*

Poikilocytes *Blood Increase* Anisopoikilocytosis of RBC. *2246*

Reticulocytes *Blood Increase* Usually in the 5% range. *2538 0433 2246*

283.00 Acquired Hemolytic Anemia (Autoimmune)

2,3-Diphosphoglycerate *Red Blood Cells Increase* Synthesis is increased in response to hypoxia. *0159*

Adenosine Deaminase *Serum Increase* Increased in hemolytic anemia. *0655 1737 2235*

Alanine Aminotransferase *Serum Increase* *0962*

Aldolase *Serum Increase* *0962*

Antinuclear Antibodies *Serum Increase* Found in a significant number of patients without other features of SLE or other rheumatic disease. *2035*

Aspartate Aminotransferase *Serum Increase* *0962*

Basophils *Blood Increase* Punctate basophilia and normoblastemia are common in severe cases. *2035 2538*

283.00 Acquired Hemolytic Anemia (Autoimmune)
(continued)

Bilirubin *Serum Increase* Although clinical jaundice is present in < 50% of patients, elevated serum bilirubin, particularly of the unconjugated fraction, is common. *2538* Increase depends on liver function and amount of hemolysis. With normal liver function, it is increased 1 mg/dL in 1-6 h to maximum in 3-12 h following hemolysis of 100 mL of blood, with hemolytic anemias. *2468*

Bilirubin, Direct *Serum Increase* Elevated if the total serum bilirubin exceeds 4 mg/dL; attributed to an associated hepatic injury permitting conjugated bilirubin to regurgitate into the general circulation. *2361 2538*

Bilirubin, Indirect *Serum Increase* There is increased indirect serum bilirubin (< 6 mg/dL because of compensatory excretory capacity of liver). *2468* Although clinical jaundice is present in < 50% of patients, elevated serum bilirubin, particularly of the unconjugated fraction, is common. *2538*

Calcium *Red Blood Cells Increase* In 19 cases of acquired autoimmune hemolysis, increased erythrocytic Ca^{++} level was observed in 6 cases. *0184*

Cold Agglutinins *Serum Increase* In hemolytic anemias. *2468*

Complement C3 *Serum Decrease* Caused by hypercatabolism. *0375 0793 1275 0509 0452*

Red Blood Cells Increase Only fractions of the complement system of proteins, principally C3 and C4 components, are detected on the red cells by antiglobulin sera having anti-C specificity. *0485 2538*

Complement C4 *Red Blood Cells Increase* Only fractions of the complement system of proteins, principally C3 and C4 components, are detected on the red cells by antiglobulin sera having anti-C specificity. *0485 2538*

Complement, Total *Serum Decrease* Low serum titers have been reported in patients with warm antibody hemolytic disease. *1804 2035*

Coombs' Test *Blood Positive* May or may not be positive, depending on the total amount of autoantibody present and its binding affinity for the red cell mass. *2538*

Coproporphyrin *Urine Increase* *0151*

Creatine Kinase *Serum Normal* *0962*

Creatinine *Serum Increase* In 72% of 11 patients hospitalized for this disorder. *0781*

Cryoglobulins *Serum Increase* Variable elevation of cryoglobulins. *2104*

Erythrocyte Survival *Red Blood Cells Decrease* Shortened survival of both the patient's own red cell population and normal donor cells. *1615 2538*

Folate *Serum Decrease* Decreased with extensive skin disease. *0299 2357 0367*

Haptoglobin *Serum Decrease* Decreased in hemoglobinemia (related to the duration and severity of hemolysis) due to extravascular hemolysis. *2467* Usually depleted; the return to normal is a valuable indicator of remission. *2538*

Hematocrit *Blood Decrease* In cases with more active hemolysis, anemia may be moderate to severe (with hematocrit's in the 10-25% range) and the reticulocyte count markedly elevated to 50% or more. *2035*

Hemoglobin *Blood Decrease* In cases with more active hemolysis, anemia may be moderate to severe and the reticulocyte count markedly elevated to 50% or more. *2035*

Hemoglobin A$_{1C}$ *Blood Decrease* Significantly lower (P < 0.0005) in patients with hemolytic anemia (n = 20) compared to patients with nonhemolytic anemia and normal controls. *1769*

Hemoglobin, Free *Serum Increase* Moderate increase when hemolysis is very rapid. *2468* Common. *2035*

Urine Increase In those patients with hyperacute hemolysis. *2538* Rarely encountered, although it is seen in occasional cases with intense hemolysis. *2035*

Immunoglobulin IgG *Red Blood Cells Increase* May be detected on the red cell surface in up to 80% of patients. *0485 2538*

Immunoglobulins *Serum Decrease* Immunoglobulin deficiency, in the form of generalized hypogammaglobulinemia or selective deficiency of one immunoglobulin, has been observed in a minority of patients, with or without associated lymphoproliferative disease. *2035*

Iron *Urine Increase* Hemosiderinuria and increased urinary iron excretion indicate recent hemoglobinemia. May occur several days after an acute intravascular hemolytic episode and persist for some time. *0964 2552*

Lactate Dehydrogenase *Serum Increase* Often increased, although not as high as in megaloblastic anemia. *2552 0962*

Lactate Dehydrogenase Isoenzymes *Serum Increase* LD_2 predominates in hemolytic, whereas LD_1 predominates in megaloblastic anemia. *2552 0962*

Leukocytes *Blood Decrease* A minority of patients will have persistent leukopenia and neutropenia. *0680* Varies widely, from slight leukopenia and neutropenia to moderately elevated total WBC counts, in the range of 20,000/μL. *2035 2538*

Blood Increase Most patients have modestly elevated counts with neutrophilia. *2538* Varies widely, from slight leukopenia and neutropenia to moderately elevated total WBC counts, in the range of 20,000/μL. *2035*

MCV *Blood Increase* Reflects increased number of reticulocytes. *0186*

Methemalbumin *Serum Increase* Low levels of hemoglobinemia and methemalbuminemia are common. *2035*

Monocytes *Blood Increase* *2538*

Neutrophils *Blood Decrease* A minority of patients will have persistent leukopenia and neutropenia. *0680 2538*

Blood Increase Most patients have modestly elevated counts. *2538*

Osmotic Fragility *Red Blood Cells Increase* May be normal with mild hemolysis. With more rapid rates of hemolysis, the cumulative curve shows increasing populations of fragile cells correlated with the appearance of spherocytosis in the peripheral blood smear. *2601 2538*

Red Blood Cells Normal Increased in some cases of secondary hemolytic anemia but it is usually normal. *2467*

Phosphate *Serum Increase* *0962*

Platelet Count *Blood Decrease* Commonly normal or slightly depressed. Severe thrombocytopenia with bleeding is encountered occasionally and has been termed the Evans' Syndrome. *0681 2538*

Reticulocytes *Blood Increase* Increased polychromasia, reflecting reticulocytosis in patients with slightly or moderately increased erythrocyte destruction. *2538* In cases with more active hemolysis, anemia may be moderate to severe (with hematocrit's in the 10-25% range) and the reticulocyte count markedly elevated to 50% or more. *2035*

Urea Nitrogen *Serum Increase* In 82% of 12 patients hospitalized for this disorder. *0781*

Uric Acid *Serum Increase* In 63% of 11 patients hospitalized for this disorder. *0781 0962*

Urobilinogen *Urine Increase* Commonly increased. *2538 2035*

Feces Increase Uniformly increased, but seldom necessary or useful for clinical purposes at present. *2538*

283.21 Paroxysmal Nocturnal Hemoglobinuria

Acetylcholinesterase *Red Blood Cells Decrease* *1443*

Albumin *Urine Increase* Has been demonstrated immediately before and after an episode of hemoglobinuria, but usually there is none between attacks. *0477 2552*

Alkaline Phosphatase *Leukocyte Decrease* Usually decreased. *2538* Often very low or absent. *1385*

Bilirubin *Serum Increase* *0433*

Bilirubin, Indirect *Serum Increase* Reflects hemolysis. *2552*

Cells *Bone Marrow Decrease* The cellularity of the marrow may be decreased and may even appear aplastic. *2538*

Complement C3 *Serum Decrease* Caused by hypercatabolism. *0375 0793 1275 0509 0452*

Serum Increase May, on occasion, be detected in the direct Coombs' test. *2538*

Coombs' Test *Blood Negative* Usually negative. *2538*

Erythrocytes *Blood Decrease* Pancytopenia is a common feature. *2538*

Haptoglobin *Serum Decrease* Absent during a hemolytic episode. *2468 0041*

Hematocrit *Blood Decrease* May be moderate or severe. *0433* Degree of anemia may vary from none to very severe. *2538*

Hemoglobin *Blood Decrease* May be moderate or severe. *0433* Degree of anemia may vary from none to very severe. *2538*

Hemoglobin Casts *Urine Increase* May be present. *2538*

Hemoglobin, Fetal *Blood Increase* Elevated levels have been reported. *1883 2538*

Hemoglobin, Free *Serum Increase* At times of active hemolysis. *0433* Increases during sleep. *2468*

Urine Increase Worse at night and remits during the day; probably observed initially in < 25% of all patients. Parallels changes in pH, circadian variation in cortisol excretion, complement levels, activation of the alternative pathway of complement, and other variable components of plasma. *1632 2538*

Iron *Serum Decrease* A remarkable amount is often lost in the urine, even in the absence of observable hemoglobinuria. *2538*

Urine Increase The excretion of iron in the urine continues between hemolytic episodes and is a simple and valuable indication of chronic hemoglobinuria. *0433* A remarkable amount is often lost in the urine, even in the absence of observable hemoglobinuria. *2538*

Bone Marrow Decrease Often absent. *2538*

Lactate Dehydrogenase *Serum Increase* Very high during active hemolysis. *2552*

Leukocytes *Blood Decrease* Pancytopenia is a common feature. *2538* Leukopenia, especially granulocytopenia, is present at some time in about 60% of patients. *0484*

MCV *Blood Decrease* Occasional microcytosis, when urinary iron loss has occurred. *2552*

Blood Increase RBC are usually macrocytic but there may be great variation in size. *2552*

Methemalbumin *Serum Increase* May be detected at times of active hemolysis. *0433 2552*

Neutrophils *Blood Decrease* Common. *0433* Leukopenia, especially granulocytopenia, is present at some time in about 60% of patients. *0484 2538*

Osmotic Fragility *Red Blood Cells Increase* Increased in symptomatic hemolytic anemia. *2467*

Red Blood Cells Normal 2552

Platelet Count *Blood Decrease* Usually decreased but shows thrombotic rather than hemorrhagic complications. *2468* Pancytopenia is a common feature. *2538* Occurs at some stage in the disease in about 66% of patients. *0484* Moderate thrombocytopenia is common. *0813*

Blood Normal May be normal or reduced. *0433* Moderate thrombocytopenia, but life span and function are normal. *0813*

Reticulocytes *Blood Increase* May be greatly increased from 20-24% depending on the severity of the hemolysis and the degree of marrow response. *0433* Count may be elevated above the level usually seen in iron deficiency. *2538* There may be relative reticulocytosis but the absolute count is often inappropriately low in relation to the severity of the anemia. *2552*

Urobilinogen *Urine Increase* Increased blood destruction. *2552*

284.01 Congenital Aplastic Anemia

Cells *Bone Marrow Decrease* Marrow is described as fatty and hypocellular or normocellular. *0695*

Erythrocyte Survival *Red Blood Cells Normal* Shortened survival has been described in some cases but earlier reports indicate no evidence of a hemolytic process. *2552*

Fat *Bone Marrow Increase* Marrow is described as fatty and hypocellular or normocellular. *0695*

Hematocrit *Blood Decrease* The anemia is normochromic or slightly macrocytic, and macrocytes and target cells may be seen in the blood. *2552*

Hemoglobin *Blood Decrease* The anemia is normochromic or slightly macrocytic, and macrocytes and target cells may be seen in the blood. *2552*

Leukocytes *Blood Decrease* In most patients, leukopenia has been due to neutropenia, but frequently all types of WBC are affected. *2552*

MCH *Blood Increase* The anemia is normochromic or slightly macrocytic, and macrocytes and target cells may be seen in the blood. *2552*

MCHC *Blood Increase* The anemia is normochromic or slightly macrocytic, and macrocytes and target cells may be seen in the blood. *2552*

MCV *Blood Increase* The anemia is normochromic or slightly macrocytic, and macrocytes and target cells may be seen in the blood. *2552*

Neutrophils *Blood Decrease* In most patients, leukopenia has been due to neutropenia, but frequently all types of WBC are affected. *2552*

Plasma Cells *Bone Marrow Increase* There may be many plasma cells and mastocytes. *0695*

Reticulocytes *Blood Decrease* May be slightly increased relatively but the absolute count is reduced. *2552*

284.90 Aplastic Anemia

2,3-Diphosphoglycerate *Red Blood Cells Increase* Synthesis is increased in response to hypoxia. *0159*

Alkaline Phosphatase *Leukocyte Increase* Usually increased in untreated disease. *2467*

Bleeding Time *Blood Increase* Reflects low platelet count. *2538* Usually moderately prolonged. *2552*

Capillary Fragility *Blood Increase* Reflects low platelet count. *2538*

Cells *Bone Marrow Decrease* Marked hypocellularity of the marrow fragments with a predominance of reticulum cells, mast cells, lymphocytoid cells, and plasma cells. Cells of the myeloid series are often grossly reduced in numbers. *0151 0415*

Clot Retraction *Blood Poor* Reflects low platelet count. *2538 2552*

Copper *Serum Increase 2467*

Erythrocytes *Blood Decrease* RBC and all cellular elements are decreased. *0151* Peripheral pancytopenia associated with hypocellular bone marrow. *0415* Invariable finding. *2538*

Bone Marrow Decrease Nucleated red cells are decreased in number, but may be the most numerous cell type. *2538 2552*

Erythrocyte Survival *Red Blood Cells Decrease* There may be evidence of premature red cell destruction. *1384* May be somewhat shortened but evidence of blood destruction is lacking. *2552 2538*

Red Blood Cells Normal Red cell survival is normal or only slightly reduced. *0999*

Erythropoietin *Serum Increase* Titers in plasma and the 24 h urinary excretion rates usually exceed those found in most other types of anemia at the same hemoglobin concentration. *2538* Activity of erythropoietin is high, in fact, higher than observed in patients with anemia of comparable severity due to other causes. *0999 0151*

Urine Increase Activity is high, in fact higher than observed in patients with anemia of comparable severity due to other causes. *0999* Titers in plasma and the 24-h urinary excretion rates usually exceed those found in most other types of anemia at the same hemoglobin concentration. *2538 0151*

Hematocrit *Blood Decrease* A severe anemia may be found at the time of presentation. The RBC are usually normocytic or slightly macrocytic. *0433* Peripheral pancytopenia associated with hypocellular bone marrow. *0415* In 100% of 20 patients hospitalized for this disorder. *0781*

Hemoglobin *Blood Decrease* A severe anemia may be found at the time of presentation. The RBC are usually normocytic or slightly macrocytic. *0433* Usually > 7 g/dL. *2552* In 100% of 20 patients hospitalized for this disorder. *0781 0151*

Hemoglobin, Fetal *Blood Increase* Returns to normal only after complete remission, and therefore is reliable indicator of complete recovery. Better prognosis in patients with higher initial level 400 mg/dL. *2467* In adults, substantial increases are rare, but in children the concentration has been reported to be as high as 1.5 g/dL. *2122 2538*

Iron *Serum Increase* Often > 200 μg/dL with 100% saturation of the iron-binding capacity. Decreased number of normal marrow cells. *0433* Increased with an almost complete saturation of iron-binding capacity. May be the first sign of erythroid suppression and is of considerable screening value in patients receiving potentially toxic drugs. *2538*

Iron-Binding Capacity, Total (TIBC) *Serum Decrease* Serum iron concentration is elevated and total capacity is reduced. *0151*

Iron Saturation *Serum Increase* Percent saturation of transferrin is increased. *0999* Almost 100% saturation. *2538*

Lactate Dehydrogenase *Serum Increase* In 42% of 21 patients hospitalized for this disorder. *0781*

284.90 Aplastic Anemia (continued)

Leukocytes *Blood   Decrease*   Counts as low as 1,000/µL are common with 70-90% lymphocytes. *0433*   Peripheral pancytopenia associated with hypocellular bone marrow. *0415*   An invariable finding. *2538   0151*

Lymphocytes *Blood   Decrease*   The absolute count is often decreased. *2538*

Blood   Normal   Production is not considered impaired. *2538*

Bone Marrow   Increase   60-100% of the nucleated cells are lymphocytes. *2552*

MCV *Blood   Increase*   Occasional macrocytosis. *0433*

Monocytes *Blood   Decrease*   Absolute monocytopenia and reduction in total circulating white cells usually occurs. *0151   2538*

Neutrophils *Blood   Decrease*   Absolute granulocytopenia invariably occurs. Counts 200/µL indicate high risk of infection. *0151* Absolute granulocytopenia is always present and is responsible for the leukopenic part of pancytopenia. *2538*   Abnormal granulation of the polymorphonuclear cells has been described. Decreased number of normal marrow cells. *0433*

Osmotic Fragility *Red Blood Cells   Normal*   RBC fragility is normal. *2552*

Platelet Count *Blood   Decrease*   Often markedly decreased. *0433*   Peripheral pancytopenia associated with hypocellular bone marrow. *0415*   Invariable finding. Many patients continue to have decreased counts for years after other abnormalities have disappeared. *2538   0151*

Protoporphyrin *Red Blood Cells   Increase   2552*

Reticulocytes *Blood   Decrease*   Percentage ranges from 0 to as high as 5%, but the absolute number is usually subnormal. Many are large and immature, possibly reflecting an increased concentration of erythropoietin and a short bone marrow transit time. *1049   0151 2538*

285.00 Sideroblastic Anemia

Alkaline Phosphatase *Leukocyte   Decrease*   Score is reduced in about 50% of the patients. *1327   2538*

Anisocytes *Blood   Increase*   Blood smear shows anisocytosis with many bizarre forms, target cells, hypochromia with pyridoxine-responsive anemia. *2467*   Prominent findings on blood smear. In hereditary x-linked sideroblastic anemia. *2552*

Basophilic Stippling *Blood   Increase*   Prominent findings on blood smear. *2552*

Bilirubin *Serum   Normal*   Rarely elevated despite the mild hemolytic anemia. *0433   1327*

Cells *Bone Marrow   Increase*   Bone marrow is characterized by intense erythroid hyperplasia, often associated with a shift to younger forms, particularly polychromatophilic normoblasts, some of which show megaloblastic nuclear changes. *2538*

Coproporphyrin *Red Blood Cells   Increase*   Conflicting reports from marked elevation to normal. *1326*

Erythrocytes *Blood   Decrease*   Reported to be low in about 80% of patients. *0433*

Ferritin *Serum   Increase   0186*

Folate *Serum   Decrease*   Reported to be low in about 80% of patients. *1462   2538*

Hematocrit *Blood   Decrease*   The anemia is normocytic or slightly macrocytic. *2538*

Hemoglobin *Blood   Decrease*   The degree of anemia is variable, ranging from concentrations as low as 5 g/dL, in severely affected boys with sex-linked sideroblastic anemia to almost normal levels in the milder cases. Older people with idiopathic or secondary forms of this disease usually have moderate anemias with concentrations ranging from 7-10 g/dL. *0433*   The anemia is normocytic or slightly macrocytic. *2538   0151*

Iron *Serum   Increase*   Characteristically normal to elevated. *0433* Increased with primary inherited sex-linked sideroblastic anemia. *0619*   Increased serum iron and reduced iron-binding capacity in > 50% of cases. *0532   0151*

Serum   Normal   Characteristically normal to elevated. *0433*

Bone Marrow   Increase   Increased in the marrow fragments and in the developing erythroblasts. *0151*   Bone marrow is hyperplastic and contains increased amounts of normoblastic iron, often forming ringed sideroblasts. *2538*

Iron-Binding Capacity, Total (TIBC) *Serum   Decrease*   Normal to low. *0433*   Associated increased serum iron and reduced iron-binding capacity in > 50% of cases. *0532*   Somewhat decreased with pyridoxine-responsive anemia. *2467*

Serum   Normal   Normal to low. *0433*

Iron Saturation *Serum   Increase*   High degree of saturation. *2538*

Leukocytes *Blood   Decrease*   Count varies from normal to leukopenic levels; when present, leukopenia is accompanied by neutropenia. Values below 2,000/µL are rare. *2538*

MCH *Blood   Decrease*   Microcytic hypochromic anemia may occur due to blood loss, increased demand or dietary inadequacy. MCH < 27 pg, MCV < 80 fL. *0532*   Reduced hemoglobin synthesis. Microcytic hypochromic anemia. *2552*

Blood   Increase   The anemia is normocytic or slightly macrocytic. *2538*

MCHC *Blood   Decrease*   Degree of anemia may vary but is usually in the range of 7-8 g/dL of hemoglobin, with a lowered MCHC. *0151*   Reduced hemoglobin synthesis. Microcytic hypochromic anemia. *2552   0532*

MCV *Blood   Decrease*   Microcytic hypochromic anemia may occur due to blood loss, increased demand or dietary inadequacy. MCH < 27 pg, MCV < 80 fL. *0532*   Reduced hemoglobin synthesis. Microcytic hypochromic anemia. *2552*

Blood   Increase   The anemia is normocytic or slightly macrocytic. *2538*

Monocytes *Blood   Increase*   Morphologically normal, but the proportion may be moderately increased. *2538*

Neutrophils *Blood   Decrease*   Leukopenia is accompanied by neutropenia. *2538*

Osmotic Fragility *Red Blood Cells   Decrease*   Tends to be decreased. *2538*

Platelet Count *Blood   Decrease*   Usually normal, but thrombocytopenia and thrombocytosis occurs in a minority of patients. *2538*

Blood   Increase   Usually normal, but thrombocytopenia and thrombocytosis occurs in a minority of patients. *2538*

Blood   Normal   Usually normal, but thrombocytopenia and thrombocytosis occurs in a minority of patients. *2538   0433*

Poikilocytes *Blood   Increase*   Blood smear shows poikilocytosis with many bizarre forms, target cells, hypochromia with pyridoxine-responsive anemia. *2467*   Prominent findings on blood smear. In hereditary x-linked sideroblastic anemia. *2552*

Protoporphyrin *Red Blood Cells   Decrease*   May be characteristically high or very low, depending upon the type of sideroblastic anemia. Usually high in idiopathic and low in hereditary. *2552   2538*

Red Blood Cells   Increase   Almost always moderately increased, and rarely it is markedly so. *1326*   Elevated (40-300 mg/dL compared to normal levels of 15-35 mg/dL) reflecting a functional block to hemoglobin synthesis. *0433*   May be characteristically high or very low, depending upon the type of sideroblastic anemia. Usually high in idiopathic and low in hereditary. *2552   2538*

Reticulocytes *Blood   Decrease*   Absolute count is usually reduced. *0151*   Inappropriately low. *2538*

Blood   Increase   Count is usually normal but may be slightly increased. *2538*

Volume *Red Blood Cells   Decrease*   Erythrocytes are formed in normal numbers but are reduced in size. *2552*

Xanthurenic Acid *Urine   Increase*   Abnormal tryptophan metabolism indicated by excessive excretion in response to loading dose of L-tryptophan has been found in pyridoxine responsive cases. *2552*

286.01 Hemophilia

AHF-Like Antigen *Plasma   Increase*   Plasma contains normal or even elevated amounts of antigenic material detected by heterologous antiserum. *2617*

Antibody Titer *Serum   Increase*   Titers of antibodies to cytomegalovirus were generally higher in hemophiliac patients than in a control group of healthy volunteers. *1378*

Beta₂-Macroglobulin *Serum   Increase*   Significantly higher. *1318*

Bleeding Time *Blood   Increase*   In severe cases. *0995*

Blood   Normal   Bleeding time and prothrombin time are not significantly prolonged. *2538   2246*

Capillary Fragility *Blood   Increase*   Occasional patients may have positive tourniquet tests. *2552*

Cholesterol *Serum   Decrease*   May be below normal in this condition. *0619*

Clotting Time *Blood Increase* May be 24 h or longer and show spontaneous irregular variations. *2552 0995 2246*

Coagulation Time *Blood Increase* In severe cases. *2552*

Creatine Kinase *Serum Increase* Increases when bleeding occurs into the muscles. Serum activity returns to normal after 10 days following treatment with cryoprecipitate. The test is useful in distinguishing between hemorrhage into the psoas muscle (raised levels) and into the hip joint only (no increase). *0619*

Erythrocytes *Urine Increase* Hematuria may persist for weeks or months. *0999* Bleeding from the kidneys is often caused by trauma, but usually the cause cannot be determined. May occasionally be due to infection. Occurs in approximately 20% of the moderate and severe cases and in 5% of the mild cases. *2538*

Factor VIII *Plasma Decrease* Varies from 0% of normal in severe to 25% in mild cases. *2552* The basic defect appears to be a failure to synthesize functional AHF. *2246* May be due to decreased or absent synthesis of factor VIII or to the synthesis of a functionally inactive factor VII molecule. *1572 0962*

Hematocrit *Blood Decrease* Presence or absence of anemia depends on the severity and frequency of bleeding. *2552*

Hemoglobin *Blood Decrease* Presence or absence of anemia depends on the severity and frequency of bleeding. *2552*

Iron-Binding Capacity, Total (TIBC) *Serum Increase* Depending upon the severity and frequency of bleeding. *2552*

Iron Saturation *Serum Decrease* Depending upon the severity and frequency of bleeding. *2552*

Lee-White Clotting Time *Blood Increase* Deficient factor VIII (AHG). *0433*

MCH *Blood Decrease* Presence or absence of anemia depends on the severity and frequency of bleeding. *2552*

MCHC *Blood Decrease* Presence or absence of anemia depends on the severity and frequency of bleeding. *2552*

MCV *Blood Decrease* Presence or absence of anemia depends on the severity and frequency of bleeding. *2552*

Partial Thromboplastin Time *Plasma Increase* The most sensitive screening test, usually prolonged if AHG levels are < 20% of normal. *0999* Always significantly prolonged in patients with 20% factor VIII. Individuals with levels ranging between 20-30% may have a PTT value either just outside or at the upper end of the normal range. *2538 0962 2246*

Platelet Count *Blood Increase* Usually normal or elevated. *2552*

Prothrombin Time *Plasma Normal* Bleeding time and prothrombin time are not significantly prolonged. *2538 2246*

Recalcification Time *Blood Increase* Greatly prolonged. *2552*

Thrombin Time *Plasma Normal* *0962 0995 2246*

Thromboplastin Generation *Blood Increase* Due to deficient function of the adsorbed plasma reagent. *2552 2538*

286.10 Christmas Disease

Bleeding Time *Blood Increase* In severe cases. *2468*

Blood Normal *2538 2246*

Clotting Time *Blood Increase* In severe deficiencies. *2538 0995 2246*

Coagulation Time *Blood Increase* In severe cases. *2468*

Creatine Kinase *Serum Increase* Increases when bleeding occurs into the muscles. Serum activity returns to normal after 10 days following treatment with cryoprecipitate. The test is useful in distinguishing between hemorrhage into the psoas muscle (raised levels) and into the hip joint only (no increase). *0619*

Erythrocytes *Urine Increase* Hematuria may persist for weeks or months. *0999* Bleeding from the kidneys is often caused by trauma, but usually the cause cannot be determined. May occasionally be due to infection. Occurs in approximately 20% of the moderate and severe cases and in 5% of the mild cases. *2538*

Factor IX *Plasma Decrease* Present in carriers in approximately half the concentration of that found in patients. *2538* Titers < 5% of normal are usual, and may be undetectable in severe cases. In mildly affected patients, values may be > 30%. *0121*

Fibrinogen *Plasma Normal* *0186*

Lee-White Clotting Time *Blood Increase* Deficient factor IX (PCT). *0433*

Partial Thromboplastin Time *Plasma Increase* In contrast to hemophilia A, the abnormality is corrected by serum but not by adsorbed plasma. *2538 0962 2246*

Prothrombin Consumption *Blood Increase* In severe cases. *2467*

Prothrombin Time *Plasma Normal* All patients have a normal test using human brain tissue factor (thromboplastin), but when ox-brain tissue factor is used, the prothrombin time is prolonged in approximately 6% of cases. *2393 2538 2246*

Thrombin Time *Plasma Normal* *2246*

Thromboplastin Generation *Blood Increase* In mild deficiency, may be the only abnormal test. *2467* In contrast to hemophilia A, the abnormality resides in the serum rather than in the adsorbed plasma. *2538*

286.20 Factor XI Deficiency

Bleeding Time *Blood Increase* Variable. *2246* In severe cases. *0995*

Blood Normal Usually normal. *2538*

Clotting Time *Blood Increase* *2246*

Coagulation Time *Blood Increase* *2468*

Factor XI *Plasma Decrease* Definitive diagnosis is by a factor XI assay using blood from a patient with established factor XI deficiency. *2538* Plasma thromboplastin antecedent (factor XI) deficiency. *2246*

Lee-White Clotting Time *Blood Increase* *0433*

Partial Thromboplastin Time *Plasma Increase* PTT or activated PTT test is prolonged and the prothrombin time normal. *2538 2246*

Prothrombin Consumption *Blood Increase* *2468*

Prothrombin Time *Plasma Normal* PTT or activated PTT test is prolonged and the prothrombin time normal. *2538 2246*

Thrombin Time *Plasma Normal* *2246*

Thromboplastin Generation *Blood Increase* The most marked abnormality is found when the patient's adsorbed plasma and serum are incubated together. *2538*

286.31 Congenital Dysfibrinogenemia

Bleeding Time *Blood Increase* Usually prolonged, but in some cases no clot forms at all. *2538*

Clot Retraction *Blood Poor* *2538*

Clotting Time *Blood Increase* The clotting time of whole blood or the recalcification time of platelet-poor plasma has usually been normal or prolonged. *2538*

Blood Normal The clotting time of whole blood or the recalcification time of platelet-poor plasma has usually been normal or prolonged. *2538*

Estrogens *Serum Normal* *2538*

Factor II *Plasma Normal* *2538*

Factor V *Plasma Normal* *2538*

Factor VII *Plasma Normal* *2538*

Factor VIII *Plasma Normal* *2538*

Factor IX *Plasma Normal* *2538*

Factor X *Plasma Normal* *2538*

Factor XIII *Plasma Normal* *2538*

Fibrinogen *Plasma Decrease* Reduced level by any technique. The discordant values suggest that abnormal fibrinogen molecules are inhibitory to coagulation of the normal fibrinogen or have a markedly delayed clotting time and are present in sufficient concentration to give a falsely low level of fibrinogen. *2538* Concentration is usually normal or only slightly depressed, but is functionally defective. *2246*

Plasma Normal In most cases determined by immunologic assays, fibrin tyrosine content, or gravimetric methods have been normal. *2538 0186*

Partial Thromboplastin Time *Plasma Increase* Variable. Even when abnormal, rarely as prolonged as the prothrombin time or the thrombin time. *2538*

Plasminogen *Serum Normal* Invariably normal. *2538*

Platelet Count *Blood Normal* *2538*

Prothrombin Time *Plasma Increase* Usually prolonged, but in some cases no clot forms at all. *2538* In many cases. *2246*

Recalcification Time *Blood Normal* The clotting time of whole blood or the recalcification time of platelet-poor plasma has usually been normal. *2538*

Reptilase Time *Blood Increase* Usually prolonged, but in some cases no clot forms at all. *2538*

286.31 Congenital Dysfibrinogenemia (continued)

Thrombin Time *Plasma Increase* Usually prolonged, but in some cases no clot forms at all. *2538* Abnormally long. *2246*

Thromboplastin Generation *Blood Normal 2538*

286.32 Factor XII Deficiency

Bleeding Time *Blood Normal* Prothrombin and bleeding times are normal. *2538 2246*

Clotting Time *Blood Increase* In severe deficiencies. *0995 2246*

Coagulation Time *Blood Increase 2468*

Factor XII *Plasma Decrease* Definitive diagnosis is made by testing against plasma from an established case. *2538* Nondetectable. *1885*

Partial Thromboplastin Time *Plasma Increase* Activated partial thromboplastin time is prolonged. *2538 2246*

Prothrombin Consumption *Blood Increase 2468*

Prothrombin Time *Plasma Normal* Prothrombin and bleeding times are normal. *2538 2246*

Thrombin Time *Plasma Normal 0433 2246*

286.33 Factor XIII Deficiency

Bleeding Time *Blood Normal 2538 2246*

Clot Solubility *Blood Poor 0433*

Clotting Time *Blood Normal 2246*

Partial Thromboplastin Time *Plasma Normal 2246*

Platelet Count *Blood Normal 2538*

Prothrombin Time *Plasma Normal 2246*

Thrombin Time *Plasma Normal 0433 2246*

286.34 Congenital Afibrinogenemia

Bleeding Time *Blood Increase* Often increased (33% of patients). *2468* Prolonged bleeding times, unrelated to thrombocytopenia, are found in some patients. *2590* Variable. *2538*

Clotting Time *Blood Increase* Corrected by the addition of normal plasma or normal fibrinogen to the patient's plasma. *2538* Infinite. *2246*

Erythrocyte Sedimentation Rate *Blood Decrease 2538*

Fibrinogen *Plasma Decrease* Undetectable by almost all physicochemical measurements or functional assays. *2538*

Lee-White Clotting Time *Blood Increase 0433*

Partial Thromboplastin Time *Plasma Increase* Corrected by the addition of normal plasma or normal fibrinogen to the patient's plasma. *2538* Infinite. *2246*

Platelet Count *Blood Decrease* Mild to moderate thrombocytopenia occurs occasionally. Count is rarely below 100,000/µL. *2590*

Prothrombin Time *Plasma Increase* Corrected by the addition of normal plasma or normal fibrinogen to the patient's plasma. *2538* Infinite. *2246*

Recalcification Time *Blood Increase* Corrected by the addition of normal plasma or normal fibrinogen to the patient's plasma. *2538*

Reptilase Time *Blood Increase* Corrected by the addition of normal plasma or normal fibrinogen to the patient's plasma. *2538 0433*

Thrombin Time *Plasma Increase* Corrected by the addition of normal plasma or normal fibrinogen to the patient's plasma. *2538* Infinite. *2246 0433*

286.35 Factor V Deficiency

Bleeding Time *Blood Increase* Slightly prolonged in approximately 33% of cases. *2538*

Blood Normal Slightly prolonged in 33% of cases. *2538 2246*

Clotting Time *Blood Increase 2538 2246*

Coagulation Time *Blood Increase* Increase in coagulation time is not corrected by administration of vitamin K. *2468*

Erythrocyte Sedimentation Rate *Blood Decrease* Nearly 0; RBC remain suspended even after 24 h. *2246*

Factor V *Plasma Decrease 2538*

Lee-White Clotting Time *Blood Increase 0433*

Partial Thromboplastin Time *Plasma Increase* Prothrombin time and partial thromboplastin time, activated or unactivated, are all prolonged. *2538 2246*

Prothrombin Consumption *Blood Increase* Increase in prothrombin consumption is not corrected by administration of vitamin K, with factor V deficiency. *2468*

Prothrombin Time *Plasma Increase* Deficient factor V (labile). *0433* Not corrected by administration of vitamin K. *2468* Prothrombin time and partial thromboplastin time, activated or unactivated, are all prolonged. *2538 2246*

Thrombin Time *Plasma Normal 0433 0995 2246*

Thromboplastin Generation *Blood Increase* Abnormal when the reaction mixture contains adsorbed plasma from the patient, but is normal when serum from the patient is used. *0995 2538 2246*

Blood Normal Abnormal when the reaction mixture contains adsorbed plasma from the patient but is normal when serum from the patient is used. *2538* Abnormal when the reaction mixture includes the serum reagent prepared for the patient. *2538* Abnormal results. *2246*

286.36 Factor X Deficiency

Bleeding Time *Blood Normal 0995 2246*

Clotting Time *Blood Increase 0995 2246*

Factor X *Plasma Decrease* True deficiency in some patients and deficiency of functional factor X in others. *2246 2538*

Lee-White Clotting Time *Blood Increase 0433*

Partial Thromboplastin Time *Plasma Increase* Prolonged. *2538 0433 2246*

Prothrombin Consumption *Blood Increase* Abnormal results. *2246*

Prothrombin Time *Plasma Increase* Not corrected by administration of vitamin K. Prolonged. *2538 2246*

Thrombin Time *Plasma Normal 0433 0995 2246*

Thromboplastin Generation *Blood Increase 2538*

286.37 Factor VII Deficiency

Bleeding Time *Blood Increase* May be abnormally long. *2246*

Blood Normal 0995 2246

Clotting Time *Blood Normal* Clotting time of recalcified plasma is normal, distinguishing this from Stuart factor deficiency. *2246 2538*

Erythrocytes *Urine Increase* Hematuria has been observed. *2246*

Factor VII *Plasma Decrease* Some patients appear to synthesize a nonfunctional variant, and other patients are truly deficient. *2246 2538*

Partial Thromboplastin Time *Plasma Normal 2538 2246*

Prothrombin Time *Plasma Increase* Usually greatly prolonged. *0035 2538 2246*

Thrombin Time *Plasma Normal 0995 2246*

Thromboplastin Generation *Blood Normal 2246*

286.38 Factor II Deficiency

Bleeding Time *Blood Normal 2246*

Clotting Time *Blood Increase 2246*

Partial Thromboplastin Time *Plasma Increase* Variable. *2246*

Prothrombin Time *Plasma Increase 0433 2246*

Thrombin Time *Plasma Normal 0433 2246*

286.40 Von Willebrand's Disease

Bleeding Time *Blood Increase* Usually prolonged 2 h after dose of 10 grains of aspirin; bleeding time is variable without this aspirin tolerance test. *2467* Prolonged. *0227* Commonly occurs in homozygotes and heterozygotes. *1389* May be detected by Dukes' method or the standard Ivy procedure. *2538 2246*

Clot Retraction *Blood Normal 2538*

Clotting Time *Blood Increase* Variable. *2246*

Factor VIII *Plasma Decrease* Characteristically reduced, usually from 20-40%. A wide range may be seen and a normal concentration is not incompatible with the diagnosis. *0433* Commonly occurs in both homozygotes and heterozygotes. *1389* Activity is usually higher than in classic hemophilia, but values of 1-5% of normal may sometimes be found. May show wide fluctuation in the same person on repeated testing. *2538* A true decrease in amount of AHF protein accompanied by a proportional or even more severe decrease in AHF-like antigens. *2617 2246 0227 0962*

Fibrinogen *Plasma Normal 0228*

Lee-White Clotting Time *Blood Normal 2467*

Partial Thromboplastin Time *Plasma Increase* May be prolonged and is related to the decreased factor VIII AHF activity. *2538* Variable. *2246 0962*

Platelet Count *Blood Decrease* Usually normal, but thrombocytopenia has been reported in some families. *0456 0962*

Blood Normal Usually normal, but thrombocytopenia has been reported in some families. *0456 2538*

Prothrombin Consumption *Blood Decrease* May be present and is related to the decreased factor VIII AHF activity. *2538*

Prothrombin Time *Plasma Normal 0962 2246*

Thrombin Time *Plasma Normal 0962 2246*

286.60 Disseminated Intravascular Coagulopathy

Alpha₂-Antiplasmin *Serum Decrease* Measured values in 9 patients with DIC. Subnormal values in 6, normal in 2 and increased in 1. *2337* Significantly decreased levels in 25 patients with acute, subacute and chronic compensated and uncompensated DIC. *2032*

Antithrombin III *Plasma Decrease* Early and significant decreases occur and therefore this may serve as a useful diagnostic test. *0203 2353*

Factor V *Plasma Decrease 2538*

Factor VIII *Plasma Decrease 2538*

Factor XIII *Plasma Decrease* Substantial depression of factor XIII concentrations developed with concomitant significant increases in the proportion and concentration of plasma high molecular weight fibrinogen complexes (HMWFC). In inverse correlation between factor XIII and percentage of HMWFC was demonstrated in the early stages of the illness. *1491*

Fibrinogen *Plasma Decrease* Substantial depression of factor XIII concentrations developed together with concomitant significant increases in the proportion and concentration of plasma high molecular weight fibrinogen complexes (HMWFC). In inverse correlation between factor XIII and percentage of HMWFC was demonstrated in the of the illness. *1491* Low or falling levels. *0433 2538*

Fibrin Split Products (FSP) *Plasma Decrease* Deposition of fibrin usually stimulates local secondary fibrinolysis producing reduced circulating plasminogen level due to consumption and a decrease in systemic fibrinolytic activity. *2538*

Plasma Increase If large amounts are present, the thrombin time will be markedly prolonged; latex agglutination test for fibrin degradation products will be positive. *2538*

Haptoglobin *Serum Decrease* Decreases in 6-10 h and lasts for 2-3 days after lysis of 20-30 mL of blood. Determination is relatively reliable and very sensitive. *2468*

Hemoglobin, Free *Serum Increase* Increases transiently with return to normal in 8 h. *2468*

Urine Increase Occurs 1-2 h after severe hemolysis and lasts 24 h. It is a transient finding and is relatively insensitive. False positive is due to myoglobinuria or to lysis of RBCs in urine with intravascular hemolysis. *2468*

Partial Thromboplastin Time *Plasma Increase* Prolonged because of consumption of clotting factors and the anticoagulant effects of fibrin degradation products. *2538*

Plasminogen *Serum Decrease* Deposition of fibrin usually stimulates local secondary fibrinolysis producing reduced circulating plasminogen level due to consumption and a decrease in systemic fibrinolytic activity. *2538*

Platelet Count *Blood Decrease* Low or falling platelet counts. *0433 2538*

Prothrombin Time *Plasma Increase* Prolonged because of consumption of clotting factors and the anticoagulant effects of fibrin degradation products. *2538 0433*

Thrombin Time *Plasma Increase* Prolonged because of consumption of clotting factors and the anticoagulant effects of fibrin degradation products. *2538*

287.00 Allergic Purpura

Albumin *Serum Decrease* Hypoalbuminemia occurs in patients with gastrointestinal involvement. *1184 2538*

Urine Increase Mild proteinuria associated with normal Addis count signifies renal involvement. *0433*

Antistreptolysin O *Serum Increase* A hemolytic streptococci can be implicated both by culture and by antistreptolysin O titers. This is an inconstant finding. *0962*

Bleeding Time *Blood Normal* Tourniquet test may be positive, but other tests of hemostasis are usually normal. *2552*

Capillary Fragility *Blood Increase* Tourniquet tests are, at times, positive. *2538 2552*

Complement, Total *Serum Normal* Usually normal. *0962*

Creatinine *Serum Increase* Increase is mild and transitory. *0433* Elevated in the presence of renal failure. *2538*

Eosinophils *Blood Increase* May be a polymorphonuclear leukocytosis and an increase in eosinophils. *2538* Slight leukocytosis and occasional eosinophilia may be seen. *0962 2552*

Erythrocyte Casts *Urine Increase* Indicate active glomerulitis. *0962* Common but often transient. *2552 2538*

Erythrocytes *Blood Decrease* The RBC is generally within normal limits except if severe gastrointestinal blood loss has occurred. *0433*

Blood Normal The RBC is generally within normal limits except if severe gastrointestinal blood loss has occurred. *0433*

Urine Increase In varying degrees signify renal involvement. *0433* An early feature of urinalysis is macroscopic hematuria. *0962*

Erythrocyte Sedimentation Rate *Blood Increase* During the acute illness. *0433* Usually elevated. *2538*

Blood Normal Unlike with other necrotizing angiitis, the ESR is often normal. *0962*

Granular Casts *Urine Increase* May be seen. *2538*

Hematocrit *Blood Decrease* Anemia is not usually present unless the hemorrhagic manifestations have been severe. *2538 0962 2552*

Blood Normal Anemia is not usually present unless the hemorrhagic manifestations have been severe. *2538 2552 0962*

Hemoglobin *Blood Decrease* Anemia is not usually present unless the hemorrhagic manifestations have been severe. *2538 0962 2552*

Blood Normal Anemia is not usually present unless the hemorrhagic manifestations have been severe. *2538 0962 2552*

Immunoglobulin IgA *Serum Increase* Found in 50% of patients. *2552*

Immunoglobulins *Serum Normal* Except for IgA, the immunoglobulins remain normal. *0962*

Iron-Binding Capacity, Total (TIBC) *Serum Increase* Anemia from blood loss may be present. *2538*

Iron Saturation *Serum Decrease* Anemia from blood loss may be present. *2538*

Leukocytes *Blood Increase* A mild leukocytosis, mainly of polymorphonuclear cells, with WBC counts of 10,000-20,000/μL is common. *0433* WBC, neutrophils, and eosinophils may be increased. *2467 2538 0962*

MCH *Blood Decrease* Anemia is not usually present unless the hemorrhagic manifestations have been severe. *2538*

MCHC *Blood Decrease* Anemia is not usually present unless the hemorrhagic manifestations have been severe. *2538*

MCV *Blood Decrease* Anemia is not usually present unless the hemorrhagic manifestations have been severe. *2538*

Neutrophils *Blood Increase* A mild leukocytosis, mainly of polymorphonuclear cells, with WBC counts of 10,000-20,000/μL common. *0433* Modest neutrophilia. *2552*

Occult Blood *Feces Positive* Stool may show blood. *2468 2552*

Platelet Count *Blood Decrease* Defect in hemostasis in drug-sensitivity allergic purpura. *0962*

Blood Normal Count is normal. *2538* Tourniquet test may be positive but other tests of hemostasis are usually normal. *2552*

Protein *Urine Increase* Urine may show hematuria and proteinuria. *2538* Proteinuria is manifest and moderate in quantity. *0962*

Urea Nitrogen *Serum Increase* Elevated in the presence of renal failure. *2538* Azotemia is a common but transient finding. *2552*

287.10   Thrombasthenia (Glanzmann's)

Bleeding Time   *Blood   Increase*   Deficient platelet factor III. *0433* Bleeding time is usually prolonged and aggregation of platelets by collagen or thrombin is abnormal. *0999*   Often marked. *2246   2552*

Capillary Fragility   *Blood   Increase*   *2246*

Clot Retraction   *Blood   Poor*   Due to platelet function abnormalities. *2246*

Clotting Time   *Blood   Normal*   *2246*

Factor IX   *Plasma   Decrease*   Deficient platelet factor III. *0433*

Partial Thromboplastin Time   *Plasma   Normal*   *2246*

Platelet Count   *Blood   Decrease*   Count is usually normal, but mild reduction may occur. *0327*

  Blood   Normal   Present in normal numbers and are morphologically normal. Deficient platelet aggregation is the most significant abnormality. *2552   0433 2538*

Prothrombin Consumption   *Blood   Increase*   *2552*

  Blood   Normal   *2246*

Prothrombin Time   *Plasma   Normal*   *2246*

Thrombin Time   *Plasma   Normal*   *2246*

Thromboplastin Generation   *Blood   Increase*   Contact activation is abnormal, resulting in abnormal TGT test. *2552*

  Blood   Normal   *2246*

287.30   Idiopathic Thrombocytopenic Purpura

Acid Phosphatase   *Serum   Increase*   13 of 15 patients had elevations. In 15 of 16 patients, serum gave higher values than plasma. *1743*   Only 2 out of 9 cases showed plasma levels to be of diagnostic value. Results of previous studies could not be reproduced successfully. *0444*   Plasma beta-glycerol acid phosphatase may be elevated in any form of thrombocytopenia due to accelerated plasma destruction. *2552*

Bleeding Time   *Blood   Increase*   *2552 2246*

Capillary Fragility   *Blood   Increase*   Positive tourniquet test. *2552 2538*

Cells   *Bone Marrow   Increase*   Normal or increased numbers of megakaryocytes, many of which are smooth in contour, are found in the bone marrow. *2538*

Clot Retraction   *Blood   Poor*   Absent or deficient due to thrombocytopenia. *2552   0433*

Clotting Time   *Blood   Normal*   *2246*

Coagulation Time   *Blood   Normal*   *2552*

Complement C3   *Serum   Normal*   In one series. *1259*

Coombs' Test   *Blood   Positive*   In chronic ITP when autoimmune hemolytic anemia and ITP occur together (Evans' syndrome). *0682*

Cryofibrinogen   *Serum   Increase*   *2035 0856 1551 2046*

Eosinophils   *Blood   Increase*   Originally thought to be common, has not been a constant finding. *1538*   Described in many patients, but has not been confirmed as a prognostic indicator. *2552   2538*

Fibrin Split Products (FSP)   *Plasma   Increase*   During the acute stage in this series. *1666*

Hematocrit   *Blood   Decrease*   An anemia from blood loss may be present, but the red blood cell morphology is normal. *0433*

Hemoglobin   *Blood   Decrease*   An anemia from blood loss may be present, but the RBC morphology is normal. *0433*

Immunoglobulin IgG   *Serum   Decrease*   Mean IgG levels were subnormal. *1259   2538*

  Serum   Increase   Children with both acute and chronic disease had significantly greater levels than normal or thrombocytopenic controls. Acute cases were elevated more than chronic. *1407*

Iron-Binding Capacity, Total (TIBC)   *Serum   Decrease*   Anemia from blood loss may be present. *2538*

Iron Saturation   *Serum   Increase*   Anemia from blood loss may be present. *2538*

LE Cells   *Blood   Increase*   1-2% of patients. *0571*

Lee-White Clotting Time   *Blood   Normal*   *2467*

Leukocytes   *Blood   Increase*   Normal or slightly elevated. *0433* Occasionally, as a result of severe bleeding. *2552*

  Blood   Normal   Normal or slightly elevated. *0433*

Lymphocytes   *Blood   Increase*   In chronic cases. *0995*   Lymphocytosis with abnormal cells resembling those found in infectious mononucleosis. *2552*

MCH   *Blood   Normal*   An anemia from blood loss may be present, but the RBC morphology is normal. *0433*

MCHC   *Blood   Normal*   An anemia from blood loss may be present, but the RBC morphology is normal. *0433*

MCV   *Blood   Increase*   Occasional moderate macrocytosis, if there has been a recent severe hemorrhage. *2552   0995*

  Blood   Normal   An anemia from blood loss may be present, but the RBC morphology is normal. *0433*

Monocytes   *Blood   Increase*   *2538*

Neutrophils   *Blood   Increase*   Shift to the left. *0995*   Usually normal, but moderate neutrophilia may occur due to severe bleeding. *2552*

Partial Thromboplastin Time   *Plasma   Normal*   *2552 2246*

Platelet Count   *Blood   Decrease*   There is a marked decrease with values under 10,000/μL in the acute form. In the chronic form a moderate thrombocytopenia with counts of 30,000-100,000/μL is present. *0433*   Usually severe at the onset; in most cases platelets are < 20,000/μL. *2538*   May be totally absent or only slightly decreased. *2552   0962*

Platelet Survival   *Blood   Decrease*   Markedly shortened. *0433* The life-span of transfused normal platelets is extremely short, sometimes only a few h. *2538*

Prothrombin Consumption   *Blood   Decrease*   Defect phase I or II blood coagulation. *2467   2552*

Prothrombin Time   *Plasma   Normal*   *0433 2552 2246*

Reticulocytes   *Blood   Increase*   Occasionally, if there has been a recent severe hemorrhage. *2552   0995*

Thrombin Time   *Plasma   Normal*   *2246*

288.00   Agranulocytosis

Albumin   *Urine   Increase*   Urine may contain traces of albumin but is otherwise normal. *2552*

Alkaline Phosphatase   *Leukocyte   Increase*   Usually increased in untreated disease. *2467*

Bleeding Time   *Blood   Normal*   Normal in most typical cases. *2552*

Coagulation Time   *Blood   Normal*   Normal in most typical cases. *2552*

Eosinophils   *Blood   Increase*   May occur. *0992*

Erythrocyte Sedimentation Rate   *Blood   Increase*   Greatly accelerated. *2552*

Globulin   *Serum   Increase*   In some patients. *0992*

Hematocrit   *Blood   Decrease*   Depending on the underlying process the patient may also manifest moderate to severe anemia. *0433*

  Blood   Normal   Typically normal; some cases have had anemia but this was most often pre-existing. *2552*

Hemoglobin   *Blood   Decrease*   Depending on the underlying process the patient may also manifest moderate to severe anemia. *0433*

  Blood   Normal   Typically normal; some cases have had anemia but this was most often pre-existing. *2552*

Leukocytes   *Blood   Decrease*   Absolute concentration of circulating neutrophils is reduced. In acute cases these cells may be virtually absent. The remaining cells may show toxic changes such as increased granulation or cytoplasmic vacuolization. *0433*   In acute fulminant form, WBC is decreased to < 2,000/μL. *2468*   Leukopenia exists when a reduction below about 4,000/μL occurs. *0151*

Lymphocytes   *Blood   Decrease*   The lymphocytes number below about 1,400/μL in children or 1,000/μL in adults. *0151*   Variable. *0992*

  Blood   Increase   Variable and may be decreased, normal or increased. *0992*

  Blood   Normal   Variable and may be decreased, normal or increased. *0992*

Metamyelocytes   *Bone Marrow   Decrease*   Characteristic lack of granulocytes, including polymorphonuclears, metamyelocytes, and myelocytes. *2552*

Monocytes   *Blood   Increase*   Sometimes occurs. Increases in the recovery. *2467*   May be relatively and absolutely increased. *2552*

Neutrophils   *Blood   Decrease*   Marked decrease or complete absence of mature granulocytes. *0433*   0-2%. May show pyknosis or vacuolization with agranulocytosis. *2468*   Counts of 500-1,000/μL have moderately increased risks, whereas below this the invasion of mucous membranes, skin and blood by microorganisms becomes increasingly frequent and severe. *0151*

  Bone Marrow   Absent   Bone marrow shows absence of cells in granulocytic series but normal erythroid and megakaryocytic series. *2468   2552*

Plasma Cells *Bone Marrow Increase* Plasma cells, lymphocytes and reticulum cells may be increased. *2552*

Platelet Count *Blood Decrease* Depending on the underlying process the patient may manifest a reduced platelet count. *0433*

289.00 Polycythemia, Secondary

Alkaline Phosphatase *Leukocyte Normal 2467*

Basophils *Blood Normal 2538*

Bilirubin *Serum Increase* Increased slightly. *0151*

Coproporphyrin *Urine Increase* Increased hemopoiesis. *0619*

Eosinophils *Blood Normal 0995*

Erythrocytes *Blood Increase* Frequently 7-10 million or more/µL when patients are first seen. *0151* Absolute erythrocytosis caused by an enhanced stimulation of RBC production. *2538*

Erythrocyte Sedimentation Rate *Blood Decrease 2231*

Erythropoietin *Serum Increase* Secondary polycythemia caused by excessive release of erythropoietin. *2538*

Hematocrit *Blood Increase 2538*

Hemoglobin *Blood Increase* May be increased less, in proportion, than the erythrocyte level because of a low MCV and MCH. *0151*

Histamine *Serum Normal 2538*

Iron *Serum Decrease 0151*

Serum Normal Usually. *1917*

Iron-Binding Capacity, Total (TIBC) *Serum Normal* Usually. *1917*

Leukocytes *Blood Normal 2538*

MCH *Blood Decrease 0151*

MCHC *Blood Decrease* Low MCHC in addition to microcytosis, especially after large hemorrhages or repeated phlebotomies. *0151*

MCV *Blood Decrease* Decreased resulting in a smaller increase in hemoglobin than usually would occur with the increased RBC count. Low MCHC and MCV, especially after large hemorrhages or repeated phlebotomies. *0151*

Metamyelocytes *Blood Increase* Are seen. *0151*

Myelocytes *Blood Increase* Occasionally seen. *0151*

Oxygen Saturation *Blood Decrease 2538*

Platelet Count *Blood Normal 2538*

pO₂ *Blood Decrease 2538*

Blood Normal 2538

Reticulocytes *Blood Increase* Percentage is usually normal, but the absolute number is increased. *0151*

Uric Acid *Serum Increase 0151 0962*

Urine Increase 0619

Urobilin *Feces Increase* Increased slightly. *0151*

Urobilinogen *Urine Increase* Increased slightly. *0151*

Vitamin B₁₂ *Serum Normal 2538*

Vitamin B₁₂ Binding Capacity *Serum Normal 2538*

Volume *Plasma Increase* Red cell mass increased. *0619*

289.40 Hypersplenism

Erythrocytes *Blood Decrease* Pancytopenia is a common feature. *2538* As much as 38% may be trapped in the enlarged spleen. *1824*

Erythrocyte Survival *Red Blood Cells Decrease* May or may not be reduced. *1824 2246*

Hematocrit *Blood Decrease* Apparent anemia is often due to expansion of plasma volume in the presence of normal RBC volume. *1824*

Hemoglobin *Blood Decrease* Apparent anemia is often due to expansion of plasma volume in the presence of normal RBC volume. *1824*

Leukocytes *Blood Decrease* Hematopoietic diseases. *2467* Pancytopenia is a common feature. *2538* Due to increased destruction and sequestration. *0214 2246*

MCV *Blood Normal* Apparent anemia is often due to expansion of plasma volume in the presence of normal RBC volume. *1824*

Neutrophils *Blood Decrease* Count may be low, even in the range of 1%, but the patient can make pus and usually is not subject to septic disease. *2538* Due to increased destruction and sequestration. *0214 2246*

Platelet Count *Blood Decrease* Pancytopenia is a common feature. *2538* As much as 50-90% of the total plasma mass may be sequestered. *0082*

Volume *Plasma Increase* When the spleen is greatly enlarged, the plasma volume and total blood volume are significantly expanded. *2538* Apparent anemia is often due to expansion of plasma volume in the presence of normal RBC volume. *1824*

289.80 Myelofibrosis

Acid Phosphatase *Serum Increase* 9 of 16 patients with myeloid metaplasia or chronic granulocytic leukemia were found to have slight but significant elevations of serum acid phos. *0129* A patient with histiocytic medullary reticulosis was found to have up to 60 X the normal upper limit, which then paralleled the activity of disease during temporary responses to therapy. *2523*

Alkaline Phosphatase *Serum Increase 0151 2538*

Leukocyte Decrease Significantly elevated in most cases but in 10% of the cases in myelofibrosis the levels were in the CML range (markedly decreased or absent). *0433* In myelofibrosis, variable with normal, high, and low figures being found. Level tends to fall as the disease progresses. *2538*

Leukocyte Increase Usually high but in 10% of cases, scores were in the CML range (markedly decreased or absent). *0433* Findings tend to be inconsistent. Generally elevated in the majority of patients. *2317* In agnogenic myeloid metaplasia, 41 of 78 patients had scores > 1.00. A significant negative correlation was found between LAP and absolute percentage of immature cells. *2167* Variable; tends to fall as the disease progresses. *2538 1563*

Anisocytes *Blood Increase* In myelofibrosis is usually pronounced. *2538*

Basophils *Blood Decrease 0532*

Blood Increase Eosinophilia and basophilia occur in 10-30% of myelofibrosis patients. *2317 0532 2538*

Coombs' Test *Blood Positive* Positive in 6 of 29 myelofibrosis patients. Positivity tends to develop in later stages of disease. *2317*

Cryofibrinogen *Serum Increase 2035 1551*

Eosinophils *Blood Increase* Eosinophils and basophils may be increased in agnogenic myeloid metaplasia. *2468* Eosinophilia and basophilia occur in 10-30% of myelofibrosis patients. *2317 0532*

Erythrocytes *Blood Decrease* Pancytopenia is a common feature. *2538*

Folate *Serum Decrease* Macrocytic anemia was reported in over 50% of the patients, the probable cause was folic acid deficiency secondary to chronic excessive cell proliferation (in myelofibrosis). *1059* Decrease with extensive skin disease *0299 2357 0367 2538*

Glutathione *Red Blood Cells Increase* RBC reduced glutathione occurred in 16 of 17 myelofibrosis patients. *2317* In myelofibrosis, usually increased. *0900*

Hematocrit *Blood Decrease* Usually there is a mild to moderate anemia with a mean Hct of 32%. *0433* Anemia mostly normochromic is found in a majority of cases. Hemoglobin < 12 g/dL occurred in 73% of cases. *2317* Anemia is present in 66% of all patients when they are first seen. Usually normochromic and moderate in degree but may become severe in advanced disease in myelofibrosis. *2538*

Hemoglobin *Blood Decrease* Usually there is a mild to moderate anemia. *0433* Anemia mostly normochromic is found in a majority of cases. 12 g/dL occurred in 73% of cases. *2317* Anemia is present in 66% of all patients when they are first seen. Usually normochromic and moderate in degree but may become severe in advanced disease in myelofibrosis. *2538*

Lactate Dehydrogenase *Serum Increase* May be elevated usually correlating with the degree of myelofibrosis or WBC elevation. *0433* Increased in every patient irrespective of the disease. The maximum rise was observed in cases of myelosclerosis, the smallest in lymphatic leukemia. *1521 2538*

Lactate Dehydrogenase Isoenzyme 5 (LD₅) *Red Blood Cells Increase* A slight mean increase was observed in hemolysates from 12 cases of agnogenic myeloid metaplasia. *2249*

Leukocytes *Blood Decrease* The WBC averages 20,000/µL but may be as high as 100,000 or as low as 1,000/µL with slight granulocytic immaturity. *0433* Pancytopenia is a common feature. *2538*

289.80 Myelofibrosis (continued)

Leukocytes (continued)

Blood Increase The WBC averages 20,000/μL, but may be as high as 100,000 or as low as 1000/μL with slight granulocytic immaturity. *0433* Elevated in about 50%, normal in 33%, and low in the remainder due to agnogenic myeloid metaplasia. *0151* Initial count was normal in 42%, increased in 47% and decreased in 12% of myelofibrosis patients. Leukopenia occurred with anemia and leukocytosis with high RBC count. *2317* Nearly always present in myelofibrosis. The most numerous cells are mature neutrophils. *2538*

Blood Normal The WBC averages 20,000/μL but may be as high as 100,000 or as low as 1,000/μL with slight granulocytic immaturity. *0433*

Lysozyme *Serum Increase* During the transition from a variety of myeloproliferative disorders to acute myeloblastic or acute myelomonocytic leukemia, there is a striking elevation in serum and urine muramidase activity. *2093*

Urine Increase During the transition from a variety of myeloproliferative disorders to acute myeloblastic or acute myelomonocytic leukemia, there is a striking elevation in serum and urine muramidase activity. *2093*

Metamyelocytes *Blood Increase* Can generally be found in myelofibrosis. *2538*

Monocytes *Blood Increase* Peripheral monocytosis is especially likely to occur in circumstances of histiocytic proliferation and increased phagocytosis as strikingly manifested in histiocytic medullary reticulosis. *1489 2538*

Myelocytes *Blood Increase* Can generally be found in myelofibrosis. *2538*

Osmotic Fragility *Red Blood Cells Decrease* Red cell osmotic fragility was decreased in 63% of myelofibrosis patients. *2317*

Platelet Count *Blood Decrease* Count ranges from 30,000-3,200,000/μL with an average of 400,000/μL. *0433* Thrombocytopenia occurred in 48% of myelofibrosis patients, mostly in the later stages. Counts > 400,000 occurred in 16% in the early stages. *2317* Pancytopenia is a common feature. *2538* In myelofibrosis as the disease progresses, may be aggravated by therapy. *2538*

Blood Increase Count ranges from 30,000-3,200,000/μL with an average of 400,000/μL. *0433* May appear large and bizarre with agnogenic myeloid metaplasia. *0151* In myelofibrosis, occurs in about 33% of cases, especially in the earlier stages, and may at times reach levels of 1,000,000/μL or higher. *2538 0532*

Prothrombin Time *Plasma Increase* Prolonged in 75% of patients with agnogenic myeloid metaplasia. *2468*

Reduced Glutathione *Red Blood Cells Increase* RBC reduced glutathione occurred in 16 of 17 myelofibrosis patients. *2317* In myelofibrosis, usually increased. *0900 2538*

Reticulocytes *Blood Increase* Greater than 1% in 75% of myelofibrosis patients; total count > 60,000/μL occurred in 51%. *2317 0151*

Uric Acid *Serum Increase* May be elevated usually correlating with the degree of myelofibrosis or WBC elevation. *0433* In myelofibrosis, secondary gout and the formation of urinary uric acid calculi are frequent consequences of the hyperuricosuria. *2538 1283 0962*

Urine Increase In myelofibrosis, secondary and the formation of urinary uric acid calculi are frequent consequences of the hyperuricemia and hyperuricosuria. *2538*

Vitamin B$_{12}$ *Serum Increase* Normal or elevated in myelofibrosis. *2317* Significantly increased in 7 cases of myelofibrosis, mean = 1,525 compared to normal, 385 pg/mL. *1990* Serum concentration is generally raised, as is the binding power, but neither of them is as high as in chronic granulocytic leukemia (in myelofibrosis). *0841 2538 0142*

Vitamin B$_{12}$ Binding Capacity *Serum Increase* Significant elevation; usually correlated with WBC in peripheral blood. *1990* In myelofibrosis, serum concentration is generally raised as is the binding power, but neither of them is as high as in chronic granulocytic leukemia. *0841 2538*

MENTAL DISORDERS

291.00 Delirium Tremens

Alanine Aminotransferase *Serum Increase* *0962*

Aldolase *Serum Increase* *0962*

Aspartate Aminotransferase *Serum Increase* Irrespective of associated hepatic disease and may arise in muscle. *0503 0962*

Bicarbonate *Serum Decrease* Respiratory alkalosis may occur. *1430*

Creatine Kinase *Serum Increase* High elevations irrespective of associated hepatic disease and may arise in muscle. *0812 0503 1942 0962*

Lactate Dehydrogenase *Serum Increase* Relatively slight elevations found in almost all patients. Perhaps of skeletal muscle origin since, like the elevated LD values of progressive muscular dystrophy, they are accompanied by increased CK. High elevations irrespective of associated hepatic disease and may arise in muscle. *0503*

Nickel *Serum Normal* Mean 2.3 (n = 35) compared with controls mean 2.6 μg/L (n = 42). *1559*

Ornithine Carbamoyl Transferase (OCT) *Serum Increase* Liver cell damage. *2467*

pCO$_2$ *Blood Decrease* Respiratory alkalosis may occur. *0962*

pH *Blood Increase* Respiratory alkalosis may occur. *0962*

Uric Acid *CSF Increase* High CSF levels of 0.9-1.3 mg/dL, with normal serum levels. *1338*

296.80 Manic Depressive Disorder

Catecholamines *Plasma Increase* Patients with a 6 month or longer history of anxiety and depression had total plasma catecholamine concentration significantly above normal. *1300*

Urine Increase Patients with a 6 month or longer history of anxiety and depression had total plasma catecholamine concentration significantly above normal. *1300*

Creatine Kinase *Serum Increase* Return towards normal following successful lithium therapy. *0619*

Norepinephrine *Plasma Increase* Usually high in patients with a 6 month or longer history of depression and anxiety, but individual patients may have a markedly low value. *1300*

Plasma Increase Usually high in patients with a 6 month or longer history of depression and anxiety, but individual patients may have a markedly low value. *1300*

Renin Activity *Plasma Increase* High resting renin activity was found in a group of manic depressives, but no relation to mood was observed. Aldosterone production rates were inappropriate for the renin activity found. *1098*

Taurine *Plasma Decrease* Mean concentration in depressed patients free of any drugs and under drug therapy was 29 ± 2 and 25 ± 3 nmol/mL platelet-free plasma respectively. Normal mean was 45 ± 4 nmol/mL. *2313*

Uric Acid *Serum Increase* Increased in both blood and CSF with a lowered CSF:blood ratio, possibly due to cellular breakdown and nucleoprotein catabolism. *2301*

Urine Increase Increased excretion in neurological and psychiatric disorders; progressive rise in urinary level following slight rise in blood, due to disturbed purine metabolism. *2301*

CSF Increase Markedly increased with decreased CSF:blood ratio, possibly due to cellular breakdown and nucleoprotein catabolism. *2301*

297.90 Paranoid States and Other Psychoses

Aldolase *Serum Increase* The increased activity of CK or aldolase or both, was generally present at the onset of a psychotic episode in acute patients and lasted about 5-10 days. Increased activities ranged from 5-50 fold above control limits. *1569*

Alpha$_1$-Antichymotrypsin *Serum Increase* Schizophrenic patients do exhibit a marked and rapid increase during acute phase reaction. *0234 0235*

Serum Normal Serum and plasma levels in acutely psychotic patients and schizophrenic patients are comparable to normals. *0234 0235*

CSF Increase Detected in the CSF of patients suffering from various psychotic and neurological disorders. *0234*

Angiotensin-Converting Enzyme (ACE) *CSF Decrease* Both treated and drug free patients had low activity when compared with controls *0148*

Aspartate Aminotransferase *Serum Increase* In 39% of 33 patients hospitalized for this disorder. *0781*

Ceruloplasmin *Serum Increase* Elevated serum copper and ceruloplasmin blood levels were reported. It is postulated that this may be an important pathognomonic feature. *0027 0065*

Cholecystokinin (CCK) *CSF Decrease* Significant decrease in cholecystokinin in untreated schizophrenics (1.4 pmol/L) compared with controls (4.0). *1440*

Copper *Serum Increase* Elevated serum copper and ceruloplasmin blood levels were reported. It is postulated that this may be an important pathognomonic feature. *0027 0065*

Creatine Kinase *Serum Increase* Increased in 24 of 37 acutely psychotic patients, some of whom had had repeated admissions. Activity was 20 X the upper limits of normal in some specimens. There were no increases in nonpsychotic psychiatric patients, but patients with toxic psychoses and with some acute brain diseases, such as brain trauma, had increased activity. *1569   0503*

Dehydroepiandrosterone (DHEA) *Serum Decrease* *0299 2356 2540*

Prolactin *Serum Decrease* Concentrations in 17 drug-free chronic schizophrenic patients correlated inversely with ratings of their psychopathology. *1279*

Prostaglandins *Serum Increase* Increased synthesis in schizophrenia. *1076*

Pyridoxine *Serum Decrease* Has been noted in schizophrenia. *2104*

Uric Acid *Serum Increase* Increased in both blood and CSF with a lowered CSF:blood ratio, possibly due to cellular breakdown and nucleoprotein catabolism. *2301* In 34% of 36 patients hospitalized for this disorder. *0781*

Urine Increase Increased excretion in neurological and psychiatric disorders; progressive rise in urinary level following slight rise in blood, due to disturbed purine metabolism. *2301*

CSF Increase Markedly increased with decreased CSF:blood ratio, possibly due to cellular breakdown and nucleoprotein catabolism. *2301*

Xanthurenic Acid *Urine Increase* Has been noted in schizophrenia. *2104*

300.00   Anxiety Neurosis

Lactic Acid *Blood Increase* Patients manifested an excessive rise in blood lactate and a lower oxygen consumption when compared with normal controls in a standard exercise test. *1182   1108*

T$_3$ Uptake *Serum Normal* *2467*

300.40   Depressive Neurosis

Catecholamines *Plasma Increase* Patients with a 6 month or longer history of anxiety and depression had total plasma catecholamine concentration significantly above normal. *1300*

Urine Decrease Documented decrease in urinary excretion of catecholamine and indolamine metabolites reported in depressed patients. Not used as a clinical tool at this time. *0433*

Urine Increase Patients with a 6 month or longer history of anxiety and depression had total plasma catecholamine concentration significantly above normal. *1300*

Cyclic Adenosine Monophosphate *Urine Decrease* Lack of primary messenger necessary to activate adenyl cyclase system resulting in decreased levels. No hormonal effect noted. *2356*

Hematocrit *Blood Decrease* Anemia is often present. *0433*

Hemoglobin *Blood Decrease* Anemia is often present. *0433*

Indolamine *Urine Decrease* Documented decrease in urinary excretion of catecholamine and indolamine metabolites reported in depressed patients. Not used as a clinical tool at this time. *0433*

Norepinephrine *Plasma Decrease* Usually high in patients with a 6 month or longer history of depression and anxiety, but individual patients may have a markedly low value. *1300*

Plasma Increase Usually high in patients with a 6 month or longer history of depression and anxiety, but individual patients may have a markedly low value. *1300*

Prostaglandins *Serum Increase* Increased synthesis in schizophrenia and depression. *1076*

Somatostatin *CSF Decrease* Low levels appear to be a state marker for episodes of depression. *0023*

Taurine *Plasma Decrease* Mean concentration in depressed patients free of any drugs and under drug therapy was 29 ± 2 and 25 ± 3 nmol/mL platelet-free plasma respectively. Normal mean was 45 ± 4 nmol/mL. *2313*

Uric Acid *Serum Increase* Increased in both blood and CSF with a lowered CSF:blood ratio, possibly due to cellular breakdown and nucleoprotein catabolism. *2301*

303.00   Acute Alcoholic Intoxication

11-Hydroxycorticosteroids *Plasma Increase* Alcohol excess in nonalcoholics. No rise in chronic alcoholics. *0619*

Aldosterone *Plasma Decrease* Decreased during ethanol intoxication, but increased greatly during hangover. *1412*

Amylase *Serum Increase* Increased in serum and urine in 8.5% of 129 patients after acute intoxication, due to changes in salivary isoenzyme, not as a result of pancreatic damage. *0178* Common as a result of vomiting and increased peptic stimulation of the pancreas. *2104*

Urine Increase Increased in serum and urine in 8.5% of 129 patients after acute intoxication, due to changes in salivary isoenzyme, not as a result of pancreatic damage. *0178*

Bicarbonate *Serum Decrease* Plasma bicarbonate ranged from 2-10 mmol/L in acidosis following alcoholic binge. *1594*

Calcium *Serum Decrease* Hypocalcemia is common in alcoholic subjects. *1394*

Serum Increase Increased following alcoholic binge of several days duration. *1594*

Cortisol *Plasma Increase* Increased following alcoholic binge of several days duration. *1594*

Creatine Kinase *Serum Increase* *1942*

Fat *Urine Increase* Significant lipuria occurred in a group of acutely intoxicated patients with neurological symptoms. *0289*

Fatty Acids, Free (FFA) *Serum Increase* Increased following alcoholic binge of several days duration. *1594*

Growth Hormone *Serum Increase* Increased following alcoholic binge of several days duration. *1594*

Hexosaminidase *Serum Increase* Elevated in 94% of cases. *1166*

Iron *Bone Marrow Increase* Iron overload shown by plasma cells containing iron in bone marrow may occur. *1594*

Lactic Acid *Blood Increase* Acidosis due to lactate and ketoacid accumulation following alcoholic binge of several days duration. *1594*

Magnesium *Serum Decrease* *2467*

Parathyroid Hormone *Serum Increase* Increased following alcoholic binge of several days duration. *1594*

pH *Blood Decrease* Severe metabolic acidosis with pH ranging between 6.96-7.28 occurred after alcoholic binge of several days duration. *1594*

Phosphate *Serum Decrease* *0619*

Serum Increase Increased following alcoholic binge of several days duration. *1594*

Pyridoxine *Serum Decrease* Has been noted in acute alcoholism. *2104*

Renin Activity *Plasma Increase* Increased more than 100%, when 1.5-2.3 g ethanol/kg body weight was ingested over a 3-h period. During hangover the increase even exceed 200%. *1412*

Xanthurenic Acid *Urine Increase* Has been noted in acute alcoholism. *2104*

303.90   Alcoholism

25-Hydroxy Vitamin D$_3$ *Serum Decrease* Lower mean value (15.0 ± 7.6 ng/mL) was found in 13 chronic alcoholics with no evidence of cirrhosis on biopsy. Normal = 23.6 ± 9.8 ng/mL. *2424*

Alanine Aminotransferase *Serum Increase* Above the normal limit (18 U/L) in 30% of 67 alcoholics, during or immediately after a heavy bout of drinking. *1781* 50% of 182 male chronic alcoholics had raised values. Highest values were found after 5-20 y of confirmed alcoholism. Patients with > 20 y duration displayed a tendency to normalization of enzyme activity. *2196*

Aldolase *Serum Decrease* *0126*

Alkaline Phosphatase *Serum Increase* Elevation occurred in 10.4% of cases. *1781* Mild elevation occurred in 80% of 5 cases with range 75-140 U/L. Maximum upper limit for normal 84 U/L. *1452* In 28% of 14 patients hospitalized for this disorder. *0781*

303.90 Alcoholism (continued)

Amylase *Serum Decrease* 20% of 182 male chronic alcoholics had decreased activity of serum pancreatic isoamylase, whereas only 6% had low total serum amylase activity. *2196*

Serum Increase Rises after gross ethanol intake (in the chronic alcoholic). *0619 2104*

Androgens *Plasma Decrease 1805*

Apolipoprotein AI *Serum Increase* Higher in drinkers than in control subjects. *1864*

Apolipoprotein AII *Plasma Increase* Higher in drinkers (+45%) than in control subjects. *1864*

Aspartate Aminotransferase *Serum Increase* 60% of 5 cases showed mild elevation, with a mean = 16 X the normal upper limit. *1452* 73% of 182 male chronic alcoholics had raised activities. Highest values were found after 5-20 y of confirmed alcoholism. Patients with 20 y duration displayed a tendency to normalization of activities. *2196* In 66% of 13 patients hospitalized for this disorder. *0781*

Bilirubin *Serum Increase* 12% of 182 male chronic alcoholics had increased concentrations. Highest values were found after 5-20 y of confirmed alcoholism. *2196*

Cadmium *Serum Increase 0126*

Calcium *Serum Decrease* Hypocalcemia is common in alcoholic subjects. *1394*

Serum Increase Increased following alcoholic binge of several days duration. *1594*

Cholesterol, High Density Lipoprotein *Serum Increase* Higher in drinkers. *1864* Increased. *0131 1519 2556*

Chylomicrons *Serum Increase* Increased. *1380 1936 1948*

Copper *Serum Increase 0998*

Coproporphyrin *Urine Increase 0619 0151*

Cortisol *Plasma Increase* Increased following alcoholic binge of several days duration. *1594*

Creatine Kinase *Serum Increase* In 21 alcoholic patients, mean values were found to be elevated to 35.1 U/L (normal value = 7.0). *1803 0503*

Fat *Urine Increase* Significant lipuria occurred in a group of acutely intoxicated patients with neurological symptoms. *0289*

Fatty Acids, Free (FFA) *Serum Increase* Increased following alcoholic binge of several days duration. *1594* Rises only after the acute ingestion of large doses of alcohol. *0962*

Follicle Stimulating Hormone (FSH) *Serum Increase* 48 male chronic alcoholics classified in 2 groups according to the presence (22) or absence (26) of clinically evident sexual disorders. The level was significantly higher in the group with sexual disorders. *2169*

Gamma Glutamyl Transferase (GGT) *Serum Increase* In 5 cases of chronic alcoholism, range 27-850 U/L. The highest activities were seen in the patients with the most extensive hepatic damage. *1452* 69% of 182 male chronic alcoholics had increased GGT activities. Highest values were found in patients with 5-20 y of alcoholism. Patients with > 20 y duration had a tendency toward normalization of enzyme activity. *2196*

Glucose *Serum Decrease* Due to depletion of glycogen stores, and an inhibitory effect of alcohol on gluconeogenesis. *0962*

Glucose Tolerance *Serum Decrease* Decrease in glucose tolerance because of inability of tissues to utilize glucose. *0619*

Gonadotropin, Pituitary *Serum Increase* 48 male chronic alcoholics classified in 2 groups according to the presence (22) or absence (26) of clinically evident sexual disorders. The level was significantly higher in the group with sexual disorders. *2169*

Growth Hormone *Serum Increase* Increased following alcoholic binge of several days duration. *1594*

Haptoglobin *Serum Increase* Mean value = 99.85 mg/dL for the alcoholic group. Normal value was 71.66 mg/dL. *0523*

Hemoglobin A₁c *Blood Increase 2539*

Iron *Bone Marrow Increase* Iron overload shown by plasma cells containing iron in bone marrow may occur. *1594*

Lactate Dehydrogenase *Serum Increase* In 42% of 14 patients hospitalized for this disorder. *0781*

Lactic Acid *Blood Increase* Acidosis due to lactate and ketoacid accumulation following alcoholic binge of several days duration. *1594* Increased in serum lactate produced from pyruvate in the presence of the increased NADH/NAD ratio. *0962*

Lipids *Serum Increase* Rise after ingestion of moderate amounts of alcohol due to increased hepatic production and release of lipoproteins. *0962*

Luteinizing Hormone (LH) *Serum Increase* The basal level of LH was significantly elevated in alcoholics with and without clinically evident sexual disorders. *2169*

Magnesium *Serum Decrease 0619*

Myoglobin *Urine Increase* Sporadic; metabolic myoglobinuria. *2467*

Ornithine Carbamoyl Transferase (OCT) *Serum Increase* Liver cell damage. *2467*

Parathyroid Hormone *Serum Increase* Increased following alcoholic binge of several days duration. *1594*

pCO₂ *Blood Decrease* Plasma bicarbonate ranged from 2-10 mmol/L in acidosis following alcoholic binge. *1594*

pH *Blood Decrease* Severe metabolic acidosis with pH ranging between 6.96 - 7.28 occurred after alcoholic binge of several days duration. *1594*

Phosphate *Serum Decrease* Occurs in about 50% of hospitalized alcoholics. *1287* An association of hypophosphatemia with chronic alcoholism was found in 11 patients studied. The hypophosphatemia was associated with low levels of RBC ATP, abnormal erythrocyte filtration, and, in at least 1 patient, with hemolytic anemia. *2342*

Serum Increase Increased following alcoholic binge of several days duration. *1594*

Phospholipids, Total *Serum Increase* Fasting serum lipid values were have been analyzed in 85 male and 10 female alcoholics of various ages in connection with an acute drinking bout and compared to control subjects. The most prominent finding was an increase in the mean concentration of triglycerides and phospholipids, most marked in the younger age groups. The elevations were moderate and most alcoholics had the same serum total lipid values as the controls. *0261*

Platelet Count *Blood Decrease* Counts as low as 20,000/μL have been recorded. Recovery to a normal count occurs within 1 week of abstinence. *0962*

Potassium *Serum Decrease* In 26 patients in whom delirium tremens developed, a continuing decrease led to hypokalemia, (mean 2.9 mmol/L) when delirium tremens started. *2449*

Pseudocholinesterase *Serum Increase 0126 0619*

Testosterone *Plasma Decrease* After abstaining from alcohol and cigarettes for one week, the testosterone levels in 30 alcoholics allowed alcohol during the second week dropped rapidly and significantly, but did not correlate with amount of alcohol ingested. *1805*

Triglycerides *Serum Increase* 19 (26%) of these male patients had serum concentrations > 150 mg/dL. *1402* 38% of the patients had a type IV hyperlipoproteinemia with elevated serum triglycerides still after 17 days of abstinence. *2472* Rise after ingestion of moderate amounts of alcohol due to increased hepatic production and release of lipoproteins. *0962*

Uric Acid *Serum Increase* Increased lactic acid concentration inhibits uric acid excretion in the distal renal tubule. Usually decreases to normal within 1 week after abstinence. *0962 1283*

Zinc *Serum Decrease* Elevated in alcoholics with normal or fatty liver and low in those with alcoholic hepatitis or cirrhosis. *0998* Statistically significant *2188 0126*

Serum Increase Elevated in alcoholics with normal or fatty liver and low in those with alcoholic hepatitis or cirrhosis. *0998*

304.90 Drug Dependence (Opium and Derivatives)

Alanine Aminotransferase *Serum Increase* This and other liver function tests are increased in 75% of patients. *2468*

Amylase *Serum Increase* Large doses of morphine or codeine will provoke a sharp rise. *2104* Increased levels were found in 19% of 91 addicts admitted after overdose. The rise was due to elevated salivary-type isoenzyme. *0178*

Aspartate Aminotransferase *Serum Increase* This and other liver function tests are usually increased in 75% of patients. *2468*

Cephalin Flocculation *Serum Increase* Cephalin flocculation or thymol turbidity tests are increased in 75% of patients. *2468*

Cholesterol *Serum Decrease* Significantly decreased in heroin addiction. *1053*

Creatine Kinase *Serum Increase* Following intravenous adulterated heroin associated with myopathy and myoglobinuria. *0619* Concentrations up to 14,000 U/L were recorded in heroin addicts. *1929*

Cyclic Adenosine Monophosphate *Plasma Decrease* Significantly decreased in heroin addiction. *1053*

Eosinophils *Blood Increase* Eosinophilia occurs in 25% of drug addicts. *2468*

Hepatitis B Surface Antigen *Serum Increase* Found in 10% of drug patients. *2468*

Lactate Dehydrogenase *Serum Increase* Markedly elevated in 4 heroin addicts after admission. Acute skeletal muscle necrosis in all 4 cases, and acute renal failure in 2 of the 4 occurred as a result of intravenous use of heroin-adulterant mixtures. *1929*

Lymphocytes *Blood Increase* Persistent absolute and relative lymphocytosis occurs with often bizarre and atypical cells that may resemble Downey cells. *2468*

Myoglobin *Serum Increase* Serum concentrations as high as 0.310 g/L were found in heroin addicts. *1929*

Urine Increase Acute myoglobinuria up to 3.25 g/L in heroin addicts. *1929*

Oxygen Saturation *Blood Decrease* Overdose. *0995*

pO₂ *Blood Decrease* Overdose. *0995*

Thymol Turbidity *Serum Increase* Thymol turbidity and cephalin flocculation are commonly increased in 75% of patients. *2468*

Thyroxine (T₄) *Serum Increase* Significantly raised in heroin addiction. *1053*

VDRL *Serum Positive* Incidence of false positive reactions is 20% in narcotic addicts. *1108*

306.10 Hyperventilation Syndrome

Calcium *Serum Decrease* Respiratory alkalosis reduces ionized Ca concentration. *2103 0995*

pCO₂ *Blood Decrease* Characteristically, the pCO₂ is reduced to 20-30 mm Hg. *0433* Respiratory alkalosis. *2103*

pH *Blood Increase* The arterial pH is raised to 7.5-7.65. *0433* Respiratory alkalosis. *2103*

Phosphate *Serum Decrease* Often decreased during prolonged hyperventilation. *0433* Respiratory alkalosis. *2103*

308.00 Stress

17-Hydroxycorticosteroids *Urine Increase* *2467*

17-Ketogenic Steroids *Urine Increase* *2467*

17-Ketosteroids *Urine Increase* *0503*

Albumin *Serum Decrease* *2467*

Aldosterone *Plasma Increase* Emotional crises or extreme anxiety elicit increased secretion in normal subjects. *2104*

Alpha₁-Globulin *Serum Increase* *2467*

Alpha₂-Globulin *Serum Increase* *2467*

Antidiuretic Hormone *Urine Increase* 50% increase with mental stress. *2092*

Catecholamines *Plasma Increase* Normal metabolic response. *2315*

Urine Increase With physical or emotional stress. *2092*

Cholesterol *Serum Increase* With mental stress. *2092* Concentrations rise during heavy stress periods. *2113*

Cholesterol, High Density Lipoprotein *Serum Normal* No change in pilot flying high performance aircraft. *0430*

Cholesterol, Very Low Density Lipoprotein *Serum Increase* Moderate increase secondary to increased secretion and decreased catabolism. *0062*

Corticotropin *Plasma Increase* Excess secretion. *2113*

Cortisol *Plasma Increase* Marked; in response to emotional stress. *2092*

Eosinophils *Blood Decrease* A drop in eosinophils with increased corticoid and epinephrine production are manifestations of stress. *2113*

Epinephrine *Plasma Increase* A drop in eosinophils with increased corticoid and epinephrine production are manifestations of stress. *2113*

Urine Increase With physical or emotional stress. *2092* Urinary excretion of epinephrine and its metabolites are rough indicators of degree of stress. *2113*

Factor VIII *Plasma Increase* Postoperative stress. *0544*

Fat *Serum Increase* A rise in blood fats is characteristic. *2113*

Fatty Acids, Free (FFA) *Serum Increase* Normal response. *2315* Fear, anxiety, or hostility elicit marked increases. *2104*

Glucocorticoids *Plasma Increase* A drop in eosinophils with increased corticoid and epinephrine production are manifestations of stress. *2113*

Glucose *Serum Increase* Decreased tolerance, with excessive peak and decreased formation of glycogen with low fasting levels and subsequent hypoglycemia. Caused by increased adrenalin as in stress and pheochromocytoma (normal return to fasting level). *2467* Normal response. *2315*

Glucose Tolerance *Serum Decrease* Decreased tolerance, excessive peak and decreased formation of glycogen with low fasting levels and subsequent hypoglycemia. Caused by increased epirephrine (normal returns to fasting level). *2467*

Growth Hormone *Serum Increase* Normal response. *0217*

Metanephrines, Total *Urine Increase* *0503*

Myoglobin *Serum Decrease* As much as 50% decrease in pilots flying high performance aircraft. *0430*

Norepinephrine *Urine Increase* With physical or emotional stress. *2092*

Prolactin *Serum Increase* *2113*

Protein *Serum Increase* Marked; with psychological stress. *2092*

Thyroxine Binding Globulin *Serum Decrease* *0062*

Triglycerides *Serum Increase* Stressful situations evoke catecholamine excretion, producing an increased circulating concentration with surprising speed. *2104*

Urea Nitrogen *Serum Increase* Increased protein catabolism (serum creatinine remains normal). *2467*

Zinc *Serum Decrease* *1443*

319.00 Mental Retardation

Cholesterol *Serum Decrease* Serum values from over 1,400 patients were significantly lower than corresponding results from normal subjects. Male patients had significantly lower results than the female patients. There appeared to be no significant correlation between serum cholesterol values and IQ, systolic or diastolic blood pressures, drugs used in treatment, presence or absence of epilepsy. *0617*

Glutamic Acid *Serum Increase* Increased glutamic acid with associated decrease in glutamine may occur in De Lange Syndrome and other mental retardation syndromes. *0493*

Glutamine *Serum Decrease* Increased glutamic acid with associated decrease in glutamine may occur in De Lange Syndrome and other mental retardation syndromes. *0493*

DISEASES OF THE NERVOUS SYSTEM

320.90 Meningitis (Bacterial)

Albumin *CSF Increase* CSF IgG and albumin are increased due to defect in the blood-CSF barrier. *0809* Often 100-200 mg/dL. *0433*

Alpha₁-Antichymotrypsin *CSF Increase* Increased in patients with meningitis or mild hemorrhage, but equal to normal in patients with encephalitis, epilepsy, degenerative disorders or diseases of the CNS. *0079*

Alpha₂-Globulin *Serum Increase* *2467*

Alpha₂-Macroglobulin *CSF Increase* *2069*

Antidiuretic Hormone *Serum Increase* Associated with excessive ADH production resulting in sodium loss. *2104*

Aspartate Aminotransferase *Serum Increase* In 70% of 14 patients hospitalized for this disorder. *0781*

Cells *CSF Increase* Increased polymorphonuclear cells are found in CSF. Mononuclear cells appear later in the disease. *0999* CSF cells are always elevated, ranging from 100-100,000/μL initially polymorphonuclear leukocytes predominate; these are replaced by lymphocytes as the inflammatory process progresses. *0151*

Chloride *Serum Decrease* The chloride content is reduced but not as dramatically as in tubercular meningitis. *0433* Slight decrease. *0503* In 33% of 18 patients hospitalized for this disorder. *0781*

CSF Decrease Characteristically reduced. *2368*

C-Reactive Protein *Serum Increase* Markedly elevated. *1337*

Creatine Kinase *Serum Increase* *0962*

Creatinine *Serum Increase* Dehydration. *0995*

320.90 Meningitis (Bacterial) (continued)

Cryofibrinogen *Serum Increase* 2035 1138

Erythrocyte Sedimentation Rate *Blood Increase* 0433

Globulin *CSF Increase* Elevated in all forms of meningeal inflammation. 2368

Glomerular Filtration Rate (GFR) *Urine Increase* Associated excess ADH may tend to accelerate GFR. 2104

Glucose *Serum Increase* In 32% of 18 patients hospitalized for this disorder. 0781

CSF Decrease CSF glucose is < 50% blood sugar. 0999 Decreased in children with transverse myelitis and mycoplasma pneumoniae meningoencephalitis. 1281 CSF/blood sugar ratios were of diagnostic and prognostic value, especially in suboptimally treated cases. 1894 Usual values < 40 mg/dL, and may be close to 0. Low CSF sugar distinguishes bacterial from viral meningitides. 0151 Usually well below 50% the blood sugar and may be entirely absent. 0962

Hematocrit *Blood Decrease* In 54% of 18 patients hospitalized for this disorder. 0781

Hemoglobin *Blood Decrease* In 66% of 18 patients hospitalized for this disorder. 0781

Immunoglobulin IgG *CSF Increase* Characteristic of brucella meningitis. Increased in acute meningitis due to impairment of blood:CSF barrier. Increases in absolute not relative amount of individual proteins are found in CSF. Little or no IgG was found to be synthesized intrathecally. A high correlation (R = 0.95) was found between plasma and CSF IgG and albumin concentrations. 0809 Increased with obstruction of the spinal canal, especially in neurosyphilis and tuberculous meningitis. 2321 0555

Immunoglobulins *CSF Increase* Early rise in CSF. 0619

Isocitrate Dehydrogenase *CSF Increase* 0619

Lactate Dehydrogenase *Serum Increase* LD and its isoenzymes are elevated, mostly due to a rise in the leukocyte fraction. Patients with increased brain LD isoenzyme usually develop neurologic sequelae or die. 0151 In 64% of 12 patients hospitalized for this disorder. 0781

CSF Increase Elevations varied from 2-100 X the normal values in 23 cases. Significantly lower levels were found in patients with viral meningitis and in CNS infection. 0720 234 specimens from 183 different children were analyzed. Activity was elevated in patients with meningitis, especially bacterial infections, and CNS leukemia. The isoenzyme pattern generally reflected the number and distribution of lymphocytes and granulocytes in the CSF. 1684

Lactate Dehydrogenase Isoenzyme 5 (LD5) *CSF Increase* LD activity varies widely from 2-100 X the normal CSF concentration. Invariably the most prominent isoenzyme. 1684

Lactate Dehydrogenase Isoenzymes *Serum Increase* LD isoenzymes are elevated, mostly due to a rise in the leukocyte fraction. Patients with increased brain isoenzyme usually develop neurologic sequelae or die. 0151

CSF Increase Slightly elevated but rise sharply in patients who die or develop neurologic sequelae. 0995

Lactic Acid *CSF Increase* CSF specimens from 60 of 62 patients with bacterial or mycoplasma etiology showed levels > 20 mg/dL. 0436

Leukocytes *Blood Increase* Generally elevated with a shift to the left. 0995 In 72% of 19 patients hospitalized for this disorder. 0781

CSF Increase Several hundred to 60,000/µL with predominantly polymorphonuclear cells present. 0151 Ranges between 500-20,000/µL, with about 90% polymorphonuclears. Counts > 25,000 suggest a ruptured brain abscess. 0962 0999 2400

Lymphocytes *CSF Increase* Lymphocytes will be more prevalent in the CSF if the disease moves into the subacute or chronic stage. Polymorphonuclear neutrophils may predominate in the early phase of an aseptic or viral meningitis. 0433

Lysozyme *CSF Increase* May be increased but clinical significance is unknown. 0995

NBT Test *Blood Positive* Mean percentage of positive neutrophils was 21.5% in 30 patients. Useful in differential diagnosis of bacterial and tubercular meningitis (all tubercular meningitis NBT scores were normal). 0391

Neutrophils *Blood Increase* In 55% of 20 patients hospitalized for this disorder. 0781 0433

CSF Increase Several hundred to 60,000/µL with predominantly polymorphonuclear cells present. 0151 Ranges between 500-20,000/µL, with about 90% polymorphonuclears. Counts > 25,000 suggest a ruptured brain abscess. 0962 0999 2400

Protein *CSF Increase* Nearly always elevated above 50 mg/dL. 2400 Ranges between 50-500 mg/dL, with an average of 200-300. 0962 Increased with obstruction of the spinal canal, especially in neurosyphilis and tuberculous meningitis. 2321 0999 0151

Rheumatoid Factor *CSF Increase* In 18 samples of CSF from patients with pneumococcal meningitis, 11 were found to be positive by the latex fixation test. 0448

Sodium *Serum Decrease* Serum concentrations below 135 mmol/L were noted on admission in 72 of 124 (58.1%) of patients. Low initial concentration and prolonged depression despite fluid restriction correlated significantly with the presence of neurologic sequelae of the disease. 0712 Associated with excessive ADH production. 2104 0062

Urine Increase Urine is almost always hypertonic to plasma 0062

Thromboplastin Generation *CSF Increase* Increased thromboplastic activity is about 145 fold more common in bacterial meningitis than in viral meningitis. 2392

Urea Nitrogen *Serum Increase* Dehydration. 0995

Uric Acid *Serum Increase* Increased in both blood and CSF with a lowered blood:CSF ratio, possibly due to cellular breakdown and nucleoprotein catabolism. 2301 In 36% of 11 patients hospitalized for this disorder. 0781

Serum Normal High CSF levels of 0.9-1.3 mg/dL, with normal serum levels. 1338

Urine Increase Increased excretion in neurological and psychiatric disorders; progressive rise in urinary level following slight rise in blood, due to disturbed purine metabolism. 2301

CSF Increase High CSF levels of 0.9-1.3 mg/dL, with normal serum levels. 1338 Markedly increased with decreased blood:CSF ratio, possibly due to cellular breakdown and nucleoprotein catabolism. 2301

323.91 Myelitis

Cells *CSF Increase* Spinal fluid may be normal or may show increased protein and cells (20-1,000/µL - lymphocytes and mononuclear cells). 2467 Increased WBCs, mononuclear, and polymorphonuclear cells are found. 0999

Glucose *CSF Decrease* Decreased in children with transverse myelitis and mycoplasma pneumoniae meningoencephalitis. 1281

Leukocytes *CSF Increase* Spinal fluid may be normal or may show increased protein and cells (20-1,000/µL--lymphocytes and mononuclear cells). 2467 Increased WBCs, mononuclear, and polymorphonuclear cells are found. 0999

Lymphocytes *CSF Increase* Spinal fluid may be normal or may show increased protein and cells (20-1,000/µL -- lymphocytes and mononuclear cells). 2467 0999

Monocytes *CSF Increase* Spinal fluid may be normal or may show increased protein and cells (20-1,000/µL - lymphocytes and mononuclear cells). 2467

Protein *CSF Increase* Increased to 45-200 mg/dL in encephalitis and myelitis. 0999

323.92 Encephalomyelitis

Alpha1-Antichymotrypsin *CSF Normal* Increased in patients with meningitis or mild hemorrhage, but equal to normal in patients with encephalitis, epilepsy, degenerative disorders or diseases of the CNS. 0079

Amylase *Serum Increase* If amylase levels are elevated, mumps or Coxsackie virus may be indicated. 0433

Antidiuretic Hormone *Serum Increase* Associated with excessive ADH production resulting in sodium loss. 2104

Cells *CSF Increase* Usually increased (< 100/µL), mostly polymorphonuclear leukocytes. After the third day cell count is > 90% lymphocytes. 2468

Chloride *CSF Increase* Usually normal or increased. 0433

Creatine Kinase *Serum Increase* Enzyme studies may help suggest certain causes, (e.g., CK is elevated with myopathy, particularly in Coxsackie A infections and leptospirosis). 0433 0962

Erythrocytes *Urine Increase* Hematuria may occur with viremia but is transient. 0433

Glomerular Filtration Rate (GFR) *Urine Increase* Associated excess ADH may tend to accelerate GFR. 2104

Immunoglobulin IgG *CSF Increase* Total protein and IgG concentration were increased. 2321

Leukocytes *Blood Decrease* The peripheral WBC reveals leukopenia at the onset of most viral infections. *0433*

CSF Increase Pleocytosis ranges from 10-500/μL. In most infections, and these are predominantly lymphocytes; however, granulocytes may prevail for 1-2 days after onset. Counts may exceed 100/μL especially in lymphocytic choriomeningitis and eastern equine encephalomyelitis. *0433*

Lymphocytes *CSF Increase* Approximately 66% of the patients show a lymphocytic pleocytosis in the spinal fluid, but in the remaining 33%, the CSF is normal. *0433*

Neutrophils *CSF Increase* Pleocytosis ranges from 10-500/μL. Granulocytes may prevail for 1-2 days after onset. Counts may exceed 100/μL especially in lymphocytic choriomeningitis and eastern equine encephalomyelitis. *0433*

Protein *CSF Increase* The protein concentration is elevated but rarely exceeds 150 mg/dL. A slight elevation is common. *0433* Total protein and IgG concentration were increased. *2321 2612*

Sodium *Serum Decrease* Associated with excessive ADH production. *2104* Serum sodium is usually less than 130 mEq/L *0062*

Urine Increase Urine is almost always hypertonic to plasma *0062*

Uric Acid *Serum Increase* Increased in both blood and CSF with a lowered blood:CSF ratio, possibly due to cellular breakdown and nucleoprotein catabolism. *2301*

Serum Normal High CSF levels of 0.9-1.3 mg/dL, with normal serum levels are seen in acute encephalitis. *1338*

Urine Increase Increased excretion in neurological and psychiatric disorders; progressive rise in urinary level following slight rise in blood, due to disturbed purine metabolism. *2301*

CSF Increase High CSF levels of 0.9-1.3 mg/dL, with normal serum levels are seen in acute encephalitis. *1338* Markedly increased with decreased blood:CSF ratio, possibly due to cellular breakdown and nucleoprotein catabolism. *2301*

324.00   Intracranial Abscess

Cells *CSF Increase* Usually < 500/μL with polymorphonuclears predominating in chronic encapsulating infections. *0999* May vary from 0 to many thousands, depending on the degree of meningitic involvement, and may be particularly high if the abscess has ruptured into the ventricles. In most chronic abscesses, the cell count is usually > 100, and the cells are usually mononuclear in the type. *0433*

Chloride *CSF Decrease* 600-750 mg/dL. *0962*

Erythrocytes *CSF Increase* *2467*

Erythrocyte Sedimentation Rate *Blood Increase* Usually elevated, as in other chronic infections, and when present with symptoms and signs of an intracranial mass lesion one should consider the possibility of brain abscess. *0433*

Glucose *CSF Increase* Elevated in lumbar CSF in all patients with subdural empyema. Moderate-marked elevation in lumbar CSF in 14 of 17 patients. *1238*

CSF Normal Usually normal; however, in the meningitic phase it may be low. *0433* Usually normal until the process extends to actively involve the meninges. *0962 0995*

Leukocytes *Blood Increase* May be normal or slightly elevated in the range of 12,000-15,000/μL. In the acute phase it may be markedly elevated with an increase in the polymorphonuclears. *0433*

Blood Normal May be normal or slightly elevated in the range of 12,000-15,000/μL. In the acute phase it may be markedly elevated with an increase in the polymorphonuclears. *0433*

CSF Increase Counts may be < 100 to several thousand in subdural empyema. *0151* Usually ranges from 50-300/μL and consists predominantly of lymphocytes. With intraventricular rupture, counts may exceed 50,000. *0962* In the range of 50-1,000/μL. *0995*

Lymphocytes *CSF Increase* Count usually ranges from 50-300/μL and consists predominantly of lymphocytes. *0962* In the range of 50-1,000/μL. *0995*

Neutrophils *Blood Increase* In the acute phase WBC may be markedly elevated with an increase in the polymorphonuclear leukocytes. *0433* Slight increase in neutrophils and lymphocytes (20-100/μL). *2467*

Protein *CSF Increase* Usually elevated, varying between 60-200 mg/dL. *0433* Raised, particularly if the abscess is near to the surface. 75-300 mg/dL. *0995 0962 2368*

CSF Normal Normal or increased. *0995*

324.10   Intraspinal Abscess

Leukocytes *CSF Increase* Usually 10-100 WBC/μL with predominantly lymphocytes present in spinal epidural abscess. *0151*

Lymphocytes *CSF Increase* Usually 1-100 WBC/μL with predominantly lymphocytes present in spinal epidural abscess. *0151*

Protein *CSF Increase* Increased (usually 100-400 mg/dL), and WBCs (lymphocytes and neutrophils) are relatively few in number. *2467*

330.00   Metachromatic Leukodystrophy

Aldolase *CSF Increase* Increased initially, then diminishes. *0078*

Arylsulfatase *Serum Decrease* Most types of leukodystrophy are associated with a basic deficiency in arylsulfatase A. *2246* Heterozygote carriers for metachromatic leukodystrophy have leukocyte arylsulfatase A concentrations of 40-60% of normal range. Patients with disease showed levels only 20% of normal value. *1190*

Liver Decrease Just at the limit of detection in 8 patients with metachromatic leukodystrophy. *2246*

Aspartate Aminotransferase *Serum Increase* Invariable in initial phases of disease. Diminishes to normal range by 4th year. *0077*

CSF Increase Increased initially, then diminishes. *0078*

Lactate Dehydrogenase *CSF Increase* Increases initially, then diminishes. *0078*

Lactic Acid *Blood Increase* Invariable in initial phases of disease. Diminishes to normal range by 4th year. *0077*

Protein *CSF Increase* Common. *0433*

330.11   Tay-Sach's Disease

Hexosaminidase *Serum Decrease* Hexosaminidase A (possessing both acetylglucosaminidase and acetylgalactosaminidase activities) is nearly absent in fetal Tay-Sach's serum. Heterozygotes have intermediate reductions in serum, leukocytes, and cultured fibroblasts. *2246 1716*

331.00   Alzheimer's Disease

5-Hydroxyindoleacetic Acid (5-HIAA) *CSF Decrease* Lower than in an aged matched control group. *1765*

Albumin *CSF Normal* No significant difference in levels compared with controls. *0372*

Ammonia *Blood Increase* Post prandial blood ammonia levels were significantly higher in 22 patients with Alzheimer's than in 37 control subjects. *0742*

Angiotensin-Converting Enzyme (ACE) *CSF Decrease* Decreased 41% of cases compared to age and sex matched controls. *2620*

Endorphin, Beta *CSF Normal* No difference from controls. *1881*

Homovanillic Acid *CSF Decrease* Lower than in an aged matched control group. *1765*

CSF Normal Level was unchanged from normal controls. *2615*

Immunoglobulin IgG *CSF Normal* No significant difference in levels compared with controls. *0372*

Oxytocin *CSF Normal* No difference from controls. *1881*

Somatostatin *CSF Decrease* Significantly lower mean CSF levels than other neurological patients. All 11 patients with Alzheimer's Disease or Parkinsons Disease dementia had levels well below 21.8 ng/ml. *2119* Significant difference from elderly normal subjects but did not differ from normal younger subjects *1881* Significantly decreased compared to other neurological patients (14.6 pg/mL versus 26.7 pg/mL) *2119*

Vasopressin *CSF Decrease* Significant decrease in arginine vasopressin compared to elderly and younger normal control subjects. *1881*

331.40   Acquired Hydrocephalus

Lactate Dehydrogenase *CSF Increase* Range of LD activity in 9 patients with hydrocephalus for shunt insertion or revision was 17-53 U/L, with normal CSF values from 3-17 U/L. *1684*

Leukocytes *CSF Normal* *1684*

331.81 Reye's Syndrome

Alanine Aminotransferase *Serum Increase* Reflects hepatic damage. *0151* High serum transaminases. *0962*

Amino Acids *Plasma Increase* Markedly elevated reflecting hepatic injury. *0435*

Ammonia *Blood Increase* Elevated in most patients. *1473* Reflects hepatic damage. *0151* Hyperammonemia results from excess waste nitrogen that overwhelms the ability of reduced ornithine transcarbamylase to detoxify the ammonia load. *2222* Increased ammonia may reflect accumulation of octopamine. *0339 0962*

Aspartate Aminotransferase *Serum Increase* 2-300 times normal values. *0416* Reflects hepatic damage *0151* High serum transaminases *0962*

Bicarbonate *Serum Decrease* Due to impaired oxidative metabolism. *0435*

Bilirubin *Serum Increase* Usually remains below 3 mg/dL. *0416* Normal or mildly elevated *0962*

Creatine Kinase *Serum Increase* Especially muscle (CPK-MM) fraction. In severely affected children. *0435* Markedly abnormal *1887*

Creatinine *Serum Increase* Markedly elevated reflecting renal injury. *0435*

Fatty Acids, Free (FFA) *Serum Increase* Commonly elevated. *0151*

Glucose *Serum Decrease* Hypoglycemia with decreased CSF glucose is common in patients < 5 years of age, but is rare in older children. *0151* Occasionally hypoglycemia. *0962* Replacement or destruction of functioning hepatic tissue may evoke hypoglycemia. *2104*

CSF Decrease Hypoglycemia with decreased CSF glucose is common in patients < 5 years of age, but is rare in older children. *0151* Low levels of glucose and protein found in the CSF *0416*

Lactate Dehydrogenase *Serum Increase* Markedly elevated reflecting hepatic injury. *0435*

Lactic Acid *Blood Increase* Due to impaired oxidative metabolism. *0435*

pCO$_2$ *Blood Decrease* Hypocapnia is common in children with this syndrome. *0151*

pH *Blood Decrease* Due to impaired oxidative metabolism. *0435* Later in disease along with decreased pCO$_2$ reflecting respiratory acidosis. *0435*

Phosphate *Serum Increase* Indicates muscle involvement. *1887*

Potassium *Serum Decrease* Hypokalemia and hyponatremia are common. *0151*

Protein *CSF Decrease* *0416* Low levels of glucose and protein found in the CSF

Prothrombin Time *Plasma Increase* May be prolonged. *0416* Reflects Hepatic damage *0151*

Sodium *Serum Decrease* Hyponatremia is common in children. *0151*

Urea Nitrogen *Serum Increase* Markedly elevated reflecting renal injury. *0435*

331.90 Cerebral and Cortical Atrophy

Acid Phosphatase *CSF Increase* Increased in lumbar CSF in relation to the degree of cerebral atrophy and duration of dementia. *2592*

Beta-Galactosidase *Serum Decrease* In cerebral atrophy due to presenile dementia and/or cerebrovascular disease. *2592*

Cholesterol *CSF Decrease* Significantly low CSF values for cholesterol and total lipids were found in a group of patients with brain atrophy in comparison with a control group. It is possible that these changes are a function of reduced brain mass or of defect in brain lipid metabolism in brain atrophy patients. *1035*

Immunoglobulin IgG *CSF Normal* Within the normal range. *2321*

Lipids *CSF Decrease* Significantly low CSF values for cholesterol and total lipids were found in a group of patients with brain atrophy in comparison with a control group. It is possible that these changes are a function of reduced brain mass or of defect in brain lipid metabolism. *1035*

Uric Acid *Serum Normal* In the chronic stage. *1338*

CSF Decrease Very low CSF levels of 0.02-0.04 mg/dL, with normal serum levels found in the chronic stage of disease. *1338*

332.00 Parkinsons's Disease

Angiotensin-Converting Enzyme (ACE) *CSF Decrease* Decreased in 27% of cases compared to matched control group. *2620* Level decrease 27% compared with an age and sex matched control group *2620*

Cholecystokinin (CCK) *CSF Decrease* Significant decreased cholecystokinin (1.9 pmol/L) versus control (4.0). *1440*

Copper *CSF Increase* Although there was considerable overlap between the 24 Parkinsonian and 34 control subjects, the former had significantly higher levels (P < 0.001). *1763*

Iron *CSF Normal* *1763*

Manganese *CSF Normal* *1763*

Somatostatin *CSF Decrease* Significantly lower mean CSF levels than other neurological patients. All 11 patients with Alzheimer's Disease or Parkinsons Disease dementia had levels well below 21.8 ng/ml. *2119* Significantly decreased in demented Parkinsonian patient *2119*

333.40 Huntington's Chorea

Alanine *Serum Decrease* 19 patients showed a significantly lower concentration of proline, alanine, valine, leucine, isoleucine, and tyrosine compared to 38 normal controls. *0534*

Alanine Aminotransferase *Serum Normal* No abnormalities in 8 patients. *0534*

Amino Acids *Plasma Decrease* 19 patients showed a significantly lower concentration of proline, alanine, valine, leucine, isoleucine, and tyrosine compared to 38 normal controls. *0534*

Aspartate Aminotransferase *Serum Normal* No abnormalities in 8 patients. *0534*

Calcium *Serum Normal* *1252*

Copper *Serum Increase* Some studies show elevated levels while others did not. *0878*

Serum Normal Some studies show elevated levels while others did not. *0878*

Creatine Kinase *Serum Normal* No abnormalities in 8 patients. *0534*

Dopamine Hydroxylase *Serum Increase* *1395*

Fatty Acids, Free (FFA) *Serum Increase* High fasting concentrations. The elevation was maintained under hypoglycemic conditions, but not in hyperglycemic states. *1816*

Globulin *Serum Increase* In 23 of 27 patients. *0303*

Homovanillic Acid *CSF Decrease* *0878*

Isocitrate Dehydrogenase *Serum Normal* No abnormalities in 8 patients. *0534*

Isoleucine *Serum Decrease* Reduced fasting plasma concentrations of leucine, isoleucine and valine. *1816* 19 patients showed a significantly lower concentration of proline, aminolevulinic acid, valine, leucine, isoleucine, and tyrosine compared to 38 normal controls. *0534*

Lactate Dehydrogenase *Serum Normal* No abnormalities in 8 patients. *0534*

Leucine *Serum Decrease* Reduced fasting plasma concentrations of leucine, isoleucine and valine. *1816* 19 patients showed a significantly lower concentration of proline, aminolevulinic acid, valine, leucine, isoleucine, and tyrosine compared to 38 normal controls. *0534*

Magnesium *Serum Normal* *1252*

Red Blood Cells Normal *0745*

Malate Dehydrogenase *Serum Normal* No abnormalities in 8 patients. *0534*

Norepinephrine *Urine Increase* *0878*

Urine Normal *1662*

Proline *Serum Decrease* 19 patients showed a significantly lower concentration of proline, alanine, valine, leucine, isoleucine, and tyrosine compared to 38 normal controls. *0534*

Protein *Serum Increase* In 23 of 27 patients. *0303*

Tryptophan *CSF Normal* In 7 patients. *2591*

Tryptophan, Free *Serum Decrease* Markedly reduced as a result of the increased concentrations of nonesterified fatty acids. In induced hypoglycemia, the difference in free tryptophan between control and diseased groups was much less severe. *1816*

Tyrosine *Serum Decrease* 19 patients showed a significantly lower concentration of proline, alanine, valine, leucine, isoleucine, and tyrosine compared to 38 normal controls. *0534*

CSF Normal In 7 patients. *2591*

Valine *Serum Decrease* Reduced fasting plasma concentrations of leucine, isoleucine and valine. *1816* 19 patients showed a significantly lower concentration of proline, aminolevulinic acid, valine, leucine, isoleucine, and tyrosine compared to 38 normal controls. *0534*

334.00 Friedreich's Ataxia

Acid Phosphatase *Serum Increase* One pair of siblings displayed a slight elevation. *1956*

Aldolase *Serum Increase* Elevated in 11 cases but markedly so in only 5 of 23 cases. *1956*

Alkaline Phosphatase *Serum Increase* One pair of siblings displayed a slight elevation. *1956*

Cholesterol *Serum Increase* In Friedreich's patients, the relative proportion of cholesterol and triglycerides was increased while the relative protein content was greatly reduced. *1091*

Lipoproteins *Serum Decrease* Their total amount of high density lipoprotein was reduced and the composition was abnormal in both Friedreich's and familial spastic ataxia. *1091*

Lipoproteins, Beta *Serum Decrease* Total amount of high density lipoprotein reduced in Friedreich's and familial spastic ataxia. *1091*

Protein *Serum Decrease* In Friedreich's patients, the relative proportion of cholesterol and triglycerides was increased while the relative protein content was greatly reduced. *1091*

Pseudocholinesterase *Serum Increase* Altered or increased in 7 of 23 patients. However, the elevation was considered to be significant in only 3. *1956*

Triglycerides *Serum Normal* Significantly higher in Friedreich's ataxia, but remained within the normal limit. *1091*

334.80 Ataxia-Telangiectasia

Alpha-Fetoprotein *Serum Increase* Present in inordinately high concentration in a majority of patients. *0151* Has been reported. *2459*

Globulin *Serum Decrease* May be decreased, resulting in increased susceptibility to infection. *0999*

Immunoglobulin IgA *Serum Decrease* About 80% of patients lack both serum and secretory IgA. *2035* Deficient in 66% of patients. *1836 2538*

Immunoglobulin IgE *Serum Decrease* Decreased or absent serum IgA and IgE causing recurrent pulmonary infections. *2467* Deficient in 80% of patients. *1836 0151*

Immunoglobulin IgG *Serum Decrease* *0999*

Serum Normal 2467

Immunoglobulin IgM *Serum Decrease* Low levels have been reported. *0151*

Serum Normal 2467

Immunoglobulins *Serum Decrease* Deficiency appears to contribute to the frequent severe infections associated with the syndrome. *2104*

Lymphocytes *Blood Decrease* T-lymphocytes and T-cell functions are regularly grossly deficient. *0151* Variable; below 1,000/μL in 33% of patients. *2552*

335.11 Familial Progressive Spinal Muscular Atrophy

Alanine Aminotransferase *Serum Increase* Elevations of serum enzymes are frequently encountered but never reach the magnitude seen in Duchenne muscular dystrophy. *0433*

Aldolase *Serum Increase* Elevations of serum enzymes are frequently encountered but never reach the magnitude seen in Duchenne muscular dystrophy. *0433*

Aspartate Aminotransferase *Serum Increase* Elevations of serum enzymes are frequently encountered but never reach the magnitude seen in Duchenne muscular dystrophy. *0433*

Creatine Kinase *Serum Increase* Elevations of CK and other serum enzymes are frequently encountered but never reach the magnitude seen in Duchenne muscular dystrophy. *0433*

Lactate Dehydrogenase *Serum Increase* Elevations of serum enzymes are frequently encountered but never reach the magnitude seen in Duchenne muscular dystrophy. *0433*

Lactate Dehydrogenase Isoenzyme 5 (LD$_5$) *Serum Increase* In rapidly destructive neurogenic atrophies such as Werdnig-Hoffmann disease a rise was noted, reflecting a temporary leakage of cytoplasmic LD$_5$ from muscle to peripheral blood. *1070*

335.20 Amyotrophic Lateral Sclerosis

5-Hydroxyindoleacetic Acid (5-HIAA) *CSF Normal 1495*

Albumin *Serum Normal 0665*

Aldolase *Serum Increase* Rises in the early stages, falling to normal later. This pattern occurs in any primary neurogenic muscular dystrophy. *0619* Normal or slightly increased. *0962*

Amino Acids *Urine Normal 0665*

Antibody Titer *Serum Increase* IgA and IgM antibodies to myelin of rabbit spinal cord. Found in 70% of patients. When IgG antimyelin antibody is present in titers greater than 1:8 it is suggestive, but not diagnostic. *1670*

Calcium *Urine Increase* Disuse atrophy with a major portion of the body immobilized. *0503*

Ceruloplasmin *Serum Normal 0665*

Creatine Kinase *Serum Normal 0962*

Creatinine *Serum Increase* Severe muscle disease. *0503*

Urine Decrease Roughly in proportion to loss of muscle mass. *0665*

Fibrinogen *Plasma Normal 0665*

Glucose Tolerance *Serum Decrease* In 30% of patients with the disease and is related to decreased muscle mass. *0665*

Homovanillic Acid *CSF Decrease 1495*

Immunoglobulin IgA *Serum Normal 0665*

Immunoglobulin IgG *Serum Normal 0665*

Immunoglobulin IgM *Serum Normal 0665*

Immunoglobulins *Serum Normal 0665*

Lactate Dehydrogenase *Serum Increase* Especially in the early stages. *0619* Slight elevations of LD are common in adults, but it is unclear whether muscular atrophy or hepatic disease is the cause. *2418*

Lactate Dehydrogenase Isoenzyme 5 (LD$_5$) *Serum Increase* In rapidly destructive progressive muscular atrophies, such as amyotrophic lateral sclerosis and Werdnig-Hoffmann disease, a rise was noted reflecting leakage of cytoplasmic LD$_5$ from muscle to peripheral blood. *1070*

Lipids *Serum Normal 0665*

Lipoproteins *Serum Normal 0665*

Phytanic Acid *Plasma Normal 0665*

Vanillylamine *Urine Normal 0665*

336.00 Syringomyelia and Syringobulbia

Protein *CSF Increase* In a minority of cases the lumbar CSF protein content is elevated in the range of 40-100 mg/dL. *0433*

CSF Normal In a minority of cases the lumbar CSF protein content is elevated in the range of 40-100 mg/dL. *0433*

340.00 Multiple Sclerosis

Albumin *Serum Decrease* 12.5% of 64 patients had concentrations < 45% of total protein. 10.9% had concentrations > 65% of total proteins. *1295*

Serum Increase 12.5% of 64 patients had concentrations < 45% of total protein. 10.9% had concentrations > 65% of total proteins. *1295*

CSF Decrease 18.7% of patients had concentrations < 45% of total proteins; 7.8% had values > 65% of total proteins. *1295*

CSF Increase 18.7% of patients had concentrations < 45% of total proteins; 7.8% had > 65% of total proteins. *1295*

Alkaline Phosphatase Isoenzymes *Serum Decrease* Preliminary studies indicate a depression of serum alk phos of intestinal origin (serum type PP2) especially in blood group O. Comparisons were made with normal sera after matching blood groups, a factor not previously taken into account. *1759*

Alpha$_1$-Globulin *Serum Increase* 7.8% of 64 patients had concentration 8% of total proteins. *1295*

CSF Increase Concentrations > 79% of total proteins found in 10.9% of cases. *1295*

340.00 Multiple Sclerosis (continued)

Alpha$_2$-Globulin *Serum Increase* Concentrations > 14% of total protein occurred in 14% of patients. *1295*

CSF Increase Values of > 8% of total proteins found in 26.5% of patients. *1295*

Alpha$_2$-Macroglobulin *CSF Normal* 2069

Alpha-Ketoglutarate *Serum Increase* High concentrations noted in these patients imply a defect in carbohydrate metabolism. *2104*

Antibody Titer *Serum Increase* IgA and IgM antibodies to myelin of rabbit spinal cord. Found in 70% of patients. When IgG antimyelin antibody is present in titers greater than 1:8 it is suggestive, but not diagnostic. *1670* Serum IgE and measles antibodies were increased more frequently in hypocomplementemic patients than in normal populations *2375*

Beta-Galactosidase *Serum Decrease* In 10 patients, mean activity was 0.163 ± 0.025 U/L at pH = 4.5, normal = 0.243 ± 0.038. *1099*

Beta-Globulin *Serum Increase* Concentration > 15% of total protein was observed in 9.3% of patients. *1295*

Cells *CSF Increase* About 50% of patients have mononuclear cells in the CSF during an acute episode in the range of 10-50 cells. *0999*

Ceruloplasmin *Serum Decrease* Slight elevation of serum copper with significant reduction of serum ceruloplasmin. *1830*

Cholesterol *CSF Increase* Raised in several neurologic diseases including multiple sclerosis. *0912*

Cholesterol Esters *CSF Increase* Significantly higher. *0912*

Complement C3 *Serum Decrease* Hypocomplementemia (fall in factor C3 related to a fall in total hemolytic activity) was found in 29.5% of the patients not on corticotherapy at the first assay, and in 36% of the patients when repeated assays were carried out. Hypocomplementemia is significantly more frequent in MS than in the normal population (0%) and in neurological patients (9.6%). *2375* Mean level was slightly lower than normal. *0068*

Complement, Total *Serum Decrease* Hypocomplementemia was found in 29.5% of the patients not on corticotherapy at the first assay, and in 36% of the patients when repeated assays were carried out. Hypocomplementemia is significantly more frequent than in the normal population (0%) and in neurological patients (9.6%). *2375*

CSF Decrease Significantly lower. *1330*

Copper *Serum Increase* Slight elevation of serum copper with significant reduction of serum ceruloplasmin. *1830*

Fat *Feces Increase* Malabsorption tests were studied in 52 patients. Fat and undigested meat fibers content were found to be abnormal in 41.6 and 40.9% respectively. *0938*

Gamma Glutamyl Transferase (GGT) *Serum Increase* 6 of 33 patients had concentrations elevated above normal (40 U/L). *0684*

Globulin *Serum Increase* Increased to > 20% of total protein in 14% of 64 patients. *1295*

CSF Increase An increase, particularly the IgG fraction, may develop. An elevation to over 15% of the total protein and an abnormal colloidal gold curve are found in more than 75% of the patients. No relationship has been drawn with degree, type or duration of disease, or any other clinical criteria. *2075* 79.3% of patients had concentrations 12% of total protein. Over 50% had concentrations > 16%, and 9.5% of cases were > 30%. *1295* 4.5-23.8% of total protein in 13 patients. *2158*

Glucose Tolerance *Serum Decrease* Many patients have impaired carbohydrate metabolism exhibited by abnormal curves. *2104*

HLA Antigens *Blood Present* HLA antigen Dw2 found in 36% of patients with this disease compared to 0% of controls. *2051* HLA-DR2 present in 55% of patients versus 23% of control *2539* Increased incidence of HLA-DR2 *1503*

Immunoglobulin IgA *Serum Increase* Levels > 388 mg/dL in 13.8% of 64 patients. *1295*

CSF Increase 35.9% of patients had CSF values > 0.6 mg/dL. *1295* Found in 5 of 45 patients. *1933*

Immunoglobulin IgD *Serum Increase* 6.4% of patients had concentrations > 29 mg/dL. *1295*

Immunoglobulin IgE *Serum Decrease* Median level was slightly lower than in controls. All other serum immunoglobulins were normal. *0068*

Serum Increase Serum IgE and measles antibodies were increased more frequently in hypocomplementemic patients than in normal populations. *2375*

Immunoglobulin IgG *Serum Increase* Levels > 1871 mg/dL in 12.3% of 64 patients. *1295*

CSF Increase Total IgG is often increased > 15 mg/dL in CSF in all forms of multiple sclerosis. *0999* Concentrations > 4 mg/dL in 77.7% of patients. *1295* Increased due to intrathecal synthesis not blood:CSF barrier damage. *1099* In 62% of cases. *1933* *2321*

Immunoglobulin IgM *Serum Increase* Levels > 161 mg/dL in 7.8% of cases; 3.1% had values 34 mg/dL. *1295*

CSF Increase Detected in CSF samples from 26.9% of patients. *1295*

Immunoglobulins *CSF Increase* 0619

Lactic Acid *Blood Increase* High concentrations noted in these patients imply a defect in carbohydrate metabolism. *2104*

Leukocytes *CSF Increase* A pleocytosis of usually not more than 25 mononuclear cells/µL can be found. *0433*

Lymphocytes *Blood Decrease* In 19 different groups of neurological diseases, absolute and relative T-lymphocyte populations were significantly decreased only in patients with acute Guillain-Barré Syndrome, active multiple sclerosis and malignant cerebral tumor. *2540*

CSF Increase Significant increase in T-lymphocytes. *1214*

Monocytes *CSF Increase* CSF shows a slight increase in mononuclear cells and normal or slightly increased protein (50% of cases). *2467*

Phospholipids, Total *Serum Decrease* Particularly in patients with evidence of recent progression. *0878*

CSF Increase Raised in patients with high total CSF proteins but lowered in chronic multiple sclerosis. *2371*

Protein *CSF Increase* A slight increase in mononuclear cells and normal or slightly increased protein (50% of cases). Diagnosis is probable if more than 20% is gamma globulin. *2467* In all forms of MS approximately 70% of patients have abnormalities of CSF proteins. *0999* Increased total protein and IgG concentration. *2321* *2612*

Pyruvate *Blood Increase* Raised levels have been reported in some cases. The cause for this has not been discovered. *0619* High concentrations noted in these patients imply a defect in carbohydrate metabolism. *2104*

Uric Acid *Serum Normal* Very low CSF levels of 0.02-0.04 mg/dL, with normal serum levels found in the chronic stage of disease. *1338*

CSF Decrease Very low CSF levels of 0.02-0.04 mg/dL, with normal serum levels found in the chronic stage of disease. *1338*

Vitamin B$_{12}$ *Serum Decrease* Malabsorption of vitamin B$_{12}$ was found in 11.9% of 52 patients. *0938*

Feces Increase Malabsorption of vitamin B$_{12}$ was found in 11.9% of 52 patients. *0938*

345.90 Epilepsy

Albumin *CSF Decrease* Slightly decreased in CSF of patients with grand mal epilepsy. *1625*

Alpha$_1$-Antichymotrypsin *CSF Normal* Increased in patients with meningitis or mild hemorrhage, but equal to normal in patients with encephalitis, epilepsy, degenerative disorders or diseases of the CNS. *0079*

Amino Acids *Urine Increase* Transient rise due to disturbed renal function during grand mal seizure. *2104*

Calcium *Serum Decrease* Up to 33% of epileptic children on long-term anticonvulsant therapy. *0619*

Serum Increase High in cases of idiopathic grand mal epilepsy. CSF calcium remained normal. This increase in serum calcium may be due to hyperparathyroidism because of low magnesium concentration. *0093*

CSF Normal 0093

Ceruloplasmin *Serum Increase* Slightly elevated (62.30 ± 6.62 mg/dL) in patients with grand mal epilepsy. *1625*

CSF Decrease Slightly decreased in grand mal epilepsy. *1625*

Creatine Kinase *Serum Increase* Especially after status epilepticus. *0619* Increases in necrosis or acute atrophy of striated muscle in status epilepticus. *2467* In 50% of 10 patients hospitalized for this disorder. *0781*

Cyclic Adenosine Monophosphate *CSF Increase* CSF concentration was measured in 62 neurological patients, 46 of whom were epileptics and 16 with CNS damage. In epileptic patients the CSF concentration was significantly elevated for 3 days after an attack when compared with those free from attacks for at least 2 weeks. *1660*

Folate *Serum Decrease* Reduced in 33 of 68 institutionalized patients with severe epilepsy. *0514*

Gamma Glutamyl Transferase (GGT) *Serum Increase* Elevated in the sera of 64 of 75 patients (85.4%) with epilepsy. Enzyme activity usually remains at a constant level, characteristic of the patients, with some peaks and depressions in activity. *0684*

Immunoglobulin IgA *CSF Decrease* Slightly decreased in grand mal epilepsy. *1625*

Immunoglobulin IgG *CSF Decrease* Slightly decreased in grand mal epilepsy. *1625* Absolute concentration and percent of total CSF protein were low. *2321*

Immunoglobulins *CSF Decrease* *0619 1625*

Iron-Binding Capacity, Total (TIBC) *Serum Decrease* Mean concentration was 123.66 ± 8.31 μg/dL in grand mal epileptic patients. *1625*

Magnesium *Serum Decrease* In idiopathic grand mal epilepsy the concentrations both in serum and CSF were significantly low just after the seizure. During interseizure period (more than 24 h) the levels increased both in the serum and CSF but in serum it still remained significantly low. *0093*

  CSF Decrease In idiopathic grand mal epilepsy the concentrations both in serum and CSF were significantly low just after the seizure. *0093*

Prealbumin *CSF Increase* Only protein to increase in CSF of epileptics. Mean concentration was 1.50 ± 0.11 mg/dL. *1625*

Pyridoxine *Serum Decrease* Has been noted in epilepsy. *2104*

Xanthurenic Acid *Urine Increase* Has been noted in epilepsy. *2104*

346.00 Migraine

5-Hydroxyindoleacetic Acid (5-HIAA) *Urine Increase* Levels are increased during acute attacks. *0996*

Endorphin, Beta *CSF Decrease* Closely correlated with severity of disease. Decreased significantly in patients with common migraine (38.5 fmol/mL) compared with healthy controls (86.1 fmol/mL). *0825*

Histamine *Serum Increase* Levels are increased during acute attacks. *0996*

  White Blood Cells Increase Mean spontaneous histamine release was increased 33.7% compared to controls. *2112*

Lipoproteins, Beta *CSF Decrease* Significantly lower (P < 0.005). *0825*

Monoamine Oxidase *Blood Increase* Platelet levels are increased during acute attacks. *0996*

Norepinephrine *Serum Increase* Levels are increased during acute attacks. *0996*

Platelet Count *Blood Increase* Increased number but depleted of their serotonin concentration. *0996*

Thromboxane B$_2$ *Serum Decrease* The patients ability to produce Thromboxane B$_2$ was reduced in both children and adults with migraine. *1245*

Vanillylamine *Urine Increase* Levels are increased during acute attacks. *0996*

356.30 Refsum's Disease

Cells *CSF Normal* High CSF protein concentration in the absence of pleocytosis has been found in all cases. *2246*

Protein *CSF Increase* High CSF protein concentration in the absence of pleocytosis has been found in all cases. *2246* Elevated in 20 patients, ranging from 55-732 mg/dL. Mean = 275, mode = 165. *0878*

357.00 Guillain-Barré Syndrome

Albumin *CSF Increase* Usually elevated between 65 and 1000 mg/dL but may not peak until four to six weeks after onset of neurologic signs. Elevation may persist for several months. Elevation is primarily albumin. *1307* IgG and Albumin increased probably result from blood/CSF barrier damage *1099*

Beta-Galactosidase *Serum Decrease* In 10 patients, mean activity was 0.163 ± 0.025 mmol/min at pH = 4.5, normal = 0.243 ± 0.038. *1099*

Bicarbonate *Serum Increase* Respiratory acidosis may occur. *0962*

Cells *CSF Normal* Characteristic findings are elevated protein concentration but no increase in number of cells in CSF. *0151*

Complement Fixation *Serum Increase* 30 patients (33%) had markedly elevated levels of complement-fixing antibody to cytomegalovirus and in 21, a 4-fold or more alteration in titer was demonstrated. *0595*

Complement, Total *CSF Increase* Oligoclonal IgG bands, specific elevation of IgM and complement activation products have been reported during the acute phase of the disease. *1307*

Erythrocyte Sedimentation Rate *Blood Increase* Moderately elevated. *0878*

Immunoglobulin IgA *CSF Increase* Early in disease. *0878*

Immunoglobulin IgG *CSF Increase* Oligoclonal IgG bands, specific elevation of IgM and complement activation products have been reported during the acute phase of the disease. *1307* IgG and Albumin increased, probably resulting from blood: CSF barrier damage *1099*

Immunoglobulin IgM *CSF Increase* Oligoclonal IgG bands, specific elevation of IgM and complement activation products have been reported during the acute phase of the disease. *1307*

Leukocytes *Blood Increase* A moderate polymorphonuclear leukocytosis. *0878*

  CSF Normal Normal cell count; usually below 10 monocytes per mL. The presence of more than 50 mononuclear cells per mL or the presence of any polymorphonuclear cells should suggest another disease. *1307*

Lymphocytes *Blood Decrease* In 19 different groups of neurological diseases, absolute and relative T-lymphocyte populations were significantly decreased only in patients with acute Guillain-Barré Syndrome, active multiple sclerosis and malignant cerebral tumor. *2540* During active phase of disease. *0878*

  CSF Increase While it is true most cases show few, if any, lymphocytes, a few show up to 20-30 cells/μL. *0878*

Neutrophils *Blood Increase* A moderate polymorphonuclear leukocytosis. *0878*

pCO$_2$ *Blood Increase* Respiratory acidosis may occur. *0962*

pH *Blood Decrease* Respiratory acidosis may occur. *0962*

Protein *CSF Increase* CSF shows albuminocytologic dissociation with normal cell count and increased protein (average, 50-100 mg/dL). Protein increase parallels increasing clinical severity; may be prolonged. *2467* Increased total protein (1.21 ± 0.274 g/L). *1099* May reach as high as 2 g/100 mL. *0878* Usually elevated between 65 and 1000 mg/dL but may not peak until 4 to 6 weeks after onset of neurological sign. Elevation may persist for several months. Primarily Albumin *1307*

357.90 Polyneuritis

Albumin *CSF Increase* CSF shows a gradual increase in protein, almost all of which is albumin in postinfectious polyneuritis, without a concomitant rise in cells. *0999*

Cells *CSF Increase* Characteristically, fewer than 10 cells/μL usually lymphocytes, are present in the CSF, and the presence of > 40/μL raises other diagnostic considerations, such as herpes simplex myelitis and poliomyelitis. *0433*

Globulin *CSF Increase* Rarely elevated. *0433*

  CSF Normal Rarely elevated. *0433*

Immunoglobulin IgA *CSF Increase* Increased amounts of immunoglobulins particularly IgA and IgM have been demonstrated. *0433*

Immunoglobulin IgM *CSF Increase* Increased amounts of immunoglobulins particularly IgA and IgM have been demonstrated. *0433*

Leukocytes *Blood Increase* A mild increase in peripheral leukocytes may occur in the early stages of the illness. *0433* In 35% of 14 patients hospitalized for this disorder. *0781*

Lymphocytes *CSF Increase* CSF showed increased protein and up to several hundred mononuclear cells in polyneuritis due to infectious mononucleosis. *2467*

Neutrophils *Blood Increase* In 53% of 13 patients hospitalized for this disorder. *0781*

357.90 Polyneuritis (continued)

Protein *CSF Increase*   From day 3-7 of the illness, over 50% of the patients will have high concentrations, frequently > 100 mg/dL. From the 2-7th week, almost all patients will have high CSF protein values. *0433 2612*

358.00 Myasthenia Gravis

Aldolase *Serum Normal 2057*

Antibody Titer *Serum Increase*   50% of patients with this disease, usually those with thymoma, have antibodies to striated muscle. At times there is an increasing titer in severe disease. Generally a titer greater than 1:60 is diagnostic. *1670*

Antinuclear Antibodies *Serum Increase*   Approximately 20% contain antinuclear factor which can occur in IgA, IgG, or IgM. *1544* There is an increased incidence of this compared to the population as a whole. *2035*

Antismooth Muscle Antibodies *Serum Increase*   There is an increased incidence of this compared to the population as a whole. *2035*

Antithyroglobulin Antibodies *Serum Increase*   Serum contains at least one form of antithyroid antibody. *2035*

Aspartate Aminotransferase *Serum Normal 2057*

Bicarbonate *Serum Increase*   Associated respiratory insufficiency. *0995*

Carcinoembryonic Antigen *Serum Increase*   18% of patients had values > 2.5 ng/mL. *2199*

Catecholamines *Urine Increase*   Some cases. *2467*

Complement, Total *Serum Decrease*   40 of 68 patients had activity below normal at some time in the course of disease. On the basis of clinical correlations, 15 patients with subnormal levels were judged to be in exacerbation. *1680 2035*

Creatine *Urine Increase*   Increased formation; myopathy. *2467*

Creatine Kinase *Serum Normal 2057*

Erythrocyte Sedimentation Rate *Blood Normal*   Complete blood count and ESR are normal. *2467*

Hematocrit *Blood Decrease*   Occasional cases of macrocytic anemia. *2467*

Hemoglobin *Blood Decrease*   Occasional cases of macrocytic anemia. *2467*

HLA Antigens *Blood Present*   HLA-DR3 present in 30% of patients versus 17% of controls. *2539*

LE Cells *Blood Increase*   Lupus erythematosus may occur in conjunction. *0995*

Lymphocytes *Blood Decrease*   17 of 32 patients had counts < 1,500/μL and 18 of the 32 did not develop sensitivity to dinitrochlorobenzene. *0003 2035*

MCH *Blood Increase*   Occasional cases of macrocytic anemia. *2467*

MCV *Blood Increase*   Occasional cases of macrocytic anemia. *2467*

Oxygen Saturation *Blood Decrease*   Associated respiratory insufficiency. *0995*

pCO$_2$ *Blood Increase*   Associated respiratory insufficiency. *0995*

pO$_2$ *Blood Decrease*   Associated respiratory insufficiency. *0995*

Rheumatoid Factor *Serum Increase*   Somewhat elevated compared to the population at large. Demonstrated in a small percentage of patients. *2035*

T$_3$ Uptake *Serum Increase*   Thyrotoxicosis may occur in conjunction with this disease. *0995*

Thyroxine (T$_4$) *Serum Increase*   Thyrotoxicosis may occur in conjunction with this disease. *0995*

Tri-iodothyronine (T$_3$) *Serum Increase*   Thyrotoxicosis may occur in conjunction with this disease. *0995*

358.80 Amyotonia Congenita

Creatine *Urine Increase*   Increased formation; myopathy. *2467 0619*

359.11 Progressive Muscular Dystrophy

17-Ketosteroids *Urine Decrease 0995*

Alanine Aminotransferase *Serum Increase*   Particularly during the early and middle stages of the disease. In the late stage of the disease when the muscle mass has been severely reduced, serum enzyme levels may be only minimally elevated. *0433 0962*

Aldolase *Serum Increase*   Serum enzymes reach extremely high levels, particularly during the early and middle stages of the disease. In the late stage of the disease when the muscle mass has been severely reduced, serum enzyme levels may be only minimally elevated. *0433*   Increases in the early stages to 10-15 X normal in 90% of cases. Levels are normal in the later and terminal stages. *0619* Strikingly elevated. *0962*

Aldosterone *Urine Normal*   The differences between the patient group and the control group for sodium and potassium in serum and urine and for urinary aldosterone were not significant. The pathologically elevated sodium:potassium ratio in skeletal muscle is not due to increased aldosterone or other causes of renal wastage of potassium. *0816*

Alkaline Phosphatase *Leukocyte Decrease*   Untreated disease. *2467*

Amino Acids *Urine Increase 0995*

Aspartate Aminotransferase *Serum Increase*   Released from breaking down muscle. Levels tend to be increased in affected young children. *0503 0433*   May have elevated levels. Usual values 145 U/L. *0503*   A marked increase in CK, LD, and AST was noted. 21 of 23 cases showed moderate-high levels of AST ranging from 24-105 U/L. *1677 0962*

Catecholamines *Urine Increase 2467*

Cholesterol, High Density Lipoprotein *Serum Normal*   Within normal limits in 15 patients with this disorder. *2328*

Cholic Acid *Serum Decrease*   In 15 patients with this disorder the serum values were usually low (0.16 μmol/L) compared with controls (1.47 μmol/L). *2328*

Creatine *Serum Increase*   Decreased transport into muscle and leakage out of muscle occur in muscular dystrophies. *2246*

Urine Increase   Urine creatine is increased; urine creatinine is decreased. These changes are less marked in limb-girdle and fascioscapulohumeral types than in the Duchenne type. May occur irregularly. *2467*   Decreased transport into muscle and leakage out of muscle occur in muscular dystrophies. *2246*   Excessive concentrations appearing in urine are newly synthesized and do not originate from muscle cells. *2104*

Creatine Kinase *Serum Increase*   Range of values up to 50 X normal upper limit with higher results in the younger patients. Abnormal results are accentuated if vasoconstriction is applied for 10 min before venesection. (Muscular atrophy of neurogenic origin shows no such increase in serum levels). *0619*   Especially Duchenne type. The most sensitive reflection of certain types of muscular dystrophy. *0812 0503*   Extremely high concentrations, particularly during the early and middle stages of the disease. In the late stage of the disease when the muscle mass has been severely reduced, may be only *0433 1677 1071 2418*

Creatinine *Urine Decrease*   Urine creatine is increased; urine creatinine is decreased. These changes are less marked in limb-girdle and fascioscapulohumeral types than in the Duchenne type. *2467*   Reduced excretion in any myopathic or neurogenic condition which decreases muscle mass. *2246 0995*

Hydroxyproline *Urine Decrease*   In boys with Duchenne type. *0878*

Lactate Dehydrogenase *Serum Increase*   Particularly during the early and middle stages of the disease. In the late stage of the disease when the muscle mass has been severely reduced, may be only minimally elevated. *0433 1677*

Lactate Dehydrogenase Isoenzyme 5 (LD$_5$) *Serum Decrease*   In 76 cases of Duchenne MD, was markedly depressed and remained low until the final stages of the disease. Abnormal isoenzyme patterns persisted over time even though the total LD value fell to normal with increasing age of patient. *1070*

Lactate Dehydrogenase Isoenzymes *Serum Increase*   Isoenzyme patterns revealed an increase in 1 (38%) and 2 (47.5%), with concomitant decrease or absence of 3, 4, 5. *1071*   In Duchenne dystrophy combined LD-1 and 2 values are 72% of total LD. Abnormal isoenzyme patterns persist with age of patient although total LD falls to normal. *1070*

Malate Dehydrogenase *Serum Increase*   In Duchenne type. *0878*

Myoglobin *Urine Increase*   Sporadic. *2467*

Nickel *Serum Normal*   Mean 2.3 (n = 10) compared with controls mean 2.6 μg/L (n = 42). *1559*

Plasma Cells *Serum Decrease*   Depressed. *2357 0659 0683*

Potassium *Serum Normal* The differences between the patients and the control group of normal boys for sodium and potassium in serum and urine were not significant. The pathologically elevated sodium:potassium ratio in skeletal muscle is not due to increased aldosterone or other causes of renal wastage of potassium. *0816*

Urine Normal The differences between the patients and the control group of normal boys for sodium and potassium in serum and urine were not significant. The pathologically elevated sodium:potassium ratio in skeletal muscle is not due to increased aldosterone or other causes of renal wastage of potassium. *0816*

Ribose *Urine Increase* Probably derived from the nucleoprotein of breaking down muscle cells. *0619*

Sodium *Serum Normal* The differences between the patient group and the group of normal boys for sodium and potassium in serum and urine were not significant. The pathologically elevated sodium:potassium ratio in skeletal muscle is not due to increased aldosterone or other causes of renal wastage of potassium. *0816*

Urine Normal The differences between the patient group and the control group for sodium and potassium in serum and urine were significant. The pathologically elevated sodium potassium ratio in skeletal muscle is not due to increased aldosterone or other causes of renal wastage of potassium. *0816*

359.21   Myotonia Atrophica

17-Ketosteroids *Urine Decrease* Primary testicular failure in males. *0878 2467*

Alanine Aminotransferase *Serum Increase* Usually normal or minimally elevated. *0433*

Aldolase *Serum Increase* Usually normal or minimally elevated. *0433* Due to cell destruction. Increased in about 20% of the patients. *2467*

Serum Normal Usually normal or minimally elevated. *0433*

Aspartate Aminotransferase *Serum Increase* Slight to moderate increase. *0503* Usually normal or minimally elevated. *0433* Increased in about 15% of the patients. *2467*

Serum Normal Usually normal in myotonic dystrophy. *2246*

Calcium *Red Blood Cells Increase* Erythrocytes from these patients accumulate calcium at a significantly higher rate than normals do. This increased rate of net accumulation appears related to an enhanced permeability of the membrane, rather than to an impairment in its active outward transport. *1827*

Cortisol *Plasma Decrease* Abnormal diurnal variation with decreased 8 A.M. values in 4 of 7 patients. *1029*

Creatine *Serum Increase* Decreased transport into muscle and leakage out of muscle occur in muscular dystrophies. *2246*

Urine Increase Decreased transport into muscle and leakage out of muscle occur in muscular dystrophies. *2246*

Creatine Kinase *Serum Increase* Slight to moderate increase. *0503* Increased in about 50% of the patients. *2467 0433*

Creatinine *Serum Increase* In severe muscle disease. *0503*

Urine Decrease Reduced excretion in any myopathic or neurogenic condition which decreases muscle mass. *2246*

Erythrocyte Sedimentation Rate *Blood Normal* Usually normal. *2467*

Globulin *Serum Decrease* *2618*

Glucose Tolerance *Serum Increase* Biphasic response was found in 19 patients (49%) compared with 12 of the control population (24%). In 9 patients (23%), the height of the 2nd peak was 20 mg/dL. *2008*

Immunoglobulin IgG *Serum Decrease* In 4 of 8 cases studied. *1158 2246*

Insulin *Serum Increase* Found in 7 of 7 patients. *1029* 80% of patients had insulin values > 2 S.D. above the normal mean during oral glucose tolerance test and 42% had high fasting plasma values. *0114* In response to glucose load, in myotonic dystrophy. *2246*

Lactate Dehydrogenase *Serum Increase* Slightly or moderately increased. *0503* In about 10% of the patients. *2467 0433*

Serum Normal Usually normal. *2246*

Lactate Dehydrogenase Isoenzyme 5 (LD$_5$) *Serum Increase* Elevation of fast moving LD in serum. *2467*

Myoglobin *Urine Increase* Metabolic defect, hereditary. *2467*

Oxygen Saturation *Blood Decrease* Respiratory muscle weakness may develop. *0361*

pCO$_2$ *Blood Increase* Respiratory muscle weakness may develop. *0361*

pO$_2$ *Blood Decrease* Respiratory muscle weakness may develop. *0361*

Prolactin *Serum Increase* Basal levels elevated in 3 of 7 patients. *1029*

359.22   Myotonia Congenita

Aspartate Aminotransferase *Serum Increase* Slight to moderate increase. *0503*

Creatine *Urine Increase* May be increased in some patients (Thomsen's disease). *2467*

Creatine Kinase *Serum Increase* Slight to moderate increase. *0503*

Lactate Dehydrogenase *Serum Increase* Slightly or moderately increased. *0503*

363.20   Inflammation of Optic Nerve and Retina

Lymphocytes *CSF Increase* CSF is normal or may show increased protein and up to 200 lymphocytes/μL. *2467*

Protein *CSF Increase* CSF is normal or may show increased protein and up to 200 lymphocytes/μL. *2467*

380.10   Otitis Externa

Leukocytes *Blood Increase* When the infection is severe and there is mild fever, an elevated WBC will occur. *0433*

381.00   Otitis Media

Eosinophils *Blood Increase* In 48% of 70 patients hospitalized for this disorder. *0781*

Erythrocyte Sedimentation Rate *Blood Increase* *0433*

Leukocytes *Blood Increase* Usually accompanied by a mild leukocytosis with the appearance of less mature forms of neutrophils. *0433* Acute exacerbations may produce elevated WBC. *0433*

Lymphocytes *Blood Increase* In 66% of 70 patients hospitalized for this disorder. *0781*

Neutrophils *Blood Decrease* In 53% of 70 patients hospitalized for this disorder. *0781*

Blood Increase Usually accompanied by a mild leukocytosis with the appearance of less mature forms of neutrophils. *0433*

DISEASES OF THE CIRCULATORY SYSTEM

Acute Rheumatic Fever

390.00   Rheumatic Fever

Adenosine Deaminase *Serum Increase* Increased. *0655 1737 2235*

Alanine Aminotransferase *Serum Normal* Usually normal unless the patient has cardiac failure with liver damage. *2467*

Albumin *Serum Decrease* Impaired hepatic synthesis. Decreased serum albumin with strikingly increased alpha$_2$ and gamma globulins. *2104*

Urine Increase Slight febrile albuminuria. Indicates mild focal nephritis. Concomitant glomerulonephritis appears in up to 2.5% of cases. *2467* . A high percentage of patients show some proteinuria. *0151*

Alpha$_1$-Globulin *Serum Increase* Moderate increase in the early stages. *0619*

Alpha$_2$-Globulin *Serum Increase* Serum proteins are altered, with decreased serum albumin and increased alpha$_2$ and gamma globulins. Streptococcus A infections do not increase alpha$_2$ globulin. *2467* Increases occur in the acute phase (parallel with the serum C-reactive protein), and fall during quiescence or following steroid therapy. *0619*

390.00 Rheumatic Fever *(continued)*

Antibody Titer *Serum Increase* Antifibrinolysin titer is increased in this disease and in recent hemolytic streptococcus infections. 1 of the 3 titers (ASO, antihyaluronidase, antifibrinolysin elevated in 95% of cases. If all are normal, a diagnosis is less likely. Antihyaluronidase titer of 1,000-1,500 follows recent streptococcus A disease and up to 4,000 with rheumatic fever. Average titer is higher in early rheumatic activity than in subsiding or inactive rheumatic fever. Increased as often as ASO and antifibrinolysin titers. *2467*

Antinuclear Antibodies *Serum Normal* *1799*

Antistreptolysin O *Serum Increase* Increased titer is found in 80% of patients within the first 2 months. Height of titer is not related to severity; rate of fall is not related to course of disease. *2467* Antibodies appear in 7 days, peak 2-4 weeks later and may remain elevated for months. Rising titer suggests infections. *2508* Titer of 250 Todd U in adults and 333 in children is considered diagnostic of preceding streptococcal infection. *1108* Increased titers develop after 2nd week and peak in 4-6 weeks. *0962*

Aspartate Aminotransferase *Serum Increase* The incidence and mechanism of occurrence is not clear. Usual values < 50 U/L. *0503* May occur as a result of chronic passive congestion in congestive heart failure or as a result of hepatotoxicity following salicylate therapy. *0962* Serum level related to severity in the early stages. *0619*

Casts *Urine Increase* Often mild abnormality of Addis count (protein, casts, RBC WBC) indicates mild focal nephritis. Concomitant glomerulonephritis appears in up to 2.5% of cases. *2467*

Catecholamines *Urine Increase* Epirephrine and norepinephrine increase in proportion to the severity of circulatory failure. Catecholamine excretion, especially norepinephrine, is significantly raised in grades 3 and 4 of hemodynamic disturbance. *2572*

Complement C3 *Serum Increase* Elevated during the acute stages of disease, coinciding with other indices of acute inflammation. *2035*

Complement, Total *Serum Decrease* In general, normal or elevated. A small number of patients have reduced levels during the acute phase without any clear relation to severity or particular clinical manifestation. *0962*

Serum Increase In general, normal or elevated. A small number of patients have reduced levels during the acute phase without any clear relation to severity or particular clinical manifestation. *0962* During the acute stage. *2035* Elevated during activity inflammation and subsides with remission. *2090*

Serum Normal In general, normal or elevated. A small number of patients have reduced levels during the acute phase without any clear relation to severity or particular clinical manifestation. *0962* During the acute stage. *2035* Elevated during activity inflammation and subsides with remission. *2090*

Synovial Fluid Decrease The early and late components of the complement system are decreased. *2300*

Copper *Serum Increase* In acute disease. *2467* Has been used as an index of disease activity. *0619* Statistically significant *2188*

Coproporphyrin *Urine Increase* *0619*

C-Reactive Protein *Serum Increase* Test is frequently positive and is not influenced by anemia, but is frequently positive with congestive heart failure of any cause. *1108* Almost always positive in the early stages of untreated disease and the most sensitive indicator of activity. Remains positive in the presence of active carditis. *0962*

Cryofibrinogen *Serum Increase* *2035 0856 1551*

Epinephrine *Urine Increase* Epirephrine and norepinephrine increase in proportion to the severity of circulatory failure. Catecholamine excretion, especially norepinephrine, is significantly raised in grades 3 and 4 of hemodynamic disturbance. *2572*

Erythrocytes *Urine Increase* Often mild abnormality of Addis count (protein, casts, RBC, WBC) indicates mild focal nephritis. Concomitant glomerulonephritis appears in up to 2.5% of cases. *2467* Moderate increase. *0151*

Erythrocyte Sedimentation Rate *Blood Decrease* May be decreased in the presence of congestive heart failure. *1108*

Blood Increase Sensitive test of rheumatic activity; returns to normal with adequate treatment with ACTH or salicylates. It may remain increased after WBC becomes normal. Becomes normal with onset of congestive heart failure even in the presence of rheumatic activity. *2467* Almost always elevated early in the course of untreated cases. May be decreased in the presence of congestive heart failure but not usually to the normal range. *1108* Typically seen in the myocarditis of rheumatic fever. *0962*

Fibrinogen *Plasma Increase* *0962*

Globulin *Serum Increase* Serum proteins are altered, with decreased serum albumin and increased alpha$_2$ and gamma globulins. *2467* *0962 2104*

Haptoglobin *Serum Increase* Conditions associated with increased ESR and alpha 2 globulin; increases in collagen disease. *2467*

Hematocrit *Blood Decrease* Anemia is common, gradually improves as activity subsides; microcytic types. Anemia may be related to increased plasma volume that occurs in early phase. *2467* Usually normochromic and normocytic and resolves without specific treatment. *1108* Anemia correlates closely with the degree of inflammation; persistence of anemia suggests continued rheumatic activity. *0962*

Hemoglobin *Blood Decrease* Anemia is common (hemoglobin usually 8-12 g/dL); gradually improves as activity subsides; microcytic type. May be related to increased plasma volume that occurs in early phase. *2467* Usually normochromic and normocytic and resolves without specific treatment. *1108* Anemia correlates closely with the degree of inflammation; persistence of anemia suggests continued rheumatic activity. *0962*

Immunoglobulin IgA *Serum Increase* Increase in the globulin fraction of the serum proteins is frequent and mainly due to an increase in IgG and IgA. *1108* Increased immunoglobulins, particularly of IgG and IgA, and elevated immune responses to streptococcal cellular and extracellular products. *2035*

Immunoglobulin IgG *Serum Increase* Increase in the globulin fraction of the serum proteins is frequent and mainly due to an increase in IgG and IgA. *1108* Increased immunoglobulins, particularly of IgG and IgA, and elevated immune responses to streptococcal cellular and extracellular products. *2035*

Immunoglobulins *Serum Increase* Increased immunoglobulins, particularly of IgG and IgA, and elevated immune responses to streptococcal cellular and extracellular products. *2035*

Lactate Dehydrogenase *Serum Increase* In some cases of acute rheumatic carditis. *0619*

Leukocytes *Blood Increase* Common leukocytosis with counts of 12,000-24,000/μL and increased percentage of polymorphonuclear cells. *0151* Increase may persist for weeks after fever subsides. Count may decrease with salicylate and ACTH therapy. *2467* Frequently present early in disease. *1108* *0962*

Urine Increase Indicates mild focal nephritis. *2467* Moderate increase in RBCs and WBCs in urine. *0151*

Synovial Fluid Increase Increased number of white cells in synovial fluid, ranging from 300-98,000/μL. *2467* 10,000-15,000/μL. *0962*

Mucoprotein *Serum Increase* *0962*

Neutrophils *Blood Increase* *2538*

Synovial Fluid Increase Increased number neutrophils, ranging from 8-98/μL. *2467*

Norepinephrine *Urine Increase* Epirephrine and norepinephrine increase in proportion to the severity of circulatory failure. Catecholamine excretion, especially norepinephrine, is significantly raised in grades 3 and 4 of hemodynamic disturbance. *2572*

Protein *Serum Increase* Increase in the globulin fraction of the serum proteins is frequent and mainly due to an increase in IgG and IgA. *1108*

Urine Increase Slight febrile albuminuria. Indicates mild focal nephritis. Concomitant glomerulonephritis appears in up to 2.5% of cases. *2467* Proteinuria may occur. *0151*

Rheumatoid Factor *Serum Normal* *2467*

Vanillylamine *Urine Increase* Increased VMA excretion was observed in cases of grade 4 hemodynamic disturbance. *2572*

VDRL *Serum Positive* Not uncommon to encounter biologic false-positive reactions. *0151*

Viscosity *Synovial Fluid Decrease* *0962*

401.00 Malignant Hypertension

17-Hydroxycorticosteroids *Urine Increase* Slightly increased. *2467*

17-Ketogenic Steroids *Urine Increase* Slightly increased. *2467*

Albumin *Urine Increase* May occur from leaking glomerular capillaries. significant proteinuria 500 mg/24h or > 1+ by qualitative estimation) occurs very rarely in benign essential hypertension; their presence suggests the malignant phase or primary renal parenchymal disease. *0433*

Aldosterone *Plasma Increase* Most patients. *0995*

Ammonia *Blood Decrease* Decreased arterial ammonia in azotemic patients, (mean = 34 mmol/L). *1853*

Bicarbonate *Serum Increase* Metabolic alkalosis may occur with potassium loss. *0962*

Catecholamines *Urine Increase* Slightly increased. *2467*

Cholesterol *Serum Increase* Mean concentration was 199.7 ± 7.5 mg/dL in 24 male patients compared to 170.9 ± 6.3 in controls. *0381*

Cholesterol Esters *Serum Increase* Mean concentration was 118.0 ± 8.4 mg/dL in 24 male patients (normal = 101.7 ± 6.3). *0381*

Erythrocytes *Urine Increase* Malignant phase of hypertension. May occur from leaking glomerular capillaries. Hematuria occurs very rarely in benign essential hypertension; its presence suggests the malignant phase or primary renal parenchymal disease. *0433*

Hematocrit *Blood Decrease* Many patients show evidence of microangiopathic hemolytic anemia. *0995*

Hemoglobin *Blood Decrease* Many patients show evidence of microangiopathic hemolytic anemia. *0995*

pCO₂ *Blood Increase* Metabolic alkalosis may occur with potassium loss. *0962*

pH *Blood Increase* Metabolic alkalosis may occur with potassium loss. *0962*

Phospholipids, Total *Serum Increase* In 24 male patients, mean concentration was 234.7 - 13.5 mg/dL compared to 204.1 ± 3.5 in normals. *0381*

Potassium *Serum Decrease* Many diseases including hyperaldosteronism are characterized by low serum concentration. *1108*

Renin Activity *Plasma Increase* Most patients. *0995 1108 0151*

Triglycerides *Serum Increase* In 24 male patients, mean concentration was 93.4 ± 6.3 mg/dL compared to 76.1 ± 3.7 in controls. *0381*

Urea Nitrogen *Serum Increase* *1853*

Vanillylamine *Urine Increase* May occur. *0995*

401.10   Essential Benign Hypertension

Albumin *Serum Decrease* *2467*

Aldolase *Serum Decrease* *0126*

Aldosterone *Plasma Increase* Decreased metabolic clearance rate. *1708*

Urine Decrease Decreased metabolic clearance rate of aldosterone. *1708*

Ammonia *Blood Decrease* Decreased arterial ammonia in azotemic patients, mean = 34 mmol/L ± 1.4. *1853*

Angiotensin-Converting Enzyme (ACE) *Serum Normal* No difference was detected between men and woman and between normotensives and hypertensives. *0608* Normal levels for 14 patients with this disorder *2041 0608 2417*

Aspartate Aminotransferase *Serum Increase* In 29% of 101 patients hospitalized for this disorder. *0781*

Beta-Glucuronidase *Urine Increase* Moderately elevated (33.7 ± 23.4 U/L). Approximately half of the values were above normal. *0885*

Bicarbonate *Serum Increase* In 59% of 98 patients hospitalized for this disorder. *0781*

Cadmium *Serum Increase* There was a high correlation between systolic and diastolic BP and cadmium levels. *0126* No association between subclinical cadmium exposure and hypertension but confirmed relationship with cigarette smoking. *0152*

Carcinoembryonic Antigen *Serum Increase* 28% of patients had values > 2.5 ng/mL. *2199*

Catecholamines *Plasma Increase* Raised plasma catecholamines in some patients with primary hypertension. *0522*

Urine Increase Up to 100 μg/24h may be excreted. *0619*

Cholesterol *Serum Increase* Frequently elevated. *0995*

Creatinine *Serum Increase* In 49% of 106 patients hospitalized for this disorder. *0781*

Epinephrine *Plasma Increase* *0765*

Glucose *Serum Increase* Significant increase in glucose and insulin response to a 75 gram oral glucose challenge. *2017*

Insulin *Serum Increase* Significant increase in glucose and insulin response to a 75 gram oral glucose *2017*

Lead *Blood Decrease* A significant correlation between high blood lead levels and high blood pressure *0152*

Potassium *Serum Decrease* Characterized by low serum concentration. *1108* Untreated hypertensive patients frequently presented with low serum concentrations unassociated with acidosis or alkalosis. *2027*

Prostaglandins *Serum Decrease* Reduced levels of A₂ in patients with essential hypertension as opposed to normal controls. *1367*

Protein *Serum Decrease* *2467*

Urine Increase May occur with accompanying renal functional impairment. *1108*

Pseudocholinesterase *Serum Increase* *0126*

Renin Activity *Plasma Decrease* Decreased in 20% of patients at diagnosis. *2467* Suppressed plasma renin activity. *0371* Can be high, low or normal. *1108*

Plasma Increase Mean level, measured after 1 h supine rest, was significantly higher in the hypertensive subjects, while the upright PRA was normal. *1211* Greater in plasma of hypertensive patients and uremic patients than in plasma of normotensive control subjects. *1310* Can be high, low or normal. *1108*

Plasma Normal Can be high, low or normal. *1108*

Urine Decrease *1362*

Sodium *Serum Decrease* Slight but highly significant depression in circulating concentration. Mean in 130 hypertensives was 137.7 mmol/L and 140.4 mmol/L in 123 normotensives. *2104*

Serum Normal Sodium homeostasis is usually maintained in gradual renal failure. *1985*

Urine Increase Significantly higher excretion in subjects with diastolic blood pressure between 95 and 109 mm Hg than in the group with diastolic blood pressure below 90 mm Hg. *0596*

Triglycerides *Serum Increase* Frequently elevated. *0995*

Urea Nitrogen *Serum Increase* *1853*

Uric Acid *Serum Increase* Found in 58% of 470 patients (27% of 333 untreated patients). Degree or occurrence of hyperuricemia did not correlate with severity of hypertension. *0275* In 54% of 102 patients hospitalized for this disorder. *0781 0962*

Zinc *Serum Decrease* *0126*

405.91   Renovascular Hypertension

Chloride *Serum Increase* Acidosis which is out of proportion to the degree of azotemia. *0962*

Cholesterol *Serum Increase* Predisposes to development of arteriosclerosis. *0992*

Creatinine *Urine Increase* Confirmatory evidence of greater water reabsorption as a cause of the decreased volume from the suspected kidney. *1108 0590*

Creatinine Clearance *Urine Decrease* Renal functional impairment. *0962*

Glomerular Filtration Rate (GFR) *Urine Decrease* Renal functional impairment. *0962*

Glucose *Serum Increase* Associated with diabetes mellitus. *0992*

Inulin Clearance *Urine Decrease* Renal functional impairment. *0962*

Lipoproteins *Serum Increase* More than 50% of the patients showed obviously abnormal profiles of serum lipoproteins, which returned to normal or near-normal when the disease was ameliorated or corrected surgically. *2446*

Osmolality *Urine Decrease* Renal functional impairment. *0962*

pH *Blood Decrease* Acidosis which is out of proportion to the degree of azotemia. *0962*

Urine Decrease Acidosis which is out of proportion to the degree of azotemia. *0962*

Renin Activity *Plasma Increase* *0992*

Sodium *Urine Decrease* A 50% or greater decrease in volume excreted and a 15% or greater decrease in sodium concentration indicated renal artery obstruction and reversible renovascular hypertension. *1108 2440*

Specific Gravity *Urine Decrease* Renal functional impairment. *0962*

Triglycerides *Serum Increase* Predisposes to development of arteriosclerosis. *0992*

Uric Acid *Serum Increase* Increased incidence of hyperuricemia. *0992*

405.91   Renovascular Hypertension (continued)

Volume *Urine Increase* A 50% or greater decrease in volume excreted and a 15% or greater decrease in sodium concentration indicated renal artery obstruction and reversible renovascular hypertension. *1108   2440*

410.90   Acute Myocardial Infarction

17-Hydroxycorticosteroids *Urine Increase 1108*

17-Ketogenic Steroids *Urine Increase 1108*

Acid Phosphatase *Serum Increase* Ten cases of acute transmural infarction were accompanied by a rise of 50-400% in serum concentration several h after onset of symptoms and lasted 3-5 days. *2078* Significant increases evident within 2-3 h and persist 3-5 days in some cases. *2104   0812*

Alanine Aminotransferase *Serum Increase* Normal or only minimally elevated. *0503* Generally parallels AST but the increase is less marked. *2467* Observed only when resulting cardiac tissue necrosis is great enough to cause a rise in AST equivalent to 150 spectrophotometric U. *2577* In 49% of 18 patients hospitalized for this disorder. *0781   0962*

Serum Normal Usually not increased unless there is liver damage due to congestive heart failure, drug therapy, etc. *2467*

Albumin *Serum Decrease* In 22% of 111 patients hospitalized for this disorder. *0781   2531*

Aldolase *Serum Increase* With cell destruction. *2467* Rises after 3 h to a peak by 24 h (2-15 X normal), falling to normal by 4-7 days. There is a semiquantitative relation between the amount of necrosis and the peak level in the serum. *0619   0962*

Alkaline Phosphatase *Serum Increase* Some patients; usually during phase of organization. *2467* Increased in conjunction with normal levels of bilirubin indicate congestive heart failure or myocardial infarction-28%, carcinoma-25%, hepatobiliary-16%, and other miscellaneous diseases. *0191*

Alpha₁-Antichymotrypsin *Serum Increase* Following myocardial infarction, a large rapid increase was noted to a maximum at day 5. *1168*

Alpha₁-Antitrypsin *Serum Increase* Showed a significant increase when compared to controls and remained elevated for 3 months after ischemic episode. *1438* Significantly elevated in patients with AMI (n = 48) compared with controls (n = 19). *0845*

Alpha₁-Glycoprotein *Serum Increase* One of the most reliable indicators of acute inflammation. *1239 1672 1866   1947 2096 2170*

Antithrombin III *Plasma Decrease* Found to be significantly diminished when measured by the Von Kaulla Method; otherwise found to show a significant increase 3 months after an acute ischemic episode. *1438* Significant decrease. *1724*

Plasma Increase Found to be significantly diminished when measured by the Von Kaulla Method; otherwise found to show a significant increase 3 months after an acute ischemic episode. *1438*

Bilirubin *Serum Normal 2467*

Calcium *Serum Normal* Plasma concentration measured in 18 patients several days after admission showed a fall in 13 cases. Correction of values to a fixed albumin level removed the apparent tendency to hypocalcemia. *2531*

Catecholamines *Plasma Increase* The adrenal medulla can release circulating catecholamines as the result either of the generalized sympathetic stress reaction or of arterial hypoxia. Patients with higher plasma levels of catecholamines and free fatty acids may have a higher incidence of severe arrhythmias, shock, and death than patients with lower levels. *1108*

Urine Increase Total urinary catecholamines were significantly elevated in the first 48 h. *0529*

Cholesterol *Serum Increase* Very significantly elevated. Mean value was 212.2 ± 15.0 mg/dL in females and 209.1 ± 4.4 in males. Normal was 168.3 ± 4.2 and 170.9 ± 6.3 in females and males, respectively. *0381* Tends to slowly decrease for a few weeks after infarction. *1108*

Cholesterol Esters *Serum Increase* Mean concentration was 134.0 ± 13.6 mg/dL compared to 92.6 ± 6.7 in women, and 129.2 ± 3.7 compared to 101.7 ± 5.6 in men. *0381*

Copper *Serum Increase* After infarction, a significant increase in serum copper and a decrease in zinc were observed. *2428* Mean concentration = 123 µg/dL in 27 patients. *2502*

Cortisol *Plasma Increase 1108*

C-Reactive Protein *Serum Increase* Appear within 24-48 h, begin to fall by the 3rd day and become negative after 1-2 weeks. *2467* Significant increase *1724*

Creatine Kinase *Serum Increase* Rises in 3 h reaching peak by 36 h (10-25 X normal), returning to normal by 4 days. Prolonged elevation indicates bad prognosis. *0619* Peak levels may be 50-100 X normal. *0812* The incidence of elevation is approximately equal to AST and LD, but is more specific. *0503* Increased in > 90% of patients when blood is drawn at appropriate time. *2467* Allows early diagnosis because increases appear within the appearance of CK-MB in the serum, the isoenzyme found only in the myocardium, is specific for myocardial damage. *0999   1264 2205*

Creatinine *Serum Increase* 9 of 22 patients showed elevations within 6 days of infarction. Initial and peak means were 0.101 ± 0.022 and 0.117 ± 0.025 µmol/L, respectively. *2530* In 59% of 98 patients at initial hospitalization for this disorder. *0781*

Cryofibrinogen *Serum Increase 2035 0856 1551 2046*

Epinephrine *Plasma Decrease* Significantly reduced the first few days. *1289*

Plasma Increase Correlates with fasting plasma free fatty acids, which are associated with increased incidence of serious arrhythmias after infarctions. *0937* Evidence for a sympathoadrenal response is found in the increased blood and urinary concentration of norepinephrine, epinephrine, or their metabolic products. *1108 1163 1451*

Urine Increase Evidence for a sympathoadrenal response is found in the increased blood and urinary concentration of norepinephrine, epinephrine, or their metabolic products. *1108* In patients developing heart failure or cardiogenic shock, the urinary level of both free catecholamines rose notably in the 1st week after infarction. in uncomplicated cases, a moderate rise in the norepinephrine level in the 1st week was associated with only a transient rise in the epinephrine level. *1163   1451*

Erythrocyte Sedimentation Rate *Blood Increase* Increased, usually by 2-3 days; peaks in 4-5 days; persists for 2-6 months. Sometimes more sensitive than WBC as it may occur before fever and persists after temperature and WBC have returned to normal. Degree of increase does not correlate with severity or prognosis. *2467* Rises slowly and may persist for weeks even though no complications are present. *0999* May be a crude indication of the extent of myocardial damage. A normal ESR during the 2nd week suggests absence of or small myocardial infarction. *0962   1108 1828*

Estrogens *Serum Increase* 34 of 35 male survivors of myocardial infarction, aged 24-48, had higher plasma concentration of estradiol than age matched controls. 29 of 35 had elevated concentration of estrone. *0669*

Factor IV *Plasma Increase* A mean of 95 ng/mL was found in 21 patients, compared to normal 16 ± 4 in controls. Patients with chest pain but without evidence of infarction had a mean of 29 ng/mL. Elevation persisted for 1 week and returned to normal. *0974*

Factor XIII *Plasma Decrease* Substantial depression developed with concomitant significant increases in the proportion and concentration of plasma high molecular weight fibrinogen complexes (HMWFC). An inverse correlation between factor XIII and percentage of HMWFC was demonstrated in the early stages of the illness. *1491*

Fatty Acids, Free (FFA) *Serum Increase* Maximum values occurred within 8 h after infarction. Patients with values > 1,200 µmol/L had increased prevalence of serious arrhythmias and disorder of conductance. *2185* Tend to rise in the first 48 h. *0529* May be partially related to pituitary-sympathoadrenal stimulation. Patients with higher plasma levels of catecholamines and free fatty acids may have a higher incidence of severe arrhythmias, shock, and death than patients with lower levels. *1108* High values (> 1,000 µmol/L) were associated with an increased incidence of serious cardiac arrhythmias after infarction. *0937   1451*

Fibrinogen *Serum Increase* Significant increase. *1724*

Plasma Increase Substantial depression of factor XIII developed with concomitant significant increases in the proportion and concentration of plasma high molecular weight fibrinogen complexes (HMWFC). An inverse correlation between factor XIII and percentage of HMWFC was demonstrated in the early stages of the illness. *1491*

Fibrin Split Products (FSP) *Plasma Increase* Clinical severity of infarction is related to the degree of elevation. Mortality rate was 22% among patients with values 20 µg/dL and 11% in those < 20 µg/dL. *1728*

Gamma Glutamyl Transferase (GGT) *Serum Increase* Usually remains in the normal range for 3-4 days, then increases to reach a peak about the 8-11th day after infarction. *0684* Activity is raised in association with anoxic damage to the liver, and also in association with recovery and repair. *0619* Increased in 50% of patients with shock or acute right heart failure, may have early peak within 48 h with rapid decline followed by later rise. *2467   0439 0675*

Glucose *Serum Increase* Glycosuria and hyperglycemia occur in up to 50% of patients. *2467* May be partially related to pituitary-sympathoadrenal stimulation. May occur in patients who are not obviously diabetic; attributed to adrenal stimulation secondary to stress and shock. *1108* Patients have higher fasting concentrations and dispose of an oral glucose load less efficiently than controls. *2104* In 70% of 119 patients hospitalized for this disorder. *0781 1451 0962*

Urine Increase Glycosuria and hyperglycemia occur in up to 50% of patients. *2467* May occur in patients who are not obviously diabetic; attributed to adrenal stimulation secondary to stress and shock. *1108*

Glucose Tolerance *Serum Decrease* Some patients will have abnormal curves when checked months later. *1108*

Haptoglobin *Serum Increase* Significant increase. *1724*

Hemagglutination Inhibition *Serum Increase* Using the passive hemagglutination reaction, a 4-fold or greater rise in antibodies to saline extracts of human heart in 46% of 50 patients was found. Highest titers and highest frequency of elevated titers occurred 2-4 weeks after onset. *1018 2035*

Hematocrit *Blood Decrease* After an initial small increase, decreased 12% until day 9 and remained constant thereafter. *2215* Significant increases in plasma volume, reflected by changes in hct. Average change was 12%. For the patients with accompanying pulmonary edema, the change was 17%. *2554*

Blood Increase Volume may be decreased, together with a slight increase in hct. *1108* After an initial small increase, decreased 12% until day 9 and remained constant thereafter. *2215 2554 0316*

Hexosaminidase *Serum Increase* Increase in total concentration (hexosaminidase A and B). *1716*

Hypoxanthine *Serum Increase* Myocardial ischemia in 18 patients resulted in an increase of coronary sinus hypoxanthine levels from 1.20 ± 0.52 mg/dL during pain. *1911*

Iron *Serum Decrease* *2538 0975*

Isocitrate Dehydrogenase *Serum Normal* Concentrations were within normal limits in assays performed within 24 h after onset of symptoms. *2260*

Lactate Dehydrogenase *Serum Increase* Rises 2-10 fold after the first 12 h and reaches a peak by 24-48 h. The increase is roughly parallel to the degree of cardiac damage and also to the serum AST. *0619* May remain elevated up to 10-14 days after onset; therefore is particularly useful when patient is first seen after sufficient time has elapsed for CK and AST to become normal. *2467* Moderate elevations in almost all patients (92-98%) with proven infarction. The complication by shock leads to higher values of AST and LD and to abnormal levels of enzymes that reflect hepatic injury (ALT, ICD). *0503* Concentrations 2,000 U/L suggest a poor prognosis. *2467 0088 0812 0191*

Urine Increase *2467*

Lactate Dehydrogenase Isoenzyme 5 (LD$_5$) *Serum Increase* Almost invariably increased, beginning 12 h after infarction and peaking after 48 h. *1390* Parallels increase of fast moving LD with peak (3-4 X normal) in 48 h and persistent elevation for up to 2 weeks. *2467*

Lactate Dehydrogenase Isoenzymes *Serum Increase* LD$_1$ is markedly increased. *1071* Increased LD$_1$ and LD$_2$. May remain elevated after total LD is normalized. In small infarctions, LD$_1$ may be increased when total LD remains normal. In acute infarction with congestive heart failure, LD$_1$ and LD$_5$ are elevated. Distinguish infarction from other diseases which elevate total LD. Heat-stable, fast moving fractions increased in infarction. *2467 0812*

Lactic Acid *Blood Increase* Patients may develop arterial and tissue hypoxia and metabolic acidosis with a decrease in arterial pH and pO$_2$, together with an increase in blood lactate concentration. *1108 0731*

Leukocytes *Blood Increase* Almost invariable. 75-90% neutrophils with only a slight shift to the left. Leukocytosis is likely to develop before fever. *2467* Patients with transmural infarcts had a significantly higher count than patients with nontransmural infarcts. *1365* Mean count was significantly elevated in 464 patients, measured, on the average, 16.8 months before the infarction occurred. Total WBC was closely related to development of infarct and to cigarette smoking. *0778 1108 0781*

Malate Dehydrogenase *Serum Increase* Elevated 2-10 X above normal in all cases of clinically proved infarction. *2443* Level rises after 6-24 h to a peak at 24-48 h (2-15 X normal), falling to normal by 5 days. The peak precedes AST and LD, and degree is similar to rise in AST. *0619* Always elevated, sometimes strikingly. *0210*

Myoglobin *Serum Increase* Very common; first appears in serum within a few h after infarction, reaching a peak before the peak of CK activity. Did not correlate with infarct size as estimated by CK. *1208*

Urine Increase Sporadic; ischemic. *2467*

Neutrophils *Blood Increase* Increase of polymorphonuclear leukocytes, with an increase in young forms. *1108* In 58% of 100 patients hospitalized for this disorder. *0781*

Nickel *Serum Decrease* Decreases occur soon after infarction (within 24 h for Caucasian males and before the 3rd day in Caucasian females and Black males), followed by a sharp rise to > 2 X normal value. *2502*

Serum Increase Decrease occurs soon after infarction (within 24 h for Caucasian males and before the 3rd day in Caucasian females and Black males), followed by a sharp rise to > 2 X normal value. *2502* Mean 5.2 µg/L (N = 33) compared with control mean of 2.6 µg/L (N = 42). *1559*

Norepinephrine *Plasma Increase* Evidence for a sympathoadrenal response is found in the increased blood and urinary concentration or norepinephrine, epinephrine, or their metabolic products. *1108 1163 1451*

Urine Increase Evidence for sympathoadrenal response is found in the increased blood and urinary concentration or norepinephrine, epinephrine, or their metabolic products. *1108* In patients developing heart failure or cardiogenic shock, the urinary level of both free catecholamines rose notably in the 1st week after infarction. In uncomplicated cases, a moderate rise in the norepinephrine level in the 1st week was associated with only a transient rise in the epinephrine level. *1163*

Oxygen Saturation *Blood Decrease* Very frequent complication; occurs in about 60% of uncomplicated cases. The intensity of hypoxemia is greatest after 2-3 days. The most intense and persisting hypoxemia was seen in patients with shock and/or acute left ventricular failure. Present even 6 months after onset in 25%. *2529* Patients may develop arterial and tissue hypoxia and metabolic acidosis with a decrease in arterial pH and pO$_2$. *1108* Arterial pO$_2$ falls, but rarely below 70 mm Hg if there is reasonable cardiovascular function. In left ventricular failure with associated pulmonary edema, the arterial pO$_2$ may fall to 50 mm Hg. *0619 0731*

pH *Blood Decrease* Slight metabolic acidosis was observed on the first day of the disease in 37% of the cases, while severe metabolic acidosis was found in 50-60% of the cases during 1 year after myocardial infarction. *2529* Patients may develop arterial and tissue hypoxia and metabolic acidosis with an increase in blood lactate concentration. *1108* Following cardiac arrest, acidosis rapidly develops, and, if not corrected, can result in the inability to defibrillate the heart in ventricular fibrillation. *0962 0731*

CSF Decrease In patients who developed severe anoxia after cardiac arrest, the normal cisternal-lumbar pH gradient was reversed, cisternal fluid was more acid (pH 6.815 vs 6.953), and cisternal potassium concentration was twice that of lumbar (6.7 vs 3.5 mmol/L). During anoxia, potassium and hydrogen ions flow from brain cells into the brain extracellular fluid. Acute changes are reflected more accurately by cisternal than by lumbar fluid. *1213*

Phospholipids, Total *Serum Increase* Mean concentration was increased to 249.5 ± 7.6 mg/L in 69 male patients, compared to 204.1 ± 3.5 in normals. *0381*

Plasma Cells *Serum Decrease* *2357 0659 0683*

Platelet Aggregation *Blood Decrease* Significantly reduced the first few days. *1289*

pO$_2$ *Blood Decrease* Very frequent complication; occurs in 60% of uncomplicated cases. The intensity of hypoxemia is greatest after 2-3 days. The most intense and persisting hypoxemia was seen in patients with shock and/or acute left ventricular failure. Present even 6 months after onset in 25%. *2529* Patients may develop arterial and tissue hypoxia and metabolic acidosis with a decrease in arterial pH and pO$_2$. *1108* Arterial pO$_2$ falls, but rarely below 70 mm Hg if there is reasonable cardiovascular function. In left ventricular failure with associated pulmonary edema, the arterial pO$_2$ may fall to 50 mm Hg. *0619 0731*

Potassium *CSF Increase* In patients who developed severe anoxia after a cardiac arrest, the cisternal K$^+$ concentration was twice that of lumbar (6.7 vs 3.5 mmol/L). During anoxia, K$^+$ and H$^+$ flow from brain cells into the brain extracellular fluid. Acute changes are reflected more accurately by cisternal than by lumbar fluid. *1213* Of 41 patients with cardiac arrest studied, 20 regained consciousness and 21 did not. In those who did not, was a significant increase in the K$^+$ concentration found in samples obtained between 40-50 min and between 50-60 min after cardiac arrest. Potassium concentration of cisternal CSF obtained soon after cardiac arrest might give an indication of the degree of cerebral damage. *2159*

410.90   Acute Myocardial Infarction   *(continued)*

Pseudocholinesterase   *Serum   Decrease*   May occur with decrease in serum albumin. *2467*

Rheumatoid Factor   *Serum   Increase*   Found in 12% of patients. *0422 0123*

Sodium   *Serum   Decrease*   Frequent hyponatremia, degree of loss seems to correlate with severity of myocardial involvement. *2104*

Triglycerides   *Serum   Increase*   Rises to peak in 3 weeks; the increase may persist for 1 year. *2467*   Mean concentration was 92.5 ± 3.5 mg/dL in 69 male patients, compared to 76.1 ± 3.7 in controls. *0381*   Tends to be moderately elevated for a few weeks following a brief decrease. *1108   0771*

Tri-iodothyronine (T$_3$)   *Serum   Decrease*   Decreased to 66% at day 9 and then returned to normal within 2 months. *2215*

Urea Nitrogen   *Serum   Increase*   In 36% of 119 patients hospitalized for this disorder. *0781*   18 of 22 patients showed elevations at some time during the study, usually within 3 days after admission. *2530   2467*

Uric Acid   *Serum   Increase*   In several studies, mean concentration ranged from 5.13 ± 1.10 to 7.32 mg/dL. Males were found to have a higher concentration (8.25 - 1.21) than females (7.16 ± 1.17) compared to normal, 3.59 ± 0.80, 3.01 ± 0.82, respectively. *2184*   Frequently occurs. *0599*   In 60% of 110 patients hospitalized for this disorder. *0781   0962*

Viscosity   *Serum   Increase*   Due to alterations in serum proteins during the acute phase of illness. *1108   1146*

Volume   *Plasma   Decrease*   Probably the result of reflex adrenergic discharge and vasoconstriction, pooling or trapping of blood, sweating, or the development of pulmonary edema. *1108*

Plasma   Increase   Significant increases in plasma volume, reflected by changes in hct. Average change was 12%. For the patients with accompanying pulmonary edema, the change was 17%. *2554*

Zinc   *Serum   Decrease*   A significant decrease was observed. *2428*   Falls immediately to low levels following a myocardial infarction, rising to the original normal level over the next 10-14 days. *0962*

413.90   Angina Pectoris

Aspartate Aminotransferase   *Serum   Normal   2467*

Bilirubin   *Serum   Normal   2467*

Creatine Kinase   *Serum   Normal   2467*

Creatinine   *Serum   Increase*   In 60% of 50 patients hospitalized for this disorder. *0781*

Erythrocyte Sedimentation Rate   *Blood   Normal*   May be helpful in distinguishing this entity from acute myocardial infarction. *0962*

Factor IV   *Plasma   Increase*   Patients with chest pain but without evidence of infarction had a mean of 29 ng/mL. Elevation persisted for 1 week and returned to normal. *0974*

Gamma Glutamyl Transferase (GGT)   *Serum   Increase*   *1016*

Lactate Dehydrogenase   *Serum   Normal*   In 89% of 75 patients hospitalized for this disorder. *0781   2467*

Lactate Dehydrogenase Isoenzyme 5 (LD$_5$)   *Serum   Normal   2467*

Uric Acid   *Serum   Increase*   In 55% of 72 patients hospitalized for this disorder. *0781*

414.00   Chronic Ischemic Heart Disease

Alpha$_2$-Globulin   *Serum   Increase*   Rapid increase occurs before the rise in the gamma fraction. *0619*

Apolipoprotein AI   *Serum   Decrease*   In each major study group mean high density lipoproteins were lower in persons with coronary heart disease than in those without the disease. The average difference was small--typically 3-4 mg/dL -- but statistically significant. *0357*

Apolipoprotein B   *Serum   Increase*   Patients with Coronary Artery Disease had increased levels. *1505*

Bicarbonate   *Serum   Increase*   In 62% of 434 patients hospitalized for this disorder. *0781*

Carcinoembryonic Antigen   *Serum   Increase*   39% of patients had values > 2.5 ng/mL. *2199*

Catecholamines   *Plasma   Increase*   Epinephrine and norepinephrine increase in proportion to the severity of circulatory failure. Catecholamine excretion, especially norepinephrine, is significantly raised in grades 3 and 4 of hemodynamic disturbance. *2572*

Urine   Increase   Epinephrine and norepinephrine increase in proportion to the severity of circulatory failure. Catecholamine excretion, especially norepinephrine, is significantly raised in grades 3 and 4 of hemodynamic disturbance. *2572*

Cholesterol   *Serum   Increase*   Studies of patients with coronary atherosclerotic heart disease and of their families have indicated a significantly higher incidence (16-44%) of elevated plasma cholesterol and/or triglyceride levels, usually classified as type II or type IV. *1108*

Copper   *Serum   Decrease*   Epidemiologic and metabolic data are consistent with the hypothesis that a metabolic imbalance in regard to zinc and copper is a major factor in the etiology of coronary heart disease. A metabolic imbalance is either a relative or an absolute deficiency of copper characterized by a high ratio of zinc to copper. The imbalance results in hypercholesterolemia and an increased mortality due to coronary heart disease. *1280*

Creatinine   *Serum   Increase*   In 58% of 312 patients hospitalized for this disorder. *0781*

Cryoglobulins   *Serum   Increase*   Variable elevation of cryoglobulins. *2104*

Epinephrine   *Urine   Increase*   Increased in proportion to the severity of circulatory failure. Catecholamine excretion is significantly raised in grades 3 and 4 of hemodynamic disturbance. *2572*

Glucose Tolerance   *Serum   Decrease*   Reported in as many as 50% of patients with coronary artery disease. *0962*

Hypoxanthine   *Serum   Increase*   Myocardial ischemia in 18 patients resulted in an increase of coronary sinus hypoxanthine levels from 1.20 ± 0.52 mg/dL during pain. *1911*

Lactic Acid   *Blood   Increase*   Early lactate production occurred frequently before angina was noted. *1911*

Lipids   *Serum   Increase*   The severity of atherosclerosis was slightly positively correlated with triglyceride concentration, especially in the younger patients and (not significantly) with plasma cholesterol concentration. Hyperlipidemia was present in 58.8% of patients. *0508*   Studies of patients with coronary atherosclerotic heart disease and of their families have indicated a significantly higher incidence (16-44%) of elevated plasma cholesterol and/or triglyceride levels, usually classified as type II or type IV. *1108*

Magnesium   *Serum   Decrease*   May occur in the course of the disease. *2107*

Norepinephrine   *Urine   Increase*   Increased in proportion to the severity of circulatory failure. Catecholamine excretion especially norepinephrine, is significantly raised in grades 3 and 4 of hemodynamic disturbance. *2572*

pH   *Blood   Increase*   In 48% of 184 patients hospitalized for this disorder. *0781*

Triglycerides   *Serum   Increase*   The severity of atherosclerosis was positively correlated with plasma concentration, especially in the younger patients (R = 0.29, P < 0.05), and (not significantly) with plasma cholesterol concentration. *0508*   Studies of patients with coronary atherosclerotic heart disease and of their families have indicated a significantly higher incidence (16-44%) of elevated plasma cholesterol and/or triglyceride levels, usually classified as type II or type IV. *1108*

Uric Acid   *Serum   Increase*   Occurs frequently. In 92 young adults with coronary heart disease, mean level was 5.13 - 0.12, ranging from 3.0-7.8 mg/dL. *0599*   In 59% of 475 patients hospitalized for this disorder. *0781   2184*

Vanillylamine   *Urine   Increase*   Increased excretion was observed in cases of grade 4 hemodynamic disturbance. *2572*

Zinc   *Serum   Increase*   Epidemiologic and metabolic data are consistent with the hypothesis that a metabolic imbalance in regard to zinc and copper is a major factor in the etiology of coronary heart disease. A metabolic imbalance is either a relative or an absolute deficiency of copper characterized by a high ratio of zinc to copper. The imbalance results in hypercholesterolemia and an increased mortality due to coronary heart disease. *1280*

415.00   Cor Pulmonale

Ammonia   *Blood   Increase*   Due to hepatic congestion. *2411*

Catecholamines   *Plasma   Increase*   Epinephrine and norepinephrine increase in proportion to the severity of circulatory failure. Catecholamine excretion, especially norepinephrine, is significantly raised in grades 3 and 4 of hemodynamic disturbance. *2572*

Urine   Increase   Epinephrine and norepinephrine increase in proportion to the severity of circulatory failure. Catecholamine excretion, especially norepinephrine, is significantly raised in grades 3 and 4 of hemodynamic disturbance. *2572*

Epinephrine   *Urine   Increase*   Increased in proportion to the severity of circulatory failure. Catecholamine excretion is significantly raised in grades 3 and 4 of hemodynamic disturbance. *2572*

Erythrocytes   *Blood   Increase*   Secondary polycythemia. *2467* Erythrocytosis, secondary to chronic hypoxemia may be prominent, especially in bronchitic patients. *1108*

Hematocrit   *Blood   Increase*   Secondary polycythemia. *2141*

Hemoglobin   *Blood   Increase*   Secondary polycythemia. *2141*

Norepinephrine   *Urine   Increase*   Increased in proportion to the severity of circulatory failure. Catecholamine excretion, especially norepinephrine, is significantly raised in grades 3 and 4 of hemodynamic disturbance. *2572*

Oxygen Saturation   *Blood   Decrease*   Acute hypoxia and hypermetabolism associated with fever and infection. *1108*

pCO$_2$ *Blood   Increase*   The degree of arterial pCO$_2$ elevation is in direct proportion to the inadequacy of alveolar ventilation in relation to metabolic production of CO$_2$. *1108*   Increased when Cor Pulmonale is secondary to chest deformities or pulmonary emphysema. *2467*

pO$_2$ *Blood   Decrease*   Acute hypoxia and hypermetabolism associated with fever and infection. *1108*

Vanillylamine   *Urine   Increase*   Increased excretion observed in cases of grade 4 hemodynamic disturbance. *2572*

Viscosity   *Serum   Increase*   An increase in blood viscosity, red blood cell mass, and blood volume is thought to further compromise the pressure-flow relationships of the constricted and restricted pulmonary vascular bed. *1108*

Volume   *Plasma   Increase*   An increase in blood viscosity, red blood cell mass, and blood volume is thought to further compromise the pressure-flow relationships of the constricted and restricted pulmonary vascular bed. *1108*

415.10   Pulmonary Embolism and Infarction

Acid Phosphatase   *Serum   Increase*   *0812*

Alanine Aminotransferase   *Serum   Increase*   Slight increase. *0962*

Aldolase   *Serum   Increase*   Moderate increase found, with no sharp peak as in myocardial infarction. *0619   0962*

Alkaline Phosphatase   *Serum   Increase*   Elevation is temporary and found at maximum value within 1-3 weeks after embolism. *0562* In 30% of 19 patients at initial hospitalization for this disorder. *0781*

Amylase   *Pleural Effusion   Increase*   *2017*   May occur *1584*

Pleural Effusion   Normal   Usually less than or equal to serum level. *2017*

Antithrombin Titer   *Blood   Decrease*   About 2% of venous thromboembolism is due to antithrombin III deficiency. *1108*

Aspartate Aminotransferase   *Serum   Increase*   Rises later and slower than after cardiac infarction. Possibly related to associated congestive failure. *0619*   Characterized by increased LD and usually by normal AST values. Incidence of elevation has varied from 0-30% and the elevations are slight to moderate. The rise is delayed for 3-5 days after onset of pain. *2467*   In a small proportion of patients with this disease slightly elevated values occur by 3 or 4 days after the bout of chest pain. *0503*   Slight increase. *0962   2474 1748*

Cold Agglutinins   *Serum   Increase*   Implicated as cause of intravascular thrombosis, but their role is neither clear nor constant. *1108*

Creatine Kinase   *Serum   Increase*   For reasons that are still unclear some cases may have high levels. *0812*

Serum   Normal   The absence of elevated CK and the presence of increased LD in conjunction with other diagnostic techniques can be used to distinguish pulmonary from myocardial infarction. *2467 0437 0962*

Cryofibrinogen   *Serum   Increase*   Implicated as a cause of intravascular thrombosis, but their role is neither clear nor constant. *1108*

Cryoglobulins   *Serum   Increase*   Implicated as a cause of intravascular thrombosis, but their role is neither clear nor constant. *1108*

Cryomacroglobulins   *Serum   Increase*   Implicated as a cause of intravascular thrombosis, but their role is neither clear nor constant. *1108*

Erythrocytes   *Pleural Effusion   Increase*   Pleural effusions in association with infarction often are bloody. *1108*   In about 10% of cases. *0503*   1000-100,000/μL *2017*

Sputum   Increase   Blood-streaked or grossly bloody sputum. *1108*

Erythrocyte Sedimentation Rate   *Blood   Increase*   Elevated in most patients. *0999*

Factor IV   *Plasma   Increase*   Markedly elevated in patients with embolic or cardiorespiratory failure. *0974*

Fibrinogen   *Plasma   Increase*   Implicated as a cause of intravascular thrombosis, but their role is neither clear nor constant. *1108 0347*

Fibrin Split Products (FSP)   *Plasma   Increase*   42% of 24 patients suspected of acute thrombophlebitis and 50% of 14 patients with documented pulmonary emboli had positive fibrinogen tests. *0347*

Glucose   *Serum   Increase*   In 44% of 21 patients at initial hospitalization for this disorder. *0781*

Pleural Effusion   Normal   Pleural Fluid = Serum level. *2017*

Lactate Dehydrogenase   *Serum   Increase*   2-4 X normal values. Increased within 24 h of onset of pain. *0503*   Combination of increased LD and a normal AST present in 60-75% of patients. *0999* Characteristically a rise of activity and in about 50% of cases no rise of AST activity. Initially considered to be diagnostic, has been shown repeatedly to be not the case. *1108*   Frequently elevated within 5 days after the embolic event. Too nonspecific to be diagnostic. *0962 2445 0781*

Serum   Normal   Values may be normal in the presence of embolism. *1108*

Pleural Effusion   Increase   Exudate. *0062*

Lactate Dehydrogenase Isoenzyme 5 (LD$_5$)   *Serum   Increase* Elevated to 8.4% of the total LD value of 736 U/L in 5 cases of pulmonary embolism. *0852*

Lactate Dehydrogenase Isoenzymes   *Serum   Increase*   LD$_3$ without hemorrhage into lung. LD$_1$, LD$_2$, LD$_3$: with hemorrhage into lung. LD$_3$ and LD$_5$, embolus with acute Cor Pulmonale causing acute congestion of liver. *2467*   There is some disagreement about whether the LD is elevated in pulmonary infarction, but elevated levels of LD$_3$ are found. *2467 0812*

Leukocytes   *Blood   Increase*   Characteristically rises to 10,000-15,000/μL, and occasionally higher. Usually a modest preponderance of polymorphonuclear cells. *1108*   Usually normal in pulmonary embolism. With pulmonary infarction there may be a relative increase in neutrophils and a leukocytosis. *0962*   In 44% of 24 patients at initial hospitalization for this disorder. *0781*

Blood   Normal   Count rarely exceeds 15,000/μL and is usually < 10,000 with little shift to left. This aids in the differential diagnosis of pulmonary embolism and pneumonia. *2126*   Usually normal with pulmonary embolism. With pulmonary infarction there may be a relative increase in neutrophils and a leukocytosis. *0962*

Neutrophils   *Blood   Increase*   In 40% of 22 patients at initial hospitalization for this disorder. *0781*   With pulmonary infarction there may be a relative increase in neutrophils and a leukocytosis. *0962*

Pleural Effusion   Increase   Predominant cell type. *2017*   Neutrophils predominate in pleural fluid *1403*

Oxygen Saturation   *Blood   Decrease*   pO$_2$ > 80 mm Hg excludes diagnosis of pulmonary embolism in almost all cases. *2126*   pO$_2$ and pCO$_2$ are both low. *1721*   Abnormal alveolar-arterial gradient for oxygen and resting hypoxemia. Arterial pO$_2$ fails to exceed 55 mm Hg following 100% oxygen breathing. *0962*

pCO$_2$ *Blood   Decrease*   Decreased pO$_2$ associated with normal or decreased pCO$_2$. *2467*   pO$_2$ and pCO$_2$ are both low. *1721*   In 62% of 19 patients at initial hospitalization for this disorder. *0781*

pH   *Blood   Increase*   May be alkaline in the acute stages. *1721* In 89% of 19 patients at initial hospitalization for this disorder. *0781*

Pleural Effusion   Decrease   Exudate (pH < 7.3). *0062*

Plasma Cells   *Serum   Decrease*   Depressed. *2357 0659 0683*

Platelet Count   *Blood   Increase*   Implicated as a cause of intravascular thrombosis, but their role is neither clear nor constant. *1108*   In 19% of 15 patients at initial hospitalization for this disorder. *0781*

pO$_2$ *Blood   Decrease*   pO$_2$ > 80 mm Hg excludes diagnosis of pulmonary embolism in almost all cases. *2126*   pO$_2$ and pCO$_2$ are both low. *1721*   Abnormal alveolar-arterial gradient for oxygen and resting hypoxemia. Arterial pO$_2$ fails to exceed 55 mm Hg following 100% oxygen breathing. *0962*   In 86% of 17 patients at initial hospitalization for this disorder. *0781*

Protein   *Pleural Effusion   Increase*   Exudative effusion in about 50% of cases. *0503*

Specific Gravity   *Pleural Effusion   Increase*   Exudate (> 1.016). *0062*

Urobilinogen   *Urine   Increase*   Hemorrhage into tissues. *2467*

420.00　Acute Pericarditis

Alanine Aminotransferase　*Serum*　*Increase*　0962

Aspartate Aminotransferase　*Serum*　*Increase*　50% incidence of slightly elevated values reported. Usual values < 48.2 U/L. *0503* Modest elevations occur. This is especially likely to happen when pericardial effusion produces venous hypertension and hepatic congestion. *1108　0962*

Cells　*Pericardial Fluid*　*Decrease*　Few lymphocytes or RBCs. *0758*

Creatine Kinase　*Serum*　*Normal*　2467

Glucose　*Pericardial Fluid*　*Normal*　Same as serum level. *0758*

Lactate Dehydrogenase　*Pericardial Fluid*　*Decrease*　Less than 60% of serum levels. *0758*

Leukocytes　*Blood*　*Decrease*　Normal or low in viral or Tuberculous Pericarditis. *0758*

　Blood　*Increase*　Usually increased in proportion to fever; normal or low in viral disease and tuberculous pericarditis; markedly increased in suppurative bacterial pericarditis. *2467* Often increased but may be within normal limits. *1108*

　Blood　*Normal*　Normal or low in viral or Tuberculous Pericarditis. *0758*

Protein　*Pericardial Fluid*　*Decrease*　Less than 50% of serum levels. *0758*

421.00　Bacterial Endocarditis

Albumin　*Serum*　*Decrease*　Mildly depressed, mean = 3.0 ± 0.1 g/dL. Lowest values found in pneumococcal infection 2.4 ± 0.4 g/dL. *1798*

　Urine　*Increase*　Almost invariably present, even when no renal lesions are found with bacterial endocarditis. *2468*

Cephalin Flocculation　*Serum*　*Increase*　Positive due to altered serum proteins and increase in gamma globulin. *2467*

Complement C3　*Serum*　*Decrease*　Decreased total C3 and C4, with conversion products of both, in subacute endocarditis. *2522* Decreased total hemolytic complement or C3 in 8 of 17 or 47% of patients tested. 7 of the 8 had evidence of renal disease. *1798*

Complement C4　*Serum*　*Decrease*　Decreased total C3 and C4, with conversion products of both, in subacute endocarditis. *2522*

Complement, Total　*Serum*　*Decrease*　Decreased total hemolytic complement in 8 of 17 or 47% of patients tested. 7 of the 8 had evidence of renal disease. *1798* Decreased total C3 and C4, with conversion products of both, in subacute endocarditis. *2522*

Coombs' Test　*Blood*　*Positive*　Rarely there is hemolytic anemia with a positive Coombs' test. *2467*

Creatinine　*Serum*　*Increase*　Elevated in patients with diffuse glomerulonephritis and chronic infective endocarditis. *0433* Increase parallels BUN elevation; higher concentration found in fatal cases than in survivors. *1798*

Cryoglobulins　*Serum*　*Increase*　Variable elevation of cryoglobulins. *2104*

Erythrocyte Casts　*Urine*　*Increase*　Found in 12% of patients. *1798* Casts are seen in the occasional patient with diffuse glomerulonephritis. *0433*

Erythrocytes　*Urine*　*Increase*　Hematuria (usually microscopic) occurs at some stage in many cases due to glomerulitis or renal infarct or focal embolic glomerulonephritis. *2467* Microscopic hematuria found in 55% of patients. *1798* Hematuria even without renal involvement *2488　0433*

Erythrocyte Sedimentation Rate　*Blood*　*Increase*　Usually elevated with a mean of 57.3 ± 3.6 mm/h. Mean ESR in survivors, 77.5, was significantly higher than in fatalities, 40.7 mm/h. *1798* Elevated in 90% of cases but is of no differential aid in the work-up of fever of unknown origin. *1108* Increased in 90% of cases. A normal ESR is useful in excluding this diagnosis. *0962　2488*

Gamma Globulin　*Serum*　*Increase*　2488

Globulin　*Serum*　*Increase*　Seen in about 50% of patients *0999* . Mean = 3.7 ± 0.1 g/dL in 125 cases of various types of infection. *1798 2104*

Hematocrit　*Blood*　*Decrease*　Anemia is more common in long-standing infection and has no specificity. *0433* Rarely there is a hemolytic anemia with a positive Coombs' test. *2467* Normocytic normochromic anemia commonly presents with mean hct = 35.5 ± 0.6%. Lowest hcts found in gram-negative (29.8 ± 3.1%) and culture-negative cases (30.4 ± 1.6%). Degree of anemia is related to duration of illness, not virulence of organism. *1798* Normochromic, normocytic anemia occurs in 60-70% of cases. *1108*

Hemoglobin　*Blood*　*Decrease*　Anemia is more common in long-standing infection and has no specificity. *0433* Rarely there is a hemolytic anemia with a positive Coombs' test. *2467* Normocytic normochromic anemia commonly present with mean hct = 35.5 ± 0.6%. Lowest hcts found in gram-negative (29.8 ±3.1%) and culture-negative cases (30.4 ± 1.6%). Degree of anemia is related to duration of illness, not virulence of organism. *1798* Normochromic, normocytic anemia occurs in 60-70% of cases. *1108*

Iron　*Serum*　*Decrease*　2467

Leukocytes　*Blood*　*Decrease*　Occasional leukopenia. *2467* Of little value in bacterial endocarditis, in which normal, high, and low counts may occur. *0962*

　Blood　*Increase*　Normal in about 50% of patients and elevated up to about 15,000/µL in the rest, with 65-85% neutrophils. Higher count indicates presence of a complication. Occasionally there is leukopenia. *2467* Only slight leukocytosis is expected in subacute cases, and even this is absent in about 50% of patients. Leukocytosis 15,000/µL is common with acute disease. *0999* Counts ranged widely; mean = 12,700 ± 600/µL. Highest in pneumococcal (17,300 ± 3,400/µL), gram-negative (16,800 ± 4,300/µL) and S. Aureus (13,900 ± 1,000/µL). *1798　0962*

　Blood　*Normal*　Normal in about 50% of patients and elevated up to about 15,000/µL in the rest. *2467 2488* May be normal, low, or elevated. Normal counts are just as prevalent as elevated counts. *1108　0590*

　CSF　*Increase*　May reach 100/µL, mostly polymorphonuclears and lymphocytes in bacterial endocarditis with embolism. *0151*

Monocytes　*Blood*　*Increase*　Elevated WBC up to about 15,000/µL in 50%. Monocytosis may be pronounced. *2467* Found in 15-20% of patients but is not correlated with the presence or number of peripheral phagocytic reticuloendothelial cells. *0488　2538*

Neutrophils　*Blood*　*Increase*　Usually increased numbers of immature granulocytes are found in the blood. *0999* Elevated WBC in 50% of patients with 65-85% neutrophils. *2467* Normal or elevated to 15,000 with 65-85% neutrophils *2488*

pCO₂　*Blood*　*Decrease*　In 14 narcotic addicts with bacterial endocarditis the arterial CO_2 tension, at 27.8 ± 1.7 mm Hg, was significantly lower than a group of narcotics with other disorders, at 40.1 ± 3.7 mm Hg. *1725*

pH　*Blood*　*Increase*　In 14 narcotic addicts with bacterial endocarditis, the blood pH, at 7.47 ± 0.01 was significantly higher than in a group of narcotics with other disorders, at 7.36 ± 0.06. *1725*

Platelet Count　*Blood*　*Decrease*　Usually normal but occasionally it is decreased; rarely purpura occurs. *2467*

　Blood　*Normal*　Usually normal but occasionally it is decreased; rarely purpura occurs. *2467*

Protein　*Urine*　*Increase*　Mild to moderate proteinuria is common as a result of joint and muscle inflammation. *0151*

　CSF　*Increase*　Slightly elevated in infection with embolism. *0151*

Rheumatoid Factor　*Serum*　*Increase*　Elevated levels of IgG and IgM rheumatoid factor were found in patients with subacute infection. *0348* 13 (24%) of 55 patients were seropositive at some point in their courses. More severe cases were more likely to develop rheumatoid factor. *2132* May be used to confirm the diagnosis. Following remission, titers fall to 0. *0962* Positive in 17 of 36 patients but did not correlate with renal failure. *1798　2035*

Thymol Turbidity　*Serum*　*Increase*　Increased due to altered serum proteins and increased gamma globulins. *2467*

Urea Nitrogen　*Serum*　*Increase*　Increased--usually 25-75 mg/dL. *2468　0433 1798*

421.91　Loeffler's Endocarditis

Eosinophils　*Blood*　*Increase*　Eosinophilia up to 70%; may be absent at first but appears sooner or later. *2467* Marked eosinophilia of the blood associated with diffuse organ infiltration by eosinophils. *1108　2538*

Immunoglobulin IgM　*Serum*　*Increase*　Especially when particulate antigenic material is present in the blood stream. *0619*

Leukocytes　*Blood*　*Increase*　Frequently increased. *2467*

422.00　Acute Myocarditis

Aspartate Aminotransferase　*Serum*　*Increase*　Marked elevation signals a poor prognosis. *1108*

Complement Fixation　*Serum*　*Increase*　Positive in helminthic myocarditis. *1108*

Creatine Kinase *Serum Increase* Elevated cardiac enzymes may be the earliest evidence of myocarditis. *1108*

Eosinophils *Blood Increase* Characteristic of helminthic myocarditis. *1108*

Lactate Dehydrogenase *Serum Increase* Elevated cardiac enzymes may be the earliest evidence of myocarditis. *1108*

Neutralizing Antibodies *Serum Increase* In viral myocarditis. *1108*

Neutrophils *Blood Decrease* Crisis is characterized by acute neutropenia and respiratory alkalosis. *1108*

pH *Blood Increase* Crisis is characterized by acute neutropenia and respiratory alkalosis. *1108*

423.10 Constrictive Pericarditis

Albumin *Serum Decrease* Decreased with normal total protein. *2467* *0999*

BSP Retention *Serum Increase* *2467*

Cold Agglutinins *Serum Increase* *2035*

Lactate Dehydrogenase *Pleural Effusion Decrease* Transudate. *0062*

Lymphocytes *Blood Decrease* *0999*

pH *Pleural Effusion Increase* Transudate (pH > 7.3). *0062*

Protein *Serum Decrease* Enteric loss of plasma protein. *2199*
Pleural Effusion Decrease Transudate secondary to increased hydrostatic pressure. (< 3 g/dL). *0062*

Specific Gravity *Pleural Effusion Decrease* Transudate (< 1.016). *0062*

Thymol Turbidity *Serum Increase* Increased in some cases. *2467*

425.40 Cardiomyopathies

Aspartate Aminotransferase *Serum Increase* Increased, often to extremely high levels; these may rise even further after recovery from shock in cobalt beer cardiomyopathy. *2467*

BSP Retention *Serum Increase* Disordered liver function in advanced cases of obliterative cardiomyopathy. *1108*

Creatine Kinase *Serum Increase* Increased, often to extremely high levels; may rise even further after recovery from shock in cobalt beer cardiomyopathy. *2467*

Eosinophils *Blood Increase* Mild to moderate eosinophilia. Marked in Loeffler's eosinophilic cardiomyopathy. *1108* *2227*

Erythrocytes *Blood Increase* Increased, often to extremely high levels; may rise even further after recovery from shock in cobalt beer cardiomyopathy. *2467*
Ascitic Fluid Increase Ascitic fluid and pericardial fluid are usually blood-stained or serous and contain leukocytes in obliterative cardiomyopathies. *1108*
Pericardial Fluid Increase Ascitic fluid and pericardial fluid are usually blood-stained or serous and contain leukocytes in obliterative cardiomyopathies. *1108*

Erythrocyte Sedimentation Rate *Blood Increase* Often elevated in Loeffler's disease. *1108*

Globulin *Serum Increase* May be found and are probably the result of hepatic insufficiency due to heart failure. *1108*

Hematocrit *Blood Decrease* A slight degree of anemia with obliterative cardiomyopathies. *1108*

Hemoglobin *Blood Decrease* A slight degree of anemia in obliterative cardiomyopathies. *1108*

Iron *Serum Decrease* Occasionally low. *1108*

Lactate Dehydrogenase *Serum Increase* Increased, often to extremely high levels; may rise even further after recovery from shock in cobalt beer cardiomyopathy. *2467*

Lactic Acid *Blood Increase* Lactic acidosis and shock in cobalt beer myopathies. *2467*

Leukocytes *Ascitic Fluid Increase* Ascitic fluid and pericardial fluid are usually blood-stained or serous and contain leukocytes in obliterative cardiomyopathies. *1108*
Pericardial Fluid Increase Ascitic fluid and pericardial fluid are usually blood-stained or serous and contain leukocytes in obliterative cardiomyopathies. *1108*

428.00 Congestive Heart Failure

^{131}I Uptake *Serum Decrease* *2104*

Serum Increase *2104*

Alanine Aminotransferase *Serum Increase* Heart failure or shock with attendant hepatic necrosis may lead to elevated values. *0503* Depending on the severity and chronicity of cardiac failure. *0433* Increased in about 12% of patients. *2467* 33% of 9 patients showed increases (range = 6.3-76.3 U/L). *1452*

Albumin *Serum Decrease* Common with cardiac fibrosis of liver. *2467* Increase in plasma volume without increase in total protein. *0619*
Urine Increase The urinalysis frequently demonstrates reversible proteinuria. *0433* Slight albuminuria (< 1 g/day) is common. *2467*

Aldosterone *Plasma Increase* In far-advanced failure, or in moderate failure under vigorous therapy with diuretics, increases in production and excretion, ranging from detectable to very striking, have been noted. *1108* Enhanced ADH and aldosterone activity. *2104*
Urine Increase May be increased in edematous states of cardiac failure. *0619* In far-advanced failure, or in moderate failure under vigorous therapy with diuretics, increases in production and excretion, ranging from detectable to very striking, have been noted. *1108*

Alkaline Phosphatase *Serum Increase* Usually elevated with cardiac cirrhosis. *0433* Mild to moderate increase (30-135 U/L) in 45% of cases. *2467* Increase in conjunction with normal levels of bilirubin indicate congestive heart failure or myocardial infarction in 28% of cases. *0191*

Alkaline Phosphatase Isoenzymes *Serum Increase* All 5 patients showed elevations of isoenzyme I. *1221*

Amino Acids *Plasma Increase* Slight increase. *0619*

Ammonia *Blood Increase* In patients with azotemia, arterial levels were elevated to 88 mmol/L. *1853*

Amylase *Serum Decrease* Possibly decreased in some cases. *0619*
Pleural Effusion Increase May occur. *1584*
Pleural Effusion Normal Usually less than or equal to serum level. *2017*

Antidiuretic Hormone *Serum Decrease* *0619*
Serum Increase Enhanced ADH and aldosterone activity. *2104*

Aspartate Aminotransferase *Serum Increase* Usually < 100 U/L. *0503* Depending on the severity and chronicity of cardiac failure. *0433* Mild elevation occurred in 33% of 9 cases, levels ranged from 11-39, with the maximum upper limit of normal at 24 U/L. *1452*

Bicarbonate *Serum Decrease* Acidosis occurs when renal insufficiency is associated or there is CO_2 retention due to pulmonary insufficiency. *2467*
Serum Increase Alkalosis occurs in uncomplicated failure; hyperventilation, alveolar-capillary block due to associated pulmonary fibrosis; hypochloremic alkalosis due to K^+ depletion. *2467*
Serum Normal *2467*

Bilirubin *Serum Increase* Depending on the severity and chronicity of cardiac failure. *0433* Frequently increased (indirect more than direct); usually 1-5 mg/dL. It usually represents combined right- and left-sided failure with hepatic engorgement and pulmonary infarcts. May suddenly rise rapidly if superimposed myocardial infarction occurs. *2467*
Urine Increase With jaundice. *2467*

Bilirubin, Indirect *Serum Increase* Unconjugated hyperbilirubinemia reflects reduced hepatic blood flow. *0151*

BSP Retention *Serum Increase* The most frequently abnormal test. It may indicate circulatory stasis as well as cellular damage. *2467* Hepatic dysfunction, often with structural damage to the liver, may result in moderate BSP retention. *1108*

Cephalin Flocculation *Serum Increase* Hepatic dysfunction, often with structural damage to the liver, may result in positive flocculation test. *1108* Positive in about 20% of cases. *2467*

Chloride *Serum Decrease* Tends to fall but may be normal before treatment. *2467*
Serum Normal Tends to fall but may be normal before treatment. *2467*
Saliva Decrease *2467*

Cholesterol *Serum Decrease* With severe hepatic congestion. *0619* *2467*

Cholesterol Esters *Serum Decrease* *2467*

Copper *Serum Increase* Statistically significant. *2188*

Creatinine *Serum Increase* Diminished renal excretion. *0619* Causes reduced blood flow leading to prerenal azotemia. *0619* *2467*

428.00 Congestive Heart Failure *(continued)*

Creatinine Clearance *Urine   Decrease*   Diminished renal excretion with severe failure. *0619*

Erythrocytes *Urine   Increase*   There are isolated RBC and WBC, hyaline and sometimes granular casts. *2467*

Pleural Effusion   Increase   May be present. *0062*

Ascitic Fluid   Increase   > 10,000 cells/μL seen in 10% of cases. *2626*

Erythrocyte Sedimentation Rate *Blood   Decrease*   May be decreased because of decreased serum fibrinogen. *2467*   As a result of decreased synthesis of fibrinogen by the liver which is passively congested. *0962   1108*

Fibrinogen *Plasma   Decrease*   Decreased secondary to impaired liver function. *1108*

Gamma Glutamyl Transferase (GGT) *Serum   Increase*   Due to anoxic damage to the liver. *0619*   All 9 patients had elevated activity, secondary to hepatic damage. Mean = 180, range = 58-568 U/L. *1452*

Globulin *Serum   Increase   2467*

Glomerular Filtration Rate (GFR) *Urine   Decrease*   With a fall in effective cardiac output, a commensurate reduction in renal blood flow generally occurs. *1108 2104*

Glucose *Serum   Decrease*   May occur if cardiac output is severely curtailed and liver congestion is marked. *0151*

Serum   Increase   Abnormal increases in the fasting blood sugar are common. *0962*

Pleural Effusion   Normal   Pleural Fluid = Serum level. *2017*

Peritoneal Fluid   Increase   High concentrations. *1831*

Granular Casts *Urine   Increase*   There are isolated RBC and WBC, hyaline and sometimes granular casts. *2467*

Hematocrit *Blood   Decrease*   Slightly decreased but red cell mass may be increased. *2467*

Hyaline Casts *Urine   Increase*   There are isolated RBC and WBC, hyaline and sometimes granular casts. *2467*

Lactate Dehydrogenase *Serum   Increase*   Increased in about 40% of patients. *2467   0433*

Lactate Dehydrogenase Isoenzyme 5 (LD$_5$) *Serum   Increase*   Elevated to 14.5% of total LD in 12 patients with passive congestion. *0852*   LD$_1$ and 5 are elevated. *2467*

Lactate Dehydrogenase Isoenzymes *Serum   Decrease*   LD$_2$ was decreased in 12 patients with passive congestion. Mean value = 28.8% of total LD (normal = 36%). *0852*

Lactic Acid *Blood   Increase*   Increased formation from glucose due to hypoxia. *0151*

Leucine Aminopeptidase *Serum   Increase*   Slight elevations were found in the sera of 9 patients. Mean for the group = 33 U/L, range = 15-62. *1452*

Leukocytes *Urine   Increase*   Occasionally WBC may be seen with hyaline or granular casts. *0433*   There are isolated RBC and WBC, hyaline and sometimes granular casts. *2467*

Pleural Effusion   Decrease   < 1000/μL. *2017*

Ascitic Fluid   Increase   Less than 1000 μL. *2626*

MCV *Blood   Increase*   Overall hypervolemia involving both plasma and red cell volume. *1669*

Monocytes *Pleural Effusion   Increase*   Predominant cell type. *2017*

Norepinephrine *Serum   Increase*   Consistently elevated. Typically average 700-800 pg/mL. *2631*

Ornithine Carbamoyl Transferase (OCT) *Serum   Increase*   Liver cell damage. *2467*

pCO$_2$ *Blood   Decrease*   Acidosis occurs when renal insufficiency is associated or there is CO$_2$ retention due to pulmonary insufficiency. *2467*

Blood   Increase   Alkalosis occurs in uncomplicated failure; hyperventilation, alveolar-capillary block due to associated pulmonary fibrosis; hypochloremic alkalosis due to potassium depletion. *2467*

pH *Blood   Decrease*   Acidosis occurs when renal insufficiency is associated or there is CO$_2$ retention due to pulmonary insufficiency, low plasma sodium, or ammonium chloride toxicity. *2467*

Blood   Increase   Occurs in uncomplicated heart failure. *2467*

Urine   Normal   2467

Plasma Cells *Serum   Decrease*   Post Surgical. *2357 0659 0683*

Potassium *Serum   Decrease*   Deficiency is common and excess is occasionally noted in patients under therapy. When failure is severe, an accelerated excretion rate may result from secondary hyperaldosteronism. *1108*   Most often due to the kaliuretic action of diuretics without adequate potassium replacement. *0962*

Serum   Increase   Deficiency is common and excess is occasionally noted in patients under therapy. *1108*   Less common than hypokalemia. A common complication in patients on potassium supplements who are not responding to their diuretics. *0962*

Serum   Normal   Normal or slightly increased (because of shift from hypochloremic alkalosis due to some diuretics. *2467*

Urine   Normal   2467

Saliva   Increase   2467

Protein *Serum   Decrease   2467*

Urine   Increase   Mild to moderate proteinuria varying from 0.5-4 g/24h is not unusual; may be greater in severe failure with a marked decrease in GFR and renal blood flow. *1108   0151*

Pleural Effusion   Decrease   Consistent with a transudate. *0186*

Ascitic Fluid   Normal   Variable amounts between 1.5-5.0 g/dL. *2626*

Prothrombin Time *Plasma   Increase*   Frequently elevated. *0433*   May be slightly increased, with increased sensitivity to anticoagulant drugs. *2467*

Pseudocholinesterase *Serum   Decrease*   Some patients. *2467*

Sodium *Serum   Decrease*   May be the result of over-vigorous use of diuretics in an already dehydrated patient who is on a sodium-restricted diet. A common hyponatremic syndrome is observed in patients who continue to have edema and clinical heart failure. Total body sodium in these patients is increased, but the amount of retained water is even greater. Is true dilutional hyponatremia. *0962*

Serum   Increase   Sodium retention. *1985*

Urine   Decrease   As the heart improves, urinary output increases but is low in sodium and has a high specific gravity. *0151*   Patients may, when renal function is intact, reduce urinary sodium concentration virtually to zero. They may retain nearly 100% of the sodium offered them. Hypervolemia and edema result. *1108*   Sodium retention. *1985   0731*

Saliva   Decrease   2467

Specific Gravity *Urine   Decrease*   May be high during the phases of salt and water retention and low during periods of diuresis. *1108*

Urine   Increase   Urine is concentrated, with specific gravity 1.020. Oliguria is a characteristic feature of right-sided failure. *2467*   May be high during the phases of salt and water retention and low during periods of diuresis. *1108*

Urea Nitrogen *Serum   Increase*   May be as high as 80-100 mg/dL as a result of prerenal azotemia. *0433*   Moderate azotemia (BUN usually < 60 mg/dL) is evident with severe oliguria; may increase with vigorous diuresis. *2467   0812 0503*

Uric Acid *Serum   Increase*   Frequently elevated from either prerenal azotemia or, more commonly, the use of diuretics *0433   1283*

Urobilinogen *Urine   Increase*   With hepatic anoxia. *0619   1108*

Volume *Plasma   Increase*   Overall hypervolemia involving both plasma and red cell volume. *1669*   May be normal or increased. *1108   0619*

Urine   Decrease   With edema. *0619*

Red Blood Cells   Increase   Overall hypervolemia involving both plasma and red cell volume. *1669*

429.40 Postcardiotomy Syndrome

Antibody Titer *Serum   Increase*   Excellent correlation between the titer of circulating antiheart antibodies and the development of this syndrome in postoperative patients. *1108   0664*

Erythrocyte Sedimentation Rate *Blood   Increase   2467*

431.00 Cerebral Hemorrhage

Alpha$_1$-Antichymotrypsin *CSF   Increase*   Increased in patients with meningitis or mild hemorrhage, but equal to normal in patients with encephalitis, epilepsy, degenerative disorders or diseases of the CNS. *0079*

Antidiuretic Hormone *Serum   Increase*   Associated with excessive ADH production resulting in sodium loss. *2104*

Aspartate Aminotransferase *CSF   Increase   2467*

Eosinophils *Blood   Increase*   In 45% of 13 patients hospitalized for this disorder. *0781*

Epinephrine *Plasma Increase* Plasma concentrations were 0.65 ± 0.11 ng/mL in subarachnoid hemorrhage patients. *0163*

Erythrocytes *CSF Increase* RBCs reach the CSF by seeping into the ventricle after hypertensive hemorrhage. CSF may remain clear if hemorrhage was small and wholly confined to the brain substance. *0999* In 75% of the patients with intracerebral hemorrhage, the CSF was either grossly bloody or xanthochromic: in 25%, the CSF was clear. *1369* All 17 patients with hemorrhagic vascular lesions had RBC counts > 5,000/μL. *2560*

Erythrocyte Sedimentation Rate *Blood Increase* *2467 0992*

Fibrinogen *Plasma Increase* The greater the degree of initial neurological deficit the greater were plasma high molecular weight fibrinogen complex (HMWFC) values, which were associated with poor clinical outcome. Values were significantly higher in patients with intracerebral hemorrhage, subarachnoid hemorrhage and cerebral embolism. *0747*

Glomerular Filtration Rate (GFR) *Urine Increase* Associated excess ADH may tend to accelerate GFR. *2104*

Glucose *Serum Increase* In 29% of 13 patients hospitalized for this disorder. *0781*

Urine Increase Transient glucosuria. *0992*

Hemoglobin, Fetal *CSF Increase* Increased percentage in CSF indicates neonatal subarachnoid hemorrhage. *0373*

Lactate Dehydrogenase *Serum Increase* In 40% of 10 patients hospitalized for this disorder. *0781 2560*

CSF Increase In the acute stage of the disease. The increase seems to be the result of blood and plasma reaching the CSF in hemorrhage. *2575* Elevated in all 27 determinations of CSF in 17 patients with hemorrhagic vascular lesions and 13 of 30 patients with nonhemorrhagic lesions. *2560*

Leukocytes *Blood Increase* Increased (15,000-20,000/μL) (higher than in cerebral occlusion, e.g., embolism, thrombosis). *2467* In 51% of 15 patients hospitalized for this disorder. *0781 0992*

CSF Increase Count will be commensurate with the amount of bleeding, 1 WBC/1,000 RBC. Increase is caused by the inflammatory reaction in the meninges and may reach levels of 500/μL. *0151*

Monocytes *CSF Increase* Mononuclear cells are increased. *0999*

Neutrophils *Blood Increase* In 45% of 13 patients hospitalized for this disorder. *0781*

Norepinephrine *Plasma Increase* Plasma concentrations were greatly increased compared to normals, cardiac catheterization patients, and patients with other illnesses. Mean for all the hemorrhagic patients was 0.94 ± 0.10 ng/mL. Patients with poor prognosis had initially higher and markedly higher follow-up concentrations than those with good prognosis. *0163*

Occult Blood *CSF Positive* In early subarachnoid hemorrhage (< 8 h after onset of symptoms), test may be positive before xanthochromia develops in CSF. *2467*

Protein *CSF Increase* Usually elevated to around 100 mg/dL with maximum levels 8-10 days after bleeding. *0151*

Sodium *Serum Decrease* Associated with excessive ADH production. *2104* Serum sodium is usually less than 130 mEq/L *0062*

Urine Increase Urine is almost always hypertonic to plasma *0062*

Uric Acid *Serum Increase* Increased in both blood and CSF with a lowered CSF:blood ratio, possibly due to cellular breakdown and nucleoprotein catabolism. *2301*

Urine Increase Increased excretion in neurological and psychiatric disorders; progressive rise in urinary level following slight rise in blood, due to disturbed purine metabolism. *2301*

CSF Increase Markedly increased with decreased CSF:blood ratio, possibly due to cellular breakdown and nucleoprotein catabolism. *2301*

434.00   Cerebral Thrombosis

Alpha₁-Antitrypsin *Serum Increase* Increased. *1866 0042 1946 1947 2129*

Antidiuretic Hormone *Serum Increase* Associated with excessive ADH production resulting in sodium loss. *2104*

Aspartate Aminotransferase *Serum Increase* Increased the following week in 50% of cases. *2467* Values may be up to 50 U/L. *0503*

Creatine Kinase *Serum Increase* Increases in 50% of patients with extensive brain infarction. Maximum levels in 3 days; increase may not appear before 2 days; levels usually < in acute myocardial infarction and remain increased for longer time; return to normal within 14 days; high mortality associated with levels > 300 U/L. *2467* 15 of 21 patients with acute stroke had raised levels at some time during the 1st week after ictus. Values ranged from 28.3-710 U/L. *0603 0639 2560*

Erythrocytes *CSF Normal* Never causes blood in the spinal fluid unless the infarct is especially congested, then a very faint xanthochromia may occur. *0992*

Fibrinogen *Plasma Increase* Significant increase was noted in cerebral thromboembolic stroke in young patients. *2127*

Fibrin Split Products (FSP) *Plasma Decrease* A decrease in fibrinolytic activity was noticed. *0112*

Glomerular Filtration Rate (GFR) *Urine Increase* Associated excess ADH may tend to accelerate GFR. *2104*

Lactate Dehydrogenase *Serum Increase* Serum elevations were less frequent and independent of those in the CSF. *2560*

CSF Increase All of the 17 patients with hemorrhagic lesions showed elevations. 13 of 30 patients with nonhemorrhagic lesions showed similar but smaller elevations in the CSF. Serum elevations were less frequent and independent of those in the CSF. *2560*

Leukocytes *CSF Increase* A slight increase is common in the 1st few days. Rarely, and for unexplained reasons, a brisk transient pleocytosis (400-2,000 polymorphonuclears/μL) occurs on the 3rd day. *0992*

Lipoproteins, Prebeta *Serum Increase* Significant rise was noticed in all patients. *0112*

Nickel *Serum Increase* Mean 5.2 (n = 33) compared with controls mean 2.6 μg/L (n = 42). *1559* Increased.

Protein *CSF Increase* The total amount may be normal, but frequently it is raised to 50-80 mg/dL. Rarely it is over 100, in which case some other diagnosis should be considered. *0992*

CSF Normal The total amount may be normal, but frequently it is raised to 50-80 mg/dL. Rarely it is over 100, in which case some other diagnosis should be considered. *0992*

Sodium *Serum Decrease* Associated with excessive ADH production. *2104* Serum sodium is usually less than 130 mEq/L. *0062*

Urine Increase Urine is almost always hypertonic to plasma *0062*

Triglycerides *Serum Increase* Significant rise noticed in all patients. *0112*

Uric Acid *Serum Increase* Increased in both blood and CSF with a lowered CSF:blood ratio, possibly due to cellular breakdown and nucleoprotein catabolism. *2301* Found in 25% of patients of both sexes with acute stroke. *1790* In 24% of 12 patients hospitalized for this disorder. *0781*

Urine Increase Increased excretion in neurological and psychiatric disorders; progressive rise in urinary level following slight rise in blood, due to disturbed purine metabolism. *2301*

CSF Increase Markedly increased with decreased CSF:blood ratio, possibly due to cellular breakdown and nucleoprotein catabolism. *2301*

434.10   Cerebral Embolism

Antidiuretic Hormone *Serum Increase* Associated with excessive ADH production resulting in sodium loss. *2104*

Aspartate Aminotransferase *Serum Increase* Increased the following week in 50% of cases. *0619* Values may be up to 50 U/L. *0503*

Creatine Kinase *Serum Increase* Peak values occur at 48 h, falling in 3-4 days. Bad prognosis is indicated by an early rise, and by its magnitude. No increase is associated with brain stem infarction and angiomata. *0619*

Erythrocytes *CSF Increase* Usually findings are the same as in cerebral thrombosis. 33% of patients develop hemorrhagic infarction, usually producing slight xanthochromia several days later; some cases may have grossly bloody CSF (10,000 RBC/μL). *2467*

Fibrinogen *Plasma Increase* The greater the degree of initial neurological deficit the greater were plasma high molecular weight fibrinogen complexes values, which were associated with poor clinical outcome. Values were significantly higher in patients with intracerebral hemorrhage, subarachnoid hemorrhage and cerebral embolism. *0747*

Glomerular Filtration Rate (GFR) *Urine Increase* Associated excess ADH may tend to accelerate GFR. *2104*

434.10 Cerebral Embolism (continued)

Glucose *Serum Normal* 2467

CSF Normal 0992

Leukocytes *CSF Increase* Septic embolism (e.g., bacterial endocarditis) may cause increased WBC, up to 200/μL with variable lymphocytes and polymorphonuclear leukocytes. 2467

Neutrophils *CSF Increase* In septic embolus, the proportion of lymphocytes and polymorphonuclears varies with the acuteness of the septic process. 0992

Protein *Serum Increase* In septic embolism. 2467

CSF Increase Elevated in septic emboli. 0992

Sodium *Serum Decrease* Associated with excessive ADH production. 2104 Serum sodium is usually less than 130 mEq/L 0062

Urine Increase Urine is almost always hypertonic to plasma 0062

Uric Acid *Serum Increase* Increased in both blood and CSF with a lowered CSF:blood ratio, possibly due to cellular breakdown and nucleoprotein catabolism. 2301 Found in 25% of patients of both sexes with acute stroke. 1790

Urine Increase Increased excretion in neurological and psychiatric disorders; progressive rise in urinary level following slight rise in blood, due to disturbed purine metabolism. 2301

CSF Increase Markedly increased with decreased CSF:blood ratio, possibly due to cellular breakdown and nucleoprotein catabolism. 2301

434.90 Brain Infarction

Alanine Aminotransferase *Serum Increase* 0962

Aldolase *Serum Increase* 0962

Alpha$_1$-Antitrypsin *Serum Increase* High molecular weight fibrinogen complexes, native fibrinogen, alpha$_1$ antitrypsin and alpha$_2$ macroglobulin were significantly increased in cerebral infarction patients. 0747

Alpha$_2$-Macroglobulin *Serum Increase* High molecular weight fibrinogen complexes, native fibrinogen, alpha$_1$ antitrypsin, and alpha$_2$ macroglobulin were significantly increased in cerebral infarction patients. 0747

Aspartate Aminotransferase *Serum Increase* Increased the following week in 50% of cases. 0619 Values may be up to 50 U/L. 0503 0962

CSF Increase Increased for some days after infarction or cerebrovascular accident without a corresponding rise in CSF ALT. 0619

Cholesterol *Serum Decrease* In all patients a significant reduction in total lipids, cholesterol, triglyceride and all lipoproteins was demonstrated after the acute cerebrovascular accident presumably due to the stress situation. 1192

Copper *Serum Increase* Abnormally high concentrations in plasma and CSF. The plasma Cu:Zn ratio was also significantly elevated. 0240

CSF Increase Patients with cerebral infarctions had abnormally high concentrations in plasma and CSF. The plasma Cu:Zn ratio was also significantly elevated. 0240

Creatine Kinase *Serum Increase* Peak values occur at 48 h, falling in 3-4 days. Bad prognosis is indicated by an early rise, and by its magnitude. No increase is associated with brain stem infarction or angiomata. 0619 0962

Factor XIII *Plasma Decrease* Substantial depression developed together with concomitant significant increases in the proportion and concentration of plasma high molecular weight fibrinogen complexes (HMWFC). An inverse correlation between factor XIII and percentage of HMWFC was demonstrated in the early stages of the illness. 1491

Fibrinogen *Plasma Increase* High molecular weight fibrinogen complexes, native fibrinogen, alpha$_1$ antitrypsin and alpha$_2$ macroglobulin were significantly increased in cerebral infarction patients. 0747 Substantial depression of factor XIII concentrations developed together with concomitant significant increases in the proportion and concentration of plasma high molecular weight fibrinogen complexes (HMWFC). An inverse correlation between factor XIII and percentage of HMWFC was demonstrated in the early stages of the illness. 1491

Lipids *Serum Decrease* In all patients a significant reduction in total lipids, cholesterol, triglyceride and all lipoproteins was demonstrated after the acute cerebrovascular accident presumably due to the stress situation. 1192

Lipoproteins *Serum Decrease* In all patients a significant reduction in total lipids, cholesterol, triglyceride and all lipoproteins was demonstrated after the acute cerebrovascular accident presumably due to the stress situation. 1192

Monocytes *CSF Increase* Mononuclear cells are increased in CSF early in the course of the disease. 0999

Protein *CSF Increase* Slight elevations of 60-75 mg/dL are found in 20% of patients. 0151

Triglycerides *Serum Decrease* In all patients a significant reduction in total lipids, cholesterol, triglyceride and all lipoproteins was demonstrated after the acute cerebrovascular accident presumably due to the stress situation. 1192

Uric Acid *Serum Increase* Increased in both blood and CSF with a lowered CSF:blood ratio, possibly due to cellular breakdown and nucleoprotein catabolism. 2301 In 36% of 115 cases of acute infarction. 1790

Urine Increase Increased excretion in neurological and psychiatric disorders; progressive rise in urinary level following slight rise in blood, due to disturbed purine metabolism. 2301

CSF Increase Markedly increased with decreased CSF:blood ratio, possibly due to cellular breakdown and nucleoprotein catabolism. 2301

435.90 Transient Cerebral Ischemia

Bicarbonate *Serum Increase* In 70% of 31 patients hospitalized for this disorder. 0781

Hematocrit *Blood Increase* In 29% of 48 patients hospitalized for this disorder. 0781

Hemoglobin *Blood Increase* In 25% of 48 patients hospitalized for this disorder. 0781

Uric Acid *Serum Increase* In 46% of 50 patients hospitalized for this disorder. 0781

440.00 Arteriosclerosis

Alpha$_2$-Macroglobulin *Serum Increase* 1438

Apolipoprotein AI *Serum Decrease* Patients with angiographically documented coronary artery disease were found to have elevated levels of Apolipoprotein B and decreased levels of A-I or A-II compared with individuals without the disease. 2221 1935 2241 An excellent predictor of this condition. 2330

Apolipoprotein AII *Plasma Decrease* Patients with angiographically documented coronary artery disease were found to have elevated levels of Apolipoprotein B and decreased levels of A-I or A-II compared with individuals without the disease. 2221 1935 2241

Apolipoprotein B *Serum Increase* Patients with angiographically documented coronary artery disease were found to have elevated levels of Apolipoprotein B and decreased levels of A-I or A-II compared with individuals without the disease. 2221 1935 2241

Bicarbonate *Serum Increase* In 56% of 67 patients hospitalized for this disorder. 0781

Cadmium *Serum Increase* The highest blood cadmium level was observed in smokers with coronary heart disc plus hypertension. 0019

Ceruloplasmin *Serum Increase* High concentrations of Zn, Cu and ceruloplasmin were found in 13 patients when compared with controls. The Zn:Cu ratio is much higher in arteriosclerotic patients than in healthy subjects. 0324

Cholesterol *Serum Increase* Correlates highly with the risk of myocardial infarction. 0992 Elevated fasting plasma concentration was frequently found in 219 male and 63 female patients. 0108 Severity of disease correlated (not significantly) with plasma cholesterol concentration. 0508 Nonfasting levels are related to the development of coronary heart disease in both men and women aged 19 years and older 0358

Cholesterol, High Density Lipoprotein *Serum Decrease* Non fasting HDL is inversely related to the development of coronary heart disease in both men and women aged 49 years and older. 0358

Copper *Serum Increase* High concentrations found in 13 patients when compared with controls. The Zn:Cu ratio is much higher in arteriosclerotic patients than in healthy subjects. 0324 Statistically significant 2188

Creatinine *Serum Increase* In 64% of 36 patients hospitalized for this disorder. 0781 May occur with kidney involvement. 0503

Cryomacroglobulins *Serum Increase* 0863

Erythrocytes *Blood Increase* True polycythemia with a considerable increase of red cell volume may occur. 1669

Factor VIII *Plasma Increase* In atherosclerosis. *0453*

Lipids *Serum Increase* Hyperlipidemia was present in 43.9% of patients with atherosclerosis of the legs. Hyperlipemia was frequently found in 219 male and 63 female patients. No significant relationship was found between uric acid and cholesterol or triglyceride. *0108* *0508*

Lipoproteins *Serum Increase* Hyperuricemia and hyperlipidemia were frequently found in 219 male and 63 female patients. No significant relationship was found between uric acid and cholesterol or triglyceride, when the males were divided into lipoprotein types it was found that those who were normolipoproteinemic or who had type IV hyperlipoproteinemia had a significantly higher mean uric acid level. *0108*

Selenium *Plasma Decrease* Low concentrations of selenium in plasma in coronary atherogenesis. *1620*

Triglycerides *Serum Increase* The severity of disease showed a slight positive correlation with plasma triglyceride concentrations, especially in the younger patients. *0508* Frequently found in 219 male and 63 female patients. No significant relationship was found between uric acid and triglyceride. *0108*

Urea Nitrogen *Serum Increase* Several mechanisms are involved. *0503* In 36% of 75 patients hospitalized for this disorder. *0781*

Uric Acid *Serum Increase* Increased in 80% of patients with elevated serum triglycerides. *2467* Frequently found in 219 male and 63 female patients. No significant relationship was found between uric acid and serum lipids. *0108* In 59% of 71 patients hospitalized for this disorder. *0781*

Volume *Red Blood Cells Decrease* RBC volume is decreased in the hypertension resulting from renal artery stenosis. *1669*

Red Blood Cells Increase True polycythemia with a considerable increase of red cell volume may occur. *1669*

Zinc *Serum Increase* High serum concentrations were found in 13 patients when compared with controls. The Zn:Cu ratio is much higher in arteriosclerotic patients than in healthy subjects. *0324*

441.00   Dissecting Aortic Aneurysm

Alanine Aminotransferase *Serum Normal* Unless complications occur. *2467*

Amylase *Serum Increase* Hyperamylasemia has been reported, although mechanism is unclear. *0653 1546*

Aspartate Aminotransferase *Serum Increase* Not helpful since modest elevations may occur in both dissection and infarction. *1108*

Serum Normal Unless complications occur. *2467*

Creatine Kinase *Serum Normal* Unless complications occur. *2467*

Erythrocyte Sedimentation Rate *Blood Increase* *2467*

Lactate Dehydrogenase *Serum Normal* Unless complications occur. *2467*

Lactate Dehydrogenase Isoenzyme 5 (LD$_5$) *Serum Normal* Unless complications occur. *2467*

Leukocytes *Blood Increase* *2467*

Occult Blood *Feces Positive* *2199*

441.50   Ruptured Aortic Aneurysm

Erythrocyte Sedimentation Rate *Blood Increase* *0186*

Hematocrit *Pleural Effusion Increase* Values approaching those found in blood are more indicative of frank hemorrhage, and such levels would be found in traumatic hemothorax or bleeding associated with pneumothorax or ruptured aortic aneurysm. *0962*

Hemoglobin *Pleural Effusion Increase* Values approaching those found in blood are more indicative of frank hemorrhage, and such levels would be found in traumatic hemothorax or bleeding associated with pneumothorax or ruptured aortic aneurysm. *0962*

Leukocytes *Blood Increase* *0186*

444.90   Arterial Embolism and Thrombosis

Acid Phosphatase *Serum Increase* Acid hyperphenylphosphatasia which lasted from 3-6 days and reached a maximum of 4.1, 5.8, and 7 U/L, respectively, was noted after each of the 3 episodes of thromboembolism. *2079* Peak activity is reached 2-3 days after onset of symptoms. *2104* *0812*

Albumin *Urine Increase* Constant finding among 31 patients. *1108*

Aspartate Aminotransferase *Serum Increase* In 38% of 37 patients hospitalized for this disorder. *0781*

Creatine Kinase *Serum Increase* *2079 0992*

Creatinine *Serum Increase* In 50% of 21 patients hospitalized for this disorder. *0781*

Erythrocyte Sedimentation Rate *Blood Increase* *2079 0992*

Lactate Dehydrogenase *Serum Increase* In 32% of 37 patients hospitalized for this disorder. *0781* *2079 0992*

Leukocytes *Blood Increase* In 47% of 46 patients hospitalized for this disorder. *0781*

Myoglobin *Urine Increase* Sporadic; ischemia. *2467* Sudden muscle damage due to ischemia, e.g., thrombosis of artery supplying a large muscle mass. *0619*

Neutrophils *Blood Increase* In 50% of 40 patients hospitalized for this disorder. *0781*

Urea Nitrogen *Serum Increase* Progressive azotemia. *1108* In 34% of 42 patients hospitalized for this disorder. *0781*

446.00   Polyarteritis-Nodosa

Albumin *Serum Decrease* Hypoalbuminemia occurs only in those patients with the nephrotic syndrome. *0962*

Urine Increase Abnormal urinalysis is far more frequent (70-80%) than azotemia (25-30%). *0433*

Alpha$_1$-Globulin *Serum Increase* Moderate increase. *0619*

Alpha$_2$-Globulin *Serum Increase* Marked increase. *0619*

Antinuclear Antibodies *Serum Increase* Infrequently seen and, when present, are in low titer. *0962* Usually absent, and when present should suggest that the arteritis is part of another disorder. *2035*

Beta-Globulin *Serum Increase* Moderate increase in some cases. *0619*

Cellular Casts *Urine Increase* Found in patients with glomerular disease. *0999* *0962*

Cholesterol *Serum Increase* Leading to nephrosis. *2467*

Cold Agglutinins *Serum Increase* Have been reported. *0962*

Complement, Total *Serum Decrease* Depression of titers may be found in early, acute phases. *0642* Subsides with remission. *2090*

Serum Increase In some patients. *0030* Possibly the result of low utilization or a rapid rate of production. *0962* Elevated during active inflammation and subsides with remission. *2090* *0999*

Coombs' Test *Blood Negative* *0642*

Creatinine *Serum Increase* With renal involvement. *0995*

Cryoglobulins *Serum Increase* Cryoglobulinemia is rarely reported, but this may reflect late collection or improper handling of specimens. *2035* Variable elevation of cryoglobulins. *2104*

Eosinophils *Blood Increase* Hallmark of patients with allergic granulomatosis and angiitis is eosinophilia > 400/μL, and usually > 1,500/μL. This degree of eosinophilia is rarely seen in patients with polyarteritis in whom the lungs are spared. *0642* Eosinophilia is almost exclusively related to the variants of necrotizing angiitis with pulmonary involvement, it is uncommonly seen in classical polyarteritis. *0962* *0999 0532 2538*

Erythrocyte Casts *Urine Increase* *0962*

Erythrocytes *Urine Increase* Abnormal urinalysis is far more frequent (70-80%) than azotemia (25-30%). *0433* Microscopic hematuria is found in patients with glomerular disease. *0999* Hematuria is likely to be intermittent. *0962*

Erythrocyte Sedimentation Rate *Blood Increase* Almost a prerequisite for diagnosis. *0433* Generally reflects the intensity of the disease activity. *0999* Almost always elevated in active untreated polyarteritis. *2035* Generally elevated (often exceeding 80 mm/h Westergren). *0962*

Globulin *Serum Increase* Frequently found *0962* *2468*

Serum Normal *2467*

Granular Casts *Urine Increase* Abnormal urinalysis is far more frequent (70-80%) than azotemia (25-30%). *0433* Hyaline and granular casts indicate renal involvement. *0151*

Hematocrit *Blood Decrease* Almost a prerequisite for diagnosis. *0433* Mild anemia is frequently present due either to blood loss or to chronic renal insufficiency. *0642* Anemia is found chiefly in cases complicated by renal insufficiency or blood loss. *0962*

446.00   Polyarteritis-Nodosa (continued)

Hemoglobin   *Blood   Decrease*   Almost a prerequisite for diagnosis. *0433*   Mild anemia is frequently present due either to blood loss or to chronic renal insufficiency. *0642*   Anemia is found chiefly in cases complicated by renal insufficiency or blood loss. *0962*

Hepatitis B Surface Antigen   *Serum   Increase*   In cases associated with hepatitis B infection the hepatitis B surface antigen is persistently detectable, usually at high titers, throughout the illness. *2035*   Found in approximately 25% of patients, independent of apparent liver involvement. *0962*

Hyaline Casts   *Urine   Increase*   Hyaline and granular casts indicate renal involvement. *0151*

Immunoglobulin IgD   *Serum   Increase*   *0619*

Immunoglobulins   *Serum   Normal*   Usually within normal limits. *2035*

Iron   *Serum   Increase*   Anemia may be due to chronic blood loss. *0642 0962*

Iron-Binding Capacity, Total (TIBC)   *Serum   Increase*   Anemia may be due to chronic blood loss. *0642 0962*

Iron Saturation   *Serum   Decrease*   Anemia may be due to chronic blood loss. *0642 0962*

Leukocytes   *Blood   Increase*   Almost a prerequisite for diagnosis. *0433*   Usually associated with leukocytosis, often 15,000/μL or more. *0999*   In about 80% of cases, there is mild leukocytosis with a shift to the left. *2035*   Polymorphonuclear leukocytosis (the result of inflammatory and necrotic lesions) occurs in the majority of patients. *0962*

Urine   Increase   Found in patients with glomerular disease. *0999*

MCH   *Blood   Decrease*   Microcytic hypochromic anemia may occur due to blood loss, increased demand or dietary inadequacy. MCH < 27 pg, MCV < 80 fL. *0532*   Mild anemia is frequently present due either to blood loss or to chronic renal failure. *0642*   Anemia is found chiefly in cases complicated by renal insufficiency or blood loss. *0962   0433*

MCHC   *Blood   Decrease*   Mild anemia is frequently present due either to blood loss or to chronic renal failure. *0642*   Anemia is found chiefly in cases complicated by renal insufficiency or blood loss. *0962 0433*

MCV   *Blood   Decrease*   Microcytic hypochromic anemia may occur due to blood loss, increased demand or dietary inadequacy. MCH < 27 pg, MCV < 80 fL. *0532*

Monocytes   *Blood   Increase*   Has been reported. *1489   2538*

Neutrophils   *Blood   Increase*   In about 80% of cases, there is mild leukocytosis with a shift to the left. *2035*

Oval Fat Bodies   *Urine   Positive*   *0186*

Platelet Count   *Blood   Increase*   Counts > 500,000/μL frequently found. *0999 0962*

Protein   *Urine   Increase*   Found in patients with glomerular disease. *0999*   With renal involvement. *0962*

Rheumatoid Factor   *Serum   Increase*   Present in some patients. *0999 2024*

Serum   Normal   Usually absent, and when present should suggest that the arteritis is part of another disorder. *2035*

Urea Nitrogen   *Serum   Increase*   With renal involvement. *0995*

446.20   Goodpasture's Syndrome

Antibody Titer   *Serum   Increase*   Glomerular and alveolar basement membrane antibodies. *1670*   Circulating antibodies to glycopeptide antigen are found in over 90% of cases. *0062*

Complement C3   *Serum   Normal*   Almost always normal. *0062*

Complement C4   *Serum   Normal*   Almost always normal. *0062*

Complement, Total   *Serum   Normal*   Almost always normal. *0062*

Creatinine   *Serum   Increase*   Progressive renal failure. *0062*

Hematocrit   *Blood   Decrease*   Secondary to prolonged pulmonary bleeding. *0062*

Hemoglobin   *Blood   Decrease*   Secondary to prolonged pulmonary bleeding. *0062*

HLA Antigens   *Blood   Present*   HLA-DR2 is twenty five times more likely in patients with this disease and caries with it a worse prognosis. *1503*

Iron   *Serum   Decrease*   Secondary to prolonged pulmonary bleeding. *0062*

Iron-Binding Capacity, Total (TIBC)   *Serum   Increase*   Secondary to prolonged pulmonary bleeding. *0062*

Iron Saturation   *Serum   Decrease*   Secondary to prolonged pulmonary bleeding. *0062*

MCHC   *Blood   Decrease*   Secondary to prolonged pulmonary bleeding. *0062*

pO2   *Blood   Decrease*   Secondary to prolonged pulmonary bleeding. *0062*

Urea Nitrogen   *Serum   Increase*   Progressive renal failure. *0062*

446.50   Cranial Arteritis and Related Conditions

Albumin   *Serum   Decrease*   In 30% of 16 patients hospitalized for this disorder. *0781*

Aldolase   *Serum   Normal*   *0186*

Alkaline Phosphatase   *Serum   Increase*   Abnormal liver test results, have been found, but biopsies have shown only minor nonspecific changes. *0557   2035*

Alpha2-Globulin   *Serum   Increase*   Parallels the rapid ESR. *2035*

Antinuclear Antibodies   *Serum   Normal*   Characteristically absent. *2035*

Aspartate Aminotransferase   *Serum   Normal*   *0186*

Complement, Total   *Serum   Increase*   In 6 patients, 50% had increased values. *2223*

Serum   Normal   *2035*

C-Reactive Protein   *Serum   Increase*   *0186*

Creatine Kinase   *Serum   Normal*   *0186*

Erythrocyte Sedimentation Rate   *Blood   Increase*   A striking elevation of ESR is characteristic. *0969*   Elevated to > 80 mm/h (Westergren) in polymyalgia rheumatica. *0151*   The only laboratory abnormality of significance is a very rapid ESR, often reaching 100 mm/h (Westergren method). *2035   0962*

Fibrinogen   *Plasma   Increase*   Parallels the rapid ESR. *2035*

Globulin   *Serum   Increase*   May occur in temporal arteritis. *2468*

Hematocrit   *Blood   Decrease*   Mild anemia is common, especially in older patients, in polymyalgia rheumatica. *0151*   Hypoproliferative anemia is common and may be significant, with Hcts in the 25-30% range. *1013*   In 30% of 16 patients hospitalized for this disorder. *0781   2035*

Hemoglobin   *Blood   Decrease*   Mild anemia is common, especially in older patients, in polymyalgia rheumatica. *0151*   Hypoproliferative anemia is common and may be significant. *1013*   In 49% of 16 patients hospitalized for this disorder. *0781   2035*

HLA Antigens   *Blood   Present*   Association noted with HLA-DR4. *1503*

Lactate Dehydrogenase   *Serum   Normal*   *0186*

LE Cells   *Blood   Normal*   *2468*

Leukocytes   *Blood   Increase*   Slightly increased with shift to the left in temporal arteritis. *2468*   In 36% of 16 patients hospitalized for this disorder. *0781*

Monocytes   *Blood   Increase*   Has been reported. *1489   2538*

Neutrophils   *Blood   Increase*   In 42% of 14 patients hospitalized for this disorder. *0781*

Protein   *CSF   Increase*   May occur due to intracerebral artery involvement. *2468*

Rheumatoid Factor   *Serum   Increase*   Present in serum in 7.5% of patients with polymyalgia rheumatica. *2468*

Serum   Normal   Characteristically absent. *2035*

446.60   Thrombotic Thrombocytopenic Purpura

Bilirubin   *Serum   Increase*   Elevated in 90% of patients. *2538*

Bilirubin, Indirect   *Serum   Increase*   In 90% of patients. *2538*

Bleeding Time   *Blood   Increase*   Varies depending upon the platelet count. *2035   2552 2246*

Capillary Fragility   *Blood   Increase*   Positive tourniquet test. *2552*

Casts   *Urine   Increase*   With kidney involvement. *0962*

Cells   *Bone Marrow   Increase*   Increased number of megakaryocytes but with marginal platelets. *2468*

Clot Retraction   *Blood   Poor*   Varies depending upon the platelet count. *2035*   Absent or deficient due to thrombocytopenia. *2552*

Clotting Time   *Blood   Normal*   *0054 2246*

Coombs' Test   *Blood   Negative*   *2552*

Blood   Positive   Rarely. *1706*

Creatinine   *Serum   Increase*   Renal function may be impaired. *0962*

Eosinophils *Blood Increase* WBC generally normal or slightly increased, often with a relative lymphocytosis and eosinophilia. *2035*

Bone Marrow *Increase* Increased numbers of young megakaryocytes and often an increase in eosinophils. *1456 2035*

Erythrocytes *Urine Increase* Gross or microscopic hematuria. *0962*

Factor V *Plasma Decrease* Slight decrease in 2 cases. *1376*

Fibrinogen *Plasma Decrease* *0556*

Glomerular Filtration Rate (GFR) *Urine Decrease* Renal function may be impaired. *0962*

Haptoglobin *Serum Decrease* May accompany elevated indirect bilirubin, indicating intravascular RBC destruction. *2552*

Hematocrit *Blood Decrease* Anemia secondary to blood loss may be present. *2035*

Hemoglobin *Blood Decrease* Anemia secondary to blood loss may be present. *2035* 5.5 g/dL in 33% of patients. *2538 2552*

Hemoglobin, Free *Serum Increase* May accompany elevated indirect bilirubin, indicating intravascular RBC destruction. *2552*

Iron-Binding Capacity, Total (TIBC) *Serum Decrease* Anemia from blood loss may be present. *2538*

Iron Saturation *Serum Increase* Anemia from blood loss may be present. *2538*

LE Cells *Blood Increase* Positive initially in 10-20% of patients. *0054*

Leukocytes *Blood Increase* Generally normal or slightly increased, often with a relative lymphocytosis, atypical lymphocytes (particularly in children), and eosinophilia. *2035 2552*

Urine Increase With kidney involvement. *0962*

Lymphocytes *Blood Increase* Often with a relative lymphocytosis, atypical lymphocytes (particularly in children), and eosinophilia. *2035 2552*

Neutrophils *Blood Increase* Leukocytosis in 50% with a shift to the left and appearance of immature granulocytes. *2552*

Partial Thromboplastin Time *Plasma Normal* *2246*

Platelet Count *Blood Decrease* Decreased count--no bleeding until 60,000/µL. *2468* Usually range 10,000-50,000. *2538*

Platelet Survival *Blood Decrease* Increased platelet destruction results in thrombocytopenia or shortened platelet survival (i.e., compensated thrombocytolytic states). *1230 2035*

Protein *Urine Increase* With kidney involvement. *0962* Proteinuria or hematuria in 90% of patients. *2538*

Prothrombin Time *Plasma Normal* *2246 0054*

Reticulocytes *Blood Increase* In most cases. *2552* Averaged 20%. *0054*

Thrombin Time *Plasma Normal* *2246*

Urea Nitrogen *Serum Increase* Renal function may be impaired. *0962* Elevated initially in 50% of patients and more terminally. *2538*

VDRL *Serum Positive* In 10% of patients (biological false-positive). *0054*

446.70 Pulseless Disease (Aortic Arch Syndrome)

Erythrocyte Sedimentation Rate *Blood Increase* May be present. *2086* Consistently elevated to high levels. *2035*

Globulin *Serum Increase* Serum proteins abnormal with increased gamma globulins, mostly composed of IgM. *2467* May be present. *2086 2035*

HLA Antigens *Blood Present* Frequency of HLA-Bw52 greater in affected Asians. *1503*

Immunoglobulin IgM *Serum Increase* Serum proteins abnormal with increased gamma globulins, mostly composed of IgM. *2467* May be present. *2086*

Leukocytes *Blood Increase* May be present. *2086* Mild. *2035*

Blood Normal Usually normal. *2467*

451.90 Phlebitis and Thrombophlebitis

Acid Phosphatase *Serum Increase* 8 of 9 female patients with thrombophlebitis of the lower extremities had elevations. Activities of 11-16.1 U/L during the acute phase of disease, a fall to borderline values of 9 U/L during convalescence, and a return to normal values of 1.6-6.5 U/L after recovery. *2080 0812*

Alkaline Phosphatase *Serum Increase* In 28% of 51 patients at initial hospitalization for this disorder. *0781*

Antithrombin III *Plasma Decrease* Significant decrease. *2025*

Antithrombin Titer *Blood Decrease* About 2% of venous thromboembolism is due to antithrombin III deficiency. *1108*

Aspartate Aminotransferase *Serum Increase* In 25% of 51 patients at initial hospitalization for this disorder. *0781*

Eosinophils *Blood Increase* In 40% of 49 patients at initial hospitalization for this disorder. *0781*

Fibrin Split Products (FSP) *Plasma Increase* 42% of 24 patients suspected of acute thrombophlebitis had positive fibrinogen tests. *0347*

Leukocytes *Blood Increase* In 28% of 51 patients at initial hospitalization for this disorder. *0781*

Neutrophils *Blood Increase* In 36% of 49 patients at initial hospitalization for this disorder. *0781*

Platelet Adhesiveness *Blood Increase* Increased in 7 cases. *2025*

Thromboglobulin, Beta *Serum Increase* Increased in 7 cases. *2025*

DISEASES OF THE RESPIRATORY SYSTEM

463.00 Acute Tonsillitis

Leukocytes *Blood Increase* Acute localized infections cause leukocytosis. *2467*

473.90 Chronic Sinusitis

Basophils *Blood Increase* *2467*

Hematocrit *Blood Increase* In 54% of 11 patients at initial hospitalization for this disorder. *0781*

Hemoglobin *Blood Increase* In 63% of 11 patients at initial hospitalization for this disorder. *0781*

Leukocytes *Blood Increase* *0062*

477.90 Hay Fever

Eosinophils *Blood Increase* May occur during the season, but its presence or absence has little diagnostic value, since it is variable. *0433* Characterized by a mild, persistent eosinophilia despite rather profound tissue involvement. *2538*

Immunoglobulin IgE *Serum Increase* Increased in atopic diseases. Occurs in about 30% of patients. *2467* During the pollen season. *0619* Allergic persons usually have values 2-6 X normal. *0999*

480.90 Viral Pneumonia

Alkaline Phosphatase *Serum Increase* In 70% of 10 patients at initial hospitalization for this disorder. *0781*

Antidiuretic Hormone *Serum Increase* Inappropriate increase. *2540*

Aspartate Aminotransferase *Serum Increase* In 80% of 10 patients at initial hospitalization for this disorder. *0781*

Bicarbonate *Serum Increase* Increased standard bicarbonate in blood. *0619*

Carcinoembryonic Antigen *Pleural Effusion Increase* Benign inflammatory effusions (tuberculosis, empyema, pneumonia) had mean activity of 6.2 ± 3.4 ng/mL, higher than effusions caused by congestive heart failure (2.9 ± 1.5 ng/mL) and other noninflammatory effusions. *1945*

Cholesterol *Serum Decrease* In 40% of 10 patients at initial hospitalization for this disorder. *0781*

Complement Fixation *Serum Positive* Complement-Fixing antibodies appear 8-9 days after onset. *1905*

Eosinophils *Blood Increase* In 32% of 15 patients at initial hospitalization for this disorder. *0781*

Pleural Effusion Increase Eosinophilia greater than 10% may be present. *0062*

Erythrocytes *Sputum Present* Sputum in acute pneumonia is rusty, blood-streaked and mucopurulent. *0999*

Glucose *Pleural Effusion Decrease* Exudate. *0062*

Hematocrit *Blood Decrease* In 49% of 16 patients at initial hospitalization for this disorder. *0781*

480.90 Viral Pneumonia (continued)

Hemoglobin *Blood Decrease* In 55% of 16 patients at initial hospitalization for this disorder. *0781*

Isocitrate Dehydrogenase *Serum Normal 2260*

Lactate Dehydrogenase *Serum Increase* In 60% of 10 patients at initial hospitalization for this disorder. *0781* The increases that did occur were in cases of viral pneumonia. *1126*

Pleural Effusion Increase Usually higher than in serum; commonly found in chronic pleural effusions and is not useful in differential diagnosis. *2467*

Lactate Dehydrogenase Isoenzyme 5 (LD$_5$) *Serum Increase* Abnormally elevated to 6.3% of the total LD value of 774 U/mL in 6 cases of lobar pneumonia. *0852*

Leukocytes *Blood Decrease* Normal or low with a relative lymphocytosis. *1905*

Blood Increase In 48% of 16 patients at initial hospitalization for this disorder. *0781*

Blood Normal Normal or low with a relative lymphocytosis. *1905*

Lymphocytes *Blood Decrease* In 52% of 15 patients at initial hospitalization for this disorder. *0781*

Blood Increase Normal or low WBC with a relative lymphocytosis. *1905* In 39% of 15 patients at initial hospitalization for this disorder. *0781*

Lymphocyte T-Cell *Blood Decrease 0793*

Neutrophils *Blood Decrease* In 52% of 15 patients at initial hospitalization for this disorder. *0781*

Blood Increase In 39% of 15 patients at initial hospitalization for this disorder. *0781*

pCO$_2$ *Blood Increase* Low pO$_2$ with normal or high pCO$_2$. *2612*

pH *Pleural Effusion Decrease* Pleural fluid pH of < 7.20 or 0.15 below arterial pH frequently occurs in parapneumonic effusions. *1403*

pO$_2$ *Blood Decrease* Low pO$_2$ with normal or high pCO$_2$. *2612*

Protein *Pleural Effusion Increase* Exudate (> 3 g/dL). *0062*

Specific Gravity *Pleural Effusion Increase* Exudate (> 1.016). *0062*

482.90 Bacterial Pneumonia

Albumin *Serum Decrease* In 50% of 17 patients at initial hospitalization for this disorder. *0781 2467*

Urine Increase Common. *2368*

Aldolase *Serum Increase 0962*

Alpha$_2$-Globulin *Serum Increase 2467*

Amylase *Pleural Effusion Normal* Usually less than or equal to serum level. *2017*

Antidiuretic Hormone *Serum Increase* Inappropriate increase. *2540*

Antistreptolysin O *Serum Increase* In group A streptococcal infections. *0962*

Aspartate Aminotransferase *Serum Increase* In 54% of 18 patients at initial hospitalization for this disorder. *0781*

Serum Normal 2467

Bilirubin *Serum Increase* Occasionally present. *0962*

Serum Normal 2467

Carcinoembryonic Antigen *Serum Increase* 47% of patients had values > 2.5 ng/mL. *2199*

Pleural Effusion Increase Benign inflammatory effusions (tuberculosis, empyema, pneumonia) had mean activity of 6.2 ± 3.4 ng/mL, higher than effusions caused by congestive heart failure (2.9 ± 1.5) and other noninflammatory effusions. *1945*

Cells *Sputum Increase* Gram's stain of sputum reveals many polymorphonuclear leukocytes, and many gram-positive cocci in pairs and singly in pneumonoccal pneumonia. *2468*

Chloride *Urine Decrease* Excretion of chlorides is decreased. *2368*

Cholesterol *Serum Decrease* Infections associated with liver damage; possibly severe pneumonia. *0619* In 45% of 17 patients at initial hospitalization for this disorder. *0781*

Complement C3 *Serum Decrease* Mean concentrations in acute infection was slightly decreased. *0449*

Copper *Serum Increase* Statistically significant. *2188*

C-Reactive Protein *Serum Increase* Nonspecific indicator of acute infection. *0186*

Cryofibrinogen *Serum Increase 2035 1138*

Eosinophils *Blood Increase 2538*

Pleural Effusion Increase Eosinophilia greater than 10% may be present. *0062*

Erythrocytes *Pleural Effusion Increase 0962*

Sputum Present Sputum in acute pneumonia is rusty, blood-streaked and mucopurulent. *0999*

Erythrocyte Sedimentation Rate *Blood Increase* Nonspecific indicator of acute infection. *0186*

Fibrin Split Products (FSP) *Plasma Increase* Elevation is much more common in fatal cases than in survivors in acute respiratory infection. *2193*

Glucose *Serum Increase* In 48% of 18 patients at initial hospitalization for this disorder. *0781*

Pleural Effusion Decrease Levels less than 3.3 mmol/L (60 mg/dL). *0174*

Granular Casts *Urine Increase* Protein, WBC, hyaline and granular casts in small amounts are common. *2467*

Hematocrit *Blood Decrease* In 40% of 19 patients at initial hospitalization for this disorder. *0781* Anemia is common in pneumococcal but not in staphylococcal pneumonia. *2368*

Hemoglobin *Blood Decrease* In 38% of 18 patients at initial hospitalization for this disorder. *0781* Anemia is common in pneumococcal but not in staphylococcal pneumonia. *2368*

Hyaline Casts *Urine Increase* Protein, WBC, hyaline and granular casts in small amounts are common. *2467*

Immunoglobulin IgE *Pleural Effusion Increase* Immunoglobulins are present in large amount. *1913*

Immunoglobulin IgG *Pleural Effusion Increase* Predominant immunoglobulin found in effusions. *1913*

Immunoglobulin IgM *Pleural Effusion Increase* Immunoglobulins are present in large amounts forming a series declining from the IgG (70% of serum concentration) to the IgM (50% of serum concentration). *1913*

Immunoglobulins *Pleural Effusion Increase* Immunoglobulins are present in large amounts forming a series declining from the IgG (70% of serum concentration) to the IgM (50% of serum concentration). *1913*

Ketones *Urine Increase* Ketones may occur with severe infection. *2467*

Lactate Dehydrogenase *Serum Increase* In some cases. *2368* In 32% of 17 patients at initial hospitalization for this disorder. *0781*

Serum Normal Normal in 45 of 50 cases of uncomplicated pneumonia. The increases that did occur were in cases of viral pneumonia. Unreliable screening methods were suggested to account for the increase in LD in pneumonia in a previous study. *1126 0619*

Pleural Effusion Increase Usually higher than in serum; commonly found in chronic pleural effusions and is not useful in differential diagnosis. *2467*

Leukocytes *Blood Decrease* Leukopenia with a shift to the left occurs in fulminating pneumococcal infections, particularly in the presence of bacteremia and in alcoholics. *0151* Normal or low WBC in aged, in overwhelming infection, or with other causative organisms such as Klebsiella pneumoniae. *2468*

Blood Increase Total count ranges from 15,000-40,000/μL or higher with a shift to the left in differential count. *0151* In 66% of 19 patients at initial hospitalization for this disorder. *0781* Already present at initial chill. *2368 0999 2468*

Urine Increase Protein, WBC, hyaline and granular casts in small amounts are common. *2467*

Pleural Effusion Increase A markedly elevated leukocyte count 10,000/μL), especially with a preponderance of neutrophils, is highly suggestive of a pyogenic infection. *0962*

Sputum Increase Sputum contains very many leukocytes with intracellular gram-positive cocci in staphylococcal pneumonia. *2468*

Lipoproteins *Pleural Effusion Increase* Pleural effusions in patients with bacterial pleurisy contain low density lipoproteins (33% of the serum LDL concentration on average) but almost no very low density lipoproteins (about 1% of the serum VLDL concentration on average). *1913*

Lipoproteins, Beta *Pleural Effusion Present* Pleural effusions in patients with bacterial pleurisy contain low density lipoproteins (33% of the serum LDL concentration on average) but almost no very low density lipoproteins (about 1% of the serum VLDL concentration on average). *1913*

Lipoproteins, Prebeta   *Pleural Effusion Decrease*   Pleural effusions in patients with bacterial pleurisy contain low density lipoproteins (33% of the serum LDL concentration on average) but almost no very low density lipoproteins (about 1% of the serum VLDL concentration on average). *1913*

NBT Test   *Blood Positive*   Elevated in 29 of 33 lobar pneumonia patients, mean = 33.5% (control mean = 5.4%). Useful in differential diagnosis of pulmonary infection and thromboembolism (3 of 55 with abnormal scores). *1024*

Neutrophils   *Blood Increase*   A polymorphonuclear leukocytosis of above 15,000/µL. However, the count may be normal and in some instances of overwhelming infection a leukopenia may be present. *0433*   In 55% of 18 patients at initial hospitalization for this disorder. *0781*

Pleural Effusion Increase   Predominant cell type. *2017*

pCO2   *Blood Decrease*   In 63% of 14 patients at initial hospitalization for this disorder. *0781*

pH   *Blood Increase*   In 91% of 14 patients at initial hospitalization for this disorder. *0781*

Pleural Effusion Decrease   Exudate (pH < 7.3). *0062*

pO2   *Blood Decrease*   Low pO2 with normal or high pCO2. *2612*   In 98% of 14 patients at initial hospitalization for this disorder. *0781*

Protein   *Urine Increase*   Protein, WBC, hyaline and granular casts in small amounts are common. *2467*

Pleural Effusion Increase   High total protein concentrations. *0368 1405*

Rheumatoid Factor   *Serum Increase*   Positive latex fixation in 22% of 50 patients. *0448*

Pleural Effusion Increase   May be present with rheumatoid disease, but may also be found in other types of pleural effusions (e.g., carcinoma, tuberculosis, bacterial pneumonia). *2467*

Specific Gravity   *Pleural Effusion Increase*   Exudate (> 1.016). *0062*

Zinc   *Serum Decrease*   Statistically significant. *2188*

483.01   Mycoplasma Pneumoniae

Antibody Titer   *Serum Increase*   IgM antibodies present in 13 of 14 patients tested. *2639*

Bilirubin   *Serum Increase*   *2538 0729*

Bilirubin, Indirect   *Serum Increase*   Occasional patients have been reported with hemolytic anemia. *0433 0729*

Cold Agglutinins   *Serum Increase*   Fourfold or greater rise in titer during the illness is considered diagnostic. *0433*   Significant titers in 50% of patients during the 2nd to 4th weeks, disappearing by the 6th to 8th weeks. *2508*   50% of patients, mostly severely ill, will develop reaction at the end of the 1st or the beginning of the 2nd week. *0151*   Elevated titers may persist for weeks or months. *2035 0715*   In over 50% of patients and is related to the *2368*

Complement Fixation   *Serum Increase*   A 4-fold or greater rise in titer of paired sera obtained during acute and convalescent phases is diagnostic of recent mycoplasma infection. *2508*   Proved to be inappropriate for the early etiological diagnosis of infections, since the high titers were distributed undifferentially among the various patient groups and many sera (38%) showed anticomplementary activity. *0352*   Demonstration of CF antibodies of IgM type in week 2 provides early specific diagnosis. *0661*

Coombs' Test   *Blood Positive*   May occur. *0151*   Direct test may be positive in convalescence. *2368*

Eosinophils   *Blood Increase*   May be observed. *0063*

Erythrocyte Sedimentation Rate   *Blood Increase*   Usually elevated. *0151 2368*

Erythrocyte Survival   *Red Blood Cells Decrease*   Occasional patients have been reported with hemolytic anemia. *0433*

Haptoglobin   *Serum Decrease*   Usually normal but, in some cases, decreases rapidly with bacteremia. *2368 0729*

Hemagglutination Inhibition   *Serum Increase*   Titer of at least 1:128 (preferably 1:512) points to the presence of a M. pneumoniae infection, especially if clinical, radiological, and laboratory data suggest a nonbacterial or mixed pneumonia. *0352*

Hematocrit   *Blood Decrease*   Occasional patients have been reported with hemolytic anemia. *0433*   Sometimes seen in convalescence. *0726 2538 0729*

Hemoglobin   *Blood Decrease*   Occasional patients have been reported with hemolytic anemia. *0433*   Sometimes seen in convalescence. *0726*

Hemoglobin, Free   *Serum Increase*   Hemolysis has been reported in severe cases. *1483 2368   2538 0729*

Indirect Fluorescent Antibodies   *Sputum Increase*   Detects antibodies in the bronchial secretions of patients with mycoplasma infection; sensitive and specific test. *0202*

Lactate Dehydrogenase   *Serum Increase*   May be elevated. *2368*

Leukocytes   *Blood Increase*   Usually below 10,000/µL but up to 20,000/µL in 10% of clinical cases. *0999*   27% of patients had counts > 10,000/µL and 5% > 15,000/µL. *0761*   Usually > 15,000/µL, peaks in the first few days unless complications develop. *2368*

Blood Normal   Counts are usually < 10,000/µL, but may go higher. *0433*

Lymphocytes   *Blood Increase*   May occur during the period of acute illness. *0151*

Neutrophils   *Blood Increase*   Slight neutrophilia occurs with counts of 60-85% neutrophils. *0151*

pH   *Pleural Effusion Decrease*   Exudate (pH < 7.3). *0062*

Platelet Count   *Blood Decrease*   *2368*

Protein   *Pleural Effusion Increase*   Rare effusion which is usually small and an exudate (> 3g/dL). *0062*

Reticulocytes   *Blood Increase*   Sometimes seen in convalescence. *0726*

Specific Gravity   *Pleural Effusion Increase*   Exudate (> 1.016). *0062*

VDRL   *Serum Positive*   False positive reactions in screening tests are common. *2368*

486.01   Resolving Pneumonia

Aspartate Aminotransferase   *Serum Increase*   In 40% of 65 patients at initial hospitalization for this disorder. *0781*

Bicarbonate   *Serum Decrease*   Respiratory alkalosis may occur. *0962*

Hematocrit   *Blood Decrease*   In 47% of 79 patients at initial hospitalization for this disorder. *0781*

Hemoglobin   *Blood Decrease*   In 42% of 79 patients at initial hospitalization for this disorder. *0781*

Lactate Dehydrogenase   *Serum Increase*   In 33% of 62 patients at initial hospitalization for this disorder. *0781*

Serum Normal   Levels were normal in 45/50 cases of uncomplicated pneumonia. Increases that did occur were in cases of viral pneumonia. Unreliable screening methods were suggested to account for the increases in a previous study. *1126*

Leukocytes   *Blood Increase*   In 51% of 79 patients at initial hospitalization for this disorder. *0781*

Lymphocytes   *Lung Tissue Increase*   In 13 patients with lymphocytic interstitial pneumonitis, lung biopsies in all cases showed diffuse interstitial infiltrations consisting of mature lymphocytes and plasma cells. *2283*

Neutrophils   *Blood Increase*   In 37% of 81 patients at initial hospitalization for this disorder. *0781*

Pleural Effusion Increase   Neutrophils predominate in pleural fluid. *1403*

Oxygen Saturation   *Blood Decrease*   Moderate to severe hypoxia and respiratory alkalosis in pneumocystis pneumonitis. *1096*   Low pO2 with normal or high pCO2. *2612*

pCO2   *Blood Decrease*   Moderate to severe hypoxia and respiratory alkalosis in pneumocystis pneumonitis. *1096*   Respiratory alkalosis may occur. *0962*   In 40% of 43 patients at initial hospitalization for this disorder. *0781*   Impaired gas diffusion and the accompanying hyperventilation results in a low pCO2, unless the defect is severe and CO2 retention occurs. *2104*

pH   *Blood Increase*   Moderate to severe hypoxia and respiratory alkalosis in pneumocystis pneumonitis. *1096*   Respiratory alkalosis may occur. *0962*   In 79% of 42 patients at initial hospitalization for this disorder. *0781*

Plasma Cells   *Lung Tissue Increase*   In 13 patients with lymphocytic interstitial pneumonitis, lung biopsies in all cases showed diffuse interstitial infiltrations consisting of mature lymphocytes and plasma cells. *2283*

pO2   *Blood Decrease*   Moderate to severe hypoxia and respiratory alkalosis in pneumocystis pneumonitis. *1096*   Low pO2 with normal or high pCO2. *2612*   In 76% of 41 patients at initial hospitalization for this disorder. *0781*

Uric Acid   *Serum Increase*   *2467*

487.10   Influenza

Acid Phosphatase   *Serum   Increase*   In some cases, even in the absence of discernible complications. *2368*

Albumin   *Urine   Increase*   Mild albuminuria will be found in most febrile conditions. *0433*   Febrile albuminuria may occur. *2368*

Aspartate Aminotransferase   *Serum   Increase*   Usually elevated. *0962*

Basophils   *Blood   Increase*   *2538*

Bilirubin   *Serum   Increase*   Hemolytic anemia. *2538 1857*

Complement Fixation   *Serum   Increase*   A very high titer is suggestive of recent infection. Recent immunization with inactivated influenza virus vaccine has little effect upon titer obtained when S antigen is used. A 4-fold or greater rise between paired sera is accepted as evidence of infection. *0433*   May become positive during the 2nd week of illness. *0962   0999*

Creatine Kinase   *Serum   Increase*   Higher in the acute stage than during the convalescence out of bed, while the controls showed higher activities when ambulant than during bed rest. *0784*

Erythrocyte Sedimentation Rate   *Blood   Increase*   *2368*

Erythrocyte Survival   *Red Blood Cells   Decrease*   Hemolytic anemia. *2538 1857*

Factor II   *Plasma   Decrease*   May be associated with defibrination resulting in platelet and coagulation factor consumption. *2538*

Factor IV   *Plasma   Decrease*   May be associated with defibrination resulting in platelet and coagulation factor consumption. *2538*

Fibrinogen   *Plasma   Decrease*   May be associated with defibrination resulting in platelet and coagulation factor consumption. *2538*

Hemagglutination Inhibition   *Serum   Increase*   May become positive during the second week of illness. *0962*   A 4-fold or greater rise in antibody level between paired sera is accepted as evidence of infection. *0433*   Appears to be more useful in detecting influenza A than complement-fixation tests (CF). 23% of cases verified by HI were missed by CF. *1867*

Hematocrit   *Blood   Decrease*   Hemolytic anemia. *2538 1857*

Hemoglobin, Free   *Serum   Increase*   Hemolytic anemia. *2538 1857*

Leukocytes   *Blood   Decrease*   Occurs in 50% of patients. *2468* Often seen early in influenza but mild leukocytosis is more common. Brisk leukocytosis 15,000/μL) suggests a secondary bacterial infection. *0999*   Leukopenia frequently associated with infectious diseases. *1077*   In many cases. *2368   2538*

Blood   Increase   Leukopenia is often seen early in influenza but mild leukocytosis is more common. Brisk leukocytosis (> 15,000/μL) suggests a secondary bacterial infection. Moderate leukocytosis (10-20,000) may occur. *0999*   Usually elevated. *0962*

Blood   Normal   Total and differential counts are within normal limits in the majority of cases. *2368*

Lymphocytes   *Blood   Decrease*   Leukopenia and lymphopenia are often seen early in influenza but mild leukocytosis is more common. *0999*   The numbers of circulating lymphocytes are sharply and regularly reduced. *2521*

Blood   Increase   The percentage of T-lymphocytes was decreased but a relative and absolute increase of non-T-lymphocytes occurred. *1152*

Neutralizing Antibodies   *Serum   Increase*   May become positive during the 2nd week of illness. *0962*   A 4-fold or greater rise in antibody level between paired sera is accepted as evidence of infection. *0433*

Neutrophils   *Blood   Decrease*   Leukopenia frequently associated with infectious diseases. *1077*

Blood   Increase   Secondary bacterial infection commonly leads to a polymorphonuclear leukocytosis in excess of 15,000/μL. *0433*

Platelet Count   *Blood   Decrease*   May be associated with defibrination resulting in platelet and coagulation factor consumption. *2538*

Prothrombin Consumption   *Blood   Increase*   May be associated with defibrination resulting in platelet and coagulation factor consumption. *2538*

491.00   Chronic Bronchitis

Alpha₁-Antichymotrypsin   *Serum   Increase*   A study of patients with emphysema, bronchitis or asthma revealed there was no deficiency similar to that of alpha₁-antitrypsin. In fact, the levels were increased in all the disease states studied. *0461*

Bicarbonate   *Serum   Increase*   In 59% of 18 patients at initial hospitalization for this disorder. *0781*

Carcinoembryonic Antigen   *Serum   Increase*   33% of patients had values > 2.5 ng/mL. *2199*

Cells   *Sputum   Increase*   *0433*

Copper   *Serum   Increase*   Statistically significant. *2188*

Eosinophils   *Blood   Increase*   Increased if there is allergic basis or component. *2467*   In 36% of 24 patients at initial hospitalization for this disorder. *0781*

Sputum   Increase   More than 3% eosinophils indicates an allergic state. *0433   1718*

Erythrocyte Sedimentation Rate   *Blood   Increase*   Present during the course of infection. *0433*

Leukocytes   *Blood   Increase*   Normal or increased. *2467*

Lymphocytes   *Sputum   Increase*   *0433*

Monocytes   *Sputum   Increase*   *0433*

Neutrophils   *Blood   Increase*   Neutrophilic cells are present only during the course of an infection. *0433*

Oxygen Saturation   *Blood   Decrease*   Tendency to decrease with the increase in dyspnea severity was apparent. *1496   1497 2335 2612*

pCO₂   *Blood   Decrease*   Can occur due to compensatory increase in ventilatory rate. *2220*

pH   *Blood   Decrease*   In 60% of 20 patients at initial hospitalization for this disorder. *0781*

Blood   Increase   Can occur due to compensatory increase in ventilatory rate. *2220*

pO₂   *Blood   Decrease*   Arterial O_2 tension in 54 patients with chronic nonspecific lung disease, indicated subnormal results to be more frequent among bronchitics (79% with hypoxemia) than among emphysematous patients (63% with hypoxemia. *1497*   Tendency to decrease witH the increase in dyspnea severity was apparent. *1496* 66% of nonasthmatic chronic lung disease patients (bronchitis and emphysema) had a mean pO_2 of 72.7 mm Hg. Bronchitics but not emphysemics showed a positive correlation between pO_2 and ventilatory performance. *2335*   In 61% of 19 patients at initial hospitalization for this disorder. *0781   2612*

Rheumatoid Factor   *Serum   Increase*   Found in 62% of patients. *0422 0123*

Zinc   *Serum   Decrease*   Statistically significant. *2188*

492.80   Pulmonary Emphysema

Alpha₁-Antitrypsin   *Serum   Decrease*   alpha₁ antitrypsin deficiency trait may account for up to 10% of emphysema cases. *1609*

Ammonia   *Blood   Increase*   Found in high percentage of patients without evidence of congestive failure or liver disease. *2104*

Carcinoembryonic Antigen   *Serum   Increase*   57% of patients had values > 2.5 ng/mL. *2199*

Eosinophils   *Sputum   Increase*   *1718*

Erythrocytes   *Blood   Increase*   Secondary polycythemia. *2467*

Hematocrit   *Blood   Increase*   Rises in later stages. *0433*

Hemoglobin   *Blood   Increase*   Rises in later stages. *0433*

Leukocytes   *Sputum   Increase*   Often infected on smear; increased WBC and epithelial debris. *0433*

Oxygen Saturation   *Blood   Decrease*   Arterial tension in 54 patients with chronic nonspecific lung disease, indicated subnormal results to be more frequent among bronchitics (79% with hypoxemia) than among emphysematous patients (63% with hypoxemia). *1497* 66% of nonasthmatic chronic lung disease patients (bronchitis and emphysema) had a mean pO_2 of 72.7 mm Hg. Bronchitics, but not emphysemics, showed a positive correlation between pO_2 and ventilatory performance. *2335   2612*

pCO₂   *Blood   Increase*   Arterial blood oxygen decreased and CO_2 increased. *2467*   Respiratory acidosis may occur. *0962*

pH   *Blood   Decrease*   Respiratory acidosis may occur. *0962*

Urine   Decrease   *2467*

Potassium   *Serum   Increase*   Rises in acidosis but total body potassium is usually depressed. *0433*

Serum   Normal   *2467*

Urine   Normal   *2467*

Sodium   *Serum   Normal*   *2467*

Urine   Decrease   *2467*

Volume   *Plasma   Increase*   Normal or increased. *2467*

Plasma   Normal   Normal or increased. *2467*

Urine   Normal   *2467*

493.10 Asthma (Intrinsic)

2,3-Diphosphoglycerate *Red Blood Cells Increase* In acute untreated attacks. *1228*

Alpha₁-Antichymotrypsin *Serum Increase* A study of patients with emphysema, bronchitis or asthma revealed there was no deficiency similar to that of alpha₁-antitrypsin. In fact, the levels were increased in all the disease states studied. *0461*

Antidiuretic Hormone *Serum Increase* In status asthmaticus. *1228*

Antismooth Muscle Antibodies *Serum Increase* In 20% of cases. *0211*

Aspartate Aminotransferase *Serum Increase* Possibly due to anoxic tissue damage in status asthmaticus. *0619* Increased in 90% of acute untreated asthma patients. *1228*

Bicarbonate *Serum Decrease* In a moderate to severe attack the partial pressure of CO_2 is reduced, while normal values are obtained for bicarbonate and pH. A condition worsens their pCO_2 and bicarbonate will rise and pH fall. *0433* May be decreased in early stages and may be increased in later stages. *2467*

Serum Increase May be decreased in early stages and increased in later stages. *2467* In 40% of 95 patients at initial hospitalization for this disorder. *0781* *0999*

Chloride *Sweat Increase* High concentrations found in sweat of chronic asthmatics and their relatives. *2275*

Complement C4 *Serum Decrease* Decreased serum concentrations of C4 and factor B were found in 3 of 15 skin-test positive asthmatic children. Confirming the involvement of complement in the pathogenesis of immediate type reaction. *1088*

Serum Normal Usually normal. *1228*

Complement, Total *Serum Normal* In the absence of any immunoglobulin deficiency, the levels of the other immunoglobulins as well as complement are within normal limits. *2035*

Copper *Serum Increase* Statistically significant. *2188*

Cortisol *Plasma Decrease* In 36 asthmatic children 8:00 A.M. plasma concentrations were compared with changes in their total eosinophil count (TEC) from 8:00 A.M. to 9:30 A.M. All children with low cortisol levels had decreases in TEC of < 2%, whereas 78% of children with normal cortisol had decreases > 15%. All children with decreases 15% had normal cortisol levels. *0232*

Plasma Normal In 36 asthmatic children 8:00 A.M. plasma concentrations were compared with changes in their total eosinophil count (TEC) from 8:00 A.M. to 9:30 A.M. All children with low cortisol levels had decreases in TEC of < 2%, whereas 78% of children with normal cortisol had decreases 15%. All children with decreases > 15% had normal cortisol levels. *0232*

Creatine Kinase *Serum Increase* Increases correlated with severity of symptoms (subjective) and objective measurement of airway obstruction. *0318* High in 38% of acute untreated asthma patients. *1228*

Eosinophils *Blood Increase* Tended to increase after bronchial provocation test but the increase did not correlate with the occurrence of the immediate type bronchial provocation test reaction. *1088* In more than 60% of patients tested. *0405* In 52 patients with active bronchial asthma (not on steroid therapy), total eosinophil counts were > 350/μL. Counts showed inverse correlation (R = -0.74) with specific airway conductance. *1072* In 55% of 122 patients at initial hospitalization for this disorder. *0781* *2538*

Sputum Increase Stained sputum is usually found to contain eosinophils; pointed elongated crystals derived from eosinophilic granules (Charcot-Leyden crystals) and spiral mucocellular bronchial casts (Curschmann's spirals) are also found. *0999* Often found; although suggestive of asthma in both allergic and infective types, they are not pathognomonic. *2035* *1718*

Glucose *Serum Increase* May be due to epinephrine or corticosteroids. *0433* May be found in corticosteroid-treated patients. *2035*

Hematocrit *Blood Increase* In 37% of 122 patients at initial hospitalization for this disorder. *0781*

Hemoglobin *Blood Increase* In 37% of 121 patients at initial hospitalization for this disorder. *0781*

Immunoglobulin IgE *Serum Normal* Elevated in most patients with allergic asthma but not in most patients with intrinsic asthma. At this time, however, the IgE level should not be used by itself to differentiate intrinsic from extrinsic asthma. Elevated in 75-81% of the children with asthma, nasal allergy, and atopic dermatitis. Elevated serum IgE concentration or blood eosinophilia, or both, was noted in 85% of the patients. *0405* Usually found in patients with allergic asthma but not with other forms. *1170* *0642*

Immunoglobulins *Serum Normal* In the absence of any immunoglobulin deficiency, the levels of the other immunoglobulins as well as complement are within normal limits. *2035*

Lactate Dehydrogenase Isoenzyme 5 (LD₅) *Serum Increase* Raised activities of LD_3 and LD_5 comprised the bulk of the increase in total activity. The increment in LD_3 activity arose from lung involvement whereas the major portion of the increment in LD_5 activity was derived from the liver. *2405*

Lactate Dehydrogenase Isoenzymes *Serum Increase* Raised activities of LD_3 and LD_5 comprised the bulk of the increase in total activity. LD_1 and LD_2 were unaltered. The increment in LD_3 activity arose from lung involvement whereas the major portion of the increment in LD-5 activity was derived from the liver in patients with asthma. *2405*

Lactic Acid *Blood Increase* Lactic acid, pyruvic acid and the lactic/pyruvic ratio are increased in some patients. *1972* Increased arterial blood lactate in acute untreated attacks. *1228*

Leukocytes *Blood Increase* In 53% of 122 patients at initial hospitalization for this disorder. *0781*

Neutrophils *Blood Increase* Modest changes in the peripheral WBC count occur along with an occasional increase in the percentage of polymorphonuclear WBC. *0433* In 38% of 122 patients at initial hospitalization for this disorder. *0781*

Oxygen Saturation *Blood Decrease* *0433* *2035*

pCO₂ *Blood Decrease* Reduced in a moderate to severe attack, while normal values are obtained for bicarbonate and pH. As the condition worsens the pCO_2 while the pH falls. *0433* pH, total plasma CO_2 and pCO_2 are decreased as a result of metabolic acidosis in status asthmaticus. *1972* In 30% of 91 patients at initial hospitalization for this disorder. *0781*

Blood Increase Reduced in a moderate to severe attack, while normal values are obtained for bicarbonate and pH. As the condition worsens the pCO_2 will rise while the pH falls. *0433* Reduction in arterial oxygen tension without concomitant elevation of arterial pCO_2 in moderately severe asthma. Elevation of pCO_2 is dependent upon total reduction in ventilation or will be seen when severe mucus plugging is present. *0433* CO_2 retention, indicating alveolar hypoventilation, has a grave prognostic significance. *0999*

Blood Normal The finding of a normal pCO_2 in a patient experiencing a severe asthmatic attack should alert the clinician to impending respiratory failure. *0433*

pH *Blood Decrease* In a moderate to severe attack; bicarbonate and pH are lowered. As the condition worsens the pCO_2 will rise while bicarbonate and pH fall. *0433* pH, total plasma CO_2 and pCO_2 are decreased as a result of metabolic acidosis in status asthmaticus. *1972*

Blood Increase In 59% of 92 patients at initial hospitalization for this disorder. *0781*

Blood Normal In moderate to severe attack. *0433*

Phosphate *Serum Decrease* In 40% of 107 patients at initial hospitalization for this disorder. *0781*

pO₂ *Blood Decrease* In general, with moderate asthma of whatever type, and even sometimes when there is no obvious distress, a modest reduction of arterial oxygen pressure to 60-70 mm Hg may be found. As an attack becomes more severe, a further reduction may yield values as low as 50-60 mm Hg. *1560* In 74% of 89 patients at initial hospitalization for this disorder. *0781* *2035* *2612*

Potassium *Serum Decrease* Hypokalemia caused by therapy or gastrointestinal fluid losses in children may intensify or induce respiratory failure by producing muscle weakness. *0433* May be found in corticosteroid-treated patients. *2035*

Pyruvate *Blood Increase* Lactic acid, pyruvic acid, and the lactic/pyruvic ratio are increased in some patients. *1972*

Rheumatoid Factor *Serum Increase* Found in 17% of patients. *0422* *0123*

Uric Acid *Serum Increase* Has been observed and is thought to be a consequence of the excessive use of sympathomimetic drugs. *0997* *0642*

494.00 Bronchiectasis

Arylsulfatase *Serum Increase* 30-50% increase in activity. *0610*

Cells *Sputum Increase* Polymorphonuclear and lymphocytic, as well as bronchial epithelial cells with varying degrees of metaplasia. *0433*

Cold Agglutinins *Serum Increase* Elevated titers may persist for weeks or months. *2035*

Erythrocyte Sedimentation Rate *Blood Increase* Nonspecific elevation seen with acute infections. *2220*

494.00 Bronchiectasis (continued)

Globulin *Serum Decrease* Seen when chronic uncontrolled infection persists. *0433* May be increased with chronic infection or decreased if congenital agammaglobulinemia is the underlying disease. *0999*

Serum Increase Seen when chronic uncontrolled infection persists. *0433* May be increased with chronic infection or decreased if congenital agammaglobulinemia is the underlying disease. *0999*

Hematocrit *Blood Decrease* When chronic uncontrolled infection persists, normochromic normocytic anemia is common. *0433*

Hemoglobin *Blood Decrease* When chronic uncontrolled infection persists, normochromic normocytic anemia is common. *0433* Leukocytosis and anemia are common. *0999*

Leukocytes *Blood Increase* During acute sepsis. *0433* Leukocytosis and anemia are common. *0999*

Blood Normal Usually normal unless pneumonitis is present. *2467*

Lymphocytes *Sputum Increase* Microscopic examination reveals polymorphonuclear and lymphocytic, as well as bronchial epithelial cells with varying degrees of metaplasia. *0433*

Neutrophils *Sputum Increase* Polymorphonuclear and lymphocytic, as well as bronchial epithelial cells with varying degrees of metaplasia. *0433*

pO$_2$ *Blood Decrease* Mild to moderate hypoxemia secondary to venous mixture with arterial blood. *2220*

495.90 Allergic Alveolitis

Eosinophils *Blood Increase* Eosinophilia is exceptional. *0433* Eosinophilia up to 45%. *2467*

Erythrocyte Sedimentation Rate *Blood Increase* *2467*

Globulin *Serum Increase* Elevation in the range of 2-3 g/dL. *0433*

Leukocytes *Blood Increase* Normal WBC; increased in presence of infection. *2467*

Neutrophils *Blood Increase* During the acute febrile episodes there is a polymorphonuclear leukocytosis of 15,000-25,000/μL. *0433*

Oxygen Saturation *Blood Decrease* Arterial blood gases show decreased pO$_2$ with either slight respiratory alkalosis or normal pH and pCO$_2$. *0433*

pH *Blood Increase* Arterial blood gases show decreased pO$_2$ with either slight respiratory alkalosis or normal pH and pCO$_2$. *0433*

pO$_2$ *Blood Decrease* Arterial blood gases show decreased pO$_2$ with either slight respiratory alkalosis or normal pH and pCO$_2$. *0433*

Precipitins *Serum Increase* Found in 17-18%, particularly against the thermophilic actinomycete M. faeni and also, against T. vulgaris and fungi such as the genus Aspergillus and Mucormycosis. *1801* *2035*

496.00 Chronic Obstructive Lung Disease

2,3-Diphosphoglycerate *Red Blood Cells Increase* Synthesis is increased. *0159*

Aldosterone *Plasma Increase* Plasma renin and aldosterone tended to have higher than normal baseline values, especially in hypercapnic patients. *0698*

Alpha$_1$-Antitrypsin *Serum Decrease* Homozygotes for alpha$_1$ antitrypsin deficiency traits usually develop chronic obstructive lung disease by age 40. Heterozygotes have levels intermediate between normals and homozygotes, and frequently develop this disease. *1609*

Alpha$_2$-Macroglobulin *Serum Decrease* *2629*

Ammonia *Blood Increase* Venous levels were significantly influenced by pH and pCO$_2$. *0538*

Bicarbonate *Serum Increase* Suggests chronic hypoventilation. *0962* In 82% of 69 patients at initial hospitalization for this disorder. *0781*

Chloride *Serum Decrease* Suggests chronic hypoventilation. *0962* In 44% of 71 patients at initial hospitalization for this disorder. *0781*

Cholesterol *Serum Decrease* Decreased in decompensated patients. Amount of decrease correlates with degree of hypoxemia. *2044*

Eosinophils *Blood Increase* In 37% of 79 patients at initial hospitalization for this disorder. *0781*

Erythrocytes *Blood Increase* Erythrocytosis, secondary to chronic hypoxemia may be prominent, especially in bronchitic patients. *1108*

Glomerular Filtration Rate (GFR) *Urine Decrease* Hypercapnic patients showed low effective renal plasma flow, impaired water and sodium excretion compared to normocapnic patients and normal controls. *0698*

Glutamic Acid *Red Blood Cells Increase* Erythrocyte l-glutamate was significantly elevated only in hypercapnic patients. *2411*

Hematocrit *Blood Decrease* Even minor degrees of anemia are poorly tolerated by patients. Because of the high incidence of peptic ulcer associated with this disease, an anemia may be due to occult or clinically evident gastrointestinal bleeding. *0962*

Blood Increase Polycythemia, suggesting a significant degree of chronic hypoxemia. *0962* In 42% of 80 patients at initial hospitalization for this disorder. *0781*

Hemoglobin *Blood Decrease* Even minor degrees of anemia are poorly tolerated by patients. Because of the high incidence of peptic ulcer associated with this disease, an anemia may be due to occult or clinically evident gastrointestinal bleeding. *0962*

Blood Increase In 25 patients with severe disease, blood hemoglobin exhibited a significant increase indicating an improved oxygen transport. In most patients a leftward shifting of the oxygen dissociation curve occurred. Hemoglobin was significantly increased in all patients, regardless of degree of hypoxia. *1092* Polycythemia, suggesting a significant degree of chronic hypoxemia. *0962* In 39% of 80 patients at initial hospitalization for this disorder. *0781*

Leukocytes *Blood Increase* In 42% of 80 patients at initial hospitalization for this disorder. *0781*

Lipids *Serum Decrease* Decreased in decompensated patients. Amount of decrease correlates with degree of hypoxemia. *2044*

Lipoproteins, Beta *Serum Decrease* Decreased in decompensated patients. Amount of decrease correlates with degree of hypoxemia. *2044*

Neutrophils *Blood Increase* In 42% of 79 patients at initial hospitalization for this disorder. *0781*

Oxygen Saturation *Blood Decrease* Greatest declines in arterial oxygen saturation occurred during sleep, with intermittent decreases as great as 44% saturation (range, 12-44% saturation). *0748* Decreased pO$_2$ associated with increased pCO$_2$. *2467*

pCO$_2$ *Blood Increase* Decreased pO$_2$ associated with increased pCO$_2$. *2467* In 10 patients with hypercapnia, mean renal net acid excretion was elevated and correlated with arterial pCO$_2$, blood pH and urinary pH. *1479* In 33% of 75 patients at initial hospitalization for this disorder. *0781*

pH *Blood Decrease* Blood pH was significantly lower in 10 patients with chronic obstructive lung disease than in normocapnic controls. Renal net acid excretion was elevated but urinary pH was not significantly raised. *1479* In 48% of 74 patients at initial hospitalization for this disorder. *0781*

pO$_2$ *Blood Decrease* Decreased pO$_2$ associated with increased pCO$_2$. *2467* Greatest declines in arterial oxygen saturation occurred during sleep, with intermittent decreases as great as 44% saturation (range = 12-44% saturation). *0748* In 82% of 70 patients at initial hospitalization for this disorder. *0781*

Potassium *Serum Decrease* Suggests a coexisting primary metabolic alkalosis. *0962*

Serum Increase When acidemia is present, may be falsely high because of potassium ions moving from the extracellular space. *0962*

Renin Activity *Plasma Increase* Plasma renin and aldosterone tended to have higher than normal baseline values, especially in hypercapnic patients. *0698*

Sodium *Urine Decrease* Hypercapnic patients showed low effective renal plasma flow, impaired water and sodium excretion compared to normocapnic patients and normal controls. *0698*

Triglycerides *Serum Decrease* Decreased in decompensated patients. Amount of decrease correlates with degree of hypoxemia. *2044*

Viscosity *Serum Increase* An increase in blood viscosity, red blood cell mass, and blood volume is thought to further compromise the pressure-flow relationships of the constricted and restricted pulmonary vascular bed. *1108*

Volume *Plasma Increase* An increase in blood viscosity, red blood cell mass, and blood volume is thought to further compromise the pressure- flow relationships of the constricted and restricted pulmonary vascular bed. *1108*

496.01 Alpha$_1$-Antitrypsin Deficiency

Alanine Aminotransferase *Serum Increase* Related to liver disease. *1636*

Albumin *Serum Decrease* Related to liver disease. *1636*

Serum Normal 2467

Alkaline Phosphatase *Serum Increase* Related to liver disease. *1636*

Alpha$_1$-Antitrypsin *Serum Decrease 2467*

Alpha$_1$-Globulin *Serum Decrease* Low alpha$_1$ globulin fraction in a patient with cirrhosis of the liver suggests the diagnosis. *0962*

Alpha$_2$-Macroglobulin *Serum Increase* Patients with all types of this disorder were found to have significantly elevated levels. *0284*

Apolipoprotein AI *Serum Increase* In patients with liver disease all apolipoproteins were elevated. *0563*

Apolipoprotein AII *Plasma Increase* In patients with liver disease all apolipoproteins were elevated. *0563*

Apolipoprotein B *Serum Increase* In patients with liver disease all apolipoproteins were elevated. *0563*

Aspartate Aminotransferase *Serum Increase* Related to liver disease. *1636*

Bicarbonate *Serum Decrease* Associated COPD. *1636*

Bile Acids *Serum Increase* In 34 patients with this disease all patients with morphological cirrhosis. *1685*

Urine Increase Excretion was increased. *0563*

Feces Increase Excretion was increased. *0563*

Bilirubin *Serum Increase* Related to liver disease. *1636*

Calcium *Serum Decrease* Related to decreased Albumin. *1636*

Chenodeoxycholic Acid *Serum Increase* In 34 patients with this disease all patients with morphological cirrhosis. *1685*

Chloride *Serum Decrease* Seen with associated hyperventilation. *1636*

Cholesterol *Serum Decrease* Related to liver disease. *1636*

Serum Increase Average 604 mg/dL. *0563*

Cholesterol Esters *Serum Decrease* Greatly depressed as was cholesterol absorption. *0563*

Cholic Acid *Serum Increase* In 34 patients with this disease all patients with morphological cirrhosis. *1685*

Complement C3 *Serum Normal 2467*

Euglobulin Clot Lysis Time *Blood Increase* Increased. *0295 2353*

Fatty Acids, Free (FFA) *Serum Normal* Normal. *0563*

Gamma Glutamyl Transferase (GGT) *Serum Increase* Related to liver disease. *1636*

Haptoglobin *Serum Normal 2467*

Hematocrit *Blood Decrease* With associated hypersplenism. *1636*

Blood Increase With associated polycythemia secondary to hypoxemia. *1636*

Hemoglobin *Blood Decrease* With associated hypersplenism. *1636*

Blood Increase With associated polycythemia secondary to hypoxemia. *1636*

Iron-Binding Capacity, Total (TIBC) *Serum Normal 2467*

Lactate Dehydrogenase *Serum Increase* Related to liver disease. *1636*

Leukocytes *Blood Decrease* With associated hypersplenism. *1636*

Lipoproteins *Serum Increase* Lipoprotein X was increased to an average of 855 mg/dL. *0563*

Platelet Count *Blood Decrease* With associated hypersplenism. *1636*

Potassium *Serum Increase* Seen with Acidosis. *1636*

Triglycerides *Serum Increase* Average 336 mg/dL. *0563*

500.00   Anthracosis

Bicarbonate *Serum Increase* CO$_2$ retention may occur. *0433*

Erythrocytes *Blood Increase* May become progressively elevated. *0433* Secondary polycythemia. *2467*

Erythrocyte Sedimentation Rate *Blood Increase* Increased ESR generally indicates secondary infection. *0433*

Hematocrit *Blood Decrease* Secondary anemia. *2467*

Blood Increase May become progressively elevated. *0433*

Hemoglobin *Blood Decrease* Secondary anemia. *2467*

Blood Increase May become progressively elevated. *0433*

Leukocytes *Blood Increase* Increased with associated infection. *2467*

Oxygen Saturation *Blood Decrease* Arterial oxygen saturation may fall. *0433*

pCO$_2$ *Blood Increase* Impaired gas exchange in established cases. *0151*

pO$_2$ *Blood Decrease* Impaired gas exchange in established cases. *0151* Arterial oxygen saturation may fall. *0433*

Rheumatoid Factor *Serum Increase* 42% of patients without associated arthritis had a positive sheep cell agglutination test, while 80% with associated rheumatoid arthritis were found to be seropositive. *0962*

501.00   Asbestosis

Bicarbonate *Serum Increase* CO$_2$ retention may occur. *0433*

Erythrocytes *Blood Increase* May become progressively elevated. *0433* Secondary polycythemia. *2467*

Pleural Effusion Increase Often blood pleural effusions. *0151*

Erythrocyte Sedimentation Rate *Blood Increase* Increased ESR generally indicates secondary infection. *0433*

Hematocrit *Blood Decrease* Secondary anemia. *2467*

Blood Increase May become progressively elevated. *0433*

Hemoglobin *Blood Decrease* Secondary anemia. *2467*

Blood Increase May become progressively elevated. *0433*

Leukocytes *Blood Increase* Increased with associated infection. *2467*

Oxygen Saturation *Blood Decrease* Arterial oxygen saturation may fall. *0433*

pCO$_2$ *Blood Decrease* Impaired gas diffusion and the accompanying hyperventilation results in a low pCO$_2$, unless the defect is severe and CO$_2$ retention occurs. *2104*

Blood Increase Impaired gas exchange in established cases. *0151*

pO$_2$ *Blood Decrease* Impaired gas exchange in established cases. *0151* Arterial oxygen saturation may fall. *0433*

Rheumatoid Factor *Serum Increase* 21% positivity. *0123 0422 0962*

502.00   Silicosis

1,25-Dihydroxy-Vitamin D$_3$ *Serum Increase 0062*

Angiotensin-Converting Enzyme (ACE) *Serum Increase* Elevated and associated with a progression of the disease. *1464 1705*

Bicarbonate *Serum Increase* CO$_2$ retention may occur. *0433*

Erythrocytes *Blood Increase* May become progressively elevated. *0433*

Erythrocyte Sedimentation Rate *Blood Increase* Increased ESR generally indicates secondary infection. *0433*

Hematocrit *Blood Decrease* Secondary anemia. *2467*

Blood Increase May become progressively elevated. *0433*

Hemoglobin *Blood Decrease* Secondary anemia. *2467*

Blood Increase May become progressively elevated. *0433*

Lactate Dehydrogenase *Serum Increase 0962*

Leukocytes *Blood Increase* Increased with associated infection. *2467*

Oxygen Saturation *Blood Decrease* Impaired gas exchange and movement of respiratory cage due to noncompliant lungs. *0151* Arterial oxygen saturation may fall. *0433*

pCO$_2$ *Blood Increase* Impaired gas exchange in established cases. *0151*

pO$_2$ *Blood Decrease* Impaired gas exchange in established cases. *0151* Impaired gas exchange and movement of respiratory cage due to noncompliant lungs. *0151* Arterial oxygen saturation may fall. *0433*

Rheumatoid Factor *Serum Increase* Positive in 15% of patients. *0123 0422 0962*

503.01   Berylliosis

Bicarbonate *Serum Increase* CO$_2$ retention may occur. *0433*

Calcium *Serum Increase 2467*

Urine Increase Hypercalciuria may occur. *0433 2467*

Erythrocytes *Blood Increase* Secondary polycythemia. *2467* May become progressively elevated. *0433*

503.01 Berylliosis (continued)

Erythrocyte Sedimentation Rate *Blood Increase* Increased ESR generally indicates secondary infection. *0433*

Globulin *Serum Increase* Occasional transient hypergammaglobulinemia. *2467*

Hematocrit *Blood Decrease* Secondary anemia. *2467*

Blood Increase Secondary polycythemia. *2467* May become progressively elevated. *0433*

Hemoglobin *Blood Decrease* Secondary anemia. *2467*

Blood Increase Secondary polycythemia. *2467* May become progressively elevated. *0433*

Leukocytes *Blood Increase* Increased with associated infection. *2467*

Oxygen Saturation *Blood Decrease* Hypoxemia is frequent. *2608* Arterial oxygen saturation may fall. *0433*

pCO$_2$ *Blood Decrease* Impaired gas diffusion and the accompanying hyperventilation results in a low pCO$_2$, unless the defect is severe and CO$_2$ retention occurs. *2104*

Blood Increase Impaired gas exchange in established cases. *0151*

pO$_2$ *Blood Decrease* Hypoxemia is frequent. *2608* Impaired gas exchange in established cases. *0151* Arterial oxygen saturation may fall. *0433*

Uric Acid *Serum Increase* *2467*

510.00 Empyema

Alpha$_1$-Antichymotrypsin *Serum Increase* A study of patients with emphysema, bronchitis or asthma revealed there was no deficiency similar to that of alpha$_1$-antitrypsin. In fact, the levels were increased in all the disease states studied. *0461*

Carcinoembryonic Antigen *Pleural Effusion Increase* Benign inflammatory effusions (tuberculosis, empyema, pneumonia) had mean activity of 6.2 ± 3.4 ng/mL, higher than effusions caused by congestive heart failure (2.9 ± 1.5) and other noninflammatory effusions. *1945*

Glucose *CSF Normal* In subdural empyema. *0186*

Pleural Effusion Decrease Levels less than 3.3 mmol/L (60 mg/dL). *0174* 0-60 mg/dL. *2017*

Leukocytes *Blood Increase* In subdural empyema. (20,000-40,000/µl) *0186* Total counts may become extremely high. *2538*

CSF Increase In subdural empyema. (50-1000/µl, 20-80% neutrophils) *0186*

Pleural Effusion Increase 25,000-100,000/µL. *2017*

Neutrophils *Pleural Effusion Increase* Very high counts occur; cells tend to degenerate, with blurred nuclei which do not stain in characteristic purple color. *1403*

Oxygen Saturation *Blood Decrease* Empyema or tuberculous effusion. *0797*

pH *Pleural Effusion Decrease* All 10 patients had a pleural fluid pH of < 7.30. Pleural fluid pH values < 7.30 are likely to result in loculation of the pleural space. *1845* May occur in non-neoplastic inflammatory pleural effusion (empyema, rheumatoid disease, tuberculosis). *0797*

pO$_2$ *Blood Decrease* Empyema or tuberculous effusion. *0797*

Protein *CSF Increase* In subdural empyema. (75-300 mg/dL) *0186*

Pleural Effusion Increase Exudate. *2017*

513.00 Abscess of Lung

Albumin *Serum Decrease* *0186*

Urine Increase Frequent. *2467*

Erythrocyte Sedimentation Rate *Blood Increase* Markedly elevated. *0433*

Hematocrit *Blood Decrease* Normochromic normocytic anemia in chronic stage. *2467*

Hemoglobin *Blood Decrease* Characteristic leukocytosis and moderate or even severe anemia. *0999* Normochromic normocytic anemia in chronic stage. *2467*

Leukocytes *Blood Increase* In most patients there is a leukocytosis in the range of 20,000-30,000/µL. The debilitated or elderly patients may fail to respond to the infection with a leukocytosis. *0433* *0999*

Neutrophils *Blood Increase* In most patients there is a leukocytosis in the range of 20,000-30,000 cells/µL. The debilitated or elderly patients may fail to respond to the infection with a leukocytosis. *0433*

514.00 Pulmonary Congestion and Hypostasis

Bicarbonate *Serum Decrease* Respiratory alkalosis may occur. *0962*

pCO$_2$ *Blood Decrease* Respiratory alkalosis may occur. *0962*

pH *Blood Increase* Respiratory alkalosis may occur. *0962*

pO$_2$ *Blood Decrease* *0503*

Protein *Pleural Effusion Decrease* Transudate (< 3 g/dL). *0503*

516.00 Pulmonary Alveolar Proteinosis

Lactate Dehydrogenase *Serum Increase* Increases when protein accumulates in lungs and drops to normal when infiltrate resolves. *2467* Values for all 12 patients were above the normal upper limit. *1518*

Oxygen Saturation *Blood Decrease* May be normal or reduced. *0151*

pCO$_2$ *Blood Decrease* Impaired gas diffusion and the accompanying hyperventilation results in a low pCO$_2$, unless the defect is severe and CO$_2$ retention occurs. *2104*

516.10 Idiopathic Pulmonary Hemosiderosis

Anisocytes *Blood Increase* Peripheral blood displays the classic changes of severe iron depletion: anisocytosis, poikilocytosis, microcytosis, and hypochromia. *2538*

Bilirubin *Urine Increase* Excretion may be increased by the increased porphyrin catabolism. *2538*

Bilirubin, Indirect *Serum Increase* Occasional findings of hemolytic type of anemia. *2467*

Carcinoembryonic Antigen *Serum Increase* *0795 2035*

Eosinophils *Blood Increase* In up to 20% of patients. *2467* Eosinophilia of moderate degree occurs in about 12% of the cases. *2538*

Erythrocytes *Urine Increase* Microscopic hematuria in some cases. Gross hematuria occurs infrequently. *2538*

Iron *Serum Decrease* Peripheral blood displays the classic changes of severe iron depletion: anisocytosis, poikilocytosis, microcytosis, and hypochromia. *2538*

Serum Normal Hypochromic microcytic anemia due to pulmonary hemorrhages with normal serum iron and iron-binding capacity. *2467*

Iron-Binding Capacity, Total (TIBC) *Serum Increase* *2538*

Serum Normal Hypochromic microcytic anemia due to pulmonary hemorrhages with normal serum iron and iron-binding capacity. *2467*

MCV *Blood Decrease* Peripheral blood displays the classic changes of severe iron depletion: anisocytosis, poikilocytosis, microcytosis, and hypochromia. *2538*

Occult Blood *Feces Positive* Stools may contain occult blood as a result of swallowed blood-laden sputum. *2538*

pCO$_2$ *Blood Decrease* Impaired gas diffusion and the accompanying hyperventilation results in a low pCO$_2$, unless the defect is severe and CO$_2$ retention occurs in primary pulmonary hemosiderosis. *2104*

Poikilocytes *Blood Increase* Peripheral blood displays the classic changes of severe iron depletion: anisocytosis, poikilocytosis, microcytosis, and hypochromia. *2538*

Urobilinogen *Urine Increase* Occasional findings of hemolytic type of anemia. *2467* Excretion may be increased by the increased porphyrin catabolism. *2538*

518.00 Pulmonary Collapse

Bicarbonate *Serum Decrease* Respiratory alkalosis may occur. *0962*

Eosinophils *Blood Increase* *0433*

Leukocytes *Blood Increase* May occur. *0433*

Oxygen Saturation *Blood Decrease* Acute massive atelectasis produces a picture of an intrapulmonary right-to-left shunt with a drop in pO$_2$. *0433*

pCO$_2$ *Blood Decrease* Acute massive atelectasis produces a picture of an intrapulmonary right-to-left shunt with a drop in pCO$_2$. *0433* Respiratory alkalosis may occur. *0962*

pH *Blood Decrease* Active massive atelectasis produces a picture of intrapulmonary right-to-left shunt with a decrease in pH. *0433*

Blood Increase Respiratory alkalosis may occur. *0962*

pO$_2$ *Blood Decrease* Acute massive atelectasis produces a picture of an intrapulmonary right-to-left shunt with a drop in pO$_2$. *0433*

518.10 Pneumomediastinum

Leukocytes *Blood Increase* Variable and nonspecific leukocytosis. *2467*

518.40 Pulmonary Edema

Creatine Kinase *Serum Increase* For reasons that are still unclear some cases may have high levels. *0812 0503*

Oxygen Saturation *Blood Decrease* Decreased pO$_2$ associated with normal or decreased pCO$_2$. *2467* Mean arterial O$_2$ tension measured in 71 patients breathing room air was 59 mm Hg. The 14 acidemic patients had markedly lower pO$_2$, all under 60 mm Hg. *0554*

pCO$_2$ *Blood Decrease* Decreased pO$_2$ associated with normal or decreased pCO$_2$. *2467*

pH *Blood Decrease* Of 71 patients breathing room air, 14 were acidemic; 35 alkalemic and 33 had a pH in the normal range. *0554*

Blood Increase Of 71 patients breathing room air, 14 were acidemic; 35 alkalemic and 33 had a pH in the normal range. The acidemic group had markedly lower pO$_2$, all under 60 mm Hg. *0554*

pO$_2$ *Blood Decrease* Decreased pO$_2$ associated with normal or decreased pCO$_2$. *2467* Mean arterial O$_2$ tension measured in 71 patients breathing room air was 59 mm Hg. The 14 acidemic patients had markedly lower pO$_2$, all under 60 mm Hg. *0554*

DISEASES OF THE DIGESTIVE SYSTEM

Diseases of the Arteries and Veins

527.90 Diseases of the Salivary Glands

Amylase *Serum Increase* Salivary gland disease: mumps, suppurative inflammation, duct obstruction due to calculus. *2467*

533.90 Peptic Ulcer, Site Unspecified

Albumin *Serum Decrease* *2467*

Alpha$_1$-Globulin *Serum Increase* May be increased. *2467*

Alpha$_2$-Globulin *Serum Increase* May be increased. *2467*

Amylase *Serum Increase* Mild-moderate elevation with active ulcer and no associated pancreatitis. Rise is directly related to the size and duration of perforation, and amount of fluid accumulated in peritoneal cavity. Free perforations not in contact with pancreas may lead to hyperamylasemia also. *2031* Extremely high values found in any condition in which the GI tract is perforated or loses viability. *2104*

Peritoneal Fluid Increase With perforation. *2467*

Angiotensin-Converting Enzyme (ACE) *Serum Increase* Significant increase regardless of whether ulceration was gastric or duodenal. *0483*

Bicarbonate *Serum Increase* Pyloric obstruction with vomiting and loss of gastric secretion results in hypochloremia, hyponatremia, hypokalemia, elevated serum pH and carbon dioxide content, and azotemia. *0962*

Duodenal Contents Decrease Bicarbonate level has been shown to be 1/2 of controls. *0949*

Calcium *Serum Increase* Due to excessive alkali intake if the antacid contains calcium, or if milk is taken in excess. *0619*

Carcinoembryonic Antigen *Serum Increase* 14% of patients had positive assay (values > 12.5 ng/mL). *0253* 45% of patients had values > 2.5 ng/mL. *0979 2199*

Chloride *Serum Decrease* May fall below 100 mmol/L in an ulcer complicated by obstruction. With persistent marked obstruction, may reach as low as 60 mmol/L. *0433* Pyloric obstruction with vomiting and loss of gastric secretion results in hypochloremia, hyponatremia, hypokalemia, elevated serum pH and carbon dioxide content, and azotemia. *0962*

Cryofibrinogen *Serum Increase* *2035 0856 1551 2046*

Erythrocyte Sedimentation Rate *Blood Increase* Elevation of the WBC, increased ESR and related phenomena are, to be expected in the event of perforation, massive hemorrhage, and toxic or infectious complications. *0962*

Blood Normal Normal in peptic ulcer, but accelerated in carcinoma of the stomach. *0962*

Gastrin *Serum Increase* Tends to be elevated in gastric ulcer and correlates with decreased acid secretion. *0151* May occur after meals. *1533*

Serum Normal Fasting concentration is generally normal despite hypersecretion of gastric acid. May occur after meals. *1533* Fasting serum concentrations are normal in patients with ordinary duodenal ulcer disease. Although the mean increase in concentration after a meal is higher in duodenal ulcer than in normal subjects, this test is not helpful diagnostically. *2199*

Glucose *Serum Decrease* A high frequency of spontaneous hypoglycemia occurs in these patients. *2104*

Glucose Tolerance *Serum Decrease* Significantly greater rise in glucose concentration and higher output of insulin was observed in patients with duodenal ulcer. *1101*

Hematocrit *Blood Decrease* A few patients will have anemia because of chronic blood loss. *0433* An ulcer that bleeds chronically will cause a varying degree of iron deficiency anemia. *0962*

Blood Normal Uncomplicated peptic ulcer is not associated with anemia. *0962*

Hemoglobin *Blood Decrease* A few patients will have anemia because of chronic blood loss. *0433* An ulcer that bleeds chronically will cause a varying degree of iron deficiency anemia. *0962*

Blood Normal Uncomplicated peptic ulcer is not associated with anemia. *0962*

Iron *Serum Decrease* An ulcer that bleeds chronically will cause a varying degree of iron deficiency anemia. *0962*

Iron-Binding Capacity, Total (TIBC) *Serum Increase* An ulcer that bleeds chronically will cause a varying degree of iron deficiency anemia. *0962*

Iron Saturation *Serum Decrease* An ulcer that bleeds chronically will cause a varying degree of iron deficiency anemia. *0962*

Lactate Dehydrogenase *Gastric Material Increase* Moderately increased activity. *0619*

Leukocytes *Blood Increase* Increased with shift to left. *2467* Elevation of the WBC, increased ESR and related phenomena are to be expected in the event of perforation, massive hemorrhage, and toxic or infectious complications. *0962*

Lipase *Serum Increase* Perforated or penetrating peptic ulcer especially with involvement of the pancreas. *2467*

Lysolecithin *Gastric Material Increase* Found to be high. *1174*

MCH *Blood Decrease* A few patients will have anemia because of chronic blood loss. *0433* An ulcer that bleeds chronically will cause a varying degree of iron deficiency anemia. *0962*

MCHC *Blood Decrease* A few patients will have anemia because of chronic blood loss. *0433* An ulcer that bleeds chronically will cause a varying degree of iron deficiency anemia. *0962*

MCV *Blood Decrease* A few patients will have anemia because of chronic blood loss. *0433* An ulcer that bleeds chronically will cause a varying degree of iron deficiency anemia. *0962*

Norepinephrine *Plasma Increase* *0271*

Pepsinogen *Serum Increase* Serum acid protease activity at pH 1.8 (pepsin) shows slightly higher levels than normal. *1604* An elevated serum concentration appears to be a subclinical marker of the ulcer diathesis in families with the autosomal dominant form of peptic ulcer disease. Elevated immunoreactive pepsinogen I (> 100 ng/mL) segregated as a dominant trait in the affected families. *1997*

pH *Blood Increase* May exceed 7.45. Complicated by obstruction. *0433* Pyloric obstruction with vomiting and loss of gastric secretion results in hypochloremia, hyponatremia, hypokalemia, elevated serum pH and CO$_2$ content, and azotemia. *0962*

Gastric Material Decrease True achlorhydria virtually excludes peptic ulcer disease. In gastric ulcer the average basal gastric secretion is decreased or normal. *0118*

Gastric Material Increase No single test of gastric secretion shows abnormal hypersecretion in more than 50% of duodenal ulcer patients. *0118 0587*

Potassium *Serum Decrease* May be < 3.5 mmol/L when complicated by obstruction. *0433* Pyloric obstruction with vomiting and loss of gastric secretion results in hypochloremia, hyponatremia, hypokalemia, elevated serum pH and carbon dioxide content, and azotemia. *0962*

533.90 Peptic Ulcer, Site Unspecified (continued)

Protein *Serum Decrease* 2467

Sodium *Serum Decrease* May be < 135 mmol/L when complicated by obstruction. 0433 Pyloric obstruction with vomiting and loss of gastric secretion results in hypochloremia, hyponatremia, hypokalemia, elevated serum pH and carbon dioxide content, and azotemia. 0962

Urea Nitrogen *Serum Increase* Pyloric obstruction with vomiting and loss of gastric secretion results in hypochloremia, hyponatremia, hypokalemia, elevated serum pH and carbon dioxide content, and azotemia. 0962

535.00 Gastritis

Albumin *Serum Decrease* May be low in patients with giant hypertrophic gastritis who exude protein into the lumen. 0433 Secondary to protein-losing enteropathy in atrophic gastroenteritis. 2104

Antibody Titer *Serum Increase* Parietal cell antibody detected by CF tests using gastric mucosal homogenate or by direct immunofluorescence on sections of gastric mucosa is present in approximately 60% of patients with idiopathic atrophic gastritis. 0583

Antithyroglobulin Antibodies *Serum Increase* With atrophic gastritis. 2199

Aspartate Aminotransferase *Serum Increase* In 33% of 37 patients at initial hospitalization for this disorder. 0781

Eosinophils *Blood Increase* Peripheral eosinophilia in eosinophilic gastritis. 2199

Gastrin *Serum Increase* Increased in chronic atrophic gastritis. 2281 The combination of high serum gastrin and low pepsinogen is commonly found in patients with atrophic gastritis. 2199 2033

Hematocrit *Blood Decrease* May be low in patients with bleeding. 0433

Hemoglobin *Blood Decrease* May be low in patients with bleeding. 0433 Hypochromic microcytic anemia due to blood loss. 2467

Hydrochloric Acid *Gastric Material Decrease* Most patients with Ménétrier's disease have achlorhydria. However, some patients may have hypersecretion. 2238 Transient hypochlorhydria or achlorhydria may be observed during episodes of acute gastritis. 2199

Iron-Binding Capacity, Total (TIBC) *Serum Increase* Anemia may be due to chronic blood loss. 0642 0962

Iron Saturation *Serum Decrease* Anemia may be due to chronic blood loss. 0642 0962

Lactate Dehydrogenase *Gastric Material Increase* Moderately increased activity. 0619

Leukocytes *Blood Increase* May be present in cases of corrosive or phlegmonous gastritis. 0433

MCH *Blood Decrease* May be low in patients with bleeding. 0433

MCHC *Blood Decrease* May be low in patients with bleeding. 0433

MCV *Blood Decrease* May be low in patients with bleeding. 0433

Blood Increase Secondary to B$_{12}$ deficiency with atrophic gastritis. 2199

Neutrophils *Blood Increase* In 40% of 36 patients at initial hospitalization for this disorder. 0781

Occult Blood *Feces Positive* Upper GI bleeding. 2199

Pepsin *Gastric Material Decrease* In Ménétrier's Disease hyposecretion is usual finding. 0407

Pepsinogen *Serum Decrease* The combination of high serum gastrin and low pepsinogen is commonly found in patients with atrophic gastritis. 2199

pH *Gastric Material Decrease* Erosive hemorrhagic gastritis appears to be due to pathologic back diffusion of hydrogen ions caused by a breakdown of the gastric mucosal barrier. 2236 Most patients with Ménétrier's disease have achlorhydria, but some may have hypersecretion. 1115 In Ménétrier's disease hyposecretion of gastric acid is usual finding 0407

Gastric Material Increase Most patients with Ménétrier's Disease have achlorhydria. However, some patients may have hypersecretion. 2238 Transient hypochlorhydria or achlorhydria may be observed during episodes of acute gastritis. 2199

Protein *Serum Decrease* An increased sensitivity of atrophic mucosa to exogenous irritants is suggested by the observation that patients with atrophic gastritis lost excessive amounts of plasma protein when they ingested ethanol. 0397 In Ménétrier's disease hypoproteinemia is often seen 0407

Feces Increase An increased sensitivity of atrophic mucosa to exogenous irritants is suggested by the observation that patients with atrophic gastritis lost excessive amounts of plasma protein when they ingested ethanol. 0397

Uropepsinogen *Urine Decrease* With atrophic gastritis. 0587

Vitamin B$_{12}$ *Serum Decrease* With atrophic gastritis. 2199

537.00 Pyloric Stenosis, Acquired

Bicarbonate *Serum Increase* Metabolic alkalosis secondary to vomiting. 0587

Chloride *Serum Decrease* Metabolic alkalosis secondary to vomiting. 0587

Hydrochloric Acid *Gastric Material Increase* Due to excess circulating gastrin. 0587

pH *Urine Increase* 2467

Gastric Material Decrease Due to excess circulating gastrin. 0587

Potassium *Serum Decrease* Secondary to vomiting. 0587

Urine Normal 2467

Sodium *Serum Decrease* Secondary to vomiting. 0587

Urine Decrease 2467

Volume *Plasma Decrease* 2467

Urine Decrease 2467

537.40 Fistula of Stomach and Duodenum

Alkaline Phosphatase *Serum Increase* Leading to secondary osteomalacia. 0619

Bicarbonate *Serum Decrease* Metabolic acidosis may occur. 0962

Carcinoembryonic Antigen *Serum Increase* Found in 15% (2.5 ng/mL). 0587

Chloride *Serum Decrease* In gastric fistula, hypokalemic, hypochloremic alkalosis may result. 2199

Fat *Feces Increase* Excessively rapid passage of intestinal contents. Increased fat in feces with gastrocolic fistula. 0619

Hematocrit *Blood Decrease* Anemia and hypoproteinemia reflect malnutrition and chronic disease. 2199

Blood Increase Will reflect the degree of hemoconcentration. 2199

Hemoglobin *Blood Decrease* Anemia and hypoproteinemia reflect malnutrition and chronic disease. 2199

Leukocytes *Blood Increase* May be elevated with sepsis. 2199

Nitrogen *Feces Increase* 0619

Occult Blood *Feces Positive* The most common presentation. False negative and positives occur. 2512

pCO$_2$ *Blood Decrease* Metabolic acidosis may occur. 0962

pH *Blood Decrease* With high output proximal small bowel or pancreatic fistulas, the patients may be acidotic, because the lost pancreatic and biliary secretions are alkaline. 2199 Metabolic acidosis may occur. 0962

Blood Increase In gastric fistula, hypokalemic, hypochloremic alkalosis may result. 2199

Potassium *Serum Decrease* Renal wasting leads to hypokalemic state. 1679 In gastric fistula, hypokalemic, hypochloremic alkalosis may result. 2199

Protein *Serum Decrease* Anemia and hypoproteinemia reflect malnutrition and chronic disease. 2199

Sodium *Serum Decrease* Small intestinal aspiration or fistula. The loss of sodium/day (430 mmol) is > the loss of chloride (270 mmol). 0619

540.90 Acute Appendicitis

Amylase *Serum Increase* 57 of 149 cases had increased concentration. Highest value was 1,480 U/L in a patient with an obstructed gangrenous appendix. 0320

Erythrocytes *Urine Increase* Small numbers are found in the urine in about 25% of patients. 2199

Erythrocyte Sedimentation Rate *Blood Increase* With abscess formation or peritonitis, the rate increases rapidly. *0962*

Blood Normal In unruptured acute appendicitis, the ESR is normal during the first 24 h, even when the appendix is suppurative or gangrenous. *0962*

Glucose *Serum Increase* In 34% of 52 patients at initial hospitalization for this disorder. *0781*

Leukocytes *Blood Increase* 96% of patients had either an abnormal total or differential count. Leukocytosis > 10,000/μL or a differential in excess of 75% neutrophils supports this clinical diagnosis. *1872* Raised total count in 42%, a raised neutrophil percentage in 93% and a raised absolute neutrophil count in 77%. *0588* In 82% of 108 patients at initial hospitalization for this disorder. *0781 2199*

Urine Increase Small numbers are found in the urine in about 25% of patients. *2199*

Lymphocytes *Blood Decrease* In 80% of 105 patients at initial hospitalization for this disorder. *0781*

Neutrophils *Blood Increase* 96% of patients had either an abnormal total or differential WBC count. Leukocytosis > 10,000/μL or a differential in excess of 75% neutrophils supports this clinical diagnosis. *1872* Raised total leukocyte count in 42%, a raised neutrophil percentage in 93% and a raised absolute neutrophil count in 77%. *0588* In 71% of 106 patients at initial hospitalization for this disorder. *0781 2199*

553.30   Hernia Diaphragmatic

Hematocrit *Blood Decrease* Microcytic anemia (due to loss of blood) may be present. *2467*

Hemoglobin *Blood Decrease* Microcytic anemia (due to loss of blood) may be present. *2467*

MCH *Blood Decrease* Microcytic anemia (due to loss of blood) may be present. *2467*

MCV *Blood Decrease* Microcytic anemia (due to loss of blood) may be present. *2467*

Occult Blood *Feces Positive* May be positive. *2467*

Oxygen Saturation *Blood Decrease* Severe hypoxia may be present. *0433* 11 out of 20 infants with congenital hernia survived. Of the 9 nonsurvivors, arterial pCO_2 levels were markedly higher (61.3 ± 15.4 mm Hg) and pO_2 levels lower (49.8 ± 14.2) than in survivors (44.3 ± 7.9, 307.9 ± 142.3, respectively). *0245*

pCO_2 *Blood Increase* 11 out of 20 infants with congenital hernia survived. Of the 9 nonsurvivors, arterial pCO_2 levels were markedly higher (61.3 + - 15.4 mm Hg) and pO_2 levels lower (49.8 ± 14.2) than in survivors (44.3 ± 7.9, 307.9 ± 142.3 respectively). *0245* Severe hypercarbia may be present. *0433*

pH *Blood Decrease* Severe acidosis may be present. *0433*

pO_2 *Blood Decrease* Severe hypoxia may be present. *0433* 11 out of 20 infants with congenital hernia survived. Of the 9 nonsurvivors, arterial pCO_2 levels were markedly higher (61.3 ± 15.4 mm Hg) and pO_2 levels lower (49.8 ± 14.2) than in survivors (44.3 ± 7.9, 307.9 ± 142.3, respectively). *0245*

555.90   Regional Enteritis or Ileitis

Alanine Aminotransferase *Serum Increase* Liver abnormalities are common. *0995*

Albumin *Serum Decrease* In 32 patients, 13 fell into a distinct group of low tryptophan sera levels. Patients in this group ate less, had lower albumin levels and greater intestinal protein loss than normal tryptophan patients. *0150* Occurs frequently and is probably due largely to the leakage of protein from the diseased gut. *2466* A reasonably accurate indication of the patient's overall condition. *2199 1160 2035*

Alkaline Phosphatase *Serum Increase* Indicates hepatic involvement. *0433* Frequently abnormal in patients who otherwise show no indication of liver disease. *2199*

Leukocyte Increase Markedly increased. *1297*

Alpha$_1$-Antichymotrypsin *Serum Increase* Serum concentrations were associated with increasing severity. *2505*

Alpha$_1$-Glycoprotein *Serum Increase* One of the most reliable indicators of acute inflammation. *1239 1672 1866 1947 2096 2170*

Angiotensin-Converting Enzyme (ACE) *Serum Decrease* Significantly depressed compared with normal controls and those with inactive disease. *0483*

Serum Normal No significant difference was noted between active Crohn's, inactive Crohn's, and normal controls. However, patients who had active disease and were receiving steroid therapy had significantly lower levels. *1710* Wide variation. *0483*

Antibody Titer *Serum Increase* Antibodies to Reticulin. *1670*

Aspartate Aminotransferase *Serum Increase* Due to associated liver disease. *0218* Liver abnormalities are common *0995*

Bile Acids *Serum Decrease* In patients with Crohn's Disease whether resected or not the postprandial level of bile acids is low. *1039*

Bilirubin *Serum Increase* Due to associated liver disease. *0218*

Calcium *Serum Decrease* *0995*

Urine Increase High levels may be found. *0282 2035*

Carcinoembryonic Antigen *Serum Increase* 14% of 58 patients had positive assay. There was no correlation between CEA concentration and extent or activity of disease, but those with elevated levels all had the disease for > 7 y, mean = 18.1 y duration. *0253* 40% of patients had values > 2.5 ng/mL. *2199 0979*

Carotene *Serum Decrease* With malabsorption. *2199*

Chenodeoxycholic Acid *Serum Normal* Fasting values were in the normal range but post prandial increase was lower than in healthy controls. *1039*

Cholic Acid *Serum Normal* Fasting values were in the normal range but post prandial increase was lower than in healthy controls. *1039*

Eosinophils *Blood Increase* *2538*

Erythrocyte Sedimentation Rate *Blood Increase* Elevation takes place during acute exacerbations. *0433* Tend to suggest that the inflammatory process is active. *2199 2035*

Fat *Feces Increase* Deficient intraluminal bile acids. *2199*

Folate *Serum Decrease* Decreased with extensive skin disease. *0299 2357 0367* Deficiency may result in anemia *0532*

Gamma Glutamyl Transferase (GGT) *Serum Increase* In the presence of pericholangitis. *2199 0619*

Globulin *Serum Decrease* May be elevated in some patients but are normal or low in others. *2199*

Serum Increase May be elevated in some patients but are normal or low in others *2199 0995*

Serum Normal May be elevated in some patients but are normal or low in others. *2199*

Haptoglobin *Serum Increase* Haptoglobin concentrations rise with increasing clinical activity of the disease, while the prealbumin fraction declines. *1510 2035*

Hematocrit *Blood Decrease* Anemia when present can be a result of iron loss or of reduced absorption of vitamin B_{12}. *0433* Anemia in approximately 70% of cases. *2035* Iron deficiency is common. *0962* Frequently moderate anemia, most often iron deficiency, but occasionally macrocytic caused by poor diet or failure to absorb vitamin B_{12} normally. *2199*

Hemoglobin *Blood Decrease* Anemia when present can be a result of iron loss or of reduced absorption of vitamin B_{12}. *0433* Anemia in approximately 70% of cases. *2035* Iron deficiency is common. *0962* Frequently moderate anemia, most often iron deficiency, but occasionally macrocytic caused by poor diet or failure to absorb vitamin B_{12} normally. *2199*

HLA Antigens *Blood Present* If associated arthritis HLA-B$_{27}$ found more frequently than control group. *1503*

Immunoglobulin IgA *Serum Increase* *0619*

Immunoglobulins *Serum Normal* Patterns vary widely within a given patient, and most workers report no consistent deviations in the mean levels of the major Ig classes (including IgE) in sera of patients compared with healthy controls. *1313 2035*

Iron *Serum Decrease* Iron deficiency is common. *0962* As a result of chronic blood loss. *2199* Iron deficiency anemia was found in 36% of 41 patients with ulcerative colitis, and 22% of 64 patients with Crohn's disease. An additional 32% and 2%, respectively, had iron deficiency with normal erythropoiesis. *2351*

Bone Marrow Decrease Iron deficiency defined by the absence of marrow hemosiderin was found with anemia in 36% of 41 patients with ulcerative colitis, and 22% of 64 with Crohn's disease. An additional 32% and 2%, respectively, had iron deficiency with normal erythropoiesis. *2351* As a result of chronic blood loss. *2199*

Iron-Binding Capacity, Total (TIBC) *Serum Increase* Frequent iron deficiency anemia. Severity depends upon rate and duration of bleeding. *2199*

Iron Saturation *Serum Decrease* Frequent iron deficiency anemia. Severity depends upon rate and duration of bleeding. *2199*

555.90 Regional Enteritis or Ileitis (continued)

Lactate Dehydrogenase *Serum Increase* Liver abnormalities are common. *0995*

Leukocytes *Blood Increase* Elevation takes place during acute exacerbations. *0433* Leukocytosis (usually mild). *2035* Tend to suggest that the inflammatory process is active. *2199*

Feces Increase Large numbers. *2199*

Lysozyme *Serum Increase* Particularly when the inflammatory process is active. *0693 2199 2035 0694*

Magnesium *Serum Decrease* Common feature of severe colitis. *2035*

MCH *Blood Decrease* Frequently moderate anemia, most often iron deficiency, but occasionally macrocytic caused by poor diet or failure to absorb vitamin B_{12} normally. *2199*

MCHC *Blood Decrease* Frequently moderate anemia, most often iron deficiency, but occasionally macrocytic caused by poor diet or failure to absorb vitamin B_{12} normally. *2199*

MCV *Blood Decrease* As a result of chronic blood loss. *2199*

Blood Increase Macrocytic anemia may occur due to vitamin B_{12} or folate deficiency. MCV > 100 fL. *0532* Macrocytic, megaloblastic anemia may indicate folic acid or vitamin B_{12} deficiency. *2199*

Monocytes *Blood Increase* Relative lymphocytopenia may occur as a result of absolute increase in monocytes and polymorphonuclear cells. *2345 2538*

Neutrophils *Blood Increase* Relative lymphocytopenia may occur as a result of absolute increase in monocytes and polymorphonuclear cells. *2345* Count increases with increasing disease activity. *1216*

Occult Blood *Feces Positive* Stools are not grossly bloody, insidious blood loss with guaiac positive stools is the rule. *0962* Chronic blood loss. *2199 0999*

Oxalate *Urine Increase* *0218*

Platelet Count *Blood Increase* May be present. *2199 2035*

Potassium *Serum Decrease* Common feature of severe colitis. *2035*

Prealbumin *Serum Decrease* Haptoglobin concentrations rise with increasing clinical activity of the disease, while the prealbumin fraction declines. *1510 2035*

Protein *Serum Decrease* Often present; due in some part to diminished intake, but mainly result from excessive enteric protein loss. *2199*

Prothrombin Time *Plasma Decrease* *0995*

Sodium *Serum Decrease* Common feature of severe colitis. *2035*

Thyroxine Binding Globulin *Serum Increase* Mean levels were high in these patients, mainly due to the high levels in female patients. *1150*

Tri-iodothyronine (T_3) *Serum Increase* The concentration was lower in the severely ill patients than in those who were mildly-moderately ill, while T_4 and TBG were not affected by the severity of the disease. *1150*

Tryptophan *Serum Decrease* In 32 patients, 13 fell into a distinct group of low tryptophan sera levels. Patients in this group ate less, had low albumin levels and greater intestinal protein loss than normal tryptophan patients. *0150*

Uric Acid *Serum Increase* *2035*

Urine Increase High levels may be found. *0282 2035*

Vitamin B_{12} *Serum Decrease* Tests may be abnormal. *0151* Frequently moderate anemia, most often iron deficiency, but occasionally macrocytic caused by poor diet or failure to absorb vitamin B_{12} normally. *2199*

Xylose Tolerance Test *Urine Normal* *2467*

556.00 Ulcerative Colitis

Alanine Aminotransferase *Serum Increase* With liver involvement. *0433*

Albumin *Serum Decrease* Deficiency may result in anemia. *0532* Occurs frequently and is probably due largely to the leakage of protein from the diseased gut. *2466* Portends a worse prognosis, probably because the degree of abnormality parallels clinical severity. *2199 1160 2035*

Alkaline Phosphatase *Serum Increase* Often increased slightly. *2467 0433*

Leukocyte Increase Markedly increased. *1297*

Alpha$_1$-Antichymotrypsin *Serum Increase* Serum concentrations were associated with increasing severity. *2505*

Alpha$_1$-Antitrypsin *Serum Increase* Increased compared to control subjects. There was a correlation between the level and disease activity. *0205*

Alpha$_1$-Globulin *Serum Increase* Serum orosomucoid was well correlated with clinical activity, intestinal protein loss, serum albumin, fractional catabolic rates of albumin, and IgG synthesis rate. *1161*

Alpha$_2$-Globulin *Serum Increase* May be increased. *2467*

Angiotensin-Converting Enzyme (ACE) *Serum Normal* Similar levels as controls. *0483*

Aspartate Aminotransferase *Serum Increase* With liver involvement. *0433*

Basophils *Blood Increase* *2538*

Beta-Globulin *Serum Decrease* *2467*

Calcium *Serum Decrease* Usually deficient. *0995*

Urine Increase High levels may be found. *0282 2035*

Carcinoembryonic Antigen *Serum Increase* Elevated in as many as 27% of patients. *2005* 11% of 61 patients had positive assays. There was no correlation between CEA and length of history, degree of activity, or extent of colonic involvement. *0253* Serial measurements done of 57 patients yield significant correlations between peak CEA concentration and disease severity and extent of colonic involvement. *0815* 31% of patients had values > 2.5 ng/mL. *0979 0795 2035 2199*

Catecholamines *Plasma Increase* Circulating levels. *0995*

Urine Increase Circulating levels. *0995*

Chloride *Serum Decrease* *0433*

Cholesterol *Serum Decrease* *0995*

Feces Increase The fecal excretion of cholesterol, coprostanol, and cholestane-38 beta, 5 alpha, 6 beta-triol was higher in these patients than in other control and patient groups. *1897*

Complement, Total *Serum Increase* Mean titer in 16 increased in 16 patients. *0752*

Coombs' Test *Blood Positive* Has been described. *2199*

Eosinophils *Blood Increase* *2538*

Erythrocyte Sedimentation Rate *Blood Increase* Often normal or only slightly increased. *2467 2035*

Folate *Serum Decrease* May be the cause of anemia. *0433*

Gamma Glutamyl Transferase (GGT) *Serum Increase* Increased with associated liver damage and correlates with other liver enzymes. *0619 0433*

Haptoglobin *Serum Increase* Haptoglobin concentrations rise with increasing clinical activity of the disease, while the prealbumin fraction declines. *1510 2035*

Hematocrit *Blood Decrease* Anemia may be due to blood loss, simple iron deficiency, deficiencies in folic acid, pyridoxine, or vitamin B_{12}. *0433* Anemia in approximately 70% of cases. *2035* Anemia secondary to colonic blood loss. Severity varies, depending on the rate and duration of bleeding. *2199*

Hemoglobin *Blood Decrease* Anemia may be due to blood loss, simple iron deficiency, deficiencies in folic acid, pyridoxine, or vitamin B_{12} (frequently 6 g/dL). *2467* Anemia in approximately 70% of cases. *2035* Anemia secondary to colonic blood loss. Severity varies, depending on the rate and duration of bleeding. *2199*

HLA Antigens *Blood Present* If associated arthritis HLA-B$_{27}$ found more frequently than control group. *1503*

Immunoglobulins *Serum Normal* Patterns vary widely within a given patient, and most workers report no consistent deviations in the mean levels of the major Ig classes (including IgE) in sera of patients compared with healthy controls. *1313 2035*

Iron *Serum Decrease* Iron deficiency defined by the absence of marrow hemosiderin was found with anemia in 36% of 41 patients. An additional 32% had iron deficiency with normal erythropoiesis. *2351* Commonly iron deficient. *2199*

Bone Marrow Decrease Iron deficiency defined by the absence of marrow hemosiderin was found with anemia in 36% of 41 patients. An additional 32% had iron deficiency with normal erythropoiesis. *2351*

Iron-Binding Capacity, Total (TIBC) *Serum Increase* Frequent iron deficiency anemia. Severity depends upon rate and duration of bleeding. *2199*

Iron Saturation *Serum Decrease* Frequent iron deficiency anemia. Severity depends upon rate and duration of bleeding. *2199*

Isocitrate Dehydrogenase *Serum Normal* *2260*

Lactate Dehydrogenase *Serum Increase* With liver involvement. *0433*

Leukocytes *Blood Increase* Leukocytosis (usually mild). *2035* Commonly associated with the more severe varieties. May be marked, with total counts as high as 40,000-50,000/μL. *2199*

Blood Normal Usually normal unless complication occurs (e.g., abscess). *2467*

Lysozyme *Serum Increase* Increased in severely affected cases. *1297 2035*

Magnesium *Serum Decrease* Common feature of severe colitis. *2035*

MCH *Blood Decrease* Anemia in approximately 70% of cases. *2035* Anemia secondary to colonic blood loss. Severity varies, depending on the rate and duration of bleeding. *2199*

MCHC *Blood Decrease* Anemia in approximately 70% of cases. *2035* Anemia secondary to colonic blood loss. Severity varies, depending on the rate and duration of bleeding. *2199*

MCV *Blood Decrease* Anemia in approximately 70% of cases. *2035* Anemia secondary to colonic blood loss. Severity varies, depending on the rate and duration of bleeding. *2199 0433*

Monocytes *Blood Increase* Relative lymphocytopenia may occur as a result of absolute increase in monocytes and polymorphonuclear cells. *2345 2538*

Neutral Sterols *Feces Increase* The fecal excretion of cholesterol, coprostanol, and cholestane-38 beta, 5 alpha, 6 beta-triol was higher in patients with ulcerative colitis than in other control and patient groups. *1897*

Neutrophils *Blood Increase* Count increases with increasing disease activity. *1216* Relative lymphocytopenia may occur as a result of absolute increase in monocytes and polymorphonuclear cells. *2345*

Occult Blood *Feces Positive* Positive for blood (gross and/or occult). *2467* Lower GI bleeding. *2199*

pH *Blood Increase* Increased progressively with increased severity of the colitis and as the lesions became more widespread. Significant differences were observed in values between the mild/moderate and severe forms and between the severe and complicated forms (toxic megacolon). *0340*

Platelet Count *Blood Increase* Most commonly in those patients having marked leukocytosis. Not associated with coagulation defects. *2199 2035*

Potassium *Serum Decrease* Serum electrolytes may show losses due to diarrhea, especially hypokalemia, which may contribute to colonic atony and may portend acute toxic dilatation. *0433* Common feature of severe colitis. *2035* Portends a worse prognosis, probably because the degree of abnormality parallels clinical severity. *2199*

Prealbumin *Serum Decrease* Haptoglobin concentrations rise with increasing clinical activity of the disease, while the prealbumin fraction declines. *1510 2035*

Protein *Serum Decrease* Fever, hypovolemia, tachycardia and hypoproteinemia are major manifestations. *0999* Malnutrition with protein deficiency. *0433 1161*

Prothrombin Time *Plasma Increase* Hypoprothrombinemia (prolonged time) is a commonly found defect in moderate or severe disease. *2199*

Pyridoxine *Serum Decrease* Anemia may be due to blood loss, simple iron deficiency, deficiencies in folic acid, pyridoxine, or vitamin B₁₂. *0433*

Rheumatoid Factor *Serum Normal* Usually negative even with associated arthritis. *2199*

Sodium *Serum Decrease* Common feature of severe colitis. *2035*

Thyroxine Binding Globulin *Serum Increase* Mean serum values were high in these patients, mainly due to the high levels in female patients. *1150*

Tri-iodothyronine (T₃) *Serum Decrease* The concentration was lower in the severely ill patients than in those who were mildly-moderately ill, while T₄ and TBG were not affected by the severity of the disease. *1150*

Uric Acid *Serum Increase* *2035*

Urine Increase High levels may be found. *0282 2035*

Vitamin B₁₂ *Serum Decrease* Anemia may be due to blood loss, simple iron deficiency, deficiencies in folic acid, pyridoxine, or vitamin B₁₂. *0433*

Volume *Plasma Decrease* Fever, hypovolemia, tachycardia and hypoproteinemia are major manifestations. *0999*

Xylose Tolerance Test *Urine Normal* *2467*

557.01 Mesenteric Artery Embolism

Acid Phosphatase *Serum Increase* Peak activity is reached 2-3 days after onset of symptoms. *2104*

Albumin *Serum Decrease* *0433*

Alkaline Phosphatase *Serum Increase* A selective elevation of the intestinal isoenzyme has been described in acute intestinal ischemia. *0433*

Alkaline Phosphatase Isoenzymes *Serum Increase* A selective elevation of the intestinal isoenzyme has been described in acute intestinal ischemia. *0433*

Amylase *Serum Increase* May occur with mesenteric infarction. *0320*

Aspartate Aminotransferase *Serum Increase* After intestinal infarction. *0619 2467 0433*

Cholesterol *Serum Decrease* *0433*

Fat *Feces Increase* Excessive fecal fat loss from recurrent ischemic damage to the intestinal mucosal function resulting in malabsorption. *1108*

Hematocrit *Blood Increase* Will reflect the hemoconcentration secondary to fluid loss into the bowel and peritoneal cavity following bowel infarction. *0433*

Lactate Dehydrogenase *Serum Increase* *0433*

Leukocytes *Blood Increase* Reflects hemoconcentration and documents the cellular response to the endotoxins released by the involved bowel. *0433* Marked increase (15,000-25,000/μL or more) with shift to the left. *2467*

Occult Blood *Feces Positive* Upper GI bleeding. *2199*

pH *Blood Decrease* Serum electrolytes usually show a depressed CO_2-combining power from the induced severe metabolic acidosis. *0433*

Phosphate *Serum Increase* Of 7 patients with massive intestinal infarction, all had elevated concentrations. *1145*

Protein *Serum Decrease* *0433*

Prothrombin Time *Plasma Increase* *0433*

Urea Nitrogen *Serum Increase* Will reflect the hemoconcentration secondary to fluid loss into the bowel and peritoneal cavity following bowel infarction. *0433*

558.90 Diarrhea

Ammonia *Urine Increase* In prolonged diarrhea. *0619*

Bicarbonate *Serum Decrease* *2467*

Bilirubin *Feces Increase* In severe diarrhea a little bilirubin may be present. *0619*

Chloride *Serum Decrease* *2467*

Urine Decrease Excessive loss, due to severe diarrhea. *0619*

Feces Increase During moderate diarrhea the output may increase to 60 mmol/day. In very severe diarrhea the fecal composition approaches that of ileal fluid, and up to 500 mmol of chloride can be lost in 24 h. *0619*

Creatinine *Serum Increase* Leading to reduced renal blood flow (prerenal azotemia). *2467*

Fat *Feces Increase* Excessively rapid passage of intestinal contents. With severe diarrhea. *0619*

Hematocrit *Blood Increase* When salt and water are lost in isotonic proportions, a contraction of the extracellular fluid compartment occurs and hemoconcentration develops. *2199*

Hemoglobin *Blood Increase* When salt and water are lost in isotonic proportions, a contraction of the extracellular fluid compartment occurs and hemoconcentration develops. *2199*

Nitrogen *Feces Increase* *0619*

pH *Blood Decrease* Tends to fall. *0619*

Urine Decrease *2467*

Potassium *Serum Decrease* Depletion may develop with any severe diarrhea. *2199*

Urine Decrease Normal or decreased. *2467*

Sodium *Serum Decrease* 60 mmol/day may be lost. *0619* Hyponatremia commonly results. *2199*

Serum Increase In osmotic diarrhea water loss is proportionately greater than that of sodium. Dehydration with hypernatremia may occur. *2199*

Urine Decrease *2467*

Urea Nitrogen *Serum Increase* Observed in patients with diarrhea and severe dehydration, who were rapidly dehydrated with concomitant fall of BUN to normal or subnormal levels. *0803*

558.90   Diarrhea (continued)

Volume   *Plasma   Decrease*   When salt and water are lost in isotonic proportions, a contraction of the extracellular fluid compartment occurs and hemoconcentration develops. *2199   2467*

Urine   Decrease   2467

560.90   Intestinal Obstruction

Albumin   *Serum   Decrease*   6% mortality in cases with > 3 g/dL; 33% mortality with < 3 g/dL. *0619*   In 35% of 42 patients at initial hospitalization for this disorder. *0781*

Serum   Normal   0619

Alkaline Phosphatase   *Serum   Increase*   In 31% of 42 patients at initial hospitalization for this disorder. *0781*

Amylase   *Serum   Increase*   Moderate hyperamylasemia without evidence of associated pancreatitis. Values > 1,850 U/L may indicate strangulated or necrotic bowel. *2031*   Often marked elevation. *2104*

Ascitic Fluid   Increase   0186

Aspartate Aminotransferase   *Serum   Increase*   In 33% of 42 patients at initial hospitalization for this disorder. *0781*

Bacteria   *Ascitic Fluid   Increase   0186*

Bicarbonate   *Serum   Increase*   Metabolic alkalosis secondary to vomiting. *2467*   In 46% of 47 patients at initial hospitalization for this disorder. *0781*

Chloride   *Serum   Decrease*   Metabolic alkalosis secondary to vomiting. *2467*

Serum   Increase   With dehydration. *2199*

Cholesterol   *Serum   Decrease*   In 39% of 42 patients at initial hospitalization for this disorder. *0781*

Creatinine   *Serum   Increase*   With dehydration. *2199*

Erythrocytes   *Ascitic Fluid   Increase*   Bloody ascitic fluid. *0186*

Glucose   *Serum   Increase*   In 42% of 46 patients at initial hospitalization for this disorder. *0781*

Hematocrit   *Blood   Increase*   Normal early, but later increased, with dehydration. *2467*

Hemoglobin   *Blood   Increase*   Normal early, but later increased, with dehydration. *2467*

Lactate Dehydrogenase   *Serum   Increase*   Increase may indicate strangulation (infarction) of small intestine. *2467*   In 32% of 42 patients at initial hospitalization for this disorder. *0781*

Leukocytes   *Blood   Decrease*   Leukopenia with left shift suggest infarction with sepsis. *0186*

Blood   Increase   May be normal in early cases of simple or strangulation obstruction. With advanced cases, may range from 12,000-15,000/μL or more. Counts of 25,000-30,000/μL or more strongly indicate vascular occlusion to the bowel as by mesenteric thrombosis. *0433*   In 40% of 47 patients at initial hospitalization for this disorder. *0781*

Neutrophils   *Blood   Increase*   In 39% of 44 patients at initial hospitalization for this disorder. *0781*

Occult Blood   *Feces   Positive*   Gross rectal blood suggests carcinoma of colon or intussusception. *2467*

Gastric Material   Positive   Positive test suggests strangulation; there may be gross blood if strangulated segment is high in jejunum. *2467*

pCO$_2$ *Blood   Decrease*   Metabolic acidosis secondary to lactic acidosis. *0186*

pH   *Blood   Decrease*   Metabolic acidosis secondary to lactic acidosis. *0186*   Reflects the course of the patient and therapy *2467*

Phosphate   *Serum   Increase   2467*

Potassium   *Serum   Decrease*   Metabolic alkalosis secondary to vomiting. *2467*

Sodium   *Serum   Increase*   Secondary to dehydration. *0995*

Urine   Increase   Specific gravity increases, with deficit of water and electrolytes unless pre-existing renal disease is present. *2467*

Specific Gravity   *Urine   Increase*   Urinalysis may be entirely normal in intestinal obstruction with the exception of relatively high specific gravity. *0433*   Increases with deficit of water and electrolytes unless pre-existing renal disease is present. Urinalysis helps rule out renal colic, diabetic acidosis, etc. *2467*

Urea Nitrogen   *Serum   Increase*   Azotemia may be striking; also with massive hemorrhage. *0503*   Increase suggests blood in intestine or renal damage. *2467*

Volume   *Urine   Decrease*   Urinary output diminishes early in the disease. *0151*

562.00   Diverticular Disease of Intestine

Carcinoembryonic Antigen   *Serum   Increase*   41% of patients had values > 2.5 ng/mL. *0979   2199*

Erythrocyte Sedimentation Rate   *Blood   Increase*   May be mildly elevated. *0433*

Hematocrit   *Blood   Decrease*   Blood loss is usually minimal but massive bleeding may occur. *2199*

Hemoglobin   *Blood   Decrease*   Blood loss is usually minimal but massive bleeding may occur. *2199*

Iron   *Serum   Decrease*   Some cases. *2199*

Iron-Binding Capacity, Total (TIBC)   *Serum   Increase*   Some cases. *2199*

MCH   *Blood   Decrease*   Some cases. *2199*

MCHC   *Blood   Decrease*   Some cases. *2199*

Occult Blood   *Feces   Positive*   May occur. *2199*

562.11   Diverticulitis of Colon

Carcinoembryonic Antigen   *Serum   Increase*   27% of patients had values > 2.5 ng/mL. *0979   0795 2035*

Erythrocytes   *Urine   Increase*   Although urinalysis may be normal hematuria may signal involvement of the bladder or ureter. *0433*

Erythrocyte Sedimentation Rate   *Blood   Increase   2467*

Iron   *Serum   Decrease*   Some cases. *2199*

Iron-Binding Capacity, Total (TIBC)   *Serum   Increase*   Some cases. *2199*

Leukocytes   *Blood   Increase*   Symptoms are chronic constipation punctuated by episodes of acute abdominal pain, fever, and leukocytosis. *0999*   Usually elevated with the appearance of less mature forms of neutrophils, but this finding might be lacking in elderly or debilitated patients *0433* . In 51% of 35 patient at initial hospitalization for this disorder. *0781   2199*

MCH   *Blood   Decrease*   Some cases. *2199*

MCHC   *Blood   Decrease*   Some cases. *2199*

Neutrophils   *Blood   Increase*   In 51% of 36 patients at initial hospitalization for this disorder. *0781*   Leukocytosis with an increase in polymorphonuclear forms. *2199*

Occult Blood   *Feces   Positive   2199*

564.20   Postgastrectomy (Dumping) Syndrome

Fat   *Feces   Increase*   Malabsorption from poor mixing and rapid transit. *0995*

Glucagon   *Plasma   Increase*   Hypoglycemia following gastrectomy, gut glucagon levels in the plasma are raised. *0619*

Glucose   *Serum   Decrease*   Rapid absorption of carbohydrate by smaller intestine leads to release of insulin which continues to act after most of the carbohydrate has been absorbed and stored. *0619*

Serum   Increase   Rapid and prolonged alimentary hyperglycemia with subsequent delayed absorption. *0995*

Urine   Increase   0619

Glucose Tolerance   *Serum   Decrease*   Characteristically the curve consists of a rise in blood glucose to between 200-300 mg/dL, 30 min after oral administration of glucose. This is followed by a rapid fall in the next hour to hypoglycemic levels, at which point symptoms occur. *0962*

Hematocrit   *Blood   Decrease*   Iron deficiency and vitamin B$_{12}$ deficiency are common following subtotal gastrectomy. *0962*

Hemoglobin   *Blood   Decrease*   Iron deficiency and vitamin B$_{12}$ deficiency are common following subtotal gastrectomy. *0962*

Iron   *Serum   Decrease*   Iron deficiency and vitamin B$_{12}$ deficiency are common following subtotal gastrectomy. *0962*

MCH   *Blood   Decrease*   Iron deficiency and vitamin B$_{12}$ deficiency are common following subtotal gastrectomy. *0962*

MCHC   *Blood   Decrease*   Iron deficiency and vitamin B$_{12}$ deficiency are common following subtotal gastrectomy. *0962*

MCV   *Blood   Decrease*   Iron deficiency and vitamin B$_{12}$ deficiency are common following subtotal gastrectomy. *0962*

Potassium   *Serum   Decrease*   Jejunal hypersecretion of water and electrolytes, especially potassium. *0995*

Vitamin B$_{12}$ *Serum   Decrease*   Iron deficiency and vitamin B$_{12}$ deficiency are common following subtotal gastrectomy. *0962*

Volume   *Plasma   Decrease*   Jejunal hypersecretion of water and electrolytes, with resultant reduced plasma volume. *0995*

567.90   Peritonitis

Albumin   *Serum   Decrease*   Increase in plasma volume without increase in total protein. *0619*

Aldosterone   *Plasma   Increase*   Increased adrenal production. *0995*

Urine   Increase   Increased adrenal production. *0995*

Amylase   *Serum   Increase*   Hyperamylasemia up to 405 U/L without appreciable pancreatic disease. *1871*

Ascitic Fluid   Increase   *0186*

Catecholamines   *Plasma   Increase*   Increased adrenal production. *0995*

Urine   Increase   Increased adrenal production. *0995*

Eosinophils   *Ascitic Fluid   Increase*   Ascites associated with eosinophilic enteritis and peritonitis has a high eosinophil count. *2199*

Erythrocytes   *Ascitic Fluid   Increase*   May be bloody. *0186*   < 10,000 cells/μL is unusual. Normally more seen *2626*

Peritoneal Fluid   Increase   Bloody ascites may be seen with tuberculous peritonitis. *2199*

Glucocorticoids   *Plasma   Increase*   Increased adrenal production. *0995*

Glucose   *Ascitic Fluid   Decrease*   Seen with tuberculous peritonitis. *0186*

Hematocrit   *Blood   Increase*   Secondary; may be increased owing to hemoconcentration from extracellular fluid loss into the peritoneal cavity. *0433*

Hemoglobin   *Blood   Increase*   May be increased owing to hemoconcentration from extracellular fluid loss into the peritoneal cavity. *0433*

Leukocytes   *Blood   Increase*   Elevated (20,000-50,000/μL) and consists predominantly of polymorphonuclear neutrophils. May not occur in the older age group and those on steroids. *0433*

Ascitic Fluid   Increase   Mean total count = 5,500/μL. *1187*   Elevated counts (> 250/μL) indicate peritoneal irritation. *0151*   > 1000 μL predominantly polymorphonuclear cells. *2626*

Lymphocytes   *Ascitic Fluid   Increase*   A high percentage suggests tuberculous peritonitis. *0151*

Monocytes   *Ascitic Fluid   Increase*   Seen with tuberculous peritonitis. *0186*

Peritoneal Fluid   Increase   Most patients have > 80% mononuclear forms. Characterize chronic inflammatory disease, especially tuberculosis. *2199*

Neutrophils   *Blood   Increase*   Secondary; WBC is elevated with a major increase in polymorphonuclear granulocytes. May not be present in the older age group and those on steroids. *0433*

Pleural Effusion   Increase   Neutrophils predominate in pleural fluid. *1403*

Ascitic Fluid   Increase   10 of 11 patients with bacterial peritonitis had counts > 250/μL. Very few patients with other diseases had comparable granulocyte counts. *1187*

Potassium   *Serum   Decrease*   Secondary to increased aldosterone production. *0995*

Protein   *Ascitic Fluid   Increase*   Often > 2.5 g/dL in ascitic fluid. *2626*

Peritoneal Fluid   Increase   Exceeds 2.5 g/dL in 85-100% of patients with tuberculous peritonitis. Exudate with protein concentration > 3.0 g/dL usually found with tuberculous and bacterial peritonitis. *2199*

Sodium   *Serum   Increase*   Secondary to increased aldosterone production. *0995*

Specific Gravity   *Peritoneal Fluid   Increase*   Exudate with specific gravity > 1.016 usually found with tuberculous and bacterial peritonitis. *2199*

Urea Nitrogen   *Serum   Increase*   Secondary; may be increased owing to hemoconcentration from extracellular fluid loss into the peritoneal cavity. *0433*

Volume   *Plasma   Decrease*   Exudation of fluid leads to reduction in effective circulating volume. *0995*

570.00   Acute and Subacute Necrosis of Liver

[131]I Uptake   *Serum   Increase*   In hepatic disease. *2104*

5'-Nucleotidase   *Serum   Increase*   Increased (although low levels have been reported with very severe liver damage), especially if intrahepatic cholestasis present. *0619*

Acid Phosphatase   *Serum   Increase*   Up to 16 U/L. *2467 0812*   With jaundice. *0169 1033*

Alanine Aminopeptidase   *Serum   Increase*   *1443*

Alanine Aminotransferase   *Serum   Increase*   A marked increase occurs which is relatively higher than the rise in AST. The level is raised in nonicteric attacks. In liver disease results of ALT and sorbitol dehydrogenase run parallel with AST results. *0619*   Sometimes reaches levels of 2,000 U/L. It falls slowly reaching normal levels in about 2-3 months, unless complications occur. *2467 0812*   Levels are higher in acute hepatitis than in obstructive jaundice. *0503*   Peak values between 200-1,500 U/L are typical. *0992*   *2576*

Albumin   *Serum   Decrease*   *2467 0619*

Serum   Normal   *2467*

Aldolase   *Serum   Increase*   Cell destruction. Normal or may be slightly increased. *2467*   *0619*

Serum   Normal   Normal or may be slightly increased. *2467*

Alkaline Phosphatase   *Serum   Increase*   Higher in obstructive jaundice than in acute hepatitis. The basis for elevation in patients with hepatobiliary disease is obscure. Increased formation by hepatic parenchymal or ductal cells, perhaps supplemented by impaired excretion, is the apparent mechanism. *0503*   Most commonly between 65-160 U/L. *0619*   Incidence of elevation is 80-100%; usual range 25-80 U/L. *0503*   *2576 0999*

Leukocyte   Increase   Markedly increased; may remain increased for years after jaundice has disappeared. *2467*

Alpha₁-Antitrypsin   *Serum   Normal*   *2467*

Alpha₁-Globulin   *Serum   Decrease*   Tend to be low in hepatocellular disease falling in parallel with serum albumin. *2339*

Alpha₁-Glycoprotein   *Serum   Increase*   It was found to have a sensitivity of 65% and a specificity of 80% with severe liver disease. *0709*

Alpha₂-Globulin   *Serum   Decrease*   Alpha and beta globulins decrease when hepatocellular failure impairs their synthesis. *0151*

Serum   Increase   If the necrosis is not too extensive there may be a slight increase. *0619*

Alpha-Fetoprotein   *Serum   Increase*   10-20% of nonmalignant liver diseases of all types have elevated serum levels, which tend to be fluctuating or transient. Steady or rising levels indicate malignancy. *2583*   Increased in hepatitis, especially in infants (when levels exceed 40 ng/mL). *0619*   Up to 40% of patients with massive hepatic necrosis. *2199   0036*

Amino Acids   *Plasma   Increase*   In acute yellow atrophy, the plasma concentration is roughly proportional to the degree of liver damage. Methionine and tyrosine show the highest increase. *0619*

Urine   Increase   In massive liver necrosis the amount present in urine is proportional to the degree of liver damage. *2104*

CSF   Increase   In massive liver necrosis the amount present in CSF is proportional to the degree of liver damage. *0619*

Ammonia   *Blood   Increase*   In acute hepatic necrosis and cirrhosis; may increase after portacaval anastomosis. *2467*

Amylase   *Serum   Decrease*   Decrease possible due to liver damage. *0619*

Antidiuretic Hormone   *Serum   Increase*   *0992*

Antithrombin III   *Plasma   Decrease*   Decreased in parenchymatous liver disease. *2353 1482*

Aspartate Aminotransferase   *Serum   Increase*   In liver diseases, may be 10-100 X normal and remain elevated for long periods of time. *0619 0812*   Higher in acute hepatitis than in obstructive jaundice. *0503*   Mean elevation in 17 cases of hepatitis was 36.5 X the normal upper limit (24 U/L). All patients showed elevation, mean = 766 U/L. *1452*

Beta-Globulin   *Serum   Decrease*   Alpha and beta globulins decrease when hepatocellular failure impairs their synthesis. *0151*

Beta-Glucuronidase   *Serum   Decrease*   Decreased. *0741 0866*

Bilirubin   *Serum   Increase*   May be > 30 mg/dL. *2467*   Rarely exceeds 15-20 mg/dL. *0999   0619*

Urine   Increase   May precede the onset of jaundice by several days *0999*

Feces   Increase   *2467*

Bilirubin, Direct   *Serum   Increase*   Normal or slight increase (< 15% of total). *2467*

Bilirubin, Indirect   *Serum   Increase*   *2467*

BSP Retention   *Serum   Increase*   Commonly observed. *0992*

Serum   Normal   In patients with ascites, BSP dye may be lost into abdomen. Results may falsely appear normal. *2467*

570.00   Acute and Subacute Necrosis of Liver
(continued)

Carcinoembryonic Antigen   *Serum   Increase*   Found in 50% of 16 patients with acute liver damage. Levels increased with increasing clinical severity. In acute damage, peak CEA occurs later than the time of maximum liver necrosis, suggesting that the rise is associated with regeneration. Higher levels occur in those patients with greater disturbance of liver function suggesting altered metabolism or excretion of CEA. *0311*

Carotene   *Serum   Decrease*   *2467*

Cholesterol   *Serum   Decrease*   Due to severe liver damage. *0619 0503*

Serum   Increase   In patients with obstructive jaundice or intrahepatic cholestasis concentration is usually elevated to 250-500 mg/dL; greater elevations occur occasionally. *0619 0503*   Greater elevations are more characteristic of hepatocanalicular jaundice (intrahepatic cholestasis) than of posthepatic jaundice. *0503*

Red Blood Cells   Increase   An increase was detected in most patients with hepatocellular disease or cholestatic jaundice but the alteration in RBC lipid content did not correlate with RBC survival. *1848*   25-50% increase in the membrane concentration, resulting in the characteristic target cell. *2552*

Complement C3   *Serum   Increase*   *2467*

Coproporphyrin   *Urine   Increase*   In liver disease, coproporphyrinuria may not indicate increased formation of the pigment, but rather its diversion from bile to urine. *0151*

Creatine Kinase   *Serum   Normal*   *2467*

Erythrocytes   *Urine   Increase*   In a few patients, slight hematuria. *0992*

Erythrocyte Sedimentation Rate   *Blood   Increase*   *2467*

Erythrocyte Survival   *Red Blood Cells   Decrease*   Decreased survival; mild to moderate hemolysis. *1849*

Estrogens   *Urine   Increase*   *2467*

Ferritin   *Serum   Increase*   Increased in acute hepatitis. Exceeded the upper limit of the normal values in most cases. *2624*   Increased in acute hepatocellular damage due to acetaminophen overdosage. *0616*

Fibrinogen   *Plasma   Decrease*   Formation is depressed in liver failure, resulting in decreased plasma levels. *0619*

Plasma   Increase   Patients with severe acute hepatic necrosis may have findings compatible with intravascular coagulation, thrombocytopenia and increased levels of fibrinogen/fibrin degradation products. *1048   2538*

Fibrin Split Products (FSP)   *Plasma   Increase*   Patients with severe acute hepatic necrosis may have findings compatible with intravascular coagulation, thrombocytopenia and increased levels of fibrinogen/fibrin degradation products. *1048   2538*

FIGLU (N-Formiminoglutamic Acid)   *Urine   Increase*   *2467*

Folate   *Serum   Decrease*   Decreased in some cases of liver disease due to inadequate intake. *2467*

Gamma Glutamyl Transferase (GGT)   *Serum   Increase*   The estimation may be useful in monitoring duration of the disease, since raised activity persists longer than do ALT or AST activities. *0619*   In acute hepatitis, elevation is less marked than that of other liver enzymes, but it is the last to return to normal. *2467   0503*

Globulin   *Serum   Decrease*   Alpha and beta globulins decrease when hepatocellular failure impairs their synthesis. *0151*

Serum   Increase   Mildly elevated due to increased gamma globulin. *0992*

Glucose   *Serum   Decrease*   Diffuse severe disease-primary or metastatic tumor. *2467*   Lowered levels result from massive hepatic necrosis or a deficiency of enzymes necessary for glycogenolysis. *0151   0619 2104*

Glucose Tolerance   *Serum   Decrease*   Decreased tolerance:excessive peak-decreased formation of glycogen with low fasting levels and subsequent hypoglycemia. *2467*   Decreased because of inability to form glycogen from administered glucose. *0619*

Haptoglobin   *Serum   Decrease*   Mild to moderate hemolysis usually occurs. *1849*

Hematocrit   *Blood   Decrease*   Mild to moderate hemolysis usually occurs. *1849*

Blood   Normal   Anemia is not a feature. *0992*

Hemoglobin   *Blood   Decrease*   Mild to moderate hemolysis usually occurs. *1849*

Blood   Normal   Anemia is not a feature. *0992*

Hemoglobin, Free   *Serum   Increase*   Mild to moderate hemolysis usually occurs. *1849*

Hepatitis B Surface Antigen   *Serum   Increase*   31 of 59 patients with acute uncomplicated hepatitis had detectable hepatitis B antigen. *0376*

Heterophil Antibody   *Serum   Increase*   May be positive but guinea pig kidney cell absorption removes the antibody. *0992*

Hexosaminidase   *Serum   Increase*   Increase in total concentration (hexosaminidase A and B). *1716*

Immunoglobulin IgA   *Serum   Increase*   Slightly increased or normal. *0992*

Immunoglobulin IgM   *Serum   Increase*   *0619*

Iron   *Serum   Increase*   The degree of increase parallels the amount of hepatic necrosis. *2467*   In acute hepatitis the serum iron level is increased, presumably due to the liberation of stored iron from necrosing liver cells. *0619*   High serum concentrations, more than can be explained by high ferritin levels are found in acute hepatitis. *2624*

Iron-Binding Capacity, Total (TIBC)   *Serum   Increase*   May be increased with hepatitis. *2467*

Isocitrate Dehydrogenase   *Serum   Increase*   *2467*

Lactate Dehydrogenase   *Serum   Increase*   Total LD is increased in 50% the cases. Relatively slight elevations or not at all. *0812 0503*   Occasionally increased. *0995   1089*

Lactate Dehydrogenase Isoenzyme 5 (LD$_5$)   *Serum   Increase*   Present in increased amounts. *0619*   Most marked increase, which occurs during prodromal stage and is greatest at time of onset of jaundice. *2467*

Lactate Dehydrogenase Isoenzymes   *Serum   Increase*   LD$_4$, LD$_5$. *0812*   Most marked increase is of LD$_5$, which occurs during prodromal stage and is greatest at time of onset of jaundice. *2467*

Lecithin   *Red Blood Cells   Increase*   25-50% increase in the membrane concentration, resulting in the characteristic target cell. *2552*

Leucine Aminopeptidase   *Serum   Increase*   Moderately increased. *0619*

Leukocytes   *Blood   Decrease*   WBC is normal or low during acute hepatitis and leukopenia may be observed. *0999*   Mild leukopenia. *0992*

Blood   Increase   Up to 50,000/µL with massive necrosis. *2467*

Lipase   *Serum   Decrease*   Lack of bile salts result in the failure to activate pancreatic lipase in the intestinal lumen. *2104*

Lipids   *Serum   Increase*   Increased in acute hepatitis. *0619*

Lymphocytes   *Blood   Decrease*   Transient. *0992*

Blood   Increase   Relative lymphocytosis. *0992*   Atypical lymphocytes varying between 2-20% is common during the acute phase. *0992*

Magnesium   *Serum   Increase*   Pathological increase in serum with liver disease. *0619   2026*

Neutrophils   *Blood   Decrease*   Transient. *0992*

Blood   Increase   May be associated with a moderate to severe neutrophilia. *2538*

Nitrogen   *Serum   Decrease*   *0619*

Ornithine Carbamoyl Transferase (OCT)   *Serum   Increase*   Liver cell damage. *2467*

Osmotic Fragility   *Red Blood Cells   Decrease*   *2467*

Phosphate   *Serum   Increase*   *2467*

Phosphoglucomutase   *Serum   Increase*   *0619*

Phospholipids, Total   *Red Blood Cells   Increase*   An increase in RBC phospholipid was detected in most patients with hepatocellular disease or cholestatic jaundice but the alteration in RBC lipid content did not correlate with RBC survival. *1848*

Plasminogen   *Serum   Decrease*   With massive necrosis. *1443*

Platelet Count   *Blood   Decrease*   Patients with severe acute hepatic necrosis may have findings compatible with intravascular coagulation, thrombocytopenia and increased levels of fibrinogen/fibrin degradation products. *1048   2538*

Protein   *Urine   Increase*   In a few patients minimal proteinuria. *0992*

Protein Bound Iodine (PBI)   *Serum   Decrease*   In severe liver disease. *2104*

Serum   Increase   *0619*

Prothrombin Time   *Plasma   Increase*   Due to poor fat absorption. *2467*   Increased time indicates degree of parenchymal damage; marked prolongation (> 20 sec) is an early reflection of massive necrosis. *0151   0433*

Pseudocholinesterase *Serum Decrease* Depression of enzyme concentration tends to be more marked in patients ill with chronic liver disease, such as cirrhosis, than in those ill with acute conditions, such as viral hepatitis, ascending cholangitis, and acute anoxic hepatomegaly. Peaks and depressions in cholinesterase activity in acute liver disease are related to the extent of hepatic parenchymal damage. *2441*

Pyruvate *Blood Increase* Very advanced liver stage. *0619*

Reticulocytes *Blood Increase* Mild. *0992*

Somatomedin *Serum Decrease* *1443*

Sulfate *Urine Decrease* Patients with liver disease often have reduced urinary sulfate. *2104*

Thymol Turbidity *Serum Increase* Active liver disease; in active hepatitis thymol turbidity becomes positive later than transaminase elevation; may remain positive after cephalin flocculation has become negative. In cirrhosis it may be normal. *2467*

Triglycerides *Serum Increase* *2467*

Tyrosine Crystals *Urine Increase* Acute yellow atrophy. *2467*

Urea Nitrogen *Serum Decrease* Abnormally low levels have been attributed to liver failure. This is not a rare finding today and its significance should not be overlooked. Values of 5 mg/dL or less observed in 1% of 16,000 determinations. *0803* *0503*

Urobilinogen *Urine Increase* Early hepatitis (usually the first 48 h, but it may persist for 1-2 days longer in some cases). Also in hepatic necrosis. *0619* May precede the onset of jaundice by several days. *0999*

Feces Increase *2467*

Vitamin A *Serum Decrease* *0619*

Vitamin B$_{12}$ *Serum Increase* The blood level may be 3-8 X the normal concentration. Predominantly the free form is increased. *0619*

Xylose Tolerance Test *Urine Abnormal* In patients with ascites, the urine level is low. *2467*

Zinc *Serum Decrease* Found to be low in patients with hepatitis. *0998*

571.20 Laennec's or Alcoholic Cirrhosis

5'-Nucleotidase *Serum Increase* Elevations ranging from 32.7-265 U/L (normal = 2-11) were observed in 36 patients. In 20 cases of Laennec's cirrhosis with acute fatty infiltration the range was 18.8-56.9. *1312*

Acid Phosphatase *Serum Increase* Up to 16 U/L in Laennec's cirrhosis. *0812* Closely parallels serum bilirubin. *2104*

Alanine Aminotransferase *Serum Increase* Ranged from 20-258 U/L (35 = maximum normal limit). *2576* Usually much lower than the AST. *0999*

Serum Normal Normal in most cases of portal cirrhosis. *2260*

Albumin *Serum Decrease* In 95 patients, there was a significant decrease in mean albumin concentration, increase in mean gamma globulins, while mean alpha and beta globulins were normal. Characteristic electrophoresis pattern revealed a lack of demarcation between beta and gamma peaks (beta-gamma bridging). *2296*

Serum Increase *0619*

Aldosterone *Plasma Increase* Increased secretion. *2104*

Urine Increase May be increased in edematous states of hepatic cirrhosis. *0619* High renal output is due to increased secretion and decreased catabolism. Renal clearance rate may be reduced. *2104*

Alkaline Phosphatase *Serum Increase* Incidence of elevation: 40%; usual range of values: 25-85 U/L; 5% incidence of values > 107 U/L. Jaundice may be absent or present. Usually normal or only mildly elevated. *0503* Associated with jaundice. *2576* *1312*

Alkaline Phosphatase Isoenzymes *Serum Increase* Alkaline phosphatase-I was the major elevated isoenzyme in 12 of 14 cases. Isoenzyme-IV was raised in 5 of the 14 patients. *1221*

Alpha$_1$-Globulin *Serum Normal* *2467*

Alpha$_2$-Globulin *Serum Increase* Moderate increase. *0619*

Serum Normal *2467*

Alpha$_2$-Macroglobulin *Serum Increase* Significantly increased. *1654*

Alpha-Fetoprotein *Serum Increase* Concentration above 30 ng/mL were found in 14% of patients. *0036*

Amino Acids *Plasma Increase* Increased amino acids (gly, glu, ser, thr, tyr, and ala) in portal cirrhosis. *2049*

Ammonia *Blood Increase* Increased in terminal portal cirrhosis. *0619*

Angiotensin-Converting Enzyme (ACE) *Serum Increase* In patients with alcoholic liver disease mean 30.8 U/mL compared with 22.8 in controls. 30% of patients had elevated levels. *0255*

Antimitochondrial Antibodies *Serum Normal* *1840*

Antinuclear Antibodies *Serum Increase* Low incidence of the autoimmune serological markers antinuclear antibody (13%) and smooth muscle antibody (13%). *0880* 7% of patients were positive (2% of controls). *1840* *2035*

Antismooth Muscle Antibodies *Serum Increase* Low incidence of the autoimmune serological markers - ANA (13%) and SMA (13%). *0880* *2035* *2528* *1840*

Aspartate Aminotransferase *Serum Increase* Consistently elevated and higher than ALT activity. *2576* 50-145 U/L. *0999*

Beta-Globulin *Serum Normal* *2467*

Bile Acids *Serum Increase* Total bile acids were elevated in all patients with alcoholic liver cirrhosis. This test was found to discriminate most efficiently between acute alcohol intoxication and liver cirrhosis. *1166* In 30 pts. with alcoholic liver cirrh. portal hypertension and bleeding esophageal varices. *1165* *0920*

Bilirubin *Serum Increase* Elevated ranging from 2.4-9.5 mg/dL. *2576* *0999*

Bilirubin, Direct *Serum Increase* Occasionally acute alcoholic disease presents with a predominant elevation in the serum conjugated bilirubin suggesting extrahepatic obstruction of the biliary system. *0999* *0151*

Bilirubin, Indirect *Serum Increase* *2199*

BSP Retention *Serum Increase* *0151*

Calcitonin *Serum Increase* Immunoreactive calcitonin was increased in relation to raised alkaline phosphatase activity. *1040*

Calcium *Serum Decrease* Low concentrations correlated well with high AST activity in 78 cirrhotic patients. *1574*

Carcinoembryonic Antigen *Serum Increase* Positive assays were obtained in 40 of 88 patients with severe alcoholic liver disease but in none of 14 patients with nonalcoholic liver disease. Values usually were lower than in colonic or pancreatic cancer. *1623* About 50% of patients with severe alcoholic liver disease have elevated (> 2.5 ng/mL) values, usually < 5 and rarely 10 ng/mL. *1624* 70% of patients had values > 2.5 ng/mL. *0979* *2199*

Cells *Bone Marrow Increase* Normal or increased. *1268*

Cephalin Flocculation *Serum Increase* *0992*

Ceruloplasmin *Serum Increase* *1654*

Cholesterol *Serum Increase* In fatty infiltration of the liver the serum concentration was significantly increased, as compared with the normal values and with the figures obtained in the cases of chronic inflammatory liver disease. *0710*

Red Blood Cells Increase 25-50% increase in the membrane concentration, resulting in the characteristic target cell. *2552*

Cold Agglutinins *Serum Increase* Elevated titers may persist for weeks or months. *2035* *2001*

Complement C3 *Serum Decrease* Low levels of C3, C4 and factor B were common with cirrhosis and confined to those cases with severe reduction in serum albumin and/or prothrombin index. *0376*

Complement C4 *Serum Decrease* Low levels of C3, C4 and factor B were common with cirrhosis and confined to those cases with severe reduction in serum albumin and/or prothrombin index. *0376*

Complement, Total *Serum Decrease* Low levels of C3, C4 and factor B were common with cirrhosis and confined to those cases with severe reduction in serum albumin and/or prothrombin index. *0376*

Erythrocyte Sedimentation Rate *Blood Increase* Extreme elevation is found. *2467* *0992*

Erythrocyte Survival *Red Blood Cells Decrease* Moderately shortened in 48 of 68 alcoholic liver disease patients. *1268* *2137* *2552* Especially in patients with predominant indirect bilirubinemia. *0722*

Factor VIII *Plasma Increase* Increased activity in alcoholic liver disease. *0911*

Fibrinogen *Plasma Normal* Fibrinolytic activity is significantly increased in advanced cirrhosis. Total fibrinogen concentration was normal. *1414*

Fibrin Split Products (FSP) *Plasma Increase* Fibrinolytic activity is significantly increased in advanced cirrhosis. Total fibrinogen concentration was normal. *1414*

Gamma Glutamyl Transferase (GGT) *Serum Increase* Increases with liver damage. *0619*

571.20   Laennec's or Alcoholic Cirrhosis (continued)

Globulin   *Serum   Increase*   In 95 patients, there was a significant increase in mean concentration, while mean alpha and beta globulins were normal. Characteristic electrophoresis pattern reveals a lack of demarcation between beta and gamma peaks (beta-gamma bridging). *2296*   Usually increased; it reflects inflammation and parallels the severity of the inflammation *2467*   Mean total globulin values were found to be lowest in the healthy subjects followed by acute viral hepatitis, primary hepatocellular carcinoma and cirrhosis in that order *0724*

Glucagon   *Plasma   Increase*   May occur. *2146*

Glucose   *Serum   Decrease*   Replacement or destruction of functioning hepatic tissue may evoke hypoglycemia. *2104*

Glucose Tolerance   *Serum   Decrease*   A diabetic curve may occur and is a reflection of endogenous insulin resistance. *0992*

Hematocrit   *Blood   Decrease*   Approximately 75% of chronic liver disease patients have anemia, usually mild. *1268 2137*

Hemoglobin   *Blood   Decrease*   Approximately 75% of chronic liver disease patients have anemia, usually mild. *1268 2137*

Immunoglobulin IgA   *Serum   Increase*   Moderate hypergammaglobulinemia, especially IgA. *0880   2035*

Immunoglobulin IgG   *Serum   Increase*   Elevated in about 50% of the patients. *1847*

Immunoglobulin IgM   *Serum   Normal*   *2467*

Insulin   *Serum   Increase*   The majority of cirrhotics demonstrated increased levels of circulating insulin due to decreased hormonal catabolism. *1178*

Iron   *Serum   Increase*   Presumably due to the liberation of stored iron from necrosing liver cells. *0619*

Liver   Increase   Iron deposition in the liver is common. *0962*

Iron-Binding Capacity, Total (TIBC)   *Serum   Decrease*   Significantly reduced. *1654   2612*

Iron Saturation   *Serum   Increase*   Moderate to marked rise in percent saturation in hepatic cirrhosis. *2612*

Isocitrate Dehydrogenase   *Serum   Normal*   Mean serum concentration was normal with portal cirrhosis. *2260*

Lactate Dehydrogenase   *Serum   Increase*   Slight increase. *0962*   High in 6 of 20 patients with portal cirrhosis. *2260*

Lactate Dehydrogenase Isoenzyme 5 (LD₅)   *Serum   Increase*   LD 4 and 5 are elevated. *0503*

Lactate Dehydrogenase Isoenzymes   *Serum   Increase*   LD 4 and 5 are elevated. *0503*

Lecithin   *Red Blood Cells   Increase*   25-50% increase in the membrane concentration, resulting in the characteristic target cell. *2552*

Leukocytes   *Blood   Decrease*   May result from hypersplenism, a direct effect of alcohol or folate deficiency. *0992*

Blood   Increase   Leukocytosis may be pronounced. *0999*

Ascitic Fluid   Increase   In 58 culture-negative patients the ascitic fluid count range was 28-1,800 and 50% of counts were > 300 WBC/µL. The percentage of polymorphonuclear leukocytes ranged from 2-98%. *1872*   In 57 uncomplicated alcoholic liver disease patients, total ascitic WBC counts were often markedly elevated. Mean = 360/µL. *1187   1282*

Lipids   *Serum   Increase*   In 28 patients, 13 showed hypercholesterolemia, 16 increased serum triglyceride and 8 increased serum phospholipid. *1045*   In fatty infiltration of the liver the serum cholesterol, triglyceride and total lipid concentrations were significantly increased, as compared with the normal values and with the figures obtained in the cases of chronic inflammatory liver disease. *0710*

Lipoproteins, Beta   *Serum   Increase*   In fatty infiltration of the liver the serum total lipid concentrations were significantly increased, as compared with the normal values and with the figures obtained in the cases of chronic inflammatory liver disease. Beta and prebeta lipoprotein were increased. *0710*

Magnesium   *Serum   Decrease*   4 of 11 patients had abnormally low concentration. Mean concentration (1.85 mmol/L) was significantly lower than the normal mean. *2469*   May occur. *2444*

Red Blood Cells   Decrease   The mean concentration (4.7 mmol/L packed cells) was significantly below normal values. *2469*

MCV   *Blood   Increase*   Occasionally mild macrocytosis, but rarely 115 fL in the absence of megaloblastic changes in marrow. Reported incidence varies from 33-65%. *2552*

Ornithine Carbamoyl Transferase (OCT)   *Serum   Increase*   Liver cell damage. *2467*

Phospholipids, Total   *Serum   Increase*   45 patients suffering from steatosis of the liver have been examined with reference to serum lipid abnormalities. 28 of the patients were chronic alcoholics. 13 patients showed hypercholesterolemia, 16 increased serum triglyceride and 8 increased serum phospholipid. *1045*

Platelet Count   *Blood   Decrease*   May result from hypersplenism, a direct effect of alcohol or folate deficiency. *0992*   Mild; in about 50% of cases. *2137*

Potassium   *Serum   Decrease*   Often present in these patients and may represent gastrointestinal losses, decreased oral intake, or increased urinary excretion through acquired renal tubular acidosis. *0999   0151*

Urine   Increase   *0151*

Protein   *Ascitic Fluid   Decrease*   Ascitic fluid is usually a transudate with protein < 3.0 g/dL and specific gravity < 1.016. However, protein may exceed 2.5 g/dL in up to 30% of patients. *2199*

Prothrombin Time   *Plasma   Increase*   Severe clotting factor deficiencies are common. *0992*

Reticulocytes   *Blood   Decrease*   Reticulocytosis can be suppressed by alcohol. *2552 1147*

Blood   Increase   Average = 8.6%, ranging from 2.3-24.6% in 16 patients. *1147*

Rheumatoid Factor   *Serum   Increase*   Found in 36% of patients. *0422 0123*

Sodium   *Serum   Decrease*   Frequent in patients with ascites or edema. *0992*

Specific Gravity   *Ascitic Fluid   Decrease*   Ascitic fluid is usually a transudate with protein < 3.0 g/dL and specific gravity < 1.016. However, protein may exceed 2.5 g/dL in up to 30% of patients. *2199*

Thymol Turbidity   *Serum   Increase*   Possibly the bile-cholesterol-phospholipid combination has a stabilizing effect on the serum proteins. *0619*

Serum   Normal   May be normal. *2467*

Thyroid Stimulating Hormone (TSH)   *Serum   Increase*   The mean serum TSH level was 3.1 µU/mL in the normals and 7.1 µU/mL in the cirrhotic patients. 15% of the hepatic patients had serum TSH values above 10 µU/mL. *1703*

Thyroxine (T₄)   *Serum   Increase*   The mean free T₄ value was significantly higher (3.3 ng/dL) than in the normal subjects (2.1 ng/dL). *1703*

Triglycerides   *Serum   Increase*   In fatty infiltration of the liver the serum cholesterol, triglyceride and total lipid concentrations were significantly increased, as compared with the normal values and with the figures obtained in the cases of chronic inflammatory liver disease. *0710*   In 28 patients, 13 showed hypercholesterolemia, 16 increased serum triglyceride and 8 increased serum phospholipid. *1045*

Tri-iodothyronine (T₃)   *Serum   Decrease*   The mean serum T₃ value, 85 ng/dL, was significantly reduced in the hepatic patients as compared to a mean serum T₃ value of 126 ng/dL in the normal subjects, while the free T₃ value was 0.28 ng/dL in both groups. The reduction of the serum total and free T₃ values were closely correlated with the degree of liver damage. *1703*

Urea Nitrogen   *Serum   Decrease*   With severe cirrhosis. *0992*

Uric Acid   *Serum   Decrease*   Serum concentration was 4.18 ± 0.25 mg/dL in 22 male patients, significantly lower than in age-matched controls, 6.44 ± 0.19. An inverse correlation (R = 0.70) was found with serum bilirubin. *1580*

Serum   Increase   Hyperuricemia resulting from depressed urinary excretion of uric acid parallels lactic acidosis. *0151*

Urobilinogen   *Urine   Normal*   Normal or increased. *2467*

Volume   *Plasma   Increase*   With nutritional cirrhosis; usually moderate and occurs in approximately 33% of the patients. *1311*   Averages 15% above normal. Hemodilution exaggerates anemia. *1268*   In 64% of patients. *1669   1108*

Urine   Decrease   With ascites and edema. *0619*

Zinc   *Serum   Decrease*   Found to be low in patients with alcoholic cirrhosis or hepatitis, and elevated in alcoholics with normal or fatty liver. *0998*

571.49   Chronic Active Hepatitis

Alanine Aminotransferase   *Serum   Increase*   Usually increased (up to 10 X normal range). *2467*   Continuing or phasic release of transaminase enzymes from damaged liver cells, depending upon the degree of hepatocellular necrosis: serum levels range from 300-1000 U/L during exacerbations. *1922*   Mild elevation. *0962*   In 90% of 15 patients at initial hospitalization for this disorder. *0781   2035*

Albumin *Serum Decrease* Active phases with hepatocellular necrosis are marked by signs of hepatic dysfunction. *2035* In 36% of 19 patients at initial hospitalization for this disorder. *0781 0962*

Alkaline Phosphatase *Serum Increase* Only slight increases. *2035* Occasionally. *0962* In 60% of 19 patients at initial hospitalization for this disorder. *0781* Moderately elevated (X 2) or normal. *0992* Approximately 90% of patients with toxic hepatocellular jaundice have elevated values. Almost always < 88 U/L and in most < 50. Approximately 5% of patients with hepatocellular jaundice may have levels of 88-135 U/L. In jaundiced patients with higher levels, posthepatic jaundice should be suspected. *0503*

Alpha₁-Antitrypsin *Serum Increase* Increased. *1866 0042 1946 1947 2129*

Serum Normal No differences with controls noted. *0700*

Alpha₂-Macroglobulin *Serum Increase* Moderate elevation. *1082 2640* Significant increase *1654*

Alpha-Fetoprotein *Serum Increase* Concentration above 30 ng/mL, were found in 58% of patients. *0036* Elevated in 42% of cases *2111 0351*

Antibody Titer *Serum Increase* Increased incidence of high titers of serum autoantibodies. *2145*

Antimitochondrial Antibodies *Serum Increase* Present in 30% of patients. *2145* Found in 10-20% of patients. *0992* Found in 66% of patients compared to 2% of controls. *1840*

Antinuclear Antibodies *Serum Increase* Raised more often than LE cell phenomenon positive. *0619* Common (20-60% of cases). *0992* Recognized by immunofluorescence, with an incidence of positive tests of 60%. *2201* 57% of patients were positive compared to 2% of controls. *1840* Increased incidence of high titers of serum autoantibodies. *2145 2035*

Antismooth Muscle Antibodies *Serum Increase* In a high percentage of cases. More frequent in HBsAg negative cases. *0992* Reaction is highly positive (an incidence of 60-70%). True incidence could be even higher if tests were done only in phases of activity. *2035* Found in about 50-66% of patients. *0962* Positive in 85% of cases. *1840 2251*

Antithrombin III *Plasma Decrease* Decreased in parenchymatous liver disease. *2353 1482*

Apolipoprotein AI *Serum Decrease* The levels of prebeta and alpha lipoprotein were decreased. *0710*

Aspartate Aminotransferase *Serum Increase* Usually increased (up to 10 X normal range). *2467* Continuing or phasic release of transaminase enzymes from damaged liver cells, depending upon the degree of hepatocellular necrosis: serum concentrations range from 145-500 U/L during exacerbations. *1922* Mild elevation. *0962* In 97% of 18 patients at initial hospitalization for this disorder. *0781 2035*

Beta₂-Macroglobulin *Serum Increase* An increased serum concentration is characteristic. *1236*

Bile Acids *Serum Increase* Postprandial levels were significantly higher. *0920*

Bilirubin *Serum Increase* Usually moderately increased (3-10 mg/dL) but rarely exceeds 20 mg/dL. *0992* Active phases with hepatocellular necrosis are marked by signs of hepatic dysfunction. *2035* In 51% of 19 patients at initial hospitalization for this disorder. *0781*

Bilirubin, Direct *Serum Increase* *0992*

Bilirubin, Indirect *Serum Increase* *0992*

BSP Retention *Serum Increase* Noted even during inactive phase of disease. *0992* Active phases with hepatocellular necrosis are marked by signs of hepatic dysfunction. *2035*

Carcinoembryonic Antigen *Serum Increase* 4 of 7 patients showed elevated values (> 12.5 ng/mL). *0253*

Ceruloplasmin *Serum Increase* Alpha₂ glycoproteins, ceruloplasmin, and transferrin were elevated. *1654*

Chenodeoxycholic Acid *Serum Increase* Degree of elevation is related to the severity of illness as judged by other biochemical and clinical parameters. Bile acids return to normal in patients who respond to therapy. *1154* 3-Beta-Hydroxy-5-Cholenoic Acid was elevated in hepatobiliary disease. Normal 0.184 mmol/L, Chronic Active Hepatitis 2.364. *2325*

Cholesterol *Serum Decrease* Significantly reduced. *0710*

Cholesterol, High Density Lipoprotein *Serum Increase* Increased. *0131 1519 2556*

Cholesterol, Very Low Density Lipoprotein *Serum Increase* Marked elevation. *0062*

Cholic Acid *Serum Increase* Degree of elevation is related to the severity of illness as judged by other biochemical and clinical parameters. Bile acids return to normal in patients who respond to therapy. *1154* Mean fasting and 3h total cholic acid conjugates were significantly higher *1183* Elevated in 80% of Patients *1039*

Complement Fixation *Serum Increase* Incidence of positivity to anticytoplasmic antibodies (titer > 8) was reported to be 27-30% in contrast to an incidence of 3-4% in controls and 7-12% in other types of liver disease. *1466 2035*

Complement, Total *Serum Decrease* Normal or mildly decreased. *0992*

Serum Normal No characteristic alterations have been reported for levels of complement or complement components. *1844 2035*

Coombs' Test *Blood Positive* Sometimes present. *2467 0992*

Fatty Acids, Free (FFA) *Serum Decrease* In 11 cases a depression of the essential fatty acid concentration (linoleic and arachidonic) was noted with concomitant elevation of oleic, palmitic, and palmitoleic acids. *0800*

Serum Increase The pattern in 11 cases of hepatitis accompanied by jaundice showed elevated levels of oleic, palmitic, and palmitoleic acids attributed to the decreased ability of the liver to desaturate the endogenous saturated and monounsaturated acids to polyunsaturated ones. *0800*

Fibrinogen *Plasma Normal* Fibrinolytic activity is increased but total fibrinogen is normal. *1414*

Fibrin Split Products (FSP) *Plasma Increase* Significantly increased. *1414*

Gamma Glutamyl Transferase (GGT) *Serum Increase* In 90% of 10 patients at initial hospitalization for this disorder. *0781*

Globulin *Serum Increase* Elevated and remain raised without normalizing late in convalescence. *2339* Levels (> 2 g/dL) common, particularly with abundant plasma cell infiltration of liver. *0992* Hyperglobulinemia is usually found Provide a good index of activity and remission; fluctuations are synchronous with those of transaminase enzymes. *1465 0999 0962*

Glucose *Serum Decrease* Replacement or destruction of functioning hepatic tissue may evoke hypoglycemia. *2104*

Glycoproteins *Serum Increase* Alpha₂ glycoproteins, ceruloplasmin, and transferrin were elevated. *1654*

Haptoglobin *Serum Decrease* The only protein to be significantly reduced. *1654*

Hematocrit *Blood Decrease* Anemia, leukopenia and thrombocytopenia occur in 40-60% of patients. *2467* Slight to moderate anemia with leukopenia and thrombocytopenia are seen, particularly in patients with splenomegaly. *2035*

Hemoglobin *Blood Decrease* Anemia, leukopenia, and thrombocytopenia occur in 40-60% of patients. *2467* Slight to moderate anemia with leukopenia and thrombocytopenia are seen, particularly in patients with splenomegaly. *2035*

Hepatitis B Surface Antigen *Serum Increase* 25-30% of patients. Occurring more frequently in men than women. *0151*

HLA Antigens *Blood Present* HLA-DR3 present in 68% of patients versus 24% of controls. *2539*

Immunoglobulin IgA *Serum Increase* In 50 patients, mean levels of all three major classes of immunoglobulin, IgG, IgM and IgA, were increased but only IgG was markedly raised. *1467 2035*

Immunoglobulin IgG *Serum Increase* Elevated levels were present in about 50% of the patients. *1847* In 50 patients, mean levels of all 3 major classes of immunoglobulin, IgG, IgM, and IgA, were increased but only IgG was markedly raised. *1467 2035*

Immunoglobulin IgM *Serum Increase* In 50 patients, mean levels of all 3 major classes of immunoglobulin, IgG, IgM and IgA, were increased but only IgG was markedly raised. *1467 2035*

Immunoglobulins *Serum Increase* Pronounced reflecting the immunological aberrations. *2035*

Iron-Binding Capacity, Total (TIBC) *Serum Increase* Alpha₂ glycoproteins, ceruloplasmin and transferrin were elevated. *1654*

LE Cells *Blood Increase* Positivity differs from that obtained in SLE, in that preparations show fewer typical LE cells and positive tests are more transient or intermittent. *1467* Found in about 50-66% of patients. *0962* Positive in 10-35% of cases. *0992 2035 0999*

Leukocytes *Blood Decrease* Anemia, leukopenia, and thrombocytopenia occur in 40-60% of patients. *2467* Slight to moderate anemia with leukopenia and thrombocytopenia are seen, particularly in patients with splenomegaly. *2035*

Lymphocyte T-Cell *Blood Decrease* *0793*

571.49 Chronic Active Hepatitis *(continued)*

Magnesium *Serum Decrease* Mean = 1.28 ± 0.18. Normal = 1.73 ± 0.13 mmol/L. *0246*

Red Blood Cells Decrease Mean RBC concentration = 3.99 ± 0.61 compared to 5.08 ± 0.25 mmol/L. *0246*

Manganese *Serum Increase* Significant P < 0.001. *2429*

pCO₂ *Blood Decrease* Reduced in a high percentage of chronic as well as acute hepatitis patients. *2104*

Plasma Cells *Serum Increase* Increased plasma cells in bone marrow and may appear in peripheral blood. *2467*

Bone Marrow Increase Plasmacytosis in the bone marrow is part of the abnormal immunological response. *1151 2035*

Platelet Count *Blood Decrease* Anemia, leukopenia, and thrombocytopenia occur in 40-60% of patients. *2467* Slight to moderate anemia with leukopenia and thrombocytopenia are seen, particularly in patients with splenomegaly. *2035*

Prothrombin Time *Plasma Increase* Often prolonged. *0992* Patients with marked prolongation, despite vitamin K replacement and a positive LE cell test, have the worst prognosis. *0962*

Thymol Turbidity *Serum Increase* Usually increased. *2467*

Zinc *Serum Decrease* Significant P < 0.001. *2429*

571.60 Biliary Cirrhosis

5'-Nucleotidase *Serum Increase* In 18 patients levels ranged from 32.7-265 U/L, mean = 127.8 ± 79.5. *1312 0151*

Alanine Aminotransferase *Serum Increase* Modestly elevated (300 U/L) in most of these patients. Values are as high or higher than those of AST. *0503* Usually only mildly elevated. *0962*

Albumin *Serum Decrease* Normal or slightly decreased early; later more markedly decreased. *2467 2238*

Alkaline Phosphatase *Serum Increase* Striking elevations. Incidence of elevation is 100%. Usual range of values 270-375 U/L. *1312 0151 0999 2035*

Alpha₂-Globulin *Serum Increase* Moderate increases. *0619*

Amino Acids *Urine Increase* Aminoaciduria, especially cystine and threonine, may be found. *2467*

Antibody Titer *Serum Increase* Increased incidence of high titers of serum autoantibodies. *2145*

Antimitochondrial Antibodies *Serum Increase* Present in > 90% of patients compared with 2-3% of obstructive bile duct patients. *2145* In almost 100% of cases, while incidence is only 10% in extrahepatic biliary obstruction. *1829* 79-94% of all cases give positive results. *0619 0962 1840*

Antinuclear Antibodies *Serum Increase* Moderate incidence (24%), but the reaction is relatively weak. *2035* Found in 40% of patients and 2% of controls. *1840* Increased incidence of high titers of serum autoantibodies. *2145 1799*

Antismooth Muscle Antibodies *Serum Increase* Occurs in up to 50% of patients. *1829* Reported incidence of 10-50%, depending on the titer selected for positivity. *0584* 40% positive. *1840 2251 2035*

Apolipoprotein AI *Serum Decrease* Low in patients with cholestatic liver disease. *0750* In 4 female patients compared with 6 age and sex matched controls. *0127*

Apolipoprotein AII *Plasma Decrease* Low in patients with cholestatic liver disease. *0750* In 4 female patients compared with 6 age and sex matched controls. *0127*

Apolipoprotein E *Plasma Decrease* Low in patients with cholestatic liver disease. *0750*

Aspartate Aminotransferase *Serum Increase* Modest elevations (usually < 145 U/L). *0503* Hepatocellular necrosis is slight as judged by low serum transaminase levels, and hepatocellular function is well preserved. *2035* Usually only mildly elevated. *0962*

Beta-Globulin *Serum Increase* Marked increase. *0619*

Beta-Glucuronidase *Serum Increase* Increased. *0741 0866*

Bilirubin *Serum Increase* Usually conjugated bilirubinemia and total concentration range from 3-20 mg/dL or higher. In the final stages, concentrations may exceed 50 mg/dL. *0992* Usually conjugated, representing posthepatic cell obstruction. At times, a large proportion may be unconjugated reflecting impaired hepatic function. *2238 0999*

Urine Increase *2467*

Bilirubin, Direct *Serum Increase* Usually conjugated bilirubinemia and total concentrations range from 3-20 mg/dL or higher. In the final stages, concentrations may exceed 50 mg/dL. *0992* Increases in the serum bilirubin, mostly of the direct fraction. *0962* Usually conjugated, representing posthepatic cell obstruction. *2238*

Bilirubin, Indirect *Serum Increase* Total concentration is usually 5-10 mg/dL but may vary between normal and 25 mg/dL. Usually conjugated and therefore represents posthepatic cell obstruction, but at times a large proportion of unconjugated bilirubin may be present in the serum as a reflection of impaired hepatic function. *2238*

Ceruloplasmin *Serum Increase* Elevated in 46 of 46 cases. *0526*

Chenodeoxycholic Acid *Serum Increase* In 15 patients with primary biliary cirrhosis 13 had increased fasting levels. *2036* Severe Cholestasis *1154*

Cholesterol *Serum Increase* Moderate to marked elevations up to 1,800 mg/dL. *0503* Marked increase in total cholesterol and phospholipids takes place, with normal triglycerides; serum is not lipemic. The increase is associated with xanthomas and xantholasmas. *2467* Hypercholesterolemia of an extreme degree (2,000 mg/dL) may be present. *0999 2035*

Cholesterol, High Density Lipoprotein *Serum Increase* In 7 female patients compared to 6 normal age matched controls. *0127 0131 1519 2556*

Cholic Acid *Serum Increase* In 15 patients with primary biliary cirrhosis 13 had increased fasting levels. *2036* Severe Cholestasis *1154*

Copper *Urine Increase* Elevated in 42 of 46 patients. A correlation was found (R = 0.68) between urinary and hepatic copper. *0526 1944*

Liver Increase Elevated in 43 of 45 patients, > 400 μg/g dry weight were found almost exclusively in patients with advanced histological disease. *0526* 8 of 13 patients had liver copper content as high as seen in patients with hepatolenticular degeneration (250 μg/g dry wt). *1944*

Cryoglobulins *Serum Increase* Found in high concentration in 90% of patients (undetectable in controls). Composed of IgM (60%), IgG-IgM (25%), and IgA-IgM (5%). *2477*

Fibrinogen *Plasma Decrease* Formation is depressed in liver failure, resulting in decreased plasma levels. *0619*

Gamma Glutamyl Transferase (GGT) *Serum Increase* Elevation is marked. *2467*

Globulin *Serum Increase* Hypergammaglobulinemia is mainly due to an elevation of IgM. *0716* Usually elevated, particularly IgM. *0962* Serum globulins (especially beta and alpha₂) are increased *2467 2238 2035*

Glucose *Serum Decrease* Replacement or destruction of functioning hepatic tissue may evoke hypoglycemia. *2104*

Hydroxyproline *Urine Normal* Not different from age matched controls. *1057*

Immunoglobulin IgA *Serum Increase* Hypergammaglobulinemia is common, involving all classes of immunoglobulins (IgG, IgA, IgM), although IgM may be selectively increased. *0151*

Immunoglobulin IgG *Serum Increase* IgG is more likely to be elevated in chronic hepatitis and cryptogenic cirrhosis, whereas IgM is high in biliary cirrhosis. *1829* Hypergammaglobulinemia is common, involving all classes of immunoglobulins (IgG, IgA, IgM), although IgM may be selectively increased. *0151*

Immunoglobulin IgM *Serum Increase* Elevated in about 80% of patients. *0992* Hypergammaglobulinemia is common, involving all classes of immunoglobulins, although IgM may be selectively increased. *0151* Hypergammaglobulinemia is mainly due to an elevation of IgM. *0716 2035 0962*

Iron-Binding Capacity, Total (TIBC) *Serum Decrease* In hepatic cirrhosis. *2612*

Iron Saturation *Serum Increase* Moderate to marked rise in percent saturation in hepatic cirrhosis. *2612*

Lipids *Serum Increase* Common. *0992*

Osteocalcin *Serum Decrease* In 15 premenopausal females with this disorder. *1057*

Phospholipids, Total *Serum Decrease* In 4 female patients compared to 6 normal age matched controls. *0127*

Serum Increase Marked increase in total cholesterol and phospholipids takes place, with normal triglycerides; serum is not lipemic. The increase is associated with xanthomas and xantholasmas. *2467*

Prothrombin Time *Plasma Increase* Laboratory findings of steatorrhea but prothrombin time is normal or restored to normal by parenteral vitamin K. *2467*

Sodium *Serum Decrease* Frequently found, especially in patients with ascites. *2104*

Thymol Turbidity *Serum Increase* Usually increased. *2467*

Thyroxine Binding Globulin *Serum Increase* *0062*

Triglycerides *Serum Increase* With time, all lipids rise, including triglycerides. *2238*

Serum Normal Marked increase in total cholesterol and phospholipids takes place, with normal triglycerides; serum is not lipemic. *2467*

Uric Acid *Serum Decrease* May occur. *2467*

Urobilinogen *Urine Increase* Urine contains urobilinogen and bilirubin. *2467*

Vitamin E (Tocopherol) *Serum Decrease* Deficiency might be expected in patients with defective fat absorption. *2104*

571.90 Cirrhosis of Liver

[131]I Uptake *Serum Increase* In hepatic disease. *2104*

5'-Nucleotidase *Serum Increase* Increased in 50% of patients. *2467*

25-Hydroxy Vitamin D$_3$ *Serum Decrease* In patients with stable cirrhosis, values were slightly depressed, mean = 18.9 ± 8.9 ng/mL. Lower normal limit = 21 ng/mL. *2077*

Adenosine Deaminase *Serum Increase* Increased. *0655 1737 2235*

Alanine Aminotransferase *Serum Increase* Values are modestly elevated (300 U/L). Much lower than the respective values for AST. In cirrhosis of the liver, even with jaundice, the moderate AST level and the lower ALT level are in contrast with the high levels of both transaminases observed in acute viral hepatitis. *0503* Slight elevation occurred in 33% of patients with cirrhosis. Values ranged from 11-77 U/L. *1452* In 52% of 48 patients at initial hospitalization for this disorder. *0781 0962 2576*

Albumin *Serum Decrease* Mean values were found to be highest in the healthy subjects followed by acute viral hepatitis, primary hepatocellular carcinoma and cirrhosis, in that order. Both the mean albumin and mean total globulin of each group, were significantly different from the respective means of the other 3 groups. *0724* Parallels functional status of parenchymal cells and may be useful for following progress of liver disease; but it may be normal in the presence of considerable liver damage. *2467* In 51% of 69 patients at initial hospitalization for this disorder. *0781*

Serum Normal Usually parallels functional status of parenchymal cells, but it may be normal in the presence of considerable liver cell damage. *2467*

Aldolase *Serum Increase* Normal or slightly increased. *0962*

Serum Normal Normal or slightly increased. *0962*

Aldosterone *Plasma Increase* Increased levels. *1887* Increased secretion *2104*

Urine Increase May be increased in edematous states of hepatic cirrhosis. *0619*

Alkaline Phosphatase *Serum Increase* Nonspecifically elevated in cirrhosis but often reaches levels exceeding 160 U/L. *0433* Average elevation in 6 cases = 3.5 X normal upper limit. *1452* In 47% of 67 patients at initial hospitalization for this disorder. *0781* 50% incidence of elevation usually in the range of 25-188 U/L in postnecrotic cirrhosis. *0503 2576*

Leukocyte Increase Slightly increased in 30% of patients. *2467*

Alpha$_1$-Antitrypsin *Serum Increase* Increased. *1866 0042 1946 1947 2129*

Alpha$_1$-Glycoprotein *Serum Increase* It was found to have a sensitivity of 65% and a specificity of 80% with severe liver disease. *0709*

Alpha$_2$-Antiplasmin *Serum Decrease* Significant decrease in hepatic cirrhosis and in several other liver diseases. Mean value of 73 ± 15% compared to 100 ± 8% for controls. *2337* Values of 4.24 and 2.56 mg/dL for compensated and decompensated liver cirrhosis compared to 6.2 mg/dL for controls. *0070 2032*

Alpha$_2$-Macroglobulin *Serum Increase* Significantly increased in patients with cryptogenic cirrhosis, alcoholic cirrhosis and chronic active hepatitis. *1654* High concentrations were found in decompensated hepatic cirrhosis, 2.8 ± 0.8 g/L compared to normal, 2.3 ± 0.6 g/L. *2064* Moderate elevation *1082*

Alpha-Fetoprotein *Serum Increase* 10-20% of nonmalignant liver diseases of all types have elevated serum concentration, which tend to be fluctuating or transient. Steady or rising levels indicate malignancy. *2583* Elevated above 10 ng/mL in 34% of cases *2111*

Amino Acids *Urine Increase* Increased in advanced cirrhosis in proportion to the degree of liver damage. *0619* Mean amino acid clearance (glycine, glumine, serine, threonine, alanine, and tyrosine) were raised in Indian childhood cirrhosis patients. *2049*

CSF Increase Increased in advanced cirrhosis in proportion to the degree of liver damage. *0619*

Ammonia *Blood Increase* Increased in liver coma and cirrhosis and with portacaval shunting of blood. *2467*

Amylase *Serum Increase* High incidence of pancreatic abnormality in patients with no clinical evidence of pancreatic acinar disease. *2406*

Urine Increase High incidence of pancreatic abnormality in patients with no clinical evidence of pancreatic acinar disease. *2406*

Pleural Effusion Normal Usually less than or equal to serum level. *2017*

Antibody Titer *Serum Increase* Increased incidence of high titers of serum autoantibodies. *2145* Patients with cirrhosis appear to have antibodies to a larger number of enteric bacteria though not higher titers to individual strains. *1829* Increased incidence of antithyroid antibodies. *2238*

Antimitochondrial Antibodies *Serum Increase* Found in 5-30% of patients with postnecrotic cirrhosis depending upon the technique used. *1829 2145*

Antinuclear Antibodies *Serum Increase* With postnecrotic cirrhosis. *0151* Increased incidence of high titers of serum autoantibodies. *2145*

Antismooth Muscle Antibodies *Serum Increase* Positive in a majority of patients with postnecrotic cirrhosis, independent of the presence of HBsAg or LE cells. *1829*

Antithrombin III *Plasma Decrease* Decreased. *2353 1482*

Antithyroglobulin Antibodies *Serum Increase* Increased incidence of antithyroid antibodies. *1115 2238*

Apolipoprotein AI *Serum Decrease* Prebeta and alpha lipoprotein were decreased. *0710*

Aspartate Aminotransferase *Serum Increase* 60-70% incidence of elevated levels. Up to 145 U/L in 65-75% of cases. *2467* Mild elevation occurred in 86% of 6 cases. Mean elevation was 2 X normal upper limit. *1452* In 89% of 69 patients at initial hospitalization for this disorder. *0781 0503 0962 2576*

Beta$_2$-Macroglobulin *Serum Increase* *2467*

Beta-Glucuronidase *Serum Increase* Increased. *0741 0866*

Bile Acids *Serum Normal* Serum bile acids did not discriminate between anicteric patients with fatty liver (n = 10) and liver cirrhosis (n = 9) and normal controls (n = 27), *0638*

Urine Increase Mean values for Bile Acids in urine: Control 1.9 μg/mL, Obstructive Jaundice μg/mL and Cirrhosis 15.14 μg/mL (compensated) and 11.84 μg/mL (compensated). *2323*

Bilirubin *Serum Increase* Usually elevated except in well-compensated liver disease. A direct bilirubin > 0.3 mg/dL means liver disease unless severe hemolysis or the rare congenital syndromes of bilirubin metabolism are present. *0433* Most is indirect unless cirrhosis is of the cholangiolitic type. Higher and more stable in postnecrotic cirrhosis; lower and more fluctuating levels occur in Laennec's cirrhosis. Terminal icterus may be constant and severe. *2467* In 54% of 68 patients at initial hospitalization for this disorder. *0781* Values range from 7.8-8 mg/dL in postnecrotic cirrhosis. *2576*

Urine Increase *2467*

Bilirubin, Direct *Serum Increase* In 87% of 29 patients at initial hospitalization for this disorder. *0781 2467*

Bilirubin, Indirect *Serum Increase* In 71% of 27 patients at initial hospitalization for this disorder. *0781 2467*

BSP Retention *Serum Increase* Sensitive index of liver function and is most useful in the absence of jaundice to follow the course of disease when the other liver function tests are normal. *2467* Decreased removal of dye in advanced cirrhosis of liver. *0619*

Calcium *Serum Decrease* Low concentrations correlated well with high AST activity in 78 cirrhotic patients. *1574* In 38% of 68 patients at initial hospitalization for this disorder. *0781*

Carcinoembryonic Antigen *Serum Increase* *0795 2035*

Serum Normal Positive assays were obtained in 40 of 88 patients with severe alcoholic liver disease but in none of 14 patients with nonalcoholic liver disease. Values usually were lower than in colonic or pancreatic cancer. *1623*

Cells *Bone Marrow Increase* Normal or increased. *1268*

571.90   Cirrhosis of Liver *(continued)*

Cephalin Flocculation *Serum Increase* *2467*

Ceruloplasmin *Serum Increase* Elevated in various forms of acute and chronic liver disease. *0931*

Chenodeoxycholic Acid *Serum Increase* 3-Beta-Hydroxy-5-cholenoic acid was elevated in hepatobiliary disease. Normal -- 0.184 mmol/L; Cirrhosis: compensated 0.433 and uncompensated 1.636. *2325*   Raised fasting levels were found in 29 of 49 patients. *2363*

Cholesterol *Serum Decrease* Significantly reduced. Prebeta and alpha lipoprotein were decreased also. *0710*   In 24% of 61 patients at initial hospitalization for this disorder. *0781*

Cholesterol Esters *Serum Decrease* Decreased esters reflect more severe parenchymal cell damage. *2467*

Cholesterol, High Density Lipoprotein *Serum Decrease* Decreased. *0131 1519 2556*

Cholic Acid *Serum Increase* Raised fasting levels were found in 19 of 49 patients (39%). *2363*   Elevated in 97% of patients. *1039*

Chylomicrons *Peritoneal Fluid Increase* Present. *1486*

Complement C3 *Serum Decrease* Low levels of C3, C4, and factor B were common with cirrhosis and confined to those cases with severe reduction in serum albumin and/or prothrombin time. *0376*

Complement C4 *Serum Decrease* Decreased C3 and C4 occasionally occur. *1120*   Low levels of C3, C4, and factor B were common with cirrhosis and confined to those cases with severe reduction in serum albumin and/or prothrombin time. *0376*

Complement, Total *Serum Decrease* Decreased C3 and C4 occasionally occurs. *1120*   Depressed in patients with chronic liver disease; does not correlate with immune phenomena, but appears to be related to impaired hepatic protein synthesis. *0151*

Copper *Serum Increase* Elevated in various forms of acute and chronic liver disease. *0931 0619*

Coproporphyrin *Urine Increase* In liver disease, coproporphyrinuria may not indicate increased formation of the pigment, but rather its diversion from bile to urine. *0151*

Creatine Kinase *Serum Normal* *0962*

Cryofibrinogen *Serum Increase* *2035 0856 1551 2046*

Erythrocytes *Blood Decrease* Anemia reflects increased plasma volume and some increased destruction of RBCs. If more severe, rule out hemorrhage in gastrointestinal tract, folic acid deficiency, excessive hemolysis, etc. *2467*

Ascitic Fluid Increase > 10,000 cells/µL seen in 1% of cases. *2626*

Erythrocyte Sedimentation Rate *Blood Increase* Extreme elevation is found. *2467*

Erythrocyte Survival *Red Blood Cells Decrease* Mild to moderate hemolysis. *1849*   Moderately shortened in 48 of 68 alcoholic liver disease patients. *1268 2137 2552*   Especially in patients with predominant indirect bilirubinemia. *0722*

Estradiol *Plasma Increase* Estradiol is the most active estrogen. *0002 0605 0046*

Estrogens *Serum Increase* Inability to conjugate estrogens. *2238*

Factor V *Plasma Decrease* Impaired hepatic synthesis. *0424*

Factor VIII *Plasma Increase* Increased activity in alcoholic liver disease. *0911*

Fat *Feces Increase* May be excessive amounts of fecal fat. *2104*

Fibrinogen *Plasma Decrease* Impaired hepatic synthesis. *0424*

Plasma Normal Fibrinolytic activity is significantly increased in advanced cirrhosis and chronic aggressive hepatitis. Total fibrinogen concentration was normal. *1414*

Fibrin Split Products (FSP) *Plasma Increase* Fibrinolytic activity is significantly increased in advanced cirrhosis and chronic aggressive hepatitis. Total fibrinogen concentration was normal. *1414 1048 2538*

Gamma Glutamyl Transferase (GGT) *Serum Increase* In inactive cases, average values are lower than in chronic hepatitis. Increases > 10-20 X in cirrhotic patients suggest superimposed primary carcinoma of the liver. *2467*   In 5 patients with cirrhosis of liver, the mean GGT elevation (132) was 4.4 X the normal upper limit. *1452*   In 79% of 34 patients at initial hospitalization for this disorder. *0781*

Saliva Increase Significantly higher (8.3 units/L) versus normal controls (5.12 U/L). *1164*

Gastrin *Serum Increase* Mean fasting concentration was elevated (41.6 ± 3.1 pmol/L) compared to normal (26.3 ± 3.4 pmol/L) in cirrhotic patients. *1341*

Globulin *Serum Increase* Hypergammaglobulinemia exceeding 3 g/dL. Suggests chronic active hepatitis or primary biliary cirrhosis. *0433*   The increase in gamma fraction is polyclonal in nature and is due first to increase in IgM fraction followed by an increase in IgG fraction. *2339*   Usually increased; it reflects inflammation and parallels the severity of the inflammation *2467*   Mean total values were found to be lowest in the healthy subjects followed by acute viral hepatitis primary hepatocellular carcinoma and cirrhosis in that order *0724*

Glucagon *Plasma Increase* Concentration was raised 2-6 fold in patients with spontaneous portal systemic shunting or surgically induced portacaval shunting. Increased levels were due to hypersecretion rather than decreased catabolism. *2147*

Glucose *Serum Decrease* Can occur with various types of liver disease. Hepatic hypoglycemia is a fasting hypoglycemia and often only relieved by food. *0962   2104*

Pleural Effusion Normal Pleural Fluid = Serum level. *2017*

Peritoneal Fluid Increase High concentrations. *1831*

Glucose-6-Phosphatase *Serum Increase* Moderate rise. *0619*

Glucose Tolerance *Serum Decrease* A diabetic-type curve may occur and is a reflection of endogenous insulin resistance. *0992*

Hematocrit *Blood Decrease* Anemia reflects increased plasma volume and some increased destruction of RBCs. *2467*   Approximately 75% of chronic liver disease patients have anemia, usually mild. *1268 2137*   In 34% of 70 patients at initial hospitalization for this disorder. *0781*

Hemoglobin *Blood Decrease* Anemia reflects increased plasma volume and some increased destruction of RBCs. *2467*   Approximately 75% of chronic liver disease patients have anemia, usually mild. *1268 2137*   In 36% of 69 patients at initial hospitalization for this disorder. *0781*

Hemoglobin, Free *Serum Increase* Mild to moderate hemolysis usually occurs. *1849*

Hexosaminidase *Serum Increase* Increase in total concentration (hexosaminidase A and B). *1716*

Immunoglobulin IgA *Serum Increase* Hypergammaglobulinemia is common, involving all classes of immunoglobulins. *0151 0433*

Immunoglobulin IgG *Serum Increase* In about 50% of the patients with cryptogenic cirrhosis, alcoholic cirrhosis, and chronic active hepatitis. *1847*   The increase in gamma fraction is polyclonal in nature and is due first to increase in IgM fraction followed by an increase in IgG fraction. *2339   1829*

Immunoglobulin IgM *Serum Increase* The increase in gamma fraction is polyclonal in nature and is due first to increase in IgM fraction followed by an increase in IgG fraction. *2339   1829*

Insulin *Serum Increase* The majority of cirrhotics demonstrated increased levels of circulating insulin due to decreased hormonal catabolism. *1178*

Iron *Serum Decrease* In 28% of 21 patients at initial hospitalization for this disorder. *0781*

Iron-Binding Capacity, Total (TIBC) *Serum Decrease* The only protein to be significantly reduced. *1654*   In 51% of 21 patients at initial hospitalization for this disorder. *0781 2612*

Iron Saturation *Serum Increase* Moderate to marked rise in percent saturation in hepatic cirrhosis. *2612*

Isocitrate Dehydrogenase *Serum Increase* Normal or slightly increased in 20% of patients. A large increase suggests a poorer prognosis. *2467*

Lactate Dehydrogenase *Serum Increase* Slight increase. *0962*   In 32% of 69 patients at initial hospitalization for this disorder. *0781 2575 1089*

Pleural Effusion Decrease Transudate. *0062*

Lactate Dehydrogenase Isoenzyme 5 (LD$_5$) *Serum Increase* LD 4 and 5 are moderately elevated. *0503*

Lactate Dehydrogenase Isoenzymes *Serum Increase* LD 4 and 5 are moderately elevated. *0503*

LE Cells *Blood Increase* Reported in about 33% of patients with postnecrotic cirrhosis at some time during their illness. Cells tended to be present during active disease and absent during remission. *1829 0151*

Leucine Aminopeptidase *Serum Increase* 92% of 25 patients had mean peak values which were moderate to highly elevated. Mean = 523 ± 204 and range = 189-900 U/L (normal = 322). *0281*

Leukocytes *Blood Decrease* Decreased with hypersplenism. *2467*

Blood Normal Usually normal with active cirrhosis. *2467*

Pleural Effusion Decrease < 500/µL. *2017*

Ascitic Fluid Increase A total WBC exceeding 300/μL with predominantly polymorphonuclear leukocytes indicates associated peritonitis. *0433* Less than 250 cells/μL. {2626}

Lipids *Serum Increase* Gross elevation noted in acute alcoholic liver injury and primary biliary cirrhosis. *0433*

Magnesium *Serum Decrease* 4 of 11 patients had abnormally low concentrations. The mean concentration for the cirrhotic patients, 1.85 mmol/L, was significantly lower than the normal mean. *2469* In 35% of 14 patients at initial hospitalization for this disorder. *0781*

Red Blood Cells Decrease The mean concentration in cirrhotic patients (4.7 mmol/L packed cells) was significantly below normal values. *2469*

Manganese *Serum Increase* Significant P < 0.001. *2429*

MCV *Blood Increase* Occasionally mild macrocytosis, but rarely 115 fL in the absence of megaloblastic changes in marrow. Reported incidence varies from 33-65%. *2552*

Monocytes *Pleural Effusion Increase* Predominant cell type. *2017*

Mucoprotein *Serum Decrease* *0503*

Nickel *Serum Decrease* Mean 1.6 (n = 18) compared with controls mean 2.6 μg/L (n = 42). *1559*

Ornithine Carbamoyl Transferase (OCT) *Serum Increase* Liver cell damage. *2467*

Partial Thromboplastin Time *Plasma Increase* Severe clotting factor deficiencies are common. *0992*

pH *Pleural Effusion Increase* Transudate (pH > 7.3). *0062*

Phosphate *Serum Decrease* Pronounced hypophosphatemic response in cirrhotic patients after glucose administration. *1287* In 40% of 68 patients at initial hospitalization for this disorder. *0781 1574*

Plasma Cells *Serum Decrease* Post Surgical. *2357 0659 0683*

Platelet Count *Blood Decrease* Patients with severe acute hepatic necrosis may have findings compatible with intravascular coagulation, thrombocytopenia and increased levels of fibrinogen/fibrin degradation products. *1048* Mild; in about 50% of cases. *2137* In 38% of 48 patients at initial hospitalization for this disorder. *0781 2538*

Blood Increase Increased in miscellaneous disease states. *2467*

Porphobilinogen *Urine Increase* Occasionally observed. *0151*

Porphyrins *Urine Increase* *2467*

Potassium *Serum Decrease* Frequent in patients with ascites and edema. *0992*

Progesterone *Plasma Increase* Raised in 36 of 50 men with liver disease compared with 20 healthy male control subjects. Significantly higher in men with nonalcoholic cirrhosis with gynaecomastic than those without. *0704*

Prolactin *Serum Increase* Found in 14% of men with liver disease. Levels unrelated to presence of gynecomastia. *0704*

Protein *Serum Decrease* Total serum protein is usually normal or decreased. *2467*

Serum Increase Increased serum globulin may cause increased total protein especially in posthepatic cirrhosis. *2467*

Pleural Effusion Decrease May cause pleural effusion by several mechanisms; most important of these is transfer of fluid from the peritoneal cavity via either direct diaphragmatic defect or lymphatics. *0216* Transudate (< 3 g/dL). *2017*

Ascitic Fluid Decrease Ascitic fluid is usually a transudate with protein < 3.0 g/dL and specific gravity < 1.016. However, protein may exceed 2.5 g/dL in up to 30% of patients. *2199* < 2.5 g/dL in ascitic fluid *2626*

Protein Bound Iodine (PBI) *Serum Decrease* In severe liver disease. *2104*

Prothrombin Time *Plasma Increase* Hypoprothrombinemia unresponsive to parenteral vitamin K is indicative of severe hepatocellular dysfunction. *0433 0962*

Pseudocholinesterase *Serum Decrease* Tends to be more marked in chronic liver disease, such as cirrhosis than in acute disorders. Sixty patients with chronic liver disease showed a serum cholinesterase range of 0.73-0.008. *2441*

Serum Increase In active cirrhosis. *0619*

Renin Activity *Plasma Increase* Increased levels. *1887*

Reticulocytes *Blood Decrease* Reticulocytosis can be suppressed by alcohol. *2552 1147*

Blood Increase Average = 8.6%, ranging from 2.3-24.6% in 16 patients. *1147*

Rheumatoid Factor *Serum Increase* Dysproteinemias and paraproteinemias present significant seropositivity. *0962*

Sodium *Serum Decrease* Characteristic. *2537* Especially in patients with ascites. *2104*

Somatomedin *Serum Decrease* *1443*

Somatomedin-C *Serum Decrease* *2634*

Specific Gravity *Pleural Effusion Decrease* Transudate (< 1.016). *0062*

Ascitic Fluid Decrease Ascitic fluid is usually a transudate with protein < 3.0 g/dL and specific gravity < 1.016. However, protein may exceed 2.5 g/dL in up to 30% of patients. *2199*

Sulfate *Urine Decrease* Patients with liver disease often have reduced urinary sulfate. *2104*

Thromboplastin Generation *Blood Increase* Reflects various abnormalities. *2467*

Thymol Turbidity *Serum Increase* Possibly the bile-cholesterol-phospholipid combination has a stabilizing effect on the serum proteins. *0619*

Serum Normal May be normal. *2467*

Thyroid Stimulating Hormone (TSH) *Serum Increase* The mean serum TSH level was 3.1 μU/mL in the normals and 7.1 μU/mL in the cirrhotic patients. 15% of the hepatic patients had serum TSH values above 10 μU/mL. *1703*

Serum Normal Patients with severe alcoholic hepatitis often are euthyroid sick with low T_3 low T_4 and elevated rT_3 and normal TSH. *0335*

Thyroxine Binding Globulin *Serum Decrease* In chronic liver disease. *0062*

Serum Increase Increased. *1887*

Thyroxine Index, Free (FTI) *Serum Increase* In 11 patients with decompensated cirrhosis, the free T_4 index and free T_4 by dialysis method and its absolute value were significantly raised, due to disturbance in the protein binding capacity. *0823*

Thyroxine (T_4) *Serum Increase* In 11 patients with decompensated cirrhosis, the free T_4 index and free T_4 by dialysis method and its absolute value were significantly raised, due to disturbance in the protein binding capacity. *0823*

Tri-iodothyronine, Reverse *Serum Increase* Patients with severe alcoholic hepatitis often are euthyroid sick with low T_3 low T_4 and elevated rT_3 and normal TSH. *0335*

Tri-iodothyronine (T_3) *Serum Increase* Mean serum reverse T_3 and free reverse T_3 (450 pg/dL) were increased in hepatic cirrhosis. *0394*

Trypsin *Serum Increase* High incidence of pancreatic abnormality in patients with no clinical evidence of pancreatic acinar disease. *2406*

Tryptophan *CSF Increase* Increased concentrations due to decreased plasma branched chain amino acids. *1733*

Tyrosine *Serum Increase* In 30 patients with alcoholic liver cirrhosis, portal hypertension and bleeding esophageal varices. *1165*

Urea Nitrogen *Serum Decrease* Often decreased (< 10 mg/dL). *2467 0376*

Serum Increase Increased with gastrointestinal hemorrhage. *2467 0812*

Uric Acid *Serum Decrease* *2467*

Serum Increase In 52% of 68 patients at initial hospitalization for this disorder. *0781*

Urobilinogen *Urine Increase* In early and recovery stages. *2467*

Urine Normal Normal or increased. *2467*

Vitamin A *Serum Decrease* *0619*

Vitamin B$_{12}$ *Serum Increase* May be 3-8 X the normal concentration. The increase is mainly in the alpha-globulin bound fraction. *0619* Markedly increased; mean = 608 pg/mL in 33 patients. *1990*

Vitamin B$_{12}$ Binding Capacity *Serum Increase* Significant elevation; usually correlated with WBC in peripheral blood. *1990*

Volume *Plasma Increase* Averages 15% above normal. Hemodilution exaggerates anemia. *1268* In 64% of patients. *1669*

Urine Decrease With ascites and edema. *0619*

Red Blood Cells Decrease 25% of patients. *1669*

Xylose Tolerance Test *Urine Normal* *2467*

Zinc *Serum Decrease* Patients had serum levels < 70 μg/dL with a mean of 53.4 $\pm$ 11 μg/dL (normal mean = 85$\pm$ μg/dL). *2567* Lower concentrations of total serum zinc (540 $\pm$ 111 mg/L), and of albumin-bound serum zinc (295 $\pm$ 113 mg/L) and a higher concentration of alpha$_2$ macroglobulin-bound zinc (245 $\pm$ 69 mg/L) were found in 28 healthy patients with decompensated hepatic cirrhosis, compared to 28 healthy subjects (835 $\pm$ 91; 679 $\pm$ 83; 156 $\pm$ 27 mg/1 respectively). *0802* Significant P < 0.001 *2429 2188 2064*

571.90   Cirrhosis of Liver (continued)

Zinc (continued)

CSF   Decrease   Mean CSF concentrations of 2.8 ± 1.8 µg/dL. Normal mean for control group was 4.0 ± 2.6 µg/dL. *2567*

572.00   Liver Abscess (Pyogenic)

Alanine Aminotransferase   *Serum   Increase*   Increases during preicteric phase to peaks 500 U/L by the time jaundice appears; then rapid fall in several days; become normal 2-5 weeks after onset of jaundice. *2467*

Serum   Normal   Transaminase levels are often normal in the absence of biliary tract infections in acute liver abscess. *0151*

Albumin   *Serum   Decrease*   Levels below 3.0 g/dL are common. *0433*   Decreased synthesis and increased catabolism of albumin cause hypoproteinemia in the majority of patients with acute liver abscess. *0151*

Alkaline Phosphatase   *Serum   Increase*   In patients with space-occupying lesions such as liver abscess, the degree of elevation may be striking (270-535 U/L) with little or no rise in the serum bilirubin values. This pattern of hepatic dysfunction is useful in the recognition of these space-occupying lesions particularly in the recognition of metastasis to the liver in patients with carcinomatosis. *0812 0503*   25-80 U/L in over 80% of cases; 80-375 U/L in 100% of cases during obstructive phase. *2467*   Elevated in 75% of cases. *2199   0433*

Alpha-Fetoprotein   *Serum   Increase*   10-20% of nonmalignant liver diseases of all types have elevated serum AFP levels, which tend to be fluctuating or transient. Steady or rising levels indicate malignancy. *2583*

Amylase   *Serum   Decrease*   Severe liver damage. *2467*

Aspartate Aminotransferase   *Serum   Increase*   May exhibit a mild to moderate elevation. *0433*   Both rise during preicteric phase to peaks 240 U/L by the time jaundice appears; then rapid fall in several days; become normal 2-5 weeks after onset of jaundice. *2467*

Serum   Normal   Transaminase levels are often normal in the absence of biliary tract infections in acute liver abscess. *0151*

Bilirubin   *Serum   Increase*   Moderate increase in about 33% of patients. Usually indicates pyogenic rather than amebic and suggests poorer prognosis because of more tissue destruction. *2467*   Elevated in 50% of cases. *2199   0433*

BSP Retention   *Serum   Normal*   BSP dye may be lost into abdomen. Results may falsely appear normal. *2467*

Cephalin Flocculation   *Serum   Increase*   *2467*

Erythrocyte Survival   *Red Blood Cells   Decrease*   Decreased RBC survival; mild to moderate hemolysis. *1849*

Gamma Glutamyl Transferase (GGT)   *Serum   Increase*   In 5 patients with liver granulomas, including miliary tuberculosis and sarcoidosis, serum GGT levels were all elevated, mean = 303, range = 116-740 U/L. *1452*

Globulin   *Serum   Increase*   *2467*

Glucose   *Serum   Decrease*   Replacement or destruction of functioning hepatic tissue may evoke hypoglycemia. *2104*

Hematocrit   *Blood   Decrease*   Mild to moderate anemia. *0433*   A mild normochromic anemia is common. *2199*

Hemoglobin   *Blood   Decrease*   Mild to moderate anemia. *0433*   A mild normochromic anemia is common. *2199*

Hemoglobin, Free   *Serum   Increase*   Mild to moderate hemolysis usually occurs. *1849*

Isocitrate Dehydrogenase   *Serum   Increase*   500-2000 U/L in 1st week; < 800 U/L after 2 weeks; slightly elevated in 3rd week. *2467*

Leucine Aminopeptidase   *Serum   Increase*   In 12 patients with granulomatous hepatitis, all showed elevated LAP levels, varying from 380-1,000 U/L, with a mean of 622 (normal = 322). *0281*

Leukocytes   *Blood   Increase*   Marked leukocytosis with WBC above 20,000/µL. *0433*   Increase in WBC due to increase in granulocytes. *2467*

Neutrophils   *Blood   Increase*   Polymorphonuclear leukocytosis in > 90% of patients; usually over 20,000/µL. *2467*

Ornithine Carbamoyl Transferase (OCT)   *Serum   Increase*   Liver cell damage. *2467*

Partial Thromboplastin Time   *Plasma   Increase*   *0433*

Platelet Count   *Blood   Decrease*   *0433*

Blood   Normal   *0433*

Protein Bound Iodine (PBI)   *Serum   Decrease*   In severe liver disease. *2104*

Prothrombin Time   *Plasma   Increase*   Increased in cases of severe liver damage due to poisons, hepatitis, cirrhosis. *2467   0433*

Pseudocholinesterase   *Serum   Decrease*   Liver diseases, especially hepatitis. Lowest level corresponds to peak of disease and becomes normal with recovery. *2467*

Sulfate   *Urine   Decrease*   Patients with liver disease often have reduced urinary sulfate. *2104*

572.20   Hepatic Encephalopathy

Albumin   *Serum   Decrease*   Marked decrease. *1733*

Alpha-Fetoprotein   *Serum   Increase*   In fulminant hepatic failure, 15 of the 64 patients (23%) had raised levels but in only 2 did they exceed 50 ng/mL. Of the 23 survivors, 11 (48%) had elevated levels. This rise was found early after the development of a grade IV coma and constitutes an encouraging prognostic sign at a time when the liver function tests and EEG are not helpful. *1655*

Ammonia   *Blood   Increase*   Elevated in most patients. *1473*   Elevated in about 60% of patients. Poor correlation between the level of blood ammonia and the depth of the hepatic coma. *0962   0339*

CSF   Increase   Elevated in most patients. *1473*

Beta-Glucuronidase   *Serum   Decrease*   Decreased. *0741 0866*

Bicarbonate   *Serum   Decrease*   Respiratory alkalosis may occur. *0962*

Bilirubin   *Serum   Increase*   *0151*

Dopamine Hydroxylase   *Serum   Decrease*   A decrease in H3-dopamine uptake was demonstrated in the blood platelets of 22 hepatic encephalopathy patients when compared to that of patients with liver cirrhosis but without hepatic encephalopathy, and controls. There was a direct correlation between the stage of hepatic encephalopathy and the decrease in H3-dopamine uptake. *1627*

Factor VII   *Plasma   Decrease*   All 7 patients with values < 8% of normal failed to regain consciousness from hepatic coma due to fulminant hepatic failure. *0821*

Fatty Acids, Free (FFA)   *Serum   Increase*   Significant elevation. *1733*   Short and medium chain fatty acids with lengths C5-C8 are often elevated in blood and CSF. *1473*   Plasma free fatty acids are commonly elevated. *0151*

CSF   Increase   Short and medium chain fatty acids with lengths C5- C8 are often elevated in blood and CSF. *1473*

Fibrinogen   *Plasma   Decrease*   Low levels of clotting factors found in fulminant hepatic failure are due to decrease in liver synthesis aggravated by increased consumption. *0821*

Glutamine   *Serum   Increase*   An end product in ammonia metabolism. *1473*

CSF   Increase   An end product in ammonia metabolism. *1473*

Isoleucine   *Serum   Decrease*   Branched chain amino acids are generally reduced. *1473*

Leucine   *Serum   Decrease*   Branched chain amino acids are generally reduced. *1473*

Methionine   *Serum   Increase*   Frequently increased and is implicated in the pathogenesis of the disorder. *1473*

Nickel   *Serum   Decrease*   Thought to be caused by hypoalbuminemia. *1559*

pCO$_2$ *Blood   Decrease*   Respiratory alkalosis may occur. *0962*

pH   *Blood   Increase*   Respiratory alkalosis may occur. *0962*

Phenylalanine   *Serum   Increase*   Consistently elevated. *1473*

Potassium   *Serum   Increase*   Decreased concentrations indirectly induce hepatic coma by its effect on ammonia metabolism. Renal production of ammonia increases in the presence of potassium deficiency. *0801*

Prothrombin Time   *Plasma   Increase*   Prolonged in liver disease. *0962*

Sodium   *Urine   Decrease*   Hyponatremia (< 130 mmol/L) occurred in 61% of patients with hepatic failure due to decompensated cirrhosis of liver. *0379*

Tryptophan   *Serum   Increase*   The only amino acid with increased CSF concentrations compared to normals and stable cirrhotics, probably attributable to increased plasma free tryptophan in hepatic coma patients. *1733*

CSF   Increase   The only amino acid with increased CSF concentrations compared to normals and stable cirrhotics, probably attributable to increased plasma free tryptophan in hepatic coma patients. *1733*

Valine   *Serum   Decrease*   Branched chain amino acids are generally reduced. *1473*

Vitamin B$_{12}$ *Serum   Increase*   May increase to 30-40 X the normal level. The increase is mainly in the free form. *0619*

572.40   Hepatic Failure

Alanine Aminopeptidase   *Serum   Increase*   *1443*

Alanine Aminotransferase   *Serum   Increase*   May be increased or normal. *0503*

Albumin   *Serum   Decrease*   *1733 0503*

Alkaline Phosphatase   *Serum   Increase*   May be normal or increased. *0503*

Alpha-Fetoprotein   *Serum   Increase*   In fulminant hepatic failure, 15 of the 64 patients (23%) had raised levels but in only 2 did they exceed 50 ng/mL. Of the 23 survivors, 11 (48%) had elevated levels. This rise was found early after the development of a grade IV coma and constitutes an encouraging prognostic sign at a time when the liver function tests and EEG are unhelpful. *1655   0503*

Amino Acids   *Urine   Increase*   *0503*

Ammonia   *Blood   Increase*   Characteristic of liver failure. *2104 0503*

Aspartate Aminotransferase   *Serum   Increase*   May be normal or increased. *0503*

Beta-Glucuronidase   *Serum   Decrease*   Decreased. *0741 0866*

Bicarbonate   *Serum   Increase*   Persistent alkalosis in patients with hepatic failure. *1775*

Bilirubin   *Serum   Increase*   May be increased or normal. *0503*

BSP Retention   *Serum   Increase*   *0503*

Cephalin Flocculation   *Serum   Increase*   *0503*

Cholesterol   *Serum   Decrease*   *0503*

Cholesterol, High Density Lipoprotein   *Serum   Increase*   Increased. *0131 1519 2556*

Creatinine   *Serum   Increase*   High values (> 1.6 mg/dL) in 22 of 50 cases of hepatic failure due to decompensated cirrhosis or attacks of acute viral hepatitis. *0379*

Erythrocytes   *Urine   Increase*   WBC, RBC, and hyaline casts were found in 26% of patients with hepatic failure due to decompensated cirrhosis or attacks of acute viral hepatitis. *0379*

Factor II   *Plasma   Decrease*   Low levels of clotting factors found in fulminant hepatic failure are due to decrease in liver synthesis aggravated by increased consumption. *0821*

Factor V   *Plasma   Decrease*   Low levels of clotting factors found in fulminant hepatic failure are due to decrease in liver synthesis aggravated by increased consumption. *0821*

Factor VII   *Plasma   Decrease*   All 7 patients with values 8% of normal failed to regain consciousness from hepatic coma due to fulminant hepatic failure. *0821*

Factor IX   *Plasma   Decrease*   *0503*

Factor X   *Plasma   Decrease*   *0503*

Fibrinogen   *Plasma   Decrease*   Low levels of clotting factors found in fulminant hepatic failure are due to decrease in liver synthesis aggravated by increased consumption. *0821*

Globulin   *Serum   Increase*   *0503*

Glomerular Filtration Rate (GFR)   *Urine   Decrease*   GFR varied from 1-24 mL/min in 25 of 43 hepatic failure patients. Only 1 of these survived. *2536*   Reduced GFR was highly significant in 6 and mild-moderate in 14 of 50 cases of hepatic failure due to decompensated cirrhosis of liver. *0379*

Glucose   *Serum   Decrease*   The incidence is low. *0503* Replacement or destruction of functioning hepatic tissue may evoke hypoglycemia. *2104*

Glucose Tolerance   *Serum   Decrease*   There is a rapid rise of the blood sugar abnormal levels and a slow return to normal. *0503*

Haptoglobin   *Serum   Decrease*   *0503*

Hippuric Acid   *Urine   Decrease*   *0503*

Hyaline Casts   *Urine   Increase*   WBC, RBC, and hyaline casts were found in 26% of patients with hepatic failure due to decompensated cirrhosis or attacks of acute viral hepatitis. *0379*

Lactate Dehydrogenase   *Serum   Increase*   May be increased or normal. *0503*

Leucine   *Urine   Increase*   *0503*

Leukocytes   *Urine   Increase*   WBC, RBC, and hyaline casts were found in 26% of patients with hepatic failure due to decompensated cirrhosis or attacks of acute viral hepatitis. *0379*

Magnesium   *Serum   Decrease*   Hypomagnesemia is common in hepatic failure. *1775*

Nickel   *Serum   Decrease*   Thought to be caused by hypoalbuminemia. *1559*

pCO$_2$ *Blood   Decrease*   Characteristic of liver failure. *2104*

pH   *Blood   Increase*   Persistent alkalosis in patients with hepatic failure. *1775*

Phosphate   *Serum   Decrease*   Hypophosphatemia may occur in hepatic failure as a result of intravenous carbohydrate feeding, gram-negative septicemia, endotoxemia, and large dose steroid treatment. *1775*

Platelet Count   *Blood   Decrease*   As a result of hypersplenism. *0503*

Prothrombin Time   *Plasma   Increase*   *0503*

Sodium   *Serum   Decrease*   In hepatic failure patients, sodium loss in urine may be high if the GFR falls below 24 mL/min. *2536* Frequently depressed in hepatic failure. Severe hyponatremic states are found in end-stage hepatic cirrhosis with uniformly poor prognosis. *1775*   Hyponatremia (< 130 mmol/L) occurred in 61% of patients with hepatic failure due to decompensated cirrhosis of liver. *0379*

Serum   Increase   Marked sodium retention (9 mmol/24h) may occur in fulminant hepatic failure when GFR exceeds 40 mL/min. *2536*

Urine   Decrease   Marked sodium retention (9 mmol/24 h) may occur in fulminant hepatic failure when GFR exceeds 40 mL/min. *2536*   Hyponatremia (< 130 mmol/L) occurred in 61% of patients with hepatic failure due to decompensated cirrhosis of liver. *0379*

Urine   Increase   In hepatic failure patients, sodium loss in urine may be high if the GFR falls below 24 mL/min. *2536*

Somatomedin-C   *Serum   Decrease*   *2634*

Thymol Turbidity   *Serum   Increase*   *0503*

Tyrosine   *Urine   Increase*   *0503*

Urea Nitrogen   *Serum   Decrease*   Only if hepatic tissue is severely damaged. *2104*

Serum   Increase   Blood levels of urea were raised in 20 cases (40%) of which in 9 cases it was > 60 mg/dL in patients with hepatic failure arising from decompensated cirrhosis or attacks of acute viral hepatitis. *0379*

Vitamin A   *Serum   Decrease*   *0503*

573.30   Toxic Hepatitis

5'-Nucleotidase   *Serum   Increase*   Six cases of toxic drug hepatitis showed activities ranging from 91.3-155.7 U/L (normal = 2-11 U/L). *1312*

Alanine Aminopeptidase   *Serum   Increase*   *1443*

Alanine Aminotransferase   *Serum   Increase*   Rises precipitously. *0433*   Levels depend upon severity. In severe toxic hepatitis, serum enzymes may be 10-20 X higher than in acute hepatitis and show a different pattern, i.e., increase in LD > AST > ALT > (acute icteric period). *2467*   Elevations in toxic hepatitis due to carbon tetrachloride occur within 24 h and may reach peaks of up to 27,000 U/L. Other toxins (chlorpromazine salicylates, azaserine and pyrazinamide) will cause smaller elevations. *2577*

Aldolase   *Serum   Increase*   Due to carbon tetrachloride and other poisons. *0619*

Alkaline Phosphatase   *Serum   Increase*   Elevated to > 3 X normal. *0433*   Found in 6 patients with toxic drug hepatitis with values of 134 ± 19.8 U/L. *1312*   Drugs particularly likely to produce this type of jaundice are chlorpromazine or organic arsenicals. Alk phos values are at least as high as in posthepatic jaundice. *0503*   Striking increase. *2104*

Alpha$_1$-Antitrypsin   *Serum   Increase*   Increased. *1866 0042 1946 1947 2129*

Alpha$_1$-Glycoprotein   *Serum   Increase*   It was found to have a sensitivity of 65% and a specificity of 80% with severe liver disease. *0709*

Alpha$_2$-Macroglobulin   *Serum   Increase*   *2640*

Alpha-Fetoprotein   *Serum   Normal*   Curiously absent. *2199*

Amylase   *Serum   Decrease*   Severe liver damage. *2467*

Antimitochondrial Antibodies   *Serum   Increase*   Especially in drug-induced hepatitis due to halothane or chlorpromazine. *1829*

Antithrombin III   *Plasma   Increase*   Elevated in the acute hepatitis following renal transplantation. *1482 2353*

573.30   Toxic Hepatitis *(continued)*

Aspartate Aminotransferase *Serum Increase* Elevations of ALT reflects acute hepatic disease somewhat more specifically than is true of AST. *0503* Usual values seen: 240-1,900 U/L. Values > 145 U/L are usual and > 240 are frequent. *0503* Concentration depend upon severity. In severe cases, (especially carbon tetrachloride poisoning), serum enzymes may be 10-20 X higher than in acute hepatitis and show a different pattern (i.e., increase in LD > AST > ALT). *2467* Elevations in toxic hepatitis due to carbon tetrachloride exposure occur within 24 h and may reach peaks of up to 13,000 U/L. Other toxins (chlorpromazine, salicylates, azaserine, and pyrazinamide) will *2577*

Beta$_2$-Macroglobulin *Serum Increase* An increased serum concentration is characteristic. *1236*

Beta-Glucuronidase *Serum Increase* Increased with extensive cell necrosis. *0741 0866*

Bilirubin *Serum Increase* *0433*

Urine Increase *2467*

Feces Decrease *2467*

Bilirubin, Direct *Serum Increase* Increased early. *2467*

Bilirubin, Indirect *Serum Increase* Increased predominantly. *2467*

BSP Retention *Serum Increase* *0503*

Cephalin Flocculation *Serum Increase* Normal or slight increase. *2467*

Cholesterol *Serum Decrease* Liver damage due to cinchophen, chloroform, carbon tetrachloride, or phosphate. *0619* Normal or mildly depressed in hepatitis; but markedly depressed in severe hepatitis. *0503*

Serum Increase *2467*

Cholesterol, Very Low Density Lipoprotein *Serum Increase* Marked elevation. *0062*

Gamma Glutamyl Transferase (GGT) *Serum Increase* Raised enzyme activity may be the only evidence of moderate liver damage due to drugs. *0619*

Glucose *Serum Decrease* Due to organic arsenic, carbon tetrachloride, chloroform, cinchophen, phosphate, alcohol, acute paracetamol poisoning. *0619* Can occur with various types of liver disease. Hepatic hypoglycemia is a fasting hypoglycemia and often only transiently relieved by food. *0962 2104*

Glucose-6-Phosphatase *Serum Increase* After liver damage with carbon tetrachloride the serum level reaches its peak values by 6 h. *0619*

Isocitrate Dehydrogenase *Serum Increase* Hepatitis of liver poisons, normal in 2-3 weeks. *2467*

Lactate Dehydrogenase *Serum Increase* LD 4 and 5 due to chemical poisoning. *0812*

Lactate Dehydrogenase Isoenzyme 5 (LD$_5$) *Serum Increase* Due to chemical poisoning. *2467*

Lactate Dehydrogenase Isoenzymes *Serum Increase* LD$_4$, LD$_5$ due to chemical poisoning. *0812*

Leucine Aminopeptidase *Serum Increase* *0503*

Manganese *Serum Increase* During acute phase increase up to four times that seen in normal subjects. *2429*

Nickel *Serum Decrease* Thought to be caused by hypoalbuminemia. *1559*

Protein *Serum Decrease* Enteric loss of plasma protein. *2199*

Prothrombin Time *Plasma Increase* Increased in cases of severe liver damage due to poisons. *2467*

Thymol Turbidity *Serum Increase* Normal or slight increase. *2467*

Thyroxine Binding Globulin *Serum Increase* Increased levels. *1887*

Urea Nitrogen *Serum Decrease* With severe damage due to hepatotoxic agents. *2104*

Urobilinogen *Urine Increase* Normal or increased during pre-icteric phase. *2467*

Urine Normal *2467*

Feces Decrease *2467*

575.00   Acute Cholecystitis

5'-Nucleotidase *Serum Increase* Slight hepatic inflammation and partial biliary obstruction. *0186*

Alanine Aminotransferase *Serum Increase* 4 of 8 patients showed elevated levels. Mean value = 44, range = 8-154 U/L. *1452* Occasionally increased. *0995* May be mildly elevated even in the absence of intrahepatic infection or common bile duct obstruction. *2199*

Albumin *Serum Decrease* *2467*

Alkaline Phosphatase *Serum Increase* Increased in some cases, even if serum bilirubin is normal. *2467* Average elevation = 3 X maximum normal limit in 75% of 8 cases studied. *1452* May be mildly elevated even in the absence of intrahepatic infection or common bile duct obstruction. *2199* In 30% of 16 patients at initial hospitalization for this disorder. *0781*

Alkaline Phosphatase Isoenzymes *Serum Increase* All 11 patients with biliary tree disease, including 5 with cholecystitis and 6 with pericholangitis, showed elevated isoenzyme I. 7 of the 11 had raised isoenzyme-IV. *1221*

Amylase *Serum Decrease* Decreased in some cases. *0619*

Serum Increase May exceed 1,000 U/L. May or may not indicate concomitant acute pancreatitis, because elevations in this range may be seen in acute cholecystitis without any changes in the pancreas. *2199 2038*

Aspartate Aminotransferase *Serum Increase* May be increased in 75% of patients. *2467* In 8 cases, 4 showed moderate elevation. The mean value for the group was 38 U/L, while the normal upper limit was 24 U/L. *1452* Occasionally increased. *0995* May be mildly elevated even in the absence of intrahepatic infection or common bile duct obstruction. *2199* In 57% of 15 patients at initial hospitalization for this disorder. *0781*

Bilirubin *Serum Increase* Mild hyperbilirubinemia occasionally occurs. *0999* Usually mild (< 4.0 mg/dL). *2199*

Serum Normal Some cases. *2467*

Urine Increase Occasionally found. *0999*

BSP Retention *Serum Increase* Increased BSP retention (some cases) even if serum bilirubin is normal. *2467*

Carcinoembryonic Antigen *Serum Increase* 23% of patients had values > 2.5 ng/mL. *2199*

Erythrocyte Sedimentation Rate *Blood Increase* Increased ESR, WBC (up to 20,000/μL) and other evidences of acute inflammatory process. *2467*

Gamma Glutamyl Transferase (GGT) *Serum Increase* In 8 patients, the mean (210 U/L) was 7.0 X the normal upper limit. *1452*

Saliva Increase Significantly higher (18.3 U/L) versus controls (5.12 U/L). *1164*

Globulin *Serum Normal* *2467*

Leucine Aminopeptidase *Serum Increase* 7 patients had raised concentrations varying from 385-450 U/L, while in those with chronic disease, only 4 of 8 cases showed mild elevation. *0281* Moderate increase. *0619*

Leukocytes *Blood Increase* Increased ESR, WBC (up to 20,000/μL) and other evidences of acute inflammatory process. *2467* During an acute attack, the count averages 12,000-15,000/μL with a neutrophilic leukocytosis and an increase in band forms. *2199* In 655% of 15 patients at initial hospitalization for this disorder. *0781*

Lipase *Serum Increase* In some cases. *2467* In 25% of cases. *2238*

Neutrophils *Blood Increase* In 60% of 15 patients at initial hospitalization for this disorder. *0781* Neutrophilic leukocytosis. *2199*

Ornithine Carbamoyl Transferase (OCT) *Serum Increase* Liver cell damage. *2467*

Protein *Serum Decrease* *2467*

Urobilinogen *Urine Increase* Usually disappears within 24-48 h after the attack subsides. *2199*

576.00   Postcholecystectomy Syndrome

Amylase *Serum Increase* If tests are performed repeatedly, immediately after attacks, some abnormalities will appear if there is an organic cause of the syndrome. *0995*

Leukocytes *Blood Increase* If tests are performed repeatedly, immediately after attacks, some abnormalities will appear if there is an organic cause of the syndrome. *0995*

Lipase *Serum Increase* If tests are performed repeatedly, immediately after attacks, some abnormalities will appear if there is an organic cause of the syndrome. *0995*

576.10   Cholangitis

5'-Nucleotidase   *Serum   Increase*   Elevated levels indicate extrahepatic obstruction. *0151*

Alanine Aminotransferase   *Serum   Increase*   With parenchymal cell necrosis and malfunction. *2467*   77% of 13 patients showed mild elevation with a mean of 46 and range of 11-96 U/L. *1452*

Alkaline Phosphatase   *Serum   Increase*   Elevation (mean = 255 U/L) observed in 100% of 13 cases. *1452*   Values indicate extrahepatic obstruction. *0151   0433*

Alkaline Phosphatase Isoenzymes   *Serum   Increase*   All 11 patients with biliary tree disease, including 5 with cholecystitis and 6 with pericholangitis, showed elevated isoenzyme I. 7 of the 11 had raised isoenzyme-IV. *1221*

Aspartate Aminotransferase   *Serum   Increase*   With parenchymal cell necrosis and malfunction. *2467*   Mean elevation of 48 U/L, twice the normal upper limit, was found in 13 cases. 77% of the patients had elevated levels. *1452*   Usually remaining < 100 U/L, but values of 240 are found, followed by a sharp drop within 48 h. *0151*   In 70% of 10 patients at initial hospitalization for this disorder. *0781*

Bilirubin   *Serum   Increase*   Values are usually in the range of 2-4 mg/dL and are uncommonly higher than 10 mg/dL. *0151*

Gamma Glutamyl Transferase (GGT)   *Serum   Increase*   A mean elevation of 249 U/L (8.3 X normal maximum) was found in 13 patients. *1452*

Glucose   *Serum   Decrease*   Often accompanies mental changes. *2199*

Leucine Aminopeptidase   *Serum   Increase*   In 13 patients, 77% showed elevations. Mean = 46 U/L, 2.1 X the normal value. *1452*

Leukocytes   *Blood   Increase*   Usually exceeds 20,000/μL in suppurative cholangitis. Marked increase, up to 30,000/μL with increase in granulocytes. *2467*   In 36% of 11 patients at initial hospitalization for this disorder. *0781   0433*

Neutrophils   *Blood   Increase*   Marked increase, up to 30,000/μL with increase in granulocytes in suppurative cholangitis. *2467*   In 36% of 11 patients at initial hospitalization for this disorder. *0781*

Platelet Count   *Blood   Decrease*   Characteristic of the acute phase. *2199*

Urobilinogen   *Urine   Increase*   With parenchymal cell necrosis and malfunction. *2467*   With infection of the biliary tract. In cholangitis very high concentrations are attained. *0619*

576.20   Extrahepatic Biliary Obstruction

5'-Nucleotidase   *Serum   Increase*   Increased in extra-hepatic biliary obstruction. *0619*

Acid Phosphatase   *Serum   Increase*   Closely parallels serum bilirubin. *2104*

Alanine Aminotransferase   *Serum   Increase*   10-100 U/L; returns to normal within 1 week after obstruction is relieved. *2467*   Increased activity in all cases of biliary tract obstruction. Common duct obstruction due to stones, pancreatitis, tumor, duct carcinoma, and leukemia nodes showed values of 64-400 U/L. Calculous biliary obstruction was associated with ALT activity of 42-45 U/L. *2576*   In obstruction due to benign or malignant disease. *2260   0962*

Aldolase   *Serum   Increase*   Normal or slightly increased. *0962*

Alkaline Phosphatase   *Serum   Increase*   Markedly increased, related to the completeness of obstruction. Up to 376 U/L in complete biliary obstruction. *2467*   Associated with increase of 53-240 U/L. Common duct obstruction due to stones had values of 53-110 U/L. *2576*   95% - 100% incidence of elevation usually ranging from 60-140 U/L. Incidence of values > 105 U/L = 40%. *0503*   May become elevated in attack in the absence of hyperbilirubinemia. *0433*

Leukocyte   Increase   Parallels alkaline phosphatase. *2467*

Alkaline Phosphatase Isoenzymes   *Serum   Increase*   10 jaundiced patients with extrahepatic biliary obstruction had elevated isoenzyme-I and 8 of the 10 had raised isoenzyme-IV. *1221*   15 of 17 patients with obstructive jaundice showed a couplet of liver isoenzymes in the alpha$_1$ and alpha$_2$ areas. Mean levels were 4.7 and 20.5 respectively. *1926*   Two main isoenzymes are present: alpha$_2$-globulin, derived directly from the liver cells, which contributed the major fraction, and the 2nd, present in smaller proportions and represents the regurgitation of bile alkaline phosphatase as a result of obstruction to the normal flow of bile. *1855*

Alpha$_2$-Globulin   *Serum   Increase*   In cholestasis, the increase in alpha$_2$ and beta globulin components correlates with the height of serum lipid values and is a useful point in distinguishing between biliary obstructive lesions and other nonobstructive types of jaundice. *2339*

Amylase   *Serum   Increase*   Occurs in calculus common duct obstruction without pancreatitis due to an increase in pancreatic isoenzyme. *2486*   Marked elevations should point to the diagnosis of acute pancreatitis of primary nature or secondary to calculus biliary tract disease. *0433*   Values > 1,000 U/L usually indicate choledocholithiasis. *0017*

Urine   Increase   Increased excretion in obstruction due to stone in common bile duct. *0619*

Antimitochondrial Antibodies   *Serum   Normal   1840*

Antinuclear Antibodies   *Serum   Increase*   Positive in 11% of patients (2% in controls). *1840*

Antismooth Muscle Antibodies   *Serum   Increase*   11% of patients were positive and 6% of controls. *1840 2251*

Aspartate Aminotransferase   *Serum   Increase*   Up to 145 U/L; returns to normal within 1 week after obstruction is relieved. *2467*   Increased activity in all cases of biliary tract obstruction. Common duct obstruction due to stones, pancreatitis, tumor, duct carcinoma, and leukemia nodes showed values of 31-193 U/L. *2576   0962*

Beta-Globulin   *Serum   Increase*   In cholestasis, the increase in alpha$_2$ and beta globulin components correlates with the height of serum lipid values and is a useful point in distinguishing between biliary obstructive lesions and other nonobstructive types of jaundice. *2339*

Bile Acids   *Urine   Increase*   Mean values for Bile Acids in urine: Control 1.9 μg/mL, Obstructive Jaundice μg/mL, Cirrhosis 15.14 μg/mL (compensated) and 11.84 (uncompensated). *2323*

Bilirubin   *Serum   Increase*   During or soon after an attack of biliary colic. Increased in about 33% of patients. *2467*

Serum   Normal   Remains normal in the presence of serum alkaline phosphatase that is markedly increased with the obstruction of one hepatic bile duct. *2467*

Urine   Increase   Values of 1-5 mg/dL are common in an episode of cholecystitis. Levels higher than 5 mg/dL are usually the result of common bile duct obstruction, particularly if there is a predominance of the direct-reacting fraction of bilirubin. *0433*   During or soon after an attack of biliary colic. Increased in about 33% of patients. *2467*

Feces   Decrease   Marked decrease. Clay colored stools. *2467*

Bilirubin, Direct   *Serum   Increase   0999*

Bilirubin, Indirect   *Serum   Increase*   Normal or slight increase. *2467*

BSP Retention   *Serum   Increase*   Normal or may later become only slightly increased. *2467*

Carcinoembryonic Antigen   *Serum   Increase*   Circulating levels are elevated in benign extrahepatic biliary tract obstruction and inflammation. *2290*   43% of patients had values > 2.5 ng/mL. *0979   2199*

Cephalin Flocculation   *Serum   Increase*   Normal or may later become only slightly increased. *2467*

Chenodeoxycholic Acid   *Serum   Increase*   3-Beta-Hydroxy-5-cholenoic acid was elevated in hepatobiliary disease. Normal = 0.184 mmol/L, Obstructive Jaundice 6.783. *2325*   Serum bile acids elevate promptly during the acute episode and indicate biliary tract disease *1154*

Cholesterol   *Serum   Increase*   Continues to rise for some time after obstruction has been established, reaching extreme heights. Persists for a long period, falling when the obstruction is relieved. *1494*   In 15 patients, (aged 16-78), compared to controls, there was an increase in total cholesterol due to an increase in the unesterified fraction. *1606*

Red Blood Cells   Increase   25-50% increase in the membrane concentration, resulting in the characteristic target cell. *2552*   An increase in RBC cholesterol and phospholipid was detected in most patients with hepatocellular disease or cholestatic jaundice but the alteration in RBC lipid content did not correlate with RBC survival. *1848*

Cholesterol, Free   *Serum   Increase*   In simple biliary obstruction the increase is greater in the free fraction. *0619*

Cholic Acid   *Serum   Increase*   Serum bile acids elevate promptly during the acute episode indicate biliary tract disease. *1154*

Creatine Kinase   *Serum   Normal   0962*

Fat   *Feces   Increase*   Deficient intraluminal bile acids. *2199*   May be excessive amounts of fecal fat. *2104*

Gamma Glutamyl Transferase (GGT)   *Serum   Increase*   Increased with obstructive jaundice. *0619*   Increase is faster and greater than that of serum alkaline phosphatase and LAP. *2467*

Globulin   *Serum   Increase*   Alpha and beta globulins increase in infection or obstructive jaundice. *0151*

576.20 Extrahepatic Biliary Obstruction (continued)

Haptoglobin *Serum Increase* Can be variable or increased. Increased in 33% of patients with obstructive biliary disease. *2467*

Isocitrate Dehydrogenase *Serum Increase* 100-500 U/L. *2467*

Serum Normal Within the normal range in patients with obstruction due to benign or malignant disease. *2260*

Lactate Dehydrogenase *Serum Increase* Slight increase. *0962* In obstruction due to benign or malignant disease. *2260*

Lactate Dehydrogenase Isoenzyme 5 (LD$_5$) *Serum Increase* Was markedly elevated in 3 cases. Mean elevation = 11.0% of total LD value. *0852*

Lactate Dehydrogenase Isoenzymes *Serum Increase* LD$_4$ was elevated to 9.3% of total LD value in 3 cases. *0852*

Lecithin *Red Blood Cells Increase* 25-50% increase in the membrane concentration, resulting in the characteristic target cell. *2552*

Leucine Aminopeptidase *Serum Increase* 9 patients with obstruction due to stones had highly elevated serum values, ranging from 48-990 U/L. *0281*

Urine Increase Moderate increase with simple obstruction. *0619*

Leukocytes *Blood Increase* Normal or increased. *0999* A moderate leukocytosis of 10,000-15,000/μL found in the majority of patients with an attack. Higher elevations in the range of 20,000-25,000/μL or the appearance of many less mature forms are indicative of complications such as suppuration or cholangitis. *0433*

Blood Normal Normal WBC. *2467*

Lipase *Serum Decrease* Lack of bile salts result in the failure to activate pancreatic lipase in the intestinal lumen. *2104*

Serum Increase Marked elevations should point to the diagnosis of acute pancreatitis of primary nature or secondary to calculus biliary tract disease. *0433*

Lipids *Serum Increase* In cholestasis, the increase in alpha$_2$ and beta globulin components correlates with the height of serum lipid values and is a useful point in distinguishing between biliary obstructive lesions and other nonobstructive types of jaundice. *2339*

Lipoproteins *Serum Increase* Alpha$_2$ and beta globulins contain lipoproteins which may be markedly increased in cholestatic lesions of the liver. *2339*

Lipoproteins, Beta *Serum Increase* *0774 0772 0773*

Mucoprotein *Serum Increase* *0503*

Occult Blood *Feces Positive* May be positive or negative in patients with extrahepatic biliary obstruction. *0999*

Ornithine Carbamoyl Transferase (OCT) *Serum Increase* Liver cell damage. *2467*

Osmotic Fragility *Red Blood Cells Decrease* Thin, flat erythrocytes are more resistant than normal cells and have decreased osmotic fragility. *0962*

Phospholipids, Total *Serum Increase* In 15 patients (aged 16-78), compared to 23 controls (aged 18-63), there was an increased in cholesterol and phospholipids and increase in phospholipid to cholesterol ratio. *1606*

Red Blood Cells Increase An increase in RBC phospholipid was detected in most patients with hepatocellular disease or cholestatic jaundice but the alteration in RBC lipid content did not correlate with RBC survival. *1848*

Prothrombin Time *Plasma Increase* Prolonged, with response to parenteral vitamin K more frequent than in hepatic parenchymal cell disease. *2467*

Thymol Turbidity *Serum Increase* Normal or may later become only slightly increased. *2467*

Triglycerides *Serum Increase* A marked and persistent elevation. The increase is of similar magnitude to that for cholesterol and phospholipid. Following relief of obstruction the triglycerides returned to normal. Associated with a clear serum and negative cold aggregation test in contrast to the changes in cases of endogenous (type IV) hypertriglyceridemia. *1606*

Urobilinogen *Urine Decrease* *2467*

Urine Increase With infection of the biliary tract. In cholangitis very high concentrations of urine urobilinogen are attained. Probably bacteria act in the proximal parts of the bile-ducts, on the bile-pigments. *0619*

Feces Decrease Marked decrease. Clay colored stools. *2467* When very high serum bilirubin levels are attained, a little bilirubin may diffuse into the bowel, resulting in the appearance of small quantities of urobilinogen in the stools. Otherwise none is detected. *0619*

Vitamin A *Serum Decrease* *0619*

Vitamin K *Serum Decrease* Due to fat malabsorption. *2104*

576.50 Spasm of Sphincter of Oddi

Amylase *Serum Increase* Obstruction of the pancreatic duct by drug-induced spasm of sphincter (e.g., opiates, codeine, methyl choline, chlorothiazide). *2467*

Lipase *Serum Increase* Obstruction of the pancreatic duct by drug-induced spasm of the sphincter (e.g.,by opiates, codeine, methyl choline). *2467*

577.00 Acute Pancreatitis

5'-Nucleotidase *Serum Increase* Six patients showed elevations ranging from 16.1-67.1 U/L (normal = 2-11). *1312*

17-Hydroxycorticosteroids *Urine Increase* May be marked; increased due to severe stress. *2467*

17-Ketogenic Steroids *Urine Increase* May be marked; increased due to severe stress. *2467*

Acid Phosphatase *Ascitic Fluid Increase* Ranged from 0.3-11.2 mmol p-nitrophenol/h/mL. *0827*

Alanine Aminotransferase *Serum Increase* 4 of 10 patients showed elevations. Values ranged from 10-50 U/L,mean = 26.5 U/L (upper limit of normal = 24 U/L). *1452 0962*

Albumin *Serum Decrease* In 66% of 21 patients at initial hospitalization for this disorder. *0781 1119*

Pleural Effusion Increase *0186*

Ascitic Fluid Increase Elevated level (> 2.9 g/dL) is characteristic. *2199*

Aldolase *Serum Increase* Other nonspecific serum enzymes may also be increased. *2467 0962*

Alkaline Phosphatase *Serum Increase* Parallels serum bilirubin. *2467* Anicteric cases had normal levels. Cases with some degree of common bile duct obstruction were all elevated. *1312* In 45% of 21 patients at initial hospitalization for this disorder. *0781*

Alpha$_1$-Antitrypsin *Serum Decrease* Decreased. *1866 0042 1946 1947 2129*

Ascitic Fluid Decrease Ranged from 15-170 mg/dL in ascites (normal serum value = 200-400 mg/dL). *0827*

Alpha$_2$-Macroglobulin *Serum Increase* *2640*

Ascitic Fluid Decrease Ascites had concentrations from 44-400 mg/dL. Normal serum level is 200-400 mg/dL. *0827*

Alpha-Glucosidase *Serum Increase* Patients with pancreatitis associated with trauma or complicated by severe necrosis, hemorrhage, or abscess also displayed greater increases. *1842*

Amino Acids *Plasma Decrease* In patients with acute hemorrhagic necrotizing pancreatitis. *1994*

Urine Increase In some patients with familial pancreatitis the urine may contain an excess amount of amino acids, especially cystine and lysine. *0433*

Amylase *Serum Decrease* Extensive marked destruction of pancreas. Decreased levels are clinically significant only in occasional cases of fulminant pancreatitis. *2467*

Serum Increase Increase begins in 3-6 h, rises to over 250 U/L within 8 h in 75% of patients, reaches maximum in 20-30 h, and may persist for 48-72 h. May be up to 40 X normal, but the height of the increase does not correlate with the severity of the disease. More than 10% of patients may have normal values even in terminal stage. *2467* Amylase isoenzyme, P3, is elevated in acute pancreatitis but not in other conditions. *0789* Rises within 24-48 h of acute onset, normalizing within 3-5 days. *2031 0827*

Serum Normal Occasionally seen; probably following a transient rise and fall, extensive necrosis or acute exacerbation of chronic pancreatitis in which the pancreas cannot produce amylase. *2031*

Urine Increase Often elevated and persists up to the 3rd day after the onset of the disease. *0433* Tends to reflect serum changes by a time lag of 6-10 h, but sometimes increased urine levels are higher and of longer duration than serum levels. *2467* Elevation has been used to diagnose acute pancreatitis in the absence of renal failure. Levels higher than 6,000 U/24h or 300 U/h are usually seen in patients with acute attacks. *0151* Increased renal clearance. *0178*

Pleural Effusion *Increase* Pleural effusions occur in about 10% of patients, with amylase commonly elevated. *1403* Elevated in primary or metastatic lung cancer, pancreatitis, or esophageal perforation. *2031* May contain very high concentration, even with normal serum level. If the concentrations are lower than the serum, pancreatitis is virtually excluded as the cause. *2199* Pleural effusion has been reported in about 6% of patients with acute pancreatitis. These effusions contain pleural fluid amylase. May occur in other conditions including metastatic carcinoma. *0503* With pancreatic pseudocyst *1405 2017*

Ascitic Fluid *Increase* Concentration in ascitic fluid is usually 1,000 U/L. *0080* Varied from 1,060-48,000 U/L in ascites. *0827* Ascites may develop, 0.5-2 liters in volume, containing increased amylase with a level higher than that of serum. *2467 2199*

Saliva *Increase* Increased alpha-amylase in parotid saliva. *0922 0080*

Antithrombin III *Plasma Decrease* In both survivors (n = 10) and fatal cases (n = 4) a high frequency of reduced values were found during the first week after admission. Values were significantly more reduced in the fatal cases. *0004*

Arylsulfatase *Ascitic Fluid Increase* Varied from 89-5170 pmol/min/mL. *0827*

Aspartate Aminotransferase *Serum Increase* No apparent correlation with damage to pancreas, serum lipase, amylase, or calcium, but there is direct correlation with the serum bilirubin level suggesting increase due to biliary obstruction. *0619* Both normal and elevated levels have been reported. Usual values = 20-700 U/L. *2467 0503* Mild elevation (mean = 36.2 U/L) in 80% of 10 cases (normal maximum = 24 U/L). *1452* In 87% of 21 patients at initial hospitalization for this disorder. *0781 0962*

Beta-Glucuronidase *Ascitic Fluid Increase* Ranged from 850-16,500 μg phenolphthalein/h/dL. *0827*

Bilirubin *Serum Increase* Seen in about 20% of patients. *0999* May be moderately elevated as a consequence of edema of the head of the pancreas with resultant obstruction of the common bile duct. *0962* In 32% of 21 patients at initial hospitalization for this disorder. *0781*

Serum Normal May be increased when pancreatitis of biliary tract origin but is usually normal in alcoholic pancreatitis. *2467*

Urine Increase Seen in about 20% of patients. *0999*

Bilirubin, Direct *Serum Increase* In 80% of 10 patients at initial hospitalization for this disorder. *0781*

Bilirubin, Indirect *Serum Increase* In 40% of 10 patients at initial hospitalization for this disorder. *0781*

Calcium *Serum Decrease* Decreased in severe cases 1-9 days after onset. Usually occurs after amylase and lipase levels have become normal. Values < 7.0 mg/dL indicates poor prognosis. *0151* Often found with a low serum albumin; when correction of serum calcium is made for hypoalbuminemia, most patients are found to be normocalcemic. *0039* Mean = 7.3 ± 1.5 mg/dL in the 12 patients (range = 4.6-9.9). The 5 patients who did not recover had the lowest concentrations. *0827* Total and ionized calcium were low or in the low normal range in 11 clearly documented case. *2509 1119 0962 2199*

Serum Increase Occasionally, in patients whose pancreatitis is related to hyperparathyroidism, it may be elevated even during the acute attack. *0433*

Carcinoembryonic Antigen *Serum Increase* May be found. *0537* 53% of patients had values > 2.5 ng/mL. *0979 0795 2035 2199*

Catecholamines *Urine Increase* May be marked; increased due to severe stress. *2467*

Cholesterol *Serum Decrease* In 42% of 21 patients at initial hospitalization for this disorder. *0781*

Chylomicrons *Serum Increase* Increased: *1380 1936 1948*

Creatine Kinase *Serum Increase* Was found to indicate a more severe or prolonged course than in cases with normal levels, but to have little diagnostic value. *1942*

Creatinine *Serum Increase* In 42% of 14 patients at initial hospitalization for this disorder. *0781*

Eosinophils *Pleural Effusion Increase* Eosinophilia greater than 10% may be present. *0062*

Epinephrine *Plasma Increase* Increased circulating epinephrine. *0619*

Erythrocytes *Pleural Effusion Increase* 1000-10,000/μL. *2017*

Ascitic Fluid Increase In hemorrhagic pancreatitis. *0186*

Ascitic Fluid Normal Variable amount noted. *2626*

Erythrocyte Sedimentation Rate *Blood Increase* *2199*

Gamma Glutamyl Transferase (GGT) *Serum Increase* Always elevated. *2467* Was elevated to a mean level of 300 U/L (10 X normal) in all 10 cases. *1452 2010*

Saliva Increase Significantly higher (15.1 U/L) versus controls (5.12 U/L). *1164*

Glucagon *Plasma Increase* Increased concentrations lead to the release of calcitonin and resultant depression of serum calcium. *0999*

Glucose *Serum Increase* Transient hyperglycemia is not rare. *2199* Often found and signifies involvement of pancreatic islet cells. *0433* Seen in about 25% of patients. *0999* In 45% of 21 patients at initial hospitalization for this disorder. *0781*

Urine Increase Routine urinalysis is usually normal but there may be glucose in the urine. *0433* Appears in 25% of the patients. *2467*

Hematocrit *Blood Decrease* *2199*

Blood Increase Occasionally because of hemoconcentration. *0433* Probably reflects intravascular volume contraction. *0962 2467*

Hemoglobin *Blood Decrease* *2199*

Blood Increase Usually normal but may be high occasionally due to hemoconcentration. *0433*

Lactate Dehydrogenase *Serum Increase* In some cases. *0619* Nonspecific serum enzymes may also be increased. *2467* In 45% of 21 patients at initial hospitalization for this disorder. *0781*

Pleural Effusion Increase Exudate. *0062*

Lactate Dehydrogenase Isoenzyme 5 (LD$_5$) *Serum Increase* Elevated to 8.3% of the total value of 861 U/L in 3 cases. Increases occurred in LD isoenzymes 4 and 5. *0852*

Lactate Dehydrogenase Isoenzymes *Serum Increase* LD$_4$ was elevated above the normal value in 3 cases. LD$_4$ comprised 8.4% of total LD of 861 U/L (= 4%). *0852*

Leucine Aminopeptidase *Serum Increase* Of 6 patients, 67% had abnormally high values, ranging from 195-455 U/L (322 = upper limit of normal). *0281* Transient moderate rise in acute but no increase in chronic pancreatitis. *0619*

Leukocytes *Blood Increase* Usually elevated. *0433* WBC is slightly to moderately increased (10,000-20,000/μL). *2467* In 60% of 21 patients at initial hospitalization for this disorder. *0781 2199*

Pleural Effusion Increase 5000-20,000/μL. *2017*

Ascitic Fluid Normal Variable *2626*

Lipase *Serum Increase* Increases in 50% of patients and may remain elevated as long as 14 days after amylase returns to normal. *2467* Usually rises in parallel with the amylase activity, reaching its peak in 72 or 96 h with a gradual fall; values > 2.0 mL of N/100 NaOH are significant. *0151* Elevated in 63%, amylase in 70%, and 83% had parallel elevation of both enzymes. *0080* Elevated in 90% of cases. *2228 0433*

Pleural Effusion Increase May contain very high concentration, even with normal serum level. If the concentration are lower than the serum, pancreatitis is virtually excluded as the cause. *2199*

Ascitic Fluid Increase May be elevated. *0080*

Lipids *Serum Increase* Transient; subsides shortly after the onset of the disease and reappears with recurrences. These features differentiate the hyperlipidemia of acute pancreatitis from pancreatitis secondarily associated with primary abnormalities of lipid metabolism. *0433* Patients with disease caused by alcohol may exhibit milky serum as a result of marked elevation of lipids. *2199*

Lipoproteins *Serum Increase* May be present. *2199*

Magnesium *Serum Decrease* Low or in the low normal range. *2509* Observed in a few patients and could partly account for the failure of hypocalcemia to respond to exogenous calcium. *2199*

Malate Dehydrogenase *Serum Increase* Slight increase. *0619* Nonspecific serum enzymes may be increased. *2467*

Methemalbumin *Serum Increase* Consistent methemalbuminemia in patients with hemorrhagic pancreatitis, whereas in patients with acute edematous pancreatitis, none could be detected in serum or ascites. *0826* Appears after 12 h, reaching peak values by 4-5 days. There is a much higher mortality in acute hemorrhagic pancreatitis than in edematous acute pancreatitis. *0619* May be present in serum in acute hemorrhagic pancreatitis and not in nonhemorrhagic pancreatitis. *2199 0962*

Ascitic Fluid Increase Ranged from 2.6-35 g/dL in the patients with hemorrhagic pancreatitis. *0827*

Neutrophils *Blood Increase* Usually elevated. *0433* In 75% of 20 patients at initial hospitalization for this disorder. *0781 2538*

Pleural Effusion Increase Predominant cell type. *2017*

Occult Blood *Feces Positive* *2199*

577.00 Acute Pancreatitis (continued)

Oxygen Saturation *Blood Decrease* Blood gases often reveal a moderate lowering of pO_2. *2199*

Parathyroid Hormone *Serum Increase* Elevated and inversely correlated with serum ionized calcium. *2509*

pH *Pleural Effusion Decrease* Exudate (pH < 7.3). *0062*

Phosphate *Serum Decrease* Low or in the low normal range. *2509* In 41% of 21 patients at initial hospitalization for this disorder. *0781*

pO$_2$ *Blood Decrease* Blood gases often reveal a moderate lowering of pO_2. *2199*

Potassium *Serum Decrease* Usually normal or only slightly depressed. *2199*

Protein *Pleural Effusion Increase* Exudate (> 3 g/dL). *0062*

Ascitic Fluid Increase Variable but often > 2.5 g/dL in ascitic fluid. *2626* Total protein varied from 1.2-6.6 g/dL *0827*

Peritoneal Fluid Increase Greater than 30 g/L in 70% of cases of pancreatic ascites. *0586*

Specific Gravity *Pleural Effusion Increase* Exudate (> 1.016). *0062*

Triglycerides *Serum Increase* Often imparts a lactescence to the serum. Elevated because of a transient inhibition to chylomicron removal from the circulation. *0962* May reach 1,000 mg/dL or higher. *2199*

Trypsin *Serum Increase* 10-40 X higher than normal. *2199*

Urea Nitrogen *Serum Increase* Not uncommon with more severe cases, especially when shock and oliguria are present. *0151* Rarely exceeds 4 mg/dL. *2199*

577.10 Chronic Pancreatitis

Alanine Aminotransferase *Serum Increase* *2199*

Albumin *Serum Decrease* In 27% of 11 patients at initial hospitalization for this disorder. *0781* Mild depression may occur. *2199*

Ascitic Fluid Increase Elevation (> 2.9 g/dL) is characteristic. *2199*

Alkaline Phosphatase *Serum Increase* Jaundice may occur not only during acute attacks but also during the silent stage. Usually due to extrahepatic cholestasis an elevated alkaline phosphatase and normal AST at the early stages tend to support this. *0433* In each of 6 male alcoholic patients with calcific disease, a marked elevation was associated with minimal elevation in serum bilirubin or BSP excretion. *2217* In 40% of 12 patients at initial hospitalization for this disorder. *0781*

Alpha$_2$-Macroglobulin *Serum Increase* *2640*

Amylase *Serum Increase* Hyperamylasemia in acute exacerbation sometimes accompanied by a transient elevation in salivary type isoamylase (S-amylase). *2456* May be found, especially if the blood is drawn early in the attack. With each succeeding episode, however, pancreatic exocrine function decreases and the likelihood of finding an elevated amylase diminishes. *0999* Usually normal during quiescent phase. Rises as chronic damage progresses, but tends to become less pronounced. May actually be normal during relapse. *2031* *2199*

Serum Normal Usually normal during quiescent phase. Rises as chronic damage progresses but tends to become less pronounced. May actually be normal during relapse. *2031* As disease progresses and more of the gland is destroyed, acute pancreatitis may occur without elevation. *2199*

Pleural Effusion Increase Pleural effusions occur in about 10% of pancreatitis patients, with amylase commonly elevated. *1403* Elevated in primary or metastatic lung cancer, pancreatitis, or esophageal perforation. *2031* Pleural fluid pH of < 7.20 or 0.15 below arterial pH frequently occurs in parapneumonic effusion *1403* With Pancreatic pseudocyst *2017* *1405*

Ascitic Fluid Increase Greatly increased in pancreatic ascites. *2199*

Saliva Decrease Salivary output, amylase, and HCO$_3$ concentration decreased in 88% of patients. *1210*

Aspartate Aminotransferase *Serum Increase* In 48% of 12 patients at initial hospitalization for this disorder. *0781* *2199*

Bicarbonate *Saliva Decrease* Salivary output, amylase, and (HCO$_3$) concentration decreased in 88% of patients. *1210* *0080*

Bilirubin *Serum Increase* *2199*

Calcium *Serum Decrease* Malnutrition is the result of the malabsorption of fat, proteins, and fat-soluble vitamins which results in low concentrations. *0433*

Carotene *Serum Decrease* With malabsorption. *2238*

Cholesterol *Serum Increase* Some cases. *0619*

Chymotrypsin *Feces Decrease* Found to be a more reliable measure of pancreatic function than trypsin activity. False-positives have been noted in 10% of controls, and normal values may occur in patients. *0052*

Eosinophils *Pleural Effusion Increase* Eosinophilia greater than 10% may be present. *0062*

Erythrocytes *Pleural Effusion Increase* 1000-10,000/μL. *2017*

Ascitic Fluid Normal Variable amount noted. *2626*

Fat *Feces Increase* The number and size of fecal fat globules correlate with the degree of steatorrhea. *0600* Deficiency intraluminal pancreatic enzymes. *2199*

Gamma Glutamyl Transferase (GGT) *Serum Increase* Increased when there is involvement of the biliary tract or active inflammation. *2467* *2010*

Glucagon *Plasma Decrease* Decreased. *0306* *0620* *0513*

Glucose *Serum Increase* Some cases. *2467* Increased circulating epinephrine. *0619* In 27% of 11 patients at initial hospitalization for this disorder. *0781*

Pleural Effusion Decrease Usually decreased in an exudate. *0062*

Glucose Tolerance *Serum Decrease* There will be a diabetic oral test in 65% of patients and frank diabetes in > 10% of patients. *2467* Of 50 patients with chronic relapsing pancreatitis, 66% had evidence of glucose intolerance. *0962*

Isocitrate Dehydrogenase *Serum Normal* *2260*

Lactate Dehydrogenase *Pleural Effusion Increase* Exudate. *0062*

Leukocytes *Blood Increase* In 27% of 11 patients at initial hospitalization for this disorder. *0781*

Pleural Effusion Increase 5000-20,000/μL. *2017*

Ascitic Fluid Normal Variable *2626*

Lipase *Serum Increase* As functioning tissue is destroyed, it is not uncommon to find only normal levels. *2238*

Serum Normal As functioning tissue is destroyed, it is not uncommon to find only normal levels. *2238*

Lipids *Serum Increase* *0619*

Feces Increase Reduced intraluminal pancreatic enzyme activity with maldigestion of lipid and protein. *0962*

Magnesium *Serum Decrease* May occur. *2444*

Neutrophils *Blood Increase* In 36% of 11 patients at initial hospitalization for this disorder. *0781*

Pleural Effusion Increase Predominant cell type. *2017* Neutrophils predominate in pleural fluid *1403*

Nitrogen *Feces Increase* *0619*

Occult Blood *Feces Positive* *2199*

pH *Pleural Effusion Decrease* Exudate (pH < 7.3). *0062*

Phospholipids, Total *Serum Increase* Increase in cholesterol, phospholipids and neutral fats. *0619*

Platelet Count *Blood Increase* *2467*

Protein *Pleural Effusion Increase* Exudate (> 3 g/dL). *0062*

Ascitic Fluid Increase Variable but often > 2.5 g/dL in ascitic fluid. *2626*

Feces Increase Reduced intraluminal pancreatic enzyme activity with maldigestion of lipid and protein. *0962*

Peritoneal Fluid Increase Greater than 30 g/L in 70% of cases of pancreatic ascites. *0586*

Sodium *Sweat Increase* Concentrations exceeded 90 mmol/L in 26% and 120 mmol/L in 6% of noncalcific pancreatitis patients. *0111*

Specific Gravity *Pleural Effusion Increase* Exudate (> 1.016). *0062*

Triglycerides *Serum Increase* Increase in cholesterol, phospholipids, and neutral fats. *0619*

Triolein ^{131}I Test *Feces Positive* Abnormal in 33% of patients. *2467*

Trypsin *Serum Increase* Mean circulatory concentration in 16 cases was 433 U/L. Normal < 100 U/L. *1678*

Vitamin A *Serum Decrease* Some cases. *0619*

Xylose Tolerance Test *Urine Abnormal* With malabsorption. *2238*

577.20 Pancreatic Cyst and Pseudocyst

Alkaline Phosphatase *Serum Increase* Increased in 10% of patients. *2467*

Amylase *Serum Increase* Laboratory findings preceding acute pancreatitis are present (mild and unrecognized in 33% of cases). Persistent increase after an acute episode may indicate formation of a pseudocyst. *2467* Persistent increase 4-6 weeks following onset of pancreatitis suggests pseudocyst. 77% of 78 patients had hyperamylasemia at diagnosis. *2031 0581*

Urine Increase Persistent increase 4-6 weeks after onset of pancreatitis suggests pseudocyst. Hyperamylasuria is usual but not invariable. *2031*

Pleural Effusion Increase 2017

Ascitic Fluid Increase Greatly increased in pancreatic ascites. *2199*

Bicarbonate *Duodenal Contents Decrease* Duodenal contents after secretin-pancreozymin stimulation usually show decreased bicarbonate content (< 70 mmol/L) but normal volume and normal content of amylase, lipase, and trypsin. *2467*

Bilirubin *Serum Increase* Serum direct bilirubin is increased (> 2 mg/dL) in 10% of patients. *2467* Occasionally elevated. *0433*

Bilirubin, Direct *Serum Increase* Increased (> 2 mg/dL) in 10% of patients. *2467*

Glucose *Serum Increase* Occasionally there is an associated elevation of the fasting blood sugar level. *0433*

Pleural Effusion Normal Pleural Fluid = Serum level. *2017*

Leukocytes *Pleural Effusion Increase* 5000-20,000/μL. *2017*

Lipase *Serum Increase* Laboratory findings preceding acute pancreatitis are present (this is mild and unrecognized in 33% of the cases). Persistent increase of serum amylase and lipase after an acute episode may indicate formation of a pseudocyst. *2467* May be elevated after recent attack of pancreatitis in pseudocyst. *0433*

Duodenal Contents Normal Duodenal contents after secretin-pancreozymin stimulation usually show decreased bicarbonate content (< 80 mmol/L) but normal volume and normal content of amylase, lipase, and trypsin. *2467*

pH *Pleural Effusion Decrease* Exudate (pH < 7.3). *0062*

Protein *Pleural Effusion Increase* Exudate. *2017*

Specific Gravity *Pleural Effusion Increase* Exudate (> 1.016). *0062*

Trypsin *Duodenal Contents Normal* Duodenal contents after secretin-pancreozymin stimulation usually show decreased bicarbonate content (< 80 mmol/L) but normal volume and normal content of amylase, lipase, and trypsin. *2467*

Volume *Duodenal Contents Normal* Duodenal contents after secretin-pancreozymin stimulation usually show decreased bicarbonate content (< 80 mmol/L) but normal volume and normal content of amylase, lipase, and trypsin. *2467*

579.00 Celiac Sprue Disease

5-Hydroxyindoleacetic Acid (5-HIAA) *Urine Increase* Abnormal tryptophan metabolism may result in elevated urinary excretion in patients with malabsorption. *2199* Slightly increased level (12-16 mg/24h). *0995*

17-Hydroxycorticosteroids *Urine Decrease* In patients with sufficient malabsorption to cause pituitary or adrenal insufficiency. *2540*

17-Ketosteroids *Urine Decrease* In patients with sufficient malabsorption to cause pituitary or adrenal insufficiency. *2540*

25-Hydroxy Vitamin D$_3$ *Serum Decrease 2238*

Albumin *Serum Decrease* Reflects possible malabsorption of protein or protein-losing enteropathy. *0962* May be diminished owing to excessive leakage of serum protein into the gut lumen. *2199*

Alkaline Phosphatase *Serum Increase* Leading to secondary osteomalacia. *0619* Suggestive of secondary hyperparathyroidism. *0433*

Amino Acids *Plasma Increase* Found in celiac disease and idiopathic steatorrhea if liver damage is also present. *0619*

Antibody Titer *Serum Increase* Antibodies to Reticulin found in 78% of cases. *1670*

Ascorbic Acid *Serum Normal 2238*

Bicarbonate *Serum Decrease* If diarrhea is severe, marked electrolyte depletion. *2199*

Feces Increase In occasional patients, significant metabolic acidosis can develop in association with bicarbonate loss in the stool. *2199*

Calcium *Serum Decrease* An indication of vitamin D and calcium malabsorption. *0962* Often decreased in patients with diarrhea and steatorrhea. *2199* In 50% of untreated patients, concentration may be less than 9 mg/dL. *2238*

Urine Decrease 2467

Feces Increase In steatorrhea. *0619*

Carcinoembryonic Antigen *Serum Increase* In adult celiac disease, 2 of 9 patients had concentrations > 12.5 ng/mL (normal < 12.5 ng/mL). *0253*

Carotene *Serum Decrease* At the time of the initial diagnosis, most patients have steatorrhea, low serum carotene levels, abnormal d-xylose absorption, and an abnormal small bowel x-ray pattern. *0999* A useful indication of fat malabsorption low levels are found in as many as 80% of patients with steatorrhea. *0962* Usually depressed in patients with sufficient intestinal involvement to produce steatorrhea. *2199 0433*

Ceruloplasmin *Serum Decrease* Moderate transient deficiencies in patients with nephrosis. *2467*

Chloride *Serum Decrease* If diarrhea is severe, marked electrolyte depletion. *2199*

Cholesterol *Serum Decrease* Malnutrition due to malabsorption. *0619* Usually depressed in patients with sufficient intestinal involvement to produce steatorrhea. *2199*

Complement C3 *Serum Decrease* Found in 28% of patients. *1614*

Copper *Serum Decrease* Plasma zinc and copper depression was found in 10 adult patients. These findings further indicate that trace metal deficiency is another common nutritional complication. *2225* Decreased in sprue and celiac disease in infants as a result of the inability to synthesize the apoprotein. *0619*

Fat *Feces Increase* Due to allergy to gluten (wheat protein). *0619* If the coefficient of fat absorption is < 93%, steatorrhea is present. *2199* In small intestinal disease. *2199*

Ferritin *Serum Decrease* The most discriminating test to distinguish between untreated celiac disease and other gastrointestinal disorders in the pediatric age group. *2229*

Folate *Serum Decrease* Patients may show a megaloblastic anemia and leukopenia secondary to folic acid or vitamin B$_{12}$ deficiency. In these instances low serum folate and B$_{12}$ levels will be found. *0433* Folic acid deficiency occurring in idiopathic steatorrhea (up to 80 mg/h). *2467 0151*

Globulin *Serum Decrease* May be diminished owing to excessive leakage of serum protein into the gut lumen. *2199*

Glucose Tolerance *Serum Increase* Flat curve in celiac disease and diseases of intestinal wall and in monosaccharide malabsorption. *0151*

Growth Hormone *Serum Decrease* Insulin-induced growth hormone is inadequate in most cases during the active phase, but returns to normal on recovery provided the diet is gluten-free. *2415*

Hematocrit *Blood Decrease* Characteristic iron-deficiency anemia. The peripheral blood smear may show hypochromia. In some cases iron-deficiency anemia may be the predominant abnormality indicative of malabsorption. *0433*

Hemoglobin *Blood Decrease* Characteristic iron-deficiency anemia. The peripheral blood smear may show hypochromia. In some cases iron-deficiency anemia may be the predominant abnormality indicative of malabsorption. *0433*

HLA Antigens *Blood Present* HLA-B8 and DRw3 are found. *0793* HLA-DR3 found in 96% of patients versus 27% of controls. *2539*

Immunoglobulin IgA *Serum Increase* May be increased. *2238*

Immunoglobulin IgM *Serum Decrease* Reported low in 37% of patients. *2238*

Indican *Urine Increase 0995*

Iron *Serum Decrease* Characteristic iron-deficiency anemia. In some cases, may be the predominant abnormality indicative of malabsorption. *0433* Very common, because the duodenal lesion usually impairs iron absorption in the untreated patient. *2199*

Iron-Binding Capacity, Total (TIBC) *Serum Increase* Characteristic iron deficiency anemia. *0433*

Iron Saturation *Serum Decrease* Characteristic iron deficiency anemia. *0433*

Leukocytes *Blood Decrease* Patients may show a megaloblastic anemia and leukopenia secondary to folic acid or vitamin B$_{12}$ deficiency. In these instances low serum folate and B$_{12}$ levels will be found. *0433* Uncommon but may occur if severe folate or vitamin B$_{12}$ deficiency is present. *2199*

579.00 Celiac Sprue Disease *(continued)*

Lymphocytes *Blood   Decrease*   Often an absolute lymphopenia due to loss of lymphocytes into the small intestine. *0962*   Uncommon but may occur if severe folate or vitamin B_{12} deficiency is present. *2199*

Magnesium *Serum   Decrease*   May occur. *2444*   Often low. 10% of untreated patients may have levels < 1 mmol/L and may have symptoms from the deficiency. *2238   2199*

MCH *Blood   Decrease*   Characteristic iron deficiency anemia. The peripheral blood smear may show hypochromia. In some cases iron deficiency anemia may be the predominant abnormality indicative of malabsorption. *0433*

MCHC *Blood   Decrease*   Characteristic iron deficiency anemia. The peripheral blood smear may show hypochromia. In some cases iron deficiency anemia may be the predominant abnormality indicative of malabsorption. *0433*

MCV *Blood   Decrease*   Characteristic of iron-deficiency anemia the peripheral blood smear may show microcytosis. In some cases iron-deficiency anemia may be the predominant abnormality indicative of malabsorption. *0433*

Blood   Increase   Macrocytic anemia may occur due to vitamin B_{12} or folate deficiency. MCV > 100 fL. *0532*

Monocytes *Blood   Increase*   *2538*

Nitrogen *Feces   Increase*   *0619*

Oxalate *Urine   Increase*   6 of 9 children with untreated disease had hyperoxaluria. *1726*

Parathyroid Hormone *Serum   Increase*   Malabsorption of calcium results in increased parathyroid hormone production and renal tubular reabsorption of phosphate decreases, leading to mild hypophosphatemia. *1287*

Phosphate *Serum   Decrease*   Low vitamin D absorption from small bowel. *0619*   Malabsorption of calcium results in increased parathyroid hormone production and renal tubular reabsorption of phosphate decreases, leading to mild hypophosphatemia. *1287   1115*

Urine   Increase   Malabsorption of calcium results in increased parathyroid hormone production and renal tubular reabsorption of phosphate decreases, leading to mild hypophosphatemia. *1287*

Platelet Count *Blood   Increase*   May be present and may reflect splenic atrophy. *2199*

Potassium *Serum   Decrease*   If diarrhea is severe, marked electrolyte depletion. *2199*

Protein *Serum   Decrease*   Defective amino acid absorption might contribute to the observed reduction in serum protein levels. *2199*   Enteric loss of plasma protein. *2199*

Prothrombin Time *Plasma   Increase*   An indication of vitamin K malabsorption. *0962*   May be prolonged in celiac sprue owing to malabsorption of vitamin K. *2199*

Pseudocholinesterase *Serum   Decrease*   May be decreased in some cases of malnutrition in which albumin is decreased. *2467*

Pyridoxine *Serum   Decrease*   Lack of B_6 results in failure to metabolize tryptophan and high concentrations of tryptophan metabolites. *2104*

Sodium *Serum   Decrease*   If diarrhea is severe, marked electrolyte depletion. *2199*

Thyroxine Binding Globulin *Serum   Decrease*   Decreased in hypoproteinemia. *2467*

Thyroxine (T$_4$) *Serum   Decrease*   Decreased in hypoproteinemia. *2467   2415*

Tri-iodothyronine (T$_3$) *Serum   Decrease*   *2415*

Triolein ^{131}I Test *Feces   Positive*   Positive test for lipid droplets in the stool, but results are inconsistent. *0962*

Urea Nitrogen *Serum   Decrease*   Impaired protein absorption. *2467*

Uric Acid *Serum   Decrease*   Slight. *2467*

Serum   Increase   *0962*

Vitamin A *Serum   Decrease*   Due to faulty fat absorption. *0619   0433*

Vitamin B$_{12}$ *Serum   Decrease*   Patients may show a megaloblastic anemia and leukopenia secondary to folic acid or vitamin B_{12} deficiency. Malabsorption. *2467*   If severe ileal disease is present, vitamin B_{12} absorption is abnormally low both with and without added intrinsic factor. *2199   0433 2538*

Vitamin E (Tocopherol) *Serum   Decrease*   Decreased. *2053*

Vitamin K *Serum   Decrease*   Due to malabsorption. *2538*

Xylose Tolerance Test *Urine   Abnormal*   The 1 h value was found to be more reliable than was fecal fat analysis in screening children for celiac disease. *0325*   One h after 5 g xylose, the blood-xylose is 20 mg/dL or more in treated disease or in cases other than celiac disease. In untreated disease, the 1 h blood-xylose is < 20 mg/dL. *0619*   Usually found at the time of initial diagnosis. *0999   2199*

Zinc *Serum   Decrease*   Depression of plasma zinc and lowered taste discrimination were observed in untreated patients. With confirmation of plasma copper depression indicates that trace metal deficiency is a common nutritional complication of adult celiac disease. *2225*

579.01 Protein-Losing Enteropathy

Albumin *Serum   Decrease*   Excessive enteric loss usually leads to the development of edema. *2104*

Alpha$_1$-Globulin *Serum   Increase*   In protein-losing enteropathy. *2467*

Alpha$_2$-Globulin *Serum   Increase*   In protein-losing enteropathy. *2467*

Calcium *Serum   Decrease*   *0503 2467*

Complement C2 *Serum   Decrease*   *1732*

Eosinophils *Blood   Increase*   Occasional eosinophilia. *2467*

Factor B *Plasma   Decrease*   *1979 2356*

Globulin *Serum   Decrease*   In protein-losing enteropathies. *2467*

Hematocrit *Blood   Decrease*   There may be a moderate anemia. *0433*

Hemoglobin *Blood   Decrease*   There may be a moderate anemia. *0433   2467*

Immunoglobulin IgG *Serum   Decrease*   *0503*

Thyroxine Binding Globulin *Serum   Decrease*   Decreased in nephrosis and other causes of marked hypoproteinemia. *2467   2104*

Thyroxine (T$_4$) *Serum   Decrease*   Decreased T$_4$ with hypoproteinemia. *2467*

579.90 Malabsorption, Cause Unspecified

25-Hydroxy Vitamin D$_3$ *Serum   Decrease*   66% of patients with malabsorption had low (< 21 ng/mL) serum concentrations. Only 1 of 31 patients had a value > 21 ng/mL and 20 had assays < 12 ng/mL. *2077*

Albumin *Serum   Decrease*   Marked hypoproteinemia. *0433*   Decreased in malabsorption syndrome. *0151   0962*

Alkaline Phosphatase *Serum   Increase*   An indication of vitamin D and calcium malabsorption. *0962   0151*

Alpha$_1$-Antichymotrypsin *Duodenal Contents   Increase*   Concentration in duodenal juice from children with malabsorption disease is elevated relative to children with pancreatic insufficiency. *1248*

Alpha$_1$-Antitrypsin *Serum   Decrease*   These conditions reduce activity. *2633*

Amino Acids *Plasma   Increase*   *0619*

Amylase *Serum   Increase*   Increased in chronic malabsorption with intestinal villous atrophy. *0619*

Ascorbic Acid *Serum   Decrease*   In steatorrhea. *0211*

Bicarbonate *Serum   Decrease*   Normal or decreased. *2467*

Calcium *Serum   Decrease*   Decreased in hypoproteinemia. *0503*   Particularly in small bowel disease. *0151*   An indication of vitamin D and calcium malabsorption. *0962*

Feces   Increase   In diarrheas of all sorts, but especially steatorrheas, large fecal calcium losses occur. One patient with steatorrhea (nontropical sprue) was observed to excrete all ingested calcium plus the amount calculated to have been derived from 8 liters of intestinal juices which are normally excreted into the tract, a deficit amounting to 500 mg of calcium daily. *1083*

Carotene *Serum   Decrease*   Decreased in malabsorption syndrome. *0151*   A useful indication of fat malabsorption low levels are found in as many as 80% of patients with steatorrhea. *0962*

Chloride *Serum   Normal*   *2467*

Cholesterol *Serum   Decrease*   Decreased in malabsorption syndrome. *0151*

Chymotrypsin *Feces   Decrease*   Found to be a more reliable measure of pancreatic function than trypsin activity. False-positives have been noted in 10% of controls, and normal values may occur in patients. *0052*

Complement C2   *Serum   Decrease*   {793} {2522}

Erythrocytes   *Blood   Decrease*   0151

Factor II   *Plasma   Decrease*   Malabsorption of fat-soluble vitamin K results in hypoprothrombinemia. 0151

Fat   *Feces   Increase*   In malabsorption syndrome. 0151   The number and size of fecal fat globules correlates with the degree of steatorrhea. 0600

Folate   *Serum   Decrease*   Particularly in small bowel disease. 0151   Macrocytic anemia may occur due to vitamin B$_{12}$ or folate deficiency. MCV > 100 fL. 0532

Glucose Tolerance   *Serum   Increase*   Flat curve in celiac disease and diseases of intestinal wall and in monosaccharide malabsorption. 0151

Hematocrit   *Blood   Decrease*   There may be moderate anemia in idiopathic hypoproteinemia. 0433

Hemoglobin   *Blood   Decrease*   Mild anemia. 0433

Indican   *Urine   Increase*   Found in several malabsorptive states as well as bacterial overgrowth. 0995

Iron   *Serum   Decrease*   0151

Iron-Binding Capacity, Total (TIBC)   *Serum   Increase*   0151

Magnesium   *Serum   Decrease*   Hypomagnesemia may occur. 2444   0151

MCH   *Blood   Decrease*   Microcytic hypochromic anemia may occur due to blood loss, increased demand or dietary inadequacy. MCH < 27 pg, MCV < 80 fL. 0532

MCV   *Blood   Decrease*   Microcytic hypochromic anemia may occur due to blood loss, increased demand or dietary inadequacy. MCH < 27 pg, MCV < 80 fL. 0532

Blood   Increase   Macrocytic anemia may occur due to vitamin B$_{12}$ or folate deficiency. MCV > 100 fL. 0532

Oxalate   *Urine   Increase*   0186

Parathyroid Hormone   *Serum   Increase*   Malabsorption of calcium results in increased parathyroid hormone production and renal tubular reabsorption of phosphate decreases, leading to mild hypophosphatemia. 1287

pH   *Urine   Decrease*   Normal or decreased. 2467

Phosphate   *Serum   Decrease*   Malabsorption of calcium results in increased parathyroid hormone production and renal tubular reabsorption of phosphate decreases, leading to mild hypophosphatemia. 1287   An indication of vitamin D and calcium malabsorption. 0962

Urine   Increase   Malabsorption of calcium results in increased parathyroid hormone production and renal tubular reabsorption of phosphate decreases, leading to mild hypophosphatemia. 1287

Potassium   *Serum   Decrease*   0151

Urine   Decrease   2467

Protein   *Serum   Decrease*   0186

Prothrombin Time   *Plasma   Increase*   An indication of vitamin K malabsorption. 0962

Pseudocholinesterase   *Serum   Decrease*   May be decreased in some cases of malnutrition in which albumin is decreased. 2467

Sodium   *Serum   Decrease*   2467 0151

Urine   Decrease   2467

Thyroxine Binding Globulin   *Serum   Decrease*   Decreased with hypoproteinemia. 2467

Thyroxine (T$_4$)   *Serum   Decrease*   Decreased with hypoproteinemia. 2467

Triolein ^{131}I Test   *Feces   Positive*   Positive test for lipid droplets in the stool, results are inconsistent. 0962

Vitamin B$_{12}$ *Serum   Decrease*   Particularly in tropical sprue and bacterial overgrowth. 0151

Vitamin B$_{12}$ Binding Capacity   *Serum   Decrease*   0151

Vitamin K   *Serum   Decrease*   Deficiency and resulting bleeding tendency is to be expected with fat malabsorption. 2104

Volume   *Plasma   Decrease*   0151

Urine   Normal   2467

Feces   Increase   Unabsorbed fats and fatty acids cause stools to be bulky and voluminous. 0151

Xylose Tolerance Test   *Urine   Abnormal*   0995

Zinc   *Serum   Decrease*   Decreased. 2297

DISEASES OF THE GENITOURINARY SYSTEM

580.00   Acute Poststreptococcal Glomerulonephritis

^{131}I Uptake   *Serum   Decrease*   In renal disease. 2104

Alanine Aminotransferase   *Urine   Increase*   Increased. 1807 1199 2534

Albumin   *Serum   Decrease*   May be low as a result of urinary loss and excessive catabolism of protein. 0995

Urine   Increase   Common although it rarely exceeds 3 g/24h. 0433   Usually occurs, with size of proteins indicating degree of glomerular damage. Albumin is nearly always present. 2545   0995

Aldosterone   *Plasma   Increase*   The decreased GFR and increased aldosterone secretion lead to retention of sodium and water with resultant hypervolemia. 1108

Urine   Decrease   Occurs in the presence of edema in children. 2468

Urine   Increase   The decreased GFR and increased aldosterone secretion lead to retention of sodium and water with resultant hypervolemia. 1108

Alkaline Phosphatase   *Urine   Increase*   0619

Alpha$_1$-Antitrypsin   *Serum   Normal*   2467

Alpha$_1$-Globulin   *Serum   Increase*   Moderate increase. 0619

Alpha$_2$-Globulin   *Serum   Increase*   There is a moderate increase appearing in the early stages. 0619

Alpha$_2$-Macroglobulin   *Serum   Increase*   2632

Ammonia   *Urine   Decrease*   Decreased in nephritis with damage to the distal renal tubules. 0619

Antistreptolysin O   *Serum   Increase*   Usually raised indicating recent streptococcal infection but may fall rapidly with the use of antimicrobials. 0151   Titer usually exhibits a rise some time during the course of the disease and may be the only evidence of antecedent beta-hemolytic streptococcal infection. 0999

Arylsulfatase   *Serum   Increase*   30-50% increase in activity. 0610

Beta-Glucuronidase   *Urine   Increase*   31 of 38 patients with active disease had elevated activities, with a mean value of 70.0 ± 50.4. Of the 38 patients with inactive glomerulonephritis, 17 had elevated activities. 1525

Bicarbonate   *Serum   Decrease*   Metabolic acidosis. 0062

Calcium   *Urine   Decrease*   Decreased excretion in acute nephritis, partly due to decreased intestinal absorption. 0619

Cells   *Urine   Increase*   36% renal epithelial cells were found in tubular nephrosis (necrosis) and in glomerulonephritis. 1411   Granular and epithelial cell casts are found. 2468

Ceruloplasmin   *Serum   Increase*   1064

Chloride   *Serum   Decrease*   Seen in azotemic or oliguric patients. 0062

Cholesterol   *Serum   Increase*   Sometimes elevated even when serum albumin is not greatly decreased. 0995

Complement C1q   *Serum   Decrease*   Particularly during diuretic phase. 0062

Complement C3   *Serum   Decrease*   Persistently low with C3 conversion products and normal C4. 2522

Serum   Increase   Particularly during diuretic phase. 0062

Complement C4   *Serum   Decrease*   Usually less than that of C3. 0277

Serum   Normal   C3 was persistently low with C3 conversion products and normal C4. 2522

Complement, Total   *Serum   Decrease*   Marked reduction coincident with development of nephritis. 0151

Copper   *Serum   Increase*   1064

Creatinine   *Serum   Increase*   Mild renal failure with plasma values of 1.5-4.0 mg/dL is very common in the initial stages. 0151   0999

Cryomacroglobulins   *Serum   Increase*   0863

Eosinophils   *Blood   Increase*   Occasionally. 2538

Erythrocyte Casts   *Urine   Increase*   Microscopic examination reveals numerous red blood cells and variable numbers of casts. Indicate bleeding from the glomerulus. 0151   0999

Erythrocytes   *Urine   Increase*   Hematuria, gross or only microscopic. May occur during the initial febrile upper respiratory infection then reappear with nephritis in 1-2 weeks. It lasts 2-12; usual duration is 2 months. 2468   Hematuria usually occurs in conjunction with proteinuria, but may occur alone in some cases. 2545   0151

580.00   Acute Poststreptococcal Glomerulonephritis
(continued)

Erythrocyte Sedimentation Rate   *Blood   Increase*   Usually moderately raised. *0151*

Factor VIII   *Plasma   Increase*   Patients who made a complete recovery upon 4 year follow-up had normal initial values, while those who developed persistent renal damage had high factor VIII values. Other coagulation factors are of no prognostic significance. *0642*

Fatty Casts   *Urine   Increase*   May appear within the first few weeks. *0995*

Fibrin Split Products (FSP)   *Plasma   Increase*   Increased (> 10 μg/mL) in 28% of acute cases. Mean value was 8.4 $\pm$ 5.6 μg/mL (Normal = 3.2 $\pm$ 1.2 μg/mL). *1325*   Raised serum or urine levels are common without other evidence of enhanced fibrinolysis. *1253*

Urine   Increase   Raised serum or urine levels are common without other evidence of enhanced fibrinolysis. *1253*

Globulin   *Serum   Increase*   *2104*

Glomerular Filtration Rate (GFR)   *Urine   Decrease*   The decreased GFR and increased aldosterone secretion lead to retention of sodium and water with resultant hypervolemia. *1108*

Glucose   *Urine   Increase*   Occasional glycosuria occurs. *0151*

Granular Casts   *Urine   Increase*   Usually present. *0151*

Haptoglobin   *Serum   Normal*   *2467*

Hematocrit   *Blood   Decrease*   Dilutional anemia. *1108*   Normocytic, normochromic anemia occurs as a result of hemodilution. *0433*

Hemoglobin   *Blood   Decrease*   Anemia is usually present, its severity varying directly with the severity of the azotemia. *0999* Slightly reduced to 11-12 g/dL as a result of dilution. *0151   1108*

Hemoglobin Casts   *Urine   Increase*   Indicate bleeding from the glomerulus. *0151*

Hexosaminidase   *Urine   Increase*   Decreased levels in urine. *2356*

Lactate Dehydrogenase   *Urine   Increase*   *2468*

Leukocytes   *Blood   Increase*   Increased neutrophils in children. *2468*

Urine   Increase   Large numbers of red and white cells are found. *0151*

Lipids   *Urine   Increase*   Lipid droplets may appear within the first few weeks. *0995*

Lipoproteins   *Serum   Increase*   More than 50% of the patients with glomerulonephritis, nephrotic syndrome and renovascular hypertension showed obviously abnormal lipoprotein profiles, which returned to normal or near-normal when the disease was ameliorated or corrected surgically. *2446*

Magnesium   *Serum   Decrease*   Majority of cases showed a fall in both serum and urinary levels, associated with hypoproteinemia and hypoalbuminemia. *1772*   Hypomagnesemia may occur in some cases. *2444*

Urine   Decrease   Majority of cases showed a fall in both serum and urinary levels, associated with hypoproteinemia and hypoalbuminemia. *1772*

Neutrophils   *Blood   Increase*   *2538*

Urine   Increase   In interstitial nephritis and nephrosclerosis patients, the percentage of polymorphonuclear granulocytes was 76-85%. *1411*

pH   *Urine   Decrease*   May occur early in the course of the illness. *0995*

Potassium   *Urine   Decrease*   *0619*

Protein   *Serum   Decrease*   Occasionally lowered with reversed A/G ratio. *0999*

Urine   Increase   Usually occurs, with size of proteins indicating degree of glomerular damage. Albumin is nearly always present. *2545*   May reach over 6-8 g/24h, but is more often below 2 g/24h. *2468   0999*

Pleural Effusion   Decrease   Pleural effusions are usually transudates (< 3 g/dL). *0062*

Sodium   *Serum   Decrease*   The decreased GFR and increased aldosterone secretion lead to retention of sodium and water with resultant hypervolemia. *1108*

Urine   Decrease   Very low (< 15 mmol/L). *0995*   Reflects avid salt reabsorption in the distal nephron. *0062*

Specific Gravity   *Urine   Increase*   May occur early in the course of the illness. *0995*

Tryptophan   *Serum   Increase*   Tyrosine and tryptophan usually rise in acute and chronic glomerulonephritis. *2104*

Tyrosine   *Serum   Increase*   Tyrosine and tryptophan usually rise in acute and chronic glomerulonephritis. *2104*

Urea Nitrogen   *Serum   Increase*   All fractions of nonprotein nitrogen increase. *0812*   Elevated in 50% of patients. *0995*

Volume   *Plasma   Increase*   Plasma volume may be as much as 50% above normal during edematous phase. *1669*   The decreased GFR and increased aldosterone secretion lead to retention of sodium and water with resultant hypervolemia. *1108*

Urine   Decrease   The disease is sometimes ushered in by oliguria which may progress to complete anuria. *0995   0619*

580.01   Glomerulonephritis (Focal)

Alanine Aminotransferase   *Urine   Increase*   Increased. *1807 1199 2534*

Albumin   *Urine   Increase*   Noted to have slight but persistent proteinuria. *0433*

Alpha$_2$-Macroglobulin   *Serum   Increase*   *2632*

Amino Acids   *Plasma   Decrease*   Mean concentration of essential amino acids and tyrosine were significantly lower, resulting in a low essential/total ratio. *1545*

Urine   Increase   May be found. *0951*

Antistreptolysin O   *Serum   Increase*   Above normal titers may occur. *1752*

Calcium   *Serum   Decrease*   Decreases as metabolic acidosis develops. *0962*

Ceruloplasmin   *Serum   Increase*   *1064*

Complement C3   *Serum   Normal*   *0419*

Copper   *Serum   Increase*   *1064*

Erythrocytes   *Urine   Increase*   Noted to have slight persistent proteinuria accompanied by microscopic hematuria. *0433*   Microscopic or massive hematuria. *0962*

Erythrocyte Sedimentation Rate   *Blood   Increase*   High ESR may be found in patients with abnormal plasma protein levels. *0962*

Glucose   *Urine   Increase*   May be found. *0951*

Hexosaminidase   *Urine   Increase*   Decreased levels in urine. *2356*

Immunoglobulin IgG   *Serum   Decrease*   May be significantly reduced. *0419*

Lymphocytes   *Urine   Increase*   May be found. *0951*

Osmolality   *Urine   Decrease*   Concentrating capacity is impaired, with urine specific gravity around 1.010. *0962*

Protein   *Urine   Increase*   May persist for years, even after other manifestations cease. *0962*

Pleural Effusion   Decrease   Pleural effusions are usually transudates (< 3 g/dL). *0062*

Specific Gravity   *Urine   Decrease*   Concentrating capacity is impaired, with urine specific gravity around 1.010. *0962*

Tryptophan   *Serum   Increase*   Tyrosine and tryptophan usually rise in acute and chronic glomerulonephritis. *2104*

Tyrosine   *Serum   Decrease*   Mean concentration of essential amino acids and tyrosine were significantly lower, resulting in a low essential/total ratio. *1545*

Serum   Increase   Tyrosine and tryptophan usually rise in acute and chronic glomerulonephritis. *2104*

Uric Acid   *Serum   Increase*   As functional loss becomes severe (GFR 50% of normal or less), there is usually a rise in serum phosphate and uric acid. *0962*

580.02   Glomerulonephritis (Minimal Change)

Alanine Aminotransferase   *Urine   Increase*   Increased. *1807 1199 2534*

Albumin   *Serum   Decrease*   Occurs as a result of heavy protein loss, especially low molecular weight plasma proteins such as albumin and transferrin in the urine. *0151*

Urine   Increase   Characterized by heavy proteinuria, consisting almost entirely of low molecular weight plasma proteins, especially albumin and transferrin. Values are > 5 g/24h. *0151*

Alpha$_2$-Macroglobulin   *Serum   Increase*   *2632*

Antistreptolysin O   *Serum   Increase*   Above normal titers may occur. *1752*

Ceruloplasmin   *Serum   Increase*   *1064*

Cholesterol   *Serum   Increase*   Usually occurs. *0151*

Complement C3   *Serum   Normal*   *1383*

Complement C4 *Serum Normal* *1383*

Copper *Serum Increase* *1064*

Erythrocytes *Urine Increase* Microscopic hematuria is seen in a minority of patients. *2544*

Fatty Casts *Urine Increase* Hyaline, granular, and fatty casts are found. *0151*

Granular Casts *Urine Increase* Hyaline, granular, and fatty casts are found. *0151*

Hexosaminidase *Urine Increase* Decreased levels in urine. *2356*

Hyaline Casts *Urine Increase* Hyaline, granular, and fatty casts are found. *0151 0433*

Immunoglobulin IgA *Serum Decrease* Usually normal or modestly decreased. *0419*

Immunoglobulin IgE *Serum Increase* May be increased. *0419*

Immunoglobulin IgG *Serum Decrease* May be profoundly depressed during relapse. *0419*

Immunoglobulin IgM *Serum Increase* May be increased. *0419*

Iron-Binding Capacity, Total (TIBC) *Serum Decrease* Decreased as a result of heavy protein loss to the urine, especially low molecular weight proteins, such as albumin and transferrin. *0151*

Plasma Cells *Serum Increase* Elevated *2357 0659 0683*

Protein *Urine Increase* Characterized by heavy proteinuria consisting almost entirely of low molecular weight plasma proteins, especially albumin and transferrin. Values are > 5 g/24h. *0151* Marked proteinuria - usually > 4.5 g/24h; usually exclusively albuminuria in children with lipoid nephrosis, but in glomerulonephritis high- and low-molecular weight proteins are present with nephrotic syndrome. *2468*

Pleural Effusion *Decrease* Pleural effusions are usually transudates (< 3 g/dL). *0062*

Tryptophan *Serum Increase* Tyrosine and tryptophan usually rise in acute and chronic glomerulonephritis. *2104*

Tyrosine *Serum Increase* Tyrosine and tryptophan usually rise in acute and chronic glomerulonephritis. *2104*

580.04   Glomerulonephritis (Membranous)

Alanine Aminotransferase *Urine Increase* Increased. *1807 1199 2534*

Albumin *Urine Increase* In excess of 3 g/24h is characteristic. *0433* Usually occurs, with size of proteins indicating degree of glomerular damage. *2545*

Alpha₂-Globulin *Urine Increase* *0995*

Alpha₂-Macroglobulin *Serum Increase* *2632*

Amino Acids *Plasma Decrease* Mean concentration of essential amino acids and tyrosine were significantly lower, resulting in a low essential/total ratio. *1545*

Antistreptolysin O *Serum Increase* Above normal titers may occur. *1752*

Ceruloplasmin *Serum Increase* *1064*

Cholesterol *Serum Increase* Occurs, but is less frequent than in minimal change glomerulonephritis. *0151*

Complement C3 *Serum Normal* Nearly always. *0419*

Complement C4 *Serum Normal* Nearly always. *0419*

Complement, Total *Serum Normal* Nearly always. *0419*

Copper *Serum Increase* *1064*

Creatinine Clearance *Urine Decrease* Progression of the disease is characterized by declining creatinine clearance. *0433*

Erythrocytes *Urine Increase* Gross hematuria is uncommon even though microscopic hematuria is observed in 40% of the patients. *0433* Hematuria usually occurs in conjunction with proteinuria, but may occur alone in some cases. *2545* Microscopic hematuria is common. *0332*

Factor B *Plasma Decrease* *1979 2356*

Glucose *Serum Increase* Chemical or overt diabetes appears more common than might be expected by chance. *0406*

Granular Casts *Urine Increase* Usually present. *0433*

Hexosaminidase *Urine Increase* Decreased levels in urine. *2356*

Hyaline Casts *Urine Increase* Usually present. *0433*

Protein *Serum Decrease* Proteinuria is nonselective, distinguishing it from minimal change glomerulonephritis. *0151* Usually occurs, with size of proteins indicating degree of glomerular damage. Albumin is nearly always present. *2545* Onset of disease was marked by proteinuria without nephrotic syndrome in 24.2% of patients. *1701*

Urine Increase Proteinuria is nonselective, distinguishing it from minimal change glomerulonephritis. *0151* Usually occurs, with size of proteins indicating degree of glomerular damage. Albumin is nearly always present. *2545* Onset of disease was marked by proteinuria without nephrotic syndrome in 24.2% of patients. *1701*

Pleural Effusion Decrease Pleural effusions are usually transudates (< 3 g/dL). *0062*

Tryptophan *Serum Increase* Tyrosine and tryptophan usually rise in acute and chronic glomerulonephritis. *2104*

Tyrosine *Serum Decrease* Mean concentration of essential amino acids and tyrosine were significantly lower, resulting in a low essential/total ratio. *1545*

Serum Increase Tyrosine and tryptophan usually rise in acute and chronic glomerulonephritis. *2104*

Urea Nitrogen *Serum Increase* Occurs late in course. *0419*

580.05   Glomerulonephritis (Membranoproliferative)

Alanine Aminotransferase *Urine Increase* Increased. *1807 1199 2534*

Alpha₂-Antiplasmin *Serum Normal* A slight decrease in patients with nephrotic syndrome, but a normal level in patients with chronic latent glomerulonephritis. *2312*

Alpha₂-Macroglobulin *Serum Increase* *2632*

Antistreptolysin O *Serum Increase* In about 40% of patients. *0331*

Ceruloplasmin *Serum Increase* *1064*

Chloride *Serum Increase* 16 patients with membranoproliferative glomerulonephritis had a mean value significantly higher than that in normal subjects or patients with nephrotic syndrome. *0598*

Complement C3 *Serum Decrease* Permanent depression of C3 is found in 60-80% of patients. *2468* Profound prolonged depression ascribed to anticomplementary factors. *0995* In 70% of cases. *0331*

Complement C4 *Serum Normal* *0277*

Complement, Total *Serum Decrease* Characteristic of membranoproliferative glomerulonephritis. *2545*

Copper *Serum Increase* *1064*

Creatinine *Serum Increase* BUN and creatinine rise as GFR decreases. *0962*

Erythrocytes *Urine Increase* *0331*

Erythrocyte Sedimentation Rate *Blood Decrease* Normal or low. *1017*

Erythrocyte Survival *Red Blood Cells Decrease* *0331*

Glomerular Filtration Rate (GFR) *Urine Decrease* BUN and creatinine rise as GFR decreases. *0962* In 50% of cases. *0331*

Hematocrit *Blood Decrease* Mild anemia which is normocytic and normochromic develops as azotemia occurs. *0962* In over 50% of the cases. *0331*

Hemoglobin *Blood Decrease* Mild anemia which is normocytic and normochromic develops as azotemia occurs. *0962* In over 50% of the cases. *0331*

Hexosaminidase *Urine Increase* Decreased levels in urine. *2356*

Phosphate *Serum Increase* As functional loss becomes severe (GFR 50% of normal or less), there is usually a rise in serum phosphate and uric acid. *0962*

Protein *Urine Increase* *0331*

Pleural Effusion Decrease Pleural effusions are usually transudates (< 3 g/dL). *0062*

Tryptophan *Serum Increase* Tyrosine and tryptophan usually rise in acute and chronic glomerulonephritis. *2104*

Tyrosine *Serum Increase* Tyrosine and tryptophan usually rise in acute and chronic glomerulonephritis. *2104*

Urea Nitrogen *Serum Increase* BUN and creatinine rise as GFR decreases. *0962*

580.40 Glomerulonephritis (Rapidly Progressive)

Alanine Aminotransferase *Urine Increase* Increased. *1807 1199 2534*

Albumin *Urine Increase* Usually occurs; with size of proteins indicating degree of glomerular damage. *2545*

Alpha$_2$-Macroglobulin *Serum Increase* *2632*

Antistreptolysin O *Serum Increase* May be found in 30% of patients without other evidence of streptococcal etiology. *2544*

Calcium *Serum Decrease* Decreases renal failure develops. *0962*

Casts *Urine Increase* *2545*

Ceruloplasmin *Serum Increase* *1064*

Complement C3 *Serum Normal* *1383*

Complement C4 *Serum Normal* *1383*

Complement, Total *Serum Normal* *0962 1383*

Copper *Serum Increase* *1064*

Creatinine *Serum Increase* Over 2.5 mg/dL at time of biopsy in all cases. *1633* BUN and creatinine rise as GFR decreases. *0962*

Erythrocyte Casts *Urine Increase* *2468*

Erythrocytes *Urine Increase* Hematuria usually occurs in conjunction with proteinuria, but may occur alone in some cases. *2545* Microscopic hematuria in 15 of 29 patients. *1633* Hematuria is usually microscopic, and it is a rather constant feature indicating activity. *0962*

Glomerular Filtration Rate (GFR) *Urine Decrease* BUN and creatinine rise as GFR decreases. *0962*

Hematocrit *Blood Decrease* Anemia which is normocytic and normochromic develops as azotemia occurs. *0962*

Hemoglobin *Blood Decrease* Anemia which is normocytic and normochromic develops as azotemia occurs. *0962*

Hexosaminidase *Urine Increase* Decreased levels in urine. *2356*

Leukocytes *Urine Increase* *2468*

Phosphate *Serum Increase* As functional loss becomes severe (GFR 50% of normal or less), there is usually a rise in serum phosphate and uric acid. *0962*

Platelet Count *Blood Decrease* Observed occasionally. *0277*

Protein *Urine Increase* Usually occurs; with size of proteins indicating degree of glomerular damage. Albumin is nearly always present. *2545* Exceeds 2.5 g/24h in 8 of 29 cases. *1633* Proteinuria is always present. *0962*

Specific Gravity *Urine Decrease* Concentrating capacity is impaired, with urine specific gravity around 1.010. *0962*

Tryptophan *Serum Increase* Tyrosine and tryptophan usually rise in acute and chronic glomerulonephritis. *2104*

Tyrosine *Serum Increase* Tyrosine and tryptophan usually rise in acute and chronic glomerulonephritis. *2104*

Urea Nitrogen *Serum Increase* Usually > 80 mg/dL. *2468* BUN and creatinine rise as GFR decreases. *0962*

Uric Acid *Serum Increase* As functional loss becomes severe (GFR 50% of normal or less), there is usually a rise in serum phosphate and uric acid. *0962*

Volume *Urine Decrease* Oliguria < 500 mL/24h was present in 20 of 29 cases and dialysis was required in 22. *1633*

581.90 Nephrotic Syndrome

[131]I Uptake *Serum Increase* Urinary loss of TBG results in lowering of most blood thyroid hormones and increased T$_3$ uptake. *0962 2104*

17-Hydroxycorticosteroids *Urine Decrease* *0503*

17-Ketogenic Steroids *Urine Decrease* *2467*

17-Ketosteroids *Urine Decrease* Marked decrease. *0503*

25-Hydroxy Vitamin D$_3$ *Serum Decrease* Range in 26 patients was 1-18.6 ng/mL, mean = 8.6 ± 1. Normal value = 21.8 ± 2.3 ng/mL. Values were inversely correlated with degree of proteinuria and directly related to serum albumin. *0882*

Albumin *Serum Decrease* Invariably reduced to < 3 g/dL, usually between 1-3 g/dL, with occasional values of < 0.5 g/dL in hypovolemia. *0151* Massive loss in urine results in low serum concentration despite increased synthesis. *2104 0962*

Urine Increase The principal protein found in the urine. Despite the fact that its concentration may be greatly reduced in the plasma. *0999* Massive loss in urine. *2104*

Aldosterone *Plasma Increase* Secretion is augmented in response to decreased plasma values. *0995* Excess contributes to the development of edema. *2104*

Urine Increase *2104*

Alkaline Phosphatase *Serum Increase* In 40% of 25 patients at initial hospitalization for this disorder. *0781*

Leukocyte Decrease Untreated disease. *2467*

Alpha$_1$-Antitrypsin *Serum Decrease* These conditions reduce activity. *2633*

Serum Increase Increased. *1866 0042 1946 1947 2129*

Alpha$_1$-Globulin *Serum Decrease* Normal or decreased. *2085*

Urine Increase Significant quantities are found. *0995*

Alpha$_2$-Antiplasmin *Serum Decrease* A slight decrease in patients with nephrotic syndrome, but a normal level in patients with chronic latent glomerulonephritis. *2312*

Alpha$_2$-Globulin *Serum Increase* There is an increase with poor separation from the beta globulin band. *0619* Hypoproteinemia is primarily due to a decrease in the albumin fraction and an increase in the alpha$_2$-globulin fraction. *0962 0433*

Alpha$_2$-Macroglobulin *Serum Increase* Marked elevations. *1692 0046* Elevations as high as 1.0 g/dL have been noted. *1355* Primarily due to decreased plasma values and selective retention of the high molecular weight protein. Increased synthesis may also be a factor. *2635*

Alpha-Fetoprotein *Serum Increase* Markedly raised maternal serum and amniotic fluid AFP levels were found in 2 cases of congenital nephrotic syndrome of the fetus. *2117*

Amino Acids *Plasma Decrease* *0619*

Antidiuretic Hormone *Serum Decrease* *0619*

Antithrombin III *Plasma Decrease* In infants this has been suggested to explain hypercoagulability. *1437 2353 1482* Greatly reduced concentration and activity. *2420*

Apolipoprotein AI *Serum Decrease* Untreated uncomplicated nephrotic syndrome is characterized by increased low (beta) and very low (prebeta) density lipoproteins and a diminution of high density (alpha) lipoprotein. Changes correlated strictly with albumin concentrat were more pronounced with albumin concentration < 20 g/L. *0833* In severe, fully developed cases, increase in low density lipoproteins with normal or decreased alpha lipoproteins has been described. *0962*

Basophils *Blood Increase* Some cases. *2467*

Beta$_2$-Macroglobulin *Serum Decrease* An increase in urine and a decrease in serum levels is seen. *1236 2220*

Urine Increase An increase in urine and a decrease in serum levels is seen. *1236*

Beta-Globulin *Serum Increase* There is a marked increase with incomplete separation from the alpha$_2$ fraction. *0619*

Urine Increase Significant quantities are found. *0995*

Beta-Glucuronidase *Urine Increase* 8 of 13 patients had activities > 30 U/L, mean for the entire group was 44.3 ± 25.3. *1525*

Butanol Extractable Iodine (BEI) *Serum Decrease* Urinary loss of TBG results in lowering of most blood thyroid hormones and increased T$_3$ uptake. *0962*

Calcium *Serum Decrease* Reduced proportionately to the fall in albumin concentration in the early stages with true hypocalcemia evident later in the disease. *1523* In 12 patients with nephrotic syndrome and 14 nephrotic patients during clinical remission, mean ionized calcium = 1.08 ± 0.10 and 1.21 ± 0.10 mmol/L ultrafiltrate respectively, significantly lower than the normal mean (1.28 ± 0.06 mmol/L). *1408* In 76% of 25 patients at initial hospitalization for this disorder. *0781*

Urine Decrease Low urinary excretion is common. *1523*

Feces Increase May be high indicating intestinal absorption. *1523*

Casts *Urine Increase* Sediment may be abnormal early in the disease before clinical signs of the syndrome become manifest, characterized by hyaline, granular, and waxy casts and plain casts with inclusions of RBC, WBC, tubular cells, and refractile fat bodies. *0962*

Ceruloplasmin *Serum Decrease* Found regularly with hypoproteinemia. *0350* Moderate transient deficiencies *2467*

Cholesterol *Serum Decrease* Normal or low cholesterol suggests poor nutrition and suggests a poor prognosis. *0186*

Serum Increase Typically elevated. *0962* In 50% of 14 patients at initial hospitalization for this disorder. *0781*

Cholesterol, High Density Lipoprotein *Serum Decrease* Decreased. *0131 1519 2556*

Cholesterol, Low Density Lipoprotein *Serum Increase* Marked elevation secondary to direct secretion by liver and decrease catabolism. *0062*

Cholesterol, Very Low Density Lipoprotein *Serum Increase* Marked elevation with uremia. *0062*

Chylomicrons *Serum Increase* Increased. *1380 1936 1948*

Copper *Serum Decrease* Found regularly with hypoproteinemia. *0350*

Creatinine *Serum Increase* In 48% of 24 patients at initial hospitalization for this disorder. *0781*

Eosinophils *Blood Increase* In 42% of 26 patients at initial hospitalization for this disorder. *0781*

Erythrocytes *Urine Increase* Microscopic hematuria is present in 33% of cases but casts are rare and there is no evidence of prior streptococcal infection. *0999*

Ascitic Fluid Increase > 10,000 cells/μL is unusual. *2626*

Erythrocyte Sedimentation Rate *Blood Increase* Due to increased fibrinogen. *0186*

Factor V *Plasma Increase* May occur. *2322*

Factor VII *Plasma Increase* May occur. *2322*

Factor VIII *Plasma Increase* May occur. *2322*

Factor X *Plasma Increase* May occur. *2322*

Factor XI *Plasma Decrease* In part due to excessive urinary loss. *2352*

Factor XII *Plasma Decrease* In part due to excessive urinary loss. *2352*

Fatty Casts *Urine Increase* *0433*

Fibrinogen *Plasma Increase* Plasma clotting factors, especially fibrinogen, have been elevated in many patients and returned to normal when remission was induced by adrenal corticosteroids. *1108 1396 2322*

Fibrinopeptide A *Plasma Increase* Marked increase. *0996*

Fibrin Split Products (FSP) *Urine Increase* The greater the degree of proteinuria the greater the level of fibrinogen degradation product in the urine. *0365*

Gamma Glutamyl Transferase (GGT) *Serum Increase* *1739*

Globulin *Serum Decrease* *2468*

Urine Increase Significant quantities are found. *0995*

Glomerular Filtration Rate (GFR) *Urine Decrease* Increased total body sodium and water occurs as a result of reduced GFR and causes the characteristic edema. *0151*

Haptoglobin *Serum Increase* Conditions associated with increased ESR and alpha$_2$-globulin. *2467*

Hemoglobin A$_{1C}$ *Blood Increase* *2539*

Immunoglobulin IgA *Serum Decrease* *2467*

Serum Increase Usually normal or elevated. *0419*

Immunoglobulin IgE *Serum Increase* Usually normal or elevated. *0419*

Immunoglobulin IgG *Serum Decrease* Higher IgM and lower IgG serum concentrations were found in nephrotic patients than in normal controls (929 ± 537 mg/dL). *2594* May be significantly reduced. *0419*

Immunoglobulin IgM *Serum Increase* Higher IgM and lower IgG serum concentrations were found in nephrotic patients than in normal controls (157 ± 108 mg/dL vs 127 ± 38 mg/dL). *2594 0419*

Serum Normal *2467*

Immunoglobulins *Serum Decrease* Usually more pronounced in children, averaging about 0.2 g/dL, which explains the high susceptibility to infection. *2104*

Urine Increase Severe urinary loss. *2104*

Iron *Serum Decrease* Probably related to loss of specific iron binding serum globulin in the urine. *0619*

Serum Increase *0619*

Iron-Binding Capacity, Total (TIBC) *Serum Decrease* Excessive loss of protein-bound iron with low total IBC. *0619 0995*

Lactate Dehydrogenase *Serum Increase* In 44% of 25 patients at initial hospitalization for this disorder. *0781 0503*

Urine Increase *2467*

Pleural Effusion Decrease Transudate. *0062*

Lactate Dehydrogenase Isoenzyme 5 (LD$_5$) *Serum Increase* May be slightly increased. *2467*

Leucine Aminopeptidase *Serum Increase* *0619*

Leukocytes *Blood Increase* In 56% of 24 patients at initial hospitalization for this disorder. *0781*

Ascitic Fluid Increase Less than 250 cells per μL. *2626*

Lipids *Serum Increase* Characteristic hyperlipidemia occurs with elevations in cholesterol, phospholipids, and triglycerides. *0151* Characterized by a great increase of all lipid constituents with both quantitative and qualitative alterations in lipoproteins. *0962*

Urine Increase All fractions increased. *2467* Lipiduria is a regular feature of the nephrotic syndrome. It is recognized in the fatty casts present in great numbers as well as in the cells which appear to be shed by the kidney. *0999*

Lipoproteins *Serum Increase* More than 50% of the patients with glomerulonephritis, nephrotic syndrome and renovascular hypertension showed obviously abnormal lipoprotein profiles, returning to normal or near-normal when the disease was ameliorated or corrected surgically. *2446 0833*

Lipoproteins, Beta *Serum Increase* Untreated uncomplicated nephrotic syndrome is characterized by increased low (beta) and very low (prebeta) density lipoproteins and a diminution of high density (alpha) lipoprotein. Changes correlated strictly with albumin concentrat were more pronounced with albumin concentration < 20 g/L. *0833* In severe, fully developed cases, increase in low density lipoproteins with normal or decreased alpha lipoproteins has been described. *0962*

Lipoproteins, Prebeta *Serum Increase* Untreated uncomplicated nephrotic syndrome is characterized by increased low (beta) and very low (prebeta) density lipoproteins and a diminution of high density (alpha) lipoprotein. Changes correlated strictly with albumin concentration and were more pronounced with albumin concentration < 20 g/L. *0833*

Lymphocytes *Blood Decrease* In 41% of 26 patients at initial hospitalization for this disorder. *0781*

Magnesium *Serum Decrease* In a majority of cases, serum levels were low with concomitant increase in urinary concentration due to massive albuminuria, as 35% of Mg is bound to albumin. *1772*

Urine Increase In a majority of cases, serum levels were low with concomitant increase in urinary concentration due to massive albuminuria, as 35% of Mg is bound to albumin. *1772*

Neutrophils *Blood Increase* In 49% of 26 patients at initial hospitalization for this disorder. *0781*

Nickel *Serum Decrease* Thought to be caused by hypoalbuminemia. *1559*

Oval Fat Bodies *Urine Increase* The lipid material is usually degenerative fatty vacuoles, neutral fat droplets, oval fat bodies, and doubly refractile fat bodies. *0962 0433*

pH *Pleural Effusion Increase* Transudate (pH > 7.3). *0062*

Phosphate *Serum Increase* In 60% of 25 patients at initial hospitalization for this disorder. *0781*

Phospholipids, Total *Serum Increase* Elevated cholesterol with lipiduria can be demonstrated; however, phospholipids and triglycerides are even more consistently and strikingly elevated. *0503* Typically elevated. *0962*

Platelet Count *Blood Increase* In 43% of 18 patients at initial hospitalization for this disorder. *0781* Mildly increased. *2322*

Protein *Urine Increase* Heavy proteinuria must be present for this diagnosis. *0999* High concentrations were observed in 19 patients, including adults and children. *2441*

Pleural Effusion Decrease Transudate secondary to decreased albumin. (< 3 g/dL). *0062*

Ascitic Fluid Decrease < 2.5 g/dL in ascitic fluid. *2626*

Protein Bound Iodine (PBI) *Serum Decrease* Urinary loss of TBG results in lowering of most blood thyroid hormones and increased T$_3$ uptake. *0962 2104*

Pseudocholinesterase *Serum Increase* 18 of 19 patients had values elevated above 12.5 U/mL. *2441*

Sodium *Urine Decrease* Results from increased aldosterone secretion and reduced GFR. *0151*

Specific Gravity *Pleural Effusion Decrease* Transudate (< 1.016). *0062*

T$_3$ Uptake *Serum Increase* Urinary loss of TBG results in lowering of most blood thyroid hormones and increased T$_3$ uptake. *0962* Low T$_4$ and raised resin uptake due to reduced TBG concentration occurs with protein loss. *2612*

Thromboplastin Generation *Blood Increase* Has been noted. *1249*

Thyroxine Binding Globulin *Serum Decrease* Urinary loss of TBG results in lowering of most blood thyroid hormones and increased T$_3$ uptake. *0962* Low T$_4$ and raised resin uptake due to reduced TBG concentration occurs with protein loss. *2612 2540 2104*

581.90   Nephrotic Syndrome *(continued)*

Thyroxine (T₄)   *Serum   Decrease*   Urinary loss of TBG results in lowering of most blood thyroid hormones and increased T₃ uptake. *0962*   Low T₄ and raised resin uptake due to reduced TBG concentration occurs with protein loss. *2612   2540*

Triglycerides   *Serum   Increase*   Elevated cholesterol with lipiduria can be demonstrated; however, phospholipids and triglycerides are even more consistently and strikingly elevated. *0503*   Typically elevated. *0962*

Tri-iodothyronine (T₃)   *Serum   Decrease*   Urinary loss of TBG results in lowering of most blood thyroid hormones and increased T₃ uptake. *0962*

Urea Nitrogen   *Serum   Decrease*   Some patients. *2467*

Serum   Increase   In 51% of 26 patients at initial hospitalization for this disorder. *0781*

Uric Acid   *Serum   Increase*   In 52% of 25 patients at initial hospitalization for this disorder. *0781*

Vitamin A   *Serum   Increase*   *0619*

Volume   *Plasma   Decrease*   In nephrotic syndrome, even with edema, blood volume is normal or decreased. *1669*

Zinc   *Serum   Decrease*   Decreased. *2297*   Associated protein loss *1893*

584.00   Acute Renal Failure

¹³¹I Uptake   *Serum   Decrease*   In renal disease. *2104*

17-Hydroxycorticosteroids   *Urine   Increase*   Both free and glucuronide fraction of 17 OHCS are elevated in acute but not chronic failure. *0219*

17-Ketogenic Steroids   *Urine   Increase*   Both free and glucuronide fraction of 17 OHCS are elevated in acute but not chronic failure. *0219*

Acid Phosphatase   *Serum   Increase*   Not related to degree of azotemia. *2467*

Amino Acids   *Plasma   Increase*   Increased total concentration due to rise in nonessential amino acids. Proline, hydroxyproline, glycine, citrulline, ornithine, were increased. Valine and tryptophan were decreased. *0533*

Ammonia   *Blood   Decrease*   Decreased arterial ammonia in azotemic patients mean = 34 mmol/L ± 1.4. *1853*

Urine   Decrease   With severe renal damage. May be < 1% of the urea nitrogen. *2104*

Amylase   *Serum   Increase*   May be increased without evidence of pancreatitis in early stage. *2468*   Mild elevation may occur with renal insufficiency but rarely more than twice the normal upper limit. *2031*

Angiotensin-Converting Enzyme (ACE)   *Serum   Decrease*   Level increased with normalization of renal function. *1970*

Aspartate Aminotransferase   *Serum   Increase*   In 63% of 11 patients at initial hospitalization for this disorder. *0781*

Beta₂-Macroglobulin   *Serum   Decrease*   An increase in urine and a decrease in serum levels is seen in disorders of renal tubular function. *1236*

Urine   Increase   An increase in urine and a decrease in serum levels is seen in disorders of renal tubular function. *1236*

Beta-Glucuronidase   *Urine   Increase*   All 8 patients revealed high values of urinary activity above the normal limit of 30 with a mean value of 148.1 ± 158.3 U/L. *0885*

Bicarbonate   *Serum   Decrease*   In 74% of 12 patients at initial hospitalization for this disorder. *0781*   Metabolic acidosis. *0787*   Falls 1-2 mmol/L each day during oliguric phase. *0277   0962*

Calcium   *Serum   Decrease*   May occur in early stage. *2468*   Hypocalcemia in acute (anuria) and chronic renal failure. *0503*   In 72% of 11 patients at initial hospitalization for this disorder. *0781*   In the range of 6.3-8.3 mg/dL. *1522*

Carcinoembryonic Antigen   *Serum   Increase*   Increased in about 50% of the patients. *2467*

Chloride   *Serum   Increase*   *2467*

Cortisol   *Plasma   Increase*   Normal or slightly elevated. *0667*

Creatine   *Serum   Increase*   High concentrations in blood and CSF have been associated with azotemia. *2104*

CSF   Increase   High concentrations in blood and CSF have been associated with azotemia. *2104*

Creatinine   *Serum   Increase*   Characteristic. *1607*   In 99% of 12 patients at initial hospitalization for this disorder. *0781   0787*

Creatinine Clearance   *Urine   Decrease*   *0619*

Cyclic Adenosine Monophosphate   *Plasma   Increase*   Elevated in uremia. *0968*

Eosinophils   *Blood   Increase*   In 32% of 12 patients at initial hospitalization for this disorder. *0781*

Erythrocyte Casts   *Urine   Increase*   Associated with active glomerulonephritis. *0433*

Erythrocytes   *Urine   Increase*   In the early stage. *2468*

Erythrocyte Survival   *Red Blood Cells   Decrease*   *0277*

Erythropoietin   *Serum   Increase*   *0277*

Fatty Acids, Free (FFA)   *Serum   Increase*   Elevated in acute renal failure, but normal or low in chronic failure. *1439*

Fibrin Split Products (FSP)   *Plasma   Increase*   In 25 patients with acute failure due to falciparum malaria, marked increase in plasma fibrinogen fibrin degradation products were observed. The other coagulation parameters were within the normal limits. *2190*

Gastrin   *Serum   Increase*   In both acute and chronic failure. *0546*

Glomerular Filtration Rate (GFR)   *Urine   Decrease*   Decreased due to reduced number of functioning glomeruli. *0619*   Decreased cortical renal blood flow was noted in acute failure due to falciparum malaria. *2190*

Glucagon   *Plasma   Increase*   Elevated 2-10 X above normal and remains essentially unchanged by dialysis. *0208*

Glucose   *Serum   Increase*   Hyperglycemia and impaired glucose tolerance are common. Elevated ratio of insulin/glucose during glucose tolerance testing is found consistently. *0787*

Glucose Tolerance   *Serum   Decrease*   Hyperglycemia and impaired glucose tolerance are common in renal failure. Elevated ratio of insulin/glucose during glucose tolerance testing is found consistently. *0787   0098*

Growth Hormone   *Serum   Increase*   Consistently occurring hypersecretion may be induced by severe uremia. *0787*

Urine   Increase   Marked elevation. *1445*

Hematocrit   *Blood   Decrease*   May fall to the low 20's. *0277*

Hemoglobin   *Blood   Decrease*   *0277*

Hemoglobin, Free   *Urine   Increase*   May appear in the urine of a patient with intravascular hemolysis or myoglobin in trauma. *0433*

Hexosaminidase   *Urine   Increase*   Extremely high values observed in acute renal failure following hypotensive episodes. *1525*

Lactate Dehydrogenase   *Serum   Increase*   In 72% of 11 patients at initial hospitalization for this disorder. *0781*

Urine   Increase   In acute tubular necrosis. *2467*

Leukocytes   *Blood   Increase*   Increased even without infection in the early stage. *2468*   In 65% of 12 patients at initial hospitalization for this disorder. *0781*   Often 10,000/μL. *0277*

Lipase   *Serum   Increase*   May be increased without evidence of pancreatitis in early stage. *2468*

Lymphocytes   *Blood   Decrease*   *0277*

Magnesium   *Serum   Increase*   Pathological increase with renal failure. *0619*

Neutrophils   *Blood   Increase*   In 74% of 12 patients at initial hospitalization for this disorder. *0781   0277*

Osmolality   *Urine   Decrease*   Manifested by oliguria, increasing serum-creatinine, a urine osmolality of < 400 mOsm/kg and a urine/plasma osmolality ratio of < 1·5. *1607*   < 350 mOsm in intrarenal acute renal failure *1595*

Urine   Increase   > 500 mOsm/kg in prerenal acute renal failure. *1595*

pCO₂   *Blood   Decrease*   Metabolic acidosis may occur. *0962*

pH   *Blood   Decrease*   Metabolic acidosis increases within 2nd week. *2468*   Mild acidosis is common. *0787   0962*

Urine   Increase   Normal or increased. *2467*

Phosphate   *Serum   Increase*   Hyperphosphatemia may occur depending on the duration and severity of disease. *0151*   In 72% of 11 patients at initial hospitalization for this disorder. *0781   0812*

Platelet Count   *Blood   Decrease*   As a consequence of peripheral destruction. *0988*

Potassium   *Serum   Decrease*   Large urinary potassium excretion may cause decreased serum concentration in diuretic stage. *2468*   May occur early in renal failure due to diarrhea, vomiting, or spontaneous potassium loss in urine. *0151*

Serum   Increase   During oliguric phase. *0277*   May occur depending on the duration and severity of the disease. *0151*   Liberated during body cell breakdown, and is not excreted completely in the urine. *0619*

Urine Decrease In acute tubular necrosis the kidney loses it ability to reabsorb sodium, and an increased concentration of urine sodium with a relative decrease in urine potassium will be noted. *0433*

Protein *Urine Increase* In the early stage. *2468*

Renin Activity *Plasma Increase* Increased in failure due to falciparum malaria. *2190*

Sodium *Serum Decrease* Often decreased, in the 2nd week. *2468*

Urine Decrease *0151*

Urine Increase In acute tubular necrosis the kidney loses its ability to reabsorb sodium, and an increased concentration of urine sodium with a relative decrease in urine potassium will be noted. *0433*

Specific Gravity *Urine Decrease* A low, fixed specific gravity indicates tubular damage. *0433*

Urine Increase May be high in the early stage. *2468*

Sulfate *Serum Increase* In metabolic acidosis accompanying renal failure. Serves as a reliable index of insufficiency. *2104*

Urea Nitrogen *Serum Increase* Rises < 20 mg/dL/day in trans­fusion reaction. Rises > 50 mg/dL/day in overwhelming infection or severe crushing injuries in early stage. Continues to rise for several days after onset of diuresis in the 2nd week. *2468* Excessive tubular reabsorption of urea and several other nonprotein nitrogen constituents may play a role in diseases producing this state. *0503* In 99% of 12 patients at initial hospitalization for this disorder. *0781* *1853*

Saliva Increase A near perfect correlation (R = 0.97) was found for saliva, plasma urea nitrogen ratios in 56 pairs of samples from patients with renal failure. The mean serum concentration before dialysis was 81.2 ± 30.9 mg/dL. In unstimulated saliva, the urea nitrogen saliva: plasma ratio remained constant at 1.3. *2125*

Uric Acid *Serum Increase* In 99% of 11 patients at initial hospitalization for this disorder. *0781*

Viscosity *Serum Increase* Significantly increased in 15 patients with acute failure due to falciparum malaria. *2190*

Volume *Plasma Decrease* Initial hypovolemia followed by hyper- or normovolemia in acute renal failure due to falciparum malaria. *2190*

Plasma Increase Initial hypovolemia followed by hyper- or normovolemia in acute renal failure due to falciparum malaria. *2190* *2467*

Urine Decrease Urine is scant in volume (often < 50 mL/day) for 2 weeks, in the early stage. Daily volume of 400 mL indicates onset of tubular recovery. Daily volume of 1,000 mL occurs in several days or < 2 weeks. *2468* Manifested by oliguria, urine osmolality of < 400 mOsm/kg and a urine/plasma osmolality ratio of < 1-5. *1607* *2467*

585.00 Chronic Renal Failure

131I Uptake *Serum Decrease* In renal disease. *2104*

1,25-Dihydroxy-Vitamin D$_3$ *Serum Decrease* *0062*

2,3-Diphosphoglycerate *Red Blood Cells Increase* Intracellular concentration is appropriately increased in response to anemia. *2538 0389*

17-Hydroxycorticosteroids *Urine Decrease* *0503*

17-Ketogenic Steroids *Urine Decrease* *0503*

Acid Phosphatase *Serum Increase* Marked increase in activity in urine, erythrocytes, and serum in the terminal stage of renal failure. *1290*

Urine Increase Activity in urine, erythrocytes, and serum was increased in patients with renal failure. Marked increases occur in all 3 specimens in the terminal stage. *1290*

Red Blood Cells Increase A 2-fold increase was found in uremic patients compared to normal controls. After hemodialysis both the serum phosphate and acid phosphatase activity were reduced. *1567* Activity in urine, erythrocytes, and serum was increased. Marked increase occurred in all 3 specimens in the terminal stage. *1290*

Alanine *Serum Decrease* Decreased. *0094 0269 2149*

Urine Increase Increases up to 4 X normal value. *0192*

Alanine Aminotransferase *Serum Increase* In 38% of 142 patients at initial hospitalization for this disorder. *0781*

Albumin *Serum Decrease* Concentrations are normal or low in chronic uremia. *1038* In 43% of 141 patients at initial hospitalization for this disorder. *0781* Tend to be diminished as a result of urinary protein loss

Urine Increase Proteinuria and granular casts suggest chronic parenchymal renal disease. *0433*

Aldosterone *Plasma Increase* Observed in some patients. *0995*

Urine Increase Observed in some patients. *0995*

Alkaline Phosphatase *Serum Increase* In 29% of 139 patients at initial hospitalization for this disorder. *0781*

Urine Increase 69% of cases showed elevation. *0817*

Alpha$_1$-Globulin *Serum Increase* Moderate increases. *0619*

Alpha$_2$-Globulin *Serum Increase* There is a moderate increase. *0619* Biochemical abnormalities are those seen in the nephrotic syndrome. *0962*

Aluminum *Serum Increase* Accumulates in all patients with renal failure. *2430*

Amino Acids *Plasma Increase* Increased total concentration due to rise in nonessential amino acids. Proline, hydroxyproline, glycine, citrulline, ornithine were increased. Valine, and tryptophan were decreased. *0533*

Urine Increase As GFR decreases, amino acid clearance and excretion increases. Increased levels of alanine (4 X normal), threonine, cystine, valine, and leucine (2-3 X normal), and proline are found in urine. *0192*

Ammonia *Blood Decrease* Decreased arterial ammonia in azotemic patients, (mean = 34 mmol/L ± 1.4). *1853*

Blood Increase Despite reduced excretion, renal failure does not usually lead to arterial excess, unless hepatic failure occurs. *2104*

Urine Decrease With severe renal damage may be < 1% of the urea nitrogen. *2104*

Amylase *Serum Increase* Patients with severe failure may have significant hyperamylasemia in the absence of clinical symptoms or signs of acute pancreatitis. *2336* Mild elevation may occur with renal insufficiency but rarely more than twice the normal upper limit. *2031*

Urine Increase In patients with severe renal insufficiency, the amylase to creatinine ratios were significantly raised. Clearance ratios of pancreatic and salivary isoamylase to creatinine changed in parallel to that of total amylase. The results suggest that in severe renal failure the loss of nephrons results in decreased fractional reabsorption of amylase in the tubules. *1779*

Angiotensin-Converting Enzyme (ACE) *Serum Increase* It is thought that an enlarged pulmonary vascular bed and accelerated cellular breakdown were the cause. *0608* Significantly higher than that of an age - matched control group *1611* Elevated regardless of severity of disease *2164*

Antinuclear Antibodies *Serum Increase* Increased in 11 of 86 patients who had never been dialyzed and 52 of 243 chronic dialysis patients. Significantly lower Hcts and WBC counts were noted with the presence of these antibodies. *1702*

Antithyroglobulin Antibodies *Serum Normal* *1617*

Arginine *Plasma Decrease* Children with mild renal insufficiency showed a significant decrease in tyrosine and arginine. *0192*

Beta$_2$-Macroglobulin *Serum Decrease* An increase in urine and a decrease in serum levels is seen in disorders of renal tubular function. *1236*

Urine Increase An increase in urine and a decrease in serum levels is seen in disorders of renal tubular function. *1236*

Beta-Globulin *Serum Normal* *2467*

Bicarbonate *Serum Decrease* Metabolic acidosis may occur. *0962* In 59% of 146 patients at initial hospitalization for this disorder. *0781*

Bilirubin *Serum Normal* Within normal limits in all 26 cases. *1421*

Cadmium *Serum Decrease* Probably due to proteinuria and a loss of cadmethionein in urine. *0019*

Calcitonin *Serum Increase* Basal plasma concentrations were increased to a mean of 185.88 ± 16.36 pg/mL. *1368*

Calcium *Serum Decrease* Falls late in renal failure, often reaching 6 mg/dL and occasionally 4 mg/dL. *0151* Usually reduced primarily as a result of diminished synthesis of active metabolites of vitamin D, particularly in the setting of high levels of intracellular phosphate. *1108* Hypocalcemia in acute (anuria) and chronic renal failure. *0503* In 47% of 142 patients at initial hospitalization for this disorder. *0781*

Urine Decrease Falls early, to < 100 mg/24h, before there is any drop in serum levels, reflecting the fall of GFR. *0151*

Sweat Increase Concentrations of Ca, Mg and phosphate in sweat were significantly elevated due to an increase in the secretion of these electrolytes in the secretory portion of the sweat gland, while that in the reabsorptive duct is normal. *1861*

Casts *Urine Increase* With renal parenchymal disease. *0838*

Catecholamines *Plasma Increase* Moderate increase. *0649*

585.00 Chronic Renal Failure (continued)

Cells *Urine Increase* Renal epithelial cells were increased to 49% of total cells in benign endemic nephropathy. *1411*

Bone Marrow Increase Tends to be moderately hypercellular. *2552 0329*

Chloride *Serum Decrease* Decreased or normal. *2467*

Serum Normal Decreased or normal. *2467*

Cholesterol *Serum Increase* May be elevated. *1038* Most studies show only a modest increase. *1108 1243*

Cholesterol, Very Low Density Lipoprotein *Serum Increase* Marked elevation with uremia. *0062*

Cortisol *Plasma Increase* Normal or slightly elevated. *0667*

Creatine *Serum Increase* High concentrations in blood and CSF have been associated with azotemia. *2104*

CSF Increase High concentrations in blood and CSF have been associated with azotemia. *2104*

Creatinine *Serum Increase* In late failure. *0151* Appears to rise more slowly in the presence of renal disease than the BUN. It is less useful than the BUN to assess effectiveness of hemodialysis in the treatment of renal failure, since it does not decrease as rapidly as BUN. *0503* In 97% of 144 patients at initial hospitalization for this disorder. *0781 0787*

Creatinine Clearance *Urine Decrease* Less than 20 mL/min. *1374*

Cyclic Adenosine Monophosphate *Plasma Increase* Elevated in uremia. *0968*

Cystine *Serum Increase* Children with renal failure showed a decrease in most amino acids but an increase in cystine and glycine. 14 of 31 children (45%) had cystine concentrations above the normal upper limit. *0192*

Epinephrine *Plasma Increase* Moderate increase. *0649*

Erythrocytes *Blood Decrease* In chronic renal insufficiency, anemia is commonly caused by a relative or absolute deficiency of red cell production. *1669*

Urine Increase With renal parenchymal disease. *0838*

Erythrocyte Sedimentation Rate *Blood Increase* Characteristic increase as a result of increased plasma fibrinogen. *0151*

Erythrocyte Survival *Red Blood Cells Decrease* Shortened to about half normal when the blood urea exceeds 200 mg/dL. *0151* Shortened RBC life span and inhibitor of heme synthesis cause anemia in renal insufficiency. *0736* Slightly to moderately reduced. *2552*

Erythropoietin *Serum Decrease* Reduced in chronic failure causing relative hypoplasia of the marrow. *0151* Decreased secretion of erythropoietin of renal origin. *1669*

Serum Increase May be elevated to varying degrees in patients with anemia associated with end-stage renal disease. The increase in erythropoietin titer was apparently not sufficient to meet the increase in demand for new RBCs created by their shortened life span and the inhibitors of heme synthesis. *0736*

Factor V *Plasma Decrease* Occasionally observed. *0151*

Factor VII *Plasma Decrease* Occasionally observed. *0151*

Factor VIII *Plasma Increase* Dramatic increase in both factor VIII/von Willebrand antigen and activity (315 ± 30% vs. 104 ± 9% in control, and 402 ± 48% activity in patients vs. 111 ± 5% controls). *2484* Increased activity has been reported. *0633*

Fatty Acids, Free (FFA) *Serum Decrease* Elevated in acute renal failure, but normal or low in chronic failure. *1439*

Fibrinogen *Plasma Increase* Usually raised about 30%, resulting in characteristic rise of ESR. *0151*

Fibrin Split Products (FSP) *Plasma Increase* Elevated levels (> 10 μg/mL) occurred in 73% of chronic nephritic patients. Mean value was 16.0 ± 5.9 μg/mL. *1325*

Gastrin *Serum Increase* Elevated; no apparent correlation with calcitonin levels. *1368* In both acute and chronic failure. *1302*

Globulin *Serum Normal* *2467*

Glomerular Filtration Rate (GFR) *Urine Decrease* BUN and creatinine rise as GFR decreases. *0962*

Glucagon *Plasma Increase* Glucagon is elevated 2-10 X above normal and remains essentially unchanged by dialysis. *0208* Fasting immunoreactive glucagon was elevated to 534 ± 2 pg/mL in chronic failure. Normal value was 113 ± 9 pg/mL. *1321 1108*

Glucose *Serum Increase* Hyperglycemia and impaired glucose tolerance are common in renal failure. Elevated ratio of insulin/glucose during glucose tolerance testing is found consistently. *0787* Increased mean plasma concentration in chronic failure. *1243*

Urine Increase With renal parenchymal disease. *0838*

Glucose-6-Phosphatase *Serum Increase* Slight rise with renal disease. *0619*

Glucose Tolerance *Serum Decrease* More than 50% of patients in late renal failure have glucose intolerance as severe as in mild diabetes but with normal fasting blood dextrose and often without glycosuria. *0151*

Glutamic Acid *Serum Decrease* Mean concentration of serine, threonine, and glutamic acid decreased with deteriorating renal function in children with renal failure. *0192*

Glycerol *Serum Increase* Increased mean plasma concentration in chronic failure. *1243*

Glycine *Serum Increase* A significant rise in mean concentration occurred in children whose GFR was < 15 mL/min/1.73 m³. 34% had values above normal upper limit. *0192*

Granular Casts *Urine Increase* Proteinuria and granular casts suggest chronic parenchymal renal disease. *0433*

Growth Hormone *Serum Increase* Increased mean plasma concentration in chronic failure. *1243* Consistently occurring hypersecretion may be induced by severe uremia. *0787 1108*

Urine Increase Marked elevation. *1445*

Hematocrit *Blood Decrease* Anemia occurs in almost all chronic patients. Uremia without anemia suggests acute renal failure. RBCs are normochromic or have slightly reduced MCHC, about 30-31. *0151* Characteristically normocytic and normochromic, and is associated with a normal or slightly decreased number of reticulocytes. *2538* Hydremia and dehydration are common. Changes will exaggerate or minimize the degree of anemia. *2552* In 89% of 146 patients at initial hospitalization for this disorder. *0781*

Hemoglobin *Blood Decrease* Anemia is characteristic of chronic failure, normal hemoglobin suggests acute failure. *0151* Normocytic and normochromic, and associated with a normal or slightly decreased number of reticulocytes. *2538* Hydremia and dehydration are common. Changes will exaggerate or minimize the degree of anemia. *2552* In 89% of 146 patients at initial hospitalization for this disorder. *0781*

Hemoglobin, Free *Serum Increase* Mild hemolysis may occur. *1669*

Hexosaminidase *Urine Increase* Urinary levels often increased in chronic renal disease and are very sensitive to degree of renal damage. *1525*

Insulin *Serum Increase* Increased basal immunoreactive insulin levels in chronic uremia may be due to prolonged half-life. *0098 1108*

Urine Increase Markedly elevated. *1445*

Iron *Serum Decrease* Normal in mild cases, but with severe failure, both hypo- and hyperferremia have been observed. *0643 0732 2552*

Serum Increase Normal in mild cases, but with severe failure, both hypo- and hyperferremia have been observed. *0643 0732 2552*

Iron-Binding Capacity, Total (TIBC) *Serum Decrease* Low in both mild and severe renal failure, with the lowest levels found in patients with poor nutritional state. *1734* In 64% of 17 patients at initial hospitalization for this disorder. *0781*

Lactate Dehydrogenase *Serum Increase* Occasional increase but to no clinically useful degree. *2467* Patients with chronic renal disease, especially those with nephrotic syndrome or hemolytic anemia, also have increased values. *0503*

Urine Increase 38% of cases showed elevation. *0817*

Pleural Effusion Decrease Transudate. *0062*

Red Blood Cells Normal Within normal limits. *1566*

Leukocytes *Blood Increase* Slight neutrophilic leukocytosis may be observed. *2552 0329* In 26% of 146 patients at initial hospitalization for this disorder. *0781*

Urine Increase With renal parenchymal disease. *0838*

Lipids *Serum Increase* Raised in late renal failure, mainly due to a rise in triglycerides; phospholipids and cholesterol are normal or slightly elevated. *0151*

Lipoproteins *Serum Increase* Characteristically increased. Type IV hyperlipoproteinemia occurs commonly secondary to renal failure. *1038* 42 of 100 patients had type IV hyperlipoproteinemia, which did not correlate with degree of disease, or age, sex, weight or diet of patient. *2557*

Lipoproteins, Beta *Serum Increase* Increased mean plasma concentration in chronic failure. *1243*

Lipoproteins, Prebeta *Serum Increase* Consistent rise in late renal failure. *0151* Increased mean plasma concentration in chronic failure. *1243*

Lymphocytes *Blood Decrease* In 66% of 141 patients at initial hospitalization for this disorder. *0781*

Lysozyme *Urine Increase* Marked increase. *1860*

Magnesium *Serum Decrease* Depletion occurs in rare instances. *1570*

Serum Increase Increases when GFR falls to < 30 mL/min. *2468* In 43% of 60 patients at initial hospitalization for this disorder. *0781*

Red Blood Cells Increase Of 15 patients with a variety of renal lesions and a wide range of BUN, 9 had elevated erythrocyte magnesium levels. Mean concentration for the whole group was significantly raised, 6.7 mmol/L packed cells. *2469*

Sweat Increase Concentrations of Ca, Mg and phosphate in sweat were significantly elevated due to an increase in the secretion of these electrolytes in the secretory portion of the sweat gland, while that in the reabsorptive duct is normal. *1861*

MCHC *Blood Decrease* Slightly reduced, to about 30-31%. *0151*

MCV *Blood Increase* Slight macrocytosis has been observed. *1421*

Metanephrines, Total *Urine Normal* Normal urinary excretion. *0649*

Monocytes *Urine Increase* 29-33% mononuclear cells found in lupus nephritis and endemic benign nephropathy. *1411*

Neutrophils *Blood Increase* Slight neutrophilic leukocytosis may be observed. *2552 0329* In 67% of 141 patients at initial hospitalization for this disorder. *0781*

Norepinephrine *Serum Increase* Moderate increase. *0649*

Osmolality *Urine Decrease* With renal parenchymal disease. *0838*

Urine Normal 250-400 mOsm/kg; becomes fixed close to plasma level of 280-295 mOsm/kg. *0186*

Osmotic Fragility *Red Blood Cells Normal* *1421*

Osteocalcin *Serum Increase* Markedly elevated. *0671*

Parathyroid Hormone *Serum Increase* Reaches 10 X normal late in renal failure. *0151* Elevated in chronic uremia. *1038* Increased nearly in all patients. May be extremely high. Rough inverse correlation with renal function. *1909* *1108*

pCO₂ *Blood Decrease* Metabolic acidosis may occur. *0962* In 63% of 31 patients at initial hospitalization for this disorder. *0781*

pH *Blood Decrease* Mild acidosis is common in renal failure. *0787* Metabolic acidosis is an invariable concomitant of chronic failure. *1108* In 31% of 31 patients at initial hospitalization for this disorder. *0781*

Urine Increase *2467*

Pleural Effusion Increase Transudate (pH > 7.3). *0062*

Phosphate *Serum Increase* Plasma levels rise late in renal failure and are unrelated to the serum calcium levels. *0151* Increases when creatinine clearance falls to approximately 25 mL/min. *2468* In 75% of 141 patients at initial hospitalization for this disorder. *0781* *0962 1393*

Sweat Increase Concentrations of Ca, Mg and phosphate in sweat were significantly elevated due to an increase in the secretion of these electrolytes in the secretory portion of the sweat gland, while that in the reabsorptive duct is normal. *1861*

Plasma Cells *Serum Decrease* Depressed. *2357 0659 0683*

Platelet Count *Blood Increase* Normal or slightly increased. However, platelet function may be severely impaired. *0329 2552*

Potassium *Serum Decrease* May occur. *0277*

Serum Increase Liberated during body cell breakdown, and is not excreted completely in the urine. *0619*

Urine Increase *2467*

Feces Increase May represent an important adaptive response. *1010*

Red Blood Cells Increase In 36 patients, a normal or high erythrocyte potassium was found. *1162*

Prolactin *Serum Increase* Significantly decreased in patients with impaired renal function, both in patients on drug therapy and in those not taking any drugs affecting plasma prolactin. No relation was found with age, sex, underlying diagnosis, or duration of uremia. *0460* Increased levels *2638*

Protein *Serum Decrease* Total protein is decreased with chronic renal insufficiency. *2468*

Urine Increase With renal parenchymal disease. *0838*

Pleural Effusion Decrease Transudate secondary to decreased albumin. (< 3 g/dL). *0062*

Protoporphyrin *Red Blood Cells Increase* May be moderately increased. *1421 2552*

Reticulocytes *Blood Decrease* Anemia is characteristically normocytic and normochromic, and is associated with a normal or slightly decreased number of reticulocytes. *2538*

Blood Increase 1-4 X normal after correction for reduced RBC. *0151* May be moderately increased. *1421 2552* Highest values (6%) observed when the BUN was 300-350 mg/dL. *2130*

Sodium *Serum Decrease* Decreased because of tubular damage with loss in urine, vomiting, diarrhea, diet restriction, etc. *2468*

Serum Increase Much less common. *0277*

Serum Normal Usually. *0277*

Urine Decrease *0151*

Urine Increase *2467*

Red Blood Cells Decrease Erythrocytes sodium values showed a wide range, from very high to very low, and the rate constant for Na⁺ efflux was found to be higher than normal. *1162*

Red Blood Cells Increase Erythrocytes sodium values showed a wide range, from very high to very low, and the rate constant for Na efflux was found to be higher than normal. *1162* In 25% of uremic patients. *2515*

Specific Gravity *Urine Decrease* With decreased renal function, specific gravity is 1.020, as renal impairment is more severe, specific gravity approaches 1.010. The test is sensitive for early loss of renal function, but a normal finding does not necessarily rule out active kidney disease. *2467*

Pleural Effusion Decrease Transudate (< 1.016). *0062*

Sulfate *Serum Increase* In metabolic acidosis accompanying renal failure. Serves as a reliable index of insufficiency. *2104*

Threonine *Serum Decrease* Mean concentration decreased with deteriorating renal function in children. *0192*

Thyroid Stimulating Hormone (TSH) *Serum Normal* *1617*

Thyroxine (T₄) *Serum Decrease* Significant decrease in total and free T₄; total T₄ mean = 5.3 ± 1.9 μg/dL. Levels were even further depleted in terminal failure. *1298* In 56% of 26 patients at initial hospitalization for this disorder. *0781* Normal or decreased *1617*

Triglycerides *Serum Increase* Endogenous VLDL triglyceride production rate was significantly raised in 13 patients who were not on dialysis treatment. *0465* Characteristically increased. Type IV hyperlipoproteinemia occurs commonly secondary to renal failure. *1038* Hypertriglyceridemia was found in 43% of patients. 20 men had values > 200 mg/dL and 23 women had 150 mg/dL or greater. *2557* Increased mean plasma concentration in chronic failure. *1243* Present in most patients whether or not they are dialyzed. *1108 0151 0099*

Tri-iodothyronine, Reverse *Serum Normal* Reverse T₃ is normal but free reverse T₃ is usually elevated. *1617*

Tri-iodothyronine (T₃) *Serum Decrease* Although mean serum total T₃ concentration was normal, 43% had low serum T₃ and 54% had low serum free T₃ concentrations. *2233* Reduced total and free T₃, mean total T₃ = 65.4 ± 17.4 ng/dL. *1298* Decreased *1617*

Urine Decrease Reduced excretion, 27 ± 44 ng/24h. *1298*

Tyrosine *Serum Decrease* Children with mild renal insufficiency showed a significant decrease in tyrosine and arginine and an increase in cystine. Tyrosine showed a linear correlation between decreasing plasma concentration and GFR (R = 0.4). *0192*

Urea Nitrogen *Serum Increase* Damage to the nephrons leads to faulty urine formation and excretion. The blood-urea begins to rise when the equivalent of one kidney lost, or when the GFR falls below 10 mL/min. *0619* In 98% of 148 patients at initial hospitalization for this disorder. *0781 1853*

Saliva Increase A near perfect correlation (R = 0.97) was found for saliva: plasma urea nitrogen ratios in 56 pairs of samples from patients with renal failure. The mean serum urea nitrogen level for renal failure patients before dialysis was 81.2 ± 30.9 mg/dL. In unstimulated saliva, the urea nitrogen saliva: plasma ratio remained constant at 1.3. *2125*

Uric Acid *Serum Increase* Increase is usually < 10 mg/dL. *2468* Rise begins very early, but is so slight that the level becomes consistently abnormal only when the GFR falls to about 15 mL/min. In late renal failure there is a further increase in fractional urate clearance so that plasma urate rises less steeply than plasma urea or creatinine. *0151* In 91% of 140 patients at initial hospitalization for this disorder. *0781*

Uric Acid Clearance *Urine Increase* Increases slightly early in renal failure and again in the late stages, causing plasma urate to rise less steeply than urea or creatinine. *0151*

Vanillylamine *Urine Normal* Normal urinary excretion. *0649*

Vitamin A *Serum Increase* *0619*

585.00 Chronic Renal Failure (continued)

Volume *Plasma Decrease* Hydremia and dehydration are common. Changes will exaggerate or minimize the degree of anemia. *2552*

Plasma Increase Hydremia and dehydration are common. Changes will exaggerate or minimize the degree of anemia. *2552*

Urine Decrease With renal parenchymal disease. *0838* Terminal chronic nephritis *0619*

588.00 Renal Dwarfism

Alkaline Phosphatase *Serum Increase* Usually elevated. *0151*

Calcium *Serum Decrease* May lead to hypocalcemia or low normal serum calcium levels. In time there will be significant parathyroid hyperplasia, and the serum calcium may become inappropriately elevated. *0999* May be quite low but is more commonly in the low-normal range. *0151*

Serum Increase May be normal or elevated. When both phosphate and calcium are high, metastatic calcifications in subcutaneous tissues and conjunctiva may develop. *0999*

Serum Normal May be normal or elevated. When both phosphate and calcium are high, metastatic calcifications in subcutaneous tissues and conjunctiva may develop. *0999*

Parathyroid Hormone *Serum Increase* *0151*

Phosphate *Serum Increase* May be normal or elevated. When both phosphate and calcium are high, metastatic calcifications in subcutaneous tissues and conjunctiva may develop. *0999*

Serum Normal May be normal or elevated. When both phosphate and calcium are high, metastatic calcifications in subcutaneous tissues and conjunctiva may develop. *0999*

588.81 Proximal Renal Tubular Acidosis

Alkaline Phosphatase *Serum Increase* Increased in Albricht-type renal tubular acidosis, as in Fanconi Syndrome, but no aminoaciduria. *0619 0503 0433 2246*

Amino Acids *Urine Increase* Found in children. *0433*

Ammonia *Urine Decrease* *2246 2552*

Bicarbonate *Serum Decrease* Low levels in the presence of alkaline urine; very low levels with acid urine. *0186* Low Bicarbonate level *2246*

Calcium *Serum Decrease* Renal tubular acidosis or Fanconi Syndrome. Must be considered in patients with osteomalacia. Normal to decreased values. *0503 2246*

Serum Increase Hypercalcemia in 5 of 17 patients with transient primary renal tubular acidosis. *1753*

Urine Increase The hypercalciuria results in nephrocalcinosis or nephrolithiasis which, in the absence of generalized aminoaciduria, aids in the differentiation of this disease from the more common De Toni-Debre-Fanconi Syndrome. *0433 0503 2246*

Chloride *Serum Increase* *2246*

Glomerular Filtration Rate (GFR) *Urine Decrease* Usually reduced. *2246*

Glucose *Urine Increase* Found in children. *0433*

Parathyroid Hormone *Serum Increase* Secondary to hypocalcemia. *0277*

pH *Blood Decrease* Tends to fall. *0619 2246*

Urine Increase Always relatively high with the gradient defect, no matter how severe the systemic acidosis. *2246*

Phosphate *Serum Decrease* Low in the early stages and increasing to normal values with increasing azotemia. *0503 0433 2246*

Urine Increase Excessive loss in urine. *2467 2246 0503*

Potassium *Serum Decrease* May be a life-threatening complication. *0433* Hydrogen ion and ammonium ion production by the renal tubule cells is diminished, with excessive loss of potassium in the urine. In any case of severe renal damage, potassium conservation may be impaired. *0619* Renal wasting leads to hypokalemic state. *1679* Normal or decreased *2645 2446*

Serum Normal Normal or decreased. *0186*

Urine Increase Renal wasting of potassium. *1679* May result in severe hypokalemic paralysis. *2246*

Sodium *Serum Decrease* Normal or decreased. *0186* Hyponatremia may develop *2246*

Serum Normal Normal or decreased. *0186*

Urine Increase *2467*

Uric Acid *Serum Decrease* Hypouricemia, secondary to increased renal clearance of uric acid, is present in some patients (children). *0433*

Urine Increase Hypouricemia, secondary to increased renal clearance of uric acid, is present in some patients (children). *0433*

Uric Acid Clearance *Urine Increase* Hypouricemia, secondary to increased renal clearance of uric acid, is present in some patients (children). *0433*

Volume *Plasma Decrease* *2467*

Urine Increase Characterized by polyuria. *2246 2467*

588.82 Distal Renal Tubular Acidosis

Beta₂-Macroglobulin *Serum Decrease* An increase in urine and a decrease in serum levels is seen. *1236*

Urine Increase An increase in urine and a decrease in serum levels is seen. *1236*

Bicarbonate *Serum Decrease* Alkaline urine regardless of bicarbonate level. *0186*

Urine Increase Alkaline urine regardless of bicarbonate level in blood. *0186*

Calcium *Serum Decrease* *0614*

Urine Increase An almost constant feature and frequently results in the formation of renal calculi. *0151 0614*

Chloride *Serum Increase* Normal anion gap. *0186*

Parathyroid Hormone *Serum Increase* Secondary to reduced calcium. *0417*

pH *Blood Decrease* *0614*

Urine Increase Cardinal clinical finding is a urine pH which is never lower than 6.0, even with severe metabolic acidosis. *0151* Inappropriately high. *0614*

Phosphate *Serum Decrease* Typical feature of Type I. *0151*

Potassium *Serum Decrease* Commonly occurs in Type I. *0151 0843*

Serum Increase Some cases. *0186*

Urine Increase Commonly occurs in Type I. *0151 0843*

Sodium *Urine Increase* Characteristic complication of metabolic acidosis. *2050*

590.00 Chronic Pyelonephritis

Alanine Aminotransferase *Urine Increase* Increased. *1807 1199 2534*

Albumin *Urine Increase* Qualitative proteinuria may be absent but if present is mild. *0433*

Alkaline Phosphatase *Urine Increase* Almost invariably elevated in a group of 10 patients. *0817*

Alpha₁-Globulin *Serum Increase* Moderate increases. *0619*

Alpha₂-Globulin *Serum Increase* Moderate increase. *0619*

Beta-Glucuronidase *Urine Increase* All 15 patients showed elevated activity (mean 61.9 ± 39.1), whereas 11 of 13 patients with inactive disease showed normal values (mean 24.0 ± 7.8 U). *0885*

Casts *Urine Increase* As in acute pyelonephritis, the leukocyte cast in the absence of other cellular casts is a most helpful finding and strongly supports the diagnosis. The urine sediment may be normal but repeated examination will usually reveal pyuria and cylindruria *0433* With Renal Parenchymal Disease *0838*

Ceruloplasmin *Serum Increase* Found in 84 patients with exacerbated disease. Raised levels indicate the amount of activity of the pathologic process and distinguishes it from glomerulonephritis. *2362*

Chloride *Serum Increase* Hyperchloremia frequently accompanies chronic pyelonephritis. *0962*

Creatinine *Serum Increase* *2468*

Creatinine Clearance *Urine Decrease* Decreased 24 h clearance. *2468*

Erythrocytes *Urine Increase* With renal parenchymal disease. *0838* Microscopic hematuria may be present *0433*

Glomerular Filtration Rate (GFR) *Urine Decrease* Decreased due to reduced filtration surface (fewer functioning glomeruli). *0619* A decrease proportional to progress of renal disease. *2468*

Glucose *Urine Increase* With renal parenchymal disease. *0838*

Haptoglobin *Serum Increase* Increased serum levels found in 84 chronic patients correlated with activity of pathologic process and distinguished it from glomerulonephritis. *2362*

Hematocrit *Blood Decrease* A normocytic, normochromic anemia may be present as in other forms of renal insufficiency. May be more severe, since chronic infection will act synergistically with renal insufficiency to depress bone marrow function. *0433*

Hemoglobin *Blood Decrease* A normocytic, normochromic anemia may be present as in other forms of renal insufficiency. May be more severe, since chronic infection will act synergistically with renal insufficiency to depress bone marrow function. *0433*

Hexosaminidase *Urine Increase* Decreased levels in urine. *2356*

Lactate Dehydrogenase *Urine Increase* Urinary activity was almost invariably elevated. *0817*

Leukocytes *Urine Increase* WBCs, bacteria, and little protein are common urinary findings. *0151*

Magnesium *Serum Decrease* Hypomagnesemia may occur. *2444*

Osmolality *Urine Decrease* With renal parenchymal disease. *0838*

Potassium *Urine Decrease* *0619*

Protein *Urine Increase* With renal parenchymal disease. *0838* Slight, usually < 3 g/24h. *0151*

Sialic Acid *Serum Increase* Increased in 84 chronic patients, correlated with activity of pathologic process and distinguished it from glomerulonephritis. *2362*

Specific Gravity *Urine Decrease* The urine is usually of low specific gravity or at least no more than isosmotic plasma. *0433*

Thyroxine (T$_4$) *Urine Increase* Urinary loss exceeds the normal mean 10-fold. *0733*

Urea Nitrogen *Serum Increase* May be elevated. *0151* *1853*

Volume *Urine Decrease* With renal parenchymal disease. *0838*

590.10 Acute Pyelonephritis

Albumin *Urine Increase* Often present but minimal in degree. *0433*

Alkaline Phosphatase *Serum Increase* Significant elevation can be found in some patients. This occurs in cases with clinical or histological evidence of severe disease, occasionally associated with papillary necrosis and gram-negative septicemia. Widespread renal inflammatory destruction results in release of enzyme from the tubular cells into the blood stream. *0753* In 29% of 13 patients at initial hospitalization for this disorder. *0781*

Alpha$_1$-Globulin *Serum Increase* Moderate increases. *0619*

Alpha$_2$-Globulin *Serum Increase* Moderate increase. *0619*

Aspartate Aminotransferase *Serum Increase* In 28% of 14 patients at initial hospitalization for this disorder. *0781*

Beta-Glucuronidase *Urine Increase* All 15 patients with active disease showed elevated activity (mean 61.9 ± 39.1 U/L), whereas 11 of 13 patients with inactive disease showed normal values (mean 24.0 ± 7.8 U/L). *0885* *1525*

Casts *Urine Increase* Generally interpreted as indicative of renal parenchymal inflammation and which in the absence of other types of cellular casts provides strong support for a diagnosis of pyelonephritis. *0433* Essentially diagnostic. *0962* With renal parenchymal disease *0838*

C-Reactive Protein *Serum Increase* Marked increase indicates an acute infection. *0186*

Creatinine *Serum Increase* In 48% of 16 patients at initial hospitalization for this disorder. *0781* *2468*

Creatinine Clearance *Urine Decrease* Decreased 24 h clearance. *2468*

Erythrocytes *Urine Increase* The finding of gross or microscopic hematuria is variable but not uncommon. *0433* With renal parenchymal disease {838}

Glomerular Filtration Rate (GFR) *Urine Decrease* Decreased due to reduced filtration surface (fewer functioning glomeruli). *0619*

Glucose *Urine Increase* With renal parenchymal disease. *0838*

Isocitrate Dehydrogenase *Serum Normal* *2260*

Lactate Dehydrogenase *Urine Increase* Increased in 25% of patients. *2467*

Leukocytes *Blood Increase* Most patients exhibit a leukocytosis of 15,000- 20,000/μL with an increase of immature neutrophils in the differential count. *0433* In 68% of 16 patients at initial hospitalization for this disorder. *0781*

Urine Increase With renal parenchymal disease. *0838*

Urine Normal Acute pyelonephritis may exist in the absence of pyuria and bacteriuria. This may occur in the patient with hematogenous dissemination of infection to the renal parenchyma without communication to urinary drainage, as in renal carbuncle or perinephric abscess. *0433* *0277*

Magnesium *Serum Decrease* May occur. *2444*

Neutrophils *Blood Increase* Most patients exhibit a leukocytosis of 15,000- 20,000/μL with an increase of immature neutrophils in the differential count. *0433* In 63% of 14 patients at initial hospitalization for this disorder. *0781*

Potassium *Urine Decrease* *0619*

Protein *Urine Increase* Usually < 2 g/24h. *0503* Proteinuria is usually mild, rarely exceeding 1.5-2.0 g/24h. *0962* With renal parenchymal disease *0838*

Specific Gravity *Urine Decrease* Urine concentrating ability is impaired relatively early. *0962*

Urea Nitrogen *Serum Increase* Uncomplicated disease does not characteristically exhibit evidence of renal insufficiency; however, a nonspecific elevation of BUN may be a reflection of volume contraction and and dehydration. *0433* In 24% of 16 patients at initial hospitalization for this disorder. *0781*

Volume *Urine Decrease* With renal parenchymal disease. *0838* *0619*

591.00 Hydronephrosis

Alanine Aminotransferase *Urine Increase* Increased. *1807* *1199* *2534*

Albumin *Urine Normal* In uninfected hydronephrosis the urine is negative. If infection supervenes, WBC and albumin are noted. *0433*

Creatinine *Serum Increase* In 70% of 10 patients at initial hospitalization for this disorder. *0781*

Erythrocytes *Blood Increase* True polycythemia with a considerable increase of red cell volume may occur. *1669*

Hematocrit *Blood Decrease* In cases of advanced renal damage elevation of the BUN and secondary anemia may be noted secondary to uremia. *0433*

Hemoglobin *Blood Decrease* In cases of advanced renal damage elevation of the BUN and secondary anemia may be noted secondary to uremia. *0433*

Leukocytes *Blood Increase* In 27% of 11 patients at initial hospitalization for this disorder. *0781*

Urine Normal In uninfected cases the urine is negative. If infection supervenes, WBC and albumin are noted. *0433*

Magnesium *Serum Decrease* Hypomagnesemia may occur. *2444*

Urea Nitrogen *Serum Increase* In cases of advanced renal damage elevation of the BUN and secondary anemia may be noted secondary to uremia. *0433* In 20% of 10 patients at initial hospitalization for this disorder. *0781*

Volume *Red Blood Cells Increase* True polycythemia with a considerable increase of red cell volume may occur. *1669*

592.00 Kidney Calculus

25-Hydroxy Vitamin D$_3$ *Serum Decrease* Significantly lower in 29 untreated patients with recurrent calcium containing kidney stones (15.8 ± 9.8 ng/mL) than in controls (23.6 ± 9.8 ng/mL). Deficiency is possible due to low milk diet followed by recurrent stone intake. *2424*

Angiotensin-Converting Enzyme (ACE) *Urine Increase* Activity was found to be significantly elevated. *0256*

Calcium *Serum Decrease* May represent presenting manifestations. *0503*

Urine Increase 35% of patients have increased urinary concentration (> 250 mg/24h in females and > 300 mg/24h in males). *2468* Increased in the majority of patients with calcareous calculi, but will be normal in patients whose primary problem is infection. *0151*

Erythrocytes *Urine Increase* Microscopic hematuria is found. *0151*

Lactate Dehydrogenase *Urine Normal* *2467*

Leukocytes *Urine Increase* Few to many WBCs and microscopic hematuria are found. *0151*

Lipoproteins, Beta *Serum Increase* With corresponding increase in beta:alpha ratio. *2416*

592.00   Kidney Calculus *(continued)*

Pyridoxine *Serum Decrease* A relationship may exist between deficient B₆ and endogenous oxalic acid production and stone formation. *2104*

Thyroxine (T₄) *Urine Decrease* In male renal calcium stone patients (20-40 y) urinary T₄ is lower than in age-matched controls. *2097*

592.10   Ureter Calculus

Albumin *Urine Increase* The urinalysis often shows no significant alteration from normal but may progress through the stages of mild pyuria to moderate pyuria with albuminuria and onto frank infection or passage of renal casts. *0433*

Erythrocyte Casts *Urine Increase* The urinalysis often shows no significant alteration from normal but may progress through the stages of mild pyuria to moderate pyuria with albuminuria and onto frank infection or passage of renal casts. *0433*

Urine Normal The urinalysis often shows no significant alteration from normal. *0433*

Erythrocytes *Urine Increase* *0277*

Leukocytes *Urine Increase* The urinalysis often shows no significant alteration from normal but may progress through the stages of mild pyuria to moderate pyuria with albuminuria and onto frank infection or passage of renal casts. *0433*

Urine Normal Children usually have no WBC in their unspun microscopic urine examination. WBC aren't always present in these lower tract obstructions even with moderate symptoms unless infection is present. *0433* Urinalysis often shows no significant alteration from normal. *0433*

593.81   Renal Infarction

Alanine Aminotransferase *Serum Increase* Increased if area of infarction is large; peak by 2nd day; return to normal by 5th day with arterial infarction of kidney. *2468*

Aspartate Aminotransferase *Serum Increase* In unilateral renal arterial infarction. Reaches a peak within several days then gradually falls. *2104* Increased if area of infarction is large; peaks by 2nd day; returns to normal by 5th day with arterial infarction of kidney. *2468*

C-Reactive Protein *Serum Increase* With large infarction. *0186*

Creatine Kinase *Serum Normal* *0186*

Erythrocytes *Urine Increase* Common. *0186*

Lactate Dehydrogenase *Serum Increase* Occasional increase but to no clinically useful degree. May be increased markedly with arterial infarction of kidneys. Peak on 3rd day; return to normal by 10th day. *2468 0503 0962*

Urine Increase May be increased markedly with arterial infarction of kidney. LD peaks on 3rd day; return to normal by 10th day. *2468 0962*

Leukocytes *Blood Increase* Increased if area of infarction is large; peaks by 2nd day; returns to normal by 5th day with arterial infarction of kidney. *2468*

Protein *Urine Increase* Common. *0186*

597.80   Urethritis

Bicarbonate *Serum Decrease* Reveals the degree of renal impairment. *0433*

Calcium *Serum Decrease* Reveals the degree of renal impairment. *0433*

Chloride *Serum Increase* Reveals the degree of renal impairment. *0433*

Creatinine *Serum Increase* Reveals the degree of renal impairment. *0433*

Leukocytes *Urine Increase* Renal impairment. *0433*

Phosphate *Serum Increase* Reveals the degree of renal impairment. *0433*

Potassium *Serum Increase* Reveals the degree of renal impairment. *0433*

Sodium *Serum Decrease* Reveals the degree of renal impairment. *0433*

Urea Nitrogen *Serum Increase* Reveals the degree of renal impairment. *0433*

599.00   Urinary Tract Infection

Angiotensin-Converting Enzyme (ACE) *Urine Increase* Activity was found to be significantly elevated. *0256*

Beta-Glucuronidase *Urine Increase* Of the 13 patients with positive bladder and negative ureteral cultures, 6 showed elevated activity. The mean value was 29.5 ± 15.7. Of 25 ureteral specimens (right or left) with negative cultures, 7 showed elevated activity (mean 25.5 ± 10.8 enzyme U). *0885*

Casts *Urine Increase* In uncomplicated acute symptomatic infections, urine sediment usually contains numbers of pus cells and WBC casts. *0962*

Erythrocyte Casts *Urine Absent* A variable number of RBCs may be present, but there are no RBC casts. *0962*

Erythrocytes *Urine Increase* A variable number of RBCs may be present, but there are no RBC casts. *0962*

Fibrin Split Products (FSP) *Plasma Increase* Elevation is much more common in fatal cases than in survivors. *2193*

Immunoglobulin IgA *Urine Increase* Mean concentration = 3.3 mg/24h. Secretory IgA locally produced in the bladder. *1237*

Leukocytes *Urine Increase* In uncomplicated acute symptomatic infections, urine sediment usually contains numbers of pus cells and WBC casts. *0962*

Neutrophils *Urine Increase* The median values for polymorphonuclear granulocytes were > 90% in bacterial renal or urinary tract disease and in polycystic kidney disease. *1411*

Protein *Urine Increase* Proteinuria to the extent of +2 (usually < 2 g/24h) occurs. *0962*

600.00   Benign Prostatic Hypertrophy

Acid Phosphatase *Serum Increase* May have slight elevations after vigorous prostatic massage. *0503* Ordinary digital rectal palpation of the prostate produced significantly raised activities in 3 of 24 patients. *0492* Elevated in 7% of 141 cases. *1647*

Albumin *Urine Increase* The urinalysis may be completely normal or may reveal albuminuria, pyuria, and hematuria as a result of obstruction with infection or stone formation. *0433*

Amylase *Serum Increase* Reported in 95% of patients with benign disease and 70% of carcinomas. Similar results have not been reported elsewhere. *0973*

Androgens *Plasma Increase* Increased testosterone; especially in older patients. *0972*

Cholesterol *Serum Increase* In patients with residual urine, nonesterified cholesterol was elevated in 42.1% and total levels in 61.4%. Patients with no residual urine had normal cholesterol. *1196*

Creatinine *Serum Increase* In 53% of 58 patients at initial hospitalization for this disorder. *0781*

Erythrocytes *Urine Increase* The urinalysis may be completely normal or may reveal albuminuria, pyuria, and hematuria as a result of obstruction with infection or stone formation. *0433*

Urine Normal The urinalysis may be completely normal or may reveal albuminuria, pyuria, and hematuria as a result of obstruction with infection or stone formation. *0433*

Gonadotropin, Pituitary *Serum Decrease* Patients with both malignant and benign prostatic disease showed lower concentrations of luteinizing hormone when compared with age-matched controls. *0971*

Hematocrit *Blood Decrease* Anemia may be present secondary to uremia. *0433*

Hemoglobin *Blood Decrease* Anemia may be present secondary to uremia. *0433*

Leukocytes *Urine Increase* The urinalysis may be completely normal or may reveal albuminuria, pyuria, and hematuria as a result of obstruction with infection or stone formation. *0433*

Urine Normal The urinalysis may be completely normal or may reveal albuminuria, pyuria, and hematuria as a result of obstruction with infection or stone formation. *0433*

Luteinizing Hormone (LH) *Serum Decrease* Patients with both malignant and benign prostatic disease showed lower concentrations when compared with age-matched controls. *0971*

Monocytes *Blood Increase* In 63% of 73 patients at initial hospitalization for this disorder. *0781*

Neutrophils *Blood Increase* In 44% of 73 patients at initial hospitalization for this disorder. *0781*

Progesterone *Plasma Increase* Increased; especially in older patients. *0972*

Protein *Urine Increase* Normal or increased. *0186*

Urine   Normal   Normal or increased. *0186*

Testosterone   *Plasma   Increase*   Increased; especially in older patients. *0972*

Urea Nitrogen   *Serum   Increase*   In 29% of 80 patients at initial hospitalization for this disorder. *0781*

Uric Acid   *Serum   Increase*   In 48% of 80 patients at initial hospitalization for this disorder. *0781*

601.00   Prostatitis

Amylase   *Serum   Increase*   Moderate increase in total concentration. *2486*

Aspartate Aminotransferase   *Serum   Increase*   In 26% of 15 patients at initial hospitalization for this disorder. *0781*

Eosinophils   *Blood   Increase*   In 45% of 13 patients at initial hospitalization for this disorder. *0781*

Isocitrate Dehydrogenase   *Serum   Normal   2260*

Leukocytes   *Urine   Increase*   Following prostatic massage the last portion of voided urine shows an increased WBC compared with the first portion. *0186*

Prostatic Fluid   Increase   Since the presence of increased number of leukocytes and oval fat bodies are seen equally in cases of chronic bacterial prostatitis and nonbacterial prostatitis, the microscopic appearance of the expressed prostatic secretions is not specifically diagnostic. *0433*   In the chronic form, prostatic fluid usually shows 10-15 WBCs (pus cells) with prostatitis. *2468*

Neutrophils   *Blood   Increase*   In 30% of 13 patients at initial hospitalization for this disorder. *0781*

Oval Fat Bodies   *Prostatic Fluid   Increase*   Since the presence of increased number of leukocytes and oval fat bodies are seen equally in cases of chronic bacterial prostatitis and nonbacterial prostatitis, the microscopic appearance of the expressed prostatic secretions is not specifically diagnostic. *0433*

pH   *Prostatic Fluid   Increase*   The pH of prostatic secretions of males with chronic bacterial prostatitis reached a mean value of 8.1 during inflammation. Values for males without inflammatory prostatic disease was 6.7. *1812*

Protein   *Prostatic Fluid   Decrease*   Average amount of protein and protein-like substance was low 28.0 g/L, range 15.0-37.7, compared to normal 42.6, range 37.5-64. *0084*

602.80   Prostatic Infarction

Acid Phosphatase   *Serum   Increase*   Sometimes to high levels. *2467   1085*

606.90   Infertility in Males

Cadmium   *Serum   Normal*   No significant difference from fertile male controls. *2247*

Copper   *Serum   Decrease*   Infertile men (n = 8) had higher mean concentrations than those of proven fertility (n = 38) The difference was statistically significant. (P < 0.01) but was of small magnitude (about 1.5 μmol). *2247*

Serum   Increase   The mean concentrations were higher than in men of proven fertility (P < 0.01) but the increases were of small magnitude. *2247*

Immunoglobulin IgA   *Semen   Positive*   20 Patients tested and 50% were positive for sperm-bound IgA. *0408*

Immunoglobulin IgG   *Semen   Positive*   20 Patients tested and 100% were positive for sperm-bound IgG. *0408*

Immunoglobulin IgM   *Semen   Negative*   20 Patients tested and 0% positive for sperm-bound IgM. *0408*

Lead   *Blood   Normal*   No significant difference from fertile male controls. *2247*

Red Blood Cells   Normal   No significant difference between fertile and infertile males. *2247*

Prolactin   *Serum   Increase*   Four patients with oligospermia were found to have slightly to moderately elevated levels. *2562*

Zinc   *Serum   Normal*   No significant difference from fertile male controls. *2247*

Red Blood Cells   Normal   No significant difference between fertile and infertile males. *2247*

620.20   Ovarian Cyst

Pregnanediol   *Urine   Increase*   Increased in luteal cysts of ovary. *2468*

Progesterone   *Plasma   Increase*   Increased in luteal cysts of ovary. *2468*

627.90   Menopausal and Postmenopausal Symptoms

17-Ketosteroids   *Urine   Decrease   2468*

Estrogens   *Urine   Decrease*   The urinary excretion of total estrogens will be below 10 μg/24h. Values above 20 μg/24h are suggestive of a pathologic process such as a granulosa cell tumor. *0433*

Follicle Stimulating Hormone (FSH)   *Serum   Increase   0433*

Gonadotropin, Pituitary   *Urine   Increase   0433 2468*

Luteinizing Hormone (LH)   *Serum   Increase   0433*

PREGNANCY, COMPLICATIONS OF PREGNANCY AND THE PUERPERIUM

630.00   Hydatidiform Mole

Alpha-Fetoprotein   *Serum   Normal*   Undetectable in 100% of patients with intact mole, but > 10 ng/mL in 18 of 23 normal pregnancies. *1613*

Carcinoembryonic Antigen   *Serum   Normal*   Only 1 of 17 patients had a value > 2.5 ng/mL in serum. In all cases, the hydatid fluid had values > 2.5 and the range was 3-40 ng/mL. *0564*

Estrogens   *Serum   Increase*   Plasma unconjugated estradiol was greater than normal in 6 of 13 patients with intact mole, ranging from 1.82-8.10 ng/mL at 15-19 weeks gestation. *1613*

Factor II   *Plasma   Decrease*   May be associated with defibrination resulting in platelet and coagulation factor consumption. *2538*

Factor IV   *Plasma   Decrease*   May be associated with defibrination resulting in platelet and coagulation factor consumption. *2538*

Fibrinogen   *Plasma   Decrease*   Decreased as a result of excess utilization due to release of tissue thromboplastin. *0619*   May be associated with defibrination resulting in platelet and coagulation factor consumption. *2538*

Fibrin Split Products (FSP)   *Plasma   Increase*   Increased circulating amounts with associated prolonged thrombin time indicate hypercoagulability. *1430*

Gonadotropin, Chorionic   *Serum   Increase*   High concentrations of chorionic gonadotropin and reduced pregnanediol indicate diagnosis. *2104*   Human chorionic somatomammotropin was > normal in 8 of 13 patients with intact mole, ranging from 10-910 ng/mL. *1613* 0.5-2,830 IU/mL and less than 200 IU/mL in 36% of the patients. *1667*

Urine   Increase   A rising titer at the end of t trimester is significant. Titers can rise to 1,000 IU/L or more. *0619*

Gonadotropin, Pituitary   *Serum   Increase   0962*

Hemoglobin, Fetal   *Blood   Increase   2467*

Partial Thromboplastin Time   *Plasma   Decrease*   Mean time was 32.9/37.1 s in patients compared to 33.6/35.9 in normal pregnancy. Associated with prolonged thrombin time and indicates hypercoagulability. *1430*

Platelet Count   *Blood   Decrease*   May be associated with defibrination resulting in platelet and coagulation factor consumption. *2538*

Pregnanediol   *Urine   Decrease*   High concentrations of chorionic gonadotropin and reduced pregnanediol suggests diagnosis. *2104*

Progesterone   *Plasma   Decrease*   High concentrations of chorionic gonadotropin and reduced pregnanediol indicate diagnosis. *2104*

Plasma   Increase   Higher progesterone concentration than found in normal pregnant women in 8 of 13 patients with intact mole, ranging from 17.5-79.2 ng/mL. *1613*

Protein Bound Iodine (PBI)   *Serum   Increase*   Occasionally increased. *2467*

Prothrombin Consumption   *Blood   Increase*   May be associated with defibrination resulting in platelet and coagulation factor consumption. *2538*

Thrombin Time   *Plasma   Increase*   Mean time was 21.1/16.6 s in patients compared to 17.6/15.9 in normal pregnancy. Prolonged time and associated reduction of partial thromboplastin time indicates hypercoagulability and high fibrinogen turnover rate. *1430*

630.00   Hydatidiform Mole   (continued)

Thyroid Stimulating Hormone (TSH)   *Serum Increase*   9 of 14 patients were hyperthyroid. Found in high concentrations in 13 preoperative patients. Close correlation with human chorionic gonadotropins suggests that the hCG molecule, when present in large amounts, stimulates thyroid function. *1044*

Thyroxine (T$_4$)   *Serum Increase*   9 of 14 patients were hyperthyroid. T$_4$ varied from 18-34 mg/dL. *1044*   In patients with gestational trophoblastic disease without signs of hyperthyroidism, the mean serum total and free T$_4$ concentrations were 43% and 92% higher than those in normal pregnancy. *1740*

Tri-iodothyronine (T$_3$)   *Serum Increase*   9 of 14 patients were hyperthyroid. Serum T$_3$ ranged from 300-800 ng/dL. Correlated closely with chorionic gonadotropins. *1044*   High in 13 of 15 patients with molar pregnancy, paralleling that of T$_4$. *2487*

633.90   Ectopic Pregnancy

Amylase   *Serum Increase*   Associated with ruptured ectopic pregnancy. *1247*   Values of 2,000 U/L have been reported. *0744* Elevated levels *2646*

Erythrocyte Sedimentation Rate   *Blood Increase*   Rises in the first 24 h *0962*

Glucose   *Serum Increase*   In 45% of 11 patients at initial hospitalization for this disorder. *0781*

Gonadotropin, Chorionic   *Serum Decrease*   82.6% of 23 women with proven ectopic pregnancies had abnormally low first trimester hCG levels. *0273*   Decreased *0001 0265 1691 2115*

Urine Decrease   Low values for the stage of pregnancy. *0619*

Hematocrit   *Blood Normal*   May be normal, even in view of acute rupture of an ectopic pregnancy, as the patient has not had time for fluid stabilization. *0433*

Lactate Dehydrogenase   *Serum Increase*   In 4 of 10 patients at initial hospitalization for this disorder. *0781*

Leukocytes   *Blood Increase*   May increase but rarely to significantly high levels. *0433*

Blood Normal   *0433*

Lipase   *Serum Normal*   Normal levels. *1887*

640.00   Threatened Abortion

Alpha-Fetoprotein   *Serum Normal*   In patients with premature labor, the majority of concentrations were significantly below the normal range, and the peak levels were achieved approximately 1 month earlier than normal. In patients whose pregnancies were terminated by abortion, the levels exhibited a significant rise within a few h after induction because of resorption of fetal elements into the maternal circulation. *1008*

Gonadotropin, Chorionic   *Serum Decrease*   Decreased. *0001 0265 0299 1691*

Urine Decrease   Low values for stage of pregnancy. Low values in early pregnancy are found in habitual abortion. *0619*

Leucine Aminopeptidase   *Serum Increase*   High prior to abortion. *0619*

Pregnanediol   *Urine Decrease*   Sometimes. *2467*

Progesterone   *Plasma Decrease*   Has been reported to be low, but is often normal prior to spontaneous abortion. *2104*

T$_3$ Uptake   *Serum Increase*   *2467*

642.40   Pre-Eclampsia

Alanine Aminotransferase   *Serum Increase*   In about 20% of patients with mild cases. *0387*   Degree of abnormality closely parallels the severity. *0472 2311 1635*

Serum Normal   Usually are not elevated. When transaminases are found to be elevated, either pronounced hepatic or marked myocardial alterations have occurred. *0433*

Albumin   *Serum Decrease*   Significantly reduced below the levels for normal pregnancy. *0433*

Urine Increase   Characteristic but may appear late in the course of the disease. Fluctuates from day to day. *0387*

Aldosterone   *Plasma Decrease*   The secretory rate is somewhat depressed, but often falls within the lower range of normal for pregnancy. In severe cases, concentration was found to be within the range for nonpregnant women (10% of that of normal pregnancy). *2495*   Significantly suppressed during the last trimester despite levels of renin substrate and progesterone that were not significantly different from those observed in normotensive pregnancy. *2507 0387*

Plasma Increase   At term, hypertensive, toxemic pregnant women had elevated aldosterone and plasma renin activity, which remained elevated > 1 week after delivery. *0066*

Plasma Normal   In hypertensive groups, plasma renin activity and aldosterone concentration were significantly suppressed during the last trimester despite levels of renin substrate and progesterone that were not significantly different from those observed in normotensive pregnancy. *2507*   During normal pregnancy, plasma levels of renin, angiotensin II, and aldosterone are increased. Paradoxically with pregnancy-induced hypertension they commonly decrease towards the normal. *1859*

Urine Decrease   The secretory rate is somewhat depressed, but often falls within the lower range of normal for pregnancy. In severe cases, concentration was found to be within the range for non-pregnant women (10% of that of normal pregnancy). *2495*   Significantly suppressed during the last trimester despite levels of renin substrate and progesterone that were not significantly different from those observed in normotensive pregnancy. *2507 0387*

Urine Increase   At term, hypertensive, toxemic pregnant women had elevated aldosterone and plasma renin activity, which remained elevated > 1 week after delivery. *0066*

Urine Normal   In hypertensive groups, plasma renin activity and aldosterone concentration were significantly suppressed during the 1st trimester despite levels of renin substrate and progesterone that were not significantly different from those observed in normotensive pregnancy. *2507*   During normal pregnancy, plasma levels of renin, angiotensin II, and aldosterone are increased. Paradoxically with pregnancy-induced hypertension, they commonly decrease towards the normal. *1859*

Alkaline Phosphatase   *Serum Increase*   May be elevated above the normal increase found in pregnancy. This is due to a rise in the heat-stable (placental) isoenzyme. *2034*   Exaggerated increases may occur and could indicate placental as well as hepatic damage. *0387*

Serum Normal   Usually not elevated. When elevated, either pronounced hepatic or marked myocardial alterations have occurred. *0433 2034*

Alkaline Phosphatase Isoenzymes   *Serum Increase*   May be elevated above the normal increase found in pregnancy, due to a rise in the heat-stable (placental) isoenzyme. *2034*

Alpha$_1$-Globulin   *Serum Increase*   Significantly elevated. *0433*

Alpha$_2$-Globulin   *Serum Increase*   Significantly elevated. *0433*

Alpha$_2$-Macroglobulin   *Serum Decrease*   Mild. *1074*

Serum Increase   Low concentration of albumin and other small proteins may stimulate almost indiscriminate synthesis of many proteins. Larger molecules cannot leak through the glomeruli and accumulate in the blood. *2287 2286   0387*

Antidiuretic Hormone   *Serum Increase*   Positive correlation between severity of toxemia and circulating ADH. *2104*

Antithrombin III   *Plasma Decrease*   Noted in one patient with severe pre-eclampsia toxemia. *0312*

Aspartate Aminotransferase   *Serum Increase*   In about 20% of patients with mild cases. *0387*   Degree of abnormality closely parallels the severity. *0472 2311 1635*

Serum Normal   Usually are not elevated. When elevated, either pronounced hepatic or marked myocardial alterations have occurred. *0433*

Bicarbonate   *Serum Decrease*   Changes in electrolytes are usually insignificant. In severe cases, the bicarbonate may be lowered. *0387*

BSP Retention   *Serum Increase*   A larger proportion of hypertensive women have increased retention than normal pregnant women, (> 5% in 45 min), but many are in the range of normal. *0387*

Cephalin Flocculation   *Serum Increase*   34 of 72 women with mild disease had abnormal reactions. *0777   0387*

Complement, Total   *Serum Increase*   Significantly higher than in late normal pregnancy. *2286 0409*

Creatinine   *Serum Decrease*   Low BUN (9 ± 2 mg/dL) and low creatinine (0.75 ± 0.2 mg/dL) in late pregnancy are indicative of toxemia. *0151*

Serum Increase If the hypertension has reached relatively severe levels, may be elevated, indicating renal damage. *0433*

Cryofibrinogen *Serum Increase* Suggest that slow, chronic, intravascular clotting is taking place. *2538 2035 1549*

Deoxycorticosterone *Plasma Decrease* Plasma concentrations averaged 10.2 ± 2.7 ng/dL, which is about half the value found in normal pregnant women. *2510 0387*

Estrogens *Serum Decrease* Average serum and urinary estrogens were reduced in pre-eclampsia compared to normal pregnancy, but there was considerable overlap in values. *2332*

Urine Decrease Average serum and urinary estrogens were reduced in pre-eclampsia compared to normal pregnancy, but there was considerable overlap in values. *2332* In a series of 794 patients, hypoglycemia had a significant association with low estriol excretion, fetal growth retardation, and perinatal mortality. *1427* In 99 pre-eclamptic patients, the incidence of subnormal concentrations was 76%. *2543* Low values were found in 36% (23 of 64) patients. *2270*

Factor VIII *Plasma Decrease* In the ratio between factor VIII-related antigen and factor VIII activity a highly significant increase was observed during the 3rd trimester. The highest ratios were associated with either a perinatal death or with the delivery of a severely growth retarded infant. *2355*

Factor X *Plasma Decrease* Factor XII was significantly higher in 12 patients than in the normal group, while factors XI and X were slightly lower. *0432*

Factor XI *Plasma Decrease* Factor XII was significantly higher in 12 patients than in the normal group, while factors XI and X were slightly lower. *0432*

Factor XII *Plasma Increase* Factor XII was significantly higher in 12 patients than in the normal group, while factors XI and X were slightly lower. *0432*

Fibrinogen *Plasma Increase* Increased by about 70% and 145% in pre-eclampsia and eclampsia, respectively. *0380*

Plasma Normal Levels of fibrinogen and of other clotting factors do not differ from those found in normal late pregnancy. *0806* In essential hypertension, the level remains more or less the same as in normal pregnancy. *0380 2538*

Liver Increase Fibrin outlining the hepatic sinusoids was found in all 12 cases; in 2 of them there were also large nodular deposits of fibrin and to a lesser extent of IgG, IgM, and C3 in areas of necrosis. *0074*

Fibrin Split Products (FSP) *Plasma Decrease* Plasma fibrinolytic activity may be more depressed than in normal pregnancy. *0250 2538*

Plasma Increase Suggest that slow, chronic, intravascular clotting is taking place. *2538* Elevated levels (> 10 μg/mL) occurred in all patients. Mean level was 35 μg/mL. *1325*

Globulin *Serum Decrease* Significantly reduced below the levels for normal pregnancy. *0433*

Glomerular Filtration Rate (GFR) *Urine Decrease* Reduced 25-30% below the rate in normal pregnancy. *2104*

Glucose *Serum Decrease* In the total series of 794 patients, hypoglycemia had a significant association with low estriol excretion, fetal growth retardation, and perinatal mortality. *1427* The patients with severe pre-eclampsia had significantly lower fasting plasma glucose levels than those with mild pre-eclampsia and normal pregnancies. *2183*

Glycoproteins *Serum Increase* Concentration of alpha$_1$ easily precipitable glycoprotein increased greatly despite large urinary losses, indicating augmented synthesis. *2287 2286*

Urine Increase Large urinary losses of alpha$_1$ easily precipitable glycoprotein. *2287 2286 0387*

Gonadotropin, Chorionic *Serum Increase* Severe cases often are associated with high urinary and serum concentrations, and mild cases are not. *1431*

Serum Normal Average serum and urinary concentrations were the same in pre-eclamptic as in normal pregnant women. *2332*

Urine Increase Severe cases often are associated with high urinary and serum concentrations, and mild cases are not. *1431*

Urine Normal Average concentrations in urine and sera were the same in pre-eclamptic as in normal pregnant women. *2332*

Hematocrit *Blood Increase* Usually thrombocytopenia and high Hct values. *0887* Hemoconcentration is an index of severity; with grave prognosis if it increases or persists. *0387*

Hemopexin *Serum Decrease* Found to be significantly lower than in normal pregnancy. *2286*

Serum Normal No change was found compared to normal late pregnancy. *0409*

Immunoglobulin IgD *Serum Decrease* Significantly lower than in normal late pregnancy. *2285*

Immunoglobulin IgG *Serum Decrease* Significantly lower than in normal late pregnancy. *0170 1073 2285*

Immunoglobulins *Serum Decrease* Decreased; may predispose to infection, especially urinary tract infections. *2286 2287 0387*

Insulin *Serum Decrease* Both the fasting plasma insulin and insulin response following glucose injection were lower in patients with severe pre-eclampsia than in those with mild pre-eclampsia or a normal pregnancy. The differences however were not statistically significant. *2183*

Iron Saturation *Serum Decrease* Found to be significantly lower than in normal pregnant women. *2286*

Serum Normal No change was found compared to normal late pregnancy. *0409*

Isocitrate Dehydrogenase *Serum Increase* Frequently increased indicating placental degeneration within previous 48 h. *0619*

Lactate Dehydrogenase *Serum Increase* Rose to a mean value of 384.1 ± 31.8 U/L in severe pre-eclampsia, over the normal value in pregnancy of 154.5 - 12.2 U/L. *2034* Usually not elevated. When transaminases are found to be elevated, either pronounced hepatic or marked myocardial alterations have occurred. *0433*

Lactic Acid *Blood Decrease* Lower in pre-eclamptic women in the 3rd trimester than in normal pregnant women. *0688*

Lipoproteins, Beta *Serum Increase* Significantly elevated. *0433* Higher than in normal late pregnancy. *1073 2286 0409 0387 2287*

Nitrogen *Urine Increase* Urinary amines are increased in hypertension resulting from pregnancy. *2623*

Oxygen Saturation *Blood Decrease* In 9 patients with severe pre-eclampsia, there was a significant increase in alveolar-to-arterial pO$_2$ difference and physiological shunt, indicating a degree of pulmonary ventilation/perfusion imbalance. *2340*

Platelet Count *Blood Decrease* Evidence of intravascular coagulation, as shown by elevated levels of fibrin degradation products and reduced platelet counts, has been found in many women. *0251* An occasional patient is mildly to moderately thrombocytopenic. *0250* Usually thrombocytopenia and high hematocrit values. *0887 2538*

Blood Normal Usually within the normal range. *2143*

pO$_2$ *Blood Decrease* In 9 patients with severe pre-eclampsia, there was a significant increase in alveolar-to-arterial pO$_2$ difference and physiological shunt, indicating a degree of pulmonary ventilation/perfusion imbalance. *2340*

Pregnanediol *Urine Decrease* Reduced compared to normal pregnant women, but there was considerable overlap in values. *2332* In 58 women with mild pre-eclampsia, mean = 29.5 mg/24h, ranging from 6-63.8. The average decrease of 40% was not found significant because of the wide range of values in both normo- and hypertensive patients. *1218*

Progesterone *Plasma Decrease* Reduced compared to normal pregnant women, but there was considerable overlap in values. *2332* In 58 women with mild pre-eclampsia, mean = 29.5 mg/24h, ranging from 6-63.8. The average decrease of 40% was not found significant because of the wide range of values in both normo- and hypertensive patients. *1218*

Protein *Serum Decrease* Significantly reduced below the levels for normal pregnancy. *0433*

Urine Increase Hypertension, edema, and proteinuria characterize toxemia of pregnancy. *0151* This diagnosis is questionable without the presence of proteinuria. Renal leakage of small molecular weight proteins is characteristic. *0387*

Renin Activity *Plasma Decrease* In hypertensive groups, plasma renin activity and aldosterone concentration were significantly suppressed during the last trimester despite levels of renin substrate and progesterone that were not significantly different from those observed in normotensive pregnancy. *2507* During normal pregnancy, plasma levels of renin, angiotensin II, and aldosterone are increased. Paradoxically with pregnancy-induced hypertension they commonly decrease towards the normal. *1859*

Plasma Increase Greater increase in pre-eclamptic than in normal pregnant women. *2309* At term, hypertensive, toxemic pregnant women had elevated aldosterone and plasma renin activity, which remained elevated > 1 week after delivery. *0066 0387*

Plasma Normal Renin activity was found to be about the same, or less, than in normotensive pregnant women. *2421 0387*

642.40 Pre-Eclampsia (continued)

Sodium *Serum Decrease* Rarely. *0387* Serum concentrations tend to decline as severity increases. *2104*

Urine Decrease Reduced to a greater extent than that of normal pregnancy. *2104*

Thymol Turbidity *Serum Normal* No abnormal results were found in a study of 20 mild and 20 severe pre-eclamptic patients. *2597* Usually normal. *0429 0387*

Thyroxine (T$_4$) *Serum Increase* The mean serum T$_4$ and free T$_4$ concentrations were significantly higher than those in normal pregnant women. *1740*

Urea Nitrogen *Serum Decrease* Low (9 ± 2 mg/dL) and low creatinine (0.75 ± 0.2 mg/dL) in late pregnancy are indicative of toxemia. *0151*

Serum Increase If the hypertension has reached relatively severe levels, may be elevated, indicating renal damage. *0433*

Uric Acid *Serum Increase* Elevations of plasma urate is an early feature of pre-eclampsia. *1899* Perinatal mortality was markedly increased when maternal plasma-urate concentration were raised, generally in associated with severe pre-eclampsia of early onset. Maternal hypertension, even severe, without hyperuricemia, was associated with an excellent prognosis for the fetus. When maternal hypertension was mild and hyperuricemia was severe, the prognosis for the fetus was poor. *1898 1283*

Serum Normal Values may or may not be elevated in severe cases. When elevated, may represent liver or kidney dysfunction. *0433*

Viscosity *Serum Increase* Apparent blood viscosity rises sharply as the hematocrit increases due to hemoconcentration. *0387*

Volume *Plasma Decrease* Hemoconcentration is an index of severity and prognosis. *0387*

Red Blood Cells Normal In 14 cases in the late stages, mean red cell volume was identical with that of normal pregnant women in the same gestational period. *0224*

642.60 Eclampsia

17-Hydroxycorticosteroids *Urine Increase* Increased due to severe stress. *2467*

17-Ketogenic Steroids *Urine Increase* Increased due to severe stress. *2467*

Alanine Aminotransferase *Serum Increase* Degree of abnormality closely parallels the severity. *1635* All 14 patients had normal activities on the day of convulsion. On the 2nd day, the test became progressively abnormal and peaked on the 5-7th day postpartum. *0500* Presumably due to ischemic damage to liver cells. *0322*

Albumin *Serum Decrease* Significantly reduced below the levels for normal pregnancy. *0433*

Urine Increase Characteristic finding. Reflects severity of disease. *0387*

Aldosterone *Plasma Increase* At term, hypertensive, toxemic pregnant women had elevated aldosterone and plasma renin activity, which remained elevated > 1 week after delivery. *0066*

Urine Decrease Less than concentrations usually found in normal pregnancy. *0619*

Alpha$_1$-Globulin *Serum Increase* Significantly elevated. *0433*

Alpha$_2$-Globulin *Serum Increase* Significantly elevated. *0433*

Amino Acids *Plasma Increase 0619*

Amylase *Serum Decrease* Severe liver damage. *2467*

Antidiuretic Hormone *Serum Increase* Positive correlation between severity of toxemia and circulating ADH. *2104*

Aspartate Aminotransferase *Serum Increase* Degree of abnormality closely parallels the severity. *1635 0472* Presumably due to ischemic damage to liver cells. *0322*

Bicarbonate *Serum Decrease* Usually reduced. Not uncommon to see values < 13.5 mmol/L. *0621*

Bilirubin *Serum Increase* Elevated in only 3 of 134 patients, and those cases were only minimally elevated. *0429* Uncommon. In 134 women, including 45 with eclampsia, only 3 had levels > 1.2 mg/dL, with 2.3 mg/dL as the highest value. *1859 0387*

Serum Normal Seldom elevated, even in severe eclampsia. *0387*

Calcium *Serum Normal 0621*

Catecholamines *Urine Increase* Increased due to severe stress. *2467*

Cephalin Flocculation *Serum Increase* 11 of 16 cases were reported to be abnormal. *2447* Higher incidence of abnormal reactions in hypertensive than in normotensive pregnancies. *0387*

Chloride *Serum Decrease* With marked edema. *0621*

Clotting Time *Blood Decrease* Markedly reduced. *1012*

Complement, Total *Serum Normal 1764*

Creatinine *Serum Decrease* Low BUN (9 ± 2 mg/dL) and low creatinine (0.75 ± 0.2 mg/dL) in late pregnancy are indicative of toxemia. *0151*

Serum Increase If the hypertension has reached relatively severe levels, may be elevated, indicating renal damage. *0433*

Estrogens *Serum Decrease 2212*

Fibrinogen *Plasma Decrease* A serious complication. *1012*

Plasma Increase Increased by about 70% and 145% in pre-eclampsia and eclampsia, respectively. *0380*

Globulin *Serum Decrease* Significantly reduced below the levels for normal pregnancy. *0433*

Glomerular Filtration Rate (GFR) *Urine Decrease* Reduced 25-30% below the rate in normal pregnancy. *2104*

Glucose *Serum Increase* Occasionally following eclamptic fit. *0621*

Glucose Tolerance *Serum Decrease* Due to either hepatic dysfunction or relative insulin resistance. *0322*

Glutathione *Serum Normal 0621*

Gonadotropin, Chorionic *Serum Increase* Not demonstrable in all cases. *2211*

Urine Increase Not demonstrable in all cases. *2211*

Hematocrit *Blood Increase* Hemoconcentration is an index of severity; with grave prognosis if it increases or persists. *0387*

Immunoglobulins *Serum Decrease* Predisposes patients to infections, especially urinary tract infections. *2286 2287 0387*

Lactic Acid *Blood Increase* Only after convulsions. *0621*

Leukocytes *Blood Increase* Intoxications due to metabolic causes can cause leukocytosis. *2467*

Lipids *Urine Increase* Lipids in the urine include all fractions. Double refractile (cholesterol) bodies can be seen. There is a high protein content. *2467*

Lipoproteins, Beta *Serum Increase* Significantly elevated. *0433*

Magnesium *Serum Decrease* Both serum and CSF concentrations were found to be low. *0093*

CSF Decrease Both serum and CSF concentrations were found to be low. *0093*

Neutrophils *Blood Increase* May be associated with a moderate to severe neutrophilia. *2538*

Nitrogen *Serum Increase* Blood-urea tends to decrease, but amino acids and unknown substances are increased. *0619*

Urine Increase Urinary amines are increased in hypertension resulting from pregnancy. *2623*

Phosphate *Serum Increase* Slight increase. *0621*

Platelet Count *Blood Decrease* Marked reduction in some patients with severe toxemia. *1012*

Pregnanediol *Urine Decrease 2467*

Progesterone *Plasma Decrease* Appears to be unrelated to the severity of the condition. *2104 2212*

Protein *Serum Decrease* Significantly reduced below the levels for normal pregnancy. *0433*

Serum Increase Secondary to hemoconcentration. *1012*

Urine Increase Hypertension, edema, and proteinuria characterize toxemia of pregnancy. *0151* As a result of hemoconcentration. *0621* Constant finding. *0387*

Prothrombin Time *Plasma Increase* Higher than normal in pregnant patients. *1012*

Renin Activity *Plasma Decrease* In hypertensive groups, plasma renin activity and aldosterone concentration were significantly suppressed during the last trimester despite levels of renin substrate and progesterone that were not significantly different from those observed in normotensive pregnancy. *2507* During normal pregnancy, plasma levels of renin, angiotensin II, and aldosterone are increased. Paradoxically with pregnancy-induced hypertension, they commonly decrease towards the normal. *1859*

Plasma Increase At term, hypertensive, toxemic pregnant women had elevated aldosterone and plasma renin activity, which remained elevated > 1 week after delivery. *0066*

Plasma Normal Average concentration and activity are slightly less than in normotensive pregnancies, but nearly all values in each group are in the same range. *0387 2421*

Sodium *Serum Decrease* Rarely. *0387* Reduced concentrations as a result of hemodilution. Averages 4-8 mmol/L lower than in normal nonpregnant women. *2104*

Urine Decrease Reduced to a greater extent than that of normal pregnancy. *2104*

Thymol Turbidity *Serum Normal* Usually normal. *0429 0387*

Urea Nitrogen *Serum Decrease* Low (9 ± 2 mg/dL) and low creatinine (0.75 ± 0.2 mg/dL) in late pregnancy are indicative of toxemia. *0151* Tends to decrease. *0619*

Serum Normal No significant increase. *0621*

Uric Acid *Serum Increase* Serial determinations to follow therapeutic response and estimate prognosis. *2467* Hyperuricemia usually precedes the development of azotemia due to reduced urate clearance. *0151* Consistently observed. *0621*

Viscosity *Serum Increase* Apparent blood viscosity rises sharply as the hematocrit increases due to hemoconcentration. *0387*

Volume *Plasma Decrease* Hemoconcentration is an index of severity and prognosis. *0387* In severe cases. *0621*

Red Blood Cells Normal In 14 cases in the late stages of eclampsia and pre-eclampsia, mean red cell volume was identical with that of normal pregnant women in the same gestational period. *0224*

650.00 Pregnancy

5'-Nucleotidase *Serum Normal* Normal in pregnancy and the postpartum period (in contrast to serum leucine aminopeptidase and alkaline phosphatase); therefore may aid in differential diagnosis of hepatobiliary disease occurring during pregnancy. *2467*

11-Hydroxycorticosteroids *Plasma Increase* Rises progressively throughout pregnancy. *2084*

17-Hydroxycorticosteroids *Urine Increase* Primarily during 3rd trimester. *0071*

17-Ketogenic Steroids *Urine Increase* *2467*

17-Ketosteroids *Urine Increase* Last trimester. *0503*

Alanine Aminopeptidase *Serum Increase* *1443*

Alanine Aminotransferase *Serum Normal* Incidence of abnormal activities is < 5%. *0387 2359*

Albumin *Serum Decrease* Decreased 22% and total globulins were unchanged. *2287 2286* Usually falls abruptly in early pregnancy and then more slowly during late. *1755* Levels decreased progressively after the first trimester *0517 0387*

Aldosterone *Plasma Increase* Among the normotensive subjects plasma renin activity, aldosterone and progesterone concentrations were elevated as early as the 6th week of gestation. While consistent, progressive, further increases were noted in renin substrate, aldosterone and progesterone during pregnancy. *2507* In hypertensive patients. *2494 0387*

Urine Increase In the 3rd trimester of normal pregnancy. *0619*

Alkaline Phosphatase *Serum Increase* Increase is due entirely to the heat stable form of the enzyme produced exclusively in the placenta. *1557* Marked increase to term *0517 0503 0387 2020*

Leukocyte Increase Increases are directly proportion to period of gestation and returned to normal after 4th week postpartum. *0081* Elevation of score has been found in high risk pregnancies due to diabetes mellitus, toxemia, renal diseases and 3rd trimester hemorrhage, but not in pregnancies complicated by cardiac disease. *1610* Activities obtained from 20 pregnant women were markedly elevated in all cases. Mean value was 187 with a range of 98-242. *1563 1424*

Alkaline Phosphatase Isoenzymes *Serum Increase* Elevation is due to circulating placental isoenzyme. *0213* Heat-stable isoenzyme progressively increases as pregnancy approaches term. If > 50% of total serum concentration is heat stable, placenta size is compatible with mature fetus in maternal serum. *2467 2020*

Alpha₁-Antichymotrypsin *Serum Increase* Many acute phase reactants are elevated during pregnancy, but pregnancy has been associated with only a slight elevation of this enzyme. *1248*

Alpha₁-Antitrypsin *Serum Increase* Increased in advanced stages. *1866 0042 1946 1947 2129* Increased in 96% in late normal pregnancy *2286 2287*

Alpha₁-Globulin *Serum Increase* Markedly increased during last 2 trimesters of pregnancy. *2468* Rises about 0.1 g/dL. *2533*

Alpha₂-Antiplasmin *Serum Normal* No significant change in pregnant woman or those taking contraceptive pills compared with age and sex related controls. *2337*

Alpha₂-Globulin *Serum Increase* Increased in last 2 trimesters of pregnancy. *2468* Rises about 0.1 g/dL. *2286*

Alpha₂-Macroglobulin *Serum Increase* *2614 2412*

Alpha-Fetoprotein *Serum Increase* In a screening study 1.2 % had raised levels. Of these 25/249 had babies with neural tube defects, an additional 13/249 had other congenital defects. *1599* Substantial increase in concentration in the maternal circulation during pregnancy *1195* Ranged from 10-80 ng/mL in 18 of 23 normal pregnancy *1575 2116*

Amino Acids *Urine Increase* During normal pregnancy increased amounts of histidine and threonine are excreted, returning to normal during lactation. *0619* Much larger quantities. *0400 2619*

Amylase *Serum Increase* Salivary amylase, present in small quantities in nonpregnant women as well as in men, show a substantial increase in concentration in the maternal circulation during pregnancy. *1195* May be associated with hyperamylasemia. *1386 1209*

Serum Normal *0323*

Androgens *Plasma Increase* Mean testosterone concentration in pregnant women with female fetuses was 597 ± 167 pg/mL, and in women with male fetuses, mean value was 828 ± 298 pg/mL, significantly higher (p = < 0.01). Increases began in week 7, reaching a maximum by 9-11. *1284*

Angiotensin-Converting Enzyme (ACE) *Serum Decrease* It is thought to be caused by enzyme consumption in the kinin system which is activated by pregnancy. *0608*

Serum Normal Levels didn't change throughout pregnancy. *0609*

Antithrombin III *Plasma Decrease* Last trimester and early postpartum. *2353 1482*

Arylsulfatase *Serum Increase* *0919 2182* 30-50% increase in serum activity *0610*

Ascorbic Acid *Serum Decrease* May be decreased, reaching lowest level in the postpartum period. *0211*

Aspartate Aminotransferase *Serum Decrease* Abnormal pyridoxal metabolism. Usual values 0-3 U/L. *0503*

Serum Normal Incidence of abnormal findings is < 5%. *0387 2359*

Basophils *Blood Decrease* *2467 0532*

Blood Increase *0532*

Beta-Globulin *Serum Increase* Slightly increased in second trimester of pregnancy. *2468* Rises progressively by about 0.3 g/dL. *0791*

Beta-Glucuronidase *Serum Increase* Increased. *0741 0866*

Urine Increase Moderately elevated (33.7 ± 23.4 U/L); approximately 50% of the values were above normal. 50% of the patients in the gestation period from 20-32 weeks showed elevated urinary enzyme activity. *0885* Mean activity in 17 patients was 35.2 U/L. Eight had values > the normal upper limit. *1525*

Bicarbonate *Serum Decrease* Decreased markedly throughout pregnancy. *0517* An effect of progesterone; slight decrease *1460*

Urine Increase Alkalosis is prevented by renal excretion of bicarbonate to offset the loss of CO₂ from the blood. *1460*

BSP Retention *Serum Increase* Abnormal retention occurs during last month of pregnancy. *2468* The rate of BSP clearance is slower in normal pregnancy, but after 60 min only 4 of 20 had more than a trace left. *2214 0387*

Calcium *Serum Decrease* Levels decreased progressively after the first trimester. *0517* Insufficient calcium, phosphorus and vitamin D ingestion *2467*

Carotene *Serum Increase* Increased. *0299 1030 1032*

Cephalin Flocculation *Serum Increase* Reported prevalence of abnormal reactions in normal pregnancy range from 0-35%, the average in 986 cases is 12%. *0387*

Ceruloplasmin *Serum Increase* Approximately twice normal at term. Mechanism not known. *2636* Normal pregnancy *0304* Increased in last trimester of pregnancy *2468*

Chloride *Serum Normal* Throughout pregnancy. *0517*

Cholesterol *Serum Increase* Third trimester of pregnancy with sustained elevations until several weeks after delivery. *0503* Increases after 8th week to maximum by 30th week in pregnancy. *2468 0913*

Chromium *Serum Decrease* Compared to non pregnant. *0966*

Cold Agglutinins *Serum Increase* Occasionally. *2468*

Complement, Total *Serum Increase* Beta-1 A-C component of complement was increased in 39% of late normal pregnancies. *2287 2286*

Serum Normal *1764*

650.00 Pregnancy (continued)

Copper *Serum Increase* During normal pregnancy the concentration in maternal serum may almost double due to increased synthesis of ceruloplasmin. Value were lower in abnormal pregnancies than in normal ones. *0304* Higher in early and late pregnancy. *0969* Approximately twice normal at term. Mechanism not known. *2636 0576*

Cortisol *Plasma Increase* Most plasma proteins decrease with the exception of alpha₁ globulins which account for elevation of protein-bound iodine and blood cortisol. *0433*

Creatine *Urine Increase* It has been suggested that renal tubular reabsorption is depressed. *0619*

Creatine Kinase *Serum Decrease* Decreased during 8th-20th week (maximum at 12th week). *2468*

Serum Increase Increased during the last few weeks and remains elevated through parturition, becoming normal approximately 5 days postpartum. *0962*

Creatinine *Serum Decrease* Slightly lower in the pregnant state than the nonpregnant state. *0433* Decreases approximately 25%, especially during first 2 trimesters. Creatinine of 1.2 mg/dL is definitely abnormal in pregnancy although normal in nonpregnant women. *2468* Level in pregnancy 0.46 mg ± 0.13 mg/dL compared to 0.67 mg ± 0.14 mg/dL for controls. *2179* Decreased markedly throughout pregnancy *0517*

Creatinine Clearance *Urine Increase* *2179*

Cryofibrinogen *Serum Increase* *0856*

Deoxycorticosterone *Plasma Increase* Plasma concentration is double the normal value in late pregnancy. *2510* *0387*

Erythrocytes *Blood Decrease* Decreased < 10-15% because of increased plasma volume during pregnancy. *2468*

Erythrocyte Sedimentation Rate *Blood Increase* Increased from the 3rd month to about 3 weeks postpartum. Due to increased fibrinogen during pregnancy. *2468* *0433*

Erythropoietin *Serum Increase* Striking increase. *1113*

Estriol *Urine Decrease* The predominant urinary estrogen during pregnancy is E3. Declining values indicate fetal jeopardy. *0002 0605 0046*

Estrogens *Serum Increase* *0484*

Urine Increase Increase from 6 months to term 100 µg/24h). *2468 0484*

Estrone *Serum Increase* Ten fold increase during pregnancy. *1177 1432 2385*

Factor II *Plasma Increase* Increased in late pregnancy. *2468*

Factor VII *Plasma Increase* Increased in late pregnancy. *2468*

Factor VIII *Plasma Increase* Increased activity has been reported. *1194*

Factor IX *Plasma Increase* Concentration rises during pregnancy. *0035*

Factor X *Plasma Increase* Normally increase as pregnancy advances. A secondary increase in XI and X may occur in the puerperium. Cord levels of all 3 factors are decreased. *0432*

Factor XI *Plasma Decrease* Decreased in late pregnancy. *2468*
Plasma Increase Factor X, XI, and XII normally increase as pregnancy advances. A secondary increase in XI and X may occur in the puerperium. Cord levels of all 3 factors are decreased. *0432*

Factor XII *Plasma Increase* Factor X, XI, and XII normally increase as pregnancy advances. A secondary increase in XI and X may occur in the puerperium. Cord levels of all 3 factors are decreased. *0432*

Fatty Acids, Free (FFA) *Serum Increase* Significant use in the 36th and 40th week of gestation. *2104*

Fibrinogen *Plasma Increase* Increases progressively as the pregnancy Moderately increased by 4th month; increased 33% by term. *2468* Rises from 0.38 g/dL to 0.58 g/dL. *1892*

FIGLU (N-Formiminoglutamic Acid) *Urine Increase* Increased in pregnancy, especially with toxemia and increased age, parity, and multiple pregnancy. *2467*

Folate *Serum Decrease* *2538*

Follicle Stimulating Hormone (FSH) *Serum Normal* Upper end of normal range. *0690*

Globulin *Serum Decrease* May decrease slightly in last trimester. *2468* Falls about 0.1 g/dL. *2533* *2286 2287*

Serum Normal Albumin was decreased and total globulins were unchanged in late normal pregnancy. *2286 2287*

Glomerular Filtration Rate (GFR) *Urine Increase* Renal plasma flow is increased during pregnancy. *2468*

Glucose *Serum Decrease* Occasionally decreased. *2468*
Serum Normal *1542*

Urine Increase The renal threshold for glucose may decrease, and some patients may show glycosuria without elevated blood sugar levels. *0433* Incidence about 35%. *0386*

Glucose Tolerance *Serum Decrease* In 124 pregnant women during the 4th quartile of pregnancy, 9-21% of women were abnormal, and using the H index, 43% would have been declared diabetic. There was no evidence of a progressive change in the glucose curve detectable by the H index nor association between actual or potential fetal morbidity. *0481*

Serum Increase Decreased formation of glycogen with low fasting levels and subsequent hypoglycemia. Normal return to fasting level. *2467* In 124 pregnant women during the 4th quartile of pregnancy, 9-21% of women were abnormal, and using the H index 43% would have been declared diabetic. There was no evidence of a progressive change in the glucose curve detectable by the H index nor association between actual or potential fetal morbidity. *0481*

Gonadotropin, Chorionic *Serum Increase* Multiple pregnancies. *0001 0265 0299 1691*

Urine Increase *0294*

Growth Hormone *Serum Normal* *2593*

Haptoglobin *Serum Decrease* Decreased 16% in late normal pregnancy. *2286 2287*

Hematocrit *Blood Decrease* Blood volume increases with a disproportionate increase in plasma volume so that the hematocrit will fall slightly as pregnancy progresses. *0433* Anemia is most often caused or aggravated by a concomitant iron deficiency. *2538 0165*

Hemoglobin *Blood Decrease* Decreases slightly to as low as 10 g/dL, with corresponding decrease of hematocrit during pregnancy. *2468* Anemia is most often caused or aggravated by a concomitant iron deficiency. *2538 0165*

Hemoglobin A₁c *Blood Increase* *0794*

Hemopexin *Serum Normal* Unchanged in late normal pregnancies. *2286 2287*

Hexosaminidase *Serum Increase* Increase in total concentration (hexosaminidase A and B). *1716*

Hippuric Acid *Urine Decrease* Reduced excretion in normal pregnancy. *1350* *0387*

Hydrochloric Acid *Gastric Material Decrease* Gastric HCl may be decreased. *2468*

Immunoglobulin IgG *Serum Increase* Progressive increase. *2286* *2287*

Immunoglobulins *Serum Decrease* Diminish during gestation and reach lowest levels in early postpartum period. *2104*

Insulin *Serum Increase* Excess of circulating insulin in the fasting state. *0811*

Iron *Serum Decrease* Progressive fall from midterm onwards, with rising total iron binding capacity. *0619* Anemia is most often caused or aggravated by a concomitant iron deficiency. *2538 0165* Reduced at term to about 35% below the mean in nonpregnant women. *1629*

Iron-Binding Capacity, Total (TIBC) *Serum Increase* In late pregnancy. *2612* In normal pregnancy, the total IBC rises to about 450 µg/dL, while the serum iron falls. *0619*

Iron Saturation *Serum Increase* Increased in 49% in late normal pregnancy. *2286 2287* Increased saturation in early pregnancy. *2612*

Isocitrate Dehydrogenase *Serum Increase* Increased in 3rd trimester. *2468* *0491*

Serum Normal Well within the normal range in term pregnancies. *2559* *1561*

Ketones *Urine Increase* *2467*

Lactate Dehydrogenase *Serum Increase* Increases variably in normal pregnancy. *0387* *0491*

Serum Normal *1561*

Lactate Dehydrogenase Isoenzyme 5 (LD₅) *Serum Increase* Mother carrying erythroblastotic child. LD₄ and LD₅. *2467* *0491*

Serum Normal *0491*

Lactate Dehydrogenase Isoenzymes *Serum Increase* Mother carrying erythroblastotic child. LD-4 and LD-5. *2467* *0491*

Serum Normal *0491*

Lactose *Urine Increase* May be present in the urine late in pregnancy, giving a positive test for reducing substances. *0433* Particularly in the afternoon during late pregnancy. *0619*

Leucine Aminopeptidase *Serum Increase* Normal early but increases steadily to > 2 X the normal value at full term. *0281* *1597*

Leukocytes *Blood Increase* During late pregnancy and labor. *2468 0433*

Lipase *Serum Decrease* Less than 50% of nonpregnant level. *0686*

Lipids *Serum Increase* Total serum lipids rise to a maximum by the 30th week, and regain prepregnancy levels by the 8th week postpartum. The increase is due to equal rises in cholesterol and phospholipids. *0619 1891*

Magnesium *Serum Decrease* Decreased progressively from early pregnancy to term. *0517*

Malate Dehydrogenase *Serum Increase* Variable increase in normal pregnancy. *0387*

Manganese *Serum Normal 0966*

MCH *Blood Normal 1113*

MCHC *Blood Normal 1113*

MCV *Blood Increase* Macrocytic anemia may occur due to vitamin B_{12} or folate deficiency. MCV > 100 fL. *0532*

Blood Normal 1113

Neutrophils *Blood Increase* Occurs almost entirely in the last trimester but is present in only about 20% of patients. *1329 2538*

Osmotic Fragility *Red Blood Cells Increase* Cells may have become more spherical due to inibition of water. *1113*

Parathyroid Hormone *Serum Increase* Decreased during midgestation and increases thereafter to clearly elevated levels. *1909*

pCO₂ *Blood Decrease* May be induced by progesterone. *1512 1460* Begins to fall early in gestation and persists at 5 mm Hg below normal until parturition. *2104*

Pepsin *Gastric Material Decrease* May be decreased. *2468*

pH *Blood Increase* Slight rise accompanies reduced alveolar pCO_2. *2104*

Gastric Material Increase May occur. *2468*

Phosphate *Serum Decrease* Levels decreased progressively after the first trimester. *0517* Sometimes a slight decline in serum concentration may occur with no serious complication *1287*

Plasma Cells *Serum Decrease* Late pregnancy. *2357 0659 0683*

Plasminogen *Serum Increase 1443*

Porphyrins *Urine Increase* May be increased. *2468*

Potassium *Serum Normal* Throughout pregnancy. *0517*

Pregnanediol *Urine Increase* Rises progressively as pregnancy progresses, with a slight fall in the last 2 weeks. Range was 26-79.4 mg/24h, with an average of 50. *1218 0850*

Progesterone *Plasma Increase* Among the normotensive subjects, concentrations were elevated as early as the 6t of gestation. While consistent, progressive, further increases were noted in renin substrate, aldosterone and progesterone during pregnancy, renin activity did not continue to rise. *2507* Mean plasma concentrations were 60% higher in twin pregnancies than in normal simplex pregnancies. *0133 1578*

Prolactin *Serum Increase* Increase in a linear pattern, related to supramaximal estrogen augmentation and is a reflection of hypertrophy and hyperplasia of pituitary lactotrophs. *1938* Mean plasma concentrations of human placental lactogen were 60% higher in twin pregnancies than in normal simplex pregnancies. *0133* Can trigger a mild to moderate increase (20-300 ng/mL). *0133*

Protein *Serum Decrease* Most plasma proteins decrease with the exception of alpha₁ globulins. *0433 1113*

Urine Increase The presence of proteinuria and pregnancy in the absence of blood pressure elevation increases perinatal mortality to at least twice the rates of patients without proteinuria. *0516*

Protein Bound Iodine (PBI) *Serum Increase* From about the 4th week until up to 6th week postpartum. *2467* Most plasma proteins decrease with the exception of alpha₁ globulins which account for elevation of protein-bound iodine and blood cortisol. *0433* In normal pregnancy the level may rise to 15 mg/dL. The level falls in threatened abortion. *0619 2104*

Protoporphyrin *Red Blood Cells Increase 0249*

Renin Activity *Plasma Increase* Highest in the first trimester and decreases thereafter. Both concentration and activity are increased. *2194* Among the normotensive subjects, activity was elevated as early as the 6th week of gestation. While consistent, progressive, further increases were noted in renin substrate, aldosterone and progesterone continue to rise. Renin activity did not continue to rise. *2507 0387*

Sodium *Serum Decrease* Average reduction in cations (chiefly sodium) was 4.7 mmol/L during pregnancy. *1690*

Serum Normal Throughout pregnancy. *0517*

T₃ Uptake *Serum Decrease* From about the 10th week of pregnancy until up to 12th week postpartum. *2467* Combination of raised T_4 and low resin uptake due to increased TBG concentration occurs in pregnancy, estrogen therapy, and oral contraceptive use. *2612*

Testosterone *Plasma Increase* Mean concentration in pregnant women with female fetuses was 597 ± 167 pg/mL, and in women with male fetuses, mean value was 828 ± 298 pg/mL, significantly higher (p = < 0.01). Increases began in week 7, reaching a maximum by 9-11. *1284 1031*

Thymol Turbidity *Serum Normal* Found to be normal in a study of 40 normal pregnant women. *2597* Usually normal. *0429 0387*

Thyroid Stimulating Hormone (TSH) *Serum Decrease 2467*

Serum Normal 1113

Thyroxine Binding Globulin *Serum Increase* Due to estrogen stimulation. *0791* Combination of raised T_4 and low resin uptake due to increased resin uptake due to increased TBG concentration occurs in pregnancy, estrogen therapy, and oral contraceptive use. *2612 2540 2104*

Thyroxine Binding Prealbumin *Serum Decrease* Decreased 27% in late normal pregnancy. *2287 2286*

Thyroxine Index, Free (FTI) *Serum Normal* Normal even though T_3 and T_4 alone are abnormal. *2467 1446*

Thyroxine (T₄) *Serum Increase* Elevation thought to be caused by an increase in T_4 binding protein secondary to high circulating-estrogen levels. *0999* Elevated in normal pregnancy, while free T_4 and free T_3 are normal. *1740* Combination of raised T_4 and low resin uptake due to increased TBG concentration occurs in pregnancy, estrogen therapy, and oral contraceptive use. *2612*

Triglycerides *Serum Increase* Steep rise. *0930*

Tri-iodothyronine (T₃) *Serum Increase* The total T_3 is elevated, thought to be caused by an increase in T_4 binding protein secondary to high circulating-estrogen levels. *0999* Elevated in normal pregnancy, while free T_4 and free T_3 are normal. *1740*

Urea Nitrogen *Serum Decrease* Slightly lower than in the nonpregnant state. *0433* 18 mg/dL is definitely abnormal in pregnancy although normal in nonpregnant women. Decreases approximately 25%, especially during first 2 trimesters. *2468* Found to be 8.7 mg ± 1.5 from the 15th week of pregnancy to term compared to 13.1 mg ± 3.0 for nonpregnant subjects. *2179* Decreased markedly throughout pregnancy *0517 0503*

Uric Acid *Serum Decrease* Averages 3.86 mg/dL in nonpregnant controls compared to 2.72 mg/dL before 16 weeks of pregnancy, 2.6 mg/dL between 17 and 28 weeks and 3.61 mg/dL after 28 weeks. May explain the observation that gout tends to improve in pregnancy. *0266* Decreased in early pregnancy but returned to normal by term. *0517*

Uropepsinogen *Urine Increase* Moderate increase in output. *0619*

Vitamin B₁₂ *Serum Decrease* Progressive decrease during pregnancy. *2467*

Vitamin E (Tocopherol) *Serum Increase* Average is about 65% higher than normal at term. *2104*

Volume *Plasma Increase* The increment averages 40% above nonpregnant values, its magnitude varying with the parity of the mother and with her body composition. *1108* Begins to increase about the 6th week and reaches a maximum between the 26-36 weeks. *0387 2538*

Urine Increase May increase up to 25% in last trimester. *2468*

Red Blood Cells Increase Red cell volume actually increases by about 20%. *2538* Although both plasma volume and RBC mass increase, plasma volume increases earlier and proportionately more, leading to relative hemodilution, the physiologic anemia of pregnancy. *1108* Increases progressively throughout pregnancy but proportionately less than does the plasma volume. *1858*

Zinc *Serum Decrease* In 84 women with complications such as abnormal labor or atonic bleeding, serum concentrations were significantly reduced during early pregnancy. Women who gave birth to immature infants delivered in the 37th week or earlier or in the 43rd week or later showed significantly lower serum zinc during early pregnancy compared to women delivered in the 40th week. *1143* Lower in early and late pregnancy *0969*

656.40 Pregnancy Complicated by Intrauterine Death

Estrogens *Urine Decrease 0619*

Gonadotropin, Chorionic *Urine Normal 2467*

Pregnanediol *Urine Decrease* Fetal death. If < 5 mg/24h then abortion is inevitable. *0619*

656.40 Pregnancy Complicated by Intrauterine Death (continued)

Progesterone *Plasma Decrease* Fetal death. If < 5 mg/24h then abortion is inevitable. *0619*

Uric Acid *Serum Increase* Perinatal mortality was markedly increased when maternal plasma-urate concentrations were raised, generally in association with severe pre-eclampsia of early onset. Maternal hypertension, even severe, without hyperuricemia, was associated with an excellent prognosis for the fetus. When maternal hypertension was mild and hyperuricemia was severe, the prognosis for the fetus was poor. *1898*

DISEASES OF THE SKIN AND SUBCUTANEOUS TISSUE

691.80 Atopic Eczema

Cyclic Adenosine Monophosphate *Lymphocytes Decrease* Individuals in the severe eczema group were shown to have a significant diminution in their unstimulated lymphocyte cAMP concentrations and absolute responses. *1770*

Eosinophils *Blood Increase* *2538*

Immunoglobulin IgE *Serum Increase* Atopic subjects tend to have moderate increases. *0619* Total serum concentration was elevated in 75-81% of the children with asthma, nasal allergy and atopic dermatitis and an elevated serum concentration or blood eosinophilia, or both, was noted in 85% of the patients. *0405* Some patients. *2035* *0642*

694.00 Dermatitis Herpetiformis

Antibody Titer *Serum Increase* Reticulin antibodies. *1670*

Eosinophils *Blood Increase* Occurs in some skin diseases. *2467* In 36% of 11 patients at initial hospitalization for this disorder. *0781* *0532* *2538*

Fat *Feces Increase* In small intestinal disease. *2199*

HLA Antigens *Blood Present* HLA antigen DR2 found in 97% of patients with this disease compared to 25% of controls. *2051* HLA-DR3 found in 77% of patients versus 20% of controls. *2539* HLA-B8 and HLA-Bw15 associated with this disease. *2191*

Lactate Dehydrogenase *Serum Increase* In 25% of 12 patients at initial hospitalization for this disorder. *0781*

Monocytes *Blood Increase* In 63% of 11 patients at initial hospitalization for this disorder. *0781*

Neutrophils *Blood Increase* In 45% of 11 patients at initial hospitalization for this disorder. *0781*

694.40 Pemphigus

Albumin *Serum Decrease* In untreated patients in the advanced stage of disease. Often drops to 25% of normal. *0743*

Alpha₁-Globulin *Serum Increase* *0151*

Alpha₂-Globulin *Serum Increase* *0151*

Antibody Titer *Serum Increase* Numerous studies have confirmed the presence of autoantibodies specific for an intercellular substance of skin and mucosa in serum from patients with active pemphigus. *0642*

Calcium *Serum Decrease* *0151*

Chloride *Serum Decrease* *0151*

Complement Fixation *Serum Increase* 50-75% of bullous pemphigoid patients have serum antibodies capable of fixing complement to the basement membrane. *2035*

Complement, Total *Serum Decrease* Cryoproteins observed in patients with pemphigus have been shown to contain IgG, complement components, and other serum proteins. *1612*

Cryoglobulins *Serum Increase* When observed in patients with pemphigus have been shown to contain IgG, complement components, and other serum proteins. Appeared in the clinically active stage and disappeared subsequent to clinical improvement. *1612*

Eosinophils *Blood Decrease* In severely ill patients the percentage, even if previously high, drops off - often to 0%. *0743*

Blood Increase Slight or absent eosinophilia in pemphigus foliaceous. *0743* Moderately increased percentage in pemphigus vulgaris. *0743* *0532* *2538*

Erythrocyte Sedimentation Rate *Blood Increase* Increased globulin, especially fibrinogen, probably accounts for the increased ESR. *0151*

Fibrinogen *Plasma Increase* *0151*

Globulin *Serum Increase* *0151*

Hematocrit *Blood Decrease* Anemia is common and may be due to inanition, serum loss and infection. *0151*

Hemoglobin *Blood Decrease* Anemia is common and may be due to inanition, serum loss and infection. *0151*

Immunoglobulin IgE *Serum Increase* Significant increase in 70% of bullous pemphigoid patients. *2035*

Immunoglobulin IgM *Serum Increase* About 70% of patients with this condition have elevated levels. *2373*

Indirect Fluorescent Antibodies *Serum Increase* Numerous studies have confirmed the presence of autoantibodies specific for an intercellular substance of skin and mucosa in serum from patients with active pemphigus. *0642*

Leukocytes *Blood Increase* Usually elevated with an increase of immature forms. *0151*

Potassium *Serum Increase* *0151*

Protein *Serum Decrease* Total serum protein may fall as low as 3.6 g/dL with a correspondingly low level of albumin. *0151* May fall to 50% of normal in untreated patients with advanced disease. *0743*

Sodium *Serum Decrease* *0151*

Volume *Plasma Increase* *0151*

695.10 Erythema Multiforme

Eosinophils *Blood Increase* Occurs in some infectious diseases. *2467* *0532*

Erythrocytes *Urine Increase* *0151*

696.10 Psoriasis

Alpha₁-Glycoprotein *Serum Increase* Elevated levels in states associated with cell proliferation. *1239 1672 1866 1947 2096 2170*

Angiotensin-Converting Enzyme (ACE) *Serum Normal* Not significantly different in Psoriatic arthritis (n = 12) from normal controls. *1443* . Normal in cutaneous Psoriasis. *2346* Levels remained normal *2346*

Dehydroepiandrosterone (DHEA) *Serum Decrease* *0299 2356 2540*

Eosinophils *Blood Increase* *2538*

Fat *Feces Increase* Steatorrhea has been reported in association with psoriasis; degree correlated with extent of involvement. *2157 0743*

Folate *Serum Decrease* Decreased with extensive skin disease. *0299 2357 0367*

HLA Antigens *Blood Present* HLA-Cw6 present in 50% of caucasian patients versus 23% of controls. *2539* HLA-B₂7 associated with psoriatic spondylitis. *2191*

Uric Acid *Serum Increase* Slight elevation may occur, especially in male patients. *1343* Increased with increased extent and severity of cutaneous lesions. *0743* Found in 30-40% of patients. *2104* Increased nucleic acid turnover. *2612* *1283*

Zinc *Serum Decrease* Decreased. *2297 0910*

706.10 Acne

Androgens *Plasma Increase* Elevated in 38% of 26 females with acne between ages 27 and 42 y. *2074* In a group of 34 women with this condition 80% had an androgen excess *2082*

Androstenedione *Serum Increase* Elevated in 38% of 26 females with acne between ages 27 and 42 y. *2074*

Dehydroepiandrosterone Sulfate (DHEA-S) *Serum Increase* Elevated in 38% of 26 females with acne between ages 27 and 42 y. *2074* Women with acne and hirsutism had increased levels compared to a group with acne only. *1020*

Ferritin *Serum Increase* 19 of 24 males had increased levels. *1387*

Hematocrit *Blood Decrease* 25% of patients with severe nodulocystic disease had mild anemia. *1387*

Hemoglobin *Blood Decrease* 25% of patients with severe nodulocystic disease had mild anemia. *1387*

Iron *Serum Decrease* Found in 75% of patients with severe nodulocystic disease. *1387*

Iron-Binding Capacity, Total (TIBC) *Serum Normal* Normal levels in 29 patients with severe nodulocystic disease. *1387*

Iron Saturation *Serum Decrease* 11 of 24 patients with severe nodulocystic disease had decreased levels. *1387*

Testosterone *Serum Increase* Elevated in 38% of 26 females with acne between ages 27 and 42 y. *2074*

Serum Normal Free and total testosterone were measured in 34 men and 14 women suffering from acne but otherwise healthy. *2294*

708.90   Urticaria

Basophils *Blood Decrease* 0532

Blood Increase 0532

Calcium *Serum Normal* In acute and chronic urticaria, mean serum values did not differ significantly from control groups. Only 7 cases had abnormal values. Abnormal calcium metabolism is not associated with urticaria and calcium treatment is not indicated. *1169*

Complement C3 *Serum Normal* Patients with hereditary angioedema have decreased levels of C1 esterase inhibitor and C4 in the presence of normal amounts of C3 and C1q. Normal values for these complement components are found in persons with allergic angioedema. *0272*

Complement C4 *Serum Decrease* Patients with hereditary angioedema have decreased levels of C1 esterase inhibitor and C4 in the presence of normal amounts of C3 and C1q. Normal values for these complement components are found in persons with allergic angioedema. *0272* Low C4 or C1 esterase confirms clinical diagnosis of hereditary angioedema. *0766*

Complement, Total *Serum Decrease* Patients with hereditary angioedema have decreased levels of C1 esterase inhibitor and C4 in the presence of normal amounts of C3 and C1q. Normal values for these complement components are found in persons with allergic angioedema. *0272* 10 of 72 patients were found to have decreased total complement hemolytic activity. *1524   0743*

Eosinophils *Blood Increase* Characterized by a mild, persistent eosinophilia despite rather profound tissue involvement. *2538* In 34% of 28 patients at initial hospitalization for this disorder. *0781*

Monocytes *Blood Increase* In 50% of 28 patients at initial hospitalization for this disorder. *0781*

Neutrophils *Blood Increase* In 28% of 28 patients at initial hospitalization for this disorder. *0781   2538*

DISEASES OF THE MUSCULOSKELETAL SYSTEM AND CONNECTIVE TISSUE

710.00   Systemic Lupus Erythematosus

5'-Nucleotidase *Serum Increase* In 2 cases elevated to 13 and 26 U/L. *1312*

Alanine Aminotransferase *Serum Increase* May be found in patients with myositis. *0433*

Albumin *Serum Decrease* Found in 50-66% of patients. *0677* Low serum concentration (2.5% g/dL) were found in 8% of 39 patients. *2081* Indicates the severity of excessive protein loss; tends to rise in the improving patient. *0782*

Serum Normal In patients with low grade activity and those in remission the serum concentration remain within the normal range. *0354* In 39 patients serum concentrations were stable throughout the course of SLE. *2081*

Urine Increase The most common abnormality ranging from mild to intermittent to nephrotic levels (> 3.56 g/24h). *0433   0962*

Aldolase *Serum Increase* May be found in patients with myositis. *0433*

Alpha₁-Antichymotrypsin *Serum Increase* Collagen vascular diseases. *1248   1168*

Alpha₁-Antitrypsin *Serum Increase* Increased. *1866 0042 1946 1947 2129   2467*

Alpha₁-Globulin *Serum Increase* Moderate increase. *0619*

Alpha₁-Glycoprotein *Serum Increase* One of the most reliable indicators of acute inflammation. *1239 1672 1866   1947 2096 2170*

Alpha₂-Globulin *Serum Increase* A less specific but frequent abnormality. *0433* Marked increase. *0619* May be elevated in lupus nephritis. *0962*

Amylase *Pleural Effusion Increase* Elevation in pleural fluid may occur. *1584*

Angiotensin-Converting Enzyme (ACE) *Serum Increase* *1398 2014*

Antibodies to dsDNA *Serum Increase* Found in 49% of cases. *2204*

Antibodies to Histones *Serum Increase* Found in 46% of cases. *2204* Found in 50% of patients. *1503* Found in 100% of patients with drug induced SLE. *0062*

Antibodies to RNP *Serum Increase* Found in 34% of cases. *2204*

Antibodies to Sjögren Syndrome A *Serum Increase* Found in 35% of cases. *2204* Found in 100% of neonatal SLE cases. *0062*

Antibodies to Sjögren Syndrome B *Serum Increase* Found in 5% of cases. *2204* 15% of cases. *1670*

Antibodies to SmAg *Serum Increase* Found in 23% of cases. *2204* Present in 30% of cases. Highly diagnostic. *1670*

Antibodies to ss-DNA *Serum Increase* Found in 42% of cases. *2204*

Antimitochondrial Antibodies *Serum Increase* 8% of patients were positive. *0619* Found in 18% of patients and 2% of controls. *1840*

Antinuclear Antibodies *Serum Increase* Present in 97.7% of patients (44 of 45) tested using immunofluorescent technique. *0321* Titers were higher in patients with nephritis than in a control group of SLE patients without nephritis but were no higher than in scleroderma. *1771* Nearly all patients with active SLE are positive. Titers vary according to the intensity of disease activity. *0999* Present in high titer but only low titers were found in other rheumatoid diseases. *1707* Appearance of antibody to DNA frequently (40% of the time) heralds an approaching clinical flare within several months. *0782* 95-100% positivity. *1799* Found in 100% of cases *2204   0713*

Serum Normal Of 165 patients with SLE a subgroup of 8 patients with active SLE yet with persistently negative tests for antinuclear factor and LE cells was identified. *0849* 10 patients with clinical signs of disease had persistently negative ANA tests. Raynaud's phenomenon, excessive hair fall and oral ulcers were frequent in this subgroup. *0728*

Synovial Fluid Increase 0962

Pleural Effusion Increase Indicates SLE. *0962*

Antismooth Muscle Antibodies *Serum Increase* Positive in 12% of patients and 6% of controls. *1840 2251*

Serum Normal Uniformly absent. *2528   2035*

Aspartate Aminotransferase *Serum Increase* May be found in patients with myositis. *0433*

Beta-Galactosidase *Serum Decrease* Mean serum concentration was 0.139 ± 0.019 mmol/min/L, compared with 0.243 ± 0.038 in controls. *1099*

Cellular Casts *Urine Increase* 0433

Cephalin Flocculation *Serum Increase* Positive; reflects nonspecific serum protein abnormalities. *0962*

Cholesterol *Serum Increase* Leading to nephrosis. *2467*

Cholesterol, High Density Lipoprotein *Serum Normal* Total lipid concentration was found to be low but HDL fraction was normal. *1435*

Chylomicrons *Synovial Fluid Increase* Chylous effusions have been reported. *1689 2012*

Coagulation Time *Blood Increase* Circulating anticoagulants are not rare but do not usually cause bleeding. *0962*

Cold Agglutinins *Serum Increase* Have been detected. *0962 2035*

Complement C1q *Serum Decrease* 2090

Complement C1r *Serum Decrease* 2090

Complement C1s *Serum Decrease* 2090

Complement C2 *Serum Decrease* 2090

Complement C3 *Serum Decrease* Concentration 63 ± 8 mg/dL in patients with subendothelial deposits, compared to 142 ± 27 mg/dL in controls. *0168* Reduced levels arise from increased catabolism and reduced synthesis which always occurs at some stage of active SLE. *1550 2198* 21 children had 52 episodes of C3 depression (mean duration 25 weeks); only 11 had active nephritis when concentrations were depressed. *2186* Especially low in patients with active nephritis. C5 is usually normal. *2090* Caused by hypercatabolism *0375 1275 0509*

Serum Increase Early in active disease the acute inflammatory response may cause increased C3 and C4 production. *1550*

Synovial Fluid Decrease Complement levels are very low. *0433*

710.00 Systemic Lupus Erythematosus *(continued)*

Complement C3 *(continued)*

Pleural Effusion *Decrease* *0062*

Pericardial Fluid *Decrease* Low or absent *0764 0877*

Complement C4 *Serum* *Decrease* Serum C4 levels was 8 ± 2 mg/dL in patients with subendothelial deposits, compared to 27 ± 6 mg/dL in patients with deposits. *0168* Reduced levels arise from increased catabolism synthesis which always occurs at some stage of active disease. *2198 1550* C4 occasionally remained depressed longer than C3, perhaps reflecting continuing subclinical disease activity. *2186* Especially low in patients with active nephritis. C5 is usually normal. *2090*

Serum *Increase* Early in active disease the acute inflammatory response may cause increased C3 and C4 production. *1550*

CSF *Decrease* Low CSF levels of C4 occur in patients with CNS involvement, due to in vivo immune reaction. *2090*

Synovial Fluid *Decrease* Complement levels are very low. *0433*

Pleural Effusion *Decrease* *0062*

Pericardial Fluid *Decrease* Low or absent *0764 0877*

Complement, Total *Serum* *Decrease* Reduced in about 75% of patients with active disease. Reduction may be correlated with the activity of the illness and varies inversely with ANA titers. *2089* Reduced levels arise from increased catabolism and reduced synthesis which always occurs at some stage of active SLE. *2198 1550* Low C1 (C1q and C1s), C2, C3, and C4 occur in active SLE. Especially low in patients with active nephritis. C5 is usually normal. *2090* Found in 80 (57%) patients. *0713* In 35 patients, 77% had decreased values. In discoid lupus, 57% had elevated levels. *2223 0999*

Serum *Increase* Normal or elevated. *0151* Early in active SLE the acute inflammatory response may cause increased C3 and C4 production. *1550* In discoid lupus, 57% had elevated levels. *2223*

CSF *Decrease* Abnormally low C4 levels. *1700*

Synovial Fluid *Decrease* May be markedly reduced below the complement level of serum. *1700* Marked decrease in synovial fluids. *1796* Low levels may occur in some patients. *2090* Compared to total protein, levels are low in 60-70% of joint effusions *0314*

Pleural Effusion *Decrease* 5 of 7 cases showed reduced levels of CH50, C1, C1 inhibitor and C2 in pleural fluid. *0854* Low complement (< 10 U/mL) in 11 of 12 patients with SLE or rheumatoid pleuritis. *1403*

Pericardial Fluid *Decrease* Low or absent *0764 0877*

Coombs' Test *Blood* *Positive* A positive test is frequently associated with active hemolysis but may be seen in individuals without markedly shortened RBC survival. *0999* Positive in 18-65% of patients in different studies, but only 10% of these manifest significant hemolysis. *0309* About 5% of patients may develop hemolytic anemia. Direct Coombs' test is almost always positive in these cases. *0962* *0713*

Copper *Serum* *Increase* Increased. *2052 1729* Increase in collagen diseases *2467 0619*

C-Reactive Protein *Serum* *Increase* C-reactive proteins and other acute phase reactants are elevated and remain elevated to some degree during periods of apparent remission. *0999* *0962*

Creatine *Serum* *Increase* Correlates well with severity of morphologic lesions. *1047*

Urine *Increase* Increased breakdown. *2467*

Creatine Kinase *Serum* *Increase* May be found in patients with myositis. *0433*

Creatinine *Serum* *Increase* Serum creatinine and BUN were increased, indicating uremia. *1269* Most reliable variable for estimation of renal involvement. *0782*

Creatinine Clearance *Urine* *Decrease* Mean decrease in clearance of 18% was accompanied by a 14% inulin clearance fall, and correlated with the prostaglandin E levels. *1269*

Cryofibrinogen *Serum* *Increase* *2035 1138 1551*

Cryoglobulins *Serum* *Increase* Increased cryoglobulins were found in patients with severe lesions and in no instance did it occur simultaneously with rheumatoid factor which was found in milder lesions. *1047* Found in 7-90% of patients in various studies; associated with disease activity especially nephritis. *0402* Variable elevations of cryoglobulins. *2104*

Erythrocyte Casts *Urine* *Increase* In lupus glomerulonephritis it is not unusual to find a sediment in which all the formed elements and casts seen in various stages. *0962*

Erythrocytes *Urine* *Increase* Levels of hematuria and proteinuria correlate well with severity of morphologic lesions. *1047* *0433* *0962*

Erythrocyte Sedimentation Rate *Blood* *Increase* Frequently and markedly elevated, even in the presence of apparently mild disease activity due to the presence of abnormal globulins. *0962* *0433 0999*

Factor B *Plasma* *Decrease* *1979 2356*

Fibrinogen *Plasma* *Increase* Frequently elevated. *0962*

Fibrin Split Products (FSP) *Plasma* *Increase* Elevated levels (> 10 µg/mL) occurred in 100% of lupus nephritis patients. Mean value was 21.4 ± 7.6 µg/mL. *1325*

Globulin *Serum* *Increase* A less specific but frequent abnormality. *0433* Serum globulin concentrations in excess of 4.0 g/dL are seen in over 50% of cases. *0999* Increase in about 70% of patients *0677* Marked increase occur in patient with proteinuria *1902 2087*

Glucose *Synovial Fluid* *Decrease* Less than 25 mg/dL, lower than blood. *0666*

Pleural Effusion *Normal* *0962*

Glycoproteins *Serum* *Increase* Have been found to be elevated but are nonspecific. *0962*

Granular Casts *Urine* *Increase* In lupus glomerulonephritis it is not unusual to find a sediment in which all the formed elements and casts seen in various stages. *0962* *0433*

Haptoglobin *Serum* *Decrease* Decreased if associated with hemolytic anemia. *2467*

Hematocrit *Blood* *Decrease* Significant anemia, usually normocytic, normochromic, found in 58% (81) of cases. *0713* The most common hematologic abnormality occurring in 57-78% of patients. May be caused by hypersplenism, iron deficiency, renal disease, drugs, antierythrocyte antibody and complement. *0309* Reflects disease activity in patients both with and without renal disease. *0782* Less than 30% in 53% of patients. *0714*

Hemoglobin *Blood* *Decrease* Anemia, usually normocytic, is present in the majority of cases and is frankly hemolytic with a positive Coombs' test in < 10% of the cases. *0433* Significant anemia, usually normocytic, normochromic, found in 58% (81) of cases. *0713* The most common hematologic abnormality occurring in 57-78% of patients. May be caused by hypersplenism, iron deficiency, renal disease, drugs, antierythrocyte antibody and complement. *0309*

Hexosamine *Serum* *Increase* Hexosamine and other acute-phase reactants are elevated and remain so to some degree during period of apparent remission. *0999* Have been found to be elevated but are nonspecific. *0962*

HLA Antigens *Blood* *Present* HLA-DR3 present in 70% of patients versus 28% of controls. *2539* HLA-DR2 and HLA-DR3 frequently associated with whites with this disease. *1503* HLA-A17, HLA-B8, HLA-DR2 and HLA-DR3 associated with this disease. *2191*

Hyaline Casts *Urine* *Increase* *0433*

Immunoglobulin IgA *Serum* *Increase* Mean concentrations were within the normal range at diagnosis (271 ± 171 mg/dL) but increased significantly to 349 ± 210 mg/dL during follow-up (P < 0.05) in 39 patients. *2081* Level decreased progressively after the first trimester *0517* Slightly elevated except in the presence of protein-losing nephropathy. *0962*

CSF *Increase* Elevation of IgG index was noted in 70% of patients, IgA index in 77% and IgM index in 100% of 13 patients when compared with 20 controls with other neurological disorders. *1887*

Immunoglobulin IgD *Serum* *Increase* *0619*

Immunoglobulin IgG *Serum* *Increase* The IgG dynamics differed from those of IgA and IgM by high mean IgG concentrations at diagnosis (1492 ± 835 mg/dL) and a significant decrease to 1195 ± 748 mg/dL during follow-up. The pattern was characterized by an inverse relation of IgA and IgG; while IgA concentrations increased significantly during follow-up, a parallel decrease in IgG occurred. *2081* Marked increase in untreated patients, 18.7 ± 5.1 g/L, with only a moderate correlation with disease activity. *1047* Slightly elevated except in the presence of protein-losing nephropathy. *0962*

CSF *Increase* Elevation of IgG index was noted in 70% of patients, IgA index in 77% and IgM index in 100% of 13 patients when compared with 20 controls with other neurological disorders. *1887*

Immunoglobulin IgM *Serum* *Increase* Increased from a mean value of 88 ± 52 mg/dL at diagnosis to 113 ± 181 mg/dL during follow-up. *2081* Slightly elevated except in the presence of protein-losing nephropathy. *0962* *0354*

CSF Increase Elevation of IgG index was noted in 70% of patients, IgA index in 77% and IgM index in 100% of 13 patients when compared with 20 controls with other neurological disorders. *1887*

Immunoglobulins *CSF Increase* *2104*

Inulin Clearance *Urine Decrease* A mean decrease of 14% was observed in 7 female patients. *1269*

Iron Saturation *Serum Decrease* *2467*

Lactate Dehydrogenase *Serum Increase* Significantly higher in patients with diffuse proliferative lupus nephritis. *1124*

Urine Increase With nephritis. *2467*

Lactate Dehydrogenase Isoenzymes *Serum Increase* Significantly higher in patients with diffuse proliferative lupus nephritis. Serum levels of total LD, LD_1 and LD_2. *1124* LD_3 and LD_4 *2467*

LE Cells *Blood Increase* Most patients will develop positive tests during their illnesses but SLE is not excluded without a positive test. *0999* The LE test was concluded to be insensitive, nonspecific, and did not correspond to clinical activity of the patient. *0820* Found in 76% (107) of 140 patients. *0713* 28 of 45 (63.5%) patients had positive results. *0321* Of 165 patients, 8 patients with active disease yet with persistently negative tests for ANA and LE cells were identified. *0849* *2087*

Synovial Fluid Increase May be present in synovial fluid. *2468*

Leukocytes *Blood Decrease* Leukopenia (< 4,000/µL) is common, and frequently is important in implicating SLE rather than infection or other inflammatory diseases which may cause similar clinical manifestations. *0433* A moderate leukopenia (1,800-4,000/µL) is seen in 70% of patients at some point in their courses and is often associated with a lymphopenia. *0999* Mild leukopenia in 68 patients (49%) with counts between 2,000-4,000/µL. *0713* Reduction in total count in almost 50% of all patients. *0309*

Urine Increase *0433*

Synovial Fluid Increase 5,000/µL. *0962* Usually low (< 5,000/µL) with a low percentage of neutrophils. *0433* Usually does not not exceed 3,000/µL. *1700*

Lipids *Serum Decrease* Total lipid concentration was found to be low but HDL fraction was normal. *1435*

Lymphocytes *Blood Decrease* Overall depression of peripheral blood leukocytes frequently with a lymphopenia and a slight shift to the left in the granulocytic series. *0433* In 158 patients with active, untreated disease, lymphopenia was present in 75%, and another 18% of those patients developed lymphopenia subsequent to disease reactivation. Lymphopenia of < 1,500 occurred more frequently than any of the preliminary criteria and it was the most prevalent initial laboratory abnormality. *1949*

Lymphocyte T-Cell *Blood Decrease* *0793*

Monocytes *Blood Increase* Was reported. *1489* *2538*

Urine Increase 29-33% mononuclear cells were found in lupus nephritis and endemic benign nephropathy. *1411*

Mucopolysaccharides *Urine Increase* Have been found to be elevated but are nonspecific. *0962*

Mucoprotein *Serum Increase* Mucoproteins and other acute-phase reactants are elevated and persist to some degree during periods of apparent remission. *0999*

Neutrophils *Blood Decrease* Reduced counts in 7 of 21 cases. 62% had a subnormal response to etiocholanolone challenge, indicating reduced marrow reserves. *1267* Present in well over 50% of patients. *0454* There is usually an overall depression of peripheral blood leukocytes, frequently with a lymphopenia and a slight shift to the left in the granulocytic series. *0433* *2538*

Synovial Fluid Decrease WBC are usually low (< 5,000/µL) with a low percentage of neutrophils. *0433*

Bone Marrow Decrease Reduced counts in 7 of 21 cases. 62% had a subnormal response to etiocholanolone challenge, indicating reduced marrow reserves. *1267*

Partial Thromboplastin Time *Plasma Increase* *0962*

pCO2 *Blood Decrease* Impaired gas diffusion and the accompanying hyperventilation results in a low pCO_2, unless the defect is severe and CO_2 retention occurs. *2104*

pH *Pleural Effusion Decrease* Exudate (pH < 7.3). *0062*

Platelet Count *Blood Decrease* Thrombocytopenia (< 100,000/µL) is common and is most frequently mild without purpura. Severe thrombocytopenia may occur, but purpura is rarely the presenting manifestation. *0433* Mild thrombocytopenia in 32 patients (23%). Purpura or bleeding noted in 5 cases. *0713* May occur, due to increased destruction. *0309*

Blood Normal Most patients have increased production and increased peripheral destruction, with a normal circulating platelet count. *0309*

Potassium *Serum Increase* Two patients with long standing disease had persistent hyperkalemia apparently due to defect in renal tubular secretion. *0527*

Precipitins *Serum Increase* Found in 15% of patients and 3% of controls. *0344*

Prostaglandins *Urine Increase* The mean pretreatment excretion of urinary immunoreactive Prostaglandin E, 42.7 ± 6.4 ng/h, was significantly higher than the value of 29.0 ± 1.9 ng/h for normal subjects. *1269*

Protein *Serum Normal* In 39 patients serum total protein and albumin concentrations were stable throughout the course of disease. *2081*

Urine Increase Levels of hematuria and proteinuria correlate well with severity of morphologic lesions. *1047* Generally precedes hematuria and red cell casts, although small degrees of renal involvement may occur without proteinuria. *0782* Changes in the amount of proteinuria do not reflect histologic changes in the kidneys. *0962*

CSF Increase In patients with neurologic symptoms. *1700*

Synovial Fluid Decrease Synovial fluid may be a transudate with low protein content (< 3 g/dL), especially in patients with asymptomatic joint effusions associated with nephritis and edema. In other patients with inflammatory joint signs, the fluid is an exudate with increased protein content (3-5 g/dL). *0433*

Synovial Fluid Increase Synovial fluid may be a transudate with low protein content (< 3 g/dL), especially in patients with asymptomatic joint effusions associated with nephritis and edema. In other patients with inflammatory joint signs, the fluid is an exudate with increased protein content (3-5 g/dL). *0433*

Prothrombin Time *Plasma Increase* A prolonged time may suggest the possibility of a circulating anticoagulant, which is particularly likely to be found in patients with a chronic false positive serologic test for syphilis. *0433*

Rheumatoid Factor *Serum Increase* Positive tests (titer of 1:80 or more) were found in 50% (61) of patients. *0713* Rheumatoid factors are present in almost 50% of patients at some time during their course, but intermittently and at low titer. *0999* In 15% of cases. *1700*

Specific Gravity *Pleural Effusion Increase* Exudate (> 1.016). *0062*

Thromboplastin Generation *Blood Increase* The type of anticoagulant most commonly found inhibits the conversion of prothrombin to thrombin and exhibits prolonged thromboplastin and prothrombin times. *0962*

Thymol Turbidity *Serum Increase* Frequently positive and reflects nonspecific serum protein abnormalities. *0962*

Urea Nitrogen *Serum Increase* Elevated, usually > 100 mg/dL. Indicates uremia. *1269* Correlates well with severity of morphologic lesions. *1047*

VDRL *Serum Positive* A persistent biologic false positive serologic test for syphilis may precede overt manifestations by many months or years. *0999* Biologic false positive results in 14% of patients. *0713* Incidence of false positive reactions is 15%. *1108*

Viscosity *Serum Increase* Modest increases may be seen, but no hyperviscosity syndromes have been reported. *2135*

Synovial Fluid Decrease Slightly decreased. *0962*

Vitamin B12 Binding Capacity *Serum Increase* Significant elevation; usually correlated with WBC in peripheral blood. *1990*

710.10 Progressive Systemic Sclerosis

Albumin *Urine Increase* Appears during renal failure. *0433* *0962*

Alpha1-Antichymotrypsin *Serum Increase* Collagen vascular diseases. *1248* *1168*

Antibodies to Centromeres *Serum Increase* Found in 10% of cases (77% with CREST syndrome). *2204*

Antibodies to dsDNA *Serum Normal* Found in 0% of cases. *2204*

Antibodies to RNP *Serum Increase* Found in 5% of cases. *2204*

Antibodies to SCL-70 *Serum Increase* Found in 23% of cases (10% with CREST syndrome). *2204*

Antibodies to Sjögren Syndrome A *Serum Increase* Found in 33% of cases. *2204*

Antibodies to Sjögren Syndrome B *Serum Increase* Found in 6% of cases. *2204*

Antibodies to SmAg *Serum Normal* Found in 0% of cases. *2204*

710.10   Progressive Systemic Sclerosis *(continued)*

Antibodies to ss-DNA   *Serum   Increase*   Found in 14% of cases. *2204*

Antibody Titer   *Serum   Increase*   The anticentromere antibody is thought to be closely associated with the CREST variant of Scleroderma. It may be a useful prognostic indicator. *1846*

Antinuclear Antibodies   *Serum   Increase*   Present in 60% of 47 serum samples in titers of 1:16 or greater. *1995*   Detected in low titer in 50-60% of cases and usually related to the nucleolar and ill-defined glycoprotein antigens. *0999*   Found in the sera of 40-90% of patients. In most cases the titers are relatively low, as compared to those found in SLE. *2035*   75-80% positivity. *1799*   Found in 58% of cases *2204   1771*

Aspartate Aminotransferase   *Serum   Increase*   Moderate to marked increase with associated myositis. *0503*

Ceruloplasmin   *Serum   Increase*   Mean level of ceruloplasmin, but not copper were raised in these patients, although both were raised in the 2 patients with the most aggressive disease. *1155*   Believed to occur as a nonspecific response (acute phase reactant). *2035*

Chylomicrons   *Serum   Increase*   Moderate increase secondary to presence of IgG or IgM that binds heparin and thereby decreases the activity of lipoprotein lipase. *0062*

Cold Agglutinins   *Serum   Increase*   Increased titer. *0186*

Complement, Total   *Serum   Decrease*   Occasionally. *2090*   In 27 patients, 44% had decreased values. *2223*

Serum   Increase   In 27 patients, 19% had increased values. *2223*

Serum   Normal   Normal in all but a few patients. *2372   2035*

Copper   *Serum   Increase*   Increased. *2052 2188 1729*

Creatine Kinase   *Serum   Increase*   Moderate to marked increase with associated myositis. *0503*

Creatinine   *Serum   Increase*   Renal function may be impaired. *0962*

Cryofibrinogen   *Serum   Increase*   Small amounts. *1112   2035   0856 1551*

Eosinophils   *Blood   Increase*   Early in the disease, the blood count is normal save for rare eosinophilia. *1700*   Eosinophilia has been observed but is uncommon. *0962*

Erythrocyte Casts   *Urine   Increase*   Appears during renal failure. *0433*

Erythrocytes   *Urine   Increase*   Appears during renal failure. *0433 0962*

Erythrocyte Sedimentation Rate   *Blood   Decrease*   Decreased in 33% of patients. *2468*

Blood   Increase   Increased in 33% of patients. *2468   0433*

Blood   Normal   Normal in 33%, decreased in 33%, and increased in 33% of patients. *2468*

Fat   *Feces   Increase*   Defects of multiple stages of digestion-absorption. *2199*

Globulin   *Serum   Increase*   Frequently found but is nonspecific. *0433*   Occurs in about 50% of patients; usually only moderate (1.4-2.0 g/dL), values of 3.5 g/dL and higher have been observed. *2035 2250*

Glomerular Filtration Rate (GFR)   *Urine   Decrease*   Renal function may be impaired. *0962*   The earliest demonstrable change in renal scleroderma. *0962*

Hematocrit   *Blood   Decrease*   A mild hypochromic microcytic anemia may be present. *0433*   Found in up to 25% of patients. *0962*

Hemoglobin   *Blood   Decrease*   A mild hypochromic microcytic anemia may be present *0433*   . Found in up to 25% of patients. *0962*

Hydroxyproline   *Urine   Increase*   Increased in some patients, especially those with active disease. *0151*

Immunoglobulin IgA   *Serum   Increase*   Usually slightly elevated. *0962   1995*

Immunoglobulin IgG   *Serum   Increase*   In most cases and in greatest measure, the increase involves IgG; less often the levels of IgA and IgM are elevated. *2035*   Usually slightly elevated. *0962 1995*

Immunoglobulin IgM   *Serum   Increase*   Usually slightly elevated. *0962   1995*

Lactate Dehydrogenase   *Serum   Increase*   Moderate to marked increase with associated myositis. *0503*

LE Cells   *Blood   Positive*   Occasionally positive. *0999*

Leukocytes   *Blood   Normal*   WBC and differential are usually normal. *0962*

MCH   *Blood   Decrease*   A mild hypochromic microcytic anemia may be present. *0433*   Found in up to 25% of patients. *0962*

MCHC   *Blood   Decrease*   A mild hypochromic microcytic anemia may be present. *0433*   Found in up to 25% of patients. *0962*

MCV   *Blood   Decrease*   A mild hypochromic microcytic anemia may be present. *0433*   Found in up to 25% of patients. *0962*

Platelet Count   *Blood   Decrease*   Has been reported. *0962*

Protein   *Urine   Increase*   In urinalysis proteinuria may be the only manifestation. *0962*   May be present for extended periods without clinical evidence of progressive renal dysfunction. *0962*   Renal involvement. *1700*

Renin Activity   *Plasma   Increase*   Extremely elevated levels are a frequent accompaniment of renal scleroderma. *0962*

Rheumatoid Factor   *Serum   Increase*   Present in 33% of sera from 47 patients with scleroderma. *1995*   25-33% of patients have positive tests. In most cases the titers have been 1:320 or less. *2035*   Almost 50% of patients have factor present in serum but it does not correlate with the existence of joint disease. *0999*

Urea Nitrogen   *Serum   Increase*   Renal function may be impaired. *0962*

VDRL   *Serum   Positive*   Occasionally there are biologic false-positive tests. *1700*

Vitamin B$_{12}$ *Serum   Decrease*   A selective vitamin B$_{12}$ deficiency only or a decrease in iron stores may be present without other obvious signs of the malabsorption syndrome. *0962*

710.20   Sjögren's Syndrome

Albumin   *Serum   Decrease*   Common. *0433*

Alpha$_1$-Antichymotrypsin   *Serum   Increase*   Collagen vascular diseases. *1248   1168*

Angiotensin-Converting Enzyme (ACE)   *Serum   Increase*   A study of 21 cases of this syndrome revealed that only 2 cases had elevated levels and these were only modest increases. *1464 1398 2014*

Serum   Normal   Raised activity isn't usually associated with this syndrome. *1464*

Antibodies to dsDNA   *Serum   Normal*   Found in 0% of cases. *2204*

Antibodies to RNP   *Serum   Increase*   Found in 5% of cases. *2204*

Antibodies to Sjögren Syndrome A   *Serum   Increase*   Found in 70% of cases. *2204*

Antibodies to Sjögren Syndrome B   *Serum   Increase*   Found in 60% of cases. *2204*

Antibodies to SmAg   *Serum   Normal*   Found in 0% of cases. *2204*

Antibodies to ss-DNA   *Serum   Normal*   Found in 0% of cases. *2204*

Antibody Titer   *Serum   Increase*   Antibodies to Reticulin. 75% of patients exhibit antibodies to salivary duct epithelium. *1670*

Antimitochondrial Antibodies   *Serum   Increase*   May occur. *2134*   Found in 18% of patients and 2% of controls. *1840*

Antinuclear Antibodies   *Serum   Increase*   Demonstrable in close to 70% of patients. *0226*   Present in about 60% (fluorescent technique). *0999*   40-75% positivity. *1799   2035*

Antismooth Muscle Antibodies   *Serum   Increase*   May occur. *2134*

Antithyroglobulin Antibodies   *Serum   Increase*   Rare. *0061*

Beta$_2$-Macroglobulin   *Serum   Increase*   Often elevated and correlates well with the degree of lymphocytic infiltration seen on biopsy. *2134*

Saliva   Increase   *0793*

Complement C3   *Serum   Decrease*   Caused by hypercatabolism. *0375 0793 1275 0509   0452*

Complement, Total   *Serum   Decrease*   Occasionally decreased, especially with cryoglobulinemia. *2090*

Coombs' Test   *Blood   Positive*   May occur. *2134*

Copper   *Serum   Increase*   Increased. *2052 2188 1729*

Cryoglobulins   *Serum   Increase*   Variable elevation of cryoglobulins. *2104*

Cryomacroglobulins   *Serum   Increase*   *0863*

Eosinophils   *Blood   Increase*   Occurs in about 25% of the patients. *2134*

Erythrocyte Sedimentation Rate   *Blood   Increase*   In approximately 66% of patients. *2134   0999*

Gamma Glutamyl Transferase (GGT) *Saliva Increase* Significantly higher (19.6 U/L) versus controls (5.12 U/L). *1164*

Globulin *Serum Increase* Hypergammaglobulinemia characterized by a diffuse increase in IgG, IgA, and IgM is found especially in those patients with the sicca complex not accompanied by a connective tissue disease. *0934* Electrophoresis shows increase globulins largely due to 7S gamma globulin. *2468* Present in most cases *0999 2035*

Hematocrit *Blood Decrease* Mild normochromic, normocytic anemia occurs in about 25% of patients. *0433* Anemia is seen in 33% of patients. *2134*

Hemoglobin *Blood Decrease* Mild normochromic, normocytic anemia occurs in about 25% of patients. *0433* Anemia is seen in 33% of patients. *2134*

HLA Antigens *Blood Present* HLA-DR3 present in 75% of patients versus 21% of controls. *2539* HLA-DR3 found found in 84% of patients with this disease compared to 24% of controls. *2051* Increased frequency of HLA-DR2 and HLA-DR3 and decrease. HLA-DR4 in primary disease and increased DR4 with normal freq. DR2 and DR3 in secondary. *1503*

Immunoglobulin IgA *Serum Increase* Hypergammaglobulinemia characterized by a diffuse increase in IgG, IgA, and IgM is found especially in those patients with the sicca complex not accompanied by a connective tissue disease. *0934 2035*

Immunoglobulin IgG *Serum Increase* The elevated globulin is usually 7S gamma globulin IgG and is not monoclonal. *0433* Hypergammaglobulinemia characterized by a diffuse increase in IgG, IgA, and IgM is found especially in those patients with the sicca complex not accompanied by a connective tissue disease. *0934 2035*

Immunoglobulin IgM *Serum Increase* Hypergammaglobulinemia characterized by a diffuse increase in IgG, IgA, and IgM is found especially in those patients with the sicca complex not accompanied by a connective tissue disease. *0934 2035*

LE Cells *Blood Increase* Found in 15-20% of patients. *2134*

Leukocytes *Blood Decrease* Occurs in about 25% of the patients. *0433* Occurs in 25% of patients. *2134*

Rheumatoid Factor *Serum Increase* Detected in > 70% of cases, regardless of the presence or absence of rheumatoid arthritis. *2134* High incidence even when not associated with a connective disease; the incidence of seropositivity is greatest in definite RA. *0962* 96% positivity. *0422 2035 0123*

710.40 Dermatomyositis/Polymyositis

Alanine Aminotransferase *Serum Increase* In general, serum enzymes correlate well with the disease activity and are useful therapeutic and prognostic indicators. *0433* Elevated at some time in nearly every patient. *0244 0962*

Aldolase *Serum Increase* Elevated at some time in nearly every patient. *0244* Released as a result of destructive myopathy. Almost invariably elevated in the acute or subacute stages. *1791 2035 0962*

Alpha₂-Globulin *Serum Increase* Commonly elevated. *0151*

Angiotensin-Converting Enzyme (ACE) *Serum Increase* *1398 2014*

Antibodies to dsDNA *Serum Increase* Found in 25% of cases of dermatomyositis. *2204*

Antibodies to RNP *Serum Normal* Found in 0% of cases. *2204*

Antibodies to SmAg *Serum Normal* Found in 0% of cases of dermatomyositis. *2204*

Antibody Titer *Serum Increase* Occasionally patients with dermatomyositis display antibodies to striated muscle. *1670*

Antinuclear Antibodies *Serum Increase* 40% of patients were ANA positive and LE cell negative. *0321* Positive in 35% of patients tested, although only 2% of patients with pure disease had detectable levels. *1791* Reported to be positive in 25%, positive only in a few cases of uncomplicated disease; positive titer in 2%, contrary to other reports. Higher titers were found in patients with other complications. *0244* Found in 82% of cases of polymyositis *2204 2035 1799*

Aspartate Aminotransferase *Serum Increase* May be increased in the absence of clinical evidence of muscle wasting. Steroid therapy causes the level to fall towards normal. *0619* Moderate to marked increase. Usual values < 145 U/L. *0503* Elevated at some time in nearly every patient. *0244* Released as a result of destructive myopathy. Almost invariably elevated in the acute or subacute stages. *1791 2035 0962*

Complement, Total *Serum Decrease* In 15 patients, 20% had decreased values. *2223*

Serum Increase Elevated during active inflammation and subsides with remission. *2090* In 15 patients, 13% had increased values. *2223*

Copper *Serum Increase* Increased. *2052 2188 1729*

Creatine *Urine Increase* Urine shows a moderate increase in creatine and a decrease in creatinine. *2467*

Creatine Kinase *Serum Increase* Elevated at some time in nearly every patient. Most consistent of the serum enzymes and correlated best with clinical course and parameters of activity. *0244* Released as a result of destructive myopathy. *1791* Almost invariably elevated in the acute stages, whereas in the clinically inactive cases or in those in remission they are often normal. *2035 2219 0962*

Creatinine *Urine Decrease* Active disease. As the urine creatine increases, so the urine creatinine falls. *0619*

Eosinophils *Blood Increase* Frequently increased. *2467*

Erythrocyte Sedimentation Rate *Blood Increase* Moderately to markedly increased; may be normal. *2467 0433 0151*

Globulin *Serum Increase* Commonly elevated. *0151 0433*

Haptoglobin *Serum Increase* Conditions associated with increased ESR and alpha 2 globulin; increases in collagen diseases. *2467*

Hematocrit *Blood Decrease* Mild anemia may be expected. *0433*

Hemoglobin *Blood Decrease* Mild anemia may be expected. *0433*

Immunoglobulin IgD *Serum Increase* *0619*

Lactate Dehydrogenase *Serum Increase* Moderate to marked increase. *0503* Elevated at some time in nearly every patient. *0244* Increased but less sensitive indicator of muscle injury. *0962* Elevation in both acute and chronic polymyositis. *1071 2575*

Lactate Dehydrogenase Isoenzyme 5 (LD₅) *Serum Increase* In cases of chronic polymyositis, a relative but mild rise was noted. *1071* May be increased, paralleling the increased LD. *2467*

Lactate Dehydrogenase Isoenzymes *Serum Increase* In cases of chronic polymyositis, a relative but mild rise was noted. *1071*

LE Cells *Blood Increase* About 5% of patients have positive test. *0151* 40% of patients were ANA positive and LE cell negative. *0321*

Leukocytes *Blood Increase* May be expected. *0433* Mild leukocytosis occurs, especially in acute cases. *0151*

Malate Dehydrogenase *Serum Increase* May be increased but offers no additional diagnostic value. *2467*

Myoglobin *Urine Increase* In severe cases. *2467*

Plasma Cells *Serum Decrease* Depressed. *2357 0659 0683*

Pseudocholinesterase *Serum Decrease* With serum albumin. *2467*

Rheumatoid Factor *Serum Increase* Positive (> 1:40) in 18 of 82 recorded (20%): including 5 patients (6%) with pure polymyositis (Type I), 4 (5%) with pure dermatomyositis (Type II), and 9 (10%) with the overlap type (Type V). *2035* Positive in 10-50% of patients. *0151* Reported to be positive in 40%. Positive only in a few cases of uncomplicated disease. Positive titer in 10% contrary to other reports. Higher titers were found in patients with other complications. *0244*

711.00 Acute Arthritis (Pyogenic)

Complement, Total *Synovial Fluid Decrease* Compared to total protein, levels are low in 60-70% of joint effusions. *0314*

Erythrocyte Sedimentation Rate *Blood Increase* *2467*

Glucose *Serum Decrease* Low in most cases. *0999*

Synovial Fluid Decrease *0650*

Lactic Acid *Synovial Fluid Increase* *0186*

Leukocytes *Blood Increase* Counts frequently exceed 50,000/μL, higher than in other types of arthritis. *0999* Elevated total WBC count. *0650* Routine blood studies should reflect the presence of a closed space infection with a polymorphonuclear leukocytosis. *0433*

Synovial Fluid Increase May vary from 10,000-300,000/μL, depending upon the stage of infection and inflammatory response. The cells are predominantly polymorphonuclear. *0433* Infected fluid is characteristically turbid or purulent, with a count of 100,000/μL or more, with a differential of 90% polymorphonuclears. *2481 2482*

711.00 Acute Arthritis (Pyogenic) *(continued)*

NBT Test *Blood Positive* NBT positive cells were found in synovial fluid of 7 of 8 patients, while only 4 showed positive peripheral blood tests. *0939*

Synovial Fluid Positive NBT positive cells were found in synovial fluid of 7 of 8 patients, while only 4 showed positive peripheral blood tests. *0939*

Neutrophils *Blood Increase* An elevated absolute neutrophil count. *0650*

Synovial Fluid Increase Increase in number, ranging from 75-100/µL. *2467*

pH *Synovial Fluid Decrease* Close correlation (R = -.92) was found between decreasing pH and increasing WBC in synovial fluid. The high WBC usually found in acute and chronic arthritis results in low pH which may contribute to the poor response to treatment with aminoglycoside antibiotics. *2482*

Protein *Synovial Fluid Decrease* 30-40% of the plasma concentration. *1958*

711.10 Mixed Connective Tissue Disease

Antibodies to dsDNA *Serum Increase* Found in 25% of cases. *2204*

Antibodies to RNP *Serum Increase* Found in 100% of cases. *2204*

Antibodies to SmAg *Serum Increase* Found in 8% of cases. *2204*

Antinuclear Antibodies *Serum Increase* Usually high titers (> 1:1000), speckled pattern. *0062*

Complement, Total *Serum Decrease* In 30% of cases. *0062*

Gamma Globulin *Serum Increase* Diffuse hypergammaglobulinemia. *0062*

Globulin *Serum Increase* Diffuse hypergammaglobulinemia. *0062*

Hematocrit *Blood Decrease* Anemia. *0062*

Hemoglobin *Blood Decrease* Anemia. *0062*

Leukocytes *Blood Decrease* Leukopenia. *0062*

Platelet Count *Blood Decrease* Thrombocytopenia. *0062*

Rheumatoid Factor *Serum Increase* Found in over 50% of cases. Titer is usually very high. *0062*

714.00 Rheumatoid Arthritis

5'-Nucleotidase *Serum Increase* May be found in up to 33% of patients with a greater increase in enzyme activity in the synovial fluid. *0619*

Synovial Fluid Increase In 58% with reduction to normal following corticosteroid therapy. *0619* Slightly increased in cases showing more advanced x-ray changes. *2320*

Acid Phosphatase *Synovial Fluid Increase* Of 155 patients with different joint disorders, patients with rheumatoid arthritis showed significantly higher levels than those with bacterial arthritis, osteoarthritis and noninflammatory joint effusions. About 70% of the patients with RA had higher concentrations than those found among the patients with nonrheumatoid diseases. *0147*

Alanine *Urine Increase* *2104*

Alanine Aminotransferase *Serum Normal* Generally normal. *0962*

Albumin *Serum Decrease* Frequent finding attributed to generalized hypermetabolism. Corticosteroid administration accentuates hypoalbuminemia. *2104 0962*

Urine Increase No abnormalities are found in the urinalysis except for proteinuria. *0433*

Alkaline Phosphatase *Serum Increase* Characteristically abnormal when the arthritis is active. *0433*

Serum Normal Generally normal. *0962*

Alpha₁-Antichymotrypsin *Serum Increase* Significant rise. *1306 0268*

Synovial Fluid Increase Significant rise. *1306 0268*

Alpha₁-Antitrypsin *Serum Increase* In patients with RA complicated by Amyloidosis. *1526*

Synovial Fluid Increase Elevated in 36 patients with involvement of the knee joint. *1953*

Alpha₁-Globulin *Serum Increase* Moderate increase. *0619*

Serum Normal Generally not significantly changed. *0962*

Alpha₁-Glycoprotein *Serum Increase* One of the most reliable indicators of acute inflammation. *1239 1672 1866   1947 2096 2170*

Alpha₂-Globulin *Serum Increase* Alpha₂ or beta globulin fractions are often elevated in the acute active phase, whereas during the chronic active phase, gamma globulin fractions are elevated. *0433* Elevation occurs in some 50% of all patients and in the majority with progressive chronic disease. *0999* Elevated and does not fall with steroid therapy. *0619*

Amino Acids *Plasma Decrease* Frequent hypoaminoacidemia. Arginine, glutamine, tyrosine, and histidine are low. *2104*

Amylase *Pleural Effusion Normal* Usually less than or equal to serum level. *2017*

Angiotensin-Converting Enzyme (ACE) *Serum Increase* *1398 2014*

Serum Normal Not significantly different (n = 48) from normal controls (n = 26). *1443*

Antibodies to Centromeres *Serum Normal* Found in 0% of cases. *2204*

Antibodies to dsDNA *Serum Increase* Found in 2% of cases. *2204 0186*

Antibodies to Histones *Serum Increase* Found in 10% of cases. *2204* Found in 15-20% of cases *0062*

Antibodies to RNP *Serum Increase* Found in 1% of cases. *2204*

Antibodies to SCL-70 *Serum Normal* Found in 0% of cases. *2204*

Antibodies to Sjögren Syndrome A *Serum Increase* Found in 4% of cases. *2204*

Antibodies to Sjögren Syndrome B *Serum Increase* Found in 1% of cases. *2204*

Antibodies to SmAg *Serum Increase* Found in 5% of cases. *2204*

Antibodies to ss-DNA *Serum Increase* Found in 4% of cases. *2204*

Antibody Titer *Serum Increase* Antibodies to Reticulin. *1670*

Antinuclear Antibodies *Serum Increase* 30 of 42 (73.2%) severely affected patients were antinuclear factor positive and 19 of them were LE cell negative. *0321* Present in serum of 10-50% of patients (depending on the technique used) but is also usually in low titer compared to that in SLE. *0999* Highly sensitive tests will detect them in 60% of patients. Titers are generally lower than in SLE; predominantly IgM. *0962* 25-60% positivity. *1799* Found in 56% of cases *2204*

Synovial Fluid Increase Occasionally positive. *0962*

Antismooth Muscle Antibodies *Serum Increase* Occasionally positive in low titer. *1829* Positive in 10% of patients. *2528 2035*

Antistreptolysin O *Serum Increase* Above normal titers may occur. *1752*

Antithrombin III *Plasma Decrease* No significant correlation between low levels and thromboembolic disease. *0238*

Apolipoprotein AI *Serum Normal* In 54 female patients found to be in normal range. *1435*

Arginine *Plasma Decrease* Frequently low. *2104*

Aspartate Aminotransferase *Serum Increase* Characteristically abnormal when the arthritis is active. *0433*

Serum Normal Generally normal. *0962*

Beta₂-Macroglobulin *Serum Increase* *2467*

Synovial Fluid Increase Increased concentration. *2302 2326*

Beta-Galactosidase *Serum Decrease* Mean serum concentration was 0.139 ± 0.019 mmol/min/L, compared with 0.243 ± 0.038 in controls. *1099*

Beta-Globulin *Serum Increase* Alpha₂ or beta globulin fractions are often elevated in the acute phase, whereas during the chronic active phase, gamma globulin fractions are elevated. *0433*

Serum Normal Generally not significantly changed. *0962*

Bicarbonate *Pleural Effusion Increase* 60-70 mm Hg. *0797*

Bile Acids *Serum Increase* In a series of 20 patients with RA and without prior causes of hepatic damage. Elevated in 80% of patients. *2625*

BSP Retention *Serum Increase* In a series of 20 patients with RA and without prior causes of hepatic damage. Elevated in 60% of patients. *2625* At times increased *0433*

Calcium *Serum Increase* After correction for hypoalbuminemia, 113/229 female and 65/135 male patients had hypercalcemia. *1251*

Serum Normal Generally normal. *0962*

Carcinoembryonic Antigen *Serum Increase* In seropositive cases. *0619*

Catecholamines *Urine Decrease* The more severe the stage and class of the arthritis, the lower the epinephrine, and the closer to normal norepinephrine values. Norepinephrine seems to reflect a compensation in catecholamine metabolism rather than adrenal cortex system influence. *1114*

Cephalin Flocculation *Serum Increase* Characteristically abnormal when the arthritis is active. *0433*

Ceruloplasmin *Serum Increase* May cause green color of plasma. *2467* Significantly raised in rheumatoid disease in both sexes. *2100*

Synovial Fluid Increase Characteristic of rheumatoid effusions. *2101*

Cholesterol *Serum Decrease* Reduced; appears to be related to the severity and activity of the disease; not affected by therapy. *0962*

Pericardial Fluid Increase High levels (2.6-5.2 mmol/L; 100 to 200 mg/dL). *0274*

Cholesterol, High Density Lipoprotein *Serum Decrease* In 54 female patients 36% reduction was noted. *1435*

Cholesterol, Low Density Lipoprotein *Serum Decrease* In 54 female patients 26% reduction was noted. *1435*

Chylomicrons *Synovial Fluid Decrease* Cylous effusions have been reported. *1689 2012*

Complement C1q *Serum Increase* *2090*

Complement C1r *Serum Decrease* {793} {2522}

Complement C2 *Serum Increase* *2090*

Complement C3 *Serum Decrease* Caused by hypercatabolism. *0375 0793 1275 0509 0452*

Serum Increase The mean plasma C3e level in these samples (3.0 ± 1.3 mg/dL) was significantly increased as compared to patients with degenerative joint disease (0.9± 0.4 mg/dL) and healthy blood donors (0.8 ± 0.5 mg/dL). C3d levels were increased by more than 2 SD in 79% of RA samples. In most RA patients, the C3d levels were higher in synovial fluid than in plasma. *1712*

Synovial Fluid Decrease Marked reduction of C1, C2, C3 and C4 in seropositive patients. Only C4 was significantly decreased in seronegative patients. *2090*

Synovial Fluid Increase The mean plasma C3e level in these samples (3.0 ± 1.3 mg/dL) was significantly increased as compared to patients with degenerative joint disease (0.9 ± 0.4 mg/dL). C3d levels were increased by more than 2 SD in 79% of RA samples. In most patients, the C3d levels were higher in synovial fluid than in plasma. *1712*

Pleural Effusion Decrease In about 5% of cases. *0062*

Pericardial Fluid Decrease Low or absent *0764 0877*

Complement C4 *Synovial Fluid Decrease* Marked reduction of C1, C2, C3, and C4 in seropositive patients. Only C4 was significantly decreased in seronegative patients. *2090*

Pleural Effusion Decrease In about 5% of cases. *0062*

Pericardial Fluid Decrease Low or absent *0764 0877*

Complement, Total *Serum Decrease* In rare instances and with a highly acute onset, may be low. *0962* In 64 patients, 19% had decreased values. *2223*

Serum Increase In 64 patients, 16% had increased values. *2223* Activity tends to be elevated in patients with mild disease, lower levels were found in seropositive than seronegative patients. *2090*

Serum Normal *0186*

Synovial Fluid Decrease Low compared to that in other types of inflammatory joint effusions, especially in relation to the total protein concentration. *0999* Whole complement activity is reduced. *1014* Intra-articular depletion of whole complement activity in the presence of normal or elevated serum levels is in proportion to the titer of rheumatoid factor in serum or synovial fluid. *2090* Marked reduction of C1, C2, C3, and C4 in seropositive patients. Only C4 was significantly decreased in seronegative patients. *2090* Low values associated with more severe disease and poorer prognosis. *0313* Compared to total protein, levels are low in 60-70% of joint effusions *0314*

Pleural Effusion Decrease Seropositive patients had decreased CH50, C1, C2, and C1 inhibitor in pleural and pericardial fluids. *0854* Low complement (< 10 U/mL) in 11 of 12 patients with SLE or rheumatoid pleuritis. *1403*

Pericardial Fluid Decrease Low or absent *0764 0877*

Copper *Serum Increase* Both serum Cu and ceruloplasmin were measured 189 RA patients and were found to be significantly elevated. An inverse relation was found between serum iron and copper and a strong direct correlation between serum antioxidant activity and ceruloplasmin. *2100* Elevated in excess of the binding capacity of ceruloplasmin, resulting in raised free copper levels. *1433*

Urine Increase Patients show an abnormal copper excretion pattern compared with nonrheumatoid subjects. *1558*

Synovial Fluid Increase Characteristic of rheumatoid effusions. *2101*

C-Reactive Protein *Serum Increase* Increased inconsistently. *2467* Nearly always abnormal and generally reflects the degree of disease activity. *2035*

Creatine *Serum Increase* *2467 0619*

Cryoglobulins *Serum Increase* Demonstrated occasionally but do not appear to have diagnostic significance. *0962* Variable elevation of cryoglobulins. *2104*

Cysteine *Urine Decrease* *2104*

Eosinophils *Blood Increase* Eosinophilia has been reported in patients with pleural or pulmonary manifestations. *0962*

Erythrocytes *Pleural Effusion Increase* *0962*

Erythrocyte Sedimentation Rate *Blood Increase* In 100 patients, correlated with disease activity and stage of disease. *1634* Nearly always abnormal and generally reflects the degree of disease activity. *2035* At times, although joint inflammation has subsided, ESR will remain accelerated because of the continued elevation of serum globulins. *0962 0999*

Blood Normal Elevated when the classic case is active, normal when the disease is quiet because of its natural course or as a result of therapy. *0433* The majority of patients who are in complete remission will have a normal ESR. *0962*

Factor B *Synovial Fluid Decrease* *1443*

Fibrinogen *Plasma Increase* Can be used to assess disease activity. *0619*

Gamma Globulin *Pericardial Fluid Increase* Gamma Globulin complexes found to be present in Rheumatoid Pericarditis. *0107*

Gamma Glutamyl Transferase (GGT) *Serum Increase* In a series of 20 patients with RA and without prior causes of hepatic damage. Elevated in 55% of patients. *2625*

Gastrin *Serum Increase* Patients tend to have higher than normal serum concentration. There appears to be poor correlation with acid secretion. *1973 2199*

Globulin *Serum Increase* Alpha$_2$ or beta globulin fractions are often elevated in the acute active phase, whereas during the chronic active phase, gamma globulin fractions are elevated. *0433* Elevation occurs in some 50% of all patients and in the majority with progressive chronic disease. *0999*

Glucose *Synovial Fluid Decrease* Normal or low. *0186* Slightly reduced glucose content *0999*

Synovial Fluid Normal Normal or low. *0186*

Pleural Effusion Decrease Concentrations are invariably < 30 mg/dL. *1403* Markedly reduced, 20 mg/dL or less, is very suggestive and virtually diagnostic of rheumatoid disease. A low level in the range of 40 mg/dL can be found in infectious processes and in malignant pleural effusions. *0962*

Pericardial Fluid Decrease With rheumatoid pericarditis a low concentration (often < 1.7 mmol/L- 30 mg/dL) is seen. *0764*

Glucose Tolerance *Serum Decrease* Characteristically depressed with active disease; easy to produce hypoglycemia if this abnormality is treated with oral hypoglycemic agents. *0433* Moderate intolerance in most patients. More severe in patients with associated infection and inflammation. *2104*

Glutamic Acid *Serum Increase* Usually the only elevated serum amino acid. *2104*

Urine Decrease *2104*

Glutamine *Serum Decrease* Frequently low. *2104*

Urine Increase *2104*

Glycine *Urine Increase* *2104*

Glycoproteins *Serum Decrease* Significant lowering of beta-2 glycoprotein concentrations found. *1305*

Haptoglobin *Serum Increase* Usually parallel the activity of the ESR. *0962*

Hematocrit *Blood Decrease* Normocytic, normochromic, or perhaps hypochromic anemia which may be severe when the disease is very active. *0433* Mild anemia occurs in approximately 40% of cases. *0999* Anemia may occur. *0532*

Hemoglobin *Blood Decrease* Normocytic, normochromic, or perhaps hypochromic anemia which may be severe when the disease is very active. *0433* Mild anemia occurs in approximately 40% of cases. *0999* Anemia may occur, hemoglobin < 13 g/dL. *0532*

Heterophil Antibody *Serum Increase* One case. *0503*

Hexosamine *Serum Increase* Usually parallel the activity of the ESR. *0962*

714.00 Rheumatoid Arthritis *(continued)*

Hexosaminidase *Urine Increase* Decreased levels in urine. *2356*

Histidine *Serum Decrease* Frequently low. *2104*

HLA Antigens *Blood Present* HLA antigen DR4 found in 54% of patients with this disease compared to 16% of controls. *2051* HLA-B$_2$7 present in 35% of patients versus 11% of controls HLA-DR4 present in 56% of patients versus 15% of controls *2539*

Immunoglobulin IgA *Serum Increase* *2467*

Saliva Increase Significantly elevated in 24% of patients. 80% of the patients with elevated IgA concentrations had keratoconjunctivitis sicca as well. *0162*

Immunoglobulin IgD *Serum Increase* *0619*

Immunoglobulin IgG *Serum Increase* *2467*

Immunoglobulin IgM *Serum Increase* *2467*

Synovial Fluid Increase Very suggestive of this disease. *0139*

Iron *Serum Decrease* Serum iron < 50 µg/dL. *0532* Seen frequently, often as a result of gastrointestinal blood loss. *0999*

Iron-Binding Capacity, Total (TIBC) *Serum Decrease* Low; rises with successful steroid therapy. *0619* Total IBC < 200-300 µg/dL. *0532*

Iron Saturation *Serum Decrease* Transferrin saturation < 20%. *0532* *2467*

Isocitrate Dehydrogenase *Serum Normal* *2260*

Lactate Dehydrogenase *Serum Increase* Characteristically abnormal when the arthritis is active. *0433* *1089*

Pericardial Fluid Increase With rheumatoid pericarditis markedly elevated. *0764*

Lactic Acid *Pleural Effusion Increase* High concentrations may be seen. *0707*

LE Cells *Blood Increase* Usually weakly reactive. *2467* Positive in up to 25% of patients. The number of cells seen in a preparation is less than in SLE. *0999* 30 of 42 (73%) severely affected patients were antinuclear factor positive and 19 were LE cell negative. *0321*

Leukocytes *Blood Decrease* Occasionally low; characteristically so in Felty's Syndrome in which granulocytes are depleted. *0999*

Blood Increase Usually normal but may be elevated or depressed. In children may be very high (70,000/µL). *0433* There may be a slight increase early in the active disease. *2467* About 25% of patients develop neutrophilic leukocytosis. These patients usually have arthritis of short duration with a high degree of activity and fever. *2154*

Blood Normal Usually normal but may be elevated or depressed. *0433* The majority of patients have normal counts. *2154*

Synovial Fluid Increase Elevated (3,000 to 60,000/µL, with an average of around 10,000/µL), with predominantly polymorphonuclear response at times of active disease. *0999* Less than 15,000/µL. *0962*

Pleural Effusion Increase 1000-20,000/µL. *2017*

Lipids *Serum Decrease* In 54 female patients plasma lipid levels were low. *1435*

Lymphocyte T-Cell *Blood Normal* Increased T$_4$/T$_8$ ratio. *0062*

MCH *Blood Decrease* Microcytic hypochromic anemia may occur due to blood loss, increased demand or dietary inadequacy. MCH < 27 pg, MCV < 80 fL. *0532*

MCV *Blood Decrease* Microcytic hypochromic anemia may occur due to blood loss, increased demand or dietary inadequacy. MCH < 27 pg, MCV < 80 fL. *0532*

Blood Increase Macrocytic anemia may occur due to vitamin B$_{12}$ or folate deficiency. MCV > 100 fL. *0532*

Monocytes *Blood Increase* Has been reported. *1489* In 41% of 91 patients at initial hospitalization for this disorder. *0781* *2538*

Pleural Effusion Increase Predominant cell type. *2017*

Neutrophils *Blood Increase* About 25% of patients develop a significant neutrophilic leukocytosis. These patients usually have arthritis of short duration with a high degree of activity and fever. *2154* In 60% of 92 patients at initial hospitalization for this disorder. *0781*

Synovial Fluid Increase Increased number, ranging from 5-96/µL. *2467*

Pleural Effusion Increase Predominant cells neutrophils or monocytes. *2017*

pCO$_2$ *Blood Decrease* Impaired gas diffusion and the accompanying hyperventilation results in a low pCO$_2$, unless the defect is severe and CO$_2$ retention occurs. *2104*

pH *Synovial Fluid Decrease* Low pH correlates with increasing WBC count (R = 0.92) in synovial fluid of acute and chronic arthritis. *2482*

Pleural Effusion Decrease 7.0-7.2 pH. *0797*

Phosphate *Serum Normal* Generally normal. *0962*

Platelet Count *Blood Increase* Counts exceeding 400,000/µL are common and correlate best with leukocytosis and highly active disease. *0962* In 46% of 40 patients at initial hospitalization for this disorder. *0781*

Prostaglandins *Synovial Fluid Increase* Prostaglandin E2 usually predominates. Concentration does not seem to correlate with clinical course of disease. *0252*

Protein *Synovial Fluid Increase* Characteristically turbid with increased protein content. *0999*

Pleural Effusion Increase Tends to produce high total protein concentration. *0368*

Pericardial Fluid Increase With rheumatoid pericarditis a high total protein is common. *0764*

Pyridoxine *Urine Decrease* Patients with active disease excrete abnormally low B$_6$ and related metabolites. *2104*

Pyrophosphate *Synovial Fluid Normal* Near normal levels. *1132*

Rheumatoid Factor *Serum Increase* The majority of rheumatoid sera give positive reactions; the incidence varies with different techniques, but at least 70%. A high degree of correlation of rheumatoid factors and subcutaneous nodules, symmetrical deforming arthritis of the hands and wrists, and various visceral manifestations of rheumatoid arthritis. *2035* Correlated with anatomical stage, class and course of disease and ESR. *0550* Low values associated with more severe disease and poorer prognosis. *0313* *0999*

Synovial Fluid Increase Low values associated with more severe disease and poorer prognosis. *0313*

Sodium *Saliva Increase* The concentrations of salivary sodium and IgA were significantly elevated in 24% of patients. 80% of the patients with elevated sodium and IgA concentrations had keratoconjunctivitis sicca as well. *0162*

Threonine *Urine Decrease* *2104*

Thymol Turbidity *Serum Increase* Characteristically abnormal when the arthritis is active. *0433*

Trypsin Inhibitor *Synovial Fluid Increase* Elevated in 36 patients with involvement of the knee joint. *1953*

Tyrosine *Serum Decrease* Frequently low. *2104*

Urea Nitrogen *Serum Increase* At times increased. Somewhat elevated (30-40 mg/dL) during active phase. *0433*

Uric Acid *Serum Increase* Slight elevation may occur, especially in male patients. *1343*

Serum Normal Generally normal. *0962*

VDRL *Serum Positive* Biologic false positive tests reported in 5-10% of patients. Those patients are more likely to have positive LE cell tests. *0962*

Viscosity *Synovial Fluid Decrease* *0962*

714.10 Felty's Syndrome

Antibodies to dsDNA *Serum Normal* Found in 0% of cases. *2204*

Antibodies to ss-DNA *Serum Increase* Found in 100% of cases. *2204*

Antinuclear Antibodies *Serum Increase* Found in 75% of cases. *2204* Positive in 100% of cases. *1799*

Complement, Total *Serum Decrease* Hypocomplementemia usually occurs. *1605*

LE Cells *Blood Increase* Positive LE test is more frequent than in rheumatoid arthritis. *2467*

Leukocytes *Blood Decrease* Leukopenia (usually due to neutropenia) occurs predisposing patients to infection. *2239*

Neutrophils *Blood Decrease* Most patients appear to have increased cell margination probably with splenic sequestration. About 33% have impaired production. *0415* Leukopenia (usually due to neutropenia) occurs predisposing patients to infection. *2239*

Rheumatoid Factor *Serum Increase* Serologic tests are positive; may be present in high titers. *2467* *2468*

714.30　Juvenile Rheumatoid Arthritis

Alanine Aminotransferase *Serum Increase* Mild elevation is common in untreated and aspirin-treated children but increases are sporadic. *1870*

Albumin *Serum Decrease* In acute systemic form. *0136*

Alpha$_2$-Macroglobulin *Serum Decrease* In acute systemic form. *0136*

Antibodies to dsDNA *Serum Increase* Found in 5% of cases. *2204*

Antibodies to RNP *Serum Increase* Found in 3% of cases. *2204*

Antibodies to Sjögren Syndrome A *Serum Normal* Found in 0% of cases. *2204*

Antibodies to Sjögren Syndrome B *Serum Normal* Found in 0% of cases. *2204*

Antibodies to ss-DNA *Serum Increase* Found in 3% of cases. *2204*

Antinuclear Antibodies *Serum Increase* Frequently found in sera from patients with pauciarticular disease and children with mild disease activity. *1993*

Found in 57% of cases. *2204* Found in 13% of cases.

Serum Normal In acute systemic form. *0136*

Antistreptolysin O *Serum Increase* Increased in 50% of cases. *0793*

Aspartate Aminotransferase *Serum Increase* Transiently but only moderately elevated in many children receiving high dosages of aspirin; decreases to normal as the dosage of salicylates is lowered. *0433* Mild elevation is common in untreated and aspirin-treated children but increases are sporadic. *1870*

Complement C3 *Serum Increase* Serum C2, C4, and C9 were elevated, but only C9 correlated well with ESR. *2090*

Synovial Fluid Decrease Synovial fluid levels C1q, C3, C4 and C9 were consistently depressed in all seropositive patients, and in 5 of 14 seronegative patients. *2090*

Complement C4 *Serum Increase* Serum C2, C3, C4, and C9 were elevated, but only C9 correlated well with ESR. *2090*

Synovial Fluid Decrease Synovial fluid levels of C1q, C3, C4, and C9 were consistently depressed in all seropositive patients and in 5 of 14 seronegative patients. *2090*

Complement, Total *Serum Decrease* In 22 patients, 32% had decreased values. *2223*

Serum Increase Serum C2, C3, C4, and C9 were elevated, but only C9 correlated well with ESR. RF positive patients tend to have lower CH50 than do RF negative patients, but both groups show increased titers during active disease. *2090* In 22 patients, 13% had increased values. *2223* Normal or increased *0136*

Serum Normal Normal or increased. *0136*

Synovial Fluid Decrease Synovial fluid levels of C1q, C3, C4, and C9 were consistently depressed in all seropositive patients and in 5 of 14 negative patients. *2090*

C-Reactive Protein *Serum Increase* In acute systemic form. *0136*

Erythrocyte Sedimentation Rate *Blood Increase* Are usually elevated moderately when inflammatory disease is severe, but is often normal in the presence of disease activity and is not a constant laboratory parameter. *0433* Moderately increased; mean = 68 mm/h, and range = 38-104 in 6 children with chronic polyarthritis. *0463*

Blood Normal Are usually elevated moderately when inflammatory disease is severe, but is often normal in the presence of disease activity and is not a constant laboratory parameter. *0433*

Ferritin *Serum Increase* Markedly increased, ranging from 120-2000 µg/dL (mean = 822) compared to normals, 35-155 µg/dL. Fluctuations correlated closely with disease activity (R = 0.954, P < 0.05). *0463*

Glucose *Synovial Fluid Decrease* *0136*

Hematocrit *Blood Decrease* Moderate anemia is common with Hct concentrations of 30-34%. *0433*

Hemoglobin *Blood Decrease* Moderate anemia is common with hemoglobin concentrations of 9-11 g/dL. *0433*

Immunoglobulin IgG *Serum Increase* Polyclonal increase. *0793*

Iron *Serum Decrease* *0136*

Iron-Binding Capacity, Total (TIBC) *Serum Decrease* *0136*

Leukocytes *Blood Increase* Usually normal but may be slightly elevated and rarely leukemoid. *0433* Leukocytosis in the range of 15,000-25,000/µL is common and distinguishes it from the adult rheumatoid arthritis. *0151* There may be a high peripheral WBC (up to 50,000/µL). *1700*

Blood Normal Usually normal but may be slightly elevated and rarely even leukemoid. *0433*

Synovial Fluid Increase *2467*

Lymphocytes *Synovial Fluid Increase* Abundant lymphocytes (sometimes > 50%) and immature lymphocytes and monocytes present in the synovial fluid. *2467* *2468*

Plasma Cells *Synovial Fluid Increase* *0793*

Rheumatoid Factor *Serum Increase* No more than 10% of patients have a positive rheumatoid factor in sera. *0151* Found in only 10-20% of children. *1700*

Serum Normal No more than 10% of patients have a positive rheumatoid factor in sera. *0151* Found in only 10-20% of children. *1700* In acute systemic form. *0136*

Synovial Fluid Normal Absent in synovial fluid. *2468*

715.90　Osteoarthritis

Angiotensin-Converting Enzyme (ACE) *Serum Normal* Not significantly different (n = 11) from normal controls (n = 26). *1443*

Aspartate Aminotransferase *Serum Increase* In 23% of 120 patients at initial hospitalization for this disorder. *0781*

Carcinoembryonic Antigen *Serum Increase* 30% of patients had values > 2.5 ng/mL. *2199*

Dopamine Hydroxylase *Serum Increase* 2 X normal value. *2037*

Synovial Fluid Increase 3 X normal value. *2037*

Erythrocyte Sedimentation Rate *Blood Increase* Occurs only during rare episodes of acute inflammation of the joints. *0962*

Blood Normal Usually normal. *0962*

Glucose *Synovial Fluid Normal* Nearly equal to blood. *0666*

Hexosaminidase *Urine Increase* *1443*

Leukocytes *Synovial Fluid Increase* Counts range from 200-2000/µL. *0151* Synovial fluid is viscid and has few white cells in degenerative joint disease. *0999*

Monocytes *Blood Increase* In 51% of 125 patients at initial hospitalization for this disorder. *0781*

Pyrophosphate *Synovial Fluid Increase* Moderately elevated levels. *1132*

Rheumatoid Factor *Serum Normal* *2467*

Viscosity *Synovial Fluid Normal* *0666*

720.00　Rheumatoid (Ankylosing) Spondylitis

Alkaline Phosphatase *Serum Increase* Elevation in 47.5% of 40 patients and in most cases was derived from bone. *1250*

Angiotensin-Converting Enzyme (ACE) *Serum Normal* Not significantly different (n = 24) from normal controls (n = 26). *1443*

Ceruloplasmin *Serum Increase* Raised significantly, with the greatest increases in the worst cases. *1155*

Cholesterol, High Density Lipoprotein *Serum Normal* Total lipid concentration was found to be low but HDL fraction was normal. *1435*

Complement C4 *Serum Increase* Mean levels of C4 and IgA were significantly elevated in patients with sporadic disease. *1273* Raised concentration of C4 and complement inactivation products. *2152*

Complement, Total *Synovial Fluid Increase* Frequently occurs. *2090*

Copper *Serum Increase* Raised significantly, with the greatest increases in the worst cases. *1155*

C-Reactive Protein *Serum Increase* 90% of cases. *0186*

Cryoglobulins *Serum Increase* Variable elevation of cryoglobulins. *2104*

Erythrocyte Sedimentation Rate *Blood Increase* Elevated in most but not in all patients with active disease. May be normal in patients who are symptomatic. *0433* Occurs in about 80% of patients but other acute phase reactants tend to be absent. *0666* *0999*

720.00 Rheumatoid (Ankylosing) Spondylitis
(continued)

Globulin *Serum Increase* Electrophoresis may show an elevation of the globulin fractions without any specific pattern. *0433* 25% of 40 Patients showed elevated and abnormal globulins, alkaline phosphatase and hemoglobin *1250*

Glucose *Synovial Fluid Decrease* Lower than blood. *0666*

Hematocrit *Blood Decrease* Anemia is occasionally present in more severe cases and is usually normocytic. *0433* Anemia occurs in < 33% of cases. *0666*

Hemoglobin *Blood Decrease* Anemia is occasionally present in more severe cases and is usually normocytic. *0433* Anemia occurs in < 33% of cases. *0666*

HLA Antigens *Blood Present* HLA antigen B_27 found in 90% of caucasian patients with this disease compared to 8% of controls. *2051* HLA-B_27 present in 90% of patients versus 8% of controls *2539*

Immunoglobulin IgA *Serum Increase* Mean levels of C4 and IgA were significantly elevated in patients with sporadic disease. *1273*

Lipids *Serum Decrease* Total lipid concentration was found to be low. *1435*

pCO₂ *Blood Increase* Impaired movement of the respiratory cage. *2612*

pO₂ *Blood Decrease* Impaired movement of the respiratory cage. *2612*

Protein *CSF Increase* Observed in 33% of patients, most often those with severe back pain. *0666*

Rheumatoid Factor *Serum Increase* Serologic tests are positive in 15% of patients with arthritis of the vertebral region in ankylosing spondylitis. *2468*

Serum Normal Occurs no more frequently than in the general population. *0666*

Viscosity *Synovial Fluid Decrease* Lower than blood. *0666*

730.00 Osteomyelitis

Albumin *Serum Decrease* *2467*

Alkaline Phosphatase *Serum Increase* In 36% of 24 patients at initial hospitalization for this disorder. *0781*

Serum Normal Normal in all 39 cases. *2464*

Alpha₂-Globulin *Serum Increase* *2467*

Aspartate Aminotransferase *Serum Increase* In 36% of 25 patients at initial hospitalization for this disorder. *0781*

Calcium *Serum Normal* Normal in all 39 cases. *2464*

Cholesterol *Serum Decrease* In 32% of 24 patients at initial hospitalization for this disorder. *0781*

C-Reactive Protein *Serum Increase* Indicates active disease. *0186*

Erythrocyte Sedimentation Rate *Blood Increase* May be elevated or normal. *2464*

Hematocrit *Blood Decrease* Patients with initial episodes tended to be more anemic and have a more marked leukocytosis than patients with recurrent disease. *2464*

Hemoglobin *Blood Decrease* Patients with initial episodes tended to be more anemic and have a more marked leukocytosis than patients with recurrent disease. *2464*

Leukocytes *Blood Increase* May be increased, especially in acute cases. *2467* Total counts may become extremely high. *2538* Patients with initial episodes tended to be more anemic and have a more marked leukocytosis than patients with recurrent disease. *2464 0151*

Blood Normal Usually normal; especially in recurrent disease. Rarely > 16,000/μL. *2464*

Monocytes *Blood Increase* In 55% of 26 patients at initial hospitalization for this disorder. *0781*

Neutrophils *Blood Increase* In 44% of 26 patients at initial hospitalization for this disorder. *0781*

Phosphate *Serum Decrease* In 24% of 25 patients at initial hospitalization for this disorder. *0781*

Serum Normal Normal in all 39 cases. *2464*

731.00 Osteitis Deformans

Acid Phosphatase *Serum Increase* Seen occasionally in advanced disease. *2104* Elevated in very advanced cases and rare in early to moderate cases. *0948 0945*

Serum Normal Normal in a high percentage of patients. *2104*

Alkaline Phosphatase *Serum Increase* Gradually rises with the extension of the disease, rising rapidly if osteogenic sarcoma develops. ACTH or cortisone causes a transitory fall, often followed by a sharp rebound increase. *0619* Marked increase directly related to severity and extent of disease. *2467* 20 cases were reported in which all patients showed elevated serum concentration. *1312 1986 0999*

Alkaline Phosphatase Isoenzymes *Serum Increase* All 7 patients had elevations of isoenzyme II. *1221*

Calcium *Serum Increase* Usually normal but immobilization of affected individuals produces a high risk of hypercalcemia. *0999 0503*

Urine Increase Excretion is frequently increased and may lead to stone formation. *0151* Common. *0999 0503*

Hydroxyproline *Urine Increase* Increase as evidence of enhanced remodeling activity. *0999*

Leucine Aminopeptidase *Serum Increase* Slightly elevated in 14% of patients. Values ranged from 8-26 U/L (22 = normal upper limit). *1452*

Osteocalcin *Serum Increase* Elevated in 53% of patients. *2535*

Phosphate *Serum Increase* Usually normal or slightly elevated. *0999 0503*

Serum Normal Normal or slightly increased. *2467*

733.00 Osteoporosis

Alkaline Phosphatase *Serum Increase* In hypermetabolic osteopenia. *0999*

Serum Normal *0433 2467*

Calcium *Serum Decrease* Hypocalcemia may be present in severe cases. *0999*

Serum Increase *2467*

Serum Normal Process is usually so gradual that homeostatic forces control the serum calcium. *1083 0433*

Urine Decrease May be increased, normal, or decreased but is not influenced by intake; calcium restriction does not produce the normal fall. *2467*

Urine Increase May be increased, normal, or decreased but is not influenced by intake; calcium restriction does not produce the normal fall. *2467 0503 0999*

Cells *Bone Marrow Increase* The iliac bone marrow specimens showed infiltrates consisting of elongated mast cells, eosinophils, plasma cells, and varying numbers of lymphocytes. *2334*

Eosinophils *Bone Marrow Increase* The iliac bone marrow specimens showed infiltrates consisting of elongated mast cells, eosinophils, plasma cells, and varying numbers of lymphocytes. *2334*

Hydroxyproline *Urine Increase* In hypermetabolic osteopenia. *0999*

Lymphocytes *Bone Marrow Increase* The iliac bone marrow specimens showed infiltrates consisting of elongated mast cells, eosinophils, plasma cells, and varying numbers of lymphocytes. *2334*

Magnesium *Serum Decrease* In severe cases. *0999*

Phosphate *Serum Normal* *2467*

Plasma Cells *Bone Marrow Increase* The iliac bone marrow specimens showed infiltrates consisting of elongated mast cells, eosinophils, plasma cells, and varying numbers of lymphocytes. *2334*

737.30 Kyphoscoliosis

Oxygen Saturation *Blood Decrease* Thoracic bellows defects; decreased pO₂ associated with increased pCO₂. *2467* Mean pCO₂ increased and pO₂ decreased with age in idiopathic scoliosis. *1206*

pCO₂ *Blood Increase* Thoracic bellows defects; decreased pO₂ associated with increased pCO₂. *2467* Mean pCO₂ increased and pO₂ decreased with age in idiopathic scoliosis. *1206*

pO₂ *Blood Decrease* Thoracic bellows defects; decreased pO₂ associated with increased pCO₂. *2467* Mean pCO₂ increased and pO₂ decreased with age in idiopathic scoliosis. *1206*

CONGENITAL ANOMALIES

753.10 Polycystic Kidney Disease

Albumin *Urine Increase* Progressive albuminuria. *0151*

Amino Acids *Plasma Decrease* Mean concentration of essential amino acids and tyrosine were significantly lower, resulting in a low essential/total ratio. *1545*

Ammonia *Blood Decrease* Decreased arterial ammonia in azotemic patients, (mean = 34 mmol/L) due to reduced synthesis by diseased kidney. *1853*

Calcium *Urine Increase* Found in nonuremic medullary cystic disease. *0151*

Creatinine *Serum Increase* Common. *0186*

Creatinine Clearance *Urine Decrease* Diminished clearance with acidosis. *0433*

Erythrocytes *Urine Increase* Progressive hematuria. *0151* Intermittent hematuria is common, and gross hematuria may be seen occasionally. *0962*

Erythropoietin *Serum Increase* Increased values were found in 49 plasma samples and 14 cyst fluids of 92 patients with renal cell carcinoma or renal cyst. Highest values were found in patients developing metastases after removal of renal carcinoma. *1609*

Hematocrit *Blood Decrease* Most of the patients show some degree of anemia. *0433* Characteristic. *0277*

Hemoglobin *Blood Decrease* Most of the patients show some degree of anemia. *0433* Characteristic anemia. *0277*

Lactate Dehydrogenase *Urine Normal* *2467*

Neutrophils *Urine Increase* The median values were higher than 90% in bacterial, renal, or urinary tract disease and in polycystic kidney disease. *1411*

Protein *Urine Increase* Usually minimal or mild. *0962*

Sodium *Serum Decrease* Renal salt wasting. *0277* *0433*

Tyrosine *Serum Decrease* Mean concentration of essential amino acids and tyrosine were significantly lower, resulting in a low essential/total ratio. *1545*

Urea Nitrogen *Serum Increase* Azotemia. *1853*

Volume *Urine Increase* Common. *0186*

Red Blood Cells Increase True polycythemia with a considerable increase of red cell volume may occur. *1669*

753.12 Medullary Cystic Disease

Calcium *Serum Decrease* Frequent, but not invariable. *0277*

Urine Increase Found in nonuremic medullary cystic disease. *0151*

Casts *Urine Normal* Normal urinary sediment. *0277*

Creatinine Clearance *Urine Decrease* Diminished with acidosis. *0433*

Hematocrit *Blood Decrease* Most of the patients show some degree of anemia. *0433* Characteristic anemia. *0277*

Hemoglobin *Blood Decrease* Most of the patients show some degree of anemia. *0433* Characteristic anemia. *0277*

pH *Blood Decrease* Characteristic acidosis. *0277*

Sodium *Serum Decrease* Renal salt wasting. *0277* *0433*

Urine Increase Characteristic renal salt wasting. *0277*

Specific Gravity *Urine Decrease* Characteristic hyposthenuria. *0277*

Urea Nitrogen *Serum Increase* Characteristic azotemia. *0277*

Volume *Urine Increase* Polyuria. *0995*

753.13 Medullary Sponge Kidney

Calcium *Urine Increase* Hypercalciuria in 19 of 36 patients tested. *0644*

pH *Urine Increase* Impaired ability to concentrate or acidify the urine maximally has been reported. *0906 0277*

Specific Gravity *Urine Decrease* Impaired ability to concentrate or acidify the urine maximally has been reported. *0906 0277*

756.40 Chondrodystrophy

Alkaline Phosphatase *Serum Decrease* Following arrest of growth in childhood, falls rapidly to adult levels. *0619*

756.51 Osteogenesis Imperfecta

Acid Phosphatase *Serum Increase* Much higher than normal in all 8 patients (37-77 U/L). *0822* *0812*

Serum Normal The levels in patients did not differ significantly from those in controls of the same age. *1135*

Alkaline Phosphatase *Serum Increase* Increase observed in 2 cases. *1312* *2467*

756.52 Osteopetrosis

Acid Phosphatase *Serum Increase* Sometimes increased. *2467*

Alkaline Phosphatase *Serum Normal* *2467*

Calcium *Serum Decrease* Moderate hypocalcemia occasionally in children. *0995*

Serum Normal *2467*

Erythrocytes *Blood Decrease* Anemia and pancytopenia. *2468*

Hematocrit *Blood Decrease* Anemia and pancytopenia. *2468*

Hemoglobin *Blood Decrease* Anemia and pancytopenia. *2468*

Leukocytes *Blood Decrease* Anemia and pancytopenia. *2468*

Lymphocytes *Blood Decrease* Relative lymphocytosis or lymphocytopenia may occur. *2468*

Blood Increase Relative lymphocytosis or lymphocytopenia may occur. *2468*

Phosphate *Serum Decrease* Occasionally in children. *0995*

Serum Normal *2467*

Platelet Count *Blood Decrease* Anemia and pancytopenia. *2468*

756.54 Polyostotic Fibrous Dysplasia

Alkaline Phosphatase *Serum Increase* In some cases. *0619* *2467 0503 1156*

756.55 Infantile Cortical Hyperostosis

Erythrocyte Sedimentation Rate *Blood Increase* Increased (Caffey's disease). *2467*

Leukocytes *Blood Increase* Increased (Caffey's disease). *2467*

758.00 Down's Syndrome

Acid Phosphatase *Serum Decrease* May be low. *2468*

Alkaline Phosphatase *Leukocyte Increase* *2467*

Cholesterol *Serum Normal* Plasma lipid levels were measured in 20 mongoloid and 16 nonmongoloid mentally retarded subjects. Significant elevations of plasma triglyceride levels were found in patients with Down's syndrome compared with mentally retarded controls. However, no significant difference was found in plasma cholesterol, phospholipid and free fatty acid levels between the mongoloids and control subjects. *1698*

Dopamine Hydroxylase *Serum Decrease* Present in abnormally low plasma concentrations although norepinephrine is not reduced. *1300*

Fatty Acids, Free (FFA) *Serum Normal* Plasma lipid levels were measured in 20 mongoloid and 16 nonmongoloid mentally retarded subjects. Significant elevations of plasma triglyceride levels were found in patients with Down's syndrome compared with mentally retarded controls. However, no significant difference was found in plasma cholesterol, phospholipid and free fatty acid concentrations between the mongoloids and control subjects. *1698*

Folate *Serum Decrease* Mean serum folate was normal in this group, these individuals displayed decreasing concentrations with age. *0828*

Red Blood Cells Decrease Red cell values were very low. *0828*

Hemoglobin, Fetal *Blood Increase* Patients with an extra G chromosome. *2467*

Iron *Serum Increase* Patients with anicteric hepatitis whose serum contained hepatitis-B surface antigen, had lower levels than controls. *0153*

Iron-Binding Capacity, Total (TIBC) *Serum Decrease* Patients with anicteric hepatitis whose serum contained HBsAg, had lower levels than controls. *0153*

MCV *Blood Increase* As a whole, the group showed an increase. Macrocytosis increased with age. *0828*

758.00 Down's Syndrome (continued)

Phospholipids, Total *Serum Normal* Plasma lipid levels were measured in 20 mongoloid and 16 nonmongoloid mentally retarded subjects. Significant elevations of plasma triglyceride levels were found in patients with Down's syndrome compared with mentally retarded controls. However, no significant difference was found in plasma cholesterol, phospholipid and free fatty acid levels between the mongoloids and control subjects. *1698*

Triglycerides *Serum Increase* Plasma lipid levels were measured in 20 mongoloid and 16 nonmongoloid mentally retarded subjects. Significant elevations of plasma triglyceride levels were found in patients with Down's syndrome compared with mentally retarded controls. However, no significant difference was found in plasma cholesterol, phospholipid and free fatty acid levels between the mongoloids and control subjects. *1698*

Uric Acid *Serum Increase* Some cases. *0619 2104*

Zinc *Serum Decrease* Decreased. *2297*

758.10 Trisomy 13

Hemoglobin, Fetal *Blood Increase* Patients with an extra D chromosome. *2467*

Blood Normal Translocation - normal mosaicism in D_1 trisomy. *2548*

758.70 Klinefelter's Syndrome (XXY)

17-Hydroxycorticosteroids *Urine Normal* Usually normal. *1090*

17-Ketogenic Steroids *Urine Normal* Usually normal. *1090*

17-Ketosteroids *Urine Decrease* May be normal or decreased. *0962*

Alkaline Phosphatase *Leukocyte Increase* *2467*

Androgens *Plasma Decrease* Testosterone reported to be low in most studies, although there is considerable overlap between normal males and Klinefelter males. Generally higher in mosaics than in pure Klinefelter patients. *1090* Quite variable but often tends to be midway between the normal male and female. *0962*

Cholesterol *Serum Increase* Hyperlipidemia found in 8 of 24 patients; in 6, only cholesterol was elevated. *1454*

Estrogens *Serum Increase* Total and free plasma concentrations of estradiol are normal or increased. Does not correlate with clinical findings such as gynecomastia or hypoandrogenicity. *1090*

Follicle Stimulating Hormone (FSH) *Serum Increase* Commonly elevated; a result of deficient testicular function. *1090* Always increased as a result of the extensive tubular disease. *0151*

Urine Increase *0619*

Glucose *Serum Increase* Mild diabetes is found in 10%. *0962*

Glucose Tolerance *Serum Decrease* Decreased 25%. *0962*

Gonadotropin, Pituitary *Serum Increase* *0962*

Urine Increase Almost invariably increased. *0151* Commonly elevated; a result of deficient testicular function. *1090 0962*

Growth Hormone *Serum Normal* Usually normal. *1090*

Lipids *Serum Increase* Hyperlipidemia found in 8 of 24 patients; in 6, only cholesterol was elevated. *1454*

Luteinizing Hormone (LH) *Serum Increase* Commonly elevated; result of deficient testicular function. *1090* May either be high or normal. *0151*

Urine Increase *0186*

Prolactin *Serum Normal* Usually normal. *1090*

Testosterone *Plasma Decrease* Reported to be low in most studies, although there is considerable overlap between normal males and Klinefelter males. Generally higher in mosaics than in pure Klinefelter patients. *1090* Quite variable but often tends to be midway between the normal male and female. *0962*

Thyroid Stimulating Hormone (TSH) *Serum Decrease* Administration of TRH revealed a decreased TSH reserve in the Klinefelter patients. *2203*

Serum Normal Usually normal. *1090*

758.80 Syndromes Due to Sex Chromosome Abnormalities

Androgens *Plasma Increase* High plasma testosterone in XYY males. *0619*

Estradiol *Plasma Decrease* In Turner's Syndrome. *0002 0605 0046*

Estrogens *Serum Decrease* In Turner's syndrome. *0503*

Urine Decrease Doesn't increase with administration of hCG. *0186*

Follicle Stimulating Hormone (FSH) *Serum Increase* In Turner's syndrome. *2467 2468*

Urine Increase In Turner's syndrome. *0619*

Gonadotropin, Pituitary *Serum Increase* In Turner's syndrome. *2468*

Urine Increase In Turner's syndrome. *0619*

Luteinizing Hormone (LH) *Serum Increase* Usually doesn't increase until puberty. *0186*

Testosterone *Plasma Increase* In XYY males. *0619*

PERINATAL DISORDERS

770.80 Respiratory Distress Syndrome

2,3-Diphosphoglycerate *Red Blood Cells Decrease* *0236*

Alpha$_1$-Antitrypsin *Serum Decrease* Decreased. *1866 0042 1946 1947 2129*

Bicarbonate *Serum Decrease* Metabolic acidosis. *0570*

Bilirubin *Serum Increase* *0702*

Complement C3 *Serum Decrease* Neonatal- Caused by hypercatabolism. *0375 0793 1275 0509 0452*

Cortisol *Plasma Decrease* 18 newborn infants of < 37 weeks gestation who developed moderate to severe disease had a significantly lower mean cord plasma cortisol concentration at birth than that observed in 67 unaffected infants of similar gestational age; mean values were 3.36 ± 0.42 and 5.58 ± 0.43 μgl/dL, respectively. *2307*

Estrogens *Serum Decrease* The average concentrations of estradiol in umbilical cord plasma from newborns with the syndrome with or without hyaline membrane disease were lower by 25% than in controls. *2306*

Lipids *Serum Increase* Plasma lipids, particularly triglycerides complexed with fibrins, were elevated several-fold in patients with adult respiratory distress. Plasma triglycerides complexed with fibrins were significantly higher in patients who died than in those who survived. *1324*

Oxygen Saturation *Blood Decrease* Impaired ventilation. *2467*

pCO$_2$ *Blood Increase* Impaired ventilation. *2467*

pH *Blood Decrease* Decreased to 7.3 or less. *2467* Acidosis is first respiratory, later also metabolic. *2061 0702*

Phospholipids, Total *Serum Decrease* *2061*

pO$_2$ *Blood Decrease* Impaired ventilation. *2467*

Potassium *Serum Increase* Increased catabolism. *2467 0702*

Prostaglandins *Serum Increase* During the acute phase, plasma concentrations of the primary prostaglandins E and F were significantly elevated. The ratio of prostaglandin E to F was reversed. *0780*

Protein *Serum Increase* *0702*

Triglycerides *Serum Increase* Plasma lipids, particularly triglycerides complexed with fibrins were elevated several-fold in patients with adult disease. Triglycerides complexed with fibrins were significantly higher in patients who died than in those who survived. *1324*

Tri-iodothyronine (T$_3$) *Serum Decrease* In preterm infants with this disorder, cord blood T_3 concentration was significantly lower than that in cord blood of babies without this disease (22 ± 2.6 vs 36 ± 5 ng/dL). There was no significant rise at 24 h of age (22 ± 2.6 vs 34.0 ± 8 ng/dL) and remained low for 3 weeks. *0006*

Urea Nitrogen *Serum Increase* Increased catabolism. *2467*

Uric Acid *Serum Increase* Higher serum concentrations during the first 3 days of life, and the urinary excretion over the period of 12-36 h of age is also higher than in the normal infants. Neonatal hyperuricemia is not due to renal retention but to increased production of uric acid. *1874*

Urine Increase Higher serum concentrations during the first 3 days of life, and the urinary excretion over the period of 12-36 h of age was also higher than in the normal infants. Neonatal hyperuricemia is not due to renal retention but to increased production of uric acid. *1874*

771.00   Congenital Rubella

Hemagglutination Inhibition *Serum Increase* The finding of antibody after 6-8 months of age may be taken as evidence of congenital rubella. *0433* Persistently elevated titers during 1st y of life. *2508*

Immunoglobulin IgM *Serum Increase* Frequently increased levels in the first 4 months of life (immunoglobulin > 20 mg/dL). Detection of rubella-specific IgM indicates congenital disease. *0433* Presence in cord blood indicates congenital rubella infection. *2508*

773.00   Hemolytic Disease of Newborn
(Erythroblastosis Fetalis)

Albumin *Serum Decrease 0433*

Ammonia *Blood Increase* There is some evidence associating hyperammonemia with the pathogenesis of kernicterus. *2104*

Bilirubin *Serum Increase* After birth, the rate of rise is a reflection of both the severity of the hemolytic process and the degree of hepatic maturity. *2538* In the severely affected group, cord blood concentration may be 10 mg/dL (of which 33-66% is direct-acting bilirubin). Peak levels may climb despite treatment, into the 30 mg/dL range (of which 66% is direct- acting bilirubin). *0433* After birth, the rate of rise is a reflection of both severity of the hemolytic process and the degree of hepatic maturity. *2538 2061*

Bilirubin, Direct *Serum Increase* Severely affected group. *0433*

Bilirubin, Indirect *Serum Increase* In mild cases on the 2nd-5th day of life, depending upon the rapidity of increase in the degree of jaundice. *0433* Concentration > 4 mg/dL in cord blood suggest severe disease. Levels of > 50 mg/dL may be seen by the 3rd day of life in untreated, severely affected infants. *2538 2061*

Serum Normal Intermediate moderately affected group: rarely a baby in this group will develop jaundice. *0433*

Coombs' Test *Blood Negative* Infant RBCs show a negative direct Coombs' test (by standard methods) with ABO erythroblastosis. *2468* Negative or only weakly positive in cases of hemolytic disease due to ABO incompatibility. *2538* Usually negative when due to anti-A antibodies. It becomes negative within a few days of effective exchange transfusion. *2468*

Blood Positive Strongly positive in infants sensitized by Rh(D) red cells and by red cells with most of the rarely involved blood group antigens. Negative or only weakly positive in cases of hemolytic disease due to ABO incompatibility. *2538* Direct test is strongly positive on cord blood RBC when due to Rh, Kel, Kidd, Duffy antibodies. *2468*

Erythrocytes *Blood Decrease* Generally parallels the fall of hemoglobin. *2061*

Erythrocyte Sedimentation Rate *Blood Increase* Of 70 infants showing accelerated rate, 49 had signs of hemolytic disease. The test was found to be very sensitive, detecting ABO incompatibilities even in absence of marked bilirubinemia. *2150*

Glucose *Serum Decrease* In the more severely affected infants. *2538 2061*

Hematocrit *Blood Decrease* Mild cases may develop mild anemia in the first 4-6 weeks of life from which they recover spontaneously. *0433* Intermediate moderately affected group will become severely anemic in the first 7-10 days of life (anemia neonatoium). *2199 2538 1742*

Hemoglobin *Blood Decrease* In mild cases, mild anemia may develop in the first 4-6 weeks of life with spontaneous recovery. Intermediate group will become severely anemic in the first 7-10 days of life (anemia neonatorum). Hemoglobin may drop below 2 g/dL and the child may die unless given a transfusion. Because hydrops fetalis is due to hepatic dysfunction, not anemia, some fetuses become hydropic with hemoglobin levels of 7-8 g/dL. Others are not hydropic with levels of 3-4 g/dL. *0433* Adult hemoglobin is increased with hemolytic disease of the newborn. *2468 2538 1742 2061*

Hemoglobin, Fetal *Blood Decrease 2468*

Immunoglobulin IgD *Serum Increase 0619*

Lactate Dehydrogenase *Serum Increase* Derived from red blood cells. *0619*

Leukocytes *Blood Increase* Increased (usually 15,000-30,000/μL) with hemolytic disease. *2468* Moderate with high polymorphonuclear percentage. *2061*

MCH *Blood Increase 2468*

MCHC *Blood Normal 2468*

MCV *Blood Increase 2468*

Neutrophils *Blood Increase 2061*

Osmotic Fragility *Red Blood Cells Increase* Increased with ABO erythroblastosis. *2468*

Platelet Count *Blood Decrease* Frequently present in the severely affected group. Although partially a result of exchange transfusion, it is predominantly caused by a reduction of marrow megakaryocytes as a result of excess erythropoiesis. Counts < 40,000/μL are not uncommon. *0433* May occur secondary to isoimmune or exchange transfusion. *2538 2061*

Prothrombin Time *Plasma Increase 2061*

Reticulocytes *Blood Increase* Counts normally 5-10% may be markedly elevated in the erythroblastic infant (up to 25-50% in severe cases). *0433* Correlates roughly with the level of hemoglobin in the cord blood, although well-compensated hemolysis may occur. *2538* Percentage is a rough indicator of prognosis. *2061*

Urobilinogen *Urine Increase* Parallels serum levels. *2468* Excess consistent with exaggerated hemolysis. *2061*

Feces Increase Parallels serum levels of indirect bilirubin. *2468*

774.40   Jaundice Due to Hepatocellular Damage
(Newborn)

Alpha-Fetoprotein *Serum Increase* Elevations occur in many cases of neonatal hepatitis and may be helpful in differentiating this condition from biliary atresia. *2609*

Bilirubin *Serum Increase 2061*
Urine Normal 2467
Feces Decrease Normal or decreased. *2467*

Bilirubin, Direct *Serum Increase* Normal or slight increase. *2467*

Bilirubin, Indirect *Serum Increase 2467*

Leucine Aminopeptidase *Serum Increase* In 12 patients with obstructive jaundice, all showed elevations, ranging from 430-990 U/L. *0281*

Partial Thromboplastin Time *Plasma Increase* Markedly prolonged. *0433*

Platelet Count *Blood Decrease 0433*

Prothrombin Time *Plasma Increase* Markedly prolonged. *0433*

Urobilinogen *Urine Normal 2467*
Feces Decrease Normal or decreased. *2467*

SIGNS AND SYMPTOMS

780.30   Convulsions

Creatine Kinase *Serum Increase* Raised levels have been reported following convulsive seizures. *0962*

Estrogens *Serum Increase* The incidence of epileptic seizures was higher in women during the high estrogen period of the menstrual cycle. Number of seizures correlated positively to estrogen/progesterone ratio and negatively to progesterone levels. *0096*

Lactic Acid *Blood Increase* In 10 patients with idiopathic seizures studied < 3 h after the seizure, arterial and CSF lactate were elevated in association with a mild arterial metabolic acidosis. *0293* May occur with febrile convulsions in children. *2178*

CSF Increase In 10 patients with idiopathic seizures studied 3 h after the seizure, arterial and CSF lactate were elevated in association with a mild arterial metabolic acidosis. The elevated CSF lactate persisted despite a return to normal of the arterial concentration in 7 patients studied between 3-6 h after the seizure. *0293* May occur with febrile convulsions in children. *2178*

Myoglobin *Urine Increase* Sporadic; exertional. *2467*

Neutrophils *Blood Increase 2538*

pH *Blood Decrease* In 10 patients with idiopathic seizures studied 3 h after the seizure, arterial and CSF lactate were elevated in association with a mild arterial metabolic acidosis. *0293*

Pregnanediol *Urine Decrease* The incidence of epileptic seizures was higher in women during the high estrogen period of the menstrual cycle. Number of seizures correlated positively to estrogen:progesterone ratio and negatively to progesterone levels. *0096*

Progesterone *Plasma Decrease* The incidence of epileptic seizures was higher in women during the high estrogen period of the menstrual cycle. Number of seizures correlated positively to estrogen:progesterone ratio and negatively to progesterone levels. *0096*

780.30 Convulsions *(continued)*

Pyruvate *Blood Increase* May occur with febrile convulsions in children. *2178*

CSF Increase May occur with febrile convulsions in children. *2178*

Uric Acid *Serum Increase* Significant increases were found in 17 patients with 2 or more grand mal seizures within 24 h. In 6 cases, concentrations were reached at which hyperuricemic renal failure may develop. *1449 1784*

780.80 Hyperhidrosis

Bicarbonate *Serum Normal* *2467*

Chloride *Serum Decrease* *2467*

Creatinine *Serum Increase* Leading to reduced renal blood flow (prerenal azotemia). *2467*

pH *Urine Normal* *2467*

Potassium *Serum Normal* *2467*

Urine Normal *2467*

Sodium *Serum Decrease* *2467*

Urine Decrease *2467*

Urea Nitrogen *Serum Increase* Salt and water depletion causes reduced renal blood flow leading to prerenal azotemia. *2467* Dehydration. *0812 0503*

Volume *Plasma Normal* *2467*

Urine Normal *2467*

785.40 Gangrene

Alanine Aminotransferase *Serum Increase* *0962*

Aldolase *Serum Increase* *0962*

Alkaline Phosphatase *Serum Increase* In 45% of 32 patients hospitalized for this disorder. *0781*

Aspartate Aminotransferase *Serum Increase* May produce slight elevations. Usual values 50 U/L. *0503* In 27% of 32 patients hospitalized for this disorder. *0781* Found with extensive necrosis *0186 0962*

Bicarbonate *Serum Increase* In 37% of 28 patients hospitalized for this disorder. *0781*

Chloride *Serum Decrease* In 39% of 28 patients hospitalized for this disorder. *0781*

C-Reactive Protein *Serum Increase* Precedes the rise in ESR; with recovery disappearance precedes the return to normal of the ESR. Also disappears when inflammatory process is suppressed by steroids or salicylates. *2467*

Creatine Kinase *Serum Increase* Found with extensive necrosis. Predominantly CPK-MM. *0186*

Cryoglobulins *Serum Increase* Marked elevation of cryoglobulins. *2104*

Lactate Dehydrogenase *Serum Increase* In 24% of 32 patients hospitalized for this disorder. *0781* Slight elevation. *0992*

Leukocytes *Blood Increase* Due to tissue necrosis. *2467* In 66% of 34 patients hospitalized for this disorder. *0781*

Neutrophils *Blood Increase* In 63% of 33 patients hospitalized for this disorder. *0781*

pCO₂ *Blood Decrease* In 22% of 13 patients hospitalized for this disorder. *0781*

pH *Blood Increase* In 74% of 13 patients hospitalized for this disorder. *0781*

pO₂ *Blood Decrease* In 63% of 11 patients hospitalized for this disorder. *0781*

Sodium *Serum Decrease* In 47% of 27 patients hospitalized for this disorder. *0781*

785.50 Shock

2,3-Diphosphoglycerate *Red Blood Cells Increase* Disturbed RBC 2,3-DPG metabolism results in reduced oxygen affinity and delivery to tissues. *0151*

17-Hydroxycorticosteroids *Urine Increase* *0164*

17-Ketogenic Steroids *Urine Increase* *2246*

Alanine Aminotransferase *Serum Increase* Heart failure or shock with attendant hepatic necrosis may lead to elevated values. *0503*

Amino Acids *Plasma Increase* In severe shock. *0619*

Amylase *Serum Increase* May be associated with hyperamylasemia. *1386*

Aspartate Aminotransferase *Serum Increase* Usual values 20-900 U/L. *0503*

Bicarbonate *Serum Decrease* Respiratory alkalosis may occur. *0962*

Catecholamines *Urine Increase* *0164*

Creatinine *Serum Increase* Causes reduced renal blood flow leading to prerenal azotemia. *2467*

Eosinophils *Blood Decrease* *2467*

Epinephrine *Plasma Increase* In patients with septicemic, traumatic or hemorrhagic shock. Plasma epinephrine and noradrenaline concentrations were increased above the normal range. *0164*

Erythrocytes *Blood Decrease* Hemoconcentration (dehydration, burns) or hemodilution (hemorrhage, crush injuries, and skeletal trauma) takes place. *2467* Disturbed RBC 2,3-DPG metabolism results in reduced oxygen affinity and delivery to tissues. *0151*

Blood Increase Hemoconcentration (e.g., dehydration, burns) or hemodilution (e.g., hemorrhage, crush injuries, and skeletal trauma) takes place. *2467*

Euglobulin Clot Lysis Time *Blood Increase* Increased in circulatory collapse. *0295 2353*

Fibrinogen *Plasma Decrease* Decreased after severe shock during operation or after trauma, as a result of excessive utilization due to release of tissue thromboplastin. *0619*

Fibrin Split Products (FSP) *Plasma Increase* Raised serum or urine levels are common without other evidence of enhanced fibrinolysis. *1253*

Urine Increase Raised serum or urine levels are common without other evidence of enhanced fibrinolysis. *1253*

Glomerular Filtration Rate (GFR) *Urine Decrease* Decreased after shock due to decreased renal blood flow. *0619*

Glucose *Serum Increase* Increased circulating epinephrine. *0619* Hyperglycemia occurs early. *2467*

Lactate Dehydrogenase *Serum Increase* 2-40 X normal values. *0503*

Lactic Acid *Blood Increase* May be of some prognostic value. *2467 0619*

Leukocytes *Blood Decrease* There may be leukopenia when shock is severe as in gram-negative bacteremia. *2467*

Blood Increase Common, especially with hemorrhage. *2467*

Metanephrines, Total *Urine Increase* *0503*

Norepinephrine *Plasma Increase* In patients with septicemic, traumatic or hemorrhagic shock, epinephrine and norepinephrine concentrations were increased above the normal range. In patients who died, plasma norepinephrine concentrations remained persistently elevated above normal while in those who survived, there was a rapid decline towards the normal range. *0164*

Oxygen Saturation *Blood Decrease* Disturbed RBC 2,3-DPG metabolism results in reduced oxygen affinity and delivery to tissues. *0151*

pCO₂ *Blood Decrease* Respiratory alkalosis may occur. *0962*

pH *Blood Increase* Respiratory alkalosis may occur. *0962*

Urea Nitrogen *Serum Increase* A decrease in plasma volume secondary to dehydration, blood loss, hypotension or shock is often referred to as prerenal azotemia. *0812 0503*

787.00 Vomiting

Ammonia *Urine Increase* Increase in urine ammonia in prolonged vomiting with associated achlorhydria and ketosis. *0619*

Bicarbonate *Serum Increase* Metabolic alkalosis. *0619*

Chloride *Urine Decrease* Excessive chloride loss, due to vomiting. *0619*

Creatinine *Serum Increase* Leading to reduced renal blood flow (prerenal azotemia). *2467*

Ketones *Serum Increase* *0619*

Urine Increase Children are more liable to develop ketosis than adults with persistent vomiting. *0619*

Neutrophils *Blood Increase* *2538*

pH *Blood Increase* Metabolic alkalosis. *0619*

Phosphate *Serum Decrease* Of 100 patients with hypophosphatemia, 12% was due to vomiting, 40% to intravenous glucose feeding, and miscellaneous or unexplained in the rest. *0190*

Potassium *Serum Decrease* Deficiency results from decreased intake of potassium, loss in the vomitus, and most important, from renal potassium wasting. *2199*

Urine Increase 0619

Sodium *Serum Increase* Resulting in relative depletion of chloride and hydrogen ions (developing metabolic alkalosis), can lead to an increase in plasma sodium concentration in the presence of gross dehydration. *0619*

Urea Nitrogen *Serum Increase* Salt and water depletion causes reduced renal blood flow leading to prerenal azotemia. *2467* Dehydration. *0812 0503*

Volume *Plasma Decrease 0619*

791.30   Myoglobinuria

11-Hydroxycorticosteroids *Urine Normal* Endocrine studies are normal. *2467*

17-Hydroxycorticosteroids *Urine Normal 2467*

17-Ketogenic Steroids *Urine Normal 2467*

Aldolase *Serum Increase* Found in paroxysmal myoglobinuria due to muscle destruction. *0619*

Aspartate Aminotransferase *Serum Increase 0619 2467*

Creatine *Serum Increase* Muscle destruction after crush injury. *0619*

Urine Increase 2467

Creatine Kinase *Serum Increase* Increases in necrosis or acute atrophy of striated muscle. *2467*

INJURY AND POISONING

829.00   Fracture of Bone

Alkaline Phosphatase *Serum Increase* Rises in proportion to the formation of new bone cells. *0812 0503*

Creatine *Urine Increase* Increased breakdown. *2467*

Fat *Serum Present* Fat globules in 42-67% of cases. *2468*

Urine Increase In 60% of cases. *2468*

Sputum Increase Fat globules found in sputum of some patients. *2468*

Fatty Acids, Free (FFA) *Serum Increase 2468*

Hemoglobin *Blood Decrease* Unexplained fall after traumatic fracture. *2468*

Lipase *Serum Increase* In 30-50% of cases. *2468*

Oxygen Saturation *Blood Decrease* Decreased arterial pO_2 associated with normal or decreased pCO_2 with associated fat embolism. *2468*

pCO_2 *Blood Decrease* Decreased arterial pO_2 associated with normal or decreased pCO_2 with associated fat embolism. *2468*

Phosphate *Serum Increase 0619 2467*

Platelet Count *Blood Decrease 2468*

pO_2 *Blood Decrease* Decreased arterial pO_2 associated with normal or decreased pCO_2 with associated fat embolism. *2468*

Triglycerides *Serum Increase* After traumatic fracture. *2468*

929.00   Crush Injury (Trauma)

17-Hydroxycorticosteroids *Urine Increase* Due to severe stress. *0995*

17-Ketogenic Steroids *Urine Increase* Due to severe stress. *0995*

Alanine Aminotransferase *Serum Increase 0962*

Aldolase *Serum Increase 0995*

Alpha$_1$-Glycoprotein *Serum Increase* One of the most reliable indicators of acute inflammation. *1239 1672 1866   1947 2096 2170*

Amylase *Serum Increase* Crush injury to abdomen resulting in contusion, rupture or hemorrhage provokes hyperamylasemia. *2104*

Aspartate Aminotransferase *Serum Increase* Slightly to moderate increase. *0503   0619 0962*

Catecholamines *Urine Increase* Due to severe stress. *0995*

Creatine *Urine Increase* Increased formation myopathy. *2467*

Creatine Kinase *Serum Increase* Raised for approximately 15 days, especially if associated arterial obstruction. *0619* Increases in necrosis or acute atrophy of striated muscle. *2467* Most reliable measure of skeletal muscle damage. *0503   0812 0962*

Epinephrine *Plasma Increase 0995*

Fat *Urine Increase 0619*

Glucose *Serum Increase 0995*

Leukocytes *Blood Increase 0995*

Lipase *Serum Increase* Activity increases in some patients sustaining severe injury to adipose tissue. *2104*

Myoglobin *Urine Increase* Sudden muscle damage. *0619*

Neutrophils *Blood Increase 0995*

Platelet Count *Blood Increase* Count rises slowly, lasting for 3 weeks in trauma. *2468*

Potassium *Serum Increase 0995*

948.00   Burns

17-Hydroxycorticosteroids *Urine Increase* Increased due to severe stress. *2467*

17-Ketogenic Steroids *Urine Increase* Increased due to severe stress. *2467*

Alanine Aminotransferase *Serum Increase* Rises soon after burn. *2104*

Albumin *Serum Decrease* Superficial burns reduce capillary membrane semipermeability and cause a disproportionate loss of albumin. *2104*

Aldolase *Serum Increase* Cell destruction. *2467*

Alpha$_1$-Antichymotrypsin *Serum Increase* Acutely burned children exhibited a rapid rise to a maximum on day 10 postburn, which remained elevated after 60 days. *1168*

Alpha$_1$-Antitrypsin *Serum Decrease* Decreased during acute phase of thermal burn. *1866 0042 1946 1947 2129*

Serum Increase Increased. *1866 0042 1946 1947 2129*

Alpha$_1$-Glycoprotein *Serum Increase* One of the most reliable indicators of acute inflammation. *1239 1672 1866   1947 2096 2170*

Amino Acids *Plasma Increase* In severe burns the peptides derived from the burnt tissues appear in the plasma. *0619*

Urine Increase Amino acids and peptides from burnt tissues are excreted in urine. *0619*

Amylase *Serum Decrease* Decreased in severe burns. *0619*

Serum Increase May be associated with hyperamylasemia. *1386*

Aspartate Aminotransferase *Serum Increase* Rises soon after burn. *2104*

Calcium *Serum Normal* On average, free or ionized calcium were in the normal range. However they were weakly correlated with the severity of burn injury. *0723*

Catecholamines *Urine Increase* Increased due to severe stress. *2467* With physical or emotional stress. *2092*

Cholesterol, Very Low Density Lipoprotein *Serum Increase* Moderate increase secondary to increased secretion and decreased catabolism. *0062*

Complement C1s *Serum Decrease* {793} {2522}

Complement C3 *Serum Decrease* Caused by hypercatabolism. *0375 0793 1275 0509   0452*

Creatine *Urine Increase* Increased breakdown. *2467*

Creatine Kinase *Serum Increase* In 8 thermal burn patients there was a significant increase (P < 0.01). *0933*

Creatinine Clearance *Urine Increase* Mean clearance in 20 burned patients, measured between the 4-35 postburn day, was 172.1 ± 48.4 mL/min/1.73 m^2. 13 patients had values > 2 S.D. above the normal. *1422*

Epinephrine *Plasma Increase* A drop in eosinophils with increased corticoid and epinephrine production are manifestations of stress. *2113*

Urine Increase With physical or emotional stress. *2092* Urinary excretion of epinephrine and its metabolites are rough indicators of degree of stress. *2113*

Factor V *Plasma Increase* Factor V and VIII may be 4-8 X normal for up to 3 months. *2468*

Factor VIII *Plasma Increase* Factor V and VIII may be 4-8 X normal for up to 3 months. *2468*

Factor B *Plasma Decrease* *1979 2356*

Fibrinogen *Plasma Decrease* Falls during first 36 h, then rises steeply for up to 3 months. *2468*

948.00 Burns (continued)

Fibrinogen (continued)

Plasma Increase Falls during the first 36 h and then rises steeply for up to 3 months. *2468*

Glomerular Filtration Rate (GFR) *Urine Increase* May rise to very high values. *1422*

Glucagon *Plasma Increase* Increased. *0306 0620 0513*

Glucose *Serum Increase* A syndrome of glycosuria, dehydration, coma, and severe glycosuria without ketosis has been recognized in patients recovering from major burns. This syndrome is distinct from the transient hyperglycemia that occurs immediately after burns or acute trauma. *2104*

Urine Increase A syndrome of glycosuria, dehydration, coma, and severe glycosuria without ketosis has been recognized in patients recovering from major burns. This syndrome is distinct from the transient hyperglycemia that occurs immediately after burns or acute trauma. *2104*

Hemoglobin, Free *Serum Increase* Intravascular hemolysis due to thermal burns; injuring RBCs. *2467*

Urine Increase Intravascular hemolysis due to thermal burns; injuring RBCs. *2467*

Hexosaminidase *Urine Increase* Decreased levels in urine. *2356*

Leukocytes *Blood Increase* Due to tissue necrosis. *2467*

Magnesium *Serum Decrease* Moderate and short-lived decrease in serum and erythrocytes occurs immediately after burn. *1335*

Red Blood Cells Decrease Moderate and short-lived decrease in serum and erythrocytes occurs immediately after burn. *1335*

Myoglobin *Serum Increase* In 8 thermal burn patients there was a significant increase (P < 0.01). *0933*

Neutrophils *Blood Increase* *2538*

Nickel *Serum Increase* Mean 7.2 (n = 3) compared with controls mean 2.6 μg/L (n = 42). *1559*

Osmotic Fragility *Red Blood Cells Increase* Increased after thermal injury. *2467*

Phosphate *Serum Decrease* Patients recovering from burns may remain hypophosphatemic and hypouricemic for months after the initial injury. *1287*

Platelet Count *Blood Decrease* Moderate thrombocytopenia is frequently present for 2-4 days following severe thermal injury to more than 10% of the body. Reduction is most pronounced in patients with sepsis. The degree of thrombocytopenia does not correlate closely with prognosis, but rising platelet levels are associated with clinical improvement. *1034 2538*

Blood Increase Count rises slowly, lasting for 3 weeks in burns and other types of trauma. *2468*

Sodium *Serum Decrease* Reduced concentration in plasma, but an increase in RBC concentration occurs even in minor burns. *2104*

Red Blood Cells Increase Reduced concentration in plasma, but an increase in RBC concentration occurs even in minor burns. *2104*

Uric Acid *Serum Decrease* Patients recovering from burns may remain hypophosphatemic and hypouricemic for months after the initial injury. *1287*

Uric Acid Clearance *Urine Increase* Significantly increased renal clearance is found. *2506*

Uropepsinogen *Urine Increase* *0619*

Viscosity *Serum Increase* Rises acutely and remains elevated for 4-5 days although hematocrit has returned to normal. *2468*

Volume *Plasma Decrease* Decreased plasma volume and blood volume follows marked drop in cardiac output. Greatest decrease occurs in first 12 h and continues at a slower rate for 6-12 h longer. In a 40% burn, plasma volume falls 25%. *2468*

958.10 Fat Embolism

Calcium *Serum Decrease* Decreased calcium correlated with leukocytosis and low hemoglobin. *1683*

Fat *Urine Increase* In 60% of cases. *2468*

Sputum Increase Fat globules found in sputum of some patients. *2468*

Fatty Acids, Free (FFA) *Serum Increase* Not of diagnostic value. *2467*

Hemoglobin *Blood Decrease* Decreased hemoglobin correlates with leukocytosis and hypocalcemia. *1683*

Leukocytes *Blood Increase* Decreased hemoglobin correlates with leukocytosis and hypocalcemia. *1683*

Lipase *Serum Increase* Increased in 30-50% of cases. *2467*

Oxygen Saturation *Blood Decrease* Decreased arterial pO$_2$ with normal or decreased pCO$_2$. *2467 2532*

pCO$_2$ *Blood Decrease* Decreased arterial PO$_2$ with normal or decreased PCO$_2$. *2467*

Platelet Count *Blood Decrease* Sometimes quite severe. *2538 2467*

pO$_2$ *Blood Decrease* Decreased arterial pO$_2$ with normal or decreased pCO$_2$. *2467 2532*

Triglycerides *Serum Increase* *2467*

984.00 Toxic Effects of Lead and Its Compounds (including Fumes)

Alanine *Urine Increase* With lead intoxication. *0889*

Aldolase *Serum Increase* *0962*

Alpha-Amino-Nitrogen *Urine Increase* With lead intoxication. *0889*

Amino Acids *Urine Increase* Results from changes in the epithelium of the proximal convoluted tubules in lead poisoning. *0151* Transient finding. *0294*

Aminolevulinic Acid *Serum Increase* In 50 cases, brain levels increased 4-fold, urine 8-fold and plasma only 2-fold compared to controls. *0487* Concentration > 20 mg/dL indicates poisoning. *0294*

Urine Increase Delta-aminolevulinic acid is increased. *2468* In 50 cases, brain levels increased 4-fold, urine 8-fold and plasma only 2-fold compared to controls. *0487* In lead poisoning. *0889*

Aminolevulinic Acid Dehydrase *Red Blood Cells Decrease* RBC concentration correlates negatively with serum lead concentration. *0294*

Basophilic Stippling *Blood Increase* Coarse basophilic stippling occurs to an extreme degree, with involvement of up to 1-2% of cells. *2538* Occurs in 60% of childhood cases. *0294*

Beta-Amino-Isobutyric-Acid *Urine Increase* A result of the nephrotoxic effect of lead. *0618*

Bilirubin *Serum Increase* Hemolytic anemia may occur. *0484*

Citrate *Urine Increase* Citraturia results from changes in the proximal convoluted tubules. *0151*

Copper *Red Blood Cells Increase* RBC concentration may increase with poisoning. *0618*

Coproporphyrin *Urine Increase* A reliable sign of intoxication and is often demonstrable before basophilic stippling. *2468* Increase in urine coproporphyrin III is associated with an increase in urine uroporphyrin and red cell protoporphyrin. *0619 0151 0889*

Red Blood Cells Increase Free erythrocyte coproporphyrin ranges from 1-20 μg/dL (Normal = 0-2 μg/dL) in lead poisoning. *0151*

Eosinophils *Blood Increase* Increases in poisoning. *2467*

Erythrocytes *Blood Decrease* Hemolytic anemia. *0484*

Urine Increase Renal damage may occur. *0889*

Erythrocyte Sedimentation Rate *Blood Increase* With arsenic and lead intoxication. *2467*

Erythrocyte Survival *Red Blood Cells Decrease* Red cell life span and osmotic fragility are decreased. *0151* Hemolysis. *0618*

Fructose *Urine Increase* Occurs as a result of changes in the epithelium of the proximal convoluted tubules. *0151*

Glucose *Urine Increase* Nephrotoxic effect of lead. *0618*

Glycine *Urine Increase* Transient increase. *0294*

Hematocrit *Blood Decrease* Acute hemolytic anemia with hemoglobinemia and hemoglobinuria occasionally occur in acute lead poisoning. *0151 0484*

Hemoglobin *Blood Decrease* Acute hemolytic anemia with hemoglobinemia and hemoglobinuria occasionally occur in acute lead poisoning. *0151 0484*

Hemoglobin A$_{1C}$ *Blood Increase* *2539*

Hemoglobin, Free *Serum Increase* With acute hemolytic crisis. *0151*

Urine Increase With acute hemolytic crisis. *0850*

Iron *Serum Increase* With hemolysis. *0618*

Lead *Blood Increase* Diagnosis of lead poisoning is confirmed by blood concentrations of 25-40 μg/DL. *2468 0151*

Urine Increase Urine lead > 80 μg/L for children and > 150 μg/L in adults indicated lead poisoning. *2468* The urine output of lead may increase to more than 100 mg/24h. This may be associated with an increased output of urine coproporphyrin III. *0619 0850*

Feces Increase Lead concentrations of > 1.1 mg/specimen constitutes lead poisoning in adults. *0151*

Leukocytes *Blood Decrease* Pancytopenia may occur. *1578*

MCH *Blood Decrease* Microcytic hypochromic anemia may occur due to blood loss, increased demand or dietary inadequacy. MCH < 27 pg, MCV < 80 fL. *0532*

MCHC *Blood Decrease* Hemolytic anemia. *0484*

MCV *Blood Decrease* Microcytic hypochromic anemia may occur due to blood loss, increased demand or dietary inadequacy. MCH < 27 pg, MCV < 80 fL. *0532* Hemolytic anemia. *0484*

Blood Increase Rare increase with poisoning. *0618*

Occult Blood *Feces Positive* Bloody diarrhea may occur. *0850*

Osmotic Fragility *Red Blood Cells Decrease* Osmotic fragility is decreased and mechanic fragility is increased. *0151*

Phosphate *Urine Increase* Results from changes in the epithelium in the proximal convoluted tubules. *0151*

Platelet Count *Blood Decrease* Pancytopenia may occur. *1578*

Porphobilinogen *Urine Normal* *1031*

Porphyrins *Urine Increase* *2467*

Protein *Urine Increase* Renal damage may occur. *0889*

CSF Increase Increased, with normal cell count in encephalopathy. *2468 0850*

Protoporphyrin *Red Blood Cells Increase* Accumulates in the erythrocytes as a result of the blocks in the synthetic process. *0151* Free erythrocyte protoporphyrin ranges from 300-3,000 mg/dL (normal = 15-60). *0151* Log of RBC protoporphyrin level closely correlated to blood level (R = 0.72) in lead-exposed workers. Especially useful in the detection of mild increases in blood lead concentrations under conditions of occupational exposure. *2366*

Reticulocytes *Blood Increase* Hemolytic anemia. *0889*

Urea Nitrogen *Serum Increase* May cause renal damage. *2084*

Uric Acid *Serum Increase* Moonshine whiskey causing 'saturnine gout'. *0619* Increased in serum due to reduced renal clearance. *0106 1283 0962*

Urine Decrease Reduced renal clearance. *0106*

Urobilinogen *Urine Increase* Possibly in some cases as evidence of increased red cell destruction. *0619 2468*

Uroporphyrin *Urine Increase* *2468*

985.00 Toxic Effects of Non-medicinal Metals

Alanine Aminotransferase *Serum Increase* Hepatotoxicity may occur with arsenicals. *1446*

Albumin *Urine Increase* Common in mercury intoxication. *0151*

Alkaline Phosphatase *Serum Increase* Hepatotoxicity may occur with arsenicals. *1446*

Arsenic *Urine Increase* Patients with chronic arsenic poisoning excrete 0.1 mg/day of arsenic. Normal values average 0.015 mg/day. *0151*

Aspartate Aminotransferase *Serum Increase* Hepatotoxicity may occur with arsenicals. *1446*

Bicarbonate *Serum Decrease* May be depressed in chronic mercury poisoning. *0618*

Bilirubin *Serum Increase* Hepatotoxicity may occur with arsenicals. *1446*

BSP Retention *Serum Increase* Hepatotoxicity may occur with arsenicals. *1446*

Calcium *Serum Increase* Highly significant hypercalciuria and decreased serum inorganic phosphate was found in a group of workers with cadmium intoxication. *2098*

Casts *Urine Increase* Nephrotoxicity may occur with therapeutic doses of arsenicals. *1514 0651 0889*

Cephalin Flocculation *Serum Increase* Hepatotoxicity may occur with arsenicals. *1446*

Cholesterol *Serum Increase* Hepatotoxic effects of arsenicals may be marked. *1446*

Coproporphyrin *Urine Increase* Increased markedly in chronic arsenic poisoning. *0151*

Creatinine *Serum Increase* Nephrotoxicity is common with therapeutic doses of arsenicals. *0811*

Eosinophils *Blood Increase* Usually 10-20% in arsenic poisoning. *0977 0811*

Erythrocytes *Blood Decrease* Pancytopenia may occur in arsenic intoxication. *0484*

Urine Increase Common in mercury poisoning. *0151* Marked hematuria may occur in arsenic intoxication. *0850 1514 0651 0889*

Erythrocyte Sedimentation Rate *Blood Increase* With arsenic and lead intoxication. *2467*

Glucose *Serum Decrease* Hepatotoxicity may occur with arsenicals. *1446*

Guanase *Serum Increase* Hepatotoxicity may occur with arsenicals. *1446*

Hematocrit *Blood Decrease* Mild to moderate anemia occurs in chronic arsenic poisoning. *0151* Pancytopenia may occur. *0484*

Hemoglobin *Blood Decrease* Mild to moderate anemia occurs in chronic arsenic poisoning. *0151*

Isocitrate Dehydrogenase *Serum Increase* Hepatotoxicity may occur with arsenicals. *1446*

Leukocytes *Blood Decrease* In chronic arsenic poisoning. *0151* Pancytopenia may occur. *0484*

Blood Increase May be caused by poisoning by chemicals, drugs, venoms, etc. (e.g., mercury, epinephrine, black widow spider). *2467* Occurs with industrial nickel exposure. *1542*

Occult Blood *Feces Positive* Bloody diarrhea occurs with arsenic and mercury poisoning. *0889*

Phosphate *Urine Increase* Highly significant hypercalciuria and decreased serum inorganic phosphate was found in a group of workers with cadmium intoxication. *2098*

Platelet Count *Blood Decrease* Pancytopenia may occur in arsenic poisoning. *0484*

Protein *Urine Increase* With renal damage in arsenic poisoning. *0811* Nephrotoxicity may occur in mercury poisoning. *1514 0651 0889*

Pyruvate *Blood Increase* Arsenic, antimony, gold, and mercury inhibit pyruvate oxidation. *0619*

Reticulocytes *Blood Increase* Values up to 18% have been observed following toxicity with arsenicals. *0977*

Sodium *Serum Decrease* May occur with established mercury poisoning. *0618*

Thymol Turbidity *Serum Increase* Hepatotoxicity may occur with arsenicals. *1446*

Urea Nitrogen *Serum Increase* Nephrotoxicity is common with therapeutic doses of arsenicals. *0811*

986.00 Toxic Effects of Carbon Monoxide

Aldolase *Serum Increase* Often elevated. *0262*

Aspartate Aminotransferase *Serum Increase* From skeletal muscle, heart muscle, and brain. *0619*

Creatine Kinase *Serum Increase* 11 of 13 cases of carbon monoxide poisoning showed elevation, often accompanied by aldolase and transaminase elevation as well. *0262*

Erythrocytes *Urine Increase* Occurs in severe cases. *0151*

Glomerular Filtration Rate (GFR) *Urine Increase* Occurs 12-24 h after exposure. *2256*

Leukocytes *Blood Increase* Occurs in severe cases. *0151*

Lipids *Urine Increase* Lipids in the urine include all fractions. Double refractile (cholesterol) bodies can be seen. There is a high protein content. *2467*

Myoglobin *Urine Increase* Sporadic; metabolic myoglobinuria. *2467 0016*

Oxygen Saturation *Blood Decrease* *2468*

pH *Blood Decrease* Markedly decreased (metabolic acidosis due to tissue hypoxia). *2468*

Phosphoglucomutase *Serum Increase* One case with serum level increased 250 X normal reported. *0619*

Protein *Urine Increase* Occurs in severe cases. *0151* Nephrotoxicity. *2084*

Urea Nitrogen *Serum Increase* Occurs in severe cases. *0151* Nephrotoxicity. *2084*

989.50 Toxic Effects of Venom

Alanine Aminotransferase *Serum Increase* Found in 6 of 14 patients admitted for bee stings. *1822*

989.50   Toxic Effects of Venom   (continued)

Aspartate Aminotransferase   *Serum   Increase*   Elevated in 9 of 17 patients admitted for wasp/bee stings. *1822   0619*

Clotting Time   *Blood   Increase*   Increased clotting time indicates severe envenomation from snake bite. *0151*

Creatine Kinase   *Serum   Increase*   14 of 17 patients admitted for wasp/bee stings showed elevated activities, indicating presence of damage to muscle fibers. *1822*

Eosinophils   *Blood   Increase*   Increases in poisoning (e.g., phosphate, black widow spider bite). *2467*

Fibrinogen   *Plasma   Decrease*   *0995*

Hematocrit   *Blood   Decrease*   A drop indicates severe envenomization following snake bite. *0151*

Hemoglobin   *Blood   Decrease*   A drop indicates severe envenomization following snake bite. *0151*

Lactate Dehydrogenase   *Serum   Increase*   Analysis of 17 patients admitted for wasp stings showed elevated LD in 8/14 cases, elevated AST and CK in 9/17 and 14/17, respectively. *1822*

Leukocytes   *Blood   Increase*   May be caused by poisoning by chemicals, drugs, or venoms. *2467*   Polymorphonuclear leukocytosis of 20,000-30,000/μL. *0995*

Myoglobin   *Urine   Increase*   Common after bites. *0619*   Sporadic elevation; metabolic myoglobinuria. *2467*

Neutrophils   *Blood   Increase*   May be caused by poisoning by chemicals, drugs, or venoms. *2467*   Polymorphonuclear leukocytosis of 20,000-30,000/μL. *0995*

Platelet Count   *Blood   Decrease*   *0995*

Protein   *Urine   Increase*   May cause nephrotoxicity. *2084   0995*

Prothrombin Time   *Plasma   Increase*   May be greatly prolonged in severe cases of snake bite. *0151*

Urea Nitrogen   *Serum   Increase*   May cause nephrotoxicity. *2084   0995*

990.00   Effects of X-Ray Irradiation

Alanine Aminotransferase   *Serum   Increase*   May be increased in cases of radiation injury, indicating major cell and tissue damage. *0151*

Alpha$_1$-Globulin   *Serum   Increase*   *0619*

Alpha$_2$-Globulin   *Serum   Increase*   *0619*

Amylase   *Serum   Increase*   Sharp rise following salivary gland irradiation. Peak values range from 9-18 X preirradiation values. Steady decline to normal within 2-3 days. *0384*

Aspartate Aminotransferase   *Serum   Increase*   May be increased in cases of radiation injury, indicating major cell and tissue damage. *0151   2467 0619*

Beta-Amino-Isobutyric-Acid   *Plasma   Increase*   Due to tissue destruction. *1556*

Bilirubin   *Serum   Increase*   Transient hyperbilirubinemia may be observed in cases of radiation injury. *0151*

Creatine   *Urine   Increase*   Due to tissue destruction. *1556*

Deoxycytidine   *Urine   Increase*   Due to tissue destruction. *1556*

Eosinophils   *Blood   Increase*   After repeated irradiation. *0134*

Erythrocytes   *Blood   Decrease*   Predominant only after large doses. *0995*

Factor VIII   *Plasma   Increase*   Increased activity after total body irradiation. *2189*

Ferritin   *Serum   Increase*   Occurs within 2 h of deep x-ray therapy. *0618*

Fibrinogen   *Plasma   Increase*   Indicates tissue damage. *0618*

Globulin   *Serum   Increase*   Some cases. *0618*

Hematocrit   *Blood   Decrease*   After large doses. *0995*

Hemoglobin   *Blood   Decrease*   After large doses. *0995*

Lactate Dehydrogenase   *Serum   Decrease*   *2467*
    Serum   Increase   May be increased in cases of radiation injury, indicating major cell and tissue damage. *0151*

Leucine Aminopeptidase   *Urine   Increase*   Toxic damage due to released metabolites. *1869*

Leukocytes   *Blood   Decrease*   Within a few h after irradiation a neutrophilic leukocytosis appears. Following this, an oscillation in the neutrophil count occurs, the rate at which it falls to the minimum being a function of the dose of radiation. *0995*

Blood   Increase   Within a few h after irradiation a neutrophilic leukocytosis appears. Following this, an oscillation in the neutrophilic count occurs, the rate at which it falls to the minimum being a function of the dose of radiation. *0995   2468*

Lymphocytes   *Blood   Decrease*   The earliest laboratory finding is lymphopenia, reaching absolute lymphocyte levels below 1,000/μL within the first 48 postexposure h in cases of radiation injury. *0151*   Lymphopenia commences immediately becoming maximal within 24-36 h. *0995   0532*

Blood   Increase   *0532*

Lysozyme   *Urine   Increase*   Often seen for over 45 days following therapy. *2360*

Neutrophils   *Blood   Decrease*   A gradual fall begins during the first 2 weeks after exposure, reaches a plateau, and may even rise slightly, followed by a steep fall to a low point at 30 days postexposure in cases of radiation injury. *0151*   Within a few h after irradiation a neutrophilic leukocytosis appears. Following this, an oscillation in the neutrophilic count occurs, the rate at which it falls to the minimum being a function of the dose of radiation. *0995*

Blood   Increase   Within a few h after irradiation a neutrophilic leukocytosis appears. Following this, an oscillation in the neutrophilic count occurs, the rate at which it falls to the minimum being a function of the dose of radiation. *0995*   Increased in electric shock. *2538*

Ornithine Carbamoyl Transferase (OCT)   *Serum   Increase*   Reflects breakdown of tissue proteins. *0290*

Platelet Count   *Blood   Decrease*   A gradual fall in the first 2 weeks postexposure and reaches a low point after 30 days in cases of radiation injury. *0151*

Properidin   *Serum   Decrease*   Reflects breakdown of tissue proteins. *0618*

Protein   *Urine   Increase*   May cause renal damage. *0618*

Prothrombin Time   *Plasma   Increase*   *0889*

Reticulocytes   *Blood   Decrease*   May decrease or disappear in the first 48 postexposure h in cases of radiation injury. *0151*

Taurine   *Urine   Increase*   Tissue destruction. *1556*

Urea Nitrogen   *Serum   Increase*   May cause renal damage. *2084*

Uric Acid   *Serum   Increase*   Reflects cellular breakdown. *0865*
    Urine   Increase   Reflects cellular breakdown. *0865*

991.60   Hypothermia

11-Hydroxycorticosteroids   *Plasma   Increase*   Increase in accidental hypothermia. *0619*

Alanine Aminotransferase   *Serum   Increase*   14 of 24 patients with accidental hypothermia showed elevated values. *1472*

Amylase   *Serum   Increase*   About 10% of cases of severe accidental hypothermia develop acute pancreatitis. *0619*

Antidiuretic Hormone   *Urine   Normal*   With cold exposure. *2092*

Aspartate Aminotransferase   *Serum   Increase*   21 of 25 patients with accidental hypothermia had raised values. *1472*   Due to hypoxia, acid-base imbalance hypotension. *1471*

Bicarbonate   *Serum   Decrease*   Especially in cases preceded by exhaustion and prolonged shivering. *0151*   Due to hypoxia, acid-base imbalance hypotension. *1471*

Creatine Kinase   *Serum   Increase*   High concentrations have been found during a study of 25 patients with accidental hypothermia. Profound cellular damage, especially in cardiac and skeletal muscle, was recorded. *1472*   In response to cold exposure. *2092*

Pleural Effusion   Increase   Due to hypoxia, acid-base imbalance hypotension. *1471*

Epinephrine   *Urine   Normal*   With cold exposure. *2092*

Fatty Acids, Free (FFA)   *Serum   Increase*   Due to hypoxia, acid-base imbalance hypotension. *1471*

Glucose   *Serum   Increase*   High, especially when preceded by shivering and exhaustion. *0151*

Kynurenic Acid   *Urine   Increase*   Possibly due to activation of tryptophan oxygenase. *0762*

Lactate Dehydrogenase   *Serum   Increase*   Due to hypoxia, acid-base imbalance hypotension. *1471*   20 of 24 patients with hypothermia had elevated concentrations. *1472*

Lactate Dehydrogenase Isoenzyme 5 (LD$_5$)   *Serum   Increase*   Due to hypoxia, acid-base imbalance hypotension. *1471*   20 of 24 patients with hypothermia had elevated concentrations. *1472*

Norepinephrine   *Urine   Increase*   With cold exposure. *2092*

Oxygen Saturation *Blood Decrease* Due to hypoxia, acid-base imbalance hypotension. *1471*

pCO₂ *Blood Decrease* pCO₂ falls as the blood pH and bicarbonate rise with falling body temperatures. *0619*

Blood Increase Due to hypoxia, acid-base imbalance hypotension. *1471*

pH *Blood Decrease* Low blood pH in the form of metabolic acidosis is found in cases of hypothermia, especially if preceded by prolonged shivering and exhaustion. *0151* Due to hypoxia, acid-base imbalance hypotension. *1471*

pO₂ *Blood Decrease* Due to hypoxia, acid-base imbalance hypotension. *1471*

Protein Bound Iodine (PBI) *Serum Decrease* Occasionally decreased. *2467* In accidental hypothermia. *0619*

Sodium *Serum Decrease* Glucose solution acts as a relatively inert extracellular fluid volume expander when the body temperature is lowered. *0619*

Thyroid Stimulating Hormone (TSH) *Serum Normal* No change observed. *1754*

Tryptophan *Serum Decrease* Decreased with cold exposure although total amino acids are unaffected. *0762*

Tyrosine *Serum Decrease* Decreased with cold exposure although total amino acids are unaffected. *0762*

Xanthurenic Acid *Urine Increase* Possibly due to activation of tryptophan oxygenase. *0762*

992.00 Heat stroke

Alanine Aminotransferase *Serum Increase* Increases (mean = 10 X normal) to a peak on the 3rd day and returns to normal by the 2nd week. Very high levels are associated with lethal outcome. *2468*

Albumin *Serum Increase* By approximately 11.6% after heat exposure for 2-11 h. *2114*

Aldosterone *Plasma Increase* Increases by 76% after 1 week of thermal stress. *0100*

Alpha₁-Glycoprotein *Serum Increase* One of the most reliable indicators of acute inflammation. *1239 1672 1866 1947 2096 2170*

Aspartate Aminotransferase *Serum Increase* Following severe heat stroke. *0619* Increased (mean = 20 X normal) peaks on 3rd day and returns to normal in 2 weeks. Very high levels are often associated with lethal outcome. *2468* In a case of malignant hyperpyrexia, the initial elevation (after 3 h) of 110 U/L was due to muscle damage. Later elevations (12-24 h) was 1,600 and 3,440 U/L reflected damage of the liver. *0541*

Serum Normal Normal in children. *0548*

Bilirubin *Serum Increase* Clinically apparent jaundice appears 24-36 h after admission. *0995*

Bleeding Time *Blood Increase* *0995*

BSP Retention *Serum Increase* In almost 50% of patients with induced fever. *0222* Without liver disease. *2467*

Calcium *Serum Decrease* Initially and consistently high phosphate levels resulted in the fall of serum calcium to 5 mg/dL after 24 h in a case of malignant hyperpyrexia. *0541*

Carotene *Serum Decrease* *2467*

Chloride *Serum Increase* Normal to high in severe cases. *0151*

Clotting Time *Blood Increase* *0995*

Creatine Kinase *Serum Increase* Biochemical estimations in a fatal case of malignant hyperpyrexia showed very high serum CK, phosphate, and potassium. *0541 0542*

Creatinine *Serum Increase* Renal failure is a common complication. *0995*

Factor VIII *Plasma Increase* Increased activity as a result of fever. *0634*

Fibrinogen *Plasma Decrease* Formation is moderately depressed in severe heat stroke. *0619*

Glucose *Serum Decrease* Has been observed. *0067*

Hemoglobin *Blood Increase* In children. *0548*

Ketones *Serum Increase* Increased ketones in blood. Carbohydrate requirement increased with fever. *0619*

Urine Increase Children are more liable to develop ketosis than adults with fever. *0619 2467*

Lactate Dehydrogenase *Serum Increase* Increases to a mean value 5 X normal by the 3rd day and returns to normal in 2 weeks. Very high levels are often associated with lethal outcome. *2468*

Serum Normal Normal in children. *0548*

Lead *Blood Increase* Increased temperature may result in mobilization of fixed lead. *0294*

Leukocytes *Blood Increase* *0995*

Lymphocytes *Blood Increase* *2467*

Monocytes *Blood Increase* *2538*

Myoglobin *Urine Increase* Sudden muscle damage. *0619* Sporadic; metabolic myoglobinuria. *2467*

Phosphate *Serum Increase* Concentrations were very high (9.5-15 mg/dL) throughout and later resulted in a fall in serum-calcium in a case of malignant hyperpyrexia. *0541* In children. *0548*

Platelet Count *Blood Decrease* Low in severe cases. *0151 0995*

Potassium *Serum Decrease* Serum K is low and Cl is high in severe cases. *0151*

Serum Increase In malignant hyperpyrexia, raised to 9.0 mmol/L (normal = 3.5-5.4 mmol/L) 2 h after the anesthetic was started. *0541*

Protein *Serum Decrease* Reduced by 15.7% after 2-11 h heat exposure. *2114*

Urine Increase *0995*

Prothrombin Time *Plasma Increase* May occur with prolonged hot weather. *1095*

Renin Activity *Plasma Increase* Plasma activity increased by 174% after 1 week of thermal stress. *0100*

Urea Nitrogen *Serum Increase* Elevated in severe cases. *0151*

Uric Acid *Serum Increase* In children. *0548*

Volume *Plasma Decrease* Reduced 13.6% after 2-11 h heat exposure. *2114*

Urine Decrease Urine volume is low in severe cases. *0151*

994.50 Exercise

17-Hydroxycorticosteroids *Urine Increase* The normal output after daily routine activity is twice the resting output. *0619* Effect most marked in well trained individuals. *0089* Response to stress of exercise. *0342*

17-Ketogenic Steroids *Urine Increase* The normal output after daily routine activity is twice the resting output. *0619* Effect most marked in well trained individuals. *0089* Response to stress of exercise. *0342*

Adenylate Kinase *Serum Increase* Observed after protracted exercise. *0589*

AHF-Like Antigen *Plasma Increase* Increased in proportion to extent. *0166*

Alanine Aminotransferase *Serum Decrease* Effect of physical training. *0804 1930*

Serum Normal No significant change after 12 min on cycle-ergometer. *0804*

Albumin *Serum Increase* Significant increase after 12 min on cycle-ergometer. *0804* Approximately 10% increase immediately, then a delayed fall. *1837*

Aldolase *Serum Increase* An effect of physical training. *1930*

Serum Normal Strenuous physical activity has no effect. *1930*

Alkaline Phosphatase *Serum Normal* Insignificant change after physical activity. *0804*

Alpha₁-Antitrypsin *Serum Increase* Significant increase within 15 min partial return by 1 day. *0985*

Serum Normal No significant change was noted. *1837*

Alpha₁-Glycoprotein *Serum Increase* One of the most reliable indicators of acute inflammation. *1239 1672 1866 1947 2096 2170*

Alpha₂-Macroglobulin *Serum Increase* Significant increase within 15 min partial return by 1 day. *0985* Approximately 5% rise immediately after. *1837*

Aminoacid Arylpeptidase *Serum Increase* With exertion. *0985*

Ammonia *Blood Increase* Tissue catabolism. *0811*

Amylase *Serum Normal* No effect even with strenuous exercise. *1838*

Aspartate Aminotransferase *Serum Increase* Three well-trained men ran 100 km at a slow speed. After the race the clinical state was good and EKG were normal, but all three subjects had a significant rise in LD, AST, and CK. *2076* Marked increase after strenuous exercise, less in trained individuals. *1930*

Serum Normal Insignificant effect after 12 min on cycle ergometer. *0804* Normal after 2 h march. *2092*

Beta₁A-Globulin *Serum Increase* Increases by approximately 14% immediately following. *1837*

994.50 Exercise (continued)

Bicarbonate *Serum Decrease* Reduced by 3 mmol/L after vigorous 30 min exercise. *0706* Decreased to 11 mmol/L with intermittent exercise. *1254*

BSP Retention *Serum Increase* Related to extent of activity. *0763*

Calcium *Serum Increase* Observed after 12 min on cycle-ergometer. *0804*

Casts *Urine Increase* Hyaline and granular; both increased with increased exercise. *1205*

Catecholamines *Urine Increase* May be increased by vigorous exercise prior to urine collection (up to 7 fold). *0212* The normal output after daily routine activity is twice the resting output. *0619*

Urine Normal After mild or moderate exercise. *2092*

Cells *Urine Increase* Epithelial cells increase with heavy exercise. *1205*

Ceruloplasmin *Serum Increase* Generally occurs within 15 min and persists for 24 h. *0985*

Chloride *Serum Increase* Vigorous exercise for 30 min results in 2 mmol/L rise. *0706*

Cholesterol *Serum Increase* Occasionally. *0342*

Serum Normal Normal, with relative reduction of unsaturated acid. *1109* *0342*

Cortisol *Plasma Decrease* Slight. *0763*

Plasma Normal Usually normal in most people. *1363*

Creatine Kinase *Serum Increase* Extent of elevation depends upon severity of exercise and conditioning of patient. *1711* Maximum effect observed the following day. *0985* *2076 2160 1930*

Creatinine *Serum Normal* The observation has been made that after intensive exercise over extended periods the urinary creatinine excretion in healthy young men is in the range of 2.5-2.7 g/24h but normal blood levels (0.6-1.2 mg/dL of serum). *0503* Observed effect with 12 min cycle-ergometer. *0804*

Urine Increase The observation has been made that after intensive exercise over extended periods the urinary creatinine excretion in healthy young men is in the range of 2.5-2.7 g/24h but normal blood levels (0.6-1.2 mg/dL of serum). *0503*

Creatinine Clearance *Urine Decrease* Decrease with heavy exercise. *1205*

Urine Increase 40% decrease with severe exercise. Mild, walking at 5.6 km/h produced 20% increase. *2092* Slight but consistent increase. *2104*

Cyclic Adenosine Monophosphate *Urine Increase* Modest increase in normal people. *0464*

Dopamine Hydroxylase *Serum Normal* No effect observed. *2520*

Epinephrine *Plasma Increase* Significant effect after physical stress. *0768*

Urine Increase If strenuous may be increased 10-fold. *0161*

Factor II *Plasma Increase* Observed effect in exercise. *1839*

Factor V *Plasma Normal* Observed effect in exercise. *1839*

Factor VIII *Plasma Increase* Striking increase in titer after exercise. *2011* In proportion to extent of exercise and antigen. *0166 0544 1839*

Fatty Acids, Free (FFA) *Serum Decrease* Approximately 15% decrease with bicycle pedalling. *0909*

Serum Increase Marked increase after strenuous exercise. *1109* Following initial depression, concentrations gradually increase during exercise. *2104*

Fibrinogen *Plasma Decrease* Observed effect in exercise. *1839*

Fibrin Split Products (FSP) *Plasma Increase* Observed effect in exercise. *1176*

Glomerular Filtration Rate (GFR) *Urine Decrease* Observed with heavy treadmill exercise. *1205*

Urine Increase Mild exercise. *1205*

Urine Normal Moderate exercise. *1205*

Glucagon *Plasma Increase* Moderate to severe exercise. *0619* May increase 20%, facilitates hepatic glycogenolysis. *0721*

Glucose *Serum Decrease* Occurs with strenuous exercise. *0067*

Serum Increase Rise due to adrenal activity. *0618*

Serum Normal Observed effect with 12 min cycle-ergometer. *0804*

Glutamate Dehydrogenase *Serum Decrease* Observed effect with 12 min cycle-ergometer. *0804*

Serum Normal Physical activity has no effect. *1930*

Glycerol *Serum Increase* Approximately 10-30% increase with bicycle pedalling. *0909*

Glycoproteins *Serum Increase* Increased alpha₁ acid glycoprotein occurs within 15 min and persists for 1 day. *0985*

Serum Normal No change was observed in alpha₁ acid glycoprotein after exercise. *1837*

Growth Hormone *Serum Increase* Effect more marked in untrained than trained athletes. *1176* *0619*

Haptoglobin *Serum Decrease* Mean effect of 18 mg/dL from pre-exercise. *2092*

Serum Increase Approximately 17% increase immediately after exercise. *1837*

Hematocrit *Blood Increase* 6% increase immediately after exercise; normal in 30 min. *1837*

Hemoglobin *Blood Increase* Mild exercise causes transient decrease in blood volume. *1031*

Blood Normal No effect with normal activity. *1134*

Hemoglobin, Free *Serum Increase* Light activity causes increase X 3-5, heavy increase X 10-13. *1930*

Urine Increase Intravascular hemolysis due to march hemoglobinuria and strenuous exercise. *2467*

Hippuran Retention *Serum Increase* During infusion (depends on extent of activity. *0763*

Immunoglobulin IgA *Serum Increase* Approximately 14% increase immediately after. *1837*

Serum Normal No observed effect 15 min or 1 day after. *0985*

Immunoglobulin IgG *Serum Increase* Approximately 10% increase immediately after. *1837*

Serum Normal No observed effect 15 min or 1 day after. *0985*

Immunoglobulin IgM *Serum Normal* No observed effect 15 min or 1 day after. *0985* No effect of exercise observed. *1837*

Insulin *Serum Decrease* If exercise strenuous. *0763*

Serum Normal No effect if of short or moderate duration. *0763*

Iron *Serum Decrease* Response to stress of exercise. *0342*

Iron Saturation *Serum Increase* Raised at 15 min, normal within 1 day. *0985* Approximately 10% increase immediately after exercise. *1837*

Ketones *Serum Increase* Effect marked in untrained individuals only. *1176* Following exercise there is no increase in ketones in trained athletes, whereas there is an increase in untrained subjects. *0619*

Lactate Dehydrogenase *Serum Increase* After a 100 km race, 3 well-trained men, showed normal EKG and good clinical states, but significant elevations in LD, AST and CK were recorded. *2076* Maximum effect observed following day. Marked increase with exercise. *2550* Exercise. *1930* *0985*

Lactate Dehydrogenase Isoenzyme 5 (LD₅) *Serum Increase* *1978*

Lactate Dehydrogenase Isoenzymes *Serum Increase* LD₃, LD₄, LD₅ increased but no change in LD₁ and LD₂. *1978*

Lactic Acid *Blood Increase* Arterial lactate increased from 5.5-20 μmole/mL. Considerable effect of exercise. *1254* *0995*

Leukocytes *Blood Increase* Mainly due to neutrophilia after exercise. *0618*

Lipoproteins, Beta *Serum Normal* No change was observed after exercise. *1837*

Lysozyme *Serum Increase* After protracted exertion. *0985*

Serum Normal No effect even with strenuous exercise. *1838*

Urine Increase Very high clearance; proximal tubular function affected. *1838*

Magnesium *Serum Normal* Observed effect with 12 min cycle-ergometer. *0804*

Malate Dehydrogenase *Serum Increase* Significant effect with exercise. *0804* Significant effect after 2 h march. *2092*

Mucoprotein *Urine Increase* Concentration of Tamm-Horsfall protein increased with decreased volume. *1118*

Myoglobin *Urine Increase* Sporadic; exertional. *2467*

Neutrophils *Blood Increase* *2538*

Norepinephrine *Plasma Increase* Significant effect after physical stress. *0768*

Urine Increase Excretion may rise up to 200-300 ng/min. *2200* If strenuous, may be increased 10 fold. *0161*

Ornithine Carbamoyl Transferase (OCT)   *Serum   Increase*   Observed to increase following exercise. *0804*   Maximum effect observed 7 days after exercise. *0985*

Osmolality   *Urine   Decrease*   Effect most marked with light exercise. *1205*

Partial Thromboplastin Time   *Plasma   Decrease*   Observed effect in exercise. *1839*

pH   *Urine   Decrease*   At all rates of exercise (acid metabolites). *1205*

   Urine   Increase   Effect noted after mild exercise. *1205*

Phosphate   *Serum   Increase*   Observed effect with 12 min cycle-ergometer. *0804*   Effect of muscular exercise. *0161*

Phospholipids, Total   *Serum   Normal*   But relative reduction of unsaturated acid. *1109*

Plasminogen   *Serum   Increase*   Observed effect in exercise. *1839*   Vigorous exercise. *1443*

Platelet Count   *Blood   Increase*   Effect of sudden exercise. *0618*

Pregnanetriol   *Urine   Increase*   Effect most marked in well trained individuals. *0089*

Prostaglandins   *Serum   Increase*   Increase of 340% (mean after exercise). *0909*

Protein   *Serum   Increase*   Significant effect with 12 min on cycle-ergometer. *0804*   9% increase immediately after exercise, normal in 30 min. *1837*

   Urine   Increase   More common with heavy exercise than mild. *1205*

Protein Bound Iodine (PBI)   *Serum   Normal*   No effect observed. *0511*

Prothrombin Time   *Plasma   Increase*   Observed effect in exercise. *1839*

Pyruvate   *Blood   Decrease*   Slight fall within 1 h and then steep drop. *0618*

   Blood   Increase   After exercise to exhaustion 1.7 X control. *1837*

Sorbitol Dehydrogenase   *Serum   Increase*   Significant effect after 2 h march. *2092*

Specific Gravity   *Urine   Decrease*   Reduced ability to concentration at all rates. *1205*

Thyroxine (T₄)   *Serum   Decrease*   Significant effect with strenuous exercise. *2092*

Trehalase   *Serum   Increase*   Observed to increase with exercise. *0804*

   Urine   Increase   Observed to increase with exercise. *0804*

Triglycerides   *Serum   Decrease*   *2104*

   Serum   Normal   With relative reduction of unsaturated acid. *1109*

Urea Nitrogen   *Serum   Decrease*   Observed effect with 12 min cycle-ergometer. *1205*

   Serum   Increase   Raised at 15 min, partial return to normal in 24 h. *0985*

   Serum   Normal   Moderate degrees of exercise will not change BUN if sufficient calories to meet the energy demand are provided. *2104*

Uric Acid   *Serum   Increase*   Marked increase with prolonged exercise. Correlates closely with serum lactic acid concentration. *2104*

Vanillylamine   *Urine   Increase*   Significant effect after physical stress. *0768*

Volume   *Urine   Decrease*   With heavy exercise. *1205*

   Urine   Increase   With mild exercise. *1205*

994.80   Effects of Electric Current

Albumin   *Urine   Increase*   Albuminuria and hemoglobinuria occurs in presence of severe burns. *2468*   Characteristic. *0995*

Aldolase   *Serum   Increase*   *0995*

Aspartate Aminotransferase   *Serum   Increase*   Indicates severe tissue damage. *2468*   Trauma following direct current countershock to convert arrhythmia to normal rhythm (from intercostal muscle damage. *0619*

Creatine Kinase   *Serum   Increase*   Rose to abnormal levels in 5 of 8 patients, while the AST values showed no rise in patients undergoing D.C. countershock. *1103*   Electrical cardiac defibrillation or countershock in 50% of patients; returns to normal in 48-72 h. *2467*   Electrocautery used within the preceding days to the test may also produce elevated levels. *0812*

Cyclic Adenosine Monophosphate   *Urine   Increase*   Mean change from 4.2 μmol/24h to 14.2 μmol/24h. *2520*

Dopamine Hydroxylase   *Serum   Normal*   *2520*

Erythrocytes   *CSF   Increase*   Bloody spinal fluid as a result of widespread vascular injury. *0995*

Hematocrit   *Blood   Increase*   Immediately following major injury. *0995*

Hemoglobin   *Urine   Increase*   In many cases, probably secondary to severe burns. *0995*

Lactate Dehydrogenase   *Serum   Increase*   *0995*

Leukocytes   *Blood   Increase*   Leukocytosis with many large immature granulocytes is common after severe shock. *0995*

Myoglobin   *Urine   Increase*   Sporadic; exertional. *2467*   Sudden muscle damage due to high-voltage electric shock. *0619   0016*

Neutrophils   *Blood   Increase*   Leukocytosis with many large immature granulocytes is common after severe shock. *0995*

pH   *Blood   Decrease*   Profound metabolic acidosis. *0995*

Potassium   *Serum   Decrease*   Unexplained acute hypokalemia leading to respiratory arrest and cardiac arrhythmias has developed in some patients between the 2nd and 4th weeks following injury. *0995*

Protein   *Urine   Increase*   May cause renal damage. *2084*

Urea Nitrogen   *Serum   Increase*   May cause renal damage. *2084*

Volume   *Plasma   Decrease*   Immediately following major injury. *0995*

ABNORMAL CONDITIONS

1013.00   Diet

131I Uptake   *Serum   Increase*   Low-iodine diets. *2104*

5-Hydroxyindoleacetic Acid (5-HIAA)   *Urine   Increase*   With ingestion of plums or pineapples; high serotonin content. *0984*

Creatinine   *Serum   Increase*   Ingestion of creatinine (roast meat). *2467*   The observation has been made that with substantial protein ingestion healthy young men have a urinary creatinine excretion in the range of 2.5-2.7 g/24h specimen but normal blood levels (0.6-1.2 mg/dL of serum). *2467 0503*

Creatinine Clearance   *Urine   Increase*   On high protein diet. *2104*

Growth Hormone   *Serum   Decrease*   Fluctuates rapidly during the day in response to nutritional factors. Generally low after food ingestion and high during a fast. *2104*

Ketones   *Urine   Increase*   High fat diets. *2467*

Lipoproteins, Beta   *Serum   Increase*   With high saturated fat and/or cholesterol diet. *0774 0772 0773*

Prostaglandins   *Serum   Increase*   With ingestion of fats. *0909*

Prothrombin Time   *Plasma   Increase*   Prolonged due to inadequate vitamin K in diet. *2467*

Triglycerides   *Serum   Increase*   With high carbohydrate diet. *2104*

Urea Nitrogen   *Serum   Decrease*   With low protein and high carbohydrate diet. *2467*

Uric Acid   *Serum   Increase*   Increased in a high-protein weight reduction diet and a diet with excess nucleoprotein (sweetbreads and liver). *2467*   With high fat diets. *2104*

Uric Acid Clearance   *Urine   Increase*   High protein and carbohydrate diets accelerate renal clearance. *2104*

Vitamin E (Tocopherol)   *Serum   Decrease*   Low concentrations indicate a diet high in unsaturated fats. *2104*

1013.01   Diet (High Sodium)

Aldosterone   *Urine   Decrease*   Reduced excretion with increased concentration of salt in diet. *1274*

Inulin Clearance   *Urine   Increase*   There was a tendency for body weight, serum sodium, exchangeable sodium, and inulin clearance to increase with increase in dietary salt. *1274*

Potassium   *Urine   Increase*   Urinary K excretion rose progressively as salt intake increased. *1274*

Renin Activity   *Plasma   Decrease*   Increased plasma volume due to high-sodium diet. *2467*   Plasma renin activity increased with decreased dietary sodium. *1274*

Sodium   *Serum   Increase*   There was a tendency for body weight, serum sodium, exchangeable sodium, and inulin clearance to increase as dietary sodium increased. *1274*

1013.02 Diet (Low Sodium)

Aldosterone *Plasma Increase* Increased secretion with a reduced salt diet. *2104*

Renin Activity *Plasma Increase* Reduced plasma volume due to low-sodium diet. *2467*

5 REFERENCES

0001 BIO-SCIENCE LABORATORIES: THE BIO-SCIENCE HANDBOOK, 12TH ED. VAN NUY, CA (1979)

0002 BIO-SCIENCE REPORTS: BIO-SCIENCE LABORATORIES; VAN NUYS, CALIF (1980)

0003 AARLI A J ET AL, ANTIBODIES AGAINST NICOTINIC ACETYLCHOLINE RECEPTOR AND SKELETAL MUSCLE IN HUMAN AND EXPERIMENTAL MYASTHENIA GRAVIS, SCAND J IMMUNOL, 4, 849 (1975)

0004 AASEN AO, KIERULF P, RUUD TE, GODAL HC, AUNE S, STUDIES ON PATHOLOGICAL PLASMA PROTEOLYSIS IN PATIENTS WITH ACUTE PANCREATITIS. A PRELIMINARY REPORT, ACTA CHIR SCAND (SUPPL), 509, 83-7 (1982)

0005 ABBASSE A A ET AL, GONADAL FUNCTION ABNORMALITIES IN SICKLE CELL ANEMIA, ANN INTERN MED, 85, 601-605 (1976)

0006 ABBASSI V ET AL, POSTNATAL TRIIODOTHYRONINE CONCENTRATIONS IN HEALTHY PRETERM INFANTS AND IN INFANTS WITH RESPIRATORY DISTRESS SYNDROME, PEDIATR RES, 11, 802-4 (1977)

0007 ABELEU G I, ALPHA-FETOPROTEIN IN ONTOGENESIS AND ITS ASSOCIATION WITH MALIGNANT TUMORS, ADV CANCER RES, 14, 295-358 (1971)

0008 ABLIN R J, SERUM PROTEINS IN PROSTATIC CANCER. III, UROLOGY, 7, 39-47 (1976)

0009 ABRAHAM J P ET AL, HEMORRHAGIC COMPLICATIONS OF POLYCYTHEMIA VERA, HENRY FORD HOSP BULL, 9, 11 (1961)

0010 ABRAMS ET AL, ANTACID INDUCTION OF PHOSPHATE DEPLETION SYNDROME IN RENAL FAILURE, WEST J MED, 120, 157-160 (1974)

0011 ABUL-FADL, THE INHIBITION OF ACID PHOSPHATASES BY FORMALDEHYDE AND ITS CLINICAL APPLICATION FOR THE DETERMINATION OF SERUM ACID PHOSPHATASES, J CLIN PATHOL, 1, 80-90 (1948)

0012 ACEVEDO H F ET AL, URINARY CHOLESTEROL. VII. THE SIGNIFICANCE OF THE EXCRETION OF NONESTERIFIED CHOLESTEROL IN PATIENTS WITH UTERINE CARCINOMAS, CANCER, 36, 1459-69 (1975)

0013 ACEVEDO H F ET AL, URINARY CHOLESTEROL. VIII. ITS EXCRETION IN WOMEN WITH OVARIAN NEOPLASMS, CANCER, 37, 2847-57 (1976)

0014 ADAMI H O ET AL, THYROID DISEASE AND FUNCTION IN BREAST CANCER PATIENTS AND NON-HOSPITALIZED CONTROLS EVALUATED BY DETERMINATION OF TSH, T_3, RT_3, AND T_4 LEVELS IN SERUM, ACTA CHIR SCAND, 144, 89-97 (1978)

0015 ADAMS E B AND MACLEOD J N, AMEBIC LIVER ABSCESS AND ITS COMPLICATIONS, MEDICINE, 56, 325-333 (1977)

0016 ADAMS E C, DIFFERENTIATION OF MYOGLOBIN AND HEMOGLOBIN IN BIOLOGICAL FLUIDS, ANN CLIN LAB SCI, 1, 208 (1971)

0017 ADAMS J T ET AL, SIGNIFICANCE OF AN ELEVATED SERUM AMYLASE, SURGERY, 63, 877-84 (1968)

0018 ADAMS RD, VANDER EECKEN HM, VASCULAR DISEASES OF THE BRAIN, ANNU REV MED, 4, 213-252 (1953)

0019 ADAMSKA-DYNIEWSKA H, BALA T, FLORCZAK H, ET AL, BLOOD CADMIUM IN HEALTHY SUBJECTS AND IN PATIENTS WITH CARDIOVASCULAR DISEASES

0020 ADLERSBERG D ET AL, URIC ACID PARTITION IN GOUT AND HEPATIC DISEASE, ARCH INTERN MED, 70, 101 (1942)

0021 ADOLPH L, LORENZ R, ENZYME DIAGNOSIS IN DISEASES OF THE HEART, LIVER AND PANCREAS;BASEL SWITZERLAND (1982)

0022 AGNA J W ET AL, PRIMARY HYPERPARATHYROIDISM ASSOCIATED WITH HYPOMAGNESEMIA, N ENGL J MED, 258, 222 (1958)

0023 AGREN H, LUNDQVIST G, LOW LEVELS OF SOMATOSTATIN IN HUMAN CSF MARK DEPRESSIVE EPISODES, PSYCHONEUROENDOCRINOLOGY, 9, 233-248 (1984)

0024 AISENBERG A C, IMMUNOLOGIC ASPECTS OF HODGKIN'S DISEASE, CANCER, 19, 385 (1966)

0025 AISENBERG A C ET AL, SERUM ALKALINE PHOSPHATASE AT THE ONSET OF HODGKIN'S DISEASE, CANCER, 26, 318 (1970)

0026 AIYATHURAI JE, ET AL, THE PROBABLE SIGNIFICANCE OF HYPERTRIGLYCERIDEMIA IN VIRAL HEPATITIS, AUST NZ J MED, 6, 529-32 (1976)

0027 AKERFELDT S, OXIDATION OF N, N-DIMETHYL-P-PHENYLENEDIAMINE BY SERUM FROM PATIENTS WITH MENTAL DISEASE, SCIENCE, 125, 117-119 (1957)

0028 AKINYANJU P A, PLASMA AND RED CELL LIPIDS IN SICKLE CELL DISEASE, ANN CLIN LAB SCI, 6, 521-4 (1976)

0029 AL-SARRAF ET AL, PRIMARY LIVER CANCER-A REVIEW, CANCER, 33, 574-582 (1974)

0030 ALARCON-SEGOVIA D, THE NECROTIZING VASCULITIDES, MED CLIN NORTH AM, 61, 241-60 (1975)

0031 ALBERT A ET AL, STUDIES ON THE BIOLOGIC CHARACTERIZATION OF HUMAN GONADOTROPINS, J CLIN ENDOCRINOL METAB, 20, 1225 (1960)

0032 ALBERTS C, VAN DER SCHOOT JB, ET AL, 67GA SCINTIGRAPHY, SERUM LYSOZYME AND ANGIOTENSIN-CONVERTING ENZYME IN PULMONARY SARCOIDOSIS, EUR J RESPIR DIS, 64, 38-46 (1983)

0033 ALDINGER K A ET AL, THYROID-STIMULATING HORMONE AND PROLACTIN LEVELS IN BREAST CANCER, ARCH INTERN MED, 138, 1638-1641 (1978)

0034 ALEEM F A ET AL, PLASMA ESTROGEN IN PATIENTS WITH ENDOMETRIAL HYPERPLASIA AND CARCINOMA, CANCER, 38, 2101-2104 (1976)

0035 ALEXANDER B ET AL, CONGENITAL SPCA DEFICIENCY: A HITHERTO UNRECOGNIZED COAGULATION DEFECT WITH HEMORRHAGE RECTIFIED BY SERUM AND SERUM FACTORS, J CLIN INVEST, 30, 596 (1951)

0036 ALEXANDER M G ET AL, ALPHA-FETOPROTEIN IN LIVER DISEASE, S AFR MED J, 53, 433-6 (1978)

0037 ALEXANIAN R, MONOCLONAL GAMMOPATHY IN LYMPHOMA, ARCH INTERN MED, 135, 62 (1975)

0038 ALHENC-GELAS F, WEARE JA, HOHNSON RL JR, ET AL, MEASUREMENT OF HUMAN CONVERTING ENZYME LEVEL BY DIRECT RADIOIMMUNOASSAY, J LAB CLIN MED, 101, 83-96 (1983)

0039 ALLAM B F ET AL, SERUM IONIZED CALCIUM IN ACUTE PANCREATITIS, BR J SURG, 64, 665-68 (1977)

0040 ALLGROVE J, ADAMI S, FRAHER L, ET AL, HYPOMAGNESAEMIA: STUDIES OF PARATHYROID HORMONE SECRETION AND FUNCTION, CLIN ENDOCRINOL (OXF), 21, 435-49 (1984)

0041 ALLISON A C AND REES W, THE BINDING OF HAEMOGLOBIN BY PLASMA PROTEINS (HAPTOGLOBINS), BR MED J, 2, 1137 (1957)

0042 ALLISON AC, STRUCTURE AND FUNCTION OF PLASMA PROTEINS, NEW YORK, PLENUM PRESS, 1 (1974)

0043 ALLOTT E N AND MCARDLE B, FURTHER OBSERVATIONS ON FAMILIAL PERIODIC PARALYSIS, CLIN SCI, 3, 229 (1938)

0044 ALPER C A & ROSEN F S, COMPLEMENT IN LABORATORY MEDICINE IN: LABORATORY DIAGNOSIS ON IMMUNOLOGIC DISORDERS, GRUNE & STRATTON NEW YORK (1975)

0045 ALSABTI E A, SERUM ALPHAFETOPROTEIN IN BLADDER CARCINOMA, ONCOLOGY, 34, 78-9 (1977)

0046 ALSEVER RN, GOTLIN RW, HANDBOOK OF ENDOCRINE TESTS IN ADULTS AND CHILDREN, YEAR BOOK MEDICAL PUBL.,INC (1978)

0047 ALTOMONTE L, ET AL, CLINICAL RHEUMATOLOGY, 3, 209-12 (1984)

0048 ALTOMONTE L, ZOLI A, SOMMELLA L, PALUMBO P, ET AL, CONCENTRATION OF SERUM BILE ACIDS AS AN INDEX OF HEPATIC DAMAGE IN SYSTEMIC LUPUS ERYTHEMATOSUS, CLIN RHEUMATOL, 3, 209-12 (1984)

0049 ALVAREZ C, RAMOS A, LIPIDS, LIPOPROTEINS AND APOPROTEINS IN SERUM DURING INFECTION, CLIN CHEM, 32/1, 142-145 (1986)

0050 ALVSAKER J O, GENETIC STUDIES IN PRIMARY GOUT: INVESTIGATIONS ON THE PLASMA LEVELS OF THE URATE-BINDING ALPHA 1 - ALPHA 2 GLOBULIN IN INDIVIDUALS FROM TWO GOUTY KINDRED, J CLIN INVEST, 47, 1254 (1968)

0051 AMBRUS CM, AMBRUS JL, COUREY N, ET AL, INHIBITORS OF FIBRINOLYSIS IN DIABETIC CHILDREN, MOTHERS, AND THEIR NEWBORN, AM J HEMATOL, 7, 245-254 (1979)

0052 AMMAN R W ET AL, DIAGNOSTIC VALUE OF FECAL CHYMOTRYPSIN AND TRYPSIN ASSESSMENT FOR DETECTION OF PANCREATIC DISEASE, AM J DIG DIS, 13, 123-46 (1968)

0053 AMMANN R W ET AL, HYPERAMYLASEMIA WITH CARCINOMA OF THE LUNG, ANN INTERN MED, 78, 521 (1973)

0054 AMOROSI E C AND ULTMANN J E, THROMBOTIC THROMBOCYTOPENIC PURPURA: REPORT OF 16 PATIENTS AND REVIEW OF THE LITERATURE, MEDICINE, 45, 139 (1966)

0055 ANDERSEN D H, CYSTIC FIBROSIS, VITAMIN A DEFICIENCY AND BRONCHIECTASIS, J PEDIAT, 15, 763 (1939)

References

0056 ANDERSEN O O ET AL, GLUCOSE TOLERANCE AND INSULIN SECRETION IN HYPERTHYROIDISM, *ACTA ENDOCRINOL*, 84, 578-87 (1977)

0057 ANDERSON ET AL, ASSOCIATION OF HYPOKALAEMIA AND HYPOPHOSPHATAEMIA, *BR MED J*, 4, 402-403 (1969)

0058 ANDERSON J A ET AL, DIAGNOSTIC VALUE OF THYROID ANTIBODIES, *J CLIN ENDOCRINOL METAB*, 27, 937 (1967)

0059 ANDERSON MJ, PEEBLES CL, MCMILLAN R, ET AL, FLUORESCENT ANTINUCLEAR ANTIBODIES AND ANTI-SS-A/RO IN PATIENTS WITH IMMUNE THROMBOCYTOPENIA SUBSEQUENTLY DEVELOPING SYSTEMIC LUPUS ERYTHEMATOSUS, *ANN INTERN MED*, 103, 548 (1985)

0060 ANDERSSEN N, THE ACTIVITY OF LACTIC DEHYDROGENASE IN MEGALOBLASTIC ANEMIA, *SCAND J HAEMATOL*, 1, 212 (1964)

0061 ANDO K, SAITO K, TAKAI T, ET AL, ANTI-T$_3$ AUTOANTIBODIES IN A CASE OF CHRONIC THYROIDITIS ASSOCIATED WITH SJÖGREN SYNDROME AND SYSTEMIC LUPUS ERYTHEMATOSUS, *J JPN SOC INT MED*, 72, 1680-5 (1984)

0062 ANDREOLI TE. CARPENTER CT. PLUM F. SMITH LH., *CECIL: ESSENTIALS OF INTERNAL MEDICINE, W.B. SAUNDERS COMPANY* (1986)

0063 ANDREWS C ET AL, AN EPIDEMIC RESPIRATORY INFECTION DUE TO MYCOPLASMA PNEUMONIAE IN A CIVILIAN POPULATION, *AM REV RESPIR DIS*, 95, 972 (1967)

0064 ANDREWS F M, OBSERVATIONS ON LACTIC DEHYDROGENASE ACTIVITY IN BLOOD OF PATIENT TREATED WITH D-PENICILLAMINE FOR RHEUMATOID ARTHRITIS, *CURR MED RES OPIN*, 2, 587-589 (1974)

0065 ANGEL C, LEACH BE, MARTENS S, COHEN M, HEATH RG, SERUM OXIDATION TESTS IN SCHIZOPHRENIC AND NORMAL SUBJECTS, *ARCH NEUROL*, 78, 500-504 (1957)

0066 ANNAT G ET AL, MATERNAL AND FETAL PLASMA RENIN AND DOPAMINE-BETA-HYDROXYLASE ACTIVITIES IN TOXEMIC PREGNANCY, *OBSTET GYNECOL*, 52, 219-24 (1978)

0067 ANONYMOUS, 52 FACTORS THAT CAN AFFECT BLOOD GLUCOSE LEVELS, *CLIN TOXICOL*, 4, 297 (1971)

0068 ANSARI K A ET AL, CIRCULATING IGE, ALLERGY AND MULTIPLE SCLEROSIS, *ACTA NEUROL SCAND*, 53, 39-50 (1976)

0069 ANSTEY L ET AL, LEUCOCYTE ALKALINE PHOSPHATASE ACTIVITY IN POLYCYTHEMIA RUBRA VERA, *BR J HAEMATOL*, 9, 91 (1963)

0070 AOKI N, YAMANAKA T, THE ALPHA 2 PLASMIN INHIBITOR LEVELS IN LIVER DISEASES, *CLIN CHIM ACTA*, 84, 99-105 (1978)

0071 APPLEBY J I ET AL, THE URINARY EXCRETION OF 17-HYDROXYCORTICOSTEROIDS IN HUMAN PREGNANCY, *J ENDOCRINOL*, 15, 310 (1957)

0072 ARCASOY A AND CAVDAR A O, CHANGES OF TRACE MINERALS (SERUM IRON, ZINC, COPPER AND MAGNESIUM) IN THALASSEMIA, *ACTA HAEMATOL (BASEL)*, 53, 341-6 (1975)

0073 ARENDS T ET AL, SERUM PROTEINS IN HODGKIN'S DISEASE AND MALIGNANT LYMPHOMA, *AM J MED*, 16, 833 (1954)

0074 ARIAS F ET AL, HEPATIC FIBRINOGEN DEPOSITS IN PRE-ECLAMPSIA. IMMUNOFLUORESCENT EVIDENCE, *N ENGL J MED*, 295, 578-82 (1976)

0075 ARMATA J ET AL, THROMBOCYTOSIS IN ACUTE LEUKEMIA, *POL MED SCI HIST BULL*, 14, 55 (1971)

0076 ARNETZ BB, THE POTENTIAL ROLE OF PSYCHOSOCIAL STRESS ON LEVELS OF HEMOGLOBIN A1C (HBA1C) AND FASTING PLASMA GLUCOSE IN ELDERLY PEOPLE, *J GERONTOL*, 39, 424-429 (1984)

0077 ARONSON S M ET AL, PROGRESSION OF AMAUROTIC FAMILY IDIOCY AS REFLECTED BY SERUM AND CEREBROSPINAL FLUID CHANGES, *AM J MED*, 24, 390 (1958)

0078 ARONSON S M ET AL, CEREBROSPINAL FLUID ENZYMES IN CENTRAL NERVOUS SYSTEM LIPIDOSIS, *PROC SOC EXP BIOL MED*, 111, 664 (1962)

0079 AROOR AR, VENKATESH A, PATTABIRAMAN TN, ANTITRYPTIC AND ANTICHYMOTRYPTIC ACTIVITIES IN CEREBROSPINAL FLUID IN HEALTH AND DISEASE, *INDIAN J MED RES*, 70, 268-274 (1979)

0080 ARVANITAKES C ET AL, DIAGNOSTIC TESTS OF EXOCRINE PANCREATIC FUNCTION AND DISEASE, *GASTROENTEROLOGY*, 74, 932-48 (1978)

0081 ASHRAF N I, LEUCOCYTE ALKALINE PHOSPHATASE IN PREGNANCY, *INDIAN J MED RES*, 64, 1272-1279 (1976)

0082 ASTER R H, POOLING OF PLATELETS IN THE SPLEEN: ROLE IN THE PATHOGENESIS OF THROMBOCYTOPENIA, *J CLIN INVEST*, 45, 645 (1966)

0083 ATA A A, PRELIMINARY INVESTIGATION OF BILHARZIAL PATIENTS FOR THE PRESENCE OF AUSTRALIA ANTIGEN USING LATEX AGGLUTINATION TEST, *EGYPT J BILHARZ*, 4, 47-51 (1978)

0084 ATANSSOV N ET AL, DISC ELECTROPHORESIS OF PROSTATIC FLUID RELATIVE MOBILITY AND MOLECULAR WEIGHT OF SOME ENZYMES AND PROTEINS, *CLIN CHIM ACTA*, 36, 213-221 (1972)

0085 AU-N'EMETH A, STRANDVIK B, *SCAND J CLIN LAB INVEST*, 44, 387-392 (1984)

0086 AUB JE ET AL, STUDIES OF CALCIUM AND PHOSPHORUS METABOLISM, III. THE EFFECTS OF THE THYROID HORMONE AND THYROID DISEASE, *CLIN INVEST*, 7 (1929)

0087 AUSTIN R F AND DESFORGES J E, HEREDITARY ELLIPTOCYTOSIS: AN UNUSUAL PRESENTATION OF HEMOLYSIS IN THE NEWBORN ASSOCIATED WITH TRANSIENT MORPHOLOGICAL ABNORMALITIES, *PEDIATRICS*, 44, 196 (1969)

0088 AUVINEN, EVALUATION OF SERUM ENZYME TESTS IN THE DIAGNOSIS OF ACUTE MYOCARDIAL INFARCTION, *ACTA MED SCAND*, 539, 7-70 (1972)

0089 AVRAMOV R ET AL, EFFECT OF EXERCISE ON THE METABOLISM OF CORTICOSTEROIDS, *CLIN CHEM*, 18, 718 (1972)

0090 AWAIS G M, SERUM LACTIC DEHYDROGENASE LEVELS IN THE DIAGNOSIS AND TREATMENT OF CARCINOMA OF THE OVARY, *AM J OBSTET GYNECOL*, 116, 1053-1057 (1973)

0091 AYVAZAIN J H AYVAZIAN L F, CHANGES IN SERUM AND URINARY URIC ACID WITH THE DEVELOPMENT OF SYMPTOMATIC GOUT, *J CLIN INVEST*, 42, 1835 (1963)

0092 AZAR H A ET AL, MALIGNANT LYMPHOMA AND LYMPHATIC LEUKEMIA ASSOCIATED WITH MYELOMA-TYPE SERUM PROTEINS, *AM J MED*, 23, 239 (1957)

0093 BABEL C S ET AL, SERUM AND CEREBROSPINAL FLUID MAGNESIUM IN EPILEPSY, *J ASSOC PHYSICIANS INDIA*, 21, 481-7. (1973)

0094 BACCHUS H, ESSENTIALS OF METABOLIC DISEASES AND ENDOCRINOLOGY, *BALTIMORE, UNIVERSITY PARK PRESS* (1976)

0095 BACH C ET AL, L'ABSENCES CONGENITALE DE B-LIPOPROTEINES: UNE NOUVELLE OBSERVATION, *ARCH FR PEDIATR*, 24, 1093 (1967)

0096 BACKSTROM T, EPILEPTIC SEIZURES IN WOMEN RELATED TO PLASMA ESTROGEN AND PROGESTERONE DURING THE MENSTRUAL CYCLE., *ACTA NEUROL SCAND*, 54, 321-347 (1976)

0097 BADRINAS F, BUENDIA E, MESTRE M, SISLO C, ET AL, [ANGIOTENSIN-CONVERTING ENZYME IN SARCOIDOSIS: DIAGNOSTIC AND PROGNOSTIC VALUE (AUTHOR'S TRANSL)], *MED CLIN (BARC)*, 77, 108-14 (1981)

0098 BAGDADE J D, DISORDERS OF CARBOHYDRATE AND LIPID METABOLISM IN UREMIA, *NEPHRON*, 14, 153 (1975)

0099 BAGDADE J D ET AL, HYPERTRIGLYCERIDEMIA - A METABOLIC CONSEQUENCE OF CHRONIC RENAL FAILURE., *N ENGL J MED*, 279, 181 (1968)

0100 BAILEY R E ET AL, ACTIVATION OF ALDOSTERONE AND RENIN SECRETION BY THERMAL STRESS, *EXPERIENTIA*, 28, 159 (1972)

0101 BAKER H, FRANK O, CLINICAL VITAMINOLOGY, *INTERSCIENCE PUBLISHERS, NEW YORK, NY* (1968)

0102 BAKER J W ET AL, ELEVATED PLASMA ANTIDIURETIC HORMONE LEVELS IN STATUS ASTHMATICUS, *MAYO CLIN PROC*, 51, 31 (1976)

0103 BAKIRI F, BENMILOUD M, VALLOTTON MB, THE RENIN-ANGIOTENSIN SYSTEM IN PANHYPOPITUITARISM: DYNAMIC STUDIES AND THERAPEUTIC EFFECTS IN SHEEHAN'S SYNDROME, *J CLIN ENDOCRINOL METAB*, 56, 1042-7 (1983)

0104 BALCERZAK S P ET AL, EFFECT OF IRON DEFICIENCY AND RED CELL AGE ON HUMAN ERYTHROCYTE CATALASE ACTIVITY, *J LAB CLIN MED*, 67, 742 (1966)

0105 BALFE J W COLE C AND WELT L G, RED CELL TRANSPORT IN PATIENTS WITH CYSTIC FIBROSIS AND IN THEIR PARENTS, *SCIENCE*, 162, 689 (1968)

0106 BALL G V ET AL, PATHOGENESIS OF HYPERURICEMIA IN SATURNINE GOUT, *N ENGL J MED*, 280, 1199 (1969)

0107 BALL GV, SCHROHENLOHER R, HESTER R, GAMMA GLOBULIN COMPLEXES IN RHEUMATOID PERICARDIAL FLUID, *AM J MED*, 58, 123 (1975)

0108 BALLANTYNE D ET AL, RELATIONSHIP OF PLASMA URIC ACID TO PLASMA LIPIDS AND LIPOPROTEINS IN SUBJECTS WITH PERIPHERAL VASCULAR DISEASE, *CLIN CHIM ACTA*, 70, 323-8 (1976)

0109 BALLARD H S AND MARCUS A J, HYPERCALCEMIA IN CHRONIC MYELOGENOUS LEUKEMIA, *N ENGL J MED*, 282, 663 (1970)

0110 BANDO K, ICHIHARA K, TOYOSHIMA H, ET AL, DECREASED ACTIVITY OF CARNOSINASE IN SERUM OF PATIENTS WITH CHRONIC LIVER DISORDERS, *CLIN CHEM*, 32/8, 1563-1565 (1986)

0111 BANK S ET AL, SWEAT ELECTROLYTES IN CHRONIC PANCREATITIS, *AM J DIG DIS*, 23, 178-81 (1978)

0112 BANSAL B C ET AL, SERUM LIPIDS, PLATELETS, AND FIBRINOLYTIC ACTIVITY IN CEREBROVASCULAR DISEASE, *STROKE*, 9, 137-9. (1978)

0113 BARBERA G J ET AL, STOOL TRYPSIN AND CHYMOTRYPSIN IN THE DIAGNOSIS OF PANCREATIC INSUFFICIENCY IN CYSTIC FIBROSIS, *AM J DIS CHILD*, 112, 536-40 (1966)

0114 BARBOSA J ET AL, PLASMA INSULIN IN PATIENTS WITH MYOTONIC DYSTROPHY AND THEIR RELATIVES, *MEDICINE*, 53, 307-323 (1974)

0115 BARLOW K A, HYPERLIPIDEMIA IN PRIMARY GOUT, *METABOLISM*, 17, 289 (1968)

0116 BARNES G R JR ET AL, A CLINICAL STUDY OF AN INSTITUTIONAL OUTBREAK OF ACUTE INFECTIOUS LYMPHOCYTOSIS, *AM J MED SCI*, 218, 646 (1949)

0117 BARNTON D F AND FINCH C H, THE DIAGNOSIS OF IRON DEFICIENCY ANEMIA, *AM J MED*, 37, 62 (1964)

0118 BARON J H, AN ASSESSMENT OF THE AUGMENTED HISTAMINE TEST IN THE DIAGNOSIS OF PEPTIC ULCER, *GUT*, 4, 243-253 (1963)

0119 BARRETT-CONNOR E ET AL, AN EPIDEMIC OF TRICHINOSIS FOLLOWING INGESTION OF WILD PIG IN HAWAII, *J INFECT DIS*, 133, 473 (1976)

0120 BARROS F ET AL, ETUDES SUR LA PARAMYLOIDOSE PORTUGAISE A FORME POLYNEURITIQUE III ALTERATIONS DES PROTEINES PLASMATIQUES, *ACTA NEUROPATHOL (SUPPL)*, 2, 101-110 (1963)

0121 BARROW E M ET AL, A STUDY OF THE CARRIER STATE FOR PLASMA THROMBOPLASTIN COMPONENT (PTC, CHRISTMAS FACTOR) DEFICIENCY, UTILIZING A NEW ASSAY PROCEDURE, *J LAB CLIN MED*, 55, 936 (1960)

0122 BARTELLONI R T ET AL, CHANGES IN INDIVIDUAL PLASMA AMINO ACID METABOLISM IN THE REGULATION OF GLUCONEOGENESIS, *METABOLISM*, 21, 67 (1972)

0123 BARTFELD H, RHEUMATOID FACTORS AND THEIR BIOLOGICAL SIGNIFICANCE. INTRODUCTION, *ANN NY ACAD SCI*, 168, 30 (1969)

0124 BARTH W F ET AL, PRIMARY AMYLOIDOSIS, *ANN INTERN MED*, 69, 787-805 (1968)

0125 BARTH W F ET AL, PRIMARY AMYLOIDOSIS. CLINICAL, IMMUNOCHEMICAL AND IMMUNOGLOBULIN METABOLISM STUDIES IN FIFTEEN PATIENTS, *AM J MED*, 47, 259-273 (1969)

0126 BARTOLIN R, BOUVENOT G, DELBOY C, JOUBERT M, CADMIUM, ZINC, PSEUDO-CHOLINESTERASE AND ALDOLASE BLOOD LEVELS IN HYPERTENSIVE AND ALCOHOLIC PATIENTS. PRELIMINARY STATISTICAL COMPUTERIZED STUDY ON 124 CASES, *SEM HOP PARIS*, 56, 1718-9 (1980)

0127 BARUCH Y, BROOK JG, EIDELMAN S, AVIRAM M, INCREASED CONCENTRATION OF HIGH DENSITY LIPOPROTEIN IN PLASMA AND DECREASED PLATELET AGGREGATION IN PRIMARY BILIARY CIRRHOSIS, *ARTERIOSCLEROSIS*, 53, 151-162 (1984)

0128 BARZEL U S ET AL, RENAL AMMONIUM EXCRETION AND URINARY PH IN IDIOPATHIC URIC ACID LITHIASIS, *J UROL*, 91, 1 (1964)

0129 BASES, ELEVATION OF SERUM ACID PHOSPHATASE IN CERTAIN MYELOPROLIFERATIVE DISEASES, *N ENGL J MED*, 266, 538-540 (1962)

0130 BASSEN F A AND KORNZWIEG A L, MALFORMATION OF THE ERYTHROCYTE IN A CASE OF ATYPICAL RETINITIS PIGMENTOSA, *BLOOD*, 5, 381 (1950)

0131 BATES HM, THE LABORATORY IN PREVENTION: HDL CHOLESTEROL AND CORONARY HEART DISEASE, *LABORATORY MANAGEMENT*, 18, 17-22 (1980)

0132 BATES HM, URINARY CYCLIC AMP IN PARATHYROID FUNCTION TESTING, *LABORATORY MANAGEMENT*, 18, 13-17 (1980)

0133 BATRA S ET AL, HUMAN PLACENTAL LACTOGEN, ESTRADIOL-17 BETA, AND PROGESTERONE LEVELS IN THE THIRD TRIMESTER AND THEIR RESPECTIVE VALUES FOR DETECTING TWIN PREGNANCY, *AM J OBSTET GYNECOL*, 131, 69-72 (1978)

0134 BAUER J D ET AL, BRAY'S CLINICAL LABORATORY METHODS, *7TH EDITION C V MOSBY CO ST LOUIS* (1968)

0135 BAUGHMAN RP, STEIN E, MACGEE J, ET AL, CHANGES IN FATTY ACIDS IN PHOSPHOLIPIDS OF THE BRONCHOALVEOLAR FLUID IN BACTERIAL PNEUMONIA AND IN ADULT RESPIRATORY DISTRESS SYNDROME, *CLIN CHEM*, 30/4, 521-523 (1984)

0136 BAUM J, JUVENILE ARTHRITIS, *AM J DIS CHILD*, 135, 557-560 (1981)

0137 BAUMAN D S ET AL, COMPARISON OF IMMUNODIFFUSION AND COMPLEMENT FIXATION TESTS IN THE DIAGNOSIS OF HISTOPLASMOSIS, *J CLIN MICROBIOL*, 2, 77-80 (1976)

0138 BAYER A S ET AL, CANDIDA MENINGITIS, *MEDICINE*, 55, 477-486 (1976)

0139 BAYLISS C E ET AL, LABORATORY DIAGNOSIS OF RHEUMATOID ARTHRITIS. PROSPECTIVE STUDY OF 85 PATIENTS, *ANN RHEUM DIS*, 34, 395-402 (1975)

0140 BAZZANO, EFFECTS OF FOLIC ACID METABOLISM ON SERUM CHOLESTEROL LEVELS, *ARCH INTERN MED*, 124, 710-713 (1969)

0141 BEAMISH M R ET AL, TRANSFERRIN IRON, CHELATABLE IRON AND FERRITIN IN IDIOPATHIC HEMOCHROMATOSIS, *BR J HAEMATOL*, 27, 219 (1974)

0142 BEARD M F ET AL, SERUM CONCENTRATIONS OF VITAMIN B_{12} IN ACUTE LEUKEMIA, *ANN INTERN MED*, 41, 323 (1954)

0143 BEARN A G ET AL, RENAL FUNCTION IN WILSON'S DISEASE, *J CLIN INVEST*, 36, 1107 (1957)

0144 BECK ET AL, BIOCHEMICAL STUDIES ON LEUCOCYTES II. PHOSPHATASE ACTIVITY IN CHRONIC LYMPHATIC LEUCEMIA, ACUTE LEUCEMIA AND MISCELLANEOUS HEMATOLOGIC CONDITIONS, *J LAB CLIN MED*, 38, 245-253 (1951)

0145 BECKER D M AND KRAMER S, THE NEUROLOGICAL MANIFESTATIONS OF PORPHYRIA: A REVIEW, *MEDICINE*, 56, 411-423 (1977)

0146 BECKER K L ET AL, CALCITONIN HETEROGENEITY IN LUNG CANCER AND MEDULLARY THYROID CANCER., *ACTA ENDOCRINOL*, 89, 89-99 (1978)

0147 BECKMAN G ET AL, ACID PHOSPHATASE ACTIVITY IN THE SYNOVIAL FLUID OF PATIENTS WITH RHEUMATOID ARTHRITIS AND OTHER JOINT DISORDERS, *ACTA RHEUM SCAND*, 17, 47-56 (1971)

0148 BECKMANN H, SAAVEDRA JM, GATTAZ WF, LOW ANGIOTENSIN-CONVERTING ENZYME ACTIVITY (KININASEII) IN CEREBROSPINAL FLUID OF SCHIZOPHRENICS, *BIOL PSYCHIATRY*, 19, 679-84 (1984)

0149 BEDE H K ET AL, FIBRINOGEN CONTENT AND FIBRINOLYTIC ACTIVITY OF BLOOD IN DIABETICS, BEFORE AND AFTER ANTIDIABETIC DRUGS, *J ASSOC PHYSICIANS INDIA*, 25, 181-5 (1977)

0150 BEEKEN W L, SERUM TRYPTOPHAN IN CROHN'S DISEASE, *SCAND J GASTROENTEROL*, 11, 735-40 (1976)

0151 BEESON-MCDERMOTT, TEXTBOOK OF MEDICINE, *14TH EDITION W B SAUNDERS CO* (1975)

0152 BEEVERS DG, CRUICKSHANK JK, YEOMAN WB, ET AL, BLOOD-LEAD AND CADMIUM IN HUMAN HYPERTENSION, *J ENVIRON PATHOL TOXICOL ONCOL*, 4, 251-60 (1980)

0153 BEISEL W R, TRACE ELEMENTS IN INFECTIOUS PROCESSES, *MED CLIN NORTH AM*, 60, 831 (1976)

0154 BELFIORE F ET AL, SERUM ACID PHOSPHATASE ACTIVITY IN DIABETES MELLITUS, *AM J MED SCI*, 266, 139-143 (1973)

0155 BELFIORE F ET AL, SERUM ENZYMES IN DIABETES MELLITUS, *CLIN CHEM*, 19, 447 (1973)

0156 BELL A, HIPPEL T, GOODMAN H, USE OF CYTOCHEMISTRY AND FAB CLASSIFICATION IN LEUKEMIA AND OTHER PATHOLOGICAL STATES, *AM J MED TECH*, 47, 437-471 (1981)

0157 BELL A, HIPPEL T, GOODMAN H, USE OF CYTOCHEMISTRY AND FAB CLASSIFICATION IN LEUKEMIA AND OTHER PATHOLOGICAL STATES, *AM J MED TECH*, 47, 437-471 (1981)

0158 BELLINGHAM AJ, DETTER JC, LENFANT C, REGULATORY MECHANISMS OF HEMOGLOBIN OXYGEN AFFINITY IN ACIDOSIS AND ALKALOSIS, *J CLIN INVEST*, 50, 700-706 (1971)

0159 BELLINGHAM AJ, DETTER JC, LENFANT C, THE RED CELL IN ADAPTATION TO ANAEMIC HYPOXIA, *CLINICS IN HAEMATOLOGY*, 3, 577-594 (1975)

0160 BELLIVEAU ET AL, LIVER ENZYMES AND PATHOLOGY IN HODGKIN'S DISEASE, *CANCER*, 34, 300-305 (1974)

0161 BELLON E M, HAEMOLYTIC ANEMIA DUE TO NALIDIXIC ACID, *LANCET*, 2, 691 (1965)

0162 BEN-ARYEH H ET AL, SIALOCHEMISTRY OF PATIENTS WITH RHEUMATOID ARTHRITIS. ELECTROLYTES, PROTEIN, AND SALIVARY IGA, *ORAL SURG*, 45, 63-70 (1978)

0163 BENEDICT C R ET AL, CLINICAL SIGNIFICANCE OF PLASMA ADRENALINE AND NORADRENALINE CONCENTRATIONS IN PATIENTS WITH SUBARACHNOID HAEMORRHAGE, *J NEUROL NEUROSURG PSYCHIATRY*, 41, 113-7 (1978)

0164 BENEDICT C R ET AL, PLASMA NORADRENALINE AND ADRENALINE CONCENTRATIONS AND DOPAMINE B HYDROXYLASE ACTIVITY IN PATIENTS WITH SHOCK DUE TO SEPTICEMIA, TRAUMA AND HEMORRHAGE, *Q J MED*, 185, 1-20 (1978)

0165 BENJAMIN F ET AL, SERUM LEVELS OF FOLIC ACID, VITAMIN B_{12} AND IRON IN ANEMIA OF PREGNANCY, *AM J OBSTET GYNECOL*, 96, 310 (1966)

0166 BENNETT B ET AL, CHANGES IN ANTIHEMOPHILIC FACTOR (AHF, FACTOR VIII) PROCOAGULANT ACTIVITY AND AHF-LIKE ANTIGEN, *J LAB CLIN MED*, 80, 256 (1972)

0167 BENNETT J M ET AL, SIGNIFICANCE OF LEUKOCYTE ALKALINE PHOSPHATASE IN HODGKIN'S DISEASE, *ARCH INTERN MED*, 121, 338 (1966)

0168 BENNETT W M ET AL, SILENT RENAL INVOLVEMENT IN SYSTEMIC LUPUS ERYTHEMATOSUS, *INT ARCH ALLERGY APPL IMMUNOL*, 55, 420-8 (1977)

0169 BENSLEY ET AL, ESTIMATION OF SERUM ACID PHOSPHATASE IN THE DIAGNOSIS OF METASTASIZING CARCINOMA, *CAN MED ASSOC J*, 58, 261-264 (1948)

0170 BENSTER B ET AL, IMMUNOGLOBULIN LEVELS IN NORMAL PREGNANCY AND PREGNANCY COMPLICATED BY HYPERTENSION, *BR J OBSTET GYNAECOL*, 77, 518-522 (1970)

0171 BERATIS N G ET AL, ALKALINE PHOSPHATASE ACTIVITY IN CULTURED SKIN FIBROBLASTS FROM FIBRODYSPLASIA OSSIFICANS PROGRESSIVA, *J MED GENET*, 13, 307-309 (1976)

0172 BERCROFT D M O ET AL, ABETALIPOPROTEINEMIC (BASSEN-KORNZWEIG SYNDROME), *ARCH DIS CHILD*, 40, 40 (1965)

0173 BERG B ET AL, URINARY EXCRETION OF HISTAMINE AND HISTAMINE METABOLITES IN LEUKEMIA, *SCAND J HAEMATOL*, 8, 63 (1971)

0174 BERGER HW, MAHER G, DECREASED GLUCOSE CONCENTRATION IN MALIGNANT PLEURAL EFFUSIONS, *AM REV RESPIR DIS*, 103, 427-429 (1971)

0175 BERGMEYER HU, GAWEHN K, GRASSL M, MYOKINASE, ADENYLATE KINASE, *BERGMEYER, HU (ED): METHODS OF ENZYMATIC ANALYSIS. NEW YORK, ACADEMIC PRESS* (1974)

0176 BERGSAGEL D E ET AL, THE TREATMENT OF PLASMA CELL MYELOMA, *ADV CANCER RES*, 10, 311 (1967)

0177 BERGSTROMM J ET AL, LACTIC ACID ACCUMULATION IN CONNECTION WITH FRUCTOSE ADMINISTRATION, *ACTA MED SCAND*, 184, 359 (1968)

0178 BERK J E, NEW DIMENSIONS IN THE LABORATORY DIAGNOSIS OF PANCREATIC DISEASE, *AM J GASTROENTEROL*, 69, 417-27 (1978)

0179 BERK P D ET AL, DEFECTIVE BSP CLEARANCE IN PATIENTS WITH CONSTITUTIONAL HEPATIC DYSFUNCTION (GILBERTS SYNDROME), *GASTROENTEROLOGY*, 63, 472 (1972)

0180 BERK P D ET AL, INBORN ERRORS OF BILIRUBIN METABOLISM, *MED CLIN NORTH AM*, 59, 817-821 (1975)

0181 BERLIN N J, DIAGNOSIS AND CLASSIFICATION OF POLYCYTHEMIA, *SEMIN HEMATOL*, 12, 339 (1975)

0182 BERMAN P H ET AL, CONGENITAL HYPERURICEMIA, AN INBORN ERROR OF PURINE METABOLISM ASSOCIATED WITH PSYCHOMOTOR RETARDATION, ATHETOSIS AND SELF-MUTILATION, *ARCH NEUROL*, 20, 44 (1969)

0183 BERNARD H R ET AL, THE PATHOLOGIC SIGNIFICANCE OF THE SERUM AMYLASE CONCENTRATION, *ARCH SURG*, 79, 311-316 (1959)

0184 BERNARD J F ET AL, HUMAN ERYTHROCYTIC CALCIUM CONCENTRATION IN HEMOLYTIC ANEMIA, *BIOMEDICINE EXPRESS*, 23, 431-33 (1975)

0185 BERNENGO M G ET AL, RELATIONSHIP BETWEEN T AND B LYMPHOCYTE VALUES AND PROGNOSIS IN MALIGNANT MELANOMA, *BR J DERMATOL*, 98, 655-62 (1978)

0186 BERNER JJ, EFFECTS OF DISEASES ON LABORATORY TESTS, *J.B. LIPPINCOTT CO, NEW YORK* (1983)

0187 BERNSTEIN JM, PARK BH, DEFECTIVE IMMUNOREGULATION IN CHILDREN WITH CHRONIC OTITIS MEDIA WITH EFFUSION, *OTOLARYNGOL HEAD NECK SURG*, 94, 334-9 (1986)

0188 BESSIS M ET AL, ETUDE COMPAREE DU PLASMOCYTOME ET DU SYNDROME DE WALDENSTRÖM, *NOUV REV FR HEMATOL*, 3, 159 (1963)

0189 BEST W R ET AL, CLINICAL VALUE OF EOSINOPHIL COUNTS AND EOSINOPHIL RESPONSE TESTS, *JAMA*, 15, 702 (1953)

0190 BETRO ET AL, HYPOPHOSPHATAESMIA AND HYPERPHOSPHATASEMIA IN A HOSPITAL POPULATION, *BR MED J*, 1, 273-276 (1972)

0191 BETRO M G, SIGNIFICANCE OF INCREASED ALKALINE PHOSPHATASE AND LACTATE DEHYDROGENASE ACTIVITIES COINCIDENT WITH NORMAL SERUM BILIRUBIN, *CLIN CHEM*, 18, 1427-1429 (1972)

0192 BETTS & GREEN, PLASMA AND URINE AMINO ACID CONCENTRATIONS IN CHILDREN WITH CHRONIC RENAL INSUFFICIENCY, *NEPHRON*, 18, 132-9 (1977)

0193 BETTS RF, SYNDROMES OF CYTOMEGALOVIRUS INFECTION, *ADV INTERN MED*, 26, 447-466 (1980)

0194 BEUTLER E, THE RED CELL INDICES IN THE DIAGNOSIS OF IRON DEFICIENCY ANEMIA, *ANN INTERN MED*, 50, 313 (1959)

0195 BEUTLER E, RED CELL METABOLISM: A MANUAL OF BIOCHEMICAL METHODS, *2ND ED. NEW YORK, GRUNE AND STRATTON* (1975)

0196 BEUTLER E, *A MANUAL OF BIOCHEMICAL METHODS, 2ND ED. NEW YORK, GRUNE AND STRATTON* (1975)

0197 BEUTLER E, HEMOLYTIC ANEMIA IN DISORDERS OF RED CELL METAB-OLISM, *NEW YORK, PLENUM PUBLISHING CO.* (1978)

0198 BEVERIDGE B R ET AL, HYPOCHROMIC ANEMIA, *Q J MED*, 34, 135 (1965)

0199 BEZWODA W R ET AL, AN INVESTIGATION INTO GONADAL DYSFUNC-TION IN PATIENTS WITH IDIOPATHIC HEMOCHROMATOSIS, *CLIN ENDOCRINOL (OXF)*, 6, 377-85 (1977)

0200 BEZWODA W, DERMAN D, BOTHWELL T, ET AL, SIGNIFICANCE OF SERUM CONCENTRATIONS OF CARCINOEMBRYONIC ANTIGEN, FERRITIN, AND CALCITONIN IN BREAST CANCER, *CANCER*, 48, 1623-8 (1981)

0201 BIANCHI R, MARIANI G, MCFARLANE A, *PLASMA PROTEIN TURNOVER. BALTIMORE, UNIVERSITY PARK PRESS* (1976)

0202 BIBERFIELD G AND STERNER G, ANTIBODIES IN BRONCHIAL SECRE-TIONS FOLLOWING NATURAL INFECTION WITH MYCOPLASMA PNEUMONIAE, *ACTA PATHOL MICROBIOL IMMUNOL SCAND*, 79B, 599-605 (1971)

0203 BICK RL, BICK MD, FEKETE LF, ANTITHROMBIN III PATTERNS IN DISSEMI-NATED INTRAVASCULAR COAGULATION, *AM J CLIN PATHOL*, 73, 577-83 (1980)

0204 BICKEL H, PROXIMAL TUBULAR DEFECTS, *RENAL DISEASE D A K BLACK (ED)* (1964)

0205 BIEMOND I, SELBY WS, JEWELL DP, KLASEN EC, ALPHA 1-ANTITRYPSIN SERUM CONCENTRATION AND PHENOTYPES IN ULCERATIVE COLI-TIS, *DIGESTION*, 29, 124-8 (1984)

0206 BIERMAN ET AL, CORRELATION OF SERUM LACTIC DEHYDROGENASE ACTIVITY WITH THE CLINICAL STATUS OF PATIENTS WITH CANCER, LYMPHOMAS, AND THE LEUKEMIAS, *CANCER RES*, 16, 660-667 (1957)

0207 BIJVOET AND DE VRIES, PLASMA-PHOSPHATE IN PAGET'S DISEASE, *J CLIN ENDOCR*, 1283-1284 (1974)

0208 BILBREY G L ET AL, HYPERGLUCAGONEMIA OF RENAL FAILURE, *J CLIN INVEST*, 53, 841 (1974)

0209 BINDER R AND GILBERT S, MURAMIDASE IN POLYCYTHEMIA VERA, *BLOOD*, 36, 228 (1970)

0210 BING R J, DIAGNOSTIC VALUE OF ACTIVITY OF MALIC DEHYDROGENASE AND PHOSPHOHEXOSE ISOMERASE, *JAMA*, 164, 647 (1957)

0211 BIOSCIENCE LAB, BIOSCIENCE HANDBOOK-SPECIALIZED DIAGNOSTIC LABORATORY TESTS, *11TH EDITION VAN NUYS CALIFORNIA* (1977)

0212 BIOSCIENCE LABORATORIES, BIOSCIENCE HANDBOOK, SPECIALIZED DIAGNOSTIC LABORATORY TESTS, *9TH EDITION VAN NUYS CALI-FORNIA* (1971)

0213 BIRKETT ET AL, SERUM ALKALINE PHOSPHATASE IN PREGNANCY:AN IMMUNOLOGICAL STUDY, *BR MED J*, 1, 1210-1212 (1966)

0214 BISHOP C R ET AL, LEUKOKINETIC STUDIES. XIV. BLOOD NEUTROPHIL KINETICS IN CHRONIC STEADY STATE NEUTROPENIA, *J CLIN INVEST*, 50, 1678 (1971)

0215 BISSETTE G, REYNOLDS GP, KILTS CD, ET AL, CORTICOTROPIN-RELEASING FACTOR-LIKE IMMUNOREACTIVITY IN SENILE DEMEN-TIA OF THE ALZHEIMER TYPE, *JAMA*, 254, 3067 (1985)

0216 BLACK L F, THE PLEURAL SPACE AND PLEURAL FLUID, *MAYO CLIN PROC*, 47, 493 (1972)

0217 BLACKARD W G, CONTROL OF GROWTH HORMONE SECRETION IN MAN, *POSTGRAD MED J*, 49, 122 (1973)

0218 BLACKLOW NR, CUKOR G, VIRAL GASTROENTERITIS, *N ENGL J MED*, 304, 397-406 (1981)

0219 BLAIR A J ET AL, THE PLASMA 17-HYDROXYCORTICOSTEROID LEVELS IN ACUTE AND CHRONIC RENAL FAILURE, *CANAD J BIOCHEM*, 39, 1617 (1961)

0220 BLAJHMAN M A ET AL, IMMUNOGLOBULINS IN WARM-TYPE AUTOIM-MUNE HAEMOLYTIC ANAEMIA, *LANCET*, 2, 340 (1969)

0221 BLANCHAER ET AL, PLASMA LACTIC DEHYDROGENASE AND PHOSPHOHEXOSE ISOMERASE IN LEUKEMIA, *BLOOD*, 13, 245-257 (1958)

0222 BLASCHKE T F ET AL, EFFECTS OF INDUCED FEVER ON SULFOBROMOPHTHALEIN KINETICS IN MAN, *ANN INTERN MED*, 78, 221 (1973)

0223 BLEICHER S J ET AL, CARBOHYDRATE METABOLISM IN PREGNANCY. V. THE INTERRELATIONS OF GLUCOSE, INSULIN AND FREE FATTY ACIDS IN LATE PREGNANCY AND POSTPARTUM, *N ENGL J MED*, 2271, 866 (1964)

0224 BLEKTA M ET AL, VOLUME OF WHOLE BLOOD AND ABSOLUTE AMOUNT OF SERUM PROTEINS IN THE EARLY STAGE OF LATE TOXEMIA OF PREGNANCY, *AM J OBSTET GYNECOL*, 106, 10-13 (1970)

0225 BLISS T L, BASAL METABOLISM IN POLYCYTHEMIA VERA, *ANN INTERN MED*, 2, 1155 (1929)

0226 BLOCH K J ET AL, SJÖGREN'S SYNDROME: A CLINICAL, PATHOLOGI-CAL, AND SEROLOGICAL STUDY OF SIXTY-TWO CASES, *MEDICINE*, 44, 187 (1965)

0227 BLOOM A ET AL, FACTOR VIII AND ITS INHERITED DISORDERS, *BR MED BULL*, 33, 219-24 (1977)

0228 BLOOM AL, THE VON WILLEBRAND SYNDROME, *SEMIN HEMATOL*, 17, 215-227 (1980)

0229 BLOOM EJ, ABRAMS DI, RODGERS G, LUPUS ANTICOAGULANT IN THE ACQUIRED IMMUNODEFICIENCY SYNDROME, *JAMA*, 256, 491 (1986)

0230 BLOOMER J R ET AL, BLOOD VOLUME AND BILIRUBIN PRODUCTION IN ACUTE INTERMITTENT PORPHYRIA, *N ENGL J MED*, 284, 17 (1971)

0231 BLUM D ET AL, SERUM ENZYMES IN THE NEONATAL PERIOD, *BIOL NEONATE*, 26, 53-57 (1975)

0232 BLUMBERG M Z ET AL, THE TOTAL EOSINOPHIL COUNT AND ADRENAL FUNCTION IN ASTHMATIC CHILDREN, *ANN ALLERGY*, 35, 377-81 (1975)

0233 BOAS G, RUBENSTEIN AH, HORWITZ D, BLIX PM, CLINICAL SIGNIFI-CANCE OF C-PEPTIDE, *EXCERPTA MEDICA INT CONGR SER*, NO. 468, 246-253 (1979)

0234 BOCK E, RAFAELSEN OJ, SCHIZOPHRENIA: PROTEINS IN BLOOD AND CEREBROSPINAL FLUID, *DAN MED BULL*, 21, 93-105 (1974)

0235 BOCK E, WEEKE B, RAFAELSON OJ, SERUM PROTEINS IN ACUTELY PSYCHOTIC PATIENTS, *J PSYCHIATR RES*, 9, 1-9 (1971)

0236 BODA D ET AL, IN VITRO EFFECTS OF INOSINE-PYRUVATE-PHOSPHATE ON P50 VALUES AND DPG CONTENTS OF FRESH AND STORED BLOOD FROM HEALTHY NEONATES, SYMPTOM-FREE PREMATURE INFANTS AND PREMATURE INFANTS WITH RESPIRATORY, *BIOL NEONATE*, 33, 25-30 (1978)

0237 BODANSKY, ACID PHOSPHATASE, *ADV CLIN CHEM*, 15, 43-147 (1972)

0238 BOEY ML, LOIZOU S, COLACO CB, ET AL, ANTITHROMBIN III IN SYS-TEMIC LUPUS ERYTHEMATOSUS, *CLIN EXP RHEUMATOL*, 2, 53-6 (1984)

0239 BOGDEN J D ET AL, EFFECT OF PULMONARY TUBERCULOSIS ON BLOOD CONCENTRATIONS OF COPPER AND ZINC, *AM J CLIN PATHOL*, 67, 251-6. (1977)

0240 BOGDEN J D ET AL, COPPER, ZINC, MAGNESIUM, AND CALCIUM IN PLASMA AND CEREBROSPINAL FLUID OF PATIENTS WITH NEURO-LOGICAL DISEASES, *CLIN CHEM*, 23, 485-9. (1977)

0241 BOGGS D R AND FAHEY J L, SERUM PROTEIN CHANGES IN MALIGNANT DISEASE. II, *J NATL CANCER INST*, 25, 1381 (1960)

0242 BOGGS D R ET AL, FACTORS INFLUENCING THE DURATION OF SUR-VIVAL OF PATIENTS WITH CHRONIC LYMPHOCYTIC LEUKEMIA, *AM J MED*, 40, 243 (1966)

0243 BOGGS D R ET AL, AN UNUSUAL PATTERN OF NEUTROPHIL KINETICS IN SICKLE CELL ANEMIA, *BLOOD*, 41, 59 (1973)

0244 BOHAN A ET AL, A COMPUTER-ASSISTED ANALYSIS OF 153 PATIENTS WITH POLYMYOSITIS AND DERMATOMYOSITIS, *MEDICINE*, 56, 255-285 (1977)

0245 BOIX-OCHOA J ET AL, THE IMPORTANT INFLUENCE OF ARTERIAL BLOOD GASES ON THE PROGNOSIS OF CONGENITAL DIAPHRAG-MATIC HERNIA, *WORLD J SURG*, 1, 783-87 (1977)

0246 BOJANOWICZ K ET AL, DISTURBANCES OF FAT, CARBOHYDRATE, MAGNESIUM AND PROTEIN BALANCE IN LIVER DISEASE, *ACTA HEPATOGASTROENTEROL*, 24, 155-61 (1977)

0247 BOKESCH V A, THE POTENTIAL ROLE OF COMPLEMENT IN DENGUE HEMORRHAGIC SHOCK SYNDROME, *N ENGL J MED*, 289, 996-1006 (1973)

0248 BOMFORD R, ANEMIA IN MYXEDEMA AND THE ROLE OF THE THYROID GLAND IN ERYTHROPOIESIS, *Q J MED*, 7, 495 (1938)

0249 BONNAR J ET AL, THE ASSESSMENT OF IRON DEFICIENCY IN PREG-NANCY, *SCOT MED J*, 14, 209 (1969)

0250 BONNAR J ET AL, COAGULATION AND FIBRINOLYTIC SYSTEMS IN PRE-ECLAMPSIA AND ECLAMPSIA, *BR MED J*, 2, 12 (1971)

0251 BONNAR J ET AL, THE ROLE OF COAGULATION AND FIBRINOLYSIS IN PREECLAMPSIA, *PERSPECT NEPHROL HYPERTENS*, 5, 85-93 (1976)

0252 BONTA I L ET AL, PROSTAGLANDINS AND CHRONIC INFLAMMATION, *BIOCHEM PHARMACOL*, 27, 1611-1624 (1978)

0253 BOOTH S N ET AL, SERUM CARCINOEMBRYONIC ANTIGEN IN CLINICAL DISORDERS, *GUT*, 14, 794-99 (1973)

0254 BORGLIN N E, SERUM GLUTAMIC-OXALOACETIC TRANSAMINASE AND-SERUM GLUTAMIC-PYRUVIC TRANSAMINASE IN TOXEMIA OF PREGNANCY, *J CLIN ENDOCRINOL METAB*, 19, 425 (1959)

0255 BOROWSKY SA, LIEBERMAN J, STROME S, SASTRE A, ELEVATION OF SERUM ANGIOTENSIN-CONVERTING ENZYME LEVEL. OCCUR-RENCE IN ALCOHOLIC LIVER DISEASE, *ARCH INTERN MED*, 142, 893-5 (1982)

0256 BORSATTI A, INCREASED URINE ANGIOTENSIN I CONVERTING ENZYME ACTIVITY IN PATIENTS WITH UPPER URINARY TRACT INFECTION, *CLIN CHIM ACTA*, 109, 211-8 (1981)

0257 BORULF S, LINDBERG T, PROTEASE INHIBITORS IN DUODENAL JUICE FROM CHILDREN WITH MALABSORPTION, *CLIN CHIM ACTA*, 112, 253-255 (1981)

0258 BOSI A, BORSOTTI M, GHELLI P, ET AL, SERUM ANGIOTENSIN-I-CON-VERTING ENZYME AND LYSOZYME LEVELS IN UNTREATED AND UNSPLENECTOMIZED PATIENTS WITH HODGKIN'S DISEASE, *ACTA HAEMATOL (BASEL)*, 71, 329-33 (1984)

0259 BOSS GR, SEEGMILLER JE, HYPERURICEMIA AND GOUT, *N ENGL J MED*, 300, 1459-1468 (1979)

0260 BOTTGER D, PROGNOSTIC SIGNIFICANCE OF LYMPHOPENIA IN PULMO-NARY SARCOIDOSIS, *Z ERKRANK ATM-ORG*, 149, 197-201 (1977)

0261 BOTTINGER L E ET AL, SERUM LIPIDS IN ALCOHOLICS, *ACTA MED SCAND*, 199, 357-61 (1976)

0262 BOUR H ET AL, LES ENZYMES DU MUSCLE AU COURS DU COMA OXYCARBONE, *SEM HOP PARIS*, 38, 3152-3157 (1962)

0263 BOWER B R AND GORDON G S, HORMONAL EFFECTS ON NON-ENDO-CRINE TUMORS, *ANNU REV MED*, 16, 83 (1965)

0264 BOYD JE, COLLINGS PL, CROFTON PM, ET AL, ALPHA 1 ANTITRYPSIN AND LUNG FUNCTION IN BRITISH COAL MINERS, *BR J IND MED*, 41, 455-8 (1984)

0265 BOYKO WL, BARRET B, DETECTION AND QUANTITATION OF THE B-SUBUNIT OF HUMAN CHORIONIC GONADOTROPIN IN SERUM BY RIA, *FERTIL STERIL*, 33, 141-150 (1980)

0266 BOYLE J A ET AL, SERUM URIC ACID LEVELS IN NORMAL PREGNANCY WITH OBSERVATIONS ON THE RENAL EXCRETION OF WATER IN PREGNANCY, *J CLIN PATHOL*, 19, 501 (1966)

0267 BRAASCH J W AND S J CAMER, PERIAMPULLARY CARCINOMA, *MED CLIN NORTH AM*, 59, 309-14 (1975)

0268 BRACKERTZ D, HAGMANN J KUEPPERS F, PROTEINASE INHIBITORS IN RHEUMATOID ARTHRITIS, *ANN RHEUM DIS*, 34, 225-230 (1975)

0269 BRADY RO, SPHINGOLIPIDOSES, *ANNU REV BIOCHEM*, 47, 687-713 (1978)

0270 BRAKMAN P ET AL, BLOOD COAGULATION AND FIBRINOLYSIS IN ACUTE LEUKEMIA, *BR J HAEMATOL*, 18, 135 (1970)

0271 BRANDSBORG O ET AL, INCREASED PLASMA NORADRENALINE AND SERUM GASTRIN IN PATIENTS WITH DUODENAL ULCER, *EUR J CLIN INVEST*, 8, 11-14 (1978)

0272 BRASHER G W ET AL, COMPLEMENT COMPONENT ANALYSIS IN ANGIOEDEMA. DIAGNOSTIC VALUE, *ARCH DERMATOL*, 111, 1140-42 (1975)

0273 BRAUNSTEIN G D ET AL, FIRST TRIMESTER CHORIONIC GONADO-TROPIN MEASUREMENTS AS AN AID IN THE DIAGNOSIS OF EARLY PREGNANCY DISORDERS, *AM J OBSTET GYNECOL*, 131, 25-32 (1978)

0274 BRAWLEY RK, VASCO JS, MORROW AG, CHOLESTEROL PERICARDITIS, *AM J MED*, 41, 235-248 (1966)

0275 BRECKINRIDGE A, HYPERTENSION IN HYPERURICEMIA, *PROC R SOC*, 59, 316-18 (1966)

0276 BREITER D N ET AL, SERUM COPPER AND ZINC MEASUREMENTS IN PATIENTS WITH OSTEOGENIC SARCOMA, *CANCER*, 42, 598-602 (1978)

0277 BRENNER B M AND RECTOR F C (EDITORS), THE KIDNEY, *W B SAUN-DERS CO*, II (1976)

0278 BRENT GA, HERSHMAN JM, REED AW, ET AL, SERUM ANGIOTENSIN-CONVERTING ENZYME IN SEVERE NONTHYROIDAL ILLNESSES ASSOCIATED WITH LOW SERUM THYROXINE CONCENTRATION, *ANN INTERN MED*, 100, 680-683 (1984)

0279 BRERETON H D ET AL, PRETREATMENT SERUM LACTATE DEHYDROGENASE PREDICTING METASTATIC SPREAD IN EWING'S SARCOMA, *ANN INTERN MED*, 83, 352-354 (1975)

0280 BRESLAU NA, MCGUIRE JL, ZERWEKH JE, HYPERCALCEMIA ASSOCI-ATED WITH INCREASED SERUM CALCITRIOL LEVELS IN THREE PATIENTS WITH LYMPHOMA, *ANN INTERN MED*, 100, 1-7 (1984)

0281 BRESSLER R ET AL, SERUM LEUCINE AMINOPEPTIDASE ACTIVITY IN HEPATOBILIARY AND PANCREATIC DISEASE, *J LAB CLIN MED*, 56, 417-430 (1960)

0282 BREUER R I ET AL, URINARY CRYSTALLOID EXCRETION IN PATIENTS WITH INFLAMMATORY BOWEL DISEASE, *GUT*, 11, 314 (1970)

0283 BRIHEIM G, FRYDEN A, TOBIASSON P, SERUM BILE ACIDS IN GILBERT'S SYNDROME BEFORE AND AFTER REDUCED CALORIC INTAKE, *SCAND J GASTROENTEROL*, 17, 877-80 (1982)

0284 BRISSENDEN JE, COX DW, ALPHA 2-MACROGLOBULIN IN PATIENTS WITH OBSTRUCTIVE LUNG DISEASE, WITH AND WITHOUT ALPHA 1-ANTITRYPSIN DEFICIENCY, *CLIN CHIM ACTA*, 128, 241-8 (1983)

0285 BROCK D J ET A, SERUM ALPHA FETOPROTEIN IN CYSTIC FIBROSIS OF THE PANCREAS, *CLIN CHIM ACTA*, 81, 101-3 (1978)

0286 BROCKLEHURST D ET AL, SERUM ALKALINE PHOSPHATASE, NUCLEO-TIDE PYROPHOSPHATASE, 5'-NUCLEOTIDASE AND LIPOPROTEIN-X IN CHOLESTASIS, *CLIN CHIM ACTA*, 67, 269-279 (1976)

0287 BROD ET AL, THE RENAL CLEARANCE OF ENDOGENOUS CREATININE IN MAN, *J CLIN INVEST*, 27, 645-654 (1948)

0288 BROD J I ET AL, SERUM ALKALINE PHOSPHATASE ISOENZYMES IN SICKLE CELL ANEMIA, *JAMA*, 232, 738-741 (1975)

0289 BRODER G, QUANTITATION AND CLINICAL SIGNIFICANCE OF URINARY FAT, *LANCET*, 2, 188 (1969)

0290 BROHULT A ET AL, EFFECTS OF ALKOXYGLYCEROLS ON THE SERUM ORNITHINE CARBAMOYL TRANSFERASE IN CONNECTION WITH RADIATION TREATMENT, *EXPERIENTIA*, 28, 146 (1972)

0291 BRONSON W R, PSEUDOHYPERKALEMIA DUE TO RELEASE OF POTAS-SIUM FROM WHITE BLOOD CELLS DURING CLOTTING, *N ENGL J MED*, 274, 369 (1966)

0292 BROOK J ET AL, LEUKOCYTE ALKALINE PHOSPHATASE LEVELS IN MULTIPLE MYELOMA, *J LAB CLIN MED*, 90, 114-117 (1977)

0293 BROOKS B R ET AL, CEREBROSPINAL FLUID ACID-BASE AND LACTATE CHANGES AFTER SEIZURES IN UNANESTHETIZED MAN. I. IDIO-PATHIC SEIZURES, *NEUROL*, 25, 935-42 (1975)

0294 BROWDER A A ET AL, THE PROBLEM OF LEAD POISONING, *MEDICINE*, 52, 121 (1973)

0295 BROWN B, *HEMATOLOGY: PRINCIPLES AND PROCEDURES 3RD ED. PHILADELPHIA, LEA AND FEBIGER* (1980)

0296 BROWN J ET AL, AUTOIMMUNE THYROID DISEASES -- GRAVE'S AND HASHIMOTO'S, *ANN INTERN MED*, 88, 379-391 (1978)

0297 BROWN J J ET AL, PLASMA RENIN IN NORMAL PREGNANCY, *LANCET*, 2, 900 (1963)

0298 BROWN JD, DAC AN N, TUBERCULOUS PERITONITIS. LOW ASCITIC FLUID GLUCOSE CONCENTRATION AS A DIAGNOSTIC AID, *AM J GASTROENTEROL*, 66, 277-282 (1976)

0299 BROWN SS, MITCHELL FL, YOUNG DS (EDS), CHEMICAL DIAGNOSIS OF DISEASE, *AMSTERDAM, ELSEVIER/NORTH-HOLLAND BIOMEDICAL PRESS* (1979)

0300 BROWNSTEIN M H AND BILLARD H S, HEPATOMA ASSOCIATED WITH ERYTHROCYTOSIS, *AM J MED*, 40, 206 (1966)

0301 BROZMANOVA E ET AL, SERUM ALKALINE PHOSPHATASE IN MALIG-NANT BONE TUMORS (OSTEOSARCOMA, CHONDROSARCOMA, FIBROSARCOMA, EWING'S SARCOMA), *NEOPLASMA*, 20, 419-425 (1973)

0302 BRUNELL P ET AL, ZOSTER IN CHILDREN, *AM J DIS CHILD*, 115, 432 (1968)

0303 BRUYN G W AND LEQUIN R M, HUNTINGTON'S CHOREA, *LANCET*, 2, 1300 (1964)

0304 BUAMAH PK, RUSSELL M, MILFORD-WARD A, ET AL, SERUM COPPER CONCENTRATION SIGNIFICANTLY LESS IN ABNORMAL PREGNANCIES, *CLIN CHEM*, 30/10, 1676-1677 (1984)

0305 BUAMAH PK, SKILLEN AW, HARRISON J, ET AL, AMNIOTIC FLUID ACETYLCHOLINESTERASE ACTIVITY AND ALPHA-FETOPROTEIN IN CHROMOSOMAL ANOMALIES AND NEURAL TUBE DEFECTS, *CLIN CHEM*, 31/4, 614-615 (1985)

0306 BUCHANAN KD, THE GASTROINTESTINAL HORMONES: GENERAL CON-CEPTS, *CLIN ENDOCRINOL METAB*, 8, 249-263 (1979)

0307 BUCHANAN T M ET AL, BRUCELLOSIS IN THE UNITED STATES, 1960-72, PART II. DIAGNOSTIC ASPECTS, *MEDICINE*, 53, 415-426 (1974)

0308 BUCKLEY, IMMUNODEFICIENCY DISEASES, *ARCH INTERN MED*, 146, 379 (1986)

0309 BUDMAN D R AND STEINBERG A, HEMATOLOGIC ASPECTS OF SYS-TEMIC LUPUS ERYTHEMATOSUS, *ANN INTERN MED*, 86, 220-229 (1977)

0310 BUEHLER BA, INHERITED DISORDERS OF AMINO ACID TRANSPORT IN RELATION TO THE KIDNEY, *ANN CLIN LAB SCI*, 11, 274-278 (1981)

0311 BULLEN A W ET AL, DIAGNOSTIC USEFULNESS OF PLASMA CARCI-NOEMBRYONIC ANTIGEN LEVELS IN ACUTE AND CHRONIC LIVER DISEASE, *GASTROENTEROLOGY*, 73, 673-78 (1977)

0312 BULLER HR, WEENINK AH, TREFFERS PE, ET AL, SEVERE ANTITHROMBIN III DEFICIENCY IN A PATIENT WITH PRE-ECLAMPSIA. OBSERVATION ON THE EFFECT OF HUMAN AT III CONCENTRATE TRANSFUSION, *SCAND J HAEMATOL*, 25, 81-6 (1980)

0313 BUNCH T W ET AL, SYNOVIAL FLUID COMPLEMENT: USEFULNESS IN DIAGNOSIS AND CLASSIFICATION OF RHEUMATOID ARTHRITIS, *ANN INTERN MED*, 81, 32-5 (1974)

0314 BUNCH TW, HUNDER GG, MCDUFFIE FC, O'BRIEN PC,ET AL, SYNOVIAL FLUID COMPLEMENT DETERMINATION AS A DIAGNOSTIC AID IN INFLAMMATORY JOINT DISEASE, *MAYO CLIN PROC*, 49, 715-720 (1974)

0315 BUNN H F ET AL, THE GLYCOSYLATION OF HEMOGLOBIN: RELEVANCE TO DIABETES MELLITUS, *SCIENCE*, 200, 21-7 (1978)

0316 BURCH G E AND DEPASQUALE N P, THE HEMATOCRIT IN PATIENTS WITH MYOCARDIAL INFARCTION, *JAMA*, 180, 62 (1962)

0317 BURCH G E ET AL, THE IMPORTANCE OF MAGNESIUM DEFICIENCY IN CARDIOVASCULAR DISEASE, *AM HEART J*, 94, 649-57 (1977)

0318 BURKI N K ET AL, SERUM CREATINE PHOSPHOKINASE ACTIVITY IN ASTHMA, *AM REV RESPIR DIS*, 116, 327-330 (1977)

0319 BURMAN K D ET AL, IONIZED AND TOTAL SERUM CALCIUM AND PARA-THYROID HORMONE IN HYPERTHYROIDISM, *ANN INTERN MED*, 84, 668-71 (1976)

0320 BURNETT W ET AL, SERUM AMYLASE AND ACUTE ABDOMINAL DIS-EASE, *BR MED J*, 2, 770 (1955)

0321 BURNHAM T K, THE IMMUNOFLUORESCENT TUMOR IMPRINT TECH-NIQUE II. THE FREQUENCY OF ANTINUCLEAR FACTORS IN CON-NECTIVE TISSUE DISEASES AND DERMATOSES, *ANN INTERN MED*, 65, 9-19 (1966)

0322 BURT R L, COMBINED AND FREE PLASMA ALPHA-AMINO NITROGEN IN NORMAL PREGNANCY AND TOXEMIA, *AM J OBSTET GYNECOL*, 65, 304 (1953)

0323 BURT R L ET AL, SERUM AMYLASE IN PREGNANCY AND THE PUERPE-RIUM, AND IN FETAL BLOOD, *OBSTET GYNECOL*, 28, 351 (1966)

0324 BUSTAMANTE J B ET AL, ZINC, COPPER AND CERULOPLASMIN IN ARTERIOSCLEROSIS, *BIOMED PHARMACOTHER*, 25, 244-5 (1976)

0325 BUTS J P ET AL, ONE-HOUR BLOOD XYLOSE TEST: A RELIABLE INDEX OF SMALL BOWEL FUNCTION, *J PEDIATR*, 92, 729-33. (1978)

0326 CADEAU B J ET AL, INCREASED INCIDENCE OF PLACENTA-LIKE ALKA-LINE PHOSPHATASE ACTIVITY IN BREAST AND GENITOURINARY CANCER, *CANCER RES*, 34, 729-32 (1974)

0327 CAEN J P ET AL, CONGENITAL BLEEDING DISORDERS WITH LONG BLEEDING TIMES AND NORMAL PLATELET COUNTS, *AM J MED*, 41, 4 (1966)

0328 CALABRESE VP, THE INTERPRETATION OF ROUTINE CSF TESTS, *VIR-GINIA MEDICAL MONTHLY*, 103, 207-209 (1976)

0329 CALLEN I R AND LIMARZ L R, BLOOD AND BONE MARROW STUDIES IN RENAL DISEASE, *AM J CLIN PATHOL*, 20, 3 (1950)

0330 CALVO R ET AL, ACUTE HEMOLYTIC ANEMIA DUE TO ANTI-I: FREQUENT COLD AGGLUTININS IN INFECTIOUS MONONUCLEOSIS, *J CLIN INVEST*, 44, 1033 (1965)

0331 CAMERON J S ET AL, MEMBRANOPROLIFERATIVE GLOMERULONE-PHRITIS AND PERSISTENT HYPOCOMPLEMENTEMIA, *BR MED J*, 4, 7 (1970)

0332 CAMERON J S ET AL, MEMBRANOUS NEPHROPATHY IN: GLOMERULO-NEPHRITIS MORPHOLOGY, NATURAL HISTORY AND TREATMENT. PT I, *KINCAID-SMITH P ET AL (EDS) JOHN WILEY & SONS*, 473 (1973)

0333 CAMP R, JONES RR, BRAIN S, ET AL, PRODUCTION OF INTRAEPIDERMAL MICROABSCESSES BY TOPICAL APPLICATION OF LEUKOTRIENE B4, *J INVEST DERMATOL*, 82, 202-4 (1984)

0334 CAMPBELL I M ET AL, ABNORMAL FATTY ACID COMPOSITION AND IMPAIRED OXYGEN SUPPLY IN CYSTIC FIBROSIS PATIENTS, *PEDI-ATRICS*, 57, 480-6. (1976)

0335 CAMPRA, JL., AND REYNOLDS, TB.,, ALCOHOLIC LIVER DISEASE: CLUE TO ACUTE AND CHRONIC CHANGES, *CONSULTANT*, 67, 69 (1985)

0336 CANDEL SAMUEL ET AL, SERUM AMYLASE AND SERUM LIPASE IN MUMPS, *ANN INTERN MED*, 25, 88-96 (1946)

0337 CANELLOS G P, CHRONIC GRANULOCYTIC LEUKEMIA, *MED CLIN NORTH AM*, 60, 1001-1018 (1976)

0338 CAPLAN A AND GROSS S, HEMATOLOGIC AND SEROLOGIC STUDIES IN CYSTIC FIBROSIS, *J PEDIAT*, 73, 540 (1968)

0339 CAPOCACCIA L ET AL, OCTOPAMINE AND AMMONIA PLASMA LEVELS IN HEPATIC ENCEPHALOPATHY, *CLIN CHIM ACTA*, 75, 99-105 (1977)

0340 CAPRILLI R ET AL, BLOOD PH: A TEST FOR ASSESSMENT OF SEVERITY IN PROCTOCOLITIS, *GUT*, 17, 763-9. (1976)

0341 CARAWAY W T, CHEMICAL AND DIAGNOSTIC SPECIFICITY OF LABORA-TORY TESTS, *AM J CLIN PATHOL*, 37, 445-459 (1962)

0342 CARAWAY W T, SOURCES OF ERROR IN CLINICAL CHEMISTRY, *STAND METH CLIN CHEM*, 5, 19 (1965)

0343 CAREY F, FORDER RA, RADIOIMMUNOASSAY OF LTB4 AND 6-TRANS LTB4: ANALYTICAL AND PHARMACOLOGICAL CHARACTERIZATION OF IMMUNOREACTIVE LTB4 IN IONOPHORE STIMULATED HUMAN BLOOD, *PROSTAGLANDINS LEUKOTRIENES MED*, 22, 57-70 (1986)

0344 CARR R I ET AL, ANTIBODIES TO BOVINE GAMMA GLOBULIN (BGG) AND THE OCCURRENCE OF A BGG-LIKE SUBSTANCE IN SYSTEMIC LUPUS ERYTHEMATOSUS SERA, *J ALLERGY CLIN IMMUNOL*, 50, 18-30 (1972)

0345 CARRE I J ET AL, IDIOPATHIC RENAL ACIDOSIS IN INFANCY, *ARCH DIS CHILD*, 29, 326 (1954)

0346 CARRELLA M ET AL, AN EVALUATION OF URINARY D-GLUCARIC ACID EXCRETION DURING ACUTE HEPATITIS IN MAN, *AM J DIG DIS*, 23, 18-22 (1978)

0347 CARRETTA R F ET AL, EARLY DIAGNOSIS OF VENOUS THROMBOSIS USING 125I-FIBRINOGEN, *J NUCL MED*, 18, 5-10 (1977)

0348 CARSON D A ET AL, IGG RHEUMATOID FACTOR IN SUBACUTE BACTE-RIAL ENDOCARDITIS: RELATIONSHIP TO IGM RHEUMATOID FAC-TOR AND CIRCULATING IMMUNE COMPLEXES, *CLIN EXP IMMUNOL*, 31, 100-3 (1978)

0349 CARTWRIGHT G E ET AL, STUDIES ON FREE ERYTHROCYTE PROTO-PORPHYRIN PLASMA IRON AND PLASMA COPPER IN NORMAL AND ANEMIC SUBJECTS, *BLOOD*, 5, 501 (1948)

0350 CARTWRIGHT GE, GUBLER CJ, BUSH JA, WINTROBE M, STUDIES ON COPPER METABOLISM. XI COPPER AND IRON METABOLISM IN THE NEPHROTIC SYNDROME, *J CLIN INVEST*, 33, 685-698 (1954)

0351 CARULLI N ET AL, ALPHA-FETOPROTEIN IN CHRONIC HEPATITIS IN: CHRONIC HEPATITIS, *GENTILINI P ET AL (ED) BASEL-KARGER*, 60-4 (1976)

0352 CARUNTU F ET AL, PASSIVE HEMAGGLUTINATION AND COMPLEMENT FIXATION REACTIONS IN THE EARLY DIAGNOSIS OF MYCOPLASMA PNEUMONIAE INFECTIONS, *VIROLOGIE*, 27, 229-35 (1976)

0353 CASASSUS P, VANNETZEL JM, TRICOT G, ET AL, HYPERCALCEMIA COMPLICATING WALDENSTRÖM'S DISEASE: A MANIFESTATION OF RICHTER'S SYNDROME, *ANN MED INTERNE (PARIS)*, 134, 130-3 (1983)

0354 CASS R M ET AL, IMMUNOGLOBULINS G, A, AND M IN SYSTEMIC LUPUS ERYTHEMATOSUS. RELATIONSHIP TO SERUM COMPLEMENT TITER, LATEX TITER, ANTINUCLEAR ANTIBODY AND MANIFESTA-TIONS OF CLINICAL DISEASE, *ANN INTERN MED*, 69, 749 (1968)

0355 CASSMER O, HORMONE PRODUCTION OF THE ISOLATED HUMAN PLA-CENTA, *ACTA ENDOCRINOL*, 45(SUPPL), 66 (1959)

0356 CASTANEDA M R AND GUERRERO G, STUDIES ON THE LEUCOCYTIC PICTURE IN BRUCELLOSIS, *J INFECT DIS*, 78, 43 (1946)

0357 CASTELLI W P ET AL, HDL CHOLESTEROL AND OTHER LIPIDS IN CORO-NARY HEART DISEASE. THE COOPERATIVE LIPOPROTEIN PHE-NOTYPING STUDY, *CIRCULATION*, 55, 767-72 (1977)

0358 CASTELLI W, GARRISON RJ, WILSON PWF, INCIDENCE OF CORONARY HEART DISEASE AND LIPOPROTEIN CHOLESTEROL LEVELS, *JAMA*, 256, 2835 (1986)

0359 CASTRO-BELLO F ET AL, HIGH SERUM GLUTAMIC ACID LEVELS IN PATIENTS WITH CARCINOMA OF THE PANCREAS, *DIGESTION*, 14, 360-63 (1976)

0360 CATTANEO R ET AL, PERIPHERAL T-LYMPHOCYTES IN JUVENILE-ONSET DIABETICS (JOD) AND IN MATERNITY-ONSET DIABETICS (MOD), *DIA-BETES*, 25, 223-6 (1976)

0361 CAUGHNEY J E AND MYRIANTHOPOULOS N C, DYSTROPHIA MYOTON-ICA AND RELATED DISORDERS, *SPRINGFIELD CC THOMAS CO* (1973)

0362 CERNY A AND KATZENSTEIN-SUTRO E, DIE PAROXYSMALE LAHMUNG, *ARCH NEUROL*, 70, 259 (1952)

0363 CHAMBERS J P ET AL, DETERMINATION OF SERUM ACID PHOSPHA-TASE IN GAUCHER'S DISEASE USING 4-METHYLUMBELLIFERYL PHOSPHATE, *CLIN CHIM ACTA*, 80, 67-77 (1977)

0364 CHAN C H, PRIMARY CARCINOMA OF THE LIVER, *MED CLIN NORTH AM*, 59, 989-994 (1975)

0365 CHAN V, YEUNG CK, CHAN TK, ANTITHROMBIN III AND FIBRINOGEN DEGRADATION PRODUCT (FRAGMENT E) IN DIABETIC NEPHROPA-THY, *J CLIN PATHOL*, 35, 661-6 (1982)

0366 CHANARIN I, THE MEGALOBLASTIC ANEMIAS, *F A DAVIS CO (PHI-LADEPHIA)* (1969)

0367 CHANARIN I, *THE MEGALOBLASTIC ANEMIAS, END ED. OXFORD, BLACKWELL SCIENTIFIC PUBLICATIONS* (1979)

0368 CHANDRASEKHAR AJ, PALATAO A, DUBIN A, ET AL, PLEURAL FLUID LACTIC ACID DEHYDROGENASE ACTIVITY AND PROTEIN CON-TENT, *ARCH INTERN MED*, 123, 48-50 (1969)

0369 CHANG S, MEASUREMENT OF COMPLEMENT OF PATIENT WITH BONE SARCOMA, *JPN J*, 37, 97-106, 67 (1967)

0370 CHANGBUMRUNG S, MIGASENA P, SUPAWAN V, ET AL, ALPHA 1-ANTITRYPSIN, ALPHA 1-ANTICHYMOTRYPSIN AND ALPHA 2-MACROGLOBULIN IN HUMAN LIVER FLUKE (OPISTHORCHIASIS), *TROPENMED PARASITOL*, 33, 195-7 (1982)

0371 CHANNICK B J ET AL, SUPPRESSED PLASMA RENIN ACTIVITY IN HYPER-TENSION, *ARCH INTERN MED*, 123, 131 (1969)

0372 CHAPEL HM ESIRI MM, WILCOCK GK, IMMUNOGLOBULIN AND OTHER PROTEINS IN THE CEREBROSPINAL FLUID OF PATIENTS WITH ALZHEIMER'S DISEASE, *J CLIN PATHOL*, 37, 697-699 (1984)

0373 CHAPLIN E R, FETAL HEMOGLOBIN IN THE DIAGNOSIS OF NEONATAL SUBARACHNOID HEMORRHAGE, *PEDIATRICS*, 58, 751-54 (1976)

0374 CHAPMAN J S AND J CLARK, COLD-PRECIPITABLE PROTEINS OF SAR-COIDOSIS SERUM, *LEVINSKY L MACHOLDA F (EDS) 5TH INTERNA-TIONAL CONF ON SARCOIDOSIS*, 198 (1971)

0375 CHAPMAN JC, REFERENCE VALUES (NORMAL RANGE) OF SEVEN PRO-TEINS IN SERUM AND EDTA PLASMA: A COMPARISON, *CAN J MED TECHNOL*, 42, 29-30 (1980)

0376 CHARLESWORTH J A ET AL, ACUTE HEPATITIS: SIGNIFICANCE OF CHANGES IN COMPLEMENT COMPONENTS, *CLIN EXP IMMUNOL*, 28, 496-501 (1977)

0377 CHASE H P ET AL, JUVENILE DIABETES MELLITUS AND SERUM LIPIDS AND LIPOPROTEIN LEVELS, *AM J DIS CHILD*, 130, 1113-7 (1976)

0378 CHASE H P ET AL, INCREASED PROSTAGLANDIN SYNTHESIS IN CHILD-HOOD DIABETES MELLITUS, *J PEDIATR*, 94, 185-89 (1979)

0379 CHATTEHEE A ET AL, RENAL FUNCTIONAL STATUS AND SERUM ELEC-TROLYTE CHANGES IN HEPATIC FAILURE, *J ASSOC PHYSICIANS INDIA*, 25, 475-82 (1977)

0380 CHATTERJEE T ET AL, STUDIES ON PLASMA FIBRINOGEN LEVEL IN PRE-ECLAMPSIA AND ECLAMPSIA, *EXPERIENTIA*, 34, 562-3 (1978)

0381 CHAUDHURI S ET AL, STUDY OF SERUM LIPIDS AND ENZYMES IN MYO-CARDIAL INFARCTION AND HYPERTENSION, *THROMB RES*, 11, 163-70 (1977)

0382 CHECK IJ, KIDD MR, STATON GW JR, SYSTEMIC AND LUNG PROTEIN CHANGES IN SARCOIDOSIS. LYMPHOCYTE COUNTS, GALLIUM UPTAKE VALUES, AND SERUM ANGIOTENSIN-CONVERTING ENZYME LEVELS MAY REFLECT DIFFERENT ASPECTS OF DISEASE ACTIVITY, *ANN NY ACAD SCI*, 465, 407-17 (1986)

0383 CHEN D S ET AL, SERUM ALPHA-FETOPROTEIN IN HEPATOCELLULAR CARCINOMA, *CANCER*, 40, 779-83 (1977)

0384 CHEN J W ET AL, RADIATION-INDUCED CHANGE IN SERUM AND URI-NARY AMYLASE LEVELS IN MAN., *RADIAT RES*, 54, 141 (1973)

0385 CHERNOFF A I, THE CLINICAL, HEMATOLOGIC AND GENETIC CHARAC-TERISTICS OF THE HEMOGLOBIN E SYNDROMES, *J LAB CLIN MED*, 47, 455 (1956)

0386 CHESLEY L C, RENAL FUNCTIONAL CHANGES IN NORMAL PREG-NANCY., *CLIN OBSTET GYNEC*, 3 (1960)

0387 CHESLEY L C, HYPERTENSIVE DISORDERS IN PREGNANCY, *APPLETON-CENTURY-CROFTS NEW YORK* (1978)

0388 CHILD, JA, SPATI B, ILLINGWORTH S, ET AL., SERUM BETA 2 MICROGLOBULIN AND C-REACTIVE PROTEIN IN THE MONITORING OF LYMPHOMAS FINDINGS IN A MULTICENTER STUDY AND EXPERI-ENCE IN SELECTED PATIENTS, *CANCER*, 45, 318-326 (1980)

0389 CHILLAR R K DESFORGES J F, RED CELL ORGANIC PHOSPHATES IN PATIENTS WITH CHRONIC RENAL FAILURE ON MAINTENANCE HAEMODIALYSIS, *BR J HAEMATOL*, 26, 549 (1974)

0390 CHIRICU TA I ET AL, URINARY 17-KETOSTEROID FRACTIONS IN YOUNG PATIENTS WITH BREAST CANCER, *ENDOCRINOLOGIE*, 16, 135-7. (1978)

0391 CHITAB M S ET AL, NITROBLUE TETRAZOLIUM TEST IN TUBERCULOUS AND PYOGENIC MENINGITIS, *INDIAN J PEDIATR*, 13, 447-50 (1976)

0392 CHODOS D D F ELY R S AND KELLY V C, PAPER ELECTROPHORESIS OF DUODENAL FLUID FROM PATIENTS WITH CYSTIC FIBROSIS, *PROC SOC EXP BIOL MED*, 99, 775 (1952)

0393 CHOPIA D AND E P CLERKEN, HYPERCALCEMIA AND MALIGNANT DIS-EASE, *MED CLIN NORTH AM*, 59, 229-39 (1977)

0394 CHOPRA T J ET AL, RECIPROCAL CHANGES IN SERUM CONCENTRA-TIONS OF 3,3',5-TRIIODOTHYRONINE (T_3) IN SYSTEMIC ILLNESSES, *J CLIN ENDOCRINOL METAB*, 41, 1043-9 (1975)

0395 CHOREMIS C ET AL, AMINO-ACID TOLERANCE CURVES AND AMINO-ACIDURIA IN COOLEY'S AND SICKLE CELL ANEMIAS, *J CLIN PATHOL*, 12, 245 (1959)

0396 CHOW D ET AL, LABORATORY DIAGNOSIS OF BENCE JONES PROTEIN-URIA IN A PATIENT WITH PLASMA CELL LEUKEMIA, *CLIN CHEM*, 81, 1683 (1975)

0397 CHOWDHURY A R ET AL, GASTROINTESTINAL PROTEIN LOSS DURING ETHANOL INGESTION, *GASTROENTEROLOGY*, 72, 37 (1977)

0398 CHOWDHURY P, BONE RC, LOURIA DB, RAYFORD PL, EFFECT OF CIGA-RETTE SMOKE ON HUMAN SERUM TRYPSIN INHIBITORY CAPACITY AND ANTITRYPSIN CONCENTRATION, *AM REV RESPIR DIS*, 126, 177-9 (1982)

0399 CHRISTENSEN N J, PLASMA CATECHOLAMINES IN LONG-TERM DIABET-ICS WITH AND WITHOUT NEUROPATHY AND IN HYPOPHYSECTOMIZED SUBJECTS, *J CLIN INVEST*, 51, 779 (1972)

0400 CHRISTENSEN P J ET AL, AMINO ACIDS IN BLOOD PLASMA AND URINE DURING PREGNANCY, *SCAND J CLIN LAB INVEST*, 9, 54 (1957)

0401 CHRISTENSSON T ET AL, SERUM LIPIDS BEFORE AND AFTER PARATHY-ROIDECTOMY IN PATIENTS WITH PRIMARY HYPERPARATHYROID-ISM, *CLIN CHIM ACTA*, 78, 411-5. (1977)

0402 CHRISTIAN C L ET AL, SYSTEMIC LUPUS ERYTHEMATOSUS. CRY-OPRECIPITATION OF SERA, *J CLIN INVEST*, 42, 823-829 (1963)

0403 CHU ET AL, COMPARATIVE EVALUATION OF SERUM ACID PHOSPHA-TASE, URINARY CHOLESTEROL, AND ANDROGENS IN DIAGNOSIS OF PROSTATIC CANCER, *UROLOGY*, 6, 291-294 (1975)

0404 CHUA ET AL, ACID PHOSPHATASE LEVELS IN BONE MARROW: VALUE IN DETECTING EARLY BONE METASTASES FROM CARCINOMA OF THE PROSTATE, *J UROL*, 103, 462-466 (1970)

0405 CHURCH J A ET AL, ROUTINE LABORATORY DETERMINATIONS IN PEDI-ATRIC ALLERGIC DISEASE, *ANN ALLERGY*, 41, 136-9 (1978)

0406 CHURG J AND EHRENREICH T, MEMBRANOUS NEPHROPATHY IN: GLO-MERULONEPHRITIS MORPHOLOGY, NATURAL HISTORY AND TREATMENT. PT. I, *KINCAID-SMITH P ET AL (EDS) JOHN WILEY & SONS*, 443 (1973)

0407 CHUSID EL, HIRSCH RL, COLCHER H, SPECTRUM OF HYPERTROPHIC GASTROPATHY, *ARCH INTERN MED*, 114, 621-628 (1964)

0408 CLARKE GN, STOJANOFF A, CAUCHI MN, ET AL, THE IMMUNOGLOBU-LIN CLASS OF ANTISPERMATOZOAL ANTIBODIES IN SERUM, *AM J REPROD IMMUNOL MICROBIOL*, 7, 143-147 (1985)

0409 CLARKE H G M ET AL, SERUM PROTEINS IN NORMAL PREGNANCY AND MILD PRE-ECLAMPSIA, *BR J OBSTET GYNAECOL*, 78, 105-109 (1971)

0410 CLAUS DR, OSMAND AP, GEWURZ H, RADIOIMMUNOASSAY OF HUMAN C-REACTIVE PROTEIN AND LEVELS IN NORMAL SERA, *J LAB CLIN MED*, 87, 120-128 (1976)

0411 CLEMENTS JA, PLATZKER ACG, TIERNERY DF, ET AL, ASSESSMENT OF THE RISK OF RESPIRATORY-DISTRESS SYNDROME BY A RAPID TEST FOR SURFACTANT IN AMNIOTIC FLUID, N ENGL J MED, 286, 1077-1081 (1972)

0412 CLERMONT ET AL, THE TRANSAMINASE TESTS IN LIVER DISEASE, MEDICINE, 46, 197-205 (1967)

0413 CLINE M J, ANEMIA IN MACROGLOBULINEMIA, AM J MED, 34, 213 (1963)

0414 CLINE M J AND BERLIN N J, ANEMIA IN HODGKIN'S DISEASE, CANCER, 16, 526 (1963)

0415 CLINE M J AND GOLDE D, IMMUNE SUPPRESSION OF HEMATOPOIESIS, AM J MED, 64, 301-309 (1978)

0416 COBERT BL, REYE'S SYNDROME, HOSPITAL MEDICINE, 89 (1986)

0417 COE F L AND FUPO J J, EVIDENCE FOR MILD REVERSIBLE HYPERPARATHYROIDISM IN DISTAL RENAL TUBULAR ACIDOSIS, ARCH INTERN MED, 135, 1485 (1975)

0418 COE JE, AIKAWA JK, CHOLESTEROL PLEURAL EFFUSION, ARCH INTERN MED, 108, 763-774 (1961)

0419 COGGINS C L ET AL, UNPUBLISHED OBSERVATIONS, US COOP STUDY OF ADULT IDIOPATHIC NEPHROTIC SYNDROME (1975)

0420 COHEN, SERUM ENZYMES DETERMINATIONS: THEIR RELIABILITY AND VALUE, MED CLIN NORTH AM, 53 (1969)

0421 COHEN A S, AMYLOIDOSIS, N ENGL J MED, 277, 522-530 (1967)

0422 COHEN A S (ED), LABORATORY DIAGNOSTIC PROCEDURES IN RHEUMATIC DISEASES, BOSTON, LITTLE, BROWN, AND CO. (1967)

0423 COHEN AJ, PHILIPS TM, KESSLER CM, CIRCULATING COAGULATION INHIBITORS IN THE ACQUIRED IMMUNODEFICIENCY SYNDROME, ANN INTERN MED, 104, 175-180 (1986)

0424 COHEN JA, KAPLAN MM, THE SGOT/SGPT RATIO-AN INDICATOR OF ALCOHOLIC LIVER DISEASE, DIG DIS SCI, 24, 835-838 (1979)

0425 COHEN M ET AL, THE SECRETION AND DISPOSITION OF CORTISOL DURING PREGNANCY, J CLIN ENDOCRINOL METAB, 78, 1976 (1958)

0426 COHEN S AND BUTCHER G A, COMMENTS ON IMMUNIZATION, MILIT MED, 134, 1191 (1969)

0427 COHEN S ET AL, LIVER DISEASE AND GALLSTONES IN REGIONAL ENTERITIS, GASTROENTEROLOGY, 60, 237 (1971)

0428 COLTART ET AL, BLOOD GLUCOSE AND INSULIN RELATIONSHIPS IN THE HUMAN MOTHER AND FETUS BEFORE ONSET OF LABOUR, BR MED J, 4, 17-19 (1969)

0429 COMBES B ET AL, DISORDERS OF THE LIVER IN PREGNANCY, PATHOPHYSIOLOGY OF GESTATION ASSALI N S & BRINKMAN C R III (EDS) NEW ACADEMIC, I, 479-522 (1972)

0430 COMENS P, REED D, METTE M, PHYSIOLOGIC RESPONSES OF PILOTS FLYING HIGH-PERFORMANCE AIRCRAFT, AVIAT SPACE ENVIRON MED, 58, 205-10 (1987)

0431 CONCANON J P ET AL, THE CEA ASSAYS IN BRONCHOGENIC CARCINOMA, AM J OF PROCTOLOGY, 34, 184 (1974)

0432 CONDIE R G, A SERIAL STUDY OF COAGULATION FACTORS XII, XI AND X IN PLASMA IN NORMAL PREGNANCY AND IN PREGNANCY COMPLICATED BY PRE-ECLAMPSIA, BR J OBSTET GYNAECOL, 83, 636-39 (1976)

0433 CONN AND CONN, CURRENT DIAGNOSIS, 4TH EDITION W B SAUNDERS & CO PHIL (1974)

0434 CONNOR T B ET AL, HYPERTENSION DUE TO UNILATERAL RENAL DISEASE: WITH A REPORT ON A FUNCTIONAL TEST HELPFUL IN DIAGNOSIS, JOHNS HOPKINS MED J, 100, 241 (1957)

0435 CONSENSUS CONFERENCE, OFFICE FOR MEDICAL APPLICATIONS OF RESEARCH, NATIONAL INSTITUTES OF HEALTH: DIAGNOSIS AND TREATMENT OF REYE'S SYNDROME, JAMA, 246, 2441-2444 (1981)

0436 CONTRONE G ET AL, CEREBROSPINAL FLUID LACTIC ACID LEVELS IN MENINGITIS, J PEDIATR, 91, 379-84 (1977)

0437 COODLEY E L, ENZYME PROFILES IN THE EVALUATION OF PULMONARY INFARCTION, JAMA, 207, 1307-1309 (1969)

0438 COOK C D ET AL, STUDIES OF RESPIRATORY PHYSIOLOGY IN CHILDREN, PEDIATRICS, 24, 181 (1959)

0439 COOK ET AL, NONUTILITY OF MEASUREMENT OF SERUM GAMMA-GLUTAMYL TRANSPEPTIDASE ACTIVITIES IN DIAGNOSIS OF MYOCARDIAL DISEASE, CLIN CHEM, 19, 774-776 (1973)

0440 COOK G C ET AL, EFFECT OF SYSTEMIC INFECTION AND RAISED SERUM IGG CONCENTRATION ON THE D-XYLOSE TEST, AM J GASTROENTEROL, 67, 570-3 (1977)

0441 COOKE ET AL, RICKETS,GROWTH, AND ALKALINE PHOSPHATASE IN URBAN ADOLESCENTS, BR MED J, 2, 293-297 (1974)

0442 COOKE W T ET AL, SERUM ALKALINE PHOSPHATASE AND RICKETS IN URBAN SCHOOL CHILDREN, BR MED J, 1, 324-327 (1973)

0443 COOKSON G H AND RIMINGTON C, PORPHOBILINOGEN, BIOCHEM J, 57, 476 (1954)

0444 COOLEY ET AL, PLASMA ACID PHOSPHATASE IN IDIOPATHIC AND SECONDARY THROMBOCYTOPENIAS, ARCH INTERN MED, 119, 345-354 (1967)

0445 COOMBES ET AL, PLASMA IMMUNOREACTIVE CALCITONIN IN PATIENTS WITH NON-THYROID TUMORS, LANCET, 1, 1080 (1974)

0446 COOMBES R C ET AL, EVALUATION OF BIOCHEMICAL MARKERS IN BREAST CANCER, PROC R SOC, 70, 843-5 (1977)

0447 COOMBS F S ET AL, RENAL FUNCTION IN PATIENTS WITH GOUT, J CLIN INVEST, 19, 525 (1940)

0448 COONROD J D ET AL, LATEX AGGLUTINATION IN THE DIAGNOSIS OF PNEUMOCOCCAL INFECTION, J CLIN MICROBIOL, 4, 168 (1976)

0449 COONROD J D ET AL, COMPLEMENT LEVELS IN PNEUMOCOCCAL PNEUMONIA, INFECT IMMUN, 18, 14-22 (1977)

0450 COOPER E H ET AL, ALPHA-GLOBULINS IN THE SURVEILLANCE OF COLORECTAL CANCER, BIOMED PHARMACOTHER, 24, 171-8 (1976)

0451 COOPER L Z ET AL, NEONATAL THROMBOCYTOPENIC PURPURA AND OTHER MANIFESTATIONS OF RUBELLA CONTRACTED IN UTERO, AM J DIS CHILD, 110, 416 (1965)

0452 COOPER N, PERSONAL COMMUNICATION, DEPARTMENT OF MOLECULAR IMMUNOLOGY, SCRIPPS CLINIC AND RESEARCH FOUNDATION, CA. (1981)

0453 COOPERBERG A A AND TEITELBAUM J I, THE CONCENTRATION OF ANTIHEMOPHILIC GLOBULIN (AHG) IN PATIENTS WITH CORONARY ARTERY DISEASE, ANN INTERN MED, 54, 899 (1961)

0454 COPELAND G D ET AL, SYSTEMIC LUPUS ERYTHEMATOSUS: A CLINICAL REPORT OF 47 CASES WITH PATHOLOGIC FINDINGS IN 18, AM J MED SCI, 236, 318 (1958)

0455 CORASH L, SHAFER B, BLAESE RM, PLATELET-ASSOCIATED IMMUNOGLOBULIN, PLATELET SIZE AND THE EFFECT OF SPLENECTOMY IN THE WISKOTT-ALDRICH SYNDROME, BLOOD, 65, 1439 (1985)

0456 CORDER M P ET AL, FAMILIAL OCCURRENCE OF VON WILLEBRAND'S DISEASE, THROMBOCYTOPENIA, AND SEVERE GASTROINTESTINAL BLEEDING, AM J MED SCI, 265, 219 (1973)

0457 CORLETTE M B ET AL, AMYLASE ELEVATION ATTRIBUTABLE TO AN OVARIAN NEOPLASM, GASTROENTEROLOGY, 74, 907-9 (1978)

0458 CORRIGAN D F ET AL, PARAMETERS OF THYROID FUNCTION IN PATIENTS WITH ACTIVE ACROMEGALY, METABOLISM, 27, 209-16 (1978)

0459 COWARD RA, DELAMORE IW, MALLICK NP, ET AL, URINARY N-ACETYL-B-D-GLUCOSAMINIDASE AS AN INDICATOR OF TUBULAR DAMAGE IN MULTIPLE MYELOMA, CLIN CHIM ACTA, 138, 293-298 (1984)

0460 COWDEN E A ET AL, HYPERPROLACTINEMIA IN RENAL DISEASE, CLIN ENDOCRINOL (OXF), 9, 241-248 (1978)

0461 COX DW, HOEPPNER VH, LEVISON H, PROTEASE INHIBITORS IN PATIENTS WITH CHRONIC OBSTRUCTIVE PULMONARY DISEASE: THE ALPHA 1-ANTITRYPSIN HETEROZYGOTE CONTROVERSY, AM REV RESPIR DIS, 113, 601-606 (1976)

0462 COX DW, SMYTH S, RISK FOR LIVER DISEASE IN ADULTS WITH ALPHA 1-ANTITRYPSIN DEFICIENCY, AM J MED, 74, 221-7 (1983)

0463 CRAFT A W ET AL, SERUM FERRITIN IN JUVENILE CHRONIC POLYARTHRITIS, ANN RHEUM DIS, 36, 271-273 (1977)

0464 CRAMER H ET AL, EFFECTS OF PROBENECID AND EXERCISE OF CEREBROSPINAL FLUID CYCLIC AMP IN AFFECTIVE ILLNESS, LANCET, 1, 1346 (1972)

0465 CRAMP D G ET AL, PLASMA TRIGLYCERIDE SECRETION AND METABOLISM IN CHRONIC RENAL FAILURE, CLIN CHIM ACTA, 76, 237-41 (1977)

0466 CRANE G G ET AL, THE ROLE OF PLASMA PROTEINS IN CHRONIC EXPANSION OF PLASMA VOLUME IN TROPICAL SPLENOMEGALY SYNDROME. III. THE INTERRELATIONSHIPS OF ALBUMIN, IMMUNOGLOBULINS AND PLASMA VOLUME, TRANS R SOC TROP MED HYG, 69, 212-20 (1975)

0467 CRAWHALL J C ET AL, ELEVATION OF SERUM CREATINE KINASE IN SEVERE HYPOKALEMIC HYPERALDOSTERONISM, CLIN BIOCHEM, 9, 237-240 (1976)

0468 CREESE BR, TEMPLE DM, THE MEDIATORS OF ALLERGIC CONTRACTION OF HUMAN AIRWAY SMOOTH MUSCLE: A COMPARISON OF BRONCHIAL AND LUNG PARENCHYMAL STRIP PREPARATIONS, CLIN EXP PHARMACOL PHYSIOL, 13, 103-11 (1986)

0469 CRIGLER J F AND NAJJAR V A, CONGENITAL FAMILIAL NON-HEMOLYTIC JAUNDICE WITH KERNICTERUS, PEDIATRICS, 10, 169 (1952)

0470 CRIPPS D J AND MCEACHERN W M, HEPATIC AND ERYTHROPOIETIC PROTOPORPHYRIA, ARCH PATHOL LAB MED, 91, 497 (1971)

0471 CRIPPS D J AND PETERS H A, STOOL PORPHYRINS IN ACUTE INTERMITTENT AND HEREDITARY COPROPORPHYRIA, ARCH NEUROL, 23, 80 (1970)

0472 CRISP W E ET AL, SERUM GLUTAMIC OXALOACETIC TRANSMINASE LEVELS IN THE TOXEMIAS OF PREGNANCY, OBSTET GYNECOL, 13, 487-497 (1959)

0473 CROCKER A C ET AL, NIEMANN-PICK DISEASE: A REVIEW OF 18 PATIENTS, MEDICINE, 37, 1-95 (1951)

0474 CROCKER AND LANDING, PHOSPHATASE STUDIES IN GAUCHER'S DISEASE, METAB CLIN EXP, 9, 341-362 (1960)

0475 CROPP G J A AND MYERS D N, PHYSIOLOGICAL EVIDENCE OF HYPERMETABOLISM IN OSTEOGENESIS IMPERFECTA, PEDIATRICS, 49, 375 (1972)

0476 CROSBY W H, THE METABOLISM OF HEMOGLOBIN AND BILE PIGMENT IN HEMOLYTIC DISEASE, AM J MED, 18, 112 (1955)

0477 CROSBY W H, PAROXYSMAL NOCTURNAL HEMOGLOBINURIA, BLOOD, 15, 505 (1960)

0478 CROUT, ET AL, SPOROTRICHOSIS ARTHRITIS, ANN INTERN MED, 86, 294 (1977)

0479 CROWLEY ET AL, A COMPARISON OF FOUR METHODS FOR MEASURING CREATINE PHOSPHOKINASE, AM J CLIN PATHOL, 53, 948-955 (1970)

0480 CUCUIANU M ET AL, INCREASED SERUM GAMMA-GLUTAMYLTRANSFERASE IN HYPERTRIGLYCERIDEMIA: COMPARISON WITH SERUM PSEUDOCHOLINESTERASE, CLIN CHIM ACTA, 71, 419-27 (1976)

0481 CUDWORTH A G ET AL, EVALUATION OF ORAL GLUCOSE TOLERANCE TEST RESULTS IN PREGNANCY, DIABETES METAB REV, 4, 89-94 (1978)

0482 CUTLER NR, KAY AD, MARANGOS PJ, BURG C, CEREBROSPINAL FLUID NEURON-SPECIFIC ENOLASE IS REDUCED IN ALZHEIMER'S DISEASE, ARCH NEUROL, 43, 153 (1986)

0483 D'ONOFRIO GM, LEVITT S, ILETT KF, SERUM ANGIOTENSIN CONVERTING ENZYME IN CROHN'S DISEASE, ULCERATIVE COLITIS AND PEPTIC ULCERATION, AUST NZ J MED, 14, 27-30 (1984)

0484 DACIE J V, THE HAEMOLYTIC ANAEMIAS, PART IV, GRUNE & STRATTON NEW YORK (1967)

0485 DACIE J V, AUTOIMMUNE HEMOLYTIC ANEMIA, ARCH INTERN MED, 135, 1293 (1975)

0486 DACIE J V (ED), SECONDARY OR SYMPTOMATIC HEMOLYTIC ANEMIAS: THE HAEMOLYTIC ANEMIAS, *GRUNE & STRATTON NEW YORK*, 908 (1967)

0487 DAGG J H ET AL, THE RELATIONSHIP OF LEAD POISONING TO ACUTE INTERMITTENT PORPHYRIA, *Q J MED*, 34, 163 (1964)

0488 DALAND G A ET AL, HEMATOLOGIC OBSERVATIONS IN BACTERIAL ENDOCARDITIS, *J LAB CLIN MED*, 48, 827 (1956)

0489 DALOVISIA J R ET AL, SUBACUTE THYROIDITIS WITH INCREASED SERUM ALKALINE PHOSPHATASE, *ANN INTERN MED*, 88, 505-507 (1978)

0490 DAMLE S R ET AL, STUDIES ON GLYCOLYTIC ENZYMES IN RELATION TO CANCER, *INDIAN J CA*, 11, 280-284 (1974)

0491 DAMMROSIO F, ENZYMES IN PREGNANCY, *ANN OBSTET GINECOL MED PERINAT*, 86 (SUPPL 12) (1964)

0492 DANIEL ET AL, RISE OF SERUM-ACID PHOSPHATASE LEVEL FOLLOWING PALPATION OF THE PROSTATE, *LANCET*, 262, 998-999 (1952)

0493 DANIEL W L ET AL, BIOCHEMICAL AND GENETIC INVESTIGATIONS OF THE DE LANGE SYNDROME, *AM J DIS CHILD*, 121, 401-5 (1971)

0494 DANIELS JC, ABNORMALITIES OF PROTEASE INHIBITORS, *SERUM PROTEIN ABNORMALITIES. DIAGNOSTIC AND CLINICAL ASPECTS*, 243-263 (1975)

0495 DANIELS JC, LARSON DL, ABSTON S, RITZMANN SE, SERUM PROTEIN PROFILES IN THERMAL BURNS, *J TRAUMA*, 14, 153-162 (1974)

0496 DANKS DM, CAMPBELL PE, WALKER-SMITH J, ET AL, MENKES' KINKY-HAIR SYNDROME, *LANCET*, 1, 1100-1103 (1972)

0497 DANKS DM, CARTWRIGHT E, STEVENS FJ, TOWNLEY RRW, MENKES' KINKY-HAIR DISEASE: FURTHER DEFINITION OF THE DEFECT IN COPPER TRANSPORT, *SCIENCE*, 179, 1140-1141 (1973)

0498 DANOVITCH S H ET AL, INTESTINAL ALKALINE PHOSPHATASE ACTIVITY IN FAMILIAL HYPOPHOSPHATASIA, *N ENGL J MED*, 278, 1253-1259 (1968)

0499 DARMADY ET AL, PROSPECTIVE STUDY OF SERUM CHOLESTEROL LEVELS DURING FIRST YEAR OF LIFE, *BR MED J*, 2, 685-688 (1972)

0500 DASS A ET AL, SERUM TRANSAMINASES IN TOXAEMIA OF PREGNANCY, *BR J OBSTET GYNAECOL*, 71, 727-734 (1964)

0501 DAUGHADAY WH, LARNER J, THE RENAL EXCRETION OF INOSITOL IN NORMAL AND DIABETIC HUMAN BEINGS, *J CLIN INVEST*, 33, 326-332 (1954)

0502 DAVIDSOHN E AND LEE C L, THE LABORATORY IN THE DIAGNOSIS OF INFECTIOUS MONONUCLEOSIS (WITH ADDITIONAL NOTES ON EPIDEMIOLOGY, ETIOLOGY, AND PATHOGENESIS), *MED CLIN NORTH AM*, 46, 225 (1962)

0503 DAVIDSOHN I, CLINICAL DIAGNOSIS BY LABORATORY METHODS, *HENRY J B (ED) 16TH EDITION PHILADELPHIA SAUNDERS* (1979)

0504 DAVIDSON ET AL, ELEVATED SERUM ACID PHOSPHATASE LEVELS WITH RECTAL CARCINOMA TUMOR, *GASTROENTEROLOGY*, 70, 114-116 (1976)

0505 DAVIDSON GP, COREY M, MORAD-HASSEL F, ET AL, IMMUNOASSAY OF SERUM CONJUGATES OF CHOLIC ACID IN CYSTIC FIBROSIS, *J CLIN PATHOL*, 33, 390-4 (1980)

0506 DAVIES SF, ROHRBACH MS, THELEN V, ET AL, ELEVATED SERUM ANGIOTENSIN-CONVERTING ENZYME (SACE) ACTIVITY IN ACUTE PULMONARY HISTOPLASMOSIS, *CHEST*, 85, 307-10 (1984)

0507 DAVIES-JONES, LACTATE DEHYDROGENASE AND GLUTAMIC OXALACETIC TRANSAMINASE OF THE CEREBROSPINAL FLUID IN TUMOURS OF THE CENTRAL NERVOUS SYSTEM, *J NEUROL NEUROSURG PSYCHIATRY*, 32, 324-327 (1969)

0508 DAVIGNON J ET AL, PLASMA LIPIDS AND LIPOPROTEIN PATTERNS IN ANGIOGRAPHICALLY GRADED ATHEROSCLEROSIS OF THE LEGS AND IN CORONARY HEART DISEASE, *CAN MED ASSOC J*, 116, 1245-50 (1977)

0509 DAVIS CA, VALLOTA EH, FORRISTAL J, SERUM COMPLEMENT LEVELS IN INFANCY: AGE RELATED CHANGES, *PEDIATR RES*, 13, 1043-1046 (1979)

0510 DAVIS JE, MCDONALD JM, JARRET L, A HIGH PERFORMANCE LIQUID CHROMATOGRAPHICAL METHODS FOR HAEMOGLOBIN A1C, *DIABETES*, 27, 102 (1978)

0511 DAVIS P J, FACTORS AFFECTING THE DETERMINATION OF THE SERUM PROTEIN-BOUND IODINE, *AM J MED*, 40, 918 (1966)

0512 DAVIS P J AND DAVIS F B, HYPERTHYROIDISM IN PATIENTS OVER THE AGE OF 60, *MEDICINE*, 53, 161-81 (1974)

0513 DAVIS PJ, AGEING AND ENDOCRINE FUNCTION, *CLIN ENDOCRINOL METAB*, 8, 153-174 (1979)

0514 DAVIS R E ET AL, SERUM PYRIDOXAL, FOLATE, AND VITAMIN B_{12} LEVELS IN INSTITUTIONALIZED EPILEPTICS, *EPILEPSIA*, 16, 463-8 (1975)

0515 DAY ET AL, SERUM PROSTATIC ACID-PHOSPHATASE LEVELS IN THE MALE PATIENTS OF A CANCER-PREVENTION CLINIC, *CANCER*, 9, 222-227 (1956)

0516 DE ALVAREZ R R, BLOOD PRESSURE, EDEMA AND PROTEINURIA IN PREGNANCY. 6. PROTEINURIA RELATIONSHIPS, *PROG CLIN BIOL RES*, 7, 169-92 (1974)

0517 DE FLAMINGH JP, VAN DER MERWE JV, A SERUM BIOCHEMICAL PROFILE OF NORMAL PREGNANCY, *S AFR MED J*, 65, 552-5 (1984)

0518 DE FRONZO R A ET AL, RENAL FUNCTION IN PATIENTS WITH MULTIPLE MYELOMA, *MEDICINE*, 57, 151-66 (1978)

0519 DE JORGE F B ET AL, BIOCHEMICAL STUDIES ON SERUM COPPER, COPPER OXIDASE, MAGNESIUM, SULFUR CALCIUM AND PHOSPHORUS IN CANCER OF THE BREAST, *CLIN CHIM ACTA*, 12, 403-6. (1965)

0520 DE MOOR ET AL, RESULTS OBTAINED FROM 75 PATIENTS OPERATED UPON FOR HYPERPARATHYROIDISM: LOW CHOLESTEROL LEVELS IN OVERT PRIMARY HYPERPARATHYROIDISM, *ANN ENDOCRINOL (PARIS)*, 616-620 (1973)

0521 DE PABLO F, EASTMAN RC, ROTH J, GORDEN P, PLASMA PROLACTIN IN ACROMEGALY BEFORE AND AFTER TREATMENT, *J CLIN ENDOCRINOL METAB*, 53, 344-52 (1981)

0522 DE QUATTRO V ET AL, RAISED PLASMA-CATECHOLAMINES IN SOME PATIENTS WITH PRIMARY HYPERTENSION, *LANCET*, 1, 806-9 (1972)

0523 DE TOROK D ET AL, QUANTITATIVE AND QUALITATIVE PLASMA PROTEIN STUDIES ON ALCOHOLICS VS NONALCOHOLICS, *ANN NY ACAD SCI*, 273, 167 (1977)

0524 DEAN G AND BARNES H D, PORPHYRIA IN SWEDEN AND SOUTH AFRICA, *S AFR MED J*, 33, 274 (1959)

0525 DECHATELET L R ET AL, ABSENCE OF MEASURABLE LEUKOCYTE ALKALINE PHOSPHATASE ACTIVITY FROM LEUKOCYTES OF PATIENTS WITH CHRONIC GRANULOCYTIC LEUKEMIA, *CLIN CHEM*, 16, 798 (1970)

0526 DEERING T B ET AL, EFFECT OF D-PENICILLAMINE ON COPPER RETENTION IN PATIENTS WITH PRIMARY BILIARY CIRRHOSIS, *GASTROENTEROLOGY*, 72, 1208-12. (1977)

0527 DEFRONZO R A ET AL, IMPAIRED RENAL TUBULAR POTASSIUM SECRETION IN SYSTEMIC LUPUS ERYTHEMATOSUS, *ANN INTERN MED*, 86, 268-71 (1977)

0528 DEFTOS LF, CATHERWOOD BD, BONE HG, ET AL, CALCITONIN: PHYSIOLOGY AND PATHOPHYSIOLOGY, *MACINTYRE I, SZELKE M (EDS) MOLECULAR ENDOCRINOLOGY.ELSEVIER/NORTH HOLLAND PRESS* (1979)

0529 DEGROOT L ET AL, SERUM ANTIGENS AND ANTIBODIES IN THE DIAGNOSIS OF THYROID CANCER, *J CLIN ENDOCRINOL METAB*, 45, 1220-23 (1977)

0530 DEISS A ET AL, HEMOLYTIC ANEMIA IN WILSON'S DISEASE., *ANN INTERN MED*, 73, 413 (1970)

0531 DELAFOSSE B ET AL, VARIATION DES ACIDES AMINES PLASMATIQUES AU COURS DES HEPATITES GRAVES AVEC ENCEPHALOPATHY, *NOUV PRESSE MED*, 6, 1207-12 (1977)

0532 DELAMORE J W ET AL, HAEMATOLOGICAL CLUES IN SYSTEMIC DISEASE, *PRACTITIONER*, 216, 27-36 (1976)

0533 DELAPORTE C ET AL, FREE PLASMA AND MUSCLE AMINO ACIDS IN UREMIC CHILDREN, *AM J CLIN NUTR*, 31, 1647-51 (1978)

0534 DELBRUCK A AND OEPEN H, MUCOPOLYSACCHARIDSTOFFWECHSEL BEI HUNTINGTONSCHER CHOREA, *HUM GENET*, 1, 105 (1964)

0535 DELK AS, DURLE PR, FLETCHER TS, ET AL, RADIOIMMUNOASSAY OF ACTIVE PANCREATIC ENZYMES IN SERA FROM PATIENTS WITH ACUTE PANCREATITIS. I. ACTIVE CARBOXYPEPTIDASE B, *CLIN CHEM*, 31/8, 1294-1300 (1985)

0536 DELREGATO J A AND SPJUT H, CANCER, *5TH EDITION C V MOSBY CO ST. LOUIS* (1977)

0537 DELWICHE R ET AL, CEA IN PANCREATITIS, *CANCER*, 31, 328 (1973)

0538 DEMEDTS M ET AL, RESPIRATORY FAILURE: CORRELATION BETWEEN ENCEPHALOPATHY, BLOOD GASES AND BLOOD AMMONIA, *RESPIRATION*, 33, 199-210 (1976)

0539 DEMISCH K ET AL, PLASMA TESTOSTERONE IN WOMEN IN LATE PREGNANCY AND AFTER DELIVERY, *J ENDOCRINOL*, 42, 477 (1968)

0540 DEMURA R ET AL, RESPONSES OF PLASMA ACTH, GH, LH AND 11-HYDROXYCORTICOSTEROIDS TO VARIOUS STIMULI IN PATIENTS WITH CUSHING'S SYNDROME, *J CLIN ENDOCRINOL METAB*, 34, 852-859 (1972)

0541 DENBOROUGH ET AL, BIOCHEMICAL CHANGES IN MALIGNANT HYPERPYREXIA, *J CLIN ENDOCR*, 1, 1137-1138 (1970)

0542 DENBOROUGH M A ET AL, MYOPATHY AND MALIGNANT HYPERPYREXIA, *LANCET*, 1, 1138 (1970)

0543 DENIS L J ET AL, LACTIC DEHYDROGENASE IN PROSTATIC CANCER, *INVEST UROL*, 1, 101-111 (1963)

0544 DENSON W K ET AL, ANTIGEN/BIOLOGICAL - ACTIVITY RATIO FOR FACTOR VIII, *LANCET*, 1, 157 (1973)

0545 DENT R I ET AL, HYPERPARATHYROIDISM: GASTRIC ACID SECRETION AND GASTRIN., *ANN SURG*, 176, 360 (1972)

0546 DENT R I ET AL, HYPERGASTRINEMIA IN PATIENTS WITH ACUTE RENAL FAILURE., *SURG FORUM*, 23, 312 (1972)

0547 DESAI M ET AL, LIPIDS AND LIPOPROTEINS IN THALASSEMIA MAJOR, *INDIAN J PEDIATR*, 13, 663 (1976)

0548 DESCHAMPS J P AND LAHRICHI M, BIOLOGICAL VALUES IN THE CHILD AND ADOLESCENT, *REFERENCE VALUES IN HUMAN CHEMISTRY G. SIEST (ED)*, 109 (1973)

0549 DEYASE S K ET AL, PLACENTAL ALKALINE PHOSPHATASE (REGAN ISOENZYME) IN CANCEROUS PATIENTS SERA, *INDIAN J CANCER*, 13, 257-61 (1976)

0550 DEZELIC G ET AL, THE PHOTOMETRIC LATEX TEST FOR RHEUMATOID FACTORS IN PATIENTS WITH RHEUMATOID ARTHRITIS. II. CLINICAL EVALUATION, *Z RHEUMATOL*, 37, 112-22 (1978)

0551 DI SANT'AGNESE P A, CYSTIC FIBROSIS OF THE PANCREAS, *JAMA*, 172, 135 (1960)

0552 DI SANT'AGNESE P A ET AL, CYSTIC FIBROSIS IN ADULTS, *AM J MED*, 66, 121-132 (1979)

0553 DIAMOND H S ET AL, HYPERURICOSURIA AND INCREASED TUBULAR SECRETION OF URATE IN SICKLE CELL ANEMIA, *AM J MED*, 59, 796-802 (1975)

0554 DIAMOND N J ET AL, ARTERIAL BLOOD GASES IN ACUTE PULMONARY EDEMA, *JACEP*, 5, 497-500 (1976)

0555 DIAZ R ET AL, ROSE BENGAL PLATE AGGLUTINATION AND COUNTER-IMMUNOELECTROPHORESIS TESTS ON SPINAL FLUID IN THE DIAGNOSIS OF BRUCELLA MENINGITIS, *J CLIN MICROBIOL*, 7, 236-7 (1978)

0556 DICKERMAN R C ET AL, THROMBOTIC THROMBOCYTOPENIC PURPURA WITH ASSOCIATED AFIBRINOGENEMIA, *J MICH STATE MED SOC*, 54, 1421 (1955)

0557 DICKSON E R ET AL, SYSTEMIC GIANT CELL ARTERITIS WITH POLYMYALGIA RHEUMATICA. REVERSIBLE ABNORMALITIES OF LIVER FUNCTION, *JAMA*, 224, 1496 (1973)

0558 DICZFALUSY E, ENDOCRINE FUNCTIONS OF THE HUMAN FETOPLACENTAL UNIT, *FED PROC*, 23, 791 (1964)

0559 DICZFALUSY E, CIRCULATING STEROIDS AND MENSTRUAL CYCLE, *VOKAER R, DEMAUBEUGE M,(EDS): SEXUAL ENDOCRINOLOGY. NEW YORK, MASSON PUBL. USA* (1978)

0560 DIETEMANN-MOLARD A, PELLETIER A, PAULI G, ET AL, PRACTICAL VALUE OF THE ASSAY OF SERUM ANGIOTENSIN CONVERTING ENZYME ACTIVITY IN SARCOIDOSIS, *REV PNEUMOL CLIN*, 40, 121-5 (1984)

0561 DIEZ-EWALD M ET AL, MECHANISMS OF HEMOLYSIS IN IRON-DEFICIENCY ANEMIA, *BLOOD*, 32, 884 (1968)

0562 DIJKMAN J H ET AL, INCREASED SERUM ALKALINE PHOSPHATASE ACTIVITY IN PULMONARY INFARCTION, *ACTA MED SCAN*, 180, 273-281 (1966)

0563 DILIBERTI JH, MCMURRY MP, CONNOR WE, ET AL, HYPERCHOLESTEROLEMIA ASSOCIATED WITH ALPHA-1 ANTITRYPSIN DEFICIENCY AND HEPATITIS: LIPOPROTEIN AND APOPROTEIN DETERMINATIONS, STEROL BALANCE AND TREATMENT, *AM J MED SCI*, 288, 81-5 (1984)

0564 DISAIA P ET AL, CARCINOEMBRYONIC ANTIGEN IN CANCER OF THE FEMALE REPRODUCTIVE SYSTEM, *CANCER*, 39, 2365-70 (1977)

0565 DISCALA V A AND KINNEY M J, EFFECTS OF MYXEDEMA ON THE RENAL DILUTING AND CONCENTRATING MECHANISM., *AM J MED*, 50, 325 (1971)

0566 DISCHE M R AND PORRO R S, THE CARDIAC LESIONS IN BASSEN-KORNZWEIG SYNDROME, *AM J MED*, 49, 568 (1970)

0567 DITZEL J, OXYGEN TRANSPORT IMPAIRMENT IN DIABETES, *DIABETES*, 25, 832-8 (1976)

0568 DITZEL J ET AL, HYPERLIPOPROTEINEMIA, DIABETES, AND OXYGEN AFFINITY OF HEMOGLOBIN, *METABOLISM*, 26, 141-50 (1977)

0569 DITZEL J ET AL, AN ADVERSE EFFECT OF INSULIN ON THE OXYGEN-RELEASE CAPACITY OF RED BLOOD CELLS IN NONACIDOTIC DIABETICS, *METABOLISM*, 27, 927-34 (1978)

0570 DIVERTIE MB, THE ADULT RESPIRATORY DISTRESS SYNDROME, *MAYO CLIN PROC*, 57, 371-8 (1982)

0571 DOAN C A ET AL, IDIOPATHIC AND SECONDARY THROMBOCYTOPENIC PURPURA, *ANN INTERN MED*, 53, 861 (1960)

0572 DOBOSZ, THE INFLUENCE OF THE DILUTION EFFECT ON SERUM CREATINE PHOSPHOKINASE ACTIVITY IN NEUROMUSCULAR DISEASES, *CLIN CHIM ACTA*, 50, 301-304 (1974)

0573 DOCHERTY I, HARROP JS, HINE KR, HOPTON MR, ET AL, MYOGLOBIN CONCENTRATION, CREATINE KINASE ACTIVITY, AND CREATINE KINASE B SUBUNIT CONCENTRATIONS IN SERUM DURING THYROID DISEASE, *CLIN CHEM*, 30/1, 42-45 (1984)

0574 DODD R, WINKLER CF, WILLIAMS ME, BUNN PA, ET AL, CALCITRIOL LEVELS IN HYPERCALCEMIC PATIENTS WITH ADULT T-CELL LYMPHOMA, *ARCH INTERN MED*, 146, 1971 (1986)

0575 DOHAN P H ET AL, EVALUATION OF URINARY CYCLIC 3'5'-ADENOSINE MONOPHOSPHATE EXCRETION IN THE DIFFERENTIAL DIAGNOSIS OF HYPERCALCEMIA, *J CLIN ENDOCRINOL METAB*, 35, 775 (1972)

0576 DOKUMOV S I, SERUM COPPER AND PREGNANCY, *AM J OBSTET GYNECOL*, 101, 217 (1968)

0577 DOLIN R ET AL, LYMPHOCYTE POPULATIONS IN ACUTE VIRAL GASTROENTERITIS, *INFECT IMMUN*, 14, 422-8 (1976)

0578 DOMINICK J C ET AL, ISOENZYMES OF ALKALINE PHOSPHATASE IN THE SERUM OF PATIENTS WITH CYSTIC FIBROSIS, *Z KINDERHEILK*, 119, 261-267 (1975)

0579 DONALDSON E M ET AL, ERYTHROPOIETIC PROTOPORPHYRIA: A FAMILY STUDY, *BR MED J*, 1, 659 (1967)

0580 DONALDSON ES, VAN NAGELL JR JR, PURSELL S, ET AL, MULTIPLE BIOCHEMICAL MARKERS IN PATIENTS WITH GYNECOLOGIC MALIGNANCIES, *CANCER*, 45, 948-53 (1980)

0581 DONALDSON L A ET AL, AMYLASE THERMOLABILITY AS A SCREENING TEST FOR PANCREATIC PSEUDOCYSTS, *BR J SURG*, 65, 413-5. (1978)

0582 DONATI R M ET AL, ERYTHROPOIESIS IN HYPOTHYROIDISM, *PROC SOC EXP BIOL MED*, 144, 78 (1973)

0583 DONIACH D ET AL, AUTOIMMUNE PHENOMENA IN PERNICIOUS ANEMIA, *BR MED J*, 1, 1374 (1963)

0584 DONIACH D ET AL, TISSUE ANTIBODIES IN PRIMARY BILIARY CIRRHOSIS, ACTIVE CHRONIC (LUPOID) HEPATITIS, CRYPTOGENIC CIRRHOSIS AND OTHER LIVER DISEASES AND THEIR CLINICAL IMPLICATIONS, *CLIN EXP IMMUNOL*, 1, 237 (1966)

0585 DONOHUGH D L, TROPICAL EOSINOPHILIA: AN ETIOLOGIC INQUIRY, *N ENGL J MED*, 269, 1357 (1963)

0586 DONOWITZ M, KERSTEIN MD, SPLIRO HM, PANCREATIC ASCITES, *MEDICINE*, 53, 183-195 (1974)

0587 DOOS W G ET AL, CEA LEVELS IN PATIENTS WITH COLORECTAL POLYPS, *CANCER*, 36, 1996-2003 (1975)

0588 DORAISWAMY N V, THE NEUTROPHIL COUNT IN CHILDHOOD ACUTE APPENDICITIS, *BR J SURG*, 64, 342-4 (1977)

0589 DORAN G R ET AL, SERUM CREATINE KINASE AND ADENYLATE KINASE IN THYROID DISEASE, *CLIN CHIM ACTA*, 35, 115 (1971)

0590 DORMER A, BACTERIAL ENDOCARDITIS: SURVEY OF PATIENTS TREATED BETWEEN 1945 AND 1956, *BR MED J*, 1, 63 (1958)

0591 DORWART BB, SCHUMACHER HR, JOINT EFFUSIONS, CHONDROCALCINOSIS AND OTHER RHEUMATIC MANIFESTATIONS IN HYPOTHYROIDISM. A CLINICOPATHOLOGIC STUDY., *AM J MED*, 59, 780-790 (1975)

0592 DOUGLAS D M CLAIREAUX A E, HODGKIN'S DISEASE IN CHILDHOOD, *ARCH DIS CHILD*, 28, 222 (1953)

0593 DOUTRE MS, BEYLOT C, BEZIAN JH, STUDIES ON T CELL SUBSETS IN CHRONIC URTICARIA BY MONOCLONAL ANTIBODIES, *IMMUNOL LETT*, 10, 49-51 (1985)

0594 DOWDING C, TH'NG KH, GOLDMAN JM, GALTON AG, INCREASED T-LYMPHOCYTE NUMBERS IN CHRONIC GRANULOCYTIC LEUKEMIA BEFORE TREATMENT, *EXP HEMATOL*, 12, 811-815 (1984)

0595 DOWLING P ET AL, CYTOMEGALOVIRUS COMPLEMENT FIXATION ANTIBODY IN GUILLAIN-BARRÉ SYNDROME, *NEUROL*, 27, 1153-6 (1977)

0596 DOYLE A E ET AL, URINARY SODIUM, POTASSIUM AND CREATININE EXCRETION IN HYPERTENSIVE AND NORMOTENSIVE AUSTRALIANS, *MED J AUST*, 2, 898-900 (1976)

0597 DRAKE T G ET AL, CHRONIC IDIOPATHIC HYPOPARATHYROIDISM; REPORT OF 6 CASES AND AUTOPSY FINDINGS IN ONE, *ANN INTERN MED*, 12, 1751 (1939)

0598 DREHER W H ET AL, HYPERCHLOREMIA ASSOCIATED WITH MEMBRANOPROLIFERATIVE GLOMERULONEPHRITIS, *NEPHRON*, 18, 321-25 (1977)

0599 DREYFUSS F, THE ROLE OF HYPERURICEMIA IN CORONARY HEART DISEASE., *DIS CHEST*, 38, 332-334 (1960)

0600 DRUMMEY G O ET AL, MICROSCOPICAL EXAMINATION OF THE STOOL FOR STEATORRHEA, *N ENGL J MED*, 264, 85-7 (1961)

0601 DUBIN A ET AL, HYPERURICEMIA IN HYPOPARATHYROIDISM, *METALS*, 5, 703-709 (1956)

0602 DUBIN I N, CHRONIC IDIOPATHIC JAUNDICE, *AM J MED*, 24, 268 (1958)

0603 DUBO H ET AL, SERUM CREATINE KINASE IN CASES OF STROKE, HEAD INJURY, AND MENINGITIS, *J CLIN ENDOCR*, 2, 743-748 (1967)

0604 DUMOULIN G, WOLF JP, HATON D, RELATIONS BETWEEN ORAL GLUCOSE LOAD AND URINARY ELIMINATION OF CALCIUM AND PHOSPHORUS IN HEALTHY MEN WITH NORMAL BODY WEIGHT, *NEPHROLOGIE*, 5, 205-7 (1984)

0605 DUSSAULT JH, MORISSETTE J, LABERGE C, BLOOD THYROXINE CONCENTRATIONS IN LOWER BIRTH-WEIGHT INFANTS, *CLIN CHEM*, 25, 2047-2049 (1979)

0606 DUTTA J K ET AL, SERUM MAGNESIUM STUDY IN CHOLERA AND NON-CHOLERIC GASTROENTERITIS, *TRANS R SOC TROP MED HYG*, 71, 263-4 (1977)

0607 DUTTA T K, CLINICAL EVALUATION OF SERUM PROTEIN-BOUND FUCOSE AS A DIAGNOSTIC AND PROGNOSTIC INDEX IN MALIGNANT TUMORS, *INDIAN J CANCER*, 13, 262-66 (1976)

0608 DUX S, ARON N, BONER G, CARMEL A, ET AL, SERUM ANGIOTENSIN CONVERTING ENZYME ACTIVITY IN NORMAL ADULTS AND PATIENTS WITH DIFFERENT TYPES OF HYPERTENSION, *ISR J MED SCI*, 20, 1138-42 (1984)

0609 DUX S, YARON A, CARMEL A, ROSENFELD JB, RENIN, ALDOSTERONE, AND SERUM-CONVERTING ENZYME ACTIVITY DURING NORMAL AND HYPERTENSIVE PREGNANCY, *GYNECOL OBSTET INVEST*, 17, 252-7 (1984)

0610 DZIALOSZYNSKI L M ET AL, SOME CLINICAL ASPECTS OF ARYL-SULFATASE ACTIVITY, *CLIN CHIM ACTA*, 15, 381-6 (1967)

0611 EALES L AND SAUNDERS S J, THE DIAGNOSTIC IMPORTANCE OF FAECAL PORPHYRINS IN THE DIFFERENTIATION OF THE PORPHYRIAS, *SOUTH AFR J LAB CLIN MED*, 40, 63 (1966)

0612 EALES L ET AL, SODIUM AND POTASSIUM BALANCE IN RELATION TO PERIODIC PARALYSIS AND IN A CASE OF PYELONEPHRITIS WITH MALIGNANT HYPERTENSION, *S AFR MED J*, 32, 251 (1958)

0613 EALES L ET AL, THE CLINICAL BIOCHEMISTRY OF THE HUMAN HEPATOCUTANEOUS PORPHYRIAS IN THE LIGHT OF RECENT STUDIES OF NEWLY IDENTIFIED INTERMEDIATES AND PORPHYRIN DERIVATIVES, *ANN NY ACAD SCI*, 244, 441 (1975)

0614 EARLEY L E AND GOLLSCHALK (EDS), DISEASES OF THE KIDNEY, *3RD EDITION LITTLE BROWN & CO BOSTON* (1974)

0615 EASTHAM AND YEOMAN, HYPOGAMMAGLOBULINAEMIA IN MYELOMA, *ACTA MED SCAND*, 166, 241-7 (1960)

0616 EASTHAM E J ET AL, SERUM FERRITIN LEVELS IN ACUTE HEPATOCELLULAR DAMAGE FROM PARACETAMOL OVERDOSAGE, *BR MED J*, 1, 750-1 (1976)

0617 EASTHAM ET AL, SERUM CHOLESTEROL IN MENTAL RETARDATION, *BR J PSYCHIATR*, 115, 1013-1017 (1969)

0618 EASTHAM R D, BIOCHEMICAL VALUES IN CLINICAL MEDICINE, *4TH EDITION WILLIAMS & WILKINS BALTIMORE MD* (1971)

0619 EASTHAM R D, BIOCHEMICAL VALUES IN CLINICAL MEDICINE, *5TH EDITION WILLIAM AND WILKINS* (1975)

0620 EASTHAM RD, BIOCHEMICAL VALUES IN CLINICAL MEDICINE, *DISTRIBUTED BY YEAR BOOK MEDICAL PUBLISHERS, INC., CHICAGO*, 6TH ED. (1978)

0621 EASTMAN AND HELLMAN, OBSTETRICS, *13TH EDITION (WILLIAMS) APPLETON-CENTURY-CROFTS NEW YORK*, 0 (1966)

0622 EBOROWICZ D ET AL, THE CORRELATION OF ROUTINE CYTOLOGY WITH THE CONTENTS OF CARCINOEMBRYONIC ANTIGEN AND ALPHA-FETOPROTEIN IN PLEURAL AND PERITONEAL EFFUSIONS, *ARCH GESCHWULSTFORSCH*, 47, 231-5 (1977)

0623 ECKFELDT JH, LEATHERMAN JW, LEVITT MD, HIGH PREVALENCE OF HYPERAMYLASEMIA IN PATIENTS WITH ACIDEMIA, *ANN INTERN MED*, 104, 362 (1986)

0624 ECONOMIDOW J ET AL, CARCINOEMBRYONIC ANTIGEN IN THYROID DISEASE, *J CLIN PATHOL*, 30, 878-80 (1977)

0625 EDITORIAL, SERUM ENZYMES IN MYOCARDIAL INFARCTION, *BR MED J*, 2, 1669-1670 (1962)

0626 EDMONDSON J W ET AL, THE RELATIONSHIP OF SERUM IONIZED AND TOTAL CALCIUM IN PRIMARY HYPERPARATHYROIDISM, *J LAB CLIN MED*, 87, 624-29 (1976)

0627 EDWARDS R ET AL, ACUTE HYPOCAPNEIC HYPOKALEMIA: AN IATROGENIC ANESTHETIC COMPLICATION, *ANESTH ANALG (CLEVE)*, 56, 786-92 (1977)

0628 EERDEKENS MW, NOUWEN EJ, POLLET DE, ET AL, PLACENTAL ALKALINE PHOSPHATASE AND CANCER ANTIGEN 125 IN SERA OF PATIENTS WITH BENIGN AND MALIGNANT DISEASES, *CLIN CHEM*, 31/5, 687-690 (1985)

0629 EFRAN M L ET AL, HYDROXYPROLINEMIA II. A RARE METABOLIC DISEASE DUE TO A DEFICIENCY OF HYDROXYPROLINE OXIDASE, *N ENGL J MED*, 272, 1299 (1965)

0630 EFREMOV GD, HUISMAN THJ, THE LABORATORY DIAGNOSIS OF THE HAEMOGLOBINOPATHIES, *CLINICS IN HAEMATOLOGY*, 3, 527-570 (1974)

0631 EFRON M L, AMINOACIDURIA, *N ENGL J MED*, 272, 1058 (1965)

0632 EGBERG N ET AL, FASTING (ACUTE ENERGY DEPRIVATION) IN MAN: EFFECT ON BLOOD COAGULATION AND FIBRINOLYSIS, *AM J CLIN NUTR*, 30, 1963-7 (1977)

0633 EGEBERG O, BLOOD COAGULATION IN RENAL FAILURE, *SCAND J CLIN LAB INVEST*, 14, 163 (1962)

0634 EGEBERG O, THE EFFECT OF UNSPECIFIC FEVER INDUCTION ON THE BLOOD CLOTTING SYSTEM, *SCAND J CLIN LAB INVEST*, 14, 471 (1962)

0635 EGEBERG O, THE BLOOD COAGULABILITY IN DIABETIC PATIENTS, *SCAND J CLIN LAB INVEST*, 15, 533 (1963)

0636 EGEBERG O, INFLUENCE OF THYROID FUNCTION IN THE BLOOD CLOTTING ACTIVITY, *SCAND J CLIN LAB INVEST*, 15, 1 (1963)

0637 EGHTEDARI A A ET AL, CIRCULATING IMMUNOBLASTS IN POLYMYALGIA RHEUMATICA, *ANN RHEUM DIS*, 35, 158-62 (1976)

0638 EINARSSON K, ANGELIN B, BJORKEM I, GLAUMANN H, THE DIAGNOSTIC VALUE OF FASTING INDIVIDUAL SERUM BILE ACIDS IN ANICTERIC ALCOHOLIC LIVER DISEASE: RELATION TO LIVER MORPHOLOGY, *HEPATOLOGY*, 5, 108-11 (1985)

0639 EISEN ET AL, SERUM CREATINE PHOSPHOKINASE ACTIVITY IN CEREBRAL INFARCTION, *NEUROL*, 18, 263-268 (1968)

0640 EISENBERG S, BLOOD VOLUME IN PATIENTS WITH ACUTE GLOMERULONEPHRITIS, *AM J MED*, 27, 241 (1959)

0641 EISNER E ET AL, COOMB'S-POSITIVE HEMOLYTIC ANEMIA IN HODGKIN'S DISEASE, *ANN INTERN MED*, 66, 258 (1967)

0642 EKBERG M R ET AL, SIGNIFICANCE OF INCREASED FACTOR VIII IN EARLY GLOMERULONEPHRITIS, *ANN INTERN MED*, 83, 337-341 (1975)

0643 EKLUND S G ET AL, ANEMIA IN UREMIA, *ACTA MED SCAND*, 190, 435 (1971)

0644 EKSTROM T ET AL, MEDULLARY SPONGE KIDNEY, *PROC THIRD INT CONR NEPHROL*, 2, 54 (1966)

0645 EL-HADDAD S ET AL, VALUE OF SERUM COPPER MEASUREMENT IN ACUTE LEUKAEMIA OF CHILDHOOD, *GAZ EGYPT PAEDIATR ASSOC*, 26, 67-72 (1977)

0646 EL-SADR W, ET AL, ACQUIRED IMMUNE DEFICIENCY SYNDROME, *DIAGN CLIN IMMUNOL*, 2, 73-85 (1984)

0647 EL-YAZIGI A, AL-SALEH I, AL-MEFTY O, CONCENTRATIONS OF AG, AL, AU, BI, CD, PB, SB, AND SE IN CEREBROSPINAL FLUID OF PATIENTS WITH CEREBRAL NEOPLASMS, *CLIN CHEM*, 30/8, 1358-1360 (1984)

0648 EL-YAZIGI A, AL-SALEH I, AL-MEFTY O, CONCENTRATIONS OF ZINC, IRON, MOLYBDENUM, ARSENIC, AND LITHIUM IN CEREBROSPINAL FLUID OF PATIENTS WITH BRAIN TUMORS, *CLIN CHEM*, 32/12, 2187-2190 (1986)

0649 ELIAS AN, VAZIRI ND, MAKSY M, PLASMA NOREPINEPHRINE, EPINEPHRINE, AND DOPAMINE LEVELS IN END-STAGE RENAL DISEASE, *ARCH INTERN MED*, 145, 1013 (1985)

0650 ELIN R J ET AL, LACK OF SPECIFICITY OF THE LIMULUS LYSATE TEST IN THE DIAGNOSIS OF PYOGENIC ARTHRITIS, *J INFECT DIS*, 137, 507-13 (1978)

0651 ELKING M P ET AL, DRUG INDUCED MODIFICATIONS OF LABORATORY TEST VALUES, *AMER J HOSP PHARM*, 25, 485 (1968)

0652 ELLIOT B A AND FLEMING A F, SOURCE OF ELEVATED SERUM ENZYME ACTIVITIES IN PATIENTS WITH MEGALOBLASTIC ERYTHROPOIESIS SECONDARY TO FOLIC ACID DEFICIENCY, *BR MED J*, 1, 626 (1965)

0653 ELLIOTT D W ET AL, A REEVALUATION OF SERUM AMYLASE DETERMINATIONS, *ARCH SURG*, 83, 130 (1961)

0654 ELLIOTT ET AL, THE RELATIVE EFFICIENCIES OF SOME SERUM-ENZYME TESTS IN THE DIAGNOSIS OF MYOCARDIAL INFARCTION, *J CLIN ENDOCR*, 1, 71-72 (1967)

0655 ELLIS G, GOLDBERG DM, A REDUCED NICTOTINAMIDE ADENINE DINUCLEOTIDE LINKED KINETIC ASSAY FOR ADENOSINE DREAMINASE ACTIVITY, *J LAB CLIN MED*, 76, 507-517 (1970)

0656 ELLIS L D ET AL, MARROW IRON: AN EVALUATION OF DEPLETED STORES IN A SERIES OF 1,322 NEEDLE BIOPSIES, *ANN INTERN MED*, 61, 44 (1964)

0657 ELLIS L D ET AL, THE EFFECT OF IRON STORES ON FERROKINETICS IN POLYCYTHEMIA, *BR J HAEMATOL*, 13, 892 (1967)

0658 ELLIS NI, LLOYD B, LLOYD RS, CLAYTON BE, SELENIUM AND VITAMIN E IN RELATION TO RISK FACTORS FOR CORONARY HEART DISEASE, *J CLIN PATHOL*, 37, 200-6 (1984)

0659 ELLMAN GL, COURTNEY KD, ANDRES V JR, ET AL, A NEW AND RAPID COLORIMETRIC DETERMINATION OF ACETYLCHOLINESTERASE ACTIVITY, *BIOCHEM PHARMACOL*, 7, 88-95 (1961)

0660 EMERSON P M AND WILKINSON J H, LACTATE DEHYDROGENASE IN THE DIAGNOSIS AND ASSESSMENT OF RESPONSE TO TREATMENT OF MEGALOBLASTIC ANEMIA, *BR J HAEMATOL*, 12, 678 (1966)

0661 EMMONS J ET AL, AN AID TO THE RAPID DIAGNOSIS OF MYCOPLASMA PNEUMONIAE INFECTIONS, *J INFECT DIS*, 179, 650 (1969)

0662 ENDE N, STUDIES OF AMYLASE IN PLEURAL EFFUSIONS AND ASCITES, *CANCER*, 13, 283-87 (1960)

0663 ENGFELDT B AND ZELLERSTROM R, OSTEODYSMETAMORPHOSIS FETALIS, *J PEDIATR*, 45, 125 (1954)

0664 ENGLE M A ET AL, POSTPERICARDIOTOMY SYNDROME. A NEW LOOK AT AN OLD CONDITION, *MOD CONCEPTS CARDIOVASC DIS*, 44, 59 (1975)

0665 ENGLE W K ET AL, METABOLIC STUDIES AND THERAPEUTIC TRIALS IN ALS, IN: MOTOR NEURON DISEASES, *NORRIS & KURLAND (EDS) NY GRUNE & STRATTON* (1969)

0666 ENGLEMAN E G AND E P ENGLEMAN, ANKYLOSING SPONDYLITIS: RECENT ADVANCES IN DIAGNOSIS AND TREATMENT, *MED CLIN NORTH AM*, 61, 347-67 (1977)

0667 ENGLERT E ET AL, METABOLISM OF FREE AND CONJUGATED 17-HYDROXY-CORTICOSTEROIDS IN SUBJECTS WITH UREMIA, *J CLIN ENDOCRINOL METAB*, 18, 36 (1958)

0668 ENSIGN D C, SERUM PHOSPHATASE IN OSTEOPETROSIS, *J LAB CLIN MED*, 32, 1541-1542 (1947)

0669 ENTRICAN J H, RAISED PLASMA ESTRADIOL AND ESTRONE LEVELS IN YOUNG SURVIVORS OF MYOCARDIAL INFARCTION, *LANCET*, 2, 487-9 (1978)

0670 EPSTEIN J H AND REDEKER A G, PORPHYRIA CUTANEA TARDA - A STUDY OF THE EFFECT OF PHLEBOTOMY, *N ENGL J MED*, 279, 1301 (1968)

0671 EPSTEIN S, TRABERG H, RAJA R, POSER J, SERUM AND DIALYSATE OSTEOCALCIN LEVELS IN HEMODIALYSIS AND PERITONEAL DIALYSIS PATIENTS AND AFTER RENAL TRANSPLANTATION, *J CLIN ENDOCRINOL METAB*, 60, 1253-6 (1985)

0672 ERSKINE KJ, TAYLOR KJ, AGNEW RA, SERIAL ESTIMATION OF SERUM ANGIOTENSIN CONVERTING ENZYME ACTIVITY DURING AND AFTER PREGNANCY IN A WOMAN WITH SARCOIDOSIS, *BR MED J*, 290, 269-70 (1985)

0673 ERSLER A J ET AL, PLASMA ERYTHROPOIETIN IN POLYCYTHEMIA, *AM J MED*, 66, 243-247 (1978)

0674 ERSLEV A J ATWATER J, EFFECT OF MEAN CORPUSCULAR HEMOGLOBIN CONCENTRATION ON VISCOSITY, *J LAB CLIN MED*, 62, 401 (1963)

0675 ERVEN L M ET AL, PATTERNS OF ENZYME ACTIVITY FOLLOWING MYOCARDIAL INFARCTION AND ISCHAEMIA, *AM J CLIN PATHOL*, 56, 614-22 (1971)

0676 ESPINOZA L R ET AL, JOINT MANIFESTATIONS OF SICKLE CELL DISEASE, *MEDICINE*, 53, 295-306 (1974)

0677 ESTES D ET AL, THE NATURAL HISTORY OF SYSTEMIC LUPUS ERYTHEMATOSUS BY PROSPECTIVE ANALYSIS, *MEDICINE*, 39, 85 (1960)

0678 ETZIONI A, BENDERLY A, LEVY J, GRIEF Z, ET AL, TRANSIENT IMMUNOREGULATORY PERTURBATION DURING THE ACUTE PHASE OF RHEUMATIC FEVER, *J CLIN LAB IMMUNOL*, 20, 7-9 (1986)

0679 EVANS A S ET AL, SPECIFICITY, SENSITIVITY, AND PERSISTENCE OF HETEROPHIL AND EB-VIRUS SPECIFIC IGM ANTIBODIES IN CLINICAL AND SUBCLINICAL INFECTIOUS MONONUCLEOSIS, *J INFECT DIS*, 132, 546 (1975)

0680 EVANS R S AND DUANE R T, ACQUIRED HEMOLYTIC ANEMIA. I. THE RELATION OF ERYTHROCYTE ANTIBODY PRODUCTION TO ACTIVITY OF THE DISEASE II. THE SIGNIFICANCE OF THROMBOCYTOPENIA AND LEUKOPENIA, *BLOOD*, 4, 1196 (1949)

0681 EVANS R S ET AL, PRIMARY THROMBOCYTOPENIC PURPURA AND ACQUIRED HEMOLYTIC ANEMIA: EVIDENCE FOR A COMMON ETIOLOGY, *ARCH INTERN MED*, 87, 48 (1951)

0682 EVANS R S ET AL, PRIMARY THROMBOCYTOPENIA PURPURA AND ACQUIRED HEMOLYTIC ANEMIA, *ARCH INTERN MED*, 122, 353 (1968)

0683 EVANS RT, WROE J, IS SERUM CHOLINESTERASE ACTIVITY A PREDICTOR OF SUCCINYL CHOLINE SENSITIVITY? AN ASSESSMENT OF FOUR METHODS, *CLIN CHEM*, 24, 1762-1766 (1978)

0684 EWEN AND GRIFFITHS, GAMMA-GLUTAMYL TRANSPEPTIDASE: ELEVATED ACTIVITIES IN CERTAIN NEUROLOGIC DISEASES, *AM J CLIN PATHOL*, 59, 2-9 (1973)

0685 EZDINLI E Z AND STUTZMAN L, CHLORAMBUCIL THERAPY FOR LYMPHOMAS, *JAMA*, 191, 444 (1965)

0686 FABIAN E ET AL, PLASMA LEVELS OF FREE FATTY ACIDS, LIPOPROTEIN LIPASE AND POST HEPARIN ESTERASE IN PREGNANCY, *AM J OBSTET GYNECOL*, 100, 904 (1968)

0687 FACCHINETTI F, COMITINI G, GENAZZANI A, ET AL, SEMINAL FLUID ANDROGEN LEVELS IN INFERTILE PATIENTS, *INT J FERTIL*, 32, 157-61 (1987)

0688 FADEL H E ET AL, HYPERURICEMIA IN PRE-ECLAMPSIA. A REAPPRAISAL, *AM J OBSTET GYNECOL*, 125, 640-7 (1976)

0689 FAHEY J L AND BOGGS D R, SERUM PROTEIN CHANGES IN MALIGNANT DISEASE, THE ACUTE LEUKEMIAS, *BLOOD*, 16, 1479 (1960)

0690 FAIMAN C ET AL, SERUM FSH AND HCG DURING HUMAN PREGNANCY AND PUERPERIUM, *J CLIN ENDOCRINOL METAB*, 28, 1323 (1968)

0691 FAIRBANKS VF, HEMOCHROMATOSIS: THE NEGLECTED DISEASE, *MAYO CLIN PROC*, 61, 296-198 (1986)

0692 FAIRLEY AND SCOTT, HYPOGAMMAGLOBULINAEMIA IN CHRONIC LYMPHATIC LEUKEMIA, *BR MED J*, 5257, 920-4 (1961)

0693 FALCHUK K R ET AL, SERUM LYSOZYME ON CROHN'S DISEASE. A USEFUL INDEX OF DISEASE ACTIVITY, *GASTROENTEROLOGY*, 69, 893 (1975)

0694 FALCHUK K R ET AL, SERUM LYSOZYME IN CROHN'S DISEASE AND ULCERATIVE COLITIS, *N ENGL J MED*, 292, 393 (1975)

0695 FANCONI G, DIE FAMILIARE PANMYELOPATHIE, *SEMIN HEMATOL*, 4, 233 (1967)

0696 FARAJ, BA CAMP VM, MURRAY DR, ET AL, PLASMA L-DOPA IN THE DIAGNOSIS OF MALIGNANT MELANOMA, *CLIN CHEM*, 32/1, 159-161 (1986)

0697 FARBER HW, MATHERS JA JR, GLAUSER FL, GALLIUM SCANS AND SERUM ANGIOTENSIN CONVERTING ENZYME LEVELS IN TALC GRANULOMATOSIS AND LYMPHOCYTIC INTERSTITIAL PNEUMONITIS, *SOUTH MED J*, 73, 1663-7 (1980)

0698 FARBER M O ET AL, STUDIES OF PLASMA VASOPRESSIN AND RENIN-ANGIOTENSIN-ALDOSTERONE SYSTEM IN CHRONIC OBSTRUCTIVE LUNG DISEASE, *J LAB CLIN MED*, 90, 373-380 (1977)

0699 FARCI P, GERIN JL, ARAGONA M, LINDSEY I, ET AL, DIAGNOSTIC AND PROGNOSTIC SIGNIFICANCE OF THE IGM ANTIBODY TO THE HEPATITIS DELTA VIRUS, *JAMA*, 255, 1443 (1986)

0700 FARGION S, KLASEN EC, LALATTA F, ET AL, ALPHA 1-ANTITRYPSIN IN PATIENTS WITH HEPATOCELLULAR CARCINOMA AND CHRONIC ACTIVE HEPATITIS, *CLIN GENET*, 19, 134-9 (1981)

0701 FARR M ET AL, LYSOZYMURIAN DIABETES, *BR MED J*, 1, 624-25 (1976)

0702 FARRELL P AND AVERY M E, HYALINE MEMBRANE DISEASE, *AM REV RESPIR DIS*, 111, 657 (1975)

0703 FARROW L J ET AL, AUTOANTIBODIES AND THE HEPATITIS-ASSOCIATED ANTIGEN IN ACUTE INFECTIVE HEPATITIS, *BR MED J*, 2, 693 (1970)

0704 FARTHING MJ, GREEN JR, EDWARDS CR, DAWSON AM, PROGESTERONE, PROLACTIN, AND GYNAECOMASTIA IN MEN WITH LIVER DISEASE, *GUT*, 23, 276-9 (1982)

0705 FAURE G, BENE MC, TAMISIER JN, GAUCHER A, ET AL, THYMULIN (FTS-ZN) INDUCED IN VITRO MODULATION OF T CELL SUBSETS MARKERS ON LYMPHOCYTES FROM RHEUMATOID ARTHRITIS AND SYSTEMIC LUPUS ERYTHEMATOSUS PATIENTS, *INT J IMMUNOPHARMACOL*, 6, 381-8 (1984)

0706 FAWCETT J R ET AL, VARIATION OF PLASMA ELECTROLYTE AND TOTAL PROTEIN LEVELS IN THE INDIVIDUAL, *BR MED J*, 2, 582 (1956)

0707 FEAGLER JR, SORENSON GD, ROSENFELD MG, ET AL, RHEUMATOID PLEURAL EFFUSION, *ARCH PATHOL LAB MED*, 92, 257-266 (1971)

0708 FEEMSTER R F, OUTBREAK OF ENCEPHALOMYELITIS IN MAN DUE TO EASTERN VIRUS OF EQUINE ENCEPHALOMYELITIS, *AM J PUBLIC HEALTH*, 28, 1403 (193)

0709 FEGER J, MEASUREMENT OF SERUM ALPHA 1-ACID GLYCOPROTEIN AND ALPHA 1-ANTITRYPSIN DESIALYLATILON IN LIVER DISEASE, *HEPATOLOGY*, 3, 356-9 (1983)

0710 FEHER J ET AL, SERUM LIPIDS AND LIPOPROTEINS IN CHRONIC LIVER DISEASE, *ACTA MED ACAD SCI HUNG*, 33, 217-23. (1976)

0711 FEIG S A ET AL, INCREASED ERYTHROCYTE CALCIUM CONTENT IN HEREDITARY SPHEROCYTOSIS, *PEDIATR RES*, 9, 928 (1975)

0712 FEIGIN R D ET AL, INAPPROPRIATE SECRETION OF ANTIDIURETIC HORMONE IN CHILDREN WITH BACTERIAL MENINGITIS., *AM J CLIN NUTR*, 30, 1482-84 (1977)

0713 FEINGLASS E J ET AL, NEUROPSYCHIATRIC MANIFESTATIONS OF SYSTEMIC LUPUS ERYTHEMATOSUS: DIAGNOSIS, CLINICAL SPECTRUM AND RELATIONSHIP TO OTHER FEATURES OF THE DISEASE, *MEDICINE*, 55, 323-339 (1976)

0714 FEINSTEIN D I AND RAPAPORT S I, ACQUIRED INHIBITORS OF BLOOD COAGULATION, *PROG HAEMOSTASIS THROMB*, 1, 75 (1972)

0715 FEIZI T, MONOTYPIC COLD AGGLUTININS IN INFECTION BY NATURE, *NATURE*, 215, 540 (1967)

0716 FEIZI T, IMMUNOGLOBULINS IN CHRONIC LIVER DISEASE, *GUT*, 9, 193 (1968)

0717 FELDMAN E B AND WALLACE S L, HYPERTRIGLYCERIDEMIA IN GOUT, *CIRCULATION*, 29, 508 (1964)

0718 FELDMAN J M, PLASMA AMINO ACIDS IN PATIENTS WITH THE CARCINOID SYNDROME, *CANCER*, 38, 2127-2131 (1976)

0719 FELDMAN JM, URINARY SEROTONIN IN THE DIAGNOSIS OF CARCINOID TUMORS, *CLIN CHEM*, 32 NO 5, 840-844 (1986)

0720 FELDMAN W E ET AL, CEREBROSPINAL FLUID LACTIC ACID DEHYDROGENASE ACTIVITY, *AM J DIS CHILD*, 129, 77-80 (1975)

0721 FELIG P ET AL, PLASMA GLUCAGON LEVELS IN EXERCISING MAN, *N ENGL J MED*, 287, 184 (1972)

0722 FELSHER B F ET AL, INDIRECT REACTING BILIRUBINEMIA IN CIRRHOSIS: ITS RELATION TO RED CELL SURVIVAL, *AM J DIG DIS*, 13, 598 (1968)

0723 FENTON JJ, JONES M, HARTFORD CE, CALCIUM FRACTIONS IN SERUM OF PATIENTS WITH THERMAL BURNS, *J TRAUMA*, 23, 863-6 (1983)

0724 FENUKU R I ET AL, SERUM ALBUMIN AND TOTAL GLOBULIN LEVELS IN COMMON LIVER DISEASES IN ACCRA (GHANA), *TROP GEOGR MED*, 30, 87-90 (1978)

0725 FERRISS J B ET AL, LOW-RENIN (PRIMARY) HYPERALDOSTERONISM. DIFFERENTIAL DIAGNOSIS AND DISTINCTION OF SUB-GROUPS WITHIN THE SYNDROME, *AM HEART J*, 95, 641-58 (1978)

0726 FERZI T ET AL, THE ROLE OF MYCOPLASMA IN HUMAN DISEASE, *PROC R SOC*, 59, 1109 (1966)

0727 FESSAS P, LOUKOPOULOS D, THE B-THALASSAEMIAS, *CLINICS IN HAEMATOLOGY*, 3, 411-435 (1974)

0728 FESSEL W J, ANA-NEGATIVE SYSTEMIC LUPUS ERYTHEMATOSUS, *AM J MED*, 64, 80-6 (1978)

0729 FIALA M ET AL, PATHOGENESIS OF ANEMIA ASSOCIATED WITH MYCOPLASMA PNEUMONIAE, *ACTA HAEMATOL (BASEL)*, 51, 297 (1974)

0730 FIELD J B AND WILLIAMS H E, ARTIFACTUAL HYPOGLYCEMIA ASSOCIATED WITH LEUKEMIA, *N ENGL J MED*, 265, 946 (1961)

0731 FILLMORE S J ET AL, BLOOD-GAS CHANGES AND PULMONARY HEMODYNAMICS FOLLOWING ACUTE MYOCARDIAL INFARCTION, *CIRCULATION*, 45, 583 (1972)

0732 FINCH C A ET AL, FERROKINETICS IN MAN, *MEDICINE*, 49, 17 (1970)

0733 FINUCANE J F ET AL, EFFECTS OF CHRONIC RENAL DISEASE ON THYROID HORMONE METABOLISM, *ACTA ENDOCRINOL*, 84, 750-8 (1977)

0734 FISELIER TJ, LIJNEN P, MONNENS L, ET AL, LEVELS OF RENIN, ANGIOTENSIN I AND II, ANGIOTENSIN-CONVERTING ENZYME AND ALDOSTERONE IN INFANCY AND CHILDHOOD, *EUR J PEDIATR*, 141, 3-7 (1983)

0735 FISHER G L ET AL, COPPER AND ZINC LEVELS IN SERUM FROM HUMAN PATIENTS WITH SARCOMAS, *CANCER*, 37, 356-63 (1976)

0736 FISHER J W ET AL, STUDIES ON THE MECHANISM OF THE ANEMIA OF RENAL INSUFFICIENCY, *REV INTERAM RADIOL*, 6, 42-9. 19-22 (1976)

0737 FISHERMAN E W ET AL, SERUM TRIGLYCERIDE AND CHOLESTEROL LEVELS AND LIPID ELECTROPHORETIC PATTERNS IN INTRINSIC AND EXTRINSIC ALLERGIC STATES, *ANN ALLERGY*, 38, 46-53 (1977)

0738 FISHMAN A ET AL, SERUM 'PROSTATIC' ACID PHOSPHATASE AND CANCER OF THE PROSTATE, *N ENGL J MED*, 255, 925-933 (1956)

0739 FISHMAN J ET AL, ESTROGEN METABOLISM IN NORMAL AND PREGNANT WOMEN, *J BIOL CHEM*, 237, 1489 (1962)

0740 FISHMAN W H ET AL, MARKERS FOR OVARIAN CANCER: REGAN ISOENZYME AND OTHER GLYCOPROTEINS, *SEMIN ONCOL*, 3, 211-216 (1975)

0741 FISHMAN WH, KATO K, ANTISS CL, GREEN S, HUMAN SERUM B-GLUCURONIDASE: ITS MEASUREMENT AND SOME OF ITS PROPERTIES, *CLIN CHIM ACTA*, 15, 435-447 (1967)

0742 FISMAN M, GORDON B, FELEKI V, HELMES E, ET AL, HYPERAMMONEMIA IN ALZHEIMER'S DISEASE, *AM J PSYCHIATRY*, 142, 71 (1985)

0743 FITZPATRICK T B ET AL (ED), DERMATOLOGY IN GENERAL MEDICINE, *MCGRAW-HILL* (1971)

0744 FLEGE J B, RUPTURED TUBAL PREGNANCY WITH ELEVATED SERUM AMYLASE LEVELS., *ARCH SURG*, 92, 397 (1966)

0745 FLEMING L W ET AL, PLASMA AND ERYTHROCYTE MAGNESIUM IN HUNTINGTON'S CHOREA, *J NEUROL NEUROSURG PSYCHIATRY*, 30, 374 (1967)

0746 FLETCHER, CARCINOEMBRYONIC ANTIGEN, *ANN INTERN MED*, 69

0747 FLETCHER A P ET AL, BLOOD COAGULATION AND PLASMA FIBRINOLYTIC ENZYME SYSTEM PATHOPHYSIOLOGY IN STROKE, *STROKE*, 7, 337-48 (1976)

0748 FLICK M R ET AL, CONTINUOUS IN-VIVO MONITORING OF ARTERIAL OXYGENATION IN CHRONIC OBSTRUCTIVE LUNG DISEASE, *ANN INTERN MED*, 86, 725-30 (1977)

0749 FLIEGNER J R, PLACENTAL FUNCTION AND RENAL TRACT STUDIES IN PRE-ECLAMPSIA WITH PROTEINURIA AND LONG-TERM MATERNAL CONSEQUENCES, *AM J OBSTET GYNECOL*, 126, 211-7 (1976)

0750 FLORE C H, GUSTAFSON A, APOLIPOPROTEINS A-I, AII AND E IN CHOLESTATIC LIVER DISEASE, *SCAND J CLIN LAB INVEST*, 45, 103-108 (1985)

0751 FOBERG U, FRYD'EN A, K'AGEDAL B, TOBIASSON P, SERUM BILE ACIDS IN GILBERT'S SYNDROME AFTER ORAL LOAD OF CHENODEOXYCHOLIC ACID, *SCAND J GASTROENTEROL*, 20, 325-9 (1985)

0752 FOGEL B J ET AL, A NOTE ON SERUM COMPLEMENT ACTIVITY WITH PARTICULAR REFERENCE TO ULCERATIVE COLITIS, *MILIT MED*, 132, 282 (1967)

0753 FOTINO, ELEVATION OF SERUM ALKALINE PHOSPHATASE IN SEVERE PYELONEPHRITIS AND OBSTRUCTIVE NEPHROPATHY, *NEPHRON*, 12, 197-210 (1974)

0754 FOULK ET AL, CONSTITUTIONAL HEPATIC DYSFUNCTION (GILBERTS DISEASE) ITS NATURAL HISTORY AND RELATED SYNDROMES, *MEDICINE*, 38, 25 (1969)

0755 FOWLER D ET AL, AMINOACIDURIA AND MEGALOBLASTIC ANEMIA, *J CLIN PATHOL*, 13, 230 (1960)

0756 FOWLER JE JR, TAYLOR G, BLOM J, STUTZMAN RE, EXPERIENCE WITH SERUM ALPHA-FETOPROTEIN AND HUMAN CHORIONIC GONADOTROPIN IN NON-SEMINOMATOUS TESTICULAR TUMORS, *J UROL*, 124, 365-8 (1980)

0757 FOWLER NO, DIFFERENTIAL DIAGNOSIS OF CARDIOMYOPATHIES, *PROG CARDIOVASC DIS*, 14, 113-128 (1971)

0758 FOWLER NO, DIFFERENTIAL DIAGNOSIS OF CARDIOMYOPATHIES, *PROG CARDIOVASC DIS*, 14, 113-128 (1971)

0759 FOWLER W, THE ERYTHROCYTE SEDIMENTATION RATE IN SYPHILIS, *BR J VENER DIS*, 52, 309-12 (1976)

0760 FOWLER W M AND PEARSON C M, DIAGNOSTIC AND PROGNOSTIC SIGNIFICANCE OF SERUM ENZYMES. II. NEUROLOGIC DISEASES OTHER THAN MUSCULAR DYSTROPHY, *ARCH PHYS MED REHABIL*, 45, 125 (1968)

0761 FOY H M ET AL, MYCOPLASMA PNEUMONIAE IN AN URBAN AREA, *JAMA*, 214, 1666 (1970)

0762 FRANCESCONI R P ET AL, HUMAN TRYPTOPHAN AND TYROSINE METABOLISM: EFFECTS OF ACUTE, EXPOSURE TO COLD STRESS, *J APPL PHYSIOL*, 33, 165 (1972)

0763 FRANCKSON J R M ET AL, LABELED INSULIN CATABOLISM AND PANCREATIC RESPONSIVENESS DURING LONG TERM EXERCISE IN MAN, *HORM METAB RES*, 3, 366 (1971)

0764 FRANCO AE, LEVINE HD, HALL AP, RHEUMATOID PERICARDITIS. REPORT OF 17 CASES DIAGNOSED CLINICALLY, *ANN INTERN MED*, 77, 837-844 (1972)

0765 FRANCO-MORSELLI R ET AL, INCREASED PLASMA ADRENALINE CONCENTRATIONS IN BENIGN ESSENTIAL HYPERTENSION, *BR MED J*, 2, 1251-4. (1977)

0766 FRANK M M ET AL, HEREDITARY ANGIOEDEMA: THE CLINICAL SYNDROME AND ITS MANAGEMENT, *ANN INTERN MED*, 84, 580-593 (1976)

0767 FRANKLIN A J, CYTOMEGALOVIRUS INFECTION PRESENTING AS ACUTE HAEMOLYTIC ANAEMIA IN AN INFANT, *ARCH DIS CHILD*, 47, 474 (1972)

0768 FRANZEN F AND EYSELK K, BIOLOGICALLY ACTIVE AMINES FOUND IN MAN THEIR BIOCHEMISTRY, PHARMACOLOGY AND PATHOPHYSIOLOGICAL IMPORTANCE, *1ST EDTION PERGAMON PRESS*, 0 (1969)

0769 FRASER, HYPOPHOSPHATASIA, *AM J MED*, 22, 730-746 (1957)

0770 FRASER DR, KOOH SW, KIND PH, HOLICK MT, ET AL, PATHOGENESIS OF HEREDITARY VITAMIN D-DEPENDENT RICKETS, *N ENGL J MED*, 289, 817-822 (1973)

0771 FREDRICKSON D S, THE ROLE OF LIPIDS IN ACUTE MYOCARDIAL INFARCTION, *CIRCULATION*, 39-40(SUPPL 4), 99 (1969)

0772 FREDRICKSON LEVY AND LEES, FAT TRANSPORT IN LIPOPROTEINS - AN INTEGRATED APPROACH TO MECHANISMS AND DISORDERS (CONTINUED), *N ENGL J MED*, 276, 215-225 (1967)

0773 FREDRICKSON LEVY AND LEES, FAT TRANSPORT IN LIPOPROTEINS - AN INTEGRATED APPROACH TO MECHANISMS AND DISORDERS (CONCLUDED), *N ENGL J MED*, 276, 273-281 (1967)

0774 FREDRICKSON LEVY AND LEES, FAT TRANSPORT IN LIPOPROTEINS - AN INTEGRATED APPROACH TO MECHANISMS AND DISORDERS (CONTINUED), *N ENGL J MED*, 276, 148-156 (1967)

0775 FRENKEL E P ET AL, ELEVATED SERUM ACID PHOSPHATASE ASSOCI-ATED WITH MULTIPLE MYELOMA, *ARCH INTERN MED*, 110, 345-349 (1962)

0776 FRENKEL J K, TOXOPLASMOSIS: MECHANISMS OF INFECTION, LABO-RATORY DIAGNOSIS AND MANAGEMENT, *CURR TOP PATHOL*, 54, 28 (1971)

0777 FRIEDBERG V, UBER DIE BEDEUTUNG DER LEBERFUNKTION-SPRUFUNGEN IN DER SCHWANGERSCHAFT, *GEBURTSH FRAUENHEILK*, 22, 109-122 (1962)

0778 FRIEDMAN G D ET AL, THE LEUKOCYTE COUNT AS A PREDICTOR OF MYOCARDIAL INFARCTION, *N ENGL J MED*, 290, 1275-78 (1974)

0779 FRIEDMAN S, EOSINOPHILIA IN SCARLET FEVER, *AM J DIS CHILD*, 49, 933 (1935)

0780 FRIEDMAN Z ET AL, ESSENTIAL FATTY ACIDS, PROSTAGLANDINS, AND RESPIRATORY DISTRESS SYNDROME OF THE NEWBORN, *PEDIAT-RICS*, 61, 341-7 (1978)

0781 FRIEDMAN, R B, AUTHORS OWN DATA GATHERED FROM PATIENTS HOSPITALIZED AT THE UNIVERSITY OF WISCONSIN HOSPITALS. DATA WAS COLLECTED ON A MINIMUM OF TEN PATIENTS FOR EACH REPORTED DISEASE-TEST ASSOCIATION. IN ALL, *UNPUB-LISHED OBSERVATIONS* (1974-1979)

0782 FRIES J F, THE CLINICAL ASPECTS OF SYSTEMIC LUPUS ERYTHEMATOSUS, *MED CLIN NORTH AM*, 61, 229-39 (1977)

0783 FRIES J F AND H R HOLMAN, SYSTEMIC LUPUS ERYTHEMATOSUS: A CLINICAL ANALYSIS, *SMITH L H JR (ED) MAJOR PROBLEMS IN INTERNAL MED PHILADELPHIA*, 5, 123 (1975)

0784 FRIMAN G, SERUM CREATINE PHOSPHOKINASE IN EPIDEMIC INFLU-ENZA, *SCAND J INFECT DIS*, 8, 13-20 (1976)

0785 FRIMPTER G W, CYSTATHIONINURIA IN A PATIENT WITH CYSTINURIA, *AM J MED*, 46, 832 (1969)

0786 FRIMPTER G W ET AL, INULIN AND ENDOGENOUS AMINO ACID RENAL CLEARANCES IN CYSTINURIA: EVIDENCE FOR TUBULAR SECRE-TION, *J CLIN INVEST*, 46, 1162 (1967)

0787 FROHLICH J ET AL, CARBOHYDRATE METABOLISM IN RENAL FAILURE, *AM J CLIN NUTR*, 31, 1541-6 (1978)

0788 FROMMER D J, DIRECT MEASUREMENT OF SERUM NON-CAERULOPLASM COPPER IN LIVER DISEASE, *CLIN CHIM ACTA*, 68, 303-7. (1976)

0789 FROST S J, A SIMPLE QUANTITATIVE INDEX OF THE P3 AMYLASE ISOENZYME IN THE DIAGNOSIS OF ACUTE PANCREATITIS, *CLIN CHIM ACTA*, 87, 23-8. (1976)

0790 FRYDEN A ET AL, DEMONSTRATION OF CEREBROSPINAL FLUID LYM-PHOCYTES SENSITIZED AGAINST VIRUS ANTIGENS IN MUMPS MEN-INGITIS, *ACTA NEUROL SCAND*, 57, 396-404 (1978)

0791 FUCHS F AND KLOPPER A, ENDOCRINOLOGY OF PREGNANCY, *HARPER AND ROW NEW YORK* (1971)

0792 FUCHS F ET AL, PROGESTERONE IN THE UTERINE VENOUS BLOOD OF WOMEN DURING THE FIRST HALF OF GESTATION, *J ENDOCRINOL*, 27, 333 (1963)

0793 FUDENBERG HH, STITES DP, CALDWELL JJ, WELLS JV, *BASIC AND CLINICAL IMMUNOLOGY, 3RD ED. LOS ALTO, CA., LANGE MEDICAL PUBLICATIONS* (1980)

0794 FUH MM, SHIEH SM, WU DA, ET AL, ABNORMALITIES OF CARBOHY-DRATE AND LIPID METABOLISM IN PATIENTS WITH HYPERTENSION, *ARCH INTERN MED*, 147, 1035-8 (1987)

0795 FULKS A ET AL, CARCINOEMBRYONIC ANTIGEN (CEA): MOLECULAR BIOLOGY AND CLINICAL SIGNIFICANCE, *BIOCHEM BIOPHYS RES COMMUN*, 417, 123 (1975)

0796 FULOP M ET AL, LACTIC ACIDOSIS IN DIABETIC PATIENTS, *ARCH INTERN MED*, 136, 987-990 (1976)

0797 FUNAHASHI A, SARKAR TK, KORY RC, PO2,PCO2, AND PH IN PLEURAL EFFUSION, *J LAB CLIN MED*, 78, 1006 (1971)

0798 FURKEM F C, SERUM MURAMIDASE IN HAEMATOLOGICAL DISORDERS, *NZ MED J*, 1, 28 (1972)

0799 FUSCO F D AND ROSEN S W, GONADOTROPIN-PRODUCING ANAPLAS-TIC LARGE CELL CARCINOMAS OF THE LUNG, *N ENGL J MED*, 275, 507 (1966)

0800 GABR Y ET AL, FATTY ACID COMPOSITION OF SERUM LIPIDS IN BILHARZIAL HEPATIC FIBROSIS AND CHRONIC ACTIVE HEPATITIS, *ACTA BIOL MED GER*, 34, 45-51 (1975)

0801 GABUZDA G J, AMMONIA METABOLISM AND HEPATIC COMA, *GASTRO-ENTEROLOGY*, 53, 806-10 (1967)

0802 GADLER H ET AL, INCREASED SERUM ALPHA-FETOPROTEIN LEVELS IN CYTOMEGALOVIRUS INFECTIONS, *SCAND J INFECT DIS*, 10, 101-5 (1978)

0803 GALLAGHER AND SELIGSON, SIGNIFICANCE OF ABNORMALLY LOW BLOOD UREA LEVELS, *N ENGL J MED*, 266, 492-495 (1962)

0804 GALTEAU M M ET AL, VARIATION PLASMATIC ENZYMES PRODUCED BY EXERCISE, *REFERENCES VALUES IN HUMAN CHEMISTRY G. SIEST (ED)*, 223 (1973)

0805 GALTON D A C, THE PATHOGENESIS OF CHRONIC LYMPHOCYTIC LEU-KEMIA, *CAN MED ASSOC J*, 94, 1005 (1966)

0806 GALTON M ET AL, COAGULATION STUDIES ON THE PERIPHERAL CIR-CULATION OF PATIENTS WITH TOXEMIA OF PREGNANCY: A STUDY FOR THE EVALUATION OF, *J REPROD MED*, 6, 89 (1971)

0807 GAMBA G, FORNASARI P MONTANI N, BIANCARDI M, ET AL, PLASMA LEVELS OF PROTEASE INHIBITORS IN ACUTE MYELOID LEUKEMIA AT THE ONSET OF THE DISEASE AND DURING ANTIBLASTIC THER-APY, *THROMB RES*, 17, 41-53 (1980)

0808 GAMKLOW R ET AL, ACTIVITY OF DELTA-1, 4-GLUCOSIDASE IN SERUM FROM PATIENTS WITH MALIGNANT TUMOR, *CANCER*, 32, 298-301 (1973)

0809 GANROT NARLIN KARIN, RELATIVE CONCENTRATIONS OF ALBUMIN AND IGG IN CEREBROSPINAL FLUID IN HEALTH AND IN ACUTE MENINGITIS, *SCAND J INFECT DIS*, 10, 57-60 (1978)

0810 GANSSLEN M ET AL, DIE HAMOLYTISCHE KONSTITUTION, *DTSCH ARCH KLIN MED*, 146, 1 (1925)

0811 GARB S, CLINICAL GUIDE TO UNDESIRABLE DRUG INTERACTIONS AND INTERFERENCES, *SPRING PUBLISHING CO NEW YORK* (1971)

0812 GARB S, LABORATORY TESTS IN COMMON USE, *6TH EDITION SPRINGER NEW YORK*, 46-121 (1976)

0813 GARDNER F H AND MURPHY S, GRANULOCYTE AND PLATELET FUNC-TIONS IN PNH, *SERIES HAEMATOL*, 5, 78 (1972)

0814 GARDNER LI, *ENDOCRINE AND GENETIC DISEASES OF CHILDHOOD AND ADOLESCENCE, W.B. SAUNDERS CO, PHILADELPHIA* (1975)

0815 GARDNER R C ET AL, SERIAL CARCINOEMBRYONIC ANTIGEN (CEA) LEVELS IN PATIENTS WITH ULCERATIVE COLITIS, *AM J DIG DIS*, 23, 129-33 (1978)

0816 GARST J B ET AL, URINARY SODIUM, POTASSIUM AND ALDOSTERONE IN DUCHENNE MUSCULAR DYSTROPHY, *J CLIN ENDOCRINOL METAB*, 44, 185-88 (1977)

0817 GAULT ET AL, CLINICAL SIGNIFICANCE OF URINARY LDH, ALKALINE PHOSPHATASE AND OTHER ENZYMES, *CAN MED ASSOC J*, 101, 208-215 (1962)

0818 GAULT M H ET AL, URINARY ENZYMES IN BENIGN AND MALIGNANT URINARY TRACT DISORDERS: ALKALINE PHOSPHATASE AND LAC-TIC ACID DEHYDROGENASE, *BR J UROL*, 39, 296-306 (1967)

0819 GAULT M H ET AL, SERUM ENZYMES IN PATIENTS WITH CARCINOMA OF LUNG: LACTIC-ACID DEHYDROGENASE, PHOSPHOHEXOSE ISOMERASE, ALKALINE PHOSPHATASE AND GLUTAMIC OXALOACETIC TRANSAMINASE, *CAN MED ASSOC J*, 96, 87-94 (1967)

0820 GAY L ET AL, LABORATORY PROCEDURES USED IN THE DIAGNOSIS OF SYSTEMIC LUPUS ERYTHEMATOSUS: A REVIEW, *AM J MED TECH*, 43, 856-63 (1977)

0821 GAZZARD B G ET AL, FACTOR VII LEVELS AS GUIDE TO PROGNOSIS IN FULMINANT HEPATIC FAILURE, *GUT*, 17, 489-91 (1976)

0822 GEBALA A, ACID HYPERPHOSPHATASIA IN THREE FAMILIES WITH OSTEOGENESIS IMPERFECTA, *LANCET*, 2, 1084 (1956)

0823 GEMBICKI M ET AL, TOTAL AND FREE THYROXINE IN PATIENTS WITH LIVER CIRRHOSIS, *POL MED SCI HIST BULL*, 15, 213-6. (1976)

0824 GENAZZANI AR, FACCHINETTI F, PETRAGLIA F, ET AL, HYPER-ENDORPHINEMIA IN OBESE CHILDREN AND ADOLESCENTS, *J CLIN ENDOCRINOL METAB*, 62, 36 (1986)

0825 GENAZZANI AR, NAPPI G, FACCHINETTI F, ET AL, PROGRESSIVE IMPAIR-MENT OF CSF BETA-EP LEVELS IN MIGRAINE SUFFERERS, *PAIN*, 18, 127-33 (1984)

0826 GEOKAS M C ET AL, METHEMALBUMIN IN THE DIAGNOSIS OF ACUTE HEMORRHAGIC PANCREATITIS, *ANN INTERN MED*, 81, 483-6 (1974)

0827 GEOKAS M C ET AL, STUDIES OF THE ASCITES FLUID OF ACUTE PAN-CREATITIS IN MAN, *AM J DIG DIS*, 23, 182-8 (1978)

0828 GERICKE G S ET AL, LEUCOCYTE ULTRASTRUCTURE AND FOLATE METABOLISM IN DOWN'S SYNDROME, *S AFR MED J*, 51, 369-74 (1977)

0829 GEWURZ H ET AL, DECREASED C1Q PROTEIN CONCENTRATIONS AND AGGLUTINATING ACTIVITY IN AGAMMAGLOBULINEMIC SYN-DROMES: AN INBORN ERROR REFLECTED IN THE COMPLEMENT SYSTEM, *CLIN EXP IMMUNOL*, 3, 437 (1968)

0830 GEYNOSO G ET AL, CEA ASSAY IN CANCER OF THE COLON AND PANCREAS AND OTHER DIGESTIVE TRACT DISORDERS, *AM J DIG DIS*, 16, 1 (1971)

0831 GHADIMI H ET AL, A FAMILIAL DISTURBANCE OF HISTIDINE METABO-LISM, *N ENGL J MED*, 265, 221 (1965)

0832 GHARIB H ET AL, SERUM LEVELS OF THYROID HORMONES IN HASHIMOTO'S THYROIDITIS, *MAYO CLIN PROC*, 47, 175-9 (1972)

0833 GHERARDI E ET AL, RELATIONSHIP AMONG THE CONCENTRATIONS OF SERUM LIPOPROTEINS AND CHANGES IN THEIR CHEMICAL COM-POSITION IN PATIENTS WITH UNTREATED NEPHROTIC SYNDROME, *EUR J CLIN INVEST*, 7, 563-70 (1977)

0834 GHOSE A C ET AL, IMMUNOGLOBULIN STUDIES IN MALARIA AND KALA-AZAR INFECTIONS, *INDIAN J MED RES*, 66, 566-9 (1977)

0835 GIANELLA RA, PATHOGENESIS OF ACUTE BACTERIAL DIARRHEAL DIS-ORDERS, *ANNU REV MED*, 32, 341-357 (1981)

0836 GIBBONS R P ET AL, MANIFESTATIONS OF RENAL CELL CARCINOMA, *UROLOGY*, 8, 201-6 (1976)

0837 GIBSON T ET AL, THE EFFECT OF ACID LOADING ON RENAL EXCRE-TION OF URIC ACID AND AMMONIUM IN GOUT, *ADV EXP MED BIOL*, 76(B), 46-55 (1977)

0838 GIFFORD R, IS THE RENIN-SODIUM PROFILE HELPFUL IN EVALUATING HYPERTENSION?, *JAMA*, 244, 35-37 (1980)

0839 GILBERT H S ET AL, PLASMA AND URINARY URATE FINDINGS IN MYELOPROLIFERATIVE DISORDERS, *J MT SINAI HOSP*, 30, 185 (1963)

0840 GILBERT H S ET AL, A STUDY OF HISTAMINE IN MYELOPROLIFERATIVE DISEASE, *BLOOD*, 28, 795 (1966)

0841 GILBERT H S ET AL, SERUM VITAMIN B$_{12}$ CONTENT AND UNSATURATED VITAMIN B$_{12}$ BINDING CAPACITY (VBBC) IN MYELOPROLIFERATIVE DISEASE: VALUE IN DIFFERENTIAL DIAGNOSIS AND AS PARAMETERS OF DISEASE, *ANN INTERN MED*, 71, 719 (1969)

0842 GILBERT M G, CUSHING'S SYNDROME IN INFANCY, *PEDIATRICS*, 46, 217 (1970)

0843 GILL J R ET AL, IMPAIRED CONSERVATION OF SODIUM AND POTASSIUM IN RENAL ACIDOSIS, *CLIN SCI*, 33, 577 (1967)

0844 GILLESPIE G, ELDER JB, SMITH IS, KENNEDY F, ET AL, AN ANALYSIS OF SPONTANEOUS GASTRIC ACID SECRETION IN NORMAL AND DUODENAL ULCER SUBJECTS: NEW CRITERION FOR THE INSULIN TEST, *GASTROENTEROLOGY*, 62, 903-911 (1972)

0845 GILUTZ H, SIEGEL Y, PARAN E, CRISTAL N, QUASTEL MR, ALPHA 1-ANTITRYPSIN IN ACUTE MYOCARDIAL INFARCTION, *BR HEART J*, 49, 26-9 (1983)

0846 GIORDANO C ET AL, GAMMA-GLOBULINS PATTERNS IN CSF OF INFLAMMATORY NEUROLOGICAL DISEASES IN TROPICAL AFRICA, *EUR NEUROL*, 17, 160-5 (1978)

0847 GIRALDO G, BETH E, KOURILSKY FM, ET AL, ANTIBODY PATTERNS TO HERPESVIRUSES IN KAPOSI'S SARCOMA: SEROLOGICAL ASSOCIATION OF EUROPEAN KAPOSI'S SARCOMA WITH CYTOMEGALOVIRUS, *INT J CANCER*, 15, 839-848 (1975)

0848 GIUSTI G, ADENOSINE DEAMINASE, *BERGMEYER, HU (ED): METHODS OF ENZYMATIC ANALYSIS. NEW YORK, ACADEMIC PRESS* (1974)

0849 GLADMAN D D ET AL, SYSTEMIC LUPUS ERYTHEMATOSUS WITH NEGATIVE LE CELLS AND ANTINUCLEAR FACTOR, *J RHEUMATOL*, 5, 142-7 (1978)

0850 GLEASON M N ET AL, CLINICAL TOXICOLOGY OF COMMERCIAL PRODUCTS, *WILLIAMS & WILKINS BALTIMORE MD* (1970)

0851 GLENNER G G ET AL, THE IMMUNOGLOBULIN ORIGIN OF AMYLOID, *AM J MED*, 52, 141-147 (1972)

0852 GLICK J H, SERUM LACTATE DEHYDROGENASE ISOENZYME AND TOTAL LACTATE DEHYDROGENASE VALUES IN HEALTH AND DISEASE, AND CLINICAL EVALUATION OF THESE TESTS BY MEANS OF DISCRIMINANT ANALYSIS, *AM J CLIN PATHOL*, 52, 320-328 (1969)

0853 GLORIEUX F AND SCRIVER C R, LOSS OF A PARATHYROID-HORMONE-SENSITIVE COMPONENT OF PHOSPHATE TRANSPORT IN X-LINKED HYPOPHOSPHATEMIC RICKETS, *SCIENCE*, 173, 997 (1972)

0854 GLOVSKY M M ET AL, REDUCTION OF PLEURAL FLUID COMPLEMENT ACTIVITY IN PATIENTS WITH SYSTEMIC LUPUS ERYTHEMATOSUS AND RHEUMATOID ARTHRITIS, *CLIN IMMUNOL IMMUNOPATHOL*, 6, 31-41 (1976)

0855 GLUECK C J LEVY R I AND FREDRICKSON D S, IMMUNOREACTIVE INSULIN, GLUCOSE TOLERANCE AND CARBOHYDRATE INDUCIBILITY IN TYPE II, III, IV, AND V HYPERLIPOPROTEINEMIA, *DIABETES*, 18, 739 (1969)

0856 GLUECK H I ET AL, COLD PRECIPITABLE FIBRINOGEN, CRYOFIBRINOGEN, *ARCH INTERN MED*, 113, 748 (1964)

0857 GLYN-JONES R, BLOOD SUGAR IN INFANTILE GASTRO-ENTERITIS, *S AFR MED J*, 49, 1474-6 (1975)

0858 GNUDI A ET AL, VARIATION OF BLOOD GLUCOSE AND SERUM GROWTH HORMONE, PROLACTIN AND INSULIN IN SUBJECTS WITH INSULIN-DEPENDENT DIABETES, *ACTA DIABETOL LAT*, 14, 119-28 (1977)

0859 GO V L W, CARCINOEMBRYONIC ANTIGEN, *CANCER*, 37, 562-66 (1976)

0860 GOEDERT JJ, BIGGAR RJ, MELBYE M, ET AL, EFFECT OF T$_4$ COUNT AND COFACTORS ON THE INCIDENCE OF AIDS IN HOMOSEXUAL MEN INFECTED WITH HUMAN IMMUNODEFICIENCY VIRUS, *JAMA*, 257, 331 (1987)

0861 GOHARA WF, RATE OF DECREASE OF GLUTAMYLTRANSFERASE AND ACID PHOSPHATASE ACTIVITIES IN THE HUMAN VAGINA AFTER COITUS, *CLIN CHEM*, 26, 254-257 (1980)

0862 GOKA AKJ. ROLSTON DDK. MATHAN VI. AND FARTHING MG, DIAGNOSIS OF GIARDIASIS BY SPECIFIC IGM ANTIBODY ENZYME-LINKED IMMUNOSORBENT ASSAY, *J CLIN ENDOCR*, II, 184 (1986)

0863 GOKCEN M, CRYOGLOBULINS BEHAVING AS COLD AGGLUTININS, *POSTGRAD MED*, 39, A68 (1966)

0864 GOLAY A, SWISLOCKI ALM, CHEN YDI, ET AL, EFFECT OF OBESITY ON AMBIENT PLASMA GLUCOSE, FREE FATTY ACID, INSULIN, GROWTH HORMONE, AND GLUCAGON CONCENTRATIONS, *J CLIN ENDOCRINOL METAB*, 63, 481 (1986)

0865 GOLD G L ET AL, HYPERURICEMIA ASSOCIATED WITH THE TREATMENT OF ACUTE LEUKEMIA, *ANN INTERN MED*, 47, 428 (1957)

0866 GOLDBARG JA, PINEDA EP, BLANKS BM, RUTENBERG AM, A METHOD FOR THE COLORIMETRIC DETERMINATION OF B-GLUCURONIDASE IN URINE, SERUM AND TISSUE: ASSAY OF ENZYMATIC ACTIVITY IN HEALTH AND DISEASE, *GASTROENTEROLOGY*, 36, 193-201 (1959)

0867 GOLDBERG A AND RIMINGTON C, DISEASES OF PORPHYRIN METABOLISM, *CHARLES C THOMAS SPRINGFIELD IL* (1962)

0868 GOLDBERG A AND RIMINGTON C, HEREDITARY COPROPORPHYRIA, *LANCET*, 1, 632 (1967)

0869 GOLDBERG D M ET AL, SERUM AMYLASE AND RELATED ENZYMES IN DIABETIC KETOACIDOSIS, *J CLIN PATHOL*, 26, 985 (1974)

0870 GOLDBERG D M ET AL, AN ASSESSMENT OF SERUM ACID ALKALINE PHOSPHATASE DETERMINATIONS IN PROSTATIC CANCER WITH A CLINICAL VALIDATION OF AN ACID PHOSPHATASE ASSAY UTILIZING ADENOSINE 3'-MONOPHOSPHATE AS SUBSTRATE, *J CLIN PATHOL*, 27, 140-147 (1974)

0871 GOLDBERG DM, *CLIN PHYSIOL*, 2, 249-68 (1984)

0872 GOLDBERG DM, THE NONINVASIVE BIOCHEMICAL DIAGNOSIS OF GASTROINTESTINAL DISEASE, WITH SPECIAL REFERENCE TO CHILDREN, *CLIN PHYSIOL BIOCHEM*, 1984, 249-68 (2)

0873 GOLDBERG D M ET AL, ELEVATION OF SERUM ALKALINE PHOSPHATASE ACTIVITY AND RELATED ENZYMES IN DIABETES MELLITUS, *CLIN BIOCHEM*, 10, 8-11 (1977)

0874 GOLDBERG M F, RETINAL VASO-OCCLUSION IN SICKLING HEMOGLOBINOPATHIES, *BIRTH DEFECTS*, 12, 475-515 (1976)

0875 GOLDBERGER J, WHEELER GA, EXPERIMENTAL PELLAGRA IN THE HUMAN SUBJECT BROUGHT ABOUT BY A RESTRICTED DIET, *PUBLIC HEALTH REPORTS*, 30, 3336-3339 (1915)

0876 GOLDBORG ET AL, A METHOD FOR THE DETERMINATION OF GAMMA GLUTAMYL TRANSPEPTIDASE IN HUMAN SERUM; ENZYMATIC ACTIVITY IN HEALTH AND DISEASE, *GASTROENTEROLOGY*, 44, 127-33 (1963)

0877 GOLDENBERG DL, LEFF G, GRAYZEL AI, PERICARDIAL TAMPONADE IN SYSTEMIC LUPUS ERYTHEMATOSUS; WITH ABSENT HEMOLYTIC COMPLEMENT ACTIVITY IN PERICARDIAL FLUID, *NEW YORK STATE JOURNAL OF MEDICINE*, 75, 910-912 (1975)

0878 GOLDENSHON E S AND APPEL S H, SCIENTIFIC APPROACH TO CLINICAL NEUROLOGY, *PHILADELPHIA LEA & FEBIGER* (1977)

0879 GOLDFARB A F ET AL, POLYCYSTIC OVARIAN DISEASE: CLINICAL CONSIDERATIONS, *J REPROD MED*, 18, 135-8 (1977)

0880 GOLDING P L ET AL, MULTISYSTEM INVOLVEMENT IN CHRONIC LIVER DISEASE: STUDIES ON THE INCIDENCE AND PATHOGENESIS, *AM J MED*, 55, 772 (1973)

0881 GOLDMAN A S ET AL, DYSGAMMAGLOBULINEMIC ANTIBODY DEFICIENCY SYNDROME, *J PEDIATR*, 70, 16 (1967)

0882 GOLDSTEIN D A ET AL, BLOOD LEVELS OF 25-HYDROXYVITAMIN D IN NEPHROTIC SYNDROME, *ANN INTERN MED*, 87, 664-667 (1977)

0883 GOLDSTEIN F ET AL, USE OF SERUM TRANSAMINASE LEVELS IN THE DIFFERENTIATION OF PULMONARY EMBOLISM AND MYOCARDIAL INFARCTION, *N ENGL J MED*, 254, 746 (1956)

0884 GOLUBJATNIKOV R ET AL, COMPARATIVE STUDY OF ANTISTREPTOLYSIN O, ANTIDEOXYRIBONUCLEASE B AND MULTI ENZYME TESTS IN STREPTOCOCCAL INFECTIONS, *HEALTH LAB SCI*, 14, 284-90 (1977)

0885 GONICK H C ET AL, URINARY B-GLUCURONIDASE ACTIVITY IN RENAL DISEASE, *ARCH INTERN MED*, 132, 63-69 (1973)

0886 GOOD R A, STUDIES ON AGAMMAGLOBULINEMIA: II. FAILURE OF PLASMA CELL FORMATION IN BONE MARROW AND LYMPH NODES OF PATIENTS WITH AGAMMAGLOBULINEMIA, *J LAB CLIN MED*, 46, 167 (1955)

0887 GOODLIN R C, SEVERE PRE-ECLAMPSIA: ANOTHER GREAT IMITATOR, *AM J OBSTET GYNECOL*, 125, 747-53 (1976)

0888 GOODMAN ET AL, SERUM GAMMA-GLUTAMYL TRANSPEPTIDASE DEFICIENCY, *J CLIN ENDOCR*, 1, 234-235 (1971)

0889 GOODMAN L S ET AL, THE PHARMACOLOGICAL BASIS OF THERAPEUTICS, *4TH EDITION MACMILLAN CO NEW YORK NY* (1970)

0890 GOODNIGHT S H JR, BLEEDING AND INTRAVASCULAR CLOTTING MALIGNANCY: A REVIEW, *ANN NY ACAD SCI*, 230, 271 (1974)

0891 GOODPASTURE H C ET AL, COLORADO TICK FEVER: CLINICAL, EPIDEMIOLOGIC AND LABORATORY ASPECTS OF 228 CASES IN COLORADO IN 1973-1974, *ANN INTERN MED*, 88, 303-310 (1978)

0892 GOODWIN R A ET AL, CHRONIC PULMONARY HISTOPLASMOSIS, *MEDICINE*, 55, 413-450 (1976)

0893 GORDEN P ET AL, HYPERURICEMIA, A CONCOMITANT OF THE CONGENITAL VASOPRESSIN-RESISTANT DIABETES INSIPIDUS IN THE ADULT: STUDIES OF URIC ACID METABOLISM AND PLASMA VASOPRESSIN, *N ENGL J MED*, 284, 1057 (1971)

0894 GORDON D A, THE EXTRARENAL MANIFESTATIONS OF HYPERNEPHROMA, *CAN MED ASSOC J*, 88, 61-67 (1963)

0895 GORDON DA, PRUZANSKI W, OGRYZLO MA, LITTLE HA, AMYLOID ARTHRITIS SIMULATING RHEUMATOID DISEASE IN FIVE PATIENTS WITH MULTIPLE MYELOMA., *AM J MED*, 55, 142-154 (1973)

0896 GORDON H H AND NITOWSKY H M, SOME STUDIES OF TOCOPHEROL IN INFANTS AND CHILDREN, *AM J CLIN NUTR*, 4, 391 (1956)

0897 GOREN R AND SIMONS L A, PLASMA CHOLESTEROL ESTERIFICATION IN HYPERTRIGLYCERIDAEMIA, *CLIN CHIM ACTA*, 74, 289-296 (1977)

0898 GORODISCHER R ET AL, HYPOPHOSPHATASIA: A DEVELOPMENTAL ANOMALY OF ALKALINE PHOSPHATASE?, *PEDIATR RES*, 10, 650-656 (1976)

0899 GOSLING ET AL, CREATINE PHOSPHOKINASE ACTIVITY DURING LITHIUM TREATMENT, *BR MED J*, 3, 327-329 (1972)

0900 GOSWITZ F ET AL, ERYTHROCYTE REDUCED GLUTATHIONE, GLUCOSE-6-PHOSPHATE DEHYDROGENASE, AND 6-PHOSPHOGLUCONIC DEHYDROGENASE IN PATIENTS WITH MYELOFIBROSIS, *J LAB CLIN MED*, 67, 615 (1966)

0901 GOTOH M, MIZUNO K, MATSUI J, KUNII N, FUKUCHI S, SERUM ANGIOTENSIN I CONVERTING ENZYME ACTIVITY IN PATIENTS WITH HYPERTHYROIDISM AND HYPOTHYROIDISM: RELATION TO RENIN AND ALDOSTERONE, *NIPPON NAIBUNPI GAKKAI ZASSHI*, 60, 835-45 (1984)

0902 GOULDER A W G ET AL, RED CELL SODIUM IN HYPERTHYROIDISM, *BR MED J*, 1, 552 (1971)

0903 GRAEFF J DE AND LAMEIJER L D, PERIODIC PARALYSIS, *AM J MED*, 39, 70 (1965)

0904 GRAHAM R C AND BERNIER G M, THE BONE MARROW IN MULTIPLE MYELOMA: CORRELATION OF PLASMA CELL ULTRASTRUCTURE AND CLINICAL STATE., *MEDICINE*, 54, 225-244 (1975)

0905 GRAIG F A ET AL, SERUM CREATINE-PHOSPHOKINASE IN THYROID DISEASE, *METABOLISM*, 12, 57-59 (1963)

0906 GRANBERG P O ET AL, RENAL FUNCTION STUDIES IN MEDULLARY SPONGE KIDNEY, *SCAND J UROL NEPHROL*, 5, 177 (1971)

0907 GRANGE JM, MITCHELL DN, KEMP M, KARDJITO T, SERUM ANGIOTENSIN-CONVERTING ENZYME AND DELAYED HYPERSENSITIVITY IN PULMONARY TUBERCULOSIS, *TUBERCLE*, 65, 117-21 (1984)

0908 GRAY C H, ACUTE PORPHYRIA, *ARCH INTERN MED*, 85, 459 (1950)

0909 GREAVES M W ET AL, THE EFFECT OF VENOUS OCCLUSION, STARVATION AND EXERCISE ON PROSTAGLANDIN ACTIVITY IN WHOLE HUMAN BLOOD, *LIFE SCI*, 11, 919 (1972)

0910 GREAVES M, BOYDE TRC, PLASMA ZINC CONCENTRATIONS IN PATIENTS WITH PSORIASIS, OTHER DERMATOSES AND VENOUS LEG ULCERATIONS, *LANCET*, 2, 1019-1020 (1967)

0911 GREEN A J AND RATNOFF O D, ELEVATED ANTIHEMOPHILIC FACTOR (AHF, FACTOR VIII) PROCOAGULANT ACTIVITY AND AHF LIKE ANTIGEN IN ALCOHOLIC CIRRHOSIS OF THE LIVER, *J LAB CLIN MED*, 83, 189 (1974)

0912 GREEN J B ET AL, THE CHOLESTEROL AND CHOLESTEROL ESTER CONTENT IN CEREBROSPINAL FLUID IN PATIENTS WITH MULTIPLE SCLEROSIS AND OTHER NEUROLOGICAL DISEASES, *J NEUROL NEUROSURG PSYCHIATRY*, 22, 117 (1959)

0913 GREEN J G, SERUM CHOLESTEROL CHANGES IN PREGNANCY, *AM J OBSTET GYNECOL*, 95, 387 (1966)

0914 GREEN O C FEFFERMAN R AND NAIR S, PLASMA GROWTH HORMONE LEVELS IN CHILDREN WITH CYSTIC FIBROSIS AND SHORT STATURE, *J CLIN ENDOCRINOL METAB*, 27, 1059 (1967)

0915 GREENBERG B H ET AL, PRIMARY TYPE V HYPERLIPOPROTEINEMIA, *ANN INTERN MED*, 87, 526-534 (1977)

0916 GREENWOOD B M ET AL, SPECKLED ANTINUCLEAR FACTOR IN AFRICAN SERA, *CLIN EXP IMMUNOL*, 7, 75 (1970)

0917 GREENWOOD B M ET AL, LYMPHOCYTE CHANGES IN ACUTE MALARIA, *TRANS R SOC TROP MED HYG*, 71, 408-10 (1977)

0918 GRIFFIN G, VARTUKARTIS JL, HORMONE SECRETING TUMORS, *IN CANCER MARKERS II, HUMANA PRESS, INC. CLIFTON, NEW JERSEY* (1982)

0919 GRIFFITHS PA, MILSOM JP, LLOYD JB, PLASMA ACID HYDROLASES IN NORMAL ADULTS AND CHILDREN, AND IN PATIENTS WITH LYSOSOMAL STORAGE DISEASES, *CLIN CHIM ACTA*, 90, 129-141 (1978)

0920 GRIGORESCU M, TAPALAGA D, DUMITRA,SCU D, ET AL, DIAGNOSTIC VALUE OF SERUM BILE ACID DETERMINATION IN CHRONIC HEPATITIS AND LIVER CIRRHOSIS, *MED INTERNE*, 18, 401-6 (1980)

0921 GRIMM RH, NEATON JD, LUDWIG W, ET AL, PROGNOSTIC IMPORTANCE OF THE WHITE BLOOD CELL COUNT FOR CORONARY, CANCER, AND ALL-CAUSE MORTALITY, *JAMA*, 254, 1932 (1985)

0922 GRIMMEL K ET AL, AMYLASE ACTIVITY OF PAROTID SALIVA IN ACUTE AND CHRONIC PANCREATITIS, *ACTA HEPATOGASTROENTEROL*, 23, 334-44 (1976)

0923 GRONHAGEN-RISKA C ET AL, THYROID HORMONES AND ACE, *ACTA MED SCAND*, 217, 260 (1985)

0924 GRONHAGEN-RISKA C, FYHRQUIST F, ET AL, THYROID HORMONES AFFECT SERUM ANGIOTENSIN I CONVERTING ENZYME LEVELS, *ACTA MED SCAND*, 217, 259-64 (1985)

0925 GROPP C ET AL, CARCINOEMBRYONIC ANTIGEN, ALPHA 1-FETOPROTEIN (AFP), FERRITIN, AND ALPHA 2-PREGNANCY ASSOCIATED GLYCOPROTEIN IN THE SERUM OF LUNG CANCER PATIENTS AND ITS DEMONSTRATION IN LUNG TUMOR TISSUES, *ONCOLOGY*, 34, 267-72 (1977)

0926 GROSS, AN HEREDITARY ENZYMATIC DEFECT IN RED BLOOD CELLS: ITS RELATION TO CERTAN DRUG INDUCED HEMOLYTIC ANEMIAS, *ANN NY ACAD SCI*, 75, 106-109 (1958)

0927 GROSS S ET AL, THE PLATELETS IN IRON-DEFICIENCY ANEMIA. I THE RESPONSE TO ORAL AND PARENTERAL IRON, *PEDIATRICS*, 34, 315 (1964)

0928 GROSSEN Y AND EALES L, PATTERNS OF FAECAL PORPHYRIN EXCRETION IN THE HEPATOCUTANEOUS PORPHYRIAS, *S AFR MED J*, 47, 2162 (1973)

0929 GROSSI CE, PRASTHOFER EF,, T-CELL IMBALANCES IN BLOOD AND LYMPH NODES FROM PATIENTS WITH ACQUIRED IMMUNE DEFICIENCY SYNDROME OR AIDS-RELATED COMPLEX

0930 GUALANDI L ET AL, PLASMA TRIGLYCERIDES IN PREGNANCY AND THE NORMAL PUERPERIUM, *BOLL SOC ITAL BIOL SPER*, 42, 825 (1966)

0931 GUBLER CJ, BROWN H, MARKOWITZ H, ET AL, STUDIES ON COPPER METABOLISM XXIII. PORTAL (LAENNEC'S) CIRRHOSIS OF THE LIVER, *J CLIN INVEST*, 36, 1208-1216 (1957)

0932 GUDJONSSON B ET AL, CANCER OF THE PANCREAS: DIAGNOSTIC ACCURACY AND SURVIVAL STATISTICS, *CANCER*, 42, 2494-2506 (1978)

0933 GUECHOT J, LIORET N, CYNOBER L, ET AL, MYOGLOBINEMIA AFTER BURN INJURY: RELATIONSHIP TO CREATINE KINASE ACTIVITY IN SERUM, *CLIN CHEM*, 32/5, 857-859 (1986)

0934 GUMPEL J M AND HOBBS J R, SERUM IMMUNE GLOBULINS IN SJÖGREN'S SYNDROME, *ANN RHEUM DIS*, 29, 681 (1970)

0935 GUNTHER H, HANDBUCH DER KRANKHEITEN DES BLUTES UND DER BLUTBILDENDEN ORGANE, *HANDBUCH DER ORGANE*, 2 (1925)

0936 GUNZ F AND BAIKIE A G, LEUKEMIA, *GRUNE & STRATTON NEW YORK*, 403 (1974)

0937 GUPTA D K ET AL, INCREASED PLASMA FREE-FATTY-ACID CONCENTRATIONS AND THEIR SIGNIFICANCE IN PATIENTS WITH ACUTE MYOCARDIAL INFARCTION, *LANCET*, 2, 1209 (1969)

0938 GUPTA J K ET AL, MULTIPLE SCLEROSIS AND MALABSORPTION, *AM J GASTROENTEROL*, 68, 560-5 (1977)

0939 GUPTA R C ET AL, NITROBLUE TETRAZOLIUM TEST IN THE DIAGNOSIS OF PYOGENIC ARTHRITIS, *ANN INTERN MED*, 80, 723-6 (1974)

0940 GUPTA RG, BEKERMAN C, SICILIAN L, OPARIL S, ET AL, GALLIUM 67 CITRATE SCANNING AND SERUM ANGIOTENSIN CONVERTING ENZYME, *RADIOLOGY*, 144, 895-9 (1982)

0941 GUSTIN M, RADERMECKER M, SIGNIFICANCE OF ELEVATED SERUM ACE IN PNEUMOLOGY, *POUMON COEUR*, 38, 339-45 (1982)

0942 GUTMAN A B, SERUM ALKALINE PHOSPHATASE ACTIVITY IN DISEASES OF THE SKELETAL AND HEPATOBILIARY SYSTEMS, *AM J MED*, 27, 875-901 (1959)

0943 GUTMAN A B AND YU T F, RENAL FUNCTION IN GOUT, *AM J MED*, 23, 600 (1957)

0944 GUTMAN A B ET AL, AN 'ACID' PHOSPHATASE OCCURRING IN THE SERUM OF PATIENTS WITH METASTASIZING CARCINOMA OF THE PROSTATE GLAND, *J CLIN INVEST*, 17, 473-478 (1938)

0945 GUTMAN A B ET AL, DETERMINATION OF SERUM 'ACID' PHOSPHATASE ACTIVITY IN DIFFERENTIATING SKELETAL METASTASES SECONDARY TO PROSTATIC CARCINOMA FROM PAGET'S DISEASE OF BONE, *AM J CANCER*, 38, 103-108 (1940)

0946 GUTMAN A B ET AL, ESTIMATION OF 'ACID' PHOSPHATASE ACTIVITY OF BLOOD SERUM, *J BIOL CHEM*, 136, 201-209 (1940)

0947 GUTMAN A B ET AL, SIGNIFICANCE OF INCREASED PHOSPHATASE ACTIVITY OF BONE AT THE SITE OF OSTEOPLASTIC METASTASES SECONDARY TO CARCINOMA OF THE PROSTATE GLAND, *AM J CANCER*, 28, 485-495 (1936)

0948 GUTMAN TYSON AND GUTMAN, SERUM CALCIUM, INORGANIC PHOSPHORUS AND PHOSPHATASE ACTIVITY IN HYPERPARATHYROIDISM, PAGET'S DISEASE, MULTIPLE MYELOMA AND NEOPLASTIC DISEASE OF THE BONES, *ARCH INTERN MED*, 57, 379-413 (1936)

0949 GUTTIERREZ LV, BARON JH, A COMPARISON OF BASAL AND STIMULATED GASTRIC ACID AND DUODENAL BICARBONATE SECRETION IN PATIENTS WITH AND WITHOUT DUODENAL ULCER DISEASE, *AM J GASTROENTEROL*, 66, 270-276 (1976)

0950 GYORKEY F, SOME ASPECTS OF CANCER OF THE PROSTATE GLAND, *METHODS IN CANCER RESEARCH BUSCH H (ED)*, 7, 279 (1973)

0951 HABIB R ET AL, THE NEPHROTIC SYNDROME IN: PEDIATRIC NEPHROLOGY, *ROYER P ET AL (EDS) W B SAUNDERS CO PHILADELPHIA*, 262 (1974)

0952 HABIB ZA, MATERNAL SERUM ALPHA-FETOPROTEIN: ITS VALUE IN ANTENATAL DIAGNOSIS OF GENETIC DISEASE AND IN OBSTETRICAL-GYNAECOLOGICAL CARE, *UPPSALA, SWEDEN, ALMQUIST & WIKSELL* (1977)

0953 HACK CE, EERENBERG-BELMER AJ, LIM UG, ET AL, LACK OF ACTIVATION OF C1, DESPITE CIRCULATING IMMUNE COMPLEXES DETECTED BY TWO C19 METHODS, IN PATIENTS WITH RHEUMATOID ARTHRITIS, *ARTHRITIS RHEUM*, 27, 40-8 (1984)

0954 HAENEL KRYSTON AND MILLS, CHLORIDE: PHOSPHATE AND HYPERCALCEMIA, *ANN INTERN MED*, 81, 270-271 (1974)

0955 HAFEZ M ET AL, CALCIUM AND PHOSPHORUS METABOLIC CHANGES IN CHILDREN WITH HEPATIC BILHARZIASIS, *GAZ EGYPT PAEDIATR ASSOC*, 23, 243-52 (1975)

0956 HAFEZ M ET AL, ANTIBODY PRODUCTION AND COMPLEMENT SYSTEM IN PROTEIN ENERGY MALNUTRITION, *J TROP MED HYG*, 80, 36-9. (1977)

0957 HAFLER DA, HEMLER ME, CHRISTENSON L, ET AL, INVESTIGATION OF IN VIVO ACTIVATED T CELLS IN MULTIPLE SCLEROSIS AND INFLAMMATORY CENTRAL NERVOUS SYSTEM DISEASES, *CLIN IMMUNOL IMMUNOPATHOL*, 37, 163-71 (1985)

0958 HAFNER GE, WUTHRICH B, GROB PJ, ET AL, CIRCULATING IMMUNE COMPLEXES, COMPLEMENT FACTORS C3, C4, C1-INHIBITOR, ALPHA-1-ANTITRYPSIN AND IMMUNOGLOBULINS IN ASTHMATIC PATIENTS, *RESPIRATION*, 41, 248-57 (1981)

0959 HAHN T J ET AL, REDUCED SERUM 25-HYDROXYVITAMIN D CONCENTRATION AND DISORDERED MINERAL METABOLISM IN PATIENTS WITH CYSTIC FIBROSIS, *J PEDIATR*, 94, 38-42 (1979)

0960 HALL R ET AL, RADIOIMMUNOASSAY OF HUMAN SERUM THYROTROPIN, *BR MED J*, 1, 582 (1972)

0961 HALLEE T J ET AL, INFECTIOUS MONONUCLEOSIS AT THE UNITED STATES MILITARY ACADEMY: A PROSPECTIVE STUDY OF A SINGLE CLASS OVER FOUR YEARS, *YALE J BIOL MED*, 47, 182 (1974)

0962 HALSTED J A, THE LABORATORY IN CLINICAL MEDICINE, *W B SAUNDERS CO* (1976)

0963 HALSTED J, HALSTED C, *THE LABORATORY IN CLINICAL MEDICINE 2ND ED- W.B. SAUNDERS CO., PHILADELPHIA* (1986)

0964 HAM T H, HEMOGLOBINURIA, *AM J MED*, 18, 990 (1955)

0965 HAMADAH K ET AL, EFFECT OF ELECTRIC CONVULSION THERAPY ON URINARY EXCRETION OF 3'5-CYCLIC ADENOSINE MONOPHOSPHATE, *BR MED J*, 3, 439 (1972)

0966 HAMBIDGE KM, DROEGEMUELLER W, CHANGES IN PLASMA AND HAIR CONCENTRATIONS OF ZINC, COPPER, CHROMIUM AND MANGANESE DURING PREGNANCY, *OBSTET GYNECOL*, 103, 666-672 (1969)

0967 HAMBURGER H, BATSAKIS J, *CLINICAL LABORATORY ANNUAL: 1982, APPLETON-CENTURY-CROFTS/NEW YORK* (1982)

0968 HAMET P ET AL, STUDIES OF THE ELEVATED EXTRACELLULAR CONCENTRATION OF CYCLIC AMP IN UREMIC MAN, *J CLIN INVEST*, 56, 339 (1975)

0969 HAMILTON C R JR AND TUMULTY P A, GIANT CELL ARTERITIS INCLUDING TEMPORAL ARTERITIS AND POLYMYALGIA RHEUMATICA, *MEDICINE*, 50, 1 (1971)

0970 HAMMETT J F ET AL, MCARDLE'S DISEASE: THREE CASES IN AN AUSTRALIAN FAMILY, *PROC AUST ASSOC NEUROL*, 4, 21-25 (1966)

0971 HAMMOND G L, SERUM FSH, LH AND PROLACTIN IN NORMAL MALES AND PATIENTS WITH PROSTATIC DISEASES, *CLIN ENDOCRINOL (OXF)*, 7, 129-35 (1977)

0972 HAMMOND G L ET AL, SERUM STEROIDS IN NORMAL MALES AND PATIENTS WITH PROSTATIC DISEASES., *CLIN ENDOCRINOL (OXF)*, 9, 113-21 (1978)

0973 HANAFY H M ET AL, INCREASED SERUM AMYLASE LEVELS IN PROSTATIC DISEASES, *UROLOGY*, 1, 372 (1973)

0974 HANDIN R I ET AL, ELEVATION OF PLATELET FACTOR FOUR IN ACUTE MYOCARDIAL INFARCTION: MEASUREMENT BY RADIOIMMUNOASSAY, *J LAB CLIN MED*, 91, 340-349 (1978)

0975 HANDJANI A M ET AL, SERUM IRON IN ACUTE MYOCARDIAL INFARCTION, *BLUT (BERLIN)*, 23, 363 (1971)

0976 HANDWEGER S ET AL, GLUCOSE TOLERANCE IN CYSTIC FIBROSIS, *N ENGL J MED*, 281, 451 (1969)

0977 HANGE F M ET AL, POSTARSPHENAMINE JAUNDICE, *JAMA*, 115, 263 (1940)

0978 HANKIN M E ET AL, AN EVALUATION OF LABORATORY TESTS FOR THE DETECTION AND DIFFERENTIAL DIAGNOSIS OF CUSHING'S SYNDROME, *CLIN ENDOCRINOL (OXF)*, 6, 185-96 (1977)

0979 HANSEN H J ET AL, CARCINOEMBRYONIC ANTIGEN (CEA) ASSAY-A LABORATORY ADJUNCT IN THE DIAGNOSIS AND MANAGEMENT OF CANCER, *HUMAN PATHOL*, 5, 139 (1974)

0980 HANSEN M ET AL, SMALL CELL CARCINOMA OF THE LUNG: SERUM CALCITONIN AND SERUM HISTAMINASE AT BASAL LEVELS AND STIMULATED BY PENTAGASTRIN, *ACTA MED SCAND*, 204, 257-261 (1978)

0981 HANSEN N E, PLASMA LYSOZYME- A MEASURE OF NEUTROPHIL TURNOVER, *SERIES HAEMATOL*, 7, 1 (1974)

0982 HANSKY J, KORMAN MG, IMMUNOASSAY STUDIES IN PEPTIC ULCER, *CLINICS IN GASTROENTEROLOGY, (ED. W. SIRCUS), W. B. SAUNDERS*, 2, 275-292 (1973)

0983 HANSSEN K F ET AL, INCREASED SERUM PROLACTIN IN DIABETIC KETOACIDOSIS: CORRELATION BETWEEN SERUM SODIUM AND SERUM PROLACTIN CONCENTRATION, *ACTA ENDOCRINOL*, 85, 372-78 (1977)

0984 HANSTEN P D, DRUG INTERACTIONS, *LEA & FEBIGER* (1971)

0985 HARALAMBIE G, BIOCHEMICAL CHANGES IN BLOOD (AT REST) INDUCED BY EXERCISE AND TRAINING, *REFERENCES VALUES IN HUMAN CHEMISTRY G. SIEST (ED)*, 243 (1973)

0986 HARBER I C ET AL, ERYTHROPOIETIC PROTOPORPHYRIA AND PHOTOHEMOLYSIS, *JAMA*, 189, 191 (1964)

0987 HARBOE M ET AL, IDENTIFICATION OF THE COMPONENTS OF COMPLEMENT PARTICIPATING IN THE ANTIGLOBULIN REACTION, *IMMUNOLOGY*, 6, 412 (1963)

0988 HARKER L A, HEMOSTASIS MANUAL, *F A DAVIS CO (PHILADEPHIA)* (1974)

0989 HARRIS C C ET AL, SERUM ALPHA-1 ANTITRYPSIN IN PATIENTS WITH LUNG CANCER OR ABNORMAL SPUTUM CYTOLOGY, *CANCER*, 38, 1655-7 (1976)

0990 HARRIS H, ERYTHROPOIETIC PROTOPORPHYRIA, *ARCH DERMATOL*, 91, 85 (1968)

0991 HARRIS-JONES J N, HYPERURICEMIA AND ESSENTIAL HYPERCHOLESTEROLEMIA, *LANCET*, 1, 857 (1957)

0992 HARRISON, PRINCIPLES OF INTERNAL MEDICINE, *5TH EDITION MCGRAW-HILL CO* (1966)

0993 HARRISON H E, THE FANCONI SYNDROME, *J CHRONIC DIS*, 7, 346 (1958)

0994 HARRISON H E ET AL, GROWTH DISTURBANCE IN HEREDITARY HYPOPHOSPHATEMIA, *AM J DIS CHILD*, 112, 290 (1966)

0995 HARRISON T R, PRINCIPLES OF INTERNAL MEDICINE, *8TH EDITION NEW YORK MCGRAW-HILL* (1977)

0996 HARRISON, T. R., *PRINCIPALS OF INTERNAL MEDICINE, MCGRAW-HILL, NEW YORK*, 10TH EDITION (1983)

0997 HARTER J G, SERUM URIC ACID LEVELS IN PATIENTS WITH BRONCHIAL ASTHMA, *J ALLERGY CLIN IMMUNOL*, 42, 88 (1968)

0998 HARTOMA T R ET AL, SERUM ZINC AND SERUM COPPER AND INDICES OF DRUG METABOLISM IN ALCOHOLICS, *EUR J CLIN PHARMACOL*, 12, 147-51 (1977)

0999 HARVEY A M ET AL, THE PRINCIPLES AND PRACTICE OF MEDICINE, *19TH EDITION APPLETON-CENTURY-CROFTS* (1976)

1000 HASTRUP B ET AL, ACID PHOSPHATASE IN NIEMANN-PICK'S DISEASE AND A THERAPEUTIC EXPERIMENT WITH CORTISONE, *ACTA MED SCAND*, 149, 287-290 (1954)

1001 HATCH F E ET AL, NATURE OF THE RENAL CONCENTRATING DEFECT IN SICKLE CELL DISEASE, *J CLIN INVEST*, 46, 336 (1967)

1002 HAUG ET AL, DIE PLASMA/SERUM-ENZYMAKTIVITATEN DER LDH,MDH,GOT,GPT BEI NEUGEBORENEN UND ERWACHSENEN, *KLIN WOCHENSCHR*, 12, 680-683 (1965)

1003 HAUGEN H N, GLUCOSE AND ACETONE AS SOURCES OF ERROR IN PLASMA CREATININE DETERMINATIONS, *SCAND J CLIN LAB INVEST*, 6, 17-21 (1954)

1004 HAUGER-KLEVENE J H ET AL, PLASMA RENIN ACTIVITY IN HYPER- AND HYPOTHYROIDISM, *J CLIN ENDOCRINOL METAB*, 34, 625 (1972)

1005 HAUTMAN R ET AL, DIAGNOSIS OF RENAL TUMOR BY GAMMA GLUTAMYLTRANSPEPTIDASE, *UROLOGY*, 7, 12-16 (1976)

1006 HAVENS W P, LEUKOCYTIC RESPONSE OF PATIENTS WITH EXPERIMENTALLY INDUCED INFECTIOUS HEPATITIS, *AM J MED SCI*, 212, 129 (1946)

1007 HAWORTH ET AL, RELATION OF BLOOD-GLUCOSE TO HAEMATOCRIT, BIRTHWEIGHT, AND OTHER BODY MEASUREMENTS IN NORMAL AND GROWTH-RETARDED NEWBORN INFANTS, *J CLIN ENDOCR*, 2, 901-905 (1967)

1008 HAY D M ET AL, MATERNAL SERUM ALPHA-FETOPROTEIN IN ABNORMAL PREGNANCIES AND DURING INDUCED ABORTION, *J REPROD MED*, 19, 75-8 (1977)

1009 HAY ID, THYROIDITIS: A CLINICAL UPDATE, *MAYO CLIN PROC*, 60, 836-843 (1985)

1010 HAYES C P AND ROBINSON R R, FECAL POTASSIUM EXCRETION IN PATIENTS ON CHRONIC INTERMITTENT HEMODIALYSIS, *TRANS AM SOC ARTIF INTERN ORGAN*, 11, 242 (1965)

1011 HAYHOE F G J ET AL, THE CYTOLOGY AND CYTOCHEMISTRY OF ACUTE LEUKEMIAS, *LONDON HER MAJESTY'S STATIONERY OFFICE* (1964)

1012 HAYNES D M, MEDICAL COMPLICATIONS DURING PREGNANCY, *MCGRAW-HILL CO BLAKISTON DIVISION NEW YORK* (1969)

1013 HEALEY L A AND WILSKE K R, ANEMIA AS A PRESENTING MANIFESTATION OF GIANT CELL ARTERITIS, *ARTHRITIS RHEUM*, 14, 27 (1971)

1014 HEDBERG H, STUDIES ON THE DEPRESSED HEMOLYTIC COMPLEMENT ACTIVITY OF SYNOVIAL FLUID IN ADULT RHEUMATOID ARTHRITIS, *ACTA RHEUM SCAND*, 9, 165 (1963)

1015 HEDBERG H, STUDIES ON SYNOVIAL FLUID IN ARTHRITIS: I. TOTAL COMPLEMENT ACTIVITY, *ACTA MED SCAND (SUPPL)*, 479 (1967)

1016 HEDWORTH-WHITTY ET AL, SERUM GAMMA-GLUTAMYL TRANSPEPTIDASE ACTIVITY IN MYOCARDIAL ISCHEMIA, *BR HEART J*, 29, 432-8 (1967)

1017 HEIDMAN R C ET AL, CHRONIC GLOMERULONEPHRITIS ASSOCIATED WITH LOW SERUM COMPLEMENT ACTIVITY (CHRONIC HYPOCOMPLEMENTEMIC GLOMERULONEPHRITIS), *MEDICINE*, 49, 207 (1970)

1018 HEINE W I ET AL, ANTIBODIES TO CARDIAC TISSUE IN ACUTE ISCHEMIC HEART DISEASE, *AM J CARDIOL*, 17, 798 (1966)

1019 HEINZ JA, O'DONNEL NJ, LOTT JA, APPARENT MITOCHONDRIAL CREATINE KINASE IN THE SERUM OF A PATIENT WITH METASTATIC CANCER TO THE LIVER, *CLIN CHEM*, 26, 1908-1911 (1980)

1020 HELD BL, NADER S, RODRIGUEZ-RIGAU LJ, ET AL, ACNE AND HYPERANDROGENISM, *J AM ACAD DERMATOL*, 10, 223 (223-226)

1021 HELLE K B ET AL, CIRCULATING DOPAMINE B HYDROXYLASE (DBH) AND CATECHOLAMINES IN A PEDIATRIC PHAEOCHROMOCYTOMA, *CLIN EXP PHARMACOL PHYSIOL*, 3, 487-91 (1976)

1022 HELLER P ET AL, GLYCOLYTIC, CITRIC ACID CYCLE, AND HEXOSEMONOPHOSPHATE SHUNT ENZYMES OF PLASMA AND ERYTHROCYTES IN MEGALOBLASTIC ANEMIA, *J LAB CLIN MED*, 55, 425 (1960)

1023 HELLER P ET AL, ENZYMES IN ANEMIA: A STUDY OF ABNORMALITIES OF SEVERAL ENZYMES OF CARBOHYDRATE METABOLISM IN THE PLASMA AND ERYTHROCYTES IN PATIENTS WITH ANEMIA, WITH PRELIMINARY OBSERVATIONS OF BONE MARROW ENZYMES, *ANN INTERN MED*, 58, 898-913 (1963)

1024 HELLUM K B, NITROBLUE TETRAZOLIUM TEST IN PULMONARY THROMBOEMBOLISM AND PNEUMONIA, *SCAND J INFECT DIS*, 9, 131-34 (1977)

1025 HEMMINGSEN L ET AL, URINARY EXCRETION OF THE TEN PLASMA PROTEINS IN PATIENTS WITH EXTRARENAL EPITHELIAL CARCINOMA, *ACTA CHIR SCAND*, 143, 177-83 (1977)

1026 HENKIN RI, ON THE ROLE OF ADRENOCORTICOSTEROIDS IN THE CONTROL OF ZINC AND COPPER METABOLISM. TRACE ELEMENT METABOLISM IN ANIMALS, *UNIVERSITY PARK PRESS, BALTIMORE*, 2, 652-655 (1974)

1027 HENKIN RI, GROWTH-HORMONE-DEPENDENT CHANGES IN ZINC AND COPPER METABOLISM IN MAN. TRACE ELEMENT METABOLISM IN ANIMALS, *UNIVERSITY PARK PRESS, BALTIMORE*, 2, 652-655 (1974)

1028 HENLE W ET AL, EPSTEIN-BARR SPECIFIC DIAGNOSTIC TESTS IN INFECTIOUS MONONUCLEOSIS, *HUMAN PATHOL*, 5, 552 (1974)

1029 HENRIKSEN O A ET AL, EVALUATION OF THE ENDOCRINE FUNCTIONS IN DYSTROPHIA MYOTONICA, *ACTA NEUROL SCAND*, 58, 178-189 (1978)

1030 HENRY JB (ED), TODD-SANFORD-DAVIDSOHN CLINICAL DIAGNOSIS AND MANAGEMENT, *LABORATORY METHODS, 16TH ED. PHILADELPHA, W.B. SAUNDER CO.* (1979)

1031 HENRY R J, CLINICAL CHEMISTRY: PRINCIPLES AND TECHNICS, *HOEBER DIVISION HARPER AND ROW NEW YORK NY* (1964)

1032 HENRY RJ, CANNON DC, WINKELMAN JW, *CLINICAL CHEMISTRY: PRINCIPLES AND TECHNICS, 2ND ED, HARPER AND ROW, HAGERSTOWN* (1974)

1033 HERBERT F K, THE ESTIMATION OF PROSTATIC PHOSPHATASE IN SERUM AND ITS USE IN THE DIAGNOSIS OF PROSTATIC CARCINOMA, *Q J MED*, 15, 221-241 (1946)

1034 HERGT K, BLOOD LEVELS OF THROMBOCYTES IN BURNED PATIENTS: OBSERVATIONS ON THEIR BEHAVIOR IN RELATION TO THE CLINICAL CONDITION OF THE PATIENT, *J TRAUMA*, 12, 599 (1972)

1035 HERISHANU Y ET AL, THE CSF LIPID CONTENT IN BRAIN ATROPHY, *J NEUROL SCI*, 26, 583-6 (1975)

1036 HERRERA M G ET AL, CUSHING'S SYNDROME, DIAGNOSIS AND TREATMENT, *AM J SURG*, 107, 144 (1964)

1037 HERSHKO ET AL, LEAD POISONING, *ARCH INTERN MED*, 144, 1970 (1984)

1038 HEUCK C C ET AL, SERUM LIPIDS IN RENAL INSUFFICIENCY, *AM J CLIN NUTR*, 31, 1547-53 (1978)

1039 HEUMAN R, SJODAHL R, TOBIASSON P, TAGESSON C, POSTPRANDIAL SERUM BILE ACIDS IN RESECTED AND NON-RESECTED PATIENTS WITH CROHN'S DISEASE, *SCAND J GASTROENTEROL*, 17, 137-40 (1982)

1040 HEYNEN C, LE CALCITONINE SERIQUE DANS LA CIRRHOSE ETHYLIQUE, *CR SOC BIOL*, 171, 690 (1977)

1041 HEYNEN C AND FRANCHIMONT, HUMAN CALCITONIN RADIOIMMUNOASSAY IN NORMAL AND PATHOLOGICAL CONDITIONS, *EUR J CLIN INVEST*, 4, 213 (1974)

1042 HICKLING R A, LEUKAEMIA AND RELATED CONDITIONS IN THE BLOOD-URIC-ACID, *LANCET*, 1, 175 (1958)

1043 HIDLE I AND SJAASTAD O, BASAL METABOLIC RATE IN PATIENTS WITH HYDROCEPHALUS. ON THE CAUSE OF LOWERED BASAL METABOLIC RATE IN MYOTONIC DYSTROPHY, *ACTA NEUROL SCAND*, 53, 237-240 (1976)

1044 HIGGINS P J, THE THYROTOXICOSIS OF HYDATIDIFORM MOLE, *ANN INTERN MED*, 83, 307-311 (1975)

1045 HILDEN M ET AL, STUDIES ON THE SERUM LIPID AND LIPOPROTEINS IN STEATOSIS OF THE LIVER, *ACTA MED SCAND*, 198, 207-12 (1975)

1046 HILL, SERUM LACTIC DEHYDROGENASE IN CANCER PATIENTS, *J NATL CANCER INST*, 18, 307-313 (1957)

1047 HILL G S ET AL, SYSTEMIC LUPUS ERYTHEMATOSUS MORPHOLOGIC CORRELATIONS WITH IMMUNOLOGIC AND CLINICAL DATA AT THE TIME OF BIOPSY, *AM J MED*, 64, 61-79 (1978)

1048 HILLENBRAND P ET AL, SIGNIFICANCE OF INTRAVASCULAR COAGULATION AND FIBRINOLYSIS IN ACUTE HEPATIC FAILURE, *GUT*, 15, 83 (1974)

1049 HILLMAN R S FINCH C A, ERYTHROPOIESIS: NORMAL AND ABNORMAL, *SEMIN HEMATOL*, 4, 327 (1967)

1050 HIRAYAMA C ET AL, SERUM CHOLESTEROL AND BILE ACID IN PRIMARY HEPATOMA, *CLIN CHIM ACTA*, 71, 21-5 (1976)

1051 HIROHATA S, HIROSE S, MIYAMOTOTO T, CEREBROSPINAL FLUID IGM, IGA, AND IGG INDEXES IN SYSTEMIC LUPUS ERYTHEMATOSUS, *ARCH INTERN MED*, 145, 1843 (1985)

1052 HO ET AL, SERUM ACID PHOSPHATASE LEVELS IN UNTREATED CARCINOMA PATIENTS, *MISSOURI MED*, 289-290 (1975)

1053 HO W K K ET AL, COMPARISON OF PLASMA HORMONAL LEVELS BETWEEN HEROIN-ADDICTED AND NORMAL SUBJECTS, *CLIN CHIM ACTA*, 75, 415-19 (1977)

1054 HOCH-LIGETI ET AL, ENZYMES IN PERIPHERAL AND BONE MARROW SERUM IN PATIENTS WITH CANCER, *CANCER*, 38, 1336-1343 (1976)

1055 HOCHMAN H I ET AL, CHLORIDE-LOSING DIARRHEA AND METABOLIC ALKALOSIS IN AN INFANT WITH CYSTIC FIBROSIS, *ARCH DIS CHILD*, 51, 390 (1976)

1056 HODGES RE, BAKER EM, *MODERN NUTRITION IN HEALTH AND DISEASE, 5TH ED (EDS. R.S. GOODHART & M.E. SHILS)*, 245 (1973)

1057 HODGSON SF, DICKSON ER, WAHNER HW, ET AL, BONE LOSS AND REDUCED OSTEOBLAST FUNCTION IN PRIMARY BILIARY CIRRHOSIS, *ANN INTERN MED*, 103, 855-860 (1985)

1058 HOEPRICH P D, INFECTIOUS DISEASES, *2ND EDITION HARPER & ROW* (1977)

1059 HOFFBRAND A V ET AL, MEGALOBLASTIC ANAEMIA IN MYELOSCLEROSIS, *Q J MED*, 37, 493 (1968)

1060 HOFFBRAND B I, HAEMOLYTIC ANEMIA IN HODGKIN'S DISEASE ASSOCIATED WITH HIGH IMMUNOGLOBULIN DEFICIENCY, *BR J CANCER*, 18, 98 (1964)

1061 HOFFBRAND B I, HODGKIN'S DISEASE AND HYPOGAMMAGLOBULINEMIA: A RARE ASSOCIATION, *BR MED J*, 1, 1156 (1964)

1062 HOLBOROW E J ET AL, SMOOTH MUSCLE AUTO-ANTIBODIES IN INFECTIOUS MONONUCLEOSIS, *BR MED J*, 3, 323 (1973)

1063 HOLDSWORTH C E ET AL, COMPARATIVE BIOCHEMICAL STUDY OF OTOSCLEROSIS AND OSTEOGENESIS IMPERFECTA, *ARCH OTOLARYNGOL HEAD NECK SURG*, 98, 336-339 (1973)

1064 HOLMBERG CG, LAURELL CB, OXIDASE REACTIONS IN HUMAN PLASMA CAUSED BY CERULOPLASMIN, *SCAND J CLIN LAB INVEST*, 3, 07 (1951)

1065 HOLTON J B ET AL, BIOCHEMICAL INVESTIGATION OF HISTIDINAEMIA, *J CLIN PATHOL*, 17, 671 (1974)

1066 HOLZEL A ET AL, AMINOACIDURIA IN GALACTOSEMIA, *BR MED J*, 1, 194 (1952)

1067 HOLZEL A ET AL, GALACTOSEMIA, *AM J MED*, 22, 703 (1957)

1068 HOMBS K S ET AL, SERUM PROLACTIN LEVELS IN UNTREATED PRIMARY HYPOPARATHYROIDISM, *AM J MED*, 64, 787-88 (1978)

1069 HONG R AND GOOD R A, LIMITED HETEROGENEITY OF GAMMA GLOBULIN IN HYPOGAMMAGLOBULINEMIA, *SCIENCE*, 156, 1102 (1967)

1070 HOOSHMAND H, SERUM LACTATE DEHYDROGENASE ISOENZYMES IN NEUROMUSCULAR DISEASES, *DIS NERVOUS SYSTEM*, 36, 607-611 (1975)

1071 HOOSHMAND H ET AL, THE USE OF SERUM LACTATE DEHYDROGENASE ISOENZYMES IN THE DIAGNOSIS OF MUSCLE DISEASES, *NEUROL*, 19, 26-31 (1969)

1072 HORN B R ET AL, TOTAL EOSINOPHIL COUNTS IN THE MANAGEMENT OF BRONCHIAL ASTHMA, *N ENGL J MED*, 292, 1152-55 (1975)

1073 HORNE C H W ET AL, SERUM ALPHA2-MACROGLOBULIN, TRANSFERRIN, ALBUMIN, AND IGG LEVELS IN PRE-ECLAMPSIA, *J CLIN PATHOL*, 23, 514-516 (1970)

1074 HORNE CHW, HOWIE PW, WEIR RJ, GOUDIE RB, EFFECT OF COMBINED OESTROGEN-PROGESTOGEN ORAL CONTRACEPTIVES ON SERUM-LEVELS OF A2-MACROGLOBULIN, TRANSFERRIN, ALBUMIN AND IGG, *LANCET*, 1, 49-51 (1970)

1075 HORNE SHW, BRIGGS JD, HOWIE, PW, KENNEDY AL, SERUM A-MACROGLOBULINS IN RENAL DISEASE AND PREECLAMPSIA, *J CLIN PATHOL*, 25, 590-593 (1972)

1076 HORROBIN D F, THE ROLES OF PROSTAGLANDINS AND PROLACTIN IN DEPRESSION, MANIA AND SCHIZOPHRENIA, *POSTGRAD MED J*, 53, 198-201 (1977)

1077 HORSFALL F L AND TAMM I (EDS), VIRAL AND RICKETTSIAL INFECTIONS OF MAN, *4TH EDITION LIPPINCOTT PHILADELPHIA* (1965)

1078 HORTON L ET AL, THE HAEMATOLOGY OF HYPOTHYROIDISM, *Q J MED*, 45, 101-23 (1976)

1079 HORTON M A ET AL, REVERSIBLE C3 HYPOCOMPLEMENTAEMIA IN MEGALOBLASTIC ANEMIA DUE TO VITAMIN B$_{12}$ DEFICIENCY, *BR J HAEMATOL*, 36, 23-7 (1977)

1080 HORWITZ D L ET AL, PROINSULIN AND C-PEPTIDE IN DIABETES, *MED CLIN NORTH AM*, 62, 723-33 (1978)

1081 HORWITZ M S AND MOORE G T, ACUTE INFECTIOUS LYMPHOCYTOSIS: AN ETIOLOGIC AND EPIDEMIOLOGIC STUDY OF AN OUTBREAK, *N ENGL J MED*, 279, 399 (1968)

1082 HOUSLEY J, A2-MACROGLOBULIN LEVELS IN DISEASE IN MAN, *J CLIN PATHOL*, 21, 27-31 (1968)

1083 HOWARD AND THOMAS, CLINICAL DISORDERS OF CALCIUM HOMEOSTASIS, *MEDICINE*, 42, 25-45 (1963)

1084 HOWARD J E AND CONNOR T B, HYPERTENSION PRODUCED BY UNILATERAL RENAL DISEASE, *ARCH INTERN MED*, 100, 62 (1962)

1085 HOWARD P J ET AL, ELEVATION OF THE ACID PHOSPHATASE IN BENIGN PROSTATIC DISEASE, *J UROL*, 94, 687-690 (1965)

1086 HOWELL R R ET AL, GLUCOSE-6-PHOSPHATASE DEFICIENCY GLYCOGEN STORAGE DISEASE. STUDIES ON THE INTERRELATIONSHIP OF CARBOHYDRATE, LIPIDS, AND PURINE ABNORMALITIES, *PEDIATRICS*, 29, 553-65 (1967)

1087 HRGOVCIC M ET AL, SERUM COPPER LEVELS IN LYMPHOMA AND LEUKEMIA: SPECIAL REFERENCE TO HODGKIN'S DISEASE, *AM J MED*, 50, 56 (1971)

1088 HSIEH K H, CHANGES OF SERUM COMPLEMENT AND EOSINOPHIL COUNT IN ANTIGEN INDUCED BRONCHOSPASM, *ANN ALLERGY*, 41, 182-5 (1978)

1089 HSIEH K M ET AL, SERUM LACTIC DEHYDROGENASE LEVELS IN VARIOUS DISEASE STATES, *PROC SOC EXPER BIOL MED*, 91, 626-630 (1956)

1090 HSUEH W A ET AL, ENDOCRINE FEATURES OF KLINEFELTER'S SYNDROME, *MEDICINE*, 57, 447-62 (1978)

1091 HUANG Y S ET AL, PLASMA LIPIDS AND LIPOPROTEINS IN FRIEDREICH'S ATAXIA AND FAMILIAL SPASTIC ATAXIA--EVIDENCE FOR AN ABNORMAL COMPOSITION OF HIGH DENSITY LIPOPROTEINS, *CAN J NEUROL SCI*, 5, 149-56. (1978)

1092 HUCKAUF H ET AL, OXYGEN AFFINITY OF HAEMOGLOBIN AND RED CELL ACID-BASE STATUS IN PATIENTS WITH SEVERE CHRONIC OBSTRUCTIVE LUNG DISEASE, *BRIT J CANCER*, 12, 129-42 (1976)

1093 HUDSON BRENDLER AND SCOTT, A SIMPLE METHOD FOR THE DETERMINATION OF SERUM ACID PHOSPHATASE, *J UROL*, 58, 89-92 (1947)

1094 HUDSON ET AL, PROSTATIC CANCER: EXTREMELY ELEVATED SERUM ACID PHOSPHATASE ASSOCIATED WITH ALTERED LIVER FUNCTION, *AM J MED*, 19, 898-901 (1955)

1095 HUFF B ET AL, SUPPLEMENT B, PHYSICIANS' DESK REFERENCE, *MEDICAL ECONOMICS INC ORADELL, NJ* (1972)

1096 HUGHES W T ET AL, SIGNS, SYMPTOMS, AND PATHOPHYSIOLOGY OF PNEUMOCYSTIS CARINII PNEUMONITIS, *NCI MONOGR*, 43, 77-88 (1976)

1097 HUIJING F ET AL, DIAGNOSIS OF GENERALIZED GLYCOGEN STORAGE DISEASE (POMPE'S DISEASE), *J PEDIATR*, 63, 984 (1963)

1098 HULLIN R P ET AL, RENIN AND ALDOSTERONE RELATIONSHIPS IN MANIC DEPRESSIVE PSYCHOSIS, *BR J PSYCHIATRY*, 131, 575-81 (1977)

1099 HULTBERG B ET AL, DIAGNOSTIC VALUE OF DETERMINATIONS OF LYSOSOMAL HYDROLASES IN CSF OF PATIENTS WITH NEUROLOGICAL DISEASE, *ACTA NEUROL SCAND*, 57, 201-15 (1978)

1100 HUME R AND GOLDBERG A, ACTUAL AND PREDICTED NORMAL RED-CELL AND PLASMA VOLUMES IN PRIMARY AND SECONDARY POLYCYTHEMIA, *CLIN SCI*, 26, 499 (1964)

1101 HUMPHREY C S, GLUCOSE TOLERANCE AND INSULIN SECRETION IN PATIENTS WITH CHRONIC DUODENAL ULCER, *BR MED J*, 4, 393 (1972)

1102 HUMPHRIES LL, ADAMS LJ, ECKFELDT JH, ET AL, HYPERAMYLASEMIA IN PATIENTS WITH EATING DISORDERS, *ANN INTERN MED*, 106, 50-52 (1987)

1103 HUNT ET AL, ENZYME CHANGES FOLLOWING DIRECT CURRENT COUNTERSHOCK, *AM HEART J*, 76, 340-344 (1968)

1104 HUNTER ET AL, ALTERED CALCIUM METABOLISM IN EPILEPTIC CHILDREN ON ANTICONVULSANTS, *BR MED J*, 4, 202-204 (1971)

1105 HUNTER G ET AL, TROPICAL MEDICINE, *5TH EDITION W B SAUNDERS PHILADELPHIA* (1976)

1106 HURLEY J R, THYROIDITIS, *DM*, 24, 13-15, 35-38 (1977)

1107 HURST D W AND MEYER O O, GIANT FOLLICULAR LYMPHOBLASTOMA, *CANCER*, 14, 753 (1961)

1108 HURST J WILLIS ED, THE HEART, *4TH EDITION MCGRAW-HILL CO* (1978)

1109 HURTER R ET AL, SOME IMMEDIATE AND LONG-TERM EFFECTS OF EXERCISE ON THE PLASMA-LIPIDS, *LANCET*, 2, 671 (1972)

1110 HUSDAN ET AL, EFFECT OF VENOUS OCCLUSION OF THE ARM ON THE CONCENTRATION OF CALCIUM IN SERUM, AND METHODS FOR ITS COMPENSATION, *CLIN CHEM*, 20, 529-532 (1974)

1111 HUSSA RO, CLINICAL UTILITY OF HUMAN CHORIONIC GONADOTROPIN AND ALPHA-SUBUNIT MEASUREMENTS, *OBSTET GYNECOL*, 60, 1-12 (1982)

1112 HUSSAN J M ET AL, SYSTEMIC SCLEROSIS AND CRYOGLOBULINEMIA, *CLIN IMMUNOL IMMUNOPATHOL*, 6, 77 (1976)

1113 HYTTEN F E AND LEITCH I, THE PHYSIOLOGY OF HUMAN PREGNANCY, *2ND EDITION BLACKWELL SCIENTIFIC PUBL OXFORD* (1971)

1114 IGARI T ET AL, CATECHOLAMINE METABOLISM IN THE PATIENTS WITH RHEUMATOID ARTHRITIS, *TOHOKU J EXP MED*, 122, 9-20 (1977)

1115 IHDE D C ET AL, CLINICAL MANIFESTATIONS OF HEPATOMA, *AM J MED*, 56, 83-91 (1974)

1116 IKAWA S, ET AL, MEASUREMENT OF THE RATIO OF PRIMARY TO TOTAL BILE ACIDS IN SERUM BY ENZYMATIC FLUOROMETRIC MICROASSAY AND ITS CLINICAL SIGNIFICANCE IN PATIENTS WITH LIVER DISEASE, *TOHOKU J EXP MED*, 145, 185-95 (1985)

1117 IKAWA S, KAWASAKI H, YAMANISHI Y, MURA T, ET AL, MEASUREMENT OF THE RATIO OF PRIMARY TO TOTAL BILE ACIDS IN SERUM BY ENZYMATIC FLUOROMETRIC MICROASSAY AND ITS CLINICAL SIGNIFICANCE IN PATIENTS WITH LIVER DISEASE, *TOHOKU J EXP MED*, 145, 185-95 (1985)

1118 IMHOF P R ET AL, EXCRETION OF URINARY CASTS AFTER THE ADMINISTRATION OF DIURETICS, *BR MED J*, 2, 199 (1972)

1119 IMRIE C W ET AL, PROCEEDINGS: HYPOCALCAEMIA OF ACUTE PANCREATITIS: THE EFFECT OF HYPOALBUMINAEMIA, *BR J SURG*, 63, 662-3 (1976)

1120 INAR S ET AL, SERUM LEVEL OF THE FOURTH COMPONENT OF COMPLEMENT IN VARIOUS DISEASES, *BIKEN J*, 10, 65-87 (1967)

1121 INDIVERI F, PIERRI I, ROGNA S, POGGI A, ET AL, ABNORMALITIES OF T CELLS ISOLATED FROM MEDIASTINAL LYMPH NODES AND PERIPHERAL BLOOD OF PATIENTS WITH LUNG CARCINOMA: DEFICIT IN PHA-INDUCED EXPRESSION OF HLA CLASS II ANTIGENS AND IN AUTOLOGOUS MIXED LYMPHOCYTE REACTIONS, *CANCER IMMUNOL IMMUNOTHER*, 22, 232-5 (1986)

1122 INGENBLEEK Y ET AL, TRIIODOTHYRONINE AND THYROID-STIMULATING HORMONE IN PROTEIN CALORIE MALNUTRITION, *LANCET*, 2, 845-8 (1975)

1123 INGENBLEEK Y ET AL, T₃ RESIN UPTAKE IN PROTEIN-CALORIE MALNUTRITION, *ACTA ENDOCRINOL*, 81, 283-7 (1976)

1124 INOUE T, OKAMURA M, AMATSU K, ET AL, SERUM LACTATE DEHYDROGENASE AND ITS ISOZYMES IN LUPUS NEPHRITIS, *ARCH INTERN MED*, 146, 548 (1986)

1125 INUTSUKA S I, PLASMA COPPER AND ZINC LEVELS IN PATIENTS WITH MALIGNANT TUMORS OF DIGESTIVE ORGANS, *CANCER*, 42, 626-31 (1978)

1126 IRANI F A ET AL, SERUM LACTIC DEHYDROGENASE IN PNEUMONIA, *SOUTH MED J*, 65, 858, 874 (1972)

1127 ISOBE T AND OSSERMAN E, PATTERNS OF AMYLOIDOSIS AND THEIR ASSOCIATION WITH PLASMA CELL DYSCRASIAS, MONOCLONAL IMMUNOGLOBULINS AND BENCE-JONES PROTEINS, *N ENGL J MED*, 290, 473 (1974)

1128 ISRAEL H L ET AL, LATEX FIXATION TESTS IN SARCOIDOSIS, *ACTA MED SCAND*, 176(SUPPL 425), 40 (1964)

1129 ITO H, TAKAGI Y, ANDO Y, KUBO A, ET AL, SERUM FERRITIN LEVELS IN PATIENTS WITH CERVICAL CANCER, *OBSTET GYNECOL*, 55, 358-62 (1980)

1130 ITOH T ET AL, STUDIES ON SERUM GASTRIN OF THE PATIENTS WITH GASTRIC CANCER, *AM J GASTROENTEROL*, 68, 56-63 (1977)

1131 JACKSON B, JOHNSTON CI, ANGIOTENSIN CONVERTING ENZYME DURING ACUTE AND CHRONIC ENALAPRIL THERAPY IN ESSENTIAL HYPERTENSION, *CLIN EXP PHARMACOL PHYSIOL*, 11, 355-9 (1984)

1132 JACOBELLI S, MCCARTY, SILCOX DC, MALL JC, CALCIUM PYROPHOSPHATE DIHYDRATE CRYSTAL DEPOSITION IN NEUROPATHIC JOINTS. FOUR CASES OF POLYARTICULAR INVOLVEMENT, *ANN INTERN MED*, 79, 340-347 (1973)

1133 JACOBS, CALCIUM AND MYOCARDIAL INFARCTION, *S A MEDICAL JOURNAL*, 48, 1553-1554 (1974)

1134 JACOBS S L AND FERNANDEZ A A, HEMOGLOBIN IN PLASMA, *STAND METH CLIN CHEM*, 6, 107 (1970)

1135 JACOBSEN J G ET AL, SERUM ACID PHOSPHATASE IN OSTEOGENESIS IMPERFECTA, *METABOLISM*, 10, 483-488 (1961)

1136 JAFFE BM, BEHRMAN HR, *METHODS OF HORMONE RADIOIMMUNOASSAY. NEW YORK, ACADEMIC PRESS* (1979)

1137 JAFFE ET AL, DIAGNOSTIC SIGNIFICANCE OF SERUM ALKALINE AND ACID PHOSPHATASE VALUES IN RELATION TO BONE DISEASE, *BULL NY ACAD MED*, 19, 831-848 (1943)

1138 JAGER B V, CRYOFIBRINOGENEMIA, *N ENGL J MED*, 266, 579 (1962)

1139 JAGWE J G ET AL, A STUDY OF SERUM URIC ACID IN ADULT PATIENTS WITH TROPICAL SPLENOMEGALY SYNDROME, *EAST AFR MED J*, 54, 74-6 (1977)

1140 JAIN V K ET AL, ESTIMATION OF COPPER IN SERUM, ERYTHROCYTE AND URINE IN PROTEIN CALORIE MALNUTRITION, *INDIAN J PEDIATR*, 13, 767-70. (1976)

1141 JAMES K, A STUDY OF THE ALPHA-2-MACROGLOBULIN HOMOLOGUES OF VARIOUS SPECIES, *IMMUNOLOGY*, 8, 55-61 (1965)

1142 JAMES K, MERRIMAN J, GRAY RS, DUNCAN LJP, HERD R, SERUM A2-MACROGLOBULIN LEVELS IN DIABETES, *J CLIN PATHOL*, 33, 163-166 (1980)

1143 JAMESON S, ZINC AND COPPER IN PREGNANCY, CORRELATIONS TO FETAL AND MATERNAL COMPLICATIONS, *ACTA MED SCAND (SUPPL)*, 593, 5-20 (1976)

1144 JAMESON S LEHFELDT H, LOW SERUM ZINC CONCENTRATIONS IN PREGNANCY, RESULTS OF INVESTIGATIONS AND TREATMENT, *ACTA MED SCAND (SUPPL)*, 593, 50-64 (1976)

1145 JAMIESON ET AL, CHANGES IN SERUM PHOSPHATE LEVELS ASSOCIATED WITH INTESTINAL INFARCTION AND NECROSIS, *SUR GYN AND OBST*, 140, 19-21 (1975)

1146 JAN K M ET AL, OBSERVATIONS ON BLOOD VISCOSITY CHANGES AFTER ACUTE MYOCARDIAL INFARCTION, *CIRCULATION*, 51, 1079 (1975)

1147 JANDL J ET AL, THE ANEMIA OF LIVER DISEASE, *J CLIN INVEST*, 34, 390 (1955)

1148 JANSSON E ET AL, COLD AGGLUTININS IN PNEUMONIA, *ACTA MED SCAND*, 175, 747 (1964)

1149 JARA P, CODOCEO R, HERNANZ A, D'IAZ MC, ET AL, SERUM PROFILE OF BILE ACIDS IN CHILDREN WITH NEONATAL HEPATITIS AND EXTRAHEPATIC BILIARY ATRESIAL, *AN ESP PEDIATR*, 20, 837-41 (1984)

1150 JARNEROT G ET AL, THE THYROID IN ULCERATIVE COLITIS AND CROHN'S DISEASE, *ACTA MED SCAND*, 199, 229-32 (1976)

1151 JARROLD R AND VILTER R W, HEMATOLOGIC OBSERVATIONS IN PATIENTS WITH CHRONIC HEPATIC INSUFFICIENCY, *J CLIN INVEST*, 28, 286 (1949)

1152 JARSTRAND C ET AL, PERIPHERAL BLOOD LYMPHOCYTE POPULATIONS IN INFLUENZA PATIENTS, *SCAND J INFECT DIS*, 9, 1-3 (1977)

1153 JATZKEWITZ H AND MEHL E, CEREBROSIDE SULPHATASE AND ARYL SULPHATASE A DEFICIENCY IN METACHROMATIC LEUKODYSTROPHY (ML), *J NEUROCHEM*, 16, 19 (1969)

1154 JAVITT N B, CHOLESTATIC JAUNDICE, *MED CLIN NORTH AM*, 59, 817-821 (1975)

1155 JAYSON M I ET AL, SERUM COPPER AND CAERULOPLASMIN IN ANKYLOSING SPONDYLITIS, SYSTEMIC SCLEROSIS, AND MORPHEA, *ANN RHEUM DIS*, 35, 443-5 (1975)

1156 JEFFREE G M, ENZYMES IN FIBROBLASTIC LESIONS, *J BONE JOINT SURG*, 54, 535-546 (1972)

1157 JEGATHEESAN ET AL, CORRELATION OF SERUM GLYCOLYTIC ENZYMES AND ACID PHOSPHATASES WITH SITES OF METASTASES IN MAMMARY CARCINOMATOSIS, *BR MED J*, 1, 831-834 (1962)

1158 JENSEN H ET AL, THE TURNOVER OF IG G AND IG M IN MYOTONIC DYSTROPHY, *NEUROL*, 21, 68 (1971)

1159 JENSEN J ET AL, BLOOD URIC ACID LEVELS IN FAMILIAL HYPERCHOLESTEROLEMIA, *LANCET*, 1, 298 (1966)

1160 JENSEN K B ET AL, ALBUMIN AND IGG TURNOVER IN ULCERATIVE COLITIS AND CROHNS DISEASE, *PLASMA PROTEIN TURNOVER. BALTIMORE, UNIVERSITY PARK PRESS* (1974)

1161 JENSEN K B ET AL, SERUM OROSOMUCOID IN ULCERATIVE COLITIS: ITS RELATION TO CLINICAL ACTIVITY, PROTEIN LOSS, AND TURNOVER OF ALBUMIN AND IGG, *SCAND J GASTROENTEROL*, 11, 177-83 (1976)

1162 JESSOP S ET AL, ERYTHROCYTE ELECTROLYTE CONTENT AND SODIUM EFFLUX IN CHRONIC RENAL FAILURE, *NEPHRON*, 18, 82-87 (1977)

1163 JEWITT D E ET AL, FREE NORADRENALINE AND ADRENALINE EXCRETION IN RELATION TO THE DEVELOPMENT OF CARDIAC ARRHYTHMIAS AND HEART FAILURE IN PATIENTS WITH ACUTE MYOCARDIAL INFARCTION, *J CLIN ENDOCR*, 1, 635-41 (1969)

1164 JIMENEZ-ALONSO J, JAIMEZ L, BARRIOS L, ET AL, SALIVARY GAMMA-GLUTAMYL TRANSFERASE ACTIVITY INTERNAL DISEASES, *ARCH INTERN MED*, 144, 1804 (1984)

1165 JOELSSON B, HULTBERG B, ALWMARK A, ET AL, TOTAL SERUM BILE ACIDS, GAMMA-GLUTAMYL TRANSFERASE, PREALBUMIN, AND TYROSINE: SENSITIVE SERUM MARKERS OF HEPATIC DYSFUNCTION IN ALCOHOLIC LIVER CIRRHOSIS, *SCAND J GASTROENTEROL*, 18, 497-501 (1983)

1166 JOELSSON B, HULTBERG B, ISAKSSON A, ET AL, TOTAL FASTING SERUM BILE ACIDS AND BETA-HEXOSAMINIDASE IN ALCOHOLIC LIVER DISEASE, *CLIN CHIM ACTA*, 31, 203-9 (1984)

1167 JOHANSSON B AND ROOS B, 5-HIAA AND HVA IN SPINAL FLUID AND HERPES ZOSTER OTICUS, *N ENGL J MED*, 285, 637 (1971)

1168 JOHANSSON BG, KINDMARK CO, TRELL EY, ET AL, SEQUENTIAL CHANGES OF PLASMA PROTEINS AFTER MYOCARDIAL INFARCTION, *SCAND J CLIN LAB INVEST*, 29 SUPPL 124, 117-126 (1972)

1169 JOHANSSON E A ET AL, FREE SERUM CALCIUM IN URTICARIA, *ACTA ALLERGOLOGICA*, 29, 25-29 (1975)

1170 JOHANSSON S G O, RAISED LEVELS OF A NEW IMMUNOGLOBULIN CLASS (IGD) IN ASTHMA, *LANCET*, 2, 951 (1967)

1171 JOHN WG, GLYCOSYLATED HAEMOGLOBIN LEVELS IN PATIENTS REFERRED FOR ORAL GLUCOSE TOLERANCE TESTS, *DIABETIC MED*, 3, 46-8 (1986)

1172 JOHNSEN T, EFFECT UPON SERUM INSULIN, GLUCOSE AND POTASSIUM CONCENTRATIONS OF ACETAZOLAMIDE DURING ATTACKS OF FAMILIAL PERIODIC HYPOKALEMIC PARALYSIS, *ACTA NEUROL SCAND*, 56, 533-41 (1977)

1173 JOHNSEN T, FAMILIAL PERIODIC PARALYSIS WITH HYPOKALEMIA, *DAN MED BULL*, 28, 1-27 (1981)

1174 JOHNSON AG, MCDERMOTT SG, LYSOLECITHIN: A FACTOR IN THE PATHOGENESIS OF GASTRIC ULCERATION?, *GUT*, 15, 710-713 (1974)

1175 JOHNSON ET AL, CLINICAL SIGNIFICANCE OF SERUM ACID PHOSPHATASE LEVELS IN ADVANCED PROSTATIC CARCINOMA, *UROLOGY*, 8, 123-126 (1976)

1176 JOHNSON R H ET AL, HUMAN GROWTH HORMONE AND KETOSIS IN ATHLETES AND NON-ATHLETES, *NATURE*, 236, 119 (1972)

1177 JOHNSON TR, MOORE WN, JEFFERIES JE, CHILDREN ARE DIFFERENT: DEVELOPMENTAL PHYSIOLOGY, *2ND ED. COLUMBUS, OHIO, ROSS LABORATORIES* (1978)

1178 JOHNSTON D G ET AL, HYPERINSULINISM OF HEPATIC CIRRHOSIS: DIMINISHED DEGRADATION OR HYPERSECRETION, *LANCET*, 1, 10-13 (1977)

1179 JONES E M M AND WILSON D C, CLINICAL FEATURES OF YELLOW FEVER CASES AT VOM CHRISTIAN HOSPITAL DURING THE 1969 EPIDEMIC ON THE JOS PLATEAU NIGERIA, *BULL WHO*, 46, 653-7 (1977)

1180 JONES J E ET AL, MAGNESIUM METABOLISM IN HYPERTHYROIDISM AND HYPOTHYROIDISM, *J CLIN INVEST*, 45, 891 (1966)

1181 JONES J W AND WAYS P, ABNORMALITIES OF HIGH DENSITY LIPOPROTEINS IN ABETALIPOPROTEINEMIA, *J CLIN INVEST*, 46, 1151 (1967)

1182 JONES M AND MELLIRSH V, A COMPARISON OF THE EXERCISE RESPONSE IN VARIOUS GROUPS OF NEUROTIC PATIENTS, AND A METHOD OF RAPID DETERMINATION OF OXYGEN IN EXPIRED AIR USING A CATHAROMETER, *PSYCHOSOM MED*, 1, 192 (1946)

1183 JONES MB, WEINSTOCK S, KORETZ RL, ET AL, CLINICAL VALUE OF SERUM BILE ACID LEVELS IN CHRONIC HEPATITIS, *DIG DIS SCI*, 26, 978-83 (1981)

1184 JONES N F ET AL, HYPOPROTEINEMIA IN ANAPHYLACTOID PURPURA, *BR MED J*, 2, 1166 (1966)

1185 JONES P A E ET AL, FERRITINEMIA IN LEUKEMIA AND HODGKIN'S DISEASE, *BR J CANCER*, 27, 212 (1973)

1186 JONES S E, AUTOIMMUNE DISORDERS AND MALIGNANT LYMPHOMA, *CANCER*, 31, 1092 (1973)

1187 JONES S R, THE ABSOLUTE GRANULOCYTE COUNT IN ASCITES FLUID, *WEST J MED*, 126, 344 (1977)

1188 JORDAN R M ET AL, CEREBROSPINAL FLUID HORMONE CONCENTRATION IN THE EVALUATION OF PITUITARY TUMORS, *ANN INTERN MED*, 85, 49-55 (1976)

1189 JORDAN RM, KENDALL JW, SEAICH JL, ET AL, CEREBROSPINAL FLUID HORMONE CONCENTRATION IN THE EVALUATION OF PITUITARY TUMORS, *ANN INTERN MED*, 85, 49-55 (1976)

1190 JORDAN T W ET AL, ENZYMIC DETECTION OF METACHROMATIC LEUKODYSTROPHY PATIENTS AND HETEROZYGOTES, *NZ MED J*, 85, 369-72 (1977)

1191 JORDON RM, KENDALL JW, DEAICH JL, CSF HORMONE CONCENTRATION IN THE EVALUATION OF PITUITARY TUMORS, *ANN INTERN MED*, 85, 49-55 (1976)

1192 JORGENSEN F S ET AL, PLASMA LIPIDS AND LIPOPROTEINS IN YOUNG PATIENTS WITH BRAIN INFARCTION, *ACTA NEUROL SCAND*, 57, 432-7 (1978)

1193 JORGENSON G, UNTERSUCHINGEN GUR GENETIK DER SARKOIDOSE, *HUTHIGS HABIL SCHRIFT GOTTINGEN HEIDELBERG GERMANY* (1965)

1194 JORPES E AND RAMGREN O, THE HAEMOPHILIA SITUATION IN SWEDEN, *ACTA MED SCAND*, 171, 23 (1962)

1195 JOSEPH J C ET AL, CHANGES IN PLASMA PROTEINS DURING PREGNANCY, *ANN CLIN LAB SCI*, 8, 130-41 (1978)

1196 JUENGST D ET AL, URINARY CHOLESTEROL EXCRETION IN MEN WITH BENIGN PROSTATIC HYPERPLASIA AND CARCINOMA OF THE PROSTATE., *CANCER*, 43, 353-359 (1979)

1197 JUMA FD, GITAU W, BWIBO NO, GACHOKA C, HAEMOGLOBIN A1C IN CHILDREN WITH SICKLE CELL DISEASE, *EAST AFR MED J*, 61, 32-34 (JAN 1984)

1198 JUNG K, DIEGO J, STROBELT V, ET AL, DIAGNOSTIC SIGNIFICANCE OF SOME URINARY ENZYMES FOR DETECTING ACUTE REJECTION CRISES IN RENAL-TRANSPLANT RECIPIENTS: ALANINE AMINOPEPTIDASE,ALKALINE PHOSPHATASE, Y-GLUTAMYLTRANSFERASE, N-ACETYL-B-D-GLUCOSAMINIDASE AND LYSOZYME, *CLIN CHEM*, 32/10, 1807-1811 (1986)

1199 JUNG K, SCHOLZ D, AN OPTIMIZED ASSAY OF ALANINE AMINOPEPTIDASE ACTIVITY IN URINE, *CLIN CHEM*, 26, 1251-1254 (1980)

1200 JUNG L C AND CAVALIERI R P, T_3 THYROTOXICOSIS DUE TO METASTATIC THYROID CARCINOMA, *J CLIN ENDOCRINOL METAB*, 36, 215 (1973)

1201 JURGA L ET AL, IMPORTANCE OF DETERMINATIONS OF SERUM HEXOKINASE, ALDOLASE, AND LACTATE DEHYDROGENASE ACTIVITIES, AND OF THE LACTATE/PYRUVATE QUOTIENT IN THE DIAGNOSIS OF MALIGNANT TUMORS, *NEOPLASMA*, 25, 95-106 (1978)

1202 JUUL, HUMAN PLASMA CHOLINESTERASE ISOENZYMES, *CLIN CHIM ACTA*, 19, 205 (1968)

1203 KABADI UM, SERUM T_3 AND REVERSE T_3 CONCENTRATIONS: INDICES OF METABOLIC CONTROL IN DIABETES MELLITUS, *DIABETES RES*, 3, 417-421 (1986)

1204 KABAKOW B ET AL, HYPERCALCEMIA IN HODGKIN'S DISEASE, *N ENGL J MED*, 256, 59 (1967)

1205 KACHADORIAN W A AND JOHNSON R E, THE EFFECT OF EXERCISE ON SOME CLINICAL MEASURES OF RENAL FUNCTION, *AM HEART J*, 82, 278 (1971)

1206 KAFER E R, IDIOPATHIC SCOLIOSIS, *J CLIN INVEST*, 58, 825-33 (1976)

1207 KAGAN I G, TRICHINOSIS: A REVIEW OF BIOLOGIC, SEROLOGIC AND IMMUNOLOGIC ASPECTS, *J INFECT DIS*, 107, 65 (1960)

1208 KAGER L ET AL, SERUM MYOGLOBIN IN MYOCARDIAL INFARCTION: THE STACCATO PHENOMENON, *AM J MED*, 62, 86-91 (1977)

1209 KAISER R ET AL, SERUM AMYLASE CHANGES DURING PREGNANCY, *AM J OBSTET GYNECOL*, 122, 283 (1975)

1210 KAKIZAKI G ET AL, A NEW DIAGNOSTIC TEST FOR PANCREATIC DISORDERS BY EXAMINATION OF PAROTID SALIVA, *AM J GASTROENTEROL*, 65, 437-46 (1976)

1211 KALBERG B E ET AL, AGE, BLOOD PRESSURE, RENIN AND URINARY ELECTROLYTES IN PRIMARY HYPERTENSION AND IN THE NORMOTENSIVE STATE, *SCAND J CLIN LAB INVEST*, 38, 319-27 (1978)

1212 KALBFLEISCH J M AND R M BIRD, CRYOFIBRINOGENEMIA, *N ENGL J MED*, 263, 881 (1960)

1213 KALIN E M, CEREBROSPINAL-FLUID ACID BASE AND ELECTROLYTE CHANGES RESULTING FROM CEREBRAL ANOXIA IN MAN, *N ENGL J MED*, 293, 1013-6. (1975)

1214 KAM-HANSEN S ET AL, B AND T LYMPHOCYTES IN CEREBROSPINAL FLUID AND BLOOD IN MULTIPLE SCLEROSIS, OPTIC NEURITIS AND MUMPS MENINGITIS, *ACTA NEUROL SCAND*, 58, 95-103 (1978)

1215 KANAI M RAY A AND GOODMAN D S, RADIOIMMUNOASSAY OF HUMAN PLASMA RETINOL-BINDING PROTEIN, *J CLIN INVEST*, 47, 2025 (1968)

1216 KANE S ET AL, INDICES OF GRANULOCYTE ACTIVITY IN INFLAMMATORY BOWEL DISEASE, *GUT*, 15, 953-99 (1974)

1217 KANESHIGE H, NONENZYMATIC GLYCOSYLATION OF SERUM IGG AND ITS EFFECT ON ANTIBODY ACTIVITY IN PATIENTS WITH DIABETES MELLITUS, *DIABETES*, 36, 822-8 (1987)

1218 KANKAANRINTA T, ON THE PREGNANEDIOL EXCRETION IN THE URINE DURING THE LAST TRIMESTER OF NORMAL AND TOXEMIC PREGNANCY, *SCAND J CLIN LAB INVEST*, 15(SUPPL), 74 (1963)

1219 KAPLAN, ALKALINE PHOSPHATASE, *N ENGL J MED*, 28, 200-202 (1972)

1220 KAPLAN ET AL, INDUCTION OF ALKALINE PHOSPHATASE BY THE OBSTRUCTED LIVER, *J CLIN INVEST*, 48, 42A (1969)

1221 KAPLAN ET AL, SEPARATION OF HUMAN SERUM-ALKALINE-PHOSPHATASE ISOENZYMES BY POLYACRYLAMIDE GEL ELECTROPHORESIS, *J CLIN ENDOCR*, 2, 1029-1031 (1969)

1222 KAPLAN ET AL, INDUCTION OF RAT LIVER ALKALINE PHOSPHATASE:THE MECHANISM OF THE SERUM ELEVATION IN BILE DUCT OBSTRUCTION, *J CLIN INVEST*, 49, 508-516 (1970)

1223 KAPLAN N M ET AL, SINGLE-VOIDED URINE METANEPHRINE ASSAYS IN SCREENING FOR PHEOCHROMOCYTOMA, *ARCH INTERN MED*, 137, 190 (1977)

1224 KAPLOWITZ N ET AL, ISOLATION OF ERYTHROCYTES WITH NORMAL PROTOPORPHYRIN LEVELS IN ERYTHROPOIETIC PORPHYRIA, *N ENGL J MED*, 278, 1077 (1968)

1225 KAPPELER R ET AL, KLINIK DER MAKROGLOBULINAMIE WALDENSTRÖM: BESCHREIBUNG VAN 21 FALLEN-UBERSICHT DER LITERATUR, *CLINICS IN GASTROENTEROLOGY, (ED. W. SIRCUS), W. B. SAUNDERS PHILADELPHIA*, 25, 54 (1958)

1226 KAPTEIN ET AL., THYROID HORMONE INDEXES, *ARCH INTERN MED*, 144, 314 (1984)

1227 KARANDANIS D, SHULMAN JA, RECENT SURVEY OF INFECTIOUS MENINGITIS IN ADULTS: A REVIEW OF LABORATORY FINDINGS IN BACTERIAL, TUBERCULOUS AND ASEPTIC MENINGITIS, *SOUTH MED J*, 69, 449-457 (1976)

1228 KARETZKY M S, BLOOD STUDIES IN UNTREATED PATIENTS WITH ACUTE ASTHMA, *AM REV RESPIR DIS*, 112, 607 (1975)

1229 KARMEN A ET AL, TRANSAMINASE ACTIVITY IN HUMAN BLOOD, *J CLIN INVEST*, 34, 126-131 (1955)

1230 KARPATKIN S ET AL, AUTOIMMUNE THROMBOCYTOPENIC PURPURA AND THE COMPENSATED THROMBOCYTOLYTIC STATE, *AM J MED*, 51, 1 (1971)

1231 KARVOUNTZIS G G ET AL, RELATION OF ALPHA-FETOPROTEIN IN ACUTE HEPATITIS TO SEVERITY AND PROGNOSIS, *ANN INTERN MED*, 80, 156-60 (1974)

1232 KASPER C K ET AL, CLINICAL ASPECTS OF IRON DEFICIENCY, *JAMA*, 191, 359 (1965)

1233 KATAYAMA I ET AL, HISTOCHEMICAL STUDY OF ACID PHOSPHATASE ISOENZYME IN LEUKEMIC RETICULOENDOTHELIOSIS, *CANCER*, 29, 157-164 (1972)

1234 KATSUNUMA T, TSUDA M, KUSUMI T, ET AL, PURIFICATION OF A SERUM DNA BINDING PROTEIN (64DP) WITH A MOLECULAR WEIGHT OF 64,000 AND ITS DIAGNOSTIC SIGNIFICANCE IN MALIGNANT DISEASES, *BIOCHEM BIOPHYS RES COMMUN*, 93, 552-557 (1980)

1235 KATTWINKEL J ET AL, THE EFFECTS OF AGE ON ALKALINE PHOSPHATASE AND OTHER SEROLOGIC LIVER FUNCTION TESTS IN NORMAL SUBJECTS AND PATIENTS WITH CYSTIC FIBROSIS, *J PEDIATR*, 82, 234 (1973)

1236 KATZMANN JA, *MAYO CLIN PROC*, 61, 752 (1986)

1237 KAUFMAN D B ET AL, SECRETORY IGA IN URINARY TRACT INFECTIONS, *BR MED J*, 4, 463-465 (1970)

1238 KAUFMAN D M ET AL, SUBDURAL EMPYEMA: ANALYSIS OF 17 RECENT CASES AND REVIEW OF THE LITERATURE., *MEDICINE*, 54, 485-498 (1975)

1239 KAWAI T, CLINICAL ASPECTS OF THE PLASMA PROTEINS, *PHILADELPHIA, J.B. LIPPINCOTT CO*, (1973)

1240 KAY AD, MILSTEIN S, KAUFMAN S, ET AL, CEREBROSPINAL FLUID BIOPTERIN IS DECREASED IN ALZHEIMER'S DISEASE, *ARCH NEUROL*, 43, 996 (1986)

1241 KAY N H ET AL, HYPOURICEMIA IN HODGKIN'S DISEASE., *CANCER*, 32, 1508 (1973)

1242 KAYDEN H J AND SILBERT R, THE ROLE OF VITAMIN E DEFICIENCY IN THE ABNORMAL AUTOHEMOLYSIS OF ACANTHOCYTES, *TRANS ASSOC AM PHYSICIANS*, 78, 334 (1965)

1243 KAYE J P ET AL, PLASMA LIPIDS IN PATIENTS WITH CHRONIC RENAL FAILURE., *CLIN CHIM ACTA*, 44, 301-305 (1973)

1244 KEAN B H ET AL, THE COMPLEMENT-FIXATION TEST IN THE DIAGNOSIS OF CONGENITAL TOXOPLASMOSIS, *AM J DIS CHILD*, 131, 21-28 (1977)

1245 KEINANEN-KIUKAANNIEMI S, KAAPA P, ET AL, DECREASED THROMBOXANE PRODUCTION IN MIGRAINE PATIENTS DURING HEADACHE-FREE PERIOD, *HEADACHE*, 24, 339-341 (1984)

1246 KELLER R T ET AL, HYPERCALCEMIA SECONDARY TO A PRIMARY HEPATOMA, *JAMA*, 193, 782 (1965)

1247 KELLEY M L, ELEVATED SERUM AMYLASE ASSOCIATED WITH RUPTURED ECTOPIC PREGNANCY, *JAMA*, 164, 406-7 (1957)

1248 KELLY UL, COOPER EH, ALEXANDER C, STONE J, THE ASSESSMENT OF ANTICHYMOTRYPSIN IN CANCER MONITORING, *BIOMED PHARMACOTHER*, 28, 209-215 (1974)

1249 KENDALL A G ET AL, NEPHROTIC SYNDROME: A HYPERCOAGULABLE STATE, *ARCH INTERN MED*, 127, 1021 (1971)

1250 KENDALL ET AL, HAEMATOLOGY AND BIOCHEMISTRY OF ANKYLOSING SPONDYLITIS, *BR MED J*, 2, 235-237 (1973)

1251 KENNEDY A C ET AL, ABNORMALITIES OF MINERAL METABOLISM SUGGESTIVE OF PARATHYROID OVERACTIVITY IN RHEUMATOID ARTHRITIS, *CURR MED RES OPIN*, 3, 345-58 (1975)

1252 KENYON F E AND HARDY S M, A BIOCHEMICAL STUDY OF HUNTINGTON'S CHOREA, *J NEUROL NEUROSURG PSYCHIATRY*, 26, 123 (1963)

1253 KERNOFF P A ET AL, NORMAL AND ABNORMAL FIBRINOLYSIS, *BR MED BULL*, 33, 239-44 (1977)

1254 KEUL J AND DOLL E, INTERMITTENT EXERCISE: METABOLITES, PO2 AND ACID-BASE EQUILIBRIUM IN THE BLOOD, *J APPL PHYSIOL*, 34, 220 (1973)

1255 KEW M C ET AL, SERUM ALPHA-FETO PROTEIN LEVELS IN ACUTE VIRAL HEPATITIS, *GUT*, 14, 939 (1973)

1256 KEYE W R ET AL, AMENORRHEA, HYPERPROLACTINEMIA AND PITUITARY ENLARGEMENT SECONDARY TO PRIMARY HYPOTHYROIDISM. SUCCESSFUL TREATMENT WITH THYROID REPLACEMENT, *OBSTET GYNECOL*, 48, 697-702 (1976)

1257 KEYS ET AL, THE CONCENTRATION OF CHOLESTEROL IN THE BLOOD SERUM OF NORMAL MAN AND ITS RELATION TO AGE, *J CLIN INVEST*, 29, 1347-53 (1950)

1258 KHAFAGY E Z ET AL, SIGNIFICANCE OF ABNORMALITIES IN URINARY NEUTRAL MUCOPOLYSACCHARIDES IN BILHARZIASIS, *EGYPT J BILHARZ*, 2, 111-6 (1975)

1259 KHALIFA A S ET AL, IMMUNOGLOBULINS IN IDIOPATHIC THROMBOCYTOPENIC PURPURA IN CHILDHOOD, *ACTA HAEMATOL (BASEL)*, 56, 205 (1976)

1260 KHALIL M ET AL, RED CELL MEMBRANE LIPIDS IN THALASSEMIA, *GAZ EGYPT PAEDIATR ASSOC*, 23, 273-80 (1975)

1261 KHAN R ET AL, BONE MARROW ACID PHOSPHATASE: ANOTHER LOOK, *J UROL*, 117, 79-80 (1977)

1262 KHAN SN, RAHMAN MA, SAMAD A, TRACE ELEMENTS IN SERUM FROM PAKISTANI PATIENTS WITH ACUTE AND CHRONIC ISCHEMIC HEART DISEASE AND HYPERTENSION, *CLIN CHEM*, 30/5, 644-648 (1984)

1263 KHANNA S K ET AL, VALUE OF LACTIC DEHYDROGENASE IN CEREBROSPINAL FLUID OF TUBERCULOUS MENINGITIS PATIENTS, *J INDIAN MED ASSOC*, 68, 4-6 (1977)

1264 KIERKEGAARD-HANSEN ET AL, CREATINE PHOSPHOKINASE DETERMINATION IN MYOCARDIAL INFARCTION, *DAN MED BULL*, 16, 53-57 (1969)

1265 KIM H ET AL, PLASMA INSULIN DISTURBANCES IN PRIMARY HYPERPARATHYROIDISM, *J CLIN INVEST*, 50, 2596-2605 (1971)

1266 KIM Y S AND PLAUT A, B-GLUCURONIDASE STUDIES IN GASTRIC SECRETIONS FROM PATIENTS WITH GASTRIC CANCER, *GASTROENTEROLOGY*, 49, 50 (1965)

1267 KIMBAL H R ET AL, MARROW GRANULOCYTE RESERVES IN RHEUMATIC DISEASES, *ARTHRITIS RHEUM*, 16, 345-352 (1973)

1268 KIMBER C ET AL, THE MECHANISM OF ANEMIA IN CHRONIC LIVER DISEASE, *Q J MED*, 34, 33 (1965)

1269 KIMBERLY R P ET AL, ELEVATED URINARY PROSTAGLANDINS AND THE EFFECTS OF ASPIRIN ON RENAL FUNCTION IN LUPUS ERYTHEMATOSUS, *ANN INTERN MED*, 89, 336-41 (1978)

1270 KING E J, THE COLORIMETRIC DETERMINATION OF PHOSPHORUS, *BIOCHEM J*, 26, 292-297 (1932)

1271 KING J S AND WARNER A, CYSTINURIA WITH HYPERURICEMIA AND METHIONINURIA: BIOCHEMICAL STUDY OF A CASE, *AM J MED*, 43, 125 (1967)

1272 KINGHORN G R, VALUE OF ERYTHROCYTE SEDIMENTATION RATE IN PRIMARY GENITAL HERPES, *BR J CLIN PRACT*, 32, 49-51 (1978)

1273 KINSELLA T D ET AL, SERUM COMPLEMENT AND IMMUNOGLOBULIN LEVELS IN SPORADIC AND FAMILIAL ANKYLOSING SPONDYLITIS, *J RHEUMATOL*, 2, 308-13 (1975)

1274 KIRKENDAL A M ET AL, THE EFFECT OF DIETARY SODIUM CHLORIDE ON BLOOD PRESSURE, BODY FLUIDS, ELECTROLYTES, RENAL FUNCTION, AND SERUM LIPIDS OF NORMOTENSIVE MAN, *J LAB CLIN MED*, 87, 411-34 (1976)

1275 KIRKPATRICK A, COMPLEMENT, *IMMUNOCHEMISTRY SYSTEM (ICS-9). FULLERTON, CALIF., BECKMAN INSTRUMENTS INC*

1276 KISHIMOTO Y, ET AL, CLINICAL SIGNIFICANCE OF FSBA IN LONGTERM OBSERVATION OF CHRONIC LIVER DISEASE, *AM J GASTROENTEROL*, 80, 136-8 (1985)

1277 KISHIMOTO Y, HIJIYA S, TAKEDA I, CLINICAL SIGNIFICANCE OF FASTING SERUM BILE ACID IN THE LONG-TERM OBSERVATION OF CHRONIC LIVER DISEASE, *AM J GASTROENTEROL*, 80, 136-8 (1985)

1278 KLECH H, KLOHN H, POHL, W, ET AL, DIAGNOSIS IN SARCOIDOSIS, SENSITIVITY AND SPECIFICITY OF 67-GALLIUM SCINTIGRAPHY SERUM ANGIOTENSIN CONVERTING ENZYME LEVELS, THORACIC READIOGRAPHY AND BLOOD LYMPHOCYTE SUBPOPULATIONS, *WIEN MED WOCHENSCHR*, 133, 425-32 (1983)

1279 KLEINMAN JE, WEINBERGER DR, ROGOL AD, ET AL, PLASMA PROLACTIN CONCENTRATIONS AND PSYCHOPATHOLOGY IN CHRONIC SCHIZOPHRENIA, *ARCH GEN PSYCHIATRY*, 39, 655-7 (1982)

1280 KLEVAY L M, CORONARY HEART DISEASE: THE ZINC/COPPER HYPOTHESIS, *AM J CLIN NUTR*, 28, 764-74 (1975)

1281 KLIMIK J J ET AL, MYCOPLASMA PNEUMONIAE MENINGOENCEPHALITIS AND TRANSVERSE MYELITIS IN PEDIATRICS, *PEDIATRICS*, 58, 133-5 (1976)

1282 KLINE M M ET AL, THE CLINICAL VALUE OF ASCITIC FLUID CULTURE AND LEUKOCYTE COUNT STUDIES IN ALCOHOLIC CIRRHOSIS, *GASTROENTEROLOGY*, 70, 408-12 (1976)

1283 KLINENBERG J R, HYPERURICEMIA AND GOUT, *MED CLIN NORTH AM*, 61, 299-312 (1977)

1284 KLINGA K ET AL, MATERNAL PERIPHERAL TESTOSTERONE LEVELS DURING THE FIRST HALF OF PREGNANCY, *AM J OBSTET GYNECOL*, 131, 60-62 (1978)

1285 KLOHN H, KLECH H, MOSTBECK A, KUMMERF, 67GA SCANNING FOR ASSESSMENT OF DISEASE ACTIVITY AND THERAPY DECISIONS IN PULMONARY SARCOIDOSIS IN COMPARISON TO CHEST RADIOGRAPHY, SERUM ACE AND BLOOD T-LYMPHOCYTES, *EUR J NUCL MED*, 7, 413-6 (1982)

1286 KNIGHT A H ET AL, SIGNIFICANCE OF HYPERAMYLASEMIA AND ABDOMINAL PAIN IN DIABETIC KETOACIDOSIS, *BR MED J*, 3, 128-131 (1973)

1287 KNOCHEL J P, THE PATHOPHYSIOLOGY AND CLINICAL CHARACTERISTICS OF SEVERE HYPOPHOSPHATEMIA, *ARCH INTERN MED*, 137, 203-220 (1977)

1288 KNOPFLE G ET AL, SERUM ALPHA1-FETOPROTEIN IN CYSTIC FIBROSIS, *EUR J PEDIATR*, 122, 241-8 (1976)

1289 KNUDSEN JB, GORMSEN J, SKAGEN K, AMTORP O, CHANGES IN PLATELET FUNCTIONS, COAGULATION AND FIBRINOLYSIS IN UNCOMPLICATED CASES OF ACUTE MYOCARDIAL INFARCTION, *THROMB HAEMOST*, 42, 1513-22 (1980)

1290 KOBAYASHI K ET AL, CLINICAL AND EXPERIMENTAL STUDIES OF ACID PHOSPHATASE IN RENAL FAILURE, *CLIN CHIM ACTA*, 173-182 (1971)

1291 KOBAYASHI K ET AL, RAPID TURNOVER SERUM PROTEINS IN FULMINANT HEPATITIS, *GASTROENTEROLOGY*, 12, 455 (1977)

1292 KOCEN R S ET AL, FAMILIAL ALPHA LIPOPROTEIN DEFICIENCY WITH NEUROLOGIC ABNORMALITIES, *LANCET*, 1, 1341 (1967)

1293 KOCH MB, GO VLW, DIMAGNO EP, CAN PLASMA HUMAN PANCREATIC POLYPEPTIDE BE USED TO DETECT DISEASES OF THE EXOCRINE PANCREAS, *MAYO CLIN PROC*, 60, 259-265 (1985)

1294 KOGA S, MIYATA Y, FUNAKOSHI A, IBAYASHI H, PLASMA APOLIPOPROTEIN A-IV LEVELS DECREASE IN PATIENTS WITH CHRONIC PANCREATITIS AND MALABSORPTION SYNDROME, *DIGESTION*, 32, 19-24 (1985)

1295 KOLAR O J ET AL, SERUM AND CEREBROSPINAL FLUID IMMUNOGLOBULINS IN MULTIPLE SCLEROSIS, *NEUROL*, 20, 1058-61 (1970)

1296 KOLARIC K ET AL, SERUM COPPER LEVELS IN PATIENTS WITH SOLID TUMORS, *TUMORI*, 61, 173-7. (1975)

1297 KOLDJAER O ET AL, INDICES OF GRANULOCYTE ACTIVITY IN ULCERATIVE COLITIS AND CROHN'S DISEASE, *DAN MED BULL*, 24, 72-76 (1977)

1298 KOLENDORF K ET AL, THE INFLUENCE OF CHRONIC RENAL FAILURE ON SERUM AND URINARY THYROID HORMONE LEVELS., *ACTA ENDOCRINOL*, 89, 80-88 (1978)

1299 KONINCKX PR, TRAPPENIERS H, VAN ASSCHE FA, PROLACTIN CONCENTRATION IN VAGINAL FLUID: A NEW METHOD FOR DIAGNOSING RUPTURED MEMBRANES, *BR J OBSTET GYNAECOL*, 88, 607-10 (1981)

1300 KOPIN I J ET AL, PLASMA LEVELS OF NOREPINEPHRINE, *ANN INTERN MED*, 88, 671-680 (1978)

1301 KOPP W L ET AL, BLOOD VOLUME AND HEMATOCRIT VALUE IN MACROGLOBULINEMIA AND MYELOMA, *ARCH INTERN MED*, 123, 394 (1969)

1302 KORMAN M G ET AL, HYPERGASTRINEMIA IN CHRONIC RENAL FAILURE, *BR MED J*, 209 (1972)

1303 KORMAN MG, STRICKLAND RG, HANSKY J, SERUM GASTRIN IN CHRONIC GASTRITIS, *BR MED J*, 2, 16-18 (1971)

1304 KORSTEN C B ET AL, CARCINOEMBRYONIC ANTIGEN ACTIVITY IN URINE OF PATIENTS WITH BLADDER CARCINOMA, *J CLIN CHEM CLIN BIOCHEM*, 14, 389-93 (1976)

1305 KOSAKA S, BETA-2 GLYCOPROTEIN I IN RHEUMATOID ARTHRITIS, *TOHOKU J EXP MED*, 122, 223 (1977)

1306 KOSAKA S, TAZAWA M, ALPHA 1 - ANTICHYMOTRYPSIN IN RHEUMATOID ARTHRITIS, *TOHOKU J EXP MED*, 119, 369-375 (1976)

1307 KOSKI CL, KHURANA R, MAYER RF, GUILLAIN-BARRE SYNDROME, *AMERICAN FAMILY PHYSICIAN*, 34, 202 (1986)

1308 KOSKINEN P, IRJALA K, VIIKARI J, SERUM FRUCTOSAMINE IN THE ASSESSMENT OF GLYCAEMIC CONTROL IN DIABETES MELLITUS, *SCAND J CLIN LAB INVEST*, 47, 285-92 (1987)

1309 KOSTINA S I, SOME PARTICULARITIES IN DIAGNOSTIC, CLINICAL PICTURE, AND THERAPY OF PULMONARY SARCOIDOSIS, *Z ERKRANK ATM-ORG*, 149, 280-82 (1977)

1310 KOTCHEN T A ET AL, MODIFICATION OF RENIN REACTIVITY BY LIPIDS EXTRACTED FROM NORMAL, HYPERTENSIVE, AND UREMIC PLASMA, *J CLIN ENDOCRINOL METAB*, 43, 971-81 (1976)

1311 KOWALSKI H J AND W H ABELMANN, THE CARDIAC OUTPUT AT REST IN LAENNECS CIRRHOSIS, *J CLIN INVEST*, 32, 1025 (1953)

1312 KOWLESSAR O D ET AL, COMPARATIVE STUDY OF SERUM LEUCINE AMINOPEPTIDASE, 5-NUCLEOTIDASE AND NONSPECIFIC ALKALINE PHOSPHATASE IN DISEASES AFFECTING THE PANCREAS, HEPATOBILIARY TREE AND BONE, *AM J MED*, 31, 231-237 (1961)

1313 KRAFT S C AND KIRSNER J B, THE IMMUNOLOGY OF ULCERATIVE COLITIS AND CROHN'S DISEASE: CLINICAL AND HUMORAL ASPECTS, *INFLAMMATORY BOWEL DISEASE LEA & FEBIGER*, 60 (1975)

1314 KRAUSS A N ET AL, METABOLIC RATE OF NEONATES WITH CONGENITAL HEART DISEASE, *ARCH DIS CHILD*, 50, 539-41 (1975)

1315 KRAVITZ S C ET AL, UREMIA COMPLICATING LEUKEMIA CHEMOTHERAPY, *JAMA*, 146, 1595 (1951)

1316 KREISBERG R A, DIABETIC KETOACIDOSIS: NEW CONCEPTS AND TRENDS IN PATHOGENESIS AND TREATMENT, *ANN INTERN MED*, 88, 681-695 (1978)

1317 KREISS JK, KASPER CK, FAHEY JL, WEAVER M, ET AL, NONTRANSMISSION OF T-CELL SUBSET ABNORMALITIES FROM HEMOPHILIACS TO THEIR SPOUSES, *JAMA*, 251, 1450-4 (1984)

1318 KREISS JK, LAWRENCE DN, KASPER CK, ET AL, ANTIBODY TO HUMAN T-CELL LEUKEMIA VIRUS MEMBRANE ANTIGENS, BETA2-MICROGLOBULIN LEVELS, AND THYMOSIN ALPHA1 LEVELS IN HEMOPHILIACS AND THEIR SPOUSES, *ANN INTERN MED*, 100, 178-182 (1984)

1319 KRUGMAN AND WARD, INFECTIOUS DISEASES, *5TH EDITION MOSBY ST LOUIS* (1973)

1320 KRUSKEMPER H L ET AL, SERUM ENZYME ACTIVITIES IN DISORDERS OF THYROID FUNCTION, *GERM MED MTH*, 14, 55-58 (1969)

1321 KUKU S F ET AL, HETEROGENEITY OF PLASMA GLUCAGON, *J CLIN INVEST*, 58, 742-50 (1976)

1322 KUMAR A ET AL, HYPERCALCEMIA IN LEUKEMIA, *INDIAN J CANCER*, 13, 277-79 (1976)

1323 KUMAR M S ET AL, THE RELATIONSHIP OF THYROID-STIMULATING HORMONE (TSH), THYROXINE (T_4), AND TRIIODOTHYRONINE (T_3) IN PRIMARY THYROID FAILURE, *AM J CLIN PATHOL*, 68, 747-51 (1977)

1324 KUNZ F ET AL, PLASMA LIPIDS, COAGULATION FACTORS, AND FIBRIN FORMATION AFTER SEVERE MULTIPLE TRAUMA, AND IN ADULT RESPIRATORY DISTRESS SYNDROME, *J TRAUMA*, 18, 115-20. (1978)

1325 KUROYANAGI T ET AL, FIBRIN DEGRADATION PRODUCTS IN RENAL DISEASES, *TOHOKU J EXP MED*, 119, 237-44 (1976)

1326 KUSCHNER J P ET AL, IDIOPATHIC REFRACTORY SIDEROBLASTIC ANEMIA: CLINICAL AND LABORATORY INVESTIGATION OF 17 PATIENTS AND REVIEW OF THE LITERATURE, *MEDICINE*, 50, 139 (1971)

1327 KUSHER J P ET AL, IDIOPATHIC REFRACTORY SIDEROBLASTIC ANEMIA. CLINICAL AND LABORATORY INVESTIGATION OF 17 PATIENTS AND REVIEW OF LITERATURE, *MEDICINE*, 50, 139 (1961)

1328 KUSHNER JP, THE ENZYMATIC DEFECT IN PORPHYRIA CUTANEA TARDA, *N ENGL J MED*, 306, 799-800 (1982)

1329 KUVIN S F AND BRECHER G, DIFFERENTIAL NEUTROPHIL COUNTS IN PREGNANCY, *N ENGL J MED*, 266, 877 (1962)

1330 KUWERT E ET AL, DEMONSTRATION OF COMPLEMENT IN SPINAL FLUID IN MULTIPLE SCLEROSIS, *ANN NY ACAD SCI*, 122, 429 (1965)

1331 KUYLENSTIERNA J, KARLBERG, B, PROSTAGLANDIN E2 AND THE RENIN-ANGIOTENSIN SYSTEM IN PRIMARY ALDOSTERONISM AND CUSHING'S SYNDROME, *PROSTAGLANDINS LEUKOTRIENES AND MEDICINE*, 17, 387-395 (1985)

1332 KWITEROVICH ET AL, NEONATAL DIAGNOSIS OF FAMILIAL TYPE-II HYPERLIPOPROTEINAEMIA, *J CLIN ENDOCR*, 1, 118-121 (1973)

1333 KYLE R A, MULTIPLE MYELOMA: REVIEW OF 869 CASES, *MAYO CLIN PROC*, 50, 29 (1975)

1334 KYLE R A AND BAYRD E O, AMYLOIDOSIS: REVIEW OF 236 CASES, *MEDICINE*, 54, 271-300 (1975)

1335 LA FARGUE P ET AL, EVOLUTION DU MAGNESIUM SERIQUE ET ERYTHROCYTAIRE CHEZ LES BRULES, *CLIN CHIM ACTA*, 80, 17-21 (1977)

1336 LACKO A G ET AL, SERUM CHOLESTEROL ESTERIFICATION IN HYPER-THYROIDISM AND HYPOTHYROIDISM, *HORM METAB RES*, 10, 147-51. (1978)

1337 LAFFERTY FW, PRIMARY HYPERPARATHYROIDISM, *ARCH INTERN MED*, 141, 1761-1766 (1981)

1338 LAHODA F ET AL, TYPING OF URIC ACID LEVEL IN CSF IN NEUROLOGI-CAL AND PSYCHIATRIC DISEASES, *ADV EXP MED BIOL*, 76(B), 256-258 (1977)

1339 LAKS MS, KAHN SE, FAVUS MJ, BERMES EW JR, CASE REPORT: CLINICAL PATHOLOGICAL CORRELATIONS IN A CASE OF PRIMARY PARATHYROID CARCINOMA, *ANN CLIN LAB SCI*, 14, 458-63 (1984)

1340 LAL ET AL, EFFECT OF RIFAMPICIN AND ISONIAZID ON LIVER FUNC-TION, *BR MED J*, 1, 148-150 (1972)

1341 LAM S K, HYPERGASTRINEMIA IN CIRRHOSIS OF LIVER, *GUT*, 17, 700-8 (1976)

1342 LAMBANA S, CLINICAL VALUE OF PROTEIN-BOUND FUCOSE IN PATIENTS WITH CARCINOMA AND OTHER DISEASES, *GANN*, 69, 379-88 (1976)

1343 LAMBERT J R ET AL, SERUM URIC ACID LEVELS IN PSORIATIC ARTHRI-TIS, *ANN RHEUM DIS*, 36, 264-267 (1977)

1344 LAMONT N M ET AL, PORPHYRIA IN THE AFRICAN, *Q J MED*, 30, 373 (1961)

1345 LAMRS C B H ET AL, SERUM ALBUMIN LEVELS IN PATIENTS WITH THE ZOLLINGER-ELLISON SYNDROME, *GASTROENTEROLOGY*, 73, 975-9 (1977)

1346 LANDAU H ET AL, GONADOTROPIN, THYROTROPIN AND PROLACTIN RESERVE IN BETA THALASSEMIA., *CLIN ENDOCRINOL (OXF)*, 9, 163-173 (1978)

1347 LANG H, CREATINE KINASE ISOENZYMES: PATHOPHYSIOLOGY AND CLINICAL APPLICATION, *BERLIN, SPRINGER-VERLAG* (1981)

1348 LANGE PH, TESTICULAR CANCER MARKERS, *IN CANCER MARKERS II, HUMANA PRESS, INC. CLIFTON, NEW JERSEY*, 262 (1982)

1349 LAPATSANIS P ET AL, PHOSPHATURIA IN THALASSEMIA, *PEDIATRICS*, 58, 885-92 (1976)

1350 LAQUEUR W ET AL, THE HIPPURIC ACID TEST IN PREGNANCY, *BR MED J*, 1, 201-202 (1946)

1351 LARSSON S D, ANEMIA AND IRON METABOLISM IN HYPOTHYROIDISM, *ACTA MED SCAND*, 157, 349 (1967)

1352 LARSSON S O, MYELOMA AND PERNICIOUS ANEMIA, *ACTA MED SCAND*, 172, 195 (1962)

1353 LARUSSA FM, LAROCCA LM, RUSCIANI L, ET AL, OKT₄/OKT8 RATIO AND SERUM BETA 2-MICROGLOBULIN IN MYCOSIS FUNGOIDES AND CHRONIC BENIGN DERMATITIS, 663

1354 LARUSSA FM, LAROCCA LM, RUSCIANI L, ET AL, OKT₄/OKT8 RATIO AND SERUM BETA 2-MICROGLOBULIN IN MYCOSIS FUNGOIDES AND CHRONIC BENIGN DERMATITIS, *EUR J CANCER CLIN ONCOL*, 22, 663-9 (1986)

1355 LAURELL C-B, JEPPSON JO, EDITED BY PUTMAN, FW, PROTEASE INHIBI-TORS IN PLASMA, *THE PLASMA PROTEINS, STRUCTURE, FUNC-TION, AND GENETIC CONTROL, ACADEMIC PRESS*, 1, 229-264 (1975)

1356 LAWRENCE D M ET AL, PLASMA TESTOSTERONE AND ANDROSTENE-DIONE LEVELS DURING MONITORED INDUCTION OF OVULATION IN INFERTILE WOMEN WITH 'SIMPLE' AMENORRHEA AND WITH THE POLYCYSTIC OVARY SYNDROME, *CLIN ENDOCRINOL (OXF)*, 5, 609-18 (1976)

1357 LAWRENCE J H AND ROSENTHAL R L, MULTIPLE MYELOMA ASSOCI-ATED WITH POLYCYTHEMIA. REPORT OF FOUR CASES, *AM J MED SCI*, 218, 149 (1949)

1358 LAWSON D H ET AL, EARLY MORTALITY IN THE MEGALOBLASTIC ANE-MIAS, *Q J MED*, 41, 1 (1972)

1359 LAWSON D, WESTCMBE P, SAGGAR B, PILOT TRIAL OF AN INFANT SCREENING PROGRAMME FOR CYSTIC FIBROSIS: MEASUREMENT OF PAROTID SALIVARY SODIUM AT FOUR MONTHS, *ARCH DIS CHILD*, 44, 715-718 (1969)

1360 LEAUTI J B ET AL, CONTRIBUTION TO THE EARLY DIAGNOSIS OF CON-GENITAL TOXOPLASMOSIS, *BIOMED PHARMACOTHER*, 27, 283-4 (1977)

1361 LEBACQ E G ET AL, HYPERCALCIURIA IN SARCOIDOSIS, *Z ERKRANK ATM-ORG*, 149, 219-23 (1977)

1362 LECHI A ET AL, DRUG CONTROL OF GOUT AND HYPERURICEMIA, *DRUGS*, 16, 158-66 (1978)

1363 LECLERCQ R AND PORTMANS J R, HORMONAL VARIATIONS DURING MUSCULAR EXERCISE IN MAN, WITH PARTICULAR REFERENCE TO PLASMA CORTISOL, *REFERENCE VALUES IN HUMAN CHEMISTRY SIEST G, KARGER, B (ED)*, 264 (1973)

1364 LEDA M ET AL, ECTOPIC PRODUCTION OF A SALIVARY TYPE AMYLASE BY ADENOCARCINOMA CELLS: DEMONSTRATION BY A CULTURE TECHNIQUE, *CLIN CHIM ACTA*, 80, 105-11 (1977)

1365 LEDWICH J R, CHEST PAIN IN THE EARLY RECOGNITION OF LARGE INFARCTS, *CAN MED ASSOC J*, 116, 38-43 (1977)

1366 LEE, AN UNUSUAL ALKALINE PHOSPHATASE ISOENZYME IN A PATIENT WITH CONCOMITANT MARKED ELEVATION OF ACID PHOSPHA-TASE WITHOUT CLINICAL EVIDENCE OF PROSTATIC CARCINOMA, *CLIN CHIM ACTA*, 71, 221-227 (1976)

1367 LEE J B, CARDIOVASCULAR-RENAL EFFECTS OF PROSTAGLANDINS, *ARCH INTERN MED*, 133, 56 (1974)

1368 LEE J C ET AL, CALCITONIN SECRETION IN RENAL FAILURE, *CALCIF TISSUE INT*, 22(SUPPL), 154-7. (1978)

1369 LEE M C ET AL, CEREBROSPINAL FLUID IN CEREBRAL HEMORRHAGE AND INFARCTION, *STROKE*, 6, 638-41 (1975)

1370 LEE Y N ET AL, PERIPHERAL B- AND T- LYMPHOCYTE COUNTS IN PATIENTS WITH SARCOMA AND BREAST CARCINOMA, *CANCER*, 40, 667-72 (1977)

1371 LEEVY C M ET AL, LIVER DISEASE OF THE ALCOHOLIC, *MED CLIN NORTH AM*, 59, 909-918 (1975)

1372 LEGGE M, DUFF GB, POTTER HC, HOETJES MM, MATERNAL SERUM ALPHA 1-ANTITRYPSIN CONCENTRATIONS IN NORMOTENSIVE AND HYPERTENSIVE PREGNANCIES, *J CLIN PATHOL*, 37, 867-9 (1984)

1373 LEHRNER L M ET AL, AN EVALUATION OF THE USEFULNESS OF AMY-LASE ISOENZYME DIFFERENTIATION IN PATIENTS WITH HYPER-AMYLASEMIA, *AM J CLIN PATHOL*, 66, 576-87 (1976)

1374 LEME C E ET AL, INTERACTION OF CALCIUM IONS WITH SERUM ALBU-MIN IN CHRONIC RENAL FAILURE, *CLIN CHIM ACTA*, 77, 287-94 (1977)

1375 LEPOW H ET AL, NON-PROSTATIC CAUSES OF ACID HYPERPHOSPHATASIA: REPORT OF A CASE DUE TO MULTPLE MYELOMA, *J UROL*, 87, 991-993 (1962)

1376 LERNER R G RAPAPORT S I AND MELTZER J, THROMBOTIC THROMBO-CYTOPENIC PURPURA: SERIAL CLOTTING STUDIES, *ANN INTERN MED*, 66, 1181 (1967)

1377 LEROY E C AND SJOERDSMA A, CLINICAL SIGNIFICANCE OF A HYDROXYPROLINE CONTAINING PROTEIN IN HUMAN PLASMA, *J CLIN INVEST*, 44, 914 (1965)

1378 LEVIN P H ET AL, HEALTH OF THE INTENSIVELY TREATED HEMOPHIL-IAC, WITH SPECIAL REFERENCES TO ABNORMAL LIVER CHEMIS-TRIES AND SPLENOMEGALY, *BLOOD*, 50, 1-9 (1977)

1379 LEVITAN R ET AL, SERUM ENZYME ACTIVITIES IN PATIENTS WITH POLY-CYTHEMIA AND MYELOFIBROSIS, *CANCER*, 13, 1218 (1960)

1380 LEVY RI, FEINLEIB M, *HEART DISEASE, W.B. SAUNDERS CO., PHILADEL-PHIA* (1980)

1381 LEW PD, DAYER JM, WOLLHEIN CB, ET AL, EFFECT OF LEUKOTRIENE B4, PROSTAGLANDIN E2 AND ARACHIDONIC ACID ON CYTOSOLIC-FREE CALCIUM IN HUMAN NEUTROPHILS, *FEBS LETT*, 166, 44-8 (1984)

1382 LEWIN K J ET AL, GASTRIC MORPHOLOGY AND SERUM GASTRIN LEVELS IN PERNICIOUS ANEMIA, *GUT*, 17, 551-60 (1976)

1383 LEWIS E J ET AL, SERUM COMPLEMENT LEVELS IN HUMAN GLOMERU-LONEPHRITIS, *ANN INTERN MED*, 75, 555 (1971)

1384 LEWIS S M, RED CELL ABNORMALITIES IN APLASTIC ANEMIA, *BR J HAEMATOL*, 8, 322 (1962)

1385 LEWIS S M ET AL, NEUTROPHIL (LEUKOCYTE) ALKALINE PHOSPHA-TASE IN PAROXYSMAL NOCTURNAL HEMOGLOBINURIA, *BR J HAEMATOL*, 11, 549 (1965)

1386 LEWISON E F, THE CLINICAL VALUE OF THE SERUM AMYLASE TEST, *SURG GYNECOL OBSTET*, 72, 202-12 (1941)

1387 LEYDON JJ, LOW SERUM IRON LEVELS AND MODERATE ANEMIA IN SEVERE NODULOCYSTIC ACNE, *ARCH DERMATOL*, 121, 214 (1985)

1388 LI CY ET AL, ACID PHOSPHATASE ISOENZYME IN HUMAN LEUKOCYTES IN NORMAL AND PATHOLOGIC CONDITIONS, *J HISTOCHEM CYTOCHEM*, 18, 473 (1970)

1389 LIAN E C AND DEYKIN D, DIAGNOSIS OF VON WILLEBRAND'S DISEASE, *AM J MED*, 60, 344-356 (1976)

1390 LIANG, VALUE OF ENZYME STUDIES AFTER PROSTATIC SURGERY, *RI MED J*, 59, 457-8,472 (1976)

1391 LIBERTINO J A AND L ZINMAN, RENAL CELL CARCINOMA, *MED CLIN NORTH AM*, 59, 293-8 (1975)

1392 LICHT A AND RACHMILEWITZ E A, MYELOFIBROSIS, OSTEOLYTIC BONE LESIONS AND HYPERCALCEMIA IN CHRONIC MYELOID LEUKEMIA, *ACTA HAEMATOL (BASEL)*, 49, 182 (1973)

1393 LICHTMAN M A AND MILLER D R, ERYTHROCYTE GLYCOLYSIS, 2,3-DPG AND ATP CONCENTRATIONS IN UREMIC SUBJECTS, *J LAB CLIN MED*, 76, 267 (1970)

1394 LIEBER C S (ED), METABOLIC EFFECTS OF ALCOHOLISM, *UNIVERSITY PARK PRESS BALTIMORE* (1977)

1395 LIEBERMAN AN ET AL, SERUM DOPAMINE BETA HYDROXYLASE IN HUNTINGTON'S DISEASE, *LANCET*, 1, 153 (1972)

1396 LIEBERMAN E ET AL, THROMBOSIS, NEPHROSIS AND CORTICOSTE-ROID THERAPY, *J PEDIATR*, 73, 320 (1968)

1397 LIEBERMAN J, COMPLEMENT COMPONENTS IN CYSTIC FIBROSIS, *LAN-CET*, 1, 1230 (1974)

1398 LIEBERMAN J, ELEVATION OF SERUM ANGIOTENSIN CONVERTING ENZYME (ACE) LEVEL IN SARCOIDOSIS, *AM J MED*, 59, 365-372 (1975)

1399 LIEBERMAN J, SASTRE A, SERUM ANGIOTENSIN-CONVERTING ENZYME: ELEVATIONS IN DIABETES MELLITUS, *ANN INTERN MED*, 93, 825-6 (1980)

1400 LIEBERMAN J, SCHLEISSNER LA, NOSAL A, ET AL, CLINICAL CORRELA-TIONS OF SERUM ANGIOTENSIN-CONVERTING ENZYME (ACE) IN SARCOIDOSIS. A LONGITUDINAL STUDY OF SERUM ACE, 67 GAL-LIUM SCANS, CHEST ROENTGENOGRAMS, AND PULMONARY FUNCTION, *CHEST*, 84, 522-8 (1983)

1401 LIEBERMAN J, SCHLEISSNER LA, NOSAL A, ET AL, CLINICAL CORRELATIONS OF SERUM ANGIOTENSIN-CONVERTING ENZYME (ACE) IN SARCOIDOSIS. A LONGITUDINAL STUDY OF SERUM ACE, 67 GALLIUM SCANS, CHEST ROENTGENOGRAMS, AND PULMONARY FUNCTION, *CHEST*, 84, 522-8 (1983)

1402 LIFTON L ET AL, ETHANOL-INDUCED HYPERTRIGLYCERIDEMIA. PREVALENCE AND CONTRIBUTING FACTORS, *AM J CLIN NUTR*, 31, 614-8. (1978)

1403 LIGHT R W, PLEURAL EFFUSIONS, *MED CLIN NORTH AM*, 61, 1339-52 (1977)

1404 LIGHT R W, PLEURAL FLUID ANALYSIS: HOW TO INTERPRET THE TESTS, *CONSULTANT*, 97 (1978)

1405 LIGHT RW, BALL WC JR, GLUCOSE AND AMYLASE IN PLEURAL EFFUSIONS, *J A M A*, 225, 257-259 (1973B)

1406 LIGHTMAN A, BRANDES JM, BINUR N, ET AL, USE OF THE SERUM COPPER/ZINC RATIO IN THE DIFFERENTIAL DIAGNOSIS OF OVARIAN MALIGNANCY, *CLIN CHEM*, 32/1, 101-103 (1986)

1407 LIGHTSEY A L ET AL, PLATELET-ASSOCIATED IMMUNOGLOBULIN G IN CHILDHOOD IDIOPATHIC THROMBOCYTOPENIC PURPURA, *J PEDIATR*, 94, 201-04 (1979)

1408 LIM P ET AL, SERUM IONIZED CALCIUM IN NEPHROTIC SYNDROME, *Q J MED*, 69, 421-26 (1976)

1409 LIN CY, YANG YM, FU YK, T CELL SUBSETS IN GLOMERULONEPHRITIS, *INT J PEDIATR NEPHROL*, 7, 63-68 (1986)

1410 LINDEMAN RD, BOTTOMLEY RG, CONNELISON RL, ET AL, INFLUENCE OF ACUTE TISSUE INJURY ON ZINC METABOLISM IN MAN, *J LAB CLIN MED*, 79, 452-460 (1972)

1411 LINDQVIST B ET AL, DIFFERENTIAL COUNT OF URINARY LEUCOCYTES AND RENAL EPITHELIAL CELLS BY PHASE CONTRAST MICROSCOPY, *ACTA MED SCAND*, 198, 505-9 (1975)

1412 LINKOLA J ET AL, RENIN-ALDOSTERONE AXIS IN ETHANOL INTOXICATION AND HANGOVER, *EUR J CLIN INVEST*, 6, 191-4 (1976)

1413 LINUMA K, IKEDA I, OGIHARA T, ET AL, RADIOIMMUNOASSAY OF METANEPHRINE AND NORMETANEPHRINE FOR DIAGNOSIS OF PHEOCHROMOCYTOMA, *CLIN CHEM*, 32/10, 1879-1883 (1986)

1414 LIPINSKI B ET AL, ABNORMAL FIBRINOGEN HETEROGENEITY AND FIBRINOLYTIC ACTIVITY IN ADVANCED LIVER DISEASE, *J LAB CLIN MED*, 90, 187-94 (1977)

1415 LIPMAN L M ET AL, RELATIONSHIP OF LONG-ACTING THYROID STIMULATOR TO THE CLINICAL FEATURES AND COURSE OF GRAVES' DISEASE, *AM J MED*, 43, 486 (1967)

1416 LIPSETT M B ET AL, HORMONAL SYNDROMES ASSOCIATED WITH NON-ENDOCRINE TUMORS, *ANN INTERN MED*, 61, 733 (1964)

1417 LISAK R P ET AL, LACK OF DIAGNOSTIC VALUE OF CREATINE PHOSPHOKINASE ASSAY IN SPINAL FLUID, *JAMA*, 199, 160-161 (1967)

1418 LOCKWOOD D H ET AL, INSULIN SECRETION IN TYPE I GLYCOGEN STORAGE DISEASE, *DIABETES*, 18, 755-8 (1969)

1419 LOEWENSTEIN M AND N ZAMCHECK, CARCINOEMBRYONIC ANTIGEN (CEA) LEVELS IN BENIGN GASTROINTESTINAL DISEASE STATES, *CANCER*, 42, 1412-8 (1978)

1420 LOEWENSTEIN M S ET AL, CARCINOEMBRYONIC ANTIGEN ASSAY OF ASCITES AND DETECTION OF MALIGNANCY, *ANN INTERN MED*, 88, 635-38 (1978)

1421 LOGE J P ET AL, CHARACTERIZATION OF ANEMIA ASSOCIATED WITH CHRONIC RENAL INSUFFICIENCY, *AM J MED*, 24, 4 (1958)

1422 LOIRAT P ET AL, INCREASED GLOMERULAR FILTRATION RATE IN PATIENTS WITH MAJOR BURNS, *N ENGL J MED*, 299, 915-919 (1978)

1423 LOKECH J J, LEUKOCYTE ALKALINE PHOSPHATASE ACTIVITY IN PATIENTS WITH MALIGNANT DISEASE, *CANCER*, 40, 1202-5 (1977)

1424 LOLIS D ET AL, LEUKOCYTE ALKALINE PHOSPHATASE ACTIVITY DURING HIGH RISK PREGNANCIES, *BR J HAEMATOL*, 39, 277-81 (1978)

1425 LOMBECK I, SCHNIPPERING HG, RITZL F, ET AL, ABSORPTION OF ZINC IN ACRODERMATITIS ENTEROPATHICA, *LANCET*, 1, 855 (1975)

1426 LONDON ET AL, ON LOW ACID PHOSPHATASE VALUES OF PATIENTS WITH KNOWN METASTATIC CANCER OF THE PROSTATE, *CANCER RES*, 14, 718-724 (1954)

1427 LONG P A ET AL, IMPORTANCE OF ABNORMAL GLUCOSE TOLERANCE (HYPOGLYCEMIA AND HYPERGLYCEMIA) IN THE AETIOLOGY OF PRE-ECLAMPSIA, *LANCET*, 1, 923-5 (1977)

1428 LONGCOPE W T ET AL, A STUDY OF SARCOIDOSIS, *MEDICINE*, 31 (1952)

1429 LOPES J ET AL, HETEROGENEITY OF 5'-NUCLEOTIDASE ACTIVITY IN LYMPHOCYTES IN CHRONIC LYMPHOCYTIC LEUKEMIA, *J CLIN INVEST*, 52, 1297 (1973)

1430 LOPEZ-LLERA M ET AL, COAGULATION AND FIBRINOLYSIS IN MOLAR PREGNANCY., *AM J OBSTET GYNECOL*, 127, 855-860 (1977)

1431 LORAINE J A, BIOASSAY OF PITUITARY AND PLACENTAL GONADOTROPINS IN RELATION TO CLINICAL PROBLEMS IN MAN, *VITAMINS HORMONES*, 14, 305-357 (1956)

1432 LORAINE JA, BELL ET, HORMONE ASSAYS AND THEIR CLINICAL APPLICATION, *NEW YORK, CHURCHILL LIVINGSTONE* (1976)

1433 LORBER A ET AL, SERUM COPPER LEVELS IN RHEUMATOID ARTHRITIS, *ARTHRITIS RHEUM*, 11, 65-71 (1968)

1434 LORBER M, ADULT-TYPE GAUCHER'S DISEASE: A SECONDARY ORDER OF IRON METABOLISM, *J MT SINAI HOSP*, 37, 404 (170)

1435 LORBER M, AVIRAM M, LINN S, ET AL, HYPOCHOLESTEROLAEMIA AND ABNORMAL HIGH-DENSITY LIPOPROTEIN IN RHEUMATOID ARTHRITIS, *BR J RHEUMATOL*, 24, 250-255 (1985)

1436 LORIA A ET AL, RED CELL LIFE SPAN IN IRON DEFICIENCY ANAEMIA, *BR J HAEMATOL*, 13, 294 (1967)

1437 LORUSSO L MINIELLO VL, FRANCIOSO G, ACETO G, ET AL, ANTITHROMBIN III IN INFANTILE NEPHROTIC SYNDROME, *BOLL SOC ITAL BIOL SPER*, 58, 1093 (1982)

1438 LOSITO R, GATTIKER H, BILODEAU G, ET AL, LEVELS OF ANTITHROMBIN III, ALPHA 2-MACROGLOBULIN, AND ALPHA 1-ANTITRYPSIN IN ACUTE ISCHEMIC HEART DISEASE, *J LAB CLIN MED*, 97, 241-50 (1981)

1439 LOSOWSKY M S ET AL, LIPID METABOLISM IN ACUTE AND CHRONIC RENAL FAILURE, *J LAB CLIN MED*, 71, 736 (1968)

1440 LOTSTRA, ET AL, REDUCED CCK LEVELS IN CSF, *ANN NY ACAD SCI*, 448, 507-17 (1985)

1441 LOTT JA, STANG JM, SERUM ENZYMES AND ISOENZYMES IN THE DIAGNOSIS AND DIFFERENTIAL DIAGNOSIS OF MYOCARDIAL ISCHEMIA AND NECROSIS, *CLIN CHEM*, 26, 1241-1250 (1980)

1442 LOUTIT J F, DISCUSSION ON THE LIFE AND DEATH OF THE RED CORPUSCLE, *PROC R SOC*, 34, 755 (1946)

1443 LOWE JR, DIXON JS, GUTHRIE JA, MCWHINNEY P, SERUM AND SYNOVIAL FLUID LEVELS OF ANGIOTENSIN CONVERTING ENZYME IN POLYARTHRITIS, *ANN RHEUM DIS*, 45, 921-4 (1986)

1444 LOWELL JR, DIAGNOSIS: FLUID AND TISSUE EXAMINATION, *PLEURAL EFFUSIONS, UNIVERSITY PARK PRESS, BALTIMORE*, 45-73 (1977)

1445 LOWY C ET AL, URINARY OF EXCRETION OF INSULIN AND GROWTH HORMONE IN SUBJECTS WITH RENAL FAILURE, *ACTA ENDOCRINOL*, 67, 85 (1971)

1446 LUBRAN M, THE EFFECTS OF DRUGS ON LABORATORY VALUES, *MED CLIN NORTH AM*, 53, 211 (1969)

1447 LUCENA ET AL, SERUM ENZYME ACTIVITY FOLLOWING CARDIAC CATHETERIZATION AND ENDOMYOCARDIAL BIOPSY, *J LAB CLIN MED*, 84, 6-19 (1974)

1448 LUETSCHER J A ET AL, ALDOSTERONE SECRETION AND METABOLISM IN HYPERTENSION AND MYXEDEMA, *J CLIN ENDOCRINOL METAB*, 23, 873 (1963)

1449 LUHDORF K ET AL, GRAND MAL PROVOKED HYPERURICEMIA, *ACTA NEUROL SCAND*, 58, 280-287 (1978)

1450 LUISI M ET AL, PLASMA STEROID DYNAMICS IN CUSHING'S SYNDROME, *ANN ENDOCRINOL (PARIS)*, 39, 107-15 (1978)

1451 LUKUMSKY P E AND OGANOV R G, BLOOD PLASMA CATECHOLAMINES AND THEIR URINARY EXCRETION IN PATIENTS WITH ACUTE MYOCARDIAL INFARCTION, *AM HEART J*, 83, 182 (1972)

1452 LUM ET AL, SERUM GAMMA-GLUTAMYL TRANSPEPTIDASE ACTIVITY AS AN INDICATOR OF DISEASE OF LIVER, PANCREAS, OR BONE, *CLIN CHEM*, 18, 358-362 (1972)

1453 LUNDBERG PO, OSTERMAN PO, WIDE L, SERUM PROLACTIN IN PATIENTS WITH HYPOTHALAMUS AND PITUITARY DISORDERS, *J NEUROSURG*, 55, 194-9 (1981)

1454 LUPPINGER K ET AL, KLINEFELTER'S SYNDROME, A CLINICAL AND CYTOGENETIC STUDY IN TWENTY-TWO CASES, *ACTA ENDOCRINOL*, 54(SUPPL), 113 (1967)

1455 LURIE B B ET AL, ELEVATED CIRCULATING CEA LEVELS IN BENIGN EXTRAHEPATIC BILIARY TRACT OBSTRUCTION AND INFLAMMATION, *JAMA*, 233, 319-25 (1975)

1456 LUSHER J M AND ZUELZER W W, IDIOPATHIC THROMBOCYTOPENIC PURPURA IN CHILDHOOD, *J PEDIATR*, 68, 971 (1966)

1457 LYBERATOS C ET AL, ERYTHROCYTE CONTENT OF FREE PROTOPORPHYRIN IN THALASSAEMIC SYNDROMES, *ACTA HAEMATOL (BASEL)*, 47, 164 (1972)

1458 LYNCH P J AND MIEDLER L J, ERYTHROPOIETIC PORPHYRIA: REPORT OF A FAMILY AND CLINICAL REVIEW, *ARCH DERMATOL*, 92, 351 (1965)

1459 LYNCH PJ, VOORHEES JJ, HARRELL ER, SYSTEMIC SPOROTRICHOSIS, *ANN INTERN MED*, 73, 23-30 (1970)

1460 LYONS H A ET AL, THE SENSITIVITY OF THE RESPIRATORY CENTER IN PREGNANCY AND AFTER THE ADMINISTRATION OF PROGESTERONE, *TRANS ASSOC AM PHYSICIANS*, 72, 173-80 (1959)

1461 MACDONALD ET AL, SERUM LACTIC DEHYDROGENASE - A DIAGNOSTIC AID IN MYOCARDIAL INFARCTION, *JAMA*, 165, 35-40 (1957)

1462 MACGIBBON B H MOLLIN D L, SIDEROBLASTIC ANAEMIA IN MAN: OBSERVATIONS ON SEVENTY CASES, *BR J HAEMATOL*, 11, 59 (1965)

1463 MACHER A, HISTOPLASMOSIS AND BLASTOMYCOSIS, *MED CLIN NORTH AM*, 14, 447-459 (1980)

1464 MACHIN ND, CHARD MD, PAICE EW, SERUM ANGIOTENSIN CONVERTING ENZYME IN SJÖGREN'S SYNDROME--A CASE REPORT AND STUDY OF 21 FURTHER CASES, *POSTGRAD MED J*, 60, 270-1 (1984)

1465 MACKAY I R, CHRONIC HEPATITIS: EFFECT OF PROLONGED SUPPRESSIVE TREATMENT AND COMPARISON OF AZATHIOPRINE WITH PREDNISOLONE, *Q J MED*, 37, 379 (1968)

1466 MACKAY I R AND LARKIN L, THE SIGNIFICANCE OF THE PRESENCE IN HUMAN SERUM OF COMPLEMENT-FIXING ANTIBODIES TO HUMAN TISSUE ANTIGENS, *AUST ANN MED*, 7, 251 (1958)

1467 MACKAY I R ET AL, AUTOIMMUNE HEPATITIS, *ANN NY ACAD SCI*, 124, 767 (1965)

1468 MACKENZIE D Y AND WOOLF L I, MAPLE SYRUP URINE DISEASE: AN INBORN ERROR OF METABOLISM OF VALINE, LEUCINE, ISOLEUCINE, ASSOCIATED WITH GROSS MENTAL DEFICIENCY, *BR MED J*, 1, 90 (1959)

1469 MACKENZIE M R AND FUDENBERG H H, MACROGLOBULINEMIA: AN ANALYSIS OF FORTY PATIENTS, *BLOOD*, 39, 874 (1972)

1470 MACKINNEY A A JR ET AL, ASCERTAINING GENETIC CARRIERS OF HEREDITARY SPHEROCYTOSIS BY STATISTICAL ANALYSIS OF MULTIPLE LABORATORY TESTS, *J CLIN INVEST*, 41, 554 (1962)

1471 MACLEAN D ET AL, SERUM ENZYME ACTIVITIES IN ACCIDENTAL HYPOTHERMIA AND HYPOTHERMIC MYXOEDEMA, *CLIN CHIM ACTA*, 52, 197 (1974)

1472 MACLEAN ET AL, SERUM-ENZYMES IN RELATION TO ELECTROCARDIOGRAPHIC CHANGES IN ACCIDENTAL HYPOTHERMIA, *J CLIN ENDOCR*, 2, 1266-1270 (1968)

1473 MADDREY W C AND WEBER F L, CHRONIC HEPATIC ENCEPHALOPATHY, *MED CLIN NORTH AM*, 59, 937-44 (1975)

1474 MADEDDU G, CASU AR, COSTANZA C, ET AL, SERUM THYROGLOBULIN LEVELS IN THE DIAGNOSIS AND FOLLOW-UP OF SUBACUTE 'PAINFUL' THYROIDITIS, *ARCH INTERN MED*, 145, 243 (1985)

1475 MADSEN S N ET AL, URINARY CYCLIC AMP RELATION TO ALBUMIN-CORRECTED SERUM CALCIUM IN HEALTHY PERSONS AND PATIENTS WITH PRIMARY HYPERPARATHYROIDISM, *ACTA MED SCAND*, 200, 195-99 (1976)

1476 MAGILL G B ET AL, SERUM LACTIC DEHYDROGENASE AND SERUM TRANSAMINASE IN HUMAN LEUKEMIA, *BLOOD*, 14, 870 (1959)

1477 MAGNUS I A, THE CUTANEOUS PORPHYRIAS, *SEMIN HEMATOL*, 5, 380 (1968)

1478 MAGNUS I A ET AL, ERYTHROPOIETIC PROTOPORPHYRIA: A NEW PORPHYRIA SYNDROME WITH SOLAR URTICARIA DUE TO PROTO-PORPHYRINAEMIA, *LANCET*, 2, 448 (1961)

1479 MAGRI G ET AL, RELATIONSHIP BETWEEN URINE ACIDIFICATION AND INTRACELLULAR PH IN RESPIRATORY ACIDOSIS, *BRONCHOPNEUMOLOGIE*, 27, 293-300 (1977)

1480 MAHAJAN R C E ET AL, SIGNIFICANCE OF SERUM LACTIC DEHYDROGENASE ENZYME IN HEPATIC AMOEBIASIS, *INDIAN J MED RES*, 63, 1006-1009 (1975)

1481 MAHARAJAN G ET AL, THYROXINE, TRIIODOTHYRONINE AND THYRO-TROPHIN LEVELS IN MENINGOCOCCAL MENINGITIS, TYPHOID FEVER AND OTHER FEBRILE CONDITIONS., *CLIN ENDOCRINOL (OXF)*, 9, 401-406 (1979)

1482 MAILE JB, *LABORATORY MEDICINE: HEMATOLOGY, 5TH ED. ST. LOUIS, C.V. MOSBY CO.* (1977)

1483 MAISEL J D ET AL, FATAL MYCOPLASMA PNEUMONIAE INFECTION WITH ISOLATION OF ORGANISMS FROM LUNG, *JAMA*, 202, 287 (1967)

1484 MAJOR R H AND LEGER L H, MARKED EOSINOPHILIA IN HODGKIN'S DISEASE, *JAMA*, 112, 2601 (1939)

1485 MAKO M E ET AL, CIRCULATING PROINSULIN IN PATIENTS WITH MATUR-ITY ONSET DIABETES, *AM J MED*, 63, 865-873 (1977)

1486 MALAGELADA JR, IBER FL, LINSCHEER WG, ORIGIN OF FAT IN CHY-LOUS ASCITES OF PATIENTS WITH LIVER CIRRHOSIS, *GASTROEN-TEROLOGY*, 67, 878-886 (1974)

1487 MALAIA LT, SHELEST AN, VOLKOV VI, ET AL, BILE ACIDS IN CORONARY ARTERIOSCLEROSIS, *KARDIOLOGIIA*, 24, 81-4 (1984)

1488 MALAIA T, ET AL, *KARDIOLOGIIA*, 24, 81-4 (1984)

1489 MALDONADO J E AND HANLON D G, MONOCYTOSIS: A CURRENT APPRAISAL, *MAYO CLIN PROC*, 40, 248 (1965)

1490 MALETTE L E HENKIN R I, ALTERED COPPER AND ZINC METABOLISM IN PRIMARY HYPERPARATHYROIDISM, *AM J MED SCI*, 272, 167-74. (1976)

1491 MALKJAERSIG N ET AL, REDUCTION OF COAGULATION FACTOR XIII CONCENTRATION IN PATIENTS WITH MYOCARDIAL INFARCTION, CEREBRAL INFARCTION, AND OTHER THROMBOEMBOLIC DISOR-DERS, *THROMB HAEMOST*, 38, 863-73 (1977)

1492 MALLETTE L E ET AL, PRIMARY HYPERPARATHYROIDISM: CLINICAL AND BIOCHEMICAL FEATURES, *MEDICINE*, 53, 127-46 (1974)

1493 MALVI ET AL, A CYTOCHEMICAL STUDY OF ACID PHOSPHATASE IN CARCINOMA OF THE CERVIX UTERI, *IND J CANCER*, 11, 81-87 (1974)

1494 MAN ET AL, THE LIPIDS OF SERUM AND LIVER IN PATIENTS WITH HEP-ATIC DISEASES, *J CLIN INVEST*, 64, 623-643 (1945)

1495 MANDELL J R ET AL, AMYOTROPHIC LATERAL SCLEROSIS: METABO-LISM OF CENTRAL MONOAMINES AND TREATMENT WITH L-DOPA, *TRANS AMER NEUROL ASSOC*, 96, 284 (1972)

1496 MANICATIDE M A ET AL, BREATHLESSNESS AND BLOOD OXYGEN TEN-SION IN PATIENTS WITH CHRONIC BRONCHITIS AND EMPHYSEMA, *MED INTERNE*, 14, 211-4 (1976)

1497 MANICATIDE M A ET AL, HYPOXEMIA IN CHRONIC BRONCHITIS AND PULMONARY EMPHYSEMA, *MED INTERNE*, 15, 41-8 (1977)

1498 MANN NP, JOHNSTON DI, TOTAL GLYCOSYLATED HAEMOGLOBIN (HBA1) LEVELS IN DIABETIC CHILDREN, *ARCH DIS CHILD*, 57, 434-7 (1982)

1499 MANROE B L ET AL, THE DIFFERENTIAL LEUKOCYTE COUNT IN THE ASSESSMENT AND OUTCOME OF EARLY-ONSET NEONATAL GROUP B STREPTOCOCCAL DISEASE, *J PEDIATR*, 91, 632-7 (1977)

1500 MANSBERGER AR JR, THE DIAGNOSTIC VALUE OF ABDOMINAL PARACENTESIS, *AM J GASTROENTEROL*, 42, 150-164 (1964)

1501 MANSFIELD CM, KIMLER BF, HENDERSON SD, ET AL, ANGIOTENSIN-I-CONVERTING ENZYME IN CANCER PATIENTS, *J CLIN ONCOL*, 2, 452-6 (1984)

1502 MANSO C ET AL, GLUTATHIONE REDUCTASE ACTIVITY IN BLOOD AND BODY FLUIDS, *J CLIN INVEST*, 37, 214-218 (1958)

1503 MANY, ALLERGY AND IMMUNOLOGY, *MKSAP VII, AMERICAN COLLEGE OF PHYSICIANS* (1986)

1504 MARBLE A, DIAGNOSES OF LESS COMMON GLYCOSURIAS, INCLUDING PENTOSURIA AND FRUCTOSURIA, *MED CLIN NORTH AM*, 31, 313 (1974)

1505 MARCOVINA S, KOTTKE BA, MAO SJT, MONOCLONAL ANTIBODIES CAN PRECIPITATE LOW-DENSITY LIPOPROTEIN.II. RADIOIMMUNOAS-SAYS WITH SINGLE AND COMBINED MONOCLONAL ANTIBODIES FOR DETERMINING APOLIPOPROTEIN B IN SERUM OF PATIENTS WITH CORONARY ARTERY DISEASE, *CLIN CHEM*, 31/10, 1659-1663 (1985)

1506 MARECEK Z ET AL, THE EFFECT OF LONG TERM TREATMENT WITH PENICILLAMINE ON THE COPPER CONTENT IN THE LIVER IN PATIENTS WITH WILSON'S DISEASE, *ACTA HEPATOGAS-TROENTEROL (STUTTG)*, 22, 292-6 (1975)

1507 MARGOLIS S AND HOMCY C, SYSTEMIC MANIFESTATIONS OF HEPATOMA, *MEDICINE*, 51, 381 (1972)

1508 MARIANI G ET AL, PATHOPHYSIOLOGY OF HYPOALBUMINEMIA ASSOCI-ATED WITH CARCINOID TUMOR, *CANCER*, 38, 854-60 (1976)

1509 MARKS C, HYPERCALCEMIA IN MALIGNANT NON-PARATHYROID DIS-EASE, *AM J SURG*, 31, 254 (1965)

1510 MARNER IL. ET AL, DISEASE ACTIVITY AND SERUM PROTEINS IN ULCER-ATIVE COLITIS, *SCAND J GASTROENTEROL*, 10, 538 (1975)

1511 MARSDED S ET AL, DETECTION OF OCCULT METASTATIC MELANOMA BY URINE CHROMATOGRAPHY, *CANCER RES*, 36, 3317-23 (1976)

1512 MARSH J C, ANALYSIS OF 106 PATIENTS WITH CHRONIC MYELOCYTIC LEUKEMIA EXAMINED IN THE UNIVERSITY OF UTAH HEMATOLOGY CLINIC, 1944-1963, *UNPUBLISHED*

1513 MARSHALL ET AL, PROSTATIC ACID PHOSPHATASE LEVELS, *UROL-OGY*, 4, 435-538 (1974)

1514 MARTIN E W, HAZARDS OF MEDICATION, A MANUAL ON DRUG INTER-ACTIONS, INCOMPATIBILITIES, CONTRAINDICATIONS AND ADVERSE EFFECTS, *LIPPINCOTT PHILADELPHIA PA* (1971)

1515 MARTIN H E ET AL, SERUM POTASSIUM, MAGNESIUM, AND CALCIUM LEVELS IN DIABETIC ACIDOSIS, *J CLIN INVEST*, 26, 217 (1947)

1516 MARTIN H E ET AL, THE FLUID AND ELECTROLYTE THERAPY OF SEVERE DIABETIC ACIDOSIS AND KETOSIS, *AM J MED*, 20, 376-388 (1956)

1517 MARTIN J V ET AL, THE ASSOCIATION BETWEEN SERUM TRIGLYCER-IDES AND GAMMA GLUTAMYL TRANSPEPTIDASE ACTIVITY IN DIA-BETES MELLITUS, *CLIN BIOCHEM*, 9, 208-11 (1976)

1518 MARTIN R J ET AL, PULMONARY ALVEOLAR PROTEINOSIS, *AM REV RESPIR DIS*, 117, 1059-62 (1978)

1519 MARX JL, THE HDL: THE GOOD CHOLESTEROL CARRIERS?, *SCIENCE*, 205, 677-679 (1979)

1520 MASON J E JR ET AL, THROMBOCYTOSIS IN CHRONIC GRANULOCYTIC LEUKEMIA: INCIDENCE AND CLINICAL SIGNIFICANCE, *BLOOD*, 44, 483 (1974)

1521 MASRY B E ET AL, LDH ISOENZYMES IN SOME HAEMOPOIETIC DIS-EASES, *HAEMATOLOGIA (BUDAP)*, 7, 405-411 (1973)

1522 MASSEY S G ET AL, DIVALENT ION METABOLISM IN PATIENTS WITH ACUTE RENAL FAILURE. STUDIES ON THE MECHANISM OF ACUTE RENAL FAILURE, *KIDNEY INT*, 5, 437 (1974)

1523 MASSRY S G ET AL, CALCIUM METABOLISM IN PATIENTS WITH NEPHROTIC SYNDROME, *AM J CLIN NUTR*, 31, 1572-80 (1978)

1524 MATHISON D A ET AL, HYPOCOMPLEMENTEMIA IN CHRONIC IDIO-PATHIC URTICARIA, *ANN INTERN MED*, 86, 534-538 (1977)

1525 MATTENHEIMER H, ENZYMES IN RENAL DISEASE, *ANN CLIN LAB SCI*, 7, 422 (1977)

1526 MAURY CP, TEPPO AM, FROSETH B, WEGELIUS O, ALPHA 1-ANTITRYP-SIN AND REACTIVE SYSTEMIC AMYLOIDOSIS, *CLIN SCI*, 64, 453-4 (1983)

1527 MAURY M, WALTI H, RICHER C, FRANCOUAL C, ET AL, SERUM ANGI-OTENSIN I-CONVERTING ENZYME ACTIVITY IN PREMATURE AND FULL-TERM INFANTS, *BIOL NEONATE*, 45, 102-4 (1984)

1528 MAUVAIS-JARVIS P ET A, BENIGN BREAST DISEASE: HORMONAL STUD-IES IN 125 CASES, *NOUV PRESSE MED*, 6, 4115-8 (1977)

1529 MAUZERALL D AND GRANICK S, THE OCCURRENCE AND DETERMINA-TION OF ALPHA-AMINOLEVULINIC ACID AND PORPHOBILINOGEN IN URINE, *J BIOL CHEM*, 219, 435 (1956)

1530 MAYO MEDICAL LABORATORIES, *INTERPRETIVE DATA FOR DIAGNOS-TIC LABORATORY TESTS. ROCHESTER, MINN* (1981)

1531 MAYR K, ASPOCK G, MAYER MH, ET AL, ANGIOTENSIN CONVERTING ENZYME IN LUNG DISEASES, *WIEN MED WOCHENSCHR*, 135, 109-13 (1985)

1532 MC CARTHY D S AND J PEPYS, ALLERGIC BRONCHOPULMONARY ASPERGILLOSIS. CLINICAL IMMUNOLOGY: (1) CLINICAL FEATURES, (2) SKIN, NASAL, AND BRONCHIAL TESTS, *CLIN ALLERGY*, 1 (1971)

1533 MC GUIGAN J E, SERUM GASTRIN IN HEALTH AND DISEASE, *AM J DIG DIS*, 22, 712-16 (1977)

1534 MC GUIGAN J E ET AL, SERUM GASTRIN CONCENTRATIONS IN PERNI-CIOUS ANEMIA, *N ENGL J MED*, 282, 358-60 (1970)

1535 MCARDLE B, FAMILIAL PERIODIC PARALYSIS, *BR MED BULL*, 12, 226 (1956)

1536 MCBEE J W ET AL, HYPOGLYCEMIA DUE TO OBSTRUCTION OF PAN-CREATIC EXCRETORY DUCTS BY CARCINOMA, *ARCH PATHOL LAB MED*, 81, 287 (1966)

1537 MCCLELLA J E ET AL, SURVIVAL TIME OF THE ERYTHROCYTE IN MYXE-DEMA AND HYPERTHYROIDISM, *J LAB CLIN MED*, 51, 91 (1958)

1538 MCCLURE P D, IDIOPATHIC THROMBOCYTOPENIC PURPURA IN CHIL-DREN: DIAGNOSIS AND MANAGEMENT, *PEDIATRICS*, 55, 68 (1975)

1539 MCCORMICK JR, THRALL RS, WARD PA, MOORE VL, ET AL, SERUM ANGIOTENSIN-CONVERTING ENZYME LEVELS IN PATIENTS WITH PIGEON-BREEDER'S DISEASE, *CHEST*, 80, 431-3 (1981)

1540 MCCUNE D J ET AL, INTRACTABLE HYPOPHOSPHATEMIC RICKETS WITH RENAL GLYCOSURIA AND ACIDOSIS (THE FANCONI SYN-DROME), *AM J DIS CHILD*, 65, 81-103 (43)

1541 MCCURDY P R AND SHERMAN A S, IRREVERSIBLY SICKLED CELLS AND RED CELL SURVIVAL IN SICKLE CELL ANEMIA, *AM J MED*, 64, 253-258 (1978)

1542 MCEVEN J ET AL, DRUGS-FALSE-POSITIVE SCREENING TESTS FOR PORPHYRIA, *BR MED J*, 1, 421 (1972)

1543 MCFADYEN I J ET AL, CIRCULATING HORMONE CONCENTRATIONS IN WOMEN WITH BREAST CANCER, *LANCET*, 1, 1100-2. (1976)

1544 MCFARLIN D E AND JOHNSON J S, STUDIES OF ANTIMUSCLE FACTOR IN MYASTHENIA GRAVIS: II. REACTIONS OF FRAGMENTS PRO-DUCED IN ENZYMATIC DIGESTION, *J IMMUNOL*, 106, 292 (1971)

1545 MCGALE E H F ET AL, QUANTITATIVE CHANGES IN PLASMA AMINO ACIDS IN PATIENTS WITH RENAL DISEASE, *CLIN CHIM ACTA*, 38, 395-403 (1972)

1546 MCGOWAN G K ET AL, DIAGNOSTIC VALUE OF PLASMA AMYLASE ESPECIALLY AFTER GASTRECTOMY., *BR MED J*, 1, 160 (1964)

1547 MCGOWAN L, BUNNAG B, ARIAS LF, MESOTHELIOMA OF THE ABDOMEN IN WOMEN. MONITORING OF THERAPY BY PERITONEAL FLUID STUDY, *GYNECOL ONCOL*, 3, 10-14 (1975)

1548 MCILROY M ET AL, GLUCOSE TOLERANCE IN VIRAL HEPATITIS, *IR J MED SCI*, 145, 3-9 (1976)

1549 MCKAY D G AND A E COREY, CRYOFIBRINOGENEMIA IN TOXEMIA OF PREGNANCY, *OBSTET GYNECOL*, 23, 508 (1964)

1550 MCKAY E J, MEASUREMENT OF COMPLEMENT AS AN AID IN DIAGNOSIS: L. NEPHRITES AND COLLAGEN DISEASE, *NZ MED J*, 87, 315-18 (1978)

1551 MCKEE P A ET AL, INCIDENCE AND SIGNIFICANCE OF CRYOFIBRINOGENEMIA, *J LAB CLIN MED*, 61, 203 (1963)

1552 MCKENNA R ET AL, NON-SPECIFIC ESTERASE POSITIVE ACUTE LEUKEMIA, *PROC AACR/ASCO*, 16, 61 (1974)

1553 MCKENZIE C G ET AL, BIOCHEMICAL MARKERS IN BRONCHIAL CARCINOMA, *BR J CANCER*, 36, 700-7 (1977)

1554 MCKINLAY I A ET AL, TRANSIENT ACUTE MYOSITIS IN CHILDHOOD, *ARCH DIS CHILD*, 51, 135-7 (1976)

1555 MCLAREN DS, EFFECTS OF VITAMIN A DEFICIENCY IN MAN, *THE VITAMINS, 2ND EDN (EDS) W.H. SEBRELL JR AND R.S. HARRIS), ACADEMIC PRESS, NY*, 1, 267-280 (1967)

1556 MCLEAN A S, EARLY ADVERSE EFFECTS OF RADIATION, *BR MED BULL*, 29, 69 (1973)

1557 MCMASTER Y ET AL, THE MECHANISM OF THE ELEVATION OF SERUM ALKALINE PHOSPHATASE IN PREGNANCY, *BR J OBSTET GYNAECOL*, 71, 735-739 (1964)

1558 MCMURRAY W ET AL, URINARY COPPER EXCRETION IN RHEUMATOID ARTHRITIS, *ANN RHEUM DIS*, 34, 340-5 (1975)

1559 MCNEELY MD, SUNDERMAN FW, NECHAY MW, LEVINE H, ABNORMAL CONCENTRATIONS OF NICKEL IN SERUM IN CASES OF MYOCARDIAL INFARCTION, STROKE, BURNS, HEPATIC CIRRHOSIS, AND UREMIA, *CLIN CHEM*, 17, 1123-1128 (1971)

1560 MCNICHOL K N AND WILLIAMS H E, SPECTRUM OF ASTHMA IN CHILDREN: I. CLINICAL AND PHYSIOLOGICAL COMPONENTS, *BR MED J*, 4, 7 (1973)

1561 MEADE B W ET AL, SERUM ENZYME ACTIVITY IN NORMAL PREGNANCY AND THE NEWBORN, *BR J OBSTET GYNAECOL*, 70, 693 (1963)

1562 MEADOR C K ET AL, CAUSE OF CUSHING'S SYNDROME IN PATIENTS WITH TUMORS ARISING FROM NONENDOCRINE TISSUE, *J CLIN ENDOCRINOL METAB*, 22, 693 (1962)

1563 MEHTA ET AL, LEUCOCYTE ALKALINE PHOSPHATASE ACTIVITY--ITS UTILITY IN DIAGNOSIS, *INDIAN J MED SCI*, 28, 12-18 (1974)

1564 MEITES S, PEDIATRIC CLINICAL CHEMISTRY, *2ND ED. WASHINGTON, D.C., AMERICAN ASSOCIATION FOR CLINICAL CHEMISTRY* (1981)

1565 MELINCOFF S M ET AL, ABNORMAL URINARY AMINO ACID PATTERNS IN ACUTE INTERMITTENT PORPHYRIA, *J LAB CLIN MED*, 53, 359 (1959)

1566 MELISSINOS K ET AL, LDH ACTIVITY OF RED CELLS IN CHRONIC RENAL FAILURE, *CLIN CHIM ACTA*, 40, 165 (1972)

1567 MELISSINOS K ET AL, STUDY OF THE ACTIVITY OF ERYTHROCYTE ACID PHOSPHATASE IN CHRONIC RENAL FAILURE, *CLIN CHIM ACTA*, 43, 195-199 (1973)

1568 MELMON K L, THE ENDOCRINOLOGIC MANIFESTATIONS OF THE CARCINOID TUMOR, *IN: TEXTBOOK OF ENDOCRINOLOGY WILLIAMS R H (ED)*, 161 (1968)

1569 MELTZER H ET AL, SERUM-ENZYME CHANGES IN NEWLY ADMITTED PSYCHIATRIC PATIENTS, *ARCH GEN PSYCHIATRY*, 21, 731-738 (1969)

1570 MENNES P ET AL, HYPOMAGNESEMIA AND IMPAIRED PARATHYROID HORMONE SECRETION IN CHRONIC RENAL DISEASE, *ANN INTERN MED*, 88, 206-209 (1978)

1571 MERCER ET AL, ACID PHOSPHATASE ISOENZYMES IN GAUCHER'S DISEASE, *CLIN CHEM*, 23, 631-635 (1977)

1572 MEYER D AND LARRIEU M J, FACTOR VIII AND IX VARIANTS, *EUR J CLIN INVEST*, 1, 425 (1971)

1573 MEYER L M ET AL, A STUDY OF CHOLINESTERASE ACTIVITY OF THE BLOOD OF PATIENTS WITH PERNICIOUS ANEMIA, *J LAB CLIN MED*, 33, 1068 (1948)

1574 MEYER M S ET AL, LOW LEVELS OF SERUM CALCIUM, PHOSPHORUS AND PLASMA 25-HYDROXY VITAMIN D IN CIRRHOSIS OF THE LIVER, *ISR J MED SCI*, 14, 725-30 (1978)

1575 MEYER O, THE ESR IN VIRAL HEPATITIS, *PEDIATRICS*, 61, 484-5 (1978)

1576 MEZZANO S, OLAVARIA F, ARDILES L, ET AL, INCIDENCE OF CIRCULATING IMMUNE COMPLEXES IN PATIENTS WITH ACUTE POSTSTREPTOCOCCAL GLOMERULONEPHRITIS AND IN PATIENTS WITH STREPTOCOCCAL IMPETIGO, *CLIN NEPHROL*, 26, 61-5 (1986)

1577 MEZZANO S, OLAVARRIA F, ARDILES L, ET AL, IN VITRO AUTORADIOGRAPHIC LOCALIZATION OF ANGIOTENSIN-CONVERTING ENZYME IN SARCOID LYMPH NODES, *CLIN NEPHROL*, 26, 61-5 (1986)

1578 MIALE J B, LABORATORY MEDICINE-HEMATOLOGY, *2ND EDITION CV MOSBY ST LOUIS MO* (1962)

1579 MIALE JB, *LABORATORY MEDICINE: HEMATOLOGY, 5TH ED. ST. LOUIS, C.V. MOSBY CO.* (1977)

1580 MICHELIS M F ET AL, HYPOURICEMIA AND HYPERURICOSURIA IN LAENNEC'S CIRRHOSIS, *ARCH INTERN MED*, 134, 681-683 (1974)

1581 MICHENER W M, HYPERURICEMIA AND MENTAL RETARDATION WITH ATHETOSIS AND SELF-MUTILATION, *AM J DIS CHILD*, 113, 195 (1967)

1582 MICHIE ET AL, MECHANISM OF HYPOCALCAEMIA AFTER THYROIDECTOMY FOR THYROTOXICOSIS, *J CLIN ENDOCR*, 1, 508-513 (1971)

1583 MIER M ET AL, ACANTHOCYTOSIS, PIGMENTARY DEGENERATION OF THE RETINA AND ATOXIC NEUROPATHY: A GENETICALLY DETERMINED SYNDROME WITH ASSOCIATED METABOLIC DISORDER, *BLOOD*, 5, 1586 (1960)

1584 MIGUERES J ET AL, VALUR THEORIQUE ET PRACTIQUE DE CERTAINS DOSAGES ENZYMATIQUES AU COURS DES EPANCHEMENTS PLEURAUX, *J FR MED CHER THORAC*, 23, 443-58 (1969)

1585 MIKKELSON W M, THE POSSIBLE ASSOCIATION OF HYPERURICEMIA AND/OR GOUT WITH DIABETES MELLITUS, *ARTHRITIS RHEUM*, 8, 853-859 (1965)

1586 MILHAUD G, CALCITONIN 1975, *BIOMED PHARMACOTHER*, 24, 159-62 (1976)

1587 MILHAUD G ET AL, EPITHELIOMA DE LA THYROIDE SECRETANT DE LA THRYROCALCITONINE, *RENDUS ACAD SCI SERIES D*, 266, 608 (1968)

1588 MILHAUD G ET AL, CALCIUM, PARATHYROID HORMONE AND THE CALCITONIN, *EXCERPTA MEDICA ACTA*, 46 (1972)

1589 MILHAUD G ET AL, RENCONTRE BIOLOGIQUE, 1975 ED, *EXPANSION SCIENTIFIC FRANC*, 125 (1975)

1590 MILL'AN N'UNEZ-CORTES J, BIOLOGICAL AND CLINICAL ASPECTS OF ALPHA 1-ANTITRYPSIN WITH SPECIAL REFERENCE TO MALIGNANT TUMOR PROCESSES, *REV ESP ONCOL*, 28, 591-641 (1981)

1591 MILLEDGE JS, CATLEY DM, ANGIOTENSIN CONVERTING ENZYME RESPONSE TO HYPOXIA IN MAN: ITS ROLE IN ALTITUDE ACCLIMATIZATION, *CLIN SCI*, 67, 453-6 (1984)

1592 MILLEDGE JS, CATLEY DM, WARD MP, ET AL, RENIN-ALDOSTERONE AND ANGIOTENSIN-CONVERTING ENZYME DURING PROLONGED ALTITUDE EXPOSURE, *J APPL PHYSIOL*, 55, 699-702 (1983)

1593 MILLER L H ET AL, HYPONATREMIA IN MALARIA, *ANN TROP MED PARASITOL*, 61, 265 (1967)

1594 MILLER P D ET AL, DEXTROSE PHOSPHORUS AND IRON METABOLISM IN ALCOHOLISM, *NUTR REV*, 36, 142-4 (1978)

1595 MILLER TR, ANDERSON RJ, LINAS SL, ET AL, URINARY DIAGNOSTIC INDICES IN ACUTE RENAL FAILURE, A PROSPECTIVE STUDY, *ANN INTERN MED*, 89, 47-50 (1978)

1596 MILLER W W ET AL, OXYGEN RELEASING FACTOR IN HYPERTHYROIDISM, *JAMA*, 211, 1824 (1970)

1597 MILLER Z B ET AL, SERUM LEVELS OF CYSTEINE AMINOPEPTIDASE, LEUCINE AMINOPEPTIDASE AND ALKALINE PHOSPHATASE IN SINGLE AND TWIN PREGNANCIES, *OBSTET GYNECOL*, 24, 707 (1964)

1598 MILOSAVLJEVIC J ET AL, DIAGNOSTIC SIGNIFICANCE OF ALPHAFETOPROTEINS IN NEONATAL HYPERBILIRUBINEMIAS AND PRIMARY CANCER OF THE LIVER IN ADULTS, *ACTA HEPATOGASTROENTEROL (STUTTG)*, 24, 30-3. (1977)

1599 MILUNSKY A, ALPERT E, RESULTS AND BENEFITS OF A MATERNAL SERUM A-FETOPROTEIN SCREENING PROGRAM, *JAMA*, 252, 1438 (1984)

1600 MINTZ D H ET AL, HYPERURICEMIA IN HYPERPARATHYROIDISM, *N ENGL J MED*, 265, 112-114 (1961)

1601 MIR M A, RENAL EXCRETION OF URIC ACID AND ITS RELATION TO RELAPSE AND REMISSION IN ACUTE MYELOID LEUKEMIA., *NEPHRON*, 19, 69-80 (1977)

1602 MIR M M ET AL, HYPOKALAEMIA IN ACUTE MYELOID LEUKAEMIA, *ANN INTERN MED*, 82, 54-57 (1975)

1603 MIRA M, STEWART PM, GEBSKI V, ET AL, CHANGES IN SODIUM AND URIC ACID CONCENTRATIONS IN PLASMA DURING THE MENSTRUAL CYCLE, *CLIN CHEM*, 30/3, 380-381 (1984)

1604 MISAKI F ET AL, ESTIMATION OF SERUM ACID PROTEASES AT PH 1.8 AND PH 3.5 IN PATIENTS WITH DUODENAL ULCER, GASTRIC ULCER AND GASTRIC CARCINOMA, *GASTROENTEROL JPN*, 12, 202-8 (1977)

1605 MISSIROLI A ET AL, INFLUENCE OF AUTOLOGOUS SERUM ON IN VITRO REACTIVITY OF PERIPHERAL LYMPHOCYTES OF PATIENTS WITH BREAST CANCER, *TUMORI*, 63, 129-35 (1977)

1606 MISTILIS S P ET AL, PLASMA LIPIDS IN EXTRA-HEPATIC BILIARY OBSTRUCTION, *AUST NZ J MED*, 5, 540-3 (1975)

1607 MITCH W E ET AL, PLASMA RENIN AND ANGIOTENSIN II IN ACUTE RENAL FAILURE, *LANCET*, 2, 328-30 (1977)

1608 MITCHELL D N ET AL, IMMUNOGLOBULIN LEVELS IN PATIENTS WITH SARCOIDOSIS, *Z ERKRANK ATM-ORG*, 149, 247-52 (1977)

1609 MITTMAN C ET AL, SMOKING AND CHRONIC OBSTRUCTIVE LUNG DISEASE IN ALPHA-1 ANTITRYPSIN DEFICIENCY, *CHEST*, 60, 214-21 (1971)

1610 MITUS W J ET AL, ALKALINE PHOSPHATASE OF MATURE NEUTROPHILS IN VARIOUS POLYCYTHEMIAS, *N ENGL J MED*, 260, 1131 (1959)

1611 MIURA H, NAKAYAMA M, SATO T, SERUM ANGIOTENSIN CONVERTING ENZYME (S-ACE) ACTIVITY IN PATIENTS WITH CHRONIC RENAL FAILURE ON REGULAR HEMODIALYSIS, *JPN HEART J*, 25, 87-92 (1984)

1612 MIYAGAWA S ET AL, CHARACTERIZATION OF CRYOPRECIPITATES IN PEMPHIGUS: DEMONSTRATION OF PEMPHIGUS ANTIBODY ACTIVITY IN CRYOPRECIPITATES USING THE IMMUNO FLUORESCENT TECHNIQUE, *J INVEST DERMATOL*, 69, 373-5 (1977)

1613 MIYAKAWA I ET AL, PLASMA LEVELS OF HUMAN CHORIONIC SOMATOMAMMOTROPIN PROGESTERONE, UNCONJUGATED OESTRADIOL AND OESTRIOL, AND ALPHA FETOPROTEIN IN PATIENTS WITH HYDATIDIFORM MOLES, *J ENDOCRINOL*, 72, 371-378 (1977)

1614 MOHAMMED I ET AL, MULTIPLE IMMUNE COMPLEXES AND HYPOCOMPLEMENTEMIA IN DERMATITIS HERPETIFORMIS AND CELIAC DISEASE, *LANCET*, 2, 487 (1976)

1615 MOLLISON P L, MEASUREMENT OF SURVIVAL AND DESTRUCTION OF RED CELLS IN HAEMOLYTIC SYNDROMES, *BR MED BULL*, 15, 59 (1959)

1616 MONCADA B, GONZALEZ-AMARO R, BARANDA ML, ET AL, IMMUNOPATHOLOGY OF POLYMORPHOUS LIGHT ERUPTION. T LYMPHOCYTES N BLOOD AND SKIN, *J AM ACAD DERMATOL*, 10, 970-3 (1984)

1617 MOORADIAN & MORLEY, ENDOCRINE DYSFUNCTION, *ARCH INTERN MED*, 144, 352 (1984)

1618 MOORE D F ET AL, MONOCLONAL GAMMAGLOBULINEMIA IN MALIGNANT LYMPHOMA, *ANN INTERN MED*, 72, 43 (1970)

1619 MOORE D L ET AL, THE SCHISTOSOMA MANSONI EGG GRANULOMA: QUANTITATION OF CELL POPULATIONS, *J PATHOL*, 121, 41 (1977)

1620 MOORE JA, NOIVA R, WELLS IC, SELENIUM CONCENTRATIONS IN PLASMA OF PATIENTS WITH ARTERIOGRAPHICALLY DEFINED CORONARY ATHEROSCLEROSIS, *CLIN CHEM*, 30/7, 1171-1173 (1984)

1621 MOORE M R ET AL, EVALUATION OF HUMAN CHORIONIC GONADOTROPIN AND ALPHA FETOPROTEIN IN BENIGN AND MALIGNANT TESTICULAR DISORDERS, *SURG GYNECOL OBSTET*, 147, 167-74 (1978)

1622 MOORE T, VITAMIN A, *ELSEVIER, AMSTERDAM, THE NETHERLANDS* (1957)

1623 MOORE T ET AL, LIVER PHYSIOLOGY AND DISEASE, *GASTROENTEROLOGY*, 63, 88 (1972)

1624 MOORE T L ET AL, CARCINOEMBRYONIC ANTIGEN ASSAY IN CANCER OF THE COLON AND PANCREAS AND OTHER DIGESTIVE TRACT DISORDERS, *AM J DIG DIS*, 16, 1-7 (1971)

1625 MORA F ET AL, AN IMMUNOLOGICAL STUDY OF NINE PROTEINS IN CSF AND SERUM OF A GROUP OF EPILEPTIC PATIENTS, *CLIN CHIM ACTA*, 80, 55-9 (1977)

1626 MOREL-MAROGER L ET AL, PATHOLOGY OF THE KIDNEY IN WALDENSTRÖM'S MACROGLOBULINEMIA: STUDY OF 16 CASES, *N ENGL J MED*, 283, 123 (1970)

1627 MORELLI A ET AL, DOPAMINE UPTAKE BY PLATELETS IN HEPATIC ENCEPHALOPATHY; EVIDENCE FOR A POSSIBLE DEPLETION OF BRAIN DOPAMINE, *ACTA HEPATOGASTROENTEROL*, 24, 405-10 (1977)

1628 MORGAN B, PROCEEDINGS: PREDICTIVE VALUE OF ACID PHOSPHATASE, *BR J CANCER*, 30, 190 (1974)

1629 MORGAN E H, PLASMA-IRON AND HAEMOGLOBIN LEVELS IN PREGNANCY, *LANCET*, I, 9 (1961)

1630 MORGAN L R ET AL, ARYLSULFATASE AND ITS RELATION TO HOMOVANILLIC ACID IN NEUROBLASTOMAS, *CLIN CHIM ACTA*, 37, 292-294 (1972)

1631 MORGANROTH J ET AL, THE BIOCHEMICAL, CLINICAL AND GENETIC FEATURES OF TYPE III HYPERLIPOPROTEINEMIA, *ANN INTERN MED*, 82, 158-174 (1975)

1632 MORLEY A A ET AL, ADRENAL STEROIDS AND HAEMOLYSIS IN PAROXYSMAL NOCTURNAL HAEMOGLOBINURIA, *LANCET*, 2, 448 (1967)

1633 MORRIN P A F ET AL, RAPIDLY PROGRESSIVE GLOMERULONEPHRITIS, *AM J MED*, 65, 446-460 (1978)

1634 MORRIS M W ET AL, THE ZETA SEDIMENTATION RATIO (ZSR) AND ACTIVITY OF DISEASE IN RHEUMATOID ARTHRITIS, *AM J CLIN PATHOL*, 68, 760-2 (1977)

1635 MORRISON J C ET AL, ENZYME LEVELS IN THE SERUM AND CEREBROSPINAL FLUID IN ECLAMPSIA, *AM J OBSTET GYNECOL*, 110, 619-624 (1971)

1636 MORSE JO, ALPHA-1-ANTITRYPSIN DEFICIENCY, *N ENGL J MED*, 299, 1045-1105 (1978)

1637 MORTIMER G, CASEY M, SERUM ACID PHOSPHATASE ACTIVITIES IN PATIENTS WITH LUNG CANCER: A BIOCHEMICAL AND IMMUNOHISTOCHEMICAL ANALYSIS OF 25 CASES, *J CLIN PATHOL*, 34, 958-62 (1981)

1638 MOSEKILDE L ET AL, DECREASED PARATHYROID FUNCTION IN HYPERTHYROIDISM, *ACTA ENDOCRINOL*, 84, 66-75 (1977)

1639 MOSES A M AND SPENCER H, HYPERCALCEMIA IN PATIENTS WITH MALIGNANT LYMPHOMA, *ANN INTERN MED*, 59, 531 (1963)

1640 MOSNAIM AD, WOLF ME, CHEVESICH J, ET AL, PLASMA METHIONINE ENKEPHALIN LEVELS. A BIOLOGICAL MARKER FOR MIGRAINE?, *HEADACHE*, 25, 259-261 (1985)

1641 MUGGIA F M ET AL, LYSOZYMURIA AND RENAL TUBULAR DYSFUNCTION IN MONOCYTIC AND MYELOMONOCYTIC LEUKEMIA, *AM J MED*, 47, 351 (1969)

1642 MULDOWNEY F P ET AL, THE TOTAL RED CELL MASS IN THYROTOXCOSIS AND MYXOEDEMA, *CLIN SCI*, 16, 309 (1957)

1643 MULLAN, SERUM ENZYMES IN DIAGNOSIS OF TETANUS, *LANCET*, 2, 505-506 (1964)

1644 MULLER W A ET AL, HYPERGLUCAGONEMIA IN DIABETIC KETOACIDOSIS: ITS PREVALENCE AND SIGNIFICANCE, *AM J MED*, 54, 52-57 (1973)

1645 MUNK P ET AL, HEMOGLOBIN-OXYGEN AFFINITY IN HYPOPHOSPHATEMIC RICKETS, *ACTA PAEDIATR SCAND*, 65, 97-9. (1976)

1646 MURDOCH J M AND SMITH C C, HEMATOLOGICAL ASPECTS OF SYSTEMIC DISEASE: INFECTION, *CLIN LAB HAEMATOL*, 1, 619 (1972)

1647 MURPHY G P ET AL, COMPARISON OF TOTAL AND PROSTATIC FRACTION SERUM ACID PHOSPHATASE LEVELS IN PATIENTS WITH DIFFERENTIATED AND UNDIFFERENTIATED PROSTATIC CARCINOMA, *CANCER*, 23, 1309-1314 (1969)

1648 MURPHY G P ET AL, ERYTHROPOIETIN LEVELS IN PATIENTS WITH RENAL TUMOR OR CYSTS, *CANCER*, 26, 191 (1970)

1649 MURPHY J R, HEMOGLOBIN CC ERYTHROCYTES: DECREASED INTRACELLULAR PH AND DECREASED $_{2}$ AFFINITY-ANEMIA, *SEMIN HEMATOL*, 13, 177 (1976)

1650 MURRAY HW, TUAZON C, ATYPICAL PNEUMONIAS, *MED CLIN NORTH AM*, 64, 507-527 (1980)

1651 MURRAY J F, ARTERIAL STUDIES IN PRIMARY AND SECONDARY POLYCYTHEMIC DISORDERS, *AM REV RESPIR DIS*, 92, 435 (1965)

1652 MURRAY R C, THE USE OF THE ABSOLUTE EOSINOPHIL COUNT IN THE DIAGNOSIS OF NEOPLASMS, *N ENGL J MED*, 248, 848 (1953)

1653 MURRAY, BJ, THE HEPATITIS B CARRIER STATE, *AMERICAN FAMILY PHYSICIAN*, 127 (1986)

1654 MURRAY-LYON I M ET AL, QUANTITATIVE IMMUNOELECTROPHORESIS OF SERUM PROTEINS IN CRYPTOGENIC CIRRHOSIS, ALCOHOLIC CIRRHOSIS, AND ACTIVE CHRONIC HEPATITIS, *CLIN CHIM ACTA*, 39, 215-220 (1972)

1655 MURRAY-LYON I M ET AL, PROGNOSTIC VALUE OF SERUM ALPHA-FETOPROTEIN IN FULMINANT HEPATIC FAILURE INCLUDING PATIENTS TREATED BY CHARCOAL HAEMOFUSION, *GUT*, 17, 576-80 (1976)

1656 MYERSON R M AND FRUMIN A M, HYPERKALEMIA ASSOCIATED WITH THE MYELOPROLIFERATIVE DISORDERS, *ARCH INTERN MED*, 106, 479 (1960)

1657 MYERSON RM, LAFAIR JS, ALCOHOLIC MUSCLE DISEASE, *MED CLIN NORTH AM*, 54, 723-730 (1970)

1658 MYGIND N, SERIAL SERUM ENZYME STUDIES IN INFECTIOUS MONONUCLEOSIS, *SCAND J INFECT DIS*, 8, 139-142 (1976)

1659 MYHRE ET AL, SERUM-LACTIC-DEHYDROGENASE ACTIVITY AND INTRAVASCULAR HAEMOLYSIS, *J CLIN ENDOCR*, 1, 355 (1970)

1660 MYLLYLA V V ET AL, CYCLIC AMP CONCENTRATION AND ENZYME ACTIVITIES OF CEREBROSPINAL FLUID IN PATIENTS WITH EPILEPSY OR CENTRAL NERVOUS SYSTEM DAMAGE, *EUR NEUROL*, 13, 123-130 (1975)

1661 N'EMETH A, STRANDVIK B, URINARY EXCRETION OF TETRAHYDROXYLATED BILE ACIDS IN CHILDREN WITH ALPHA 1-ANTITRYPSIN DEFICIENCY AND NEONATAL CHOLESTASIS, *SCAND J CLIN LAB INVEST*, 44, 387-92 (1984)

1662 NACHOLD B S JR AND KIRSCHNER N, THE METABOLISM OF ADRENALIN AND NORADRENALINE IN PATIENTS WITH BASAL GANGLIA DISEASE, *NEUROL*, 13, 753 (1963)

1663 NAEIJE R ET AL, A LOW T_3 SYNDROME IN DIABETIC KETOACIDOSIS, *CLIN ENDOCRINOL (OXF)*, 8, 467-72 (1978)

1664 NAFF G B BYERS P H, POSSIBLE IMPLICATION OF COMPLEMENT IN ACUTE GOUT, *J CLIN INVEST*, 46, 1099 (1967)

1665 NAGAKI K, HIRAMATSU S, INAI S, SASAKI A, THE EFFECT OF AGING ON COMPLEMENT ACTIVITY (CH50) AND COMPLEMENT PROTEIN LEVELS, *J CLIN LAB IMMUNOL*, 3, 45-50 (1980)

1666 NAGASAWA T ET AL, FIBRONOGEN/FIBRIN DEGRADATION PRODUCTS IN SERUM OF PATIENTS WITH ITP, *THROMB HAEMOST*, 35, 628 (1976)

1667 NAGATAKI S ET AL, THYROID FUNCTION IN MOLAR PREGNANCY, *J CLIN ENDOCRINOL METAB*, 44, 254-63 (1977)

1668 NAGAWA S, KUMIN S, NITOWSKY HM, HUMAN HEXOSAMINIDASE ISOENZYMES: CHROMATOGRAPHIC SEPARATION AS AN AID TO HETEROZYGOTE IDENTIFICATION, *CLIN CHIM ACTA*, 75, 181-191 (1977)

1669 NAJEAN Y ET AL, BLOOD VOLUME IN HEALTH AND DISEASE, *CLIN LAB HAEMATOL*, 6, 543-64 (1977)

1670 NAKAMURA RM, CLINICAL LABORATORY CONCEPTS AND METHODS, *IMMUNOPATHOLOGY* (1974)

1671 NAKAMURA RM, DITO WR, NICHOLS WS, ET AL, *SYMPOSIUM ON RECENT PROGRESS IN DIAGNOSTIC LABORATORY IMMUNOLOGY, SAN DIEGO, CA* (1981)

1672 NAKAMURA RM, DITO WR, TUCKER ES III, IMMUNOASSAYS IN THE CLINICAL LABORATORY, *NEW YORK, ALAN R. LISS, INC.* (1979)

1673 NAKAMURA Y, TAKEDA T, ISHII M, ET AL, ELEVATION OF SERUM ANGIOTENSIN-CONVERTING ENZYME ACTIVITY IN PATIENTS WITH HYPERTHYROIDISM, *J CLIN ENDOCRINOL METAB*, 55, 931-4 (1982)

1674 NAKAMURA R M, DITO W R, TUCKER E S, *CLINICAL LABORATORY ASSAYS NEW YORK, MASSON PUBLISHING USA, INC* (1983)

1675 NAKANO I, FUNAKOSHI A, KIMURA T, ET AL, ELEVATED LEVELS OF SERUM PANCREATIC SECRETORY TRYPSIN INHIBITOR (PSTI) IN PATIENTS WITH MALABSORPTION SYNDROME, *GASTROENTEROL JPN*, 21, 617-22 (1986 DEC)

1676 NANKERVES G A AND M KUMAR, DISEASES PRODUCED BY CYTOMEGALOVIRUSES, *MED CLIN NORTH AM*, 62, 1021-35 (1978)

1677 NARAYANAN I ET AL, MUSCULAR DYSTROPHY. PART I: SERUM ENZYMES IN THE DUCHENNE MUSCULAR DYSTROPHY AND NEUROMUSCULAR DISORDERS, *INDIAN J MED RES*, 62, 598-604 (1974)

1678 NARDI G L ET AL, SERUM TRYPSIN, *N ENGL J MED*, 2658, 797-8 (1958)

1679 NARDONE D A ET AL, MECHANISMS IN HYPOKALEMIA: CLINICAL CORRELATION, *MEDICINE*, 57, 435-46 (1978)

1680 NASTUK W L ET AL, CHANGES IN SERUM COMPLEMENT ACTIVITY IN PATIENTS WITH MYASTHENIA GRAVIS, *PROC SOC EXP BIOL MED*, 105, 177 (1960)

1681 NEALE ET AL, EFFECTS OF INTRAHEPATIC AND EXTRAHEPATIC INFECTION ON LIVER FUNCTION, *BR MED J*, 1, 382-387 (1966)

1682 NEELY C L ET AL, LACTIC ACID DEHYDROGENASE ACTIVITY AND PLASMA HEMOGLOBIN ELEVATIONS IN SICKLE CELL DISEASE, *AM J CLIN PATHOL*, 52, 167-169 (1969)

1683 NELSON C S, REVIEW OF FAT EMBOLISM: SPECIAL REFERENCE TO CARDIAC AND PULMONARY FAT EMBOLECTOMY, *SHOEMAKER W C ET AL (ED) CURRENT TOPICS IN CRITICAL CARE MEDICINE*, 153-60 (1976)

1684 NELSON P V ET AL, DIAGNOSTIC SIGNIFICANCE AND SOURCE OF LACTATE DEHYDROGENASE AND ITS ISOENZYMES IN CEREBROSPINAL FLUID OF CHILDREN WITH A VARIETY OF NEUROLOGIC DISORDERS, *J CLIN PATHOL*, 28, 828-833 (1975)

1685 NEMETH A, SAMUELSON K, STRANDVIK B, SERUM BILE ACIDS AS MARKERS OF JUVENILE LIVER DISEASE IN ALPHA 1-ANTITRYPSIN DEFICIENCY, *J PEDIATR GASTROENTEROL NUTR*, 1, 479-83 (1982)

1686 NEUGUT AI, JOHNSEN CM, FINK DJ, SERUM CHOLESTEROL LEVELS IN ADENOMATOUS POLYPS AND CANCER OF THE COLON, *JAMA*, 255, 365 (1986)

1687 NEUMANN ET AL, DISTINCT ALKALINE PHOSPHATASE IN SERUM OF PATIENT WITH LYMPHATIC LEUKEMIA AND INFECTIOUS MONONUCLEOSIS, *SCIENCE*, 186, 151-3 (1974)

1688 NEVALAINEN TJ, ESKOLA JU, AHO AJ, ET AL, IMMUNOREACTIVE PHOSPHOLIPASE A2 IN SERUM IN ACUTE PANCREATITIS AND PANCREATIC CANCER, *CLIN CHEM*, 31/7, 1116-1120 (1985)

1689 NEWCOMBE DS, COHEN AS, CHYLOUS SYNOVIAL EFFUSION IN RHEUMATOID ARTHRITIS, *AM J MED*, 38, 156-164 (1965)

1690 NEWMAN R L, SERUM ELECTROLYTES IN PREGNANCY, PARTURITION, AND PUERPERIUM, *OBSTET GYNECOL*, 10, 51-55 (1957)

1691 NICHOLS INSTITUTE, *PROFESSIONAL SERVICES. SAN PEDRO, CALIF.* (1979)

1692 NICKEL K, DHEA-S-NEW FROM BIO-SCIENCE, *BIO-SCIENCE REPORTS: BIO-SCIENCE LABORATORIES; VAN NUYS, CALIF* (1980)

1693 NIEJADLIK D C, HYDROXYPROLINE, *J POSTGRAD MED*, 51, 213-6 (1972)

1694 NIEJADLIK ET AL, GLUCOSE MEASUREMENTS AND CLINICAL CORRELATIONS, *JAMA*, 224, 1734-1736 (1973)

1695 NIELSEN K, COELIAC DISEASE: ALPHA-1-ANTITRYPSIN CONTENTS IN JEJUNAL MUCOSA BEFORE AND AFTER GLUTEN-FREE DIET, *HISTOPATHOLOGY*, 8, 759-64 (1984)

1696 NIGHTINGALE S ET AL, THE HAEMATOLOGY OF HYPERTHYROIDISM, *Q J MED*, 185, 35-47 (1978)

1697 NIK SI'C-IVAN CI'C M, ORESKOVI'C M, THE ROLE OF ALPHA-1-ANTITRYPSIN IN PATIENTS WITH LARYNGEAL CARCINOMA, *LARYNGOL RHINOL OTOL (STUTTG)*, 62, 246-8 (1983)

1698 NISHIDA Y ET AL, HYPERLIPIDEMIA IN PATIENTS WITH DOWN'S SYNDROME, *ARTERIOSCLEROSIS*, 26, 369-72 (1977)

1699 NISHIOKA K ET AL, THE COMPLEMENT SYSTEM IN TUMOR IMMUNITY: SIGNIFICANCE OF ELEVATED LEVELS OF COMPLEMENT IN TUMOR BEARING HOSTS, *ANN NY ACAD SCI*, 276, 303-15 (1976)

1700 NO AUTHOR, PRIMER ON THE RHEUMATIC DISEASES, *THE ARTHRITIS FOUNDATION*, 0 (7)

1701 NOEL L H ET AL, LONG-TERM PROGNOSIS OF IDIOPATHIC MEMBRANOUS GLOMERULONEPHRITIS, *AM J MED*, 66, 82-89 (1979)

1702 NOLPH K ET AL, ANTIBODIES TO NUCLEAR ANTIGENS IN PATIENTS WITH RENAL FAILURE, *J LAB CLIN MED*, 91, 559-567 (1978)

1703 NOMURA S ET AL, REDUCED PERIPHERAL CONVERSION OF THYROXINE TO TRIIODOTHYRONINE IN PATIENTS WITH HEPATIC CIRRHOSIS, *J CLIN INVEST*, 56, 643-52 (1975)

1704 NORDIN BEC, PEACOCK M, AARON J, ET AL, OSTEOPOROSIS AND OSTEOMALACIA, *CLIN ENDOCRINOL METAB*, 9, 177-205 (1980)

1705 NORDMAN H, KOSKINEN H, ET AL, INCREASED ACTIVITY OF SERUM ANGIOTENSIN-CONVERTING ENZYME IN PROGRESSIVE SILICOSIS, *CHEST*, 86, 203-7 (1984)

1706 NORKIN S A ET AL, THROMBOTIC THROMBOCYTOPENIC PURPURA IN SIBLINGS, *AM J MED*, 43, 294 (1967)

1707 NOTMAN D D ET AL, PROFILES OF ANTINUCLEAR ANTIBODIES IN SYSTEMIC RHEUMATIC DISEASES, *ANN INTERN MED*, 83, 464-469 (1975)

1708 NOWACZNSKI W ET AL, A DECREASED METABOLIC BENIGN ESSENTIAL HYPERTENSION, *J CLIN INVEST*, 50, 2184 (1971)

1709 NOWAK J ET AL, B AND T LYMPHOCYTES IN VIRAL HEPATITIS, *POL MED SCI HIST BULL*, 15, 149-54 (1975)

1710 NUNEZ-GORNES JF, TEWKSBURY DA, SERUM ANGIOTENSIN-CONVERTING-ENZYME IN CROHN'S DISEASE, *AM J GASTROENTEROL*, 75, 384-5 (1981)

1711 NUTTALL ET AL, CREATINE KINASE AND GLUTAMIC OXALACETIC TRANSAMINASE ACTIVITY IN SERUM: KINETICS OF CHANGE WITH EXERCISE AND EFFECT OF PHYSICAL CONDITIONING, *J LAB CLIN MED*, 71, 847-854 (1968)

1712 NYDEGGER U E ET AL, CIRCULATING COMPLEMENT BREAKDOWN PRODUCTS IN PATIENTS WITH RHEUMATOID ARTHRITIS. CORRELATION BETWEEN PLASMA C3D, CIRCULATING IMMUNE COMPLEXES, AND CLINICAL ACTIVITY, *J CLIN INVEST*, 59, 862-8 (1977)

1713 NYDICK ET AL, VARIATIONS IN SERUM GLUTAMIC OXALOACETIC TRANSAMINASE ACTIVITY IN EXPERIMENTAL AND CLINICAL CORONARY INSUFFICIENCY, PERICARDITIS AND PULMONARY INFARCTION, *CIRCULATION*, 15, 324-334 (1957)

1714 NYLAND H AND NAESS A, T LYMPHOCYTES IN PERIPHERAL BLOOD FROM PATIENTS WITH NEUROLOGICAL DISEASES, *ACTA NEUROL SCAND*, 58, 272-279 (1978)

1715 NYULASSY S ET AL, SUBACUTE (DE QUERVAIN'S) THYROIDITIS: ASSOCIATION WITH HLA-BW35 ANTIGEN AND ABNORMALITIES OF THE COMPLEMENT SYSTEM, IMMUNOGLOBULINS AND OTHER SERUM PROTEINS, *J CLIN ENDOCRINOL METAB*, 45, 270-4- (1977)

1716 O'BRIEN J S ET AL, TAY-SACH'S DISEASE: DETECTION OF HETEROZYGOTES AND HOMOZYGOTES BY HEXOSAMINIDASE ASSAY, *N ENGL J MED*, 283 1970, 15 (1970)

1717 O'BRIEN JF, MACROAMYLASE, *MAYO CLIN PROC*, 61, 669 (1986)

1718 O'CONNELL J M ET AL, SPUTUM EOSINOPHILIA IN CHRONIC BRONCHITIS AND ASTHMA, *RESPIRATION*, 35, 65-72 (1978)

1719 O'LEARY J A AND FELDMAN M, SERUM COPPER ALTERATIONS IN GENITAL CANCER, *SURG FORUM*, 21, 411-2 (1970)

1720 O'SHEA G, PLASMA ESTRIOLS, *CAN J MED TECHNOL*, 41, E132-E134 (1979)

1721 OAKLEY C, THE DIAGNOSIS OF ACUTE PULMONARY EMBOLISM, *BR J HOSP MED*, 18, 15-24 (1977)

1722 OCKERMAN P A, GLUCOSE GLYCEROL AND FREE FATTY ACIDS IN GLYCOGEN STORAGE DISEASE TYPE I: BLOOD LEVELS IN THE FASTING AND NON-FASTING STATE, *CLIN CHIM ACTA*, 12, 370-82 (1965)

1723 OCKERMAN P A AND KOHLIN P, HYDROLASES IN PLASMA IN GAUCHER'S DISEASE, *CLIN CHEM*, 15, 61 (1969)

1724 OEHLER G, BUDINGER M, HEINRICH D, ET AL, ANTITHROMBIN III CHANGES FOLLOWING MYOCARDIAL INFARCT, *KLIN WOCHENSCHR*, 62, 832-6 (1984 SEP)

1725 OGBUAWA O ET AL, BACTERIAL ENDOCARDITIS IN NARCOTIC ADDICTS: ANALYSIS OF ARTERIAL BLOOD GASES, *SOUTH MED J*, 71, 813-4. (1978)

1726 OGILVIE D ET AL, URINARY OUTPUTS OF OXALATE, CALCIUM, AND MAGNESIUM IN CHILDREN WITH INTESTINAL DISORDERS. POTENTIAL CAUSE OF RENAL CALCULI, *ARCH DIS CHILD*, 51, 790-95 (1976)

1727 OKABE T, YAMAGATA K, FUJISAWA M, ET AL, INCREASED ANGIOTENSIN-CONVERTING ENZYME IN PERIPHERAL BLOOD MONOCYTES FROM PATIENTS WITH SARCOIDOSIS, *J CLIN INVEST*, 75, 911-4 (1985)

1728 OKUNO T ET AL, VALUE OF DETERMINATION OF SERUM FIBRIN-FIBRINOGEN DEGRADATION PRODUCTS IN ACUTE MYOCARDIAL INFARCTION, *AM J CLIN PATHOL*, 61, 155-9 (1974)

1729 OLATUNBOSUN DA, ISAACS-DODEYE WA, ET AL, SERUM COPPER IN SICKLE-CELL ANEMIA, *LANCET*, 1, 285-286 (1975)

1730 OLIVER ET AL, REDUCTION OF SERUM-LIPID AND URIC-ACID LEVELS BY AN ORALLY ACTIVE ANDROSTERONE, *J CLIN ENDOCR*, 1, 1321-1323 (1962)

1731 OLIVO J ET AL, STUDIES OF PROTEIN-BINDING OF TESTOSTERONE IN PLASMA IN DISORDERS OF THYROID FUNCTION, *J CLIN ENDOCRINOL METAB*, 31, 539 (1970)

1732 OLUSI S O ET AL, COMPLEMENT COMPONENTS IN CHILDREN WITH PROTEIN-CALORIE MALNUTRITION, *TROP GEOGR MED*, 28, 323-28 (1976)

1733 ONO J ET AL, TRYPTOPHAN AND HEPATIC COMA, *GASTROENTEROLOGY*, 74, 196-200 (1978)

1734 OOI B S ET AL, SERUM TRANSFERRIN LEVELS IN CHRONIC RENAL FAILURE, *NEPHRON*, 9, 200-7 (1972)

1735 OPPE ET AL, CALCIUM AND PHOSPHORUS LEVELS IN HEALTHY NEWBORN INFANTS GIVEN VARIOUS TYPES OF MILK, *J CLIN ENDOCR*, 1, 1045-1048 (1968)

1736 ORDONEZ-LLANOS J, RODRIGUEZ-ESPINOSA J, ET AL, ANTIBODY BINDING SERUM T_3 IN A PATIENT WITH HEPATOCARCINOMA, *J ENDOCRINOL INVEST*, 7, 123-7 (1984)

1737 ORFANOS AP, NAYLOR EW, GUTHRIE R, MICROMETHOD FOR ESTIMATING ADENOSINE DEAMINASE ACTIVITY IN DRIED BLOOD SPOTS ON FILTER PAPER, *CLIN CHEM*, 24, 591-594 (1978)

1738 ORGEL H A, GENETIC AND DEVELOPMENTAL ASPECTS OF IGE, *PEDIATR CLIN NORTH AM*, 22, 17 (1975)

1739 ORLOWSKI M, THE ROLE OF GAMMA-GLUTAMYL TRANSPEPTIDASE IN THE INTERNAL DISEASES CLINIC, *ARCH IMMUNOL THER EXP (WARSZ)*, 11, 1-61 (1963)

1740 OSATHANONDH R ET AL, TOTAL AND FREE THYROXINE AND TRIIODOTHYRONINE IN NORMAL AND COMPLICATED PREGNANCY, *J CLIN ENDOCRINOL METAB*, 42, 98-104 (1976)

1741 OSEI KWAME, FALKO JM, CHRONIC HYPONATREMIA ASSOCIATED WITH DIABETIC AMYOTROPHY, *ARCH INTERN MED*, 146, 534 (1986)

1742 OSKI F A AND NAIMAN J L, HEMATOLOGIC PROBLEMS IN THE NEWBORN, *2ND EDITION SAUNDERS PHILADELPHIA* (1972)

1743 OSKI F A ET AL, USE OF THE PLASMA ACID PHOSPHATASE VALUE IN THE DIFFERENTIATION OF THROMBOCYTOPENIC STATES, *N ENGL J MED*, 268, 1423-1431 (1963)

1744 OSSERMAN E F, PLASMA-CELL MYELOMA: II. CLINICAL ASPECTS, *N ENGL J MED*, 261, 952, 1006 (1959)

1745 OSSERMAN E F, AMYLOIDOSIS AND PLASMA CELL DYSCRASIA, *FOURTH INTERNATIONAL SYMPOSIUM*, 283 (1965)

1746 OSSERMAN E F AND LAWLOR D P, SERUM AND URINARY LYSOZYME (MURAMIDASE) IN MONOCYTIC AND MONOMYELOCYTIC LEUKEMIA, *J EXP MED*, 124, 921 (1966)

1747 OSTERGAARD PA, ALPHA-1-ANTITRYPSIN LEVELS AND CLINICAL SYMPTOMS IN FORTY-EIGHT CHILDREN WITH SELECTIVE IGA DEFICIENCY, *EUR J PEDIATR*, 142, 276-8 (1984)

1748 OSTROW B AND J M EVANS, SGOT IN PULMONARY EMBOLIZATION, *CLIN RES*, 4, 155 (1956)

1749 OSTROW ET AL, SERUM GLUTAMIC-OXALOACETIC TRANSAMINASE IN CORONARY ARTERY DISEASE, *CIRCULATION*, 14, 790-799 (1956)

1750 OUDART J L AND REY M, PROTEINURIE, PROTIENEMIE ET TRANSAMINASEMIES DANS 23 CAS DE FIEVRE JAUNE CONFIRMIE, *BULL WHO*, 42, 95-102 (1970)

1751 OUYANG A, COHEN S, MILK-ALKALI SYNDROME, *HOSPITAL MEDICINE*, 37 (1985)

1752 OWEN C A, MAYO-MEDICAL LABORATORIES HANDBOOK, *MAYO MED LAB ROCHESTER MN* (1977)

1753 OWEN E E AND VERNER J V, RENAL TUBULAR DISEASES WITH MUSCLE PARALYSIS AND HYPOKALEMIA, *AM J MED*, 28, 8 (1960)

1754 OYAMA T ET AL, EFFECT OF ETHER, THIOPENTINE ANESTHESIA AND SURGERY ON PLASMA THYROID-STIMULATING HORMONE (TSH) LEVELS IN MAN, *BR J ANAESTH*, 44, 841 (1972)

1755 PAABY P, CHANGES IN SERUM PROTEINS DURING PREGNANCY, *BR J OBSTET GYNAECOL*, 67, 43 (1960)

1756 PADDOCK R K AND SMITH S E, THE PLATELETS IN PERNICIOUS ANEMIA, *AM J MED SCI*, 198, 372 (1939)

1757 PADOVA J ET AL, HYPERURICEMIA IN DIABETIC KETOACIDOSIS, *N ENGL J MED*, 267, 530-534 (1962)

1758 PAGLIGRA A S AND GOODMAN A D, ELEVATION OF PLASMA GLUTAMATE IN GOUT, ITS POSSIBLE ROLE IN THE PATHOGENESIS OF HYPERURICEMIA, *N ENGL J MED*, 281, 767 (1969)

1759 PAHPIHA ET AL, SERUM ALKALINE PHOSPHATASE IN PATIENTS WITH MULTIPLE SCLEROSIS, *CLIN GENET*, 7, 77-82 (1975)

1760 PAHWA ET AL., HTLV-III INFECTION IN CHILDREN, *JAMA*, 255, 2301 (1986)

1761 PAKARINEN A, HAMMOND GL, VIHKO R, SERUM PREGNENOLONE, PROGESTERONE, 17 ALPHA HYDROXYPROGESTERONE, ANDROSTENEDIONE, TESTOSTERONE, 5 ALPHA DIHYDROTESTOSTERONE AND ANDROSTERONE DURING PUBERTY IN BOYS, *CLIN ENDOCRINOL (OXF)*, 11, 465-474 (1979)

1762 PAL B, GRIFFITHS ID, KATRAK, A, JUNGLEE D, SALIVARY AMYLASE AND PANCREATIC ENZYMES IN SJÖGREN'S SYNDROME, *CLIN CHEM*, 33/2, 305-307 (1987)

1763 PALL HS, ET AL, RAISED CEREBROSPINAL-FLUID COPPER CONCENTRATIONS IN PARKINSON'S DISEASE, *LANCET*, 2, 238 (1987)

1764 PALL R H AND KANTOR F S, SERUM COMPLEMENT IN ECDAMPTOGENIC TOXEMIA, *AM J OBSTET GYNECOL*, 95, 530 (1966)

1765 PALMER AM, SIMS NR, BOWEN DM, NEARY D, ET AL, MONOAMINE METABOLITE CONCENTRATIONS IN LUMBAR CEREBROSPINAL FLUID OF PATIENTS WITH HISTOLOGICALLY VERIFIED ALZHEIMER'S DEMENTIA, *J NEUROL NEUROSURG PSYCHIATRY*, 47, 481-484 (1984)

1766 PALMER ET AL, THE CHLORIDE-PHOSPHATE RATIO IN HYPER-CALCEMIA, *ANN INTERN MED*, 80, 200-204 (1974)

1767 PALOYAN D ET AL, CARCINOEMBRYONIC ANTIGEN LEVELS IN PANCRE-ATIC CARCINOMA, *AM SURG*, 43, 410 (1977)

1768 PANTEGHINI M, PAGANI F, CUCCIA C, ACTIVITY OF SERUM ASPARTATE AMINOTRANSFERASE ISOENZYMES IN PATIENTS WITH ACUTE MYOCARDIAL INFARCTION, *CLIN CHEM*, 33/1, 67-71 (1987)

1769 PANZER S, KRONIK G, LECHNER K, BETTELHEIM P, ET AL, GLYCOSY-LATED HEMOGLOBINS (GHB): AN INDEX OF RED CELL SURVIVAL, *BLOOD*, 59, 1348-50 (1982)

1770 PARKER C W ET AL, LEUKOCYTE AND LYMPHOCYTE CYCLIC AMP RESPONSES IN ATOPIC ECZEMA, *J INVEST DERMATOL*, 68, 302-6 (1977)

1771 PARKER M D ET AL, COMPARISON OF THE COMPLEMENT-FIXING ACTIV-ITY OF ANTINUCLEAR ANTIBODIES IN LUPUS NEPHRITIS, MIXED CONNECTIVE TISSUE DISEASE, AND SCLERODERMA, *ARTHRITIS RHEUM*, 19, 857-61 (1976)

1772 PARMAR V P ET AL, A STUDY OF MAGNESIUM SERUM AND URINE IN ACUTE NEPHRITIS AND NEPHROTIC SYNDROME IN CHILDHOOD, *INDIAN J PEDIATR*, 13, 701-06 (1976)

1773 PARRISH RW, WILLIAMS JD, DAVIES BH, SERUM BETA-2 MICROGLOBU-LIN AND ANGIOTENSIN-CONVERTING ENZYME ACTIVITY IN SAR-COIDOSIS, *THORAX*, 37, 936-40 (1982)

1774 PARSON H A ET AL, ERYTHROKINETIC STUDIES IN THALASSEMIA TRAIT, *J LAB CLIN MED*, 56, 866 (1960)

1775 PARSONS V ET AL, USE OF DIALYSIS IN THE TREATMENT OF RENAL FAILURE IN LIVER DISEASE, *POSTGRAD MED J*, 51, 515-20 (1975)

1776 PARTIN JR, HURD II HP, GAUCHER'S DISEASE, *HOSPITAL MEDICINE*, 155 (1986)

1777 PASCUAL R S ET AL, USEFULNESS OF SERUM LYSOZYME MEASURE-MENT IN DIAGNOSIS AND EVALUATION OF SARCOIDOSIS, *N ENGL J MED*, 289, 1074-75 (1973)

1778 PASSAMONTE, HYPOURICEMIA, *ARCH INTERN MED*, 144, 1570 (1984)

1779 PASTERNACK A ET AL, CLEARANCE RATIOS OF AMYLASE AND ISOAMYLASE TO CREATININE IN RENAL DISEASE, *CLIN NEPHROL*, 9, 25-8. (1978)

1780 PATEL AR, SHAH PC, VOHRA RM, HART WL, SHAH JR, SERUM FERRITIN LEVELS IN HEMATOLOGIC MALIGNANT NEOPLASMS, *ARCH PATHOL LAB MED*, 104, 509-112 (1980)

1781 PATEL S ET AL, SERUM ENZYME LEVELS IN ALCOHOLISM AND DRUG DEPENDENCY, *J CLIN PATHOL*, 28, 414-417 (1975)

1782 PATTERSON R ET AL, SERUM IMMUNOGLOBULIN LEVELS IN PULMO-NARY ALLERGIC ASPERGILLOSIS AND CERTAIN OTHER LUNG DIS-EASES WITH SPECIAL REFERENCE TO IGE, *AM J MED*, 54 (1973)

1783 PATTON R B AND HORN R C, PRIMARY LIVER CARCINOMA, *CANCER*, 17, 757-768 (1967)

1784 PAULSON G W, ELEVATION OF SERUM URIC ACID LEVELS IN PATIENTS WITH SEIZURES, *OHIO STATE MED J*, 9, 245-52 (1978)

1785 PAVLOVIC-KENTERA V ET AL, ERYTHROPOIETIN LEVELS IN PATIENTS WITH ACUTE LEUKEMIA., *HAEMATOL*, 10, 455-62 (1976)

1786 PAVRI K M ET AL, IMMUNOGLOBULIN E IN SERA OF PATIENTS OF DEN-GUE HAEMORRHAGIC FEVER, *INDIAN J MED RES*, 66, 537-43 (1977)

1787 PAXTON J W ET AL, URINARY EXCRETION OF 17-OXOSTEROIDS IN HEREDITARY COPROPORPHYRIA, *CLIN SCI*, 49, 441 (1975)

1788 PAYNE ET AL, CORRECTION OF PLASMA CALCIUM MEASUREMENTS, *BR MED J*, 1, 393 (1974)

1789 PAZZI P, ARLOTTI A, STABELLINI G, ET AL, CLINICAL VALUE OF SERUM CONCENTRATION OF TOTAL BILE ACIDS IN CHRONIC HEPATOPA-THIES, *MINERVA MED*, 76, 105-12 (1985)

1790 PEARCE J ET AL, URIC ACID AND PLASMA LIPIDS IN CEREBROVASCU-LAR DISEASE. PART I., *BR MED J*, 4, 78-80 (1969)

1791 PEARSON C M AND A BOHAN, THE SPECTRUM OF POLYARTERITIS AND DERMATOMYOSITIS, *MED CLIN NORTH AM*, 61, 439-57 (1977)

1792 PEARSON H A, ERYTHROKINETIC STUDIES IN THALASSEMIA TRAIT, *J LAB CLIN MED*, 56, 866 (1960)

1793 PEARSON H A ET AL, SCREENING FOR THALASSEMIA TRAIT BY ELEC-TRONIC MEASUREMENT OF MEAN CORPUSCULAR VOLUME, *N ENGL J MED*, 288, 351 (1973)

1794 PEJME J, INFECTIOUS MONONUCLEOSIS, *ACTA MED SCAND*, 413 (1964)

1795 PEKAREK R S ET AL, SERUM ZINC, IRON, AND COPPER CONCENTRA-TIONS DURING TYPHOID FEVER IN MAN: EFFECT OF CHLORAM-PHENICOL THERAPY, *CLIN CHEM*, 21, 528-32 (1975)

1796 PEKIN T J ET AL, SYNOVIAL FLUID FINDINGS IN SYSTEMIC LUPUS ERYTHEMATOSUS, *ARTHRITIS RHEUM*, 13, 777-85 (1970)

1797 PELKONEN R ET AL, HYDROXYPROLINEMIA, *N ENGL J MED*, 283, 451 (1970)

1798 PELLETIER L L ET AL, INFECTIVE ENDOCARDITIS: A PREVIEW OF 125 CASES FROM THE UNIVERSITY OF WASHINGTON HOSPITALS, 1963-1972, *MEDICINE*, 56, 287-313 (1977)

1799 PELTIER A P & ESTER D, PATHOBIOLOGY ANNUAL, *APPLETON-CEN-TURY-CROFTS NEW YORK* (1972)

1800 PENNY R ET AL, SERUM FOLLICULAR-STIMULATING HORMONE AND LUTEINIZING HORMONE AS MEASURED BY RADIOIMMUNOASSAY CORRELATED WITH SEXUAL DEVELOPMENT IN HYPOPITUITARY SUBJECTS, *J CLIN INVEST*, 51, 74 (1972)

1801 PEPYS J, HYPERSENSITIVITY DISEASES OF THE LUNGS DUE TO FUNGI AND ORGANIC DUSTS, *MONOGR ALLERGY*, 4 (1969)

1802 PERILLIE P E ET AL, SIGNIFICANCE OF CHANGES IN SERUM MURAMIDASE ACTIVITY IN MEGALOBLASTIC ANEMIA, *N ENGL J MED*, 277, 10-2 (1967)

1803 PERKOFF G T ET AL, REVERSIBLE ACUTE MUSCULAR SYNDROME IN CHRONIC ALCOHOLISM, *N ENGL J MED*, 274, 1277-1285 (1966)

1804 PERRIN K J ET AL, QUANTITATION OF C3 PROACTIVATOR (PROPERDIN FACTOR B) AND OTHER COMPLEMENT COMPONENTS IN DISEASES ASSOCIATED WITH A LOW C3 LEVEL, *CLIN IMMUNOL IMMU-NOPATHOL*, 2, 16 (1973)

1805 PERSKY H ET AL, THE EFFECT OF ALCOHOL AND SMOKING ON TES-TOSTERONE FUNCTION AND AGGRESSION IN CHRONIC ALCOHOLICS, *AM J PSYCHIATRY*, 134, 621-5 (1977)

1806 PERTSEMLIDIS D ET AL, PHEOCHROMACYTOMA, *ANN SURG*, 169, 376 (1969)

1807 PETERS JE, REHFELD N, SCHNEIDER I, ET AL, ABGRENZUNG VON NIEREN-UND SERUMFRAKTION DER ALANINAMINOPEPTIDASE, *CLIN CHIM ACTA*, 24, 314-315 (1969)

1808 PETERS S P ET AL, GAUCHER'S DISEASE: A REVIEW, *MEDICINE*, 56, 425-42. (1977)

1809 PETTERSSON T ET AL, T AND B LYMPHOCYTES IN PLEURAL EFFU-SIONS, *CHEST*, 73, 49-51 (1978)

1810 PETTINGALE K W ET AL, SERUM PROTEIN CHANGES IN BREAST CAN-CER: A PROSPECTIVE STUDY, *J CLIN PATHOL*, 30, 1048-52 (1977)

1811 PEZZOLI G, PANERAI AE, GIULIO AD, ET AL, METHIONINE-ENKEPHALIN, SUBSTANCE P, AND HOMOVANILLIC ACID IN THE CSF OF PARKIN-SONIAN PATIENTS, *NEUROL*, 34, 516 (1984)

1812 PFAU A ET AL, THE PH OF THE PROSTATIC FLUID IN HEALTH AND DISEASE: IMPLICATIONS OF TREATMENT IN CHRONIC BACTERIAL PROSTATITIS, *J UROL*, 119, 384 (1978)

1813 PHILIP R N ET AL, A COMPARISON FOR SEROLOGIC METHODS FOR DIAGNOSIS OF ROCKY MOUNTAIN SPOTTED FEVER, *AM J EPIDEMOL*, 105, 56-67 (1977)

1814 PHILLIPS R W ET AL, ELEVATION OF LEUCINE AMINOPEPTIDASE IN DISSEMINATED MALIGNANT DISEASE, *CANCER*, 26, 1006-1012 (1970)

1815 PHILLIPS RC, WASNER CK, SCLERODERMA, CURRENT UNDERSTAND-ING OF PATHOGENESIS AND MANAGEMENT, *POSTGRAD MED*, 70, 153-168 (1981)

1816 PHILLIPSON O T ET AL, PLASMA GLUCOSE, NON-ESTERIFIED FATTY ACIDS AND AMINO ACIDS IN HUNTINGTON'S CHOREA, *CLIN SCI*, 52, 311-8 (1977)

1817 PICK A I, DIAGNOSTIC SIGNIFICANCE OF CEA CONCENTRATIONS, *AM J PROCTOL*, 28, 37, 77. (1977)

1818 PICKERING NJ, BRODY JI, FINK GB, FINNEGAN JO,ET AL, THE BEHAVIOR OF ANTITHROMBIN III, ALPHA 2 MACROGLOBULIN, AND ALPHA 1 ANTITRYPSIN DURING CARDIOPULMONARY BYPASS, *AM J CLIN PATHOL*, 80, 459-64 (1983)

1819 PIERACH CL, WEIMER MK, CARDINAL RA, ET AL, RED BLOOD CELL PORPHOBILINOGEN DEAMINASE IN THE EVALUATION OF ACUTE INTERMITTENT PORPHYRIA, *JAMA*, 257, 60 (1987)

1820 PIERONI, CHLORIDE-PHOSPHATE RATIO IN HYPERCALCEMIA, *N ENGL J MED*, 291, 531-532 (1974)

1821 PILHEN J A ET AL, SERUM PROTEINS IN PULMONARY TUBERCULOSIS, *DIS CHEST*, 41, 174 (1962)

1822 PIN LIM ET AL, ELEVATED SERUM ENZYMES IN PATIENTS WITH WASP/BEE STING AND THEIR CLINICAL SIGNIFICANCE, *CLIN CHIM ACTA*, 66, 405-409 (1976)

1823 PIPER D ET AL, GASTRIC JUICE LACTIC ACIDOSIS IN THE PRESENCE OF GASTRIC CARCINOMA, *GASTROENTEROLOGY*, 58, 766 (1970)

1824 PITNEY W R, THE TROPICAL SPLENOMEGALY SYNDROME, *TRANS R SOC TROP MED HYG*, 62, 717 (1968)

1825 PITNEY W R ET AL, OBSERVATIONS ON THE BOUND FORM OF VITAMIN B_{12}IN HUMAN SERUM, *J BIOL CHEM*, 207, 143 (1954)

1826 PITNEY W R ET AL, COLD HAEMAGLUTININS ASSOCIATED WITH SPLE-NOMEGALY IN NEW GUINEA, *VOX SANG*, 14, 438 (1968)

1827 PLISHKER G A ET AL, MYOTONIC MUSCULAR DYSTROPHY: ALTERED CALCIUM TRANSPORT IN ERYTHROCYTES, *SCIENCE*, 200, 323-25 (1978)

1828 PLOTZ M, SEDIMENTATION RATE IN MYOCARDIAL INFARCTION, *AM J MED SCI*, 224, 23 (1952)

1829 PLOTZ P H, AUTOIMMUNITY IN HEPATITIS, *MED CLIN NORTH AM*, 59, 869-876 (1975)

1830 PLUM CM, HANSEN SE, STUDIES ON VARIATIONS IN SERUM COPPER AND SERUM COPPER OXIDASE ACTIVITY TOGETHER WITH STUD-IES ON THE COPPER CONTENT OF THE CEREBROSPINAL FLUID, WITH PARTICULAR REFERENCE TO THE VARIATIONS IN MULTIPLE SCLEROSIS, *ACTA PSYCHIATR SCAND*, 35, 41-78 (1960)

1831 POLAK M, TORESS DA COSTA AC, DIAGNOSTIC VALUE OF THE ESTIMA-TION OF GLUCOSE IN ASCITIC FLUID, *DIGESTION*, 8, 347-352 (1973)

1832 POLLAD V E ET AL, QUANTITATIVE HISTOCHEMISTRY OF THE NEPH-RON, IV. ALKALINE PHOSPHATASE AND LACTIC DEHYDROGENASE ACTIVITIES IN RENAL TUBULAR DISEASES, *J CLIN INVEST*, 39, 1386-1393 (1960)

1833 POLLET DE, NOUWEN EJ, SCHELSTRAETE JB, ET AL, ENZYME-ANTIGEN IMMUNOASSAY FOR HUMAN PLACENTAL ALKALINE PHOSPHA-TASE IN SERUM AND TISSUE EXTRACTS AND ITS APPLICATION AS A TUMOR MARKER, *CLIN CHEM*, 31/1, 41-45 (1985)

1834 POLLEY M J AND BEARN A G, ANNOTATION: CYSTIC FIBROSIS CUR-RENT CONCEPTS, *J MED GENET*, 11, 249 (1974)

1835 POLLYCOVE M ET AL, CLASSIFICATION AND EVOLUTION OF PATTERNS OF ERYTHROPOIESIS IN POLYCYTHEMIA VERA AS STUDIED BY IRON KINETICS, *BLOOD*, 28, 807 (1966)

1836 POLMAR S H ET AL, IMMUNOGLOBULIN E IN IMMUNOLOGIC DEFI-CIENCY DISEASES, *J CLIN INVEST*, 51, 326 (1972)

1837 POORTMANS J R, SERUM PROTEIN DETERMINATION DURING SHORT EXHAUSTIVE PHYSICAL ACTIVITY, *J APPL PHYSIOL*, 30, 190 (1971)

1838 POORTMANS J R, EFFECT OF EXERCISE ON THE RENAL CLEARANCE OF AMYLASE AND LYSOZYME IN HUMANS, *CLIN SCI*, 43, 115 (1972)

1839 POORTMANS J R, BODY FLUIDS FLUCTUATIONS INDUCED BY PHYSICAL ACTIVITIES, *REFERENCES VALUES IN HUMAN CHEMISTRY G. SIEST (ED)*, 255 (1973)

1840 POPPER H & SCHAFFNER F (EDS), PROGRESS IN LIVER DISEASE, *GRUNE & STRATTON NEW YORK*, 3 (1970)

1841 PORATH A ET AL, SERUM CHOLINESTERASE IN TETANUS, *ANAESTHESIA*, 32, 1009-11 (1977)

1842 PORTER WH, JENNINGS JR. CD, WILSON HD, MEASUREMENT OF A-GLUCOSIDASE ACTIVITY IN SERUM FROM PATIENTS WITH CYSTIC FIBROSIS OR PANCREATITIS, *CLIN CHEM*, 32/4, 652-656 (1986)

1843 POSEY L E ET AL, URINE ENZYME ACTIVITIES IN PATIENTS WITH TRANSITIONAL CELL CARCINOMA OF THE BLADDER, *CLIN CHIM ACTA*, 74, 7-10 (1977)

1844 POTTER B J ET AL, SERUM COMPLEMENT IN CHRONIC LIVER DISEASE, *GUT*, 14, 451 (1973)

1845 POTTS D E ET AL, PLEURAL FLUID PH IN PARAPNEUMONIC EFFUSIONS, *CHEST*, 70, 328-31 (1976)

1846 POWELL FC, WINKELMANN RK ET AL, THE ANTICENTROMERE ANTIBODY: DISEASE SPECIFICITY AND CLINICAL SIGNIFICANCE, *MAYO CLIN PROC*, 59, 700-706 (1984)

1847 POWELL L W ET AL, CIRRHOSIS OF THE LIVER: A COMPARATIVE STUDY OF THE FOUR MAJOR AETIOLOGICAL GROUPS, *MED J AUST*, 1, 941-50 (1971)

1848 POWELL L W ET AL, THE RELATIONSHIP OF RED CELL MEMBRANE LIPID CONTENT TO RED CELL MORPHOLOGY AND SURVIVAL IN PATIENTS WITH LIVER DISEASE, *AUST NZ J MED*, 5, 101-7 (1975)

1849 POWELL L W ET AL, HAEMOLYSIS IN LIVER DISEASE: RELATIONSHIP TO ERYTHROCYTE MEMBRANE FUNCTION, SERUM BILIRUBIN CONCENTRATION AND PLASMA ELECTROLYTE DISTURBANCES, *AUST NZ J MED*, 6, 3-6 (1976)

1850 POWELL L W ET AL, RELATIONSHIP BETWEEN SERUM FERRITIN AND TOTAL BODY IRON STORES IN IDIOPATHIC HAEMOCHROMATOSIS, *GUT*, 19, 538-42 (1978)

1851 POWERS RD, SERUM CHEMISTRY ABNORMALITIES IN ADULT PATIENTS WITH SEIZURES, *ANN EMERG MED*, 14, 416-20 (1985)

1852 PREECE M J AND RICHARDSON J A, THE EFFECT OF MILD DEHYDRATION ON ONE-HOUR CREATININE CLEARANCE RATES, *NEPHRON*, 9, 106 (1972)

1853 PREUSS H G ET AL, AMMONIA METABOLISM IN RENAL FAILURE, *ANN INTERN MED*, 65, 54-61 (1966)

1854 PREUSS H G ET AL, ELECTROLYTE AND ACID-BASE DISTURBANCES IN DIABETES MELLITUS, *COMPR THER*, 4, 20-23 (1978)

1855 PRICE AND SAMMONS, THE NATURE OF THE SERUM ALKALINE PHOSPHATASES IN LIVER DISEASES, *J CLIN PATHOL*, 27, 392-398 (1974)

1856 PRINZ RA, SANDBERG L, SERUM LEVELS OF ALPHA-1-ANTITRYPSIN IN PANCREATIC ISLET CELL TUMORS, *J MED*, 15, 177-83 (1984)

1857 PRIOSKY B, INFECTIOUS DISEASE AND AUTOIMMUNE HEMOLYTIC ANEMIA: AUTOIMMUNIZATION AND THE AUTOIMMUNE HEMOLYTIC ANEMIAS, *WAVERLY BALTIMORE*, 147 (1969)

1858 PRITCHARD J A, CHANGES IN BLOOD VOLUME DURING PREGNANCY AND DELIVERY, *ANESTHESIOLOGY*, 26, 393-399 (1965)

1859 PRITCHARD J A MACDONALD P C, OBSTETRICS, *15TH EDITION (WILLIAMS) APPLETON-CENTURY-CROFTS NEW YORK* (1971)

1860 PROCKOP D J AND DAVIDSON W D, A STUDY OF URINARY AND SERUM LYSOZYME IN PATIENTS WITH RENAL DISEASE, *N ENGL J MED*, 240, 269 (1964)

1861 PROMPT C A ET AL, HIGH CONCENTRATION OF SWEAT CALCIUM, MAGNESIUM AND PHOSPHATE IN CHRONIC RENAL FAILURE, *NEPHRON*, 20, 4-9 (1978)

1862 PROUT, CHEMICAL TESTS IN THE DIAGNOSIS OF PROSTATIC CARCINOMA, *JAMA*, 209, 1699-1700 (1969)

1863 PROUT G R ET AL, ALTERATIONS IN SERUM LACTIC DEHYDROGENASE AND ITS FOURTH AND FIFTH ISOZYMES IN PATIENTS WITH PROSTATIC CARCINOMA, *J UROL*, 94, 451 (1965)

1864 PUCHOIS P, FONTAN M, GENTILINI J, ET AL, SERUM APOLIPOPROTEIN A-II, A BIOCHEMICAL INDICATOR OF ALCOHOL ABUSE, *CLIN CHIM ACTA*, 185, 185-189 (1984)

1865 PUDENZ R H ET AL, THE ROLE OF POTASSIUM IN FAMILIAL PERIODIC PARALYSIS, *JAMA*, 111, 2253 (1938)

1866 PUTNAM FW (ED), THE PLASMA PROTEINS: STRUCTURE, FUNCTIONS AND GENETIC CONTROL, *NEW YORK, ACADEMIC PRESS*, 1-3 (1977)

1867 PYHALA R ET AL, THE VALUE OF COMPLEMENT FIXATION AND HAEMAGGLUTINATION INHIBITION TESTS IN THE DIAGNOSIS OF INFLUENZA A, *ACTA VIROL (PRAHA)*, 20, 66-69 (1976)

1868 QUIMBY GF, BONNICE CA, BURSTEIN SH, ET AL, ACTIVE SMOKING DEPRESSES PROSTAGLANDIN SYNTHESIS IN HUMAN GASTRIC MUCOSA, *ANN INTERN MED*, 104, 616-619 (1986)

1869 RAAB W P, THE DIAGNOSTIC VALUE OF URINARY ENZYME DETERMINATIONS, *CLIN CHEM*, 18, 5 (1972)

1870 RACHELEFSKY G S ET AL, SERUM ENZYME ABNORMALITIES IN JUVENILE RHEUMATOID ARTHRITIS, *PEDIATRICS*, 58, 730-36 (1976)

1871 RAFFENSPERGER E C, ELEVATED SERUM PANCREATIC ENZYME VALUES WITHOUT PRIMARY INTRINSIC DISEASE, *ANN INTERN MED*, 35, 342 (1951)

1872 RAFTERY A T, THE VALUE OF THE LEUCOCYTE COUNT IN THE DIAGNOSIS OF ACUTE APPENDICITIS, *BR J SURG*, 63, 143-4 (1976)

1873 RAGANATI M ET AL, ADENOSINE DEAMINASE ACTIVITY IN SERUM OF CHILDREN WITH DIFFERENT DISEASES, *PEDIATRIA (NAPOLI)*, 84, 247-52 (1976)

1874 RAIVIO K O, NEONATAL HYPERURICEMIA, *J PEDIATR*, 88, 625-30 (1976)

1875 RAMACHANDRAN S ET AL, PH OF AMOEBIC LIVER PUS, *TRANS R SOC TROP MED HYG*, 70, 159-60 (1976)

1876 RAMAEKERS L H ET AL, ACUTE LYMPHOPENIA, STRESS, AND PLASMA CORTISOL, *ARCH DIS CHILD*, 50, 555-9 (1975)

1877 RAMIREZ A ET AL, DAILY URINARY CATECHOLAMINE PROFILE IN MARASMUS AND KWASHIORKOR, *AM J CLIN NUTR*, 31, 41-5 (1978)

1878 RAMU G ET AL, PLASMA FIBRINOGEN LEVELS AND FIBRINOLYTIC ACTIVITY IN LEPROMATOUS LEPROSY, *J ASSOC PHYSICIANS INDIA*, 25, 133-8 (1977)

1879 RAR V ET AL, BLOOD HISTAMINE AND HISTAMINASE IN LEPROSY PATIENTS - A SHORT COMMUNICATION, *INDIAN J MED RES*, 66, 978-982 (1977)

1880 RASI V, IKKALA E, TORSTILA I, PLASMA BETA-THROMBOGLOBULIN IN ACUTE MYOCARDIAL INFARCTION, *THROMB RES*, 25, 203-12 (1982)

1881 RASKIND MA, PESKIND ER, LAMPE TH, ET AL, CEREBROSPINAL FLUID VASOPRESSIN, OXYTOCIN, SOMATOSTATIN, AND B-ENDORPHIN IN ALZHEIMER'S DISEASE, *ARCH GEN PSYCHIATRY*, 43, 382 (1986)

1882 RASMUSSEN K, PHOSPHOETHANOLAMINE AND HYPOPHOSPHATASIA, *DAN MED BULL*, 15, 1 (1968)

1883 RASSIGA-PIDOT A L ET AL, PAROXYSMAL NOCTURNAL HEMOGLOBINURIA WITH ELEVATED FETAL HEMOGLOBIN, *BLOOD*, 43, 233 (1974)

1884 RATNER ET AL, TRANSAMINASE IN CORONARY ARTERY DISEASE, *CAN MED ASSOC J*, 76, 720-725 (1957)

1885 RATNOFF O D AND COLOPY J E, A FAMILIAL HEMORRHAGIC TRAIT ASSOCIATED WITH A DEFICIENCY OF A CLOT-PROMOTING FRACTION OF PLASMA, *J CLIN INVEST*, 34, 602 (1955)

1886 RATNOFF O D AND HOLLAND T R, COAGULATION COMPONENTS IN NORMAL AND ABNORMAL PREGNANCIES, *ANN NY ACAD SCI*, 75, 626 (1959)

1887 RAVEL R., *CLINICAL LABORATORY MEDICINE 4TH ED*, YEARBOOK MEDICAL PUBLISHERS, INC. CHICAGO (1984)

1888 RAWAT M AND VIJAYVARGIYA R, SERUM COPPER ESTIMATION IN LYMPHOMAS, *INDIAN J MED RES*, 66, 815-19. (1977)

1889 RAYFIELD E J ET A, IMPAIRED CARBOHYDRATE METABOLISM DURING A MILD VIRAL ILLNESS, *N ENGL J MED*, 289, 618 (1973)

1890 RAZ R ET AL, SERUM AND URINARY URIC ACID IN INFECTIOUS HEPATITIS, *ISR J MED SCI*, 13, 1219-21 (1977)

1891 REBOUND P ET AL, THE INFLUENCE OF NORMAL PREGNANCY AND THE POSTPARTUM STATE ON PLASMA PROTEINS AND LIPIDS, *AM J OBSTET GYNECOL*, 86, 820 (1963)

1892 REBOUND P ET AL, PLASMA PROTEINS AND LIPIDS DURING PREGNANCY AND POSTPARTUM, *ANN BIOL CLIN*, 25, 383 (1967)

1893 RECAN L AND RIGGS P S, THYROID FUNCTION IN NEPHROSIS, *J CLIN INVEST*, 31, 789 (1952)

1894 REDDI Y R ET AL, CEREBROSPINAL FLUID AND BLOOD SUGAR RATIO IN HEALTH AND DISEASE: DIAGNOSTIC AND PROGNOSTIC SIGNIFICANCE IN INTRACRANIAL INFECTIONS, *INDIAN J PEDIATR*, 12, 401 (1975)

1895 REDDY B S ET AL, FECAL BILE ACIDS AND NEUTRAL STEROLS IN PATIENTS WITH FAMILIAL POLYPOSIS, *CANCER*, 39, 1694-8 (1976)

1896 REDDY B S ET AL, METABOLIC EPIDEMIOLOGY OF COLON CANCER. FECAL BILE ACIDS AND NEUTRAL STEROLS IN COLON CANCER PATIENTS WITH ADENOMATOUS POLYPS, *CANCER*, 39, 2533-9 (1977)

1897 REDDY B S ET AL, FECAL BILE ACIDS AND CHOLESTEROL METABOLITES OF PATIENTS WITH ULCERATIVE COLITIS, A HIGH-RISK GROUP FOR DEVELOPMENT OF COLON CANCER, *CANCER RES*, 37, 1697-701 (1977)

1898 REDMAN C W ET AL, PLASMA-URATE MEASUREMENTS IN PREDICTING FETAL DEATH IN HYPERTENSIVE PREGNANCY, *LANCET*, 1, 1370-3 (1976)

1899 REDMAN C W ET AL, PLASMA URATE AND SERUM DEOXYCYTIDYLATE DEAMINASE MEASUREMENTS FOR THE EARLY DIAGNOSIS OF PRE-ECLAMPSIA, *BR J OBSTET GYNAECOL*, 84, 904-8 (1977)

1900 REED JS, BOYER JL, VIRAL HEPATITIS, EPIDEMIOLOGIC, SEROLOGIC AND CLINICAL MANIFESTATION, *DM*, 25, 1-61 (1979)

1901 REEMTSMA K ET AL, CYSTIC FIBROSIS OF THE PANCREAS, INTESTINAL ABSORPTION OF FAT AND FATTY ACID LABELED WITH I 131, *PEDIATRICS*, 22, 525 (1958)

1902 REES E G ET AL, SERUM PROTEINS IN SYSTEMIC LUPUS ERYTHEMATOSUS, *BR MED J*, 5155, 795 (1959)

1903 REEVES B, SIGNIFICANCE OF JOINT FLUID URIC ACID LEVELS IN GOUT, *ANN RHEUM DIS*, 24, 569-571 (1965)

1904 REEVES ET AL, DIFFERENTIAL DIAGNOSIS OF HYPERCALCEMIA BY THE CHLORIDE PHOSPHATE RATIO, *AM J SURG*, 130, 166-171 (1975)

1905 REICHMAN RC, DOLIN R, VIRAL PNEUMONIAS, *MED CLIN NORTH AM*, 64, 491-506 (1980)

1906 REIF A E ET AL, ACID PHOSPHATASE ISOZYMES IN CANCER OF THE PROSTATE, *CANCER*, 31, 689-699 (1973)

1907 REINER ET AL, ACID PHOSPHATASE ACTIVITY IN HUMAN NEOPLASMS, *CANCER*, 10, 563-576 (1957)

1908 REINSTONE SM, PURCELL RH, NEW METHODS FOR THE SERODIAGNOSIS OF HEPATITIS A, *GASTROENTEROLOGY*, 78, 1092-1094 (1980)

1909 REISS E AND CANTERBURY J, BLOOD LEVELS OF PARATHYROID HORMONE IN DISORDERS OF CALCIUM METABOLISM, *ANNU REV MED*, 24, 217-232 (1973)

1910 REJTHAR A ET AL, PROGNOSTIC SIGNIFICANCE OF AN ENHANCED NUMBER OF T LYMPHOCYTES IN CHRONIC LYMPHATIC LEUKEMIA, *NEOPLASMA*, 25, 141-4 (1978)

1911 REMME W J ET AL, CHANGES IN PURINE NUCLEOSIDE CONTENT IN HUMAN MYOCARDIAL EFFLUX DURING PACING-INDUCED ISCHEMIA, *RECENT ADV STUD CARDIAC STRUCT METAB*, 12, 409-13 (1976)

1912 RENNIE ET AL, THE CLINICAL SIGNIFICANCE OF SERUM TRANSAMINASE IN INFECTIOUS MONONUCLEOSIS COMPLICATED BY HEPATITIS, *N ENGL J MED*, 257, 547-553 (1957)

1913 RERABEK J E, LOW DENSITY LIPOPROTEINS AND IMMUNOGLOBULINS IN HUMAN PLEURAL EFFUSIONS, *CLIN CHIM ACTA*, 76, 363-9 (1977)

1914 RESKE SN, DROPP J, HECK I, MATTERN H, ET AL, REDUCTION OF REGURGITATION IN AORTIC INSUFFICIENCY BY INHIBITION OF THE RENIN-ANGIOTENSIN CONVERTING ENZYME, *NUKLEARMEDIZIN*, 23, 241-5 (1984)

1915 RESNICK H, LAPP NL, MORGAN WKC, SERUM TRYPSIN INHIBITOR CONCENTRATIONS IN COAL MINERS WITH RESPIRATORY SYMPTOMS, *JAMA*, 215, 1101-1105 (1971)

1916 RESNITZKY P ET AL, OSMOTIC FRAGILITY OF PERIPHERAL BLOOD LYMPHOCYTES IN CHRONIC LYMPHATIC LEUKEMIA AND MALIGNANT LYMPHOMA, *BLOOD*, 51, 645-51 (1978)

1917 REYNAFARIE C ET AL, THE POLYCYTHEMIA OF HIGH ALTITUDE: IRON METABOLISM AND RELATED STUDIES, *BLOOD*, 14, 433 (1959)

1918 REYNAFARJE C AND RAMOS J, THE HEMOLYTIC ANEMIA OF HUMAN BARTONELLOSIS, *BLOOD*, 17, 562 (1961)

1919 REYNOLDS C, URINE GLUCOSE MEASUREMENT IN THE MANAGEMENT OF DIABETES MELLITUS, *COMPR THER*, 4, 13-19 (1978)

1920 REYNOLDS LR, DIAGNOSTIC PROCEDURES IN ENDOCRINOLOGY, *DIVISION OF ENDOCRINOLGY, UNIVERSITY OF KENTUCKY MEDICAL CENTER* (1977)

1921 REYNOLDS M D ET AL, COPPER-RESISTANT SERUM ACID PHOSPHATASE I. METHOD AND VALUES IN HEALTH AND DISEASE, *CANCER RES*, 16, 943-950 (1959)

1922 REYNOLDS T B ET AL, LUPOID HEPATITIS, *ANN INTERN MED*, 61, 650 (1964)

1923 REYNOLDS, LR, *DIAGNOSTIC PROCEDURES IN ENDOCRINOLOGY. LEXINGTON, KY., DIV. OF ENDOCRINOLOGY* (1977)

1924 RHOADS C P ET AL, OBSERVATIONS ON ETIOLOGY AND TREATMENT OF ANEMIA ASSOCIATED WITH HOOKWORM INFECTION, *MEDICINE*, 13, 317 (1934)

1925 RHOADS GG, DAHLEN G, BERG K, ET AL, LP (A) LIPOPROTEIN AS A RISK FACTOR FOR MYOCARDIAL INFARCTION, *JAMA*, 256, 2540 (1986)

1926 RHONE ET AL, ISOENZYMES OF LIVER ALKALINE PHOSPHATASE IN SERUM OF PATIENTS WITH HEPATOBILIARY DISORDERS, *CLIN CHEM*, 19, 1142-1147 (1973)

1927 RICH ET AL, SALICYLATE HEPATOTOXICITY IN PATIENTS WITH JUVENILE RHEUMATOID ARTHRITIS, *ARTHRITIS RHEUM*, 16, 1-9 (1973)

1928 RICHENS, DISTURBANCE OF CALCIUM METABOLISM BY ANTICONVULSANT DRUGS, *BR MED J*, 4, 73-76 (1970)

1929 RICHTER ET AL, ACUTE MYOGLOBINURIA ASSOCIATED WITH HEROIN ADDICTION, *JAMA*, 216, 1172-1176 (1971)

1930 RICHTERICH R, CLINICAL CHEMISTRY-THEORY AND PRACTICE, *CLIN CHEM* (1969)

1931 RICKLES F F AND O'LEARY D S, THE ROLE OF THE COAGULATION SYSTEM IN THE PATHOPHYSIOLOGY OF SICKLE CELL DISEASE, *ARCH INTERN MED*, 133, 465 (1974)

1932 RIDDLE M C AND STURGIS C C, BASAL METABOLISM IN CHRONIC MYELOGENOUS LEUKEMIA, *ARCH INTERN MED*, 39, 255 (1927)

1933 RIDDOCH D AND THOMPSON R A, IMMUNOGLOBULIN LEVELS IN THE CEREBROSPINAL FLUID, *BR MED J*, 1, 396 (1970)

1934 RIEDLER ET AL, HYPOPHOSPHATAEMIA IN SEPTICAEMIA:HIGHER INCIDENCE IN GRAM-NEGATIVE THAN IN GRAM-POSITIVE INFECTIONS, *BR MED J*, 1, 753-756 (1969)

1935 RIESEN WF, ET AL, ARTERIOSCLEROSIS, 37, 197 (1980)

1936 RIFKIND BM, LEVY RI, *HYPERLIPIDEMIA: DIAGNOSIS AND THERAPY. NEW YORK, GRUNE & STRATTON* (1977)

1937 RIFKIND D ET AL, URINARY EXCRETION OF IRON-BINDING PROTEIN IN THE NEPHROTIC SYNDROME., *N ENGL J MED*, 265, 115-118 (1961)

1938 RIGG L A ET AL, PATTERN OF INCREASE IN CIRCULATING PROLACTIN LEVELS DURING HUMAN GESTATION, *AM J OBSTET GYNECOL*, 129, 454-6 (1977)

1939 RILEY V, BREAST CANCER PATIENTS: SUBSTANCE IN BLOOD CAUSING ACCELERATION OF ERYTHROCYTE SEDIMENTATION RATE., *SCIENCE*, 191, 86-88 (1976)

1940 RIMINGTON C, THE EXCRETION OF PORPHYRIN-PEPTIDE CONJUGATES IN PORPHYRIA VARIEGATA, *CLIN SCI*, 43, 299 (1972)

1941 RIMMINGTON C AND MILES R A, A STUDY OF THE PORPHYRINS EXCRETED IN THE URINE BY A CASE OF CONGENITAL PORPHYRIA, *BIOCHEM J*, 50, 202 (1951)

1942 RINDERKNECHT H ET AL, SERUM CREATINE PHOSPHOKINASE IN ACUTE PANCREATITIS, *CLIN BIOCHEM*, 3, 165-170 (1970)

1943 RITCHIE AW, JAMES K, MICKLEM HS, CHISHOLM GD, LYMPHOCYTE SUBSETS IN RENAL CARCINOMA--A SEQUENTIAL STUDY USING MONOCLONAL ANTIBODIES, *BR J UROL*, 56, 140-8 (1984)

1944 RITLAND S ET AL, HEPATIC COPPER CONTENT, URINARY COPPER EXCRETION, AND SERUM CERULOPLASMIN IN LIVER DISEASE, *SCAND J GASTROENTEROL*, 12, 81-8 (1977)

1945 RITTGERS R H ET AL, CARCINOEMBRYONIC ANTIGEN LEVELS IN BENIGN AND MALIGNANT EFFUSIONS, *ANN INTERN MED*, 88, 631-34 (1978)

1946 RITZMANN SE, DANIELS JC, SERUM PROTEIN ABNORMALITIES, DIAGNOSTIC AND CLINICAL ASPECTS, *BOSTON, LITTLE, BROWN, AND CO.* (1975)

1947 RITZMANN SE, TUCKER ES III, PROTEIN ANALYSIS IN DISEASE-CURRENT CONCEPTS, *WORKSHOP MANUAL, CHICAGO, AMERICAN SOCIETY OF CLINICAL PATHOLOGISTS* (1979)

1948 RITZMANN SE, TUCKER ES III,, ELECTROPHORESIS ASSAYS, *SPITTELL JA, JR. (ED.): CLINICAL MEDICINE. HAGERSTOWN, MD., HARPER AND ROW* (1980)

1949 RIVERO S J ET AL, LYMPHOPENIA IN SYSTEMIC LUPUS ERYTHEMATOSUS. CLINICAL, DIAGNOSTIC, AND PROGNOSTIC SIGNIFICANCE, *ARTHRITIS RHEUM*, 21, 295-305 (1978)

1950 ROBBOY S J ET AL, MECHANISM OF ASPERGILLUS-INDUCED MICROANGIOPATHIC HEMOLYTIC ANEMIA, *ARCH INTERN MED*, 128, 790 (1971)

1951 ROBERTS EA, COX DW, MEDLINE A, WANLESS IR, OCCURRENCE OF ALPHA-1-ANTITRYPSIN DEFICIENCY IN 155 PATIENTS WITH ALCOHOLIC LIVER DISEASE, *AM J CLIN PATHOL*, 82, 424-7 (1984)

1952 ROBERTS ET AL, ANTENATAL FACTORS ASSOCIATED WITH NEONATAL HYPOCALCAEMIC CONVULSIONS, *J CLIN ENDOCR*, 2, 809-811 (1973)

1953 ROBINSON AD, BOYDEN KN, HENDRICKSON SM, MUIRDEN KD, ANTITRYPSIN ACTIVITY AND ENZYME INHIBITORS IN THE RHEUMATOID JOINT, *J RHEUMATOL*, 8, 547-54 (1981)

1954 ROBINSON ET AL, CLINICAL SIGNIFICANCE OF INCREASED SERUM 'ACID' PHOSPHATASE IN PATIENTS WITH BONE METASTASES SECONDARY TO PROSTATIC CARCINOMA, *J UROL*, 42, 602-618 (1939)

1955 ROBINSON H ET AL, A COMPARISON OF FASTING PLASMA INSULIN AND GROWTH HORMONE CONCENTRATIONS IN MARASMIC, KWASHIORKOR, AND UNDERWEIGHT CHILDREN., *PEDIATR RES*, 11, 637-640 (1977)

1956 ROBINSON N ET AL, SERUM ENZYMES IN FRIEDREICH'S ATAXIA, *BRAIN*, 88, 131 (1965)

1957 ROCHER H D ET AL, DIAGNOSIS OF PRIMARY AND SECONDARY HYPERPARATHYROIDISM, *WORLD J SURG*, 1, 709-20 (1977)

1958 RODNAN GP, PRIMER ON THE RHEUMATIC DISEASES, *J A M A*, 224, 661-812 (1973)

1959 RODNIGHT R ET AL, URINARY DIMETHYLTRYSTAMINE AND PSYCHIATRIC SYMPTOMATOLOGY AND CLASSIFICATION, *PSYCHO MED*, 6, 649-57 (1976)

1960 ROE T F ET AL, THE PATHOGENESIS OF HYPERURICEMIA IN GLYCOGEN STORAGE DISEASE, TYPE I., *PEDIATR RES*, 11, 664-669 (1977)

1961 ROELS OA, *THE VITAMINS, 2ND EDN., (EDS W.H. SEBRELL, JR. AND R.S. HARRIS) ACADEMIC PRESS, NY*, 1 (1967)

1962 ROHATGI PK, KUZMOWYCH TV, ASSESSMENT OF ACTIVITY IN CHRONIC SARCOIDOSIS: USEFULNESS OF SERUM ANGIOTENSIN CONVERTING ENZYME AND GALLIUM SCAN, *RESPIRATION*, 49, 140-6 (1986)

1963 ROHATGI, PK, SIGNIFICANCE OF SERUM ANGIOTENSIN-CONVERTING ENZYME AND GALLIUM SCAN IN NONINVASIVE DIAGNOSIS OF SARCOIDOSIS, *EUR J RESPIR DIS*, 62, 223-30 (1981)

1964 ROHRBACH MS, DEREMEE RA, MEASUREMENT OF ANGIOTENSIN CONVERTING ENZYME ACTIVITY IN SERUM IN THE DIAGNOSIS AND MANAGEMENT OF SARCOIDOSIS, *CLINICAL LABORATORY ANNUAL: 1982, APPLETON-CENTURY-CROFTS/NEW YORK*, 1, 435-453 (1982)

1965 ROLA-PLESZCZYNSKI M, CHAVAILLAZ PA, LEMAIRE I, STIMULATION OF INTERLEUKIN 2 AND INTERFERON GAMMA PRODUCTION BY LEUKOTRIENE B4 IN HUMAN LYMPHOCYTE CULTURES, *PROSTAGLANDINS LEUKOTRIENES AND MEDICINE*, 23, 207-10 (1986)

1966 ROMER FK, ANGIOTENSIN-CONVERTING ENZYME IN NEWLY DETECTED SARCOIDOSIS. WITH SPECIAL REFERENCE TO ENZYME LEVELS IN PATIENTS WITH ERYTHEMA NODOSUM, *ACTA MED SCAND*, 208, 437-43 (1980)

1967 ROMER FK, ANGIOTENSIN-CONVERTING ENZYME AND ITS ASSOCIATION WITH OUTCOME IN LUNG CANCER, *BR J CANCER*, 43, 135-42 (1981)

1968 ROMER FK, AHLBOM G, JENSEN JU, RELATIONSHIP BETWEEN ANGIOTENSIN-CONVERTING ENZYME AND LYSOZYME IN SARCOIDOSIS, *EUR J RESPIR DIS*, 63, 330-6 (1982)

1969 ROMER FK, EMMERTSEN K, SERUM ANGIOTENSIN-CONVERTING ENZYME IN MALIGNANT LYMPHOMAS, LEUKAEMIA AND MULTIPLE MYELOMA, *BR J CANCER*, 42, 314-8 (1980)

1970 ROMER FK, SCHMITZ O, ANGIOTENSIN-CONVERTING ENZYME ACTIVITY IN RENAL DISORDERS: INFLUENCE OF DISEASE PATTERN, HEMODIALYSIS AND TRANSPLANTATION, *CLIN NEPHROL*, 21, 178-83 (1984)

1971 RON M, BELLER U, ORI J, BEN-DAVID M, PALTI Z, ELEVATED CEREBROSPINAL FLUID PROLACTIN CONCENTRATION IN WOMEN WITH PSEUDOTUMOR CEREBRI, *SOUTH MED J*, 75, 807-8 (1982)

1972 RONCORONI A J ET AL, METABOLIC ACIDOSIS IN STATUS ASTHMATICUS, *RESPIRATION*, 33, 85-94 (1976)

1973 ROONEY P J ET AL, SERUM IMMUNOREACTIVE GASTRIN IN RHEUMATOID ARTHRITIS, *ANN RHEUM DIS*, 35, 246 (1976)

1974 ROPES M W AND W BAUER, SYNOVIAL FLUID CHANGES IN JOINT DISEASE, *HARVARD UNIVERSITY PRESS BOSTON* (1956)

1975 ROSAHN P D AND PEARCE L, THE BLOOD CYTOLOGY IN UNTREATED AND TREATED SYPHILIS, *AM J MED SCI*, 187, 88 (1934)

1976 ROSE D P ET AL, PLASMA THYROID-STIMULATING HORMONE AND THYROXINE CONCENTRATIONS IN BREAST CANCER, *CANCER*, 41, 666-9 (1978)

1977 ROSE DP, PRUITT BT, PLASMA PROLACTIN LEVELS IN PATIENTS WITH BREAST CANCER, *CANCER*, 48, 2687-91 (1981)

1978 ROSE L I ET AL, SERUM ENZYMES AFTER MARATHON RUNNING, *J APPL PHYSIOL*, 35, 355 (1970)

1979 ROSE NR, FRIEDMAN H, *MANUAL OF CLINICAL IMMUNOLOGY, AMERICAN SOCIETY FOR MICROBIOLOGY, 2ND ED* (1980)

1980 ROSEN BARBARA, MULTIPLE MYELOMA: A CRITICAL REVIEW, *MED CLIN NORTH AM*, 59, 375-86 (1975)

1981 ROSEN FS, ALPER CA, PENSKY J, ET AL, GENETICALLY DETERMINED HETEROGENEITY OF THE C1 ESTERASE INHIBITOR IN PATIENTS WITH HEREDITARY ANGIONEUROTIC EDEMA, *J CLIN INVEST*, 50, 2143-2149 (1971)

1982 ROSENBACH L M AND XEFTERIS E D, ERYTHROCYTOSIS ASSOCIATED WITH CARCINOMA OF THE KIDNEY, *JAMA*, 176, 136 (1961)

1983 ROSENBERG M ET AL, CLINICAL AND IMMUNOLOGIC CRITERIA FOR THE DIAGNOSIS OF ALLERGIC BRONCHOPULMONARY ASPERGILLOSIS, *ANN INTERN MED*, 86, 405-414 (1977)

1984 ROSENBERG S A ET AL, LYMPHOSARCOMA, *ANN INTERN MED*, 53, 877 (1960)

1985 ROSENHEIN M L, SODIUM, *LANCET*, 2, 505 (1951)

1986 ROSENKRANTZ J A ET AL, PAGET'S DISEASE (OSTEITIS DEFORMANS), *ARCH INTERN MED*, 90, 610-633 (1952)

1987 ROSENLUND M ET AL, DIETARY ESSENTIAL FATTY ACIDS IN CYSTIC FIBROSIS, *PEDIATRICS*, 59, 428-32 (1977)

1988 ROSENTHAL A ET AL, HEMOBLOBIN-OXYGEN EQUILIBRIUM IN CYSTIC FIBROSIS, *PEDIATRICS*, 59, 919-26 (1976)

1989 ROSENTHAL R, BLOOD COAGULATION IN LEUKEMIA AND POLYCYTHEMIA, *J LAB CLIN MED*, 34, 1321 (1949)

1990 ROSNER F AND SCHREIBER Z, SERUM VITAMIN B_{12} AND VITAMIN B_{12} BINDING CAPACITY IN CHRONIC MYELOGENOUS LEUKEMIA AND OTHER DISORDERS, *AM J MED SCI*, 263, 473-480 (1972)

1991 ROSNER F ET AL, LEUKOCYTE ALKALINE PHOSPHATASE FLUCTUATIONS WITH DISEASE STATUS IN CHRONIC GRANULOCYTIC LEUKEMIA, *ARCH INTERN MED*, 130, 892-894 (1972)

1992 ROSSE F AND WALDMAN T A, A COMPARISON OF SOME PHYSICAL AND CHEMICAL PROPERTIES OF ERYTHROPOIESIS-STIMULATING FACTORS FROM DIFFERENT SOURCES, *BLOOD*, 24, 739 (1964)

1993 ROSSEN R D ET AL, CIRCULATING IMMUNE COMPLEXES AND ANTINUCLEAR ANTIBODIES IN JUVENILE RHEUMATOID ARTHRITIS, *ARTHRITIS RHEUM*, 20, 1485-90 (1977)

1994 ROTH E, ZOCH G, SCHULZ F, ET AL, AMINO ACID CONCENTRATIONS IN PLASMA AND SKELETAL MUSCLE OF PATIENTS WITH ACUTE HEMORRHAGIC NECROTIZING PANCREATITIS, *CLIN CHEM*, 31/8, 1305-1309 (1985)

1995 ROTHFIELD N F ET AL, SERUM ANTINUCLEAR ANTIBODIES IN PROGRESSIVE SYSTEMIC SCLEROSIS (SCLERODERMA), *ARTHRITIS RHEUM*, 11, 607-17 (1968)

1996 ROTHWELL ET AL, LACTATE DEHYDROGENASE ACTIVITIES IN SERUM AND PLASMA, *CLIN CHEM*, 22, 1024-1026 (1976)

1997 ROTTER J I ET AL, DUODENAL-ULCER DISEASE ASSOCIATED WITH ELEVATED SERUM PEPSINOGEN I, *N ENGL J MED*, 300, 63-66 (1979)

1998 ROTTINO A ET AL, BEHAVIOR OF TOTAL SERUM COMPLEMENT IN HODGKIN'S DISEASE AND OTHER MALIGNANT LYMPHOMAS, *BLOOD*, 14, 246-53 (1959)

1999 ROZENSZAJIN L, LEIBOVICH M, SHOHAM D, EPSTEIN J, THE ESTERASE ACTIVITY IN MEGALOBLASTS, LEUKAEMIC AND NORMAL HAEMATOPOIETIC CELLS, *BR J HAEMATOL*, 14, 605-610 (1968)

2000 ROZNER F, GORFIEN PC, ERYTHROCYTE AND PLASMA ZINC AND MAGNESIUM IN HEALTH AND DISEASE, *J LAB CLIN MED*, 72, 213-219 (1968)

2001 RUBIN H AND SOLOMON A, COLD AGGLUTININS OF ANTI-I SPECIFICITY IN ALCOHOLIC CIRRHOSIS, *VOX SANG*, 12, 227 (1967)

2002 RUBINSTEIN A, NOVICK BE, SICKLICK MJ, ET AL, CIRCULATING THYMULIN AND THYMOSIN-ALPHA 1 ACTIVITY IN PEDIATRIC ACQUIRED IMMUNE DEFICIENCY SYNDROME: IN VIVO AND IN VITRO STUDIES, *J PEDIATR*, 109, 422 (1986)

2003 RUDDERS R A, B LYMPHOCYTE SUBPOPULATIONS IN CHRONIC LYMPHOCYTIC LEUKEMIA, *BLOOD*, 47, 229-35 (1976)

2004 RUDZKI C ET AL, CHRONIC INTRAHEPATIC CHOLESTASIS OF SARCOIDOSIS, *AM J MED*, 59, 373-87 (1975)

2005 RULE A H E ET AL, TUMOR-ASSOCIATED (CEA-REACTING) ANTIGEN IN PATIENTS WITH INFLAMMATORY BOWEL DISEASE, *N ENGL J MED*, 287, 24 (1972)

2006 RUNDLES R A ET AL, SERUM PROTEINS IN LEUKEMIA, *AM J MED*, 16, 842 (1954)

2007 RUSH TJ, BETTS RF, SAXINGER C, COWELL SA, ET AL, NORMAL T CELL SUBSETS IN HOMOSEXUAL MEN LIVING IN A COMMUNITY WITHOUT ENDEMIC AIDS, *AM J MED*, 81, 584-90 (1986)

2008 RUSSELL D ET AL, BIPHASIC RESPONSE ON ORAL GLUCOSE TOLERANCE TESTING IN MYOTONIC DYSTROPHY, *ACTA NEUROL SCAND*, 53, 226-8 (1976)

2009 RUSSELL ET AL, SERUM TRANSAMINASES DURING SALICYLATE THERAPY, *BR MED J*, 2, 428-429 (1971)

2010 RUTENBURG A M ET AL, SERUM GAMMA-GLUTAMYL TRANSPEPTIDASE ACTIVITY IN HEPATOBILIARY PANCREATIC DISEASE, *GASTROENTEROLOGY*, 45, 43-8 (1963)

2011 RUZZA C R, THE EFFECT OF EXERCISE ON THE EFFECT OF ANTIHEMOPHILIC GLOBULIN IN HUMAN BLOOD, *J PHYSIOL*, 156, 128 (1961)

2012 RYAN WE, ELLEFSON RD, WARD LE, CLINICAL CONFERENCE:LIPID SYNOVIAL EFFUSION. UNIQUE OCCURRENCE IN SYSTEMIC LUPUS ERYTHEMATOSUS, *ARTHRITIS RHEUM*, 16, 759-764 (1973)

2013 RYDEN KIRKISH AND MCCANN, EVALUATION OF SERUM IONIC CALCIUM MEASUREMENT IN A GENERAL HOSPITAL POPULATION, *AM J CLIN PATHOL*, 66, 634-638 (1966)

2014 RYDER KW, JAY SJ, JACKSON SA, HOKE SR, CHARACTERIZATION OF A SPECTROPHOTOMETRIC ASSAY FOR ANGIOTENSIN CONVERTING ENZYME, *CLIN CHEM*, 27, 530-534 (1981)

2015 RYDER KW, JAY SJ, KIBLAWI SO, HULL MT, SERUM ANGIOTENSIN CONVERTING ENZYME ACTIVITY IN PATIENTS WITH HISTOPLASMOSIS, *JAMA*, 249, 1888-9 (1983)

2016 RYNES R I ET AL, INTRAARTICULAR ACTIVATION OF THE COMPLEMENT SYSTEM IN PATIENTS WITH JUVENILE RHEUMATOID ARTHRITIS, *ARTHRITIS RHEUM*, 19, 161 (1976)

2017 SABIN SA, PULMONARY DISEASE, *IN: KELLER LB, ET AL, CLINICAL INTERNAL MEDICINE, LITTLE BROWN AND COMPANY*, 100-107 (1979)

2018 SACHS B ET AL, ESSENTIAL FRUCTOSURIA: ITS PATHOPHYSIOLOGY, *AM J DIS CHILD*, 63, 252 (1942)

2019 SACKETT, MODIFICATION OF BLOOR'S METHOD FOR THE DETERMINATION OF CHOLESTEROL IN WHOLE BLOOD OR BLOOD SERUM, *J BIOL CHEM*, 64, 203-205 (1925)

2020 SADOVSKY E ET AL, AN ALKALINE PHOSPHATASE SPECIFIC TO NORMAL PREGNANCY, *OBSTET GYNECOL*, 26, 211 (1965)

2021 SAFA AM, VAN ORDSTRAND HS, PLEURAL EFFUSION DUE TO MULTIPLE MYELOMA, *CHEST*, 64, 246-248 (1973)

2022 SAHI T ET AL, SERUM LIPIDS AND PROTEINS IN LACTOSE MALABSORPTION, *AM J CLIN NUTR*, 30, 476-81 (1977)

2023 SAIFER A, RAPID SCREENING METHODS FOR THE DETECTION OF INHERITED AND ACQUIRED AMINOACIDOPATHIES, *ADV CLIN CHEM*, 14, 140-199 (1971)

2024 SAIRANEN E ET AL, PERIARTERITIS NODOSA. A TEN-YEAR FOLLOW-UP OF TEN CASES, *ACTA MED SCAND*, 191, 501-4 (1972)

2025 SAKAGUCHI S, FURUTA Y, KAMEDA T, HAEMOPATHOLOGICAL CHANGES IN RECURRENT DEEP VENOUS THROMBOSIS OF THE EXTREMITIES, *J CARDIOVASC SURG (TORINO)*, 23, 117-22 (1982)

2026 SALAH I A ET AL, LEVELS OF SOME SERUM ENZYMES IN PATIENTS WITH SCHISTOSOMIASIS, *J TROP MED HYG*, 79, 270-4 (1976)

2027 SALAKA L A, SERUM ELECTROLYTES IN HYPERTENSION IN NIGERIANS, *CLIN CHIM ACTA*, 34, 105 (1971)

2028 SALIH S T ET AL, EOSINOPHILIA IN SCHISTOSOMA MANSONI INFECTION, *EAST AFR MED J*, 54, 421-4 (1977)

2029 SALKIE, TOO MANY TESTS?, *J CLIN ENDOCR*, 2, 915-916 (1971)

2030 SALT H B ET AL, ON HAVING NO BETA-LIPOPROTEIN: A SYNDROME COMPRISING A-BETA-LIPOPROTEINEMIA, ACANTHOCYTOSIS AND STEATORRHEA, *LANCET*, 2, 325 (1960)

2031 SALT W B II ET AL, AMYLASE - ITS CLINICAL SIGNIFICANCE: A REVIEW OF THE LITERATURE., *MEDICINE*, 55, 269-290 (1976)

2032 SAMAMA MM, SCHLEGEL N, CAZENAVE B, ET AL, ALPHA 2 ANTIPLASMIN ASSAY: AMIDOLYTIC AND IMMUNOLOGICAL METHOD. CRITICAL EVALUATION, *SYNTHETIC SUBSTRATES IN CLINICAL BLOOD COAGULATION ASSAYS*, 93-101 (1980)

2033 SAMLOFF I M AND WALSH J H, UNPUBLISHED OBSERVATIONS

2034 SAMMOUR M G ET AL, SERUM AND PLACENTAL LACTIC DEHYDROGENASE AND ALKALINE PHOSPHATASE ISOENZYMES IN NORMAL PREGNANCY AND IN PRE-ECLAMPSIA, *ACTA OBSTET GYNECOL SCAND*, 54, 393-400 (1975)

2035 SAMTER M ED, IMMUNOLOGICAL DISEASES, *3RD EDITION LITTLE BROWN AND CO* (1978)

2036 SAMUELSON K, ALY A, JOHANSSON C, NORMAN A, SERUM AND URINARY BILE ACIDS IN PATIENTS WITH PRIMARY BILIARY CIRRHOSIS, *SCAND J GASTROENTEROL*, 17, 121-8 (1982)

2037 SANCHEZ-MARTIN M ET AL, DOPAMINE BETA HYDROXYLASE IN HUMAN SYNOVIAL FLUID, *EXPERIENTIA*, 33, 650-51 (1977)

2038 SANCHEZ-UBEDA R ET AL, THE SIGNIFICANCE OF PANCREATITIS ACCOMPANYING ACUTE CHOLECYSTITIS, *ANN SURG*, 144, 44 (1956)

2039 SANDBERG A A ET AL, STUDIES ON LEUKEMIA I. URIC ACID EXCRETION, *BLOOD*, 11, 154 (1956)

2040 SANDLER M ET AL, PROSTAGLANDINS IN AMINE-PEPTIDE SECRETING TUMOURS, *LANCET*, 2, 1053 (1968)

2041 SANDRON D, LECOSSIER D, GRODET A, BASSET G, ET AL, DIAGNOSTIC, PROGNOSTIC AND DEVELOPMENTAL VALUE OF SERUM ANGIOTENSIN CONVERTING ENZYME IN SARCOIDOSIS, *ANN MED INTERNE (PARIS)*, 135, 46-50 (1984)

2042 SANDSTEAD H, MODERN NUTRITION IN HEALTH AND DISEASE, 5TH ED (EDS. R.S. GOODHART & M.E. SHILS), 596 (1973)

2043 SANDSTEAD HH, SHUKRY AS, PRASAD AS, ET AL, KWASHIORKOR IN EGYPT. I. CLINICAL AND BIOCHEMICAL STUDIES WITH SPECIAL REFERENCE TO PLASMA ZINC AND SERUM LACTIC DEHYDROGENASE, *AM J CLIN NUTR*, 17, 15-26 (1965)

2044 SANTOS P G ET AL, LES LIPIDES PLASMATIQUE DANS L'INSUFFISANCE RESPIRATOIRE: RELATION AVEC L'HYPERCAPNIE ET L'HYPOXEMIE, *BRIT J CANCER*, 12, 179-83 (1976)

2045 SAOJI A ET AL, ELECTROPHORESIS AND IMMUNO ELECTROPHORESIS IN LEPROSY, *LEPR INDIA*, 50, 161-5 (1978)

2046 SAPIRA J D AND B M DOMM, CRYOFIBRINOGENEMIA AND CIRRHOSIS OF THE LIVER, *TEX REP BIOL MED*, 25, 156 (1967)

2047 SARCIONE E J ET AL, FERRITIN SYNTHESIS BY SPLENIC TUMOR TISSUE OF HODGKIN'S DISEASE, *EXPERIENTIA*, 31, 1334-5 (1975)

2048 SARLES H, LAUGIER R, ALCOHOLIC PANCREATITIS, *CLIN GASTROENTEROL*, 10, 401-415 (1981)

2049 SARNE A S ET AL, RENAL CLEARANCES OF AMINO ACIDS IN INDIAN CHILDHOOD CIRRHOSIS AND PORTAL CIRRHOSIS, *INDIAN J PEDIATR*, 13, 713-18 (1976)

2050 SARTORIUS O W ET AL, THE RENAL REGULATION OF ACID-BASE BALANCE IN MAN, *J CLIN INVEST*, 28, 423 (1949)

2051 SASAYUKI T, GRUMET FC, MCDEVITT HO, THE ASSOCIATION BETWEEN GENES IN THE MAJOR HISTOCOMPATIBILITY COMPLEX AND DISEASE SUSCEPTIBILITY, *ANNU REV MED*, 28, 425-452 (1977)

2052 SASS-KORTSAK A, COPPER METABOLISM, *ADV CLIN CHEM*, 8, 1-67 (1965)

2053 SAUBERLICH HE, DOWDY RP, SKALA JH, LABORATORY TESTS FOR THE ASSESSMENT OF NUTRITIONAL STATUS, *CRC PRESS, CLEVELAND, OHIO* (1974)

2054 SAUDEK C D ET AL, ABNORMAL GLUCOSE TOLERANCE IN BETA THALASSEMIA MAJOR, *METABOLISM*, 26, 43-52 (1977)

2055 SAVAGE J M ET AL, RENIN AND BLOOD PRESSURE IN CHILDREN WITH RENAL SCARRING AND VESICO-URETERIC REFLUX, *LANCET*, 2, 441-4 (1978)

2056 SAXE AW, HOLLINGER MA, ESSAM T, EFFECT OF BILIRUBIN ON THE SPECTROPHOTOMETRIC AND RADIONUCLIDE ASSAY FOR SERUM ANGIOTENSIN-CONVERTING ENZYME, *RES COMMUN CHEM PATHOL PHARMACOL*, 51, 129-36 (1986)

2057 SCADDING GK, HAVARD CW, PATHOGENESIS AND TREATMENT OF MYASTHENIA GRAVIS, *BR MED J*, 283, 1008-1012 (1981)

2058 SCANNI A ET AL, SERUM COPPER AND CERULOPLASMIN LEVELS IN PATIENTS WITH NEOPLASIAS LOCALIZED IN THE STOMACH, LARGE INTESTINE OR LUNG, *TUMORI*, 63, 175-80. (1977)

2059 SCHACHNER AND BRENNAN, AN ACUTE ELEVATION OF SERUM INORGANIC PHOSPHATE IN CARDIO-VASCULAR COLLAPSE, *VIRGINIA MEDICAL MONTHLY*, 97, 758-759 (1970)

2060 SCHACHTER J ET AL, LYMPHOGRANULOMA VENEREUM. I COMPARISON OF THE FREI TEST, COMPLEMENT-FIXATIOUS TEST, AND ISOLATION OF THE AGENT, *J INFECT DIS*, 120, 372 (1969)

2061 SCHAFFER A J AND AVERY M E, DISEASES OF THE NEWBORN, *4TH EDITION W B SAUNDERS & CO PHIL* (1977)

2062 SCHAFFER ET AL, COMPARISON OF ENZYME, CLINICAL RADIOGRAPHIC AND RADIONUCLIDE METHODS OF DETECTING BONE METASTASES FROM CARCINOMA OF THE PROSTATE, *RADIOLOGY*, 121, 431-434 (1976)

2063 SCHECHTER AN, BUNN HF, WHAT DETERMINES SEVERITY IN SICKLE CELL DISEASE?, *N ENGL J MED*, 306, 295-6 (1982)

2064 SCHECHTER P J ET AL, DISTRIBUTION OF SERUM ZINC BETWEEN ALBUMIN AND ALPHA 2 MACRO GLOBULIN IN PATIENTS WITH DECOMPENSATED HEPATIC CIRRHOSIS, *EUR J CLIN INVEST*, 6, 147-50 (1976)

2065 SCHELP F P ET AL, SERUM PROTEINASE INHIBITORS AND OTHER SERUM PROTEINS IN PROTEIN-ENERGY MALNUTRITION, *BR J NUTR*, 38, 31-8 (1977)

2066 SCHELP F P ET AL, ALTERATIONS OF HUMAN SERUM PROTEINS AND OTHER BIOCHEMICAL PARAMETERS AFTER FIVE TO TEN DAYS OF UNTREATED ACUTE FALCIPARUM MALARIA, *TROPENMED PARASITOL*, 28, 319-22 (1977)

2067 SCHELP FP, THANANGKUL O, SUPAWAN V, ET AL, SERUM PROTEINASE INHIBITORS AND ACUTE-PHASE REACTANTS FROM PROTEIN-ENERGY MALNUTRITION CHILDREN DURING TREATMENT, *AM J CLIN NUTR*, 32, 1415-1422 (1979)

2068 SCHERNTHANER G, SCHWARZER C, KUZMITS R, ET AL, INCREASED ANGIOTENSIN-CONVERTING ENZYME ACTIVITIES IN DIABETES MELLITUS: ANALYSIS OF DIABETES TYPE, STATE OF METABOLIC CONTROL AND OCCURRENCE OF DIABETIC VASCULAR, *J CLIN PATHOL*, 37, 307-12 (1984)

2069 SCHLIEP G, FELGENHAUER K, THE A2-MACROGLOBULIN LEVEL IN CEREBROSPINAL FLUID; A PARAMETER FOR THE CONDITION OF THE BLOOD-CSF CARRIER, *J NEUROL*, 207, 171-181 (1974)

2070 SCHLOESSER L L ET AL, THROMBOCYTOSIS IN IRON DEFICIENCY ANEMIA, *J LAB CLIN MED*, 66, 107 (1965)

2071 SCHMID R AND HAMMAKER L, METABOLISM AND DISPOSITION OF C14 BILIRUBIN IN CONGENITAL NONHEMOLYTIC JAUNDICE, *J CLIN INVEST*, 42, 1720 (1963)

2072 SCHMID R ET AL, PORPHYRIN CONTENT OF BONE MARROW AND LIVER IN THE VARIOUS FORMS OF PORPHYRIA, *ARCH INTERN MED*, 93, 167 (1954)

2073 SCHMID R ET AL, ERYTHROPOIETIC (CONGENITAL) PORPHYRIA: A RARE ABNORMALITY OF THE NORMOBLASTS, *BLOOD*, 10, 416 (1955)

2074 SCHMIDT JB, SPONA J, THE LEVELS OF ANDROGEN IN SERUM IN FEMALE ACNE PATIENTS, *ENDOCRINOL EXP*, 19, 17 (1985)

2075 SCHMIDT R ET AL, THE COURSE OF MULTIPLE SCLEROSIS WITH EXTREMELY HIGH GAMMA GLOBULIN VALUES IN THE CSF, *EUR NEUROL*, 15, 241-8 (1977)

2076 SCHNOHR P, ENZYME CONCENTRATIONS IN SERUM AFTER PROLONGED PHYSICAL EXERCISE, *DAN MED BULL*, 21, 68-71 (1974)

2077 SCHOEN M S ET AL, SIGNIFICANCE OF SERUM LEVEL OF 25-HYDROXYCHOLECALCIFEROL IN GASTROINTESTINAL DISEASE, *AM J DIG DIS*, 23, 137-42 (1978)

2078 SCHOENFELD ET AL, ACID PHOSPHATASE IN SERUM: INCREASE IN ACUTE MYOCARDIAL INFARCTION, *SCIENCE*, 139, 51-52 (1963)

2079 SCHOENFELD ET AL, INCREASED SERUM PHOSPHATASE AFTER ARTERIAL EMBOLISM, *AM HEART J*, 67, 92-94 (1964)

2080 SCHOENFELD M R ET AL, ACID HYPERPHENYLPHOSPHATASIA IN THROMBOPHLEBITIS AND PULMONARY EMBOLISM, *ANN INTERN MED*, 57, 468-471 (1962)

2081 SCHOENFELD Y ET AL, IMMUNOGLOBULIN CHANGES IN SLE, *CLIN IMMUNOL IMMUNOPATHOL*, 39, 99-101 (1977)

2082 SCHOLL GM, WU CH, LEYDEN J, ANDROGEN EXCESS IN WOMEN WITH ACNE, *OBSTET GYNECOL*, 64, 683 (1984)

2083 SCHONELL M E ET AL, FAILURE TO DIFFERENTIATE PULMONARY INFARCTION BY BIOCHEMICAL TESTING, *BR MED J*, 1, 1146 (1966)

2084 SCHREINER G C ET AL, TOXIC NEPHROPATHY: ADVERSE RENAL EFFECTS CAUSED BY DRUGS AND CHEMICALS, *JAMA*, 191, 849 (1965)

2085 SCHREINER G E, THE NEPHROTIC SYNDROME IN: DISEASES OF THE KIDNEY, *2ND EDITION LITTLE BROWN & CO M B STRAUSS & L G WELT (EDS)*, 503 (1971)

2086 SCHRIRE V AND R A ASHERSON, ARTERITIS OF THE AORTA AND ITS MAJOR BRANCHES, *Q J MED*, 33, 439 (1964)

2087 SCHULMAN L E ET AL, SEROLOGIC ABNORMALITIES IN SYSTEMIC LUPUS ERYTHEMATOSUS, *J CHRONIC DIS*, 16, 889 (1963)

2088 SCHUMACHER HR JR, LABORATORY DIAGNOSIS OF DEGENERATIVE JOINT DISEASE, *ANN CLIN LAB SCI*, 5, 242-247 (1975)

2089 SCHUR P H ET AL, IMMUNOLOGIC FACTORS AND CLINICAL ACTIVITY IN SYSTEMIC LUPUS ERYTHEMATOSUS, *N ENGL J MED*, 278, 533 (1968)

2090 SCHUR P H ET AL, COMPLEMENT IN RHEUMATIC DISEASES, *BULL RHEUM DIS*, 26, 666-73 (1971)

2091 SCHWARTZ J F ET AL, BASSEN-KORNZWEIG SYNDROME: DEFICIENCY OF SERUM BETA-LIPOPROTEIN, *ARCH NEUROL*, 8, 438 (1963)

2092 SCHWARTZ M K, INTERFERENCES IN DIAGNOSTIC BIOCHEMICAL PROCEDURES, *ADV CLIN CHEM*, 16, 1 (1973)

2093 SCHWARTZ M K ET AL, LABORATORY AIDS TO DIAGNOSIS: ENZYMES, *CANCER (SUPPL)*, 37, 542 (1976)

2094 SCHWARTZ M K, ROLE OF TRACE ELEMENTS IN CANCER, *CANCER RES*, 35, 3481-87. (1975)

2095 SCHWARTZ TB, RYAN WG, *THE YEAR BOOK OF ENDOCRINOLOGY. CHICAGO, YEAR BOOK MEDICAL PUBLISHERS, INC* (1979)

2096 SCHWICK H-G, HAUPT H, CHEMISTRY AND FUNCTION OF HUMAN PLASMA PROTEINS, *ANGEW CHEM*, 191, 87-99 (1980)

2097 SCHWILLE P O ET AL, URINARY THYROXINE IN RATS FED VARIOUS DIETS AND IN RENAL CALCIUM STONE-FORMING PATIENTS, *EUR UROL*, 2, 196-9 (1976)

2098 SCOTT R ET AL, HYPERCALCIURIA RELATED TO CADMIUM EXPOSURE, *UROLOGY*, 11, 462-65 (1978)

2099 SCOTT R, CUNNINGHAM C, MCLELLAND A, ET AL, THE IMPORTANCE OF CADMIUM AS A FACTOR IN CALCIFIED UPPER URINARY TRACT STONE DISEASE--A PROSPECTIVE 7-YEAR STUDY, *BR J UROL*, 54, 584-9 (1982)

2100 SCUDDER P R ET AL, SERUM COPPER AND RELATED VARIABLES IN RHEUMATOID ARTHRITIS, *ANN RHEUM DIS*, 37, 67-70 (1978)

2101 SCUDDER P R ET AL, SYNOVIAL FLUID COPPER AND RELATED VARIABLES IN RHEUMATOID AND DEGENERATIVE ARTHRITIS, *ANN RHEUM DIS*, 37, 71-72 (1978)

2102 SEAL U S ET AL, RESPONSE OF SERUM CHOLESTEROL AND TRIGLYCERIDES TO HORMONE TREATMENT AND THE RELATION OF PRETREATMENT VALUES TO MORTALITY IN PATIENTS WITH PROSTATIC CANCER, *CANCER*, 38, 109-107 (1976)

2103 SEAMONDS B ET AL, DETERMINATION OF IONIZED CALCIUM IN SERUM BY USE OF AN ION-SELECTIVE ELECTRODE, *CLIN CHEM*, 18, 155 (1972)

2104 SEARCY R L, DIAGNOSTIC BIOCHEMISTRY, *MCGRAW-HILL* (1969)

2105 SEED J R ET AL, THE PRESENCE OF AGGLUTINATING ANTIBODY IN THE IGM IMMUNOGLOBULIN FRACTION OF RABBIT ANTISERUM DURING EXPERIMENTAL AFRICAN TRYPANOSOMIASIS, *PARASITOLOGY*, 59, 283 (1969)

2106 SEEDAT, EFFECT OF POTASSIUM ON BLOOD-SUGAR AND PLASMA-INSULIN LEVELS IN PATIENTS UNDERGOING PERITONEAL DIALYSIS AND HAEMODIALYSIS, *J CLIN ENDOCR*, 2, 1166-1169 (1968)

2107 SEELIG M S ET AL, MAGNESIUM INTERRELATIONSHIPS IN ISCHEMIC HEART DISEASE: A REVIEW, *AM J CLIN NUTR*, 27, 59 (1974)

2108 SEINO Y ET AL, HYPERGASTRINEMIA IN HYPERTHYROIDISM, *J CLIN ENDOCRINOL METAB*, 43, 852-55 (1976)

2109 SEIP M ET AL, SERUM CHOLESTEROL AND TRIGLYCERIDES IN CHILDREN WITH ANEMIA, *SCAND J HAEMATOL*, 19, 503-8 (1977)

2110 SEITANIDIS B ET AL, SERUM IMMUNOGLOBULIN LEVELS IN WHITE PATIENTS WITH SICKLE CELL DISEASE., *CLIN CHIM ACTA*, 37, 531-532 (1972)

2111 SELL S, HEPATOCELLULAR CANCER MARKERS, *IN CANCER MARKERS II, HUMANA PRESS, INC. CLIFTON, NEW JERSEY* (1982)

2112 SELMAJ K, HISTAMINE RELEASE FROM LEUCOCYTES DURING MIGRAINE ATTACK, *CEPHALAGIA*, 4, 97-100 (1984)

2113 SELYE H, THE STRESS OF LIFE, *3RD EDITION MCGRAW-HILL NEW YORK* (1978)

2114 SENAY L C JR AND CHRISTENSEN M L, CHANGES IN BLOOD PLASMA DURING PROGRESSIVE DEHYDRATION, *J APPL PHYSIOL*, 20, 1136 (1965)

2115 SEPP'AL'A M, RANTA T, RUTANEN EM, ET AL, IMPROVED DIAGNOSIS OF PREGNANCY-RELATED GYNAECOLOGICAL EMERGENCIES BY RAPID HUMAN CHORIONIC GONADOTROPIN BETA-SUBUNIT ASSAY, *BR J OBSTET GYNAECOL*, 88, 138-40 (1981)

2116 SEPPALA M, FETAL PATHOPHYSIOLOGY OF HUMAN AFP, *GUT*, 14, 939 (1977)

2117 SEPPALA M ET AL, CONGENITAL NEPHROTIC SYNDROME: PRENATAL DIAGNOSIS AND GENETIC COUNSELLING BY ESTIMATION OF AMNIOTIC FLUID AND MATERNAL SERUM ALPHA-FETOPROTEIN, *LANCET*, 2, 123-5 (1976)

2118 SEQUEIRA W, STINAR D, SERUM ANGIOTENSIN-CONVERTING ENZYME LEVELS IN SARCOID ARTHRITIS, *ARCH INTERN MED*, 146, 125 (1986)

2119 SERBY M, RICHARDSON SB, TWENTE S, ET AL, CSF SOMATOSTATIN IN ALZHEIMER'S DISEASE, *NEUROBIOLOGY OF AGING*, 5, 187-189 (1984)

2120 SERJEANT GR, GALLOWAY RE, GUERI MC, SERUM-COPPER IN SICKLE-CELL ANEMIA, *LANCET*, II, 891 (1970)

2121 SERNO Y ET AL, HYPOGASTRINEMIA IN HYPOTHYROIDISM, *AM J DIG DIS*, 23, 189-91 (1978)

2122 SHAHIDI N T ET AL, ALKALI-RESISTANT HEMOGLOBIN IN APLASTIC ANEMIA OF BOTH ACQUIRED AND CONGENITAL TYPES, *N ENGL J MED*, 266, 177 (1962)

2123 SHAMBAUGH G E ET AL, INSULIN RESPONSE DURING TULAREMIA IN MAN, *DIABETES*, 16, 369 (1967)

2124 SHANNON ET AL, AN ULTRASTRUCTURAL STUDY OF ACID PHOSPHATASE ACTIVITY IN NORMAL, ADENOMATOUS AND HYPERPLASTIC (CHIEF CELL TYPE) HUMAN PARATHYROID GLANDS, *AM J PATH*, 77, 493 (1974)

2125 SHANNON I L ET AL, HUMAN PAROTID SALIVA UREA IN RENAL FAILURE AND DURING DIALYSIS, *ARCH ORAL BIOL*, 22, 83-86 (1977)

2126 SHARMA G V ET AL, PULMONARY EMBOLISM: THE GREAT IMITATOR, *DM*, 22, 16-21 (1976)

2127 SHARMA S C ET AL, PLATELET ADHESIVENESS, PLASMA FIBRINOGEN, AND FIBRINOLYTIC ACTIVITY IN YOUNG PATIENTS WITH ISCHAEMIC STROKE, *J NEUROL NEUROSURG PSYCHIATRY*, 41, 118-21 (1978)

2128 SHARP GC, MIXED CONNECTIVE TISSUE DISEASE, *BULL RHEUM DIS*, 25, 828-831 (1974-1975)

2129 SHARP HL, ALPHA-1-ANTITRYPSIN DEFICIENCY, *HOSP PRACT*, 83-96 (1971)

2130 SHAW A B AND SCHOLES M C, RETICULOCYTOSIS IN RENAL FAILURE, *LANCET*, 1, 799 (1967)

2131 SHAW N F H ET AL, HISTIDINEMIA, *J PEDIATR*, 63, 720 (1963)

2132 SHEAGREN J N ET AL, RHEUMATOID FACTOR IN BACTERIAL ENDOCARDITIS, *ARTHRITIS RHEUM*, 19, 887-90 (1976)

2133 SHEARMAN R P, SOME ASPECTS OF THE URINARY EXCRETION OF PREGNANEDIOL IN PREGNANCY, *BR J OBSTET GYNAECOL*, 64, 1 (1959)

2134 SHEARN M A, SJÖGREN'S SYNDROME, *MED CLIN NORTH AM*, 61, 271-82 (1977)

2135 SHEARN M A ET AL, SERUM VISCOSITY IN THE RHEUMATIC DISEASES AND MACROGLOBULINEMIA, *ARCH INTERN MED*, 112, 684-687 (1963)

2136 SHEEHY T AND MONTALVO G, THE ESCAPE PHENOMENON OF POLYCYTHEMIA VERA: ITS RELATION TO HEMORRHAGE AND THROMBOSIS IN THE DISEASE, *AM J MED SCI*, 243, 105 (1962)

2137 SHEEHY T W AND BERMAN A, THE ANEMIA OF CIRRHOSIS, *J LAB CLIN MED*, 56, 72 (1960)

2138 SHEFFER A ET AL, SERUM COMPLEMENT LEVELS IN SARCOIDOSIS, *LEVINSKY L MACHOLDA F (EDS) 5TH INTERNATIONAL CONF ON SARCOIDOSIS*, 195 (1971)

2139 SHELDON S ET AL, PLASMA CATECHOLAMINES IN HYPOTHYROIDISM AND HYPERTHYROIDISM, *J CLIN ENDOCRINOL METAB*, 36, 587-9 (1973)

2140 SHELL, THE ASSESSMENT OF MYOCARDIAL INFARCTION WITH SERUM ENZYME DETERMINATIONS, *W VIRGINIA MED J*, 70, 54-55 (1974)

2141 SHEPS SG, KIRKPATRICK RA, HYPERTENSION, *MAYO CLIN PROC*, 50, 709-720 (1975)

2142 SHER A ET AL, IMMUNE RESPONSES DURING HUMAN SCHISTOSOMIASIS MANSONI. II. OCCURRENCE OF EOSINOPHIL-DEPENDENT CYTOTOXIC ANTIBODIES IN RELATION TO INTENSITY AND DURATION OF INFECTION, *AM J TROP MED HYG*, 26, 909-16 (1977)

2143 SHER G ET AL, PREGNANCY, PRE-ECLAMPSIA, AND DISSEMINATED INTRAVASCULAR COAGULATION, *S AFR MED J*, 49, 1197 (1975)

2144 SHERLOCK S, PRIMARY BILIARY CIRRHOSIS, *AM J MED*, 65, 217-219 (1978)

2145 SHERLOCK S ET AL, IMMUNOLOGICAL DISTURBANCE IN DISEASES OF LIVER AND THYROID, *PROC R SOC*, 70, 851-7 (1977)

2146 SHERWIN R ET AL, HYPERGLUCAGONEMIA IN LAENNEC'S CIRRHOSIS: THE ROLE OF PORTAL SYSTEMIC SHUNTING, *N ENGL J MED*, 290, 239-42 (1974)

2147 SHERWIN R S ET AL, HYPERGLUCAGONEMIA IN CIRRHOSIS: ALTERED SECRETION AND SENSITIVITY TO GLUCAGON, *GASTROENTEROLOGY*, 74, 1224-8 (1978)

2148 SHERWIN RW, WENTWORTH DN, CUTLER JA, ET AL, SERUM CHOLESTEROL LEVELS AND CANCER MORTALITY IN 361 662 MEN SCREENED FOR THE MULTIPLE RISK FACTOR INTERVENTION TRIAL, *JAMA*, 257, 943 (1987)

2149 SHIH V, LABORATORY TECHNIQUES FOR THE DETECTION OF HEREDITARY METABOLIC DISORDERS, *BOCA RATON, FLA., CRC PRESS* (1973)

2150 SHILO R ET AL, REEVALUATION OF THE POLYVINYLPYRROLIDONE SEDIMENTATION TEST IN THE DIAGNOSIS OF ABO HEMOLYTIC DISEASE OF THE NEWBORN, *VOX SANG*, 31, 16-24 (1976)

2151 SHIMAMURA J ET AL, NON-PANCREATIC HYPERAMYLASEMIA IN PANCREATIC CANCER, *GASTROENTEROLOGY*, 68, 985 (1975)

2152 SHIRROCK R D ET AL, RAISED LEVELS OF COMPLEMENT INACTIVATION PRODUCTS IN ANKYLOSING SPONDYLITIS, *J RHEUMATOL*, 1, 428 (1974)

2153 SHOHET S B AND NESS P M, HEMOLYTIC ANEMIAS: FAILURE OF THE RED CELL MEMBRANE, *MED CLIN NORTH AM*, 60, 913-932 (1976)

2154 SHORT C L BAUER W AND W E REYNOLDS, RHEUMATOID ARTHRITIS, *HARVARD UNIVERSITY PRESS* (1957)

2155 SHRIFRINE M FISHER G L, CERULOPLASMIN LEVELS IN SERA FROM HUMAN PATIENTS WITH OSTEOSARCOMA, *CANCER*, 38, 244-8. (1976)

2156 SHUSTER F ET AL, DISSOCIATION OF SERUM BILIRUBIN AND ALKALINE PHOSPHATASE IN INFECTIOUS MONONUCLEOSIS, *JAMA*, 209, 267-268 (1969)

2157 SHUSTER S ET AL, SMALL INTESTINE IN PSORIASIS, *BR MED J*, 3, 445-506 (1967)

2158 SIEMES H ET AL, OLIGOCLONAL GAMMA-GLOBULIN BANDING OF CEREBROSPINAL FLUID IN PATIENTS WITH SUBACUTE SCLEROSING PANENCEPHALITIS. COMPARISON OF THE ELECTROPHORETIC PATTERN WITH THAT IN MULTIPLE SCLEROSIS AND CONGENITAL, *J NEUROL SCI*, 32, 395-409 (1977)

2159 SIEMKOWICZ E ET AL, CHANGES IN CISTERNAL FLUID POTASSIUM CONCENTRATION FOLLOWING CARDIAC ARREST, *ACTA NEUROL SCAND*, 55, 137-44 (1977)

2160 SIEST G ET AL, PLASMA ENZYMES-PHYSIOLOGICAL AND ENVIRONMENTAL VARIATIONS, *REFERENCE VALUES IN HUMAN CHEMISTRY G. SIEST (ED)*, 28 (1973)

2161 SIGURDSSON ET AL, CALCIUM ABSORPTION AND EXCRETION IN THE GUT IN ACROMEGALY, *CLIN ENDOCRINOL (OXF)*, 2, 187-192 (1973)

2162 SILVERBERG J AND VOLPE R, RHEUMATOID FACTORS IN GRAVE'S DISEASE, *ANN INTERN MED*, 88, 216-217 (1978)

2163 SILVERSTEIN E ET AL, ELEVATED SERUM AND SPLEEN ANGIOTENSIN CONVERTING ENZYME AND SERUM LYSOZYME IN GAUCHER'S DISEASE, *CLIN CHIM ACTA*, 74, 21-26 (1977)

2164 SILVERSTEIN E, BRUNSWICK J, RAO TK, FRIEDLAND J, INCREASED SERUM ANGIOTENSIN-CONVERTING ENZYME IN CHRONIC RENAL DISEASE, *NEPHRON*, 37, 206-10 (1984)

2165 SILVERSTEIN E, SCHUSSLER GC, FRIEDLAND J, ELEVATED SERUM ANGIOTENSIN-CONVERTING ENZYME IN HYPERTHYROIDISM, *AM J MED*, 75, 233-6 (1983)

2166 SILVERSTEIN H, A RAPID PROTEIN TEST FOR ACOUSTIC NEURINOMA, *ARCH OTOLARYNGOL HEAD NECK SURG*, 95, 202-203 (1972)

2167 SILVERSTEIN M N ET AL, LEUKOCYTE ALKALINE PHOSPHATASE IN AGNOGENIC MYELOID METAPLASIA, *AM J CLIN PATHOL*, 61, 307 (1974)

2168 SILVIS S E ET AL, THROMBOCYTOSIS IN PATIENTS WITH LUNG CANCER, *JAMA*, 211, 1852 (1970)

2169 SIMIONESCU L ET AL, THE HORMONAL PATTERN IN ALCOHOLIC DISEASE. I. LUTEINIZING HORMONE (LH), FOLLICLE-STIMULATING HORMONE (FSH) AND TESTOSTERONE, *ENDOCRINOLOGIE*, 15, 45-9 (1977)

2170 SIMMONS P, PLASMA PROTEIN-DIAGNOSTICS, *BEHRING DIAGNOSTICS, SOMERVILLE, N.J.* (1974)

2171 SIMON E R ET AL, INCUBATION HEMOLYSIS AND RED CELL METABOLISM IN ACANTHOCYTOSIS, *J CLIN INVEST*, 43, 1311 (1964)

2172 SIMON ET AL, CLINICAL INTERPRETATION OF TOTAL SERUM AND PROSTATIC ACID PHOSPHATASE LEVEL, *JAMA*, 171, 125-129 (1959)

2173 SIMON G, MORIOKA S, SNYDER DK, INCREASED SERUM AND URINARY N-ACETYL-B-D-GLUCOSAMINIDASE ACTIVITY IN HUMAN HYPERTENSION: EARLY INDICATOR OF RENAL DYSFUNCTION, *CLIN EXP HYPERTENS (A)*, A6(4), 879-896 (1984)

2174 SIMON RP, NEUROSYPHILIS: AN UPDATE, *WEST J MED*, 134, 87-91 (1981)

2175 SIMONE J V ET AL, BLOOD COAGULATION IN THYROID DYSFUNCTION, *N ENGL J MED*, 273, 1057 (1965)

2176 SIMONE J V ET AL, INITIAL FEATURES AND PROGNOSIS IN 363 CHILDREN WITH ACUTE LYMPHOCYTIC LEUKEMIA, *CANCER*, 36, 2099-108 (1975)

2177 SIMONS L A ET AL, TYPE V HYPERLIPOPROTEINAEMIA RE-VISITED: FINDINGS IN A SYDNEY POPULATION, *AUST NZ J MED*, 5, 210-9 (1975)

2178 SIMPSON H, CSF ACID-BASE STATUS AND LACTATE AND PYRUVATE CONCENTRATIONS AFTER SHORT (< 30 MINUTES) FIRST FEBRILE CONVULSIONS IN CHILDREN, *ARCH DIS CHILD*, 52, 837-843 (1977)

2179 SIMS K A H ET AL, SERIAL STUDIES OF RENAL FUNCTION DURING PREGNANCY AND THE PUERPERIUM IN NORMAL WOMEN, *J CLIN INVEST*, 37, 1764 (1958)

2180 SINGER F R ET AL, HYPERCALCEMIA IN RETICULUM CELL SARCOMA WITHOUT HYPERPARATHYROIDISM OR SKELETAL METASTASES, *ANN INTERN MED*, 78, 365 (1973)

2181 SINGER K ET AL, THE LIFE SPAN OF THE MEGALOCYTE AND THE HEMOLYTIC SYNDROME OF PERNICIOUS ANEMIA, *J LAB CLIN MED*, 33, 1068 (1948)

2182 SINGH J, TRAVELLA D, DIFERRANTE N, MEASUREMENTS OF ARYLSULFATASES A AND B IN HUMAN SERUM, *J PEDIATR*, 86, 574-576 (1975)

2183 SINGH M M, CARBOHYDRATE METABOLISM IN PRE-ECLAMPSIA, *BR J OBSTET GYNAECOL*, 83, 124-31 (1976)

2184 SINGH V ET AL, PROGNOSTIC VALUE OF SERUM URIC ACID IN PATIENTS OF ACUTE MYOCARDIAL INFARCTION, *J INDIAN MED ASSOC*, 59, 97-9 (1977)

2185 SINGH V S ET AL, SERUM FREE FATTY ACIDS AND ARRHYTHMIAS AFTER ACUTE MYOCARDIAL INFARCTIONS, *J POSTGRAD MED*, 23, 19-24 (1977)

2186 SINGSEN B H ET AL, SYSTEMIC LUPUS ERYTHEMATOSUS IN CHILDHOOD CORRELATIONS BETWEEN CHANGES IN DISEASE ACTIVITY AND SERUM COMPLEMENT LEVELS, *J PEDIATR*, 89, 358-59 (1976)

2187 SINHA S ET AL, SERUM CALCIUM AND MAGNESIUM IN DIFFERENT TYPES OF LEPROSY, *LEPR INDIA*, 50, 54-56 (1978)

2188 SINHA SN, GABRIELI ER, SERUM COPPER AND ZINC LEVELS IN VARIOUS PATHOLOGIC CONDITIONS, *AM J CLIN PATHOL*, 54, 570-577 (1970)

2189 SISE H S ET AL, BLOOD COAGULATION FACTORS IN TOTAL BODY IRRADIATION, *BLOOD*, 18, 702 (1961)

2190 SITPRIJA V ET AL, RENAL FAILURE IN MALARIA: A PATHOPHYSIOLOGIC STUDY, *NEPHRON*, 18, 277-87 (1977)

2191 SJEJGAARD,A. AND RYDER,L.P., ASSOCIATION BETWEEN HLA AND DISEASE, *IN: DAUSSET, J. AND SVEJGAARD A.; HLA AND DISEASE; WILLIAMS AND WILKINS, BALT.*, 46-71 (1977)

2192 SJOGREN U, AMOEBOID MOVEMENT CONFIGURATION AND MITOTIC INDICES OF LYMPHOID CELLS FROM CHILDREN WITH ACUTE LYMPHOBLASTIC LEUKAEMIA, *LYMPHOLOGY*, 9, 69-71 (1976)

2193 SKANSBERG P, PROGNOSTIC VALUE OF BLOOD PLATELET COUNTS, COAGULATION FACTORS AND SERUM FIBRIN/FIBRINOGEN DEGRADATION PRODUCTS (FDP) IN ACUTE INFECTIONS, *SCAND J INFECT DIS*, 10, 61-65 (1978)

2194 SKINNER S L ET AL, ANALYSIS OF CHANGES IN THE RENIN-ANGIOTENSIN SYSTEM DURING PREGNANCY, *CLIN SCI*, 42, 479-488 (1972)

2195 SKOOTSKY SA, ROSOVE MH, LANGLEY MB, IMMUNE THROMBOCYTOPENIA AND RESPONSE TO SPLENECTOMY IN CHRONIC LIVER DISEASE, *ARCH INTERN MED*, 146, 555 (1986)

2196 SKUDE G ET AL, AMYLASE, HEPATIC ENZYMES AND BILIRUBIN IN SERUM OF CHRONIC ALCOHOLICS, *ACTA MED SCAND*, 201, 53-58. (1977)

2197 SKUDE G ET AL, SERUM ISOAMYLASE PATTERN IN OBSTRUCTIVE PANCREATIC DISEASE, *SCAND J GASTROENTEROL*, 12, 673-6 (1977)

2198 SLAVINSKIE Z, DECREASED SYNTHESIS OF SERUM COMPLEMENT (C3) IN HYPOCOMPLEMENTEMIC SLE, *CLIN EXP IMMUNOL*, 11, 21-9 (1972)

2199 SLEISENGER M H AND FORTRAN J S, GASTROINTESTINAL DISEASE, *W B SAUNDERS CO PHILADELPHIA* (1978)

2200 SLOB S ET AL, THE EFFECT OF ACUTE NOISE EXPOSURE ON THE EXCRETION OF CORTICOSTEROIDS, ADRENALIN AND NORADRENALIN IN MAN, *INTERNAT ARCH ARBEITS MED*, 31, 225 (1973)

2201 SMALLEY M J ET AL, ANTINUCLEAR FACTORS AND HUMAN LEUCO-CYTES: REACTION WITH GRANULOCYTES AND LYMPHOCYTES, *AUST ANN MED*, 17, 28 (1968)

2202 SMALLRIDGE RC, RODGERS J, VERMA PS, SERUM ANGIOTENSIN-CONVERTING ENZYME. ALTERATIONS IN HYPERTHYROIDISM, HYPO-THYROIDISM, AND SUBACUTE THYROIDITIS, *JAMA*, 250, 2489-93 (1983)

2203 SMALS A G ET AL, THE PITUITARY-THYROID AXIS IN KLINEFELTER'S SYNDROME, *ACTA ENDOCRINOL*, 84, 72-9 (1977)

2204 SMEENK R, WESTGEEST T, SWAAK T, ANTINUCLEAR ANTIBODY DETER-MINATION: THE PRESENT STATE OF DIAGNOSTIC AND CLINICAL RELEVANCE, *SCAND J RHEUMATOL*, SUPPL. 56, 78-92 (1985)

2205 SMITH A F, DIAGNOSTIC VALUE OF SERUM C-K IN A CORONARY CARE UNIT, *LANCET*, 2, 178-82 (1967)

2206 SMITH AND SPEICHER, *CHOOSING EFFECTIVE LABORATORY TESTS, W B SAUNDERS COMPANY, PHILADEPHIA* (1983)

2207 SMITH C E ET AL, SEROLOGICAL TESTS IN THE DIAGNOSIS AND PROG-NOSIS OF COCCIDIOIDOMYCOSIS, *AM J HYG*, 52, 1 (1950)

2208 SMITH C H, FAMILIAL BLOOD STUDIES IN CASES OF MEDITERRANEAN (COOLEY'S) ANEMIA, *AM J DIS CHILD*, 65, 681 (1943)

2209 SMITH EK, MANAGING CONGENITAL ADRENAL HYPERPLASIA, *CLIN CHEM NEWS*, 35 (1980)

2210 SMITH ET AL, CLOFIBRATE, SERUM ENZYMES, AND MUSCLE PAIN, *BR MED J*, 2, 86-88 (1970)

2211 SMITH G V, THE ANTERIOR PITUITARY-LIKE HORMONE IN LATE PREG-NANCY TOXEMIA, *AM J OBSTET GYNECOL*, 38, 618 (1939)

2212 SMITH G V ET AL, ESTROGEN AND PROGESTIN METABOLISM IN PREG-NANT WOMEN, WITH ESPECIAL REFERENCE TO PRE-ECLAMPTIC TOXEMIA AND THE EFFECT OF HORMONE ADMINISTRATION, *AM J OBSTET GYNECOL*, 39, 405 (1940)

2213 SMITH J, THE PLASMA PHOSPHATASE IN RICKETS AND SCURVY, *ARCH DIS CHILD*, 7, 149-158 (1932)

2214 SMITH J A, THE PHENOLTETRACHLORPHTHALEIN TEST OF LIVER FUNCTION IN THE TOXEMIAS OF PREGNANCY, *AM J OBSTET GYNECOL*, 8, 298-312 (1924)

2215 SMITH S J ET AL, LOWERING OF SERUM 4,4',5-TRIIODOTHYRONINE THY-ROXINE RATIO IN PATIENTS WITH MYOCARDIAL INFARCTION; RELA-TIONSHIP WITH EXTENT OF TISSUE INJURY, *EUR J CLIN INVEST*, 8, 99-102 (1978)

2216 SMITH TF, MYCOPLASMA PNEUMONIAE INFECTIONS: DIAGNOSIS BASED ON IMMUNOFLUORESCENCE TITER OF IGG AND IGM ANTIBODIES, *MAYO CLIN PROC*, 61, 830-831 (1986)

2217 SNAPE W J ET AL, MARKED ALKALINE PHOSPHATASE ELEVATION WITH PARTIAL COMMON BILE DUCT OBSTRUCTION DUE TO CALCIFIC PANCREATITIS, *GASTROENTEROLOGY*, 70, 70-73 (1976)

2218 SNAPPER I ET AL, DETERMINATION OF BENCE-JONES PROTEIN IN URINE, *JAMA*, 173, 1137-9 (1959)

2219 SNEHALATHA ET AL, CREATINE PHOSPHOKINASE LEVEL IN NEURO-MUSCULAR DISORDERS EFFECT OF DILUTION AND DIALYSIS, *CLIN CHIM ACTA*, 44, 229-235 (1973)

2220 SNIDER GL, PATHOGENESIS OF EMPHYSEMA AND CHRONIC BRONCHI-TIS, *MED CLIN NORTH AM*, 65, 647-651 (1981)

2221 SNIDERMAN A, ET AL, *PROC NAT ACAD SCI (USA)*, 77, 604 (1980)

2222 SNODGRASS P J ET AL, UREA-CYCLE ENZYME DEFICIENCIES AND AN INCREASED NITROGEN LOAD PRODUCING HYPERAMMONEMIA IN REYE'S SYNDROME, *N ENGL J MED*, 294, 855-60 (1976)

2223 SNYDERMAN R AND MCCARTY G A, CLINICAL USEFULNESS OF HEMO-LYTIC COMPLEMENT DETERMINATION, *IN: CLINICAL ASPECTS OF THE COMPLEMENT SYSTEM OPFERKUCH ET AL (ED)* (1976)

2224 SOBOL RE, O'CONNOR DT, ADDISON J, ET AL, ELEVATED SERUM CHROMOGRANIN A CONCENTRATIONS IN SMALL-CELL LUNG CAR-CINOMA, *ANN INTERN MED*, 105, 698-700 (1986)

2225 SOLOMONS N W ET AL, ZINC NUTRITION IN CELIAC SPRUE, *AM J CLIN NUTR*, 29, 371-5 (1976)

2226 SOMER T, HYPERVISCOSITY SYNDROME IN PLASMA CELL DYSCRA-SIAS, *ADV MICROCIRC*, 6, 1 (1975)

2227 SOMERS K AND FOWLER J N, ENDOMYOCARDIAL FIBROSIS. CLINICAL DIAGNOSIS, *CARDIOLOGIA*, 52, 25 (1968)

2228 SONG H ET AL, USEFULNESS OF SERUM LIPASE, ESTERASE, AND AMY-LASE ESTIMATIONS IN THE DIAGNOSIS OF PANCREATITIS. A COM-PARISON, *CLIN CHEM*, 16, 264 (1970)

2229 SOUROUJON M, ASHKENAZI A, LUPO M, SERUM FERRITIN LEVELS IN CELIAC DISEASE, *AM J CLIN PATHOL*, 77, 82-6 (1982)

2230 SOUTHERN P M AND SANFORD J P, RELAPING FEVER: A CLINICAL AND MICROBIOLOGICAL REVIEW, *MEDICINE*, 48, 129 (1967)

2231 SOX HC, LIANG MIT, THE ERYTHROCYTE SEDIMENTATION RATE, *ANN INTERN MED*, 104, 515-523

2232 SPATI B, CHILD JA, KERRUISH SM, ET AL, BEHAVIOR OF SERUM B_2-MICROGLOBULIN AND ACUTE PHASE REACTANT PROTEINS IN CHRONIC LYMPHOCYTIC LEUKAEMIA: A MULTICENTRE STUDY, *ACTA HAEMATOL (BASEL)*, 64, 79-86 (1980)

2233 SPECTOR D A ET AL, THYROID FUNCTION AND METABOLIC STATE IN CHRONIC RENAL FAILURE, *ANN INTERN MED*, 85, 724-30 (1976)

2234 SPELLACY W N ET AL, PLASMA INSULIN IN NORMAL LATE PREGNANCY, *N ENGL J MED*, 268, 988 (1963)

2235 SPENCER N, HOPKINSON DA, HARRIS H, ADENOSINE DEAMINASE POL-YMORPHISM IN MAN, *ANN HUM GENET*, 32, 9-14 (1968)

2236 SPERANZA V ET AL, PROGRESS IN THE TREATMENT OF ACUTE GAS-TRODUODENAL MUCOSAL LESIONS (AGML), *WORLD J SURG*, 1, 35-44 (1977)

2237 SPILBERG I ET AL, THE ARTHRITIS OF SARCOIDOSIS, *ARTHRITIS RHEUM*, 12, 126 (1969)

2238 SPIRO H M, CLINICAL GASTROENTEROLOGY, *1ST EDITION NEW YORK MACMILLAN* (1970)

2239 SPIVAK J L, FELTY'S SYNDROME: AN ANALYTICAL REVIEW, *JOHNS HOPKINS MED J*, 141, 156-62. (1977)

2240 SRICHAIKUL T ET AL, FERROKINETICS IN PATIENTS WITH MALARIA: HAEMOGLOBIN SYNTHESIS AND NORMOBLASTS IN VITRO, *TRANS R SOC TROP MED HYG*, 70, 244-6 (1976)

2241 SRINIVASAN SR, FREEDMAN DS, BERENSON GS, ARE PLASMA APOLI-POPROTEINS HELPFUL AS MARKERS OF CORONARY ARTERY DIS-EASE?, *INTERNAL MEDICINE FOR THE SPECIALIST*, 8, 195 (1987)

2242 SRIVASTAVA ET AL, BENIGN TUMOURS OF THE BREAST WITH SPECIAL REFERENCE TO CELLULAR ENZYMATIC ACTIVITY, *INDIAN J CAN-CER*, 13, 215-219 (1976)

2243 SRIVASTAVA ET AL, CLINCO-PATHOLOGICAL STUDY OF MALIGNANT BREAST TUMORS WITH SPECIAL REFERENCE TO CELLULAR ENZY-MATIC ACTIVITY, *INDIAN J CANCER*, 13, 220-226 (1976)

2244 STABILE BE, BRAUNSTEIN GD, PASSARO E JR, SERUM GASTRIN AND HUMAN CHORIONIC GONADOTROPIN IN THE ZOLLINGER-ELLISON SYNDROME, *ARCH SURG*, 115, 1090-5 (1980)

2245 STABILE BE, PASSARO E JR, CARLSON HE, ELEVATED SERUM PROLAC-TIN LEVEL IN THE ZOLLINGER-ELLISON SYNDROME, *ARCH SURG*, 116, 449-53 (1981)

2246 STANBURY J B ET AL, THE METABOLIC BASIS OF INHERITED DISEASE, *MCGRAW-HILL NEW YORK 3RD EDITION* (1972)

2247 STANWELL-SMITH R, THOMPSON SG, HAINES AP, ET AL, A COMPARA-TIVE STUDY OF ZINC, COPPER, CADMIUM, AND LEAD LEVELS IN FERTILE AND INFERTILE MEN, *FERTIL STERIL*, 40, 670 (1983)

2248 STARKWEATHER ET AL, ALTERATIONS OF SLDH ISOENZYMES DURING THERAPY DIRECTED AT LUNG CANCER, *J LAB CLIN MED*, 68, 314 (1968)

2249 STARKWEATHER W H ET AL, ALTERATIONS OF ERYTHROCYTE LAC-TATE DEHYDROGENASE IN MAN, *BLOOD*, 26, 63-73 (1965)

2250 STAVA Z, SERUM PROTEINS IN SCLERODERMA, *DERMATOLOGICA*, 117, 147 (1958)

2251 STEFFANINI M (ED), PROGRESS IN CLINICAL PATHOLOGY, *GRUNE & STRATTON NEW YORK*, 3 (1970)

2252 STEIN ET AL, HYPOPHOSPHATEMIA IN ACUTE ALCOHOLISM, *AM J MED SCI*, 252, 112/78-117/83 (1966)

2253 STEIN I D ET AL, LACTATE DEHYDROGENASE IN MEGALOBLASTIC ANE-MIA, *J LAB CLIN MED*, 74, 331-339 (1969)

2254 STEIN J A, ACUTE INTERMITTENT PORPHYRIA, *MEDICINE*, 49, 1 (1970)

2255 STEINBERG, WM, GOLDSTEIN SS, DAVIS ND, ET AL, DIAGNOSTIC ASSAYS IN ACUTE PANCREATITIS, *ANN INTERN MED*, 102, 576-580 (1985)

2256 STEINER S ET AL, RENAL FUNCTION AND PROTEIN ELIMINATION OF HUMAN SUBJECTS DURING CARBON MONOXIDE EXPOSURE, *HELV MED ACTA*, 36, 39 (1972)

2257 STEINITZ H ET AL, ESSENTIELLE FRUCTOSURIE, *SCHWEIZ MED WOCHENSCHR*, 93, 751 (1963)

2258 STEINKAMP R C ET AL, LONG TERM EXPERIENCE WITH THE USE OF P32 IN THE TREATMENT OF CHRONIC LYMPHOCYTIC LEUKEMIA, *J NUCL MED*, 4, 92 (1963)

2259 STEMMERMANN G N, AN HISTOLOGIC AND HISTOCHEMICAL STUDY OF FAMILIAL OSTEOECTASIA, *AM J PATHOL*, 48, 641-648 (1966)

2260 STERKEL R L ET AL, SERUM ISOCITRIC DEHYDROGENASE ACTIVITY WITH PARTICULAR REFERENCE TO LIVER DISEASE, *J LAB CLIN MED*, 52, 176 (195)

2261 STERLING K ET AL, FREE THYROXINE IN HUMAN SERUM: SIMPLIFIED MEASUREMENT WITH THE AID OF MAGNESIUM PRECIPITATION, *J CLIN INVEST*, 45, 153 (1966)

2262 STERNLIEB I, LABORATORY DIAGNOSIS OF HEPATOLENTICULAR DEGENERATION, *LABORATORY DIAGNOSIS OF LIVER DISEASES, WARREN H. GREEN CO., ST. LOUIS, MO*, 189-192 (1968)

2263 STEWART ET AL, A CASE OF BENIGN PROSTATIC HYPERTROPHY WITH RECENT INFARCTS AND ASSOCIATED HIGH SERUM ACID PHOS-PHATASE, *J UROL*, 63, 128-131 (1950)

2264 STOCKLEY RA, AFFORD SC, THE INTERACTION OF CIGARETTE SMOKE SOLUTION WITH ALPHA 1-ANTITRYPSIN: EFFECT ON INHIBITORY CAPACITY, ELECTROPHORETIC MOBILITY AND IMMUNOLOGICAL MEASUREMENT, *CLIN SCI*, 64, 223-30 (1983)

2265 STOCKS A E AND MARTIN F I R, PITUITARY FUNCTION IN HAEMOCHRO-MATOSIS, *AM J MED*, 45, 839 (1968)

2266 STOCKS A E AND POWELL L, PITUITARY FUNCTION IN IDIOPATHIC HEMOCHROMATOSIS AND CIRRHOSIS OF THE LIVER., *LANCET*, 2, 298-300 (1972)

2267 STOLBACH ET AL, ECTOPIC PRODUCTION OF AN ALKALINE PHOSPHA-TASE ISOENZYME IN PATIENTS WITH CANCER, *N ENGL J MED*, 281, 757-762 (1974)

2268 STOLBACH L L ET AL, CORRELATION OF REGAN ISOENZYME AND HCG IN SERUM AND MALIGNANT EFFUSIONS OF PATIENTS WITH OVA-RIAN CANCER, *PROC AM ASSOC CAN RES*, 78 (1974)

2269 STOREY EL, MACK U, POWELL LW, HALLIDAY JW, USE OF CHRO-MATOFOCUSING TO DETECT A TRANSFERRIN VARIANT IN SERUM OF ALCOHOLIC SUBJECTS, *CLIN CHEM*, 31/9, 1543-1545 (1985)

2270 STRAND A, THE FUNCTION OF THE PLACENTA AND PLACENTAL INSUF-FICIENCY WITH ESPECIAL REFERENCE TO THE DEVELOPMENT OF PROLONGED FOETAL DISTRESS, *ACTA OBSTET GYNECOL SCAND*, 45, 125-230 (1966)

2271 STRAND L J ET AL, DECREASED RED CELL UROPORPHYRINOGEN I SYNTHETASE ACTIVITY IN INTERMITTENT ACUTE PORPHYRIA, *J CLIN INVEST*, 51, 2530 (1972)

2272 STRAND V, TALAL N, ADVANCES IN THE DIAGNOSIS AND CONCEPT OF SJÖGREN'S SYNDROME (AUTOIMMUNE EXOCRINOPATHY), *BULL RHEUM DIS*, 30, 1046-1052 (1980)

2273 STRANDJORD ET AL, THE DIAGNOSIS OF ACUTE MYOCARDIAL INFARCTION ON THE BASIS OF HEAT-STABLE SERUM LACTIC DEHYDROGENASE, *J LAB CLIN MED*, 57-58, 962 (1961)

2274 STRANDVIK B, SAMUELSON K, FASTING SERUM BILE ACID LEVELS IN RELATION TO LIVER HISTOPATHOLOGY IN CYSTIC FIBROSIS, *SCAND J GASTROENTEROL*, 20, 381-4 (1985)

2275 STRAUSS A ET AL, EXOCRINE DISORDER IN ASTHMATICS: DEMONSTRATION OF HIGH SWEAT CHLORIDE LEVELS IN CHRONIC PATIENTS AND THEIR RELATIVES, *ALLERGOL IMMUNOPATHOL (MADR)*, 6, 19-24 (1978)

2276 STRAUSS R G ET AL, HEMATOLOGIC EFFECTS OF PHENYTOIN THERAPY DURING PREGNANCY, *CARDIOVASC CLINC*, 9, 682-5 (1978)

2277 STREMPLE AND WATSON, SERUM CALCIUM, SERUM GASTRIN, AND GASTRIC ACID SECRETION BEFORE AND AFTER PARATHYROIDECTOMY FOR HYPERPARATHYROIDISM, *SURGERY*, 75, 841-852 (1974)

2278 STRICKLAND G T AND LEW M, WILSON'S DISEASE - CLINICAL LABORATORY MANIFESTATIONS IN 40 PATIENTS., *MEDICINE*, 54, 113-138 (1975)

2279 STRICKLAND G T ET AL, HYPERSPLENISM IN WILSON'S DISEASE., *GUT*, 13, 220 (1972)

2280 STRICKLAND GT, LEU M, WILSON'S DISEASE CLINICAL AND LABORATORY MANIFESTATIONS IN 40 PATIENTS, *MEDICINE*, 54, 113-137 (1975)

2281 STRICKLAND R E ET AL, A REAPPRAISAL OF THE NATURE AND SIGNIFICANCE OF CHRONIC ATROPHIC GASTRITIS, *AM J DIG DIS*, 18, 426-40 (1973)

2282 STRIFE CF, HUG G, CHUCK G, MCADAMS AJ, ET AL, MEMBRANOPROLIFERATIVE GLOMERULONEPHRITIS AND ALPHA 1-ANTITRYPSIN DEFICIENCY IN CHILDREN, *PEDIATRICS*, 71, 88-92 (1983)

2283 STRIMLAN C V ET AL, LYMPHOCYTIC INTERSTITIAL PNEUMONITIS. REVIEW OF 13 CASES, *ANN INTERN MED*, 88, 616-21 (1978)

2284 STROBER W PETER G AND SCHWARTZ R H, ALBUMIN METABOLISM IN CYSTIC FIBROSIS, *J PEDIAT*, 73, 540 (1968)

2285 STUDD J W W, IMMUNOGLOBULINS IN NORMAL PREGNANCY, PRE-ECLAMPSIA AND PREGNANCY COMPLICATED BY THE NEPHROTIC SYNDROME, *BR J OBSTET GYNAECOL*, 78, 786-790 (1971)

2286 STUDD J W W ET AL, SERUM PROTEIN CHANGES IN THE PRE-ECLAMPSIA-ECLAMPSIA SYNDROME, *BR J OBSTET GYNAECOL*, 77, 796-801 (1970)

2287 STUDD J W W ET AL, A STUDY OF SERUM PROTEIN CHANGES IN LATE PREGNANCY AND IDENTIFICATION OF THE PREGNANCY ZONE PROTEIN USING ANTIGEN ANTIBODY CROSSED IMMUNOELECTROPHORESIS, *BR J OBSTET GYNAECOL*, 77, 42-51 (1970)

2288 STUDDY PR, LAPWORTH R, BIRD R, ANGIOTENSIN-CONVERTING ENZYME AND ITS CLINICAL SIGNIFICANCE--A REVIEW, *J CLIN PATHOL*, 36, 938-47 (1983)

2289 STURGEON P FINCH C A, ERYTHROKINETICS IN COOLEY'S ANEMIA, *BLOOD*, 12, 64 (1959)

2290 STUTZMAN F L ET AL, BLOOD SERUM MAGNESIUM IN PORTAL CIRRHOSIS AND DIABETES MELLITUS, *J LAB CLIN MED*, 26, 215 (1953)

2291 SUFRIN G, HORMONES IN RENAL CANCER, *J UROL*, 117, 433-8 (1977)

2292 SUFRIN G ET AL, ADENOSINE DEAMINASE ACTIVITY IN PATIENTS WITH RENAL ADENOCARCINOMA, *CANCER*, 40, 796-802 (1977)

2293 SUFRIN G ET AL, ADENOSINE DEAMINASE ACTIVITY IN PATIENTS WITH CARCINOMA OF THE BLADDER, *J UROL*, 119, 343 (1978)

2294 SULTAN C, OLIEL V, AUDRAN F, MEYNADIER J, FREE AND TOTAL PLASMA TESTOSTERONE IN MEN AND WOMEN WITH ACNE, *ACTA DERM VENEREOL (STOCKH)*, 66, 301-4 (1986)

2295 SUN FF, MCGUIRE JC, METABOLISM OF ARACHIDONIC ACID BY HUMAN NEUTROPHILS. CHARACTERIAZATION OF THE ENZYMATIC REACTIONS THAT LEAD TO THE SYNTHESIS OF LEUKOTRIENE B4, *BIOCHEM BIOPHYS RES COMMUN*, 794, 56-64 (1984)

2296 SUNDERMAN F W ET AL, CLINICAL APPLICATIONS OF THE FRACTIONATION OF SERUM PROTEINS BY PAPER ELECTROPHORESIS, *AM J CLIN PATHOL*, 27, 125-8 (1957)

2297 SUNDERMAN FW JR, CURRENT STATUS OF ZINC DEFICIENCY IN THE PATHOGENESIS OF NEUROLOGICAL, DERMATOLOGICAL AND MUSCULOSKELETAL DISORDERS, *ANN CLIN LAB SCI*, 5, 132-145 (1975B)

2298 SUSKIND R ET AL, COMPLEMENT ACTIVITY IN CHILDREN WITH PROTEIN-CALORIE MALNUTRITION, *AM J CLIN NUTR*, 29, 1089-92 (1976)

2299 SUZUKI S ET AL, HISTAMINE CONTENTS OF BLOOD PLASMA AND CELLS IN PATIENTS WITH MYELOGENOUS LEUKEMIA, *CANCER*, 28, 384 (1971)

2300 SVARTMAN M ET AL, IMMUNOGLOBULINS AND COMPLEMENT COMPONENTS IN THE SYNOVIAL FLUID OF PATIENTS WITH ACUTE RHEUMATIC FEVER, *J CLIN INVEST*, 56, 111 (1975)

2301 SWAROOP A K ET AL, URIC ACID LEVELS IN NEUROLOGICAL AND PSYCHIATRIC DISORDERS., *NEUROL INDIA*, 24, 100-103 (1976)

2302 SWEDLUND HA, HUNDER GG, GLEICH GJ, ALPHA 1-ANTITRYPSIN IN SERUM AND SYNOVIAL FLUID IN RHEUMATOID ARTHRITIS, *ANN RHEUM DIS*, 33, 162-164 (1974)

2303 SWEENEY J D, PATTERNS OF PORPHYRIN EXCRETION IN SOUTH AFRICAN PORPHYRIC PATIENTS, *SOUTH AFR J LAB CLIN MED*, 9, 182 (1963)

2304 SWEENEY V P ET AL, ACUTE INTERMITTENT PORPHYRIA: INCREASED ALA-SYNTHETASE ACTIVITY DURING AN ACUTE ATTACK, *BRAIN*, 93, 369 (1970)

2305 SWEETIN ET AL, REVISED NORMAL RANGES FOR SIX SERUM ENZYMES: FURTHER STATISTICAL ANALYSIS AND THE EFFECTS OF DIFFERENT TREATMENTS OF BLOOD SPECIMENS, *CLIN CHIM ACTA*, 48, 49-63 (1973)

2306 SYBULSKI S ET AL, UMBILICAL CORD PLASMA ESTRADIOL LEVELS IN RELATION TO COMPLICATION OF PREGNANCY AND NEWBORN AND TO CORTISOL LEVELS, *BIOL NEONATE*, 27, 302-7 (1974)

2307 SYBULSKI S ET AL, RELATIONSHIP BETWEEN CORTISOL LEVELS IN UMBILICAL CORD PLASMA AND DEVELOPMENT OF THE RESPIRATORY DISTRESS SYNDROME IN PREMATURE NEWBORN INFANTS, *AM J OBSTET GYNECOL*, 125, 239-43 (1976)

2308 SYKES S, DENNIS PM, ELECTRORADIOIMMUNOASSAY: A SENSITIVE METHOD FOR THE QUANTITATION OF ALPHA-FETOPROTEIN, *CLIN CHIM ACTA*, 79, 309-316 (1977)

2309 SYMONDS E M ET AL, CHANGES IN THE RENIN-ANGIOTENSIN SYSTEM IN PRIMIGRAVIDAE WITH HYPERTENSIVE DISEASE OF PREGNANCY, *BR J OBSTET GYNAECOL*, 83, 643-650 (1975)

2310 SZASZ G, A KINETIC PHOTOMETRIC METHOD FOR SERUM GAMMA-GLUTAMYL TRANSPEPTIDASE, *CLIN CHEM*, 15, 124-136 (1969)

2311 SZINNYAI M ET AL, TRANSAMINASE-UTERSUCHUNGEN BEI FRUHER UND SPATER SCHWANGERSCHAFTOXIKOSE, *ZENTRALBL GYNAKOL*, 84, 1675-1678 (1962)

2312 TABERNER DA, ACQUIRED ALPHA 2-ANTIPLASMIN DEFICIENCY IN PATIENTS WITH GLOMERULARPROTEINURIA, *THROMB HAEMOST*, 46, 389 (1981)

2313 TACHIKI ET AL, A RAPID COLUMN CHROMATOGRAPHIC PROCEDURE FOR THE ROUTINE MEASUREMENT OF TAURINE IN PLASMA OF NORMALS AND DEPRESSED PATIENTS, *CLIN CHIM ACTA*, 75, 455-65 (1977)

2314 TADDERNI L AND WATSON C J, THE CLINICAL PORPHYRIAS, *SEMIN HEMATOL*, 5, 335 (1968)

2315 TAGGART P ET AL, SUPPRESSION BY OXPRENOLOL OF ADRENERGIC RESPONSE TO STRESS, *LANCET*, 2, 256 (1972)

2316 TAKACS O ET AL, DISTRIBUTION OF SERUM AMYLASE ISOENZYMES IN CYSTIC FIBROSIS HOMOZYGOTES AND HETEROZYGOTES, *ACTA PAEDIATR HUNG*, 18, 21-6 (1977)

2317 TAKACSE-NAGAY L ET AL, DEFINITION OF CLINICAL FEATURES AND DIAGNOSIS OF MYELOFIBROSIS, *CLIN LAB HAEMATOL*, 4, 291-308 (1977)

2318 TAKAHASHI H, HATTORI A, SHIBATA A, PROFILE OF BLOOD COAGULATION AND FIBRINOLYSIS IN CHRONIC MYELOPROLIFERATIVE DISORDERS, *TOHOKU J EXP MED*, 138, 71-80 (1982)

2319 TAKAHASHI K ET AL, PATHOLOGICAL, HISTOCHEMICAL AND ULTRASTRUCTURAL STUDIES ON SEA-BLUE HISTIOCYTES AND GAUCHER-LIKE CELLS IN ACQUIRED LIPIDOSIS OCCURRING IN LEUKEMIA, *ACTA PATHOL JPN*, 27, 775-97 (1977)

2320 TAKALA I ET AL, THE ACTIVITIES OF PLASMA MEMBRANE MARKER ENZYMES IN RHEUMATOID SYNOVIAL TISSUES AND FLUIDS, *SCAND J RHEUMATOL*, 6, 33-36 (1977)

2321 TAKASE S AND YOSHIDA M, QUANTITATIVE DETERMINATION OF IMMUNOGLOBULINS IN CEREBROSPINAL FLUID, *TOHOKU J EXP MED*, 98, 189 (1969)

2322 TAKEDA Y AND CHEN A Y, FIBRINOGEN METABOLISM AND DISTRIBUTION IN PATIENTS WITH THE NEPHROTIC SYNDROME, *J LAB CLIN MED*, 70, 678 (1967)

2323 TAKIKAWA H, BEPPU T, SEYAMA Y, URINARY CONCENTRATIONS OF BILE ACID GLUCURONIDES AND SULFATES IN HEPATOBILIARY DISEASES, *GASTROENTEROL JPN*, 19, 104-9 (1984)

2324 TAKIKAWA H, BEPPU T, SEYAMA Y, OBINATA K, ET AL, SERUM CONCENTRATIONS OF GLUCURONIDATED AND SULFATED BILE ACIDS IN CHILDREN WITH CHOLESTASIS, *BIOCHEM MED METAB BIOL*, 33, 381-6 (1985)

2325 TAKIKAWA H, OTSUKA H, BEPPU T, SEYAMA Y, DETERMINATION OF 3 BETA-HYDROXY-5-CHOLENOIC ACID IN SERUM OF HEPATOBILIARY DISEASES--ITS GLUCURONIDATED AND SULFATED CONJUGATES, *BIOCHEM MED METAB BIOL*, 33, 393-400 (1985)

2326 TALAL N, GREY HM, ZVAIFLER N, ET AL, ELEVATED SALIVARY AND SYNOVIAL FLUID BETA 2-MICROGLOBULIN IN SJÖGREN'S SYNDROME AND RHEUMATOID ARTHRITIS, *SCIENCE*, 187, 1196-1198 (1975)

2327 TALWAR K K ET AL, SERUM LEVELS OF THYROTROPIN, THYROID HORMONES AND THEIR RESPONSE TO THYROTROPIN RELEASING HORMONE IN INFECTIVE FEBRILE ILLNESSES, *J CLIN ENDOCRINOL METAB*, 44, 398-403 (1977)

2328 TANAKA K, TAKESHITA K, SUGANUMA I, KASAGI S, LOW SERUM CHOLIC ACID CONCENTRATION OF DUCHENNE MUSCULAR DYSTROPHY, *BRAIN DEV*, 5, 511-3 (1983)

2329 TARANTINO A ET AL, SERUM COMPLEMENT PATTERN IN ESSENTIAL MIXED CRYOGLOBULINEMIA, *CLIN EXP IMMUNOL*, 32, 77-85 (1978)

2330 TASSI G, NAVA AM, BETTONCELLI G, DOTTI A, ET AL, DETERMINATION OF SERUM ANGIOTENSIN-CONVERTING ENZYME IN SARCOIDOSIS, *RIC CLIN LAB*, 14, 621-7 (1984)

2331 TATSUMURA T ET AL, CLINICAL SIGNIFICANCE OF FUCOSE LEVELS IN GLYCOPROTEIN FRACTION OF SERUM IN PATIENTS WITH MALIGNANT TUMORS, *CANCER RES*, 37, 4101-3 (1977)

2332 TAYLOR H C JR ET AL, HORMONE FACTORS IN THE TOXEMIAS OF PREGNANCY, WITH SPECIAL REFERENCE TO QUANTITATIVE ABNORMALITIES OF PROLAN AND ESTROGENS IN THE BLOOD AND URINE, *AM J OBSTET GYNECOL*, 37, 980 (1939)

2333 TAYLOR W, URINARY EXCRETION OF METABOLITES OF STEROID HORMONES BY MEN WITH CANCER OF THE STOMACH, *J STEROID BIOCHEM*, 7, 929-34 (1976)

2334 TE VELDE J ET AL, THE EOSINOPHILIC FIBROHISTIOCYTIC LESION OF THE BONE MARROW. A MASTOCELLULAR LESION IN BONE DISEASE, *VIRCHOWS ARCH PATHOL ANAT*, 377, 277-85 (1978)

2335 TECULESCU D ET AL, VENTILATORY IMPAIRMENT AND HYPOXEMIA IN CHRONIC NON-SPECIFIC LUNG DISEASE, *BULL EUR PHYSIOPATHOL RESPIR*, 12, 735-45 (1976)

2336 TEDESCO F J ET AL, SERUM AMYLASE DETERMINATIONS AND AMYLASE TO CREATININE CLEARANCE RATIOS IN PATIENTS WITH CHRONIC RENAL INSUFFICIENCY, *GASTROENTEROLOGY*, 71, 594-8 (1976)

2337 TEGER-NILSSON AC, FRIBERGER P, GYZANDER E, DETERMINATION OF FAST-ACTING PLASMIN INHIBITOR (ALPHA 2 - ANTIPLASMIN) IN PLASMA FROM PATIENTS WITH TENDENCY TO THROMBOSIS AND INCREASED FIBRINOLYSIS, *HAEMOSTASIS*, 7, 155-157 (1978)

2338 TELLIS CJ, PUTNAM JS, PULMONARY DISEASE CAUSED BY NON-TUBERCULOSIS MYCOBACTERIA, *MED CLIN NORTH AM*, 64, 433-446 (1980)

2339 TELOH H A, SERUM PROTEINS IN HEPATIC DISEASE, *ANN CLIN LAB SCI*, 8, 127-128 (1978)

2340 TEMPLETON A A ET AL, ARTERIAL BLOOD GASES IN PRE-ECLAMPSIA, *BR J OBSTET GYNAECOL*, 84, 290-3. (1977)

2341 TEREE R M AND KLEIN L, HYPOPHOSPHATASIA: CLINICAL AND METABOLIC STUDIES, *PEDIATRICS*, 72, 41 (1968)

2342 TERRITO AND TANAKA, HYPOPHOSPHATEMIA IN CHRONIC ALCOHOLISM, *ARCH INTERN MED*, 134, 445-447 (1974)

2343 TERRY P B ET AL, FALSE-POSITIVE COMPLEMENT-FIXATION SEROLOGY IN HISTOPLASMOSIS. A RETROSPECTIVE STUDY, *JAMA*, 239, 2453-6 (1978)

2344 THALER MS, KLAUSNER RD, COHEN HJ, MEDICAL IMMUNOLOGY, *PHILADELPHIA, J.B. LIPPINCOTT CO*, (1977)

2345 THAYER W R ET AL, THE SUBPOPULATIONS OF CIRCULATING WHITE BLOOD CELLS IN INFLAMMATORY BOWEL DISEASE, *GASTROENTEROLOGY*, 71, 379-84 (1976)

2346 THESTRUP-PEDERSEN K, ROMER FK, JENSEN JH, ET AL, SERUM ANGIOTENSIN-CONVERTING ENZYME IN SARCOIDOSIS AND PSORIASIS, *ARCH DERMATOL RES*, 277, 16-18 (1985)

2347 THOMAS E D ET AL, HOMOZYGOUS HEMOGLOBIN C DISEASE, *AM J MED*, 18, 832 (1955)

2348 THOMMESEN P ET AL, HISTIOCYTOSIS X. I. ERYTHROCYTE SEDIMENTATION RATE CORRELATED TO PROGNOSIS AND EXTENT OF DISEASE, *ACTA RADIOLOGICA (STOCKHOLM)*, 16, 538-44 (1977)

2349 THOMPSON ET AL, HEREDITARY HYPERPHOSPHATASIA, *AM J MED*, 47, 209-219 (1969)

2350 THOMPSON R H S AND JOHNSON R E, BLOOD PYRUVATE IN VITAMIN B$_1$ DEFICIENCY, *BIOCHEM J*, 29, 694 (1935)

2351 THOMSON A B R ET AL, IRON DEFICIENCY IN INFLAMMATORY BOWEL DISEASE, *AM J DIG DIS*, 23, 705-9 (1978)

2352 THOMSON C ET AL, CHANGES IN BLOOD COAGULATION AND FIBRINOLYSIS IN THE NEPHROTIC SYNDROME, *Q J MED*, 43, 399 (1974)

2353 THOMSON JM, *BLOOD COAGULATION AND HAEMOSTASIS, 2ND ED. NEW YORK, CHURCHILL LIVINGSTONE* (1980)

2354 THORLING E B THORLING K, THE CLINICAL USEFULNESS OF SERUM COPPER DETERMINATIONS IN HODGKIN'S DISEASE. A RETROSPECTIVE STUDY OF 241 PATIENTS FROM 1963-1973, *CANCER*, 38, 225-31 (1976)

2355 THORNTON C A ET AL, FACTOR VIII-RELATED ANTIGEN AND FACTOR VIII COAGULANT ACTIVITY IN NORMAL AND PRE-ECLAMPTIC PREGNANCY, *BR J OBSTET GYNAECOL*, 84, 919-23 (1977)

2356 TIETZ NW, *CLINICAL GUIDE TO LABORATORY TESTS. W.B. SAUNDERS CO., PHILADELPHIA* (1983)

2357 TIETZ NW (ED), *FUNDAMENTALS OF CLINICAL CHEMISTRY, 2ND ED. W.B. SAUNDERS CO. PHILADELPHIA* (1976)

2358 TILKIAN, CONOVER, TILKIAN, *CLINICAL IMPLICATIONS OF LABORATORY TESTS 3RD ED, THE CV MOSBY CO. ST. LOUIS* (1983)

2359 TINDALL V R ET AL, AN ASSESSMENT OF CHANGES IN LIVER FUNCTION DURING NORMAL PREGNANCY USING A MODIFIED BROMSULPHTHALEIN TEST, *BR J OBSTET GYNAECOL*, 72, 717 (1965)

2360 TISCHENDORF F W ET AL, HEAVY LYSOZYMURIA AFTER X-IRRADIATION OF THE SPLEEN IN HUMAN CHRONIC MYELOCYTIC LEUKEMIA, *NATURE*, 235, 274 (1972)

2361 TISDALE W A ET AL, THE SIGNIFICANCE OF THE DIRECT-REACTING FRACTION OF SERUM BILIRUBIN IN HEMOLYTIC JAUNDICE, *AM J MED*, 26, 214 (1959)

2362 TISHKOV I ET AL, DIAGNOSTIC VALUE OF CERULOPLASMIN, HAPTOGLOBIN AND SIALIC ACID IN CHRONIC PYELONEPHRITIS, *INT UROL NEPHROL*, 8, 155-9 (1976)

2363 TOBIASSON P, BOERYD B, SERUM CHOLIC AND CHENODEOXYCHOLIC ACID CONJUGATES AND STANDARD LIVER FUNCTION TESTS IN VARIOUS MORPHOLOGICAL STAGES OF ALCOHOLIC LIVER DISEASE, *SCAND J GASTROENTEROL*, 15, 657-63 (1980)

2364 TODD D, OBSERVATIONS ON THE AMINOACIDURIA IN MEGALOBLASTIC ANEMIA, *J CLIN PATHOL*, 12, 238 (1959)

2365 TOMAR R H AND D KOLCHINS, COMPLEMENT COAGULATION: SERUM B$_1$C-B$_1$A IN DISSEMINATED INTRAVASCULAR COAGULATION, *THROMB DIATH HAEMORRH*, 27, 389 (1972)

2366 TOMOKUNI K ET AL, ERYTHROCYTE PROTOPORPHYRIN TEST FOR OCCUPATIONAL LEAD EXPOSURE, *ARCH ENVIRON HEALTH*, 30, 588-90 (1975)

2367 TONZ O, THE CONGENITAL METHAEMOGLOBINAEMIAS, *S. KARGER, BASEL* (1968)

2368 TOP F H AND WEHRELE P F (EDS), COMMUNICABLE AND INFECTIOUS DISEASES, *7TH EDITION C V MOSBY CO ST LOUIS* (1972)

2369 TOTH J ET AL, EOSINOPHIL PREDOMINANCE IN HODGKIN'S DISEASE, *Z KREBSFORSCH*, 89, 107-11 (1977)

2370 TOUNTAS Y, SPAROS L, THEODROPOULOS C, ET AL, ALPHA 1-ANTITRYPSIN AND CANCER OF THE PANCREAS, *DIGESTION*, 31, 37-40 (1985)

2371 TOUR TELLOTTE W E AND HAERER A F, LIPIDS IN CEREBROSPINAL FLUID, *ARCH NEUROL*, 20, 605 (1969)

2372 TOWNES A S, COMPLEMENT LEVELS IN DISEASE, *JOHNS HOPKINS MED J*, 120, 337 (1967)

2373 TRIMARCHI F, BENVENGA S, FENZI G, ET AL, IMMUNOGLOBULIN BINDING OF THYROID HORMONES IN A CASE OF WALDENSTRÖM'S MACROGLOBULINEMIA, *J CLIN ENDOCRINOL METAB*, 54, 1045-50 (1982)

2374 TRONGONE L ET AL, CEA ASSAY IN THE FOLLOW-UP OF PATIENTS WITH EXTRA-GASTROINTESTINAL MALIGNANCIES, *BULLETIN DU CANCER*, 63, 495-504 (1976)

2375 TROUILLAS P ET AL, MULTIPLE SCLEROSIS WITH REDUCED AND WITH NORMAL LEVELS OF COMPLEMENT IN THE BLOOD. CLINICAL AND GENETIC CORRELATION, *REV NEUROL (PARIS)*, 132, 684-704 (1976)

2376 TSCHANZ ET AL, PLASMA ALKALINE PHOSPHATASE, *CLIN BIOCHEM*, 7, 68-80 (1974)

2377 TSO S C AND HUA A, ERYTHROCYTES IN HEPATOCELLULAR CARCINOMA: A COMPENSATORY PHENOMENON, *BR J HAEMATOL*, 28, 497 (1974)

2378 TSUCHIDA Y ET AL, ALPHA-FETOPROTEIN, PREALBUMIN, ALBUMIN, ALPHA 1 ANTITRYPSIN AND TRANSFERRIN AS DIAGNOSTIC AND THERAPEUTIC MARKERS FOR ENDODERMAL SINUS TUMORS, *J PEDIATR SURG*, 13, 25-9 (1978)

2379 TSVETKOVA V, DAILY FLUCTUATIONS IN THE PLASMA CORTISOL LEVEL OF CHILDREN WITH RHEUMATOID ARTHRITIS BEFORE AND AFTER TREATMENT WITH TETRACOSACTRIN CORTROSYN DEPOT' AND CORTICOSTEROID HORMONES, *CURR MED RES OPIN*, 4, 477-84 (1977)

2380 TUCHMAN ET AL, ELEVATION OF SERUM ACID PHOSPHATASE IN GAUCHER'S DISEASE, *J MT SINAI HOSP*, 23, 227-229 (1956)

2381 TUCHMAN ET AL, HIGH ACID PHOSPHATASE LEVEL INDICATING GAUCHER'S DISEASE IN PATIENT WITH PROSTATISM, *JAMA*, 164, 2034-2035 (1957)

2382 TUCHMAN ET AL, STUDIES OF THE NATURE OF THE INCREASED SERUM ACID PHOSPHATASE IN GAUCHER'S DISEASE, *AM J MED*, 27, 959-962 (1959)

2383 TUCKER ES III, NAKAMURA RM, DITO WR, NICHOLS WS, TEST COMPENDIUM, *SCRIPPS-MILES IMMUNOLOGY REFERECE LABORATORY, SAN DIEGO, CALIF* (1981)

2384 TUDHOPE G R & WILSON G M, ANEMIA IN HYPOTHYROIDISM INCIDENCE, PATHOGENESIS AND RESPONSE TO TREATMENT, *Q J MED*, 29, 513 (1960)

2385 TULCHINSKY D, RYAN KJ, MATERNAL-FETAL ENDOCRINOLOGY, *PHILADELPHIA, W.B. SAUNDERS* (1980)

2386 TURANEN E M ET AL, CARCINOEMBRYONIC ANTIGEN IN GYNECOLOGIC TUMORS, *CANCER*, 42, 581-90 (1978)

2387 TURK J L AND BRYCESON A D M, IMMUNOLOGICAL PHENOMENA IN LEPROSY AND RELATED DISEASES, *ADV IMMUNOL*, 13, 209 (1971)

2388 TURKINGTON R W ET AL, INSULIN SECRETION IN THE DIAGNOSIS OF ADULT-ONSET DIABETES MELLITUS, *JAMA*, 240, 833-6 (1978)

2389 TURNBULL A ET AL, IRON METABOLISM IN PORPHYRIA CUTANEA TARDA AND IN ERYTHROPOIETIC PROTOPORPHYRIA, *Q J MED*, 42, 341 (1973)

2390 TURNER A ET AL, HAIRY CELL LEUKEMIA: A REVIEW, *MEDICINE*, 57, 477-500 (1978)

2391 TURNER MW, HULME B, THE PLASMA PROTEINS: AN INTRODUCTION, *LONDON, PITTMAN MEDICAL & SCIENTIFIC PUBLISHING CO. LTD* (1971)

2392 TUTUARIMA JA, HISCHE EAH, VAN TROTSENBURG L, ET AL, THROMBOPLASTIC ACTIVITY OF CEREBROSPINAL FLUID IN NEUROLOGICAL DISEASE, *CLIN CHEM*, 31/1, 99-100 (1985)

2393 TWOMEY J J ET AL, STUDIES ON THE INHERITANCE AND NATURE OF HEMOPHILIA B, *AM J MED*, 46, 372 (1969)

2394 TWOMEY J J ET AL, RHEUMATOID FACTOR AND TUMOR-HOST INTERACTION, *PROC NAT ACAD SCI (USA)*, 73, 2106-8 (1976)

2395 TYSON ET AL, GAUCHER'S DISEASE (WITH ELEVATED SERUM ACID PHOSPHATASE LEVEL) MASQUERADING AS CIRRHOSIS OF THE LIVER, *AM J MED*, 37, 156-158 (1964)

2396 UCHIYAMA T, HATTORI T, WANO Y, TSUDO M, ET AL, CELL SURFACE PHENOTYPE AND IN VITRO FUNCTION OF ADULT T-CELL LEUKEMIA CELLS, *DIAGN CLIN IMMUNOL*, 1, 150-4 (1983)

2397 UDALL JN, DIXON M, NEWMAN AP, WRIGHT JA, ET AL, LIVER DISEASE IN A1-ANTITRYPSIN DEFICIENCY, *JAMA*, 253, 2679 (1985)

2398 ULTMANN J E, CLINICAL FEATURES AND DIAGNOSIS OF HODGKIN'S DISEASE, *CANCER*, 9, 297 (1966)

2399 ULTMANN J E ET AL, THE CLINICAL IMPLICATIONS OF HYPOGAMMAGLOBULINEMIA IN PATIENTS WITH CHRONIC LYMPHOCYTIC LEUKEMIA AND LYMPHOCYTIC LYMPHOSARCOMA, *ANN INTERN MED*, 51, 501 (1959)

2400 UNDERMAN H E ET AL, BACTERIAL MENINGITIS, *DM*, 24, 19-27 (1978)

2401 UNDERWOOD J C ET AL, PERSISTENT DIARRHEA AND HYPOALBUMINEMIA ASSOCIATED WITH CYTOMEGALOVIRUS ENTERITIS, *BR MED J*, 1, 1029-30 (1976)

2402 URA N, SHIMAMOTO K, TANAKA S, ET AL, URINARY EXCRETIONS OF KININASE I AND KININASE II ACTIVITIES IN ESSENTIAL HYPERTENSION. A SENSITIVE AND SIMPLE METHOD FOR ITS KININ-DESTROYING CAPACITY, *J CLIN HYPERTENS*, 1, 15-22 (1985)

2403 URBANIAK W J ET AL, CIRCULATING LYMPHOCYTE SUBPOPULATIONS IN HASHIMOTO'S THYROIDITIS, *CLIN EXP IMMUNOL*, 15, 345 (1973)

2404 URELES A L, DIAGNOSIS AND TREATMENT OF MALIGNANT CARCINOID SYNDROME, *JAMA*, 229, 10 (1974)

2405 USHER D J ET AL, SERUM LACTATE DEHYDROGENASE ISOENZYME ACTIVITIES IN PATIENTS WITH ASTHMA, *THORAX*, 29, 685-689 (1974)

2406 VACCA J B ET AL, PANCREATIC EXOCRINE FUNCTION IN DIABETES MELLITUS AND CIRRHOSIS OF THE LIVER, *J LAB CLIN MED*, 52, 176 (1958)

2407 VAKIL B J ET AL, SERUM CREATINE PHOSPHOKINASE IN TETANUS, *J ASSOC PHYSICIANS INDIA*, 24, 417-421 (1976)

2408 VALENTINE WN, PAGLIA EE, TARTAGLIA AP, GILSANZ F, HEREDITARY HEMOLYTIC ANEMIA WITH INCREASED RED CELL ADENOSINE TRIPHOSPHATE, *SCIENCE*, 195, 783-785 (1977)

2409 VALLEE B L ET AL, MAGNESIUM DEFICIENCY TETANY SYNDROME IN MAN, *N ENGL J MED*, 262, 155 (1960)

2410 VAN DEMMELEN C K V AND KLASSEN C H L, CYANOCOBALAMIN-DEPENDENT DEPRESSION ON THE SERUM ALKALINE PHOSPHATASE LEVEL IN PATIENTS WITH PERNICIOUS ANEMIA, *N ENGL J MED*, 271, 541 (1964)

2411 VAN DEN BERGH M ET AL, ELEVATION IN ERYTHROCYTE-L-GLUTAMATE IN CHRONIC HYPOXIA AND HYPERCAPNIA, *BRIT J CANCER*, 12, 177-78 (1976)

2412 VAN DIEIJEN-VISSER MP, SALEMANS T, ET AL, GLYCOSYLATED SERUM LPROTEINS AND GLYCOSYLATED HAEMOGLOBIN IN NORMAL PREGNANCY, *ANN CLIN BIOCHEM*, 23, 661-6 (1986)

2413 VAN NAGELL J R ET AL, CARCINOEMBRYONIC ANTIGEN IN CARCINOMA OF THE UTERINE CERVIX, *CANCER*, 42, 2428-2434 (1978)

2414 VAN PEENEN ET AL, THE EFFECT OF MEDICATION ON LABORATORY TEST RESULTS, *AM J CLIN PATHOL*, 52, 666 (1969)

2415 VANDERSCHUEREN-LODEWEYCKX M ET AL, DECREASED SERUM THYROID HORMONE LEVELS AND INCREASED TSH RESPONSE TO TRH IN INFANTS WITH CELIAC DISEASE, *CLIN ENDOCRINOL (OXF)*, 6, 361-67 (1977)

2416 VARALAKSHMI G ET AL, BLOOD LIPIDS IN RENAL STONE DISORDER, *INDIAN J MED RES*, 66, 840-46 (1977)

2417 VARDI J, KISCH E, BORNSTEIN N, ET AL, CSF RENIN ACTIVITY IN HYPERTENSIVE AND NORMOTENSIVE PATIENTS, *SCHWEIZ ARCH NEUROL NEUROCHIR PSYCHIATR*, 129, 347-52 (1981)

2418 VASSELLA F ET AL, THE DIAGNOSTIC VALUE OF SERUM CREATINE KINASE IN NEUROMUSCULAR AND MUSCULAR DISEASE, *PEDIATRICS*, 35, 322-330 (1965)

2419 VAZIRI ET AL, NEPHROTIC SYNDROME, *ARCH INTERN MED*, 144, 1803 (1984)

2420 VAZIRI ND, PAULE P, TOOHEY J, HUNG E, ET AL, ACQUIRED DEFICIENCY AND URINARY EXCRETION OF ANTITHROMBIN III IN NEPHROTIC SYNDROME, *ARCH INTERN MED*, 144, 1802-3 (1984)

2421 VEDRA B, DAS RENIN-ANGIOTENSIN-ALDOSTERON-SYSTEM IN DER PATHOGENESE DER GESTOSEODEMS, *DIE SPATGESTOSE RIPPMANN E T (ED) BASED SCHWABE*, 152-156 (1970)

2422 VEENEMA R J ET AL, BONE MARROW ACID PHOSPHATASE: PROGNOSTIC VALUE IN PATIENTS UNDERGOING RADICAL PROSTATECTOMY, *J UROL*, 117, 81-82 (1977)

2423 VEJJAJIVA, SERUM CREATINE KINASE AND PHYSICAL EXERCISE, *BR MED J*, 1, 1653-1654 (1965)

2424 VELENTZAS C ET AL, ABNORMAL VITAMIN D LEVELS, *ANN INTERN MED*, 86, 198 (1977)

2425 VENDSALU A, STUDIES ON ADRENALINE AND NORADRENALINE IN HUMAN PLASMA, *ACTA PHYSIOL SCAND*, 49(SUPPL 173), 1 (1966)

2426 VENTURA S ET AL, LA PORFIRIA ERITROPOIETICA. NOTA. I. IL COMPORTAMENTO DEL RICAMBIO PORFIRINICO, *HAEMATOLOGICA (PAVIA)*, 44, 993 (1959)

2427 VERHAGEN H ET AL, INCREASE OF SERUM COMPLEMENT LEVELS IN CANCER PATIENTS WITH PROGRESSING TUMORS, *CANCER*, 38, 1608-13 (1976)

2428 VERSIECK J ET AL, INFLUENCE OF MYOCARDIAL INFARCTION ON SERUM MANGANESE, COPPER, AND ZINC CONCENTRATION, *EXPERIENTIA*, 31, 280-1. (1975)

2429 VERSIECK J, BARBIER F, SPEECKE A, HOSTE J, MANGANESE, COPPER, AND ZINC CONCENTRATIONS IN SERUM AND PACKED BLOOD CELLS DURING ACUTE HEPATITIS, CHRONIC HEPATITIS, AND POSTHEPATIC CIRRHOSIS, *CLIN CHEM*, 20, 1141-5 (1974)

2430 VERSIECK J, CORNELIS R, NORMAL LEVELS OF TRACE ELEMENTS IN HUMAN BLOOD, PLASMA OR SERUM, *ANAL CHIM ACTA*, 116, 217-254 (1980)

2431 VIJ SC, ET AL, SERUM MAGNESIUM, COPPER AND IRON LEVELS IN INFANTILE CIRRHOSIS, *INDIAN J PEDIATR*, 12, 411 (1975)

2432 VINCENT ET AL, CARCINOEMBRYONIC ANTIGEN IN PATIENTS WITH CARCINOMA OF THE LUNG, *I THORAC CARD SURG*, 66, 320-7 (1973)

2433 VINKE B AND DONKER A J M, THE NEUTROPENIC (PANCYTOPENIC?) TYPE OF BACILLARY DYSENTERY, *ACTA TROP (BASEL)*, 23, 81 (1966)

2434 VISVIKIS S, DUMON MF, STEINMENTZ J, ET AL, PLASMA APOLIPOPROTEINS IN TANGIER DISEASE, AS STUDIED WITH TWO-DIMENSIONAL ELECTROPHORESIS, *CLIN CHEM*, 33/1, 120-122 (1987)

2435 VITTO J ET AL, FURTHER EVALUATION OF THE SIGNIFICANCE OF URINARY HYDROXYPROLINE DETERMINATIONS IN THE DIAGNOSIS OF THYROID DISORDERS, *CLIN CHIM ACTA*, 22, 583 (1968)

2436 VLADUTIU A O ET AL, DOUBLE SPIKE IN THE ELECTROPHEROGRAM OF A MYELOMA SERUM, FROM BENCE JONES PROTEIN, *CLIN CHEM*, 23, 67-73 (1975)

2437 VOIGHT D ET AL, UBER DIE BLUTKONZENTRATIONEN DER LEUKOZYTEN UND THROMBOCYTEN BER EISENMANGEL, *BLUT (BERLIN)*, 14, 267 (1967)

2438 VOLLER A ET AL, SEROLOGICAL INDICES IN TANZANIA: II. ANTINUCLEAR FACTOR AND MALARIAL INDICES IN POPULATIONS LIVING AT DIFFERENT ALTITUDES, *J TROP MED HYG*, 75, 136 (1972)

2439 VOLPE R ET AL, THE PATHOGENESIS OF GRAVE'S DISEASE AND HASHIMOTO'S THYROIDITIS, *CLIN ENDOCRINOL (OXF)*, 3, 239 (1974)

2440 VON STUDNITZ W ET AL, URINARY EXCRETION OF PHENOLIC ACIDS IN HUMAN SUBJECTS ON A GLUCOSE DIET, *CLIN CHIM ACTA*, 9, 224 (1958)

2441 VORHAUS ET AL, SERUM CHOLINESTERASE IN HEALTH AND DISEASE, *AM J MED*, 15, 707-711 (1953)

2442 VYAS GN, STITES DP, BRECHER G, *LABORATORY DIAGNOSIS OF IMMUNOLOGIC DISORDERS, NEW YORK, GRUNE & STRATTON* (1975)

2443 WACKER ET AL, METALLOENZYMES AND MYOCARDIAL INFARCTION, *N ENGL J MED*, 255, 449 (1956)

2444 WACKER W E C ET AL, MAGNESIUM METABOLISM, *N ENGL J MED*, 278, 712 (1968)

2445 WACKER W ET AL, A TRIAD FOR THE DIAGNOSIS OF PULMONARY EMBOLISM AND INFARCTION, *JAMA*, 178, 108-113 (1961)

2446 WADA M ET AL, SERUM LIPID AND LIPOPROTEIN ABNORMALITIES IN MAJOR CLINICAL ENTITIES OF RENAL DISEASE, *CONTRIB NEPHROL*, 9, 61-8. (1978)

2447 WADE L J ET AL, THE CEPHALIN-CHOLESTEROL FLOCCULATION TEST, 30, 6-13 (1945)

2448 WADMAN S K ET AL, THREE NEW CASES OF HISTIDINEMIA: CLINICAL AND BIOCHEMICAL DATA, *ACTA PAEDIATR SCAND*, 56, 485 (1967)

2449 WADSTEIN J ET AL, DOES HYPOKALAEMIA PRECEDE DELIRIUM TREMENS, *LANCET*, 2, 549-50 (1978)

2450 WAGENER D ET AL, TOTAL SERUM HAEMOLYTIC COMPLEMENT ACTIVITY, ESR AND PLASMA FIBRINOGEN AS INDICATORS OF THE STAGE IN HODGKIN'S DISEASE, *EUR J CLIN INVEST*, 7, 289-294 (1977)

2451 WAGER O, IMMUNOLOGICAL ASPECTS OF LEPROSY WITH SPECIAL REFERENCE TO AUTOIMMUNE DISEASE, *BULL WHO*, 41, 793 (1969)

2452 WAHLIN A, ROOS G, HOLM J, T-CELL SUBSETS IN MULTIPLE MYELOMA. IMPACT OF CYTOSTATIC TREATMENT, *BLUT (BERLIN)*, 51, 291-5 (1985)

2453 WAISMAN H A ET AL, AMINO ACID METABOLISM IN PATIENTS WITH ACUTE LEUKEMIA, *PEDIATRICS*, 10, 653 (1952)

2454 WAJIMA T ET AL, LOW LEUKOCYTE ALKALINE PHOSPHATASE ACTIVITY IN SICKLE CELL ANEMIA, *J LAB CLIN MED*, 72, 980 (1968)

2455 WAJSMAN W R ET AL, EVALUATION OF BIOLOGICAL MARKERS IN BLADDER CANCER, *J UROL*, 114, 879-93 (1975)

2456 WAKABAYASHI A ET AL, SERUM AMYLASE ISOZYMES IN PATIENTS WITH CHRONIC PANCREATITIS WITH HYPERAMYLASEMIA, *GASTROENTEROL JPN*, 12, 269-74 (1977)

2457 WALDENSTROM J, STUDIEN UEBER PORPHYRIE, *ACTA MED SCAND*, 82(SUPPL) (1937)

2458 WALDENSTROM J G AND HAEGER-ARONSEN B, THE LIVER IN PORPHYRIA AND CUTANEA TARDA, *ANN INTERN MED*, 53, 286 (1960)

2459 WALDMAN T A AND MCINTYRE K R, SERUM AFP LEVELS IN PATIENTS WITH ATAXIA-TELANGIECTASIA, *LANCET*, 2, 1112 (1972)

2460 WALDMAN T A ET AL, THE PROTEINURIA OF CYSTINOSIS: ITS PATTERN AND PATHOGENESIS, *CYSTINOSIS J D SCHULMAN (ED)*, 72-249 (1973)

2461 WALDMANN T A AND BRADLEY J E, POLYCYTHEMIA SECONDARY TO A PHEOCHROMOCYTOMA WITH PRODUCTION OF AN ERYTHROPOIESIS STIMULATING FACTOR TUMOR, *PROC SOC EXP BIOL MED*, 108, 425 (1962)

2462 WALDMANN T ET AL, ALBUMIN METABOLISM IN PATIENTS WITH LYMPHOMA, *J CLIN INVEST*, 42, 171 (1963)

2463 WALDMANN TA, MCINTIRE KR, SERUM ALPHA-FETOPROTEIN LEVELS IN PATIENTS WITH ATAXIA-TELANGIECTASIA, *LANCET*, 2, 1112-1115 (1972)

2464 WALDVAGEL F A ET AL, OSTEMYELITIS: A REVIEW OF CLINICAL FEATURES, THERAPEUTIC CONSIDERATIONS AND UNUSUAL ASPECTS. I, *N ENGL J MED*, 282, 198 (1970)

2465 WALKOFF A ET AL, ROTORS SYNDROME: A DISTINCT INHERITABLE PATHOPHYSIOLOGIC ENTITY, *AM J MED*, 60, 173 (1976)

2466 WALL A J AND KIRSNER J B, ULCERATIVE COLITIS AND CROHN'S DISEASE OF THE COLON: SYMPTOMS, SIGNS, AND LABORATORY ASPECTS, *INFLAMMATORY BOWEL DISEASE LEA & FEBIGER*, 101 (1975)

2467 WALLACH J, INTERPRETATION OF DIAGNOSTIC TESTS, *2ND EDITION LITTLE, BROWN AND CO. BOSTON* (1974)

2468 WALLACH JACQUES, INTERPRETATION OF DIAGNOSTIC TESTS, *3RD EDITION LITTLE BROWN AND CO. BOSTON* (1978)

2469 WALLACH S ET AL, PLASMA AND ERYTHROCYTE MAGNESIUM IN HEALTH AND DISEASE, *J LAB CLIN MED*, 59, 195-209 (1962)

2470 WALLAERT B, RAMON P, FOURNIER, E, TONNEL AB, ET AL, BRONCHOALVEOLAR LAVAGE, SERUM ANGIOTENSIN-CONVERTING ENZYME, AND GALLIUM-67 SCANNING IN EXTRATHORACIC SARCOIDOSIS, *CHEST*, 82, 553-5 (1982)

2471 WALLENTIN L ET AL, STUDIES ON PLASMA LIPID AND PHOSPHOLIPID COMPOSITION IN PERNICIOUS ANEMIA BEFORE AND AFTER SPECIFIC TREATMENT, *ACTA MED SCAND*, 201, 161-5 (1977)

2472 WALLERSTEDT S ET AL, SERUM LIPIDS AND LIPOPROTEINS DURING ABSTINENCE AFTER HEAVY ALCOHOL CONSUMPTION IN CHRONIC ALCOHOLICS, *SCAND J CLIN LAB INVEST*, 37, 599-604 (1977)

2473 WALSH C H ET AL, A STUDY OF PITUITARY FUNCTION IN PATIENTS WITH IDIOPATHIC HEMOCHROMATOSIS, *J CLIN ENDOCRINOL METAB*, 43, 866-72 (1976)

2474 WALSH ET AL, SERUM TRANSAMINASE IN PULMONARY DISEASE AND MULTIPLE INFARCTIONS, *ANN INTERN MED*, 46, 1105-1112 (1957)

2475 WALSH P N ET AL, PLATELET COAGULANT ACTIVITIES AND SERUM LIPIDS IN TRANSIENT CEREBRAL ISCHEMIA, *N ENGL J MED*, 295, 854-8 (1976)

2476 WALTER J E, THE SIGNIFICANCE OF ANTIBODIES IN CHRONIC HISTOPLASMOSIS BY IMMUNOELECTROPHORETIC AND COMPLEMENT FIXATION TEST, *AM REV RESPIR DIS*, 99, 50 (1969)

2477 WANDS J R ET AL, CIRCULATING IMMUNE COMPLEXES AND COMPLEMENT ACTIVATION IN PRIMARY BILIARY CIRRHOSIS, *N ENGL J MED*, 298, 233-37 (1978)

2478 WANEBO H J AND CLARKSON B D, ESSENTIAL MACROGLOBULINEMIA, *ACTA MED SCAND*, 170(SUPPL 367), 110 (1961)

2479 WANNEMACHER R W ET AL, EFFECT OF GLUCOSE INFUSION ON THE CONCENTRATION OF INDIVIDUAL SERUM FREE AMINO ACIDS DURING SANDFLY FEVER IN MAN, *AM J CLIN NUTR*, 30, 573-8. (1977)

2480 WARD A M ET AL, ACUTE-PHASE REACTANT PROTEIN PROFILES: AN AID TO MONITORING LARGE BOWEL CANCER BY CEA AND SERUM ENZYMES, *BR J CANCER*, 35, 170 (1977)

2481 WARD J R AND S ATCHESON, INFECTIOUS ARTHRITIS, *MED CLIN NORTH AM*, 61, 313-29 (1977)

2482 WARD T T ET AL, ACIDOSIS OF SYNOVIAL FLUID CORRELATES WITH SYNOVIAL FLUID LEUKOCYTOSIS, *AM J MED*, 64, 933-6. (1978)

2483 WARDENER N E, RENAL HEMODYNAMICS IN PRIMARY POLYCYTHEMIA, *LANCET*, 2, 204 (1951)

2484 WARRELL R P ET AL, INCREASED FACTOR VIII/VON WILLEBRAND FACTOR ANTIGEN AND VON WILLEBRAND FACTOR ACTIVITY IN RENAL FAILURE, *AM J MED*, 66, 226-228 (1978)

2485 WARSHAW A L, ON THE CAUSE OF RAISED SERUM AMYLASE IN DIABETIC KETOACIDOSIS, *LANCET*, 1, 929 (1977)

2486 WARSHAW D L ET AL, CHARACTERISTIC ALTERATIONS OF SERUM ISOENZYMES OF AMYLASE IN DISEASES OF LIVER, PANCREAS, SALIVARY GLAND, LUNG, AND GENITALIA, *J SURG RES*, 22, 362-9 (1977)

2487 WARTOFSKY L ET AL, STUDIES ON THE NATURE OF THYROIDAL SUPPRESSION DURING ACUTE FALCIPARUM MALARIA: INTEGRITY OF PITUITARY RESPONSE TO TRH AND ALTERATIONS IN SERUM T_3 AND REVERSE T_3, *J CLIN ENDOCRINOL METAB*, 44, 85-90 (1977)

2488 WASHINGTON JA, THE ROLE OF THE MICROBIOLOGY LABORATORY IN THE DIAGNOSIS AND ANTIMICROBIAL TREATMENT OF INFECTIVE ENDOCARDITIS, *MAYO CLIN PROC*, 57, 22-32 (1982)

2489 WASI P AND BLOCK M, THE MECHANISM OF THE DEVELOPMENT OF ANEMIA IN UNTREATED CHRONIC LYMPHATIC LEUKEMIA, *BLOOD*, 17, 597 (1961)

2490 WASI P, NA-NAKORN S, POOTRAKUL SN, THE ALPHA THALASSAEMIAS, *CLINICS IN HAEMATOLOGY*, 4, 383-410 (1974)

2491 WASSERMAN L R AND GILBERT H S, SURGICAL BLEEDING IN POLYCYTHEMIA VERA, *ANN NY ACAD SCI*, 115, 122 (1964)

2492 WASSERMAN L R ET AL, BLOOD OXYGEN STUDIES IN PATIENTS WITH POLYCYTHEMIA AND IN NORMAL SUBJECTS, *J CLIN INVEST*, 28, 60 (1940)

2493 WATANABE H, QUANTIFICATION OF INDIVIDUAL SERUM BILE ACIDS IN PATIENTS WITH LIVER DISEASES USING HIGH-PERFORMANCE LIQUID CHROMATOGRAPHY, *HEPATOGASTROENTEROLGY*, 31, 168-71 (1984)

2494 WATANABE M ET AL, SECRETION RATE OF ALDOSTERONE IN NORMAL PREGNANCY, *J CLIN INVEST*, 42, 42 (1963)

2495 WATANABE M ET AL, ALDOSTERONE SECRETION RATES IN ABNORMAL PREGNANCY, *J CLIN ENDOCRINOL METAB*, 25, 1665-1670 (1965)

2496 WATKINSON ET AL, PLASMA ACID PHOSPHATASE IN CARCINOMA OF THE PROSTATE AND THE EFFECT OF TREATMENT WITH STILBOESTROL, *BR MED J*, 2, 492-495 (1944)

2497 WATSON C J, PORPHYRIN METABOLISM IN THE ANEMIAS, *ARCH INTERN MED*, 99, 323 (1957)

2498 WATSON C J, THE PROBLEM OF PORPHYRIA - SOME FACTS AND QUESTIONS, *N ENGL J MED*, 263, 1205 (1960)

2499 WATSON C J ET AL, A SIMPLE TEST FOR URINARY PORPHOBILINOGEN, *PROC SOC EXP BIOL MED*, 47, 393 (1941)

2500 WAXMAN A D ET AL, ISOLATED ACTH DEFICIENCY IN ACUTE INTERMITTENT PORPHYRIA, *ANN INTERN MED*, 70, 317 (1969)

2501 WAYS P ET AL, RED CELL AND PLASMA LIPIDS IN ACANTHOCYTOSIS, *J CLIN INVEST*, 42, 1248 (1963)

2502 WEBB J ET AL, ANALYSIS BY PATTERN RECOGNITION TECHNIQUES OF CHANGES IN SERUM LEVELS OF 14 TRACE METALS AFTER ACUTE MYOCARDIAL INFARCTION, *EXPER MOLEC PATHOL*, 25, 322-31 (1976)

2503 WECHSLER M ET AL, THE CANCER ASSOCIATED ANTIGEN TEST AS AN INDEX TO FAILURE OF COMPLETE REMOVAL OF UROLOGIC CANCER, *J UROL*, 109, 699 (1973)

2504 WEEKE B, FLENBORG EW, JACOBSEN L, ET AL, IMMUNOCHEMICAL QUANTITATION OF 18 SERUM PROTEINS IN SERA FROM PATIENTS WITH CYSTIC FIBROSIS: CONCENTRATIONS CORRELATED TO CLASS OF FIBROBLAST METACHROMASIA, CLINICAL AND RADIOLOGICAL LUNG SYMPTOMS, *DAN MED BULL*, 23, 155-160 (1976)

2505 WEEKE B, JARNUM S, SERUM CONCENTRATION OF 19 SERUM PROTEINS IN CROHN'S DISEASE AND ULCERATIVE COLITIS, *GUT*, 12, 197-302 (1972)

2506 WEINBERGER A ET AL, INCREASED URIC ACID CLEARANCE IN PATIENTS WITH BURNS, *BIOMED PHARMACOTHER*, 27, 277-8 (1977)

2507 WEINBERGER M H ET AL, SEQUENTIAL CHANGES IN THE RENIN-ANGIOTENSIN-ALDOSTERONE SYSTEMS AND PLASMA PROGESTERONE CONCENTRATION IN NORMAL AND ABNORMAL HUMAN PREGNANCY, *PERSPECT NEPHROL HYPERTENS*, 5, 263-9 (1976)

2508 WEINSTEIN A J AND FARKAS S, SEROLOGIC TESTS IN INFECTIOUS DISEASES: CLINICAL UTILITY AND INTERPRETATION, *MED CLIN NORTH AM*, 62, 1099-1118 (1978)

2509 WEIR G C ET AL, THE HYPOCALCEMIA OF ACUTE PANCREATITIS, *ANN INTERN MED*, 83, 185-189 (1975)

2510 WEIR R J ET AL, ANGIOTENSIN, ALDOSTERONE, AND DOC IN HYPERTENSIVE DISEASE OF PREGNANCY, *SCOT MED J*, 18, 64 (1973)

2511 WEISS SH, GOEDERT JJ, SARNGADHARAN MG, ET AL, SCREENING TEST FOR HTLV-III (AIDS AGENT) ANTIBODIES, *JAMA*, 253, 221 (1985)

2512 WELCH C E AND HEDBERG S E, POLYPOID LESIONS OF THE GASTROINTESTINAL TRACT, *2ND EDITION W B SAUNDERS CO* (1975)

2513 WELCH K M ET AL, SERUM CREATINE PHOSPHOKINASE IN MOTOR NEURON DISEASE, *NEUROL*, 22, 697-701 (1972)

2514 WELLS SA, DILLEY WG, FARNDON JA, ET AL, EARLY DIAGNOSIS AND TREATMENT OF MEDULLARY THYROID CARCINOMA, *ARCH INTERN MED*, 145, 1248 (1985)

2515 WELT L G ET AL, AN ION TRANSPORT DEFECT IN ERYTHROCYTES FOR UREMIC PATIENTS, *ARCH INTERN MED*, 126, 827 (1970)

2516 WENHAM PR, ET AL, MULTIPLE FORMS OF GAMMA-GLUTAMYLTRANSFERASE: A CLINICAL STUDY, *CLIN CHEM*, 31, 569-73 (1985)

2517 WENHAM PR, HORN DB, SMITH AF, MULTIPLE FORMS OF GAMMA-GLUTAMYLTRANSFERASE: A CLINICAL STUDY, *CLIN CHEM*, 31, 569-73 (1985)

2518 WEST ET AL, SERUM ENZYMOLOGY IN THE DIAGNOSIS OF MYOCARDIAL INFARCTION AND RELATED CARDIOVASCULAR CONDITIONS, *MED CLIN NORTH AM*, 50, 171 (1966)

2519 WESTERMAN M P ET AL, HYPOCHOLESTEROLAEMIA AND ANAEMIA, *BR J HEMATOL*, 31, 87-94 (1975)

2520 WETTESBERG L ET AL, PLASMA DOPAMINE-B-HYDROXYLASE ACTIVITY IN HYPERTENSION AND VARIOUS NEUROPSYCHIATRIC DISORDERS, *SCAND J CLIN LAB INVEST*, 30, 283 (1972)

2521 WHEELOCK E F ET AL, THE PARTICIPATION OF LYMPHOCYTES IN VIRAL INFECTIONS, *ADV IMMUNOL*, 16, 124 (1973)

2522 WHICHER J T, THE VALUE OF COMPLEMENT ASSAYS IN CLINICAL CHEMISTRY, *CLIN CHEM*, 24, 7-22 (1978)

2523 WHITE ET AL, HISTIOCYTIC MEDULLARY RETICULOSIS WITH PARALLEL INCREASES IN SERUM ACID PHOSPHATASE AND DISEASE ACTIVITY, *CANCER*, 37, 1403-1411 (1976)

2524 WHITE R H R ET AL, CLINICOPATHOLOGICAL STUDY OF NEPHROTIC SYNDROME IN CHILDHOOD, *LANCET*, 1, 1353 (1970)

2525 WHITEHEAD ET AL, THE COMBINED EFFECT OF A HALOGENATED DERIVATIVE AND X-RAYS ON THE GROWTH OF CERTAIN EXPERIMENTAL TUMORS, *CANCER RES*, 14, 418-422 (1954)

2526 WHITFIELD ET AL, SERUM GAMMA-GLUTAMYL TRANSPEPTIDASE ACTIVITY IN LIVER DISEASE, *GUT*, 13, 702-708 (1972)

2527 WHITMORE ET AL, SERUM PROSTATIC ACID PHOSPHATASE LEVELS IN PROVED CASES OF CARCINOMA OR BENIGN HYPERTROPHY OF THE PROSTATE, *CANCER*, 9, 228-233 (1956)

2528 WHITTINGHAM S ET AL, SMOOTH MUSCLE AUTOANTIBODY (SMA) IN AUTOIMMUNE HEPATITIS, *GASTROENTEROLOGY*, 51, 499 (1966)

2529 WIDOMSKA-CZEKAJSKA T, BLOOD OXYGENATION AND DISTURBANCES OF THE ACID-BASE EQUILIBRIUM IN MYOCARDIAL INFARCTION, *COR VASA*, 18, 1-10. (1976)

2530 WIENER K, URAEMIA AND HYPERURICAEMIA IN ACUTE MYOCARDIAL INFARCTION, *CLIN CHIM ACTA*, 73, 45-50 (1976)

2531 WIENER K, PLASMA CALCIUM IN ACUTE MYOCARDIAL INFARCTION, *ANN CLIN BIOCHEM*, 14, 553-54 (1977)

2532 WILDSMITH J A ET AL, SEVERE FAT EMBOLISM: A REVIEW OF 24 CASES, *SCOT MED J*, 23, 141-8 (1978)

2533 WILKIN P, STUDY OF THE PHYSICAL FACTORS THAT DETERMINE PERMEABILITY OF THE PLACENTA, *BULL FED GYNEC OBSTET FRANCE*, 9, 33 (1957)

2534 WILKINSON JH, THE PRINCIPLES AND PRACTICE OF DIAGNOSTIC ENZYMOLOGY, *YEARBOOK MEDICAL PUBLISHERS, INC., CHICAGO* (1976)

2535 WILKINSON MR, WAGSTAFFE C, DELBRIDGE L, ET AL, SERUM OSTEOCALCIN CONCENTRATIONS IN PAGET'S DISEASE OF BONE, *ARCH INTERN MED*, 146, 268 (1986)

2536 WILKINSON S P, ABNORMALITIES OF SODIUM EXCRETION AND OTHER DISORDERS OF RENAL FUNCTION IN FULMINANT HEPATIC FAILURE, *GUT*, 17, 501-5 (1976)

2537 WILKINSON S P ET AL, RENAL RETENTION OF SODIUM IN CIRRHOSIS AND FULMINANT HEPATIC FAILURE, *POSTGRAD MED J*, 51, 527-31 (1975)

2538 WILLIAMS J W ET AL, HEMATOLOGY, *2ND EDITION MCGRAW-HILL NY* (1977)

2539 WILLIAMS JW, ET AL, HEMATOLOGY 3RD EDITION, *MCGRAW-HILL NY*, 3RD ED (1983)

2540 WILLIAMS R H, TEXTBOOK OF ENDOCRINOLOGY, *5TH ED PHILADELPHIA, SAUNDERS* (1974)

2541 WILLS M R, VALUE OF PLASMA CHLORIDE CONCENTRATION AND ACID-BASE STATUS IN THE DIFFERENTIAL DIAGNOSIS OF HYPERPARATHYROIDISM FROM OTHER CAUSES OF HYPERCALCEMIA, *J CLIN PATHOL*, 24, 219 (1971)

2542 WILLS M R AND MCGOWAN G K, PLASMA CHLORIDE LEVELS IN HYPERPARATHYROIDISM AND OTHER HYPERCALCEMIC STATES, *BR MED J*, 1, 1153 (1964)

2543 WILMORE D W ET AL, IMPAIRED GLUCOSE FLOW IN BURNED PATIENTS WITH GRAM-NEGATIVE SEPSIS, *SURG GYNECOL OBSTET*, 143, 720-4 (1976)

2544 WILSON C B AND DIXON F J, ANTIGLOMERULAR BASEMENT MEMBRANE ANTIBODY INDUCED GLOMERULONEPHRITIS, *KIDNEY INT*, 3, 74 (1973)

2545 WILSON C B ET AL, GLOMERULONEPHRITIS, *DM*, 22, 18-27 (1976)

2546 WILSON D M ET AL, RENAL URATE EXCRETION IN PATIENTS WITH WILSON'S DISEASE., *KIDNEY INT*, 4, 331-336 (1973)

2547 WILSON M ET AL, COMPARISON OF THE COMPLEMENT FIXATION, INDIRECT IMMUNOFLUORESCENCE, AND INDIRECT HEMAGGLUTINATION TESTS FOR MALARIA, *AM J TROP MED HYG*, 24, 755-59 (1975)

2548 WILSON M G AND MELNYK J, TRANSLOCATION: NORMAL MOSAICISM IN D TRISOMY, *PEDIATRICS*, 40, 842 (1967)

2549 WINAWER S J ET AL, SCREENING FOR COLON CANCER, *GASTROENTEROLOGY*, 70, 783 (1976)

2550 WINSTEN S, COLLECTION AND PRESERVATION OF SPECIMENS, *STAND METH CLIN CHEM*, 5, 1 (1965)

2551 WINSTON R M ET AL, ENZYMATIC DIAGNOSIS OF MEGALOBLASTIC ANEMIA, *BR J HAEMATOL*, 19, 587 (1970)

2552 WINTROBE M M ET AL, CLINICAL HEMATOLOGY, *7TH EDITION* (1974)

2553 WITHERS K L, LEUKAEMOID REACTIONS IN DISSEMINATED NON-REACTIVE TUBERCULOSIS: A REVIEW OF THE LITERATURE WITH REPORT OF A CASE, *MED J AUST*, 2, 142 (1964)

2554 WITTEVEEN S A ET AL, THE INFLUENCE OF PLASMA VOLUME CHANGES ON ENZYMATIC ESTIMATION OF INFARCT SIZE, *RECENT ADV STUD CARDIAC STRUCT METAB*, 12, 401-7 (1976)

2555 WITTS L J ET AL, CHRONIC GRANULOCYTIC LEUKEMIA COMPARISON OF RADIOTHERAPY AND BUSULPHAN THERAPY. REPORT OF THE MEDICAL RESEARCH COUNCIL'S WORKING PARTY FOR THERAPEUTIC TRIALS IN LEUKAEMIA, *BR MED J*, 1, 201 (1968)

2556 WITZTUM J, SCHONFELD G, HIGH DENSITY LIPOPROTEINS, *DIABETES*, 28, 326-336 (1979)

2557 WOCHOS D N ET AL, SERUM LIPIDS IN CHRONIC RENAL FAILURE, *MAYO CLIN PROC*, 51, 660-64 (1976)

2558 WOLF P L & WILLIAMS D, PRACTICAL CLINICAL ENZYMOLOGY, *JOHN WILEY & SONS INC* (1973)

2559 WOLFSON S K AND WILLIAMS-ASHMAN H G, ISOCITRIC AND 6-PHOSPOGLUCONIC DEHYDROGENASES IN HUMAN BLOOD SERUM, *PROC SOC EXP BIOL MED*, 96, 231 (1957)

2560 WOLINTZ A H ET AL, SERUM AND CEREBROSPINAL FLUID ENZYMES IN CEREBROVASCULAR DISEASE, *ARCH NEUROL*, 20, 54-61 (1969)

2561 WOLKOFF A W ET AL, INHERITANCE OF THE DUBIN-JOHNSON SYNDROME, *N ENGL J MED*, 288, 113 (1973)

2562 WONG T W, JONES T M, HYPERPROLACTINEMIA AND MALE INFERTILITY, *ARCH PATHOL LAB MED*, 108, 35-39 (1984)

2563 WOODARD, FACTORS LEADING TO ELEVATIONS IN SERUM ACID GLYCEROPHOSPHATASE, *CANCER*, 5, 236-241 (1952)

2564 WOODARD, THE CLINICAL SIGNIFICANCE OF SERUM ACID PHOSPHATASE, *AM J MED*, 27, 902-910 (1959)

2565 WOODARD ET AL, THE SIGNIFICANCE OF PHOSPHATASE FINDINGS IN CARCINOMA OF PROSTATE, *J UROL*, 57, 158-171 (1947)

2566 WOODARD H Q, CHANGES IN BLOOD CHEMISTRY ASSOCIATED WITH CARCINOMA METASTATIC TO BONE, *CANCER*, 6, 1219-1227 (1953)

2567 WOODBURY J ET AL, CEREBROSPINAL FLUID AND SERUM LEVELS OF MAGNESIUM, ZINC, AND CALCIUM IN MAN, *NEUROL*, 18, 700 (1968)

2568 WOODRUFF A W ET AL, THE ANAEMIA OF KALA AZAR, *BR J HAEMATOL*, 22, 319 (1972)

2569 WOODRUFF A W ET AL, ANEMIA IN AFRICAN TRYPANOSOMIASIS AND BIG SPLEEN DISEASE IN UGANDA, *TRANS R SOC TROP MED HYG*, 67, 329 (1973)

2570 WOODY M C ET AL, HISTIDINEMIA, *AM J DIS CHILD*, 110, 606 (1965)

2571 WORLD HEALTH ORGANIZATION, TOXOPLASMOSIS, *WHO TECH REP SER*, 431, 3 (1966)

2572 WOYDA J ET, FREE ADRENALINE, NORADRENALINE AND VANILLYLMANDELIC ACID EXCRETION WITH 24-HOUR URINE IN PATIENTS WITH CHRONIC CIRCULATORY FAILURE, *POL MED SCI HIST BULL*, 15, 425-30 (1975)

2573 WROBLEWSKI, CLINICAL SIGNIFICANCE OF SERUM ENZYME ALTERATIONS ASSOCIATED WITH MYOCARDIAL INFARCTION, *AM HEART J*, 54, 219-224 (1957)

2574 WROBLEWSKI, THE SIGNIFICANCE OF ALTERATIONS IN LACTIC DEHYDROGENASE ACTIVITY OF BODY FLUIDS IN THE DIAGNOSIS OF MALIGNANT TUMORS, *AM J MED SCI*, 234, 27-39 (1957)

2575 WROBLEWSKI, THE CLINICAL SIGNIFICANCE OF ALTERATIONS IN LACTIC DEHYDROGENASE ACTIVITY OF BODY FLUIDS, *AM J MED SCI*, 234, 301-312 (1957)

2576 WROBLEWSKI, THE SIGNIFICANCE OF ALTERATIONS IN SERUM ENZYMES IN THE DIFFERENTIAL DIAGNOSIS OF JAUNDICE, *ARCH INTERN MED*, 100, 635-641 (1957)

2577 WROBLEWSKI, THE CLINICAL SIGNIFICANCE OF ALTERATIONS IN TRANSAMINASE ACTIVITIES OF SERUM AND OTHER BODY FLUIDS, *ADV CLIN CHEM*, 1, 313 (1958)

2578 WROBLEWSKI, INCREASING CLINICAL SIGNIFICANCE OF ALTERATIONS IN ENZYMES OF BODY FLUIDS, *ANN INTERN MED*, 50, 62-68 (1959)

2579 WROBLEWSKI ET AL, LACTIC DEHYDROGENASE ACTIVITY IN BLOOD, *PROC SOC EXP BIOL MED*, 90, 210-213 (1955)

2580 WROBLEWSKI ET AL, SERUM GLUTAMIC PYRUVIC TRANSAMINASE IN CARDIAC AND HEPATIC DISEASE, *PROC SOC EXP BIOL MED*, 91, 569-571 (1956)

2581 WROBLEWSKI ET AL, SERUM LACTIC DEHYDROGENASE ACTIVITY IN ACUTE TRANSMURAL MYOCARDIAL INFARCTION, *SCIENCE*, 123, 1122-1123 (1956)

2582 WYNGAARDEN J B, URIC ACID, *THE ENCYCLOPEDIA OF MEDICINE SURGERY SPECIALTIES*, 341 (1955)

2583 YACHMAN ET AL, CLINICAL SIGNIFICANCE OF THE HUMAN ALPHA-FETO PROTEIN, *ANN CLIN LAB SCI*, 8, 84-90 (1978)

2584 YAM, CLINICAL SIGNIFICANCE OF THE HUMAN ACID PHOSPHATASE, *AM J MED*, 56, 604-616 (1974)

2585 YAM ET AL, LEUKEMIC RETICLOENDOTHELIOSIS, *ARCH INTERN MED*, 130, 248-256 (1972)

2586 YAM L T ET AL, TARTRATE-RESISTANT ACID PHOSPHATASE ISOENZYME IN THE RETICULUM CELLS OF LEUKEMIC RETICLOENDOTHELIOSIS, *N ENGL J MED*, 284, 357-360 (1971)

2587 YAM L T ET AL, IMPAIRED MARROW GRANULOCYTE RESERVE AND LEUKOCYTE MOBILIZATIONS IN LEUKEMIA RETICULOENDOTHELIOSIS, *ANN INTERN MED*, 87, 444-446 (1977)

2588 YAM LT, LI CY, CROSBY WH, CYTOCHEMICAL IDENTIFICATION OF MONOCYTES AND GRANULOCYTES, *AM J CLIN PATHOL*, 55, 183-290 (1971)

2589 YAMADA T ET AL, ACTIVATION OF THE KALLIKREIN-KININ SYSTEM IN ROCKY MOUNTAIN SPOTTED FEVER, *ANN INTERN MED*, 88, 764-766 (1978)

2590 YAMAGATA S ET AL, A CASE OF CONGENITAL AFIBRINOGENEMIA AND REVIEW OF REPORTED CASES IN JAPAN, *TOHOKU J EXP MED*, 96, 15 (1968)

2591 YATES C M ET AL, LYSOSOMAL ENZYMES, AMINO ACID AND ACID METABOLITES OF AMINES IN HUNTINGTON'S CHOREA, *CLIN CHIM ACTA*, 44, 139 (1973)

2592 YATES C M ET AL, LYSOSOMAL ENZYMES IN CEREBRAL ATROPHY, *CLIN CHIM ACTA*, 71, 215-219 (1976)

2593 YEN S S C ET AL, GROWTH HORMONE LEVELS IN PREGNANCY, *J CLIN ENDOCRINOL METAB*, 27, 1341 (1967)

2594 YEN T S ET AL, HUMORAL COMPONENTS OF IMMUNOLOGICAL RESPONSE IN NEPHROTIC SYNDROME, *CHIN J MICROBIOL*, 10, 21-7 (1977)

2595 YENDT ET AL, DETECTION OF PRIMARY HYPERPARATHYROIDISM, WITH SPECIAL REFERENCE TO ITS OCCURRENCE IN HYPERCALCIURIC FEMALES WITH NORMAL OR BORDERLINE SERUM CALCIUM, *CAN MED ASSOC J*, 98, 331-336 (1968)

2596 YEO KHJ, WHITAU WJ, 125 I RADIOIMMUNOASSAY FOR 17 ALPHA-HYDROXYPROGESTERONE IN PLASMA, FOR DIAGNOSING AND MANAGING CONGENITAL ADRENAL HYPERPLASIA, *CLIN CHEM*, 31/3, 454-456 (1985)

2597 YLOSTALO P, LIVER FUNCTION IN HEPATOSIS OF PREGNANCY AND PRE-ECLAMPSIA WITH SPECIAL REFERENCE TO MODIFIED BROMSULPHTHALEIN, *ACTA OBSTET GYNECOL SCAND*, 49, 1-53 (1970)

2598 YOKOYAMA M ET AL, AMYLASE-PRODUCING LUNG CANCER, *CANCER*, 40, 766-72 (1977)

2599 YONEZAWA S, SATO E, KAKINOKI T, OHI Y, ALPHA 1-ANTITRYPSIN AND ANTITHROMBIN III IN ATROPHIC NEPHRONS OF CHRONIC PYELO-NEPHRITIS, *ACTA PATHOL JPN*, 32, 193-8 (1982)

2600 YOTSUMOTO H, IMAI Y, KUZUYA N, UCHIMURA H, ET AL, INCREASED LEVELS OF SERUM ANGIOTENSIN-CONVERTING ENZYME ACTIVITY IN HYPERTHYROIDISM, *ANN INTERN MED*, 96, 326-8 (1982)

2601 YOUNG L E AND MILLER G, DIFFERENTIATION BETWEEN CONGENITAL AND ACQUIRED FORMS OF HEMOLYTIC ANEMIA, *AM J MED SCI*, 226, 664 (1953)

2602 YOUSUFI MA A ET AL, HETEROGENEITY OF AMYLASE IN DIABETES MELLITUS, *J A M A*, 27, 393-4. (1977)

2603 YU T F, SECONDARY GOUT ASSOCIATED WITH MYELOPROLIFERATIVE DISEASES, *ARTHRITIS RHEUM*, 8, 765 (1965)

2604 YU T F ET AL, PLASMA AND URINARY AMINO ACIDS IN PRIMARY GOUT WITH SPECIAL REFERENCE TO GLUTAMINE, *J CLIN INVEST*, 48, 885 (1969)

2605 ZAMCHECK N, CARCINOEMBRYONIC ANTIGEN. QUANTITATIVE VARIATIONS IN CIRCULATING LEVELS IN BENIGN AND MALIGNANT DIGESTIVE TRACT DISEASES, *ADVAN INT MED*, 19, 420 (1974)

2606 ZANIEWSKI M, JORDAN JR PH, YIP B, ET AL, SERUM GASTRIN LEVEL IS INCREASED BY CHRONIC HYPERCALCEMIA OF PARATHYROID OF PARATHYROID OR NONPARATHYROID ORIGIN, *ARCH INTERN MED*, 146, 478 (1986)

2607 ZANNOS-MARICLEA L ET AL, RELATIONSHIP BETWEEN TOCOPHEROLS AND SERUM LIPID LEVELS IN CHILDREN WITH BETA-THALASSEMIA MAJOR, *AM J CLIN NUTR*, 31, 259-63 (1978)

2608 ZECK R T AND D CUGELL, DIFFUSE INFILTRATIVE LUNG DISEASE, *MED CLIN NORTH AM*, 61, 1251-66 (1977)

2609 ZELTZER P M, ALPHA FETOPROTEIN IN THE DIFFERENTIATION OF NEONATAL HEPATITIS AND BILIARY ATRESIA: CURRENT STATUS AND IMPLICATIONS FOR THE PATHOGENESIS OF THESE DISORDERS, *J PEDIATR SURG*, 13, 381-7 (1978)

2610 ZENER AND HARRISON, SERUM ENZYME VALUES FOLLOWING INTRA-MUSCULAR ADMINISTRATION OF LIDOCAINE, *ARCH INTERN MED*, 134, 48-49 (1974)

2611 ZICCARDI RJ, COOPER NR, DEVELOPMENT OF AN IMMUNOCHEMICAL TEST TO ASSESS C1 INACTIVATOR FUNCTION IN HUMAN SERUM AND ITS USE FOR THE DIAGNOSIS OF HEREDITARY ANGIOEDEMA, *CLIN IMMUNOL IMMUNOPATHOL*, 15, 465-471 (1980)

2612 ZILVA J F & PANNALL P, CLINICAL CHEMISTRY IN DIAGNOSIS AND TREATMENT, *2ND ED YEAR BOOK MED PUBL CHICAGO* (1975)

2613 ZILVA J F ET AL, PLASMA PHOSPHATE AND POTASSIUM LEVELS IN THE HYPERCALCEMIA OF MALIGNANT DISEASE, *J CLIN ENDOCRINOL METAB*, 36, 1019 (1973)

2614 ZILVERSMIT DB, DIETSCHY JA, GOTTO AM, ONTKO JA, EDS. BALTIMORE, WAVERLY, *IN DISTURBANCES IN LIPID AND LIPOPROTEIN METABOLISM*, 69-81 (1978)

2615 ZIMMER R, TEELKEN AW, TRIELING WB, WEBER W, ET AL, Y-AMI-NOBUTYRIC ACID AND HOMOVANILLIC ACID CONCENTRATION IN THE CSF OF PATIENTS WITH SENILE DEMENTIA OF ALZHEIMER'S TYPE, *ARCH NEUROL*, 41, 602 (1984)

2616 ZIMMERMAN H J ET AL, LACTIC DEHYDROGENASE ACTIVITY IN HUMAN SERUM, *J LAB CLIN MED*, 48, 607-616 (1956)

2617 ZIMMERMAN T S ET AL, IMMUNOLOGIC DIFFERENTIATION OF CLASSIC HEMOPHILIA (FACTOR VIII DEFICIENCY) AND VON WILLEBRAND'S DISEASE WITH OBSERVATION ON COMBINED DEFICIENCIES OF ANTIHEMOPHILIC FACTOR AND PROACCELERIN (FACTOR V) AND, *J CLIN INVEST*, 50, 244 (1971)

2618 ZINNEMAN H H AND ROTSTEIN J, A STUDY OF GAMMA GLOBULIN IN DYSTROPHICA MYOTONICA, *J LAB CLIN MED*, 47, 907 (1956)

2619 ZINNEMAN H H ET AL, URINARY AMINO ACIDS IN PREGNANCY, FOLLOWING PROGESTERONE AND ESTROGEN-PROGESTERONE, *J CLIN ENDOCRINOL METAB*, 27, 397 (1967)

2620 ZUBENKO GS, VOLICER L, DIRENFELD LK, ET AL, CEREBROSPINAL FLUID LEVELS OF ANGIOTENSIN-CONVERTING ENZYME IN ALZHEIMER'S DISEASE, PARKINSON'S DISEASE AND PROGRESSIVE SUPRANUCLEAR PALSY, *BRAIN RES*, 328, 215-21 (1985)

2621 ZUCKER M D ET AL, ELEVATION OF SERUM ACID GLYCEROPHOSPHATASE ACTIVITY IN THROMBOCYTOSIS, *J LAB CLIN MED*, 59, 760-770 (1963)

2622 ZUSMAN J ET AL, HYPERPHOSPHATEMIA, HYPERPHOSPHATURIA, AND HYPOCALCEMIA IN ACUTE LYMPHOBLASTIC LEUKEMIA, *N ENGL J MED*, 289, 1335-40 (1973)

2623 ZUSPAN F P ET AL, URINE AMINE EXCRETION IN PREGNANCY-INDUCED HYPERTENSION, *PERSPECT NEPHROL HYPERTENS*, 5, 339-47 (1976)

2624 ZUYDERHOUDT F M ET AL, AN ENZYME LINKED IMMUNOASSAY FOR FERRITIN IN HUMAN SERUM AND RAT PLASMA AND THE INFLUENCE OF THE IRON IN SERUM FERRITIN ON SERUM IRON MEASUREMENT, DURING ACUTE HEPATITIS, *CLIN CHIM ACTA*, 88, 37-44 (1978)

2625 ALTOMONTE, L., ET. AL., SERUM CONCENTRATION OF BILE ACIDS IN THE DIAGNOSIS OF LIVER LESTIONS IN RHUEMATOID ARTHRITIS, *MINERVA MED.*, 73(24), 1695-1698 (1982)

2626 BABB, R.R., ASCITES: DIFFERENTIAL DIAGNOSIS AND TREATMENT, *HOSPT. MED.*, 129-155 (APRIL 198)

2627 BATELLE, D., AND DURTZMAN, N.A., DISTAL RENAL TUBULAR ACIDOSIS: PATHOGENESIS AND CLASSIFICATION, *AM. J. KID. DIS.*, 1, 328-344 (1982)

2628 BEUTNER, E.H., ET. AL., CLINICAL SIGNS OF SERA AND SKIN IN BULLOUS DISEASE, *INT. J. DERM.*, 24, 406 (SEPT. 198)

2629 BURNETT, D. AND STOCKLEY, R.A., SERUM AND SPUTUM ALPHA-2 MACROGLOBULIN IN PATIENTS WITH CHRONIC OBSTRUCTIVE AIRWAYS DISEASE, *THORAX*, 36, 512-516 (1981)

2630 CHAMPEYROUX, J., MOINADE, S., AND GENTAU, C., ALPHA-2 MACROGLOBULINEMIE CHEXZ LES DIABETIQUES AYANT UNE RETINOPATHIE (LTR), *LA NOUV. PRESSE. MED.*, 8, 135 (1979)

2631 FRANCIS, CATECHOLAMINE LEVELS IN CHF, *CARDIOVASCULAR REPORTS AND REVIEWS*, 6(4), 445 (APRIL 198)

2632 HEDFORS, E., KISNER, S., AND NORBERG, D., SERUM LEVEL AND URINARY EXCRETION OF ALPHA-2 MACROGLOBULIN IN PATIENTS WITH RENAL DISEASE, *ACTA. MED. SCAND.*, 190, 347-351 (1971)

2633 HEIDELBERGER, K.P., ALPHA-1 ANTITRYPSIN DEFICIENCY: A REVIEW 1963-1975, *ANN. CLIN. LAB. SCI.*, 6:110 (1976)

2634 HINTZ, HUMAN SOMATOMEDIN PLASMA BINDING PROTEINS, *IN SOMATOMEDIN AND RELATED PEPTIDES*, G. GIORDANO (EDITOR), *EXERPTA MEDICA*, 143 (1979)

2635 KLUTHE, R., HAGEMANN, U., AND KLEINE, N., THE TURNOVER OF ALPHA-2 MACROGLOBULIN IN NEPHROTIC SYNDROME, *VOX. SANG.*, 12, 308-311 (1967)

2636 MARKOWITZ, H., ET.AL., STUDIES IN COPPER METABOLISM: XIV, *J. CLIN INVEST.*, 34, 1498-1508 (1955)

2637 MCBLACK, P., DIAGNOSIS OF PITUITARY TUMOR, *HOSPT. MED.*, 43-69 (OCT. 1985)

2638 MCCARTY, K.S. AND DODSON, C.E., PITUITARY PATHOLOGY ASSOCIATED WITH ABNORMALITIES OF PROLACTIN SECRETION, *CLIN. OBSTET. GYNECOL.*, 23, 367 (1980)

2639 MERTZ, L.E. ET. AL., TICKS, SPIROCHETES AND NEW DIAGNOSTIC TESTS FOR LYME DISEASE, *MAYO CLINIC PROC.*, 60(6), 402-406 (JUNE 1985)

2640 MIESCH, F., BIETH, J., AND METAIRS, P., THE ALPHA-2 ANTITRYPSIN AND ALPHA-2 MACROGLOBULIN CONTENT AND THE PROTEASE INHIBITING CAPACITY OF NORMAL AND PATHOLOGICAL SERA, *CLIN. CHIM. ACTA.*, 31, 231-241 (1971)

2641 MONTOYE, H.J., EPSTEIN, F.H., AND KJELSBERG, M.O., RELATIONSHIP BETWEEN SERUM CHOLESTEROL AND BODY FATNESS, *AM. J. CLIN. NUTR.*, 18, 397-406 (1966)

2642 RODA, A., ET. AL., SERUM PRIMARY BILE ACIDS IN GILBERT'S SYNDROME, *GASTROENTEROLOGY*, 82(1), 77-83 (1982)

2643 SHIMADA, M., MIYASHIMAKI, AND YAVATA, Y., INCREASED CALCIUM UPTAKE IN THE RED CELLS OF UNSPLENECTOMIZED PATIENTS WITH HEREDITARY SPHEROCYTOSIS, *CLIN. CHIM. ACTA.*, 142(2), 183-192 (1984)

2644 SHUSTER, J., GOLD, P., PRILICK, BETA-2 MICROGLOBULIN LEVELS IN CANCEROUS AND OTHER DISEASE STATES, *CLIN. CHIM. ACTA.*, 67, 307-313 (1976)

2645 STINEBAUGH BT, ET. AL., PATHOGENESIS OF DISTAL RENAL TUBULAR ACIDOSIS, *KIDNEY INT.*, 17, 1-7 (1981)

2646 WEINSTEIN, A., ET. AL., ANTIBODIES TO NATIVE DNA AND SERUM COMPLEMENT (C3) LEVELS: APPLICATIONS TO DIAGNOSIS AND CLASSIFICATION OF SYSTEMIC LUPUS ERYTHEMATOSUS, *AM. J. MED.*, 74,206 (1983)